a LANGE medical book

T0383331

CURRENT
Diagnosis & Treatment
Pediatrics

TWENTY-SEVENTH EDITION

Edited by

Maya Bunik, MD, MPH
Professor, Department of Pediatrics
Section of General Pediatric Academic Medicine
University of Colorado School of Medicine
Associate Chief Medical Officer-Ambulatory
Children's Hospital Colorado

Mark J. Abzug, MD
Professor and Vice Chair for Academic Affairs,
Department of Pediatrics
Section of Pediatric Infectious Diseases and Epidemiology
University of Colorado School of Medicine and
Children's Hospital Colorado

Myron J. Levin, MD
Professor, Departments of Pediatrics and Medicine
Section of Pediatric Infectious Diseases and Epidemiology
University of Colorado School of Medicine and
Children's Hospital Colorado

Teri L. Schreiner, MD
Associate Professor, Department of Pediatrics
Section of Child Neurology
Director, Neuroimmunology Center for Children
University of Colorado School of Medicine and
Children's Hospital Colorado

and Associate Authors

The Department of Pediatrics at the University of Colorado School of Medicine
is affiliated with Children's Hospital Colorado

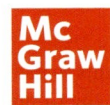

McGraw Hill

ISBN 978-1-265-73989-8
MHID 1-265-73989-7
ISSN 0093-8556

Notice

Medicine is an ever-changing science. As new research and clinical experience broaden our knowledge, changes in treatment and drug therapy are required. The authors and the publisher of this work have checked with sources believed to be reliable in their efforts to provide information that is complete and generally in accord with the standards accepted at the time of publication. However, in view of the possibility of human error or changes in medical sciences, neither the authors nor the publisher nor any other party who has been involved in the preparation or publication of this work warrants that the information contained herein is in every respect accurate or complete, and they disclaim all responsibility for any errors or omissions or for the results obtained from use of the information contained in this work. Readers are encouraged to confirm the information contained herein with other sources. For example and in particular, readers are advised to check the product information sheet included in the package of each drug they plan to administer to be certain that the information contained in this work is accurate and that changes have not been made in the recommended dose or in the contraindications for administration. This recommendation is of particular importance in connection with new or infrequently used drugs.

This book was set in Minion Pro by KnowledgeWorks Global Ltd.
The editors were Timothy Y. Hiscock, Kathleen Saylor, and Peter J. Boyle.
The production supervisor was Catherine H. Saggese.
The digital production manager was Priscilla Beer.
Project management was provided by Revathi Viswanathan, KnowledgeWorks Global Ltd.

This book is printed on acid-free paper.

Dedicated to Dr. Bill Hay who carried this book through many years with his humility, great expertise, passion, and superb editorial leadership.

Dr. Bill Hay, now a retired Professor at the University of Colorado, was previously Director of the Child Maternal Health Program, the Early Life Exposures Program, and the Neonatal-Perinatal Clinical Translational Research Center of the Colorado Clinical and Translational Sciences Institute. He also served as Scientific Director of the Perinatal Research Center. His research focused on maternal nutrition and metabolism, placental nutrient transport and metabolism, fetal physiology, and fetal and neonatal nutrition and metabolism. A major emphasis of his research was on intrauterine growth restriction and how this condition programs fetal and neonatal growth and development. He was continuously funded for this research by National Institutes of Health (NIH) for his entire career. He served on many NIH study sections (three as Chair) as well as President of the Perinatal Research Society, the Western Society for Pediatric Research, and, most importantly, the American Pediatric Society. He also translated his basic research findings into clinical studies of nutrition to the preterm infant, aiming to emulate the nutrition of the normally growing human fetus of the same gestational age. As a PI and Program 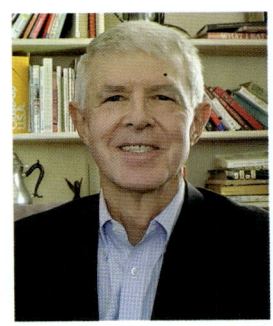 Director and Research Mentor of the NICHD T32 Training Program in Perinatal Medicine and Biology and Program Director of the Department of Pediatrics NICHD K12 Child Health Research Career Development Program GB assisted in mentoring well over 30 trainees at the fellow and junior faculty level. Having worked in the NICU for 43 years Bill taught countless residents and provided exemplary care for many thousands of infants and their families.

His expertise in nutrition of the preterm infant was recognized by receiving the American Academy of Pediatrics (AAP) Nutrition Award (now named after Samuel J. Fomon). Bill is also recognized nationally and internationally for his expertise in disorders of glucose metabolism in neonates. He was honored with many lectureships nationally and internationally. His educational accomplishments were noted by awards such as the WSPR Joseph W. St. Geme Jr. Education Award. His research and review publications number over 400, including two editions of his own book, Neonatal Nutrition and Metabolism.

Bill joined the Current Diagnosis and Treatment—Pediatrics (CDT-P) editorial team for the 8th edition. Henry Kempe, the original author, encouraged Bill to take this on early in his career. Later, it was Bill Hathaway, who had collaborated on research projects with Marilyn Manco-Johnson and Bill Hay, who got Bill to join the CDT-P editorial team. After Bill Hathaway retired, Bill Hay took over as lead editor, a position he held through the 25th edition, spanning 40 years. Bill had the privilege of collaborating with many truly exceptional editors, including Jessie Groothuis, Myron Levin, Anthony Hayward, Judy Sondheimer, Robin Deterding, Mark Abzug, and most recently Maya Bunik. For Bill Hay, CDT-P was always the banner that he carried and promoted in recognition of Henry Kempe, his first Chair and mentor and remarkable leader in academic pediatrics.

Contents

4. Adolescence   79

Amy E. Sass, MD, MPH
Molly J. Richards, MD

5. Adolescent Substance Use Disorders   115

Jesse Hinckley, MD, PhD
Clifford Costello, DO
Paritosh Kaul, MD
Diane Straub, MD, MPH

6. Eating Disorders   129

Francisco Prada, MD
Eric J. Sigel, MD

7. Child & Adolescent Psychiatric Disorders & Psychosocial Aspects of Pediatrics   141

Kelly Glaze, PsyD
Kimberly Kelsay, MD
Ayelet Talmi, PhD

15. Skin   362

Lori D. Prok, MD
Carla X. Torres-Zegarra, MD

16. Eye   385

Lauren Mehner, MD, MPH
Jennifer Lee Jung, MD

17. Oral Medicine & Dentistry   429

Anne R. Wilson, DDS, MS
Abidin Hakan Tuncer, DDS, DMD, MPH, FSCD
Chaitanya P. Puranik, BDS, MS, MDentSci, PhD
Katherine L. Chin, DDS, MS

18. Ear, Nose, & Throat   440

Patricia J. Yoon, MD
Melissa A. Scholes, MD
Brian W. Herrmann, MD

19. Respiratory Tract & Mediastinum   468

Paul Stillwell, MD
Emily M. DeBoer, MD
Jordana Hoppe, MD
Paul Houin, MD

20. Cardiovascular Diseases   512

John S. Kim, MD
Dale Burkett, MD
Roni Jacobsen, MD
Johannes Von Alvensleben, MD

21. Gastrointestinal Tract 569

David Brumbaugh, MD
Glenn T. Furuta, MD
Edward J. Hoffenberg, MD
Gregory E. Kobak, MD
Robert E. Kramer, MD
Nathalie Nguyen, MD
Seth Septer, DO
Mary Shull, MD
Jason Soden, MD
Thomas Walker, MD

22. Liver & Pancreas 609

Ronald J. Sokol, MD
Julia M. Boster, MD, MSCS
Amy G. Feldman, MD, PhD
Jacob A. Mark, MD
Cara L. Mack, MD
Shikha S. Sundaram, MD, MSCI

23. Fluid, Electrolyte, & Acid–Base Disorders & Therapy 656

Melisha G. Hanna, MD, MS
Margret E. Bock, MD, MS

24. Kidney & Urinary Tract 666

Margret E. Bock, MD, MS
Eliza D. Blanchette, MD, MS
Melisha G. Hanna, MD, MS

25. Neurologic & Muscular Disorders 691

Ricka Messer, MD, PhD
Elizabeth Troy, MD
Diana Walleigh, MD
Melissa Wright, MD, PhD

Authors

Jordan K. Abbott, MD, MA
Associate Professor of Pediatrics, Section of Pediatric
    Allergy and Immunology, University of Colorado School
    of Medicine and Children's Hospital Colorado
Chapter 33: Immunodeficiency

Abigail Angulo, MD, MPH
Associate Professor, Department of Pediatrics, Section of
    Developmental Pediatrics, University of Colorado School
    of Medicine and Children's Hospital Colorado
Chapter 3: Child Development and Behavior

Aubrey Armento, MD, CAQSM
Assistant Professor, Department of Orthopedics, University
    of Colorado School of Medicine, Sports Medicine Center,
    Children's Hospital Colorado Orthopedics Institut
Chapter 27: Sports Medicine

Edwin J. Asturias, MD
The Jules Amer Chair in Community Pediatrics at Children's
    Hospital Colorado
Professor of Pediatrics and Epidemiology
Section of Pediatric Infectious Diseases and Epidemiology,
    University of Colorado School of Medicine
Center for Global Health | Colorado School of Public Health
Chapter 40: Infections: Viral & Rickettsia

Lalit Bajaj, MD, MPH/MSPH
Professor, Pediatrics, Section of Emergency Medicine,
    Chief Quality, Equity Outcomes Officer, Children's
    Hospital Colorado, University of Colorado School
    of Medicine
Chapter 1: Advancing the Quality and Safety of Care

Peter R. Baker II, MD
Associate Professor, Department of Pediatrics, Section
    of Clinical Genetics and Metabolism, University of
    Colorado School of Medicine and Children's Hospital
    Colorado
Chapter 36: Inborn Errors of Metabolism

Sarah Bartz, MD
Associate Professor, Department of Pediatrics, Section of
    Pediatric Endocrinology, Clinical Lead for Colorado
    Springs Pediatric Endocrinology, University of Colorado
    School of Medicine and Children's Hospital Colorado
Chapter 34: Endocrine Disorders

Eliza D. Blanchette, MD, MS
Assistant Professor, Department of Pediatrics, Section
    of Pediatric Nephrology, University of Colorado and
    Children's Hospital Colorado
Chapter 24: Kidney & Urinary Tract

Margret E. Bock, MD, MS
Associate Professor, Department of Pediatrics, Section of
    Pediatric Nephrology, Clinic Medical Director, Medical
    Director, Kidney Transplantation
*Chapter 23: Fluid, Electrolyte, & Acid-Base Disorders and
    Treatment*
Chapter 24: Kidney & Urinary Tract

Juri Boguniewicz, MD
Assistant Professor, Departments of Pediatrics and
    Medicine, Section of Pediatric Infectious Diseases and
    Epidemiology, University of Colorado School of Medicine
    and Children's Hospital Colorado
Chapter 43: Infections: Parasitic & Mycotic

Mark Boguniewicz, MD
Professor, Department of Pediatrics, Section of Pediatric
    Allergy-Immunology, University of Colorado School
    of Medicine and National Jewish Medical and Research
    Center
Chapter 38: Allergic Disorders

Julia M. Boster, MD, MSCS
Assistant Professo of Pediatrics, Department of Pediatrics,
    Section of Pediatric Gastroenterology, Hepatology and
    Nutrition, University of Colorado School of Medicine
    and Children's Hospital Colorado
Chapter 22: Liver and Pancreas

Cortney Braund, MD
Assistant Professor, Department of Pediatrics, Section of
    Pediatric Emergency Medicine, University of Colorado
    School of Medicine and Children's Hospital Colorado
Chapter 12: Emergencies & Injuries

Meghan Breheney, MD
Assistant Professor, Department of Pediatrics, Section of
    Developmental Pediatrics, University of Colorado School
    of Medicine and Children's Hospital Colorado
Chapter 3: Child Development and Behavior

David Brumbaugh, MD
Associate Professor, Department of Pediatrics, Section of Pediatric Gastroenterology, Hepatology and Nutrition, Digestive Health Institute, Center for Celiac Disease, University of Colorado School of Medicine and Children's Hospital Colorado
Chapter 21: Gastrointestinal Tract

Dale Burkett, MD
Assistant Professor, Department of Pediatrics, Section of Cardiology, University of Colorado School of Medicine and Children's Hospital Colorado
Chapter 20: Cardiovascular Diseases

Alice Campbell, MT (ASCP)
Department of Pathology and Laboratory Medicine, Children's Hospital Colorado
Chapter 46: Chemistry & Hematology Reference Intervals

Jessica R. Cataldi, MD, MSCS
Associate Professor, Department of Pediatrics, Section of Pediatric Infectious Diseases and Epidemiology, University of Colorado School of Medicine and Children's Hospital Colorado
Chapter 10: Immunization

Christina Chambers, MD
Assistant Professor, Department of Pediatrics, Section of Pediatric Endocrinology, University of Colorado School of Medicine and Children's Hospital Colorado
Chapter 34: Endocrine Disorders

Christine M. Chan, MD
Associate Professor of Clinical Practice, Department of Pediatrics, Section of Pediatric Endocrinology, University of Colorado School of Medicine and Children's Hospital Colorado
Chapter 34: Endocrine Disorders

Rohini Chakravarthy, MD, MPH
Assistant Professor of Pediatrics
Pediatric Hematology/Oncology & Stem Cell Transplantation
University of Chicago Medicine & Biological Sciences
Comer Children's Hospital
Chapter 31: Neoplastic Disease

Antonia Chiesa, MD
Associate Professor, Department of Pediatrics, University of Colorado School of Medicine, Kempe Child Protection Team, Kempe Center for the Prevention and Treatment of Child Abuse and Neglect and Children's Hospital Colorado
Chapter 8: Child Abuse & Neglect

Jason Child, PharmD
Co-Director, Antimicrobial Stewardship, Department of Pharmacy, University of Colorado Skaggs School of Pharmacy and Pharmaceutical Sciences
Chapter 39: Antimicrobial Therapy

Katherine L. Chin, DDS, MS
Associate Clinical Professor, Department of Pediatric Dentistry, University of Colorado School of Dental Medicine and Children's Hospital Colorado
Chapter 17: Oral Medicine & Dentistry

Christine Cho, MD
Associate Professor, of Clinical Practice, Department of Pediatrics, Section of Pediatric Allergy and Clinical Immunology, University of Colorado School of Medicine and Children's Hospital Colorado
Chapter 38: Allergic Disorders

Amy C. Clevenger, MD, PhD
Associate Professor, Department of Pediatrics, Section of Pediatric Critical Care Medicine, University of Colorado School of Medicine and Children's Hospital Colorado
Chapter 14: Critical Care

Erin Cobry, MD
Assistant Professor Barbara Davis Center for Diabetes, Department of Pediatrics
Chapter 35: Diabetes Mellitus

Clifford Costello, DO
Fellow, Department of Pediatrics, Section of Adolescent Medicine, University of Colorado School of Medicine and Children's Hospital Colorado
Chapter 5: Substance Use

Ronina A. Covar, MD
Professor, Department of Pediatrics, Section of Pediatric Allergy-Immunology, University of Colorado School of Medicine and National Jewish Medical and Research Center
Chapter 38: Allergic Disorders

Melanie Cree-Green, MD, PhD
Associate Professor, Department of Pediatrics, Section of Pediatric Endocrinology, Director, multi-disciplinary PCOS clinic, University of Colorado School of Medicine and Children's Hospital Colorado
Chapter 34: Endocrine Disorders

Angela S. Czaja, MD, MSc, PhD
Professor, Department of Pediatrics, Section of Pediatric Critical Care Medicine, University of Colorado School of Medicine and Children's Hospital Colorado
Chapter 14: Critical Care

Matthew F. Daley, MD
Associate Professor, Department of Pediatrics, University of Colorado School of Medicine and Children's Hospital Colorado, Senior Investigator, Institute for Health Research, Kaiser Permanente Colorado
Chapter 10: Immunization

Richard C. Dart, MD, PhD
Professor, Department of Surgery, Director, Rocky Mountain Poison and Drug Center, Denver Health and Hospital Authority, University of Colorado School of Medicine and Children's Hospital Colorado
Chapter 13: Poisoning

Shanlee Davis, MD, PhD
Associate Professor, Department of Pediatrics, Section of Pediatric Endocrinology, Director of the eXtraOrdinary Kids Turner Syndrome Clinic, University of Colorado School of Medicine and Children's Hospital Colorado
Chapter 34: Endocrine Disorders

Sayan De, MD
Assistant Professor, Department of Orthopedic Surgery, University of Colorado School of Medicine and Children's Hospital Colorado
Chapter 26: Orthopedics

Emily M. DeBoer, MD
Associate Professor, Department of Pediatrics, Section of Pediatric Pulmonology and Sleep Medicine, University of Colorado School of Medicine and Children's Hospital Colorado
Chapter 19: Respiratory Tract & Mediastinum

Liliane K. Diab, MD
Assistant Professor, Department of Pediatrics, Section of Pediatric Nutrition, Clinical Director, Growth and Parenting, University of Colorado School of Medicine, Children's Hospital Colorado
Chapter 11: Normal Childhood Nutrition & Its Disorders

Melkon G. DomBourian, MD
Assistant Professor, Department of Pediatrics, Section of Pediatric Pathology, Medical Director, Core Lab & Point of Care Testing | Associate Medical Director, Transfusion Medicine Services, University of Colorado School of Medicine and Children's Hospital Colorado
Chapter 46: Chemistry & Hematology Reference Intervals

Jessica Duis, MD
Assistant Professor, Department of Pediatrics, Section of Clinical Genetics and Metabolism, University of Colorado School of Medicine, Director, Special Care Clinic, Children's Hospital Colorado
Chapter 37: Genetics & Dysmorphology

Cullen M. Dutmer, MD
Associate Professor, Department of Pediatrics, Section of Pediatric Allergy and Immunology, University of Colorado School of Medicine and Children's Hospital Colorado
Chapter 33: Immunodeficiency

Vanessa Fabrizio, MD, MS
Assistant Professor, Department of Pediatrics, Section of Pediatric Hematology, Oncology, and Bone Marrow Transplant, Center for Cancer and Blood Disorders, University of Colorado School of Medicine and Children's Hospital Colorado
Chapter 31: Neoplastic Disease

Amy G. Feldman, MD, PhD
Associate Professo of Pediatrics, Department of Pediatrics, Section of Pediatric Gastroenterology, Hepatology and Nutrition, University of Colorado School of Medicine and Children's Hospital Colorado
Chapter 22: Liver and Pancreas

David M. Fleischer, MD
Professor, Department of Pediatrics, Section of Pediatric Allergy and Clinical Immunology, University of Colorado School of Medicine and Children's Hospital Colorado
Chapter 38: Allergic Disorders

David Fox, MD
Associate Professor, Department of Pediatrics, Section of General Academic Pediatrics, University of Colorado and Children's Hospital Colorado
Chapter 9: Ambulatory and Community Pediatrics

C. Rashaan Ford, MD
Assistant Professor, Department of Pediatrics, University of Colorado School of Medicine, Kempe Child Protection Team, Kempe Center for the Prevention and Treatment of Child Abuse and Neglect and Children's Hospital Colorado
Chapter 8: Child Abuse & Neglect

Brigitte I. Frohnert, MD, PhD
Associate Professor, Department of Pediatrics, Barbara Davis Center for Childhood Diabetes, University of Colorado School of Medicine
Chapter 35: Diabetes Mellitus

Glenn T. Furuta, MD
Professor of Pediatrics, Section of Pediatric
 Gastroenterology, Hepatology and Nutrition, Digestive
 Health Institute, Director Gastrointestinal Eosinophil
 Disease Program—National Jewish Health, University of
 Colorado School of Medicine and Children's Hospital
 Colorado
Chapter 21: Gastrointestinal Tract

James Gaensbauer, MD, MScPH
Associate Professor, Department of Pediatric and Adolescent
 Medicine, Division of Infectious Diseases, Mayo Clinic
Chapter 42: Infections: Bacterial & Spirochetal
Chapter 43: Infections: Parasitic & Mycotic

Jeffrey L. Galinkin, MD
Anesthesiologist, US Anesthesia Partners, Greenwood
 Village, Colorado
Chapter 32: Palliative Care & Pain Medicine

Timothy Price Garrington, MD
Professor, Department of Pediatrics, Section of Pediatric
 Hematology, Oncology, and Bone Marrow Transplant,
 Center for Cancer and Blood Disorders, University of
 Colorado School of Medicine and Children's Hospital
 Colorado
Chapter 31: Neoplastic Disease

Kelly Glaze, PsyD
Assistant Professor, Department of Psychiatry, University
 of Colorado School of Medicine and Children's Hospital
 Colorado
*Chapter 7: Child & Adolescent Psychiatric Disorders &
 Psychosocial Aspects of Pediatrics*

Ryan J. Good, MD
Associate Professor, Department of Pediatrics, Section of
 Pediatric Critical Care Medicine, University of Colorado
 School of Medicine and Children's Hospital Colorado
Chapter 14: Critical Care

Brian S. Greffe, MD
Professor Emeritus of Pediatrics, Department of Pediatrics,
 Section of Pediatric Hematology, Oncology, and Bone
 Marrow Transplant, Center for Cancer/Blood Disorders,
 University of Colorado School of Medicine and Children's
 Hospital Colorado
*Chapter 32: Pain Management & Pediatric Palliative &
 End-of-Life Care*

Matthew A. Haemer, MD, MPH
Professor, Department of Pediatrics, Section of Pediatric
 Nutrition, Associate Director - Clinical Nutrition
 Fellowship for Physicians, Medical Director Lifestyle
 Medicine Level 1, University of Colorado School of
 Medicine, Children's Hospital Colorado
Chapter 11: Normal Childhood Nutrition & Its Disorders

Melisha G. Hanna, MD, MS
Associate Professor, Department of Pediatrics, Section
 of Pediatric Nephrology, Medical Director, Pediatric
 Dialysis Unit, University of Colorado School of Medicine
 and Children's Hospital Colorado
*Chapter 23: Fluid, Electrolyte, & Acid-Base Disorders and
 Treatment*
Chapter 24: Kidney & Urinary Tract

Pia J. Hauk, MD
Professor, Department of Pediatrics, Section of Pediatric
 Allergy and Immunology, University of Colorado School
 of Medicine and National Jewish Medical and Research
 Center
Chapter 33: Immunodeficiency

Andrew S. Haynes, MD
Assistant Professor, Department of Pediatrics, Section
 of Pediatric Infectious Diseases and Epidemiology,
 University of Colorado School of Medicine and Children's
 Hospital Colorado
Chapter 39: Antimicrobial Therapy

Louise Helander, MBBS
Assistant Professor of Medicine, Director to Red Cell
 Antigen Molecular Testing, Children's Hospital Colorado
 Medical Director, Clin Immune Cell and Gene Therapy
 University of Colorado, School of Medicine
Chapter 46: Chemistry & Hematology Reference Intervals

Brian W. Herrmann, MD
Associate Professor, Department of Otolaryngology, Head
 and Neck Surgery, Division of Pediatric Otolaryngology,
 University of Colorado School of Medicine and Children's
 Hospital Colorado
Chapter 18: Ear, Nose, Throat

Jesse Hinckley, MD, PhD
Assistant Professor, Department of Psychiatry, University of
 Colorado School of Medicine
Chapter 5: Substance Use

Edward J. Hoffenberg, MD
Professor, Department of Pediatrics, Section of Pediatric
 Gastroenterology, Hepatology and Nutrition, Digestive
 Health Institute, University of Colorado School of
 Medicine and Children's Hospital Colorado
Chapter 21: Gastrointestinal Tract

Jordana Hoppe, MD
Associate Professor, Department of Pediatrics, Section of
 Pediatric Pulmonary Medicine, University of Colorado
 School of Medicine and Children's Hospital Colorado
Chapter 19: Respiratory Tract & Mediastinum

Paul Houin, MD
Assistant Professor of Clinical Practice, Department of Pediatrics, Section of Pediatric Pulmonology and Sleep Medicine, University of Colorado School of Medicine and Children's Hospital Colorado
Chapter 19: Respiratory Tract & Mediastinum

Stephanie Hsu, MD, PhD
Associate Professor Department of Pediatrics, Section of Pediatric Endocrinology, University of Colorado School of Medicine and Children's Hospital Colorado
Chapter 34: Endocrine Disorders

Roni Jacobsen, MD
Associate Professor, Departments of Pediatrics and Internal Medicine, Sections of Pediatric and Adult Cardiology, University of Colorado School of Medicine and Children's Hospital Colorado
Chapter 20: Cardiovascular Diseases

Monika Jelic, MD
Postgraduate Fellow, Departments of Pediatrics and Medicine, Section of Pediatric Infectious Diseases and Epidemiology, University of Colorado School of Medicine and Children's Hospital Colorado
Chapter 43: Infections: Parasitic & Mycotic

Jennifer Lee Jung, MD
Assistant Professor, Department of Ophthalmology, University of Colorado School of Medicine and Children's Hospital Colorado
Chapter 16: Eye

Paritosh Kaul, MD
Adjunct Professor, Department of Pediatrics, Section of Adolescent Medicine, University of Colorado School of Medicine and Professor, Department of Pediatrics, Section of Adolescent Medicine, Medical College of Wisconsin
Chapter 5: Substance Use

Kimberly Kelsay, MD
Associate Professor, Department of Psychiatry, University of Colorado School of Medicine and Children's Hospital Colorado
Chapter 7: Child & Adolescent Psychiatric Disorders & Psychosocial Aspects of Pediatrics

Sheryl J. Kent, PhD
Associate Professor of Clinical Practice, Anesthesiology, University of Colorado School of Medicine and Children's Hospital Colorado, Aurora, Colorado
Chapter 32: Palliative Care & Pain Medicine

John S. Kim, MD
Associate Professor, Department of Pediatrics, Section of Pediatric Cardiology, University of Colorado School of Medicine and Children's Hospital Colorado
Chapter 20: Cardiovascular Diseases

Nancy A. King, MSN, RN, CPNP
Senior Instructor, Department of Pediatrics, Section of Pediatric Hematology, Oncology, and Bone Marrow Transplant, Center for Cancer/Blood Disorders, University of Colorado School of Medicine and Children's Hospital Colorado
Chapter 32: Palliative Care & Pain Medicine

Gregory E. Kobak, MD
Senior Instructor of Pediatrics, Section of Pediatric Gastroenterology, Hepatology and Nutrition, Digestive Health Institute, University of Colorado Denver and Children's Hospital Colorado
Chapter 21: Gastrointestinal Tract

Aaina Kochhar, MD
Assistant Professor, Department of Pediatrics, Section of Clinical Genetics and Metabolism, University of Colorado School of Medicine and Children's Hospital Colorado
Chapter 37: Genetics & Dysmorphology

Robert E. Kramer, MD
Professor, Department of Pediatrics, Section of Pediatric Gastroenterology, Hepatology and Nutrition, Digestive Health Institute, University of Colorado School of Medicine and Children's Hospital Colorado
Chapter 21: Gastrointestinal Tract

Austin A. Larson, MD
Associate Professor, Department of Pediatrics, Section of Clinical Genetics and Metabolism, University of Colorado School of Medicine and Children's Hospital Colorado
Chapter 36: Inborn Errors of Metabolism

Jean M. Mulcahy Levy, MD
Associate Professor, Department of Pediatrics, Section of Pediatric Hematology, Oncology, and Bone Marrow Transplant, Center for Cancer and Blood Disorders, Morgan Adams Foundation Pediatric Brain Tumor Research Program, University of Colorado School of Medicine and Children's Hospital Colorado
Chapter 31: Neoplastic Disease

Michele Loi, MD
Associate Professor, Department of Pediatrics, Section of Pediatric Critical Care Medicine, University of Colorado School of Medicine and Children's Hospital Colorado
Chapter 14: Critical Care

Christine E. MacBrayne, PharmD, MSCS
Department of Pharmacy, University of Colorado Skaggs School of Pharmacy and Pharmaceutical Sciences
Chapter 39: Antimicrobial Therapy

Cara L. Mack, MD
Professor of Pediatrics, Division Chief-Pediatric Gastroenterology, Hepatology & Nutrition Medical College of Wisconsin and Children's Wisconsin
Chapter 22: Liver & Pancreas

Kelly Maloney, MD
Professor, Department of Pediatrics, Section of Pediatric Hematology, Oncology, and Bone Marrow Transplant, Center for Cancer/Blood Disorders, University of Colorado School of Medicine and Children's Hospital Colorado
Chapter 31: Neoplastic Disease

Jacob A. Mark, MD
Assistant Professor of Pediatrics, Department of Pediatrics, Section of Pediatric Gastroenterology, Hepatology and Nutrition, University of Colorado School of Medicine and Children's Hospital Colorado
Chapter 22: Liver and Pancreas

Stephanie W. Mayer, MD
Associate Professor, Department of Orthopedic Surgery, University of Colorado
Sports Medicine and Hip Preservation
Team Physician, Colorado Avalanche Hockey Club, University of Denver, University of Colorado
Chapter 27: Sports Medicine

Elizabeth J. McFarland, MD
Professor, Department of Pediatrics, Section of Pediatric Infectious Diseases and Epidemiology,
University of Colorado School of Medicine and Children's Hospital Colorado
Chapter 41: Human Immunodeficiency Virus Infection

Christopher McKinney, MD
Associate Professor, Department of Pediatrics, Section of Pediatric Hematology, Oncology and bone Marrow transplant, Center for Cancer and Blood disorders, University of Colorado School of Medicine and Children's Colorado
Chapter 30: Hematologic Disorders

Naomi J. L. Meeks, MD
Associate Professor, Department of Pediatrics, Section of Clinical Genetics and Metabolism, University of Colorado School of Medicine and Children's Hospital Colorado
Chapter 37: Genetics & Dysmorphology

Lauren Mehner, MD, MPH
Assistant Professor, Department of Ophthalmology, University of Colorado School of Medicine and Children's Hospital Colorado
Chapter 16: Eye

Ricka Messer, MD, PhD
Associate Professor, Department of Pediatrics, Section of Child Neurology, Director, Pediatric Neurohospitalist Program, Medical Director of Clinical Informatics for Neurology, University of Colorado School of Medicine and Children's Hospital Colorado
Chapter 25: Neurologic & Muscular Disorders

Scott Miller, MS
Research Assistant, Department of Orthopedic Surgery, University of Colorado School of Medicine and Children's Hospital Colorado
Chapter 26: Orthopedics

Nathalie Nguyen, MD
Associate Professor, Department of Pediatrics, Section of Pediatric Gastroenterology, Hepatology and Nutrition, Digestive Health Institute, Center for Celiac Disease, University of Colorado School of Medicine and Children's Hospital Colorado
Chapter 21: Gastrointestinal Tract

Hai Nguyen-Tran, MD
Assistant Professor, Departments of Pediatrics and Medicine, Section of Pediatric Infectious Diseases and Epidemiology, University of Colorado School of Medicine and Children's Hospital Colorado
Chapter 42: Infections: Bacterial & Spirochetal

Daniel Nicklas, MD
Associate Professor of Pediatrics, Director of Primary Care Education, Children's Hospital Colorado Residency Program, University of Colorado and Children's Hospital Colorado
Chapter 9: Ambulatory and Community Pediatrics

Yosuke Nomura, MD
Instructor, Department of Pediatrics, Section of Pediatric Infectious Diseases and Epidemiology, University of Colorado School of Medicine and Denver Health Medical Center
Chapter 42: Infections: Bacterial & Spirochetal

Rachelle Nuss, MD
Professor, Department of Pediatrics, Section of Pediatric Hematology, Oncology, and Bone Marrow Transplant, Sickle Cell Center, University of Colorado School of Medicine and Children's Hospital Colorado
Chapter 30: Hematologic Disorders

Ann-Christine Nyquist, MD, MSPH
Professor, Department of Pediatrics, Section of Pediatric Infectious Diseases and Epidemiology, University of Colorado School of Medicine and Chief Epidemiology Officer, Children's Hospital Colorado
Chapter 1: Advancing the Quality & Safety of Care
Chapter 44: Sexually Transmitted Infections

Sean T. O'Leary, MD, MPH
Professor, Department of Pediatrics, Section of Pediatric Infectious Diseases and Epidemiology, University of Colorado School of Medicine and Children's Hospital Colorado
Chapter 10: Immunization

Daniel Olson, MD, PhD
Associate Professor, Department of Pediatrics, Sections of Pediatric Infectious Diseases and Epidemiology, University of Colorado School of Public Health, Center for Global Health, and Children's Hospital Colorado
Chapter 40: Infections: Viral & Rickettsial

Sarah K. Parker, MD
Associate Professor, Department of Pediatrics, Section of Pediatric Infectious Diseases and Epidemiology, Medical Director of Antimicrobial Stewardship, University of Colorado School of Medicine and Children's Hospital Colorado
Chapter 39: Antimicrobial Therapy

Aaron Powell, MD
Assistant Professor, Department of Physical Medicine and Rehabilitation Medicine, University of Colorado School of Medicine and Children's Hospital Colorado
Chapter 28: Rehabilitative Medicine

Francisco Prada, MD
Fellow, Department of Pediatrics, Section of Adolescent Medicine, University of Colorado School of Medicine and Children's Hospital Colorado
Chapter 6: Eating Disorders

Laura E. Primak, RD, CNSC
Professional Research Assistant/Dietitian, Department of Pediatrics, Section of Pediatric Nutrition, School of Medicine Nutrition Electives Coordinator, University of Colorado School of Medicine and Children's Hospital Colorado
Chapter 11: Normal Childhood Nutrition & Its Disorders

Lori D. Prok, MD
Professor of Dermatology, Pediatric Dermatology and Dermatopathology, University of Colorado School of Medicine, Children's Hospital Colorado
Chapter 15: Skin

Chaitanya P. Puranik, BDS, MS, MDentSci, PhD
Assistant Professor, Department of Pediatric Dentistry, University of Colorado School of Dental Medicine and Children's Hospital Colorado
Chapter 17: Oral Medicine & Dentistry

Suchitra Rao, MBBS, MSCS
Associate Professor, Department of Pediatrics, Section of Pediatric Infectious Diseases and Epidemiology, and Hospital Medicine University of Colorado School of Medicine and Associate Medical Director, Infection Prevention and Control, Children's Hospital Colorado
Chapter 45: Travel Medicine

Marian Rewers, MD, PhD
Professor, Department of Pediatrics, Clinical Director, Barbara Davis Center for Childhood Diabetes, University of Colorado School of Medicine
Chapter 35: Diabetes Mellitus

Ann Reynolds, MD
Professor, Department of Pediatrics, Section of Developmental Pediatrics, Medical Director of Developmental Pediatrics, University of Colorado School of Medicine and Children's Hospital Colorado
Chapter 3: Child Development and Behavior

Jason T. Rhodes, MD, MS
Associate Professor, Department of Orthopedic Surgery, Director Cerebral Palsy Program, University of Colorado School of Medicine and The Children's Hospital, Adjunct Associate Professor, Department of Mechanical and Materials Engineering, University of Denver
Chapter 26: Orthopedics

Molly J. Richards, MD
Associate Professor, Department of Pediatrics, Section of Developmental Pediatrics, University of Colorado School of Medicine and Children's Hospital Colorado
Chapter 4: Adolescence

Laura Rochford, MD
Instructor, Department of Pediatrics, Section of Pediatric Emergency Medicine, University of Colorado School of Medicine and Children's Hospital Colorado
Chapter 12: Emergencies & Injuries

Barry H. Rumack, MD
Professor Emeritis of Emergency Medicine and Pediatrics, University of Colorado School of Medicine, Rocky Mountain Poison and Drug Center
Chapter 13: Poisoning

Christopher Ruzas, MD
Assistant Professor, Department of Pediatrics, Section of Pediatric Critical Care Medicine, University of Colorado School of Medicine and Children's Hospital Colorado
Chapter 14: Critical Care

Margarita Saenz, MD
Associate Professor of Clinical Practice, Department of Pediatrics, Section of Clinical Genetics and Metabolism, University of Colorado School of Medicine and Children's Hospital Colorado
Chapter 37: Genetics & Dysmorphology

Cristina Sarmiento, MD
Assistant Professor, Department of Physical Medicine and Rehabilitation Medicine, University of Colorado School of Medicine and Children's Hospital Colorado
Chapter 28: Rehabilitative Medicine

Amy E. Sass, MD, MPH
Associate Professor, Department of Pediatrics, Section of Adolescent Medicine, University of Colorado School of Medicine and Children's Hospital Colorado
Chapter 4: Adolescence

Melissa A. Scholes, MD
Associate Professor, Department of Otolaryngology, Head and Neck Surgery, Division of Pediatric Otolaryngology, University of Mississippi Medical Center and Children's of Mississippi
Chapter 18: Ear, Nose, Throat

Seth Septer, DO
Associate Professor, Department of Pediatrics, Section of Pediatric Gastroenterology, Hepatology and Nutrition, Digestive Health Institute, University of Colorado School of Medicine and Children's Hospital Colorado
Chapter 21: Gastrointestinal Tract

Animesh Sharma, MD
Assistant Professor, Departments of Pediatrics and Endocrinology, University of Colorado School of Medicine and Children's Hospital Colorado, Aurora, Colorado
Chapter 34: Endocrine Disorders

Mary Shull, MD
Assistant Professor, Department of Pediatrics, Section of Pediatric Gastroenterology, Hepatology and Nutrition, Digestive Health Institute, Center for Celiac Disease, University of Colorado School of Medicine and Children's Hospital Colorado
Chapter 21: Gastrointestinal Tract

Eric J. Sigel, MD
Professor, Department of Pediatrics, Section of Adolescent Medicine, University of Colorado School of Medicine and Children's Hospital Colorado
Chapter 6: Eating Disorders

Austin Skinner, BS
Medical Student, Kansas City University College of Osteopathic Medicine
Chapter 26: Orthopedics

Christiana Smith, MD, MSC
Associate Professor, Department of Pediatrics, Sections of Adolescent Medicine and Section of Infectious Diseases and Epidemiology, University of Colorado School of Medicine and Children's Hospital Colorado
Chapter 41: Human Immunodeficiency Virus Infection
Chapter 44: Sexually Transmitted Infections

Danielle Smith, MD
Associate Professor of Clinical Practice, Department of Pediatrics, Section of Neonatology, University of Colorado School of Medicine and Children's Hospital Colorado
Chapter 2: The Newborn Infant

Jason Soden, MD
Associate Professor, Department of Pediatrics, Section of Pediatric Gastroenterology, Hepatology and Nutrition, Digestive Health Institute, University of Colorado School of Medicine+D91 and Children's Hospital Colorado
Chapter 21: Gastrointestinal Tract

Jennifer B. Soep, MD
Associate Professor, Department of Pediatrics, Section of Pediatric Rheumatology, University of Colorado School of Medicine and Children's Hospital Colorado
Chapter 29: Rheumatic Diseases

Ronald J. Sokol, MD
Distinguished Professor of Pediatrics, and Vice Chair, Department of Pediatrics, Head Section of Pediatric Gastroenterology, Hepatology and Nutrition, Director, Colorado Clinical Translational Sciences institute, University of Colorado School of Medicine and Children's Hospital Colorado
Chapter 22: Liver and Pancreas

Paul Stillwell, MD
Senior Instructor, Department of Pediatrics, Section of Pediatric Pulmonology and Sleep Medicine, University of Colorado School of Medicine and Children's Hospital Colorado
Chapter 19: Respiratory Tract & Mediastinum

Diane Straub, MD, MPH
Professor, Department of Pediatrics, Section of Adolescent Medicine, University of Colorado School of Medicine and Children's Hospital Colorado
Chapter 5: Substance Use

Shikha S. Sundaram, MD, MSCI
Professo of Pediatrics,, Department of Pediatrics, Section of Pediatric Gastroenterology, Hepatology and Nutrition, University of Colorado School of Medicine and Children's Hospital Colorado
Chapter 22: Liver and Pancreas

Alex Tagawa, BS
Research Coordinator Department of Orthopedic Surgery, University of Colorado School of Medicine and Children's Hospital Colorado
Chapter 26: Orthopedics

Ayelet Talmi, PhD
Professor, Departments of Psychiatry and Pediatrics, Director of Integrated Behavioral Health, Pediatric Mental Health Institute, Director, Project CLIMB, Co-Director, Harris Program in Infant Mental Health, University of Colorado School of Medicine, and Children's Hospital Colorado
Chapter 7: Child & Adolescent Psychiatric Disorders & Psychosocial Aspects of Pediatrics

Janet A. Thomas, MD
Professor, Department of Pediatrics, Section of Clinical Genetics and Metabolism, University of Colorado School of Medicine and Children's Hospital Colorado
Chapter 36: Inborn Errors of Metabolism

Carla X. Torres-Zegarra, MD
Associate Professor, Departments of Dermatology and Pediatrics, University of Colorado and Children's Hospital Colorado
Chapter 15: Skin

Elizabeth Troy, MD
Assistant Professor, Department of Pediatrics, Section of Child Neurology, University of Colorado School of Medicine and Children's Hospital Colorado
Chapter 25: Neurologic & Muscular Disorders

Meghan Treitz, MD
Associate Professor, Department of Pediatrics, Section of General Academic Pediatrics, University of Colorado School of Medicine and Children's Hospital Colorado
Chapter 9: Ambulatory and Community Pediatrics

Abidin Hakan Tuncer, DDS, DMD, MPH, FSCD
Assistant Professor, Department of Pediatric Dentistry, School of Dental Medicine and Children's Hospital Colorado
Chapter 17: Oral Medicine & Dentistry

Karin VanBaak, MD, CAQSM
Assistant Professor, Department of Family Medicine and Orthopedics, University of Colorado School of Medicine, UC Health Family Medicine Clinic – Boulder, CU Sports Medicine and Performance Center
Chapter 27: Sports Medicine

Johan L. K. Van Hove, MD, PhD, MBA
Professor, Department of Pediatrics, Section of Clinical Genetics and Metabolism, University of Colorado School of Medicine and Children's Hospital Colorado
Chapter 36: Inborn Errors of Metabolism

Johannes Von Alvensleben, MD
Associate Professor, Department of Pediatrics, Section of Pediatric Cardiology, University of Colorado School of Medicine and Children's Hospital Colorado
Chapter 20: Cardiovascular Diseases

Thomas Walker, MD
Professor of Pediatrics, Section of Pediatric Gastroenterology, Hepatology and Nutrition, Digestive Health Institute, University of Colorado School of Medicine and Children's Hospital Colorado
Chapter 21: Gastrointestinal Tract

Diana Walleigh, MD
Assistant Professor, Department of Pediatrics, Section of Child Neurology, University of Colorado School of Medicine and Children's Hospital Colorado
Chapter 25: Neurologic & Muscular Disorders

George Sam Wang, MD
Associate Professor, Department of Pediatrics, Emergency Medicine/Medical Toxicology, University of Colorado School of Medicine
Chapter 13: Poisoning

Michael Wang, MD
Professor, Department of Pediatrics, Section of Pediatric Hematology, Oncology, and Bone Marrow Transplant, Center for Cancer/Blood Disorders, University of Colorado School of Medicine and Children's Hospital Colorado
Chapter 30: Hematologic Disorders

Joshua T.B. Williams, MD
Associate Professor, General Pediatrician, Ambulatory Care Services, Denver Health & Hospital Authority, Denver, Colorado
Chapter 10: Immunization

Anne R. Wilson, DDS, MS
Professor and Delta Dental of Colorado Endowed Chairperson, Department of Pediatric Dentistry, University of Colorado School of Dental Medicine and Children's Hospital Colorado
Chapter 17: Oral Medicine & Dentistry

Pamela E. Wilson, MD
Associate Professor, Department of Physical Medicine and Rehabilitation Medicine, University of Colorado School of Medicine and Children's Hospital Colorado
Chapter 28: Rehabilitative Medicine

Melissa Wright, MD, PhD
Assistant Professor, Department of Pediatrics, Section of Child Neurology, University of Colorado School of Medicine and Children's Hospital Colorado
Chapter 25: Neurologic & Muscular Disorders

Patricia J. Yoon, MD
Associate Professor, Department of Otolaryngology, Head and Neck Surgery, Division of Pediatric Otolaryngology, University of Colorado School of Medicine and Children's Hospital Colorado
Chapter 18: Ear, Nose, Throat

Preface

The 27th edition of *Current Diagnosis & Treatment: Pediatrics (CDTP)* features practical, up-to-date, well-referenced information on the care of children from birth through infancy and adolescence. *CDTP* emphasizes the clinical aspects of pediatric care while also covering important underlying principles. *CDTP* provides a guide to diagnosis, understanding, and treatment of the medical problems of all pediatric patients in an easy-to-use and readable format.

INTENDED AUDIENCE

Like all Lange medical books, *CDTP* provides a concise, yet comprehensive source of current information. Students will find *CDTP* an authoritative introduction to pediatrics and an excellent source for reference and review. *CDTP* provides excellent coverage of The Council on Medical Student Education in Pediatrics (COMSEP) curriculum used in pediatric clerkships. Residents in pediatrics (and other specialties) will appreciate the detailed descriptions of diseases as well as diagnostic and therapeutic procedures. Pediatricians, family practitioners, nurses, nurse practitioners, physician assistants, and other health care providers who work with infants, children, and adolescents will find *CDTP* a useful reference on management of pediatric medicine.

COVERAGE

Forty-six chapters cover a wide range of topics, including neonatal medicine, child development and behavior, emergency and critical care medicine, and diagnosis and treatment of specific disorders according to major problems, etiologies, and organ systems. A wealth of tables and figures along with photographs in select chapters provides quick access to important information, such as acute and critical care procedures in the delivery room, the office, the emergency room, and in-hospital critical care units; anti-infective agents; drug dosages; immunization schedules; differential diagnosis; and developmental disorders.

NEW TO THIS EDITION

The 27th edition of *CDTP* has been revised comprehensively by the editors and contributing authors. We also included photographs where helpful in certain chapters. Continued efforts involved streamlining the contents of the book by condensing text into tables, eliminating wordy text, and updating references. New references and up-to-date and useful websites have been added, facilitating access to the original material and material that goes beyond the confines of the textbook. As editors and practicing pediatricians, we have tried to ensure that each chapter reflects the needs and realities of day-to-day practice.

ACKNOWLEDGMENTS

The editors would like to thank Robin Pence, RN, at Children's Hospital Colorado, who produced the cover photograph of Dr. William Hay and the infant, Teckla Olivares. We appreciate Dr. Teri Schreiner, Associate Professor, Pediatric Neurology, for her expertise and for joining us on the editor team as a successor for Dr. Hay.

Maya Bunik, MD, MPH
William W. Hay Jr., MD
Myron J. Levin, MD
Mark J. Abzug, MD
Teri Schreiner, MD, MPH

Aurora, Colorado
April 2024

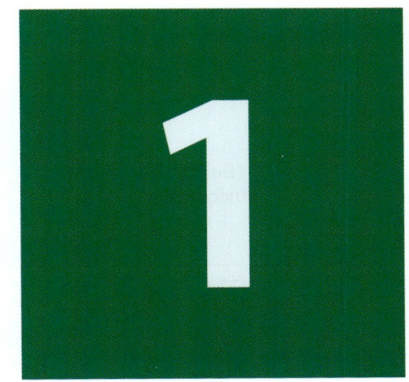

Advancing the Quality & Safety of Care

Lalit Bajaj, MD, MPH/MSPH
Ann-Christine Nyquist, MD, MSPH

INTRODUCTION

Hippocrates' famous dictum *primum non nocere* 2500 years ago may have been the earliest declaration of the importance of patient safety, but the Institute of Medicine's (IOM) 1999 landmark report *To Err Is Human* galvanized the current focus on eliminating preventable harm from health care. Its most quoted statistic, between 44,000 and 98,000 Americans die every year because of medical error, was based on studies of hospital mortality in Colorado, Utah, and New York, and extrapolated to an annual estimate for the country. The IOM follow-up publication, *Crossing the Quality Chasm*, said, "Health care today harms too frequently, and routinely fails to deliver its potential benefits.... Between the health care we have and the care we could have lies not just a gap, but a chasm." These two reports serve as central elements in an advocacy movement that has engaged stakeholders across the continuum of our health care delivery system and has changed the nature of how we think about the quality and safety of the care we provide and receive.

In 1966, Avedis Donabedian reviewed the then scant literature on the methods for assessing the quality of medical care and noted, "it seems likely that there will never be a single comprehensive criterion by which to measure the quality of patient care." The subsequent IOM landmark publication, *Crossing the Quality Chasm*, offers an elegant definition of the word "quality" as it applies to health care. They defined six domains of health care quality: (1) SAFE—free from preventable harm; (2) EFFECTIVE—optimal clinical outcomes; doing what we should do, not what we should not do according to the evidence; (3) EFFICIENT—without waste of resources—human, financial, or supplies/equipment; (4) TIMELY—without unnecessary delay; (5) PATIENT/FAMILY CENTERED—according to the wishes and values of patients and their families; and (6) EQUITABLE—eliminating disparities in outcomes between patients of different race, gender, and socioeconomic status.

Since the publication of these two seminal reports, multiple stakeholders who have been concerned about the effectiveness, safety, and cost of health care in the United States and, indeed throughout the world, have accelerated their individual and collective involvement in analyzing and improving care. In the United States, numerous governmental agencies, large employer groups, health insurance plans, consumers/patients, health care providers, and delivery systems are among the key constituencies calling for and working toward better and safer care at lower cost. Similar efforts are occurring internationally. Indeed, the concept of the Triple Aim (Care, Health, Cost) has been widely accepted as an organizing framework for considering the country's overall health care improvement goals.

Committee on Quality Health Care in America, Institute of Medicine: *Crossing the Quality Chasm: A New Health System for the 21st Century*. Washington, DC: National Academy Press; 2001.
Donabedian A: Evaluating the quality of medical care. Milbank Q 2005;83(4):691–729 [PMID: 16279964].
Kohn L, Corrigan JM: *To Err Is Human: Building a Safer Health System*. Washington, DC: National Academy Press; 2000.

CURRENT CONTEXT

Transformation of the health care industry is being driven by at least four converging factors: (1) the recognition of serious gaps in the safety and quality of care we provide (and receive), (2) the unsustainable increases in the cost of care as a percent of the national economy, (3) the aging of the population, and (4) the increased role of health care information technology as a potential tool to improve care. These factors are impacting health care organizations as well as individual practitioners in numerous ways that can also be traced to expectations regarding transparency and increasing accountability for results. As depicted in Figure 1–1, the Quadruple Aim (advancing the original concept of the Triple Aim) includes the simultaneous goals of achieving

*IHI Quadruple Aim

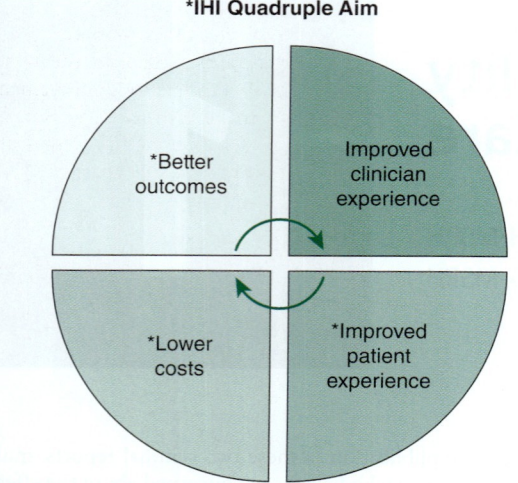

▲ **Figure 1–1.** Quadruple Aim.

better care (outcomes/experience) for individual patients and families, better health status for the population, and lower overall cost of care and enhancing the experience of the health care workforce. Practitioners and trainees (and health care workers in general) must adapt to a new set of priorities that focus attention on new goals to extend our historic focus on the doctor-patient relationship and autonomous physician decision-making. These new imperatives are evidence-based medicine, advancing safety, and reducing unnecessary expense. Increasingly there is the recognition that we need to continually address the resiliency and wellness of our health care workforce if we are to achieve our patient-oriented goals. Staff must be safe, both physically and psychologically, and programs to address these concepts must be a focus of health care systems around the country. Finally, in the aftermath of widespread protests over racism and advocacy for social justice in the United States and globally during 2020, there is greater recognition of the need to address pervasive health care and health disparities and inequities. As leaders of health care systems and communities assume responsibility to address these gaps in care, we expect to see that longstanding but modest efforts with limited impact toward the domain of equity will be spread and strengthened. This work will require efforts not only inside our health care system but even more so at the interfaces between health systems, schools, communities, payers, and government.

The impact of health care quality improvement is increasingly influencing clinical practice and the delivery of pediatric care. This chapter provides a summary of some of the central elements of health care quality improvement and patient safety and offers resources for the reader to obtain additional information and understanding about these topics.

External influences are driving many of these changes. Six key national organizations central to the changes occurring:

1. Center for Medicare and Medicaid Services (CMS, Department of Health and Human Services)—www.cms.gov
   CMS oversees federally funded health care programs of the United States, including Medicare, Medicaid, and other related programs. CMS and the Veterans Affairs Divisions together now provide funding for nearly $1.2 trillion of the total $3.8 trillion the United States spent in 2018 on health care expense https://www.cms.gov/medicare/payment/prospective-payment-systems/acute-inpatient-pps/hospital-acquired-condition-reduction-program-hacrp. CMS has payment mechanisms that withhold payment for the costs of preventable complications of care and gives incentives to providers for achieving better outcomes for their patients, primarily in its Medicare population. The agency has also enabled and advocated for greater transparency of results and makes available on its website comparative measures of performance for its Medicare population. CMS is also increasingly utilizing its standards under which hospitals and other health care provider organizations are licensed to provide care as tools to ensure greater compliance with these regulations. It has instituted a Hospital-Acquired Condition (HAC) Reduction program (https://www.cms.gov/medicare/payment/prospective-payment-systems/acute-inpatient-pps/hospital-acquired-condition-reduction-program-hacrp) that targets a range of conditions, with payment reductions from Medicare based on rates of occurrence. CMS can generate comparative national data only for its Medicare population because it, unlike Medicaid, is a single federal program with a single financial database. Because the Medicaid program functions as 51 state-federal partnership arrangements, patient experience and costs are captured in 51 separate state-based program databases. However, state Medicaid programs have been growing to create incentives to hospitals that care for a disproportionate amount of Medicaid patients such as the Delivery System Reform Incentive programs. CMS also has leveraged legislation to publish Medicaid measures that can be applied to the pediatric community primarily in the outpatient setting.

2. National Quality Forum (NQF)—www.qualityforum.org
   NQF is a private, not-for-profit organization whose members include consumer advocacy groups, health care providers, accrediting bodies, employers and other purchasers of care, and research organizations. Its mission is to "drive measurable health improvements" so that "every person experiences high-value care and optimal outcomes." The NQF promotes improvement in the quality of American health care primarily through defining priorities for improvement, approving consensus standards and metrics for performance reporting, and educational efforts. The NQF, for example, has endorsed a list of 29

"serious reportable events" in health care that include events related to surgical or invasive procedures, products or device failures, patient protection, care management, environmental issues, radiologic events, and potential criminal events (https://www.qualityforum.org/Topics/SREs/Serious_Reportable_Events.aspx). This list and the CMS list of HACs are both being used by insurers to reduce payment to hospitals/providers as well as to require reporting to state agencies for public review. In 2012, NQF released a set of 44 measures for the quality of pediatric care, largely representing outpatient preventive services and management of chronic conditions, and population-based measures applicable to health plans, for example, immunization rates and frequency of well-child care.

3. Leapfrog—www.leapfroggroup.org

Leapfrog is a group of large employers who seek to use their purchasing power to influence the health care community to achieve big "leaps" in health care safety and quality. It promotes transparency and issues public reports of how well individual hospitals meet their recommended standards, including computerized physician-order entry, intensive care unit (ICU) staffing models, and rates of health care–associated infections (HAIs). There is some evidence that meeting these standards is associated with improved hospital quality and/or mortality outcomes. In 2020, nine pediatric hospitals are part of this group.

4. Agency for Healthcare Research and Quality (AHRQ)—www.ahrq.gov

AHRQ is currently one of 12 agencies within the US Department of Health and Human Services. Its primary mission is to produce evidence to make health care safer and support health services research initiatives that seek to improve the quality of health care in the United States. AHRQ's core competencies include Health Systems Research, Practice Improvement, and Data and Analytics. Its activities extend well beyond the support of research and now include the development of measurements of quality and patient safety, reports on disparities in performance, measures of patient safety culture in organizations, and promotion of tools to improve care. The collaboration between federal agencies is best described as AHRQ is funding research and creating tools for patient safety interventions, the Centers for Disease Control and Prevention (CDC) researches and translates best practices into clinical guidelines and tracking systems (ie, National Healthcare Safety Network [NHSN]), and CMS uses its pay-for-performance regulatory power to provide financial incentives and penalties.

5. Specialty society boards

Specialty society boards, for example, the American Board of Pediatrics (ABP), along with other specialty certification organizations, have responded to the call for greater accountability to consumers by enhancing their maintenance of certification (MOC) programs (https://www.abp.org/content/maintenance-certification-moc). All trainees, and an increasing proportion of active practitioners, are now subject to the requirements of the MOC program, including participation in quality improvement activities in the diplomat's clinical practice. The Board's mission is focused on assuring the public that certificate holders have been trained according to their standards and meet continuous evaluation requirements in six areas of core competency: patient care, medical knowledge, practice-based learning and improvement, interpersonal and communication skills, professionalism, and systems-based practice. These same competencies are required of residents in training programs as certified by the Accreditation Council on Graduate Medical Education (ACGME). Providers need not only to be familiar with the principles of quality improvement and patient safety, but also must demonstrate having implemented quality improvement efforts within their practice settings. The American Board of Medical Specialties is addressing significant concerns with respect to the MOC program and in May 2021 requested comment on their proposed new guidelines for member boards to certify their physicians. The overall framework requiring professionalism, lifelong learning, and continuous improvement in care is retained in the new proposed ABMS guidelines despite likely changes to the existing structure over the next several years.

The American Academy of Pediatrics has its own several programs to support pediatricians in their pursuit of ongoing certification, and more importantly, ongoing improvement in practice. An example would be the Council on Quality Improvement and Patient Safety that is designed to define, implement, disseminate evidence-based practices for effective, equitable and safe clinical care using quality improvement (https://www.aap.org/en/community/aap-councils/council-on-quality-improvement-and-safety/).

6. The Joint Commission (TJC)—www.jointcommission.org

TJC is a private, nonprofit agency licensed to accredit health care provider organizations, including hospitals, nursing homes, and other health care provider entities in the United States as well as internationally. Its mission is to continuously improve the quality of care through evaluation, education, and enforcement of regulatory standards. Since 2003, TJC has annually adopted a set of National Patient Safety Goals designed to help advance the safety of care provided in all health care settings. Examples include the use of two patient identifiers to reduce the risk of care being provided to an unintended patient; the use of a universal protocol for preventing wrong site, wrong procedure, and wrong person surgery; and adherence to hand hygiene recommendations to reduce the risk of spreading HAIs. These goals often become regulatory standards with time and widespread adoption. Failure to meet these standards can result in actions against the licensure of the health care provider, or more commonly, require corrective action plans, measurement to demonstrate improvement, and resurveying depending on the severity of findings. The TJC publishes a monthly journal on quality and safety, available at https://www.jointcommission.org/resources/for-consumers/the-joint-commission-journal-on-quality-and-patient-safety/.

Finally, ongoing governmental impacts on quality and safety will likely be subject to modifications in any future US government changes to the Patient Protection and Affordable Care Act (PPACA) enacted by the US government in 2010. This federal health care legislation sought to provide near-universal access to health care through discounted health care exchanges that supplemented the existing, largely employer-based system. Changes in payment mechanisms for health care will continue irrespective of what happens to the PPACA, and current and future providers' practices will be economically, structurally, and functionally impacted by these emerging trends. Furthermore, changes in the funding and structure of the US health care system may ultimately also result in changes in other countries. Many countries have single-payer systems for providing health care to their citizens and often are leaders in defining new strategies for health care improvement.

Agency for Healthcare Research and Quality: www.ahrq.gov. Accessed January 30, 2024.

American Board of Pediatrics: https://www.abp.org. Accessed January 30, 2024.

Berwick D, Nolan T, Whittington J: The triple aim: care, health, and cost. Health Aff (Millwood) 2008;27(3):759–769. doi:10.1377/hlthaff.27.3.759 [PMID: 18474969]. https://pubmed.ncbi.nlm.nih.gov/18474969/. Accessed January 30, 2024.

Center for Medicare and Medicaid Services: www.cms.gov. Accessed January 30, 2024.

CMS list of Hospital-Acquired Conditions: https://www.cms.gov/medicare/payment/prospective-payment-systems/acute-inpatient-pps/hospital-acquired-condition-reduction-program-hacrp. Accessed January 30, 2024.

Connors E, Gostin L: Health care reform—a historic moment in US social policy. JAMA 2010;303(24):2521–2522. doi:10.1001/jama.2010.856 [PMID: 20571019]. https://pubmed.ncbi.nlm.nih.gov/20571019/. Accessed January 30, 2024.

Hawkins RE, Weiss KB: Commentary: building the evidence base in support of the American Board of Medical Specialties maintenance of certification program. Acad Med 2011;86(1):67. doi:10.1097/ACM.0b013e318201801b [PMID: 21191200]. https://pubmed.ncbi.nlm.nih.gov/21191200/. Accessed January 30, 2024.

Jha A, Oray J, Ridgway A, Zheng J, Eptein A: Does the Leapfrog program help identify high-quality hospitals? Jt Comm J Qual Patient Saf 2008;34(6):318–325 [PMID: 18595377].

Leapfrog: www.leapfroggroup.org. Accessed January 30, 2024.

Miller T, Leatherman S: The National Quality Forum: a "me-too" or a breakthrough in quality measurement and reporting? Health Aff (Millwood) 1999;18(6):233–237 [PMID: 10650707].

National Health Expenditure Data: https://www.cms.gov/medicare/payment/prospective-payment-systems/acute-inpatient-pps/hospital-acquired-condition-reduction-program-hacrp. Accessed January 30, 2024.

NQF 29 Serious Reported Events List: https://www.qualityforum.org/Topics/SREs/Serious_Reportable_Events.aspx. Accessed January 30, 2024.

https://www.qualityforum.org/Publications/2012/01/Child_Health_Quality_Measures_2010_Final_Report.aspx. Accessed January 30, 2024.

Rosenthal M: Beyond pay for performance—emerging models of provider-payment reform. New Engl J Med 2008;359:1197–1200 [PMID: 18799554].

Shekelle P et al: Advancing the science of patient safety. Ann Intern Med 2011;154(10):693–696 [PMID: 21576538].

Straube B, Blum JD: The policy on paying for treating hospital-acquired conditions: CMS officials respond. Health Aff (Millwood) 2009;28(5):1494–1497 [PMID: 19738268].

The Joint Commission: www.jointcommission.org. Accessed January 30, 2024.

STRATEGIES & MODELS FOR QUALITY IMPROVEMENT (QI)

While there are many approaches to improving the quality of care in health care settings, the following represent three common tools for conducting clinical improvement work. The Model for Improvement (MFI) is emphasized because of its ease of adoption and because it is the foundation for most improvement efforts included in the Maintenance of Certification program of the ABP. Briefer summaries of Lean and Six Sigma methods are also included, with listings of resources where the reader can find additional information.

MODEL FOR IMPROVEMENT

Widely taught and promoted by the Boston-based educational and advocacy organization the Institute for Healthcare Improvement (IHI), the MFI is grounded in three simple questions that guide the work of the improvement leader and team. The model's framework includes an Aim statement, a measurement strategy, and then the use of rapid cycle changes to achieve the aim. The IHI website, www.ihi.org, has an extensive resource library, and hosts an "Open School" that includes a quality improvement (QI)/patient safety modular curriculum for health professions students and their faculty at www.ihi.org/openschool.

AIM STATEMENT

The Aim statement answers the question, "What do we want to accomplish?" The measure question is "How will we know that a change is an improvement?" and the change component is focused on "What changes can we make that will result in improvement?" This model is represented in Figure 1–2.

Aim statements are a *written* description of what the team's improvement goal is and include information on who comprises the patient population and a time frame within which the improvement will be achieved. They identify a

Model for Improvement

> What are we trying to accomplish?
>
> How will we know that a change is an improvement?
>
> What changes can we make that will result in an improvement?

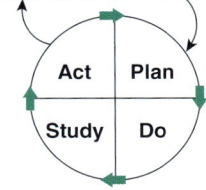

▲ **Figure 1–2.** Model for improvement. (Reproduced with permission from Langley G, Moen R, Nolan K, et al: *The Improvement Guide: AIM Model for Improvement.* San Francisco, CA: Jossey-Bass; 2009.)

"stretch" but achievable improvement target goal and, often, some general statement regarding how the improvement will be achieved. Aim statements are sometimes characterized using the mnemonic SMAART: Specific, Measurable, Achievable, Actionable, Relevant, and Timely. Aim statements should be unambiguous and understandable to stakeholders and are most likely to be achieved if they are aligned with the strategic goals of the team or organization.

For example, the following statement meets the criteria for a SMAART Aim statement: "We will reduce the frequency of emergency department visits and hospitalizations for patients with asthma seen at E Street Pediatrics by 25% by December 31, 2022," whereas this next statement does not: "We will improve the care for patients with asthma by appropriately prescribing indicated medications and better educating families in their use."

The first example provides a specific, measurable goal, a time frame, and clarity with respect to who the patients are.

A 25% reduction in ED/inpatient asthma visits will require a change in the system for asthma care delivery for the entire population of children with asthma; that extent of level of improvement is a stretch, but it is much more achievable than a goal would be if it were set to "eliminate" such encounters. The second example is unclear in terms of the measure for improvement, the time frame for the goal to be met, and even the population in question. The statement provides some sense of processes that could be utilized to improve asthma care but is missing needed specificity.

MEASURES

Specific measures provide a means to assess whether the improvement effort is on track. Three types of measures are useful. *Outcome measures* answer questions concerning the health care impact for the patients, such as how has their health status changed? *Process measures* are related to the health care delivery system itself. They answer questions about how the system is performing. *Balancing measures* seek to identify potential unintended consequences that are related to the improvement effort being undertaken. Examples are helpful to contextualize these conceptual definitions.

Table 1–1 reflects some examples of types of measures that might be employed in an asthma QI initiative.

One might argue that adherence to a treatment plan (third process measure) is an outcome of the work of the practice/practitioner prescribing the medication. It is more consistent, however, to consider the translation of the treatment plan into action as a part of the process of care, and that the health status or outcome measure will be improved by fully improving the measured processes of care, including patient adherence to the treatment plan.

Measures are essential elements of any improvement work. It is a good idea to choose a manageable (4–6) number of measures, all of which can be obtained with limited or no

Table 1–1. Examples of types of measures used in an asthma QI initiative.

Outcome Measures	Process Measures	Balancing Measures
Percent of children with asthma in the practice seen in the ED or hospitalized for asthma in the past 6 months	Proportion of children with an asthma severity assessment in their medical record in the past year	Average difference in the time between the last office patient's scheduled appointment time and the actual office close time
Percent of children with persistent asthma in the practice with fewer than 5 missed school days due to asthma in the past year	Percent of children with persistent asthma, of any severity, prescribed a controller medication at their most recent visit	Staff satisfaction with their job
	Percent of children prescribed a controller medication who report taking their medicine	
	Percent of children in a practice asthma registry provided with a complete asthma action plan in the past 12 months	

extra effort, and with a mix of outcome, process, and balancing measures. Ideally, the best process measures are those that are directly linked to the outcome goal. The hypothesis in this specific example would be that assessing asthma severity and appropriately using controller medications and action plans would all contribute to reducing the number or frequency of missed school days and the need for ED/hospital utilization.

It is important to note that measurement in the setting of an improvement project is different from measurement in a research study. Improvement projects require "just enough" data to guide the team's continuing efforts. Often, the result seen in a sequence of 10 patients is enough to tell you whether a particular system is functioning consistently or not. For example, considering the first process measure in Table 1–1, if in the last 10 patients seen with asthma, only 2 had their asthma severity documented, how many more charts need be checked to conclude that the system is not functioning as intended and that changes are needed? Other measures may require larger sample sizes, especially when assessing the impact of care changes on a population of patients with a particular condition. See Randolph's excellent summary for a fuller description of measurement for improvement (https://www.pediatric.theclinics.com/article/S0031-3955(09)00066-2/pdf).

CHANGES & IDEAS

Once the team's aim is established and the measures are selected, the third component of the MFI focuses on what changes in the system must be made that will result in the targeted improvements. To answer the question "What changes will result in improvement?" the improvement team should incorporate "Plan-Do-Study (or check)-Act" cycles, typically referred to as PDSA cycles. The cycles include the following steps.

- *Plan*: What will we do that will likely improve the process measures linked to the outcome target goal? Who will do it? Where? When? How? How will the data be collected?
- *Do*: Implementation of the planned change(s). *TIP!* It is good to make the change cycles as small as possible, for example, trying a new process on the next five patients being seen by one provider as opposed to wide-scale implementation of a new chart documentation form across an entire clinic.
- *Study (or check)*: Once the small test of change is tried, its results are assessed. How many times did the process work as planned for the five patients included in the cycle?
- *Act*: Based on the results of the study of the cycle, recommendations are made as to what the next steps ought to be to achieve the goal. At this point, the cycle then resumes and planning begins for the next cycle.

Over the course of an improvement effort, multiple tests of change might be implemented for any or all the process

measures felt to be likely to impact the outcome measures relevant to the project.

The MFI has been used by improvement teams across numerous health care settings around the world. Further information about the model and examples can be found at www.ihi.org/openschool or in *The Improvement Guide* (Langley et al).

The IHI Open School modules are an excellent online resource for clinicians interested in learning more about the fundamentals of quality improvement and patient safety. These educational lessons are free of charge to health professional students, residents, and university faculty members, and for a modest subscription fee to other clinicians. They are also free to health care practitioners in the low resource countries and settings. An excellent original resource on implementing this model in clinical practice is in Berwick's summary article from 1998.

Berwick D: The science of improvement. JAMA 2008:299(10): 1182–1184 [PMID: 18334694].
Berwick DM: Developing and testing changes in delivery of care. Ann Intern Med 1998;128:651–656 [PMID: 9537939].
Langley G, Moen R, Nolan K, Nolan T, Norman C, Provost L: *The Improvement Guide: AIM Model for Improvement*. San Francisco, CA: Jossey-Bass; 2009:24.
Randolph G, Esporas M, Provost L, Massie S, Bundy D: Model for improvement—Part Two: measurement and feedback for quality improvement efforts. Pediatr Clin North Am 2009;56(4): 779–798 [PMID: 19660627].

LEAN

An increasingly popular method for driving improvement efforts in health care settings is Lean or Lean processing. Lean is grounded in industrial engineering and early thinking about Lean processes is credited to the Toyota Manufacturing Company in Japan. Although the crossover to health care from manufacturing is a relatively recent phenomenon, numerous hospitals and health care delivery settings, including individual clinics, have benefited from the application of these principles to their clinical operations. Lean improvement methods focus on reducing errors and variability in repetitive steps that are part of any process. In health care, examples of repeated processes would include how patients are registered and their information obtained; and how medications are ordered, compounded, distributed, and administered.

Lean is a philosophy of continuous improvement. It is grounded in recognizing that the way we do things today is merely current state. With time, effort, focus, and long-term thinking, we can create a future state that is better than the status quo. It does so by focusing on identifying the value of all steps in any process and eliminating those steps that do not contribute to the value sought by the customer, or in health care, the patient/family. In doing so, improvements in outcomes, including cost and productivity, and in clinical measures of effectiveness can be realized. See Young et al for an early critical assessment of the incorporation of Lean into health care settings.

Four categories describe the essential elements of Toyota's adoption of Lean as a management strategy. These four categories are (1) *philosophy* (emphasize long-term thinking over short-term gain); (2) *process* (eliminate waste through very defined approaches including an emphasis on process flow and the use of pull systems to reduce overproduction, for example); (3) *people/partners* (respect, challenge, and grow staff); and (4) *problem solving* (create a culture of continuous learning and improvement).

Several hospitals have fully integrated Lean management as a primary basis for their organizational approach to improvement and are featured in a White Paper published by the IHI in 2005.

Going Lean in Health Care, Innovation Series White Paper. Institute for Healthcare Improvement: 2005. https://www.ihi. org/resources/white-papers/going-lean-health-care. Accessed January 30, 2024.

Liker JK: *The Toyota Way*. Madison, WI: McGraw-Hill; 2004.

Young TP, McClean SI: A critical look at Lean Thinking in healthcare. BMJ Qual Saf Health Care 2008;17:382–386 [PMID: 18842980].

SIX SIGMA

A third quality improvement methodology also arose in the manufacturing industry. Motorola is generally credited with promoting Six Sigma as a management strategy designed to reduce the variability in its processes and thereby reducing the number of defects in its outputs. Organizations adopting Six Sigma as an improvement strategy utilize measurement-based strategies that focus on process improvement and variation reduction to eliminate defects in their work and to reduce cycle times, thereby increasing profitability and enhancing customer satisfaction. Sigma is the statistical measure of standard deviation, and Motorola adopted Six Sigma as a performance indicator, promoting consistency of processes to have fewer than 3.4 defects per million opportunities. This performance goal has since become the common descriptor for this approach to improvement both in manufacturing and in service industries, including health care. Similar to Lean, the translation of business manufacturing strategies into health care has various challenges, but there are many processes that repeatedly occur in health care that can be routinized and made more consistent. Many health care processes fail far more frequently than 3.4 times per million opportunities. Consider pharmacy dispensing errors, medication ordering or administration errors, and patient-scheduling errors, just to name a few. These are a few of many examples of processes that could potentially benefit from the kind of rigorous analysis that is integral to the Six Sigma approach.

In a typical Six Sigma structured improvement project, there are five phases generally referred to as DMAIC: (1) Define (what is the problem, what is the goal?), (2) Measure (quantify the problem and improvement opportunity), (3) Analyze (use of observations and data to identify causes), (4) Improve (implementation of solutions based on data analysis), and finally, (5) Control (sustainable change).

One of the central aspects of Six Sigma as an improvement strategy is its defined focus on understanding the reasons for defects in any process. By understanding these drivers, it is then possible to revise the approach to either the manufacturing process or the service functions to reduce these errors and failures.

Lean-Six Sigma is a newer entity that draws from both methodologies to simplify the improvement work where possible but retain the rigorous statistical method that is a hallmark of Six Sigma projects. Lean focuses on where time is lost in any process and can identify opportunities to eliminate steps or reduce time. Six Sigma aims to reduce or eliminate defects in the process, thereby resulting in a higher quality product through a more efficient and lower cost process.

Regardless of the method used, improvement happens because an organization, team, or individual sets a goal to improve a current process through systematic analysis of the way things are done now, and then implements planned changes to see how they impact the outputs or outcomes.

For additional information on Lean and Six Sigma, see www.isixsigma.com (Accessed January 30, 2024) or https://asq.org/quality-resources/six-sigma (Accessed January 30, 2024).

Pande P, Holpp L: *What Is Six Sigma?* New York, NY: McGraw Hill; 2002.

PRINCIPLES OF PATIENT SAFETY (INCIDENT REPORTING, JUST CULTURE, DISCLOSURE, FMEA, RCA, RELIABILITY, DATA, & CHECKLISTS)

Safe patient care avoids preventable harm; it is a care that does not cause harm as it seeks to cure. The list of adverse events that are considered preventable is evolving. As mentioned earlier, both CMS and NQF have endorsed lists of various complications of care as being never events or serious reportable events for which providers are often now not reimbursed, and which are increasingly reportable to the public through various state transparency programs.

A national network of Children's Hospitals has been active since 2012, collaborating on a shared aim of eliminating serious harm in their now more than 145 organizations. Initially funded as a Hospital Engagement Network by the Center for Medicare and Medicaid Innovation program, Children's Hospitals Solutions for Patient Safety merge approaches to achieving reliability in evidence-based prevention practices (bundles) with safety practices at both staff and leadership levels to reducing serious safety events (SSEs) and HACs in general. Numerous hospitals have demonstrated dramatic reductions in the occurrence rates of both HACs and SSEs with the following interventions: (1) implementation of structured processes to improve consistency of prevention processes, (2) education and reinforcement of principles of patient safety culture designed to improve communication and reduce error, (3) effective, structured cause analyses after SSEs, and (4) data systems, including both human resources and information technology to support the ongoing focus on improved process reliability and continuous reductions in harm.

Irrespective of one's views about whether various complications are entirely preventable at the current state of science or not, these approaches reflect a changing paradigm that is impacting many aspects of health care delivery. Transparency of results is increasingly expected. Perspectives and data on how these kinds of efforts are impacting actual improvement in outcomes are mixed.

Given these trends, health care providers need to have robust systems for measuring and improving the safety of care provided to patients, as well as the safety of employees and staff in health care roles. The methods for improving quality reviewed earlier are frequently used to reduce harm, just as they can be used to improve effectiveness or efficiency. For example, hospitals attempting to reduce infections have successfully used these types of process improvement approaches to improve antibiotic use prior to surgical procedures or to improve hand hygiene practices.

Common patient safety tools include

Incident-reporting systems: Efforts to advance safety in any organization require a clear understanding of the kinds of harm occurring within that organization, as well as the kinds of near-misses that are occurring. These reporting systems can range from a simple paper reporting form to a telephone hotline to a computerized database that is available to staff (and to potential patients/families) within the organization. Events are traditionally graded according to the severity of harm that resulted from the incident. One example is the NCC MERP Index, which grades events from A (potential to cause harm) to I (resulting in patient death). Errors recognized represent only a fraction of the actual errors and near-misses that are present in the system. Incident-reporting systems depend on people recognizing the error or near-miss, being comfortable reporting it, knowing how and when to report, and then actually doing so. It is no surprise therefore that estimates for how frequently incidents that could or should be reported into incident-reporting systems range from 1.5% to 30% depending on the type of adverse or near-miss event. Trigger tools (either manual chart reviews for indications of adverse events, or automated reports from

electronic medical records) have been used to increase the recognition of episodes of harm in health care settings.

Just culture: The effectiveness of incident-reporting systems is highly dependent on the culture of the organization within which the reporting is occurring. Aviation industry safety-reporting systems are often highlighted for their successes in promoting reporting of aviation events that might have led to accidents. The Aviation Safety Reporting System (ASRS) prioritizes confidentiality to encourage reporting and protects reporters from punishment, with certain limitations when they report incidents, even if related to nonadherence to aviation regulations. Although the system is voluntary, as of 2019 more than 1.7 million reports have been submitted and used by the Federal Aviation Administration to improve air travel safety.

In health care, the variable recognition of adverse events as well as fear about reprisal for reporting events both work to reduce the consistent reporting of events. The concept of just culture has been promoted as a strategy to increase the comfort of staff members to report the occurrence of errors or near-misses, even if they may have done something incorrectly. See the work of David Marx and the Just Culture Community for more information on how to evaluate error to support reporting and safer practices in organizations. A great deal of information about just culture principles is available at https://www.justculture.com/.

Failure modes and effects analyses (FMEA): An FMEA is a systematic methodology used to proactively identify ways in which any process might fail and then prioritize strategies for reducing the risk or impact of identified potential failures. In conducting an FMEA, which all hospitals are required to do annually, a team will carefully describe and analyze each step in a particular process, consider what and how anything might go wrong, why it would happen, and what the impact would be of such failures. Like Lean and Six Sigma, the FMEA has been adopted into health care from its origins in military and industrial settings. The FMEA is an effective method for identifying strategies to reduce risks in health care settings, thereby protecting patients if interventions are put into place as a result of the analysis. A tool to use in conducting an FMEA is available from the IHI at https://www.ihi.org/resources/tools/failure-modes-and-effects-analysis-fmea-tool.

Root-cause analyses (RCAs) (post-event reviews): As contrasted with the proactive FMEA process, an RCA is a retrospective analysis of an adverse occurrence (or near-miss) that has already happened. It too is a systematic process that allows a team to reach an understanding of why certain things occurred, what systems factors and human factors contributed to the occurrence, and what defects in the system might be changed to reduce the likelihood of recurrence. Key to an effective RCA process, and similar to the principles discussed above related to just culture, RCAs are designed not to ask who was at fault, but rather what system reasons contributed to the event. Why, not who, is the essential question to be asked. The answer to the question "why did this occur" almost invariably results in a combination of factors, often illustrated by a series of pieces of Swiss cheese where the holes all line up. Taken from the writings of James Reason, the Swiss Cheese Model illustrates the many possible system failures that can contribute to an error and contributes to identifying potential system changes that reduce the risk of error recurrence. Strategies for approaching retrospective RCA and the causes of human and system error are available at http://www.ncbi.nlm.nih.gov/pmc/articles/pmc1117770. The use of retrospective review processes to learn from adverse events is frequently now referred to as Safety 1 approach to health care improvement. Increasingly, safety experts are focusing on Safety 2, which is a complementary strategy oriented to learning from situations "when things go right," and designing systems for reliability using approaches common in the field of human factors engineering. A few selected reading materials for the interested learner are listed as follows.

Communication and team training: Because failures of communication are the most common identified factors in the analysis of reported serious health care events, many health care organizations have incorporated tools from other industries, particularly aviation, to enhance patient safety. As a result of the knowledge gained through analysis of tragic aviation accidents, the airline industry implemented methods like crew resource management training to ensure that communication among cockpit team members is effective and clear, thereby reducing risk of air accidents. Similar methods have been used to train teams in operating rooms, delivery rooms, and other team-based settings. Most of these curricula include a few common elements: introductions to be sure all team members know one another's name, promoting the likelihood of speaking up; leader clarity with team members about the expectation that all will speak up if anyone has a concern; and structured language and other tools like verbal read-back of critical information to ensure clarity in interpersonal or interdisciplinary communications. Such training also seeks to flatten the hierarchy, making it more likely that potential risks or problems will be identified and effectively addressed. Common tools used in promoting effective team communication include structured language like SBAR (Situation, Background, Assessment, and Recommendation), taken from the Navy, to promote clarity of communication.

Several resources exist in the public domain to support better teamwork and communication. One good place to start is the TeamSTEPPS program from the Agency for Healthcare Research and Quality. It can be found at http://teamstepps.ahrq.gov/.

Ashley L, Armitage G, Neary M, Hoolingsworth G: A practical guide to failure mode and effects analysis in health care: making the most of the team and its meetings. Jt Comm J Qual Patient Saf 2010;36(8):351–358 [PMID: 20860241].

Children's Hospitals Solutions for Patient Safety: http://www.solutionsforpatientsafety.org. Accessed January 30, 2024.

Hollnagel E: A Tale of Two Safeties. http://erikhollnagel.com/A%20Tale%20of%20Two%20Safeties.pdf. Accessed January 30, 2024.

http://www.ihi.org/resources/Pages/Tools/FailureModesandEffectsAnalysisTool.aspx. Accessed January 30, 2024.

Incident Reporting Systems: http://www.nccmerp.org/. Accessed January 30, 2024.

Marx D: *A Primer for Health Care Executives: Patient Safety and the "Just Culture."* New York, NY: Columbia University; 2011.

Reason J: Human error: models and management. BMJ 2000;320:768–770. doi:10.1136/bmj.320.7237.768:2000 [PMID: 10720363].

Reference on 29 Serious Reportable Events NQF: https://www.qualityforum.org/Topics/SREs/Serious_Reportable_Events.aspx. Accessed January 30, 2024.

Shekelle P et al: Advancing the science of patient safety. Ann Intern Med 2011;154(10):693–696 [PMID: 21576538].

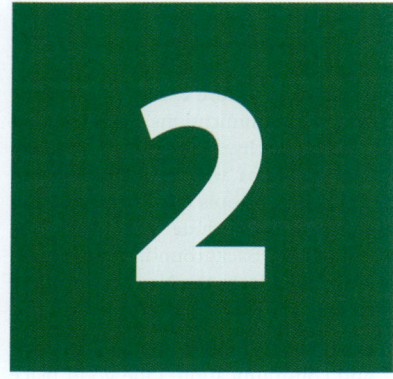

The Newborn Infant

Danielle Smith, MD

INTRODUCTION

The newborn period is defined as the first 28 days of life. In practice, however, sick or very immature infants may require neonatal care for many months. There are four levels of newborn care, ranging from level 1 for basic care of well newborns to level 4 that includes availability of pediatric subspecialists, pediatric surgery, and cardiac surgery.

THE NEONATAL HISTORY

The newborn medical history has three key components:

1. Maternal and paternal medical and genetic history
2. Maternal past obstetric history
3. Current antepartum and intrapartum obstetric history

The mother's medical history includes chronic medical conditions, medications taken during pregnancy, unusual dietary habits, smoking history, substance use history, occupational exposure to chemicals or infections of potential risk to the fetus, and any social history that might increase the risk for parenting challenges. Family illnesses and a history of congenital anomalies with genetic implications should be sought. The past obstetric history includes maternal age, gravidity, parity, blood type, and pregnancy outcomes. The current obstetric history includes the results of procedures during the current pregnancy such as ultrasound, amniocentesis, screening tests (rubella antibody, hepatitis B surface antigen [HBsAg], serum quadruple screen for genetic disorders, HIV [human immunodeficiency virus]), and antepartum tests of fetal well-being (eg, biophysical profiles, nonstress tests, or Doppler assessment of fetal blood flow patterns). Pregnancy-related maternal complications such as urinary tract infection, pregnancy-induced hypertension, eclampsia, gestational diabetes, vaginal bleeding, and preterm labor should be documented. Significant peripartum

events include duration of ruptured membranes, maternal fever, fetal distress, meconium-stained amniotic fluid, type of delivery (vaginal or cesarean section), anesthesia and analgesia used, reason for operative or forceps delivery, infant status at birth, resuscitative measures, and Apgar scores.

ASSESSMENT OF GROWTH & GESTATIONAL AGE

It is important to know the infant's gestational age because normal behavior and possible medical problems can be predicted on this basis. The date of the last menstrual period is the best indicator of gestational age with early fetal ultrasound providing supporting information.

Commonly accepted definitions of term and preterm gestation are as follows:

- Term infants: delivery at or beyond 37 weeks' gestation
- Preterm infants: delivery before 37 weeks' gestation
    - Late preterm infants: delivery between 34 and 37 weeks' gestation
    - Extremely preterm infant: delivery before 28 weeks' gestation

Postnatal physical characteristics and neurologic development are also clues to gestational age. The Ballard examination uses physical and neurologic criteria of maturity to estimate gestational age (https://perinatology.com/calculators/Ballard.htm). Adding the scores assigned to each neonatal physical and neuromuscular sign yields a score corresponding to gestational age.

Birth weight and gestational age are plotted on standard grids to determine whether the birth weight is appropriate for gestational age (AGA), small for gestational age (SGA, also known as intrauterine growth restriction [IUGR]), or large for gestational age (LGA). Birth weight for gestational age in normal neonates varies with gender, race, maternal nutrition, access to obstetric care, and environmental factors such as altitude, smoking, and drug and alcohol use. Whenever possible, standards for newborn weight and gestational age based on local or regional data should be used. Birth weight related to gestational age is a screening tool that should be supplemented by clinical data when entertaining a diagnosis of IUGR or excessive fetal growth. These data include the infant's physical examination and other factors such as parental size and the birth weight–gestational age of siblings.

An important distinction, particularly in SGA infants, is whether a growth disorder is symmetrical (weight, length, and occipitofrontal circumference [OFC] all ≤ 10%) or asymmetrical (only weight ≤ 10%). Asymmetrical growth restriction implies a problem late in pregnancy such as pregnancy-induced hypertension or placental insufficiency. Symmetrical growth restriction implies an event of early pregnancy: chromosomal abnormality, drug or alcohol use, or congenital viral infections. SGA infants, when compared with AGA infants of the same gestational age, have increased morbidity and mortality rates. In general, the outlook for normal growth and development is better in asymmetrically growth-restricted infants whose intrauterine brain growth has been spared.

Knowledge of birth weight in relation to gestational age allows anticipation of some neonatal problems. LGA infants are at risk for birth trauma. LGA infants of diabetic mothers (IDMs) are also at risk for hypoglycemia, polycythemia, congenital anomalies, cardiomyopathy, hyperbilirubinemia, and hypocalcemia. SGA infants are at risk for fetal distress during labor and delivery, polycythemia, hypoglycemia, and hypocalcemia.

EXAMINATION AT BIRTH

The extent of the newborn physical examination depends on the condition of the infant and the setting. Examination in the delivery room consists largely of observation plus auscultation of the chest and inspection for congenital anomalies and birth trauma. Major congenital anomalies occur in 1.5% of live births and account for 20%–25% of perinatal and neonatal deaths. The Apgar score (Table 2–1) should be recorded at 1 and 5 minutes of age. In severely depressed infants, scores can be recorded at 20 minutes of age. Although the 1- and 5-minute Apgar scores alone have almost no predictive value for long-term outcome, serial scores provide a useful description of the severity of perinatal depression and the response to resuscitative efforts.

Skin color is an indicator of cardiac output because of the normal high blood flow to the skin. Stress that triggers a catecholamine response redirects cardiac output away from the skin to preserve oxygen delivery to more critical organs. Cyanosis and pallor are thus two useful signs suggestive of inadequate cardiac output. Cyanosis can be difficult to assess in dark-skinned neonates; therefore, the oral mucosa should be examined for evidence of central cyanosis, and early use of pulse oximetry in the delivery room is recommended if there is a question of cyanosis.

Skeletal examination at delivery serves to detect obvious congenital anomalies and to identify birth trauma, particularly in LGA infants or those born after a protracted second stage of labor where a fractured clavicle or humerus might be found.

The placenta and umbilical cord should be examined at delivery. The number of umbilical cord vessels should be determined. Normally, there are two arteries and one vein. In 1% of deliveries (5%–6% of twin deliveries), the cord has only one artery and one vein. This minor anomaly slightly increases the risk of associated defects such as chromosomal abnormalities and renal, cardiovascular, and musculoskeletal anomalies. The placenta should be examined at delivery. The placental examination includes identification of membranes and vessels (particularly in multiple gestations) as well as placental infarcts or clots (placental abruption) on the maternal side.

Table 2–1. Evaluation of the newborn infant—Apgar score.

	Clinical Characteristic	0	1	2
A = Appearance	Color	Blue, pale	Body pink with blue extremities	Body and extremities pink
P = Pulse	Heart rate	Absent	< 100 beats/min	> 100 beats/min
G = Grimace	Response to catheter in nares	No response	Grimace	Cough, sneeze
A = Activity	Muscle tone	Limp	Some flexion	Active motion
R = Respiratory effort	Respiratory effort	Absent	Slow, irregular	Good, crying

Add points to generate total score. Normal: 7–10. Requires immediate resuscitation: 0–3.

EXAMINATION IN THE NURSERY

The purpose of the newborn physical examination is to identify abnormalities that might influence the infant's well-being and to evaluate for any acute illness or difficulty in the transition from intrauterine to extrauterine life. Start with observation, then auscultation of the chest, and then palpation of the abdomen. Examination of the eyes, ears, throat, and hips should be performed last, as these maneuvers are most disturbing to the infant. The heart rate should range from 120 to 160 beats/min and the respiratory rate from 30 to 60 breaths/min. Systolic blood pressure on day 1 ranges from 50 to 70 mm Hg and increases steadily during the first week of life. An irregularly irregular heart rate, usually caused by premature atrial contractions, is common, benign, and usually resolves in the first days of life.

Approximately 15%–20% of healthy newborns have one minor anomaly (a common variant that would not influence the infant's well-being, eg, a unilateral transverse palmar crease or a single umbilical artery). Those with a minor anomaly have a 3% risk of an associated major anomaly. Other common minor anomalies requiring no special investigation in healthy infants include preauricular pits, a shallow sacral dimple without other cutaneous abnormality within 2.5 cm of the anus, and three or fewer café au lait spots in a white infant or five or fewer in an African-American infant.

Skin

Observe for bruising, petechiae (common over the presenting part), meconium staining, and jaundice. Visible jaundice in the first 24 hours is never normal and generally indicates either a hemolytic process or a congenital hepatitis, either of which requires further evaluation. Peripheral cyanosis is commonly present when the extremities are cool or the infant is polycythemic. Generalized cyanosis merits immediate evaluation. Pallor may be caused by acute or chronic blood loss or by acidosis. In dark-skinned infants, pallor and cyanosis should be assessed in the lips, mouth, and nail beds. Plethora suggests polycythemia. Dry skin with cracking and peeling of the superficial layers is common in postterm infants. Edema may be generalized (hydrops) or localized (eg, on the dorsum of the feet in Turner syndrome). Check for birthmarks such as capillary hemangiomas and slate gray nevi over the back and buttocks. There are many benign skin eruptions such as milia, miliaria, erythema toxicum, and pustular melanosis that are present in the newborn period. See Chapter 15 for a more in-depth description of these conditions.

Head

Check for cephalohematoma (a swelling over one or both parietal bones that is contained within suture lines) and caput succedaneum (edema of the scalp over the presenting part that crosses suture lines). Subgaleal hemorrhages (beneath the scalp) are uncommon but can cause extensive blood loss into this large potential space, resulting in hypovolemic shock (see section Birth Trauma). Skull fractures may be linear or depressed and may be associated with cephalohematoma. Check for the presence and size of the fontanelles. The anterior fontanelle varies from 1 to 4 cm in any direction; the posterior fontanelle should be less than 1 cm. A third fontanelle is a bony defect along the sagittal suture in the parietal bones and may be seen in genetic syndromes, such as trisomy 21. Sutures should be freely mobile but are often overriding just after birth.

Face

Unusual facies may be associated with a specific syndrome. Bruising from birth trauma (especially with face presentation) and forceps application should be identified. Face presentation may cause soft tissue swelling around the nose and mouth and significant facial distortion. Facial nerve palsy is most obvious during crying; the unaffected side of the mouth moves normally, giving an asymmetric grimace.

Eyes

Subconjunctival hemorrhages are a frequent result of birth trauma. Less commonly, a corneal tear (presenting as a clouded cornea), or a hyphema (a layering of blood in the anterior chamber of the eye) may occur. Ophthalmologic consultation is indicated in such cases. Extraocular movements should be assessed. Occasional uncoordinated eye movements are common, but persistent irregular movements are abnormal. The iris should be inspected for abnormalities such as speckling (Brushfield spots seen in trisomy 21) and colobomas. Retinal red reflexes should be present and symmetrical. Dark spots, unilateral blunted red reflex, absent reflex, or a white reflex all require ophthalmologic evaluation. Leukocoria can be caused by glaucoma (cloudy cornea), cataract, or tumor (retinoblastoma). Infants with suspected or known congenital viral infection should have a retinoscopic examination with pupils dilated to look for chorioretinitis.

Nose

Examine the nose for size and shape. In utero compression can cause deformities. Because infants younger than 1 month are obligate nose breathers, any nasal obstruction (eg, bilateral choanal atresia or stenosis) can cause respiratory distress. Purulent nasal discharge at birth suggests congenital syphilis ("snuffles").

Ears

Malformed or malpositioned (low-set or posteriorly rotated) ears are often associated with other congenital anomalies. Preauricular pits and tags are common minor variants and may be familial. Any external ear abnormality may be associated with hearing loss.

Mouth

Epithelial (Epstein) pearls are benign keratin-filled cysts along the gum margins and at the junction of the hard and soft palates. Bohn's nodules are mucus gland cysts that commonly occur along the alveolar ridge. Both types of lesions resolve spontaneously within the first weeks after birth. Natal teeth may be present and sometimes must be removed to prevent their aspiration. Check the integrity and shape of the palate for clefts and other abnormalities. A small mandible and retraction of the tongue with cleft palate is seen with Pierre Robin sequence and can present as respiratory difficulty as the tongue occludes the airway; prone positioning can be beneficial. A prominent tongue can be seen in trisomy 21 and Beckwith-Wiedemann syndrome. Excessive oral secretions suggest esophageal atresia or a swallowing disorder.

Neck

Redundant neck skin or webbing, with a low posterior hair line, is seen in Turner syndrome. Cervical sinus tracts may be seen as remnants of branchial clefts. Check for masses: midline (thyroglossal duct cysts), anterior to the sternocleidomastoid (branchial cleft cysts), within the sternocleidomastoid (hematoma and torticollis), and posterior to the sternocleidomastoid (cystic hygroma).

Chest & Lungs

Check for fractured clavicles (crepitus, bruising, and tenderness). Check air entry bilaterally and the position of the mediastinum by locating the point of maximum cardiac impulse and assessment of heart tones. Decreased breath sounds with respiratory distress and a shift in the heart tones suggests pneumothorax (tension) or a space-occupying lesion (eg, diaphragmatic hernia). Pneumomediastinum causes muffled heart sounds. Expiratory grunting and decreased air entry are observed in hyaline membrane disease.

Heart

Cardiac murmurs are common in the first hours and are most often benign; conversely, severe congenital heart disease in the newborn infant may be present with no murmur at all. The two most common presentations of heart disease in the newborn infant are (1) cyanosis and (2) congestive heart failure with abnormalities of pulses and perfusion. In hypoplastic left-sided heart disease and critical aortic stenosis, pulses are diminished at all sites. In aortic coarctation and interrupted aortic arch, pulses are diminished in the lower extremities.

Abdomen

Check for tenderness, distention, and bowel sounds. If polyhydramnios was present or excessive oral secretions are noted, pass a soft catheter into the stomach to rule out esophageal atresia. Most abdominal masses in the newborn infant are associated with kidney disorders (eg, multicystic or dysplastic, and hydronephrosis). When the abdomen is relaxed, normal kidneys may be felt but are not prominent. Absence of abdominal musculature (prune belly syndrome) may occur in association with renal abnormalities. The liver and spleen are superficial in the neonate and can be felt with light palpation. A distended bladder may be seen as well as palpated above the pubic symphysis.

Genitalia & Anus

Male and female genitals show characteristics according to gestational age. In the female infant during the first few days, a whitish vaginal discharge with or without blood is normal. Check the patency and location of the anus.

Skeleton

Check for obvious anomalies such as absence of a bone, clubfoot, fusion or webbing of digits, and extra digits. Examine for hip dislocation by attempting to dislocate the femur posteriorly and then abducting the legs to relocate the femur noting a clunk as the femoral head relocates. Look for extremity fractures and for palsies (especially brachial plexus injuries) and evidence of spinal deformities (eg, scoliosis, cysts, sinuses, myelomeningocele). Arthrogryposis (multiple joint contractures) results from chronic limitation of movement in utero that may result from lack of amniotic fluid or from congenital neuromuscular disease.

Neurologic Examination

Normal newborns have reflexes that facilitate survival (eg, rooting and sucking reflexes), and sensory abilities (eg, hearing and smell) that allow them to recognize their mother soon after birth. Although the retina is well developed at birth, visual acuity is poor (20/400) because of a relatively immobile lens. Acuity improves rapidly over the first 6 months, with fixation and tracking becoming well developed by 2 months.

Observe the newborn's resting tone. Term newborns should exhibit flexion of the upper and lower extremities and symmetrical spontaneous movements. Extension of the extremities should result in spontaneous recoil to the flexed position. Assess the character of the cry; a high-pitched cry with or without hypotonia may indicate disease of the central nervous system (CNS) such as hemorrhage or infection, a congenital neuromuscular disorder, or systemic disease. Check the following newborn reflexes:

1. *Sucking reflex*: The newborn sucks in response to a nipple in the mouth; observed by 14 weeks' gestation.
2. *Palmar grasp*: Evident with the placement of the examiner's finger in the newborn's palm; develops by 28 weeks' gestation and disappears by age 4 months.

3. *Moro (startle) reflex*: Hold the infant supine while supporting the head. Allow the head to drop 1–2 cm suddenly. The arms will abduct at the shoulder and extend at the elbow with spreading of the fingers. Adduction with flexion will follow. This reflex develops by 28 weeks' gestation (incomplete) and disappears by age 3 months.

CARE OF THE WELL NEONATE

The primary responsibility of the level 1 nursery is care of the well neonate—promoting mother–infant bonding, establishing feeding, and teaching the basics of newborn care. Staff must monitor infants for signs and symptoms of illness, including temperature instability, change in activity, refusal to feed, pallor, cyanosis, early or excessive jaundice, tachypnea, respiratory distress, delayed (beyond 24 hours) first stool or first void, and bilious vomiting.

Several preventive measures are routine in the normal newborn nursery. Prophylactic erythromycin ointment is applied to the eyes within 1 hour of birth to prevent gonococcal ophthalmia. Vitamin K (1 mg) is given intramuscularly or subcutaneously within 4 hours of birth to prevent hemorrhagic disease of the newborn.

All infants should receive hepatitis B vaccine. Both hepatitis B vaccine and hepatitis B immune globulin (HBIG) are administered if the mother is positive for HBsAg. If maternal HBsAg status is unknown, vaccine should be given before 12 hours of age, maternal blood should be tested for HBsAg, and HBIG should be given to the neonate before 7 days of age if the test is positive.

Cord blood collected from infants at birth can be used for blood typing and Coombs testing if the mother is type O or Rh-negative to help assess the risk for development of jaundice.

Bedside glucose testing should be performed in infants at risk for hypoglycemia (IDMs, preterm, SGA, LGA, or stressed infants). Values below 45 mg/dL should be confirmed by laboratory blood glucose testing and treated.

State-sponsored newborn genetic screens (for inborn errors of metabolism such as phenylketonuria [PKU], galactosemia, sickle cell disease, hypothyroidism, congenital adrenal hyperplasia, and cystic fibrosis) are performed prior to discharge, after 24–48 hours of age if possible. In many states, a repeat test is required at 8–14 days of age because the PKU test may be falsely negative when obtained before 48 hours of age. Not all state-mandated screens include the same panel of diseases. Many states now include an expanded screen that tests for other inborn errors of metabolism such as fatty acid oxidation defects and amino or organic acid disorders. Some states also screen for severe combined immunodeficiency syndrome.

Infants should routinely be positioned supine to minimize the risk of sudden infant death syndrome (SIDS). Prone positioning is contraindicated unless there are compelling clinical reasons for that position. Bed sharing with adults and prone positioning are associated with increased risk of sudden unexpected infant death.

FEEDING THE WELL NEONATE

A neonate is ready for feeding if he or she (1) is alert and vigorous, (2) has no abdominal distention, (3) has good bowel sounds, and (4) has a normal hunger cry. These signs usually occur within 6 hours after birth, but fetal distress or traumatic delivery may prolong this period. The healthy full-term infant should be allowed to feed every 2–5 hours on demand. The first breast-feeding should occur within 1 hour from birth if mother and baby are clinically stable. For formula-fed infants, the first feeding usually occurs by 3 hours of life. The feeding volume generally increases from 0.5–1 oz per feeding initially to 1.5–2 oz per feeding on day 3. By day 3, the average full-term newborn takes about 100 mL/kg/day of milk (Table 2–2).

A wide range of infant formulas satisfy the nutritional needs of most neonates. Breast milk is the standard on which formulas are based (see Chapter 11). Despite low concentrations of several vitamins and minerals in breast milk, bioavailability is high. All necessary nutrients, vitamins, minerals, and water are provided by human milk for the first 6 months of life except vitamin K (1 mg IM is administered at birth) and vitamin D (400 IU/day for all infants beginning shortly after birth). Advantages of breast milk include (1) immunologic, antimicrobial, and anti-inflammatory factors such as immunoglobulin A (IgA) and cellular, protein, and enzymatic components that decrease the incidence of upper respiratory and gastrointestinal (GI) infections; (2) possible decreased frequency and severity of childhood eczema and asthma; (3) improved mother-infant bonding; and (4) improved neurodevelopmental outcome.

Although 85% of mothers in the United States start by breast-feeding, only about 50% continue to do so at 6 months. Hospital practices that facilitate successful initiation of breast-feeding include rooming-in, nursing on demand, and avoiding unnecessary supplemental formula. Nursery staff must be trained to recognize problems associated with breast-feeding and provide help and support for mothers in the hospital. An experienced professional should observe and assist with several feedings to document good latch-on.

American Academy of Breastfeeding Medicine: www.bfmed.org. Accessed April 2023.
Jullien S: Sudden infant death syndrome prevention. BMC Pediatr 2021 Sep 8;21(Suppl 1):320 [PMID: 34496779].

CIRCUMCISION

Circumcision is an elective procedure to be performed only in healthy, stable infants. The procedure has medical benefits, including prevention of urinary tract infections, decreased

Table 2–2. Guidelines for successful breast-feeding.

	First 8 h	First 8–24 h	Day 2	Day 3	Day 4	Day 5	Day 6 Onward
Milk supply	Mother may be able to express a few drops of milk.		Milk should come in between the second and fourth days.			Milk should be in. Breasts may be firm or leak milk.	Breasts should feel softer after feedings.
Baby's activity	Baby is usually wide-awake in the first hour of life. Put baby to breast within 30 min after birth.	Babies may not wake up on their own to feed and should be woken up.	Baby should be more cooperative and less sleepy.	Baby will display early feeding cues such as rooting, lip smacking, and hands to face.			Baby should appear satisfied after feedings.
Feeding routine	Baby may go into a deep sleep 2–4 h after birth.	Baby should be fed every 1–4 h or as often as wanted—at least 8–12 times a day.				May go one longer interval (up to 5 h between feeds) in a 24-h period.	
Baby's urine output		Baby must have a minimum of one wet diaper in the first 24 h.	Baby must have at least one wet diaper every 8–11 h.	Increase in wet diapers (up to four to six) in 24 h.	Baby's urine should be light yellow.	Baby should have six to eight wet diapers per day of colorless or light yellow urine.	
Baby's stool		Baby may have a very dark (meconium) stool.	Baby may have a very dark second (meconium) stool.	Baby's stools should be in transition from black-green to yellow.		Baby should have three or four yellow, seedy stools a day.	The number of stools may decrease gradually after 4–6 wk.

incidence of penile cancer, and decreased incidence of sexually transmitted diseases (including HIV). Most parental decisions regarding circumcision are religious and social, not medical. The risks of circumcision include local infection, bleeding, removal of too much skin, and urethral injury. The combined incidence of complications is less than 1%. Local anesthesia is safe and effective and should always be used. Techniques allowing visualization of the glans throughout the procedure (Plastibell and Gomco clamp) are preferred to blind techniques (Mogen clamp) as occasional amputation of the glans has occurred with the latter technique. Circumcision is contraindicated in infants with genital abnormalities. A coagulation screen should be performed prior to the procedure in infants with a family history of serious bleeding disorders.

HEARING SCREENING

Normal hearing is critical to normal language development. Significant bilateral hearing loss is present in 1–3 per 1000 well neonates and in 2–4 per 100 neonates in the intensive care unit population. Infants should be screened for hearing loss by auditory brainstem-evoked responses or evoked otoacoustic emissions as early as possible because up to 40% of hearing loss will be missed by risk analysis alone. Primary care providers and parents should be advised of the possibility of hearing loss and offered immediate referral in suspect cases. With the use of universal screening, the average age at which hearing loss is confirmed has dropped from 24–30 to 2–3 months. If remediation is begun by 6 months, language and social development are commensurate with physical development.

SCREENING FOR CRITICAL CONGENITAL HEART DISEASE

Screening for critical congenital heart disease (CCHD) is standard practice in newborn nurseries. The goal of screening is to identify newborn infants with structural heart disease significant enough to require intervention within the first year of life prior to symptoms developing. Newborn infants are screened by pulse oximetry on the second day of life. A failed screen is defined as: any oxygen saturation measure is less than 90%; oxygen saturation is less than 95% in the right hand and foot on three measures, each separated by 1 hour, or a greater than 3% absolute difference exists in oxygen saturation between the right hand and foot on three measures, each separated by 1 hour. Infants who fail the screen are evaluated by echocardiogram prior to hospital discharge. CCHD screening targets the following primary cardiac lesions: hypoplastic left heart syndrome, pulmonary atresia, tetralogy of Fallot, total anomalous pulmonary venous return, transposition of the great arteries, tricuspid atresia, and truncus arteriosus.

EARLY DISCHARGE OF THE NEWBORN INFANT

Discharge at 24–36 hours of age is safe and appropriate for some newborns if there are no contraindications (Table 2–3) and if a follow-up visit within 48 hours is ensured. Most infants with cardiac, respiratory, or infectious disorders are identified in the first 12–24 hours of life. The exception may be the infant for whom maternal intrapartum antibiotic prophylaxis for maternal group B streptococcal (GBS) colonization or infection was indicated. The Centers for Disease Control and Prevention (CDC) and the American Academy of Pediatrics (AAP) recommend that such infants be observed in hospital for at least 48 hours if their mothers received no or inadequate intrapartum antibiotic prophylaxis or cefazolin. Hospital observation beyond 24 hours may not be necessary for well-appearing full-term infants whose mothers received adequate intrapartum chemoprophylaxis and for whom ready access to medical care can be ensured if needed. Other problems, such as jaundice and breast-feeding problems, typically occur after 48 hours and can usually be dealt with on an outpatient basis.

Table 2–3. Contraindications to early newborn discharge.

Contraindications to early newborn discharge
1. Jaundice ≤ 24 h
2. High risk for infection (eg, maternal chorioamnionitis); discharge allowed after 24 h with a normal transition
3. Known or suspected narcotic addiction or withdrawal
4. Physical defects requiring evaluation
5. Oral defects (clefts, micrognathia)
Relative contraindications to early newborn discharge (infants at high risk for feeding failure, excessive jaundice)
1. Prematurity or early-term infant (< 38 weeks gestation)
2. Birth weight < 2700 g (6 lb)
3. Infant difficult to arouse for feeding; not demanding regularly in nursery
4. Medical or neurologic problems that interfere with feeding (Down syndrome, hypotonia, cardiac problems)
5. Twins or higher multiples
6. ABO blood group incompatibility or severe jaundice in previous child
7. Mother whose previous breast-fed infant gained weight poorly
8. Mother with breast surgery involving periareolar areas (if attempting to nurse)

Table 2–4. Guidelines for early outpatient follow-up evaluation.

History
Rhythmic sucking and audible swallowing for at least 10 min total per feeding?
Infant wakes and demands to feed every 2–3 h (at least 8–10 feedings per 24 h)?
Do breasts feel full before feedings, and softer after?
Are there at least 6 noticeably wet diapers per 24 h?
Are there yellow bowel movements (no longer meconium)—at least 4 per 24 h?
Is infant still acting hungry after nursing (frequently sucks hands, rooting)?
Physical assessment
Weight, unclothed: should not be more than 8%–10% below birth weight
Extent and severity of jaundice
Assessment of hydration, alertness, general well-being
Cardiovascular examination: murmurs, brachial and femoral pulses, respirations

The AAP recommends a follow-up visit within 48 hours for all newborns discharged before 72 hours of age. Infants who are small or late preterm—especially if breast-feeding—are at particular risk for inadequate intake; the early visit is especially important for these infants. Suggested guidelines for the follow-up interview and physical examination are presented in Table 2–4. The optimal timing of discharge must be determined in each case based on medical, social, and financial factors.

Benitz WE; Committee on Fetus and Newborn, American Academy of Pediatrics: Hospital stay for healthy term newborn infants. Pediatrics 2015 May;135(5):948–953 [PMID: 25917993]
Centers for Disease Control and Prevention Congenital Heart Defects: https://www.cdc.gov/ncbddd/heartdefects/hcp.html. Accessed May 2023.
Zeitler M, Rayala B: Neonatal circumcision. Prim Care 2021 Dec; 48(4):597–611 [PMID: 34752272].

COMMON PROBLEMS IN THE TERM NEWBORN

NEONATAL JAUNDICE

▶ General Considerations

Sixty-five percent of newborns develop visible jaundice with a total serum bilirubin (TSB) level higher than 6 mg/dL during the first week of life. Approximately 8%–10% of newborns develop excessive hyperbilirubinemia. Extremely high and potentially dangerous TSB levels are rare but can cause kernicterus, characterized by injury to the basal ganglia and brainstem.

Bilirubin is produced by the breakdown of heme (iron protoporphyrin) in the reticuloendothelial system and bone marrow. Heme is cleaved by heme oxygenase to iron, which is conserved; carbon monoxide, which is exhaled; and biliverdin, which is converted to bilirubin by bilirubin reductase. This unconjugated bilirubin is bound to albumin and carried to the liver, where it is taken up by hepatocytes. In the presence of the enzyme uridyl diphosphoglycyronyl transferase (UDPGT; glucuronyl transferase), bilirubin is conjugated to one or two glucuronide molecules. Conjugated bilirubin is then excreted through the bile to the intestine. In the presence of normal gut flora, conjugated bilirubin is metabolized and excreted in the stool. Absence of gut flora and slow GI motility, both characteristics of the newborn, cause stasis of conjugated bilirubin in the intestinal lumen, where mucosal β-glucuronidase removes the glucuronide molecules and leaves unconjugated bilirubin to be reabsorbed (enterohepatic circulation). Excess accumulation of bilirubin in blood depends on both the rate of bilirubin production and the rate of excretion. It is best determined by comparing an hour-specific TSB level to a standard curve of TSB concentration by age in hours. Serum bilirubin can be fractionated to quantify an unconjugated and conjugated component. Most of the neonatal jaundice presenting in the first week of life is due to unconjugated hyperbilirubinemia and is the focus of the following discussion. Jaundice due to conjugated hyperbilirubinemia is seen in some congenital infections, intrahepatic cholestasis, or extrahepatic obstruction of the biliary tract.

1. Physiologic Jaundice

ESSENTIALS OF DIAGNOSIS & TYPICAL FEATURES

▶ Visible jaundice appearing after 24 hours of age.

▶ Total bilirubin rises by < 5 mg/dL (86 mmol/L) per day.

▶ Peak bilirubin occurs at 3–5 days of age, with a total bilirubin of no more than 15 mg/dL (258 mmol/L).

▶ Visible jaundice resolves by 1 week in the full-term infant and by 2 weeks in the preterm infant.

Factors contributing to physiologic jaundice in neonates include low UDPGT activity, relatively high red cell mass, absence of intestinal flora, slow intestinal motility, and increased enterohepatic circulation of bilirubin in the first days of life.

2. Pathologic Unconjugated Hyperbilirubinemia

Pathologic unconjugated hyperbilirubinemia can be grouped into two main categories: overproduction of bilirubin or

Table 2–5. Causes of pathologic unconjugated hyperbilirubinemia.

Overproduction of bilirubin
1. Hemolytic causes of increased bilirubin production (reticulocyte count elevated)
   a. Immune-mediated: positive direct antibody (DAT, Coombs) test
      • ABO blood group incompatibility, Rh incompatibility, minor blood group antigen incompatibility
   b. Nonimmune: negative direct antibody (DAT, Coombs) test
      • Abnormal red cell shapes: spherocytosis, elliptocytosis, pyknocytosis, stomatocytosis
      • Red cell enzyme abnormalities: glucose-6-phosphate dehydrogenase deficiency, pyruvate kinase deficiency, hexokinase deficiency, other metabolic defects
   c. Patients with bacterial or viral sepsis
2. Nonhemolytic causes of increased bilirubin production (reticulocyte count normal)
   a. Extravascular hemorrhage: cephalohematoma, extensive bruising, intracranial hemorrhage
   b. Polycythemia
   c. Exaggerated enterohepatic circulation of bilirubin: bowel obstruction, functional ileus
   d. Breast-feeding–associated jaundice (inadequate intake of breast milk causing exaggerated enterohepatic circulation of bilirubin)

Decreased rate of conjugation
1. Crigler-Najjar syndrome (rare, severe)
   a. Type I glucuronyl transferase deficiency, autosomal-recessive
   b. Type II glucuronyl transferase deficiency, autosomal-dominant
2. Gilbert syndrome (common, milder)
3. Hypothyroidism

decreased conjugation of bilirubin (Table 2–5). The TSB is a reflection of the balance between these processes. Visible jaundice with a TSB greater than 5 mg/dL before 24 hours of age is most commonly a result of significant hemolysis.

A. Increased Bilirubin Production

1. Antibody-mediated hemolysis (Coombs test–positive)

A. ABO BLOOD GROUP INCOMPATIBILITY—This finding can accompany any pregnancy in a type O mother. Hemolysis is usually mild, but the severity is unpredictable because of variability in the amount of naturally occurring maternal anti-A or anti-B IgG antibodies. Although 15% of pregnancies are "setups" for ABO incompatibility (mother O, infant A or B), only 33% of infants in such cases have a positive direct Coombs test and less than 10% of these infants develop jaundice that requires therapy. Since maternal antibodies may persist for several months after birth, the newborn may become progressively more anemic over the first few weeks of life, occasionally to the point of requiring transfusion.

B. Rʜ-ɪsᴏɪᴍᴍᴜɴɪᴢᴀᴛɪᴏɴ—This hemolytic process is less common, more severe, and more predictable than ABO incompatibility. The severity increases with each immunized pregnancy. Most Rh-disease can be prevented by giving high-titer Rho (D) immune globulin to the Rh-negative woman after invasive procedures during pregnancy or after miscarriage, abortion, or delivery of an Rh-positive infant. Affected neonates are often anemic at birth, and continued hemolysis rapidly causes hyperbilirubinemia and worsening anemia. The most severe form of Rh-isoimmunization, erythroblastosis fetalis, is characterized by life-threatening anemia, generalized edema, and fetal or neonatal heart failure. Without antenatal intervention, fetal or neonatal death often results. The cornerstone of antenatal management is transfusion of the fetus with Rh-negative cells, either directly into the umbilical vein or into the fetal abdominal cavity. Phototherapy is usually started in these infants upon delivery, with exchange transfusion frequently needed. Intravenous immune globulin (IVIG) given to the infant as soon as the diagnosis is made may decrease the need for exchange transfusion. Ongoing hemolysis occurs until all maternal antibodies are gone; therefore, these infants require monitoring for 2–3 months for recurrent anemia.

2. Nonimmune hemolysis (Coombs test–negative)

A. Hᴇʀᴇᴅɪᴛᴀʀʏ sᴘʜᴇʀᴏᴄʏᴛᴏsɪs—This condition is the most common of the red cell membrane defects and causes hemolysis by decreasing red cell deformability. Affected infants may have hyperbilirubinemia severe enough to require exchange transfusion. Splenomegaly may be present. Diagnosis is suspected by peripheral blood smear and family history (see Chapter 30).

B. G6PD ᴅᴇғɪᴄɪᴇɴᴄʏ—This condition is the most common red cell enzyme defect causing hemolysis, especially in infants of African, Mediterranean, or Asian descent. Although the disorder is X-linked, female heterozygotes are also at increased risk of hyperbilirubinemia due to X-chromosome inactivation. Their increased bilirubin production is further exaggerated by a decreased rate of bilirubin conjugation. Since G6PD enzyme activity is high in reticulocytes, neonates with a large number of reticulocytes may have falsely normal enzyme tests. A low G6PD level should always raise suspicion. Repeat testing in suspect cases with initially normal results is indicated at 3 months of age (see Chapter 30).

3. Nonhemolytic increased bilirubin production—Enclosed hemorrhage, such as cephalohematoma, intracranial hemorrhage, or extensive bruising in the skin, can lead to jaundice. Polycythemia leads to jaundice by increased red cell mass, with increased numbers of cells reaching senescence daily. Bowel obstruction, functional or mechanical, leads to an increased enterohepatic circulation of bilirubin.

B. Decreased Rate of Conjugation

1. UDPGT deficiency: Crigler-Najjar syndrome type I (complete deficiency, autosomal recessive) and type II (partial deficiency, autosomal dominant)—These rare conditions result from mutations in the UDPGT gene that cause complete or nearly complete absence of enzyme activity. Both can cause severe unconjugated hyperbilirubinemia, bilirubin encephalopathy, and death if untreated. In type II, the enzyme can be induced with phenobarbital, which may lower bilirubin levels by 30%–80%. Liver transplantation is curative.

2. Gilbert syndrome—This is a common mild autosomal dominant disorder characterized by decreased hepatic UDPGT activity caused by genetic polymorphism at the promoter region of the UDPGT gene. Approximately 9% of the population is homozygous, and 42% is heterozygous for this abnormality. Affected individuals tend to develop hyperbilirubinemia in the presence of conditions that increase bilirubin load and are more likely to have prolonged neonatal jaundice and breast-milk jaundice.

C. Hyperbilirubinemia Caused by Unknown or Multiple Factors

1. Racial differences—Asians (23%) are more likely than whites (10%–13%) or African Americans (4%) to have a peak neonatal TSB greater than 12 mg/dL (206 mmol/L). It is likely that these differences result from racial variations in prevalence of UDPGT gene polymorphisms or associated G6PD deficiency.

2. Prematurity—Premature infants often have poor enteral intake, delayed stooling, and increased enterohepatic circulation, as well as a shorter red cell life. Infants at 35–36 weeks' gestation are 13 times more likely than term infants to be readmitted for hyperbilirubinemia.

3. Breast-feeding and jaundice

A. Bʀᴇᴀsᴛ-ᴍɪʟᴋ ᴊᴀᴜɴᴅɪᴄᴇ—Unconjugated hyperbilirubinemia lasting until 2–3 months of age is common in breast-fed infants. Moderate unconjugated hyperbilirubinemia for 6–12 weeks in a thriving breast-fed infant without evidence of hemolysis, hypothyroidism, or other disease strongly suggests this diagnosis.

B. Bʀᴇᴀsᴛ-ғᴇᴇᴅɪɴɢ–ᴀssᴏᴄɪᴀᴛᴇᴅ ᴊᴀᴜɴᴅɪᴄᴇ—This common condition has also been called "lack-of-breast-milk" jaundice. Breast-fed infants have a higher incidence (9%) of elevated unconjugated serum bilirubin levels compared to formula-fed infants (2%). The pathogenesis is probably poor enteral intake and increased enterohepatic circulation. Excessive jaundice should be considered a possible sign of failure to establish an adequate milk supply. The best way to evaluate successful breast-feeding is to monitor the infant's weight, urine, and stool output (see Table 2–2). If intake is inadequate, the infant should receive supplemental formula and the mother should be instructed to nurse more frequently and to use an electric breast pump every 2 hours to enhance milk production. Consultation with a lactation specialist should be considered. Because hospital discharge of normal newborns occurs before the milk supply is established and before jaundice peaks, a follow-up visit 2 days after discharge is recommended by the AAP to evaluate adequacy of intake and degree of jaundice.

3. Bilirubin Toxicity

Unconjugated bilirubin anion is the agent that causes bilirubin neurotoxicity. It is unknown whether there is a fixed level of bilirubin above which brain damage always occurs. The blood-brain barrier has a role in protecting the infant from brain damage, but its integrity is impossible to measure clinically. Albumin binds unconjugated bilirubin, which is protective against bilirubin neurotoxicity. The amount of albumin available to bind the unconjugated bilirubin anion and the presence of other anions that may displace bilirubin from albumin-binding sites are important factors to consider.

The risk of bilirubin encephalopathy is small in healthy, term neonates even at bilirubin levels of 25–30 mg/dL (430–516 mmol/L). Risk depends on the duration of hyperbilirubinemia, the concentration of serum albumin, associated illness, acidosis, and the concentrations of anions such as sulfamethoxazole and ceftriaxone that compete for albumin-binding sites. Premature infants are at greater risk than term infants because of the greater frequency of associated illness affecting the integrity of the blood-brain barrier, reduced albumin levels, and decreased affinity of albumin-binding sites. For these reasons, the "exchange level" (the level at which bilirubin encephalopathy is thought likely to occur) in premature infants may be lower than that of a term infant.

4. Acute Bilirubin Encephalopathy

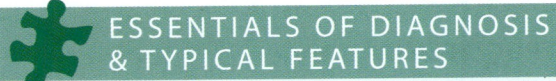

ESSENTIALS OF DIAGNOSIS & TYPICAL FEATURES

- ► Lethargy, poor feeding.
- ► Irritability, high-pitched cry.
- ► Arching of the neck (retrocollis) and trunk (opisthotonos).
- ► Apnea, seizures, and coma (late).

The term acute bilirubin encephalopathy describes the signs and symptoms of evolving brain injury in the newborn. Newborn infants with evolving acute bilirubin encephalopathy may be described as "sleepy and not interested in feeding."

Although these symptoms are nonspecific, they are also the earliest signs of acute bilirubin encephalopathy and should trigger, in the jaundiced infant, a detailed evaluation of the birth and postnatal history, feeding and elimination history, an urgent assessment for signs of bilirubin-induced neurologic dysfunction (BIND), and a TSB and albumin measurement. Currently the most sensitive means of assessing neurotoxicity may be the auditory brainstem-evoked response, which shows predictable, early effects of bilirubin toxicity.

5. Chronic Bilirubin Encephalopathy (Kernicterus)

ESSENTIALS OF DIAGNOSIS & TYPICAL FEATURES

- ► Extrapyramidal movement disorder (choreoathetoid cerebral palsy).
- ► Gaze abnormality, especially limitation of upward gaze.
- ► Auditory disturbances (deafness, failed auditory brainstem-evoked response with normal evoked otoacoustic emissions, auditory neuropathy, auditory dyssynchrony).
- ► Dysplasia of the enamel of the deciduous teeth.

Kernicterus is an irreversible brain injury characterized by choreoathetoid cerebral palsy and hearing impairment. Intelligence is probably normal but may be difficult to assess because of associated hearing, communication, and coordination problems. The diagnosis is clinical, but magnetic resonance imaging (MRI) scanning of the brain is nearly diagnostic if it shows abnormalities isolated to the globus pallidus, the subthalamic nuclei, or both.

Evaluation of Hyperbilirubinemia

Because most newborns are discharged at 24–48 hours of age, before physiologic jaundice peaks and before maternal milk supply is established, a predischarge TSB or a transcutaneous bilirubin (TcB) measurement is recommended to help predict which infants are at risk for severe hyperbilirubinemia. In all infants, an assessment of risk for severe hyperbilirubinemia should be performed before discharge (Table 2–6). The greater the number of risk factors, the greater the likelihood of developing severe hyperbilirubinemia. As recommended by the AAP, follow-up within 24–48 hours for all infants discharged before 72 hours of age is imperative. Visual estimation of the bilirubin level is inaccurate. TSB should be interpreted based on the age of the infant in hours at the time of sampling. Term infants with a TSB level greater

Table 2–6. Factors affecting the risk of severe hyperbilirubinemia in infants 35 or more weeks gestation (in approximate order of importance).

Predischarge TSB or TcB level close to the phototherapy threshold
Jaundice observed in the first 24 h
Blood group incompatibility with positive direct Coombs test or other known hemolytic disease (eg, G6PD deficiency)
Gestational age 35–36 wk
Previous sibling required phototherapy
Cephalohematoma or significant bruising
Exclusive breast-feeding, particularly if weight loss is excessive
Jaundice observed before discharge
Macrosomic infant of a diabetic mother

G6PD, glucose-6-phosphate dehydrogenase; TcB, transcutaneous bilirubin; TSB, total serum bilirubin.

than the 95th percentile for age in hours have a 40% risk of developing significant hyperbilirubinemia.

Infants with visible jaundice on the first day of life or who develop excessive jaundice require further evaluation. The minimal evaluation consists of the following:

- Feeding and elimination history
- Birth weight and percent weight change since birth
- Examination for sources of excessive heme breakdown
- Assessment of blood type, Coombs testing, complete blood count (CBC) with smear, serum albumin, and TSB
- G6PD test if jaundice is otherwise unexplained and in African-American infants with severe jaundice
- Fractionated bilirubin level in infants who appear ill, those with prolonged jaundice, acholic stool, hepatosplenomegaly, or dark urine to evaluate for cholestasis

Treatment of Unconjugated Hyperbilirubinemia

A. Phototherapy

Phototherapy is the most common treatment for unconjugated hyperbilirubinemia. It is relatively noninvasive and safe. Intensive phototherapy should decrease TSB by 30%–40% in the first 24 hours. The infant's eyes should be shielded to prevent retinal damage.

Phototherapy is started electively when the TSB is approximately 6 mg/dL (102 mmol/L) lower than the predicted exchange level for that infant. AAP guidelines for phototherapy and exchange transfusion in infants of 35 or more weeks' gestation are available online through BiliTool (https://bilitool.org). Hyperbilirubinemic infants should be fed by mouth, if possible, to decrease enterohepatic bilirubin circulation. Although phototherapy has been shown to decrease the need for exchange transfusion, its long-term benefits, if any, in infants with less severe jaundice are unknown.

B. Exchange Transfusion

Although most infants with unconjugated hyperbilirubinemia can be treated with phototherapy, bilirubin levels within 2 mg/dL of the double volume exchange threshold require rapid escalation of care. Infants should be admitted to a neonatal intensive care unit where exchange transfusion can be performed before irreversible neurologic damage occurs. Intensive phototherapy should be instituted immediately, during transport to the hospital if possible. As TSB nears the potentially toxic range, serum albumin should be determined. Albumin administration (1 g/kg) will aid in binding and removal of bilirubin during exchange transfusion, as well as afford some neuroprotection while preparing for the procedure.

Double-volume exchange transfusion (~160–200 mL/kg body weight) is most often required in infants with extreme hyperbilirubinemia secondary to Rh isoimmunization, ABO incompatibility, or hereditary spherocytosis. The procedure decreases serum bilirubin acutely by approximately 50% and removes about 80% of sensitized or abnormal red blood cells and offending antibody so that ongoing hemolysis is decreased. Exchange transfusion is also indicated in any infant with TSB above 30 mg/dL, in infants with signs of encephalopathy, or when intensive phototherapy has not lowered TSB by at least 0.5 mg/dL/h after 4 hours. The decision to perform exchange transfusion should be based on TSB, not on the unconjugated fraction of bilirubin.

Exchange transfusion is invasive, potentially risky, and infrequently performed. It should therefore be performed at a referral center. Mortality is 1%–5% and is greatest in the smallest, most immature, and unstable infants. Sudden death during the procedure can occur in any infant. There is a 5%–10% risk of serious complications such as necrotizing enterocolitis (NEC), infection, electrolyte disturbances, or thrombocytopenia.

Kemper AR et al: Clinical practice guideline revision: management of hyperbilirubinemia in the newborn infant 35 or more weeks of gestation. Pediatrics 2022 Sep 1;150(3):e2022058859. doi: 10.1542/peds.2022-058859 [PMID: 35927462].

HYPOGLYCEMIA

ESSENTIALS OF DIAGNOSIS & TYPICAL FEATURES

- ▶ Blood glucose < 40 mg/dL at birth to 4 hours or < 45 mg/dL at 4–24 hours of age.
- ▶ LGA, SGA, preterm, and stressed infants at risk.
- ▶ May be asymptomatic.
- ▶ Infants can present with lethargy, poor feeding, irritability, or seizures.

General Considerations

Glucose concentration decreases in the immediate postnatal period, to as low as 30 mg/dL in many healthy infants at 1–2 hours after birth. Concentrations below 40 mg/dL after the first feeding are considered hypoglycemic. By 3 hours, the glucose concentration in normal full-term infants stabilizes at 45 mg/dL or greater. The two groups of full-term newborn infants at highest risk for hypoglycemia are IDMs and growth-restricted infants.

A. Infants of Diabetic Mothers

The IDM has abundant glucose stores in the form of glycogen and fat but develops hypoglycemia because of hyperinsulinemia induced by maternal and fetal hyperglycemia. Increased energy supply to the fetus from the maternal circulation results in a macrosomic infant. The IDM is at increased risk for multiple neonatal problems, including trauma during delivery; cardiomyopathy (asymmetrical septal hypertrophy) that may present with murmur, respiratory distress, or cardiac failure; and microcolon that causes symptoms of low intestinal obstruction. Other neonatal problems include hypercoagulability and polycythemia, a combination that predisposes the infant to large vein thromboses (especially the renal vein). IDMs are often immature for their gestational age and are at increased risk for surfactant deficiency, hypocalcemia, feeding difficulties, and hyperbilirubinemia.

B. Intrauterine Growth-Restricted Infants

The intrauterine growth-restricted (IUGR) infant has reduced glucose stores in the form of glycogen and body fat and is prone to hypoglycemia. In addition, marked hyperglycemia and a transient diabetes mellitus–like syndrome occasionally develop, particularly in the very premature IUGR infant. The latter problems usually respond to adjustment in glucose intake, although insulin is sometimes needed transiently.

C. Other Causes of Hypoglycemia

Hypoglycemia occurs in disorders with islet cell hyperplasia, including Beckwith-Wiedemann syndrome, and genetic forms of hyperinsulinism. Hypoglycemia also occurs in certain inborn errors of metabolism such as glycogen storage disease and galactosemia. Endocrine causes of hypoglycemia include adrenal insufficiency and hypopituitarism, which should be suspected in the setting of hypoglycemia and micropenis. Hypoglycemia also occurs in infants with birth asphyxia, hypoxia, and bacterial or viral sepsis. Premature infants are at risk for hypoglycemia due to decreased glycogen stores.

Clinical Findings & Monitoring

The signs of hypoglycemia in the newborn infant may be nonspecific and subtle: lethargy, poor feeding, irritability, tremors, jitteriness, apnea, and seizures. IDMs and IUGR infants with polycythemia are at greatest risk for symptomatic hypoglycemia. Hypoglycemia due to increased insulin is the most severe and most resistant to treatment. Hypoglycemia in hyperinsulinemic states can develop within the first 30–60 minutes of life.

Blood glucose can be measured by heel stick using a bedside glucometer. All infants at risk should be screened, including IDMs, IUGR infants, premature infants, and any infant with suggestive symptoms. All low or borderline values should be confirmed by laboratory measurement of blood glucose concentration. It is important to continue surveillance of glucose concentration until the baby has been on full enteral feedings without intravenous supplementation for 24 hours. Relapse of hypoglycemia thereafter is unlikely.

Infants with hypoglycemia requiring IV glucose infusions for more than 5 days should be evaluated for less common disorders, including inborn errors of metabolism, hyperinsulinemic states, and deficiencies of counterregulatory hormones.

Treatment

Therapy is based on the provision of enteral or parenteral glucose. Treatment guidelines are shown in Table 2–7. Enteral glucose is the preferred treatment for an asymptomatic hypoglycemic infant who is vigorous and able to orally feed. Oral dextrose gel can be used to supplement an oral feeding and has been shown to decrease mother-infant separation and promote full breast-feeding at discharge. In hyperinsulinemic states, glucose boluses should be avoided and a higher glucose infusion rate used. Glucose infusion should be increased gradually as needed from a starting rate of 6 mg/kg/min and weaned slowly once the infant is normoglycemic.

Prognosis

The prognosis of hypoglycemia is good if therapy is prompt. CNS sequelae are more common in infants with hypoglycemic seizures and in neonates with persistent hyperinsulinemic hypoglycemia. Hypoglycemia may potentiate brain injury after perinatal depression and should be avoided.

Blanco CL, Kim J: Neonatal glucose homeostasis. Clin Perinatol 2022 Jun;49(2):393–404 [PMID: 35659093].

Rozance PJ, Wolfsdorf JI: Hypoglycemia in the newborn. Pediatr Clin North Am 2019 Apr;66(2):333–342 [PMID: 30819340].

Table 2–7. Hypoglycemia: suggested therapeutic regimens.

Screening Test[a]	Presence of Symptoms	Action
30–45 mg/dL	No symptoms of hypoglycemia	Draw blood glucose[b]; if the infant is alert and vigorous, feed; follow with frequent glucose monitoring. Consider 40% oral glucose gel (0.5 mL/kg) to supplement feeding.
		If the infant continues to have blood glucose < 40 mg/dL or is unable to feed, provide intravenous glucose at 6 mg/kg/min ($D_{10}W$ at 3.6 mL/kg/h).
< 45 mg/dL	Symptoms of hypoglycemia present	Draw blood glucose[b]; provide bolus of $D_{10}W$ (2 mL/kg) followed by an infusion of 6 mg/kg/min (3.6 mL/kg/h).
< 30 mg/dL	With or without symptoms of hypoglycemia	Draw blood glucose[b]; provide bolus of $D_{10}W$ followed by an infusion of 6 mg/kg/min.
		If IV access cannot be obtained immediately, an umbilical vein line should be used.

[a]Rapid bedside determination.
[b]Laboratory confirmation.

RESPIRATORY DISTRESS IN THE TERM NEWBORN INFANT

ESSENTIALS OF DIAGNOSIS & TYPICAL FEATURES

► Tachypnea (respiratory rate > 60 breaths/min).
► Intercostal and sternal retractions.
► Expiratory grunting.
► Cyanosis in room air.

General Considerations

Respiratory distress is one of the most common symptom complexes of the newborn. It may result from airway, pulmonary, cardiac, and other causes (Table 2–8). Chest radiography, arterial blood gases, and pulse oximetry are useful in assessing the cause and severity of the distress. Most of the noncardiopulmonary causes can be ruled out by history, physical examination, and a few simple laboratory tests. The most common pulmonary causes of respiratory distress in the full-term infant are transient tachypnea, aspiration syndromes, congenital pneumonia, and pneumothorax.

A. Transient Tachypnea (Retained Fetal Lung Fluid)

Respiratory distress is typically present at birth, usually associated with a mild to moderate oxygen requirement (25%–50% O_2). The infant is usually full term or late preterm, non-asphyxiated, and born following a short labor or cesarean section without labor. The pathogenesis of the disorder is

related to delayed clearance of fetal lung fluid via the circulation and pulmonary lymphatics. The chest radiograph shows perihilar streaking and fluid in interlobar fissures. Resolution usually occurs within 12–24 hours.

Table 2–8. Causes of respiratory distress in the term newborn.

Airway anomalies/obstruction
    Choanal atresia
    Vocal cord paralysis
    Pierre-Robin sequence
    Subglottic stenosis
Primary pulmonary disease
    Transient tachypnea
    Aspiration syndromes
        Amniotic fluid
        Blood
        Meconium
    Pneumonia
    Pneumothorax
    Surfactant deficiency
    Surfactant dysfunction
    Pleural effusion
    Mass lesions
        Congenital adenomatoid malformation
        Congenital diaphragmatic hernia
        Bronchopulmonary sequestration
    Alveolar capillary dysplasia
Congenital heart disease
    Cyanotic lesions
    Left-sided outflow tract obstruction
    Right-sided outflow tract obstruction
    Total anomalous pulmonary venous return
Other causes
    Neuromuscular disorders
    Central nervous system injury
    Skeletal dysplasia

B. Aspiration Syndromes

Aspiration syndromes typically occur in full-term or late preterm infants with fetal distress prior to delivery or depression at delivery. Blood or meconium may be present in the amniotic fluid. Aspiration of meconium most commonly occurs in utero when the stressed infant gasps. Respiratory distress is present from birth, often accompanied by coarse breath sounds. Pneumonitis may cause an increasing oxygen need and may require intubation and ventilation. The chest radiograph shows coarse asymmetric infiltrates, hyperexpansion, and, in the worst cases, lobar consolidation. In some cases, because of secondary surfactant deficiency, the radiograph shows a diffuse homogeneous infiltrate pattern. Infants who aspirate are at risk of pneumothorax because of uneven aeration with segmental overdistention and are at risk for persistent pulmonary hypertension (see Cardiac Problems in the Newborn Infant).

C. Congenital Pneumonia

The lungs are the most common site of infection in the neonate. Infections usually ascend from the genital tract before or during labor, with vaginal or rectal flora the most likely agents (especially group B streptococci and *Escherichia coli*). Infants of any gestational age, with or without a history of prolonged rupture of membranes, chorioamnionitis, or maternal antibiotic administration, may be affected. Respiratory distress may begin at birth or may be delayed for several hours. The chest radiograph may resemble that of retained lung fluid or surfactant deficiency. Rarely, there may be a lobar infiltrate or pleural effusion. Congenital pneumonia may be complicated by systemic sepsis.

Shock, poor perfusion, absolute neutropenia (< 2000/mL), and elevated C-reactive protein or procalcitonin level provide supportive evidence for pneumonia. Gram stain of tracheal aspirate may be helpful. Because no signs or laboratory findings can confirm a diagnosis of pneumonia, obtaining a blood culture and treatment with broad spectrum antibiotics should be considered in all term newborn with respiratory distress.

D. Spontaneous Pneumothorax

Spontaneous pneumothorax occurs in 1% of all deliveries. Risk is increased by interventions such as positive-pressure ventilation (PPV) in the delivery room. Respiratory distress (primarily tachypnea) is present from birth and typically is mild. Breath sounds may be decreased on the affected side; heart tones may be shifted toward the opposite side and may be distant. The chest radiograph shows the pneumothorax. Treatment usually consists of supplemental oxygen and watchful waiting. Drainage by needle thoracentesis or tube thoracostomy is occasionally required.

E. Other Respiratory Tract Causes

Other respiratory tract causes of respiratory distress are rare. Bilateral choanal atresia should be suspected if there is no air movement when the infant breathes through the nose. These infants have good color and heart rate while crying at delivery but become cyanotic and bradycardic when they resume normal nasal breathing. Other causes of upper airway obstruction usually produce some degree of stridor or poor air movement despite good respiratory effort.

Pleural effusion is likely in hydropic infants. Space-occupying lesions cause a shift of the mediastinum with asymmetrical breath sounds and are apparent on chest radiographs. Many are associated with severe respiratory distress. Other rare causes of respiratory distress in term newborns include surfactant protein deficiencies resulting in surfactant dysfunction and alveolar capillary dysplasia. These disorders present with severe respiratory distress shortly after birth. Many can be identified with targeted genetic testing.

▶ Treatment

Whatever the cause, neonatal respiratory distress is treated with supplemental oxygen sufficient to maintain a Pao_2 of 60–70 mm Hg and an oxygen saturation by pulse oximetry (Spo_2) of 92%–96%. Oxygen should be warmed, humidified, and delivered through an air blender. An umbilical or peripheral arterial line should be considered in infants requiring more than 45% fraction of inspired oxygen (Fio_2) by 4–6 hours of life to allow frequent blood gas determinations. Noninvasive monitoring with pulse oximetry should also be used.

Supportive treatment includes IV glucose, and, unless infection can be ruled out, blood cultures should be obtained and broad-spectrum antibiotics started. Other specific testing should be done as indicated by the history and physical examination. In most cases, a chest radiograph, blood gas measurements, CBC, and blood glucose determination allow a diagnosis.

Intubation and mechanical ventilation should be undertaken if there is respiratory failure, commonly defined as a Pao_2 less than 60 mm Hg and greater than 60% Fio_2, a $Paco_2$ greater than 60 mm Hg, or repeated apnea.

▶ Prognosis

Most respiratory conditions of the full-term infant are acute and resolve in the first several days. Meconium aspiration and congenital pneumonia carry a mortality rate of up to 10% and can produce significant long-term pulmonary morbidity. Mortality has been reduced by use of high-frequency oscillatory ventilation and inhaled nitric oxide for treatment of pulmonary hypertension. Only rarely is extracorporeal membrane oxygenation (ECMO) needed as rescue therapy.

Chowdhury N, Giles BL, Dell SD: Full-term neonatal respiratory distress and chronic lung disease. Pediatr Ann 2019 Apr 1; 48(4):e175–e181 [PMID: 30986319].

HEART MURMURS

Heart murmurs are common in the first days of life and do not usually signify structural heart problems (see also Cardiac Problems in the Newborn Infant). If a murmur is present at birth, it should be considered a valvular problem until proved otherwise because the common benign transitional murmurs (eg, patent ductus arteriosus) are not audible until minutes to hours after birth.

If an infant is not cyanotic, well-perfused, and in no respiratory distress, with palpable and symmetrical pulses (right brachial pulse no stronger than the femoral pulse), a murmur first hard sometime after birth is most likely transitional. Transitional murmurs are soft (grade 1–3/6), heard at the left upper to midsternal border, and generally loudest during the first 24 hours. If the murmur persists beyond 24 hours of age, blood pressure in the right arm and a leg should be determined. If there is a difference of more than 15 mm Hg (arm > leg) or if the pulses in the lower extremities are difficult to palpate, the infant should be evaluated for coarctation of the aorta. If there is no difference, the infant can be discharged home with follow-up in 2–3 days for auscultation and evaluation for signs of congestive failure. If signs of congestive failure or cyanosis are present, the infant should be referred for evaluation immediately. If the murmur persists without these signs, the infant can be referred for elective evaluation at age 2–4 weeks.

BIRTH TRAUMA

Most birth trauma is associated with difficult delivery (eg, large fetus, abnormal presenting position, or fetal distress requiring rapid extraction). The most common injuries are soft tissue bruising, fractures (clavicle, humerus, or femur), and cervical plexus palsies. Skull fracture, intracranial hemorrhage (primarily subdural and subarachnoid), and cervical spinal cord injury can also occur.

Fractures are often diagnosed by the obstetrician, who may feel or hear a snap during delivery. Clavicular fractures may cause decreased spontaneous movement of the arm, with local tenderness and crepitus. Humeral or femoral fractures usually cause tenderness and swelling over the shaft with a diaphyseal fracture, and always cause limitation of movement. After 8–10 days, callus is visible on radiographs. Treatment in all cases is gentle handling, with immobilization for 8–10 days.

Brachial plexus injuries may result from traction as the head is pulled away from the shoulder during delivery. Injury to the C5–C6 roots is most common (Erb-Duchenne palsy). The arm is limp, adducted, and internally rotated, extended, and pronated at the elbow, and flexed at the wrist (so-called waiter's tip posture). Grasp is present. If the lower nerve roots (C8–T1) are injured (Klumpke palsy), the hand is flaccid. If the entire plexus is injured, the arm and hand are flaccid, with associated sensory deficit. Early treatment for brachial plexus injury is conservative because function usually returns over several weeks. Referral should be made to a physical therapist so that parents can be instructed on range-of-motion exercises, splinting, and further evaluation if needed. Return of function begins in the deltoid and biceps, with recovery by 3 months in most cases.

Spinal cord injury can occur at birth, especially in difficult breech extractions with hyperextension of the neck, or in midforceps rotations when the body fails to turn with the head. Infants are flaccid, quadriplegic, and without respiratory effort at birth. Facial movements are preserved. The long-term outlook for such infants is poor.

Facial nerve palsy is sometimes associated with forceps use but more often results from in utero pressure of the baby's head against the mother's sacrum. The infant has asymmetrical mouth movements and eye closure with poor facial movement on the affected side. Most cases resolve spontaneously in a few days to weeks.

Subgaleal hemorrhage into the large potential space under the scalp (Figure 2–1) is associated with repeated attempts at vacuum extraction. It can lead to hypovolemic shock and death from blood loss and coagulopathy triggered by consumption of clotting factors, an emergency requiring rapid replacement of blood and clotting factors.

INFANTS OF MOTHERS WITH SUBSTANCE USE DISORDERS

Current studies estimate that 10% of women use alcohol during pregnancy, depending on the population studied and the methods of ascertainment. Other drugs commonly used in pregnancy are tobacco, marijuana, cocaine, and methamphetamine. The American College of Obstetricians and Gynecologists recommends universal drug screening during prenatal care using a validated screening tool. Because mothers may use multiple substances, it is difficult to pinpoint which drug is causing morbidity observed in a newborn infant. Early hospital discharge makes recognition of affected infants based on physical findings and abnormal behavior difficult. Except for alcohol, a birth defect syndrome has not been defined for any substance of abuse.

1. Cocaine & Methamphetamine

Cocaine and methamphetamine are often used in association with other drugs such as tobacco, alcohol, and marijuana. These stimulants can cause maternal hypertension, decreased uterine blood flow, fetal hypoxemia, uterine contractions, and placental abruption. Rates of stillbirth, placental abruption, symmetric IUGR, and preterm delivery are increased in users. Although no specific malformation complex or withdrawal syndrome is described for cocaine and methamphetamine abuse, infants may show irritability, tremors, increased stress response, and poor state regulation.

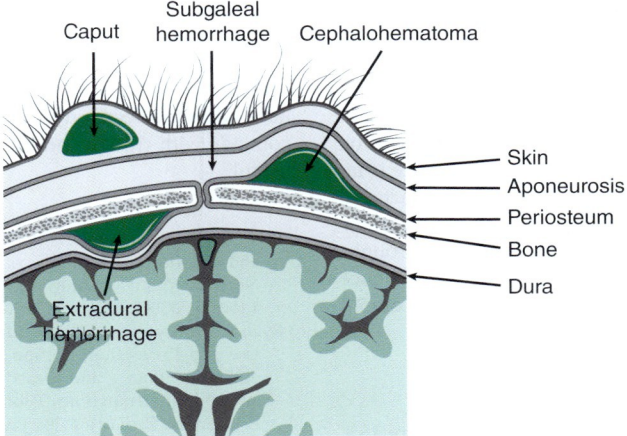

▲ **Figure 2–1.** Sites of extracranial bleeding in the newborn.

Children of mothers who use methamphetamines are at particularly high risk for neglect and abuse. Social services evaluation is important to assess the home environment for these risks. The risk of SIDS is three to seven times higher in infants of users (0.5%–1% of exposed infants) than in those of nonusers. The risk may be lessened by environmental interventions such as avoidance of tobacco smoke and supine infant positioning.

2. Opioids

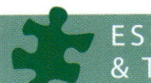

ESSENTIALS OF DIAGNOSIS & TYPICAL FEATURES

► CNS—irritability, hyperactivity, hypertonicity, incessant high-pitched cry, tremors, seizures.
► GI—vomiting, diarrhea, weight loss, poor feeding, incessant hunger, excessive salivation.
► Metabolic and respiratory—nasal stuffiness, sneezing, yawning, sweating, hyperthermia.
► Often IUGR.

▶ Clinical Findings

Withdrawal signs seen in infants born to opioid-using mothers, whether heroin, prescription pain medication, methadone, or other opioids are similar and referred to as neonatal opioid withdrawal syndrome (NOWS). These symptoms include problems with feeding and sleep, fever, increased tone, tremors, and seizures. Symptoms usually begin within 1–3 days of life. The symptoms in infants born to methadone-maintained mothers may be delayed in onset,

more severe, and more prolonged than those seen with heroin use. The clinical picture of NOWS is typical enough to suggest a diagnosis even if a maternal history of opioid use has not been obtained. Confirmation should be made with maternal and newborn toxicology screening.

▶ Treatment

If opioid abuse or withdrawal is suspected, the infant is not a candidate for early discharge. A serial scoring system should be used to objectively diagnose NOWS and quantify the severity of symptoms. Supportive treatment includes swaddling the infant and providing a quiet, dimly lit environment, minimizing procedures, and disturbing the infant as little as possible. Specific treatment should be used when the infant has severe symptoms. No single drug has been identified as optimally effective, but oral morphine or methadone are first-line agents. Phenobarbital may be used for increased irritability, particularly in patients who were exposed to multiple drugs. Treatment can be tapered over several days to 2 weeks, as tolerated. It is also important to review maternal tests for HIV, hepatitis B, and hepatitis C, as all are common in intravenous drug users.

▶ Prognosis

These infants often have chronic neurobehavioral handicaps; however, it is difficult to distinguish the effects of in utero drug exposure from those of the environment. Infants of opioid abusers have a four- to fivefold increased risk of SIDS.

3. Alcohol

Alcohol is the only recreational drug of abuse that is clearly teratogenic, and prenatal exposure to alcohol is the most common preventable cause of mental retardation. Prevalence estimates of fetal alcohol syndrome (FAS) in the United States range from 0.5 to 2 per 1000 live births with up to 1 in 100 having lesser effects (fetal alcohol spectrum disorders). The effects of alcohol on the fetus and newborn are determined by the degree and timing of ethanol exposure and by the maternal, fetal, and placental metabolism of ethanol, which is likely genetically determined. Although there is no clear evidence that minimal amounts of alcohol are harmful, there is no established safe dose. Fetal growth and development are adversely affected if drinking continues throughout the pregnancy, and infants can occasionally experience withdrawal similar to that associated with maternal opioid abuse.

4. Tobacco Smoking

The fetus is exposed to nicotine concentrations that are 15% higher than in maternal blood. Smoking has a negative effect on fetal growth rate. The more the mother smokes, the greater is the degree of IUGR. There is a twofold increase in low birth weight even in light smokers (< 10 cigarettes per day). Infants exposed to nicotine prenatally are also at increased risk for preterm labor and SIDS. Smoking during pregnancy has been associated with irritability, hypertonicity, hyperexcitability, and tremors in the newborn.

5. Marijuana

Marijuana does not appear to be teratogenic, and although a mild abstinence-type syndrome has been described, infants exposed to marijuana in utero rarely require treatment. Long-term neurodevelopmental problems, particularly increased impulsivity and hyperactivity and problems in abstract and visual reasoning, have been noted.

6. Other Drugs

Other drugs with potential effects on the newborn fall in two categories. First are drugs to which the fetus is exposed because of therapy for maternal conditions. The human placenta is relatively permeable, particularly to lipophilic solutes. If possible, maternal drug therapy should be postponed until after the first trimester to avoid teratogenic effects. Drugs with potential fetal toxicity include antineoplastics, antithyroid agents, warfarin, lithium, and angiotensin-converting enzyme inhibitors. Anticonvulsants, especially high-dose or multiple-drug therapy, may be associated with craniofacial abnormalities. Selective serotonin reuptake inhibitors (SSRIs), benzodiazepines, and antipsychotic medications appear to be generally safe, and risk should be balanced against the risk of untreated psychiatric conditions in the mother. However, up to 33% of infants exposed to SSRIs in utero experience signs of withdrawal during the first days of life. Phenobarbital may be used for severe irritability in cases of SSRI withdrawal.

In the second category are drugs transmitted to the infant in breast milk. Most drugs taken by the mother achieve some concentration in breast milk, although they usually do not present a problem to the infant. If the drug is one that could have adverse effects on the infant, timing breast-feeding to coincide with trough concentrations in the mother may be useful.

Patrick SW, Barfield WD, Poindexter BB; Committee on Fetus and Newborn, Committee on Substance Use and Prevention: Neonatal opioid withdrawal syndrome. Pediatrics 2020 Nov; 146(5):e2020029074 [PMID: 33106341].

Ryan SA, Ammerman SD, O'Connor ME; Committee on Substance Use and Prevention; Section on Breastfeeding: Marijuana use during pregnancy and breastfeeding: implications for neonatal and childhood outcomes. Pediatrics 2018 Sep;142(3):e20181889. Erratum in: Pediatrics. 2018 Aug 27 [PMID: 30150209].

MULTIPLE BIRTHS

ESSENTIALS OF DIAGNOSIS & TYPICAL FEATURES

► Monochorial twins
  • Always monozygous (identical twins) and same sex.
  • Can be diamniotic or monoamniotic.
  • Risk for twin-to-twin transfusion and higher risk of congenital anomalies, neurodevelopmental problems, and cerebral palsy.

► Dichorial twins
  • Either dizygous (fraternal twins) or monozygous (identical twins); same sex or different sex.
  • Can have growth restriction due to abnormal placental implantation.
  • Not at risk for twin transfusion syndrome; less risk for anomalies and neurodevelopmental problems than monochorial twins.

Race, maternal parity, and maternal age affect the incidence of dizygous (fraternal), but not monozygous (identical), twinning. Drugs used to induce ovulation, such as clomiphene citrate and gonadotropins, increase the incidence of dizygotic or polyzygotic twinning. The incidence of malformations is increased in monozygous twins and may affect only one of the twins. If a defect is found in one twin, the other should be examined carefully for lesser degrees of the same defect.

Early transvaginal ultrasound and examination of the placenta after birth can help establish the type of twinning. Two amnionic membranes and two chorionic membranes are found in all dizygous twins and in one-third of monozygous twins even when the placental disks appear to be fused into one. A single chorionic membrane always indicates monozygous twins. The rare monochorial, monoamniotic situation (1% of twins) is especially dangerous, with a high risk of antenatal cord entanglement and death of one or both twins. Close fetal surveillance is indicated, and preterm delivery is often elected.

► Complications of Multiple Births

A. Intrauterine Growth Restriction

There is some degree of IUGR in most multiple pregnancies, especially after 32 weeks, although it is usually not clinically significant with two exceptions. First, in monochorial twin pregnancy an arteriovenous shunt may develop between the twins (known as twin-twin transfusion syndrome). The twin on the venous side (recipient) becomes plethoric and larger than the smaller anemic twin (donor), who may ultimately die or be severely growth restricted. The occurrence of polyhydramnios in the larger twin and severe oligohydramnios in the smaller may be the first sign of this problem. Second, discordance in size (birth weights that are significantly different) can also occur when separate placentas are present if one placenta develops poorly because of a poor implantation site. In this instance, no fetal exchange of blood takes place but the growth rates of the two infants are different.

B. Preterm Delivery

Length of gestation tends to be inversely related to the number of fetuses. The mean age at delivery for singletons is 38.8 weeks, for twins 35.3 weeks, for triplets 32.2 weeks, and for quadruplets 29.9 weeks. There is an increased incidence of cerebral palsy in multiple births, more so with monochorial than dichorial infants. Prematurity is the main cause of increased mortality and morbidity in twins, although in the case of monochorial twins, intravascular exchange through placental anastomoses also increases the risk substantially.

C. Obstetric Complications

Polyhydramnios, pregnancy-induced hypertension, premature rupture of membranes, abnormal fetal presentations, and prolapsed umbilical cord occur more frequently in women with multiple fetuses. Multiple pregnancies should always be identified prenatally with ultrasound examinations; doing so allows the obstetrician and pediatrician or neonatologist to plan management jointly. Because neonatal complications are usually related to prematurity, prolongation of pregnancy significantly reduces neonatal morbidity.

▼ NEONATAL INTENSIVE CARE

PERINATAL RESUSCITATION

Perinatal resuscitation refers to the steps taken by the obstetrician to support the infant during labor and delivery and the resuscitative steps taken by the pediatrician after delivery. Intrapartum support includes maintaining maternal blood pressure, maternal oxygen therapy, positioning the mother to improve placental perfusion, readjusting oxytocin infusions or administering a tocolytic if appropriate, minimizing trauma to the infant, obtaining all necessary cord blood samples, and completing an examination of the placenta. The pediatrician or neonatologist focuses on temperature support, initiation and maintenance of effective ventilation, maintenance of perfusion and hydration, and glucose regulation.

A number of conditions associated with pregnancy, labor, and delivery place the infant at risk for birth asphyxia: (1) maternal diseases such as diabetes, pregnancy-induced hypertension, heart and renal disease, and collagen-vascular disease; (2) fetal conditions such as prematurity, multiple births, growth restriction, and fetal anomalies; and (3) labor and delivery conditions, including fetal distress with or without meconium in the amniotic fluid, and administration of anesthetics and opioid analgesics.

Physiology of Birth Asphyxia

Birth asphyxia can be the result of (1) acute interruption of umbilical blood flow (eg, prolapsed cord with cord compression), (2) premature placental separation, (3) maternal hypotension or hypoxia, (4) chronic placental insufficiency, and (5) failure to perform resuscitation properly.

The neonatal response to asphyxia follows a predictable pattern. The initial response to hypoxia is an increase in respiratory rate and a rise in heart rate and blood pressure. Respirations then cease (primary apnea) as heart rate and blood pressure begin to fall. The initial period of apnea lasts 30–60 seconds. Gasping respirations (3–6/min) then begin, while heart rate and blood pressure gradually decline. Secondary or terminal apnea then ensues, with further decline in heart rate and blood pressure. The longer the duration of secondary apnea, the greater is the risk for hypoxic organ injury. A cardinal feature of the defense against hypoxia is the underperfusion of certain tissue beds (eg, skin, muscle, kidneys, and GI tract), which allows maintenance of perfusion to core organs (ie, heart, brain, and adrenals).

Response to resuscitation also follows a predictable pattern. During the period of primary apnea, almost any physical stimulus causes the infant to initiate respirations. Infants in secondary apnea require PPV. The first sign of recovery is an increase in heart rate, followed by an increase in blood pressure with improved perfusion. The time required for rhythmic, spontaneous respirations to occur is related to the duration of the secondary apnea. For each minute past the last gasp, approximately 2 minutes of PPV is required before gasping begins and 4 minutes is required to reach rhythmic breathing. Spinal and corneal reflexes return later, and muscle tone gradually improves over the course of several hours.

Delivery Room Management

When asphyxia is anticipated, a resuscitation team of at least two persons should be present: one to manage the airway and one to monitor the heartbeat and provide assistance.

A. Steps in the Resuscitative Process

1. Dry the infant well and place under a radiant heat source. Do not allow the infant to become hyperthermic.

2. Position the infant to open the airway. Gently suction the mouth, then the nose.

3. Quickly assess the infant's condition. The best criteria are the infant's respiratory effort (apneic, gasping, or regular) and heart rate (> 100 or < 100 beats/min). A depressed heart rate—indicative of hypoxic myocardial depression—is the single most reliable indicator of the need for resuscitation.

4. Infants who are breathing and have heart rates more than 100 beats/min usually require no further intervention other than supplemental oxygen if persistently cyanotic. Infants with heart rates less than 100 beats/min and apnea or irregular respiratory efforts should be stimulated gently. The infant's back should be rubbed and/or heels flicked.

5. If the infant fails to respond to tactile stimulation within a few seconds, begin bag and mask ventilation, using a soft mask that seals well around the mouth and nose. Adequacy of ventilation is assessed by observing expansion of the infant's chest accompanied by an improvement in heart rate, perfusion, and color. An oximeter probe should be placed on the infant's right hand.

6. Most neonates can be resuscitated effectively with bag-and-mask ventilation. If the infant does not respond to bag and mask ventilation, reposition the head (slight extension), reapply the mask to achieve a good seal, consider suctioning the mouth and the oropharynx, and try ventilating with the mouth open. An increase in peak pressure should also be attempted, but if the infant does not respond within 30 seconds, intubation is appropriate. Failure to respond to intubation and ventilation can result from (1) mechanical causes, (2) profound asphyxia with myocardial depression, and (3) inadequate circulating blood volume. Very few neonates (~0.1%) require either cardiac compressions or drugs during resuscitation. Almost all newborns respond to ventilation if done effectively. All resuscitations in term infants should begin using room air. Oxygen concentration can be increased

using an oxygen blender during PPV. It is not expected for the preductal (right hand) oxygen saturation to reach 90% until 10 minutes of age. The use of 100% oxygen may increase the risk of post-resuscitative oxidative injury without any improvement in efficacy.

7. If mechanical causes are ruled out and the heart rate remains less than 60 beats/min after intubation and effective PPV for 30 seconds, cardiac compressions should be initiated. Chest compressions should be synchronized with ventilation at a 3:1 ratio (90 compressions and 30 breaths/min). Electronic cardiac monitoring should be used to monitor the heart rate when chest compressions are administered.

8. If drugs are needed, the drug and dose of choice is epinephrine 1:10,000 solution given via an umbilical venous line. If volume loss is suspected, normal saline should be administered through an umbilical vein line.

B. Continued Resuscitative Measures

The appropriateness of continued resuscitative efforts should be reevaluated in infants who do not respond to initial measures. In current practice, resuscitative efforts are made even in apparent stillbirths (ie, infants whose Apgar score at 1 minute is 0–1). Modern resuscitative techniques have led to improved survival in such infants, with 60% of survivors showing normal development. Although it is clear that resuscitation of these infants should be performed, subsequent continued support depends on the response to resuscitation. If the Apgar score does not improve markedly in the first 10 minutes of life, the mortality rate and the incidence of severe developmental handicaps among survivors are high.

C. Special Considerations

1. Delayed cord clamping—Current recommendations for neonatal resuscitation include that cord clamping should be delayed for at least 30–60 seconds for most vigorous term and preterm newborns. In cases where placental circulation is compromised (placental abruption, umbilical cord compression or avulsion), the umbilical cord should be clamped immediately and the initial steps of resuscitation begun.

2. Preterm infants

A. Minimizing heat loss improves survival. Prewarmed towels should be available. The environmental temperature of the delivery suite should be raised to more than 25°C (especially for infants weighing < 1500 g). An occlusive skin cover such as a gallon-sized food-grade plastic bag with an opening to slip over the infant's head and an exothermic blanket should be used to minimize heat loss in the extremely low birth weight (< 1000 g) infant.

B. The lungs of preterm infants are especially prone to injury from PPV due to volutrauma. For this reason, if possible, the infant's respiratory efforts should be supported with nasal continuous positive airway pressure (CPAP) rather than PPV. If PPV is needed, a T-piece resuscitation device should be used to allow precise and consistent regulation of pressure delivery. Resuscitation in the preterm should begin with a blended oxygen concentration of 30% with titration to achieve target oxygen saturations.

C. In the infant of extremely low gestational age, immediate intubation for administration of surfactant should be considered.

D. Volume expanders should be infused slowly to minimize rapid swings in blood pressure, especially important in the extremely low birth weight infant.

3. Narcotic depression—In the case of opioid administration to the mother within 4 hours of delivery, institute resuscitation as described earlier. The use of naloxone is not recommended during neonatal resuscitation due to insufficient evidence of safety and efficacy.

4. Meconium-stained amniotic fluid—Resuscitation of the infant should proceed with the same initial steps as an infant born without meconium-stained amniotic fluid.

5. Universal precautions—In the delivery suite, universal precautions should always be observed.

Treatment of the Asphyxiated Infant

Asphyxia is manifested by multiorgan dysfunction, seizures, neonatal encephalopathy, and metabolic acidemia. The infant with significant perinatal hypoxia and ischemia is at risk for dysfunction of multiple end organs (Table 2–9). The organ of greatest concern is the brain.

The features of neonatal encephalopathy are decreased level of consciousness, poor tone, decreased spontaneous movement, periodic breathing or apnea, and seizures. Brainstem signs (oculomotor and pupillary disturbances, absent gag reflex) may also be present. The severity and duration of clinical signs correlate with the severity of the insult. Other evaluations helpful in assessing severity in the full-term infant include electroencephalogram (EEG) and MRI which, particularly with diffusion-weighted imaging, is useful in the early evaluation of infants with perinatal asphyxia. A markedly abnormal EEG with voltage suppression and slowing evolving into a burst-suppression pattern is associated with severe clinical symptoms. MRI may show perfusion defects and areas of ischemic injury on diffusion-weighted imaging.

Management is directed at supportive care and treatment of specific abnormalities. Fluids should be restricted initially to 40-60 mL/kg/day; oxygenation should be maintained with mechanical ventilation if necessary; blood pressure should be supported with judicious volume expansion (if hypovolemic) and vasopressor support; and glucose should be in the normal range of 45–100 mg/dL. Hypocalcemia, coagulation abnormalities, and metabolic acidemia should be corrected and seizures treated. Therapeutic hypothermia initiated within 6 hours of birth has been shown to improve outcome at 24 months and 6–7 year follow-up of infants with moderate encephalopathy.

Birth Asphyxia: Long-Term Outcome

Fetal heart rate tracings, cord pH, and 1-minute Apgar scores are imprecise predictors of long-term outcome. Apgar scores of 0–3 at 5 minutes in full-term infants are associated with an increased risk of death in the first year of life. The risks of mortality and morbidity increase with more prolonged depression of the Apgar score. The single best predictor of outcome is the severity of clinical neonatal encephalopathy (severe symptomatology including coma carries a 75% chance of death and a 100% rate of neurologic sequelae among survivors). The major sequela of neonatal encephalopathy is cerebral palsy with or without cognitive delay and epilepsy. Prolonged seizures refractory to therapy, markedly abnormal EEG, and MRI scan with evidence of major ischemic injury are associated with poor neurodevelopmental outcome.

Table 2–9. Signs and symptoms caused by asphyxia.

Neonatal encephalopathy, seizures
Respiratory distress due to aspiration or secondary surfactant deficiency, pulmonary hemorrhage
Persistent pulmonary hypertension
Hypotension due to myocardial dysfunction
Transient tricuspid valve insufficiency
Anuria or oliguria due to acute tubular necrosis
Feeding intolerance; necrotizing enterocolitis
Elevated aminotransferases due to liver injury
Adrenal insufficiency due to hemorrhage
Disseminated intravascular coagulation
Hypocalcemia
Hypoglycemia
Persistent metabolic acidemia
Hyperkalemia

Bonifacio SL, Hutson S: The term newborn: evaluation for hypoxic-ischemic encephalopathy. Clin Perinatol 2021 Aug;48(3):681–695 [PMID: 34353587].

Weiner GM, Zaichkin J: Updates for the neonatal resuscitation program and resuscitation guidelines. Neoreviews 2022 Apr 1;23(4): e238–e249 [PMID: 35362042].

THE PRETERM INFANT

Premature infants comprise most high-risk newborns. The preterm infant faces a variety of physiologic handicaps:

1. The ability to coordinate sucking, swallowing, and breathing is not achieved until 34–36 weeks' gestation. Therefore, enteral feedings must be provided by gavage.

2. Lack of body fat stores causes decreased ability to maintain body temperature and may predispose to hypoglycemia.

3. Pulmonary immaturity–surfactant deficiency is associated with structural immaturity in infants younger than 26 weeks' gestation. This condition is exacerbated by the combination of noncompliant lungs and an extremely compliant chest wall, causing inefficient respiratory mechanics.

4. Immature respiratory control leads to apnea and bradycardia.

5. Persistent patency of the ductus arteriosus compromises pulmonary gas exchange because of overperfusion and edema of the lungs.

6. Immature cerebral vasculature and structure predisposes to subependymal and intraventricular hemorrhage, and periventricular leukomalacia (PVL).

7. Impaired substrate absorption by the GI tract compromises nutritional management.

8. Immature renal function complicates fluid and electrolyte management.

9. Increased susceptibility to infection.

10. Immaturity of metabolic processes predisposes to hypoglycemia and hypocalcemia.

1. Delivery Room Care

See section Perinatal Resuscitation.

2. Care in the Nursery

A. Thermoregulation

Maintaining stable body temperature is a function of heat production and conservation balanced against heat loss. Heat production in response to cold stress occurs through voluntary muscle activity, involuntary muscle activity (shivering), and thermogenesis not caused by shivering. Newborns produce heat mainly through the last of these three mechanisms. This metabolic heat production depends on the quantity of brown fat, which is very limited in the preterm infant. In addition to decreased heat production in preterm infants, heat loss is accelerated because of a high ratio of surface area to body mass, reduced insulation by subcutaneous tissue, and water loss through the immature skin.

The thermal environment should be regulated carefully. The infant can be kept warm in an isolette, in which the air is heated and convective heat loss is minimized, or on an open bed with a radiant heat source. Ideally, the infant should be kept in a neutral thermal environment, allowing the infant to maintain a stable core body temperature with a minimum of metabolic heat production through oxygen consumption. A neutral thermal environment can be obtained by maintaining an abdominal skin temperature of 36.5°C. The appropriate neutral thermal environment depends on the infant's size, gestational age, and postnatal age. Generally, when infants reach 1700–1800 g, they are able to maintain temperature while bundled in an open crib.

B. Monitoring the High-Risk Infant

At a minimum, equipment to monitor heart rate, respirations, and blood pressure should be available. Oxygen saturation is assessed continuously using pulse oximetry, correlated with arterial oxygen tension (PaO_2) as needed. Transcutaneous PO_2 and PCO_2 can also be used to assess oxygenation and ventilation in sicker infants. Arterial blood gases, electrolytes, glucose, calcium, bilirubin, and other chemistries must be measured on small volumes of blood. Early in the care of a sick preterm infant, the most efficient way to sample blood for tests and monitor blood pressure is through an umbilical arterial line. Once the infant is stable and the need for frequent blood samples is reduced (usually 4–7 days), the umbilical arterial line should be removed. All indwelling lines are associated with potential morbidity from thrombosis, infection, and bleeding.

C. Fluid and Electrolyte Therapy

Fluid requirements in preterm infants are a function of (1) insensible losses (skin and respiratory tract), (2) urine output, (3) stool output (< 5% of total), and (4) other losses, such as nasogastric (NG) losses. In most circumstances, the fluid requirement is determined largely by insensible losses plus urine losses. The major contribution to insensible water loss is evaporative skin loss. The rate of water loss is a function of gestational age (body weight and skin thickness and maturity), environment (losses are greater under a radiant warmer than in an isolette), and the use of phototherapy. Respiratory losses are minimal when humidified oxygen is used. The renal contribution to water requirement is influenced by the limited ability of the preterm neonate either to concentrate the urine and conserve water or to excrete a water load.

Electrolyte requirements are minimal for the first 24–48 hours until there is significant urinary excretion. Basal requirements thereafter are as follows: sodium, 3 mEq/kg/day; potassium, 2 mEq/kg/day; chloride, 2–3 mEq/kg/day; and bicarbonate, 2–3 mEq/kg/day. In the infant younger than 30 weeks gestation, sodium and bicarbonate losses in the urine are often elevated, thereby increasing the infant's requirements.

Initial fluid management after birth varies with the infant's size and gestation. Infants weighing more than 1200 g should start at 80–100 mL/kg/day of $D_{10}W$. Those weighing less should start at 100–120 mL/kg/day of either $D_{10}W$ or D_5W (infants < 800 g and born before 26 weeks' gestation often become hyperglycemic on $D_{10}W$ at these infusion rates). The most critical issue in fluid management is monitoring of body weight, urine output, fluid and electrolyte intake, serum electrolytes, and glucose to allow fairly precise determination of the infant's water, glucose, and electrolyte needs. Parenteral nutrition should be started early, preferably on the first day, and continued until an adequate enteral intake is achieved.

D. Nutritional Support

The average caloric requirement for the growing premature infant is 120 kcal/kg/day. Desired weight gain is 15–20 g/kg/day for infants younger than 35 weeks, and 15 g/kg/day for those older than 35 weeks; linear and head circumference growth should average 1 cm/wk. Infants initially require IV glucose infusion to maintain blood glucose concentration in the range of 60–100 mg/dL. Infusions of 5–7 mg/kg/min (~80–100 mL/kg/day of $D_{10}W$) are usually needed. Nutritional support in the very low-birth-weight infant should be started as soon as possible after birth, with parenteral alimentation solutions containing 3–4 g/kg/day of amino acids (Table 2–10). Small-volume trophic feeds with breast milk or 20 kcal/oz premature formula should be started by gavage at 10% or less of the infant's nutritional intake as soon as possible, generally within the first few days after birth. The infant can then be slowly advanced to full caloric needs over 5–7 days. Even extremely small feedings can enhance intestinal readiness to accept larger feeding volumes. Intermittent bolus feedings are preferred because these appear to stimulate the release of gut-related hormones and may accelerate maturation of the GI tract, although in the extremely low-birth-weight infant (< 1000 g) or the postsurgical neonate, continuous-drip feeds are sometimes better tolerated.

In general, long-term nutritional support for infants of very low birth weight consists either of breast milk supplemented to increase protein, caloric density, and mineral content or infant formulas modified for preterm infants. In these formulas, protein concentrations and caloric concentrations are relatively high and increased calcium and phosphorus are provided to enhance bone mineralization. Success of feedings is assessed by timely passage of feeds out of the stomach without emesis, an abdominal examination free of distention, and a normal stool pattern.

When the preterm infant approaches term age, the nutritional source for the bottle-fed infant can be changed to a transitional formula until age 6–9 months. These formulas are designed for premature infants after hospital discharge and have higher caloric density and increased calcium and phosphorus compared to term infant formulas. Additional iron supplementation (2–4 mg/kg/day) is recommended for premature infants, beginning at 2 weeks to 2 months of age, depending on gestational age and number of previous transfusions. Infants who are treated with erythropoietin (epoetin alfa) for anemia of prematurity require a higher dosage of iron (4–6 mg/kg/day). Iron overload is a possibility in multiply transfused sick preterm infants; such infants should be evaluated with serum ferritin levels prior to beginning iron supplementation.

Embleton N et al. Enteral Nutrition in Preterm Infants (2022): A Position Paper from the ESPGHAN Committee on Nutrition and Invited Experts. J Pediatr Gastroenterol Nutr 2023 Feb 1; 76(2):248–268 [PMID: 36705703].

Table 2–10. Use of parenteral alimentation solutions.

	Volume (mL/kg/day)	Carbohydrate (g/dL)	Protein (g/kg)	Lipid (g/kg)	Calories (kcal/kg)
Peripheral: short-term (7–10 days)					
Starting solution	100–150	$D_{10}W$	3	1	56–84
Target solution	150	$D_{12.5}W$	3–4	3	80–110
Central: long-term (> 10 days)					
Starting solution	100–150	$D_{10}W$	3	1	56–84
Target solution	130	$D_{12.5}$–$D_{15}W$	3–4	3	80–110

Notes
1. Advance dextrose in central hyperalimentation as tolerated per day as needed to achieve appropriate weight gain, as long as blood glucose remains normal, keeping glucose as 40%–60% of total calories administered.
2. Advance lipids by 0.5–1.0 g/kg/day as long as triglycerides are normal. Use 20% concentration.
3. Total water should be 100–150 mL/kg/day, depending on the child's fluid needs.

Monitoring
1. Blood glucose two or three times a day when changing dextrose concentration, then daily.
2. Electrolytes daily, then twice a week when the child is receiving a stable solution.
3. Every 1–2 weeks: blood urea nitrogen and serum creatinine; total protein and serum albumin; serum calcium, phosphate, magnesium, direct bilirubin, and CBC with platelet counts.
4. Triglyceride level after 24 hours at 2 g/kg/day and 24 hours at 3 g/kg/day, then every other week.

3. Apnea in the Preterm Infant

ESSENTIALS OF DIAGNOSIS & TYPICAL FEATURES

▶ Respiratory pause of sufficient duration to result in cyanosis or bradycardia.

▶ Most common in infants born before 34 weeks gestation; onset before 2 weeks of age.

▶ Methylxanthines (eg, caffeine) provide effective treatment.

▶ General Considerations

Apnea is defined as a respiratory pause lasting more than 20 seconds. Shorter respiratory pauses associated with cyanosis or bradycardia also qualify as significant apnea. Periodic breathing, which is common in full-term and preterm infants, is defined as regularly recurring ventilatory cycles interrupted by short pauses *not* associated with bradycardia or color change. By definition, apnea of prematurity is not associated with a predisposing factor and is a diagnosis of exclusion. A variety of processes may precipitate apnea (Table 2–11) and should be considered before a diagnosis of apnea of prematurity is established.

Apnea of prematurity is the most frequent cause of apnea. Most apnea of prematurity is mixed apnea characterized by a centrally (brainstem) mediated respiratory pause preceded or followed by airway obstruction. Apnea of prematurity is the result of immaturity of both the central respiratory regulatory

Table 2–11. Causes of apnea in the preterm infant.

Temperature instability—both cold and heat stress
Response to passage of a feeding tube
Gastroesophageal reflux
Hypoxemia
    Pulmonary parenchymal disease
    Patent ductus arteriosus
    Anemia
Infection
    Sepsis (viral or bacterial)
    Necrotizing enterocolitis
Metabolic causes
    Hypoglycemia
Intracranial hemorrhage
Posthemorrhagic hydrocephalus
Seizures
Drugs (eg, morphine)
Apnea of prematurity

centers and protective mechanisms that aid in maintaining airway patency.

▶ Clinical Findings

Onset is typically during the first 2 weeks of life. The frequency of spells gradually increases with time. Pathologic apnea should be suspected if spells are sudden in onset, unusually frequent, or very severe. Apnea at birth or on the first day of life is unusual but can occur in the nonventilated preterm infant. In the full-term or late preterm infant, presentation at birth suggests neuromuscular abnormalities of an acute (asphyxia, birth trauma, or infection) or chronic (eg, congenital hypotonia or structural CNS lesion) nature.

All infants—regardless of the severity and frequency of apnea—require a minimum screening evaluation, including a general assessment of well-being (eg, tolerance of feedings, stable temperature, normal physical examination), a check of the association of spells with feeding, measurement of Pao_2 or Sao_2, blood glucose, hematocrit, and a review of the drug history. Infants with severe apnea of sudden onset require more extensive evaluation for primary causes, especially infection.

▶ Treatment

Any underlying cause should be treated. If the apnea is due simply to prematurity, symptomatic treatment is dictated by the frequency and severity of apneic spells. Spells frequent enough to interfere with other aspects of care (eg, feeding) or severe enough to cause cyanosis or bradycardia necessitating significant intervention or bag and mask ventilation require treatment. Caffeine citrate is the drug of choice. Side effects of caffeine are generally mild and include tachycardia and occasional feeding intolerance. Nasal CPAP, by treating the obstructive component of apnea, is effective in some infants. Intubation and ventilation can eliminate apneic spells but carry the risks associated with endotracheal intubation. Although many preterm infants are treated medically for possible reflux-associated apnea, there is little evidence to support this intervention. If suspected, a trial of continuous drip gastric or transpyloric feedings can be helpful as a diagnostic and therapeutic intervention.

▶ Prognosis

In most premature infants, apneic and bradycardic spells cease by 34–36 weeks postmenstrual age. Spells that require intervention resolve prior to self-resolving episodes. In infants born at less than 28 weeks' gestation, episodes may continue past term. Apneic and bradycardic episodes in the nursery are not predictors of later SIDS, although the incidence of SIDS is slightly increased in preterm infants. Thus, home monitoring in infants who experienced apnea in the nursery is rarely indicated.

4. Hyaline Membrane Disease

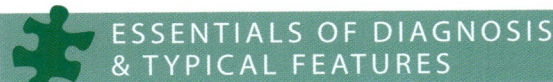

ESSENTIALS OF DIAGNOSIS & TYPICAL FEATURES

▶ Tachypnea, cyanosis, and expiratory grunting.

▶ Poor air movement despite increased work of breathing.

▶ Chest radiograph showing hypoexpansion and air bronchograms.

▶ General Considerations

The most common cause of respiratory distress in the preterm infant is hyaline membrane disease. The incidence increases from 5% of infants born at 35–36 weeks gestation to more than 50% of infants born at 26–28 weeks gestation. This condition is caused by a deficiency of surfactant production as well as surfactant inactivation by protein leak into airspaces. Surfactant decreases surface tension in the alveolus during expiration, allowing the alveolus to remain partly expanded and maintain a functional residual capacity. The absence or inactivation of surfactant results in poor lung compliance and atelectasis. The infant must expend a great deal of effort to expand the lungs with each breath, and respiratory failure ensues. Antenatal administration of corticosteroids to the mother is an important strategy to accelerate lung maturation. Infants whose mothers were given corticosteroids more than 24 hours prior to preterm birth are less likely to have hyaline membrane disease and have a lower mortality rate.

▶ Clinical Findings

Infants with hyaline membrane disease show all the clinical signs of respiratory distress. On auscultation, air movement is diminished despite vigorous respiratory effort. The chest radiograph demonstrates diffuse bilateral atelectasis, causing a ground-glass appearance. Major airways are highlighted by the atelectatic air sacs, creating air bronchograms. In the unintubated child, doming of the diaphragm and hypoinflation occur.

▶ Treatment

Supplemental oxygen, nasal CPAP, early intubation for surfactant administration and ventilation, and placement of umbilical artery and vein lines are the initial interventions required. In stable infants, a trial of nasal CPAP at 5–7 cm H_2O pressure is routinely attempted prior to intubation and surfactant administration. Indications for mechanical ventilation include respiratory acidosis, progressive hypoxia, and apnea. Surfactant replacement can be used both in the delivery room as prophylaxis for infants born before 26 weeks gestation and with established hyaline membrane disease as rescue, preferably within 2–4 hours of birth. Surfactant therapy decreases both the mortality rate in preterm infants and air leak complications of the disease. During the acute course, ventilator settings and oxygen requirements are significantly lower in surfactant-treated infants than in controls. A total of two to three doses given 8–12 hours apart may be necessary. As the disease evolves, proteins that inhibit surfactant function leak into the air spaces, making surfactant replacement less effective.

For patients requiring mechanical ventilation, a ventilator that can deliver breaths synchronized with the infant's respiratory efforts (synchronized intermittent mandatory ventilation) and accurately deliver a preset tidal volume should be used. Alternatively, pressure-limited ventilation with measurement of exhaled tidal volumes can be used. High-frequency ventilators are available for rescue of infants doing poorly on conventional ventilation. Extubation to nasal CPAP should be done as early as possible to minimize lung injury and evolution of chronic lung disease.

5. Chronic Lung Disease in the Premature Infant

▶ General Considerations

Chronic lung disease, defined as respiratory symptoms, oxygen requirement, and chest radiograph abnormalities at 36 weeks postmenstrual age, occurs in about 20% of preterm infants ventilated for surfactant deficiency. The incidence is higher at lower gestational ages and in infants exposed to chorioamnionitis prior to birth. The development of chronic lung disease is a function of lung immaturity at birth, inflammation, and exposure to high oxygen concentrations and ventilator volutrauma. Surfactant replacement therapy or early nasal CPAP has diminished the severity of chronic lung disease. Chronic lung disease results in significant morbidity secondary to reactive airway symptoms and hospital readmissions during the first 2 years of life for intercurrent respiratory infection.

▶ Treatment

Long-term supplemental oxygen, mechanical ventilation, and NIPPV including nasal CPAP are the primary therapies for chronic lung disease of the premature infant. Diuretics, inhaled β_2-adrenergics, inhaled corticosteroids, and systemic corticosteroids are used as adjunctive therapy. The use of systemic corticosteroids remains controversial. Although a decrease in lung inflammation can aid in weaning from ventilator support, there are data associating dexamethasone use in the first week of life with an increased incidence of cerebral palsy. This risk must be balanced against the higher risk of neurodevelopmental handicap in infants with severe chronic lung disease. There is likely a point in the course of these infants at which the benefit of using systemic corticosteroids for the shortest amount of time at the lowest dose possible outweighs the risk of continued mechanical ventilation. After hospital discharge, some infants will require oxygen at home, and some will continue to manifest pulmonary symptomatology into adolescence.

Sweet DG et al: European Consensus Guidelines on the Management of Respiratory Distress Syndrome: 2022 Update. Neonatology 2023;120(1):3–23. doi: 10.1159/000528914. Epub 2023 Feb 15 [PMID: 36863329; PMCID: PMC10064400].

6. Patent Ductus Arteriosus

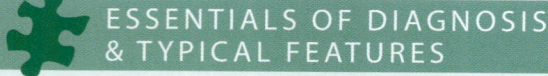

ESSENTIALS OF DIAGNOSIS & TYPICAL FEATURES

► Hyperdynamic precordium.
► Widened pulse pressure.
► Hypotension.
► Presence of a systolic heart murmurs in many cases.

General Considerations

Clinically significant patent ductus arteriosus usually presents on days 3–7 as respiratory distress from hyaline membrane disease is improving. Presentation can be as early as days 1 or 2, especially in infants born before 28 weeks' gestation and in those who have received surfactant-replacement therapy. Signs include a hyperdynamic precordium, increased peripheral pulses, and a widened pulse pressure, with or without a systolic machinery type heart murmur. Early presentations are sometimes manifested by systemic hypotension without a murmur or hyperdynamic circulation. These signs are often accompanied by an increased need for respiratory support and metabolic acidemia. The presence of patent ductus arteriosus is confirmed by echocardiography.

Treatment

Treatment of patent ductus arteriosus is by medical or surgical ligation. Intravenous indomethacin and ibuprofen, either oral or IV, are the most common treatments for a hemodynamically significant PDA. Ibuprofen has a lower risk of side effects such as transient oliguria and necrotizing enterocolitis compared to indomethacin. For infants that remain symptomatic, the ductus may be closed by cardiac catheterization or surgical ligation.

Hamrick SEG et al. Patent Ductus Arteriosus of the Preterm Infant. Pediatrics. 2020 Nov;146(5):e20201209[PMID: 33093140]

7. Necrotizing Enterocolitis

ESSENTIALS OF DIAGNOSIS & TYPICAL FEATURES

► Feeding intolerance with gastric residuals or vomiting.
► Bloody stools.
► Abdominal distention and tenderness.
► Pneumatosis intestinalis on abdominal radiograph.

General Considerations

Necrotizing enterocolitis (NEC) is the most common acquired GI emergency in the newborn. It is most common in preterm infants, with an incidence of 10% in infants less than 1500 g. In full-term infants, it occurs in association with polycythemia, congenital heart disease, and birth asphyxia. The pathogenesis is multifactorial. Ischemia, immaturity, microbial dysbiosis (proliferation of pathogenic bacteria with less colonization with beneficial or commensal bacteria), and genetics are all thought to play a role. In up to 20% of affected infants, the only risk factor is prematurity. IUGR infants with a history of absent or reversed end-diastolic flow in the umbilical artery prior to delivery have abnormalities of splanchnic flow after delivery and an increased risk of NEC. Although there are no proven strategies to prevent NEC, use of trophic feedings, breast milk, and cautious advancement of feeds, as well as probiotic agents, may provide some protection.

Clinical Findings

The most common presenting sign is abdominal distention. Other signs are vomiting, increased gastric residuals, heme positive stools, abdominal tenderness, temperature instability, increased apnea and bradycardia, decreased urine output, and poor perfusion. There may be an increased white blood cell count with an increased band count or, as the disease progresses, absolute neutropenia. Thrombocytopenia often occurs along with stress-induced hyperglycemia and metabolic acidosis. Diagnosis is confirmed by the presence of pneumatosis intestinalis (air in the bowel wall) or biliary tract air on a plain abdominal radiograph. There is a spectrum of disease, and milder cases may exhibit only distention of bowel loops with bowel wall edema.

▶ Treatment

A. Medical Treatment

NEC is managed with bowel rest, NG decompression of the gut, maintenance of oxygenation, mechanical ventilation if necessary, and IV fluids to replace third-space GI losses. Enough fluid should be given to restore good urine output. Other measures include broad-spectrum antibiotics (usually ampicillin, a third-generation cephalosporin or an aminoglycoside, and, possibly, additional anaerobic coverage), close monitoring of vital signs, and serial physical examinations and laboratory studies (blood gases, white blood cell count, platelet count, and radiographs).

B. Surgical Treatment

Surgery is needed in less than 25% of cases. Indications for surgery are evidence of perforation (free air present on a left lateral decubitus or cross-table lateral film), a fixed dilated loop of bowel on serial radiographs, abdominal wall cellulitis, or deterioration despite maximal medical support. All of these are indicative of necrotic bowel. Necrotic bowel is removed and ostomies are created, although occasionally a primary end-to-end anastomosis may be performed. Reanastomosis in infants with ostomies is performed after the disease resolves and the infant is bigger (usually > 2 kg and after 4–6 weeks).

▶ Course & Prognosis

Infants treated medically or surgically should not be refed until the disease is resolved (normal abdominal examination and resolution of pneumatosis), usually after 7–10 days. Nutritional support during this time should be provided by total parenteral nutrition.

Death occurs in 10% of cases. Long-term prognosis among survivors is determined by the amount of intestine lost. Infants with short bowel require long-term support with IV nutrition (see Chapter 21). Late strictures—about 3–6 weeks after initial diagnosis—occur in 8% of patients whether treated medically or surgically and generally require operative management. Infants with surgically managed NEC have an increased risk of poor neurodevelopmental outcome.

Neu J. Prevention of Necrotizing Enterocolitis. Clin Perinatol 2022 Mar;49(1):195–206 [PMID: 35210001].

8. Anemia in the Premature Infant

▶ General Considerations

In the premature infant, the hemoglobin concentration reaches its nadir at about 8–12 weeks and is 2–3 g/dL lower than that of the full-term infant. The lower nadir in premature infants appears to be the result of decreased erythropoietin response to the low red cell mass. Symptoms of anemia include poor feeding, lethargy, increased heart rate, poor weight gain, and, perhaps, periodic breathing.

▶ Treatment

Transfusion is not indicated in an asymptomatic infant simply because of a low hematocrit. Most infants become symptomatic if the hematocrit drops below 20%. Infants on ventilators and supplemental oxygen are usually maintained with hematocrits above 25%–30%. Alternatively, infants can be treated with erythropoietin. Use of erythropoietin may increase the rate and severity of retinopathy of prematurity and should be used judiciously. Delayed cord clamping 1–2 minutes after birth, if possible, can significantly decrease the need for future transfusion.

German KR, Juul SE. Neonatal Anemia. Curr Pediatr Rev 2023; 19(4):388–394 [PMID: 36411551].

9. Intraventricular Hemorrhage

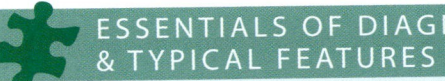

ESSENTIALS OF DIAGNOSIS & TYPICAL FEATURES

- ▶ Large bleeds cause hypotension, metabolic acidosis, and altered neurologic status; smaller bleeds can be asymptomatic.
- ▶ Routine cranial ultrasound scanning is essential for diagnosis in infants born before 32 weeks gestation.

▶ General Considerations

Periventricular and intraventricular hemorrhage occur almost exclusively in premature infants. The incidence is 15%–25% in infants born before 31 weeks gestation and weighing less than 1500 g. The highest incidence occurs in infants of the lowest gestational age (< 26 weeks). Bleeding most commonly occurs in the subependymal germinal matrix (a region of undifferentiated cells adjacent to or lining the lateral ventricles) and can extend into the ventricular cavity. The proposed pathogenesis is presented in Figure 2–2. The critical event is ischemia with reperfusion injury to the capillaries in the germinal matrix in the immediate perinatal period, in the face of immature cerebral pressure autoregulation. This pathogenetic scheme applies also to intraparenchymal bleeding (venous infarction in a region rendered ischemic) and to PVL (ischemic white matter injury in a water-shed region of arterial supply). CNS complications in preterm infants are more frequent in infants exposed to intrauterine and postnatal infection, implying involvement of inflammatory mediators in the pathogenesis of brain injury.

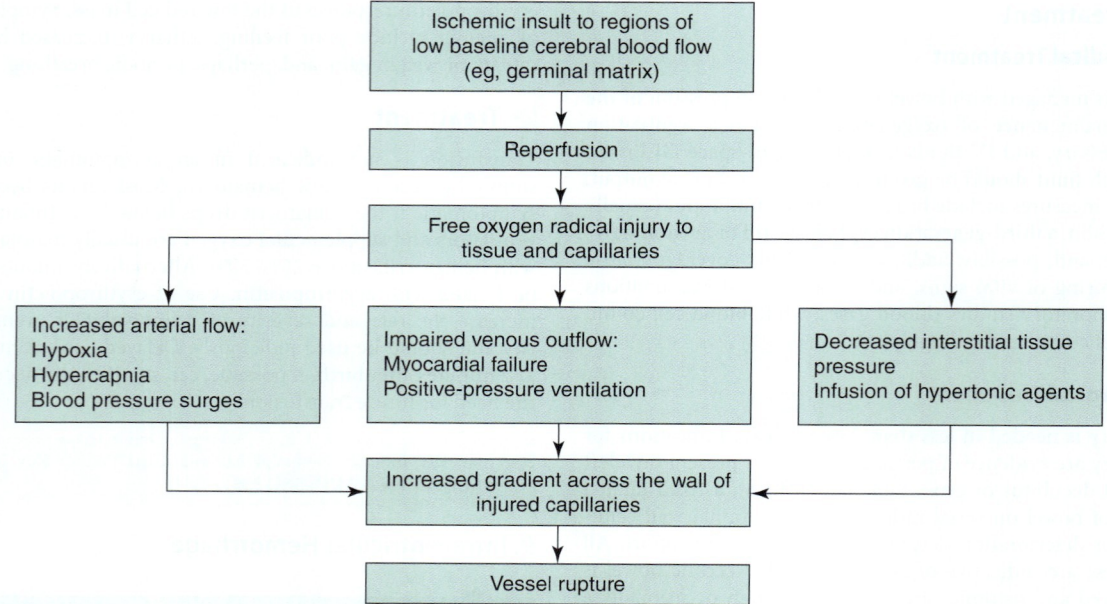

▲ **Figure 2–2.** Pathogenesis of periventricular and intraventricular hemorrhage.

Although the incidence and severity of intracranial bleeding in premature infants have decreased, strategies to prevent this complication are still needed. Maternal antenatal corticosteroids appear to decrease the risk of intracranial bleeding. Magnesium sulfate administered to the mother appears to reduce the rate of cerebral palsy, although not the rate of IVH. The route of delivery may be important, as infants delivered by cesarean section have a decreased rate of intracranial bleeding. Postnatal preventive strategies are less effective. Early indomethacin administration may have some benefit in minimizing bleeding, especially in males, with unclear influence on long-term outcome.

Clinical Findings

Up to 50% of hemorrhages occur before 24 hours of age, and virtually all occur by the fourth day. The clinical syndrome ranges from rapid deterioration (coma, hypoventilation, decerebrate posturing, fixed pupils, bulging anterior fontanelle, hypotension, acidosis, or acute drop in hematocrit), to a more gradual deterioration with more subtle neurologic changes, to absence of any specific physiologic or neurologic signs.

The diagnosis can be confirmed by real-time ultrasound scan. Routine scanning should be done at 10–14 days in all infants born before 29 weeks' gestation. Hemorrhages are graded as follows: grade I, germinal matrix hemorrhage only; grade II, intraventricular bleeding without ventricular enlargement; grade III, intraventricular bleeding with

ventricular enlargement; or grade IV, intraparenchymal bleeding. Follow-up ultrasound examinations are scheduled based on the results of the initial scan. Infants with no bleeding or germinal matrix hemorrhage require only a single follow-up scan at age 4–6 weeks to look for PVL. An infant with blood in the ventricular system is at risk for posthemorrhagic ventriculomegaly. This is usually the result of impaired absorption of cerebrospinal fluid (CSF), but it can also occur secondary to obstructive phenomena. Infants with intraventricular bleeding and ventricular enlargement should be followed every 7–10 days until ventricular enlargement stabilizes or decreases.

Treatment

During acute hemorrhage, supportive treatment should be provided to avoid further cerebral ischemia. Progressive posthemorrhagic hydrocephalus is treated initially with a subgaleal shunt. When the infant is large enough, this can be converted to a ventriculoperitoneal shunt.

Prognosis

No deaths occur as a result of grades I and II hemorrhages. Grades III and IV hemorrhages carry a mortality rate of 10%–20%. Posthemorrhagic ventricular enlargement is rarely seen with grade I hemorrhages but is seen in 54%–87% of grades II–IV hemorrhages. Very few of these infants will require a ventriculoperitoneal shunt. Long-term neurologic sequelae are seen slightly more frequently in infants with grades I and II hemorrhages than in preterm infants without bleeding. In infants with grades III and IV hemorrhages, severe sequelae occur in 20%–25% of cases, mild sequelae in 35% of cases, but no sequelae in 40% of cases. Severe PVL, large parenchymal bleeds, especially if bilateral, and progressive hydrocephalus increase the risk of neurologic sequelae. It is important to note that extremely low-birth-weight infants without major ultrasound findings also remain at increased risk for both cerebral palsy and cognitive delays. Recent reports using quantitative MRI scans demonstrate that subtle gray and white matter findings not seen with ultrasound are prevalent in preterm survivors and are predictive of neurodevelopmental handicap.

Boyd SM, Tapawan SJ, Badawi N, Popat H: Protecting the brain of the micropreemie. Semin Fetal Neonatal Med 2022 Jun; 27(3):101370 [PMID: 35752599].

10. Retinopathy of Prematurity

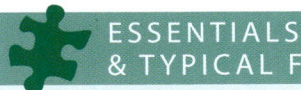

ESSENTIALS OF DIAGNOSIS & TYPICAL FEATURES

► Risk of severe retinopathy is greatest in the most immature infants.

► Diagnosis depends on screening eye examinations in at-risk preterm infants.

► Examination evaluates stage of abnormal retinal vascular development, extent of retinal detachment, and distribution and amount of retina involved.

Retinopathy of prematurity occurs in the incompletely vascularized premature retina. The incidence of retinopathy is highest in infants of the lowest gestational age, with an incidence of 66% in infants weighing less than 1250 g, but only 6% have retinopathy severe enough to warrant intervention. The condition appears to be triggered by an initial injury to the developing retinal vessels. After the initial injury, normal vessel development may follow or abnormal vascularization may occur due to excessive vascular endothelial growth factor (VEGF), with ridge formation on the retina. Lability in oxygen levels with periods of hypoxia/hyperoxia likely potentiates this progression. The frequency of retinopathy progressing to the need for treatment can be diminished by careful monitoring of the infant's oxygen saturation levels. The process can regress or may progress, with growth of fibrovascular tissue into the vitreous associated with inflammation, scarring, and retinal folds or detachment. The disease is graded by stages of abnormal vascular development and retinal detachment (I–V), by the zone of the eye involved (1–3, with zone 1 being the posterior region around the

macula), and by the amount of the retina involved in "clock hours" (eg, a detachment in the upper, outer quadrant of the left eye would be defined as affecting the left retina from 12 to 3 o'clock).

Initial eye examination should be performed at 31 weeks postmenstrual age or at 4 weeks of age, whichever is earlier, in infants born at 30 weeks' gestation or less. Follow-up occurs at 1- to 3-week intervals, depending on the findings, until the retina is fully vascularized. Laser therapy is used in infants with progressive disease at risk for retinal detachment. Although this treatment does not always prevent retinal detachment, it reduces the incidence of poor outcomes based on visual acuity and retinal anatomy. An alternative therapy is intravitreal bevacizumab, an anti-VEGF monoclonal antibody, which may prove superior to laser therapy for severe Zone I and II retinopathy of prematurity.

11. Discharge & Follow-up of the Premature Infant

A. Hospital Discharge

Criteria for discharge of the premature infant include maintaining normal temperature in an open crib, adequate oral intake, acceptable weight gain, and absence of apnea and bradycardia spells requiring intervention. Factors such as support for the mother at home and stability of the family situation play a role in the timing of discharge. Home nursing visits and early physician follow-up can be used to hasten discharge. Additionally, the AAP recommends that preterm infants have a period of observation in an infant car seat, preferably their own, before hospital discharge, with careful positioning to mimic optimal restraint as would occur in the car, to see that they do not have obstructive apnea or desaturation for periods up to 90–120 minutes.

B. Prognosis and Follow-up

With advances in obstetric and maternal care, survival of infants born after 28 weeks gestation or weighing as little as 1000 g at birth is now better than 90%. Survival at gestational age 25 weeks ranges from 75%–85%, at 24 weeks' gestation from 60%–70%, and at 23 weeks from 35%–55%. Antenatal steroid treatment increases survival and decreases major morbidity and can be considered for pregnancies as early as 22 weeks' gestation if parents desire full intervention.

These high rates of survival come with some morbidity. Major neurologic sequelae, including cerebral palsy, cognitive delay, and hydrocephalus, occur in 10%–25% of survivors with birth weight less than 1500 g. Infants with birth weights less than 1000 g also have an increased rate of lesser disabilities, including learning, behavioral, and psychiatric problems. Risk factors for neurologic sequelae include seizures, grade III or IV intracranial hemorrhage, PVL, ventricular dilation, white matter abnormalities on term-equivalent MRI examinations, severe IUGR, poor early head growth, need for mechanical ventilation, chronic lung disease, and NEC.

Maternal fever and chorioamnionitis are associated with an increased risk of cerebral palsy. Other morbidities include chronic lung disease and reactive airway disease, resulting in increased severity of respiratory infections and hospital readmissions in the first 2 years; retinopathy of prematurity with associated loss of visual acuity and strabismus; hearing loss; and growth failure. All these issues require close multidisciplinary outpatient follow-up. Infants with residual lung disease are candidates for monthly palivizumab (Synagis) injections during their first winter after hospital discharge to prevent infection with respiratory syncytial virus. Routine immunizations should be given at the appropriate chronologic age and should not be age-corrected for prematurity.

THE LATE PRETERM INFANT

The rate of preterm births in the United States has increased by more than 30% in the past 30 years, so that preterm infants now comprise 10%–11% of all births. Late preterm births, those from 34 0/7 to 36 6/7 weeks' gestation, have increased the most and now account for over 70% of all preterm births. This is in part due to changes in obstetric practice, with increases in inductions of labor and cesarean sections, as well as a rise in multiple births and increasing demand for cesarean section "at maternal request."

Compared with term infants, late preterm infants have higher prevalence of acute neonatal problems, including respiratory distress, temperature instability, hypoglycemia, kernicterus, apnea, seizures, feeding problems, and rehospitalization after discharge. The respiratory issues are caused by delayed clearance of lung fluid or surfactant deficiency, or both, and can progress to respiratory failure requiring mechanical ventilation, persistent pulmonary hypertension, and even ECMO support. Feeding issues are caused by immature coordination of suck and swallow, which can interfere with bottle feeding and cause failure to establish successful breast-feeding, putting the infant at risk for excessive weight loss and dehydration. These infants are nearly five times as likely as full-term infants to require either supplemental IV fluids or gavage feedings. Related both to feeding issues and immaturity, late preterm infants have at least four times the risk of developing a bilirubin level above 20 mg/dL when compared with infants born after 40 weeks. Rehospitalizations due to jaundice, proven or suspected infection, feeding difficulties, and failure to thrive are much more common than in term infants. Long-term development may also be adversely affected, with some large population-based studies showing a higher incidence of cerebral palsy, developmental delay, and behavioral and emotional disturbances compared with term infants.

Late preterm infants, even if similar in size to their term counterparts, should be considered preterm rather than near term and require closer in-hospital monitoring after birth. Although they may feed reasonably well for the first day or two, they often fail to increase feeding volume and become sleepier and less interested in feeding as they lose weight and become jaundiced. Discharge of these newborns should be delayed until they have demonstrated reliable and appropriately increasing intake and absence of other issues such as hypothermia, hypoglycemia, or apnea. Following nursery discharge, close outpatient follow-up is indicated, generally within 48–72 hours, to ensure continued adequate intake and weight gain.

CARDIAC PROBLEMS IN THE NEWBORN INFANT

STRUCTURAL HEART DISEASE

1. Cyanotic Presentations

ESSENTIALS OF DIAGNOSIS & TYPICAL FEATURES

- ▶ Cyanosis, initially without associated respiratory distress.
- ▶ Failure to increase PaO_2 with supplemental oxygen.
- ▶ Chest radiograph with decreased lung markings suggests right heart obstruction, while increased lung markings suggest transposition or pulmonary venous obstruction.

▶ General Considerations

The causes of cyanotic heart disease in the newborn are transposition of the great vessels, total anomalous pulmonary venous return, truncus arteriosus (some types), tricuspid atresia, and pulmonary atresia or critical pulmonary stenosis. Many are diagnosed antenatally by ultrasound.

▶ Clinical Findings

Infants with these disorders present with early cyanosis. The hallmark of many of these lesions is cyanosis without associated respiratory distress. In most of these infants, tachypnea develops over time either because of increased pulmonary blood flow or secondary to metabolic acidemia from progressive hypoxemia. Diagnostic aids include comparing the blood gas or oxygen saturation in room air to that in 100% FiO_2. Failure of PaO_2 or SaO_2 to increase suggests cyanotic heart disease. **Note:** A PaO_2, if feasible, is the preferred measure. Saturation in the newborn may be misleadingly high despite pathologically low PaO_2 due to the left-shifted oxyhemoglobin dissociation curve seen with fetal hemoglobin. Other useful aids are chest radiography, electrocardiography (ECG), and echocardiography.

Transposition of the great vessels is the most common form of cyanotic heart disease presenting in the newborn. Examination may reveal a systolic murmur and single S_2. Chest radiograph shows cardiomegaly and a narrow mediastinum with normal or increased lung markings. There is little change in PaO_2 or SaO_2 with supplemental oxygen. Total anomalous pulmonary venous return, in which venous return is obstructed, presents early with severe cyanosis and respiratory failure because of severe pulmonary edema. The chest radiograph typically shows a small to normal heart size with marked pulmonary edema. Infants with right-sided heart obstruction (pulmonary and tricuspid atresia, critical pulmonary stenosis, and some forms of truncus arteriosus) have decreased lung markings on chest radiographs and, depending on the severity of hypoxia, may develop metabolic acidemia. Those lesions with an underdeveloped right-sided heart will have left-sided predominance on electrocardiography. Although tetralogy of Fallot is the most common form of cyanotic heart disease, the obstruction at the pulmonary valve is often not severe enough to result in cyanosis in the newborn. In all cases, diagnosis can be confirmed by echocardiography.

2. Acyanotic Presentations

ESSENTIALS OF DIAGNOSIS & TYPICAL FEATURES

► Most newborns with symptomatic acyanotic heart disease have left-sided outflow obstruction.
► Differentially diminished pulses (coarctation) or decreased pulses throughout (aortic atresia).
► Metabolic acidemia.
► Chest radiograph showing large heart and pulmonary edema.

► General Considerations

Newborn infants who present with serious acyanotic heart disease usually have congestive heart failure secondary to left-sided outflow tract obstruction. Infants with left-to-right shunt lesions (eg, ventricular septal defect) may have murmurs in the newborn period, but clinical symptoms do not occur until pulmonary vascular resistance drops enough to cause significant shunting and subsequent congestive heart failure (usually at 3–4 weeks of age).

► Clinical Findings

Infants with left-sided outflow obstruction generally do well in the first days of life until the ductus arteriosus—the source of all or some of the systemic flow—narrows. Tachypnea,

tachycardia, congestive heart failure, and metabolic acidosis develop. On examination, these infants have abnormal pulses. In aortic atresia (hypoplastic left-sided heart syndrome) and stenosis, all peripheral pulses are diminished. In aortic coarctation, differential pulses (diminished or absent in the lower extremities) are evident, and SpO_2 and blood pressure may be lower in the legs than in the right upper extremity. Chest radiographic films in these infants show a large heart and pulmonary edema. Diagnosis is confirmed with echocardiography.

3. Treatment of Cyanotic & Acyanotic Lesions

Early stabilization includes supportive therapy as needed (eg, IV glucose, oxygen, ventilation for respiratory failure, and pressor support). Specific therapy includes infusions of prostaglandin E_1 to maintain ductal patency. In some cyanotic lesions (eg, pulmonary atresia, tricuspid atresia, and critical pulmonary stenosis) in which lung blood flow is ductus-dependent, this improves pulmonary blood flow and PaO_2 by allowing shunting through the ductus to the pulmonary artery. In left-sided outflow tract obstruction, systemic blood flow is ductus-dependent; prostaglandins improve systemic perfusion and acidosis. Further specific management—including palliative surgical and cardiac catheterization procedures—is discussed in Chapter 20. Neurodevelopmental outcome with congenital heart disease depends on the lesion, associated defects and syndromes, severity of neonatal presentation, and complications related to palliative and corrective surgery.

PERSISTENT PULMONARY HYPERTENSION

ESSENTIALS OF DIAGNOSIS & TYPICAL FEATURES

► Onset of symptoms on day 1 of life.
► Hypoxia with poor response to high concentrations of inspired oxygen.
► Right-to-left shunts through the foramen ovale, ductus arteriosus, or both.
► Most often associated with parenchymal lung disease.

► General Considerations

Persistent pulmonary hypertension of the newborn (PPHN) results when the normal decrease in pulmonary vascular resistance after birth does not occur. Most affected infants are full term or postterm, and many have experienced perinatal asphyxia. Other clinical associations include meconium aspiration syndrome, hyaline membrane disease, perinatal depression, neonatal sepsis, chronic intrauterine hypoxia, and pulmonary hypoplasia.

There are three underlying pathophysiologic mechanisms of PPHN: (1) vasoconstriction due to perinatal hypoxia related to an acute event such as sepsis or asphyxia; (2) prenatal increase in pulmonary vascular smooth muscle development; and (3) decreased cross-sectional area of the pulmonary vascular bed associated with lung hypoplasia (eg, diaphragmatic hernia).

▶ Clinical Findings

PPHN is characterized by onset on the first day of life, usually from birth. Respiratory distress is prominent, and Pao_2 is usually poorly responsive to high concentrations of inspired oxygen. Many infants have associated myocardial depression with systemic hypotension. Echocardiography reveals right-to-left shunting at the level of the ductus arteriosus or foramen ovale, or both. The chest radiograph may show lung infiltrates related to associated pulmonary pathology (eg, meconium aspiration or hyaline membrane disease). If the majority of right-to-left shunting is at the ductal level, pre- and postductal differences in Pao_2 and Sao_2 will be observed.

▶ Treatment

Therapy for PPHN involves treatment of associated multiorgan dysfunction. Specific therapy is aimed at both increasing systemic arterial pressure and decreasing pulmonary arterial pressure to reverse the right-to-left shunting through fetal pathways. First-line therapy includes oxygen and ventilation (to reduce pulmonary vascular resistance) and crystalloid infusions (10–30 mL/kg) to improve systemic pressure. With compromised cardiac function, systemic pressors can be used as second-line therapy. Metabolic acidemia should be corrected because acidemia exacerbates pulmonary vasoconstriction. Pulmonary vasodilation can be enhanced using inhaled nitric oxide. High-frequency oscillatory ventilation has proved effective in many of these infants, particularly those with severe associated lung disease, by improving lung expansion and recruitment. In cases in which conventional therapy is failing (poor oxygenation despite maximum support), ECMO is used. The lungs are essentially at rest during ECMO, and with resolution of pulmonary hypertension infants are weaned from ECMO back to ventilator therapy. Approximately 10%–15% of survivors of PPHN have significant neurologic sequelae, with cerebral palsy or cognitive delays. Other sequelae such as chronic lung disease, sensorineural hearing loss, and feeding problems have also been reported.

ARRHYTHMIAS

Irregularly irregular heart rates, commonly associated with premature atrial contractions and less commonly with premature ventricular contractions, are common in the first days of life in well newborns. These arrhythmias are typically benign. Clinically significant bradyarrhythmias are seen in association with congenital heart block. Heart block can be seen in an otherwise structurally normal heart (associated with maternal lupus or other autoimmune conditions) or with structural cardiac abnormalities. In the absence of fetal hydrops, the bradyarrhythmia is often well tolerated. Cardiac pacing may be required if there are symptoms of inadequate cardiac output.

Tachyarrhythmias can be either wide complex (ventricular tachycardia) or narrow complex (supraventricular tachycardia) on ECG. Supraventricular tachycardia is the most common neonatal tachyarrhythmia and may be a sign of structural heart disease, myocarditis, left atrial enlargement, aberrant conduction pathways, or may be an isolated event. Acute treatment is ice to the face to induce a vagal response, and if unsuccessful, IV adenosine. Multiple doses of adenosine may be needed. Long-term prophylactic antiarrhythmic therapy is generally indicated; cardiology consultation is suggested. Cardioversion is rarely needed for supraventricular tachycardia but is needed acutely for hemodynamically unstable ventricular tachycardia.

Singh Y, Lakshminrusimha S: Pathophysiology and management of persistent pulmonary hypertension of the newborn. Clin Perinatol 2021 Aug;48(3):595–618 [PMID: 34353582].

GASTROINTESTINAL & ABDOMINAL SURGICAL CONDITIONS IN THE NEWBORN INFANT

ESOPHAGEAL ATRESIA & TRACHEOESOPHAGEAL FISTULA

ESSENTIALS OF DIAGNOSIS & TYPICAL FEATURES

▶ Polyhydramnios.

▶ Excessive drooling and secretions; choking with attempted feeding.

▶ Unable to pass an orogastric tube to the stomach.

▶ General Considerations

Esophageal atresia is characterized by a blind esophageal pouch with or without a fistulous connection between the proximal or distal esophagus and the trachea (see also Chapter 21). In 85% of infants, the fistula is between the distal esophagus and the airway. Polyhydramnios is common because of high GI obstruction. Incidence is approximately 1 in 3000 births.

Clinical Findings

Infants present in the first hours of life with copious secretions, choking, cyanosis, and respiratory distress. Diagnosis is confirmed with chest radiograph after careful placement of an NG tube to the point at which resistance is met. The tube will be seen radiographically in the blind pouch. If a tracheoesophageal fistula is present to the distal esophagus, gas will be present in the bowel. In esophageal atresia without tracheoesophageal fistula, no gas is seen in the bowel.

Treatment

The NG tube in the proximal pouch should be placed on low intermittent suction to drain secretions and prevent aspiration. The head of the bed should be elevated to prevent reflux of gastric contents through the distal fistula into the lungs. IV glucose and fluids should be provided and oxygen administered as needed. Definitive treatment is surgical, and the technique used depends on the distance between the segments of esophagus. If the distance is short, the fistula can be ligated and the ends of the esophagus anastomosed. If the ends of the esophagus cannot be brought together, the initial surgery is fistula ligation and a feeding gastrostomy tube. Echocardiography should be performed prior to surgery to rule out a right-sided aortic arch (for which a left-sided thoracotomy would be preferred).

Prognosis

Prognosis is determined primarily by the presence or absence of associated anomalies, particularly cardiac, and low birth weight. Mortality is highest when the infant is less than 2000 g and has a serious associated cardiac defect. Vertebral, anal, cardiac, renal, and limb anomalies may be observed (VACTERL association). Evaluation for associated anomalies should be initiated early.

Kunisaki SM, Foker JE: Surgical advances in the fetus and neonate: esophageal atresia. Clin Perinatol 2012;39(2):349361 [PMID: 22682384].

INTESTINAL OBSTRUCTION

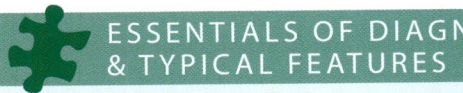

ESSENTIALS OF DIAGNOSIS & TYPICAL FEATURES

- ► Infants with high intestinal obstruction present soon after birth with emesis.
- ► Bilious emesis suggests intestinal malrotation with midgut volvulus until proven otherwise.
- ► Low intestinal obstruction is characterized by abdominal distention and late onset of emesis, often with delayed or absent stooling.

General Considerations

Intestinal obstruction is the most common surgical emergency in neonates. Obstructive lesions are most commonly caused by bowel atresias, which are often caused by an ischemic event during development. Approximately 30% of cases of duodenal atresia are associated with Down syndrome. Meconium ileus is a distal small bowel obstruction caused by viscous meconium produced in utero and may be the presenting symptom of cystic fibrosis. In contrast to meconium ileus, meconium plug syndrome, the most common (1 in 500 live births) cause of lower intestinal obstruction, is a transient functional obstruction of the large bowel. Hirschsprung disease is caused by a failure of neuronal migration to the myenteric plexus of the distal bowel. The distal bowel lacks ganglion cells, causing a lack of peristalsis in that region with a functional obstruction.

Malrotation with midgut volvulus is a surgical emergency that appears in the first days to weeks as bilious vomiting without distention or tenderness. If malrotation is not treated promptly, torsion of the intestine around the superior mesenteric artery can lead to necrosis of the entire small bowel. For this reason, bilious vomiting in the neonate always demands immediate attention and evaluation.

Clinical Findings

A history of polyhydramnios is common, and bile staining of the amniotic fluid can easily be confused with thin meconium staining. The higher the location of the obstruction in the intestine, the earlier the infant will develop vomiting and the less prominent the abdominal distention will be. Lower intestinal obstruction presents with abdominal distention and later onset of emesis. Diagnosis of intestinal obstructions depends on plain abdominal radiographs with either upper GI series (high obstruction suspected) or contrast enema (lower obstruction apparent) to define the area of obstruction. Table 2–12 summarizes the findings expected.

Infants with meconium ileus, an obstruction of the distal ileum from thick inspissated meconium, are presumed to have cystic fibrosis, although infants with pancolonic Hirschsprung disease, colon pseudo-obstruction syndrome, or colonic dysgenesis or atresia may also present with meconium impacted in the distal ileum. Definitive testing for cystic fibrosis by the sweat chloride test or genetic testing should be performed. Intestinal perforation in utero can result in meconium peritonitis with residual intra-abdominal calcifications. Many perforations are completely healed at birth. If the infant has no signs of obstruction or ongoing perforation, no immediate evaluation is needed.

Low intestinal obstruction may present with delayed stooling (> 24 hours in term infants is abnormal) with mild distention. Causes of lower intestinal obstruction include meconium plug syndrome, Hirschsprung's disease and small left colon syndrome. Patients with delayed passage of

Table 2–12. Intestinal obstruction.

Site of Obstruction	Clinical Findings	Plain Radiographs	Contrast Study
Duodenal atresia	Down syndrome (30%–50%); early vomiting, sometimes bilious	"Double bubble" (dilated stomach and proximal duodenum, no air distal)	Not needed
Malrotation and volvulus	Bilious vomiting with onset anytime in the first few weeks	Dilated stomach and proximal duodenum; paucity of air distally (may be normal gas pattern)	UGI shows displaced duodenojejunal junction with "corkscrew" deformity of twisted bowel
Jejunoileal atresia, meconium ileus	Bilious gastric contents > 25 mL at birth; progressive distention and bilious vomiting	Multiple dilated loops of bowel; intra-abdominal calcifications if in utero perforation occurred (meconium peritonitis)	Barium or osmotic contrast enema shows micro-colon; contrast refluxed into distal ileum may demonstrate and relieve meconium obstruction (successful in about 50% of cases)
Meconium plug syndrome; Hirschsprung disease	Distention, delayed stooling (> 24 h)	Diffuse bowel distention	Barium or osmotic contrast enema outlines and relieves plug; may show transition zone in Hirschsprung disease; delayed emptying (> 24 h) suggests Hirschsprung disease

UGI, upper gastrointestinal contrast study.

meconium and radiographic findings of gaseous distention should undergo a contrast enema to diagnose (and treat) meconium plug syndrome. If no plug is found, a rectal biopsy is required to rule out Hirschsprung disease.

Imperforate anus is generally apparent on physical examination, although a rectovaginal fistula with a mildly abnormal appearing anus can occasionally be confused with a normal exam. High imperforate anus in males may be associated with rectourethral or rectovesical fistula, with meconium "pearls" seen along the median raphe of the scrotum and meconium being passed via the urethra.

▶ Treatment

Orogastric suction to decompress the bowel, IV glucose, fluid and electrolyte replacement, and respiratory support as necessary should be instituted. Antibiotics are usually indicated in the setting of bowel distention due to risk of bacterial translocation. The definitive treatment for these conditions (with the exception of meconium plug syndrome, small left colon syndrome, and some cases of meconium ileus) is surgical.

▶ Prognosis

Up to 10% of infants with meconium plug syndrome are subsequently found to have cystic fibrosis or Hirschsprung disease. For this reason, it is appropriate to consider a sweat chloride test and rectal biopsy in all these infants before discharge, especially the infant with meconium plug syndrome who is still symptomatic after contrast enema.

In duodenal atresia associated with Down syndrome, the prognosis depends on associated anomalies (eg, heart defects) and the severity of prestenotic duodenal dilation and

subsequent duodenal dysmotility. Otherwise, these conditions usually carry an excellent prognosis after surgical repair.

Rich BS, Bornstein E, Dolgin SE: Intestinal atresias. Pediatr Rev 2022 May 1;43(5):266–274. doi: 10.1542/pir.2021-005177 [PMID: 35490204].

ABDOMINAL WALL DEFECTS

1. Omphalocele

Omphalocele is a membrane-covered herniation of abdominal contents into the base of the umbilical cord; the incidence is 2 per 10,000 live births. More than 50% of cases have either an abnormal karyotype or an associated syndrome. The sac may contain liver and spleen as well as intestine. Prognosis varies with the size of the lesion, the presence of pulmonary hypoplasia and respiratory insufficiency, and the presence of associated abnormalities.

At delivery, the omphalocele should be covered with a sterile dressing soaked with warm saline to prevent fluid loss. NG decompression is performed, and IV fluids and glucose are given. If the contents of the omphalocele will fit into the abdomen and can be covered with skin, muscle, or both, primary surgical closure is done. If not, staged closure is performed, with placement of a Gore-Tex patch over the exposed contents and gradual coverage of the patch by skin over days to weeks. A large ventral hernia is left, which is repaired in the future.

2. Gastroschisis

In gastroschisis, the uncovered intestine extrudes through a small abdominal wall defect to the right of the umbilical cord. There is no membrane or sac and no liver or spleen outside the abdomen. Gastroschisis is associated with intestinal atresia in approximately 10%–20% of infants and with IUGR. The prevalence of gastroschisis has been increasing worldwide over the past 20 years, from 0.03% to 0.1%. Environmental factors, including use of illicit drugs such as methamphetamine and cocaine and cyclooxygenase inhibitors such as aspirin and ibuprofen during pregnancy, may be involved. Young maternal age is also strongly linked to the occurrence of gastroschisis.

Therapy initially involves placing the bowel or the lower half of the infant into a Silastic bowel bag to decrease fluid and electrolyte losses as well as to conserve heat. IV fluids, antibiotics, and low intermittent gastric suction are required. The infant is placed right side down to preserve bowel perfusion. Subsequent therapy involves replacement of the bowel into the abdominal cavity. This is done as a single primary procedure if the amount of bowel to be replaced is small. If the amount of bowel is large or if the bowel is significantly dilated, staged closure with placement of a Silastic silo and gradual reduction of the bowel into the underdeveloped abdominal cavity over several days is preferred. Perioperatively, third-space fluid losses may be extensive; fluid and electrolyte therapy must be monitored carefully. Bowel motility may be slow to return if the bowel was dilated, thickened, matted together, and covered with a fibrinous "peel" at delivery. Prolonged intravenous nutrition is often required, but long-term outcome is very good.

Lakshminarayanan B, Lakhoo K: Abdominal wall defects. Early Hum Dev 2014;90(12):917–920 [PMID: 25448781].

DIAPHRAGMATIC HERNIA

ESSENTIALS OF DIAGNOSIS & TYPICAL FEATURES

▶ Respiratory distress from birth.

▶ Poor breath sounds; flat or scaphoid abdomen.

▶ Bowel loops seen in the chest with mediastinal shift to opposite side on chest radiograph.

This congenital malformation consists of herniation of abdominal organs into the hemithorax (usually left-sided) through a posterolateral defect in the diaphragm. The incidence overall is 1 in 2500 births. It is usually diagnosed antenatally by ultrasound, and if so, delivery should occur at a perinatal center. If undiagnosed antenatally, it should be suspected in any infant with severe respiratory distress, poor breath sounds, and a scaphoid abdomen. The rapidity and severity of presentation depend on several factors: the degree of pulmonary hypoplasia

resulting from lung compression by the intrathoracic abdominal contents in utero; degree of associated pulmonary hypertension; and associated anomalies, especially chromosomal abnormalities and congenital cardiac defects. Affected infants are prone to development of pneumothorax during attempts at ventilation of the hypoplastic lungs.

Treatment includes intubation, mechanical ventilation, and decompression of the GI tract with an orogastric tube. An IV infusion of glucose and fluid should be started. Chest radiograph confirms the diagnosis. Surgery to reduce the abdominal contents from the thorax and close the diaphragmatic defect is delayed until after the infant is stabilized and pulmonary hypertension and lung compliance have improved, usually after 24–48 hours. Both pre- and postoperatively, pulmonary hypertension may require therapy with high-frequency oscillatory ventilation, inhaled nitric oxide, pressors, or ECMO. Survival depends on the severity of the defect and resulting pulmonary hypoplasia, ranging from 20% for the most severe case to greater than 70% for patients with mild defects. Many of these infants have ongoing problems with pulmonary hypertension and severe gastroesophageal reflux and are at risk for neurodevelopmental problems, behavior problems, hearing loss, and poor growth.

GASTROINTESTINAL BLEEDING

▶ Upper Gastrointestinal Bleeding

Upper GI bleeding sometimes occurs in the newborn nursery but is rarely severe. Old blood ("coffee-grounds" material) in the stomach of the newborn may be either swallowed maternal blood or infant blood from gastritis or stress ulcer. Bright red blood from the stomach is most likely from acute bleeding due to gastritis or iatrogenic from trauma related to an NG tube. Treatment generally consists of gastric lavage to obtain a sample for Apt testing or blood typing to determine if it is mother's or baby's blood and antacid medication. If the volume of bleeding is large, intensive monitoring, fluid and blood replacement, and endoscopy are indicated. Coagulation studies should also be sent, and vitamin K administration confirmed or repeated.

▶ Lower Gastrointestinal Bleeding

Rectal bleeding in the newborn is less common than upper GI bleeding and is associated with infections, milk protein intolerance, or, in ill infants, NEC. An abdominal radiograph should be obtained to rule out pneumatosis intestinalis or other abnormalities in gas pattern suggesting inflammation, infection, or obstruction. If the radiograph is negative, the examination is benign, and infection is considered unlikely, a protein hydrolysate or elemental formula should be tried. The nursing mother should be instructed to avoid all cow milk protein products in her diet. If the amount of rectal bleeding is large or persistent, endoscopy may be needed.

Boyle JT: Gastrointestinal bleeding in infants and children. Pediatr Rev 2008;29:39 [PMID: 18245300].

GASTROESOPHAGEAL REFLUX

Physiologic regurgitation is common in infants. Reflux is pathologic and should be treated when it results in failure to thrive owing to excessive regurgitation, poor intake due to dysphagia, or chronic respiratory symptoms of wheezing and recurrent pneumonias suggestive of aspiration. Diagnosis is clinical, with confirmation by pH probe or impedance study. Barium radiography is helpful to rule out anatomic abnormalities causing delayed gastric emptying but is not diagnostic of pathologic reflux.

Most antireflux therapies have not been studied systematically in infants, especially in premature infants, and there is little correlation between clinical symptoms and documented gastroesophageal reflux events when studied. Treatment modalities have included thickened feeds for those with frequent regurgitation and poor weight gain and positioning in a prone or left-side-down position for 1 hour after a feeding, although this may increase risk for SIDS. Gastric acid suppressants such as ranitidine or lansoprazole can also be used, especially if there is associated irritability; however, these may be associated with an increased incidence of NEC and invasive infections in the young and/or premature infant. Prokinetic agents such as erythromycin or metoclopramide are of little benefit and have significant side effects. Because most infants improve by 12–15 months of age, surgery is reserved for the most severe cases.

Chabra S, Peeples ES: Assessment and management of gastroesophageal reflux in the newborn. Pediatr Ann 2020 Feb 1;49(2): e77–e81 [PMID: 32045486].

INFECTIONS IN THE NEWBORN INFANT

There are three major routes of perinatal infection: (1) blood-borne transplacental infection of the fetus (eg, cytomegalovirus [CMV], rubella, and syphilis); (2) ascending infection with disruption of the barrier provided by the amniotic membranes (eg, bacterial infections after 12–18 hours of ruptured membranes); and (3) infection on passage through an infected birth canal or exposure to infected blood at delivery (eg, herpes simplex, hepatitis B, HIV, and bacterial infections). Some perinatal pathogens may infect via more than one of these routes.

Susceptibility of the newborn infant to infection is related to immaturity of the immune system at birth. This feature applies particularly to the preterm neonate. Passive protection against some organisms is provided by transfer of IgG across the placenta, particularly during the third trimester of pregnancy. Preterm infants, especially those born before 30 weeks' gestation, do not receive the full amount of passively acquired antibody.

BACTERIAL INFECTIONS

1. Bacterial Sepsis

ESSENTIALS OF DIAGNOSIS & TYPICAL FEATURES

► Most infants with early-onset sepsis present at < 24 hours of age.

► Respiratory distress is the most common presenting symptom.

► Hypotension, acidemia, and neutropenia are associated clinical findings.

► The presentation of late-onset sepsis is more subtle.

► General Considerations

The incidence of early-onset (< 3 days) neonatal bacterial infection is 1–2 in 1000 live births. If rupture of the membranes occurs more than 24 hours prior to delivery, the infection rate increases to 1 in 100 live births. If early rupture of membranes with chorioamnionitis occurs, the infection rate increases further to 1 in 10 live births. Regardless of membrane rupture, infection rates are five times higher in preterm than in full-term infants.

► Clinical Findings

Early-onset bacterial infections appear most commonly on day 1 of life, the majority by 12 hours of age. Respiratory distress due to pneumonia is the most common presenting sign. Other features include unexplained low Apgar scores without fetal distress, poor perfusion, and hypotension. Late-onset bacterial infection (> 3 days of age) presents in a more subtle manner, with poor feeding, lethargy, hypotonia, temperature instability, altered perfusion, new or increased oxygen requirement, and apnea. Late-onset bacterial sepsis is more often associated with meningitis or other localized infections.

Low total white count, absolute neutropenia (< 1000/mL), and elevated ratio of immature to mature neutrophils all suggest neonatal bacterial infection. Thrombocytopenia is another common feature. Other laboratory findings are hypoglycemia or hyperglycemia, unexplained metabolic acidosis, and elevated C-reactive protein and procalcitonin. Definitive diagnosis is made by positive cultures from blood, CSF, or other body fluids.

Early-onset infection is most often caused by group B β-hemolytic streptococci (GBS) and gram-negative enteric pathogens (eg, *E coli*). Other organisms to consider are nontypeable *Haemophilus influenzae*, enterococcus, *Staphylococcus aureus*, other streptococci, and *Listeria monocytogenes*. Late-onset sepsis is caused by coagulase-negative staphylococci (most common in infants with indwelling central venous lines), *S aureus*, GBS, *Enterococcus*, and gram-negative organisms, in addition to *Candida* species (see section Fungal Sepsis).

► **Treatment**

A high index of suspicion is important in diagnosis and treatment of neonatal infection. Infants with risk factors (rupture of membranes > 18 hours, maternal chorioamnionitis, prematurity) need to be carefully observed for signs of infection. Evaluation with a CBC and differential and blood and CSF cultures are indicated in infants with clinical signs of early sepsis. Initial broad-spectrum antibiotic coverage for early onset sepsis should include ampicillin plus a third-generation cephalosporin or an aminoglycoside. Treatment for late onset sepsis in hospitalized neonates should generally be expanded to include staphylococcal coverage. The duration of treatment for proven sepsis is 10–14 days of IV antibiotics. In sick infants, the essentials of good supportive therapy should be provided: IV glucose and nutritional support, volume expansion and pressors as needed, and oxygen and ventilator support.

► **Prevention**

Prevention of early-onset neonatal GBS infection has been achieved with intrapartum administration of penicillin given 4 or more hours prior to delivery, with overall rates of infection now at 0.3–0.4 cases per 1000 live births. Current clinical guidelines are to perform a vaginal and rectal GBS culture at 36–37 weeks' gestation in all pregnant women. Prophylaxis with penicillin or ampicillin is given during labor to GBS-positive women, those who had GBS bacteriuria during the current pregnancy, those who had a previous infant with invasive GBS disease, and those who have unknown GBS status at delivery in the presence of any of the following risk factors for infection: preterm labor and/or premature rupture of membranes prior to 37 weeks gestation, maternal intrapartum temperature equal to or greater than 38.0°C. or amniotic membrane rupture equal to or greater than 18 hours. Secondary prevention of early-onset GBS infections in newborns involves laboratory evaluation and empiric antibiotics for patients at increased risk for GBS infection based on risk factors, whether or not their mothers received adequate antibiotic prophylaxis prior to delivery. Clinical guidelines for intrapartum antibiotic prophylaxis and empiric treatment of the newborn are available from the CDC (https://www.cdc.gov/groupbstrep/guidelines/index.html).

2. Meningitis

Any newborn with bacterial sepsis is at risk for meningitis. The workup for any newborn with possible signs of CNS infection should include a lumbar puncture because blood cultures can be negative in neonates with meningitis. The presence of seizures should increase the suspicion for meningitis. Diagnosis is suggested by a CSF protein level higher than 150 mg/dL, glucose less than 30 mg/dL, leukocytes of more than 20/μL, and a positive Gram stain. The diagnosis is confirmed by culture. The most common organisms are GBS and gram-negative enteric bacteria. Although sepsis can be treated with antibiotics for 10–14 days, meningitis requires 14–21 days. Gram-negative infections, in particular, are difficult to eradicate, and may relapse. The mortality rate of neonatal meningitis is approximately 10%, with significant neurologic morbidity present in one-third of the survivors.

3. Pneumonia

The respiratory system can be infected in utero, on passage through the birth canal, or postnatally. Early-onset neonatal infection is usually associated with pneumonia. Pneumonia should also be suspected in older neonates with a recent onset of tachypnea, retractions, and cyanosis. In infants already receiving respiratory support, an increase in the requirement for oxygen or ventilator support, perhaps with a change in the character of tracheal secretions, may indicate pneumonia. Not only common bacteria but also viruses (CMV, respiratory syncytial virus, adenovirus, influenza, herpes simplex, parainfluenza) and *Chlamydia trachomatis* can cause pneumonia. In infants with preexisting respiratory disease, intercurrent pulmonary infections contribute to the development of chronic lung disease.

4. Urinary Tract Infection

Infection of the urine is uncommon in the first days of life. Urinary tract infection in the newborn can occur in association with genitourinary anomalies and is usually caused by gram-negative enteric pathogens or enterococci. Urine should always be evaluated as part of the workup for later-onset infection. Culture should be obtained either by suprapubic aspiration or bladder catheterization. Antibiotic IV therapy is continued for 3–5 days if the blood culture is negative and clinical signs resolve quickly, and then completed with oral medications. Evaluation for genitourinary anomalies with an ultrasound examination and a voiding cystourethrogram should be done in most neonates with urinary tract infections.

5. Omphalitis

A normal umbilical cord stump atrophies and separates at the skin level. A small amount of purulent material at the base of the cord is common and can be minimized by keeping the cord open to air and dry. The cord can become colonized with streptococci, staphylococci, or gram-negative organisms that can cause local infection. Omphalitis is diagnosed when redness and edema develop in the soft tissues around the stump. Local and systemic cultures should be obtained. Treatment is with broad-spectrum IV antibiotics, usually nafcillin or vancomycin, a third-generation cephalosporin, and anaerobic coverage with metronidazole as the infection may be polymicrobial. Complications are determined by the degree of infection of the cord vessels and include septic thrombophlebitis, hepatic abscess, necrotizing fasciitis, and portal vein thrombosis. Surgical consultation should be obtained because of the potential for necrotizing fasciitis.

6. Conjunctivitis

Neisseria gonorrhoeae may colonize an infant during passage through an infected birth canal. Gonococcal ophthalmitis presents at 3–7 days with copious purulent conjunctivitis. The diagnosis can be suspected when gram-negative intracellular diplococci are seen on a Gram-stained smear and confirmed by culture. Treatment for non-disseminated disease is with IV or IM ceftriaxone, given once. For disseminated disease (sepsis, arthritis, or meningitis), cefotaxime or ceftriaxone for 7–14 days is preferred. Prophylaxis at birth is with 0.5% erythromycin ointment. Infants born to mothers with known gonococcal disease should also receive a single dose of ceftriaxone.

Chlamydia trachomatis is another important cause of conjunctivitis, appearing at 5 days to several weeks of age with conjunctival congestion, edema, and minimal discharge. The organism is acquired at birth after passage through an infected birth canal. Acquisition occurs in 50% of infants born to infected women, with a 25%–50% risk of conjunctivitis. Prevalence in pregnancy is over 10% in some populations. Diagnosis is by isolation of the organism or by rapid antigen detection tests. Treatment is with oral erythromycin for 14 days or oral azithromycin for 3 days.

Dhudasia MB, Flannery DD, Pfeifer MR, Puopolo KM: Updated guidance: prevention and management of perinatal group B *Streptococcus* infection. Neoreviews 2021 Mar;22(3):e177–e188 [PMID: 33649090].

FUNGAL SEPSIS

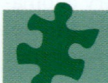

ESSENTIALS OF DIAGNOSIS & TYPICAL FEATURES

▶ Risk factors include low birth weight, indwelling central lines, and multiple antibiotic exposures.

▶ Colonization with *Candida* species is common; systemic infection occurs in 5%–7% of infants.

▶ Presents with often subtle clinical deterioration, thrombocytopenia, and hyperglycemia.

With the survival of smaller, sicker infants, infection with *Candida* species has become more common. Infants of extremely low birth weight with central lines who have had repeated exposures to broad-spectrum antibiotics are at highest risk. Infection is more common in the smallest and least mature infants; up to 20% in infants 24 weeks gestation, and 7% overall in those less than 1000 g.

Clinical features of fungal sepsis can be indistinguishable from those of late-onset bacterial sepsis. Thrombocytopenia or hyperglycemia may be the earliest and only indications. Deep organ involvement (eg, renal, eye, or endocarditis) is commonly associated with systemic candidiasis. Treatment is with intravenous fluconazole or deoxycholate amphotericin B. Prophylaxis with fluconazole can be used for those infants at highest risk, eg, those with central venous lines and receiving parenteral nutrition in units with high candidiasis rates. Prophylaxis with fluconazole diminishes intestinal colonization with yeast and decreases the frequency of systemic disease, with an overall reduction in invasive *Candida* disease of 83%, from 9% to 1.6%, without significant adverse effects or resistance to fluconazole. Nystatin prophylaxis may also be effective but has been less rigorously tested.

CONGENITAL INFECTIONS

ESSENTIALS OF DIAGNOSIS & TYPICAL FEATURES

▶ Can be acquired in utero, perinatally, and postnatally.

▶ Can be asymptomatic in the newborn period.

▶ Clinical symptom complexes include IUGR, chorioretinitis, cataracts, cholestatic jaundice, thrombocytopenia, skin rash, and brain calcifications.

▶ Diagnosis can be confirmed using polymerase chain reaction (PCR) testing, antigen and antibody studies, and culture.

1. Cytomegalovirus Infection

Cytomegalovirus (CMV) is the most common virus transmitted in utero, affecting approximately 1% of all newborns (see also Chapter 40). Symptomatic disease in the newborn period occurs in 10% of these congenitally infected infants, with a spectrum of findings including hepatosplenomegaly, petechiae and "blueberry muffin" spots, growth restriction, microcephaly, direct hyperbilirubinemia, thrombocytopenia, intracranial calcifications, and chorioretinitis. More than half of these infants will develop long-term sequelae, including sensorineural deafness in 30% or more. Sensorineural hearing loss also occurs in 10%–15% of infants with asymptomatic infection. Transmission of CMV can occur during either primary or reactivated maternal infection; the risk of symptomatic neonatal disease is highest when the mother acquires infection in the first half of pregnancy. Diagnosis in the neonate should be confirmed by culture or polymerase chain reaction (PCR) testing of urine or saliva. Oral valganciclovir therapy for 6 months is recommended for neonates with moderate-severe symptomatic congenital infection, particularly infections affecting the CNS, to prevent progression of hearing loss and, possibly, improve neurodevelopmental outcome. Infection can also be acquired during delivery and postnatally through blood transfusion or ingestion of CMV-infected breast milk. These infections generally cause no symptoms or sequelae, although hepatitis, pneumonia, hematologic abnormalities, and sepsis presentations may occur in compromised seronegative premature infants.

2. Rubella

Congenital rubella infection occurs as a result of maternal rubella infection during pregnancy (see also Chapter 40). The risk of fetal infection and congenital defects is as high as 80%–85% in mothers infected during the first trimester, but after 12 weeks gestation the risk of congenital malformation decreases markedly. Features of congenital rubella syndrome include microcephaly and encephalitis; cardiac defects; cataracts, retinopathy, and microphthalmia; growth restriction, hepatosplenomegaly, thrombocytopenia, and purpura; and deafness. Affected infants can be asymptomatic at birth but develop clinical sequelae during the first year of life as the viral infection is persistent due to an inadequate immune response. The diagnosis should be suspected in cases of a characteristic clinical illness in the mother (rash, adenopathy, and arthritis) confirmed by a detection of serum rubella-specific IgM or stable/increasing rubella-specific IgG in the infant or by positive culture or PCR of pharyngeal or nasal secretions in the infant. Congenital rubella is now rare in industrialized countries because of widespread immunization but still occurs due to the presence of unimmunized individuals and widespread travel.

3. Varicella

Congenital varicella syndrome is rare (1%–2% after maternal varicella infection acquired during the first 20 weeks of pregnancy) and may include limb hypoplasia, cutaneous scars, microcephaly, cortical atrophy, chorioretinitis, and cataracts. Perinatal exposure (5 days before to 2 days after delivery) can cause severe to fatal disseminated varicella in the infant. If maternal varicella infection develops within this perinatal risk period, the newborn should receive varicella-zoster immune globulin (or IVIG if varicella-zoster immune globulin is unavailable). If this has not been done, subsequent illness can be treated with IV acyclovir.

Hospitalized premature infants of at least 28 weeks gestation whose mothers have no history of chickenpox—and all infants younger than 28 weeks gestational age regardless of maternal history—should receive varicella immune globulin following any postnatal exposure.

4. Toxoplasmosis

Toxoplasmosis is caused by the protozoan *Toxoplasma gondii* (see also Chapter 43). Maternal infection occurs in 0.1%–0.5% of pregnancies and is usually asymptomatic. It is estimated that between 1 in 1000 and 1 in 10,000 infants are infected via *in utero* transmission. Maternal infection occurs due to exposure to cat feces and ingestion of raw or undercooked meat. Fetal injury is most likely to occur when maternal infection occurs in the first trimester.

Seventy–ninety percent of congenital infected newborns are initially asymptomatic but are at risk of subsequent developmental delay, visual impairment, and learning disabilities within months to years. Among newborns with clinical illness, findings may include growth restriction, chorioretinitis, seizures, jaundice, hydrocephalus, microcephaly, intracranial calcifications, hepatosplenomegaly, adenopathy, cataracts, maculopapular rash, thrombocytopenia, and pneumonia. Serologic diagnosis is based on a positive toxoplasma-specific IgA, IgE, or IgM in the first 6 months of life, a rise in serial IgG levels compared to the mother's, or persistent IgG positivity beyond 12 months. Infants with suspected infection should have eye and auditory examinations and a computed tomographic (CT) scan of the brain. Organism isolation from placenta or cord blood and PCR tests on amniotic fluid or CSF are also available for diagnosis. Spiramycin treatment of primary maternal infection is used to try to reduce transmission to the fetus. Neonatal treatment using pyrimethamine and sulfadiazine with folinic acid can improve long-term outcome.

5. Parvovirus B19 Infection

Parvovirus B19 is a small, nonenveloped, single-stranded DNA virus that causes erythema infectiosum (fifth disease) in children. Transmission to the mother is primarily by respiratory secretions. The virus replicates initially in erythroid progenitor cells and induces cell-cycle arrest, resulting in severe fetal anemia, myocarditis, and nonimmune hydrops; fetal death occurs in approximately 3%–6%. Resolution of the hydrops may occur in utero, either spontaneously or after fetal transfusion. Mothers who have been exposed may have specific serologic testing and serial ultrasound, Doppler examinations, and percutaneous umbilical cord blood sampling to assess for anemia. If the fetus survives, the long-term outcome is good with no late effects from the infection.

6. Congenital Syphilis

Rates of transplacental fetal infection with *Treponema pallidum* are 60%–100% in the setting of maternal primary or secondary syphilis, ~40% in early latent maternal infection, and less than 8% in late latent maternal infection (see also Chapter 42). Transmission to the fetus increases with increasing gestational age at time of maternal infection and is rare before 18 weeks' gestation. Fetal infection can result in stillbirth or prematurity. Findings of early congenital syphilis (presentation before age 2 years) include mucocutaneous lesions, lymphadenopathy, hepatosplenomegaly, bony changes, and hydrops, although newborn infants are often asymptomatic. Late manifestations (after 2 years of age) in untreated infants involve the CNS, bones and joints, teeth, eyes, and skin. An infant should be evaluated for congenital syphilis if he or she has proven or probable congenital syphilis, defined as a suggestive examination, serum quantitative nontreponemal titer more than fourfold the mother's, positive darkfield or fluorescent antibody test of body fluids, or birth to a mother with positive nontreponemal and treponemal tests but without documented adequate treatment (parenteral penicillin G), including the expected fourfold decrease in nontreponemal antibody titer. Infants of mothers treated less than 1 month before delivery also require evaluation. Evaluation should include physical examination, a quantitative nontreponemal serologic test for syphilis, CBC, CSF examination (cell count, protein, and Venereal Disease Research Laboratory test), and long bone radiographs. Treatment in most cases is aqueous penicillin G (50,000 U/kg every 8–12 hours) or procaine penicillin G (50,000 U/kg IM daily) for 10 days.

7. Congenital Zika Infection

The Zika virus is a mosquito-borne virus that generally causes a mild and self-limited infection. Congenital Zika syndrome is a constellation of congenital anomalies including microcephaly, intracranial calcifications or other brain abnormalities or ocular anomalies associated with maternal Zika infection during pregnancy. The risk of complications to the fetus in women with confirmed Zika infection during pregnancy is 5%–10%. Zika testing is recommended in infants born to mothers with laboratory evidence of Zika infection during pregnancy and infants who have clinical features of congenital Zika infection with maternal history of possible exposure to Zika (travel to areas with high prevalence of infection). Both molecular (blood PCR) and immunologic (IgM) testing should be done directly on infant blood (not cord blood) within the first few days of birth; PCR testing of urine and PCR and IgM testing of CSF are also recommended. There is no treatment for congenital Zika infection.

Moodley A, Payton KSE: The term newborn: congenital infections. Clin Perinatol 2021 Aug;48(3):485–511 [PMID: 34353577].

PERINATALLY ACQUIRED INFECTIONS

1. Herpes Simplex

Herpes simplex virus infection is usually acquired at birth during transit through an infected birth canal (see also Chapter 40). The mother may have either primary or reactivated secondary infection. Primary maternal infection, because of the high titer of organisms and the absence of antibodies, poses the greatest risk to the infant. The risk of neonatal infection with vaginal delivery in this setting is 25%–60%. Seventy-five percent of mothers with primary herpes at the time of delivery are asymptomatic. The risk to an infant born to a mother with recurrent herpes simplex is much lower (< 2%). Time of presentation of localized (skin, eye, or mouth) or disseminated disease (pneumonia, shock, or hepatitis) in the infant is usually 5–14 days of age. CNS disease presents later, at 14–28 days, with lethargy, fever, and seizures. In about 45% of patients, localized skin, eye, and mouth disease is the first indication of infection. Another 30% present with CNS disease, whereas the remaining 25% have disseminated or multiorgan disease that may be indistinguishable from bacterial sepsis. Herpes infection should be considered in neonates with sepsis syndrome, negative bacterial culture results, and liver dysfunction or coagulopathy. Herpes simplex virus also should be considered as a causative agent in neonates with fever, irritability, and abnormal CSF findings, especially in the presence of seizures. PCR testing of vesicles, nasopharynx, conjunctivae, anus/rectum, blood, and CSF is performed for diagnosis (culture of mucosal sites and vesicular lesions can be performed, if available); testing may be falsely negative in the CSF early in the course.

Acyclovir is the drug of choice for neonatal herpes infection. Localized disease is treated for 14 days, and a 21-day course is used for disseminated or CNS disease. Prompt initiation of therapy improves survival of neonates with CNS and disseminated disease and prevents the spread of localized disease. Infants born to mothers with a history of herpes simplex virus infection, but no active lesions, can be observed closely after birth, and do not need to be isolated. Recommendations for laboratory evaluation and treatment of infants born to mothers with active lesions are complex and depend on maternal history of infection and specific maternal serologic testing and neonatal virologic testing. Detailed clinical guidelines are available in the AAP *Red Book/Report of the Committee on Infectious Diseases*.

The prognosis is good for localized skin and mucosal disease that does not progress, although skin recurrences are common. The mortality rate for disseminated herpes is high (approximately 30%), with significant morbidity among survivors of both disseminated and CNS infections despite treatment. Infants with neonatal herpes simplex virus infections (skin/mucosal disease, disseminated, or CNS) should receive long-term oral acyclovir for 6 months after completion of intravenous treatment to prevent recurrences.

2. Hepatitis B & C

Infants become infected with hepatitis B at the time of birth; intrauterine transmission is rare. Clinical illness is rare in the neonatal period, but infants born to positive mothers are at risk of becoming chronic HBsAg carriers and developing chronic active hepatitis and hepatocellular carcinoma. The presence of HBsAg should be determined in all pregnant women. If the result is positive, the infant should receive HBIG and hepatitis B vaccine as soon as possible after (and within 12 hours of) birth, followed by two subsequent vaccine doses at 1 and 6 months of age. If HBsAg has not been tested prior to birth, the test should be run after delivery and hepatitis B vaccine given within 12 hours after birth. If the mother is subsequently found to be positive, HBIG should be given as soon as possible (preferably within 48 hours, but not later than 1 week after birth). Subsequent vaccine doses should be given at 1 and 6 months of age. In premature infants born to HBsAg-positive mothers, vaccine and HBIG should be given within 12 hours of birth, but a subsequent three-dose hepatitis B vaccine series should be given beginning at 1 month of age.

Perinatal transmission of hepatitis C occurs in about 5% of infants born to mothers who carry the virus; maternal coinfection with HIV increases the risk of transmission. Up to 12–18 months of age, PCR can be used to detect perinatal transmission. After 18 months, presence of hepatitis C antibodies in the infant strongly suggests that infection has occurred.

3. Enterovirus Infection

Enterovirus infections occur most frequently in the late summer and early fall, and neonatal infection is generally acquired in the perinatal period. There is often a history of maternal fever, abdominal pain, diarrhea, and/or rash in the week prior to delivery. Illness appears in the newborn in the first 2 weeks of life and is most commonly characterized by fever, lethargy, irritability, diarrhea, and/or rash. More severe forms occasionally occur, especially if infection occurs before 1 week of age, including meningoencephalitis, myocarditis, hepatitis, pneumonia, shock, and disseminated intravascular coagulation. Diagnosis is best confirmed by PCR of throat, rectum, blood, and/or CSF. Treatment consists primarily of supportive care. The prognosis is good in most cases, except those with severe hepatitis, myocarditis, or disseminated disease, which carry high mortality rates.

4. HIV Infection

HIV can be acquired in utero or at the time of delivery, or it can be transmitted postpartum via breast milk (see also Chapter 41). Testing for HIV should be performed in all pregnant women. Without treatment, transmission of virus occurs in 13%–39% of births to infected mothers, mostly at the time of delivery. The combination of maternal zidovudine treatment during pregnancy and of the infant for the first 6 weeks of life, elective cesarean delivery in cases of elevated maternal viral loads, and avoidance of breast-feeding can lower transmission to 1%–2%. With maternal virologic suppression using combination antiretroviral therapy, transmission rates of less than 1%–2% are achieved. In cases of unknown HIV status at presentation in labor, rapid HIV testing should be performed, and, if positive, intrapartum maternal treatment and postpartum neonatal treatment should be offered. The risk of transmission is increased in mothers with advanced disease, high viral loads, low CD4 counts, and intrapartum events such as chorioamnionitis and prolonged membrane rupture that increase exposure of the fetus to maternal blood. Newborns who are HIV infected are usually asymptomatic. Perinatally exposed infants require serial testing to determine their infection status (Chapter 41).

American Academy of Pediatrics: In: Kimberlin DW et al (eds): *Red Book: 2021 Report of the Committee on Infectious Diseases.* 32nd ed. American Academy of Pediatrics; 2021.

HEMATOLOGIC DISORDERS IN THE NEWBORN INFANT

BLEEDING DISORDERS

Bleeding in the newborn infant may result from inherited clotting deficiencies (eg, factor VIII deficiency) or acquired disorders—hemorrhagic disease of the newborn (vitamin K deficiency), disseminated intravascular coagulation, liver failure, and isolated thrombocytopenia.

1. Vitamin K Deficiency Bleeding of the Newborn

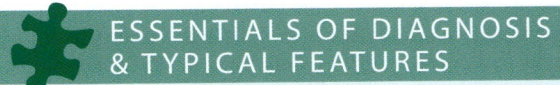

ESSENTIALS OF DIAGNOSIS & TYPICAL FEATURES

- ▶ Frequently exclusively breast fed, otherwise clinically well infant.
- ▶ Bleeding from mucous membranes, GI tract, skin, or internal (intracranial).
- ▶ Prolonged prothrombin time (PT), relatively normal partial thromboplastin time (PTT), normal fibrinogen, and platelet count.

Bleeding is caused by the deficiency of the vitamin K–dependent clotting factors (II, VII, IX, and X). Bleeding occurs in 0.25%–1.7% of newborns who do not receive vitamin K prophylaxis after birth, generally in the first 5 days to 2 weeks in an otherwise well infant. There is an increased risk in exclusively breastfed infants and infants of mothers receiving therapy with anticonvulsants that interfere with vitamin K metabolism. Early vitamin K deficiency bleeding (0–2 weeks) can be prevented by either parenteral or oral vitamin K administration, whereas late disease (onset 2 weeks to 6 months) is most effectively prevented by administering parenteral vitamin K. Sites of ecchymoses and surface bleeding include the GI tract, umbilical cord, circumcision site, and nose, although devastating intracranial hemorrhage can occur. Coagulation studies reveal a prolonged PT with normal PTT and fibrinogen level. Treatment consists of 1 mg of vitamin K SC or IV. IM injections should be avoided in infants who are actively bleeding. Such infants may require factor replacement in addition to vitamin K administration.

2. Thrombocytopenia

> ### ESSENTIALS OF DIAGNOSIS & TYPICAL FEATURES
>
> ▶ Generalized petechiae; oozing at cord or puncture sites.
> ▶ Thrombocytopenia, often marked (platelets < 10,000–20,000/mL).
> ▶ In an otherwise well infant, suspect isoimmune thrombocytopenia.
> ▶ In a sick or asphyxiated infant, suspect disseminated intravascular coagulation.

Infants with thrombocytopenia have generalized petechiae and platelet counts less than 150,000/mL. Neonatal thrombocytopenia can be isolated in a seemingly well infant or may occur in association with a deficiency of other clotting factors in a sick infant. The differential diagnosis for thrombocytopenia is presented in Table 2–13. Treatment of neonatal thrombocytopenia is transfusion of platelets (10 mL/kg of platelets increases the platelet count by ~70,000/mL). Indications for transfusion in the full-term infant are clinical bleeding or a total platelet count less than 10,000–20,000/mL.

Isoimmune (alloimmune) thrombocytopenia is analogous to Rh-isoimmunization, with a human platelet antigen HPA-1a (in 80%) or HPA-5b (in 15%) negative mother and an HPA-1a– or HPA-5b–positive fetus. Transplacental passage of IgG antibody leads to platelet destruction. Treatment includes platelet transfusion for active bleeding and IVIG infusions. Twenty to thirty percent of infants with isoimmune thrombocytopenia will experience intracranial hemorrhage,

Table 2–13. Differential diagnosis of neonatal thrombocytopenia.

Disorder	Clinical Tips
Immune Passively acquired antibody; idiopathic thrombocytopenic purpura, systemic lupus erythematosus, drug-induced	Proper history, maternal thrombocytopenia
Isoimmune sensitization to HPA-1a antigen	No rise in platelet count from random donor platelet transfusion. Positive antiplatelet antibodies in baby's serum, sustained rise in platelets by transfusion of mother's platelets

Infections
  Bacterial infections
  Congenital viral infections
	Sick infants with other signs consistent with infection

Syndromes
  Absent radii
  Fanconi anemia
	Congenital anomalies, associated pancytopenia

DIC	Sick infants, abnormalities of clotting factors
Giant hemangioma	
Thrombosis	Hyperviscous infants, vascular catheters
High-risk infant with respiratory distress syndrome, pulmonary hypertension, etc	Isolated decrease in platelets is not uncommon in sick infants even in the absence of DIC (localized trapping)

DIC, disseminated intravascular coagulation; HPA, human platelet antigen.

half of them before birth. Antenatal therapy of the mother with IVIG with or without steroids may reduce this risk.

Infants born to mothers with idiopathic thrombocytopenic purpura are at low risk for serious hemorrhage despite thrombocytopenia, and treatment is usually unnecessary. If bleeding does occur, IVIG can be used in addition to platelet transfusion.

ANEMIA

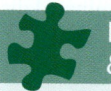

> ### ESSENTIALS OF DIAGNOSIS & TYPICAL FEATURES
>
> ▶ Hematocrit < 40% at term birth.
> ▶ Acute blood loss—signs of hypovolemia, normal reticulocyte count.

► Chronic blood loss—pallor without hypovolemia, elevated reticulocyte count.

► Hemolytic anemia—accompanied by excessive hyperbilirubinemia.

The newborn infant with anemia from acute blood loss presents with signs of hypovolemia: tachycardia, poor perfusion, and hypotension. The initial hematocrit may be normal and fall after volume replacement. Anemia from chronic blood loss is evidenced by pallor without signs of hypovolemia, with an initially low hematocrit and reticulocytosis.

Anemia can be caused by hemorrhage, hemolysis, or failure to produce red blood cells. Anemia occurring in the first 24–48 hours of life is the result of hemorrhage or hemolysis. Hemorrhage can occur in utero (fetoplacental, fetomaternal, or twin-to-twin), perinatally (cord rupture, placenta previa, placental abruption, or incision through the placenta at cesarean section), or internally (intracranial hemorrhage, cephalohematoma, or ruptured liver or spleen). Hemolysis is caused by blood group incompatibilities, enzyme or membrane abnormalities, infection, and disseminated intravascular coagulation, and is accompanied by significant hyperbilirubinemia.

Initial evaluation should include a review of the perinatal history, assessment of the infant's volume status, and a complete physical examination. A Kleihauer-Betke test for fetal cells in the mother's circulation can be done. A CBC, blood smear, reticulocyte count, and direct and indirect Coombs tests should be performed. This simple evaluation should suggest a diagnosis in most infants. Many infants tolerate anemia quite well due to the increased oxygen availability in the extrauterine environment; however, treatment with erythropoietin or transfusion might be needed if the infant develops signs of cardiopulmonary compromise. Additionally, if blood loss is the cause of the anemia, early supplementation with iron will be needed. It is important to remember that hemolysis related to blood group incompatibility can continue for weeks after birth. Serial hematocrits should be followed because late transfusion may be needed.

POLYCYTHEMIA

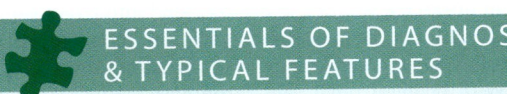

ESSENTIALS OF DIAGNOSIS & TYPICAL FEATURES

► Hematocrit > 65% (venous) at term.

► Plethora, tachypnea, retractions.

► Hypoglycemia, irritability, lethargy, poor feeding.

Table 2–14. Organ-related symptoms of hyperviscosity.

Central nervous system	Irritability, jitteriness, seizures, lethargy
Cardiopulmonary	Respiratory distress secondary to congestive heart failure, or persistent pulmonary hypertension
Gastrointestinal	Vomiting, heme-positive stools, distention, necrotizing enterocolitis
Renal	Decreased urinary output, renal vein thrombosis
Metabolic	Hypoglycemia
Hematologic	Hyperbilirubinemia, thrombocytopenia

Polycythemia in the newborn is manifested by plethora, cyanosis, respiratory distress with tachypnea and oxygen need, hypoglycemia, poor feeding, emesis, irritability, and lethargy. Hyperbilirubinemia is expected. The consequence of polycythemia is hyperviscosity with decreased perfusion of the capillary beds. Clinical symptomatology can affect several organ systems (Table 2–14). Deep vein or artery thrombosis is a severe complication. Screening can be done by measuring a capillary (heel stick) hematocrit. If the value is greater than 68%, a peripheral venous hematocrit should be measured.

Elevated hematocrits occur in 2%–5% of live births. Delayed cord clamping is the most common cause of benign neonatal polycythemia. Although 50% of polycythemic infants are AGA, the prevalence of polycythemia is greater in the SGA and LGA populations. Other causes of increased hematocrit include (1) twin-twin transfusion, (2) maternal-fetal transfusion, and (3) chronic intrauterine hypoxia.

Treatment should be considered for symptomatic infants. Treatment for asymptomatic infants based strictly on hematocrit is not indicated as there is no proven long-term benefit for neurodevelopmental outcome. Treatment for symptomatic infants is isovolemic partial exchange transfusion with normal saline, effectively decreasing the hematocrit.

Watchko JF: Common hematologic problems in the newborn nursery. Pediatr Clin North Am 2015 Apr;62(2):509–524 [PMID: 25836711].

RENAL DISORDERS IN THE NEWBORN INFANT

Renal function and the speed of maturation after birth depend on postmenstrual age (see also Chapter 24). Creatinine can be used as a clinical marker of glomerular filtration rate. Creatinine at birth reflects the maternal level and should decrease slowly over the first 3–4 weeks. An increasing serum creatinine is never normal.

The ability to concentrate urine and retain sodium also depends on gestational age. Infants born before 28–30 weeks' gestation are compromised in this respect and can easily become dehydrated and hyponatremic. Preterm infants also have increased bicarbonate excretion and are prone to developing metabolic acidosis.

RENAL FAILURE

ESSENTIALS OF DIAGNOSIS & TYPICAL FEATURES

▶ Clinical setting—birth depression, hypovolemia, hypotension, shock.

▶ Low or delayed urine output (< 1 mL/kg/h).

▶ Rising serum creatinine, hyperkalemia, metabolic acidosis, fluid overload.

Renal failure is most commonly seen in the setting of birth asphyxia, hypovolemia, or shock from any cause. The normal rate of urine flow is 1–3 mL/kg/h. After a hypoxic or ischemic insult, acute tubular necrosis may ensue. Typically, 2–3 days of anuria or oliguria is associated with hematuria, proteinuria, and a rise in serum creatinine. The period of anuria or oliguria is followed by a period of polyuria and then gradual recovery. During the polyuric phase, excessive urine sodium and bicarbonate losses may be seen.

The initial management is restoration of the infant's volume status. Thereafter, restriction of fluids to insensible water loss (40–60 mL/kg/day) without added electrolytes, plus milliliter-for-milliliter urine replacement, should be instituted. Serum and urine electrolytes and body weights should be followed frequently. These measures should be continued through the polyuric phase. Hyperkalemia, which may become life-threatening, may occur in this situation despite the lack of added IV potassium. If the serum potassium reaches 7 mEq/L, therapy should be started with glucose and insulin infusion. Nebulized albuterol, IV Lasix, and binding resins per rectum may also be used to quickly decrease serum potassium levels. Calcium chloride (20 mg/kg bolus) and correction of metabolic acidosis with bicarbonate are also helpful in the acute management of arrhythmias resulting from hyperkalemia.

Peritoneal dialysis is occasionally needed for the management of neonatal acute renal failure and for removal of waste products and excess fluid. Hemodialysis, although possible, is difficult due to the small blood volume of the infant and problems with vascular access. Although most acute renal failure in the newborn resolves, ischemic injury severe enough to result in acute cortical necrosis and chronic renal failure can occur. Such infants are also at risk of developing hypertension.

URINARY TRACT ANOMALIES

Abdominal masses in the newborn are most frequently caused by renal enlargement. Most common is a multicystic or dysplastic kidney, followed by congenital hydronephrosis. Chromosomal abnormalities and syndromes with multiple anomalies frequently include renal abnormalities. The first step in diagnosis is an ultrasound. In pregnancies complicated by oligohydramnios, renal agenesis or bladder outlet obstruction secondary to posterior urethral valves should be considered. Only bilateral disease or disease in a solitary kidney is associated with oligohydramnios, significant morbidity, and death. Such infants will generally also have pulmonary hypoplasia, and present with pulmonary rather than renal insufficiency.

Ultrasonography identifies many infants with renal anomalies (most often hydronephrosis) prior to birth. Postnatal evaluation of infants with hydronephrosis should include renal ultrasound at about 1 week of age and, depending on the severity of the antenatal findings, possibly a voiding cystourethrogram. Earlier postnatal ultrasound might underestimate the severity of the hydronephrosis due to low glomerular filtration rates in the first days of life, although cases in which oligohydramnios or severe renal abnormality are suspected will be accurately diagnosed even on the first day of life. Voiding cystourethrogram is indicated to determine the severity of vesicoureteral reflux in the setting of significant hydronephrosis.

RENAL VEIN THROMBOSIS

ESSENTIALS OF DIAGNOSIS & TYPICAL FEATURES

▶ History of IDM, birth depression, dehydration.

▶ Hematuria, oliguria.

▶ Thrombocytopenia, polycythemia.

▶ Renal enlargement on examination.

Renal vein thrombosis occurs most often in dehydrated, polycythemic newborns. At particular risk is the IDM with polycythemia. Thrombosis is unilateral in 70%, usually begins in intrarenal venules, and can extend into larger veins and the vena cava. Hematuria, oliguria, thrombocytopenia, and possibly an enlarged kidney raise suspicion for this diagnosis. With bilateral renal vein thrombosis, anuria ensues. Diagnosis can be confirmed with an ultrasound examination that includes Doppler flow studies of the kidneys. Treatment involves correcting the predisposing condition. Systemic heparinization or the use of thrombolytics for this condition is controversial. Prognosis for a full recovery is uncertain.

Many infants will develop significant atrophy of the affected kidney, and some develop systemic hypertension. All require careful follow-up.

Stein D, McNamara E: Congenital anomalies of the kidneys and urinary tract. Clin Perinatol 2022 Sep;49(3):791–798 [PMID: 36113935].

NEUROLOGIC PROBLEMS IN THE NEWBORN INFANT

SEIZURES

ESSENTIALS OF DIAGNOSIS & TYPICAL FEATURES

▶ Usual onset at 12–48 hours.

▶ Seizure types include subtle (characterized by variable findings), tonic, and multifocal clonic.

▶ Most common causes include hypoxic-ischemic encephalopathy, intracranial bleeds, and infection.

Newborns rarely have well-organized tonic-clonic seizures because of their incomplete cortical organization and a preponderance of inhibitory synapses. The most common type of seizure is characterized by a constellation of findings, including horizontal deviation of the eyes with or without jerking; eyelid blinking or fluttering; sucking and other oral-buccal movements; swimming or bicycling movements; and desaturation and apneic spells. Strictly tonic or multifocal clonic episodes are also seen.

▶ Clinical Findings

The differential diagnosis of neonatal seizures is presented in Table 2–15. Most neonatal seizures occur between 12 and 48 hours of age. Later-onset seizures suggest meningitis, benign familial seizures, or hypocalcemia. Information regarding antenatal drug use, the presence of birth asphyxia or trauma, and family history (regarding inherited disorders) should be obtained. Physical examination focuses on neurologic features, concurrent signs of infection, dysmorphic features, and intrauterine growth. Screening workup should include blood glucose, ionized calcium, and electrolytes in all cases. Further workup depends on diagnoses suggested by the history and physical examination. In most cases, a lumbar puncture should be done. Hemorrhages, perinatal stroke, and structural disease of the CNS can be addressed with brain imaging (ultrasound, CT, MRI). Metabolic workup should be pursued when appropriate. EEG should be done; the presence of spike discharges must be noted and the background wave pattern

Table 2–15. Differential diagnosis of neonatal seizures.

Diagnosis	Comment
Hypoxic-ischemic encephalopathy	Most common cause (40%), onset in first 24 h
Intracranial hemorrhage	Up to 15% of cases, periventricular/intraventricular hemorrhage, subdural or subarachnoid bleeding
Ischemic stroke	20% of cases
Infection	< 5% of cases
Hypoglycemia	Small for gestational age, IDM
Hypocalcemia, hypomagnesemia	Infant of low birth weight, IDM
Hyponatremia	Rare, seen with SIADH
Disorders of amino and organic acid metabolism, hyperammonemia	Associated acidosis, altered level of consciousness < 5% of cases
Pyridoxine dependency	Seizures refractory to routine therapy; cessation of seizures after administration of pyridoxine
Developmental defects	Congenital brain malformations, chromosomal syndromes
Drug withdrawal	
Genetic causes of neonatal onset epilepsy	Up to 10% of cases
Benign familial neonatal seizures	

IDM, infant of a diabetic mother; SIADH, syndrome of inappropriate secretion of antidiuretic hormone.

evaluated. Correlation between EEG changes and clinical seizure activity is sometimes absent making a prolonged EEG with video monitoring a useful tool.

▶ Treatment

Adequate ventilation and perfusion should be ensured. Hypoglycemia should be treated immediately with a 2-mL/kg infusion of $D_{10}W$ followed by IV glucose infusion. Other treatments such as calcium or magnesium infusion and antibiotics are indicated to treat hypocalcemia, hypomagnesemia, and suspected infection. Electrolyte abnormalities should be corrected. Intravenous phenobarbital is the first line agent used to stop seizures in neonates. Other medications include fosphenytoin, levetiracetam, and midazolam.

▶ Prognosis

Outcome is related to the underlying cause of the seizure. In general, seizures that are difficult to control carry a poor prognosis for normal development. Seizures resulting from hypoglycemia, infection of the CNS, some inborn errors of metabolism, and developmental defects also have a high rate of poor outcome. Seizures caused by hypocalcemia or isolated subarachnoid hemorrhage generally resolve without sequelae.

HYPOTONIA

One should be alert to the diagnosis of congenital hypotonia when a mother has polyhydramnios and a history of poor fetal movement. The newborn may present with poor respiratory effort and birth asphyxia. For a discussion of causes and evaluation, see Chapter 25.

INTRACRANIAL HEMORRHAGE AND STROKE

1. Primary Subarachnoid Hemorrhage

Primary subarachnoid hemorrhage is the most common type of neonatal intracranial hemorrhage. In the full-term infant, it can be related to trauma of delivery, whereas subarachnoid hemorrhage in the preterm infant can be seen in association with germinal matrix hemorrhage. Clinically, these hemorrhages can be asymptomatic or can present with seizures and irritability on day 2, or rarely, a massive hemorrhage with a rapid downhill course. Seizures associated with subarachnoid hemorrhage are very characteristic—usually brief, with a normal examination interictally. Diagnosis can be suspected on lumbar puncture and confirmed with CT scan or MRI. Long-term follow-up is uniformly good.

2. Subdural Hemorrhage

Subdural hemorrhage is related to birth trauma; the bleeding is caused by tears in the veins that bridge the subdural space. Most commonly, subdural bleeding is from ruptured superficial cerebral veins, with blood over the cerebral convexities. These hemorrhages can be asymptomatic or may cause seizures, with onset on days 2–3 of life, and vomiting, irritability, and lethargy. Associated findings include retinal hemorrhages and a full fontanelle. The diagnosis is confirmed by CT scan or MRI. Specific treatment entailing needle drainage of the subdural space is rarely necessary. Most infants survive; 75% are normal on follow-up.

3. Neonatal Stroke

Focal cerebral ischemic injury can occur in the context of intraventricular hemorrhage in the premature infant and hypoxic-ischemic encephalopathy. Neonatal stroke has also been described in the context of underlying disorders of thrombolysis, maternal drug use (cocaine), a history of infertility, preeclampsia, prolonged membrane rupture, and chorioamnionitis. In some cases, the origin is unclear. The injury often occurs antenatally. The most common clinical presentation of an isolated cerebral infarct is seizure and

diagnosis can be confirmed acutely with diffusion-weighted MRI scan. The most frequently described distribution is that of the middle cerebral artery. Treatment is directed at controlling seizures. Use of anticoagulants and thrombolytics is controversial. Long-term outcome is variable, ranging from near normal to hemiplegia and cognitive deficits.

Soul JS: Acute symptomatic seizures in term neonates: etiologies and treatments. Semin Fetal Neonatal Med 2018 Jun;23(3): 183–190 [PMID: 29433814].
Srivastava R, Kirton A. Perinatal stroke: a practical approach to diagnosis and management. Neoreviews 2021 Mar;22(3):e163–e176 [PMID: 33649089].

METABOLIC DISORDERS IN THE NEWBORN INFANT

HYPERGLYCEMIA

Hyperglycemia may develop in preterm infants, particularly those of extremely low birth weight who are also SGA. Glucose concentrations may exceed 200–250 mg/dL, particularly in the first few days of life. This transient diabetes-like syndrome usually lasts approximately 1 week.

Management may include simply reducing glucose intake while continuing to supply IV amino acids to prevent protein catabolism with resultant gluconeogenesis and worsened hyperglycemia. Intravenous insulin infusions may be needed in infants who remain hyperglycemic despite glucose infusion rates of less than 5–6 mg/kg/min, but caution should be used as hypoglycemia is a frequent complication.

HYPOCALCEMIA

ESSENTIALS OF DIAGNOSIS & TYPICAL FEATURES

► Irritability, jitteriness, seizures (see also Chapter 34).
► Normal blood glucose.
► Possible dysmorphic features and congenital heart disease (DiGeorge syndrome).

Calcium concentration in fetal plasma is higher than that of the neonate or adult and decreases in all infants in the immediate newborn period. Hypocalcemia is usually defined as a total serum concentration less than 7 mg/dL although the physiologically active fraction, ionized calcium, should be measured whenever possible, and is usually normal even when total calcium is as low as 6–7 mg/dL. An ionized calcium level above 0.9 mmol/L (1.8 mEq/L; 3.6 mg/dL) is not likely to be detrimental.

Clinical Findings

The clinical signs of hypocalcemia and hypocalcemic tetany include a high-pitched cry, jitteriness, tremulousness, and seizures. Hypocalcemia tends to occur at two different times in the neonatal period. Early-onset hypocalcemia occurs in the first 2 days of life and has been associated with prematurity, maternal diabetes, asphyxia, and rarely, maternal hypoparathyroidism. Late-onset hypocalcemia occurs at approximately 7–10 days and is observed in infants receiving modified cow's milk rather than infant formula (high phosphorus intake), in infants with hypoparathyroidism (DiGeorge syndrome, 22q11 deletion), or in infants born to mothers with severe vitamin D deficiency. An evaluation for hypomagnesemia should be performed in cases of hypocalcemia that are resistant to treatment and treated if identified.

Treatment

A. Oral Calcium Therapy

Oral administration of calcium salts, often along with vitamin D, is the preferred method of treatment for chronic forms of hypocalcemia resulting from hypoparathyroidism (see Chapter 34).

B. Intravenous Calcium Therapy

IV calcium therapy is usually needed for infants with symptomatic hypocalcemia or an ionized calcium level below 0.9 mmol/L. Several precautions must be observed when calcium is given intravenously. The infusion must be given slowly so that there is no sudden increase in calcium concentration of blood entering the right atrium, which could cause severe bradycardia and even cardiac arrest. Furthermore, the infusion must be observed carefully, because an IV infiltrate containing calcium can cause full-thickness skin necrosis requiring grafting. For these reasons, IV calcium therapy should be given judiciously and through a central venous line if possible. IV administration of 10% calcium gluconate may be given as a bolus or continuous infusion. Ten percent calcium chloride may result in a larger increment in ionized calcium and greater improvement in mean arterial blood pressure in sick hypocalcemic infants. *Note:* Calcium salts cannot be added to IV solutions that contain sodium bicarbonate because they precipitate as calcium carbonate.

Prognosis

The prognosis is good for neonatal seizures entirely caused by hypocalcemia that is promptly treated.

INBORN ERRORS OF METABOLISM

ESSENTIALS OF DIAGNOSIS & TYPICAL FEATURES

► Altered level of consciousness (poor feeding, lethargy, seizures) in a previously well-appearing infant (see also Chapter 36).

► Tachypnea without hypoxemia or distress.

► Hypoglycemia, respiratory alkalosis, metabolic acidosis.

► Recurrent "sepsis" without proven infection.

Each individual inborn error of metabolism is rare, but collectively they have an incidence of 1 in 1000 live births. Expanded newborn genetic screening aids in the diagnosis of these disorders; however, many infants will present prior to these results being available. These diagnoses should be entertained when infants who were initially well present with sepsis-like syndromes, recurrent hypoglycemia, seizures, altered levels of consciousness, or unexplained acidosis (suggestive of organic acidemias).

In the immediate neonatal period, urea cycle disorders present as an altered level of consciousness (coma) secondary to hyperammonemia. A clinical clue that supports this diagnosis is hyperventilation with primary respiratory alkalosis, along with low blood urea nitrogen. The other major diagnostic category to consider in infants with altered consciousness is severe and unremitting acidemia secondary to organic acidemias.

QUALITY ASSESSMENT & IMPROVEMENT IN THE NEWBORN NURSERY & NICU

Quality improvement initiatives are critical for NICUs to provide the best care possible for patients. Individual units can benchmark their care through participation in multicenter databases such as the Vermont Oxford Network or Children's Hospitals Neonatal Consortium, in which many NICUs submit data. These data can form the framework for strategies to improve performance in areas in a unit that are below network standards. Examples of initiatives include lowering the incidence of central line-associated bacteremia, decreasing the incidence of ventilator-associated pneumonia, and structured feeding protocols to decrease the incidence of NEC.

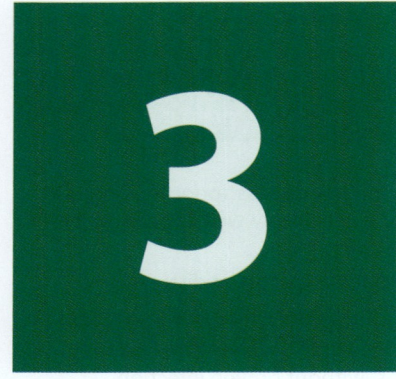

Child Development & Behavior

Ann Reynolds, MD

Abigail Angulo, MD, MPH

Meghan Breheney, MD

INTRODUCTION

This chapter provides an overview of typical development, identifies developmental variations, and discusses several developmental disorders. It does not cover typical development in the newborn period or adolescence (see Chapters 2 and 4, respectively). It addresses behavioral variations that reflect the spectrum of normal development, along with developmental and behavioral disorders and their treatment. The developmental principle of ongoing change and maturation is integral to the daily practice of pediatrics. The medical home is the optimal setting to understand and enhance typical development and to address variations, delays, and deviations as they may occur in the life trajectory of the child and the family.

NORMAL DEVELOPMENT

Typically developing children follow a trajectory of increasing physical size and increasing complexity of function, especially during the first 5 years of life. The child triples his or her birth weight within the first year and achieves two-thirds of his or her adult brain size by age 2½–3 years of age. The child progresses from a totally dependent infant at birth to a mobile, verbal person who can express his or her needs and desires by age 2–3 years. In the ensuing 3 years, the child further develops the capacity to interact with peers and adults, achieves considerable verbal and physical prowess, and prepares to enter the academic world of learning and socialization.

It is critical for the clinician to identify disturbances in development during these early years as there are windows of opportunity to intervene and effectively address developmental challenges.

Early developmental milestones have been recently updated by the Centers for Disease Control and Prevention (CDC) and the American Academy of Pediatrics (AAP) with the goal of providing evidence-informed guidelines for surveillance and providing clinicians with firm expectations for developmental progress. Many of the traditional milestones have been adjusted to align with the age at which most children would be expected to achieve this milestone. Milestones that coincide with health supervision visits were also included. It is important to consider the range of normal around a milestone but also to know when a clinician should consider further evaluation and intervention. These new guidelines provide surveillance recommendations and eliminate the need for a "watch and wait" mentality. The updated guidelines can be found on the CDC website referenced below. Selected milestones are included here for specific illustrations.

THE FIRST 2 YEARS

From a motor perspective, children develop in cephalocaudal and mediolateral directions. They can lift their heads with good control at 4 months, sit independently at 9 months, take first steps at 15 months, and run by 24 months. The child learning to walk has a wide-based gait at first. Next, he or she walks with legs closer together, the arms move medially, a heel-toe gait develops, and the arms swing symmetrically by 24 months.

Clinicians often focus on gross motor development, but an appreciation of fine motor development and dexterity, particularly the grasp, can be instructive not only in monitoring normal development but also in identifying deviations in development. The grasp begins as a raking motion involving the ulnar aspect of the hand by age 9 months. The immature pincer grasp develops by age 12 months, utilizing the most lateral finger, the thumb. Most young children have symmetrical movements. Children should not have a significant hand preference before 1 year of age and typically develop handedness between 18 and 30 months. Early handedness may provide clues to neurologic injury.

Communication is important from birth, particularly the nonverbal, reciprocal interactions between infant and caregiver. By age 4 months, these interactions begin to include melodic vowel sounds called *cooing* and reciprocal vocal play between parent and child. Babbling, which adds consonants to vowels, begins by age 9 months, and the repetition of sounds such as "da-da-da-da" is facilitated by the child's increasing oral muscular control. The child then moves into a stage of having needs met by using individual words to represent objects or actions. It is common at this age for children to express wants and needs by pointing to objects or using other gestures. Children usually have 5 comprehensible words by 18 months; by age 2 years, they are putting 2–3 words into flexible phrases. By 30 months, children will use about 50 words. The acquisition of expressive vocabulary expands significantly between 12 and 24 months of age. As they age, children become more understandable, with approximately 75% of speech understandable at 3 years and about 100% understandable by 4 years. As a group, males and children who are bilingual tend to develop expressive language more slowly during that time, though still within the typical time frame. Gender and exposure to multiple languages should never be used as an excuse for failing to refer a child who has significant delay in the acquisition of speech and language for further evaluation. Exposure to multiple languages during infancy can enhance future acquisition skills (priming the brain for the distinct sounds for each language) and support social development of the child.

Receptive language usually develops more rapidly than expressive language. Word comprehension begins to increase at age 9 months, and by age 12 months the child's receptive vocabulary may be as large as 20–100 words. After age 18 months, both expressive vocabulary and receptive language increase dramatically, and by the end of the second year, there is typically a quantum leap in language development. Children begin to put verbs into phrases and focus much of their language on describing their new abilities, for example, "I go out," by 30 months old. They begin to incorporate prepositions, such as "I" and "you" into speech and ask "why?" and "what?" questions more frequently.

In the first year of life, the infant's perception of reality revolves around their self and what they can see or touch. The infant follows the trajectory of an object through the field of vision, but before age 6 months the object ceases to exist once it leaves the infant's field of vision. At age 7–10 months, the infant gradually develops the concept of object permanence, or the realization that objects exist even when not seen. The concept attaches first to the image of the primary caregiver because of his or her emotional importance and is a critical part of attachment behavior (see below).

In the first year of life, there is a bidirectional attachment process called *bonding*. The caregivers learn to be aware of and to interpret the infant's cues, which reflect the infant's needs. More sensitive emotional and social interaction develops. This is seen in the mirroring of facial expressions by the primary caregiver and infant and in their mutual engagement. Basic trust versus mistrust is another way of describing the reciprocal interaction that characterizes this stage. Turn-taking games, such as repeating cooing sounds, which occur by 6 months, are a pleasure for both the parents and the infant and are an extension of mirroring behavior. They also represent an early form of imitative behavior, which is important in later social and cognitive development. More sophisticated games, such as peek-a-boo, become meaningful at approximately age 9 months. The infant's thrill at the reappearance of the face that vanished momentarily demonstrates the emerging understanding of object permanence. Age 9 months is also a critical time in the attachment process as this is when separation anxiety and stranger anxiety become marked. The infant is able to appreciate change in his/her environment. This can provoke fear and anxiety. In stranger anxiety, the infant analyzes the face of a stranger, detects the mismatch with previous schemata or what is familiar, and responds with fear or anxiety. In separation anxiety, the child perceives the difference between the primary caregiver's presence and his or her absence by remembering the schema of the caregiver's presence. Perceiving the inconsistency in the caregiver's absence, the child first becomes uncertain and then anxious and fearful. This begins at age 9 months, reaches a peak at 15 months, and disappears by the end of 2 years in a relatively orderly progression as central nervous system (CNS) maturation facilitates the development of new skills. Children may be comforted by a visual substitute, such as a comfort item, during a caregiver's absence.

Once the child can walk independently, he or she can move away from the parent and explore the environment. Although the child uses the parent as "home base," returning frequently for reassurance, he or she has now taken a major step toward independence. This is the beginning of mastery over the environment and an emerging sense of autonomy. The "terrible twos" and the frequent self-asserting use of "no" are the child's attempt to develop a better idea of what is or might be under his or her control. As children develop a sense of self, they begin to understand the feelings of others and develop empathy. They hug another child who is in perceived distress or become concerned when one is hurt. This realization helps them to inhibit their own aggressive behavior. Children also begin to understand right and wrong and parental expectations. They recognize that they have done something "bad" and may signify that awareness with expressions such as "uh oh." They also take pleasure in their accomplishments and become more aware of their bodies.

Play is an important behavior at this stage. Play is a very complex process whose purpose can include the practice and rehearsal of roles, skills, and relationships; a means of revisiting the past; a means of actively mastering a range of experiences; and a way to integrate the child's life experiences into understanding of their environment. Play involves emotional development (affect regulation and individual identification and roles), cognitive development (nonverbal and verbal function and executive functioning and creativity), and social/motor development (motor coordination, frustration tolerance, and social interactions such as turn taking). Play has a developmental progression. The typical 12-month-old engages in the game of peek-a-boo, which is a form of social interaction. During the next several months, although children engage in increasingly complex social interactions and imitation, their play is primarily solitary. However, they begin to engage in symbolic play such as by drinking from a toy cup and then by giving a doll a drink from a toy cup. By age 2 years, children begin to engage in parallel play (engaging in behaviors that are imitative of a peer). This form of play gradually evolves into more interactive or collaborative play by age 3–4 years and is also more thematic in nature. There are wide variations in the development of play, reflecting cultural, educational, and socioeconomic variables. Nevertheless, the development of play does follow a sequence that can be assessed and can be informative in the evaluation of the child.

Brain maturation sets the stage for toilet training. After 18 months, toddlers have the sensory capacity for awareness of a full rectum or bladder and are physically able to control bowel and urinary tract sphincters. They also take great pleasure in their accomplishments, particularly in appropriate elimination, if it is reinforced positively. Children must be given some control over when elimination occurs. If parents impose severe restrictions, the achievement of this developmental milestone can become a battle between parent and child. The development of bowel control encompasses a more generalized theme of socialized behavior.

AGES 2–4 YEARS

The 2- to 4-year-old stage begins when language ability allows the child to understand the symbolic world and differentiate reality from fantasy imperfectly. For example, they may be terrified of dreams. Cause-effect relationships are confused with temporal ones or interpreted with respect to themselves. For example, children may focus their understanding of divorce on themselves ("My father left because I was bad" or "My mother left because she didn't love me"). Illness and the need for medical care are also commonly misinterpreted at this age. The child may make a mental connection between a sibling's illness and a recent argument, a negative comment, or a wish for the sibling to be ill. The child may experience significant guilt unless the caregivers are aware of these misperceptions and take time to address them directly.

At this age, children also endow inanimate objects with human feelings. They also assume that humans cause or create all natural events. For instance, when asked why the sun sets, they may say, "The sun goes to his house" or "It is pushed down by someone else." Magical thinking blossoms between ages 3 and 5 years as symbolic thinking incorporates more elaborate fantasy. Children test new experiences in fantasy, both in their imagination and in play. In their play, children often create magical stories and novel situations that reflect issues with which they are dealing, such as aggression, relationships, fears, and control. Children often invent imaginary friends at this time, and nightmares or fears of monsters are common. At this stage, other children become important in facilitating play, such as in a preschool group. Play gradually becomes more cooperative with shared fantasies.

EARLY SCHOOL YEARS: AGES 5–7 YEARS

Attendance at kindergarten at age 5 years marks an acceleration in the separation-individuation theme initiated in the preschool years. The child is ready to relate to peers in a more interactive manner. The brain has reached 90% of its adult weight. Sensorimotor coordination abilities are maturing and facilitating pencil-and-paper tasks and sports, both part of the school experience. Cognitive abilities are still at the preoperational stage, and children focus on one variable in a problem at a time. However, most children have mastered conservation of length by age 5½ years, conservation of mass and weight by 6½ years, and conservation of volume by 8 years.

By first grade, there is more pressure on the child to master academic tasks—recognizing numbers, letters, and words and learning to write. Concrete operations typically begin after age 6 years, when the child can perform mental operations concerning concrete objects that involve manipulation of more than one variable. The child can order, number, and classify because these activities are related to concrete objects in the environment and because these activities are stressed in early schooling. The reality of cause-effect relationships is better understood. Fantasy and imagination are still strong and are reflected in themes of play.

MIDDLE CHILDHOOD: AGES 7–11 YEARS

From 7 to 11 years of age, children devote most of their energies to school and peer group interactions. For the 7-year-old child, the major developmental tasks are achievement in school and acceptance by peers. Academic expectations intensify, become more abstract, and require the child to concentrate on and process increasingly complex auditory and visual information. Children with learning disabilities or problems with attention, organization, and impulsivity may have difficulty with academic tasks. This may subsequently lead to negative reinforcement from teachers, peers, and even parents. Such children may develop a poor self-image manifested as behavioral difficulties. The pediatrician must evaluate potential learning disabilities in any child who is not developing adequately at this stage or who presents with emotional or behavioral problems. The developmental status of school-aged children is not documented as easily as that of younger children because of the complexity of the milestones. In the school-aged child, the quality of the response, the attentional abilities, and the child's emotional approach to the task can make a dramatic difference in success at school. The clinician must consider all these aspects in the differential diagnosis of learning disabilities and behavioral disorders.

Dixon SD, Stein MT: *Encounters With Children: Pediatric Behavior and Development.* 4th ed. St. Louis, MO: Mosby-Year Book; 2006.

Feldman HM, Elias ER, Blum NJ, Jimenez M, Stancin T: *Developmental-Behavioral Pediatrics.* 5th ed. Elsevier; 2022. https://www.cdc.gov/ncbddd/actearly/milestones/index.html.

Squires J, Bricker D: *Ages and Stages Questionnaires.* 3rd ed. Baltimore, MD: Brookes Publishing; 2009.

Voigt RG, Macias MM, Myers SM, Tapia CD (eds): *Developmental and Behavioral Pediatrics.* 2nd ed. Itasca, IL: American Academy of Pediatrics; 2018.

Zubler JM et al: Evidence-informed milestones for developmental surveillance tools. Pediatrics 2022 Mar 1;149(3):e2021052138 [PMID: 35132439].

BEHAVIORAL & DEVELOPMENTAL VARIATIONS

Variations in children's behavior reflect a blend of intrinsic biological characteristics and the environments with which the children interact. Often identified as complaints by parents, such normal variations in behavior reflect each child's unique, individual biologic and temperament traits and the parents' responses. There are no cures for these behaviors, but management strategies can enhance the parents' understanding of the child and the child's relationship to the environment.

Hagan Jr JF, Shaw JS, Duncan PM (eds): *Bright Futures: Guidelines for Health Supervision of Infants, Children, and Adolescents.* 4th ed. Elk Grove Village, IL: American Academy of Pediatrics; 2017.
Voigt RG, Macias MM, Myers SM, Tapia CD (eds): *Developmental and Behavioral Pediatrics.* 2nd ed. Itasca, IL: American Academy of Pediatrics; 2018.

NORMALITY & TEMPERAMENT

Variations in temperament and behavior are not as straightforward as delays in developmental milestones and there is often overlap between physiologic and behavioral signs. Labeling such variations as disorders is generally not productive. Temperament is the style with which the child interacts with the environment. It is a genetically influenced behavioral disposition that is stable over time. Temperament is sometimes thought of as being the "how" of behavior as distinguished from the "why" (motivation) and the "what" (ability). The influence of temperament is bidirectional: The effect of a particular experience will be influenced by the child's temperament, and the child's temperament will influence the responses of others in the child's environment.

The perceptions and expectations of parents must be considered when a child's behavior is evaluated. A child whom one parent might describe as hyperactive might not be characterized as such by the other parent. This truism can be expanded to include all the dimensions of temperament. Thus, the concept of "goodness of fit" comes into play. For example, if the parents want and expect their child to be predictable but that is not the child's temperamental style, the parents may perceive the child as being bad or having a behavioral disorder rather than as having a developmental variation. An appreciation of this phenomenon is important because the physician may be able to enhance the parents' understanding of the child and influence their responses to the child's behavior. When there is goodness of fit, there will be more harmony and a greater potential for healthy development not only of the child but also of the family. When goodness of fit is not present, tension and stress can result in parental anger, disappointment, frustration, and conflict with the child.

All models of temperament seek to identify intrinsic behavioral characteristics that lead the child to respond to the world in particular ways. One child may be highly emotional and another may be impassive in response to a variety of experiences, stressful or pleasant. The clinician must recognize that each child brings some intrinsic, biologically based traits to his or her environment and that such characteristics are neither good nor bad, right nor wrong, normal nor abnormal; they are simply part of the child. Thus, as one looks at variations in development, one should abandon the illness model and consider this construct as an aid to understanding the nature of the child's behavior and its influence on the parent-child relationship.

Caring for Your School Age Child: Ages 5 to 12. American Academy of Pediatrics; 2015.
DePauw SSW, Mervield I: Temperament, personality, and developmental psychopathology: a review of the conceptual dimensions underlying childhood traits. Child Psychiatry Hum Dev 2010;41:313–329 [PMID: 20238477].
How to Understand Your Child's Temperament. Healthychildren.org.
Nigg JT: Temperament and developmental psychopathology. J Child Psychol Psychiatr 2006;47:395–422 [PMID: 16492265].

ENURESIS & ENCOPRESIS

ESSENTIALS OF DIAGNOSIS & TYPICAL FEATURES

▶ Enuresis: A child older than 5 years with urine incontinence at least twice a week for 3 months.

▶ Encopresis: A child older than 4 years with episodes of bowel incontinence occurring monthly for at least 3 months.

▶ The child generally has no underlying pathology to which the incontinence can be attributed. Most cases of encopresis, however, are secondary to constipation.

Enuresis and encopresis are common childhood problems encountered by primary care providers. Bedwetting is particularly common with about 20% of children in the first grade occasionally wetting the bed and 4% wetting the bed two or more times a week. Enuresis is more common in boys than in girls. In a recent large US study, the prevalence of enuresis among boys 7 and 9 years was 9% and 7%, respectively, and among girls at those ages, 6% and 3%, respectively. Approximately 1%–3% of children experience encopresis. Overall, encopresis/constipation accounts for 3% of referrals to pediatricians' offices. What is more striking, however, is that constipation and enuresis often co-occur; when they co-occur, the constipation needs to be dealt with before the enuresis can be addressed.

ENURESIS

Enuresis is defined as repeated urination into the clothing during the day and into the bed at night by a child who is chronologically and developmentally older than 5 years at least twice a week for 3 months. Enuresis has been categorized by the International Children's Continence Society as monosymptomatic or non-monosymptomatic. **Monosymptomatic enuresis** is uncomplicated nocturnal enuresis (NE). Monosymptomatic enuresis reflects a delay in achieving nighttime continence and reflects a delay in the maturation of the urologic and neurologic systems. Specifically, there is a delay in the communications between the frontal lobes, locus coeruleus, pons, sacral voiding center, and the bladder and rectum. There is no underlying organic problem. Complicated or non-monosymptomatic enuresis often involves NE and daytime incontinence and often reflects an underlying disorder. This is discussed in greater detail below.

Most children are continent at night within 2 years of achieving daytime control. However, 15.5% of 7.5-year-old children wet the bed but only about 2.5% meet the criteria for enuresis. With each year of age, the frequency of bedwetting decreases: by 15 years only about 1%–2% of children continue to have NE. This occurs more commonly among boys than girls.

The causes for NE are varied and interrelated. Genetic factors are strongly implicated, as enuresis tends to run in families. The etiology of NE is not completely understood but based on current knowledge, there are three primary reasons: higher threshold for arousal from sleep when the bladder is full, overproduction of urine from decreased production of desmopressin or a resistance to antidiuretic hormone, and decreased bladder functional capacity.

The evaluation of a child with NE involves a complete history and physical examination to rule out any anatomical abnormalities, underlying pathology, or the presence of constipation. In addition, every child with NE should undergo a urinalysis including a specific gravity. A urine culture should be obtained, especially in girls.

Treatment involves education and the avoidance of judgement or shame. A variety of behavioral strategies have been employed such as limiting liquids before sleep and awakening the child at night so that he/she can go to the toilet. Central to this simple strategy is consistency on the parents' part and the need for the child to be completely awake. If this simple approach is unsuccessful, the use of bedwetting alarms is suggested. Every time the alarm goes off, the child should go to the toilet and void. Therapy needs to be continued for at least 3 months, be used every night, and involve the parents as active partners to ensure the child fully wakes up. The alarm system, which is a form of cognitive behavioral therapy, has been found to cure two-thirds of affected children. The most common cause of failure of this intervention is parental inconsistency.

While behavioral strategies should be the first line of treatment, medications can be helpful if further intervention is needed. Desmopressin acetate (DDAVP), an antidiuretic hormone analogue, has been used successfully. DDAVP decreases urine production. Imipramine, a tricyclic antidepressant, also has been used successfully to control NE, although the mechanism of action is not understood. However, potential adverse side effects, including the risk of death with an overdose, suggest that imipramine should be used only as a last resort. Unfortunately, when such medications are stopped, there is a very high relapse rate.

Daytime incontinence or **non-monosymptomatic enuresis** is more complicated than NE. Daytime continence is achieved by 70% of children by 3 years of age and by 90% of children by 6 years. When this is not the case, one needs to consider underlying pathology, including cystitis, diabetes insipidus, diabetes mellitus, seizure disorders, neurogenic bladder, anatomical abnormalities of the urinary tract system such as urethral obstruction, constipation, and psychological stress and child maltreatment. A complete history and physical examination must be obtained, along with a diary that includes daily records of voiding and fecal elimination. Treatment must be directed at the underlying pathology and often requires the input of pediatric subspecialists. Following diagnosis, family support and education are essential.

ENCOPRESIS

Encopresis is described in the *Diagnostic and Statistical Manual of Mental Disorders*, 5th Edition (DSM-5) as the repeated passage of stool into inappropriate places (such as in the underpants) by a child who is chronologically or developmentally older than 4 years. It occurs at least once a month for 3 months and is not attributable to the physiologic effects of a substance or another medical condition other than constipation. In rare instances, children have severe toilet phobia and so do not defecate into the toilet. It is critical to note that more than 90% of cases of encopresis result from constipation. Thus, in the evaluation of a child with encopresis, one must rule out underlying pathology associated with constipation (see Chapter 21) while at the same time addressing functional and behavioral issues. Conditions associated with constipation include metabolic disorders such as hypothyroidism, neurologic disorders such as cerebral palsy or tethered cord, and anatomical abnormalities of the anus. In addition, children who have been continent can also develop encopresis as a response to stress or child maltreatment.

The prevalence of encopresis is somewhat difficult to ascertain as it is a subject often kept secret by the family and the child. However, some authors report that 1%–3% of children ages 4–11 years of age suffer from encopresis. The highest prevalence is between 5 and 6 years of age.

A complete history and physical examination should be performed, including examination of the spine. A rectal examination may be considered. An abdominal radiograph can be helpful in determining the degree of constipation and whether there is obstruction. Assuming no gastrointestinal abnormalities, initial intervention starts with treatment of constipation. Subsequently education, support, and guidance around evacuation are essential, including behavioral strategies such as having the child sit on the toilet after meals to take advantage of the gastrocolic reflex. Caregivers should avoid punishment or shame. Helping the child to clean himself and his clothing in a nonjudgmental, nonpunitive manner is more productive than criticism and reproach.

When medical management of constipation is indicated, oral medication or an enema for "bowel cleanout" followed by oral medications should be used. A bowel regimen needs to be established with the goal of the child achieving continence and defecating in the toilet on a regular basis. The child should be encouraged to have a daily bowel movement. The use of fiber, laxatives, and stool softeners can be helpful. Ensuring adequate daily water intake is also important. Consultation with a gastroenterologist should be considered in more refractory cases.

Nevéus T, Fonseca E, Franco I, Kawauchi A, Kovacevic L, Nieuwhof-Leppink A: Management and treatment of nocturnal enuresis-an updated standardization document from the International Children's Continence Society. J Pediatr Urol 2020;16:10–19 [PMID: 32278657].

Rajindrajith S, Devanarayana NM, Thapar N, Benninga MA: Functional fecal incontinence in children: epidemiology, pathophysiology, evaluation, and management. J Pediatr Gastroenterol Nutr 2021 Jun 1;72(6):794–801. doi: 10.1097/MPG.0000000000003056 [PMID: 33534361].

▼ COMMON DEVELOPMENTAL CONCERNS

COLIC

 ESSENTIALS OF DIAGNOSIS & TYPICAL FEATURES

► An otherwise healthy infant aged 2–3 months seems to be in pain, cries for > 3 hours a day, for > 3 days a week, for > 3 weeks ("rule of threes").

Infant colic is characterized by severe and paroxysmal crying that occurs mainly in the late afternoon. The infant's knees are drawn up, and its fists are clenched, the facies appear strained, and there is minimal response to attempts at soothing. Although colic has traditionally been attributed to gastrointestinal disturbances, this has never been proven. Others have suggested that colic reflects a disturbance in the infant's sleep-wake cycling or an infant state regulation disorder. In any case, colic is a behavioral sign or symptom that begins in the first few weeks of life and peaks at age 2–3 months. In about 30%–40% of cases, colic continues into the fourth and fifth months.

A *colicky infant* is healthy and well fed but cries for more than 3 hours a day, for more than 3 days a week, and for more than 3 weeks—commonly referred to as the "rule of threes." The important word in this definition is "healthy." Thus, before the diagnosis of colic can be made, the pediatrician must rule out diseases that might cause crying including undetected corneal abrasion, urinary tract infection, and unrecognized traumatic injuries, including child abuse. Gastroesophageal reflux is often suspected as a cause of colicky crying in young infants. There has been little evidence of an association of colic with allergic disorders. Some attempts have been made to eliminate gas with simethicone and to slow gut motility with dicyclomine. Simethicone has not been shown to ameliorate colic and dicyclomine has been associated with apnea in infants and is contraindicated.

Infants have different behavioral states: a crying state, a quiet alert state, an active alert state, a transitional state, and a state of deep sleep. The crying state and the transitional state are most pertinent to colic. During transition from one state to another, infant behavior may be more easily influenced. Once an infant is in a stable state (eg, crying), it becomes more difficult to change (eg, to soothe). How these transitions are accomplished is probably influenced by the infant's temperament and neurologic maturity. Some infants move from one state to another easily; other infants are resistant to change.

Another factor to be considered in evaluating the colicky infant is the feeding and handling behavior of the caregiver. Colic is a behavioral phenomenon that involves interaction between the infant and the caregiver. Different caregivers perceive and respond to crying behavior differently. If the caregiver is not sensitive to or knowledgeable about the infant's cues and rhythms, the infant's ability to organize and self-soothe or respond to the caregiver's attempts at soothing may be compromised. Alternatively, if the temperament of an infant with colic is understood and the rhythms and cues deciphered, crying can be anticipated and the caregiver can intervene before the behavior becomes "organized" in the crying state and more difficult to extinguish.

► Management

1. Parents need to be educated about the developmental characteristics of crying behavior and made aware that crying increases normally into the second month and abates by the third to fourth month.

2. Parents need reassurance, based on a complete history and physical examination, that the infant is not sick. A discussion of the differential/potential causes and why they have been ruled out can be helpful. Although these behaviors are stressful, they are normal variants and are usually self-limited.

3. For parents to effectively soothe and comfort the infant, they need to understand the infant's cues. The pediatrician (or nurse) can help by observing the infant's behavior and devising interventions aimed at calming both the infant and the parents. Rhythmic stimulation such as gentle swinging or rocking, soft music, drives in the car, or walks in the stroller may be helpful, especially if the parents are able to anticipate the onset of crying. Another approach is to change the feeding habits so that the infant is not rushed, has ample opportunity to burp and if necessary, can be fed more frequently to decrease gastric distention.

4. Medications such as dicyclomine should not be used because of the risk of adverse reactions and overdosage. A trial of famotidine or a proton pump inhibitor might be of help if proven gastroesophageal reflux is contributing to the child's discomfort.

5. For colic that is refractory to behavioral management, a trial of changing the feedings and eliminating cow's milk from the formula or from the mother's diet if she is nursing may be indicated. The use of whey hydrolysate formulas for formula-fed infants has been suggested. There is conflicting evidence regarding the use of probiotics to treat infant colic.

6. There is no conclusive evidence for complementary and alternative interventions to treat colic. Furthermore, herbal remedies have potential for toxicity and neurologic impairment, compounded by lack of knowledge of appropriate dosing in children. The same holds true for the use of chiropractic interventions and reflexology.

Bellaïche M, Levy M, Jung C: Treatments for infant colic. J Pediatr Gastroenterol Nutr 2013;57(Suppl 1):S27–S30.

Biagoli E et al: Pain-relieving agents for infantile colic. Cochrane Database Syst Rev 2016 Sep 16;9:CD009999 [PMID: 27631535].

Cabanillas-Barea S et al: Systematic review and meta-analysis showed that complementary and alternative medicines were not effective for infantile colic. Acta Paediatr 2023 Jul;112(7):1378–1388. doi: 10.1111/apa.16807. Epub 2023 May 8 [PMID: 37119443].

Cohen-Silver J, Ratnapalan S: Management of infantile colic: a review. Clin Pediatr (Phila) 2009;48:14–17 [PMID: 18832537].

Schreck BA et al: Probiotics for the treatment of infantile colic: a systemic review. J Pharm Pract 2017 Jun;30(3):366–374 [PMID: 26940647].

Shamir R et al: Infant crying, colic, and gastrointestinal discomfort in early childhood: a review of the evidence and most plausible mechanisms. J Pediatr Gastroenterol Nutr 2013 Dec;57(Suppl 1): S1–S45 [PMID: 24356023].

FEEDING DISORDERS IN INFANTS & YOUNG CHILDREN

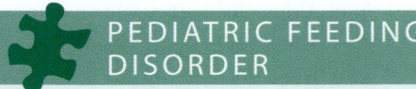

PEDIATRIC FEEDING DISORDER

▶ Inadequate or disordered intake of food associated with dysfunction in one or more of the following Areas:

Medical

- Fatigue secondary to a chronic disease
- Pain associated with feeding
- Craniofacial structure

Nutrition

- Inadequate calories
- Inadequate intake of nutrients
- Poor appetite

Feeding Skills for Age

- Poor oral-motor skills
- Poor fine motor skills

Psychosocial/Behavioral

- Behavioral issues relating to parent-child interaction issues
- Behavioral issues relating to child sensory issues
- Anxiety/hyperarousal affecting child's appetite and behavior

Feeding problems are common in children, and yet there are no widely accepted diagnostic criteria. Feeding problems can present in various ways, including oral-motor dysfunction (gagging, trouble with chewing and/or swallowing, and aspiration), fine motor skill deficits, cardiopulmonary disorders leading to fatigue, gastrointestinal disturbances causing pain or discomfort, sensory hypersensitivity, anxiety/hyperarousal, and psychosocial issues. Children with medical or developmental conditions are more likely to experience feeding problems. Infants and young children may refuse to eat if the rhythm of the feeding experience with the caregiver is not harmonious. The infant who needs to burp more frequently or who needs time between bites may develop feeding problems if these issues are not easily recognized by the caregiver. Children may develop a negative association with feeding if it is uncomfortable (child who had an esophageal atresia repair and has a stricture), painful (infant with severe oral candidiasis or child with eosinophilic esophagitis), anxiety provoking (choking or aspiration), or novel (new or unfamiliar food). Children who have required nasogastric feedings or who have required periods of fasting and intravenous nutrition in the first 1–2 months of life are more likely to display food refusal behavior upon introduction of oral feedings.

Avoidant/restrictive food intake disorder (ARFID) is a new diagnosis created in DSM-5. ARFID is characterized by poor intake or limited variety of food leading to weight loss, poor growth, nutrient deficiency, requirement of greater than 50% of calories from nutritional supplements, and/or psychosocial dysfunction. Restricted food intake cannot be due to distorted body image seen in anorexia and bulimia. The overlap of ARFID with pediatric feeding disorder leads to some controversy regarding the ARFID diagnosis. As ARFID is a new diagnosis, evaluation tools and treatments are emerging but still need more research. (See Chapter 6.)

The typical developmental and interactive feeding stages through which a child and caregiver normally progress are homeostasis (0–2 months), attachment (2–6 months), and separation and individuation (6 months to 3 years). During the first stage, feeding can be accomplished most easily when the caregiver allows the infant to determine the timing, amount, and pacing of food intake. During the attachment phase, allowing the infant to control the feeding permits the parent to engage the infant in a positive manner. This paves the way for the separation and individuation phase. When a disturbance occurs in the parent-child interaction at any of these developmental stages, difficulty in feeding may ensue, with both the parent and the child contributing to the dysfunctional interaction.

► **Evaluation**

History of feeding environment and behavior: When attempting to sort out the factors contributing to food refusal, it is essential first to obtain a complete history, including social history, caregiver's expectations for the child's intake and perceptions about the function of the child's behavior. This includes frequency of refusal, caregiver response to food refusal, taste and texture of rejected foods, the environment in which the child eats, and timing of meals and snacks. In addition, provider should evaluate for any evidence of pain or discomfort associated with eating (dental pain, GERD, dysphagia, choking or gagging, constipation, etc), and onset of feeding challenges and any stressors that occurred at that time.

Dietary intake: Providers should ask about calories, nutritional value, and variety of foods.

Physical examination: Exam with emphasis on growth and weight gain; neurologic, anatomic, or physiologic abnormalities affecting feeding (poor trunk tone could affect the child's ability to sit upright when feeding without using arms for support making it difficult to independently feed herself); developmental level; evidence of anxiety or depression; and observation of oral-motor function and feeding interaction if possible.

► **Management**

A multidisciplinary approach is recommended in the assessment and treatment of feeding problems in children. Consider a feeding evaluation by a team including an occupational therapist, speech therapist, feeding behavior specialist, dietician (including 3-day diet record), and/or medical provider with expertise in feeding and nutrition. Also consider a swallow study if there is a history of choking or gagging, or nutrition labs if the child has a limited diet predisposing them to dietary insufficiency. If failure to gain weight or weight loss are present, an evaluation for failure to thrive would be indicated. See Chapter 9.

The goals of treatment of the child with feeding challenges are to establish a pattern of eating that is harmonious with the goals of the family or caregivers. Guidelines to accomplishing these goals include (1) establish a comprehensive diagnosis that considers all factors contributing to poor feeding; (2) monitor the feeding interaction and ensure appropriate weight gain; (3) monitor the developmental progress of the child and the changes in the family dynamics that facilitate optimal weight gain and

psychosocial development; and (4) provide support to the family as they work on feeding with their child including education about variations in styles of eating, food preferences, temperament, need for a calm environment in which to eat, temperament, anxiety, rigidity or need for sameness in food choices, and ways of processing olfactory, gustatory, and tactile stimuli.

Goday PS et al: Pediatric feeding disorder: consensus definition and conceptual framework. J Pediatr Gastroenterol Nutr 2019;68(1):124–129.
Kambanis PE, Thomas JJ: Assessment and treatment of avoidant/restrictive food intake disorder. Curr Psychiatry Rep 2023 Feb;25(2):53–64. doi: 10.1007/s11920-022-01404-6. Epub 2023 Jan 14 [PMID: 36640211].
Morris N, Knight RM, Bruni T, Sayers L, Drayton A: Feeding disorders. Child Adolesc Psychiatr Clin N Am 2017;26(3), 571–586. doi:10.1016/j.chc.2017.02.011 [PMID: 28577610].

SLEEP DISORDERS

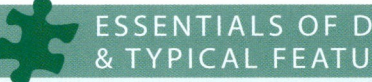

ESSENTIALS OF DIAGNOSIS & TYPICAL FEATURES

► Children aged < 12 years:
- Difficulty initiating or maintaining sleep that is viewed as a problem by the child or caregiver.
- Bedtime resistance or need for caregiver intervention to initiate sleep or to go back to sleep.
- May be characterized by its severity, chronicity, frequency, *and* associated impairment in daytime function in the child *or* family.
- May be due to a primary sleep disorder or occur in association with other sleep, medical, or psychiatric disorders.

► Adolescents:
- Difficulty initiating or maintaining sleep, early morning awakening, nonrestorative sleep, or a combination of these problems.

Sleep problems impact quality of life and are considered a public health problem. Poor sleep in children is associated with maladaptive daytime behaviors, poorer developmental outcome, greater parental stress, obesity, insulin resistance, alterations in sympathetic tone, and immune dysfunction. Sleep is a complex physiologic process influenced by intrinsic biologic properties, temperament, cultural norms and expectations, and environmental conditions. Between 20% and 40% of children experience sleep disturbances at some point in the first 4 years of life. The percentage decreases to 10%–12% in school-aged children. The most common sleep disorder encountered by pediatricians is insomnia, difficulty initiating and maintaining sleep. Parasomnias refer to abnormalities of arousal, partial arousal, and transitions between stages of sleep. Other sleep disorders include sleep-disordered breathing (covered in greater depth in Chapter 19), restless legs syndrome (RLS)/periodic limb movement disorder (PLMD), narcolepsy, and circadian rhythm disturbances. Narcolepsy, benign neonatal sleep myoclonus, and nocturnal frontal lobe epilepsy will be covered in Chapter 25. DSM-5 no longer differentiates between primary and secondary insomnia to acknowledge the importance of managing sleep issues no matter what the perceived cause, and to recognize the bidirectional and interactive effects between sleep issues and co-occurring conditions such as attention-deficit/hyperactivity disorder (ADHD), anxiety, and depression.

Sleep is controlled by two mechanisms: homeostatic drive, that is, the increase in pressure to fall asleep over the course of the day, and circadian drive to be alert. This drive for alertness increases over the course of the morning, dips in the early afternoon, and then rises again to the highest levels several hours before bedtime. This increase in alertness prior to bedtime is often called the "forbidden zone," because it may be more difficult to fall asleep during this period. This is very important to consider when attempting to have a child fall asleep earlier than their usual bedtime. If the child typically falls asleep at 10 and the caregiver would like the child to fall asleep at 8:00, they may be asking the child to fall asleep when their body is most alert. The change would need to be made gradually. There also are two different biological clocks. The first is the circadian rhythm, the daily sleep-wake cycle. The second is an ultradian rhythm that occurs several times per night, the stages of sleep. Sleep stages vary over the course of the night and cycle every 50–60 minutes in infants to about every 90 minutes in adolescents. The daily circadian clock is longer than 24 hours. Environmental cues entrain the sleep-wake cycle into a 24-hour cycle. The cues include light-dark, ambient temperature, core body temperature, noise, social interaction, hunger, pain, and hormone production. Without the ability to perceive these cues (ie, blindness), a child might have difficulty entraining a 24-hour sleep-wake cycle.

Two major sleep stages have been identified clinically and with the use of polysomnography: rapid eye movement (REM) and nonrapid eye movement (NREM) sleep. In REM sleep, muscle tone is relaxed, the sleeper may twitch and grimace, and the eyes move erratically beneath closed lids. REM sleep occurs throughout the night but is increased during the latter half of the night. NREM sleep is divided into three stages. In the process of falling asleep, the individual enters stage N1, light sleep, characterized by reduced body movements, slow eye rolling, and sometimes opening and closing of the eyelids. Stage N2 sleep is characterized by slowing eye movements, slowing respirations and heart rate, and relaxation of the muscles. Most mature individuals spend about half of their sleep time in this stage. Stage N3 is slow-wave sleep during which the body is relaxed, breathing is slow and shallow, and the heart rate is slow. The deepest NREM sleep occurs during the first 1–3 hours after going to sleep. Most parasomnias occur during deep NREM sleep. Dreams and nightmares that occur later in the night occur during REM sleep.

Sleep is clearly a developmental phenomenon. Infants are not born with a sleep-wake cycle. REM sleep is more common than NREM sleep in newborns and decreases by 3–6 months of age. Sleep patterns slowly mature throughout infancy, childhood, and adolescence until they become adult like. Newborns sleep 10–19 hours per day in 2- to 5-hour blocks. Over the first year of life, the infant slowly consolidates sleep into a 9- to 12-hour block at night and naps gradually decrease to one per day by about 12 months. Most children stop napping between 3 and 5 years of age. In 2015, the National Sleep Foundation published recommendations for the total number of hours of sleep per day in different age groups: 1- to 2-year-olds—11–14 hours per day; 3- to 5-year-olds—10–13 hours per day; 6- to 13-year-olds—9–11 hours per day. Adolescents need 9–9½ hours per night but often only get 7–7¼ hours per night. This is complicated by an approximate 1- to 3-hour sleep phase delay in adolescence that is due to physiologic changes in hormonal regulation of the circadian system. Often, adolescents are not tired until 2 hours after their typical bedtime but still must get up at the same time in the morning. Some school districts have implemented later start times for high school students because of this phenomenon.

PARASOMNIAS

Parasomnias include both NREM arousal disorders such as confusional arousals, night terrors, sleeptalking (somniloquy), and sleepwalking (somnambulism), and REM-associated sleep disorders which are beyond the scope of this chapter.

▶ Night Terrors & Sleepwalking

Night terrors commonly occur within 2 hours after falling asleep, during the deepest stage of NREM sleep, and are often associated with sleepwalking. They occur in about 3% of children and most cases occur between ages 3 and 8 years. During a night terror, the child may sit up in bed screaming, thrashing about, and exhibiting rapid breathing, tachycardia, and sweating. The child is often incoherent and unresponsive to comforting. The episode may last up to ½ hour, after which the child goes back to sleep and has no memory of the event the next day. Management of night terrors consists of reassurance of the parents plus measures to avoid stress, irregular sleep schedule, or sleep deprivation, which prolongs deep sleep when night terrors occur. Scheduled awakening (awakening the child 30–45 minutes before the time the night terrors usually occur) has been used in children with nightly or frequent night terrors, but there is little evidence that this is effective.

Sleepwalking also occurs during slow-wave/deep sleep and is common between 4 and 8 years of age. It is often associated with other complex behaviors during sleep. It is typically benign except that injuries can occur while the child is walking around. Steps should be taken to ensure that the environment is free of obstacles and that doors to the outside are locked. Parents may also wish to put a bell on their child's door to alert them that the child is out of bed. As with night terrors, steps should be taken to avoid stress and sleep deprivation.

▶ Nightmares

Nightmares are frightening dreams that occur during REM sleep, typically followed by awakening, which usually occurs in the latter part of the night. The peak occurrence is between ages 3 and 5 years, with an incidence between 25% and 50%. A child who awakens during these episodes is usually alert. He or she can often describe the frightening images, recall the dream, and talk about it during the day. The child seeks and will respond positively to parental reassurance. The child will often have difficulty going back to sleep and will want to stay with their parents. Nightmares are usually self-limited and do not require treatment. They can be associated with stress, trauma, anxiety, sleep deprivation that can cause a rebound in REM sleep, and medications that increase REM sleep.

INSOMNIA

Insomnia includes difficulty initiating sleep and staying asleep. It can result in daytime fatigue for both the parents and the child, parental discord about management, and disruption of family routines.

Several factors contribute to these disturbances. The quantity and timing of feeds in the first year of life will influence nighttime awakening. Most infants beyond age 6 months can go through the night without being fed. Thus, under normal circumstances, night waking for feeds is probably a learned behavior and is a function of the child's arousal and the parents' response to that arousal.

Bedtime habits can influence both sleep onset and night waking. If the child learns that going to sleep is associated with calming activities such as rocking, singing, reading, sucking on a pacifier or bottle, or nursing, going back to sleep after nighttime arousal without these calming strategies may be difficult. This is called sleep-onset association disorder and is often the reason for night waking. Every time that the child gets to the light sleep portion of the sleep-wake cycle, he or she may wake up. This is usually brief and not remembered the next morning, but for the child who does not have strategies for returning to sleep independently, getting back to sleep may require the same caregiver interventions. Night waking occurs in 40%–60% of infants and young children.

Parents need to set limits for the child while acknowledging the child's individual biologic rhythms. They should resist the child's attempts to put off bedtime or to engage them during nighttime awakenings. The goal is to establish clear bedtime rituals, to put the child to bed while still awake, and to create a dark, quiet, secure bedtime environment.

The child's temperament is another factor contributing to sleep. It has been reported that children with low sensory thresholds and less rhythmicity (regulatory disorder) are more prone to night waking. Night waking often starts at about 9 months around the onset of separation anxiety. Parents should receive anticipatory guidance prior to that time so that they know how to reassure their child without making the interaction prolonged or pleasurable. Finally, psychosocial stressors and changes in routine can play a role in night waking.

Insomnia is common in children with complex medical conditions and neurologic, developmental, and psychiatric disorders.

Sleep hygiene education and cognitive behavioral therapy for insomnia are considered first-line treatments for pediatric insomnia.

SLEEP-DISORDERED BREATHING

Sleep-disordered breathing or obstructive sleep apnea is characterized by obstructed breathing during sleep accompanied by loud snoring, chest retractions, morning headaches, dry mouth, and daytime sleepiness. Obstructive sleep apnea occurs in 1%–3% of preschoolers. It has its highest peak in childhood between the ages of 2 and 6 years. It has been associated with daytime behavioral disorders, including ADHD. (See Chapter 19.)

RESTLESS LEGS SYNDROME & PERIODIC LIMB MOVEMENT DISORDER

Restless legs syndrome (RLS) and periodic limb movement disorder (PLMD) are common disorders in adults and frequently occur together. The frequency of these disorders in children is about 2%. RLS is associated with an uncomfortable sensation in the lower extremities that occurs at night when trying to fall asleep, is relieved by movement, and is sometimes described by children as "creepy-crawly" or "itchy bones." PLMD is stereotyped, repetitive limb movements often associated with a partial arousal or awakening. These disorders have been associated with iron deficiency. A diagnosis of RLS is generally made by history, and a diagnosis of PLMD can be made with a sleep study. Caffeine, nicotine, antidepressants, and other drugs have been associated with RLS and PLMD. The medical evaluation includes obtaining a serum ferritin and C-reactive protein (CRP) level as ferritin can be falsely elevated during inflammation. If the CRP is normal and the ferritin is less than 30–50 ng/mL, treatment with ferrous sulfate should be considered. Medications have been studied for treatment of RLS and PLMD in adults but not in children.

▶ Management of Sleep Disorders

BEARS is a mnemonic that has been recommended for screening for sleep problems in primary care: **B**edtime resistance, **E**xcessive daytime sleepiness, **A**wakening during the night, **R**egularity and duration of sleep, **S**leep-disordered breathing. Screening for the quality and quantity of sleep at every well-child visit has been recommended as parents may not necessarily bring up sleep issues or be aware of what constitutes poor sleep. Once a problem with sleep is identified, a complete medical and psychosocial history should be obtained, and a physical examination performed. A detailed sleep history and sleep diary should be completed by both parents. Assessment for allergies, lateral neck films, and polysomnography may be indicated to complete the evaluation, especially if sleep-disordered breathing is suspected. It is important to consider disorders such as gastroesophageal reflux, which may cause discomfort or pain when recumbent. Dental pain or eczema may cause nighttime awakening. It is also important to make sure that any medications that the child is taking do not interfere with sleep.

The key to treatment of children who have difficulty going to sleep or who awaken during the night and disturb others is for the physician and parents to understand normal sleep patterns, daytime and nighttime habits that promote sleep, responses that inadvertently reinforce undesirable sleep behavior, and the child's individual temperament traits. The **ABCs** of **SLEEPING** were developed by Allen et al (2016) as a mnemonic for typical recommendations offered to improve sleep: **A**ge-appropriate **B**edtimes and wake times with **C**onsistency, **S**chedules and routines, **L**ocation (quiet, dark, cool environment), **E**xercise and diet, no **E**lectronics in the bedroom or before bed, **P**ositivity (positive home environment), **I**ndependence when falling asleep, **N**eeds of child met during the day, equals **G**reat sleep. Good sleep hygiene includes discontinuing any activities that are stimulating in the hour before bedtime. It is also important to dim lights and avoid blue light during the "wind down" time. Red night lights are less likely to interfere with sleep. Apps are available to decrease blue light and increase red/orange light at night on computers, phones, and tablets. Exposure to light and physical activity during the day are helpful and it is important to ask about caffeine ingestion. Many recommendations for improving sleep in pediatric patients have limited evidence base.

There is little evidence regarding pharmacologic management of sleep disorders in children. Non-pharmacologic interventions should be tried first. While the role for melatonin in children with typical development is unclear, there is mounting evidence that it can be effective in children with visual impairments, developmental disabilities, and autism spectrum disorders (ASDs). Medications such as clonidine are often used for sleep disorders, especially in children with ADHD and ASD, but there are little data to support its use.

Allen SL et al: ABCs of SLEEPING: a review of the evidence behind pediatric sleep practice recommendations. Sleep Med Rev 2016;29:1–14 [PMID: 26551999].

American Academy of Sleep Medicine: http://sleepeducation.org//.

Badin et al: Insomnia: the sleeping giant of pediatric public health. Curr Psychiatry Rep 2016;18:47 [PMID: 26993792].

Braam W, Smits MG, Didden R, Korzilius H, Van Geijlswijk IM, Curfs LM: Exogenous melatonin for sleep problems in individuals with intellectual disability: a meta-analysis. Dev Med Child Neurol 2009;51(5):340–349 [PMID: 19379289].

Economou NT, Ferini-Strambi L, Steiroopoulos P: Sleep-related drug therapy in special conditions: children. Sleep Med Clin 2018;13(2):251–262 [PMID: 29759275].

Meltzer LJ, Mindell JA. Systematic review and meta-analysis of behavioral interventions for pediatric insomnia. J Pediatr Psychol 2014 Sep;39(8):932–448. doi: 10.1093/jpepsy/jsu041. Epub 2014 Jun 19. Erratum in: J Pediatr Psychol 2015 Mar;40(2): 262–265 [PMID: 24947271].

National Sleep Foundation: http://www.sleepforkids.org/http://www.sleepfoundation.org.

TEMPER TANTRUMS & BREATH-HOLDING SPELLS

 ESSENTIALS OF DIAGNOSIS & TYPICAL FEATURES

► Behavioral responses to stress, frustration, and loss of control.

► Tantrum—child may throw him- or herself on the ground, kick, scream, or strike out at others.

► Breath-holding spell—child engages in a prolonged expiration that is reflexive and may become pale or cyanotic.

► Rule out underlying organic disease in children with breath-holding spells (eg, CNS abnormalities, Rett syndrome, seizures).

1. Temper Tantrums

Temper tantrums are common between ages 12 months and 4 years, occurring about once a week in 50%–80% of children in this age group. The child may throw themselves on the ground, kick and scream, strike out at people or objects in the room, and hold their breath. These behaviors are often a reflection of immaturity as the child strives to accomplish age-appropriate developmental tasks and has difficulty because of inadequate motor and language skills, impulsiveness, or parental restrictions.

Some children tolerate frustration well, can persevere at tasks, and cope easily with difficulties; others have much more difficulty dealing with experiences beyond their developmental level. Parents can minimize tantrums by understanding the child's temperament and what he or she is trying to communicate. Parents must also be committed to supporting the child's drive to master his or her feelings.

► Management

Appropriate caregiver intervention can help the child to overcome their frustrations and grow developmentally.

Several suggestions can be offered to parents and physicians to help manage tantrums:

1. Minimize the need to say "no" by "child-proofing" the environment so that fewer restrictions need to be enforced.

2. Use distraction when frustration increases; direct the child to other, less frustrating activities; and reward the positive response.

3. Present options within the child's capabilities so that he or she can achieve mastery and autonomy.

4. Fight only those battles that need to be won and avoid those that arouse unnecessary conflict.

5. Do not abandon the preschool child when a tantrum occurs. Stay nearby during the episode without intruding.

6. Do not use negative terms when the tantrum is occurring. Instead, point out that the child is out of control and give praise when he or she regains control.

7. Never let a child hurt him- or herself or others.

8. Do not "hold a grudge" after the tantrum is over, but do not grant the child's demands that led to the tantrum.

9. Seek to maintain an environment that provides positive reinforcement for desired behavior. Do not overreact to undesired behavior but set reasonable limits and provide responsible direction for the child.

10. Approximately 5%–20% of young children have severe temper tantrums that are frequent and disruptive. Such tantrums may result from a disturbance in the parent-child interaction, lack of limit setting, and permissiveness. They may be part of a larger behavioral or developmental disorder or may emerge under adverse socioeconomic conditions, in circumstances of maternal depression and family dysfunction, or when the child is in poor health. Referral to a psychologist or psychiatrist is appropriate while the pediatrician continues to support and work with the family.

2. Breath-Holding Spells

Whereas temper tantrums can be frustrating to parents, breath-holding spells can be terrifying. The name for this behavior may be a misnomer in that it connotes prolonged inspiration. In fact, breath-holding occurs during expiration and is reflexive—not volitional—in nature. It is a paroxysmal event occurring in 0.1%–5% of healthy children from age 6 months to 6 years. The spells usually start during the first year of life, often in response to anger or a mild injury. The child is provoked or surprised, starts to cryand then falls silent in the expiratory phase of respiration. This is followed by a color change (either pallor or cyanosis). The spell may resolve spontaneously, or the child may lose consciousness, urinary continence and have abnormal movements including tonic posturing, opisthotonus, and myoclonic jerks. Rarely a spell progresses to asystole or a seizure.

▶ Management

For the child with frequent spells, underlying disorders such as seizures, orthostatic hypotension, obstructive sleep apnea, abnormalities of the CNS, tumors, familial dysautonomia, and Rett syndrome (almost exclusively in girls) need to be considered. An association exists among breath-holding spells, pica,

and iron deficiency anemia. These conditions can be ruled out on the basis of the history, physical examination, and laboratory studies. Once it has been determined that the child is healthy, the focus of treatment is behavioral. Caregivers should be taught to handle the spells in a matter-of-fact manner and monitor the child for any untoward events. The reality is that parents cannot completely protect the child from upsetting and frustrating experiences and should not try to do so. Just as in temper tantrums, parents need to help the child control his or her responses to frustration. Parents need to be careful not to be too permissive and submit to the child's every whim for fear the child might have a spell.

If loss of consciousness occurs, the child should be placed on his or her side to protect against head injury and aspiration. Maintaining a patent oral airway is essential, but cardiopulmonary resuscitation should be avoided unless asystole ensues.

Daniels et al: Assessment, management and prevention of temper tantrums. J Am Acad Nurse Pract 2012;24(10):569–573 [PMID: 23006014].

Leung AKC, Leung AAM, Wong AHC, Hon KL: Breath-holding spells in pediatrics: a narrative review of the current evidence. Curr Pediatr Rev 2019;15(1):22–29. doi: 10.2174/157339631466 6181113094047 [PMID: 30421679].

▌ WELL-CHILD SURVEILLANCE & SCREENING

The AAP Periodicity Schedule provides guidelines for surveillance and screening at well-child visits. Surveillance is a procedure for recognizing children at risk for a developmental disorder and involves asking parents if they have concerns about their child's development. Screening involves the use of standardized tools to clarify risk. The goal of screening is to optimize the child's development. However, it also demonstrates to the parent the interest their primary care provider has not only for the child's physical well-being but also for the child's developmental and psychosocial well-being. Comprehensive evaluations are done by a specialist and involve a more definitive evaluation of a child's development.

Surveillance should occur at all well-child visits. Screening of development should occur at 9, 18, and 30 months. A 30-month visit is not part of the standard well-child visit schedule and may not be reimbursed. Therefore, screening may occur at 24 months instead. Screening should increase in frequency when the child is at risk for developmental delay (eg, known genetic disorders, primary care provider (PCP) or, or parent concern for developmental delay, etc). It is also recommended that autism-specific screening should occur at the 18- and 24-month visits. Because children with ASD often experience a regression or plateau in skills between 12 and 24 months of age, some children may be missed by a single screen at 18 months. Similarly, if there is increased risk for ASD (eg, positive family history), increased frequency of screening is recommended. The Screening Tool for Autism in Toddlers and Young Children (STAT) is a second line screening tool for children who were found to have concerns for ASD on first-line screener such as the Modified Checklist for Autism in Toddlers, Revised with Follow-Up (MCHAT-R/F). The STAT includes direct interaction with the child and was designed to differentiate children with ASD from children with developmental delay. The measure and training can be found at http://stat.vueinnovations.com/about. Clinicians should keep in mind that if they are administering a screen because they are concerned and the child passes the screen, they should still schedule an early follow-up visit to ensure that appropriate developmental progress has been made and that there are no further concerns.

Committee on Practice and Ambulatory Medicine; Bright Futures Periodicity Schedule Workgroup: 2016 Recommendations for preventive pediatric health care. Pediatrics 2016;137(1):1–3.

Hagan JF, Shaw JS, Duncan PM (eds): *Bright Futures: Guidelines for Health Supervision of Infants, Children, and Adolescents*. 4th ed. Elk Grove Village, IL: American Academy of Pediatrics; 2017.

http://stat.vueinnovations.com/about.

https://downloads.aap.org/AAP/PDF/periodicity_schedule.pdf

https://www.cdc.gov/ncbddd/actearly/milestones/index.html.

Zubler JM et al: Evidence-informed milestones for developmental surveillance tools. Pediatrics 2022 Mar 1;149(3): e2021052138 [PMID: 35132439].

DEVELOPMENTAL DISORDERS

Developmental disorders include abnormalities in one or more aspects of development, such as language, motor, visual-spatial, attention, and social abilities. Problems with development are often noted by parents when a child does not meet typical motor and language milestones. However, mild developmental disorders are often not noted until the child is of school age. Developmental disorders may also include difficulties with behavior or attention. ADHD is the most common neurodevelopmental disorder. ADHD occurs in 2%–8% of school-aged children and may occur in combination with a variety of other learning or developmental issues.

Many biological and psychosocial factors influence a child's performance on developmental tests. In the assessment of the child, it is important to document adverse psychosocial factors, such as neglect or poverty, which can negatively influence developmental progress. Many of the biological factors that influence development are genetic.

The diagnostic criteria for developmental disorders are found in the DSM-5-TR. The term *mental retardation* has been replaced by *intellectual disability* (ID). The diagnostic criteria for ASDs changed dramatically in DSM-5 with some changes in the criteria for ADHD. There are also subtle changes to communication disorders, specific learning disorders, and motor disorders. These can be found at the following website: https://www.psychiatry.org/psychiatrists/practice/dsm/educational-resources/dsm-5-fact-sheets.

Evaluation

The neurodevelopmental evaluation must focus on (1) defining the child's level of developmental abilities in a variety of domains, including language, motor, visual-spatial, attention, and social abilities; (2) attempting to determine the etiology of the child's developmental delays; and (3) planning a treatment program. These objectives are ideally achieved by a multidisciplinary team that may include a medical provider, a psychologist, a speech or language therapist, an occupational therapist, and an educational specialist. This type of evaluation is ideal but not always readily available. Many times, an individual medical provider or psychologist can determine if a child meets criteria for a developmental disorder, which is more cost effective than a multidisciplinary team evaluation.

Medical & Neurodevelopmental Examination

Medical history should include the mother's pregnancy, labor, and delivery to identify conditions that might compromise the child's CNS function. This includes prenatal exposures to toxins, medications, alcohol, drugs, smoking, and infections; maternal chronic illness; complications of pregnancy or delivery; and neonatal course. Problems such as poor weight gain, chronic illnesses, hospitalizations, and maltreatment can interfere with typical development. Major illnesses or hospitalizations should be discussed. Any CNS problems, such as trauma, infection, or encephalitis, should be documented. The presence of metabolic diseases and exposure to environmental toxins such as lead should be determined. Chronic diseases such as chronic otitis media, hyper- or hypothyroidism, and chronic renal failure can impact typical development. The presence of motor or vocal tics, seizures, and gastrointestinal or sleep disturbances should be documented. In addition, parents should be questioned about any motor, cognitive, or behavioral regression.

The physician should review and document the child's developmental milestones. The physician should also review temperament, difficulties with sleep or feeding, tantrums, poor attention, impulsivity, hyperactivity, anxiety/fears, and aggression. When asking questions about problematic behaviors, it is important to have the parent describe the behavior including frequency and duration. It is also important to try to determine triggers of the behavior and consequences or potential reinforcers of the behavior (ABC—antecedent/behavior/consequence).

A detailed history of school-related events should be recorded, including previous special education support, evaluations through the school, history of repeating grades, difficulties with specific academic areas, problems with peers, and the teacher's impressions of the child's difficulties, particularly related to problems with attention, impulsivity, or hyperactivity. Input from teachers can be invaluable and should be sought prior to the evaluation.

An important aspect of medical history is a detailed family history of emotional or behavioral problems, learning disabilities, ASD, ID, or psychiatric disorders. Parental learning strengths and weaknesses, temperament difficulties, or attentional problems may be passed on to the child (eg, dyslexia).

The neurodevelopmental examination should include a careful assessment of dysmorphic features such as epicanthal folds, palpebral fissure size, shape and length of the philtrum, low-set or posteriorly rotated ears, prominent ear pinnae, unusual dermatoglyphics (e.g., a single transverse palmar crease), hyperextensibility of the joints, syndactyly, clinodactyly, or other anomalies. A detailed physical and neurologic examination needs to be carried out with an emphasis on both soft and hard neurologic findings. Soft signs can include motor incoordination, which can be related to handwriting problems and academic delays in written language or drawing. Visual-motor coordination abilities can be assessed by having the child write, copy shapes and designs, or draw a person.

The child's growth parameters, including height, weight, and head circumference, need to be assessed. Normal hearing and visual acuity should be documented or evaluated. Cranial nerve abnormalities and oral-motor coordination problems need to be noted. The examiner should watch closely for motor or vocal tics or stereotypies. Both fine and gross motor abilities should be assessed. Tandem gait, ability to balance on one foot, and coordinating a skip should be evaluated based on age. Fine motor coordination can be noted when watching a child stack blocks or draw.

The developmental aspects of the examination can include an assessment of auditory processing and perceptual ability with simple tasks, such as two- to fivefold directions, assessing right and left directionality, memory for a series of spoken words or digit span, and comprehension of a graded paragraph. In assessing expressive language abilities, the examiner should look for difficulties with word retrieval, formulation, articulation, and adequacy of vocabulary. Visual-perceptual abilities can be assessed by simple visual memory tasks, puzzles, or object assembly, and evaluating the child's ability to decode words or organize math problems. Visual-motor integration and coordination can be assessed with handwriting, design copying, and drawing a person. Throughout the assessment, the clinician should pay special attention to the child's ability to focus attention and concentrate, and to other aspects of behavior or affect, such as evidence of depression or anxiety.

Additional questionnaires and checklists—such as the Child Behavior Checklist by Achenbach; ADHD scales such as the Conners' Parent/Teacher Rating Scale; Vanderbilt ADHD Diagnostic Parent/Teacher Rating Scales; and the Swanson, Nolan, and Pelham Questionnaire-IV—can be used to help with this assessment.

Referral of family to community resources is critical, as is a medical home.

American Academy of Pediatrics Council on Children With Disabilities: Care coordination in the medical home: integrating health and related systems of care for children with special health care needs. Pediatrics 2005;116:1238 [PMID: 16264016].

Voigt RG, Macias MM, Myers SM, Tapia CD (eds): *Developmental and Behavioral Pediatrics*. 2nd ed. Itasca, IL: American Academy of Pediatrics; 2018.

ATTENTION-DEFICIT/HYPERACTIVITY DISORDER

ADHD is a common neurodevelopmental disorder that may affect about 9%–10% of children and 2.5% of adults. It is associated with a triad of symptoms: inattention, hyperactivity, and impulsivity. DSM-5 describes three ADHD subtypes: hyperactive-impulsive, inattentive, and combined. To be classified according to one or another of these subtypes, the child must exhibit six or more of the symptoms listed in Table 3–1. These symptoms need to be present in two or more settings, cause impairment in academic or social functioning and be present prior to the age of 12. A diagnosis is allowed in children with ASD, and symptom thresholds are lower in adolescents 17 and older and in adults (only five symptoms required from each category).

Most children with ADHD have a combined type with symptoms of inattention as well as hyperactivity and impulsivity. Girls

Table 3–1. Attention deficit/hyperactivity disorder.

Diagnostic Criteria:
Inattention and/or hyperactivity that interferes with everyday functioning. These symptoms have to be present in more than one setting (typically home and school for young children), not explained by developmental delay, and was present before 12 years of age.

1) Inattention: (at least 6 of the following symptoms in individuals less than 17. For those older than 17, only need 5 symptoms)
   a. Makes senseless mistakes or problems paying attention to specifics
   b. Difficulty maintaining attention to tasks (schoolwork or play)
   c. Difficulty paying attention when being spoken to
   d. Difficulty following through on instructions or difficulty completing tasks such as schoolwork, chores or work duties
   e. Difficulty organizing tasks and activities
   f. Avoids or is reluctant to engage in difficult tasks requiring sustained concentration or mental effort
   g. Difficulty with organization and often loses necessary objects like phones, wallets, school materials
   h. Easily distracted
   i. Frequently forgetful in daily activities
2) Hyperactivity/Impulsivity: (at least 6 of the following symptoms in individuals less than 17. For those older than 17, only need 5 symptoms)
   a. frequently moves their hands and/or body (fidgets)
   b. frequently has difficulty staying seated when that is expected
   c. frequently runs and/or climbs on tables, furniture etc. in settings where this is not expected
   d. Difficulty playing quietly
   e. Constantly moving or on the go. Can be described as "driven by a motor"
   f. Talks out of turn and has difficulty remaining quiet
   g. Calls out answers without being called on
   h. Has trouble waiting their turn
   i. Frequently interrupts or has difficulty with personal space boundaries with others

have a higher prevalence of the inattentive subtype; boys have a higher prevalence of the hyperactive subtype. Although symptoms begin in early childhood, they can diminish between ages 10 and 25 years. Hyperactivity declines more quickly, and impulsivity and inattentiveness often persist into adolescence and adulthood. ADHD may co-occur with other psychiatric conditions, such as mood disorder in approximately 20% of patients, conduct disorders in 20%, and oppositional defiant disorder in up to 40%. Up to 25% of children with ADHD seen in a referral clinic have tics or Tourette syndrome, additionally. Conversely, well more than 50% of individuals with Tourette syndrome also have ADHD. ADHD also can co-occur with learning disabilities.

ADHD has substantial genetic underpinings. There is strong evidence that ADHD is a disorder involving multiple genes. ADHD is also associated with a variety of genetic disorders including fragile X syndrome, Williams syndrome, Angelman syndrome, XXY syndrome (Klinefelter syndrome), and Turner syndrome. Fetal alcohol syndrome (FAS) is also strongly associated with ADHD. CNS trauma, CNS infections, prematurity, and a difficult neonatal course with brain injury are also be associated with ADHD. Metabolic problems such as hyperthyroidism can sometimes cause ADHD. These organic causes of ADHD should be considered in the evaluation of any child presenting with attentional problems, hyperactivity, or impulsivity. However, in most children who have ADHD, the cause remains unknown. Additionally, other causes of inattention and/or hyperactivity should also be considered. Particularly inattention and hyperactivity can occur with obstructive sleep apnea. Children with anxiety, learning disabilities, or language impairment can also present with inattention.

▶ Management

The treatment of ADHD varies depending on the complexity of the individual case, including comorbid disorders such as anxiety, sleep disorders, and learning disabilities. It is important to educate the family regarding the symptoms of ADHD and to clarify that it is a neurologic disorder which makes the symptoms difficult for the child to control. However, behavior modification techniques usually help these children and should include structure and consistency in daily routine, positive reinforcement whenever possible, and time-out for negative behaviors. A variety of educational interventions can be helpful, including preferential seating in the classroom, a system of consistent positive behavior reinforcement, consistent structure, the repetition of information when needed, and the use of instruction that incorporates both visual and auditory modalities. Many children with ADHD have significant social difficulties. Social skills training can be helpful. Individual counseling is beneficial in alleviating poor self-esteem, oppositional behavior, and conduct problems. In children younger than 6, a trial of behavioral therapy is recommended before considering medication treatments.

Stimulant medications (methylphenidate and amphetamine preparations) are considered first-line medication for the treatment of ADHD. They are available in short- and long-acting preparations and in tablet, capsule, liquid, and dermal patch forms. Alternative medications for the treatment of ADHD include extended-release clonidine or guanfacine, which are α_2-adrenergic presynaptic agonists and atomoxetine, a norepinephrine reuptake inhibitor. These medications can also be used as an adjunct therapy to stimulant medications. It should be noted that the stimulants are rapidly acting while alpha agonists and atomoxetine take more time for effect (ie, 2–4 weeks). A recent CDC study found that 6 out of 10 children between the ages of 2 and 17 with ADHD were taking medication for ADHD.

Seventy to 90% of children with ADHD and average intellectual abilities respond well to stimulant medications. Stimulants enhance both dopamine and norepinephrine neurotransmission, which seems to improve impulse control, attention, and hyperactivity. The main side effects of methylphenidate and dextroamphetamine include appetite suppression and resulting weight loss, as well as sleep disturbances. Some individuals experience increased anxiety, particularly with higher doses of stimulant medications. Stimulants may either exacerbate motor tics (30% of patients) or improve tics (10% of patients).

Atomoxetine is a selective inhibitor of the presynaptic norepinephrine transporter, which increases norepinephrine and dopamine, and has a similar side-effect profile to the stimulants as well as side effects associated with antidepressants. Alpha agonists stimulate postsynaptic alpha-2A adrenergic receptors enhancing signals in the prefrontal cortex. Side effects of alpha agonist include sedation, dizziness, and constipation.

Cardiovascular effects of stimulant medications have undergone significant scrutiny over the past several years and do not appear to increase the risk of sudden death, especially in children without any underlying risk. Prior to beginning a stimulant medication, it is recommended that clinicians obtain any history of syncope, palpitations, chest pain, and family history of sudden death prior to age 30 that may predispose a child to sudden death. Stimulant products and atomoxetine should generally not be used in patients with serious heart problems or in those for whom an increase in BP or HR would be problematic. Consultation with the child's cardiologist would be indicated prior to initiating stimulant use. The US Food and Drug Administration (FDA) includes this statement in the labeling of stimulants: "sudden death has been reported in association with CNS stimulant treatment at usual doses in children and adolescents with structural cardiac abnormalities or other serious heart problems." The FDA has recommended that patients treated with ADHD medications should be monitored for changes in HR or BP.

Children with autism and developmental disabilities may be at increased risk for side effects with stimulants. Because of this risk, the Society of Developmental and Behavioral Pediatrics has published medication guidelines for the treatment of "complex ADHD" (ADHD co-occurring with one or more learning, neurodevelopmental or psychiatric disorders). These guidelines can be found in the references below.

ADHD CDC: http://www.cdc.gov/ncbddd/adhd/guidelines.html.

Attention Deficit Disorder Association: http://www.add.org.

American Psychiatric Association: *Diagnostic and Statistical Manual of Mental Disorders.* 5th ed., text rev. https://doi.org/10.1176/appi.books.9780890425787.

Barbaresi W et al: Society for Developmental and Behavioral Pediatrics Clinical Practice Guideline for the Assessment and Treatment of Children and Adolescents With Complex Attention-Deficit/Hyperactivity Disorder. J Dev Behav Pediatr 2020 Feb/Mar;41:S35–S57 [PMID: 31996577].

Children and Adults With Attention Deficit/Hyperactivity Disorder: http://www.chadd.org.

FDA Drug Safety Communication: http://www.fda.gov/Drugs/DrugSafety/ucm277770.htm.

Feldman HM, Reif MI: Attention-deficit hyperactivity disorder in children and adolescents. New Eng J Med 2014;370:838–846 [PMID: 24571756].

Questions and Answers: Safety of Pills for Treating ADHD: http://www.aap.org/healthtopics/adhd.cfm.

Wolraich M et al: Subcommittee on Attention-Deficit/Hyperactivity Disorder; Steering Committee on Quality Improvement and Management: ADHD: clinical practice guideline for the diagnosis, evaluation, and treatment of attention-deficit/hyperactivity disorder in children and adolescents. Pediatrics 2019;144(4):e20192528. 10.1542/peds.2019-2528 [PMID: 22003063].

AUTISM SPECTRUM DISORDERS

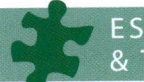

ESSENTIALS OF DIAGNOSIS & TYPICAL FEATURES

► Two core features:
  • Persistent deficits in social communication and social interaction across multiple contexts.
  • Restricted, repetitive patterns of behavior, interests, or activities.

Autism spectrum disorder (ASD) is a neurologic disorder characterized by (1) persistent difficulty with social communication and social interaction across multiple contexts and (2) restricted, repetitive patterns of behavior, interests, or activities. Table 3–2 lists the DSM-5 TR criteria for diagnosis of ASD. Features of ASD are typically present prior to 3 years of age, but some features may not be present until social demands become greater and may be difficult to recognize in an individual who has learned compensatory strategies. As with any disorder, the typical features must cause "clinically significant impairment" in function. As ASD and ID may be diagnosed in the same individual, social communication function should be impaired in relation to the individual's "general developmental level." Severity is now specified as level I: "requiring support," level II: "requiring substantial support," and level III: "requiring very substantial support."

Table 3–2. Autism spectrum disorder.

A. Difficulty with Social Communication (all 3 criteria should be met)
  1. Difficulty engaging in shared interaction with others. This can range from complete lack of initiation of social interactions to difficulty initiating and sustaining interactions and conversations.
  2. Difficulty with nonverbal communication used to promote social interaction. This can range from lack of facial expression, gestures and eye contact to difficulty integrating verbal and nonverbal communication.
  3. Difficulty with relationships with others. This can range from lack of interest in peers, to difficulty making friends, to difficulty adjusting behavior to different situations.
B. Restricted, repetitive patterns of behavior, interests, or activities (at least 2 of 4 criteria should be met)
  1. Stereotyped or repetitive movements, use of objects, or speech such as moving hands back and forth, lining up or sorting objects, or echolalia.
  2. Rigid thinking, routines or rituals such as significant difficulty with transitions or changes, severely limited food choices (only eating one brand of pretzels), need to walk in the house through the garage instead of the front door.
  3. Restricted interests that are not typical in intensity or type of focus. Examples include: Intensity of interest interferes with activities of daily living or accessing learning or social environment such as child who only plays one game on the playground, only talks about one specific topic even when conversation partner is ready to move to another topic or is not interested, or distraction by special interest interferes with attending to school work.
  4. Over or under sensitivity to sensory experiences such as loud noises, textures, or pain; or an unusual interest in sensory experiences such as textures, smell, deep pressure, or movement.

ASDs are relatively common, occurring in approximately 1 in 36 children based on surveillance data on 8-year-olds in 2020 (approximately 2.7% of children: 4% of boys and 1% of girls). This is consistent with previous data showing that autism is more prevalent in males by a ratio of about 4:1. About 31% of children with ASD also have an ID.

The genetics of ASD are complex. ASD is a heterogeneous disorder for which single gene disorders are not commonly found. About 4000 susceptibility genes for neurodevelopmental conditions have been identified. These genes often have variable penetrance and expression, as well as "pleiotropy" (one genotype associated with different neuropsychiatric or physical phenotypes such as ASD, seizures, or schizophrenia). In addition, epigenetics, gene-gene interactions, and gene-environment interactions may also play a role. A rare presumably pathogenic genetic variant can be found in 10%–30% of individuals with ASD or in up to 30%–40% who have had a "thorough clinical genetics evaluation" or have "complex autism," the term used for children with co-occurring microcephaly, seizures, dysmorphic features, or major congenital anomalies. This percentage may increase as newer techniques such as whole-exome sequencing become more widely used.

Parents of one child with ASD of unknown etiology have a 7%–23% chance of having a second child with ASD. The prevalence is higher if the second child is male, or the affected child is female. The concordance rate among monozygotic twins is high but not absolute, and there is an increased incidence of speech, language, reading, attention, and affective disorders in family members of children with ASD.

▶ Evaluation & Management

Children with ASD are often not diagnosed until age 3–4 years, when their differences in reciprocal social interaction and communication become more apparent. However, atypical communication and behavior can often be recognized in the first 12–18 months of life. The most common early characteristics are a consistent failure to orient to one's name, regard people directly, use gestures, and to develop speech. Even if one of these skills is present, it is often diminished in frequency, inconsistent, or fleeting. Sharing affect or enjoyment is an important precursor to social interaction. By 16–18 months a child should have "joint attention," with a caregiver. This is usually accomplished by shifting eye gaze, pointing, or saying "look." Toddlers should regularly point to get needs met ("I want that") and to show ("look at that") by 1 year of age. By 18 months, a toddler should be able to follow a point, imitate others, and engage in functional play (using toys in the way that they are intended to be used, such as rolling a car, throwing a ball, or feeding a baby doll).

There is mounting evidence that a diagnosis of ASD can be made reliably by age 14 months and is typically stable over time. However, there are a small percentage of children who have been diagnosed with ASD who no longer meet criteria after age 3. In addition, emerging evidence shows that about 9% of children diagnosed with ASD at a young age do not meet criteria for ASD in early adulthood. No longer meeting criteria for an ASD diagnosis by adulthood is associated with early intervention, higher cognitive scores at age 2, and a decrease in repetitive behaviors as they mature. Because there is evidence that a diagnosis made at 14–18 months is stable at age 3 and that early intervention is particularly important for children with ASD, the M-CHAT-R/F was designed for children 16–30 months of age. It is a parent report measure with 20 yes/no questions. There are clinician-administered follow-up questions for those who screen positive. Just under 50% of children who screen positive initially (M-CHAT-R/F score ≥ 3) and after follow-up (M-CHAT-R/F score ≥ 2) will go on to be diagnosed with an ASD; however, 95% will have some type of developmental concern. The Screening Tool for Autism in Toddlers and Young Children (STAT) is a second-line screening tool. For a review of early ASD screening tests, see Hyman et al, 2020.

An autism-specific screen is recommended at 18 months and at 24–30 months to verify symptoms and screen for a regression. Screening at 18 months alone could miss many of these children.

When behaviors raising concern for ASD are noted, the primary care provider should complete a thorough history and examination as discussed in the previous section on developmental disorders and the child should be referred to a team of specialists experienced in the assessment of ASD. At the same time, the child should be referred to a local early intervention program and to a speech and language pathologist to begin therapy as soon as possible. If the diagnostic features are clearly present, a primary care provider may make a diagnosis of ASD using DSM-5 criteria to start autism-specific treatments as soon as possible. All children with ASD should have a formal audiology evaluation. A chromosomal microarray (CMA) and a DNA for fragile X syndrome are currently considered first-tier tests in children with ASD. Second-tier tests such as whole exome sequencing (WES), whole genome sequencing (WGS), and autism gene panels (comprised of ~4000 genes associated with ASD and other neurodevelopmental disorders) are being used more frequently. Rare gene variants are considered to play a causal role in 10%–30% of individuals with ASD, and combinations of common gene variants are considered causal in 15%–50%. Discussion of the recurrence risk for ASD is important. In families with one child with ASD of unknown etiology, the recurrence risk is at least 4%–14%. A more detailed description of genetic workup is beyond the scope of this chapter (see the references below). Metabolic screening, lead level, and thyroid studies may also be done if indicated by the history and physical examination. Routine screening for metabolic disorders has been suggested including screening for mitochondrial disorders if there is evidence of an abnormal neurologic examination or lactic acidosis. An evaluation by a clinical geneticist should be considered. A Wood's lamp examination for tuberous sclerosis should also be considered. Neuroimaging is not routinely indicated even in the presence of mild/relative macrocephaly. Neuroimaging should be considered if microcephaly, moderate or greater macrocephaly, atypical regression, or focal neurologic signs are noted. Retrospective studies have found that approximately 20%–30% of children with ASD have a history of a plateau or loss of skills (usually only language and/or social skills) between 12 and 24 months of age. However, prospective longitudinal studies of high-risk infant siblings who are later diagnosed with ASD have found that more will have a subtle regression/plateau in skills. This is found when the study evaluates skills that are present prior to 12 months of age: eye contact, social interest, and response to name. The loss is often gradual, fluctuating, and can co-occur with atypical development. It usually occurs before the child attains a vocabulary of 10 words. If a child presents with regression, he or she may be referred to a child neurologist. Metabolic testing, magnetic resonance imaging (MRI) of the brain, and an overnight electroencephalogram (EEG) to rule out electrical status epilepticus of sleep should be considered when there is a history of regression, especially if the regression is atypical (occurs after 30 months, includes regression in motor skills, or multiple clear episodes of regression are reported).

Early, intensive (up to 25 hours per week) behavioral intervention for children with ASD is indicated for optimal cognitive and adaptive function. The cost of care and/or supports for an individual with ASD over a lifetime is estimated to be $1.4–2.4 million per person. Intervention prior to 2.5–3.5 years of age can reduce lifetime costs by up to two-thirds. Naturalistic training models for children with ASD implemented before age 3 result in 90% of children attaining functional use of language compared to 20% who begin intervention after age 5. Interventions should include parent training and involvement in treatment, and ongoing assessment, program evaluation and adjustment as needed. Interventions focus on communication, social interaction, and play skills that can be generalized in a naturalistic setting. Functional use of language leads to better behavioral and medical outcomes. Repetitive behaviors that are calming or enjoyable should not be targeted for treatment unless they are interfering significantly with day-to-day function.

The Early Start Denver Model (ESDM) is one model for early intervention that has been tested and shown significant improvement over standard of care community intervention. There are many models for this type of intervention and much variability in what is available in different areas of the country. Families should be encouraged to find a model that best suits the needs of the child and the family.

One role of the primary care provider is to ensure that medical concerns such as sleep problems, feeding problems with limited diet, and constipation often accompanied by withholding are addressed (Table 3–3). Any worsening of behavior in a child with autism may be secondary to unrecognized medical issues such as pain from a dental abscess or esophagitis. Practice pathways for primary care providers for management of multiple co-occurring conditions in children with ASD have

Table 3–3. Co-occurring conditions in children with ASD.

	Prevalence (%)
Sleep problems	50–80
Feeding/limited diet	70–90
Gastrointestinal problems	50–80
Obesity	~23
Seizures	7–38
Anxiety disorders	~22–84
Attention-deficit/hyperactivity disorder (ADHD)	~30–50
Irritability, aggression, dysregulation	~20–50
Self-injurious behavior	~30
Pica	~25
Wandering	~30
Dental	Very little data

been developed. A practice pathway for the identification, evaluation, and management of insomnia in children with ASDs stresses the importance of screening for sleep issues in children with ASD and interviewing around comorbid medical conditions that may impact sleep. Individualizing behavior strategies/sleep hygiene for the child with ASD is also very important, often requiring creativity and flexibility to adapt strategies used for children with typical development. In addition, psychiatric comorbidities such as anxiety and ADHD are common in children with ASD and should be addressed by the PCP or a specialist. Psychopharmacologic management may be needed to address issues with attention, hyperactivity, anxiety, irritability, aggression, and other behaviors that have a significant impact on daily function. Multiple recent reviews of psychopharmacologic treatments are available. A clinical practice pathway for evaluation and medication choice for ADHD symptoms in children with ASD has also been developed. Children with ASD are less likely to respond to stimulants than children with typical development and are more likely to have side effects requiring discontinuation of the stimulants. Smaller stimulant doses and non-stimulants such as guanfacine should be considered especially in children younger than 5 years, children with IQ less than 50–70, severe anxiety, unstable mood, or low weight/poor appetite. A practice pathway for the management of irritability and problem behavior (aggression toward property, self, or others) in children with ASD was published in 2016. The pathway includes evaluation for conditions that may contribute to irritability and problem behavior: medical (sleep problems, medication side effects, and management of pain or discomfort associated with gastrointestinal, dental, or other medical conditions); impairment in ability to communicate; psychiatric (anxiety, depression); environmental stressors (psychosocial, inadequate educational and behavioral supports, change in routine); and unintentional reinforcement (attention, task avoidance, removal from overwhelming sensory stimuli, or tangible reward such as giving a snack to calm the child). A functional behavioral assessment (FBA) is helpful to characterize the behavior, and to identify the antecedent and consequence associated with the behavior. Strategies to improve behavior include reinforcing positive behavior, providing supports in the environment to assist with tolerance of triggers, providing replacement behaviors for negative behaviors, and avoiding reinforcement. Risperidone and aripiprazole are the only medications that have an FDA indication for treatment of irritability and aggression in children with ASD. The practice pathway recommended consideration of clonidine, guanfacine and N-acetylcysteine prior to atypical antipsychotics when there were no significant safety concerns necessitating urgent use of atypical antipsychotics. These medications have limited evidence for safety and efficacy but appear to have fewer long-term side effects.

Anxiety is common in children with ASD with approximately 40% having at least one anxiety disorder. Anxiety can be difficult to diagnose in children with ASD due to difficulty with communication and insight/recognition of feelings and due to some overlap with symptoms of ASD. Anxiety in children with ASD can present with irritability/externalizing behaviors and with dysregulation or symptoms that mimic ADHD. A recent review of diagnosis and management of anxiety in children with ASD recommended using feedback from multiple sources such as the child, parent, clinician, therapists, and school personnel when evaluating for the presence of an anxiety disorder. Randomized controlled trials (RCTs) for treating anxiety in children with ASD show efficacy with cognitive behavioral therapy. There have been few RCTs for medications to treat anxiety in children with ASD; and the results are conflicting. Selective serotonin reuptake inhibitors (SSRIs) may be used, but clinicians should start with low doses and increase slowly while monitoring for behavioral activation. α-agonists, propranolol, and hydroxyzine can sometimes be helpful as well although there are little data to support their use. Many complementary and alternative (CAM) treatments for autism have been proposed. As many as 33% of families use special diets and 54% of families use supplements for their child with ASD based on data from the Interactive Autism Network. Most have limited evidence regarding safety and efficacy. The review of CAM prepared by the AAP Task Force on Complementary and Alternative Medicine and the Provisional Section on Complementary, Holistic, and Integrative Medicine is particularly valuable.

AAP Autism Tool Kit: Autism: caring for children with autism spectrum disorders: a resource toolkit for clinicians, 2012. www.aap.org/autism.

American Psychiatric Association: *Diagnostic and Statistical Manual of Mental Disorders*. 5th ed., text rev., 2022. https://doi.org/10.1176/appi.books.9780890425787.

Autism Speaks publishes many toolkits for families: http://www.autismspeaks.org.

Barbaresi W et al: Society for Developmental and Behavioral Pediatrics Clinical Practice Guideline for the Assessment and Treatment of Children and Adolescents With Complex Attention-Deficit/Hyperactivity Disorder. J Dev Behav Pediatr 2020 Feb/Mar;41:S35–S57 [PMID: 31996577].

Deb S et al: Randomised controlled trials of antidepressant and anti-anxiety medications for people with autism spectrum disorder: systematic review and meta-analysis. BJPsych Open 2021;7(6). doi: org/10.1192/bjo.2021.1003 [PMID: 34593083].

FDA Center for Safety and Applied Nutrition: http://www.cfsan.fda.gov/%7Edms/ds-warn.html.

First Signs (educational site on autism): http://firstsigns.org.

Golnik A, Scal P, Wey A, Gaillard P: Autism-specific primary care medical home intervention. J Autism Dev Disord 2012; 42(6):1087–1093 [PMID: 21853373].

Hanen Centre (information on family-focused early intervention programs): http://www.hanen.org.

http://www.cdc.gov/ncbddd/autism/data.html.

Hyman SL, Levy SE, Myers SM; AAP Council on Children With Disabilities, Section on Developmental and Behavioral Pediatrics: Identification, evaluation, and management of children with autism spectrum disorder. Pediatrics 2020;145(1):e20193447. doi.org/10.1542/peds.2019-3447 [PMID: 31843864].

Kemper KJ, Vohra S, Walls R; Task Force on Complementary and Alternative Medicine; Provisional Section on Complementary, Holistic, and Integrative Medicine: The use of complementary and alternative medicine in pediatrics. Pediatrics 2008;122;1374–1386 [PMID: 19047261].

Maenner M et al: Prevalence and characteristics of autism spectrum disorder among children aged 8 years—Autism and Developmental Disabilities Monitoring Network, 11 Sites, United States, 2020. MMWR Surveill Summ 2023 Mar 24;72(2):1–14. doi: 10.15585/mmwr.ss7202a1 [PMID: 36952288].

Mahajan R et al; Autism Speaks Autism Treatment Network Psychopharmacology Committee: Clinical practice pathways for evaluation and medication choice for attention-deficit/hyperactivity disorder symptoms in autism spectrum disorders. Pediatrics 2012 Nov;130(Suppl 2):S125–S138. doi: 10.1542/peds.2012-0900J [PMID: 23118243].

Malow BA et al; Sleep Committee of the Autism Treatment Network: A practice pathway for the identification, evaluation, and management of insomnia in children and adolescents with autism spectrum disorders. Pediatrics 2012 Nov;130(Suppl 2):S106–S124. doi: 10.1542/peds.2012-0900I [PMID: 23118242].

M-CHAT-RF/Validation: http://pediatrics.aappublications.org/content/early/2013/12/18/peds.2013-1813.full.pdf+html.

McGuire K et al: Irritability and problem behavior in autism spectrum disorder: a practice pathway for pediatric primary care. Pediatrics 2016;137(Suppl 2):A136–S148 [PMID: 26908469].

NCCAM sponsors and conducts research using scientific methods and advanced technologies: http://nccam.nih.gov/. [The National Center for Complementary and Alternative Medicine (NCCAM) was established in 1998.]

Ng-Cordell E, Wardell V, Stewardson C, Kerns CM: Anxiety and trauma-related disorders in children on the autism spectrum. Curr Psychiatry Rep 2022 Mar;24(3):171–180. doi: 10.1007/s11920-022-01331-6. Epub 2022 Mar 4 [PMID: 35244867].

Vasa RA et al: Assessment and treatment of anxiety in youth with autism spectrum disorders. Pediatrics 2016;137(Suppl 2):S115–S123 [PMIID: 26908467].

Vorstman JAS, Parr JR, Moreno-De-Luca D, Anney RJL, Nurnberger JI Jr, Hallmayer JF: Autism genetics: opportunities and challenges for clinical translation. Nat Rev Genet 2017 Jun;18(6):362–376 [PMID: 28260791].

INTELLECTUAL DISABILITY

The field of developmental disabilities has been evolving and redefining the constructs of disability and using new terms to reflect that evolution. The term *mental retardation* is considered demeaning; therefore, the term *intellectual disability* (ID) is used. DSM-5-TR uses the diagnosis *intellectual disability* (intellectual developmental disorder) and emphasizes the need for evaluation of adaptive function in addition to cognitive testing (IQ) to make this diagnosis.

Recently, a rethinking of the construct of disability has emerged that shifts the focus from limitations in intellectual functioning and adaptive capability (a person-centered trait) to a human phenomenon with its source in biologic or social factors and contexts. The current view is a social-ecological conception of disability that articulates the role of disease or disorder leading to impairments in structure and function, limitations in activities, and restriction in participation in personal and environmental interactions. The term *intellectual disability* reflects an appreciation of the humanness and potential of the individual. The diagnostic criteria currently remain the same.

It is important to acknowledge that significant delays in the development of language, motor skills, attention, abstract reasoning, visual-spatial skills, and academic or vocational achievements are associated with ID. Deficits on standardized testing in cognitive and adaptive functioning greater than two standard deviations below the mean for the population are considered to fall in the range of ID. The most common way of reporting the results of these tests is by using an intelligence quotient (IQ). The IQ is a statistically derived number reflecting the ratio of age-appropriate cognitive function and the child's actual level of cognitive function. Several accepted standardized measurement tools, such as the Wechsler Intelligence Scale for Children, fifth edition, can be used to assess these capacities. To receive a diagnosis of ID, a child must not only have an IQ of 70 or less but must also demonstrate adaptive skills more than two standard deviations below the mean. Adaptive function refers to the child's ability to function in his or her environment and can be measured by a parent or teacher interview using an instrument such as the Vineland Adaptive Behavior Scales or the Adaptive Behavior Assessment System. While some aspects of cognitive functioning may be slightly higher than a standard score of 70, the DSM 5-TR specifically states that the diagnosis would not be appropriate for individuals with substantially higher scores. Cognitive function tends to predict academic success and adaptive function tends to predict level of independence in daily living skills. Levels of severity ranging from mild to profound, are based on adaptive function which determines the level of supports needed.

Global Developmental Delay (GDD) is the diagnosis used for children with significant delays in at least two developmental domains (cognitive, speech and language, gross and fine motor, social, or daily living skills). This diagnosis is typically used in children younger than 5 years due to poor predictive validity of cognitive testing prior to age 5–6 years. The diagnosis of GDD is also used in children older than 5 who cannot adequately participate in standardized testing. Approximately two-thirds of children diagnosed with GDD in early childhood will go on to carry the diagnosis of ID after the age of 5.

The prevalence of ID is approximately 1%–3% in the general population and may vary by age. Mild levels of ID are more common and more likely to have a sociocultural cause than more severe levels. Poverty, deprivation, or a lack of exposure to a stimulating environment can contribute to developmental delays and poor performance on standardized tests.

▶ **Evaluation**

Children who present with developmental delays should be evaluated by a multidisciplinary team as described at the beginning of this section. The Bayley Scales of Infant Development, fourth edition, is a standardized developmental test for children 0–3½ years of age, based on normative data. For children older than 3 years, standardized cognitive testing—such as the Wechsler Preschool and Primary Scale of Intelligence, fourth edition; the Wechsler Intelligence Scale for Children, fifth edition; the Stanford-Binet V; or the Differential Abilities Scale, second edition—should be administered to assess cognitive function over a broad range of abilities, including verbal and nonverbal scales. For the nonverbal patient, a scale such as the Leiter, third edition, will assess skills that do not involve language. A full psychological evaluation in school-aged children should include an emotional assessment if psychiatric or emotional problems are suspected. Such problems are common in children with developmental delays or ID.

The evaluation of a child with ID or GDD should include a complete medical and family history; as well as a physical examination, including head circumference, neurologic examination, dysmorphology examination, and skin examination for neurocutaneous stigmata. Clinicians should also screen for co-occurring conditions such as sleep problems, feeding problems, obesity, gastrointestinal disorders, and behavioral and psychiatric conditions. Families should be offered a genetics evaluation. Expert consensus recommends fragile X molecular genetic testing and CMA as the initial workup for ID/GDD unless the child's phenotype suggests more targeted testing, as in the case of Down or Williams syndrome. If there is a family history of multiple miscarriages suggesting a possible balanced translocation, a karyotype is recommended in addition to CMA. In children with ID/GDD, CMA will be positive about 15%–20% of the time and Fragile X testing will be positive in about 2%. Families should be counseled about the possibility of CMA finding a copy number variation of unknown clinical relevance or one with clinical relevance unrelated to ID/GDD. A child with an abnormal result should receive genetic counseling from a medical geneticist or certified genetic counselor. Second-tier testing may include nonsyndromic X-linked ID genes and high-density X-CMA in males, and MECP2 deletion, duplication, and sequencing in females or testing with a targeted ID gene panel. Whole-exome sequencing may also be considered in patients for whom there is a high index of suspicion that a cytogenetic etiology exists but whose workup has been negative. An audiology evaluation should be completed, even if a child passed a hearing evaluation at birth. An ophthalmology examination should also be considered. An EEG should be considered if there are any concerns for seizures or a regression in skills.

Neuroimaging should be considered in patients with microcephaly, macrocephaly, seizures, loss of psychomotor skills, or specific neurologic signs such as spasticity, dystonia, ataxia, or abnormal reflexes. A lead level should be considered in children who frequently put toys or other nonfood items in their mouth. Thyroid function studies should be carried out in any patient who exhibits clinical features associated with hypothyroidism.

Screening for Inborn Errors of Metabolism (IEM) has a relatively low yield (0%–5%) in children who present with developmental delay or ID. Most patients with IEM will be identified by newborn screening or present with specific indications for more focused testing, such as failure to thrive, recurrent unexplained illnesses, plateauing or loss of developmental skills, coarse facial features, cataracts, recurrent coma, abnormal sexual differentiation, arachnodactyly, hepatosplenomegaly, deafness, structural hair abnormalities, muscle tone changes, and skin abnormalities. However, treatable forms of IEMs may present later or without regression or plateau. There are currently 89 "treatable" types of IEM. Treatments may target improvement in symptoms, slowing progression of the disease, or providing support during an illness. While controversy over cost-benefit of screening for rare diseases exists, van Karnebeek et al proposed a two-tiered approach to screening for treatable IEM, which is based on "availability, affordability, yield, and invasiveness." Tier 1 tests or "nontargeted screening tests" include blood tests for lactate, ammonia, plasma amino acids, total homocysteine, acylcarnitine profile, copper, ceruloplasmin, and urine tests for organic acids, purines and pyrimidines, creatine metabolism, oligosaccharides, and glycosaminoglycans. Testing for 7- and 8-dehydrocholesterol to screen for Smith-Lemli Opitz syndrome and screening for congenital disorders of glycosylation may also be included in first-tier testing. Second-tier testing usually comprises tests that are the only tests for one disease or are more invasive such as tests of cerebrospinal fluid. AAP guidelines for tier 1 tests are somewhat different and include blood tests for plasma amino acids, total homocysteine, and acylcarnitine profile and urine tests for organic acids, purines and pyrimidines, creatine metabolism, oligosaccharides, and mucopolysaccharides. An app has been developed, which is helpful for identifying appropriate tests for treatable etiologies of ID/GDD.

Serial follow-up of patients is important as the physical and behavioral phenotype changes over time and diagnostic testing improves with time. Although cytogenetic testing may have been negative 10 years earlier, advances in high-resolution techniques may now reveal an abnormality that was not identified previously. A stepwise approach to diagnostic testing may also be more cost-effective, so that the test most likely to be positive is done first.

▶ Management

Once a diagnosis of ID is made, treatment should include a combination of individual therapies, such as speech and language therapy, occupational therapy and/or physical therapy, special education support, behavioral therapy or counseling, and medical intervention, which may include psychopharmacology. To illustrate how these interventions work together, two disorders are described in detail in the next section.

Moeschler JB, Shevell M; Committee on Genetics: Comprehensive evaluation of the child with intellectual disability or global developmental delays. Pediatrics 2014 Sep;134(3):e903–e918 [PMID: 25157020].

Purugganan O: Intellectual disabilities. Pediatr Rev 2018 Jun;39(6): 299–309 [PMID: 29858292].

The Arc of the United States (grassroots advocacy organization for people with disabilities): http://www.thearc.org.

van Karnebeek CD, Shevell M, Zschocke J, Moeschler JB, Stockler S: The metabolic evaluation of the child with an intellectual developmental disorder: diagnostic algorithm for identification of treatable causes and new digital resource. Mol Genet Metab 2014 Apr;111(4):428–438 [PMID: 24518794]. www.treatable-id.org.

SPECIFIC FORMS OF INTELLECTUAL DISABILITY & ASSOCIATED TREATMENT ISSUES

1. Fragile X Syndrome

The most common inherited cause of ID is fragile X syndrome, which is caused by a trinucleotide expansion within the fragile X mental retardation I (FMR1) gene (see Chapter 37). Fragile X syndrome includes a broad range of symptoms. Children with fragile X syndrome often present with developmental delays, social anxiety, hyperactivity, and difficult behavior in early childhood. Most males will have ID with symptoms such as gaze aversion, perseverative language, hand biting, and significant hypersensitivity to environmental stimuli. About 20% of males with fragile X syndrome meet criteria for an ASD. Girls are usually less affected by the syndrome because they have a second X chromosome that produces FMR1 protein. However, due to random X inactivation, the phenotype in girls varies greatly from no symptoms to moderate ID. Approximately 30% of girls with the full mutation have cognitive deficits and a greater proportion have ADHD and anxiety. Prominent ears; long, thin face; prominent jaw and forehead; joint hyperextensibility; and macroorchidism (in boys) are common; however, approximately 30% of children with fragile X syndrome may not have these features. The diagnosis should be suspected in any child with behavioral problems and developmental delays. As boys move into puberty, macroorchidism becomes more obvious, and facial features can become more elongated. Medical conditions commonly associated with fragile X syndrome include seizures, strabismus, otitis media, gastroesophageal reflux, mitral valve prolapse, and hip dislocation.

▶ Management

A variety of therapies are helpful for individuals with fragile X syndrome. Speech and language therapy can decrease oral hypersensitivity, improve articulation, enhance verbal output and comprehension, and stimulate abstract reasoning skills. Because approximately 10% of boys with the syndrome will be nonverbal at age 5 years, the use of augmentative communication techniques may be helpful. Occupational therapy can be helpful in providing techniques for calming hyperarousal to stimuli and in improving the child's fine and gross motor coordination and motor planning. If the behavioral problems are severe, it can be helpful to involve a behavioral psychologist who emphasizes positive reinforcement, time-outs, consistency in routine, and the use of both auditory and visual modalities, such as a picture schedule, to help with transitions and new situations.

Psychopharmacology can also be useful to treat ADHD, aggression, anxiety, or severe mood instability. Clonidine or guanfacine may be helpful in low doses to treat hyperarousal, tantrums, or hyperactivity. Stimulant medications such as methylphenidate and dextroamphetamine are usually beneficial by age 5 years and occasionally earlier. Relatively low doses are used because irritability is often a problem with higher doses.

Anxiety may also be a significant problem and the use of an SSRI is often helpful. SSRIs may also decrease aggression or moodiness, although in approximately 25% of cases, an increase in agitation or activation may occur. Aggression may become a significant problem in childhood or adolescence for individuals with fragile X syndrome. In addition to behavioral management, medication may be needed. Clonidine, guanfacine, or an SSRI may decrease aggression, and sometimes an atypical antipsychotic may be needed.

Clinical trials have begun in adults and children with fragile X syndrome to evaluate targeted treatments such as metabotropic glutamate receptor 5 antagonists and γ-aminobutyric acid (GABA) agonists. These medications have shown promising results in mouse models of fragile X syndrome.

An important component of management is genetic counseling. Parents should meet with a genetic counselor after the diagnosis of fragile X syndrome is made because there is a high risk that other family members are carriers or may be affected by the syndrome. A detailed family history is essential. Female carriers have a 50% risk of having a child with the fragile X mutation. Male carriers are at risk for developing fragile X-associated tremor/ataxia syndrome (FXTAS), a neurodegenerative disorder, as they age.

It is also helpful to refer a newly diagnosed family to a parent support group. Educational materials and parent support information may be obtained on the National Fragile X Foundation website.

Fragile X Research Foundation: http://www.fraxa.org.

Hersh JH, Saul RA; Committee on Genetics: Health supervision for children with fragile X syndrome. Pediatrics 2011;127(5): 994–1006 [PMID: 21518720].

Lozano R, Azarang A, Wilaisakditipakorn T, Hagerman RJ: Fragile X syndrome: a review of clinical management. Intractable Rare Dis Res 2016 Aug;5(3):145–157 [PMID: 27672537].

National Fragile X Foundation: http://www.FragileX.org.

van Karnebeek CD, Bowden K, Berry-Kravis E: Treatment of neurogenetic developmental conditions: from 2016 into the future. Pediatr Neurol 2016 Dec;65:1–13 [PMID: 27697313].

2. Fetal Alcohol Spectrum Disorders

Alcohol exposure in utero is associated with a broad spectrum of developmental problems, ranging from learning disabilities to severe ID. *Fetal alcohol spectrum disorders* (FASD) is an umbrella term describing the range of effects that can occur in an individual exposed to alcohol prenatally. The prevalence of FASD is about 1%–5%. Thus, physicians should always ask about alcohol (and other drug) intake during pregnancy when evaluating a child presenting with developmental delays. Features associated with FASD include facial anomalies, including short palpebral fissures (≤ 10th percentile), thin upper lip, and smooth philtrum (lip/philtrum guide is available for some races/ethnicities); poor prenatal or postnatal growth (height or weight ≤ 10th percentile); CNS abnormalities including poor brain growth (head circumference ≤ 10th percentile), morphogenesis, or neurophysiology (recurrent nonfebrile seizures with no other known etiology); neurobehavioral impairment; and major congenital cardiac, skeletal, renal, ocular, or auditory malformations or dysplasias. See Chapter 37 for more information.

New clinical consensus guidelines for the diagnosis or FASD were published in 2016 by Hoyme et al (Table 3–4). The new guidelines include definitions for prenatal alcohol exposure and neurobehavioral dysfunction, an updated definition of alcohol related birth defects, a dysmorphology rating system, and a lip/philtrum guide. The guidelines provide criteria for documented prenatal alcohol exposure (see reference). The AAP's position is that no amount of alcohol during pregnancy is considered safe.

The differential diagnosis includes disorders with overlapping features like Cornelia de Lange, 22q11.2 deletion syndrome, 15q duplication syndrome, Noonan syndrome, Dubowitz syndrome, and exposure to other teratogens such as valproic acid.

▶ Management

There are currently no evidence-based interventions for children with FASD. This is likely due to small sample sizes in some studies and a lack of high-quality studies. Individuals with FASD typically have significant difficulty with complex cognitive tasks and executive function (planning, conceptual set shifting, affective set shifting, response inhibition, and fluency). They process information slowly. They may do well with simple tasks but have difficulty with more complex tasks. They have difficulty with attention and short-term memory. They are also at risk for social difficulties and mood disorders. Functional classroom assessments can be a very helpful part of a complete evaluation. Structure is very important for individuals with FASD. Types of structure that may be helpful are visual structure (color-code each content area), environmental structure (keep work area uncluttered, avoid decorations), and task structure (clear beginning, middle, and end). Psychopharmacologic intervention may be needed to address issues such as attention and mood. Most children with FASD will not have improvement in ADHD symptoms with stimulants, but a subset will respond. Amphetamines may be more effective than methylphenidate.

Table 3–4. Fetal alcohol spectrum disorders (FASD).

FASD Diagnoses	Clinical Features Required	Confirmed Prenatal Exposure
Fetal alcohol syndrome	1) At least 2 of 3 specified facial anomalies[a] 2) Poor prenatal or postnatal growth[b] 3) At least 1 CNS abnormality[c] 4) Neurobehavioral impairment	±
Partial fetal alcohol syndrome (with known exposure)	1) At least 2 of 3 specified facial anomalies[a] 2) Neurobehavioral impairment	+
Partial fetal alcohol syndrome (without known exposure)	1) At least 2 of 3 specified facial anomalies[a] 2) Growth deficiency or CNS abnormality[b,c] 3) Neurobehavioral impairment	–
Alcohol-related neurodevelopmental disorder	Neurobehavioral impairment (cannot be made before 3 y of age)	+
Alcohol-related birth defects	One major congenital malformation[d]	+

[a]Facial anomalies: short palpebral fissures (≤ 10th percentile), thin upper lip, and smooth philtrum (lip/philtrum guide is available for some races/ethnicities).
[b]Poor prenatal or postnatal growth (height or weight ≤ 10th percentile).
[c]Central nervous system (CNS) abnormalities: poor brain growth (head circumference ≤ 10th percentile), morphogenesis, or neurophysiology (recurrent nonfebrile seizures with no other known etiology).
[d]Major congenital anomalies, malformations, or dysplasias: cardiac, skeletal, renal, ocular, or auditory.

Betts JL et al: Interventions for improving executive functions in children with foetal alcohol spectrum disorder (FASD): a systematic review. Campbell Syst Rev 2022 Nov 3;18(4):e1258. doi: 10.1002/cl2.1258 [PMID: 36908848].

FASD: http://www.cdc.gov/ncbddd/fasd/facts.html.

FASD Center for Excellence: http://www.fasdcenter.samhsa.gov/.

Hilly C, Wilson PH, Lucas B, McGuckian TB, Swanton R, Froude EH: Effectiveness of interventions for school-aged-children and adolescents with fetal alcohol spectrum disorder: a systematic review and meta-analysis. Disabil Rehabil 2023 May 9:1–26. doi: 10.1080/09638288.2023.2207043. Epub ahead of print [PMID: 37158227].

Hoyme HE et al: Updated clinical guidelines for diagnosing fetal alcohol spectrum disorders. Pediatrics 2016 Aug;138(2) [PMID: 27464676].

Ordenewitz L et al: Evidence-based interventions for children and adolescents with fetal alcohol spectrum disorders—a systematic review. Eur J Paediatr Neurol 2021;33:50–60 [PMID: 34058625].

Ritfeld GJ, Kable JA, Holton JE, Coles CD: Psychopharmacological treatments in children with fetal alcohol spectrum disorders: a review. Child Psychiatry Hum Dev 2021 Jan 27. doi: 10.1007/s10578-021-01124-7. Epub ahead of print [PMID: 33502703].

Williams JF, Smith VC; Committee on Substance Abuse: Fetal alcohol spectrum disorders, American Academy of Pediatrics Clinical Report. Pediatrics 2015;136(5):e1395–e1406 [PMID: 26482673].

WEB RESOURCES FOR FAMILIES

Center for Parent Information & Resources: https://www.parentcenterhub.org/.

Family Voices (website devoted to children and youth with special health care needs): http://www.familyvoices.org.

Hanen Centre (information on family-focused early intervention programs): http://www.hanen.org.

The Arc of the United States (grassroots advocacy organization for people with disabilities): http://www.thearc.org.

Adolescence

Amy E. Sass, MD, MPH

Molly J. Richards, MD

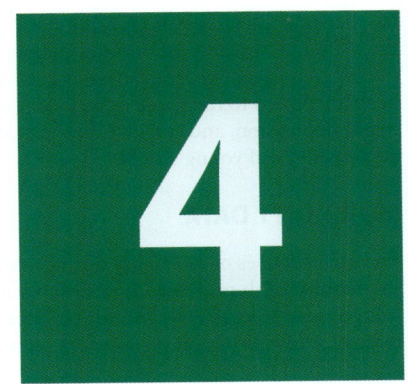

INTRODUCTION

The Centers for Disease Control and Prevention (CDC) and World Health Organization define adolescence as the phase of life between childhood and adulthood, usually between the ages of 10 and 19 years. Adolescence is a period of rapid physical, emotional, cognitive, and social development. There is considerable variability in the pace of adolescent development, and chronological age may be a poor indicator of physical, physiologic, and emotional maturity. Most teenagers complete puberty by age 16–18 years; in Western society, however, for educational and cultural reasons, the adolescent period is prolonged to allow for further psychosocial development before the individual assumes adult status. The transition to adulthood often continues through ages 20–24 years (young adulthood). The developmental passage from childhood to adulthood includes the following steps: (1) completing puberty and somatic growth; (2) developing socially, emotionally, and cognitively, and moving from concrete to abstract thinking; (3) establishing an independent identity and separating from the family; and (4) preparing for a career or vocation.

EPIDEMIOLOGY

Adolescents and young adults make up 13% of the population of the United States. Several important public health and social problems can greatly affect morbidity and mortality during these years. The most common causes of illness, injury, and death in adolescents are preventable. Cultural and environmental factors are critical in challenging or supporting an adolescent's health. The behavioral patterns established during the developmental periods of adolescence help determine young people's current health status and their risk for developing chronic diseases in adulthood.

MORTALITY DATA

In 2021, there were 13,407 deaths among adolescents aged 15–19 years, representing a rate of 62.2 per 100,000 and an 8% increase since 2020. The three leading causes of death of adolescents aged 15–19 years in 2021 were unintentional injury (37.9%), homicide (20.6%), and suicide (17.5%). The primary cause of unintentional injury death was motor vehicle crashes (62%), followed by poisoning (20%), which includes prescription drug overdoses. In the United States, the fatal crash rate per mile driven for 16- to 19-year-olds was nearly three times the rate for drivers ages 20 and older, with the highest risk for death at ages 16–17 years. Since 2000, deaths from opioid overdose have increased by over twofold among 15- to 24-year-olds. Homicide deaths were predominantly attributable to firearms (95%), and firearms were also a leading mechanism of suicide death (51%).

The mortality rate of adolescents differs by gender, with the rate significantly higher among males aged 15–19 compared to females (88 vs 35.1 per 100,000, respectively, in 2021). This reflects gender differences in the top three leading causes of death of adolescents. Among adolescent males, homicide was the leading cause of death in 2021 (2383 deaths), followed by motor vehicle crashes (1984 deaths), suicide (1780 deaths), and poisonings/overdoses (1220). Among adolescent females, motor vehicle crashes were the leading cause of death in 2021 (954 deaths), followed by suicide (563 deaths), poisoning/overdose (599 deaths), and homicide (375 deaths).

The risk of injury-related death differs significantly by race and ethnicity. In 2021, Blacks 10–19 years of age were 20 times more likely to die by homicide than white and Asian American/Pacific Islander youths and six times more likely than Hispanic youths. Death by suicide was more than twice as likely among Black and American Indian/Alaska Native youths than white youths, reflecting historic disparities that increase risk in marginalized populations. Youth suicide has become an increasingly prominent public health issue; the national suicide rate among people aged 10–19 years, overall, increased by 70% between 2007 and 2019. This has been attributed to increases in serious psychological distress, major depression, and suicidal thoughts and attempts among adolescents and young adults.

MORBIDITY DATA

The major causes of morbidity during adolescence are related to mental health or behavior (substance use, sexually transmitted infections [STIs], and unintended pregnancy). Risk-taking behavior in some areas is considered normal in adolescence, but certain types of behavior can have adverse and potentially long-term consequences. High-risk behavior in one area is frequently associated with problems in another.

The major causes of morbidity during adolescence often correlate with poverty. In 2019, almost one in five (18%) adolescents was living in families with incomes below the federal poverty line, with significant racial and ethnic disparities: 27% of non-Hispanic black children, nearly 21% of Hispanic children, and 21% of non-Hispanic American Indian/Alaska Native children live in poverty, compared to 8.3% of non-Hispanic white children. Single-parent families are particularly vulnerable to poverty. In 2019, 60% of children living in a female-headed household experienced poverty, compared with 8.4% of children living in a male-headed household and 6.4% of children living in two-parent families. Adolescents living in poverty have worse academic outcomes, are more likely to suffer from behavioral health problems and engage in high-risk behaviors, and are also less likely to have access to health care.

Centers for Disease Control and Prevention, National Center for Health Statistics: National Vital Statistics System, Mortality 2018–2021 on CDC WONDER Online Database, released in 2023. http://wonder.cdc.gov/mcd-icd10-expanded.html. Accessed March 14, 2023.
https://www.iihs.org/topics/fatality-statistics/detail/teenagers#yearly-snapshot.
Miron O, Yu KH, Wilf-Miron R, Kohane IS: Suicide rates among adolescents and young adults in the United States, 2000–2017. JAMA 2019 Jun 18;321(23):2362–2364. doi: 10.1001/jama.2019.5054 [PMID: 31211337].
Murphy SL, Xu JQ, Kochanek KD, Arias E, Tejada-Vera B: Deaths: final data for 2018. National Vital Statistics Reports; vol 69, no 13. Hyattsville, MD: National Center for Health Statistics; 2020.

PROVIDING A MEDICAL HOME FOR ADOLESCENTS

The American Academy of Pediatrics (AAP) developed the primary care medical home (PCMH) as a model of delivering primary care with the goal of addressing health promotion, acute care and chronic condition management in a coordinated and family-centered manner. Adolescent and young adults enrolled in PCMHs are more likely to receive multiple preventive services, including immunizations, screening for STIs, and contraception counseling. PCMHs that provide care for adolescents also often provide access to co-located behavioral health care and programming for the promotion of health care transition from adolescence to adulthood. Unfortunately, although many adolescents can identify a source for health care, only about half have access to a PCMH, with less access among minorities, those living in poverty, and those with multiple special health care needs. Adolescents, therefore, frequently receive care within a variety of delivery systems with varying access to comprehensive care or specialty care and from a variety of providers with diverse levels of training in adolescent care. They are often seen in pediatric clinics that may not be geared toward teens, making them feel less comfortable and less likely to continue regular care. Many only seek acute health care in urgent care or emergency room settings. Adolescents respond positively to settings and services that are adolescent-friendly and that communicate sensitivity to their age and progressing autonomy and offer developmentally appropriate, inclusive health information and educational materials.

Martone C et al: Adolescent access to patient-centered medical homes. J Pediatr 2019 Oct;213:171–179. doi: 10.1016/j.jpeds.2019.06.036. Epub 2019 Aug 6 [PMID: 31399246].

RELATING TO THE ADOLESCENT PATIENT

Adolescence is one of the physically healthiest periods in life. The challenge of caring for most adolescents lies not in managing complex organic disease, but in accommodating the cognitive, emotional, and psychosocial changes that influence health behavior. An adolescent may initially present as guarded but this is often a result of negative past experiences in a health care setting, such as feeling intimidated, judged, or unheard. It is beneficial for providers to be aware of and effectively manage any implicit biases they may have toward adolescents and adolescent health issues. The primary care provider should create a safe space for the adolescent to discuss health concerns openly. The following tips can be helpful to establish rapport with the adolescent:

1. Remember that the adolescent is your primary patient. Introduce yourself to the adolescent first and address your questions directly to the adolescent. This can be a significant change for adolescents and their families from a pediatric model in which providers engage mostly with parents/guardians. This is an important transition though may be initially challenging for both the adolescent and caregivers.

2. Show genuine interest in the adolescent, as a person and as a patient, and point out positive behaviors and

accomplishments. It is important to take a "strength-based approach," acknowledging strengths of the adolescent and not only focusing on negative behaviors.

3. Treat adolescent concerns seriously and take time to listen. Providers often get frustrated with teenagers' nonspecific somatic complaints. Discussing, exploring, and validating these complaints often reveals the primary underlying concerns that need to be addressed, including both physical and psychological issues. A shared decision-making approach often yields a more productive and cost-effective encounter.

4. Use a developmentally oriented approach. While it is important to cover sensitive topics, the provider should consider the patient's age and cognitive and psychological developmental stages. Asking questions in a developmentally appropriate manner will likely yield more useful information.

THE STRUCTURE OF THE VISIT

The Interview

It is important to introduce yourself (with your preferred pronouns) and describe your role on the adolescent care team. This is a good opportunity to ask the adolescent what name and pronouns they prefer. Then, ask a few neutral, nonpersonal questions to start to establish rapport and defuse anxiety. Describing a plan for the visit is helpful, so adolescents and caregivers know what to expect, especially if it is their first time in a specific health care setting (eg, "Today it looks like you are coming in for a sports physical. Is that correct? We'll start out talking all together about your medical history and any concerns you may have. Then, I will ask to speak with you alone, as we like to spend some individual time with all our patients.") Having the adolescent and parent/guardian complete a health history questionnaire prior to the start of the appointment is useful to identify health concerns and collect past medical and surgical historical data, medication use and medication allergies, family history of medical and psychiatric problems, and a review of systems. The questionnaire should also contain social history questions that assess healthy and risky behaviors. Adolescents often report health concerns and behaviors on a questionnaire that they may not articulate verbally. Ideally, the adolescent should complete the questionnaire privately without the parent/guardian seeing the responses, particularly about confidential risk behaviors. Although individual time with adolescents is important, caregivers remain crucial to supporting teens' health and psychosocial development. They offer vital information about the home environment, school, medical and family history, and other issues that adolescents may not know or offer. Providers should spend time talking with caregivers and may give them their own questionnaires.

Confidentiality

Confidentiality is an essential component of adolescent health care and an important part of the provider-patient relationship. Adolescents are more likely to disclose sensitive information, have positive perceptions of care, feel more actively involved in their own health care, and return for future care if physicians assure confidentiality. Despite the importance of confidentiality, many teens do not identify their primary care physicians as sources of confidential care.

While caregivers are integral to a comprehensive visit, beginning in early adolescence providers should routinely spend at least part of each visit alone with each patient to convey to young patients and their families that this is a standard part of adolescent health care. This emphasizes independent provider-patient relationships, an important step in the transition process to the adult model of care. It is essential to discuss the importance of confidentiality with teens and their caregivers as well as the limits of confidentiality, for example life-threatening concerns. Although parents have complex views regarding adolescent confidentiality, studies have shown that they support there being opportunities for adolescents to openly communicate with their providers alone. It is helpful to address confidentiality at the beginning of the visit, by speaking to the teen and caregivers together (eg, "When I talk with Sarah alone, everything we discuss is private, except if there is a safety concern. If Sarah is at risk of hurting herself or hurting someone else, or if someone is hurting her, I will share the information to protect Sarah's safety. Do you have questions about this?").

When talking with adolescents alone it is important to remind adolescents that sensitive issues are discussed because they are important for health. It can be helpful to introduce sensitive topics before asking specific questions (eg, "I am going to ask some questions about your sexual health. Are you okay with that?").

Maslyanskaya S, Alderman EM: Confidentiality and consent in the care of the adolescent patient. Pediatr Rev 2019;40(10):508–516 [PMID: 31575802].

The HEEADSSS Assessment

Health care providers who see adolescents must be able and willing to take a developmentally appropriate psychosocial history. The HEEADSSS (Home, Education/employment, Eating/Exercise Activities, Drugs, Sexuality, Suicide/depression and Safety) assessment acronym is useful for organizing this history (Table 4–1). Ideally, sensitive aspects of the history should be obtained with the adolescent alone. Providers may need to be flexible with history taking to allow for this to happen after the parent/guardian leaves the examination room. Although many of these questions assess for risk behaviors, it is important to highlight strengths and give attention to positive behaviors.

Table 4–1. HEEADSSS assessment.

	Questions	Reasons
Home and environment	Where do you live, and who lives there with you? Any changes in your family recently? Could you talk with anyone in your family if you were stressed? Have you ever run away from home?	Home life has an important impact on an adolescent's ability to succeed. It is important to know whether they live in a safe and supportive environment. Stress at home and running away from home can be high risk indicators.
Education and employment	Are you in school? What are you good at in school? What do you like about school? What is hard for you? What grades do you get? How much school did you miss last year? Have you ever been suspended or expelled? Do you feel safe in school? How do you get along with your teachers/peers? Have you been involved with bullying? What are your future plans/goals?	School is likely the primary social venue in the adolescent's life. Problems in school, academically or socially, can be an indicator of other issues (medical and/or psychosocial). Future goals and plans can be important motivators in high-risk behavior change. Some providers begin with school questions first as these may be less sensitive than questions about home.
Eating and Exercise	When and what do you eat during the day and how do you move your body? Have you been trying to gain or lose weight? Why?	Exercise and nutrition are important for adolescent health, but it is essential to screen for extreme behaviors that may influence health (binge eating, eating disorders)
Activities	Tell me about your relationships with friends. What do you (or your friends) do for fun? Are you involved in any extracurricular activities or activities in your community? Do you have a job? How many hours a week do you work? Do you play sports or exercise? What activities do you do and how often? How many hours of screen time do you have per day?	Disengagement and withdrawal can be a sign of other problems.
Drugs	Many young people experiment with marijuana, drugs, smoking cigarettes, vaping or drinking alcohol. Have you or your friends ever tried them? What did you try? What was your experience? How often do you use these things? Do you ever drive under the influence of drugs or alcohol or ride with an driver who is intoxicated?	Positive answers can lead to more in-depth evaluation of use (see Chapter 5).
Sexuality/ Relationships	Are you attracted to guys, girls, both, or neither? How do you describe the people you are attracted to? Are you in a romantic relationship or have you been in one in the past? Tell me about your partner. Do you feel you have a healthy relationship? How do you define a healthy relationship? How do you define sex? Have you (or your friends) had sex? How do you feel about it?	It is important to normalize sexual feelings even in the absence of sexual activity. Teens who are not having sex can still have conversations about sexuality, including masturbation. It is important to avoid assumptions about patients' sexual orientation and to be nonjudgmental about sexual practices.
Suicide/ depression	Have you had long periods of time where you felt down, depressed, or irritable? Have you ever thought about death, dying, or suicide?	Psychosocial history should reveal indicators of depression.
Safety	Do you feel safe at home and in school? In the past year has anyone physically hurt you? Have you been in any fights or seen any fights? Have you been involved with the law? Do you or anyone you know have access to weapons/ firearms? Have you ever been pressured or forced to have sex when you didn't want to?	Issues with safety or concern about safety can greatly influence a youth's social functioning and mental health

HEEADSSS, Home, Education/employment, Eating/exercise, Activities, Drugs, Sexuality, Suicide/depression, and Safety.

Physical Examination

A complete physical examination should be conducted at annual health supervision visits (Table 4–2). Examinations can be uncomfortable for adolescents, and this should be addressed by discussing why it is important, especially when doing sensitive parts of the examination. Adolescents should be allowed to have a support person in the room during the examination (eg, a parent/guardian). Chaperones may be needed for parts of the physical examination (breasts, genitals); the AAP recommends chaperones for genital exams but also states the use of a chaperone should be a shared decision between patient and physician. Attempts should be made to keep the examination as discrete as possible by keeping any parts of the body that are not being examined covered by a sheet, gown, or clothing.

A pictorial chart of sexual development (Figures 4–1 and 4–2) is useful for showing the patient how development is proceeding and what changes to expect. It can be helpful for adolescents to know that puberty progresses in a predictable order, but that the rate of progression is variable. This discussion is particularly useful in counseling teenagers who lag behind their peers in physical development.

Table 4–2. Physical examination of adolescents.

A complete physical examination is included as part of every health supervision visit. The following examination components are especially important in the adolescent patient:

Vital signs: Measure and plot height, weight, and BMI on CDC clinical growth charts (http://www.cdc.gov/growthcharts/clinical_charts.htm). Measure BP and evaluate according to age and height percentiles to determine the degree of hypertension per the National Heart, Lung, and Blood Institute BP tables for children and adolescents (https://www.nhlbi.nih.gov/files/docs/guidelines/child_tbl).

Skin: Inspect for acne, acanthosis nigricans, atypical nevi, tattoos, piercings, and signs of abuse or self-inflicted injury.

Spine: Examine back for scoliosis with Adam's forward bend test (also assess for leg length discrepancy).

Breast
Female: Assess SMR. Conduct clinical breast examination for breast disorders if there is a reported concern.
Male: Examine breasts if inspection shows breast hypertrophy and gynecomastia or other breast pathology is suspected.

Genitalia
Female: Perform visual inspection of external genitalia to assess SMR, anatomic and skin abnormalities, and signs of STIs (warts, vesicles, pathologic vaginal discharge).
Male: Perform visual inspection for circumcision status, SMR, and signs of STIs (warts, vesicles, penile discharge). Examine testicles for abnormalities (hydroceles, hernias, varicoceles, or masses).

BMI, body mass index (height [cm]/weight [kg^2]); BP, blood pressure; CDC, Centers for Disease Control and Prevention; SMR, sexual maturity rating; STI, sexually transmitted infection.

GUIDELINES FOR ADOLESCENT PREVENTIVE SERVICES

ADOLESCENT SCREENING

The AAP's *Bright Futures: Guidelines for Health Supervision of Infants, Children, and Adolescents* cover health screening and guidance, immunization, and health care delivery. The goals of these guidelines are to (1) deter adolescents from participating in behaviors that jeopardize health; (2) detect physical, emotional, and behavioral problems early and intervene promptly; (3) reinforce and encourage behaviors that promote healthful living; and (4) provide immunization against infectious diseases. The guidelines recommend that adolescents between ages 11 and 21 years have annual routine health visits. Table 4–3 lists the current adolescent screening guidelines from the AAP, the U.S. Department of Health and Human Services, and the CDC.

Recommendations for Preventive Pediatric Health Care; Bright Futures/American Academy of Pediatrics: https://downloads.aap.org/AAP/PDF/periodicity_schedule.pdf. Accessed June 1, 2021.
Sexually Transmitted Infections Treatment Guidelines, 2021: https://www.cdc.gov/std/treatment-guidelines/adolescents.htm. Accessed June 1, 2021.
U.S. Preventive Services Task Force, Published Recommendations: https://www.uspreventiveservicestaskforce.org/uspstf/topic_search_results?topic_status=P&age_group%5B%5D=9&type%5B%5D=5&searchterm=. Accessed June 1, 2021.

PROMOTING HEALTHY BEHAVIORS

Motivational Interviewing

A role of a pediatric provider is to screen for unhealthy behaviors and promote healthy behaviors. Providers may report feeling frustrated with adolescents if they are perceived as resistant to change. Motivational interviewing (MI) has been shown to be an effective tool for changing several health behaviors in adolescents, including tobacco use, substance use, and control of type 1 diabetes. It is a counseling style that guides patients toward behavior change by helping to resolve ambivalence. Adolescents may know that certain behaviors are bad for them (smoking, drug use, unprotected sex, eating disordered behaviors, etc) but also have reasons they do not want to change (sense of improved mood with marijuana use, use with peers, desire for weight loss, etc) and/or are not confident in their ability to change. MI promotes collaboration between provider and patient, with the patient ultimately deciding what goals the adolescent would like to achieve and how to achieve them.

MI starts with a provider assessing a patient's motivation and readiness for change (Table 4–4). These questions provide the patient the opportunity to tell the provider why it

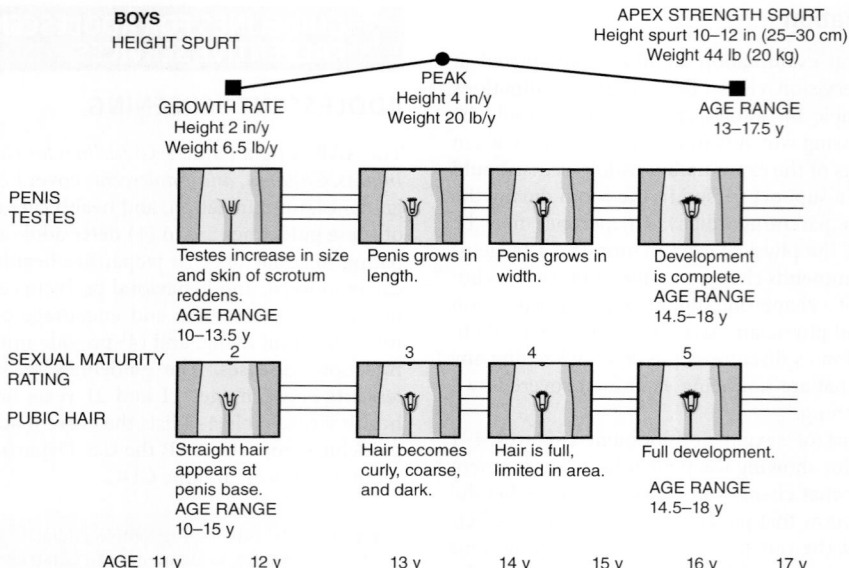

▲ **Figure 4–1.** Adolescent male sexual maturation and growth: relationship among height, penis and testes development, and pubic hair growth.

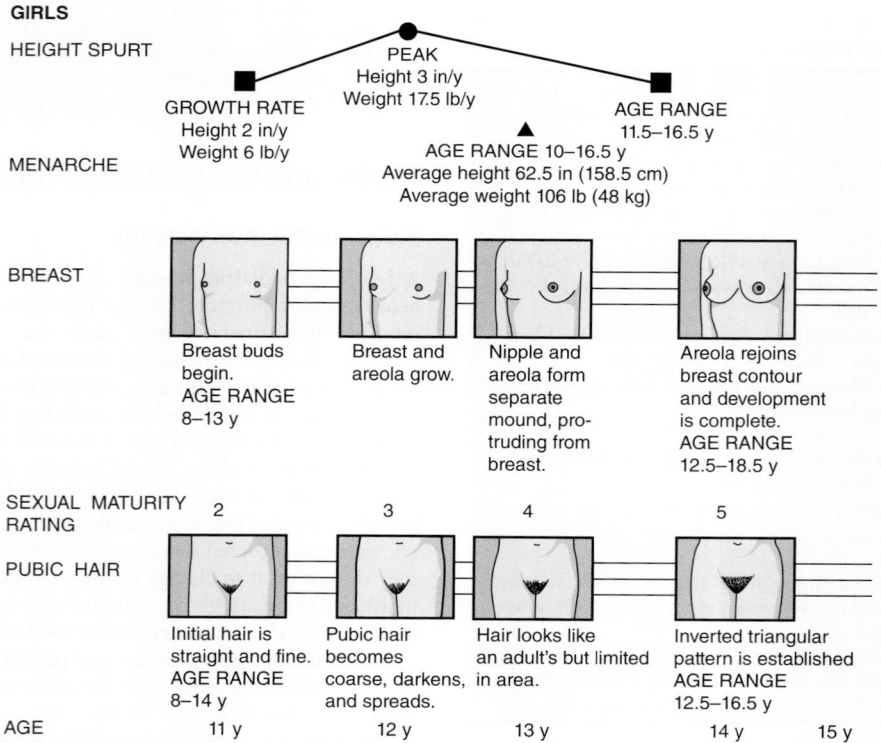

▲ **Figure 4–2.** Adolescent female sexual maturation and growth: relationship among height, breast development, menstruation, and pubic hair growth.

Table 4–3. Adolescent screening guidelines.

	AAP	USPSTF	CDC
Cardiovascular (CV)			
Blood pressure	Check annually.	Current evidence is insufficient to assess the balance of benefits and harms of screening for high blood pressure in children and adolescents.	
Lipid levels	Universal screening with lipid panel once at ages 9–11 y and once at ages 17–21 y. Selective screening at age 12–16 y if new knowledge of RFs (myocardial infarction, angina, coronary artery bypass graft/stent/angioplasty, sudden cardiac death in parent, grandparent, aunt, or uncle, male < 55 y, female < 65 y).	Current evidence is insufficient to assess the balance of benefits and harms of screening for lipid disorders in children and adolescents age ≤ 20 y.	
General Health			
Obesity	Screen BMI annually.	Screen children aged ≥ 6 y for obesity and refer as appropriate for comprehensive, intensive behavioral intervention to promote improvement in weight status.	
Diabetes	Risk-based screening for type 2 diabetes adolescents with (BMI > 85th percentile for age and sex, weight for height > 85th percentile, or weight >120% of ideal for height) and with one or more RFs (maternal history of DM during child's gestation, FH of T2DM, high-risk ethnic group, signs of insulin resistance (dyslipidemia, hypertension, polycystic ovarian syndrome, acanthosis nigricans).		
Scoliosis	Females at age 10 and 12 y. Males once at age 13 or 14 y.	Current evidence is insufficient to assess the balance of benefits and harms of screening for adolescent idiopathic scoliosis in children and adolescents aged 10–18 y.	
Anemia	Screen all nonpregnant women every 5–10 y, starting in adolescence with Hgb or HCT. Assess RFs for anemia (diet low in iron-rich foods, history of iron deficiency anemia, excessive menstrual bleeding, poverty, food insecurities) annually. Screen those with RFs with Hgb or HCT at minimum.		

(Continued)

Table 4–3. Adolescent screening guidelines. (*Continued*)

	AAP	USPSTF	CDC
Behavioral Health			
Depression	Screen youth ≥ 12 y using the PHQ2 or other tools available in the GLAD-PC toolkit: http://www.glad-pc.org/.	Screen adolescents aged 12–18 y for major depressive disorder. Screening should be implemented with adequate systems in place to ensure accurate diagnosis, effective treatment, and appropriate follow-up.	
Substance use	Screen youth ≥ 11 y with CRAFFT screening tool: http://www.ceasar-boston.org/CRAFFT/index.php.	Current evidence is insufficient to assess the balance of benefits and harms of screening for unhealthy drug use in adolescents.	
Tobacco use	Screen youth ≥ 11 y.	Clinicians should provide interventions, including education or brief counseling, to prevent initiation of tobacco use among school-aged children and adolescents.	
Sexually Transmitted Diseases			
Chlamydia Trachomatis	Per USPSTF.	Screen sexually active females ≤ 24 y.	Screen all sexually active women < 25 y, and MSM at least annually (including pharyngeal, urine, rectal testing on basis of sexual behavior and anatomic site of exposure). Consider screening sexually active young men with a high prevalence of chlamydial infections (e.g., adolescent service clinics, correctional facilities, and STD clinics).
Neisseria Gonorrhoeae	Per USPSTF.	Screen sexually active females ≤ 24 y.	Screen all sexually active women < 25 y and MSM at least annually (including pharyngeal, urine, rectal testing on basis of sexual behavior and anatomic site of exposure).
HIV	Per USPSTF.	Screen adolescents > 15 y and younger adolescents if RFs for infection present.[a]	HIV screening should be discussed and offered to all adolescents. Frequency of repeat screenings should be based on the patient's sexual behaviors and the local disease prevalence.
Syphilis	Per USPSTF.	Screen for syphilis infection in people who are at increased risk for infection (MSM, persons living with HIV, history of incarceration, history of commercial sex work, geography, race/ethnicity, male < 29 y).	Screen sexually active MSM at least annually.

AAP, American Academy of Pediatrics; BMI, body mass index; CDC, Centers for Disease Control and Prevention; DM, diabetes mellitus; FH, family history; HCT, hematocrit; HDL, high-density lipoprotein; Hgb, hemoglobin; HIV, human immunodeficiency virus; HSV, herpes simplex virus; MSM, men who have sex with men; RF, risk factor; STD, sexually transmitted disease; T2DM, type 2 diabetes mellitus; USPSTF, US Preventive Services Task Force.
[a]History of STDs, multiple sex partners, inconsistent condom use, sex work, illicit drug use, patients seeking care in high-prevalence settings (eg, clinics located in higher-prevalence geography [prevalence ≥ 1%], STD clinics, correctional facilities, homeless shelters, tuberculosis clinics, clinics serving MSM, adolescent clinics with high STD rates).

Table 4–4. Motivational interviewing skills.

Skill	Description
Assess Motivation and Commitment to Change	
Ask open-ended questions	Tell me about…., Describe for me…., Tell me more….
Explore patients' reason for change	"Have you ever tried to quit? Why did you try to quit? Do you see yourself smoking marijuana in 5 y? Why not?
Evoke change talk and reflect it back	"What are the good things about smoking marijuana? What are the not-so-good things about smoking marijuana?" When you look at this list of pros and cons, what do you think?"
Assess importance	On a scale from 0 to 10, how important do you think it is for you to stop smoking marijuana? (Unless they say 0, can respond "Why do you feel it is that important?")
Assess readiness and confidence	On a scale from 0 to 10, how ready do you think you are to stop smoking marijuana? How confident are you that you can stop smoking marijuana? (Based on answers, can assess barriers to readiness/confidence.)
Affirm and accept	Affirmations are statements that provide positive feedback about goal-oriented behaviors or personal characteristics or strengths, reinforcing autonomy and self-efficacy. "I can see that you are upset about being here, but I'd like to tell you that I am impressed that you chose to come here anyway."
Listen reflectively	Reflective listening shows that you are listening and understanding. Patient: "I know it really upsets my parents, but it just isn't that big a deal." Provider: "You don't think it's such a big deal, but you know that your parents are really worried about you and it sounds like you feel badly about that."
Express empathy	"You've worked hard on this problem and it's frustrating you that it's not much better yet."
Develop discrepancies	"You do not want to quit marijuana because most of your friends smoke and you think it helps you relax, and, at the same time, you know it makes your parents angry and you want to play football and are worried it will get you in trouble with your coach."
Roll with resistance	Accept patients' statements of resistance rather than confronting them directly: Patient: "Most of the people I know get high. Why do we even have to talk about it?" Provider: "It's hard to figure out why we have to talk about it when it is all around you. Kind of makes you wonder how you could be the only one who is having problems with pot."
Avoid righting reflex	Avoid the desire to fix things, direct persuasion, and confrontation.
Support self-efficacy	Increase patient perception about his/her skills, resources, and abilities that the patient may access to achieve desired goals. "You say you quit before so you may have good ideas about how to do it again. Tell me what they are."
Encourage autonomy	Convey that responsibility for making change resides with the patient or parent who must decide if, how, and when change will occur.
Encourage self-direction	Patient: "I know I made a mistake, but the hoops that they are making me jump through are getting ridiculous." Provider: "You don't like what others are asking you to do, but so far you are choosing to follow-through with what they are asking. It takes a lot of fortitude to do that. Tell me what motivates you."

is important to change, rather than telling the provider convincing reasons why it is not important to make changes. This "change talk" is a hallmark of MI. The provider should avoid asking the adolescent why it is *not* important, as that will put the patient in the position of indicating reasons the adolescent cannot or does not want to change. Other components of MI are to "roll with resistance" and resist the "righting reflex." Providers often seek to fix problems or challenge patients' stated barriers, causing patients to come up with new reasons they cannot make changes. If the provider is the

only one arguing in favor of change, patients and families can become even more entrenched in not changing. Instead of progressing into this conflictual stance, the provider should focus on the patient's own individual goals and reflect on the patient's challenges. Developing discrepancies is another MI strategy. This can be done by asking a patient about specific health goals and the future and how the teen feels these goals align with current health and/or behaviors (eg, failing school and wanting to go to medical school; vaping and wanting to be an athlete). Supporting self-efficacy and using the patient's solutions to break down barriers to change are important, as they will bring longer lasting change. Most essential is for the provider to listen reflectively, avoid confrontation, and roll with resistance.

The guiding principles of MI are to express empathy and meet patients where they are in the process of change, as many patients are ambivalent. It can be frustrating to see patients putting their health at risk, but it is important, when appropriate, to meet patients where they are in their readiness to change. This allows them to find their internal motivations, encourages autonomy, and establishes collaboration between patients and providers in achieving healthy and attainable goals. MI seeks to progress through stages of change (precontemplative, contemplative, preparation, action), but with the understanding that the provider cannot force a patient into a stage that the teen is not ready for. Instead of imposing goals and being disappointed or frustrated when these goals are not accomplished, a patient needs to make goals independently if motivated to do so, even if the goals seem insignificant to the provider. It is acceptable to take time to work through this process as long as there is no acute danger. In situations of medical or psychiatric instability, MI is not an appropriate tool.

Naar S, Mariann S: *Motivational Interviewing With Adolescents and Young Adults*. 2nd ed. New York, NY: The Guildford Press; 2021.

TRANSITION TO ADULT CARE

It is important for health care providers to have a process for transitioning primary and subspecialty medical care of adolescents to adult providers. This process should incorporate education, guidance, and stepwise planning. Patients should be actively involved in this process to maximize their self-efficacy. The AAP clinical report, "Supporting the Health Care Transition From Adolescence to Adulthood in the Medical Home" describes the Six Core Elements, a structured process that can be customized for use (Table 4–5). The final step of transition occurs when the provider implements an adult care model or the patient transfers to an adult medical home provider. Direct communication between pediatric and adult providers is essential for a smooth transition, especially in the case of patients with special needs.

White PH, Cooley WC; Transitions Clinical Report Authoring Group; American Academy of Pediatrics; American Academy of Family Physicians; American College of Physicians: Supporting the health care transition from adolescence to adulthood in the medical home. Pediatrics 2018 Nov;142(5):e20182587. doi: 10.1542/peds.2018-2587. Epub 2018 Oct 22. Erratum in: Pediatrics 2019 Feb;143(2) [PMID: 30348754].

Table 4–5. Transition to adult care.

Transition Policy and Monitoring/Tracking Transition Readiness
- Discuss policies addressing transition with patients and families early and regularly. This can be accomplished with handouts and direct conversations.
- Assess patients regularly for transition readiness (often with use of checklists).
- Document patient readiness and steps needed to achieve successful transition (eg, ability to schedule appointments, obtain medications, know medications and doses).
- Track progress on transition preparedness/readiness.

Transition Planning
- Educate and communicate with families about transition process and differences between pediatric and adult models of care.
- Patient must be the driver of transition process.
- Health care team should empower and encourage youth to assume increasing responsibility for their own health care as their development progresses.

Transfer of Care
- Develop transition plan which includes needed readiness skills and medical summary.
- Communicate with new clinician.

GROWTH & DEVELOPMENT

PUBERTY

Puberty is defined as the time when a child develops secondary sexual characteristics and reproductive function. Pubertal growth and physical development are a result of activation of the hypothalamic-pituitary-gonadal axis in late childhood. Before puberty, pituitary and gonadal hormone levels are low. It is estimated that at least 50% of pubertal timing is determined by genetics, including ethnicity. Nutrition and general health can also affect the pubertal process. Teenagers began entering puberty earlier in the last century because of better nutrition and socioeconomic conditions.

At onset of puberty, inhibition of gonadotropin-releasing hormone (GnRH) in the hypothalamus is removed, allowing pulsatile production of GnRH, which signals release of the gonadotropins, luteinizing hormone (LH), and follicle-stimulating hormone (FSH) from the anterior pituitary. In early to middle adolescence, pulse frequency and amplitude of LH and FSH secretion increase, stimulating the gonads to produce estrogen or testosterone.

In females, FSH stimulates ovarian maturation, granulosa cell function, and estradiol secretion. LH is important in ovulation, corpus luteum formation, and progesterone secretion. Initially, estradiol inhibits the release of LH and FSH. Eventually, estradiol becomes stimulatory, and the secretion of LH and FSH becomes cyclic. Estradiol levels progressively increase, resulting in maturation of the female genital tract and breast development.

In males, LH stimulates the interstitial cells of the testes to produce testosterone. FSH stimulates the production of spermatocytes in the presence of testosterone. The testes also produce inhibin, a Sertoli cell protein that inhibits the secretion of FSH. During puberty, circulating testosterone levels increase more than 20-fold. Levels of testosterone correlate with the physical stages of puberty and the degree of skeletal maturation.

PHYSICAL GROWTH

A teenager's weight almost doubles in adolescence, and height increases by 15%–20%. During puberty, major organs double in size, except for lymphoid tissue, which decreases in mass. Before puberty, there is little difference in the muscular strength of boys and girls. Muscle mass and muscle strength both increase during puberty, with maximal strength lagging the increase in mass by many months. Boys attain greater mass and strength, and strength continues to increase into late puberty. In boys, the lean body mass increases from 80% to 85% of body weight to approximately 90% at maturity, and muscle mass doubles between 10 and 17 years. In contrast, the lean body mass decreases in girls from approximately 80% of body weight in early puberty to approximately 75% at maturity. Skeletal maturation correlates well with growth and pubertal development. Motor coordination lags growth in stature and musculature, but it continues to improve as strength increases.

There is great variability in the timing and onset of puberty and growth, and psychosocial development does not always parallel physical changes. Chronologic age, therefore, may be a poor indicator of physiologic and psychosocial development. The pubertal growth spurt begins nearly 2 years earlier in girls than in boys. Girls reach peak height velocity between ages 11½ and 12 years, and boys between ages 13½ and 14 years. Linear growth at peak velocity is 9.5 cm/y ± 1.5 cm in boys and 8.3 cm/y ± 1.2 cm in girls. Pubertal growth lasts about 2–4 years and continues longer in boys than in girls. By age 11 years in girls and age 12 years in boys, 83%–89% of ultimate height is attained. An additional 18–23 cm in females and 25–30 cm in males is achieved during late pubertal growth. Following menarche, height rarely increases more than 5–7.5 cm. Males' ability to grow 2 more years prior to peak height velocity and their greater average velocity allows them to leave puberty an average of 13 cm taller than females despite their entering puberty at similar heights.

SEXUAL MATURATION

Sexual maturity rating (SMR) is useful for categorizing genital development. Figures 4–1 and 4–2 show the chronologic development of pubic hair growth, penis, and testis development in boys and breast maturation in girls and age ranges

of normal development. SMR 1 is prepuberty and SMR 5 is adult maturity. In SMR 2, pubic hair is sparse, fine, nonpigmented, and downy; in SMR 3, the hair becomes pigmented and curly and increases in amount; and in SMR 4, the hair is adult in texture but limited in area. The appearance of pubic hair precedes axillary hair by more than 1 year.

Although the first measurable sign of puberty in girls is the beginning of the height spurt, the first conspicuous sign is usually development of breast buds between 8 and 11 years. A large longitudinal study reported a median age of thelarche of 8.8 years for black, 9.3 years for Hispanic, and 9.7 years for Caucasian and Asian girls. Higher body mass index (BMI) was associated with earlier attainment of SMR 2. Although breast development usually precedes growth of pubic hair, the order may be reversed. Female breast development follows a predictable sequence. Small, raised breast buds appear in SMR 2. In SMR 3, the breast and areolar tissue generally enlarge and become elevated. The areola and nipple form a separate mound from the breast in SMR 4, and in SMR 5, the areola assumes the same contour as the breast. A common concern for girls at this time is whether the breasts will be of the right size and shape, especially because initial breast growth is often asymmetrical. The growth spurt may precede breast and pubic hair development by approximately 1 year. Girls gain their peak height velocity during SMR 2, at an average age of 11.5 years. Girls who mature early will reach peak height velocity sooner and attain their final height earlier. Girls who mature later will attain a greater final height because of the longer period of growth before the growth spurt ends. Final height is related to skeletal age at onset of puberty as well as genetic factors. The height spurt correlates more closely with breast developmental stages than with pubic hair stages. In the United States, the average age at menarche is 12.5 and usually occurs during SMR 3 or 2 years after breast budding. The range is variable, from 9 to 15 years, and depends on many factors including race and ethnicity as well as nutrition and genetics.

The first sign of puberty in the male (SMR 2) is an increase in testicular volume to 4 mL or 2.5 cm in the long axis, accompanied by reddening and thickening of the scrotal skin; these changes usually occur between ages 10 and 12 years. Pubic hair development may be the earliest noticeable sign of puberty and may appear anytime between ages 10 and 15 years. The penis begins to grow significantly a year or so after the onset of testicular and pubic hair development. In SMR 3, the penis lengthens, and in SMR 4, the penis enlarges in overall size and the scrotal skin becomes pigmented. The first ejaculation, along with evidence of spermarche, usually occurs at in SMR 3. The height spurt begins at age 11 years but increases rapidly between ages 12 and 13 years, with the peak height velocity reached at age 13½ years (SMR 3–4). As with girls, there are racial and ethnic differences in pubertal onset. Mean ages for genital development are 10.14 years for non-Hispanic white boys, 9.14 years for black boys, and 10.04 years for Hispanic boys. The average length of time for genital development is 3 years but can range from 2 to 5 years, and the average age at completion is 15 years. Development of axillary hair, deepening of the voice, and the development of chest hair in boys usually occur in mid-puberty, about 2 years after onset of growth of pubic hair. Facial and body hair begin to increase at age 16–17 years. The duration of pubertal development lasts longer in boys than girls and may not be completed until age 18 years.

Biro FM et al: Age of menarche in a longitudinal US cohort. J Pediatr Adolesc Gynecol 2018;31(4):339–345 [PMID: 29758276].
Herman-Giddens ME et al: Secondary sexual characteristics in boys: data from the Pediatric Research in Office Settings Network. Pediatrics 2012;130(5):e1058e1068 [PMID: 23085608].

PSYCHOSOCIAL DEVELOPMENT

Adolescence is a period of progressive individuation and separation from the family. Adolescents must learn who they are, decide what they want to do, and identify their personal strengths and weaknesses. Because of the rapidity of physical, emotional, cognitive, and social growth during adolescence, it is useful to divide psychological development into three phases (Table 4–6). Early adolescence is roughly from 10 to 13 years of age; middle adolescence is from 14 to 16 years; and late adolescence is from 17 years and later.

Early Adolescence

Early adolescence is characterized by rapid growth and development of secondary sex characteristics. Body image, self-concept, and self-esteem fluctuate dramatically. Concerns about how personal growth and development deviate from that of peers may be significant. Although there is a certain curiosity about sexuality, young adolescents generally feel more comfortable with peers who identify as the same gender. Peer relationships become increasingly important. Young teenagers still think concretely and cannot easily conceptualize about the future. They may have vague and unrealistic professional goals, such as becoming a movie star or professional athlete.

Middle Adolescence

During middle adolescence, as rapid pubertal development subsides, teenagers become more comfortable with their new bodies. Intense emotions and wide swings in mood are typical. Although some teenagers go through this experience relatively peacefully, others struggle. Cognitively, the middle adolescent moves from concrete thinking to formal operations and abstract thinking. With this new mental power comes a sense of omnipotence and a belief that the world can be changed by merely thinking about it. Sexually active teenagers may believe they do not need to worry about using contraception because they can't get pregnant ("it won't happen to me"). With the onset of abstract thinking, teenagers

Table 4–6. Stages of adolescent psychosocial development.

Stages of Adolescence	Cognitive Development	Social-Emotional Development
Early adolescence: ~10–13 y	• Growing capacity for abstract thought • Interested in present, limited thought to future • Intellectual interests expand • Deeper moral thinking	• Struggle with sense of identity • Worries about being normal, feels awkward about self and body • Realize parents aren't perfect; increased conflict with parents • Desire for independence • Tendency to return to "childish" behavior especially when stressed • Moodiness • Rule and limit testing • Greater interest in privacy
Middle adolescence: ~14–16 y	• Continued growth of capacity for abstract thought • Greater capacity for setting goals • Interest in moral reasoning • Thinking about meaning of life	• Intense self-involvement • Continued adjustment to changing body and worries about being normal • Distance from parents, drive for independence • Peers gain importance • Feelings of love and passion
Late adolescence: ~ ≥ 17 y	• Ability to think ideas through • Ability to delay gratification • Examination of inner experiences • Increased concern for future • Continued interest in moral reasoning	• Firmer sense of identity • Increased emotional stability • Increased concern for others • Increased independence and self-reliance • Peer relationships remain important • Development of more serious relationships

Data from American Academy of Child and Adolescent's Facts for Families (2017).

begin to see themselves as others see them and may become extremely self-centered. Because they are establishing their own identities, relationships with peers and others are narcissistic. Experimenting with different self-images is common. As sexuality increases in importance, adolescents may begin dating and experimenting with sex. Peers determine the standards for identification, behavior, activities, and clothing and provide emotional support, intimacy, empathy, and the sharing of guilt and anxiety during the struggle for autonomy. The struggle for independence and autonomy is often a stressful period for both teenagers and parents.

Late Adolescence

During late adolescence, the young person generally becomes less self-centered and more caring for others. Social relationships shift from the peer group to the individual. Dating becomes much more intimate. In 2021, 16% of adolescents in 9th grade reported having sexual intercourse, and 48% by 12th grade. Abstract thinking allows older adolescents to think more realistically about their plans for the future. This is a period of idealism; older adolescents have rigid concepts of what is right or wrong.

Gender Identity and Expression

Gender identity is one's internal sense of who one is. The identity may be male, female, somewhere in between, a combination of both, or neither (ie, not conforming to a binary conceptualization of gender). Self-recognition of gender identity develops over time, and, for some people, gender identity can be fluid and shifting. Gender expression refers to the wide array of ways people display their gender through clothing, hair styles, mannerisms, or social roles. A gender nonconforming person expresses one's gender(s) differently from how family, culture, or society expects the individual to behave, dress, and act. A transgender person has deep awareness that one's gender identity differs from the sex that was assigned at birth. This incongruence may lead to gender dysphoria, which includes a strong desire to be of the identified gender(s) and is associated with significant psychological distress or impairment in social, occupational, or other areas of functioning. Transition is the process of shifting toward a gender role different from that assigned at birth, which can include social transition, such as new names, pronouns, and clothing, and/or medical transition, such as hormone therapy and gender affirming surgery.

Sexual Orientation and Sexuality

In addition to rapid physical changes during puberty, adolescence is also characterized by emotional and sexual changes during which sexual discovery, exploration, and experimentation are part of the process of incorporating sexuality into one's identity. Sexual orientation is the preferred term used when referring to a person's sexual identity in relation to the gender(s) to which they are attracted. Typically, sexual orientation emerges before or early in adolescence. Individuals who self-identify as heterosexuals are attracted to people of the opposite gender, homosexual individuals self-identify as being attracted to people of the same gender, and bisexual adolescents report attraction to both genders. Generally, self-identified homosexual people are referred to as "gay" if male and "lesbian" if female. Some people who have same-sex attractions or relationships may identify as "queer." Some people, for a range of personal, social, or political reasons, may choose not to self-identify with these or any labels. Sexuality and identity formation are dynamic processes and adolescents who struggle with their sexual attractions are referred to as "questioning." Overall, adolescents who self-identify as lesbian, gay, bisexual, transgender, queer, or questioning (LGBTQ+) comprise a sexual minority population.

Heterosexism is the societal expectation that heterosexuality is the norm and that LGBTQ+ youth are "abnormal." Some LGBTQ+ youth may feel that it is necessary to hide their sexuality from family and friends, and this nondisclosure can be ultimately damaging to a developing self-image. For LGBTQ+ people, coming out is the process of self-identifying and self-acceptance that entails the sharing of their identity with others. Coming out can be an incredibly personal and transformative lifelong process. As health care providers, it is critical to respect where each person is within the process of self-identification; it is up to each person to decide if and when and to whom to come out or disclose. Parents' and other family members' reactions to a young person "coming out" or declaring his or her self-identified sexuality vary; parental rejection of sexual minority youth is, unfortunately, common.

Although many LGBTQ+ youth are resilient, they are a vulnerable population and experience many health disparities. Population studies and public health data demonstrate that sexual minority youth are at increased risk of tobacco and substance abuse, being victims of violence including bullying and physical and sexual abuse, STI and HIV acquisition, school avoidance and failure, depression and suicide, homelessness, and other crises. As part of providing culturally effective care to reduce health disparities experienced by sexual minority youth, providers should ask their patients what their preferred pronouns are pertaining to their gender identity and encourage adolescents to discuss any questions they have about their sexual orientation and/or sexual behaviors. Providers will optimize opportunities to learn about youth's behaviors by creating an accepting environment and providing nonjudgmental and confidential care. For transgender youth, providers should affirm feelings of gender dysphoria and provide referrals to qualified mental health and medical professionals for information about gender transition. Providers can also be sources of support for parents and family members of sexual minority youth. Organizations such as the AAP (healthychildren.org) and PFLAG (www.pflag.org) provide valuable resources. Local LGBTQ+ and sexual health advocacy organizations are additional resources for sexual minority youth and their families.

Centers for Disease Control and Prevention: 2021 Youth Risk Behavior Survey Data. www.cdc.gov/yrbs. Accessed May 1, 2023.

Rafferty J; Committee on Psychosocial Aspects of Child and Family Health; Committee on Adolescence; Section on Lesbian, Gay, Bisexual, and Transgender Health and Wellness: Ensuring comprehensive care and support for transgender and gender-diverse children and adolescents. Pediatrics 2018 Oct;142(4):e20182162. Epub 2018 Sep 17 [PMID: 30224363].

Society for Adolescent Health and Medicine: Promoting health equality and nondiscrimination for transgender and gender-diverse youth. J Adolesc Health 2020;66(6):761–765 [PMID: 32473724].

Society for Adolescent Health and Medicine: Recommendations for promoting the health and well-being of lesbian, gay, bisexual, and transgender adolescents: a position paper of the Society for Adolescent Health and Medicine. J Adolesc Health 2013;52(4):506–510 [PMID: 23521897].

ADOLESCENT GYNECOLOGY & REPRODUCTIVE HEALTH

BREAST EXAMINATION

Screening clinical breast examinations are not recommended for breast cancer screening in women younger than 25 years per the American College of Obstetricians and Gynecologists (ACOG). Breast self-examination, self-inspection of a woman's breasts on a regular, repetitive basis for the purpose of detecting breast cancer, is no longer recommended. In contrast, breast self-awareness, defined as a woman's awareness of the normal appearance and feel of her breasts and being attuned to changes or potential problems that should prompt medical attention, is recommended. Young women can be educated by their primary care provider about normal breast physiology and changes during puberty as well as signs and symptoms that may represent a breast problem such as pain, a mass, new onset of nipple discharge, or redness in their breasts.

If a patient has a breast complaint and a breast exam is necessary, the examination begins with inspection of the breasts for symmetry and SMR stage. Asymmetrical breast development is common in young adolescents and is generally transient, although 25% of women may continue to have asymmetry as adults. Organic causes of breast asymmetry include unilateral breast hypoplasia, amastia, absence of the pectoralis major muscle, and unilateral juvenile hypertrophy, in which there is rapid overgrowth of breast tissue usually immediately after thelarche. Next, with the patient supine and the ipsilateral arm placed behind the head, the examiner palpates the breast tissue using flat finger pads in concentric circles starting at the outer borders of the breast tissue along the sternum, clavicle, and axilla and then moving in toward the areola. The areola should be compressed gently to check for nipple discharge. Supraclavicular and infraclavicular and axillary regions should be palpated for lymph nodes.

BREAST MASSES

ESSENTIALS OF DIAGNOSIS & TYPICAL FEATURES

► Primary breast cancer during adolescence is exceptionally rare.

► Fibroadenomas are the most common breast masses.

► Typical features of fibroadenomas include 2–3 cm, nontender, rubbery, smooth, well-circumscribed, mobile mass.

Most breast masses in adolescents are benign (Tables 4–7 and 4–8). Rare malignancies in adolescent girls include juvenile secretory carcinoma, intraductal carcinoma, rhabdomyosarcoma, malignant cystosarcoma phyllodes, and metastatic tumor.

Table 4–7. Breast masses in adolescent females.

Common
Fibroadenoma
Fibrocystic changes
Breast cysts (including subareolar cysts)
Breast abscess or mastitis
Fat necrosis (after trauma)
Less common (benign)
Lymphangioma
Hemangioma
Intraductal papilloma
Juvenile papillomatosis
Giant fibroadenoma
Neurofibromatosis
Nipple adenoma or keratoma
Mammary duct ectasia
Intramammary lymph node
Lipoma
Hematoma
Hamartoma
Galactocele
Rare (malignant or malignant potential)
Juvenile secretory carcinoma
Intraductal carcinoma
Cystosarcoma phyllodes
Sarcomas (fibrosarcoma, malignant fibrous histiocytoma, rhabdomyosarcoma)
Metastatic cancer (hepatocellular carcinoma, lymphoma, neuroblastoma, rhabdomyosarcoma)

Table 4–8. Characteristics and management of breast lesions in adolescent females.

Fibroadenoma	2- to 3-cm, rubbery, well-circumscribed, mobile, nontender. Commonly found in upper outer quadrant of the breast. Management is observation.
Giant juvenile fibroadenoma	Large, > 5 cm fibroadenoma with overlying skin stretching and dilated superficial veins. Benign but requires excision for confirmation of diagnosis and for cosmetic reasons.
Breast cysts	Usually caused by ductal ectasia or blocked Montgomery tubercles, both of which can have associated nipple discharge. Ultrasound can help differentiate from solid mass. Most resolve spontaneously.
Fibrocystic changes	More common with advancing age after adolescence. Mild swelling and palpable nodularity in upper outer quadrants. Associated with cyclic premenstrual mastalgia.
Abscess	Often associated with overlying mastitis and/or purulent nipple discharge. Culture abscess material and/or nipple discharge before starting antibiotics.
Cystosarcoma phyllodes	Large, rapidly growing tumor associated with overlying skin changes, dilated veins, and skin necrosis. Requires excision. Most often benign but can be malignant.
Intraductal papilloma	Palpable intraductal tumor, which is often subareolar with associated nipple discharge, but may be in the periphery of the breast in adolescents. Requires surgical excision.
Juvenile papillomatosis	Rare breast tumor characterized by a grossly nodular breast mass described as having a "Swiss-cheese" appearance. Requires surgical excision.
Fat necrosis	Localized inflammatory process in the breast; typically follows trauma (sports or seat belt injuries). Subsequent scarring may be confused with changes similar to those associated with malignancy.

Retrospective studies indicate that biopsies of breast masses in adolescents most commonly show fibroadenoma (67%), fibrocystic change (15%), and abscess or mastitis (3%).

1. Fibroadenoma

Fibroadenomas are the most common breast masses of adolescent girls. Fibroadenomas are composed of glandular and fibrous tissue. They are typically nontender and diagnosed clinically based on examination findings of rubbery, smooth, well-circumscribed, mobile masses most often in the upper outer quadrant of the breast, although fibroadenomas can be found in any quadrant. Ten to twenty-five percent of girls will have multiple or bilateral lesions. Fibroadenomas are typically slow growing, with an average size 2–3 cm. They may remain static in size for months to years, with 10%–40% completely resolving during adolescence. The dense fibroglandular tissue of the adolescent breast may cause false-positive results on standard mammograms. Thus, ultrasonography is the best imaging modality with which to evaluate a breast mass in an adolescent if further evaluation beyond clinical examination is necessary. Fibroadenomas less than 5 cm can be monitored for growth or regression over 3–4 months. Further evaluation will be dictated by the course, with semiannual clinical examinations for a few years followed by annual examinations for a mass that is regressing. Patients with concerning breast masses including fibroadenomas that are larger than 5 cm, undiagnosed breast masses that are enlarging or have overlying skin changes, and any suspicious breast mass in a patient with a history of previous malignancy should be referred to a breast care specialist.

2. Fibrocystic Breast Changes

Fibrocystic breast changes are much more common in adults than adolescents. Symptoms include mild swelling and palpable nodularity, most commonly in the upper outer quadrants. Mastalgia is typically cyclic, usually occurring just before menstruation. Reassuring the young woman about the benign nature of the process may be all that is needed. Nonsteroidal anti-inflammatory drugs (NSAIDs) such as ibuprofen or naproxen sodium help alleviate symptoms. Oral contraceptive pills (OCPs) can also be beneficial. Supportive bras may provide symptomatic relief. Studies have shown no association between methylxanthine and fibrocystic breasts; however, some women report reduced symptoms when they discontinue caffeine.

3. Breast Abscess and Nipple Piercing

ESSENTIALS OF DIAGNOSIS & TYPICAL FEATURES

► Common causes of mastitis and breast abscess during adolescence include manipulation of periareolar hair and nipple piercing, with subsequent infection with normal skin flora.

► Typical features include breast pain and overlying erythema and warmth.

► Breast ultrasound may be helpful to differentiate between mastitis and breast abscess.

Although breastfeeding is the most common cause of mastitis, shaving or plucking periareolar hair, nipple piercing, and trauma during sexual activity are predisposing factors in teenagers. The most common causative organisms are normal skin flora. The female with a breast abscess usually complains of unilateral breast pain, and examination reveals overlying inflammatory changes. The examination may be misleading in that the infection may extend deeper into the breast than suspected. *Staphylococcus aureus* is the most common pathogen. β-Hemolytic streptococci, *Escherichia coli*, and *Pseudomonas aeruginosa* have also been implicated. Fluctuant abscesses should be incised and drained and fluid cultured. Antimicrobial coverage for *S aureus* (including consideration of methicillin-resistant strains) should be given initially (generally orally, unless infection is severe), and the patient should be monitored closely for response to therapy until culture and susceptibility test results are available.

Healing time after nipple piercing is 3–6 months. Health risks associated with nipple piercing, in addition to breast abscess, include allergic reactions to jewelry, keloid scar formation, and risk of hepatitis B and C and HIV acquisition. Complications associated with abscess formation secondary to nipple piercing include endocarditis, cardiac valve injury, cardiac prosthesis infection, metal foreign-body reaction in the breast tissue, and recurrent infection.

NIPPLE DISCHARGE & GALACTORRHEA

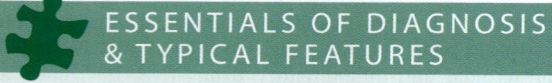

ESSENTIALS OF DIAGNOSIS & TYPICAL FEATURES

▶ Bloody or serosanguineous discharge may indicate a duct problem; milky nipple discharge is typical of galactorrhea.

▶ Galactorrhea is typically benign and caused by chronic nipple stimulation, certain prescription psychiatric drugs, or illicit drug use.

Ductal ectasia is a common cause of nipple discharge in the developing breast and is associated with dilation of the mammary ducts, periductal fibrosis, and inflammation. It can present with bloody, brown, or sticky multicolored nipple discharge and/or a cystic breast mass, usually in the subareolar region. Blocked ducts and fluid collections usually resolve spontaneously but can become infected, producing mastitis. Patients should be counseled to watch for erythema, warmth, and tenderness indicating mastitis. Oral antibiotics covering skin flora should be initiated if infection is suspected. Serous or serosanguineous nipple discharge is common and can be associated with fibrocystic breast changes. Montgomery tubercles, small glands located at the outer aspect

of the areola, can drain clear or brownish fluid through an ectopic opening on the areola and may be associated with a small subareolar mass. These lesions and discharge typically resolve spontaneously. Intraductal papillomas arising from proliferation of ductal cells projecting into the duct lumen are a rare cause of bloody or serosanguineous nipple discharge and can also present with a subareolar or peripheral mass. These lesions are associated with increased risk of malignancy in adults.

Galactorrhea is distinguishable from other causes of nipple discharge by its milky character and tendency to involve both breasts. It is usually benign. The most common causes include chronic stimulation or irritation of the nipple, medications and illicit drugs (Table 4–9), pregnancy, childbirth, or abortion. Prolactin-secreting tumors (prolactinomas) and hypothyroidism are common pathologic causes of galactorrhea during adolescence. Less commonly, tumors of the hypothalamus and/or pituitary, both benign (eg, craniopharyngiomas) and malignant (eg, metastatic disease); infiltrative diseases of the hypothalamus (eg, sarcoidosis); and pituitary stalk damage (eg, section due to head trauma or surgery or compression) cause hyperprolactinemia and galactorrhea by interfering with secretion of dopamine or its delivery to the hypothalamus. Stimulation of the intercostal nerves (eg, chest wall surgery or herpes zoster infection), renal failure (decreased prolactin clearance), polycystic ovarian syndrome, and emotional or physical stress can also cause hyperprolactinemia which can induce galactorrhea.

▶ Clinical Findings

Breast ultrasonography can be helpful in determining the cause of nipple discharge and breast masses. Depending on additional history and examination findings, evaluation may include a pregnancy test, prolactin level, and thyroid function studies. If there is a question as to whether the

Table 4–9. Medications and herbs associated with galactorrhea.

Anticonvulsants (valproic acid)
Antidepressants (selective serotonin reuptake inhibitors, tricyclic antidepressants)
Anxiolytics (alprazolam)
Antihypertensives (atenolol, methyldopa, reserpine, verapamil)
Antipsychotics
Typical (haloperidol, phenothiazine, pimozide)
Atypical (risperidone, olanzapine, molindone)
Antiemetics (prochlorperazine)
Herbs (anise, blessed thistle, fennel, fenugreek seed, nettle)
Hormonal contraceptives
Isoniazid
Illicit drugs (amphetamines, cannabis, opiates)
Motility agents (metoclopramide)
Muscle relaxants (cyclobenzaprine)

discharge is true galactorrhea, fat staining of the discharge can be confirmatory. Elevated TSH confirms the diagnosis of hypothyroidism. Elevated prolactin and normal TSH, often accompanied by amenorrhea, in the absence of medication known to cause hyperprolactinemia suggests a hypothalamic or pituitary tumor and magnetic resonance imaging (MRI) of the brain and consultation with a pediatric endocrinologist are indicated.

▶ Treatment

Observation with serial examination is recommended for nipple discharge associated with a breast mass unless a papilloma is suspected based on presence of bloody or serosanguineous nipple discharge with or without a subareolar or peripheral mass. The latter entity requires further evaluation and excision by a breast surgeon. For galactorrhea, treating the underlying cause is usually effective. Galactorrhea due to hypothyroidism should be treated with thyroid hormone replacement. An alternative medication can be prescribed in cases of medication-induced galactorrhea. Adolescents with galactorrhea without a breast mass who have normal prolactin and TSH levels can be followed clinically and counseled about supportive measures such as avoidance of nipple stimulation, stress reduction, and keeping a menstrual calendar to monitor for oligomenorrhea, which might indicate a systemic hormonal problem such as hyperprolactinemia or thyroid disease. In many cases, symptoms resolve spontaneously, and no underlying diagnosis is made. Medical management of prolactinomas with dopamine agonists such as bromocriptine is the favored approach.

GYNECOMASTIA

ESSENTIALS OF DIAGNOSIS & TYPICAL FEATURES

- ▶ Gynecomastia is common in males during puberty and may last 1–3 years.
- ▶ Typical features include a palpable fibroglandular mass located concentrically beneath the nipple-areolar complex. It may be unilateral or bilateral.
- ▶ Clinical observation is appropriate; however, further evaluation may be necessary for atypical cases including prepubertal gynecomastia, eccentric position, rapid breast enlargement, presence of testicular mass, or prolonged persistence.

Gynecomastia, benign subareolar glandular breast enlargement, affects up to 65% of adolescent males. It typically appears at least 6 months after the onset of secondary sex characteristics, with peak incidence during SMR stages 3 and 4. Breast tissue enlargement usually regresses within 1–3 years, and persistence beyond age 17 years is uncommon. Approximately half of young men with gynecomastia have a positive family history of gynecomastia. The pathogenesis of pubertal gynecomastia has long been attributed to a transient imbalance between estrogens that stimulate proliferation of breast tissue and androgens which antagonize this effect. Alterations in estrogen-androgen ratio induced by leptin has been implicated, as levels are higher in healthy nonobese adolescent males with gynecomastia compared to controls.

▶ Clinical Findings

Palpation of the breasts is necessary to distinguish adipose tissue (pseudogynecomastia) from glandular tissue found in true gynecomastia, which is palpable as a fibroglandular mass located concentrically beneath the nipple-areolar complex. Gynecomastia is bilateral in almost two-thirds of patients. Findings that indicate more serious disease include hard or firm breast tissue, unilateral breast growth, eccentric masses outside of the nipple-areolar complex, and overlying skin changes. A genitourinary examination is needed to evaluate pubertal SMR, testicular volume and masses, or irregularities of the testes.

In the absence of abnormalities on history or physical examination, clinical monitoring of male gynecomastia for 12–18 months is sufficient. Laboratory evaluation is warranted if the patient is prepubertal, appears under-virilized, has an eccentric breast mass, has rapid progression of breast enlargement, has a testicular mass, or has persistence of gynecomastia beyond the usual observation period. Initial laboratory evaluation includes thyroid function tests and testosterone, estradiol, human chorionic gonadotropin (hCG), and LH levels. Additional studies, depending on preliminary findings, include karyotype, liver and renal function studies, and dehydroepiandrosterone sulfate (DHEAS) and prolactin levels. Any patient with a testicular mass or laboratory results suggesting possible tumor, such as high serum testosterone, hCG, or estradiol, should have a testicular ultrasound. Further evaluation includes adrenal or brain imaging if a prolactin-secreting pituitary tumor or adrenal tumor is suspected.

▶ Differential Diagnosis

Gynecomastia may be drug-induced (Table 4–10). Testicular, adrenal, or pituitary tumors, Klinefelter syndrome, secondary hypogonadism, partial or complete androgen insensitivity syndrome, hyperthyroidism, or chronic diseases (eg, cystic fibrosis, ulcerative colitis, liver disease, renal failure, and AIDS) leading to malnutrition may be associated with gynecomastia. Breast cancer in the adolescent male is extraordinarily rare.

Table 4–10. Drugs associated with gynecomastia.

	Examples
Antiandrogens	Cyproterone, finasteride, flutamide, ketoconazole, nilutamide, spironolactone
Antineoplastic and immunomodulators	Alkylating agents, bleomycin, cisplatin, cyclosporine, imatinib, methotrexate, nitrosourea, vincristine
Antiulcer drugs	Cimetidine, metoclopramide, omeprazole, ranitidine
Cardiovascular drugs	Amiodarone, angiotensin-converting enzyme inhibitors, calcium channel blockers, digitoxin, reserpine, spironolactone
Drugs of abuse	Alcohol, amphetamines, marijuana, opiates
Hormones	Anabolic androgenic steroids, estrogens, testosterone, chorionic gonadotropin
Infectious agents	Antiretrovirals, ketoconazole, isoniazid, metronidazole
Psychoactive medications	Diazepam, tricyclic antidepressants, haloperidol, atypical antipsychotics, phenothiazines

▶ **Treatment**

If gynecomastia is idiopathic, reassurance about the common and benign nature of the process can be given. Resolution may take up to 2 years. Surgery is reserved for those with persistent severe breast enlargement and/or significant psychological trauma. In cases of drug-induced gynecomastia, the inciting agent should be discontinued if possible. The patient should be referred to an endocrinologist or oncologist if pathologic etiologies are diagnosed.

Guss CE, Divasta AD: Adolescent gynecomastia. Pediatr Endocrinol Rev 2017;14(4):371–377 [PMID: 28613047].

Khaja A, DeSilva N: The female adolescent breast: disorders of development. Curr Opin Obstet Gynecol 2019;31(5):293–297 [PMID: 31356237].

Practice Bulletin Number 179: Breast cancer risk assessment and screening in average-risk women. Obstet Gynecol 2017 Jul;130(1):e1–e16 [PMID: 28644335].

GYNECOLOGIC CARE & GYNECOLOGIC DISORDERS IN ADOLESCENCE

▶ **Physiology of Menstruation**

The ovulatory menstrual cycle is divided into three consecutive phases: follicular (days 1–14), ovulatory (midcycle), and luteal (days 16–28). During the follicular phase, pulsatile gonadotropin-releasing hormone from the hypothalamus stimulates anterior pituitary secretion of FSH and LH. Under the influence of FSH and LH, a dominant ovarian follicle emerges by day 5–7 of the menstrual cycle, and the other follicles become atretic. Rising estradiol levels produced by the maturing follicle cause proliferation of the endometrium. By the midfollicular phase, FSH begins to decline secondary to estradiol-mediated negative feedback, while LH continues to rise as a result of estradiol-mediated positive feedback.

Rising LH initiates progesterone secretion and luteinization of the granulosa cells of the follicle. Progesterone in turn further stimulates LH and FSH. This leads to the LH surge, which causes the follicle to rupture and expel the oocyte. During the luteal phase, LH and FSH gradually decline. The corpus luteum secretes progesterone, and the endometrium enters the secretory phase in response to rising levels of estrogen and progesterone, with maturation 8–9 days after ovulation. If pregnancy and placental hCG release do not occur, luteolysis begins; estrogen and progesterone levels decline, and the endometrial lining is shed as menstrual flow approximately 14 days after ovulation. In the first 2 years after menarche, most cycles (50%–80%) are anovulatory. Between 10% and 20% of cycles are anovulatory for up to 5 years after menarche.

▶ **Pelvic Examination**

Pelvic examination in an adolescent may be considered part of the evaluation of abdominal or pelvic pain, intra-abdominal or pelvic mass, abnormal vaginal bleeding or other menstrual disorders, and/or pathologic vaginal discharge. The American Cancer Society published an updated guideline for cervical cancer screening for average-risk individuals in 2020, which includes the recommendation to begin screening at age 25 years, rather than the previous recommendation of 21 years. Pregnancy during adolescence does not alter screening guidelines. Per the 2021 CDC STI guidelines, HIV-infected female adolescents should have cervical screening cytology obtained 1 year after onset of sexual activity (but no later than age 21 years) using conventional liquid-based cytology and, if the results are normal, annually thereafter. After 3 years of consecutive normal cytology results, the screening interval can be increased to every 3 years. Co-testing (cytology and human papillomavirus [HPV] test) is not recommended for individuals aged 30 years or younger.

Sensitive counseling and age-appropriate education about the purpose of the examination, pelvic anatomy, and the components of the examination should occur in an unhurried manner to alleviate apprehension. Diagrams and models may facilitate discussion. The adolescent may request to have a family member present for reassurance; however, in many instances an adolescent will request that the examination occur confidentially. Having another female staff member present as a chaperone and support for the adolescent may be helpful; a female staff chaperone should be present with male examiners.

Table 4–11. Items for pelvic examination.

General	Gloves, good light source, appropriate-sized speculums, sterile cotton applicator swabs, large swabs to remove excess bleeding or discharge, patient labels, hand mirror for patient education
Wet prep of vaginal discharge	pH paper, microscope slides and cover slips, NaCl and KOH solutions
Pap smear	Pap smear liquid media or slides with fixative; cervical spatula and endocervical cytologic brush; or broom for collection
STI testing	Gonorrhea and *chlamydia* test media with specific collection swabs
Bimanual examination	Gloves, water-based lubricant

Table 4–12. Diagnostic tests and procedures performed during speculum vaginal examination.

Vaginal pH	Use applicator swab to sample vaginal discharge adherent to the wall or in the vaginal pool if a speculum is in place; immediately apply it to pH paper for reading.
Saline and KOH wet preparations	Sample discharge as above with different swabs, smear small sample on glass slide, apply small drop of saline or KOH and immediately cover with coverslip, and evaluate under microscope.
Pap smear[a]	Gently remove excessive discharge from surface of cervix. Exocervical cells are sampled with a spatula by applying gentle pressure on the cervix with the spatula while rotating it around the cervical os. Endocervical cells are sampled by gently inserting the cytologic brush into the cervical os and rotating it. Both cell types are collected by the broom when it is centered over the cervical os and rotated.
STI testing[a]	Insert specific test swabs (eg, Dacron for most *Chlamydia* test media) into the cervical os and rotate to obtain endocervical samples for *chlamydia* and gonorrhea, or if using approved test for vaginal collection, insert the swab into the vagina and rotate, touching the vaginal wall. Vaginal testing for *Trichomonas vaginalis* is also available.

STI, sexually transmitted infection.
[a]Refer to manufacturer instructions for sample collection and processing.

The pelvic examination begins by placing the patient in the dorsal lithotomy position after equipment and supplies are ready (Table 4–11). Patients with orthopedic or other physical disabilities require accommodation for proper positioning and comfort. The examiner inspects the external genitalia, noting sexually maturity rating; estrogenization of the vaginal mucosa (moist, pink, and more elastic mucosa); shape of the hymen; the size of the clitoris (2–5 mm wide is normal); any unusual rashes or lesions on the vulva such as folliculitis from shaving, warts, or other skin lesions; and genital piercing or body art. It can be helpful to ask an adolescent if she has any questions about her body during the inspection as she might have concerns that she was too shy to ask (eg, normalcy of labial hypertrophy). In cases of alleged sexual abuse or assault, the presence of any lesions, including lacerations, bruises, scarring, or synechiae near the hymen, vulva, or anus should be noted.

The patient should be prepared for insertion of the speculum to help her remain relaxed. The speculum should be inserted into the vagina posteriorly with a downward direction to avoid the urethra. It can be helpful to do a one-finger digital vaginal examination prior to placing a speculum to identify the position of the cervix and can give the patient an appreciation for the sensation she can expect with placement of the speculum. Warming the speculum with tap water prior to insertion can be more comfortable for the patient and also provide lubrication. Simultaneously touching the inner aspect of the patient's thigh or applying gentle pressure to the perineum away from the introitus while inserting the speculum helps distract attention from the placement of the speculum. The vaginal walls and cervix are inspected for anatomical abnormalities, inflammation, and lesions, and the quantity and quality of discharge adherent to the vaginal walls and pooled in the vagina are noted. The presence of a cervical ectropion, extension of the endocervical columnar epithelium outside the cervical os onto the face of the cervix,

is commonly observed in adolescents as erythema surrounding the cervical os.

Specimens are obtained in the following order: vaginal pH, saline and KOH wet preparations, cervical cytology (Pap) screening if indicated, and vaginal swabs for gonorrhea and *Chlamydia trachomatis* (Table 4–12). The speculum is then removed, and bimanual examination is performed with one or two fingers in the vagina and the other hand on the abdomen to palpate the uterus and adnexa for size, position, and tenderness.

▶ **Menstrual Disorders**

1. Amenorrhea

Primary amenorrhea is defined as having no menstrual periods in the presence of secondary sex characteristics by age 15 years. In the adolescent who has achieved menarche, *secondary amenorrhea* is defined as the absence of menses for three consecutive cycles or for 6 months in a patient with irregular cycles.

A. Evaluation of Primary and Secondary Amenorrhea

In evaluating amenorrhea, it is helpful to consider anatomical levels of possible abnormalities from the hypothalamus to the genital tract (Table 4–13).

A stepwise approach, using clinical history, growth charts, physical examination, and appropriate laboratory

Table 4–13. Differential diagnosis of amenorrhea by anatomic site of cause.

Hypothalamic-pituitary axis
Hypothalamic suppression
  Chronic disease
  Stress
  Malnutrition
  Strenuous athletics
  Drugs (haloperidol, phenothiazines, atypical antipsychotics)
Central nervous system lesion
  Pituitary lesion: adenoma, prolactinoma
  Craniopharyngioma, brainstem, or parasellar tumors
  Head injury with hypothalamic contusion
  Infiltrative process (sarcoidosis)
  Vascular disease (hypothalamic vasculitis)
Congenital conditions[a]
  Kallmann syndrome (anosmia)
Ovaries
Gonadal dysgenesis[a]
  Turner syndrome (XO)
  Mosaic (XX/XO)
Injury to ovary
  Autoimmune disease (oophoritis)
  Infection (mumps)
  Toxins (alkylating chemotherapeutic agents)
  Irradiation
  Trauma, torsion (rare)
Polycystic ovary syndrome
Ovarian failure
Uterovaginal outflow tract
Müllerian dysgenesis[a]
  Congenital deformity or absence of uterus, uterine tubes, or vagina
Imperforate hymen, transverse vaginal septum, vaginal agenesis, agenesis of the cervix[a]
Androgen insensitivity syndrome (absent uterus)[a]
Uterine lining defect
  Asherman syndrome (intrauterine synechiae postcurettage or endometritis)
  Tuberculosis, brucellosis
Defect in hormone synthesis or action (virilization may be present)
Adrenal hyperplasia[a]
Cushing disease
Adrenal tumor
Ovarian tumor (rare)
Drugs (steroids, ACTH)

ACTH, adrenocorticotropic hormone.
[a]Indicates condition that usually presents as primary amenorrhea.

studies will allow providers to determine the etiology of amenorrhea in most adolescents. Evaluation begins with a thorough developmental and sexual history. Establishing a pubertal timeline including age at thelarche, adrenarche, growth spurt, and menarche is helpful in evaluating pubertal development. Although there can be variations in the onset, degree, and timing of these stages, the progression of stages is predictable. Adrenal androgens are largely responsible for axillary and pubic hair. Estrogen is responsible for breast development; maturation of the external genitalia, vagina, and uterus; and menstruation. Lack of development suggests pituitary or ovarian failure or gonadal dysgenesis. Determining the patient's gynecologic age (time in years and months since menarche) is helpful in assessing the maturity of the hypothalamic-pituitary-ovarian axis. A menstrual history includes date of last menstrual period (LMP), frequency and duration of periods, amount of bleeding, and premenstrual symptoms. Irregular menstrual cycles are common in the first 1–2 years after menarche. Two-thirds of adolescents with a gynecologic age more than 2 years have regular menstrual cycles.

Relevant components of the past medical and surgical histories include neonatal history, treatment for malignancies, presence of autoimmune disorders or endocrinopathies, and current medications (prescribed and over-the-counter). Family history includes age at menarche of maternal relatives, familial gynecologic or fertility problems, autoimmune diseases, or endocrinopathies. A review of systems should focus on symptoms of hypothalamic-pituitary disease such as weight change, headache, visual disturbance, galactorrhea, polyuria, and/or polydipsia. A history of cyclic abdominal and/or pelvic pain in a mature adolescent with amenorrhea may indicate an anatomic abnormality such as an imperforate hymen. Acne and hirsutism are clinical markers of androgen excess. Both hypo- and hyperthyroidism can cause menstrual irregularities, and changes in weight, quality of skin and hair, and stooling pattern may indicate a thyroid problem. A confidential social history should include sexual activity; contraceptive use; possibility of pregnancy; and use of nicotine, drugs, or alcohol. The patient should also be questioned about major stressors, symptoms of depression and anxiety, dietary habits including any disordered eating or weight-loss behaviors, and athletic participation.

A thorough physical examination should include the components listed in Table 4–14. If there is no other reason to do a pelvic or bimanual examination, the presence of the uterus can be assessed by pelvic ultrasonography. Ultrasound provides evaluation of pelvic anatomy and possible genital tract obstruction, measurement of the endometrial stripe thickness as an indicator of estrogen stimulation, and identification of ovarian cysts or masses.

Figure 4–3 illustrates an approach to the laboratory and radiologic evaluation of primary or secondary amenorrhea. Initial studies should include a urine pregnancy test, complete

Table 4–14. Components of the physical examination for amenorrhea.

General appearance	Syndromic features (eg, Turner syndrome with webbed neck, shield chest, widely spaced nipples, increased carrying angle of the arms)
Anthropometrics	Height, weight, BMI and percentiles for age, vital signs (HR, BP)
Ophthalmologic	Visual field cuts, papilledema
Neck	Thyromegaly
Breast	SMR staging, galactorrhea
Abdomen	Masses
Genital	SMR staging, estrogenization of vaginal mucosa (pink and moist vs thin red mucosa of hypoestrogenization), hymenal patency, clitoromegaly (length > 10 mm)
Pelvic and bimanual	Vaginal depth by insertion of a saline moistened applicator swab into the vagina or by bimanual examination (normal > 2 cm); palpation of the uterus and ovaries by bimanual examination
Skin	Acne, hirsutism, acanthosis nigricans

BMI, body mass index; BP, blood pressure; HR, heart rate; SMR, sexual maturity rating.

blood count, TSH, prolactin, and FSH. If there is evidence of hyperandrogenemia (acne, hirsutism) and polycystic ovary syndrome (PCOS) is suspected, total and free testosterone should be obtained. Additional androgen testing including DHEAS, androstenedione, and 17-hydroxyprogesterone can be considered for the evaluation of androgen-secreting tumors and 21-hydroxylase deficiency. If systemic illness is suspected, a urinalysis and a chemistry panel (including renal and liver function tests) and erythrocyte sedimentation rate should be obtained. If short stature and delayed puberty are present, a bone age and karyotype should be done.

If pelvic examination or ultrasonography reveals normal female external genitalia and pelvic organs and the patient is not pregnant, the patient should be given a challenge of oral medroxyprogesterone, 10 mg daily for 10 days. Positive response to the progestin challenge with withdrawal bleeding is suggestive of the presence of an estrogen-primed uterus.

Elevated serum prolactin indicates a possible prolactin-secreting tumor. Prolactin testing is sensitive and can be elevated with stress, eating, or sexual intercourse. A mildly elevated test should be repeated prior to MRI of the brain for a prolactinoma. Elevated FSH indicates ovarian insufficiency or gonadal dysgenesis and a karyotype for Turner

syndrome or Turner mosaic should be obtained. Autoimmune oophoritis should be assessed by antiovarian antibodies if the chromosome analysis is normal. Normal or low serum gonadotropins indicate hypothalamic suppression and functional amenorrhea if the patient's weight is normal and there is a reasonable explanation such as vigorous exercise. Functional amenorrhea, although relatively common, is a diagnosis of exclusion. Low serum gonadotropin concentration can also be caused by malnutrition as in anorexia nervosa, endocrinopathies, and chronic diseases or by a central nervous system tumor.

If the physical examination or ultrasound reveals an absent uterus, chromosomal analysis and serum testosterone should be obtained to differentiate between mullerian dysgenesis and androgen insensitivity. Mullerian dysgenesis or Mayer-Rokitansky-Küster-Hauser (MRKH) syndrome is the congenital absence of the vagina with variable uterine development. These women have normal serum testosterone levels. Pelvic MRI is helpful to clarify the nature of the vaginal agenesis and to differentiate it from low-lying transverse vaginal septum, agenesis of the uterus and vagina, and imperforate hymen. Individuals with androgen insensitivity are phenotypically female but have an absent upper vagina, uterus, and fallopian tubes; a male karyotype; and an elevated serum testosterone (normal range for males).

The management of primary or secondary amenorrhea depends on the underlying pathology. Hormonal treatment is used in patients with hypothalamic, pituitary, and ovarian causes. Surgical repair may be required in patients with outflow tract anomalies.

B. Polycystic Ovary Syndrome

ESSENTIALS OF DIAGNOSIS & TYPICAL FEATURES

▶ Typical features of polycystic ovary syndrome (PCOS) include menstrual irregularities, signs of hyperandrogenism (eg, hirsutism and moderate to severe acne), and overweight or obesity.

▶ The primary laboratory abnormality is an elevated free testosterone level.

▶ Obese adolescents with PCOS should be screened for lipid abnormalities, glucose intolerance and/or type 2 diabetes, fatty liver disease, obstructive sleep apnea, and depression and anxiety.

PCOS is the most common endocrine disorder of reproductive-aged women, affecting 6%–15% of women of reproductive age. PCOS is characterized by ovarian dysfunction, disordered gonadotropin secretion, and hyperandrogenism,

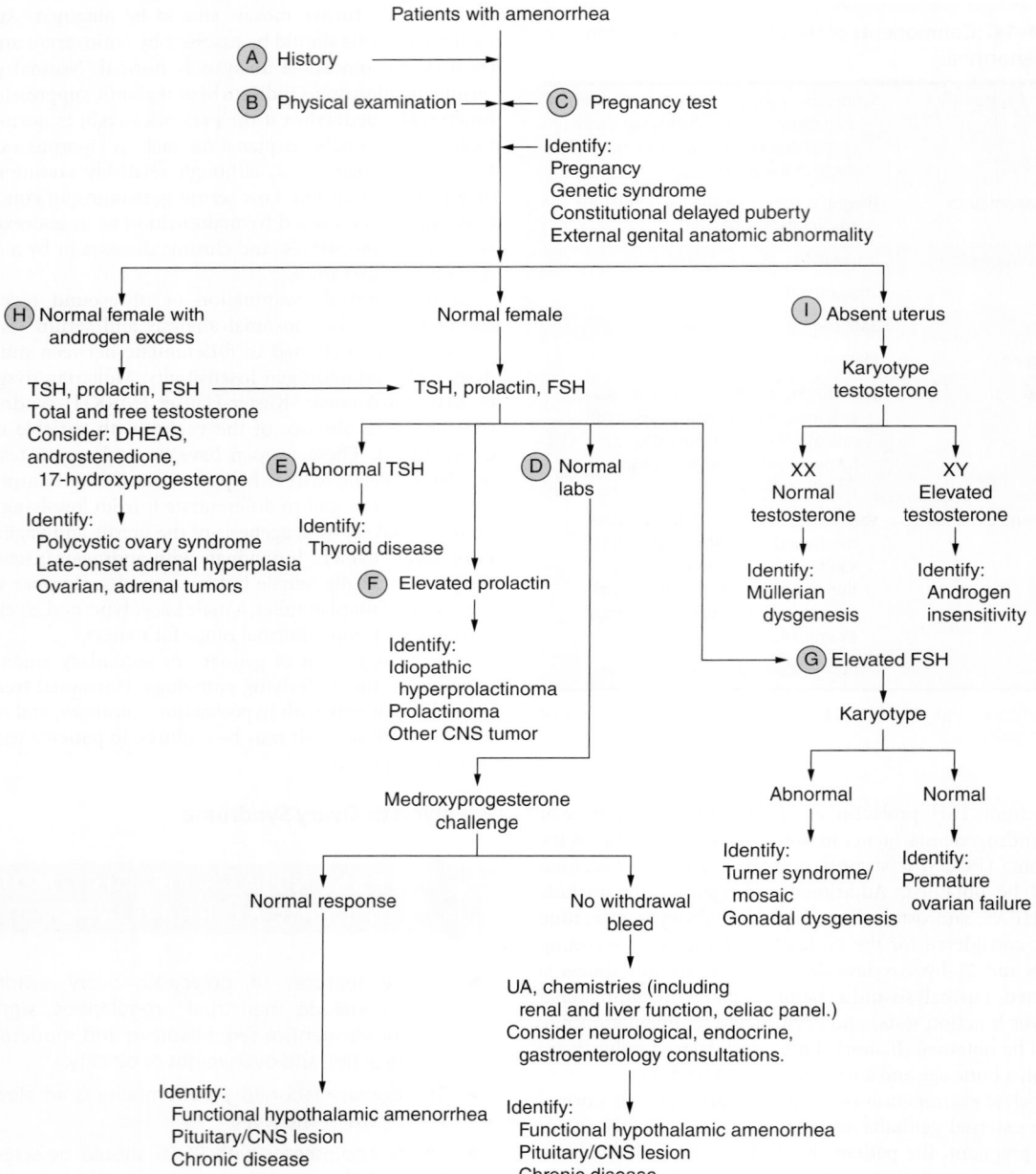

▲ **Figure 4–3.** Evaluation of primary amenorrhea and secondary amenorrhea. CNS, central nervous system; DHEAS, dehydroepiandrosterone sulfate; FSH, follicle-stimulating hormone; TSH, thyroid-stimulating hormone; UA, urine analysis.

which cause irregular periods, hirsutism, and acne. Many adolescents with PCOS are overweight and the association of PCOS with insulin resistance in adults is well established. Adolescents with PCOS are at increased risk for obesity-related morbidities including type 2 diabetes mellitus; cardiovascular disease including dyslipidemia; fatty liver disease; obstructive sleep apnea; low self-esteem, depression, and anxiety; and adult reproductive health problems including infertility and endometrial cancer.

Hyperandrogenemia occurs during normal puberty and also as a function of prolonged anovulatory cycles as the hypothalamic-pituitary-ovarian axis matures during the first few years of typical pubertal development. The normalcy of this hyperandrogenemia confounds the diagnosis of PCOS in early adolescence if adult criteria of evidence of chemical hyperandrogenemia are applied. Therefore, many experts recommend avoiding testing androgen levels until at least 1 year after menarche for symptomatic adolescents. The current diagnostic criteria for PCOS in adolescents include clinical signs and symptoms of androgen excess, increased androgen levels, and exclusion of other causes of hyperandrogenemia in the setting of oligomenorrhea.

▶ Evaluation

Standard laboratory evaluation for PCOS includes assessment of total and free testosterone levels. If other etiologies of hyperandrogenemia and virilization such as androgen-secreting tumors or late-onset congenital adrenal hyperplasia are suspected, additional androgen testing should include DHEAS, androstenedione, and a first morning 17-hydroxyprogesterone. Urine cortisol or a dexamethasone suppression test is performed if Cushing syndrome is suspected. If the patient is overweight and/or has acanthosis nigricans, a fasting lipid panel and glucose testing are recommended. A 2-hour oral glucose tolerance test (OGTT) to evaluate for impaired glucose tolerance should also be considered as a normal fasting glucose may be falsely reassuring. A hemoglobin A_{1C} test may also be considered with or as an alternative to OGTT. Additionally, as obstructive sleep apnea, depression, and anxiety have been associated with the diagnosis of PCOS, clinicians should screen for these comorbidities. A pediatric endocrinologist can assist in further evaluation and management of significantly elevated androgens and possible endocrinopathies.

▶ Treatment

Encouraging lifestyle changes that will promote weight loss is a primary goal of therapy for PCOS in adolescence. Weight loss is associated with improved menstrual regulation, decreased symptoms of hyperandrogenemia, and improved obesity-related comorbidities. Use of combination hormonal contraceptives will improve menstrual regularity and reduce risk of endometrial hyperplasia, decrease ovarian and

adrenal androgen production, and increase sex hormone–binding globulin (SHBG). There are no current guidelines for the use of metformin to treat PCOS in adolescents; however, it is prescribed for impaired glucose tolerance or type 2 diabetes. Metformin will improve the frequency of ovulation; therefore, contraception should also be prescribed for sexually active teens.

2. Dysmenorrhea

ESSENTIALS OF DIAGNOSIS & TYPICAL FEATURES

► The majority of adolescent girls experience primary dysmenorrhea.

► Typical features include lower abdominal cramps radiating to the lower back and thighs and nausea and/or vomiting starting a few days before the onset of menses and lasting a few days into the period.

► Use of scheduled NSAIDs and contraceptives to suppress ovulation are mainstays of treatment.

Dysmenorrhea or pain with menstrual periods is the most common gynecologic complaint of adolescents, with up to 90% of menstruating adolescents reporting some symptoms and 15% describing their symptoms as severe. The prevalence of dysmenorrhea increases with gynecologic age due to its association with ovulatory cycles. Dysmenorrhea can be designated as primary or secondary depending on the absence or presence of underlying pelvic pathology (Table 4–15). Potent prostaglandins are the mediators of dysmenorrhea, producing uterine contractions, tissue ischemia, and hypersensitivity of pain fibers in the uterus.

▶ Evaluation

In addition to a gynecologic and sexual history, an accurate characterization of the pain (timing with menses, intensity, duration, use of pain medications) is important in determining functional impairment. The pelvic examination can usually be deferred in non–sexually active adolescents with probable primary dysmenorrhea.

▶ Treatment

Adolescents should be encouraged to keep track of their menstrual cycles using a calendar to predict when a period is imminent, thereby allowing for more proactive use of NSAIDs 1–2 days before the start of the anticipated period or with the first indication of discomfort. NSAIDs are typically continued for an additional 2–3 days after onset of pain. Recommended medications are ibuprofen 400–600 mg

Table 4–15. Dysmenorrhea in the adolescent.

	Etiology	Onset and Duration	Symptoms	Pelvic Examination	Treatment
Primary Dysmenorrhea[a]					
Primary	Excessive amount of prostaglandin F$_2\alpha$, which attaches to myometrium, causing uterine contractions, hypoxia, and ischemia. Also, directly sensitizes pain receptors.	Begins just prior to or with the onset of menstrual flow and lasts 1–2 days. Typically does not start until 1–2 y after menarche, when cycles are more regularly ovulatory.	Lower abdominal cramps radiating to lower back and thighs. Associated nausea, vomiting, and diarrhea due to excess prostaglandins.	Typically unnecessary for diagnosis.	Start NSAIDs at first signs of discomfort and continue as directed through the first few days of period. If pain persists after 3 mo of scheduled NSAID use, consider suppressing ovulation with hormonal contraceptives.
Secondary Dysmenorrhea[b]					
Infection	Often due to an STI such as *chlamydia* or gonorrhea.	Recent onset of pelvic pain. Can also have chronic pain with prolonged untreated infection.	Pelvic pain, excessive or irregular menstrual bleeding, unusual vaginal discharge.	Mucopurulent or purulent discharge from cervical os, cervical friability, cervical motion, uterine or adnexal tenderness, positive wet prep for bacterial vaginosis, positive test for STI.	Appropriate antibiotics.
Endometriosis	Ectopic implants of endometrial tissue in pelvis or abdomen; may result from retrograde menstruation. Definitive diagnosis requires laparoscopy.	Generally starts > 2 y after menarche, is not significantly responsive to standard NSAID and suppression of ovulation therapies, and worsens through time.	Cyclic or acyclic chronic pelvic pain.	Mild to moderate tenderness typically in the posterior vaginal fornix or along the uterosacral ligaments.	Suppression of ovulation with combined hormonal contraceptive methods. Continuous use may provide additional control. If pain persists, refer to a gynecologist for further evaluation of chronic pelvic pain and consideration of gonadotropin-releasing hormone agonists.
Complication of pregnancy	Spontaneous abortion, ectopic pregnancy.	Acute onset.	Pelvic or abdominal pain associated with vaginal bleeding following missed menstrual period.	Positive hCG, enlarged uterus, or adnexal mass.	Pelvic US if hemodynamically stable to evaluate for intrauterine pregnancy. Immediate obstetric or surgical consult with concern for ectopic pregnancy.
Congenital anomalies	Outflow tract anomalies: imperforate hymen, transverse or longitudinal vaginal septum, septate uterus.	Onset at menarche.	Cyclic pelvic or abdominal pain which can become chronic.	Imperforate hymen may be visible on external examination. Pelvic US for general anatomy. Pelvic MRI is most sensitive and specific test for septums.	Gynecology consult for further evaluation and management.

(Continued)

Table 4–15. Dysmenorrhea in the adolescent. (*Continued*)

	Etiology	Onset and Duration	Symptoms	Pelvic Examination	Treatment
Pelvic adhesions	Previous abdominal surgery or pelvic inflammatory disease.	Delayed onset after surgery or PID.	Abdominal pain, may or may not be associated with menstrual cycles; possible alteration in bowel pattern.	Variable.	Gynecology consult for possible lysis of adhesion.

DMPA, depot medroxyprogesterone acetate; hCG, human chorionic gonadotropin; MRI, magnetic resonance imaging; NSAID, nonsteroidal anti-inflammatory drug; PID, pelvic inflammatory disease; STI, sexually transmitted infection; US, ultrasound.
[a]No pelvic pathology.
[b]Underlying pathology present.

every 6 hours or naproxen 500 mg twice a day. If the patient does not respond to NSAIDs, suppression of ovulation with combined oral contraceptive (COCs) pills or other combined hormonal contraceptives such as the transdermal patch or intravaginal ring can be effective. COCs and the intravaginal ring can also be used continuously for extended cycling to decrease the frequency of menstrual periods. This is accomplished by skipping the placebo pill week and immediately starting a new package of birth control pills or skipping the standard 1-week break after removal of the intravaginal ring and immediately placing a new ring. Depot medroxyprogesterone acetate (DMPA) and long-acting reversible contraceptives (LARCs) including the etonogestrel implant and levonorgestrel intrauterine device (IUD) are also effective and may be preferable for patients who may have challenges with adherence. If patients have persistent symptoms despite use of a contraceptive for suppression of ovulation and scheduled NSAIDs, further evaluation for secondary dysmenorrhea is indicated. A pelvic examination, pelvic imaging with ultrasonography or MRI, and diagnostic laparoscopy may be necessary for diagnosis. Secondary dysmenorrhea is more likely to be associated with chronic pelvic pain, midcycle pain, dyspareunia, and metrorrhagia.

3. Abnormal Uterine Bleeding

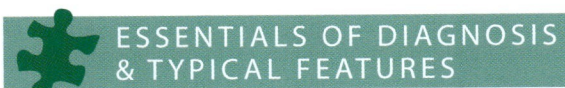

ESSENTIALS OF DIAGNOSIS & TYPICAL FEATURES

▶ Typical features include heavy menstrual bleeding for longer than 7 days or blood loss that exceeds 80 mL per menses.

▶ The severity is categorized according to hemodynamic status and degree of anemia and classified as mild, moderate, or severe.

▶ Acute management depends on the severity and its specific etiology and typically consists of hormonal management.

Abnormal uterine bleeding (AUB) describes any aberration of menstrual volume, regulation, frequency, and duration. Examples of AUB include periods that are characterized by heavy menstrual bleeding (HMB) such as menorrhagia (prolonged bleeding that occurs at regular intervals) and menometrorrhagia (heavy prolonged bleeding that occurs irregularly and more frequently than normal). The differential diagnosis of common and less common etiologies in adolescence are listed in Table 4–16.

▶ Evaluation

In addition to a menstrual and sexual history, the bleeding pattern should be characterized by cycle length, duration, and quantity of bleeding (eg, number of soaked pads or tampons in 24 hours, number of menstrual accidents). Bleeding for longer than 7 days or blood loss that exceeds 80 mL per menses is considered abnormal. The patient should be assessed for symptoms of anemia including fatigue, lightheadedness, syncope, and tachycardia, and for other abnormal bleeding (gingivae, stool, easy bruising). Physical examination includes an assessment of hemodynamic stability with orthostatic heart rate and blood pressure measurements. Mucous membranes and skin should be evaluated for pallor; the heart for tachycardia and murmur; the abdomen for organomegaly; and the external genitalia for signs of trauma or congenital anomalies. If the patient has never been sexually active and the external examination is normal, a pelvic examination is usually unnecessary. In a sexually experienced female, a pelvic and bimanual examination to examine the vagina, cervix, and adnexa may be helpful. Initial laboratory studies should include a pregnancy test, complete blood cell count, prothrombin time, partial thromboplastin

Table 4–16. Differential diagnosis of AUB in adolescents.

Condition	Examples
Anovulation	
Sexually transmitted infections	Cervicitis, pelvic inflammatory disease
Pregnancy complications	Ectopic, miscarriage
Bleeding disorders	von Willebrand disease, platelet function abnormalities, thrombocytopenia, coagulopathy
Endocrine disorders	Hypo-/hyperthyroidism, hyperprolactinemia, adrenal insufficiency, PCOS
Anatomic abnormalities	Congenital anomalies, ovarian cysts or tumors, cervical polyps
Trauma	Vaginal laceration
Foreign body	Retained tampon
Chronic illness	Liver, renal, inflammatory bowel, lupus
Malignancy	Leukemia
Drugs	Contraception, anticoagulants

AUB, abnormal uterine bleeding; PCOS, polycystic ovary syndrome.

time, TSH, fibrinogen level, and iron studies. If the patient has signs of hemodynamic compromise potentially requiring blood transfusion, blood type and cross-match should be obtained. Among adolescents with HMB, up to 20% are reported to have an underlying bleeding disorder. Evaluation for underlying bleeding disorders such as von Willebrand deficiency should be considered for patients who endorse any of the following: insignificant wounds that lead to prolonged bleeding; heavy, prolonged, or recurrent bleeding after surgery or dental procedures; epistaxis > 10 minutes in duration or requiring medical attention; unexplained bleeding from the gastrointestinal tract; HMB with iron deficiency; postpartum hemorrhage; and/or a family history of bleeding disorders. Abnormalities in platelet function and/or aggregation can also be considered with consultation with a pediatric hematologist. For patients suspected of having PCOS, total and free testosterone, DHEAS and androstenedione should be measured. For sexually experienced females, cervical or vaginal or urine-based testing for *C trachomatis* and gonorrhea should be obtained.

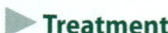 **Treatment**

The goals of treatment include (1) establishment and/or maintenance of hemodynamic stability, (2) correction of acute or chronic anemia, (3) resumption of normal menstrual cycles, (4) prevention of recurrence, and (5) prevention

of long-term consequences of anovulation. Management depends on the severity and specific etiology (Table 4–17). Many different hormonal regimens have been shown to be successful in controlling AUB; however, there is little evidence to support one regimen over another in the adolescent population. It is important to determine whether the patient has any medical contraindications to estrogen use, as monophasic COCs containing 30–50 mcg of ethinyl estradiol with potent progestins, norgestrel or levonorgestrel, are recommended when an oral regimen can be started, and intravenous IV conjugated estrogen is often used in settings with rapid blood loss and/or severe anemia (see Table 4–17). Once acute menstrual bleeding is stopped and the patient is transitioned to an oral maintenance regimen to continue to suppress bleeding, it is important to remind adolescents and their families that adherence with medications to control bleeding and treat anemia is imperative. Historically, COCs have been used with a daily multidose tapered regimen to manage heavy menstrual bleeding. It is becoming more common to use a combination of COCs and norethindrone acetate (eg, one COC and 10 mg norethindrone acetate per day) to manage menorrhagia as this regimen is often successful and the side effects from taking higher daily doses of estrogen are reduced. Heavy menstrual bleeding should be treated until the anemia is resolved and often for an additional 6 months or longer if there is an underlying problem such as a platelet function abnormality or von Willebrand disease. For patients with contraindications to the use of exogenous estrogens, there are progestin-only and nonhormonal (antifibrinolytic) therapies available for acute management and maintenance treatment of AUB (Table 4–18). Patients with severe anemia and/or those with rapid blood loss that does not stop with initial hormonal management may require blood transfusion and consultation by hematology and gynecology for consideration of a procedural intervention to control bleeding.

4. Mittelschmerz

Mittelschmerz is midcycle discomfort resulting from ovulation. The cause of the pain is unknown but irritation of the peritoneum due to spillage of fluid from the ruptured follicular cyst at the time of ovulation has been suggested. The patient presents with a history of midcycle, unilateral dull or aching abdominal pain lasting a few minutes to as long as 8 hours. Rarely, the pain mimics that of acute appendicitis, torsion or rupture of an ovarian cyst, or ectopic pregnancy. The patient should be reassured and treated symptomatically.

5. Premenstrual Syndrome & Premenstrual Dysphoric Disorder

It is estimated that 51%–86% of adolescent women experience some premenstrual symptoms. Premenstrual syndrome (PMS) is a cluster of physical and psychological symptoms that occur during the luteal phase of the menstrual cycle and

Table 4–17. Management of AUB for patients without medical contraindications to estrogen.

	Mild	Moderate	Severe
Hgb value (g/dL)	Hgb > 12 (outpatient management)	Hgb 9–12 (outpatient management)	Hgb < 9 (emergency room, inpatient management)
Acute treatment	Menstrual calendar; iron supplementation (ferrous sulfate 325 mg po qd). Consider hormonal management.	Monophasic 30–35 mcg COC bid until bleeding stops, then decease to 1 pill qd. Continue active pill qd (skip placebo pills) until Hct > 30%. Alternative option is 1 COC and 5 mg NETA qd until Hct > 30%. (Stop NETA when taking placebo pills.) Daily iron supplementation with both approaches. Advise patient to call office if bleeding hasn't stopped within 24 h. Follow-up appointment 7 days.	Assess hemodynamic stability and treat appropriately. Consider blood transfusion for severe symptomatic anemia and/or rapid blood loss. Conjugated estrogen, 25 mg IV every 4–6 h, up to 48 h. Provide scheduled IV antiemetic. When bleeding stops, stop IV estrogen and start COC taper with monophasic 30–35 mcg pill PO qid (or tid), then taper as below. Alternative oral option is 1 COC and NETA 10 mg PO qd. If bleeding doesn't improve, hematology and gynecology consultations for possible antifibrinolytic and procedural intervention. Discharge criteria: hemodynamically stable, Hgb and Hct stable, bleeding stopped, patient tolerating oral regimen. Taper: One 30–35 mcg COC PO qid until bleeding stops, then decrease to tid for 2 days (up to 7 days), then bid for 2 days (up to 7 days), then qd (skip placebo pills) until Hct > 30%. PO antiemetic 2 h prior to COC dose as needed for nausea. Regimen requires excellent adherence. Advise patient to call office if bleeding resumes; may need to stop taper and revert back to dose frequency that stopped bleeding. Follow-up appointment 7 days.
Long-term management	Monitor menstrual calendar and Hgb. Follow-up in 2–3 mo.	Iron supplementation. Monitor Hgb closely for improvement. May need to revert to bid COC dosing if bleeding persists. If bleeding controlled, cycle with COCs (28 days pack) or other combined hormonal contraceptive agent for minimum 3–6 mo.	Iron supplementation. Recheck Hgb/Hct at follow-up visit and/or if bleeding resumes. Goal to have normalization of Hgb/Hct prior to next period. Consider ongoing menstrual management with combined hormonal contraceptive for minimum 6–12 mo. Levonorgestrel intrauterine system has an indication for menorrhagia management.

AUB, abnormal uterine bleeding; bid, twice daily (every 12 hours); COC, combined oral contraceptive pill; Hct, hematocrit; Hgb, hemoglobin; IV, intravenous; NETA, norethindrone acetate; PO, by mouth; qd, daily; qid, four times per day (every 6 hours); tid, three times per day (every 8 hours).

resolve with menstruation. Physical symptoms include bloating, breast tenderness, fatigue, headache, myalgia, increased appetite, and food craving. Emotional symptoms may include fatigue, mood lability, anxiety, depression, irritability, hostility, sleep dysfunction, and impaired social function. PMS can be diagnosed when at least one disabling physical or psychological symptom is documented prospectively for at least two consecutive menstrual cycles, is restricted to the luteal phase of the menstrual cycle, resolves by the end of menses, results in functional impairment, and is not an exacerbation of another underlying disorder. Severe PMS with functional impairment affects 1.8%–5.8% of women of reproductive age and is classified in the *Diagnostic and Statistical Manual of Mental Disorders*, Fifth Edition, as premenstrual dysphoric disorder (PMDD). The clinical diagnosis of PMDD requires

a combination of a minimum of five physical and psychological symptoms in the majority of cycles that must be present in the final week before onset of menses, start to improve within a few days after the onset of menses, and become minimal or absent in the week post-menses.

The pathophysiology of PMS is not well understood; however, there is evidence of dysregulation of serotonergic activity and/or of GABAergic receptor functioning during the luteal phase of the menstrual cycle with heightened sensitivity to circulating progesterone metabolites. PMS and PMDD are highly associated with unipolar depressive disorder and anxiety disorders, such as obsessive-compulsive disorder, panic disorder, and generalized anxiety disorder. During adolescence, it may be difficult to determine if the affective symptoms represent a mood or anxiety disorder,

Table 4–18. Progesterone-only hormone regimens for management of AUB.

Hormone	Tapering Regimen
Norethindrone acetate	5–10 mg PO every 4 h until bleeding stops, then qid for 4 days, then tid for 3 days, then bid for 2 days–2 wk, then qd. Advise patient to call office if bleeding resumes; may need to stop taper and revert to dose frequency that stopped bleeding. Follow-up appointment 7 days. Once anemia improved, can stop NETA for 5-7 days for menses. Can continue NETA 5 mg PO qd for menstrual suppression and patient can determine the length of each suppressed cycle (eg, 21 days of NETA followed by 5–7 days off for menses if monthly periods are desired, or extended cycling with 90 days NETA and then 5–7 days off for menses.) If contraception is needed, consider levonorgestrel intrauterine system placement, etonogestrel contraceptive implant placement, or DMPA 150 mg IM q12wk. If patent experiences breakthrough bleeding with these methods, NETA 2.5–5 mg qd can be used for suppression.
Medroxyprogesterone	10 mg PO every 4 h (max 80 mg) until bleeding stops, then qid for 4 days, then tid for 3 days, then bid for 2 days–2 wk, then qd. Once anemia improved, can stop medication and allow for period. Consider transitioning to NETA as above for ongoing menstrual suppression or to a progesterone-only contraceptive method if contraception is needed.

AUB, abnormal uterine bleeding; bid, twice daily (every 12 hours); DMPA, depot medroxyprogesterone acetate; DUB, dysfunctional uterine bleeding; IM, intramuscular; NETA, norethindrone acetate; PO, by mouth; qd, daily; qid, four times per day (every 6 hours); tid, three times per day (every 8 hours).

a premenstrual exacerbation of a psychiatric disorder, or simple PMS.

Current treatment for PMS in adolescence is based on findings from adult studies and includes lifestyle recommendations and pharmacologic agents that suppress the rise and fall of ovarian steroids or augment serotonin. Proven effective interventions include education about pathophysiology, lifestyle changes (eg, increasing physical activity and smoking cessation), stress reduction, and cognitive behavioral therapy. If contraception or cycle control is important, a combined hormonal contraceptive pill may be beneficial. The pill containing 20 mcg ethinyl estradiol and 3 mg drospirenone has been shown to be therapeutic in adult women with PMDD. If these interventions do not adequately control symptoms, luteal phase or continuous administration of selective serotonin reuptake inhibitors (SSRIs) can be considered. SSRIs are increasingly used as first-line therapy for PMS and PMDD in adults, and a recent Cochrane review in severe adult PMS determined that SSRIs administered continuously or during the luteal phase were effective in reducing premenstrual symptoms. Although SSRIs are not approved by the Food and Drug Administration (FDA) for treatment of PMS or PMDD in adolescents, case reports indicate that adolescents with PMDD respond well to luteal phase dosing of fluoxetine at the standard adult dosage of 20 mg/day.

6. Ovarian Cysts

Functional ovarian cysts account for the majority of benign ovarian tumors in postpubertal adolescents and are a result of the normal process of ovulation. They may be asymptomatic or may cause menstrual irregularities or pelvic pain. Large cysts can cause constipation or urinary frequency. Follicular cysts are the most common functional cysts. They are usually unilateral, less than 3 cm in diameter, and resolve spontaneously in 1–2 months. Cyst pain occurs as the diameter of the cyst increases, stretching the overlying ovarian cortex and capsule. If the patient's discomfort is tolerable, she can be reexamined monthly and observed for resolution. Hormonal contraceptive products that suppress ovulation can be started to prevent additional cysts from forming. Patients with cysts should be counseled about the signs and symptoms of ovarian and/or tubal torsion, which are serious complications. Adnexal torsion presents with the sudden onset of pain, nausea, and vomiting. Low-grade fever, leukocytosis, and development of peritoneal signs with rebound and guarding can be found. Torsion is a surgical emergency due to the risk of ischemia and death of the ovary. Patients should be referred to a gynecologist for potential laparoscopy if a cyst has a solid component and measures more than 6 cm by ultrasonography, if there are symptoms or signs of hemorrhage or torsion, or if the cyst fails to regress within 2 months.

Corpus luteum cysts occur less commonly and may be large, 5–10 cm in diameter. The patient with a corpus luteum cyst may have associated amenorrhea, or as the cyst becomes atretic, heavy vaginal bleeding. There may be bleeding into the cyst or rupture with intraperitoneal hemorrhage. To determine whether bleeding is self-limited, serial hematocrit measurements and ultrasounds can be used. If the patient is stable, hormonal contraception that suppresses ovulation can be started to prevent additional cyst formation and the patient may be monitored for 3 months for resolution. Laparoscopy may be indicated if the cyst is larger than 6 cm or if there is severe pain or hemorrhage.

Borzutzky C, Jaffray J: Diagnosis and management of heavy menstrual bleeding and bleeding disorders in adolescents. JAMA Pediatr 2020 Feb 1;174(2):186–194 [PMID: 31886837].

Committee on Adolescent Health Care: The Initial Reproductive Health Visit: ACOG Committee Opinion, Number 811. Obstet Gynecol 2020 Oct;136(4):e70–e80 [PMID: 32976378].

Committee on Adolescent Health Care: Screening and Management of Bleeding Disorders in Adolescents With Heavy Menstrual Bleeding: ACOG Committee Opinion, Number 785. Obstet Gynecol. 2019 Sep;134(3):e71–e83 [PMID: 31441825].

Fontham ETH et al: Cervical cancer screening for individuals at average risk: 2020 guideline update from the American Cancer Society. CA Cancer J Clin 2020 Sep;70(5):321–346. Epub 2020 Jul 30 [PMID: 32729638].

Gordon CM et al: Functional hypothalamic amenorrhea: an Endocrine Society Clinical Practice Guideline. J Clin Endocrinol Metab 2017;102(5):1413–1439 [PMID: 28368518].

Ryan SA: The treatment of dysmenorrhea. Pediatr Clin North Am 2017;64(2):331–342 [PMID: 28292449].

Teede HJ et al; International PCOS Network: Recommendations from the international evidence-based guideline for the assessment and management of polycystic ovary syndrome. Fertil Steril 2018 Aug;110(3):364–379 [PMID: 30033227].

Workowski KA et al: Sexually Transmitted Infections Treatment Guidelines, 2021. MMWR Recomm Rep 2021 Jul 23;70(4):1–187 [PMID: 34292926].

CONTRACEPTION

According to the CDC 2021 Youth Risk Behavior Survey, 30% of high school students reported having had sexual intercourse and 21% reported being currently sexually active. Forty-eight percent reported not using a condom during their latest intercourse. Most young people have sex for the first time at about the age of 18, but do not marry until their middle or late twenties. This means that young adults are at higher risk of unwanted pregnancy and STIs for nearly a decade. A sexually active female who does not use contraceptives has almost a 90% chance of becoming pregnant within a year.

▶ Contraception Evaluation and Counseling

Talking with teenagers about sexual intercourse and its implications can help teens make informed decisions regarding engaging in sexual activity. The AAP endorses a comprehensive approach to sexuality education that incorporates encouraging abstinence while providing appropriate risk reduction counseling regarding sexual behaviors. Counseling should include discussions about confidentiality, STI

Table 4–19. Effectiveness for contraceptive methods (%).

	Perfect Use	Typical Use
No method	15	15
Spermicides	84	79
Withdrawal	96	80
Internal (female) condom	95	79
External (male) condom	98	77
Oral contraceptive pill	99.7	93
Contraceptive patch	99.7	93
Vaginal ring	99.7	93
Medroxyprogesterone acetate injection	99.8	96
Hormonal IUD	99.7	99.6
Copper IUD	99.4	99.2
Etonogestrel Implant	99.9	99.9

prevention and testing, and contraceptive methods including abstinence and emergency contraception (Table 4–19). The CDC provides the useful *Guide to Taking a Sexual History*, which covers the "five Ps" of sexual health: *p*artners, *p*ractices, *p*rotection from STIs, *p*ast history of STIs, and *p*revention of pregnancy (http://www.cdc.gov/std/treatment/SexualHistory.pdf).

Evaluation of an adolescent female requesting contraception should include a review of current and past medical conditions, current medications and allergies, menstrual history, confidential social history including sexual history, and family medical history. Important components of a sexual history include age at first intercourse, number of partners in lifetime, history of STIs and pelvic inflammatory disease (PID), condom use, current and past use of other contraceptives and reasons for discontinuation, and pregnancy history and outcomes. It is helpful to have a baseline weight, height, BMI, and blood pressure. A pelvic examination is not necessary before initiating contraception. However, if the woman is sexually active and has missed menstrual periods or has symptoms of pregnancy, a pregnancy test is warranted. STI screening (if asymptomatic) or diagnostic testing (if symptomatic) should be offered to sexually experienced women.

The goals of counseling adolescents about contraception include promoting safe and responsible sexual behavior through delaying initiation of sexual activity, reinforcing consistent condom use for those who are sexually active, and discussing other contraceptive options to provide protection from unwanted pregnancy. Encouraging adolescents to use contraception when they do engage in sexual intercourse does not lead to higher rates of sexual activity. MI can be used to address ambivalence and discrepancies among adolescents' sexual and contraceptive behaviors, their sexual and relationship values, and future life goals. Providers should familiarize themselves with their state policies regarding the ability of minors to consent for sexual and reproductive health care services (accessible at http://www.guttmacher.org and http://www.adolescenthealthlaw.org).

Providers should consider the adolescent's lifestyle, potential challenges to compliance, need for confidentiality, previous experiences with contraception and reasons for discontinuation, and any misconceptions regarding contraceptive options. Barriers to health care access including transportation and financial limitations should be identified. Prescribing contraception for other medical reasons (eg, management of dysmenorrhea) can create opportunities for providers and adolescent patients to make parents aware of the use of the medication while maintaining confidentiality around sexual behaviors.

Advantages, disadvantages, potential side effects, and instructions for use of contraceptive methods in a concise and age-appropriate manner should be reviewed with adolescent patients. Written instructions that are clear and at an appropriate educational level can also be helpful. Teens need to be reminded that hormonal contraception will not protect them from STI transmission (including HIV infection), and condoms need to be used consistently. Encouraging teens to be creative about personal reminders such as setting a cell phone alarm to take a pill can help with adherence. Teens often discontinue birth control for nonmedical reasons or minor side effects and should be encouraged to contact their providers if any questions or concerns arise to avoid unintentional pregnancy. Follow-up visits every few months may improve adherence and also provide opportunities for further reproductive health education and STI screening.

► Barrier Methods

All sexually active adolescents should be counseled to use condoms correctly and consistently with all intimate behaviors (oral, vaginal, and anal intercourse). Condoms offer protection against STIs by providing a mechanical barrier. Polyurethane condoms can be used by adolescents with an allergy to latex. Spermicides containing nonoxynol-9 are no longer recommended, as exposure to spermicide can cause genital irritation which may facilitate the acquisition of STIs including HIV. Patients should be counseled to use water-based lubricants with condoms.

Vaginal barrier methods include the female condom, diaphragm, and cervical cap. The female condom is a polyurethane vaginal pouch that can be used as an alternative to the male condom. Female condoms have lower efficacy in preventing pregnancy and STIs and are more expensive than male condoms. Diaphragms and cervical caps may not be feasible for adolescents as they require prescription, professional fitting, and skill with insertion, and they do not prevent STIs.

► Hormonal Contraceptives

1. Mechanism of Action

The primary mechanism of action for combined hormonal contraceptives containing estrogen and progestin (OCPs, transdermal patch, intravaginal ring) is inhibition of ovulation. Thickening of the cervical mucus also makes sperm penetration more difficult, and atrophy of the endometrium diminishes the chance of implantation. The primary mechanisms by which pregnancy is prevented by progestin-only methods (pills, DMPA, and etonogestrel implant) include cervical mucous thickening and thinning of the endometrial lining, and variable inhibition of ovulation.

Starting all hormonal birth control methods during the menstrual period (either first day of bleeding or first Sunday of bleeding) produces the most reliable suppression of ovulation. Conventional OCPs, transdermal patches, and intravaginal rings typically require that the adolescent wait for her next period to begin before starting. Data show that many women who receive prescriptions or even samples of medication never begin the prescribed method. Furthermore, these women could become pregnant while waiting to start. "Quick Start" is an alternative approach to starting contraception that allows the patient to begin contraception on the day of the appointment regardless of menstrual cycle day, following a negative pregnancy test. This approach has been studied in adolescent women and increases adherence with the method of choice.

2. Absolute and Relative Contraindications

The World Health Organization's (WHO) publication, *Improving Access to Quality Care in Family Planning: Medical Eligibility Criteria for Contraceptive Use* is an evidence-based guide providing criteria for initiating and continuing contraceptive methods based on a risk assessment of an individual's characteristics or preexisting medical conditions. Absolute and relative contraindications to using combined hormonal birth control pills, listed in Table 4–20, can be extended to other combined hormonal products that contain estrogen and progestins, including the transdermal patch and intravaginal ring. The CDC publication, *US Medical Eligibility Criteria for Contraceptive Use,* adapted from the WHO publication, allows consideration of use of combined hormonal contraceptive products in women who are receiving anticoagulation therapy.

Patients should be assessed for possible risk factors for venous thromboembolic events (VTEs) prior to initiating any contraceptive product containing estrogen. The risk of VTE for reproductive-aged women is extremely low

Table 4–20. Contraindications to combined oral contraceptive (COC) pills.

Absolute contraindications
Pregnancy
Breast-feeding (within 6 wk of childbirth)
Hypertension SBP > 160 mm Hg or DBP > 100 mm Hg
History of thrombophlebitis; current thromboembolic disorder, cerebrovascular disease, or ischemic heart disease
Known thrombogenic mutations (factor V Leiden; prothrombin mutation; protein S, protein C, and antithrombin deficiencies)
Systemic lupus erythematosus
Complicated valvular heart disease (with pulmonary hypertension; atrial fibrillation; history of bacterial endocarditis)
Diabetes with nephropathy; retinopathy; neuropathy
Liver disease: active viral hepatitis; severe cirrhosis; tumor (hepatocellular adenoma or hepatoma)
Breast cancer (current)
Migraine headaches with aura
Major surgery with prolonged immobilization
Relative contraindications
Postpartum (first 3 wk)
Breast-feeding (6 wk–6 mo following childbirth)
Hypertension (adequately controlled HTN; any history of HTN where BP cannot be evaluated; SBP 140–159 mm Hg or DPB 90–99 mm Hg)
Migraine headache without aura (for continuation of COC)
Breast cancer history with remission for 5 y
Active gallbladder disease or history of COC-induced cholestasis
Use of drugs that affect liver enzymes (rifampin, phenytoin, carbamazepine, barbiturates, primidone, topiramate, oxcarbazepine, lamotrigine, ritonavir-boosted protease inhibitors)

BP, blood pressure; DBP, diastolic blood pressure; HTN, hypertension; SBP, systolic blood pressure.

(1–5/10,000 woman-years for nonpregnant women not using contraceptive products containing estrogen). The use of estrogen increases the risk of VTE for nonpregnant women (3–15/10,000 woman-years); however, pregnancy markedly increases the risk of VTE (5–20/10,000 woman-years in pregnancy and 40–65/10,000 woman-years postpartum). In light of the low population risk of VTE, it is not cost-effective to screen all reproductive-aged women for inherited thrombophilia (factor V Leiden, prothrombin mutation, protein S, protein C, and antithrombin deficiencies).for personal and family history of VTE. If testing identified a specific defect in a close relative who had VTE, the adolescent should be tested for that defect prior to initiating a product containing estrogen. If results of testing in family members is unknown but the family history is highly suggested of inherited thrombophilia, testing the adolescent for all inherited thrombophilic disorders prior to initiating estrogen should be considered. Additionally, if testing is indicated but not possible, providers should consider alternative contraceptive products that do not contain estrogen.

3. Combined Hormonal Methods

A. Oral Contraceptive Pills

Combined oral contraceptive (COC) pills are the most commonly used contraceptive method in the adolescent age group. COC pills are also utilized for noncontraceptive indications (Table 4–21). All COC pills contain estrogen (ethinyl estradiol). "Low-dose" COC pills contain 20–35 mcg of ethinyl estradiol per pill. There are a variety of progestins used in COC pills, most made from testosterone with differing androgenic profiles. Drospirenone is a progestin derived from spironolactone that possesses anti-androgenic and anti-mineralocorticoid activity. This formulation has appeal for use with patients who have PCOS but should not be prescribed for patients with risk of hyperkalemia (those who have renal, hepatic, or adrenal insufficiency or take certain medications including angiotensin-converting enzyme inhibitors and angiotensin II receptor antagonists). Extended cycle regimens are available to decrease menstrual frequency from twelve cycles a year to four cycles per year, and chewable COCs exist for those who cannot swallow pills.

In general, COC pill side effects are mild and improve or lessen during the first 3 months of use. Table 4–22 shows the more common estrogenic, progestogenic, and combined (estrogenic and progestogenic) effects of COC pills. These symptoms can also be observed with the other combined hormonal methods. If a patient taking contraceptive pills has persistent minor side effects for more than 3 months, a different type of COC can be tried to achieve the hormonal effects desired (eg, decreasing the estrogen content or changing progestin). Breakthrough bleeding is a common side effect in the first few months of COC use and generally resolves without intervention. If breakthrough bleeding is persistent, possible etiologies such as missed pills, pregnancy, infection, or interaction with other medications should be ruled out.

Table 4–21. Noncontraceptive health benefits of oral contraceptive pills.

Protection against life-threatening conditions
Ovarian cancer
Endometrial cancer
Pelvic inflammatory disease
Ectopic pregnancy
Morbidity and mortality due to unintended pregnancies
Alleviate conditions affecting quality of life
Iron deficiency anemia
Benign breast disease
Dysmenorrhea
Irregular menstrual cycles
Functional ovarian cysts
Premenstrual syndrome
Acne

Table 4–22. Estrogenic, progestenic, and combined effects of COCs by system.

System	Estrogen Effects	Progestin Effects	Estrogen and Progestin Effects
General		Bloating	Cyclic weight gain due to fluid retention
Cardiovascular	Hypertension		Hypertension
Gastrointestinal	Nausea; hepatocellular adenomas	Increased appetite and weight gain; increased LDL cholesterol levels; decreased HDL cholesterol levels; decreased carbohydrate tolerance; increased insulin resistance	
Breast	Increased breast size	Increased breast tenderness or breast size	Breast tenderness
Genitourinary	Leukorrhea; cervical eversion or ectopy		
Hematologic	Thromboembolic complications, including pulmonary emboli (rare), deep venous thrombosis, cerebrovascular accident, or myocardial infarction (rare)		
Neurologic			Headaches
Skin	Telangiectasia, melasma	Acne, oily skin	
Psychological		Depression, fatigue, decreased libido	

COC, combined oral contraceptive pill; HDL, high-density lipoprotein; LDL, low-density lipoprotein.
Reproduced with permission from Hatcher RA: *Contraceptive Technology*, 20th ed. New York: Ardent Media; 2011.

For women who have spotting or bleeding before completing the active hormonal pills, increasing the progestin content will provide more endometrial support. For those with continued spotting or bleeding after the period, increasing the estrogen content will provide more endometrial support.

B. Transdermal Patch

The contraceptive transdermal patch releases 20 mcg of ethinyl estradiol and 150 mcg of norelgestromin daily. One patch is worn for 7 days and changed weekly for 3 consecutive weeks. The patch is an attractive alternative to COC pills for adolescents who have difficulty remembering to take a pill every day. As with other estrogen-containing contraceptive products, patients should be advised to avoid smoking and consider planned discontinuation of these methods around major surgery and prolonged immobilization. In clinical trials, the most common side effects include breast pain and swelling, headache, nausea, and skin irritation. The patch may be less effective in women weighing more than 90 kg and those with skin conditions preventing absorption.

C. Intravaginal Ring

There are two intravaginal ring contraceptive systems. One releases on average 0.12 mg of etonogestrel and 0.015 mg of ethinyl estradiol daily and must remain in place in the vagina continuously for 3 weeks (21 days) followed by a 1-week

(7-day) vaginal ring-free interval during which there will be withdrawal bleeding. A new ring is inserted exactly seven days after removal. The other ring releases on average 0.15 mg of segesterone acetate and 0.013 mg of ethinyl estradiol daily and must remain in place in the vagina continuously for 3 weeks (21 days) followed by a 1-week (7-day) vaginal ring-free interval during which there is withdrawal menstrual bleeding. When the ring is removed from the vagina, it can be washed with mild soap and water, dried with a clean cloth towel or paper towel and stored in the case provided until it is reinserted exactly seven days after removal. One vaginal ring provides contraception for thirteen 28-day cycles. This ring not been adequately studied in females with a BMI greater than 29 kg/m². In clinical trials, more common side effects included vaginitis and vaginal discharge, headache, weight gain, and nausea.

4. Progestin-Only Methods

A. Oral Contraceptive Pills

Progestin-only pills (POPs) do not contain estrogen. They are used in women with contraindications to estrogen-containing products, for example, inherited risk factors for thrombophilia, or unacceptable estrogen-related side effects with COC pills. The efficacy of POPs in preventing pregnancy is slightly less than with COC pills. They require strict adherence and must be taken daily at the same time (within 3 hours) due to the shorter half-life of the progestin. The main side effect of POPs is unpredictable menstrual patterns. The need for strict adherence and the possibility of breakthrough bleeding may make POPs a less desirable method for teens.

B. Injectable Hormonal Contraception

DMPA, or Depo-Provera, is a long-acting injectable progestin contraceptive. It is injected into the gluteal or deltoid muscle every 12 weeks at a dose of 150 mg. The first injection should be given during the first 5 days of the menstrual cycle to ensure immediate contraceptive protection. The quick-start method may also be used with DMPA following a negative pregnancy test. Adolescents who have been sexually active within the previous 2 weeks of administration of DMPA using the quick-start method should be informed of the chance of pregnancy and instructed to return for a repeat pregnancy test 2 weeks after receiving DMPA. With a failure rate of less than 0.3%, its long-acting nature that reduces adherence issues, reversibility, and lack of estrogen-related side effects, DMPA is an attractive contraceptive option for many adolescents. The hypoestrogenic state that results from DMPA suppression of the hypothalamic-pituitary-ovarian axis reduces the normal effect of estrogen to inhibit bone resorption. The FDA issued a black box warning that long-term (>2 years) use of DMPA was a cause of decreased bone density, a particular concern as adolescence is the critical time of peak bone accretion. Current recommendations are that long-term use of DMPA should be limited to situations in which other contraceptive methods are inadequate. Although DMPA use is associated with decreased bone density, studies show that bone mineral density recovers after stopping DMPA. There are no studies that address whether decreased bone density from adolescent DMPA use increases the risk of osteoporosis and fractures in adulthood. The consensus of experts is that the advantages of DMPA generally outweigh the theoretical risks of fractures later in life. As with every other contraceptive method, providers need to help patients weigh the pros and cons of initiating and continuing with this method of contraception. Adolescents using DMPA should be counseled to take adequate dietary calcium (1300 mg/day) and vitamin D (400 IU/day), avoid tobacco smoking and have regular weight-bearing physical activity for overall bone health. Other adverse effects of DMPA include unpredictable menstrual patterns, weight gain (typically 5 lb/y for the first 2 years of use), and mood changes.

C. Contraceptive Implant

Adolescents most commonly use short-acting hormonal contraceptive methods described above. Unfortunately, these methods have relatively high failure rates (see Table 4–19) and low continuation rates. LARCs, which include the contraceptive implants and IUDs, have lower rates of failure and discontinuation. In one study comparing 1-year continuation

rates for short-acting contraceptives versus LARCs, the continuation rate for short-acting methods was 55% versus 86% for LARCs. The pregnancy rate associated with use of short-acting contraceptives was 22 times higher than the rate of unintended pregnancy associated with the use of LARCs. Adolescents should be encouraged to consider LARCs as the best reversible methods for preventing unintended pregnancy, rapid repeat pregnancy, and abortion.

Nexplanon is a single-rod implant LARC that contains the progestin etonogestrel. Nexplanon also contains barium sulfate which makes it radiopaque. Nexplanon is placed subdermally and provides highly effective contraception for four years, with failure rates less than 1%. Nexplanon suppresses ovulation and thickens cervical mucous like DMPA but does not suppress ovarian estradiol production or induce a hypoestrogenic state. Therefore, the risk of decreased bone density is less than that associated with DMPA. Placement should occur during the first 5 days of the menstrual period or at any time if a woman is correctly using a different hormonal contraceptive method. Proper timing minimizes the likelihood that the implant is placed during an early pregnancy or in a nonpregnant woman too late to inhibit ovulation in the first cycle of use. Irregular menstrual bleeding is the single most common reason for stopping use in clinical trials. On average, the volume of bleeding is similar to the woman's typical menstrual periods, but the schedule of bleeding is irregular and unpredictable. Other side effects include headache, weight gain, acne, breast pain, and emotional lability. Return to fertility is rapid following removal. The efficacy of Nexplanon has not been formally defined in women with BMIs greater than 130% ideal and could theoretically be less in these women. The etonogestrel implant is not recommended for women who chronically take medications that are potent hepatic enzyme inducers because etonogestrel levels may be substantially reduced.

D. Hormone-Containing Intrauterine Devices

Intrauterine devices (IUDs) are LARCs approved for use in nulliparous and parous teens. They have high efficacy, with failure rates of less than 1%. Four IUDs release the progestin levonorgestrel: Mirena, which releases 20 mcg of levonorgestrel per day and is approved for contraception for up to 8 years; Liletta, which releases 18.6 mcg/day initially and declines progressively to 12.6 mcg/day at 3 years after insertion and is approved for contraception for up to 8 years; Kyleena, which has a release rate of 17.5 mcg/day after 24 days, declining to 7.4 mcg/day after 5 years and is approved for contraception for up to 5 years; and Skyla, which releases an average of 6 mcg/day and is approved for contraception for up to 3 years. The levonorgestrel IUDs have many contraceptive actions including thickening of cervical mucous, inhibiting sperm capacitation and survival, suppressing the endometrium, and suppression of ovulation in some women. Given that the contraceptive effect of levonorgestrel in the

IUDs is mainly due to its local effect versus systemic absorption, ovulation is not always suppressed, and cysts related to normal ovulation can occur. In addition to pregnancy prevention, women with IUDs report reduced symptoms of dysmenorrhea and reduced pain from endometriosis. Irregular bleeding is common in the first few months following insertion because endometrial suppression takes several months to evolve. Bleeding is then markedly decreased and secondary amenorrhea can occur. Other side effects include abdominal and/or pelvic pain, acne, ovarian cysts, and headache. Cramping is common during insertion and spontaneous expulsion can occur. Uterine perforation during insertion is an uncommon risk.

A common misconception about IUD use is that it increases the risk of PID. Current research shows that the risk of PID is increased above baseline only for the first 20 days after insertion. IUD use has also not been shown to increase the risk of tubal infertility or ectopic pregnancy. Contraindications to IUD placement include pregnancy, PID, postabortion sepsis within the past 3 months, current STI, purulent cervicitis, undiagnosed abnormal vaginal bleeding, malignancy of the genital tract, uterine anomalies, leiomyomata distorting the uterine cavity that prevent insertion, and allergy to any component of the IUD. Adolescents should be screened for STIs prior to insertion of an IUD.

▶ Non-hormonal Intrauterine Devices

The copper T 380A IUD, ParaGard, does not contain hormones. It provides contraception for up to 10 years by release of copper ions which inhibit sperm migration and by development of a sterile inflammatory reaction which is toxic to sperm and ova and prevents implantation. Menstrual pain and heavy bleeding are the most common reasons for discontinuation. Patients with disorders of copper metabolism (Wilson disease) should not use a copper-containing IUD.

▶ Emergency Contraception

Emergency contraception (EC) is the only contraceptive method designed to prevent pregnancy after unprotected or underprotected intercourse (Table 4–23). Indications for EC include unprotected vaginal intercourse, failure of contraceptive methods (broken condoms, missing three or more active COC pills, detached contraceptive patch, removed vaginal ring, or late DMPA injection), and sexual assault. EC medications include products labeled and approved for use as EC by the FDA (levonorgestrel; ulipristal acetate) and "off-label" use of COC pills (the Yuzpe method).

Levonorgestrel EC is a one-pill progesterone-only regimen that contains 1.5 mg of levonorgestrel, taken immediately after unprotected intercourse. The exact mechanism of levonorgestrel EC is unknown but is thought to inhibit ovulation, disrupt follicular development, or interfere with the maturation of the corpus luteum. EC is not teratogenic and

Table 4–23. Emergency contraception regimens.

Progestin-Only	Dose: Once
Plan B One-Step, Take Action, Next Choice One Dose, My Way	1 pill
Ulipristal Acetate	**Dose: Once**
Ella	1 pill
Estrogen and Progestin	**Dose: Repeat in 12 h**
Ovral, Ogestrel	2 white pills
Levlen, Nordette	4 orange pills
Lo/Ovral, Low-Ogestrel, Levora, Quasense, Cryselle	4 white pills
Jolessa, Portia, Seasonale, Trivora	4 pink pills
Triphasil, Tri-Levlen	4 yellow pills
Seasonique	4 light blue-green pills
Enpresse	4 orange pills
Alesse, Lessina, Levlite	5 pink pills
Aviane	5 orange pills
Lutera	5 white pills

does not interrupt a pregnancy that has already implanted in the uterine lining. Therefore, pregnancy testing before use is not required. It is recommended that patients take these products within 72 hours of unprotected intercourse. Efficacy diminishes with time from the event: 90% effective if used within 24 hours, 75% effective within 72 hours, and approximately 60% within 120 hours; thus, patients should be counseled to take the medication as soon as possible following unprotected intercourse or contraception failure. EC, available without a prescription, could potentially prevent approximately 80% of unintended pregnancies and should be part of anticipatory guidance given to sexually active adolescents. A follow-up appointment should be conducted 10–14 days after administration of EC for pregnancy testing, STI screening, and counseling regarding reproductive health and contraceptive use.

If an approved EC medication is not available, certain COC pills containing levonorgestrel or norgestrel can also be used for EC in a two-dose regimen separated by 12 hours; this approach is known as the Yuzpe method (see Table 4–23). An antiemetic drug taken 30 minutes prior to pills containing estrogen may help control nausea. A pregnancy test is not required prior to prescription and administration.

Ulipristal, marketed as Ella, is a single pill containing 30 mg of ulipristal acetate that is available by prescription only and can be used within 120 hours after unprotected intercourse. Ulipristal binds to the human progesterone receptor and prevents binding of progesterone. Unlike levonorgestrel EC, a pregnancy test must be performed to exclude existing pregnancy before taking ulipristal because of the risk of fetal loss if used in the first trimester. Patients should be counseled that a pregnancy test is indicated if their period is more than 7 days later than expected after taking ulipristal and that they should return for evaluation of the rare occurrence of ectopic pregnancy if severe abdominal pain occurs 3–5 weeks after use.

Finally, insertion of ParaGard (copper IUD) within 5 days of unprotected intercourse is an additional method of emergency contraception available in the U.S.

Centers for Disease Control and Prevention: 2021 Youth Risk Behavior Survey Questionnaire. www.cdc.gov/yrbs. Accessed May 1, 2023.

Committee on Adolescence: Contraception and adolescents. Pediatrics 2014;134:e1257–e1281 [PMID: 17974753].

Grubb LK, Powers M; Committee on Adolescence: Emerging issues in male adolescent sexual and reproductive health care. Pediatrics 2020;145(5):e20200627 [PMID: 32341182].

Hatcher RA et al: Contraceptive efficacy. In: Hatcher RA et al (eds): *Contraceptive Technology*. 21st ed. New York, NY: Ayer Company Publishers; 2018.

Marcell AV, Burstein GR; Committee on Adolescence: Sexual and reproductive health care services in the pediatric setting. Pediatrics 2017 Nov;140(5):e20172858 [PMID: 29061870].

Menon S; Committee on Adolescence: Long-acting reversible contraception: specific issues for adolescents. Pediatrics 2020 Aug;146(2):e2020007252. doi: 10.1542/peds.2020-007252. Epub 2020 Jul 20 [PMID: 32690806].

Practice Committee of the American Society for Reproductive Medicine: Combined hormonal contraception and the risk of venous thromboembolism: a guideline. Fertil Steril 2017;107(1):43–51 [PMID: 27793376].

World Health Organization: *Medical Eligibility Criteria for Contraceptive Use*. 5th ed. Geneva: World Health Organization, Reproductive Health and Research, Family and Community Health; 2015 [PMID: 26337268].

PREGNANCY

In the United States, approximately 456,000 women younger than 20 years become pregnant every year. Of all pregnancies in adolescent mothers, it is estimated that 18%–35% involve fathers younger than 20 years at the time of birth. Most teen pregnancies are unintended. Both the teenage pregnancy rate and birth rate in the United States have steadily declined over the past two decades, which has been attributed to improved access to contraceptives and increased use of LARCs. In 2018, the birth rate for adolescents, 17.4 births per 1000 women, was the lowest it has ever been for all racial and ethnic groups since the peak rate of 61.8 in 1991. However, racial and ethnic disparities persist, with the pregnancy rate among non-Hispanic white teens less than half that among non-Hispanic blacks and Hispanics. Lower socioeconomic status and lower maternal education are risk factors for teen pregnancy regardless of racial or ethnic group. Approximately 60% of adolescent pregnancies result in live births, 25% end in abortion, and 15% in miscarriage.

Presentation

Pregnancy is the most common cause of secondary amenorrhea and should be considered as a cause of even one missed period. The level of denial about the possibility of pregnancy is high and adolescents with undiagnosed pregnancies may present with abdominal pain, nausea or vomiting, breast tenderness, urinary frequency, dizziness, or other nonspecific symptoms. In addition to denial, difficult social situations can contribute to delays in diagnosis and in seeking prenatal care. Young, newly pregnant adolescents may fear violence from their partner or abandonment by their family. Clinicians should have a low threshold for suspecting pregnancy and obtaining pregnancy tests.

Diagnosis

Enzyme-linked immunosorbent assay test kits specific for the β-hCG subunit and sensitive to less than 50 mIU/mL of serum hCG can be performed on urine (preferably the day's first voided specimen, because it is more concentrated) in less than 5 minutes and are accurate by the expected date of the missed period in almost all patients. Serum radioimmunoassay, also specific for the β-hCG subunit, is accurate within 7 days after fertilization and is helpful in ruling out ectopic pregnancy or threatened abortion, as the quantitative result of this assay can be tracked over time and compared to normal ranges for gestational age. Serum hCG doubles approximately every 2 days in the first 6–7 weeks of the pregnancy, and a gestational sac is identifiable using transvaginal ultrasonography at hCG levels of 1000–2000 mIU/mL.

Pregnancies are dated from the first day of the LMP. The estimated due date can be calculated by adding 7 days to the LMP, subtracting 3 months and adding 1 year. Pregnancy dating calendars are widely available. In the absence of an accurate LMP, ultrasonography for confirmation of the presence of an intrauterine pregnancy and accurate dating can be obtained.

A speculum examination is not mandatory at the time of pregnancy diagnosis for an asymptomatic adolescent. If there is vaginal spotting or bleeding, unusual vaginal discharge, symptoms of STI, pelvic pain, or abdominal pain, a speculum examination is required. The differential diagnosis includes infection, miscarriage, ectopic pregnancy, and other disorders of early pregnancy. An 8-week gestational age uterus is about the size of an orange, and a 12-week uterus is about the size of a grapefruit on bimanual examination. The uterine fundus is just palpable at the symphysis pubis at a gestational age of 12 weeks, midway between the symphysis and umbilicus at 16 weeks and, typically, at the umbilicus at 20 weeks. If the uterus is smaller than expected for pregnancy dates, possible diagnoses include inaccurate dates, false-positive test, ectopic pregnancy, or incomplete or missed abortion. A uterus that is larger than expected may be caused by inaccurate dates, twin gestation, molar pregnancy, or a corpus luteum cyst of pregnancy.

Management

1. Counseling at the Time of Pregnancy Testing

When an adolescent presents for pregnancy testing, it is helpful before performing the test to find out what she hopes the result will be and what she thinks she will do if the test is positive. The diagnosis of pregnancy may be met with shock, fear, anxiety, happiness, or, most likely, a combination of emotions. It is important to provide confidential, nonjudgmental counseling that includes the full range of pregnancy options, including unbiased discussion of the adolescent's options to continue or terminate the pregnancy. The adolescent should be supported in the decision-making process and referred to appropriate resources and services. Pediatricians should be familiar with local laws and policies impacting the pregnant adolescent and access to abortion care, especially for minor adolescents, as well as laws that seek to limit health care professionals' provision of unbiased pregnancy options counseling and referrals, whether for abortion care or continuation of pregnancy. Pediatricians who choose not to provide comprehensive options counseling should promptly refer pregnant adolescent patients to a health care professional who will offer developmentally appropriate options counseling that includes the full range of pregnancy options.

It is helpful to offer confidential follow-up care in 1 week while a pregnant adolescent is considering her options. Avoiding a decision reduces the adolescent's options and may result in poor pregnancy outcomes. Providers can help ensure that the patient obtains prenatal care if she has chosen to continue the pregnancy. In addition, counseling about healthful diet; folic acid supplementation (400 mcg/day); and avoiding alcohol, tobacco, and other drugs is important.

2. Pregnancy Outcomes

Young maternal age, low maternal pre-pregnancy weight, poor weight gain during pregnancy, delay in prenatal care, maternal depression, exposure to domestic violence, and low socioeconomic status contribute to low birth weight and increased neonatal mortality. Poor nutritional status of some teenagers, substance abuse, and high incidence of STIs also play a role in poor outcomes. Teenagers are at greater risk than adults for preeclampsia, eclampsia, iron deficiency anemia, cephalopelvic disproportion, prolonged labor, premature labor, and maternal death. Good family support, early prenatal care, and good nutrition can positively impact several of these problems.

Psychosocial consequences for the teenage mother include risks of not graduating from high school or participating in higher education, lower income status and dependence on public assistance, and faster rate of subsequent childbearing. Pregnant teenagers and teenage parents require additional support from their medical providers. Multidisciplinary clinics that provide medical care to both the young mother and her infant in the same appointment; offer breastfeeding and nutrition education; and provide behavioral health care, social work support and parenting education are particularly beneficial. Adolescent mothers tend to be more negative and authoritative when disciplining their children, and they may have inadequate knowledge of normal behavior and development. Providers can help by educating the adolescent mother during routine visits regarding appropriate discipline and expectations for her child's behavior.

Approximately 17% of births in adolescents are repeat births. Postpartum contraceptive counseling and follow-up may help prevent additional pregnancies. Combined hormonal contraceptive options can be started 6 weeks after delivery in non–breast-feeding adolescents; progestin-only methods can be started immediately postpartum, even in breast-feeding adolescents.

Ectopic Pregnancy

In the United States, approximately 2% of pregnancies are ectopic. Adolescents have the highest mortality rate from ectopic pregnancy, most likely related to delayed diagnosis. Risk factors for ectopic pregnancy include history of PID or STIs (including repeat infections with *C trachomatis*) and cigarette smoking. Conception while on progestin-only methods of contraception also increases the risk of ectopic pregnancy because of the progestin-mediated decrease in tubal motility.

The classic presentation is missed menstrual period, abdominal pain, and vaginal bleeding. A urine pregnancy test is usually positive by the time of presentation. The patient may have abdominal or pelvic tenderness, adnexal tenderness, and/or an adnexal mass on examination. The uterus is typically either normal sized or slightly enlarged. Diagnosis is based on serial serum quantitative hCG levels and transvaginal ultrasound. Patients should be referred urgently to an obstetrician gynecologist for management to avoid a ruptured ectopic pregnancy. Ruptured ectopic pregnancy often presents with shock and an acute surgical abdomen and is a surgical emergency.

ACOG Practice Bulletin No. 191: Tubal ectopic pregnancy. Obstet Gynecol 2018;131(2):e65–e77 [PMID: 29232273].

American Academy of Pediatrics Committee on Adolescence: Options counseling for the pregnant adolescent patient. Pediatrics 2022;150(3):e2022058781 [PMID: 35739621].

Martin JA, Hamilton BE, Osterman MJK: Births in the United States, 2019. NCHS Data Brief 2020 Oct;(387):1–8 [PMID: 33054913].

Powers ME, Takagishi J; Committee on Adolescence, Council on Early Childhood: Care of adolescent parents and their children. Pediatrics 2021 May;147(5):e2021050919. doi: 10.1542/peds.2021-050919 [PMID: 33903162].

Adolescent Substance Use Disorders

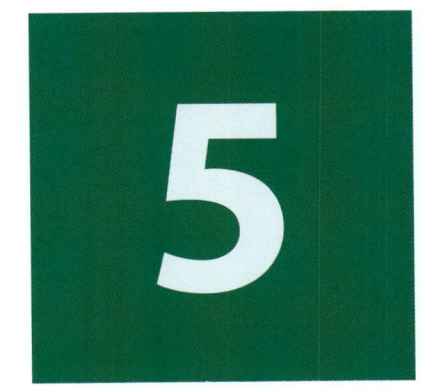

Jesse Hinckley, MD, PhD

Clifford Costello, DO

Paritosh Kaul, MD

Diane Straub, MD, MPH

Adolescence is a vital period of neurodevelopment, and youth are particularly vulnerable to the neurodevelopmental consequences of substance use problems. Adolescence is also a time when many youth experiment with substance use, and more than 90% of individuals with substance use disorders (SUDs) started using substances by the age of 18 years. While most adolescents who experiment with substance use do not develop an SUD, many youth with frequent use do experience substance use problems, recently conceptualized as pre-addiction by McLellan et al.

Adolescents with substance use problems are particularly at risk of accidental injury and physical or sexual violence related to substance use, in addition to risk of overdose and death. Further, an estimated 14% of 12- to 18-year-old youth will meet *Diagnostic and Statistical Manual of Mental Disorders*, 5th Edition (DSM-5) criteria for a SUD (see section Diagnosis). Across the lifespan, SUDs are among the costliest health problems in the United States, with an annual economic impact of $249 billion for alcohol and $193 billion for other non-tobacco substance use. SUDs are also a contributing factor to the leading causes of morbidity and mortality among adolescents and young adults. In fact, adolescent-onset SUDs have been shown to prospectively predict early mortality.

McLellan AT, Koob GF, Volkow ND: Preaddiction—a missing concept for treating substance use disorders. JAMA Psychiatry 2022;79(8):749–751 [PMID: 35793096].

Thorpe HHA, Hamidullah S, Jenkins BW, Khokhar JY: Adolescent neurodevelopment and substance use: receptor expression and behavioral consequences. Pharmacol Ther 2020;206:107431 [PMID: 31706976].

EPIDEMIOLOGY

ESSENTIALS OF ADOLESCENT SUBSTANCE USE EPIDEMIOLOGY

► Nicotine, alcohol, and marijuana are the most commonly used substances in adolescence, with a dramatic increase in vaping since being systematically tracked in 2017.

► Illicitly manufactured fentanyl is ubiquitous in the street drug market, often in combination with other drugs, resulting in unintentional exposure and a dramatic increase in adolescent and young adult opioid overdose deaths.

The best source of information on the epidemiology of substance use among American adolescents is the Monitoring the Future (MTF) study, an annual cross-sectional survey that tracks substance use–related behaviors in school youth in the United States, since its onset in 1975. This study probably understates the magnitude of the problem of SUD because it excludes high-risk adolescent groups—school dropouts, runaways, and those in the juvenile justice system. Table 5–1 includes the epidemiology of commonly abused mood-altering substances by agent from the 2022 MTF study, collected from 31,438 American 8th, 10th, and 12th graders.

Table 5–1. Epidemiology, pharmacology, and physiologic effects of commonly abused mood-altering substances by agent.

Substance	Epidemiology[a]	Pharmacology	Intoxication	Withdrawal	Chronic Use
Alcohol (ethanol)	Lifetime use: 61.6% 12th, 41.4 10th, 23.1 8th graders; Past 30 days use: 28.4% 12th, 13.6 10th, 6.0% 8th graders; Daily use: 1.5% 12th, 0.4% 10th, 0.1% 8th graders	Depressant; 10 g/drink Drink: 12-oz beer, 4-oz wine, 1½-oz liquor; one drink increases blood level by approximately 0.025 g/dL (varies by weight)	Legal: 0.05–0.1 g/dL (varies by state) Mild (< 0.1 g/dL): disinhibition, euphoria, mild sedation, and impaired coordination Moderate (0.1–0.2 g/dL): impaired mentation and judgment, slurred speech, ataxia Severe: > 0.3 g/dL: confusion, stupor > 0.4 g/dL: coma, depressed respiration	Mild: headache, tremors, nausea and vomiting ("hangover") Severe: fever, sweaty, seizure, agitation, hallucination, hypertension, tachycardia Delirium tremens (chronic use)	Hepatitis, cirrhosis, cardiac disease, Wernicke encephalopathy, Korsakoff syndrome
Marijuana (cannabis)	Lifetime use: 38.3% 12th, 24.2% 10th, 11.0% 8th graders; Past 30 days use: 20.2% 12th, 12.1% 10th, 5.0% 8th graders; Daily use: 6.3% 12th, 2.1% 8th graders	THC; 4%–6% in marijuana; 20%–30% in hashish	Low: euphoria, relaxation, impaired thinking. High: mood changes, depersonalization, hallucinations Toxic: panic, delusions, paranoia, psychosis	Irritability, disturbed sleep, tremor, nystagmus, anorexia, diarrhea, vomiting	Cough, gynecomastia, low sperm count, infertility, amotivational syndrome, apathy
Cocaine	Lifetime use: 2.4% 12th, 0.8% 10th, 0.8% 8th graders; Past 30 days use: 0.8% 12th, 0.2% 10th, 0.3% 8th graders; Daily use: 0.2% 12th graders	Stimulant; releases biogenic amines; concentration varies with preparation and route of administration	Hyperalert, increased energy, confident, insomnia, anxiety, paranoia, dilated pupils, tremors, seizures, hypertension, arrhythmia, tachycardia, fever, dry mouth Toxic: coma, psychosis, seizure, myocardial infarction, stroke, hyperthermia, rhabdomyolysis	Drug craving, depression, dysphoria, irritability, lethargy, tremors, nausea, hunger	Nasal septum ulceration, epistaxis, lung damage, intravenous drug use
Opioids (heroin, morphine, codeine, methadone, opium, fentanyl, meperidine, propoxyphene)	Lifetime use (heroin/non-heroin opioids): 0.5%/3.2% 12th, 0.5% 10th, 0.4% 8th graders; Past 30 days use: 0.3%/0.7% 12th, 0.2% 10th, 0.2% 8th graders; Daily use: 0.1%/0.0% 12th graders	Depressant; binds central opioid receptor; variable concentrations with substance	Euphoria, sedation, impaired thinking, low blood pressure, pinpoint pupil, urinary retention Toxic: hypotension, arrhythmia, depressed respiration, stupor, coma, seizure, death	Only after > 3 wk of regular use: drug craving, rhinorrhea, lacrimation, muscle aches, diarrhea, anxiety, tremors, hypertension, tachycardia	Intravenous drug use: cellulitis, endocarditis, embolisms, HIV
Amphetamines	Lifetime use: 5.3% 12th, 5.4% 10th, 6.0% 8th graders; Past 30 days use: 1.3% 12th, 1.3% 10th, 1.9% 8th graders; Daily use: 0.2% 12th graders	Stimulant; sympathomimetic	Euphoria, hyperalert state, hyperactive, hypertension, arrhythmia, fever, flushing, dilated pupils, tremor, ataxia, dry mouth	Lethargy, fatigue, depression, anxiety, nightmares, muscle cramps, abdominal pain, hunger	Paranoia, psychosis

Drug	Prevalence of use	Mechanism/class	Clinical effects	Withdrawal	Chronic/psychiatric effects
MDMA (ecstasy)	Lifetime use: 3.0% 12th, 1.4% 10th, 1.2% 8th graders; Past 30 days use: 0.9% 12th, 0.3% 10th, 0.2% 8th graders; Daily use: 0.1% 12th graders	Stimulant, psychedelic; releases serotonin, dopamine, and norepinephrine; inhibits reuptake of neurotransmitters; increases dopamine synthesis; inhibits MAO	Enhanced empathy, euphoria, increased energy and self-esteem, tachycardia, hypertension, increased psychomotor drive, sensory enhancement, illusions, difficulty concentrating and retaining information, headaches, palpitations, flushing, hyperthermia Toxic: frank psychosis, coma, seizures, intracranial hemorrhage, cerebral infarction, asystole, pulmonary edema, multisystem organ failure, acute renal or hepatic failure, ARDS, DIC, SIADH, death	None	Paranoid psychosis
GHB (liquid ecstasy)	Lifetime use < 0.1% in 12-17 years[b]	Depressant, endogenous CNS transmitter; influences dopaminergic activity, higher levels of GABA-B activity	10 mg/kg: sleep 30 mg/kg: memory loss 50 mg/kg: general anesthesia Toxic: CNS and respiratory depression, aggressiveness, seizures, bradycardia, apnea	Only after chronic use with dosing every 3 h. Early: mild tremor, tachycardia, hypertension, diaphoresis, moderate anxiety, insomnia, nausea, vomiting Progressive: confusion, delirium, hallucinations, autonomic instability, death	Wernicke-Korsakoff syndrome
Sedative-hypnotics (barbiturates, benzodiazepines, methaqualone)	Lifetime use: 3.6% 12th graders; Past 30 days use: 1.1% 12th; Daily use: 0.1% 12th graders	Depressant	Sedation, lethargy, slurred speech, pinpoint pupils, hypotension, psychosis, seizures Toxic: stupor, coma, cardiac arrest, seizure, pulmonary edema, death	Only after weeks of use: agitation, delirium, psychosis, hallucinations, fever, flushing, hyper-/hypotension, death	Paranoia
Hallucinogens (LSD, peyote, mescaline, mushrooms, nutmeg, jimson weed)	Lifetime use: 7.1% 12th, 3.4% 10th, 2.0% 8th graders; Past 30 days use: 1.4% 12th, 0.7% 10th, 0.5% 8th graders; Daily use: 0.0% 12th graders	Inhibition of serotonin release	Illusions, depersonalization, hallucination, anxiety, paranoia, ataxia, dilated pupils, hypertension, dry mouth Toxic: coma, terror, panic, "crazy feeling"	None	Flashbacks
Phencyclidine	Lifetime use < 0.1% in 12-17 years[b]	Dissociative anesthetic	Low dose (< 5 mg): illusions, hallucinations, ataxia, hypertension, flushing Moderate dose (5–10 mg): hyperthermia, salivation, myoclonus High dose (> 10 mg): rigidity, seizure, arrhythmia, coma, death	None	Flashbacks

(Continued)

Table 5–1. Epidemiology, pharmacology, and physiologic effects of commonly abused mood-altering substances by agent. (*Continued*)

Substance	Epidemiology[a]	Pharmacology	Intoxication	Withdrawal	Chronic Use
Inhalants (toluene, benzene, hydrocarbons, and fluorocarbons)	Lifetime use: 5.8% 12th, 7.5% 10th, 9.8% 8th graders; Past 30 days use: 0.7% 12th, 1.2% 10th, 1.9% 8th graders; Daily use: 0.1% 12th graders	Stimulation progressing to depression	Euphoria, giddiness, impaired judgment, ataxia, rhinorrhea, salivation, hallucination Toxic: respiratory depression, arrhythmia, coma, stupor, delirium, sudden death	None	Permanent damage to nerves, liver, heart, kidney, brain
Nicotine (cigarettes/ smokeless tobacco/vaping)	Lifetime use: 16.8%/10.3%/38.8% 12th, 10.2%/5.8%/28.2% 10th, 6.1%/3.9%/17.0% 8th graders; Past 30 days use: 4.0%/3.2%/20.7% 12th, 1.7%/2.5%/14.2% 10th, 0.8%/1.2%/7.1% 8th graders; Daily use: 1.6%/1.1%/6.2% 12th, 0.7%/0.7%/3.3% 10th, 0.3%/0.3%/1.2% 8th graders	Releases dopamine, 1 mg nicotine per cigarette	Relaxation, tachycardia, vertigo, anorexia	Drug craving, irritability, anxiety, hunger, impaired concentration	Permanent damage to lung, heart, cardiovascular system
Anabolic steroids[c]	Lifetime use: 1.5% 12th, 0.9% 10th, 1.6% 8th graders; Past 30 days use: 1.3% 12th, 0.3% 10th, 0.5% 8th graders; Daily use: 0.4% 12th graders	Bind steroid receptor Stacking: use many types simultaneously Pyramiding: increase dosage	Increased muscle bulk, strength, endurance, increased drive, hypogonadism, low sperm count, gynecomastia, decreased libido, virilization, irregular menses, hepatitis, early epiphysial closure, aggressiveness	Drug craving, dysphoria, irritability, depression	Tendon rupture, cardiomyopathy, atherosclerosis, peliosis hepatis (orally active C17 derivatives of testosterone are especially hepatotoxic)

ARDS, acute respiratory distress syndrome; CNS, central nervous system; DIC, disseminated intravascular coagulation; GABA, γ-aminobutyric acid; GHB, γ-hydroxybutyrate; HIV, human immunodeficiency virus; LSD, lysergic acid diethylamide; MAO, monoamine oxidase; MDMA, methylenedioxymethamphetamine; SIADH, syndrome of inappropriate secretion of antidiuretic hormone; THC, δ-9-tetrahydrocannabinol.

[a]Data from 31,438 US 8th, 10th, and 12th graders in 2022 (Miech RA, Johnston LD, Patrick ME, O'Malley PM, Bachman JG, Schulenberg JE: Monitoring the Future National Survey Results on Drug Use, 1975–2022: Secondary School Students. Ann Arbor MI: Institute for Social Research, The University of Michigan; 2023. http://monitoringthefuture.org/results/publications/monographs. Accessed March 26, 2023.)

[b]Substance Abuse and Mental Health Services Administration. (2021). Key substance use and mental health indicators in the United States: Results from the 2020 National Survey on Drug Use and Health (HHS Publication No. PEP21-07-01-003, NSDUH Series H-56). Rockville, MD: Center for Behavioral Health Statistics and Quality, Substance Abuse and Mental Health Services Administration. Retrieved from https://www.samhsa.gov/data/.

[c]Despite conventional assumptions, scientific studies show that anabolic steroids do not improve aerobic athletic performance and improve strength only in athletes trained in weightlifting before they begin using steroids and who continue to train and consume a high-protein diet.

Nicotine vaping has become one of the top forms of substance use among teens. Among 8th and 10th grade students, respectively, nicotine vaping in the past 30 days (7.1% and 14.2%) topped alcohol (6.0% and 13.6%) and cannabis (5.0% and 12.1%) use, and in 12th grade students, nicotine vaping (20.7%) was below alcohol (28.4%) but similar to cannabis (20.2%) use. Among young adults 19–30, since 2017 when vaping was first recorded in the MTF study, nicotine vaping prevalence nearly tripled from 6% to 16%, with marijuana vaping increasing from 6% to 12%. The growth in use of vape devices and electronic cigarettes (e-cigarettes) has been largely driven by marketing and advertising by e-cigarette companies. E-cigarettes are battery-operated devices designed to heat liquid into an aerosol that users inhale. The aerosol can contain nicotine, glycerol, propylene glycol, formaldehyde, cadmium, benzoic acid, lead, cannabis, chromium, nickel, different flavors, and other chemicals. Pod-based e-cigarettes that use a salt-based nicotine made popular by Juul Labs have added to the availability of this product.

Several notable trends have emerged in marijuana use. By the ages of 18–22, daily use rates rise rapidly; recent use among this age group is the highest it has been in decades. Multiple factors have likely contributed to this increase, including increasing legalization of both medical and nonmedical adult (> 21 years old) marijuana in states across the country, despite it remaining illegal federally; illegal market sources and state-regulated sales leading to widespread availability; mass commercialization of high-potency products; and a vast array of products appealing to youth, such as marijuana-infused candy and baked items.

Cannabis plants contain more than 100 cannabinoids. Delta-9-tetrahydrocannabinol (Δ9-THC) and cannabidiol (CBD) are the two primary cannabinoids, with Δ9-THC being intoxicating. Marijuana flower potency has increased since the early 1990s from approximately 3%–4% THC to 14% currently, with some flowers as high as 30%, and concentrates typically as high as 40%–90%. Cannabis plants are processed to generate multiple types of products, including plant form ("flower"), sinsemilla (seedless flowers with higher THC content), hashish (compressed and screened dried flowers more potent than dried flowers), and concentrates/extracts (cannabinoids, especially THC, chemically extracted from the plant resulting in a more potent product). These types of marijuana can be smoked (hand-rolled cigarettes, blunts, bongs, pipes, bowls), inhaled (vaporizers, e-cigarettes, dab pens or rigs, pipes), ingested orally (candy, baked items, beverages, gel caps, pills), or absorbed transdermally (oils, lotions, creams, patches, salves).

Under the Controlled Substances Act, cannabis is divided into marijuana and hemp, both derived from the cannabis plant. Hemp-derived products contain no more than 0.3% Δ9-THC levels and are classified as supplements under federal law, which means there is minimal Food and Drug Administration (FDA) regulation. Recently, broad-spectrum hemp-derived products have included high levels of Δ8-THC, a psychoactive cannabinoid that can produce similar effects to Δ9-THC, and other cannabinoids previously produced at comparatively low concentrations in the cannabis plant. Finally, there are synthetic cannabinoids on the illicit market that can be 10–200 times more potent than THC and therefore have potential for more serious adverse events such as psychosis and fatal overdose.

The dramatic opioid epidemic in adults has been well documented, but the impact on adolescents and young adults has been equally unprecedented, driven largely by the increased prevalence of illicitly manufactured fentanyl use. In the last decade, annual drug overdose deaths in youth increased 2.3-fold; during this same timeframe, fentanyl-involved deaths increased 23.5-fold. In comparison to adults, adolescents and young adults are more likely to seek out and are more likely to be exposed to fentanyl. Fentanyl is ubiquitous in the illicit drug market, often in combination with other drugs, resulting in unintentional exposure and potential for fatal overdose with minimal prior opioid use.

Friedman J et al: Trends in drug overdose deaths among US adolescents, January 2010 to June 2021. JAMA 2022 Apr 12;327(14):1398–1400. doi: 10.1001/jama.2022.2847 [PMID: 35412573].

Hinckley JD, Bhatia D, Ellingson J, Molinero K, Hopfer C: The impact of recreational cannabis legalization on youth: the Colorado experience. Eur Child Adolesc Psychiatry 2022 Apr 15. doi: 10.1007/s00787-022-01981-0 [PMID: 354288970].

Miech RA, Johnston LD, Patrick ME, O'Malley PM, Bachman JG, Schulenberg JE:. Monitoring the Future National Survey Results on Drug Use, 1975–2022: Secondary School Students. Ann Arbor, MI: Institute for Social Research, The University of Michigan; 2023. http://monitoringthefuture.org/results/publications/monographs. Accessed March 26, 2023.

Patrick ME, Schulenberg JE, Miech RA, Johnston LD, O'Malley PM, Bachman JG: Monitoring the Future Panel Study annual report: National data on substance use among adults ages 19 to 60, 1976–2021. Monitoring the Future Monograph Series. University of Michigan Institute for Social Research: Ann Arbor, MI. doi:10.7826/ISR-UM.06.585140.002.07.0001.2022.

Substance Abuse and Mental Health Services Administration (SAMHSA). Preventing Marijuana Use Among Youth. SAMHSA Publication No. PEP21-06-01-001. Rockville, MD: National Mental Health and Substance Use Policy Laboratory. Substance Abuse and Mental Health Services Administration; 2021.

MORBIDITY AND MORTALITY ASSOCIATED WITH SUBSTANCE USE

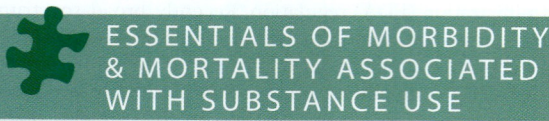

ESSENTIALS OF MORBIDITY & MORTALITY ASSOCIATED WITH SUBSTANCE USE

▶ Misuse of substances may cause acute problems, with alcohol, opioids, sedative-hypnotics, and stimulants posing a risk of lethal overdose.

▶ Intoxication is a primary contributor to the leading causes of death among adolescents.

▶ Substance misuse may cause acute exacerbations of mental health problems, including psychosis and increased risk of suicide, and worsen long-term mental health.

Physiologic effects of and signs and symptoms associated with commonly misused substances are presented in Tables 5–1 and 5–2. Acute substance use may result in injury or death. Overdose on alcohol, opioids, or sedative-hypnotics induces potentially lethal respiratory depression. This risk is higher with fentanyl, combining fentanyl with stimulants, or the combined use of more than one central depressant. Overdose of cocaine and, in some cases, methamphetamine may also result in acute cardiotoxicity, including life-threatening arrhythmias and myocardial infarction, even in youth. Inhalants, in particular, are neurotoxic and pose a risk of lethal overdose. Methamphetamine, ecstasy, and hallucinogen intoxication may also cause dysphoric delusions and hallucinations that typically resolve with drug metabolism. Though less common, cannabis may also induce psychosis in youth. Of concern, some cases of substance-induced psychosis may be refractory to treatment, even with prolonged abstinence. Certain modes of substance use also pose a risk of acute injury and death, including electronic cigarette and vaping associated lung injury (EVALI) and burns caused from the use of torches to vaporize high-concentrate cannabis (ie, wax, shatter, or dabs) or other substances. Acute and chronic medical complications associated with substance use are summarized in Table 5–1.

In addition to the morbidity and mortality associated with the direct physiologic consequences of substance use, alcohol and other mood-altering substance use is a major contributor to other leading causes of death among adolescents in the United States, including gun violence, homicide, suicide, and motor vehicle collisions. Substance misuse and SUD are also associated with increased risk-taking behaviors and increased risk of unintentional injury, interpersonal violence including sexual assault, and other types of potentially traumatic events. While intoxication contributes to increased risk, the behaviors and environment associated with obtaining and using substances also exposes adolescents to risk of harm.

Comorbid Mental Health Disorders

Though some substances may induce psychosis or altered mental status, the misuse of substances more commonly exacerbates preexisting mental health disorders. The most common comorbid disorders include major depressive disorder, generalized anxiety and other anxiety disorders, attention deficit/hyperactivity disorder (ADHD), trauma- and stressor-related disorders including posttraumatic stress disorder (PTSD), and behavioral disorders including conduct or oppositional defiant disorder. There is a bidirectional relationship between substance use and mental health disorders. Substance use may worsen underlying psychopathology and decrease mental health treatment engagement and compliance. Conversely, mental health problems also increase motivation to misuse substances, often in an attempt to self-medicate. States of intoxication and withdrawal also mimic mental health symptoms and may be difficult to differentiate. Thus, clinicians should screen all youth for both substance use and mental health problems. Integrated treatment of comorbid substance use and mental health disorders is central to optimizing treatment outcomes of either disorder.

Supplements

Supplements, many of which are minimally regulated and widely available, are also misused by adolescents, though not commonly for intoxicating purposes. Many athletes use ergogenic (performance-enhancing) supplements in an attempt to gain a competitive advantage. The most popular products are anabolic-androgenic steroids and steroid hormone precursors, creatine, human growth hormone (GH), and protein supplements. Adverse effects of anabolic-androgenic steroids, which increase lean body mass and lessen muscle breakdown, include acne, liver tumors, hypertension, premature closure of the epiphysis, ligamentous injury, and precocious puberty. Female youth may experience virilization, whereas steroids may cause gynecomastia and testicular atrophy in male youth. Creatine improves performance in brief, high-intensity exercises; misuse causes dehydration and muscle cramps and may be nephrotoxic. GH increases lean body mass through stimulating bone and cartilage growth and muscle development, as well as increasing utilization of fat. However, use of GH is not associated with increased strength nor enhanced physical performance. Potential risks include coarsening of facial features and cardiovascular disease. Excess consumption of protein supplements, often utilized to enhance recovery after strength conditioning, is also not associated with improved strength and may provoke renal failure in the presence of underlying renal dysfunction.

Table 5–2. Signs and symptoms associated with commonly abused mood-altering substances by organ/system.

Eyes/pupils	
Mydriasis	Amphetamines, MDMA, or other stimulants; cocaine; glutethimide; jimson weed; LSD. Withdrawal from alcohol and opioids
Miosis	Alcohol, barbiturates, benzodiazepines, opioids, PCP
Nystagmus	Alcohol, barbiturates, benzodiazepines, inhalants, PCP
Conjunctival injection	LSD, marijuana
Lacrimation	Inhalants, LSD. Opioid withdrawal
Cardiovascular	
Tachycardia	Stimulants, including amphetamines, MDMA, cocaine; LSD; marijuana; PCP. Alcohol, barbiturate, benzodiazepine withdrawal
Hypertension	Stimulants, including amphetamines, MDMA, cocaine; LSD; marijuana; PCP. Alcohol, barbiturate, benzodiazepine withdrawal Amphetamines, MDMA, or other stimulants; cocaine; LSD; marijuana; PCP. Withdrawal from alcohol, barbiturates, benzodiazepines
Hypotension	Barbiturates, opioids. Orthostatic: marijuana. Withdrawal from depressants
Arrhythmia	Amphetamines, MDMA, or other stimulants; cocaine; inhalants; opioids; PCP
Respiratory	
Depression	Opioids, antidepressants, GHB
Pulmonary edema	Opioids, stimulants
Core body temperature	
Elevated	Amphetamines, MDMA, or other stimulants; cocaine; PCP. Withdrawal from alcohol, barbiturate, benzodiazepine, opioid withdrawal
Decreased	Alcohol, barbiturates, benzodiazepines, opioids, GHB
Peripheral nervous system response	
Hyperreflexia	Amphetamines, MDMA, or other stimulants; cocaine; LSD; marijuana; methaqualone; PCP. Withdrawal from alcohol, barbiturates, benzodiazepines
Hyporeflexia	Alcohol, barbiturates, benzodiazepines, inhalants, opioids
Tremor	Amphetamines or other stimulants, cocaine, LSD. Alcohol, barbiturate, benzodiazepine, opioid withdrawal
Ataxia	Alcohol, amphetamines, MDMA, or other stimulants; barbiturates; benzodiazepines; inhalants; LSD; PCP; GHB
Central nervous system response	
Hyperalertness	Amphetamines, MDMA, or other stimulants; cocaine
Sedation, somnolence	Alcohol, barbiturates, benzodiazepines, inhalants, marijuana, opioids, GHB
Seizures	Alcohol; amphetamines, MDMA, or other stimulants; cocaine; inhalants; methaqualone; opioids (particularly meperidine, propoxyphene). Alcohol, barbiturate, benzodiazepine, opioid withdrawal
Hallucinations	Amphetamines, MDMA, or other stimulants; cocaine; inhalants; LSD; marijuana; PCP. Alcohol, barbiturate, benzodiazepine, opioid withdrawal
Gastrointestinal	
Nausea, vomiting	Alcohol, amphetamines or other stimulants, cocaine, inhalants, LSD, opioids, peyote, GHB. Withdrawal from alcohol, barbiturates, benzodiazepines, cocaine, opioids

GHB, γ-hydroxybutyrate; LSD, lysergic acid diethylamide; MDMA, methylenedioxymethamphetamine (ecstasy); PCP, phencyclidine hydrochloride.

Ganson KT et at: Legal performance-enhancing substances and substance use problems among young adults. Pediatrics 2020 Sep;146(3):e20200409. doi: 10.1542/peds.2020-0409 [PMID: 32868471].

Hinckley JD, Riggs P: Integrated treatment of adolescents with co-occurring depression and substance use disorder. Child Adolesc Psychiatr Clin N Am 2019 Jul;28(3):461–472. doi: 10.1016/j.chc.2019.02.006 [PMID: 31076120].

Mason MJ et al: Psychiatric comorbidity and complications. Child Adolesc Psychiatr Clin N Am 2016 Jul;25(3):521–532. doi: 10.1016/j.chc.2016.02.007 [PMID: 27338972].

Robinson ZD et al: Cooccurring psychiatric and substance use disorders. Child Adolesc Psychiatr Clin N Am 2016 Oct;25(4): 713–722. doi: 10.1016/j.chc.2016.05.005 [PMID: 27613347].

PREVENTION OF MISUSE & PROGRESSION TO SUD

ESSENTIALS OF ADOLESCENT SUBSTANCE USE PREVENTION

▶ Identifying and addressing risk factors while promoting protective factors are key in preventing the development of a substance use disorder (SUD) in youth.

▶ Prevention strategies for adolescent substance use include primary efforts targeting the general population, secondary efforts targeting high-risk youth, and tertiary efforts targeting youth who show early signs of substance use.

Experimentation with and initiation of regular substance use typically begins during adolescence. Transition into emerging adulthood is also a time of transition to regular substance use and misuse for youth. Older adolescents and emerging adults aged 18–25 years are more likely to engage in binge drinking; nicotine, cigarette, cannabis use, and vaping; prescription drug misuse; and use of illicit substances. During this developmental period, youth are also more likely than other age groups to think that regular substance use is not harmful and, for cannabis, may even be helpful. Simultaneously, youth are less likely to recognize substance-related losses or recognize symptoms of a SUD. Thus, primary care providers (PCPs) play a vital role in detection of substance use and prevention of progression to misuse and SUD.

▶ Risk Factors

Transition from experimentation to regular use and then developing a SUD typically occurs in youth with multiple risk factors (Table 5–3). Individual risk factors include those

Table 5–3. Risk factors for adolescent substance misuse and use disorders.

Category		Risk Factor
Individual		
	Demographic	Male
		Rural community
		Single
		Gender or sexual minority
	Neurodevelopmental	Impulsivity
		Increased reward-seeking
		Impaired emotional regulation
	Mental health	Disruptive behavior disorders
		Comorbid mental health disorders
		History of trauma or childhood maltreatment
		Behavioral addiction
	Substance use	Early initiation of substance use
		Previous exposure to vaping
		Low perceived risk
Family		Parental substance use
		Substance-using family members
		Favorable parental attitudes toward substance use
		Poor supervision or negligence
		High family conflict
		Poor maternal psychological control
		Low parental education
		Familial rejection of gender or sexual identity
Socioeconomic		Availability
		Friends who engage in substance use
		Societal norms and laws favoring substance use
		Lack of school connectedness or achievement
		Membership in college fraternity/ sorority
		Homeless
		Unsupervised access to money

that are not modifiable (demographic), as well as factors that may be modified through therapeutic, prevention, and skills-based intervention strategies (neurodevelopmental, mental health, and substance use). Neurodevelopmental risk factors may evolve over time as reward pathways (limbic and dopaminergic systems) and cognitive and decision-making functions (frontal lobe) continue to mature through adolescence and young adulthood. Modifiable family risk factors primarily target family connectedness and parenting and supervision strategies. Similarly, some socioeconomic risk factors may be mitigated through psychosocial interventions (peer group, school connectedness, access to money). Other risk factors, including availability and societal norms and laws, may better be addressed through governmental processes (eg, legislation and regulatory rule-making).

Protective Factors

While mitigating risk factors may prevent the initiation of problematic substance use, interventions should also focus on enhancing and developing protective factors (Table 5–4). Individual protective factors may be developed through psychosocial and skills-based interventions that increase emotional competence, self-efficacy and self-worth, and views about physical and mental health. Family-based interventions may not only reduce risk factors, but also develop and strengthen protective factors including connectedness or attachment and parenting skills including supervision. It is also important to consider the role of schools in developing socioeconomic protective factors by increasing connectedness and engagement, as well as self-efficacy in school, work, and social settings.

Prevention

Due to the potential long-term medical complications related to SUD in adolescents, prevention has been a public health priority since the 1980s. While a comprehensive community-based approach is ideal, many schools and communities continue to use programs with little evidence for effectiveness. Pediatric health care providers are important advocates for and educators of the community and government about developmentally appropriate evidence-based programs.

Primary-level or universal programs focus on preventing the initiation of substance use and are aimed at all members of a given population. While the previous school of thought was to direct services to those with high-risk factors for SUD, the larger population of those with lower-risk factors actually account for a much higher percentage of substance misuse, a phenomenon known as the "Prevention Paradox." Therefore, universal prevention aimed at general populations likely has a greater overall benefit. The Drug Awareness and Resistance Education (D.A.R.E.) program is a familiar example of a primary prevention program that attempted to educate elementary and middle school students about the adverse consequences of substance abuse and enable them to resist peer pressures. This program continues to be utilized in school systems, despite data indicating its lack of effectiveness.

Secondary-level or selective programs target populations at increased risk for substance use. Their aim is to prevent progression from initiation to continuance and maintenance, relying on individualized intervention to reduce risk and enhance protective factors (see Tables 5–3 and 5–4). Alateen, which supports children of alcoholic parents, typifies secondary level prevention.

Tertiary-level or indicated prevention programs target young people who have been identified as substance abusers. Their aim is to prevent the morbid consequences of substance use. One example is the identification of adolescents who misuse alcohol and drugs at parties and providing them with a safe ride home. Because prevention is more effective when targeted at reducing initiation of substance use than at decreasing use or associated morbidity, tertiary prevention is the least effective approach.

At the policy level, several evidence-based programs have been shown to reduce morbidity and mortality of adolescent SUD, particularly SUD associated with alcohol misuse. Alcohol taxes and fees have been linked to a reduction in underage drinking. Law enforcement approaches such as sobriety checkpoints and setting a legal blood alcohol content (BAC) have reduced the rate of alcohol-related traffic crashes and injuries amongst adults and adolescents. Additionally, policies such as raising the minimum legal drinking age to 21 years old, zero tolerance laws to those under 21 years old with any measurable BAC, and civil social host liability laws have also improved these outcomes.

Table 5–4. Protective factors for adolescent substance use disorders.

Category	Protective Factor
Individual	Emotional and moral competence Self-efficacy Optimism High level of mindfulness Strong beliefs against substance use Desire to maintain health Strong religious beliefs Positive social orientation
Family	Strong bonding and attachment Family engagement and support High parental awareness and monitoring Parental disapproval of substance use
Socioeconomic	School connectedness Peers who do not use Engagement in structured activities

Harrop E et al: Evidence-based prevention for adolescent substance use. Child Adolesc Psychiatr Clin N Am 2016 Jul;25(3):387–410 [PMID: 27338963].

Lynam D et al: Project DARE: no effects at 10-year follow-up. J Consult Clin Psychol 1999;67(4):590–593 [PMID: 10450631].

Nawi A et al: Risk and protective factors of drug abuse among adolescents: a systematic review. BMC Public Health 2021 Nov 13; 21:2088.

Substance Abuse and Mental Health Services Administration: Substance Misuse Prevention for Young Adults. Publication No. PEP19-PL-Guide-1 Rockville, MD: National Mental Health and Substance Use Policy Laboratory. Substance Abuse and Mental Health Services Administration; 2019.

EVALUATION OF SUBSTANCE USE

ESSENTIALS OF ADOLESCENT SUBSTANCE USE EVALUATION

▶ The SBIRT model is an effective approach for early identification and treatment of adolescent SUD.

▶ Validated screening tools can be used in the primary care setting to quickly and accurately identify youth who may be at risk for SUD.

▶ Brief in-office interventions, such as motivational interviewing, can be effective in promoting a personalized plan for behavioral change.

▶ Referral to subspecialty treatment programs may be necessary for youth who require more attentive and specialized care.

▶ Pharmacologic screening for substance use is not recommended in the office setting, although it can be used as a tool in the residential or intensive treatment setting.

Office-Based Screening, Brief Intervention, & Referral to Treatment (SBIRT)

Early detection and treatment of SUD during adolescence is critical to preventing morbidity and mortality, including progression of SUD into adulthood. The recent rise in substance-related overdose deaths among youth highlights the urgency of early detection and intervention for adolescent SUD. Early intervention during the first decade of use is associated with a reduction in SUD later in life and may significantly reduce hospital-based SUD care utilized in adulthood. Youth who receive treatment are also more likely to attain a high school diploma and maintain job placement. While fewer than 10% of youth with SUD receive treatment, it is estimated that 90% of youth who would benefit are engaged in settings, such as school, where they could be screened and engaged.

To address the gap in youth receiving SUD treatment, the American Academy of Pediatrics (AAP) recommended implementation of universal substance use screening, brief intervention, and referral to treatment (SBIRT) starting at 12 years old. The three main goals of the integrated, algorithm-based SBIRT screening model are to (1) determine whether teens have used any alcohol or drugs; (2) determine where adolescents are on the substance use spectrum; and (3) initiate a brief discussion with teenage patients about substance use and provide them with education, advice, and resources within a motivational interviewing (MI) model. SBIRT may be adapted to multiple treatment settings and the level of provider expertise, from general practitioners and emergency providers to behavioral health professionals. A recent review of SBIRT implementation in 1266 sites found rates of youth screening positive for potential substance use problems ranging from 4.4%–5.3% in school-based and primary care settings to 91.8% in juvenile justice programs, strongly supporting the accessibility of youth at risk of or with substance use problems across settings.

Screening

There are several effective tools that can be used to identify adolescents at risk for SUD (Box 5–1). The S2BI (Screening to Brief Intervention) and BSTAD (Brief Screener for Tobacco, Alcohol, and other Drugs) are examples of validated screening tools that can be used in the primary care setting. These tools are designed to be quick and easy, can be administered online by a patient or clinician (https://nida.nih.gov/s2bi/, https://nida.nih.gov/bstad/), and can help providers identify patients who may need further assessment or intervention. The CRAFFT+N (https://crafft.org/) is another validated screener for adolescents aged 12–21 that can further assess risk behavior associated with substance use. The AUDIT (Alcohol Use Disorders Identification Test) was developed by the WHO specifically to assess for alcohol consumption and related problems in the primary care setting.

BOX 5–1. Screening Resources

- AUDIT https://nida.nih.gov/sites/default/files/audit.pdf
- BSTAD https://nida.nih.gov/bstad/
- S2BI https://nida.nih.gov/s2bi/
- CRAFFT+N https://crafft.org/

Brief Intervention

Utilizing the SBIRT framework, clinicians should provide individualized feedback in the form of a brief intervention, a 5- to 15-minute conversation specific to the screening results. When a youth does not use substances regularly, the clinician provides praise, normalizes that most youth do not use substances, and provides education about potential harms of substance use to encourage preventing or delaying the onset of use. Up-to-date knowledge about the harms of substance use is particularly important as youth are exposed to information primarily through peers and social media. The National Institute on Drug Abuse (https://nida.nih.gov) and the National Harm Reduction Coalition (https://harmreduction.org) provide numerous resources for clinicians, caregivers and other adults, and youth.

For youth who report regular substance use, the goal is to engage and empower the youth to be responsible for change. MI has been shown to be an effective part of in-office treatment for adolescent SUD. Based on the principle of empathy, MI is designed to help patients explore their ambivalence about substance use and build motivation for change.

Table 5–5. Stages of change and intervention tasks.

Patient Stage	Motivation Tasks
Precontemplation	Create reservation, increase the patient's awareness of risks and problems with current patterns of use
Contemplation	Assist the patient with assessing relative risks and benefits of changing substance use; focus on reasons to change and risks of not changing; strengthen the patient's self-efficacy for changing current use
Determination	Assist the patient with determining the best course of action to change substance use from among available alternatives
Action	Assist the patient with establishing a clear plan of action toward changing substance use
Maintenance	Assist the patient with identifying and implementing strategies to prevent relapse
Relapse	Assist the patient with renewing the process of change starting at contemplation

Providers who use this approach create a non-judgmental and supportive environment to encourage healthy behavior change. This has been shown to be effective in reducing substance use and risk behavior amongst adolescents. One advantage of MI is that it can be done in a short period of time, which is important in the primary care setting. Clinicians should consider the construct presented in Table 5–5. In theory, individuals pass through this series of stages while changing problem behaviors. To be maximally effective, providers should tailor their counseling messages to the patient's stage of readiness to change.

The use of MI techniques such as "chunk-check-chunk" or "elicit-provide-elicit" can be particularly helpful. These techniques involve asking open-ended questions or a readiness ruler to elicit the patient's perspective, providing information or feedback in a concise and targeted way, and then returning to the patient's perspective to explore their readiness for change. Another technique that can be utilized after open-ended questions are reflections, which involve actively listening to the patient and reflecting back their thoughts and feelings in a nonjudgmental way. Reflections help the patient explore their ambivalence towards substance use, build rapport with the healthcare provider, and ultimately increase the likelihood the patient makes a behavioral change. Overall, this patient-centered strategy of harm reduction focuses on the risk behaviors identified during intake and aims to meet youth where they are, recognize their inherent strengths and motivation to be well, respect their rights, and create a collaborative and personalized health promotion strategy.

Referral to Treatment

Providing resources and referrals to a subspecialty level of care for substance use is an important aspect of screening and management. Patients with moderate to severe SUDs, clinically significant substance-related problems, co-occurring mental health disorders, or interest in a higher level of care are candidates for substance use treatment programs. Across the United States, there is a dearth of substance use treatment programs, with some regions having minimal resources. PCPs can utilize the SAHMSA treatment finder (https://find-treatment.gov/, 1-800-662-HELP) to find resources within their area.

There are many different levels of subspecialty care for adolescent substance use, ranging from outpatient counseling to inpatient detoxification and residential rehabilitation. The appropriate level of care for a patient depends on severity and complexity of the disorder, as well as individual needs and circumstances. Key elements of an effective adolescent drug treatment program include assessment, a comprehensive and integrated treatment approach, family involvement, a developmentally appropriate program, engagement and retention of teens, qualified staff, gender and cultural competence, continuing care, and satisfactory treatment outcomes.

Well-established psychosocial treatments such as family-based therapy, cognitive behavioral therapy, and multi-component approaches remain the most effective methods of treatment. For most adolescents, the family is a central system in their development. An example of an intensive outpatient program may utilize contingency management, a behavioral intervention that involves providing incentives or rewards to patients for achieving specific treatment goals, such as abstaining from substance use or attending counseling sessions. In addition to therapy, new advances in adjunctive treatments such as pharmacotherapy, exercise, mindfulness, and recovery-oriented educational centers may also have some clinical utility.

Youth may not be readily accepting of a referral for several reasons, including lack of insight into substance-related losses and symptoms of SUD. Youth may also be defiant about substance use, necessitating the clinician come alongside rather than confront the youth. Similarly, nearly all youth experience perceived positives of substance use, including "self-medication" of comorbid mental health problems or escape from other stressors. Thus, it is not uncommon for youth to fear giving up substance use. Other barriers to youth engaging in treatment include stigma and confidentiality. Engaging the youth in the spirit of MI allows the clinician to present the referral in a way that empowers the youth to make change. This approach also enhances facilitators of treatment engagement, notably having a positive experience with providers, education and awareness, and openness and emotional expression. Youth with previous attempts at help-seeking are also more likely to engage in treatment. Presenting a referral to an outpatient program as a consultation or conversation with a specialist is less intimidating for many youth. Ultimately, clinicians should provide resources and refer youth to treatment if clinically indicated, even if the youth is precontemplative and does not want to reduce their substance use.

Hunt D, Fischer L, Sheedy K, Karon S: Substance use screening, brief intervention, and referral to treatment in multiple settings: evaluation of a national initiative. J Adolesc Health 2022;71(4S):S9–S14. doi: 10.1016/j.jadohealth.2022.03.002 [PMID: 36122975].

Miller WR, Rollnick S: *Motivational Interviewing: Helping People Change*. New York, NY: Guilford Press; 2023.

Roberts E, Martinez J: Harm Reduction Approach, 2016. https://harmreduction.org/wp-content/uploads/2017/07/Webinar-HReduxn_092716.pdf. Accessed June 20, 2019.

Substance Abuse and Mental Health Services Administration: Evidence Supporting the Effectiveness of an SBIRT. https://www.samhsa.gov/sites/default/files/sbirtwhitepaper_0.pdf. Accessed July 7, 2021.

Substance Abuse and Mental Health Services Administration (SAMHSA). (2019). SBIRT: Screening, Brief Intervention, and Referral to Treatment.

▶ Diagnosis

The American Psychiatric Association *Diagnostic and Statistical Manual of Mental Disorders*, 5th Edition, Text Revision (DSM-5-TR) outlines diagnostic criteria for SUD (Box 5–2). An SUD diagnosis is made for a specific class of substance: alcohol; cannabis; phencyclidine or other hallucinogens; inhalants; opioids; sedatives, hypnotics, or anxiolytics; stimulants; tobacco; and other or unknown substances. Providers may seek to further clarify the diagnosis by replacing the substance class with the specific misused substance, such as heroin use disorder or methamphetamine use disorder, consistent with the International Statistical Classification of Disease and Related Health Problem 10th revision (ICD-10) codes.

The DSM-5 combines substance abuse and dependence into one diagnosis, with severity determined by the number of diagnostic criteria manifested by the individual. Specifiers may be included to provide further diagnostic clarity, including "in early remission" (no criteria met for 3–11 months) and "in sustained remission" (no criteria met for 12 months or longer). For opioid use disorder, the specifier "on maintenance therapy" is used to designate if an individual is receiving agonist medications. The DSM-5 also outlines criteria for states of intoxication and withdrawal for each class of substance, except for hallucinogens and inhalants (no withdrawal state) and tobacco (no intoxication state). While DSM-5 does not propose a caffeine use disorder, states of intoxication and withdrawal are well defined.

More recently, the term *abuse* has been de-emphasized in substance use treatment as stigmatizing, with clinicians encouraged to refer to such use by its diagnosis or as problematic use or misuse. Clinicians are also encouraged to use

BOX 5–2. Substance Use Disorder Criteria

DSM-5-TR criteria for substance use disorders can be categorized as impaired control, social impairment, risky use, and pharmacologic effects.

Impaired control
- Using more than intended (larger amounts or over a longer time)
- Spending a large amount of time and effort to obtain and use
- Having a desire to or having unsuccessfully tried to cut back
- Having strong cravings or urges to use

Social impairment
- Failing to fulfill responsibilities at school, home, or work
- Giving up important activities or responsibilities
- Having relationship and social problems

Risky use
- Using in physically unsafe situations
- Knowing that use is causing or worsening physical or mental health problems

Pharmacologic effects
- Needing to use increased amounts to reach the same effect (tolerance)
- Experiencing withdrawal or continuing to use to avoid withdrawal

The severity of the substance use disorder is determined by the number of symptoms:
- Mild: 2-3 symptoms
- Moderate: 4-5 symptoms
- Severe: 6 or more symptoms

person-first language, for example referring to a youth as having an alcohol use disorder or misusing alcohol rather than as an alcoholic. Such efforts are meant to reduce stigma and encourage help-seeking and treatment engagement.

▶ Pharmacologic Screening

While the AAP recommends screening for substance use during routine visits, the use of pharmacological screening for substance use detection and treatment is controversial. The AAP recommends testing under certain circumstances (eg, an inexplicably obtunded patient in the emergency department) but discourages routine screening for the following reasons: (1) voluntary screening is rarely truly voluntary owing to the negative consequences for those who decline to participate; (2) infrequent users or individuals who have not used substances recently may be missed; (3) confronting adolescents with SUD with objective evidence of their use has little or no effect on behavior; and (4) the role of health care providers is to provide counseling and treatment, not law enforcement, that is, drug testing for the purpose of detecting illegal use. If testing is to be performed, the provider should discuss the plan for screening with the patient, explain the reasons for it, and obtain informed consent. The AAP does not consider parental request and permission sufficient justification for involuntary screening of mentally competent minors.

When laboratory screening is indicated, it can be conducted by a variety of methods that provide different windows of detection and may be more or less effective depending on

Table 5–6. Pharmacologic screening for adolescent substance use.

Substance	Urine Detection Time[a]	Blood Detection Time[1]	Saliva Detection Time[a]	Potential False-Positive Substances
Alcohol	12–24 h	10–12 h	1–5 days	None
Cannabis	3–30 days	2 days	24–48 h	NSAIDs
Cocaine	2–3 days	1–2 days	1–2 days	Lidocaine, novocaine, diltiazem
Methamphetamine	3–5 days	1–2 days	1–2 days	Nasal decongestants
MDMA (Ecstasy)	3–4 days	1–2 days	1–2 days	Cold medications, antibiotics
Heroin	3–4 days	6–8 h	1–2 days	Codeine, morphine, poppy seeds
LSD	1–4 days	2–4 h	1–4 days	None
PCP	7–14 days	48–72 h	1–3 days	Dextromethorphan, diphenhydramine, ketamine

LSD, lysergic acid diethylamide; MDMA, methylenedioxymethamphetamine (ecstasy); NSAIDs, nonsteroidal anti-inflammatory drugs; PCP, phencyclidine hydrochloride.
[a]Detection time in the biologic specimen type after last use of the substance.

the substance being detected. Blood tests provide the shortest window of detection and are heavily utilized in emergency and acute intoxication settings, while urine, saliva, and hair testing can generally provide information about a longer window of detection (Table 5–6). Available laboratory methods include immunoassay screening, gas chromatography-mass spectrometry (GC-MS), and liquid chromatography-mass spectrometry (LC-MS). GC-MS and LC-MS are substance specific and confirmatory, whereas immunoassays may cross-react with a number of medications and substances (false positives; see Table 5–6) and may not detect other substances within the same class (false negatives). While specific testing modalities can more accurately detect the presence of a substance, they cannot provide information on the quantity and frequency of use. Interpretation of results can be further complicated by false positives resulting from a patient's passive exposure to illicit substances. Home drug-testing products are available and can be procured online; however, these products have limitations and potential risks. The AAP recommends that home (and school-based) drug testing not be implemented until its safety and efficacy can be established.

While routine in-office point-of-care testing is not recommended to aid in diagnosis or monitoring treatment progression, pharmacologic testing can be used as part of a comprehensive treatment plan for adolescent SUD. More complex testing methodology is frequently used in subspecialty levels of care, in many types of treatment plans. In combination with behavioral intervention and pharmacotherapy, voluntary pharmacologic testing can aid in an individual treatment plan. It is important to create and maintain a nonjudgmental space if testing is incorporated in a patient's treatment plan, as relapse and positive tests may play an important part in overall treatment and recovery.

American Psychiatric Association: *Diagnostic and Statistical Manual of Mental Disorders*, Fifth Edition, Text Revision (DSM-5-TR). Washington, DC; 2022.

Levy S, Siqueira LM: Committee on substance abuse: testing for drugs of abuse in children and adolescents. Pediatrics 2014;133(6):e1798–e1807 [PMID: 24864184].

U.S. Department of Health & Human Services. Substance Abuse and Mental Health Services Administration (SAMHSA): Drug Testing Resources. Feb 2023. http://www.samhsa.gov/workplace/drg-testing-resources.

TREATMENT

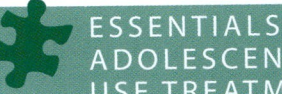

ESSENTIALS OF ADOLESCENT SUBSTANCE USE TREATMENT

▶ The SBIRT model can be used to diagnose and treat SUDs in the outpatient setting with motivational interviewing, cognitive behavioral therapy, the "five A's" for tobacco cessation, and other integrated behavioral interventions.

▶ Pharmacotherapy such as nicotine replacement therapy (NRT) and buprenorphine for opioid use disorder can also be implemented in the outpatient setting. Addiction medicine subspecialists can be consulted for assistance with an integrated treatment approach.

▶ Patients with severe SUDs or comorbidities can be referred for higher levels of substance use treatment and detoxification.

Table 5–7. "Five A's" for tobacco cessation.

Ask about tobacco use from all patients
Advise all tobacco users to quit
Assess willingness and motivation for tobacco user to make a quit attempt
Assist in the quit attempt
Arrange for follow-up

Reproduced from Treating Tobacco Use and Dependence: 2008 Update. Content last reviewed February 2020. Agency for Healthcare Research and Quality, Rockville, MD. https://www.ahrq.gov/prevention/guidelines/tobacco/index.html.

Office-Based Treatment

The primary care office can serve as a crucial entry point for identifying and treating adolescent substance use. By offering and providing confidential healthcare services, PCPs can utilize the brief intervention within the SBIRT model as an effective treatment for reducing substance use and progression to SUD. MI, cognitive behavioral therapy, and goal-setting strategies can be effective office-based treatments, with follow-up support to sustain behavioral change and prevent relapse.

For nicotine use disorder and smoking cessation specifically, an easy guideline for providers is the "five A's" for tobacco cessation (Table 5–7), published by the US Public Health Service and endorsed by the AAP.

Relapse should be regarded as a normal part of quitting nicotine use (and other substance use), rather than evidence of personal failure or a reason to forgo further attempts. Patients who exhibit nicotine dependency can be referred to community smoking cessation programs, including "smoking quit lines." The AAP and the World Health Organization recommend against the use of e-cigarettes as a cessation aid or nicotine dependence treatment for adolescents.

The use of pharmacotherapy in combination with behavioral interventions has been shown to be an effective approach to adolescent substance use. Pharmacotherapy for nicotine use includes nicotine replacement therapy (NRT) in the form of gum or patches, available over-the-counter as a first-line treatment for tobacco use disorder. Varenicline, a partial nicotine receptor agonist, and bupropion, an antidepressant, have both been shown to reduce cravings and symptoms of withdrawal. Other emerging medications for SUD include naltrexone and acamprosate, used in the treatment of alcohol use disorder to reduce the pleasurable effects of alcohol as well as cravings. Health care providers who work with adolescents should be familiar with these medications and consider incorporating them into their treatment plans in conjunction with behavioral intervention.

Buprenorphine is an opioid partial agonist approved for the treatment of opioid use disorder in patients 16 years or older. Effective in reducing opioid use and risk of overdose and increasing treatment retention, buprenorphine can be initiated both in inpatient and outpatient settings. The Consolidated Appropriations Act (2023) permits any provider with a schedule III DEA license to prescribe buprenorphine for opioid use disorder. Protocols are available to guide initiation of buprenorphine at low and high doses based on an individual's opioid history, physical examination, and withdrawal symptoms, in either the office-based or even home settings. PCPs can co-manage opioid use disorders with addiction specialists who can provide additional support for complex cases. In circumstances where a youth is misusing fentanyl and at high-risk of overdose, it is vital for the PCP to consider initiating buprenorphine and prescribe a naloxone kit while awaiting intake at substance use treatment programs.

SUDs can be complex and require an integrative multidisciplinary approach. PCPs can work collaboratively with subspecialty SUD providers to develop comprehensive treatment plans that may include behavioral interventions, pharmacotherapy, and/or support groups. Coordinated, evidenced-based care provided by PCPs and addiction specialists can facilitate achievement of long-term recovery.

Barclay RP et al: Integrated care for pediatric substance abuse. Child Adolesc Psychiatr Clin N Am 2016 Oct;25(4):769–777. doi: 10.1016/j.chc.2016.05.007 [PMID: 27613351].

National Institute on Drug Abuse. 2021, December 2. Overview. http://nida.nih.gov/publications/research-reports/medications-to-treat-opioid-addiction/overview. Accessed April 17, 2023.

Thomasius R, Paschke K, Arnaud N: Substance-use disorders in children and adolescents. Dtsch Arztebl Int 2022 Jun 24;119(25):440–450. doi: 10.3238/arztebl.m2022.0122 [PMID: 35635442].

U.S. Department of Human & Health Services. Substance Abuse and Mental Health Services Administration (SAMHSA). Removal of DATA Waiver (X-Waiver) Requirement. https://www.samhsa.gov/medications-substance-use-disorders/removal-data-waiver-requirement. Accessed March 2023.

Eating Disorders

Francisco Prada, MD

Eric J. Sigel, MD

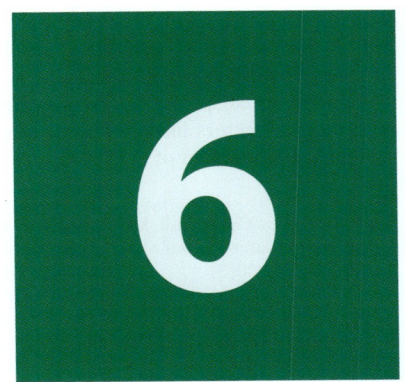

INTRODUCTION

Adolescents as well as younger children engage in disordered eating behavior at an alarming rate, and many develop partial or full-blown eating disorders (EDs). The spectrum of EDs includes anorexia nervosa (AN), bulimia nervosa (BN), binge-eating disorder (BED), other specified feeding or eating disorder (OSFED), and avoidant/restrictive food intake disorder (ARFID). These disorders are best defined in a biopsychosocial context.

ETIOLOGY

There is strong evidence for a genetic basis for EDs. The incidence of AN is 7% in first-degree relatives of anorexic patients compared with 1%–2% in the general population. The concordance rate in monozygotic twins is 55% compared with 7% in dizygotic twins. Twin studies estimate the heritability of AN as 33%–84% and BN as 28%–83%.

There is evidence of altered serotonergic and dopaminergic function and alterations in neuropeptides and gut peptides in AN and BN. It remains unclear whether abnormalities of neurotransmitters contribute to the development of EDs or are a consequence of the physiologic changes associated with the disorders. Patients with BN or BED appear to have a blunted serotonin response to eating and satiety. With decreased satiety, patients continue to eat, leading to a binge. Treatment with selective serotonin reuptake inhibitors (SSRIs) tends to equilibrate satiety regulation. Adiponectin is elevated in AN, although it is unclear whether this is merely secondary to malnutrition. Cholecystokinin is decreased in BN, perhaps contributing to the lack of post-ingestion satiety that perpetuates a binge. Ghrelin, a gut peptide, is elevated in patients with AN, and it does not decrease normally after a meal in these patients. Obestatin, a gut peptide that inhibits appetite, is elevated in AN as well.

Leptin physiology is deranged in patients with AN. These abnormalities may mediate energy changes that affect the hypothalamic-pituitary axis and play a role in perpetuating AN. Leptin levels increase excessively as individuals with AN regain weight. The abnormally high levels of leptin may contribute to the difficulty AN patients have when trying to regain weight, as higher leptin levels signal the body to decrease energy intake.

Traditional psychological theory has suggested many environmental factors that might promote the development of EDs. Enmeshment of mother with daughter to the point that the teenager cannot develop her own identity (a key developmental marker of adolescence) may be a predisposing factor. The teenager may cope by asserting control over food, as she senses her lack of control in the developmental realm. A second theory is related to puberty. Some teenagers may fear or dislike their changing bodies. By restricting food intake, they lose weight, stop menstruating, and effectively reverse pubertal development. Related, emerging literature demonstrates that transgender youth may use food restriction and compensatory behaviors to control pubertal development. It is generally recognized that ED diagnoses are more common in trans youth compared to cisgender youth. The largest study showed that 17% of transgender American college youth reported past year ED diagnoses.

Society has promoted the message that being thin or muscular is necessary for attractiveness and success. The ease of access to diet products—foods and diet pills—as well as internet instructions (proanorexia sites and social media) makes it simple for adolescents to embark on a quest for thinness or muscularity.

Importantly, the SARS CoV-2 pandemic created a surge in mental health issues in adolescents, with a substantial increase in the prevalence of EDs and prolonged wait times prior to initiating treatment. Theories as to why the pandemic was associated with an increase in eating disordered behavior include (1) disruption to daily routine, including constraints on physical activity that may have increased weight and body shape concerns; (2) increased exposure to ED-specific or anxiety-provoking media that may have increased ED risk; and (3) elevated stress and social isolation that may have promoted the development of EDs.

Genetic predisposition, environmental factors, and psychological factors likely combine to create a milieu that promotes development of EDs.

Bulik CM, Slof-Op't Landt MC, van Furth EF, Sullivan PF: The genetics of anorexia nervosa. Annu Rev Nutr 2007;27:263–275 [PMID: 17430085].

Campbell IC, Mill J, Uher R, Schmidt U: Eating disorders, gene-environment interaction, and epigentics. Neurosci Biobehav Rev 2011;35:784–793 [PMID: 20888360].

Coelho JS, Suen J, Clark BA, Marshall SK, Geller J, Lam PY: Eating disorder diagnoses and symptom presentation in transgender youth: a scoping review. Curr Psychiatry Rep 2019 Oct 15; 21(11):107 [PMID: 31617014].

Duffy ME, Henkel KE, Joiner TE: Prevalence of self-injurious thoughts and behaviors in transgender individuals with eating disorders: a national study. J Adolesc Health 2019;64(4): 461–466. https://doi.org/10.1016/j.jadohealth.2018.07.016 [PMID: 30314865].

Grzelak T et al: Neurobiochemical and psychologic factors influencing the eating behaviors and attitudes in anorexia nervosa. J Physiol Biochem 2017;73(2):297–305 [PMID: 27924450].

Rodgers RF et al: The impact of the COVID-19 pandemic on eating disorder risk and symptoms. Int J Eat Disord 2020 Jul;53(7):1166–1170. doi: 10.1002/eat.23318 [Epub 2020 Jun 1] [PMID: 32476175].

Warren MP: Endocrine manifestations of eating disorders. J Clin Endocrin Metab 2011;96(2):333 [PMID: 21159848].

INCIDENCE

EDs are the third most common chronic illness of adolescent girls in the United States The incidence has been increasing steadily in the United States since the 1930s. Although ascertaining exact incidence is difficult, most studies show that 1%–2% of teenagers develop AN and 2%–4% develop BN. Males typically comprise about 10% of patients with EDs.

Preadolescents with EDs, in comparison to teenagers with EDs, are more likely to be male and present with rapid weight loss and lower percentile body weight and are less likely to engage in bulimic behaviors. Prepubertal patients often have associated psychiatric diagnoses.

Hornberger LL, Lane MA; AAP the Committee on Adolescence: Identification and management of eating disorders in children and adolescents. Pediatrics 2021;147(1):e2020040279 [PMID: 33386343].

Kann L et al: Centers for Disease Control and Prevention (CDC): youth risk behavior surveillance—United States 2013. MMWR Surveill Summ 2014 Jun 13;63(SS-4):39–41. http://www.cdc.gov/mmwr/pdf/ss/ss6304.pdf [PMID: 24918634].

Lindvall Dahlgren C, Wisting L: Transitioning from DSM-IV to DSM-5: a systematic review of eating disorder prevalence assessment. Int J Eat Disord 2016;49(11):975–999 [PMID: 27528542].

PREDISPOSING FACTORS & CLINICAL PROFILES

Children involved in gymnastics, figure skating, and ballet—activities that emphasize thin bodies—are at higher risk for AN than are children in sports that do not emphasize body image. Adolescents who believe that being thin represents the ideal frame for a female, those who are dissatisfied with their bodies, and those with a history of dieting are at increased risk for EDs. Sudden changes in dietary habits, such as becoming vegetarian, may be a first sign of anorexia, especially if the change is abrupt and without good reason.

The typical bulimic patient tends to be impulsive and engages in risk-taking behavior such as alcohol use, drug use, and sexual experimentation. Bulimic patients often have an appropriate weight for height or are slightly overweight. They have average academic performance. Youth with diabetes have an increased risk of BN. In males, wrestling predisposes to BN, and same sex orientation is associated with binge eating.

Striegel-Moore RH, Bulik CM: Risk factors for eating disorders. Am Psychol 2007;62:181 [PMID: 17469897].

Vo M, Lau J, Rubinstein M: Eating disorders in adolescent and young adult males: presenting characteristics. J Adolesc Health 2016;59(4):397–400 [PMID: 27287963].

ANOREXIA NERVOSA

 ESSENTIALS OF DIAGNOSIS & TYPICAL FEATURES: ANOREXIA NERVOSA

Diagnostic criteria for AN, adapted from the *Diagnostic and Statistical Manual of Mental Disorders,* Fifth Edition (DSM-5), are:

► Restriction of energy intake relative to requirements leading to low body weight in the context of age, sex, physical health, and developmental trajectory.

► Strong fear of gaining weight or becoming fat, even though underweight.

► Disturbance in the way one's body weight or shape is experienced, undue influence of body weight or shape on self-evaluation, or denial of the seriousness of current low body weight.

https://www.nationaleatingdisorders.org/anorexia-nervosa

There are two major types of AN. In the restricting type, patients do not regularly engage in binge eating or purging. In the binge-purge type, AN is combined with binge eating or purging, or both. Distinguishing between the two is important as they carry different implications for prognosis and treatment. Patients may not demonstrate all features of AN, but may exhibit some of the deleterious symptoms associated with AN.

▶ Clinical Findings

A. Symptoms and Signs

Patients may show some typical AN behaviors, such as reduction in dietary fat and intense concern with body image, even before weight loss or amenorrhea occurs. Recognition of early symptoms and signs is important because early intervention may prevent the full-blown syndrome from developing.

Diagnosing AN can be challenging because adolescents may try to conceal their illness. Assessing the patient's body image is essential to determining the diagnosis. Table 6–1 lists screening questions that help tease out a teenager's perceptions of body image. Other diagnostic screening tools (eg, EDs inventory) assess a range of eating and dieting behaviors. Parental observations are critical in determining whether a patient has expressed dissatisfaction over body habitus and describing weight loss techniques the child has used. If the teenager is unwilling to share his or her concerns about body image, the clinician may find clues to the diagnosis by carefully considering other presenting symptoms or signs. Weight loss from a baseline of normal body weight is an obvious red flag for the presence of an ED. Additionally, AN should be considered in anyone with secondary amenorrhea who has lost weight.

Physical symptoms and signs are usually secondary to weight loss and proportional to the degree of malnutrition. The body effectively goes into hibernation, becoming functionally hypothyroid (euthyroid sick) to save energy. Body temperature decreases, and patients report being cold. Bradycardia develops, especially in the supine position, postulated to be due to increased vagal tone and energy conservation. Dizziness, light-headedness, and syncope may occur as a result of orthostasis and hypotension. Left ventricular mass is decreased, stroke volume is compromised, and peripheral resistance is increased, contributing to left ventricular systolic dysfunction. Patients can develop prolonged QTc syndrome and increased QT dispersion (irregular QT intervals), putting them at risk for cardiac arrhythmias. Peripheral circulation is reduced. Hands and feet may be blue and cool. Hair thins, nails become brittle, and skin becomes dry. Lanugo develops as a primitive response to starvation. The gastrointestinal (GI) tract may be affected; inability to take in normal quantities of food, early satiety, and gastroesophageal reflux can develop as the body adapts to reduced intake. The normal gastrocolic reflex may be lost due to lack of stimulation by food, causing bloating and constipation. Delayed gastric emptying may develop. Nutritional rehabilitation improves gastric emptying and dyspeptic symptoms in AN restricting type, but not in those who vomit. Neurologically, patients may experience decreased cognition, inability to concentrate, increased irritability, and depression, which may be related to structural brain changes and decreased cerebral blood flow.

Determining body mass index (BMI) is critical for assessing degree of malnutrition. A gown-only weight after urination is the most accurate way to assess weight. Patients tend to wear bulky clothes and may hide weights in their pockets or drink excessive fluid (water-loading) to trick the practitioner. BMI below the 25th percentile indicates risk for malnutrition and below the 5th percentile indicates significant malnutrition. Median body weight (MBW) for height, calculated using the 50th percentile of BMI for age and sex, should be determined, as it serves both as the denominator to determine what percent weight an individual is and to provide a general goal weight during recovery. Any individuals less than 75% MBW are deemed severely malnourished and often warrant medical admission.

A combination of malnutrition and stress causes hypothalamic hypogonadism. The hypothalamic-pituitary-gonadal axis shuts down, directing finite energy resources to vital functions. This may be mediated by the effect of low serum leptin levels on the hypothalamic-pituitary axis. Pubertal development and skeletal growth may be interrupted, and adolescents may experience decreased libido. Amenorrhea, an important clinical sign that the body is malnourished, occurs for two reasons. The hypothalamic-pituitary-ovarian axis shuts down under stress, causing hypothalamic amenorrhea. In addition, when weight loss is significant, there is insufficient adipose tissue needed to convert estrogen to its activated form. Resumption of menses occurs only when both body weight and body fat increase. An adolescent needs about 17% body fat to restart menses and 22% body fat to initiate menses if primary amenorrhea is present. Approximately 73% of postmenarchal patients resume menstruating if they reach 90% of MBW. Some evidence suggests that

Table 6–1. Screening questions to help diagnose anorexia and bulimia nervosa.

How do you feel about your body?
Are there parts of your body you might change?
When you look at yourself in the mirror, do you see yourself as overweight, underweight, or satisfactory?
If overweight, how much do you want to weigh?
If your weight is satisfactory, has there been a time when you were worried about being overweight?
If overweight (underweight), what would you change?
Have you ever been on a diet?
What have you done to help yourself lose weight?
Do you count calories or fat grams?
Do you keep your intake to a certain number of calories?
Have you ever used nutritional supplements, diet pills, or laxatives to help you lose weight?
Have you ever made yourself vomit to get rid of food or lose weight?

target weight gain for return of menses is approximately 1 kg higher than the weight at which menses ceased.

B. Laboratory Findings

All organ systems may suffer some degree of damage in the anorexic patient, related to both severity and duration of illness (Table 6–2). Initial screening should include complete blood count with differential; serum levels of electrolytes, blood urea nitrogen, creatinine, phosphorus, calcium, magnesium, and thyroid-stimulating hormone; liver function tests; and urinalysis. Increase in lipids, likely due to abnormal liver function, is seen in 18%, with subsequent return to normal once weight is restored. An electrocardiogram (ECG) should be performed because significant ECG abnormalities may be present, most importantly prolonged QTc syndrome. Bone densitometry should be done if illness persists for 6 months, as patients begin to accumulate risk for osteoporosis.

Differential Diagnosis

If the diagnosis is unclear (ie, the patient has lost a significant amount of weight but does not have typical body image distortion or fat phobia), the clinician must consider the differential diagnosis for weight loss in adolescents. This includes inflammatory bowel disease, diabetes, hyperthyroidism, malignancy, depression, and chronic infectious disease such as human immunodeficiency virus (HIV). Less common diagnoses include adrenal insufficiency and malabsorption syndromes such as celiac disease. The history and physical examination should direct specific laboratory and radiologic evaluation.

Table 6–2. Laboratory findings: anorexia nervosa.

Increased blood urea nitrogen and creatinine secondary to renal insufficiency
Decreased white blood cells, platelets, and less commonly red blood cells and hematocrit secondary to bone marrow suppression or fat atrophy of the bone marrow
Increased AST and ALT secondary to malnutrition
Increased cholesterol, thought to be related to altered fatty acid metabolism
Decreased alkaline phosphatase secondary to zinc deficiency
Low- to low-normal thyroid-stimulating hormone and thyroxine
Decreased follicle-stimulating hormone, luteinizing hormone, estradiol, and testosterone secondary to shutdown of hypothalamic pituitary-gonadal axis
Abnormal electrolytes related to hydration status
Decreased phosphorus
Decreased insulin-like growth factor
Increased cortisol
Decreased urine specific gravity in cases of intentional water intoxication

ALT, alanine aminotransferase; AST, aspartate aminotransferase.

Complications (Table 6–3)

A. Short-Term Complications

1. Early satiety—Patients may have difficulty tolerating even modest quantities of food when intake increases; this usually resolves after the patients adjust to larger meals. Gastric emptying is poor. Pancreatic and biliary secretion is diminished.

2. Superior mesenteric artery syndrome—As patients become malnourished, the fat pad between the superior mesenteric artery and the duodenum shrinks and compression of the transverse duodenum may cause obstruction and vomiting, especially with solid foods. The upper GI series shows to-and-fro movement of barium in the descending and transverse duodenum proximal to the obstruction. Treatment involves a liquid diet or nasoduodenal feedings until restoration of the fat pad has occurred coincident with weight gain.

3. Constipation—Patients may be very constipated. Two mechanisms contribute—loss of the gastrocolic reflex and loss of colonic muscle tone. Typically, stool softeners are not effective because the colon has decreased peristaltic amplitude. Agents that induce peristalsis, such as bisacodyl, as well as osmotic agents, such as polyethylene glycol-electrolyte solution (MiraLax), are helpful. Constipation can persist for up to 6–8 weeks after refeeding. Occasionally, enemas are required.

4. Refeeding syndrome—Described in section Treatment.

5. Pericardial effusion—The degree of malnutrition correlates with increasing prevalence of pericardial effusion. One study demonstrated that 22% of those with AN had silent pericardial effusion, with 88% of effusions resolving after weight restoration.

B. Long-Term Complications

1. Osteoporosis—Approximately 50% of females with AN have reduced bone mass at one or more sites. The lumbar spine has the most rapid turnover and is the area likely to be affected first. Teenagers are particularly at risk as they accrue 40% of their bone mineral during adolescence. Low body weight is most predictive of bone loss. The causes of osteopenia and osteoporosis are multiple. Estrogen and testosterone are essential to potentiate bone development. Bone minerals begin to resorb without estrogen. Elevated cortisol levels and decreased insulin-like growth factor-1 also contribute to bone resorption. Amenorrhea is highly correlated with osteoporosis; as few as 6 months of amenorrhea is associated with osteopenia or osteoporosis. Males have similar bone loss related to their degree of malnutrition, likely due to decreased testosterone and elevated cortisol.

The most effective treatment for bone loss in females is regaining of sufficient weight and body fat to restart the menstrual cycle. Studies do not support the use of hormone replacement therapy delivered orally to improve bone

Table 6–3. Complications of anorexia and bulimia nervosa by mechanism.

Cardiovascular	**Hematologic**
Bradycardia (WL/MN)	Leukopenia (WL/MN)
Postural hypotension (WL/MN, SIV, LX)	Anemia (WL/MN)
Arrhythmia, sudden death (WL/MN, SIV, LX)	Thrombocytopenia (WL/MN)
Congestive heart failure (during refeeding) (WL/MN)	↓ ESR (WL/MN)
Pericardial effusion (WL/MN)	Impaired cell-mediated immunity (WL/MN)
Mitral valve prolapse (WL/MN)	**Metabolic**
ECG abnormalities (prolonged QT, low voltage, T-wave abnormalities, conduction defects) (WL/MN)	Dehydration (WL/MN, SIV, LXA, DU)
Endocrine	Acidosis (LXA)
↓ LH, FSH (WL/MN)	Alkalosis (SIV)
↓ T_3, ↑ rT_3, ↓ T_4, TSH (WL/MN)	Hypokalemia (SIV, LXA, DU)
Irregular menses (WL/MN, B/P)	Hyponatremia (SIV, LXA, DU, WL/MN)
Amenorrhea (WL/MN)	Hypochloremia (SIV)
Hypercortisolism (WL/MN)	Hypocalcemia (WL/MN, SIV)
Growth retardation (WL/MN)	Hypophosphatemia (WL/MN)
Delayed puberty (WL/MN)	Hypomagnesemia (WL/MN)
Decreased libido (WL/MN)	Hypercarotenemia (WL/MN)
Gastrointestinal	**Neurologic**
Dental erosion (SIV)	Cortical atrophy-white and gray matter (WL/MN)
Parotid swelling (SIV)	Peripheral neuropathy (WL/MN)
Esophagitis, esophageal tears (SIV)	Seizures (WL/MN, SIV, LXA)
Delayed gastric emptying (WL/MN, SIV)	Thermoregulatory abnormalities (WL/MN)
Gastric dilation (rarely rupture) (SIV)	↓ REM and slow-wave sleep (All)
Pancreatitis (WL/MN)	**Renal**
Constipation (WL/MN, LXA)	Hematuria (WL/MN)
Diarrhea (LXA)	Proteinuria (WL/MN)
Superior mesenteric artery syndrome (WL/MN)	↓ Renal concentrating ability (WL/MN, DU)
Hypercholesterolemia (WL/MN)	Enuresis (WL/MN)
↑ Liver function tests (fatty infiltration of the liver) (WL/MN)	**Skeletal**
	Osteopenia (WL/MN)
	Fractures (WL/MN)

B/P, binge-purge; DU, diuretic abuse; ECG, electrocardiogram; ESR, erythrocyte sedimentation rate; FSH, follicle-stimulating hormone; LH, luteinizing hormone; LXA, laxative abuse; REM, rapid eye movement; rT_3, resin triiodothyronine uptake; SIV, self-induced vomiting; T_3, triiodothyronine; T_4, thyroxine; TSH, thyroid-stimulating hormone; WL/MN, weight loss/malnutrition.

recovery; however, one randomized controlled trial demonstrated that physiologic doses of estrogen delivered transdermally over 18 months did improve bone density. Clinicians may consider transdermal estrogen treatment if patients are recalcitrant to intervention and do not restore weight in a timely manner. Bisphosphonates show moderate effectiveness in adults with AN, but not in adolescents. The use of dehydroepiandrosterone in combination with oral contraceptive pills is shown to maintain bone mineral density in adolescents with AN compared to controls, though this treatment approach has not been adopted as standard of care. Loss of bone mineral density also occurs in males with AN; however, less is known about treatment of bone loss in males except that regaining weight to a healthy range is important to stop further bone loss.

2. Brain changes—As malnutrition becomes pronounced, brain tissue—both white and gray matter—is lost, with a compensatory increase in cerebrospinal fluid in the sulci and ventricles. Follow-up studies of weight-recovered anorexic patients show a persistent loss of gray matter, although white matter returns to normal. Functionally, there does not seem to be a direct relationship between cognition and brain tissue loss, although studies have shown a decrease in cognitive ability and decreased cerebral blood flow in very malnourished patients.

Fazeli PK, Klibanski A: Effects of anorexia nervosa on bone metabolism. Endocr Rev 2018 Dec;39(6):895–910 [PMID: 30165608].

Frank GKW: Advances from neuroimaging studies in eating disorders. CNS Spectr 2015;20(4):391–400 [PMID: 25902917].

Golden NH et al: Update on the medical management of eating disorders in adolescents. J Adolesc Health 2015;56:370–375 [PMID: 25659201].

Kastner S, et al: Echocardiographic findings in adolescents with anorexia nervosa at beginning of treatment and after weight recovery. Eur Child Adolesc Psychiatry 2012 Jan;21(1):15–21 [PMID: 22086424].

Misra M et al: Physiologic estrogen replacement increases bone density in adolescent girls with anorexia nervosa. J Bone Miner Res 2011 Oct;26(10):2430–2438 [PMID: 21698665].

Nagata J et al: Assessment of sex differences in bone deficits among adolescents with anorexia nervosa. Int J Eat Disord 2017 Apr;50(4):352–358 [PMID: 27611361].

Sachs KV, Harnke B, Mehler PS, Krantz MJ: Cardiovascular complications of anorexia nervosa: a systematic review. Int J Eat Disord 2016 Mar;49(3):238–248 [PMID: 26710932].

C. Mortality

Patients with EDs are at a higher risk of death than the general population and those with AN have the highest risk of dying among those with EDs. Meta-analysis estimates the standardized mortality ratio associated with AN to be 5.9. Death in anorexic patients occurs due to suicide, abnormal electrolytes, and cardiac arrhythmias.

▶ Treatment

A. General Approach

Factors that determine treatment interventions are severity and duration of illness, specific disease manifestations, previous treatment approaches and outcomes, program availability, financial resources, and insurance coverage. Options include outpatient management, partial hospitalization programs, inpatient medical or psychiatric hospitalization, and residential treatment. The key to determining level of intervention is the degree of malnutrition, rapidity of weight loss, degree of medical compromise, and presence of life-threatening electrolyte abnormalities. No absolute criteria determine level of intervention. The practitioner must examine the degree of medical compromise and consider immediate risks and the potential for an individual to reverse the situation on his or her own. As treatment is costly and patients may not have insurance benefits that adequately cover the costs, parents and practitioners may face profound dilemmas as to how to best provide treatment. However, EDs are now legally recognized in many states as a parity mental health diagnosis similar to the other biologically based mental health illnesses, which has increased the ease of obtaining insurance coverage.

A multidisciplinary approach is most effective and should include medical monitoring, nutrition therapy, and individual and family psychotherapy by experienced practitioners. Family therapy is an important means of helping families understand the development of the disease and addressing issues that may be barriers to recovery. Both individual and family psychotherapy is encouraged in most treatment programs, and recovery without psychotherapy is unusual. The average length of psychotherapy is roughly 6–9 months, although some individuals continue therapy for extended periods. Adjunctive modalities include art and horticulture therapy, therapeutic recreation, and massage therapy.

Manualized family therapy, which gives power and control over eating back to parents, is the most utilized therapeutic approach for adolescents with AN. Treatment is prescribed for 20 weekly sessions and delivered by a trained therapist, resulting in good or intermediate outcomes in 90% of treated adolescents. The first 10 weeks empower parents, putting them in control of their child's nutrition and exercise and instructing them to supervise each meal. Sessions 11–16 return control over eating to the adolescent. Finally, sessions 17–20 occur when the patient is maintaining a healthy weight and shifts the focus away from the ED, examining instead the impact that the ED has had on establishing a healthy adolescent identity.

Careful instruction in nutrition helps the teenager and family dispel misconceptions, identify realistic nutritional goals, and normalize eating. Initially, nutrition education may be the most important intervention as the teenager slowly works through fears of fat-containing foods and weight gain. The teenager begins to trust the nutrition therapist and restore body weight, eventually eating in a well-balanced, healthy manner.

Regardless of which level of treatment intervention a patient begins, an overriding goal is to help the patient achieve a healthy body weight. Ideally, a dietician is part of the treatment team and can help determine the goal/target weight. Often MBW and target weight are similar, though if growth records reveal a patient has consistently developed at the 25th percentile BMI, as an example, then it may be reasonable to set a target weight for the 25th percentile BMI.

B. Inpatient Treatment

Table 6–4 lists criteria for hospital admission for patients with EDs that are generally used in the medical community.

Table 6–4. Criteria for hospitalization for eating disordered patients.

One or more of the following justify hospitalization:
1. Body weight: < 75% median body weight.
2. Dehydration
3. Electrolyte disturbance (hypokalemia, hyponatremia, hypophosphatemia)
4. ECG abnormalities (prolonged QTC, severe bradycardia)
5. Physiologic Instability
   Supine heart rate < 45 beats/min
   Symptomatic hypotension or syncope
   Hypothermia
6. Failure of outpatient management
7. Acute food refusal
8. Uncontrolled bingeing and purging
9. Acute medical complications of malnutrition (syncope, seizures, cardiac failure, pancreatitis)
10. Comorbid psychiatric or medical condition that prohibits or limits appropriate outpatient treatment (severe depression, suicidal ideation, obsessive-compulsive disorder, type 1 diabetes)

It is usually quite difficult for a patient who is losing weight rapidly (> 2 lb/wk) to reverse the weight loss because the body is in a catabolic state.

Goals of hospitalization include arresting weight loss and stabilizing hemodynamics. Nutrition is the most vital inpatient medicine. Studies suggest that meal plans can begin with as high as 1750 kcal regardless of baseline intake. Meal plans should be well balanced with appropriate proportions of carbohydrate, protein, and fat. Oral meals are usually tolerated, although it is important to be supervised by medical staff. If the patient resists, nasogastric alimentation can be used. Aside from caloric needs, the clinician needs to consider the patient's hydration. Dehydration should be corrected slowly, with the oral route usually adequate. Aggressive intravenous fluid administration should be avoided because left ventricular mass is compromised and a rapid increase in volume may not be tolerated. Regulating fluid intake is important because water intoxication can contribute to abnormal electrolytes and falsified weights.

During the initial introduction of food, the clinician should monitor the patient for refeeding syndrome, a phenomenon that occurs if caloric intake is increased too rapidly. Indications of refeeding syndrome are decreased serum phosphorus (as the body resumes synthesis of adenosine triphosphate), decreased serum potassium (as increased insulin causes K^+ to shift from extracellular fluid into K^+-depleted cells), and, rarely, edema related to fluid shifts or congestive heart failure. Although specific guidelines do not exist, many practitioners begin phosphorus supplementation if patients are severely malnourished (< 70% MBW) or their intake has been consistently less than 500 kcal/day. Caloric intake can be increased 250 kcal/day as long as refeeding syndrome does not occur. Weight goals vary depending on programmatic approach. Typically, intake is adjusted to achieve a goal of 0.1–0.25 kg/day weight gain.

Overnight monitoring for bradycardia is helpful in assessing degree of metabolic compromise. Usually, the more rapid and severe the weight loss, the worse the bradycardia. Improving bradycardia correlates with weight recovery. Orthostatic hypotension is most severe around hospital day 4, improving steadily and correcting by the third week of nutritional rehabilitation. An ECG should be obtained due to risk for prolonged QTc syndrome and junctional arrhythmias related to the severity of bradycardia.

It usually takes 1–2 weeks to reach the initial goals of hospitalization—steady weight gain, toleration of oral diet without signs of refeeding syndrome, improved bradycardia (heart rate > 45 beats/min), and correction of orthostasis. Specific weight criteria are used by many programs for considering discharge. This depends partly on admission weight, but ideally a patient gains at least 5% of MBW. Some programs set discharge at achievement of 80%, 85%, or 90% MBW. Patient outcomes are improved with discharge at a higher body weight; some evidence suggests that patients do better if discharged at 95% MBW. Anecdotally, relapse rates are high if patients are discharged at less than 75% MBW.

C. Pharmacotherapy

Practitioners frequently use psychotropic medications for treatment of AN, despite lack of evidence confirming efficacy. Several open-label trials suggest that atypical antipsychotics (risperidone, olanzapine, quetiapine) may be helpful. One review found that olanzapine (2.5–15 mg/day) was associated with improved body weight, decreased delusional thinking, improvement in body image, and decreased agitation and premeal anxiety. However, a randomized controlled trial did not show any difference in outcomes between risperidone and placebo.

SSRIs repeatedly have been shown to not be helpful in the initial therapy of AN. A recent study showed that use of SSRIs may decrease bone mineral density when used in malnourished patients. However, once the patient has achieved approximately 85% MBW, SSRIs (fluoxetine, citalopram, or sertraline) may help prevent relapse.

Zinc deficiency is common in AN, and several studies support its use as a supplement during the initial phases of treatment. Because zinc deficiency adversely affects neurotransmitters, administering zinc helps restore neurotransmitter action to baseline. Additionally, zinc may restore appetite and improve depressive mood. Zinc should be administered for approximately 2 months from the beginning of therapy, with at least 14 mg of elemental zinc daily. Because of global nutritional deficits, a multivitamin with iron is also recommended daily. Symptomatic treatment for constipation and reflux should be used appropriately until symptoms resolve.

D. Outpatient Treatment

A range of treatment modalities are available, including partial hospitalization programs (8–11 hours per day, 5–7 days per week), intensive outpatient programs (3 hours per day, 2–3 days per week), and routine outpatient care. Youth may transition from an inpatient medical stay to a less intensive outpatient program. Alternatively, they may begin treatment at one of these outpatient treatment levels initially, as not all patients with AN require inpatient treatment, especially if signs are recognized early. Ideally, regardless of the level required, treatment should employ a multidisciplinary team approach. Manualized family-based treatment is ideal for the outpatient setting if a trained therapist is available. Appropriate nutrition counseling is vital in guiding a patient and family through the initial stages of recovery. As the nutrition therapist is working at increasing the patient's caloric intake, a practitioner needs to monitor the patient's weight and vital signs. Often, activity level needs to be decreased to help reverse the catabolic state. A reasonable weight gain goal may be 0.2–0.5 kg/wk. If weight loss persists, careful monitoring of vital signs, including supine heart rate, is important in determining whether an increased level of care is needed. Concomitantly, the patient should be referred to a psychotherapist and, if indicated, assessed by a psychiatrist.

E. Treatment Goals and Outcomes

Goals of treatment include reaching a healthy body weight, elimination of medical sequelae, and resumption of menses. Symptoms can wax and wane over an extended period for several years. Approximately 50% of adolescents recover in a relatively short period of time. Thirty percent may take several years to get back to a state of health, although symptoms may reappear on occasion. About 20% of adolescents can go on to develop chronic, unremitting AN.

DiVasta AD, Feldman HA, O'Donnell JM: Effect of exercise and antidepressants on skeletal outcomes in adolescent girls with anorexia nervosa. J Adolesc Health 2017 Feb;60(2):229–232 [PMID: 27939877].

Garber AK et al: A systematic review of approaches to refeeding in patients with anorexia nervosa. Int J Eat Disord 2016 Mar;49(3):293–310 [PMID: 26661289].

Jada K, Djossi SK, Khedr A, Neupane B, Proskuriakova E, Mostafa JA: The pathophysiology of anorexia nervosa in hypothalamic endocrine function and bone metabolism. Cureus 2021 Dec 20;13(12):e20548. doi: 10.7759/cureus.20548 [PMID: 35103128].

Jowik K, Tyszkiewicz-Nwafor M, Słopień A: Anorexia nervosa—what has changed in the state of knowledge about nutritional rehabilitation for patients over the past 10 years? A review of literature. Nutrients 2021 Oct 27;13(11):3819. doi: 10.3390/nu13113819 [PMID: 34836075].

Keshaviah A et al: Re-examining premature mortality in anorexia nervosa: a meta-analysis redux. Compr Psychiatry 2014 Nov;55(8):1773–1784 [PMID: 25214371].

BULIMIA NERVOSA

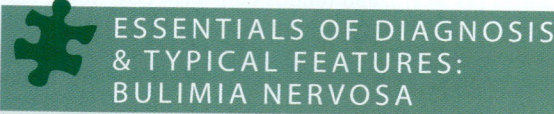

ESSENTIALS OF DIAGNOSIS & TYPICAL FEATURES: BULIMIA NERVOSA

Diagnostic criteria for BN are:

► Recurrent episodes of binge eating, characterized by both of the following:

- Eating in a discrete period an amount of food that is larger than most people would eat during a similar period under like circumstances.

- A sense of lack of control during the episode (eg, feeling that one cannot stop eating or control what or how much one is eating).

► Recurrent inappropriate compensatory behavior to prevent weight gain (eg, self-induced vomiting; misuse of laxatives, diuretics, or other products; excessive exercise; fasting).

► Binge eating and inappropriate compensatory behaviors occur at least once a week for 3 months (on average).

https://www.nationaleatingdisorders.org/bulimia-nervosa

Binge eating refers to either eating excessive amounts of food during a normal mealtime or having a meal that lasts longer than usual. Bulimic individuals feel out of control while eating, unable or unwilling to recognize satiety signals. Any type of food may be eaten in a binge, although typically it includes carbohydrates or junk food. Extreme guilt is often associated with the episode. At some point, either prior to or during a binge, bulimic individuals often decide to purge as a means of preventing weight gain. The most common ways to purge are self-induced vomiting, exercise, and laxative use. Some individuals will vomit multiple times during a purge episode after using large amounts of water to cleanse their system. This can induce significant electrolyte abnormalities such as hyponatremia and hypokalemia, which may put the patient at acute risk for arrhythmia or seizure. Other methods of purging include diuretics, diet pills, cathartics, and nutritional supplements that promote weight loss.

Diagnosing BN can be difficult unless the teenager is forthcoming, or parents or caregivers can supply direct observations. Bulimic patients are usually average or slightly above average in body weight and have no physical abnormalities. Screening all teenagers for body image concerns is crucial. If the teenager expresses concern about being overweight, the clinician should screen the patient about dieting methods. Asking whether patients have binged, feel out of control while eating, or cannot stop eating can clarify the diagnosis. Parents may report that significant amounts of food are missing or disappearing more quickly than normal. If the physician is suspicious, direct questioning about all the ways to purge should follow. Indicating first that the behavior is not unusual can make questioning less threatening and more likely to elicit a truthful response. For example, the clinician might say, "Some teenagers who try to lose weight make themselves vomit after eating. Have you ever considered or done that yourself?" (See Table 6–1 for additional screening questions.)

► Clinical Findings

A. Symptoms and Signs

Symptoms are related to the mechanism of purging. GI problems are most prominent. Abdominal pain is common. Gastroesophageal reflux occurs as the lower esophageal sphincter becomes compromised due to repetitive vomiting. Frequent vomiting may also cause esophagitis or gastritis, as the mucosa is irritated by acid exposure. Early satiety, involuntary vomiting, and complaints that food is "coming up" on its own are frequent. Hematemesis and esophageal rupture have been reported. Patients may report diarrhea or constipation, especially if laxatives have been used. Sialadenitis (parotid pain and enlargement) may be caused by frequent vomiting. Erosion of dental enamel results from increased oral acid exposure during vomiting. Because comorbid depression is common in BN, patients may report difficulty sleeping, decreased energy, or decreased motivation. Light-headedness or syncope may develop secondary to dehydration.

It is important to note that most purging methods are ineffective. When patients binge, they may consume thousands of calories. Digestion begins rapidly, and although the patient may be able to vomit some food, much is actually digested and absorbed. Laxatives work in the large intestine, leading to fluid and electrolyte loss, but consumed calories are still absorbed from the small intestine. Use of diuretics may result in decreased fluid weight and electrolyte imbalance.

On physical examination, bulimic patients may be dehydrated and have orthostatic hypotension. Sialadenitis, tooth enamel loss, dental caries, and abdominal tenderness are the most common findings. Abrasion of the proximal interphalangeal joints may occur secondary to scraping the fingers against teeth while inducing vomiting. Rarely, a heart murmur is heard, which may be due to mitral valve prolapse. Irreversible cardiomyopathy can develop secondary to ipecac use.

B. Laboratory Findings

Electrolyte disturbances are common. The method of purging results in specific abnormalities. Vomiting causes metabolic alkalosis, hypokalemia, and hypochloremia. Laxatives cause metabolic acidosis, hypokalemia, and hypochloremia. Diuretic use may lead to hypokalemia, hyponatremia, hypocalcemia, and metabolic alkalosis. Amylase may be increased secondary to chronic parotid stimulation.

▶ Complications

A. Short-Term Complications

Complications in normal-weight bulimic patients are related to the mechanisms of purging (see section Symptoms and Signs). Other complications include esophageal rupture, acute or chronic esophagitis, and, rarely, Barrett esophagitis. Chronic vomiting can lead to metabolic alkalosis, and laxative abuse may cause metabolic acidosis. Diet pill use can cause insomnia, hypertension, tachycardia, palpitations, seizures, and sudden death.

Some patients who abuse laxatives may become chronically dehydrated. The renin-angiotensin-aldosterone axis is activated, and the level of antidiuretic hormone is elevated to compensate. These hormones do not normalize immediately when laxatives are stopped, and fluid retention of up to 10 kg/wk may result. This puts patients at risk for congestive heart failure and can frighten them as their weight increases dramatically. This problem often resolves on its own with diuresis that often occurs after 7–10 days.

B. Mortality

The mortality rate in bulimic patients is similar to that in anorexic patients. Death usually results from suicide or electrolyte derangements.

▶ Treatment

Treatment of BN depends on the frequency of binging and purging and the severity of biochemical and psychiatric derangement. If K^+ is less than 3.0 mEq/L, inpatient medical admission is warranted. Typically, extracellular K^+ is spared at the expense of intracellular K^+, so a patient may become hypokalemic several days after the serum K^+ concentration appears to be corrected. Usually, cessation of purging is sufficient to correct K^+ concentration and is the recommended intervention for K^+ above 3.0 mEq/L. If K^+ is 2.5–2.9 mEq/L, oral supplementation is suggested, and if K^+ is less than 2.5 mEq/L, intravenous therapy is recommended. Supplements can be stopped once K^+ levels are more than 3.5 mEq/L. Total body K^+ can be assumed to be normal when serum K^+ corrects and remains normal 2 days after supplements are stopped.

Hospitalization of bulimic patients is recommended if there has been failure of outpatient management. The binge-purge cycle is addictive and can be difficult for patients to interrupt on their own. Hospitalization can offer a forced break from the cycle, allowing them to normalize their eating, interrupt the addictive behavior, and regain the ability to recognize satiety signals.

Outpatient management can be pursued if patients are medically stable. Cognitive-behavioral therapy is crucial to help bulimic patients understand their disease. Nutrition therapy offers patients ways to regulate eating patterns so that they can avoid the need to binge. Medical monitoring should be done to check electrolytes periodically, depending on the purging method used.

SSRIs are generally helpful in treating the binge-purge cycle. Fluoxetine has been studied most extensively; a dose of 60 mg/day is most efficacious in teenagers. Other SSRIs appear to be effective as well and may be used in patients experiencing side effects of fluoxetine. GI symptoms should be treated when indicated. The pain and swelling of enlarged parotid glands can be helped by sucking on tart candy and application of warm compresses.

Goals of treatment are to interrupt the binge/purge cycle and achieve remission.

Crow SJ: Pharmacologic treatment of eating disorders. Psychiatr Clin North Am 2019 Jun;42(2):253–262 [PMID: 31046927].

Hail L, LeGrange D: Bulimia nervosa in adolescents: prevalence and treatment challenges. Adolesc Health Med Ther 2018 Jan;9:11–16 [PMID: 29379324].

Mehler PS: Medical complications of bulimia nervosa and their treatments. Int J Eat Disord (0276–3478) 2011 Mar;44(2):95 [PMID: 21312201].

Steinhausen HC, Weber S: The outcome of bulimia nervosa: findings from one-quarter century of research. Am J Psychiatry 2009;166:1331–1341 [PMID: 19884225].

BINGE-EATING DISORDER

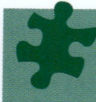

ESSENTIALS OF DIAGNOSIS & TYPICAL FEATURES: BINGE-EATING DISORDER

Diagnostic criteria for BED are:

► Recurring episodes of binge eating:
  • Eating significantly more food in a short period than most people would eat under similar circumstances.
  • Episodes marked by feelings of lack of control.
► Binge eating is associated with marked distress.
► Binge eating occurs at least once a week over 3 months (on average).

https://www.nationaleatingdisorders.org/sites/default/files/ResourceHandouts/MultiPageRGB.pdf

Clinical Findings

A. Symptoms and Signs

Most adults who have binge-eating disorder (BED), which has a prevalence of 2%–4%, develop symptoms during adolescence. BED most often is found in overweight or obese individuals. Eighteen percent of such patients report binging at least once in the past year. Patients with BED have an increased incidence of depression and substance abuse. The possibility of BED should be raised for any significantly overweight patient. Specific questionnaires are available for evaluating patients suspected of BED.

B. Laboratory Findings

The clinician should assess causes and complications of obesity, and laboratory evaluation should include thyroid function tests and lipid profile.

Treatment

A combination of cognitive-behavioral therapy and antidepressant medication has been helpful in treating BED in adults. In adults, fluoxetine and citalopram help decrease binge episodes, improve depressive symptoms, and, possibly, decrease appetite. Although their use for BED in adolescents has not been studied, this evidence suggests that SSRIs may be helpful. Studies have shown that lisdexamfetamine dimesylate, at a dose of 50 mg in adults, as well as topiramate led to statistically significant decreases in binge eating episodes; these medications have not been studied for BED in adolescents. As BED has been recognized only recently, outcomes have not been studied and little is known regarding long-term prognosis.

Bello NT, Yeomans BL: Safety of pharmacotherapy options for bulimia nervosa and binge eating disorder. Expert Opin Drug Saf 2018;17(1):17–23. doi:10.1080/14740338.2018.1395854 [PMID: 29108432].

Reas DL, Grilo CM: Pharmacological treatment of binge eating disorder: update review and synthesis. Expert Opin Pharmacother 2015;16(10):1463–1478. doi:10.1517/14656566.2015.1053465 [PMID: 26044518].

OTHER SPECIFIED FEEDING OR EATING DISORDERS

Other specified feeding or eating disorders (OSFED) is a catch all category for a variety of ED behaviors that do not meet full criteria for AN, BN, BED, or ARFID (see the next section). Patients exhibit feeding or eating behaviors that cause clinically significant distress and impairment but do not meet full criteria for the classic ED diagnostic categories.

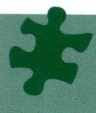

ESSENTIALS OF DIAGNOSIS & TYPICAL FEATURES: OTHER SPECIFIED FEEDING OR EATING DISORDERS

► A person must present with feeding or eating behaviors that cause clinically significant distress and impairment, but do not meet the full criteria for any of the other disorders.
► The following represent the different types of OSFEDs:
  • Atypical anorexia nervosa: All AN criteria are met, except despite significant weight loss, the individual's weight is within or above the normal range.
  • Bulimia nervosa (of low frequency and/or limited duration): All of the BN criteria are met, except that the binge eating and inappropriate compensatory behavior occurs at a lower frequency and/or for less than 3 months.

- BED (of low frequency and/or limited duration): All BED criteria are met, except at a lower frequency and/or for less than 3 months.
- Purging disorder: Recurrent purging behavior to influence weight or shape in the absence of binge eating.
- Night eating syndrome: Recurrent episodes of night eating, such as eating after awakening from sleep or excessive food consumption after the evening meal. The behavior is not better explained by environmental influences or social norms or another mental health disorder (eg, BED) and causes significant distress/impairment.

▶ Disturbance not explained by lack of available food or culturally sanctioned practice.

▶ Eating disturbance does not occur exclusively during AN or BN, and there is no disturbance in experience of one's body weight or shape.

▶ Eating disturbance not attributable to concurrent medical condition or explained by a different mental disorder, or, when eating disturbance occurs in the context of another condition or disorder, severity of eating disturbance exceeds that associated with the other condition or disorder.

▶ Clinical Findings

Pertinent clinical findings are directly related to the type of disordered eating behaviors exhibited. For example, a patient who has lost 60 pounds in 6 months, but who remains overweight, may have atypical AN and exhibit many of the physical findings of AN: bradycardia, orthostasis, dizziness, etc. Similarly, a patient who meets criteria for purging disorder—with self-induced vomiting as the purging behavior—may manifest electrolyte changes, sialadenitis, and/or gastric issues like BN. Clinical and laboratory assessment should be guided by the mechanism of maladaptive behavior engaged in by the patient.

AVOIDANT/RESTRICTIVE FOOD INTAKE DISORDER

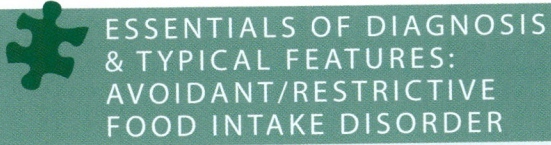

ESSENTIALS OF DIAGNOSIS & TYPICAL FEATURES: AVOIDANT/RESTRICTIVE FOOD INTAKE DISORDER

▶ Diagnostic criteria for ARFID are:

▶ Eating or feeding disturbance (including lack of interest in eating, avoidance due to sensory characteristics of food, concern for aversive consequences of eating) demonstrated by failure to meet appropriate nutritional and/or energy needs and associated with one or more of:

- Weight loss (or failure to achieve expected weight gain or faltering growth).
- Nutritional deficiency.
- Dependence on enteral feeding or oral nutritional supplementation.
- Interference with psychosocial functioning.

The hallmark feature of ARFID is avoidance or restriction of oral food intake, in the absence of criteria for AN (body image disturbance, fear of weight gain/body fat). For teenagers, food avoidance may be associated with more generalized emotional difficulties that do not meet diagnostic criteria for anxiety or depression. Though the epidemiology of ARFID is not well established, one study of 8- to 13-year-olds showed that 3.2% reported some features of ARFID. Another study revealed that 45% of those diagnosed with ARFID had a comorbid psychiatric diagnosis. Similar health effects to AN may be found in youth with ARFID, depending on the degree of malnutrition and how an individual became malnourished.

Bourne L, Bryant-Waugh R, Cook J, Mandy W: Avoidant/restrictive food intake disorder: a systematic scoping review of the current literature. Psychiatry Res 2020 Jun;288:112961. doi: 10.1016/j.psychres.2020.112961 [Epub 2020 Apr 4] [PMID: 32283448].
Iron-Segev S et al: Feeding, eating, and emotional disturbances in children with avoidant/restrictive food intake disorder (ARFID). Nutrients 2020;12(11):3385. doi:10.3390/nu12113385 [PMID: 33158087].
Kambanis PE et al: Prevalence and correlates of psychiatric comorbidities in children and adolescents with full and subthreshold avoidant/restrictive food intake disorder. Int J Eat Disord 2020 Feb;53(2):256–265. doi: 10.1002/eat.23191 [Epub 2019 Nov 8] [PMID: 31702051].

PROGNOSIS, QUALITY ASSESSMENT, AND OUTCOMES METRICS

Outcome in EDs, especially AN, has been studied extensively. Prior metrics generally defined remission or recovery as being at a healthy body weight with return of menses. As diagnostic criteria for AN changed, a US national collaborative effort that included 14 ED programs defined AN recovery based on reaching at least 90% median BMI, without consideration of return of menses. Most studies have focused on specific inpatient treatment programs, and few have evaluated less ill patients who do not need hospitalization. About 40%–50% of AN patients receiving treatment recover, 20%–30% have intermittent relapses, and 20% have chronic, unremitting illness.

As time from initial onset of illness lengthens, the recovery rate decreases and mortality associated with AN and BN increases. A study from the Swedish ED registry revealed that 55% of the participants were in remission and approximately 85% were within a healthy weight range at the end of treatment (15 months on average). The US national collaborative showed that 65% of patients with AN demonstrated recovery at 1 year, with higher BMI at baseline the most significant predictor of recovery.

The course of AN often includes significant weight fluctuations over time, and it may be a matter of years until recovery is certain. The BN course often includes relapses of binging and purging, although bulimic patients initially recover faster than do anorexic patients. Up to 50% of anorexic patients may develop bulimia, as well as major psychological complications, including depression, anxiety, and substance abuse disorders. Bulimic patients also develop similar psychological illness but rarely develop anorexia. Long-term medical sequelae, aside from low body weight and amenorrhea, have not been systematically studied, although AN is known to have multiple medical consequences, including osteoporosis and structural brain changes.

For all EDs, it is unclear whether age at onset affects outcome, but shorter length of time between symptom onset and therapy tends to improve outcome. Favorable outcomes have been found with varying treatment modalities, including brief medical hospitalization and long psychiatric or residential hospitalization. Higher discharge weight, as well as more rapid weight gain during inpatient treatment (> 0.8 kg/wk), seems to improve the initial outcome. It is difficult to compare treatment regimens because numbers are small and the type of patient and illness varies among studies. No existing studies compare outpatient to inpatient treatment or the effects of partial hospitalization on recovery.

Forman SF et al: Predictors of outcome at 1 year in adolescents with DSM-5 restrictive eating disorders: report of the National Eating Disorders Quality Improvement Collaborative. J Adolescent Health 2014;55(6):750–756 [PMID: 25200345].

Lindstedt K, Kjellin L, Gustafson SA: Adolescents with full or subthreshold anorexia nervosa in a naturalistic sample—characteristics and treatment outcome. J Eat Disord 2017 Mar; 5(1):4 [PMID: 28265410].

Lund BC et al: Rate of inpatient weight restoration predicts outcome in anorexia nervosa. Int J Eat Disord 2009;42(4): 301–305 [PMID: 19107835].

RESOURCES FOR PRACTITIONERS & FAMILIES

Web Resources

Academy for Eating Disorders: (The Academy for Eating Disorders [AED] is a global, multidisciplinary professional organization that provides cutting-edge professional training and education; inspires new developments in eating disorders research, prevention, and clinical treatments; and is the international source for state-of-the-art information in the field of eating disorders.) www.aedweb.org. Accessed June 14, 2021.

Eating Disorder Hope: Detailed information for patients and families about eating disorders, and treatment centers, and individual providers. https://www.eatingdisorderhope.com.

National Eating Disorders Association: (Information available to help individuals/families locate resources and treatment for eating disorders around the world.) http://www.nationaleating-disorders.org/. Accessed June 14, 2021.

Child & Adolescent Psychiatric Disorders & Psychosocial Aspects of Pediatrics

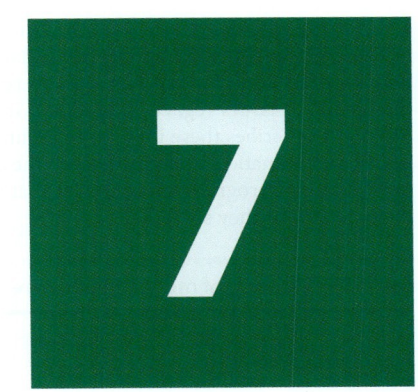

Kelly Glaze, PsyD

Kimberly Kelsay, MD

Ayelet Talmi, PhD

INTRODUCTION

Pediatric primary care settings are often the first entry points for identification of mental and behavioral health issues for the 14%–20% of affected children and adolescents. Beyond addressing identified and diagnosable mental health conditions, pediatric primary care settings are tasked with (1) prevention and health promotion, (2) screening and surveillance, (3) early identification, (4) risk and crisis evaluation and triage, (5) initiating treatment for low acuity issues, and (6) triage and referral around complex behavioral health and psychosocial issues for the child, their family, and the environments in which the child interacts.

Primary care providers see approximately 75% of children with psychiatric disturbances, and half of all pediatric office visits involve behavioral, psychosocial, or educational concerns. Parents and children often prefer discussing these issues with pediatric providers who they already know and trust. As a result, pediatric primary care providers play an important role in the prevention, identification, initiation, management, and coordination of mental health issues, in addition to providing behavioral and developmental care and support for children and adolescents. Many factors contribute the fact that only 15%–25% of children with diagnosable disorders have access to and are seen by mental health specialists: the shortage of mental health providers, particularly in rural regions and for medically underserved communities, the stigma attached to receiving mental health services, chronic underfunding for behavioral/mental health services, institutional barriers within the public mental health system, and disparate insurance benefits. In contrast, more than 78,000 board-certified pediatricians and innumerable mid-level pediatric providers are in a unique position to identify issues affecting the emotional health of children and to initiate treatment or referrals to other providers.

Emotional problems that develop during childhood and adolescence can significantly impact development and may continue into adulthood. In fact, most adult psychiatric disorders involve childhood onset. Many disorders do not present as an all-or-none phenomenon, but rather progress from less severe concerns, such as adjustment problems or perturbations in functioning, to significant disturbances and severe disorders. The chronicity of these disorders provides many opportunities for pediatricians to evaluate and manage emotional problems and behavioral conditions early on when improvement can be achieved with less intensive interventions. These opportunities, when missed, can result in downward spiral of school and social difficulties, poor employment opportunities, poverty in adulthood, and increased health care utilization and costs as adults. These outcomes are even more pronounced for children and adolescents from underserved, low socio-economic backgrounds.

Pediatricians and other primary care providers may be the first, or only, medical professional to identify a behavioral/mental health problem. Pediatricians working in specialty care settings, hospitalists, and intensivists will also encounter and need to treat children and adolescents with emotional and behavioral problems. This chapter reviews prevention, surveillance, and screening for mental and behavioral health concerns; situations that may arise in the context of such assessments; psychiatric illnesses commonly identified and diagnosed during childhood or adolescence; current treatment recommendations; and indications for referral to mental health professionals.

MODELS OF CARE ENCOMPASSING BEHAVIORAL HEALTH IN THE PRIMARY CARE SETTING

Mental health, behavior, and development are routinely addressed in the context of pediatric primary care. The continuum of behavioral health services in primary care settings spans from providing anticipatory guidance around development, behavior, and social-emotional well-being to implementing screening processes, identifying concerns, and making external referrals (eg, routine pediatric care), to utilizing external rapid response consultation (eg, consultation model), and/or providing on-site services to address the identified issues (eg, co-located and integrated models). Table 7–1 describes these models. In addition, practices may utilize a combination of elements from the models to develop individualized programs and services that meet the needs of the populations they serve.

PREVENTION, EARLY IDENTIFICATION, & DEVELOPMENTAL CONTEXT

Developmental contexts and the environments in which children and adolescents grow up play a significant role in their development and well-being. Environments provide access to resources, relationships, and support in addition to being settings for learning, growth, and development. Longitudinal

Table 7–1. Models of mental health care in pediatric primary care.

	Routine Care/Referral	Outside Consultation	Co-Location	Integrated/Collaborative Care
Model Description	Surveillance and recommended routine screening Anticipatory guidance Patient referral to specialty mental health and developmental services when needs identified	Various models may include telephone or electronic consultation with option of subsequent 1–2 telepsychiatry or in-person visits with a BH provider	BH provider in same physical space as primary care provider, often with an office on-site BH provider has scheduled appointments to see patients identified with BH needs	BH provider available for in the moment consultation or patient care Operates as a member of the primary care team
Advantages	No change necessary in routine practice No added cost	Rapid response Preferred access to BH providers Consultations may improve provider knowledge and comfort No waitlist	Can care for acute, high needs patients within practice Convenience of being seen for physical and BH in one setting Warm handoffs between primary care and BH providers Patients are more likely to follow through with BH providers to whom they are introduced by their primary care providers Less stigma for patients	No waitlist Ability to address the full continuum of BH needs from prevention and health promotion to early identification, consultation, intervention, and referral Direct communication between providers including shared health records BHC can manage and follow up on referrals Patient sees primary care provider and BHC provide team-based care Provider knowledge and comfort of BH care often improves with co-management of case
Disadvantages	Limited time for providers to discuss anticipatory BH needs or address identified issues when screen or surveillance reveals problems Practice must manage referrals and follow-up on referral outcomes Referral follow through ≤ 10% No mechanism to improve provider knowledge and comfort of BH issues Poor communication between BH system and primary care due to regulatory and systemic barriers	Practice responsible for managing referrals to mental health systems as recommended by consultant There must be a structure to pay for system (eg, state funding, pediatric practice fee, grant funding)	BH often becomes "full," and new patients must wait for slots to open Direct communication between providers not built into model, including challenges in documentation and transfer of information about the patient Limited ability to improve provider knowledge and comfort of BH issues	Most severe patients referred to external BH system Costs of hiring BH staff (typically can be covered through billing, institutional support, grant funding, and optimization of health utilization practices)

BH, behavioral health; BHC, behavioral health clinician.

and retrospective research studies link specific early mental health interventions with good health, stable relationships, increased earnings in adulthood, and improved outcomes for the children of participants while adverse experiences in childhood are linked to significant, lifelong health problems (eg, substance use, cardiovascular disease, or depression), lower quality of life, and decreased lifespan. Understanding social determinants of health helps providers attend to the needs of individual children and their families in the context of complex experiences and environments.

However, the major threats to the health of children living in the United States increasingly arise from problems that cannot be adequately addressed by the practice model alone. These problems include unacceptably high infant and maternal morbidity and mortality rates in communities of color, increasing rates of intentional and unintentional injuries, childhood obesity, substance misuse and dependency, behavioral and developmental consequences of inadequate access to care, exposure to family and community violence, sexually transmitted diseases, unplanned pregnancies, and lack of a medical home. Today's community pediatrician seeks to provide a far more realistic and complete clinical picture by taking responsibility for all children in a community, facilitating access to preventive and curative services, and understanding the determinants and consequences of child health and illness, as well as the effectiveness of services provided.

Bright Futures is a national health promotion and disease prevention initiative that addresses children's health needs in the context of family and community. *Bright Futures in Practice: Mental Health* provides numerous guidelines, tools, and strategies for improving mental health identification, assessment, initiation, management, and coordination.

Prevention and early intervention programs are showing promise in helping to reduce risk for patients and their families. Evidenced-based and promising programs and strategies include, but are not limited to:

- **HealthySteps:** www.healthysteps.org
- **Parent–Child Interaction Therapy (PCIT):** www.pcit.org
- **Triple P (Positive Parenting Program):** www.triplep-america.com
- **Nurse-Family Partnership:** www.nursefamilypartnership.org
- **Incredible Years:** www.incredibleyears.com
- **Strengthening Families for Parents and Youth:** www.extension.iastate.edu/sfp
- **The Safe Environment for Every Kid (SEEK):** http://umm.edu/programs/childrens/services/child-protection/seek-project
- **Child Parent Psychotherapy (CPP):** https://childparent-psychotherapy.com/

- **Bright Futures:** https://brightfutures.aap.org
- **Centers for Disease Control and Prevention, Injury Prevention & Control: Division of Violence Prevention:** https://www.cdc.gov/violenceprevention/index.html
- **The Center of Excellence for Infant and Early Childhood Mental Health Consultation:** https://www.samhsa.gov/iecmhc
- **Zero to Three:** http://www.zerotothree.org
- **The Heckman equation and other resources regarding early intervention return on investments:** https://heckmanequation.org/

LIFESTYLE RECOMMENDATIONS

Proper screening, assessment, diagnosis, and treatment are fundamental aspects of practice. In addition, it is equally important that primary care providers are familiar with and aware of factors that can help promote both physical and mental health. Many studies demonstrate clear physical and behavioral health benefits from regular exercise, optimal nutrition, meditation, yoga, and participation in prosocial activities. Other contributing factors that directly impact overall health include adequate sleep and the use of relaxation and mindfulness techniques. The American Academy of Pediatrics (AAP) recommends engaging families in conversations to encourage consumption of fruits and vegetables, avoid sugar-containing drinks, encourage physical activity, and make a family plan around limiting screen time. While these guidelines focus on physical health, successful implementation and adherence depend on the relationships and environments in which children live.

Summary of the Pediatrician's Role

Pediatric primary care providers are on the frontlines of behavioral health care, often being the first to identify and address concerns and issues related to social-emotional health and well-being, healthy relationships, adverse experiences and environments, and mental wellness. See Table 7–2 for a summary of these functions.

IDENTIFICATION & ASSESSMENT DURING HEALTH SUPERVISION VISITS

Approaches to identify problems include surveillance, screening, and assessment. *Surveillance* consists of the following elements: checking in, eliciting concerns, asking open-ended questions, listening for red flags, identifying risk factors, and monitoring closely over time. Like vital signs, which represent an essential component of the physical evaluation, the essential components of the primary care surveillance for mental health concerns should generally include a review of the youth's general functioning in

Table 7–2. The pediatric primary care provider's role in mental health.

Role	Specific Activities
Prevention/health promotion	Provide anticipatory guidance on social-emotional, behavioral, and developmental topics Screen and address social risk factors on intake Screen and refer for early socioemotional risk
Identification	Shared family concern Clinical concerns and behavioral observations Surveillance Screening
Assessment	Interview and physical Assessment tools Comorbid conditions
Initiation	Education about condition and treatment options Continued collaboration and assessment with family Refer to behavioral health services for further evaluation Refer for therapy Start medication
Management	Monitor condition for improvement Monitor for side effects Provide guidance on treatment and management
Coordination	With social work, therapist, psychologist, psychiatrist, and/or navigators/care coordinators/case managers
Collaboration	With behavioral health service providers, child protective services, local schools, and community entities and resources

Table 7–3. PSYCH: a tool for opening discussion regarding behavioral health surveillance.

Parent-child interaction	How are things going with you and your parents? Or, in early childhood: What's it like to take care of your baby/toddler?
School	How are things going in school (or childcare); ask about academics, behaviors, and social interactions?
Youth	How are things going with peer relationships/friendships (how does child get along with same-aged peers)?
Casa	How are things going at home (including siblings, family stresses, and relationship with parents)?
Happiness	How would you describe your mood? How would you describe your child's mood?

different aspects of their life. Five questions forming the mnemonic PSYCH provide a tool for opening discussion of surveillance topics (Table 7–3).

Many pediatric practices are challenged by lack of continuity in primary care providers across childhood and adolescence and insufficient visit time for in-depth surveillance. Typically, families spend only a few minutes of in-person time with their pediatric provider during routine health supervision visits. Surveillance activities are further hampered by not being allowable as separate and billable services under current Medicaid and insurance reimbursement plans, in contrast to formal screening, which is billable and reimbursable. Given limited time available during pediatric visits and the fact that only 18% of parents who report elevated behavior problems in children tell their providers about it, surveillance should be paired with universal screening for development, mental health, behavior, psychosocial, and environmental risk factors. *Screening*

involves using standardized instruments to identify areas of risk, delay, or concern. Newborn hearing, vision, and developmental screenings are common in today's pediatric practice. However, the morbidity associated with developmental, emotional, and psychosocial problems necessitates routinely and universally conducting social-emotional and psychosocial screening to identify the presence of symptoms of emotional, behavioral, or relationship disorders and those environmental factors that negatively influence development. Screening tools are brief, easy to use, and can be administered as a questionnaire or using an interview format. Many common screening instruments are also available in digital format allowing for electronic administration (eg, iPad/tablet or through a patient portal) and integration within electronic health records. While all screening questionnaires require review and acknowledgment by the primary care provider, a positive screen warrants additional inquiry and possible referral for a more thorough assessment. Newer methods of eliciting social-emotional and behavior concerns have been developed (see below for resources and links to access common screening tools). Helpful information can also be obtained from broad screening checklists and symptom-specific questionnaires such as depression or anxiety self-report inventories. Questions can be incorporated into the general pediatric office screening forms or specific questionnaires can be used. Beyond identification, successful screening requires attention to appropriate referrals, referral uptake and completion, and communication back to the referring entity regarding the results of the evaluation. These activities often require additional care coordination resources that could be provided by nonmedical staff such as family navigators and community health workers. Pediatric primary care providers need information about eligibility for services and community referrals to successfully monitor and address behavioral and developmental issues.

TOOLS FOR MENTAL HEALTH SCREENING IN THE PRIMARY CARE OFFICE SETTING

Given the low rates of identification of psychosocial problems using pediatric surveillance, the use of standardized, validated screening tools has become standard practice. Typically, broad screeners that elicit information regarding multiple domains are employed first and are followed by targeted screens to address symptomatology, severity, impairment, and context of specific psychosocial problems.

Targeted Screening Tools & Assessment Measures

As with broad screening tools, targeted screening or assessment instruments can be very valuable due to standardization and ability to assess current symptoms and severity. They can also be useful for following or reassessing a patient's progress after initiation of treatment. A few common resources are listed below. Additional screening tools are listed in Table 7–4.

> Resources for obtaining screening tools:
> http://www.brightfutures.org/mentalhealth/pdf/tools.html
> https://www.nncpap.org/
> https://www.psychiatry.pitt.edu/research/investigator-resources/
>   assessment-instruments

Assessment of Behavioral & Emotional Signs & Symptoms

When an emotional/behavioral problem is mentioned by the patient or caregivers, elicited by an interview, or identified by a screening instrument, a more comprehensive assessment and plan for triage is needed. Regardless of access to behavioral health services, the pediatric provider should engage in a meaningful conversation about the findings from screening processes and be integrally involved in follow-up plans. Response to screening results and additional assessment is required to determine appropriate referral resources, safety planning, need for immediate attention or action in the clinic, and follow-up appointments and services. Examples of more thorough questions and observations are given in Table 7–5. Targeted assessment screening tools are also useful in determining severity, comorbidity, and context of impairment.

Situations Requiring Emergent or More Extensive Psychiatric Assessment

If there is any concern about safety, the provider must evaluate risk by assessing danger to self (eg, suicidal ideation, plans, or attempts), danger to others (eg, assault, aggression, or homicidal ideation) as well as risk and protective factors.

SUICIDE RISK IN CHILDREN & ADOLESCENTS

ESSENTIALS OF DIAGNOSIS & TYPICAL FEATURES

► Suicide: Death caused by self-injurious behavior with intent to die because of the behavior.

► Nonfatal suicidal behaviors occur on a continuum from suicidal preparatory acts that occur prior to injury or harm (eg, notes, massing medicines) to suicide attempts that are nonfatal to self-injurious behaviors without intent to die.

► Suicidal thoughts occur on a continuum from passive thoughts of death to passive thoughts of suicide to active thoughts about planning with the goal to die.

► Common risk factors: history of prior suicide attempt(s), mental health diagnoses, substance use, social isolation, family history of suicide, access to lethal means, and stigma and/or barriers related to accessing mental health care.

► Common protective factors: supportive social network, sense of responsibility to family or others, school engagement, spirituality, and fears of death due to perceived pain to self-and/or suffering inflicted on others because of the death.

Different populations experience different risk factors and disparities, including access to appropriate health care. American Indian/Alaska Native youth have the highest suicide rates, and the once low suicide rates for black youth have increased faster than any other group. There has also been an increase in suicide rates for female Hispanic youth, and risk is higher for American-born Hispanic youth. Data are limited on rates of suicide among LGBTQ youth, but a recent survey by the Trevor Project found an alarming 45% considered suicide in the last year with rates highest among LGBTQ American Indian/Alaska Native and black youth. While LGBTQ youth experience increased risk, high social support from family and LGBTQ-affirming school and community environments acts as important protective factors. Suicide is most associated with a psychiatric disorder and can occur in youth with minimal apparent risk factors who experience a stressful event or perceived loss or failure. In addition to depression and bipolar disorder, other disorders that can increase risk for suicide include psychotic disorders, substance use disorders, posttraumatic stress disorder (PTSD), panic attacks, and conduct disorder. Behavioral risks include aggression, sleep difficulties, irritability, intoxication at the time of the attempt, a history of previous suicide

Table 7–4. Screening tools for primary care settings.

Screening Tool	Area/Domains	Age Range	Notes
Ages and Stages Questionnaire, Third Edition (ASQ-3)	Developmental: Communication, gross motor, fine motor, problem solving, personal-social	1 mo–5.5 y	Parent-completed questionnaire available in Arabic, Chinese, English, French Spanish, and Vietnamese: https://agesandstages.com/
Ages and Stages Questionnaire, Second Edition Socio-Emotional (ASQ: SE-2)	Social-emotional development: Self-regulation, compliance, social communication, adaptive functioning, autonomy, affect, interaction with people	1–72 mo	Parent-completed questionnaire available in English, French, Korean, and Spanish: https://agesandstages.com/
Modified Checklist of Autism in Toddlers (M-CHAT)	Developmental: 20-item screener that detects risk for autism diagnosis	16 and 30 mo	Parent-completed questionnaire available in English, Spanish: https://mchatscreen.com
Strengths and Difficulties Questionnaires (SDQs)	General behavioral health: Emotional symptoms, conduct problems, hyperactivity/inattention, peer relationship problems, prosocial behavior	2–17 y	Parent-, teacher-, or child-completed questionnaire available in 89 languages: http://www.sdqinfo.org
Pediatric Symptoms Checklist (PSC)	Cognitive, emotional, and behavioral problems	Preschool to 17 y	Parent- or child-completed questionnaire available in English and Spanish: http://www.brightfutures.org/mentalhealth/pdf/professionals/ped_sympton_chklst.pdf
Pediatric Intake Form/Family Psychosocial Screen	Psychosocial: Parental depression, substance use, domestic violence, parental history of abuse, social supports	Adults	Provider-completed screen available in English: https://www.brightfutures.org/mentalhealth/pdf/professionals/ped_intake_form.pdf
WE CARE (Well-child care, Evaluation, Community resources, Advocacy, Referral, Education)	Psychosocial: Parental educational attainment, employment, child care, risk of homelessness, food security, household heat, and electricity	Adults	Parent-completed questionnaire available in English: https://sirenetwork.ucsf.edu/tools-resources/resources/we-care
Patient Health Questionnaire 9 (PHQ-9) modified for teens	Depression and suicide	11–17 y	Child-completed questionnaire available in English and Spanish: https://www.aacap.org/App_Themes/AACAP/docs/member_resources/toolbox_for_clinical_practice_and_outcomes/symptoms/GLAD-PC_PHQ-9.pdf
CRAFFT	Substance abuse	12–21 y	Clinician interview and youth-completed questionnaire available in several languages: https://crafft.org/get-the-crafft/
Vanderbilt Assessment Scales	Attention deficit/hyperactivity disorder	6–12 y	Parent- and teacher-completed questionnaire available in English and Spanish: https://www.nichq.org/sites/default/files/resource-file/NICHQ_Vanderbilt_Assessment_Scales.pdf
Center for Epidemiologic Studies Depression Scale for Children (CES-DC)	Depression	6–17 y	Child-completed questionnaire available in English: https://www.brightfutures.org/mentalhealth/pdf/professionals/bridges/ces_dc.pdf
Self-report for Childhood Anxiety-Related Emotional Disorders (SCARED)	Childhood anxiety disorders: General anxiety disorder, separation anxiety disorder, panic disorder, social phobia, school phobia	8–18 y	Parent- and child-completed questionnaire available in 12 languages: https://www.pediatricbipolar.pitt.edu/resources/instruments
Edinburgh Postnatal Depression Scale (EPDS)	Pregnancy-related depression and anxiety	Adult mothers	Self-completed questionnaire: https://www.aap.org/en/patient-care/screening-technical-assistance-and-resource-center/screening-tool-finder/edinburgh-postpartum-depression-scale-epds/

(Continued)

Table 7–4. Screening tools for primary care settings. (*Continued*)

Screening Tool	Area/Domains	Age Range	Notes
Survey of Wellbeing of Young Children	Developmental milestones, behavioral/emotional development, and family risk factors	2-60 months All ages	https://pediatrics.tuftsmedicalcenter.org/The-Survey-of-Wellbeing-of-Young-Children/Overview
Bright Futures Toolkit	Numerous guidelines, tools, and other resources for identifying mental health concerns		Tools for health professionals and families: https://www.brightfutures.org/mentalhealth/pdf/tools.html

Table 7–5. Possible topics for discussion and observation when assessing psychosocial problems.

Developmental history
1. Review the landmarks of psychosocial development
2. Summarize the child's temperamental traits
3. Review stressful life events and the child's reactions to them
   a. Separations from primary caregivers or close family members
   b. Losses
   c. Marital conflict, family violence, divorce
   d. Illnesses, injuries, and hospitalizations
   e. Moves, household changes
   f. School transitions
   g. Traumatic events
   h. Financial changes (eg, employment issues) that impact daily living environment
   i. Resource issues including food insecurity, housing instability, and inability to make ends meet
4. Obtain details of past mental health problems and their treatment

Family history
1. Marital/relationship history
   a. Overall satisfaction with the marriage/partnership
   b. Conflicts or disagreements within the relationship
   c. Quantity and quality of time together away from children
   d. Whether the child comes between or is a source of conflict between the parents
   e. Marital history prior to having children
2. Parenting history
   a. Feelings about parenthood
   b. Whether parents feel united in parenting the child
   c. "Division of labor" in parenting
   d. Parental energy or stress level
   e. Sleeping arrangements
   f. Privacy
   g. Attitudes about discipline
   h. Interference with discipline from outside the family (eg, ex-spouses, grandparents)
3. Stresses on the family
   a. Problems with employment
   b. Financial problems
   c. Resource needs
   d. Changes of residence or household composition
   e. Illness, injuries, and deaths

4. Family history of mental health problems and treatment
   a. Depression? Who?
   b. Bipolar Disorder? Who?
   c. Suicide attempts? Who?
   d. Psychiatric hospitalizations? Who?
   e. "Nervous breakdowns"? Who?
   f. Substance abuse or problems? Who?
   g. Nervousness or anxiety? Who?
   h. Other concerns about behavior or mental health problems in family members? Who?

Observation of the parents
1. Do they agree on the existence of the problem or concern?
2. Are they uncooperative or antagonistic about the evaluation?
3. Do the parents appear depressed or overwhelmed?
4. Can the parents present a coherent picture of the problem and their family life?
5. Do the parents accept some responsibility for the child's problems, or do they blame forces outside the family and beyond their control?
6. Do they appear burdened with guilt about the child's problem?

Observation of the child
1. Does the child acknowledge the existence of a problem or concern?
2. Does the child want help?
3. Is the child uncooperative with the assessment?
4. What is the child's predominant mood or attitude?
5. What does the child wish could be different (eg, "three wishes")?
6. Does the child display unusual behavior (activity level, mannerisms, fearfulness)?
7. What is the child's apparent cognitive level?

Observation of parent-child interaction
1. Do the parents show concern about the child's feelings?
2. Does the child control or disrupt the joint interview?
3. Do the parents set appropriate limits?
4. Does the child respond to parental limits and control?
5. Do the parents inappropriately answer questions addressed to the child?
6. Is there obvious tension between family members?

Data from other sources
1. Observations by staff
2. School (teacher, nurse, social worker, counselor, day care provider)
3. Department of social services
4. Other caregivers: grandparents, etc

attempts, or nonsuicidal self-injury. Youth may also be more susceptible than adults when exposed to the suicide of others; suicide clusters are common. Exposure through media and social media (eg, *13 Reasons Why*) has also been associated with increases in suicide attempts and suicides. Other risk factors beyond the youth's control include a history of trauma, adoption, loss, familial suicide, and parental mental health problems. Protective factors include healthy connections to peers, supported engagement in communities such as school, athletics, employment, religious or cultural activities, and supportive family relationships. Skills such as problem solving, emotional regulation, and support seeking are also protective.

Most young people who attempt suicide provide some indication of their distress or their tentative plans and show signs of dysphoric mood (anger, irritability, anxiety, or depression). For those who are screened, there is often a history of elevated distress reported on a screening instrument. Over 60% make comments such as, "I wish I were dead" or "I just can't deal with this any longer" within the 24 hours prior to death. In one study, nearly 70% of subjects experienced a crisis event such as a loss (eg, rejection by a girlfriend or boyfriend), public shaming, a failure, or an arrest prior to dying by suicide.

Assessment of Suicide Risk

Routine screening for children 12 and older includes questions regarding suicide. If a child or adolescent expresses suicidal thinking, the treating provider must assess for (1) the presence of an active plan, (2) intent to carry out that plan, (3) access to lethal means, and (4) history of previous suicide attempts. The Columbia Lighthouse Project provides screens to assess suicide risk and online training in how to use the tools appropriately. **Suicidal ideation accompanied by any plan warrants immediate referral for a psychiatric crisis assessment.** This can usually be accomplished at the nearest hospital emergency room.

Assessment of suicide risk calls for a high index of concern and a direct interview with the patient and caregivers. When a patient's immediate safety is at risk, providers can break the youth's wishes for confidentiality. In addition to the risk factors above, high-risk factors include self-injurious behavior, a suicide note, and a viable plan for suicide with the availability of lethal means, close personal exposure to suicide, conduct disorder, and substance abuse. The immediacy of events, such as loss, exposure to suicide, or upcoming punishments/negative consequences, are important to consider, as is the level of distress related to these events or to chronic or acute symptoms (eg, depression, panic, psychosis, poor sleep, and pain). A view of death as a relief from the pain in the youth's life indicates high risk. With ubiquitous social networking technologies and the presence of digital profiles, posting distress messages electronically and aggression in the form of cyber-bullying are important to identify and discuss when conducting risk assessments and obtaining information about relationships, supports, and sources of stress.

Intervention: Immediate Steps When Risk Is Suspected

Suicidal ideation and any suicide attempt must be considered a potentially life-threatening issue. The patient should not be left alone, and the treating provider should express concern while conveying a desire to help. If a behavioral health clinician (BHC) is embedded in the practice, the BHC can aid in evaluating the patient. Either the provider or the BHC should meet with the patient and the family, both alone and together, and listen carefully to their concerns and perceptions. It is helpful to explicitly state that with the assistance of mental health professionals, solutions can be found. The practice should err on the side of caution in deciding whether further referral or an emergency evaluation is indicated. While the practice may not have the expertise or time to determine full suicide risk, primary care providers can determine if further evaluation is indicated. Most patients who express suicidal ideation and all who have made a suicide attempt should be referred for urgent crisis evaluation and possible hospitalization. Referral for further assessment is always appropriate under these circumstances.

Pediatric providers should have a practice-specific algorithm for suicidal youth. The algorithm should include the steps to be taken for youth who need to be sent to an emergency room, youth who need an urgent or routine referral, or youth who will be followed in the practice. The algorithm should specify who in the practice is responsible for each step and primary care providers should be aware and involved in treatment planning. This should include who will call for emergency transport, if indicated, and who will flag a patient's record to ensure follow-up with care recommendations. Additionally, the primary care practice will need to follow up and document the outcome of the emergency assessment (eg, triage for crisis evaluation, safety planning, hospitalization, community referrals) in the patient's record and schedule a follow-up visit in the primary care setting as soon as is feasible given the disposition.

Prevention

Suicide prevention efforts include heightened awareness in the community and schools to identify at-risk individuals, and increased access to services, including hotlines and culturally appropriate counseling services. Restricting access to firearms is a critical factor, as firearms are responsible for 52% of deaths due to suicide among youth ages 15–24 in the United States. Other prevention methods include instructing families to lock up all medications, removing access to sharp objects (eg, knives, tools), and ensuring that other common mechanisms are not accessible. Many families are not aware that overdoses of over-the-counter medications such as acetaminophen can be lethal. Safety planning includes providing families with information and resources for crisis lines, mobile crisis assessment, and local community mental health resources to address urgent or emergent situations. Many school districts around the country have implemented programs in which anyone who has a concern about an individual's safety can make an anonymous report. It is important to have an open dialogue about suicide as 2019 data revealed almost 20% of youth seriously considered suicide and 16% made a plan. This is always critical, and even more salient in communities that have recently experienced a death by suicide. Prevention efforts must also carefully consider the needs of minoritized youth. To address increasing rates of suicide, efforts must address disparities in access to care, exposure to violence, and systemic barriers and inequities that can increase youth suicide risk. Finally, the treating provider should be aware of his or her own emotional reactions to dealing with suicidal adolescents and their families. Providers may be reluctant to increase family stress or go against their will by requiring an emergency evaluation. Providers may feel concerned about precipitating suicide through direct and frank discussions of suicidal risk, yet research suggests the opposite. Acknowledging and directly addressing suicide has been found to *reduce* suicidal ideation, particularly for adolescents who experience decreased distress after communicating with an adult and improved access to care. Reviewing difficult cases with colleagues, developing formal or informal relationships with psychiatrists, and attending workshops on assessment and management of depression and suicidal ideation can decrease the anxiety and improve competence for primary care providers.

HIGH-RISK PATIENTS & HOMICIDE

Youth Who Engage in Aggressive & Violent Behaviors

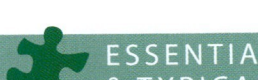

ESSENTIALS OF DIAGNOSIS & TYPICAL FEATURES

► Behaviors that deliberately hurt or threaten others and are outside of age or developmental norms.

► Can be associated with increased risk for suicide.

► Common risk factors: history of violent behavior, history of trauma, substance use, social isolation, access to firearms or other weapons, and family history of violence.

The tragic increase in teenage violence, including school shootings, is of particular concern to health professionals, as well as to society at large. There is strong evidence that screening and initiation of interventions by primary care providers can make a significant difference in violent behavior in youth. Although the prediction of violent behavior remains a difficult and imprecise endeavor, providers can support and encourage several important prevention efforts.

Most of the increase in youth violence, including suicides and homicides, involves the use of firearms. Thus, the presence of firearms in the home, the method of storage and safety measures taken when present, and access to firearms outside the home should be explored regularly with all adolescents as part of their routine medical care. Families should be encouraged to ask about the presence of and access to firearms as a matter of course, particularly when children are spending time in other people's homes, including friends and family members.

It is important to note that violent behavior is often associated with suicidal impulses. In the process of screening for violent behavior, suicidal ideation should not be overlooked. Any comment about wishes to be dead or hopelessness should be taken seriously and assessed immediately.

Interventions for caregivers include encouraging caregivers to be aware of their child's school attendance and performance. Parents should be encouraged to take an active role and learn about their children's friends, be aware of who they are going out with, where they will be, what they will be doing, and when they will be home. Communities and school districts nationwide have increased their efforts to identify and intervene with students whom teachers, peers, or parents recognize as having difficulty.

Threats & Warning Signs Requiring Immediate Consultation

All threats that children make can be alarming, and it is important to respond to serious and potentially lethal threats. These threats should be taken with the utmost seriousness, and caregivers should involve a mental health provider immediately. Such threats include threats/warnings of hurting or killing someone or oneself, threats to run away from home, and/or threats to damage or destroy property.

Factors Associated With Increased Risk of Violent and/or Dangerous Behavior

Not all threats signify imminent danger. There are several potential predictors to consider when assessing violent behavior, such as history of violence or aggressive behavior, including uncontrollable anger outbursts; access to firearms or other weapons; history of bringing a weapon to school; and family history of violent behaviors. In addition, children who witness abuse and violence at home and/or have a pre-occupation with themes and acts of violence (eg, TV shows, movies, music, violent video games) are also at high risk of such behavior. Victims of abuse (ie, physical, sexual, and/or emotional) are more susceptible to feeling shame, loss, and rejection, and this difficulty can further exacerbate an underlying mood, anxiety, or conduct disorder. Children who have been abused are more likely to be perpetrators of bullying and engage in verbal and physical intimidation toward peers. Substance use is another major factor frequently associated with violent, aggressive, and/or dangerous behavior, particularly because it impacts judgment and is often associated with decreased inhibition and increased impulsivity. Socially isolated children also carry a high risk for violent and dangerous behavior. These include children with little to no adult supervision, poor connection with peers, and little to no involvement in extracurricular activities. These individuals may be more likely to seek out deviant peer groups for a sense of belonging.

How Adults Can Respond to Concerns of Violence and/or Dangerous Behavior

If a provider, parent, or trusted adult (eg, teacher, coach, clergy) suspects that a child is at risk for violent and/or dangerous behavior, the most important intervention is to talk with the child immediately about the alleged threat and/or behavior. One should consider the child's past behavior, personality, and current stressors when evaluating the seriousness and likelihood of them engaging in a destructive or dangerous behavior. If the child is already connected to mental health services, their provider should be contacted immediately. If they are not reachable, the caregivers should take the child to the nearest emergency room or crisis center to evaluate safety and potential need for hospitalization. It is always acceptable to contact local police for assistance, especially if harm to others or lethal means are suspected. Other indications that warrant a crisis evaluation include a child refusing to talk, being argumentative, responding defensively, or continuing to express violent or dangerous thoughts or plans. Continuous, face-to-face adult supervision is essential while awaiting professional intervention. After evaluation, it is imperative to follow up with recommendations from mental health provider(s) to ensure safety and ongoing management.

Tips for Adults on How to Talk With Children About Violence

Talking about violence and personal safety is a necessary component of child rearing given the rise in violence in public places, including schools, communities, and places of worship. Adults are encouraged to be honest, address *the child's* concerns at an age-appropriate level, act as a trusted source

of information, and provide reassurance of **their** safety. Some reputable national websites that provide guidance on how to talk with children about violence and threats to personal safety include:

- **AAP How to Talk With Children About Tragedies:** https://www.healthychildren.org/English/family-life/Media/Pages/Talking-To-Children-About-Tragedies-and-Other-News-Events.aspx
- **NCTSN Age-Related Responses to Trauma:** https://www.nctsn.org/sites/default/files/resources//age_related_reactions_to_traumatic_events.pdf
- **APA Coping Following Shooting**: https://www.apa.org/topics/violence/school-shooting
- **AACAP Facts for Families:** https://www.aacap.org/AACAP/Families_and_Youth/Facts_for_Families/FFF-Guide/Childrens-Threats-When-Are-They-Serious-065.aspx
- **American Psychological Association Warning Signs of Youth Violence:** https://www.apa.org/topics/physical-abuse-violence/youth-warning-signs

A. Civil Commitment and Involuntary Mental Health "Holds"

If a risk assessment indicates a need for inpatient hospitalization, it is optimal if the patient and guardian consent to this care. In a situation in which the guardian is unwilling or unable to give consent for emergency room assessment, crisis evaluation, or inpatient hospitalization of a child or adolescent, an involuntary mental health "hold" may become necessary.

The terminology used to describe civil commitment law and involuntary treatment vary by state, as do the criteria for applying these laws. Most states define a process that can be initiated by individuals defined by the state (often providers, police officers, and certified mental health professionals) with reason to believe the patient is at acute risk to seriously harm themselves or others or is gravely disabled (in the case of children this often means no longer able to eat or perform self-care activities necessary for acute health). The process prevents the individual from leaving the emergency room or hospital for a brief, defined time (often 72 hours). During that time, a formal evaluation to determine safety must be completed. During this allotted time, if an individual is deemed to be safe, they can be discharged prior to 72 hours, or the patient or family can agree to care voluntarily. Specific forms must be completed and signed by designated professionals, and the patient and family must be informed of their rights. Since mental health holds revoke the civil rights of a patient or their guardian, it is critical to implement the procedure correctly. Providers should familiarize themselves with state laws regulating this process and with clinic and institutional policies and procedures. To learn more about state requirements for mental health holds visit the Treatment Advocacy Center (https://www.treatmentadvocacycenter.org).

Patients who have a medical condition(s) requiring urgent or emergent treatment do not require a mental health hold if they refuse treatment. In these cases, the primary team/provider should conduct a capacity evaluation to determine the patient's ability to understand the risks, benefits and alternatives of treatment if the patient is of age to provide consent. Laws regarding minors' ability to legally consent for care for specific medical conditions vary widely among states.

B. Mandatory Reporting of Abuse or Neglect or Threat to Others

Mandatory reporting of suspected physical or sexual abuse or neglect to the local human services agency is discussed in greater detail in Chapter 8. The "Tarasoff rule" refers to a California legal case that led to a "duty to protect." Laws vary by state and often require providers to warn potential victims when plans are disclosed to them about serious threats to harm specific individuals or to perform harmful acts at specific sites. Under such circumstances, providers may contact police, warn the individual (or site) by phone, and consider involuntary civil commitment of the potential perpetrator if harm appears likely. These protective efforts must be clearly documented and should include the clinical rationale to reduce potential liability.

Youth Mental Health & the COVID-19 Pandemic

The devastating impact of the coronavirus disease-19 (COVID-19) pandemic on child and adolescent mental health is well established with recent estimates suggesting difficulties likely *doubled* among youth globally. A 2021 survey conducted by the Centers for Disease Control and Prevention indicates 44% of high school students in the United States reported persistent sadness and hopelessness and 37% reported poor mental health in the last year. Prolonged stress, social isolation, and limited access to care exacerbated prepandemic trends, particularly in communities of color and for those living in poverty who face greater psychosocial inequities. To draw attention to this growing crisis and inform policy and advocacy efforts, the American Academy of Child and Adolescent Psychiatry, the AAP, and the Children's Hospital Association issued a *Declaration of a National Emergency in Child and Adolescent Mental Health*. The current unprecedented need for mental health treatment demands innovative solutions across the continuum of care, and pediatric primary care offers an important access point for youth and families. From universal screening to integrated behavioral health services, medical practices are uniquely positioned to address the mental health crisis in a trusted setting families routinely utilize. To inform these

efforts, the AAP developed an excellent resource for pediatric providers outlining key considerations and practices, *Interim Guidance on Supporting the Interim Emotional and Behavioral Health Needs of Children, Adolescents, and Families During the COVID-19 Pandemic*. This and additional resources are listed below:

- **AAP Declaration of National Emergency**: https://www.aap.org/en/advocacy/child-and-adolescent-healthy-mental-development/aap-aacap-cha-declaration-of-a-national-emergency-in-child-and-adolescent-mental-health/
- **AAP Guidance on Supporting Emotional & Behavioral Needs During COVID-19**: https://www.aap.org/en/pages/2019-novel-coronavirus-covid-19-infections/clinical-guidance/interim-guidance-on-supporting-the-emotional-and-behavioral-health-needs-of-children-adolescents-and-families-during-the-covid-19-pandemic/
- **Surgeon General Youth Mental Health Guidance:** https://www.hhs.gov/surgeongeneral/priorities/youth-mental-health/index.html
- **SAMHSA Guidelines for Youth Behavioral Health Crisis Care:** https://store.samhsa.gov/product/national-guidelines-child-and-youth-behavioral-health-crisis-care/pep22-01-02-001

Diagnostic Formulation & Interpretation of Findings

A mental status examination (MSE) is the mental health provider's equivalent to the physical examination. It includes some standard aspects to help evaluate an individual, including observation of an individual's overall cognitive, emotional, and behavioral presentation including any areas of clinical concern (eg, suicidal thinking, hallucinations). Depending on the presenting problem, pediatricians may choose to document a complete MSE or a focused MSE. Refer to standard elements of MSE (Table 7–6).

Diagnosis, the final product of an assessment, starts with a description of the presenting problem and is evaluated within the context of the child's age, developmental abilities, history of adverse experiences and stressors impacting the child and the family, and functioning of the family system. In the absence of integrated mental health providers, the primary care provider uses the information gathered to distinguish among possible explanations for the emotional or behavioral problem(s) (Table 7–7).

While a diagnosis is not necessary to refer a patient to a mental health provider, it is important to identify any diagnosis that may be addressed within the primary care setting, such as attention-deficit/hyperactivity disorder (ADHD), mild anxiety, mild-moderate depression, and mild adjustment disorders. Diagnoses are made when symptoms fit criteria for a disorder, when a child's functioning is impaired in

Table 7–6. Standard elements of mental status examination.

Category	Description	Questions to Ask/Observations to Document
General appearance	Physical presentation, attitude, and how the child carries themselves (observation, interaction).	Does the child look their age? Document physical size compared to peers, dysmorphic features, grooming, cooperation, level of distress, and quality of interaction.
Eye contact	Quality of eye contact in context (observation, interaction).	Observe and document quality of eye contact, eg, good, fair, or poor. Is gaze fixed?
Psychomotor activity	Overall energy and physical movement (observation).	Document whether activity level is normal, slowed, or increased.
Musculoskeletal	Gait, range of motion (extremities), abnormal movements (observation and directed tasks).	Document gait and the presence of any rigidity, ataxia, tics, or other abnormal movements.
Speech/language	Rate, volume, tone, articulation, coherence, and spontaneity; appropriate naming and word usage (observation).	Observe and document pattern and quality of speech.
Mood/affect	Subjective (child's stated mood); objective (clinician's observation of affect), and how well the two correspond (observation, direct questioning, and optional self-report questionnaire).	Is the child able to identify their mood- happy, sad, angry, and anxious? Is the child's affect congruent with mood? What is the observed range of affect?
Thought process; associations	Rate, relevance, and reasoning (observation).	Are the child's thoughts goal-directed, logical, tangential, or circumferential? How does the child reason and problem solve? Is thought process concrete or does the child demonstrate abstract reasoning?
Thought content	Content of what the child is saying (observation).	Does the child express suicidal or homicidal ideation, and if so, is there intent and a plan? Does the child experience obsessions? Does the child experience perceptual abnormalities such as hallucinations or illusions?
Attention span	Child's ability to stay on task, focus, and concentrate (observation).	Does the child have an age-appropriate attention span? Is the child able to stay on task or are they easily distracted?
Insight; judgment	Child's psychological understanding of his/her situation; ability to make safe and appropriate choices based on situation (observation and response to directed questions).	What is the child's capacity for insight into his/her situation (intact, poor, impaired)?
Orientation	Awareness of oneself, location, date, and reason for care (observation and response to directed questions).	Does the child know where he/she is, the date, who he/she is, who the parents are?
Fund of knowledge; memory	Common knowledge, ability to recall long-term events and recent details (observation and response to directed questions).	Response to direct questions about current events and memory.
Cognition	Intelligence	Results of cognitive testing (from outside source), assessment of intellectual capacity based on interaction, and other sources of information (average, below average, above average for age and level of education).

major domains of life, such as learning, peer relationships, family relationships, authority relationships, and recreation, or when substantial deviation from typical developmental trajectories occurs. Providers may need to obtain collateral information to further assess symptoms, such as teacher reports when assessing symptoms of ADHD. Symptoms can occur across several diagnoses, and children experience a high rate of comorbidity, necessitating providers to carefully consider a differential diagnosis.

Identifying and discussing the diagnosis is often the starting point for initiating treatment. The provider's interpretation of the presenting problem and diagnosis in the context

Table 7–7. Behavior health diagnostic formulation tool.

The behavior falls within the range of normal given the child's developmental level.

The behavior is a temperamental variation.

The behavior is related to central nervous system impairment (eg, prematurity, exposure to toxins in utero, seizure disorder, or genetic disorders).

The behavior is a normal reaction to stressful circumstances (eg, medical illness, change in family structure, or loss of a loved one).

The behavior is related to relationship problems within the family.

The problem is complicated or exacerbated by an underlying medical condition.

The problem reaches the threshold for a diagnosis.

Some combination of the above.

Table 7–8. When to consider consultation with a psychotherapist or referral to a child and adolescent psychiatrist.

Diagnostic clarification

Further assessment

Medication evaluation outside of primary care

Psychopharmacologic consultation for prescribing pediatricians

Individual, family, or group psychotherapy is needed

Clinical complexity including psychotic symptoms (hallucinations, paranoia) or bipolar disorder

Chronic medical regimen nonadherence

of current family circumstances and available resources and supports enhances referral uptake, engagement in treatment, and coordinated care. The interpretive process includes the following components:

1. Psychoeducation: An explanation of how the presenting problem or symptom reflects a suspected cause, and typical outcomes both with and without intervention.

2. A discussion of interventions including the following options:
   a. Close monitoring
   b. Counseling provided by the primary care provider or integrated mental health provider
   c. Initiation of medication
   d. Referral to a mental health professional outside of the primary care clinic
   e. Some combination of the above

3. A discussion of the parent's and patient's response to the diagnosis and potential interventions.

A joint plan involving the provider, caregivers, and child is then negotiated to address symptoms and developmental needs while considering the family structure and stresses. This can occur within one visit or over the course of several visits. If an appropriate plan cannot be developed or if the provider feels that further diagnostic assessment is required, referral to a mental health practitioner is recommended.

A. Referral of Patients to Mental Health Professionals

Primary care providers often refer patients to a child and adolescent psychiatrist or other qualified mental health professional for diagnostic clarification, ongoing treatment, or if a specialist is preferred to initiate or manage medication (Table 7–8). The local branches of the American Academy of Child and Adolescent Psychiatry (AACAP) and the American Psychological Association (APA) and state chapters are often able to provide a list of mental health professionals who

are trained in the evaluation and treatment of children and adolescents. There are also several levels of care between involuntary inpatient psychiatric hospitalization and outpatient treatment including: day treatment hospitalization, home-based services, intensive outpatient, and primary care management. For academic difficulties not associated with behavioral difficulties, a child educational psychologist or multidisciplinary learning disorder team may be most helpful in assessing for learning disorders and potential remediation. For cognitive difficulties associated with head trauma, epilepsy, or brain tumors, a referral to a pediatric neuropsychologist may be indicated. The presence of drug or alcohol misuse in adolescent patients may require referral to community resources specializing in the treatment of these addictive disorders.

In many states, patients who are publicly insured or do not have mental health insurance coverage may receive assessment and treatment services at their local mental health center. Patients with private mental health insurance typically need to contact their insurance company for a list of local mental health professionals trained in the assessment and treatment of children and adolescents who are on their insurance panel. The referring primary care provider or staff should assist the family by providing information to connect with the appropriate resources and services. Systems of care with co-located mental health providers also remove barriers and improve access and care. After a referral is made, the medical home should arrange a follow-up visit to monitor if the family established care and troubleshoot any barriers. Pediatricians who feel comfortable implementing the recommendations of a mental health professional with whom they have a collaborative relationship should consider remaining involved in the management and coordination of treatment.

B. Other Resources

Many states have a Child Psychiatry Access Program. These are often funded through the states or Health Resources and Services Administration (HRSA) to provide primary care providers with rapid access to a child psychiatrist. This support ranges from prompt phone consultations regarding clinical questions, consultation visits with complex patients, connection to ECHO (Extension for Community Healthcare Outcomes) learning opportunities—typically delivered through online learning communities around specific topics—and support for connecting families to resources. Many programs also have information about local resources, algorithms, and medications posted on their website. The National Network of Child Psychiatry Access programs has links to each program by state and has posted many of the resources from various state programs (https://www.nncpap.org/).

PSYCHIATRIC DISORDERS OF CHILDHOOD & ADOLESCENCE

A psychiatric disorder is defined as a characteristic cluster of signs and symptoms (emotions, behaviors, thought patterns, and mood states) that are associated with subjective distress or maladaptive behavior. This definition presumes that the symptoms are of such intensity, persistence, and duration that the ability to adapt to life's challenges is compromised.

The *Diagnostic and Statistical Manual of Mental Disorders*, 5th Edition, Text Revision (DSM-5-TR™), the formal reference text for psychiatric disorders, describes the criteria for each of the mental illnesses, including those that begin in childhood and adolescence.

Special Considerations in Prescribing Psychotropic Medications

Each primary care provider must establish their comfort level in prescribing psychotropic medications as part of a treatment regimen. Table 7–9 includes commonly prescribed psychotropic medications and their indications. More complete information regarding medical treatment is detailed throughout this chapter. In addition, The Center for Medicare and Medicaid Services (CMS) has a helpful website with dosing information for psychotropic medications, however this was last updated in 2015: https://www.cms.gov/Medicare-Medicaid-Coordination/Fraud-Prevention/Medicaid-Integrity-Program/Education/Pharmacy-Toolkits.

ATTENTION-DEFICIT/HYPERACTIVITY DISORDER

Inattentive, Hyperactive/Impulsive, & Combined Presentation

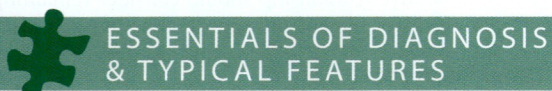

ESSENTIALS OF DIAGNOSIS & TYPICAL FEATURES

- ▶ Significant impairment in attention or concentration.
- ▶ And/or significant hyperactivity and impulsivity more than that expected for age.
- ▶ Must be present in two or more settings.

Table 7–9. Psychoactive medications (other than medications approved for ADHD[a] and movement disorders[b]) approved by the FDA for use in children and adolescents.

Drug	Indication	Minimum Age for Which Approved (y)
SSRIs		
Escitalopram (Lexapro)	Depression	≥ 12
Fluvoxamine	OCD	≥ 8
Fluoxetine (Prozac)	Depression OCD	≥ 12 ≥ 6
Sertraline (Zoloft)	OCD	≥ 6
SNRIs		
Duloxetine	Generalized anxiety disorder	≥ 7
TCAs		
Clomipramine[c] (Anafranil)	OCD	≥ 10
Imipramine[c] (Norpramin)	Enuresis	≥ 6
Atypical antipsychotics		
Aripiprazole (Abilify)	Bipolar disorder Schizophrenia Aggression and autism	≥ 10 ≥ 13 ≥ 6
Asenapine (Saphris)	Bipolar I disorder	≥ 10
Lurasidone (Latuda)	Schizophrenia Bipolar I depression	≥ 13 ≥ 10
Olanzapine (Zyprexa)	Bipolar disorder Schizophrenia	≥ 10 ≥ 13
Paliperidone (Invega)	Schizophrenia	≥ 12
Quetiapine (Seroquel, XR)	Bipolar disorder Schizophrenia	≥ 10 ≥ 13
Risperidone (Risperdal)	Bipolar disorder Schizophrenia Aggression and autism	≥ 10 ≥ 13 ≥ 6
Ziprasidone (Geodon)	Bipolar disorder Schizophrenia	≥ 10 ≥ 13
Other mood stabilizer		
Lithium) (eskalith, litho-bid, lithium citrate, lithium carbonate)	Bipolar Disorder	≥ 12
Olanzapine-Fluoxetine (Symbyax)	Bipolar I depression	≥ 10

ADHD, attention-deficit/hyperactivity disorder; FDA, Food and Drug Administration; OCD, obsessive-compulsive disorder; SSRI, serotonin selective reuptake inhibitor; SNRI, serotonin norepinephrine reuptake inhibitor; TCA, tricyclic antidepressant.

[a]ADHD medication guide can be found at http://www.adhdmedicationguide.com/.

[b]Use of pimozide in the treatment of movement disorders is discussed in Chapter 25.

[c]Not recommended for use as an antidepressant.

General Considerations

ADHD is one of the most seen and treated psychiatric conditions in children and adolescents. Although there is no definitive cause or cure for this disorder, with adequate screening and monitoring, it can be identified and effectively treated and managed.

Identification & Diagnosis

Symptoms of ADHD fall into two categories: hyperactive and impulsive, or inattentive. If a child has a significant number of symptoms in both categories, a diagnosis of ADHD, combined presentation is given. Accurate diagnosis includes obtaining information regarding symptoms and functional impairment from two sources, typically parents and teachers. Functional impairment is required across at least two settings. Standardized forms in the public domain such as Vanderbilt parent and teacher evaluation and follow-up forms for youth aged 6–12 years, the ADHD rating Scale IV for children 3–5 years and the SNAP IV for youth 6–18 years are helpful in this process. It is important to keep in mind that intermittent symptoms of hyperactivity and/or inattention without functional impairment do not warrant a diagnosis of ADHD.

Not all hyperactivity and/or inattention can be attributed to ADHD. Some of the most common psychiatric conditions that have similar presenting problems to ADHD include mood disorder (ie, bipolar and depression), anxiety disorders, oppositional defiant disorder (ODD), adjustment disorder, and PTSD. Learning disorders and other neurodevelopmental disorders can present with symptoms suggestive of ADHD. There are also several medical diagnoses with presenting problems like ADHD, including head injury, hyperthyroidism, fetal alcohol syndrome, and lead toxicity. Inadequate nutrition and sleep deprivation, including poor quality of sleep, can also cause inattention. It is important to have the correct diagnosis prior to initiating treatment.

Treatment

For children diagnosed with ADHD younger than 6, behavioral therapy is the first line of treatment.

Medication can be very helpful for school-age children and adolescents with ADHD. Stimulants are the most effective and most commonly prescribed medications for ADHD. Approximately 75% of children with ADHD experience symptom improvement when given stimulant medications. Children with ADHD who do not respond favorably to one stimulant may respond to a stimulant from the other class (amphetamines vs methylphenidate stimulants). Children and adolescents with ADHD without prominent hyperactivity (ADHD, predominantly inattentive presentation) are also likely to be responsive to stimulant medications. When stimulants are not well tolerated or effective, nonstimulants may be used as an alternative. Among nonstimulant medications,

selective noradrenergic reuptake inhibitors (ie, atomoxetine, viloxazine) and central α_{2A}-adrenergic receptor agonists (ie, guanfacine and clonidine) have FDA approval for the treatment of ADHD in children. The ADHD Medication Guide is an extremely useful, up-to-date site with FDA dosing, administration, and length of action information: http://www.adhdmedicationguide.com/.

A device placed on the forehead overnight to stimulate the trigeminal nerve has FDA approval for treatment of children aged 7–12 years who are not also being treated with medication. The effect of treatment with the external trigeminal nerve stimulation (ETNS) system is mild and did not separate from placebo until 4 weeks. Side effects include appetite increase, sleep difficulties, teeth clenching, headache, and fatigue. EndeavorRx® is a video game with FDA approval for ADHD. The treatment involves 25 minutes of game time/day, 5 days/week. Differential improvement was demonstrated with a computerized continuous performance test. Parent and clinician ratings of ADHD symptoms in the intervention group did not differ from the control group.

Other Considerations

A large majority of children and adolescents with ADHD are not formally diagnosed, and of those who are diagnosed, only 55% receive ongoing treatment. ADHD comorbidities are common and include anxiety disorders, mood disorders, ODD, conduct disorder, and tic disorder. While stimulant medication, the first-line treatment for ADHD, has the potential for abuse, individuals who are treated for ADHD are significantly less likely to abuse substances compared to those who have not been treated.

Special Considerations Regarding the Use of Stimulant Medication

Common adverse events include anorexia, weight loss, abdominal distress, headache, insomnia, dysphoria and tearfulness, irritability, lethargy, mild tachycardia, and mild elevation in blood pressure. Less common side effects include interdose rebound of ADHD symptoms, anxiety, tachycardia, hypertension, depression, mania, and psychotic symptoms. Reduced growth velocity can occur; however, there is evidence of catch up and ultimate height is not usually compromised. Young children are at increased risk for side effects from stimulant medications. Additive stimulant effects are seen with sympathomimetic amines (ephedrine and pseudoephedrine). Although there is no evidence that stimulants increase tics, clinicians may find rare individuals experience an increase in tics with dose adjustments.

Reports of sudden death and serious cardiovascular adverse events among children taking stimulant medication raised concerns about their safety. The labels for methylphenidate and amphetamine medications note reports of stimulant-related deaths in patients with heart problems and advised against using these products in individuals with known serious structural abnormalities of the heart, cardiomyopathy, or serious heart rhythm abnormalities. Insufficient data continue to confirm whether taking stimulant medication causes cardiac problems or sudden death. The FDA advises providers to conduct a thorough physical examination, paying close attention to the cardiovascular system, and to collect information about the patient's history and any family history of cardiac problems. If this scrutiny suggests a problem, providers should consider a screening electrocardiogram (ECG). Caution should also be taken if there is a personal or family history of substance misuse, as these medications can be abused. Formulations such as the methylphenidate transdermal patch or lisdexamfetamine are more difficult to abuse. Students attending college/university may be at increased risk to divert their stimulants to peers. Stimulants should be used with caution in individuals with psychotic disorders, as they can significantly worsen psychotic symptoms. Likewise, stimulants should be used with caution in individuals with bipolar disorder as they can worsen mood dysregulation.

Initial medical screening should include observation for involuntary movements and measurement of height, weight, pulse, and blood pressure, and should be recorded every 3–4 months and at times of dosage increases. Abnormal movements such as motor tics should be assessed at each visit.

Prognosis

Research indicates that 60%–85% of those diagnosed with ADHD in childhood continue to carry the diagnosis into adolescence and those who don't meet full criteria for ADHD may still have functional impairment. While many develop skills to cope with their symptoms in a manner that does not require medication, about one-third of adults previously diagnosed with ADHD in childhood require ongoing medication management.

ANXIETY DISORDERS

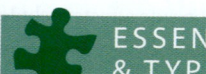

ESSENTIALS OF DIAGNOSIS & TYPICAL FEATURES

▶ Fear or anxiety that is excessive or persisting beyond developmentally appropriate period.

▶ Fear or anxiety is accompanied by behavioral disturbances or physical manifestations.

▶ Symptoms cause functional impairment or significant distress.

Anxiety is described as the anticipation of future threat, and fear is described as the emotional response to real or perceived threat. Both are protective emotions, part of the normal repertoire of children. Distinguishing developmentally appropriate fears and anxiety from those associated with anxiety disorders can be challenging and requires knowledge of normative development. Generally, fears or anxiety that persist beyond the expected developmental period or cause significant distress or impairment in functioning suggest an anxiety disorder. Some anxiety disorders are more likely to be precipitated by stress, but many are not. An anxious temperament can be identified as early as infancy, and children with such temperaments are more likely to develop anxiety disorders, especially if they are living with caregivers who are anxious. Community-based studies of school-aged children and adolescents suggest that nearly 10% of children have some type of anxiety disorder. According to the CDC, this number has been increasing in the past decade. Anxiety disorders are important to identify and treat early as untreated disorders often persist or evolve into other anxiety disorders.

Identification & Diagnosis

Comorbidity is common with anxiety disorders. Children with one anxiety disorder are likely to have another anxiety disorder and have increased risk for other psychiatric disorders such as depression. Carefully screening children with an anxiety disorder helps ensure that another disorder is not missed. In addition, children with anxiety presenting to a pediatrician are more likely to present with a physical complaint, such as headaches or abdominal pain than with identified anxiety (Table 7–10). While medical causes of

Table 7–10. Signs and symptoms of anxiety in children.

Psychological
Fears and worries
Increased dependence on home and parents
Avoidance of anxiety-producing stimuli
Decreased school performance
Increased self-doubt and irritability
Frightening themes in play and fantasy
Psychomotor
Motoric restlessness and hyperactivity
Sleep disturbances
Decreased concentration
Ritualistic behaviors (eg, washing, counting)
Psychophysiologic
Autonomic hyperarousal
Dizziness and lightheadedness
Palpitations
Shortness of breath
Flushing, sweating, dry mouth
Nausea and vomiting
Panic
Headaches and stomach aches

anxiety are rare, it is important to not misdiagnose a physical symptom as anxiety, for example, to ascribe the gastrointestinal (GI) upset of inflammatory bowel disease to anxiety. Screening should also assess for medications and substances that can cause anxiety or present similarly. Such substances include caffeine, marijuana, amphetamines, cocaine, and alcohol. Medications that have been associated with anxiety include steroids, tacrolimus, angiotensin-converting enzyme inhibitors, anticholinergics, dopamine agonists, β-adrenergic agonists, thyroid medications, and procaine derivatives. Medical illnesses that can lead to symptoms suggestive of anxiety include those associated with hyperthyroid states, hypoglycemia, hypoxia, and, more rarely, pheochromocytoma.

► Treatment

Treatment must be tailored to the developmental age of the child. Treatment of younger children focuses on helping parents understand their child's symptoms, developing skills to help their child manage distress, while also helping parents tolerate their child's distress. As soon as children have the developmental capacity to engage in assessing their own anxiety and in learning coping strategies, they are incorporated into therapy.

Cognitive behavioral therapy (CBT) with exposure has the most evidence for the successful treatment of anxiety. Exposure refers to planned progressive presentation of low- to mid-level anxiety-provoking stimulus. The aim is to desensitize the child to the stimulus (eg, an event—separation, going to school, thunderstorms; an object or thing—bugs, the dark) while providing strategies to manage anxiety during exposure. CBT can be delivered in group settings or with an individual child and caregivers. The basic goals include helping children identify and quantify anxiety symptoms, identify maladaptive cognitions, learn cognitive and behavioral coping strategies to begin exposures to situations or items associated with medium- to low-level anxieties. Caregivers also learn these skills to help children or youth practice in settings outside the therapy office. The goal is to enable the child to face the specific situation(s) or stimuli that causes distress or dysfunction, experience a decrease in anxiety, respond in a more adaptive manner, and resume typical functioning.

When anxiety symptoms do not remit with cognitive, behavioral, and environmental interventions, and continue to significantly affect daily functioning, psychopharmacologic agents may be helpful. There is evidence that selective serotonin reuptake inhibitors (SSRIs) are effective in treating anxiety disorders in children as young as 6 years. Pediatricians should be aware that these medications do not have FDA approval for this indication and should inform patients/caregivers regarding off-label use. The anxiolytic effect of SSRIs can be as rapid as a few days. Pediatricians are discouraged from prescribing benzodiazepines, despite their rapid onset. The risk/benefit ratio is unacceptable, given the high risk for

dependency and iatrogenic substance abuse for the developing brain. Antihistamines (ie, hydroxyzine), β-blockers, and α-agonists are alternatives that can be used on a scheduled or as-needed based and usually are better tolerated without concern for physiologic dependence. Refer to medication used for treatment of depressive disorders (Table 7–11) as they are commonly used in the treatment for anxiety as well.

► Prognosis

Early treatment of anxiety disorders can be very effective and decreases the risk for negative impact on developmental trajectories or the development of other psychiatric disorders. The standard of care is CBT for milder cases and a combination of CBT/antidepressant for more severe cases or cases that do not respond to CBT alone.

Anxiety disorders tend to wax and wane during childhood. Patients who present with more severe anxiety symptoms often develop several anxiety disorders during adolescence and are at risk for depression, substance misuse, and other negative developmental outcomes. Parenting style and caregiver anxiety may contribute to increased anxiety in children. Treatment of caregiver anxiety disorders, when present, often improves the outcome of the child's anxiety disorder.

1. Separation Anxiety

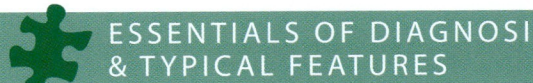

ESSENTIALS OF DIAGNOSIS & TYPICAL FEATURES

► Persistent excessive worry about losing or being separated from attachment figures, due to harm, illness, or death befalling either the attachment figure or the patient.

► Reluctance or refusal to separate from or leave the attachment figure(s) or sleep away from home or without the attachment figure(s).

► Fear of being home or in other settings without the attachment figure(s).

► Can be accompanied by physical complaints when separation occurs or is anticipated.

► General Considerations

Very young children may not be symptomatic until the separation is imminent or occurring and may not experience anticipatory fears related to separation. As children get older, they may experience fears in anticipation of separations, particularly around routine separations such as going to preschool/school or at bedtime. Additionally, specific fears such as fears of kidnapping, parents getting into car accidents, and being separated due to natural

Table 7–11. Antidepressant information.

Drug Name and class	Dosage Form	Usual Starting Dose for Adolescent	Increase Increment (After ~4 wk)	RCT Evidence in Kids	FDA Depression Approved for Children?	Editorial Comments
Fluoxetine (Prozac) SSRI	10, 20, 40 mg 20 mg/5 mL	5–10 mg/day (60 mg max)[a]	10–mg[b]	Yes	Yes (over age 8)	Long half-life, no side effects from a missed dose. More potential drug-drug interactions.
Sertraline (Zoloft) SSRI	25, 50, 100 mg 20 mg/mL	12.5–25 mg/day (200 mg max)[a]	25–50 mg[b]	Yes	No	May cause more GI upset, more potential side effects when stopping.
Escitalopram (Lexapro) SSRI	5, 10, 20 mg 5 mg/5 mL	2.5–5 mg/day (20 mg max)[a]	5–10 mg[b]	Yes	Yes (for adolescents)	The active isomer of citalopram, less potential for drug-drug interactions.
Citalopram (Celexa) SSRI	10, 20, 40 mg 10 mg/5 mL	5–10 mg/day (40 mg max)[a]	10–20 mg[b]	Yes	No	Few drug interactions for SSRI.
Bupropion (Wellbutrin) miscellaneous	75, 100 mg 100, 150, 200 mg SR forms 150, 300 mg XL forms	75 mg/day (later can dose BID until reach formulations for once daily dosing) (6/mg/kg or not to exceed 3-400 mg max)[a]	75–100 mg[b]	No	No	Also 3rd- or 4th-line treatment for ADHD. Potential for increasing seizure risk.
Mirtazapine (Remeron) SNRI	15, 30, 45 mg	7.5–15 mg/day (45 mg max)[a]	15 mg[b]	No	No	Sedating, increases appetite.
Venlafaxine (Effexor) SNRI	25, 37.5, 50, 75, 100 mg 37.5, 75, 150 mg ER forms	37.5 mg/day (225 mg max)[a]	37.5–75 mg[b]	No (May have higher SI risk than others for children)	No	Only recommended for older adolescents. Withdrawal symptoms can be severe.
Duloxetine (Cymbalta) SNRI	Delayed release (DR) 20, 30, 60 mg	20–30 mg	30 mg after 2 weeks	Yes	Yes	Doses higher than 60 mg daily are rarely more effective.

[a]Recommend low starting dose for young children and children and adolescents with anxiety, who may be more sensitive to brief increase in anxiety
[b]If starting at the lowest dose to decrease side effect, may increase again in 1–2 weeks.

disasters may emerge. Behaviors associated with separation anxiety also vary by age; young children are more likely to present with difficulties around bedtimes while other separations, such as school, sleep overs, and camp, may be the focus of anxiety for older children. In addition to appearing anxious, children with separation anxiety can appear sad, aggressive, or experience physical symptoms when facing anxiety-provoking separation. Separation anxiety disorder is more prevalent in younger children (4% 6-month prevalence compared with 1.6% 6-month prevalence in adolescence).

▶ Identification & Diagnosis

Anxiety about separation from attachment figures is typical in early childhood development. Separation anxiety disorder must be distinguished from normal development, occur for more than 4 weeks and lead to impairment or significant distress.

Treatment

Parents or caregivers must be involved in treatment to ensure they understand the nature of the disorder, the importance of not accommodating avoidant behaviors, can tolerate their child's distress, and develop supportive routines that promote optimal separations. Clinical treatment of separation anxiety includes CBT that is modified to address the developmental level of the child. Children who do not respond to therapy may require medication such as an SSRI. Children younger than school age are generally not treated with medication.

Other Considerations

The differential for separation anxiety is broad and includes other anxiety disorders, mood disorders, ODD, conduct disorder, psychotic disorder, and personality disorders. Pediatricians are likely to encounter children with school refusal, a common behavioral manifestation of separation anxiety. It is important to recognize and intervene early with school refusal as the longer a child is out of school, the more difficult it is to help the child return. Symptoms of school refusal often include physical symptoms and or behavioral outbursts as school time approaches. Parents often notice symptoms abate on the weekend, vacations, or if the child is no longer expected to attend school. Mild cases may be handled with the help of the pediatrician's office, but more severe cases may require a mental health specialist.

School refusal can also be related to other anxiety disorders, learning disorders, mood disorders, psychotic disorders, ODD, conduct disorder, and environmental stressors such as bullying, traumatic events, or poor student teacher fit. Identifying the etiology of school refusal helps providers appropriately target the level and type of intervention.

Prognosis

Separation anxiety often abates by adolescence but may persist or manifest again in adulthood. Adolescents who experienced separation anxiety disorder in childhood are at increased risk of developing other disorders.

2. Selective Mutism Disorder

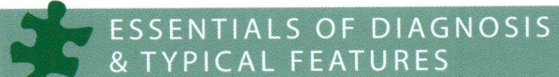

ESSENTIALS OF DIAGNOSIS & TYPICAL FEATURES

▶ Consistent failure to speak in social settings (such as school) where speaking is expected, despite speaking in other settings.

General Considerations

Selective mutism affects less than 1% of children and is more common in younger children. Symptoms may be present before age 5 but usually do not manifest until the child enters school and is expected to speak to children and adults outside their family. It is also more common among children who are bilingual.

Identification & Diagnosis

Children with selective mutism usually speak with close family members and may also speak with close friends or peers. They may be quite outgoing within a familiar setting but are often inhibited when in unfamiliar settings. They may be comfortable in social roles and interactions that do not require verbal communication. Children with selective mutism can become angry and aggressive when facing a demand to speak. Screening for selective mutism is useful as families may not be aware of the problem or may not appreciate how it interferes with functioning at school. To meet criteria for selective mutism, symptoms must interfere with function in school, work, or social communication, and must last longer than 1 month, not including the first month of school. Symptoms cannot be due to a neurodevelopmental disorder, learning disorder, autism spectrum disorder, language or communication disorders, or psychotic disorders. However, children with selective mutism have higher rates of language and communication disorders.

Treatment

Selective mutism can be perplexing for parents and teachers as the child's engagement in speaking can vary significantly across settings. Treatment therefore usually begins with psychoeducation. Children with selective mutism can be difficult to engage due to their inhibition and refusal to speak, so clinicians must be adept at using both verbal and nonverbal methods to form an alliance with the child. Behavioral interventions (eg, contingency management, shaping, and systematic desensitization) combined with CBT make use of exposures aimed at increasing verbal interactions. Patients with more severe symptoms, or symptoms that do not respond to therapy, may benefit from an antidepressant (ie, SSRI).

Other Considerations

The differential diagnosis includes other disorders that can interfere with verbal communication, such as autism spectrum disorders, language and communication disorders, and psychotic disorders. Children with selective mutism can have other comorbid anxiety disorders, such as social anxiety disorder, separation anxiety, and specific phobia.

Recognition and treatment of selective mutism is critical as this behavior becomes increasingly entrenched the longer a child avoids verbal communication in settings outside of the family. Children with untreated selective mutism are at risk for depression, school difficulties, relational disruptions, social anxiety disorder, and substance use disorders as adolescents.

3. Specific Phobias

ESSENTIALS OF DIAGNOSIS & TYPICAL FEATURES

► Excessive fear or worry about a certain thing, experience, or situation.
► The thought about or exposure to this trigger causes excessive anxiety.

▶ General Considerations

Most specific phobias have onset before 10 years of age. Specific phobias are common, impacting 5% of children and 16% of adolescents. Simple phobias often lessen over time while more severe, persistent forms can be debilitating.

▶ Identification & Diagnosis

A specific phobia is an intense fear of a particular object, experience, or situation that persists for at least 6 months. This object or situation is a cause of great distress nearly every time the individual anticipates or is exposed to the stimulus. The perceived harm or threat is well out of proportion to the actual stimulus. To handle the distress, the child avoids the object or situation, therefore reinforcing the anxiety. The distress caused by the stimulus can also present as a panic attack, fainting, or irritability. Young children may present with increased clinginess.

▶ Treatment

The mainstay of treatment for specific phobias is CBT with imaginal or in vivo exposure aimed at reducing anxiety or fear of the phobic stimulus.

▶ Other Considerations

Children commonly experience more than one specific phobia and as the number of phobias increases, so does the degree of impairment. The differential diagnosis includes other anxiety disorders, trauma and stress-related disorders, eating disorders, schizophrenia, and other psychotic disorders.

Significant childhood separation events are associated with later onset of phobia. Addressing specific phobia is important as untreated specific phobias have one of the higher rates of stability over time among childhood anxiety disorders.

4. Panic Disorder

ESSENTIALS OF DIAGNOSIS & TYPICAL FEATURES

► Recurrent, unexpected panic attacks, described as an abrupt onset of intense fear, that crescendos over the course of minutes and is accompanied by physical symptoms.

▶ General Considerations

Panic disorder is more likely to present after the onset of puberty with a prevalence rate of 2%–3% during adolescence. Unlike many other anxiety disorders, there is more likely to be a stressor preceding the onset of panic disorder. Children who experience separation anxiety disorder are at increased risk of developing panic disorder.

▶ Identification & Diagnosis

The physical symptoms of panic disorder are symptoms of a surge in the adrenergic system and include palpitations, sweating, shortness of breath, choking, chest pain or tightness, GI distress, dizziness or associated feelings, chills or heat, numbness, or tingling. Cognitive symptoms can include feelings of unreality and fear of going crazy or of dying. To meet criteria for a panic attack, at least four of the above symptoms must be present. At least one attack must be followed by anticipatory fear of having another attack in the subsequent month which may lead to maladaptive behavior. Youth with panic disorder are most likely to present to the pediatrician with fears related to physical symptoms of autonomic arousal, such as a fear that there is something wrong with their heart. Adolescents are less likely than adults to report panic attacks, and thus specific questions or questionnaires should be used when adolescents present with anxiety. To meet the criteria of panic disorder, at least two panic attacks must be unexpected (ie, occur without an identifiable trigger); however, once panic attacks are cued or paired with an event or trigger, it can be difficult for children and adolescents to recall un-cued panic attacks. Panic disorder can be debilitating as youth can go to extensive lengths to avoid cues.

▶ Treatment

CBT for youth with panic disorder focuses on the cognitions associated with the panic attack as well as the physiologic distressing symptoms. Exposure targets may include situations that trigger panic attacks or some of the physiologic symptoms experienced during an attack. The frequency of treatment can vary depending on the acuity of the patient, with lower levels of care provided during weekly outpatient therapy and higher levels provided several times a week through intensive outpatient treatment programs or daily in psychiatric day treatment programs. Patients who do not respond to therapy alone may benefit from an antidepressant such as an SSRI. Other nonbenzodiazepine medication options include antihistamines (eg, hydroxyzine) and occasionally off-label use of β-blockers or low-dose atypical antipsychotics. Benzodiazepines have been used with adults but are discouraged for use with youth in the primary care setting.

Other Considerations

The differential diagnosis of panic attacks includes a physical cause of panic symptoms, which must be ruled out when appropriate. Youth who avoid going out in public by themselves should be diagnosed with agoraphobia in addition to panic disorder. Although panic disorder increases the risk of developing a substance abuse disorder, withdrawal of some substances can also lead to panic symptoms. For adolescents who are actively using substances, this can be difficult to distinguish. Panic attacks can present as part of other anxiety disorders and are cued by the underlying fear or anxiety, such as public performance in social anxiety disorder or anticipation of an event in generalized anxiety disorder (GAD). The diagnosis given is the underlying disorder with the specifier of panic attacks, for example, social anxiety disorder with panic attacks. Panic disorder is also higher among individuals with other anxiety disorders, depression, and bipolar disorder.

Prognosis

Panic symptoms and panic disorder are both important to recognize and treat. Untreated panic disorder has the highest rate of persistence over time among childhood anxiety disorders. Individuals with panic symptoms that occur in the context of another disorder are at increased risk of developing depression.

5. Agoraphobia

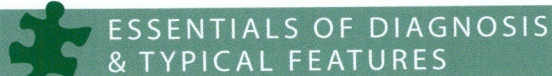

ESSENTIALS OF DIAGNOSIS & TYPICAL FEATURES

▶ An excessive fear of being in two or more of the following situations: public transportation, open spaces, enclosed spaces, lines or crowds, or outside the home alone.

▶ The situation almost always or always causes persistent fear or anxiety that is disproportionate to the actual danger posed by the situation and lasts more than 6 months.

▶ Avoidance of situations that increase fear, anxiety, or the possibility of panic attacks.

General Considerations

Agoraphobia can be debilitating. In children and adolescents, it is more likely to present as school refusal than fear of the other situations listed below. Children and adolescents may be reluctant to report symptoms, so careful screening is warranted for children with anxiety or children who are refusing to attend school. In community samples, agoraphobia is more likely to occur in later adolescence; 1.7% of adolescents suffer from agoraphobia, but this may be an underestimate because of the difficulty of assessing youth. Like panic disorder, initial symptoms often are triggered by a stressful event.

Identification & Diagnosis

The most well-known fear associated with agoraphobia is fear of open spaces, including shopping centers, grocery stores, and other public settings. For individuals with agoraphobia, other situations can also trigger intense fear, such as using public transportation, standing in line or being in a crowd, and being in an enclosed space or outside the home alone. Individuals with agoraphobia experience two or more of these fears that last for over 6 months and lead to distress or impairment. Full panic disorder symptoms do not have to be present to meet criteria for agoraphobia, which can occur with or without panic attacks.

Treatment

Treatment of individuals with agoraphobia can be very challenging, as treatment typically requires leaving home. Online treatments are available, but efficacy data are limited. The current standard remains CBT with exposure, and SSRI for individuals who do not respond to treatment or are severely impacted by agoraphobia.

Other Considerations

The differential diagnosis includes other anxiety disorders, PTSD, depression, and medical conditions. For example, adolescents with postural orthostatic tachycardia syndrome (POTS) may fear leaving the house due to a fear of fainting. Similarly, individuals with inflammatory bowel disease may fear having an episode of diarrhea outside the home.

Prognosis

Individuals with agoraphobia are at risk for comorbid disorders including other anxiety disorders and depression, and males have a high incidence of substance misuse.

6. Generalized Anxiety Disorder

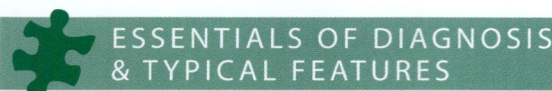

ESSENTIALS OF DIAGNOSIS & TYPICAL FEATURES

▶ Multiple, intense, disproportionate, or irrational worries, often about future events.

▶ Worry is accompanied by other symptoms.

▶ The worry is difficult to control.

General Considerations

Individuals with generalized anxiety disorder (GAD) often recall a lifetime of anxiety, but studies utilizing a nonclinically referred population or community sample find GAD rarely presents before adolescence; the prevalence of GAD in adolescence is 0.9%. Potential reasons for this discrepancy include that the symptoms of anxiety may not meet full criteria for GAD at an earlier age, or symptoms may be underestimated by caregivers. Individuals who develop GAD at an early age are more likely to have greater impairment. The differential diagnosis of symptoms of anxiety is presented in Table 7–12.

Identification & Diagnosis

Young children with generalized anxiety often worry about their competence or performance while older youth may worry about additional issues such as family finances or being on time. Worry and anxiety that is not pathologic must be distinguished from the worries or anxieties of GAD. In addition, children with GAD experience at least one symptom of fatigue, restlessness or poor concentration, irritability, feeling on edge, or sleep disturbance. GAD can also be accompanied by other somatic symptoms, and the pediatrician is more likely to encounter children with GAD who present with symptoms of GI difficulties or headaches. To meet criteria for GAD, the symptoms must cause significant distress or disturbance of function and be present for at least 6 months.

Treatment

As with other anxiety disorders psychotherapy is the first-line treatment, with the possible addition of an SSRI or similar agent if the response is insufficient.

Table 7–12. Differential diagnosis of symptoms of anxiety.

- **Normal developmental anxiety**
  A. Stranger anxiety (5 mo–2½ y, with a peak at 6–12 mo)
  B. Separation anxiety (7 mo–4 y, with a peak at 18–36 mo)
  C. The child is fearful or even phobic of the dark and monsters (3–6 y)
- **"Appropriate" anxiety**
  A. Anticipating a painful or frightening experience
  B. Avoidance of a reminder of a painful or frightening experience
  C. Child abuse
- **Anxiety disorder (see Table 7–11), with or without other comorbid psychiatric disorders**
- **Substance abuse**
- **Medications and recreational drugs**
  A. Caffeinism (including colas and chocolate)
  B. Sympathomimetic agents
  C. Idiosyncratic drug reactions
- **Hypermetabolic or hyperarousal states**
  A. Hyperthyroidism
  B. Pheochromocytoma
  C. Anemia
  D. Hypoglycemia
  E. Hypoxemia
- **Cardiac abnormality**
  A. Dysrhythmia
  B. High-output state
  C. Mitral valve prolapsed

Other Considerations

It can be challenging to distinguish GAD from other anxiety disorders. Substance-induced anxiety should be considered with adolescents who experience a sudden onset of anxiety.

Prognosis

The combination of medication and therapy can be very effective for treating youth with GAD. Individuals with GAD are at increased risk for depression.

7. Social Anxiety Disorder

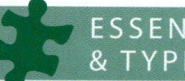

ESSENTIALS OF DIAGNOSIS & TYPICAL FEATURES

▶ Excessive worrying in social settings.

▶ Inability to perform in front of others as expected for age.

▶ Avoidance of events or settings that are social in nature or involve large groups.

General Considerations

Social anxiety disorder is characterized by significant, persistent fear in social settings, or performance situations. The disorder results in overwhelming anxiety and inability to function when exposed to unfamiliar people and/or scrutiny. This is usually a problem for older children and adolescents.

Identification & Diagnosis

Anxiety symptoms in children with social anxiety disorder are related specifically to the social setting and not better explained by another anxiety disorder. Common manifestations of this disorder include consistent avoidance of social functions and persistent somatic complaints that occur in a social setting and resolve in the absence of social exposure. The symptoms significantly disrupt the child's—and frequently the family's—life, and caregivers often describe a pattern of overly accommodating their child's avoidance and/or incentivizing their child to attend routine social, extracurricular, or family functions.

Treatment

Like the other anxiety disorders, the mainstay of treatment for social anxiety disorder is CBT. The goal is to modify behavior and diminish anxiety in social settings through specific cognitive and behavioral techniques. As with other anxiety disorders, if ongoing CBT is not effective at mitigating anxiety, psychopharmacologic agents may be helpful. SSRIs are the only class of medication to have demonstrated efficacy for children with social anxiety disorder.

Other Considerations

Children with social anxiety disorder are at increased risk for depression and school avoidance. They can also experience panic attacks, and there is high comorbidity between substance use disorders and anxiety disorders, especially social anxiety disorder.

Prognosis

Early age of onset, more severe avoidance, and the presence of panic symptoms are all predictors of persistence over time. Treatment with CBT or a combination of CBT and medication can be effective for most youth with social anxiety disorder.

OBSESSIVE-COMPULSIVE & RELATED DISORDERS

General Considerations

Obsessive-compulsive and related disorders is a broad term to describe disorders with shared features (ie, obsessions and compulsions) and includes hoarding disorder, body dysmorphic disorder (BDD), trichotillomania (hair pulling) disorder, excoriation (skin picking) disorder, and obsessive-compulsive disorder (OCD). Anxiety disorders and depression are common co-morbid disorders. Pediatricians might be the first providers to assess trichotillomania, excoriation disorder, or BDD to rule out medical causes and assigning the correct diagnosis can help youth access treatment in a timely manner.

Identification & Diagnosis

Distinguishing developmentally appropriate behaviors from those associated with these disorders can be challenging and requires knowledge of normative development. For example, many young children twirl or play with their hair or occasionally pick at a scab, but do not pick (as in excoriation disorder) or pull (as in trichotillomania) to the point of causing significant distress or impairment. The cognitive transition to thinking more about others is accompanied by a normative drive towards self-comparison and youth often find slight or non-existent flaws in themself. When youth spend time thinking or engaging in behaviors to minimize this flaw and this impacts their ability to function (such as go to school) or causes significant distress, BDD should be considered. Children often like to collect things or have a difficult time getting rid of possessions, but when this begins to cause significant distress or intrude on their (or the family's) function, hoarding should be considered. Hoarding symptoms often begin between ages 11 and 15 years and may be more amenable to treatment if addressed early.

Treatment

While treatment can differ depending on the disorder, parents, or caregivers generally play an important role. CBT, habit reversal therapy, cognitive skills training, and acceptance and commitment therapy can be effective depending on the disorder, although hoarding disorder is typically more difficult to treat. Indicated medications also vary by disorder and given the lack of evidence other than SSRIs for OCD and BDD, treatment should be undertaken with consultation with a child and adolescent psychiatrist. Parents may be tempted to help youth with BDD obtain minor surgery to address a flaw but should be aware that these youth often find another body "flaw" to focus on.

Other Considerations

OCD, BDD, and hoarding disorder all have specifiers regarding the level of insight the patient has into their disorder. Poor insight is indicative of worse prognosis.

Obsessive-Compulsive Disorder

ESSENTIALS OF DIAGNOSIS & TYPICAL FEATURES

▶ Recurrent obsessive thoughts, impulses, or images that are experienced as intrusive at times.

▶ Repetitive compulsive behaviors or mental acts are performed to prevent or reduce distress stemming from obsessive thoughts.

▶ Obsessions and compulsions cause marked distress, are time-consuming, and interfere with normal routines.

▶ General Considerations

Onset often occurs during childhood, and untreated OCD can have a lifelong course. Males have an earlier age of onset, with childhood cases usually occurring before the age of 10 years. OCD often leads to avoidance of situations that trigger obsessions, and for children and adolescents, this can interfere with development.

▶ Identification & Diagnosis

The obsessions that lead to OCD are defined as recurrent, persistent, intrusive thoughts, urges, or images that cause significant distress. The individual tries to avoid, suppress, or ignore the obsessions or to mitigate them through action or thought. The obsessions and compulsions of OCD consume more than 1 h/day. Obsessions vary by individuals but tend to cluster into the following groups: intrusive "forbidden" images such as sexual, aggressive, or religiously taboo images, thoughts of contamination, need for symmetry, fears of harming others, and fears of harm to oneself or loved ones. Individuals often experience more than one cluster, and types of obsessions can change over time. In addition to compulsive symptoms, youth who are experiencing obsessions may also experience symptoms of panic, depression, irritability, and suicidality. Sudden onset of symptoms should alert pediatricians to screen for group A streptococcal infections, as pediatric autoimmune disorders associated with these infections have been implicated in the development of OCD for some children.

Caregivers can often identify children who have compulsions, but obsessions can be difficult to recognize because they are experienced internally. Youth who recognize that obsessions and compulsions are strange may not spontaneously reveal symptoms unless specifically asked.

▶ Treatment

Many individuals with OCD feel that their symptoms are "crazy," or alternatively, they do not want to consider giving up their compulsions as they feel these will lead to intense distress. Psychoeducation is an important first step in treatment of OCD to help put symptoms in perspective and outline treatment progression. OCD is best treated with a combination of CBT specific to OCD and with medications in more severe cases. SSRIs are effective in diminishing OCD symptoms, but higher doses—occasionally above maximum recommended daily dose—may be needed. Fluoxetine, fluvoxamine, and sertraline have FDA approval for the treatment of pediatric OCD. The tricyclic antidepressant (TCA) clomipramine has FDA approval for the treatment of OCD in adults. Severe cases have been treated with gamma knife brain surgery interrupting the circuit involved in OCD. Some individuals have benefitted from other nonpharmacologic interventions such as neurofeedback and transcranial magnetic stimulation (TMS); however, they are not FDA approved for this condition.

▶ Other Consideration

In addition to increased risk of other related disorders, youth with OCD are at increased risk for comorbid anxiety, ADHD, depression, and tics. The differential diagnosis includes all the above as well as eating disorders, psychotic disorders, and obsessive-compulsive personality disorder. The perseveration of children with autism spectrum disorders can also be confused with OCD.

▶ Prognosis

The combination of CBT plus medication is most effective for patients who do not respond to either treatment alone. It is important to recognize and treat OCD early, as early age of onset and greater impairment are predictors of poor prognosis.

▶ Posttraumatic Stress Disorder

ESSENTIALS OF DIAGNOSIS & TYPICAL FEATURES

▶ Arousal and reactivity such as hypervigilance, difficulty concentrating, and sleep disturbance.

▶ Avoidance of reminders of the trauma.

▶ Negative changes in thoughts and mood.

▶ Flashbacks to a traumatic event such as nightmares, intrusive thoughts, or repetitive play.

▶ Follows traumatic events such as exposure to violence, physical or sexual abuse, natural disasters, car accidents, dog bites, and unexpected personal tragedies.

General Considerations

Factors that predispose individuals to the development of PTSD include proximity to the traumatic event or loss, history of exposure to trauma, preexisting depression or anxiety disorder, being abused by a caregiver, witnessing a threat to a caregiver, or an unstable social situation. PTSD can develop in response to natural disasters, terrorism, motor vehicle crashes, and significant personal injury, in addition to physical, sexual, and emotional abuse. Natural disasters, such as hurricanes, fires, flooding, and earthquakes, create situations in which large numbers of affected individuals are at heightened risk for PTSD. Witnessing events through electronic media does not qualify as exposure to traumatic events.

Long overdue attention is now being paid to the substantial effects of family and community violence on the psychological development of children and adolescents. Abused children are especially likely to develop PTSD and to suffer wide-ranging symptoms and impaired functioning. As many as 25% of young people exposed to violence develop symptoms of PTSD and children with some symptoms of PTSD can suffer significant distress and functional impairment, even when not meeting full criteria for PTSD.

Identification & Diagnosis

Children and adolescents with PTSD typically show persistent fear, anxiety, and hypervigilance. Children may regress developmentally, experience fears of strangers, the dark, and being alone, and avoid reminders of traumatic events. For young children with magical thinking, this can involve avoiding objects or events that may not be obviously linked to the traumatic experience. Children and adolescents with PTSD are often more irritable and can experience detachment and diminished interest in activities. They reexperience elements of the trauma in the form of nightmares and flashbacks. In the symbolic play of children with PTSD, one can often notice repetition of some aspects of the traumatic event. A subset of children experiences dissociative symptoms such as feeling detached or unreal. The adjusted criteria for PTSD in children under 6 reflect developmental differences in emotional and behavioral symptom presentation. Symptoms must be present for at least 1 month to meet criteria and can present months after the event.

Treatment

Before considering treatment, it is critical to ensure that the child is living in a safe environment. If there is concern regarding current or past abuse, this must be reported to child welfare and/or law enforcement. Treatment of patients with PTSD includes psychoeducation regarding the nature of trauma, the disorder, and the varied symptoms that parents may not recognize as related to PTSD. The child needs support, reassurance, and empathy, and the primary caregiver may also need additional help to provide this. Individual and family psychotherapy are central features of treatment interventions. Treatments differ based on age, chronicity of trauma, and access to treatment. Young children may benefit from therapy focused on strengthening the parent-child relationship whereas other treatments focus on creating a developmentally appropriate trauma narrative to help the child understand and process their experience. Trauma-focused cognitive behavioral therapy (TF-CBT) has the most evidence for treatment of children and adolescents with PTSD while treatments such as eye movement desensitization and reprocessing therapy (EMDR) have more limited evidence. Pediatricians can help the family establish or maintain daily routines as much as possible, especially after a trauma or disaster disrupts the family's functioning. In the case of media coverage of a disaster or event, children's viewing should be avoided or limited.

For children with severe and persistent symptoms, medication may be indicated in addition to psychotherapy. Children who have lived in abusive environments for an extended period or have been exposed to multiple traumas are more likely to require treatment with medications. Currently, there are no medications with FDA approval for treating PTSD in children. Child psychiatrists may choose medications to target specific symptoms (eg, anxiety, depression, nightmares, and aggression). Some of the medications used to treat children with PTSD include antiadrenergic agents (clonidine, guanfacine, or propranolol), mood stabilizers, antidepressants, and second-generation antipsychotics.

Other Considerations

Growing evidence supports a connection between traumatic experiences in childhood and problems in adulthood, including health problems, substance misuse, personality disorders, and mood disorders. It is important to treat PTSD not only to relieve the suffering of youth with PTSD but also to mitigate long-term negative sequelae.

Many of the symptoms of PTSD can be mistaken for other disorders such as depression, anxiety, primary substance abuse, ADHD, learning disorders, ODD, bipolar disorder, and even psychosis in severe cases. All behavioral health assessments should include inquiries related to traumatic events. It is important not to miss trauma-related etiology as this may change treatment focus. Traumatic events may not lead to PTSD but may cause grief, an adjustment disorder, depression, or an acute stress disorder (same criteria as PTSD but symptoms last < 1 month). Children with PTSD may have comorbid diagnoses that require treatment. This diagnostic complexity often requires the assistance of the child psychiatrist or other mental health provider.

Prognosis

The best prognostic indicator for children exposed to trauma is a supportive relationship with a caregiving adult.

Frequently, caregivers exposed to trauma also have PTSD and need treatment to support their child's recovery. Timely access to therapy enhances prognosis. Children with more severe PTSD may require intermittent therapy to identify and treat symptoms that emerge during different stages of development. The National Child Traumatic Stress Network offers additional resources and information on evidence-based treatments: https://www.nctsn.org.

ADJUSTMENT DISORDERS

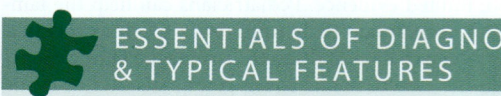

ESSENTIALS OF DIAGNOSIS & TYPICAL FEATURES

► The precipitating event or circumstance is identifiable.
► Symptoms appear within 3 months of the onset of the stressor.
► Does not persist more than 6 months after the stressor has terminated.

General Considerations

The most common and most disturbing stressors in the lives of children and adolescents are the death of a loved one, marital discord, separation and divorce, family illness, a change of residence or school setting, experiencing a traumatic event, and, for adolescents, peer-relationship problems. These stressors naturally have a significant impact on children and adolescents.

Identification & Diagnosis

When faced with stress, children can experience many different symptoms, including changes in mood, changes in behavior, anxiety symptoms, and physical complaints. When the reaction is out of proportion to the stressor and a decline in functioning is noted, a diagnosis of adjustment disorder is likely. The two main categories of adjustment disorders include disturbance in emotions (ie, depression and anxiety) and/or conduct.

Treatment

The mainstay of treatment involves genuine empathy and assurance to the caregivers and the patient that the emotional or behavioral change is a predictable consequence of the stressful event. This validates the child's reaction and encourages the child to talk about the stressful occurrence and its aftermath. Caregivers are encouraged to help with appropriate expression of feelings, while defining boundaries for behavior that prevent the child from feeling out of control and ensure safety of self and others. Maintaining or reestablishing routines can also alleviate distress and help children and adolescents adjust to changing circumstances by increasing predictability and decreasing distress about the unknown.

Other Considerations

When symptoms emerge in reaction to an identifiable stressor but are severe, persistent, or disabling, mood disorders, anxiety disorders, and conduct disorders should be considered.

Prognosis

The duration of symptoms in adjustment reactions depends on the severity of the stress, the child's personal sensitivity to stress and vulnerability to anxiety, depression, and other psychiatric disorders, and the available support system.

MOOD DISORDERS

1. Depression

ESSENTIALS OF DIAGNOSIS & TYPICAL FEATURES

► Dysphoric mood, mood lability, irritability, or loss of interest or pleasure, persisting for weeks to months at a time
► Characteristic neurovegetative signs and symptoms (eg, changes in sleep, appetite, concentration, and activity levels).
► Can include worthlessness and hopelessness.

General Considerations

The incidence of depression in children increases with age, from 1% to 3% before puberty to around 9% for adolescents, and this is likely even higher in patients seen in primary care. Over the course of adolescence, 20% of individuals will experience depression. The rate of depression in females approaches adult levels by age 15, and the lifetime risk of depression ranges from 10% to 25% for women and 5% to 12% for men. The sex incidence is equal in childhood, but with the onset of puberty, the rates of depression for females begin to exceed those for males. The incidence of depression in children is higher when other family members have been affected by depressive disorders.

Identification & Diagnosis

Clinical depression can be defined as a persistent state of unhappiness or misery that interferes with pleasure or productivity. Children and younger adolescents are more likely to present with an irritable mood state and older adolescents with a sad mood like adults. Typically, a child or adolescent with depression begins to look unhappy and may make comments such as "I have no friends," "life is boring," "there is nothing I can do to make things better," or "I wish I were dead." Behavior patterns change from baseline and can include social isolation, deterioration in schoolwork, loss of interest in usual activities, anger, and irritability. Sleep and appetite patterns commonly change, and the child may complain of tiredness and nonspecific pain such as headaches, stomach aches, or musculoskeletal pains.

Clinical depression is typically identified by asking about the symptoms. Adolescents are often more accurate than their caregivers in describing their own mood state. When several depressive symptoms cluster together over time, are persistent (≥ 2 weeks), and cause impairment, a major depressive disorder may be present. When depressive symptoms are of lesser severity but have persisted for 1 year or more, a diagnosis of dysthymic disorder should be considered. Milder symptoms of short duration in response to some stressful life event may be consistent with a diagnosis of adjustment disorder with depressed mood. Table 7–13 describes some symptoms of depression as they may appear in children and adolescents.

The AAP recommends annual screening for depression in children aged 12 and older using a standardized measure. The Patient Health Questionnaire-9 modified for adolescents (PHQ-A) is a commonly used validated self-report rating scale that is easily used in primary care to assist in assessment

Table 7–13. Clinical manifestations of depression in children and adolescents.

Depressive Symptom	Clinical Manifestations
Anhedonia	Loss of interest and enthusiasm in play, socializing, school, and usual activities; boredom; loss of pleasure
Dysphoric mood	Tearfulness; sad, downturned expression; unhappiness; slumped posture; quick temper; irritability; anger
Fatigability	Lethargy and tiredness; no play after school
Morbid ideation	Self-deprecating thoughts, statements; thoughts of disaster, abandonment, death, suicide, or hopelessness
Somatic symptoms	Changes in sleep or appetite patterns; difficulty in concentrating; bodily complaints, particularly headache, and stomachache

Table 7–14. Targets to improve depression.

Positive lifestyle changes (improve sleep hygiene, exercise, nutrition)
Positive parenting
Increase supports at school
Address stressors
Support positive peer relationships

and monitoring response to treatment and is available in the public domain.

Treatment

Treatment varies by severity level. Children and adolescents with mild depression should receive close monitoring over several weeks and psychoeducation that includes caregivers. The treatment team (patient, caregiver, and provider) may be able to identify targets for change that may improve depression. See Table 7–14.

Treatment for moderate to severe depression includes developing a comprehensive plan to treat the depressive episode, help the family to respond effectively to the patient's emotional needs, and build supports within the school setting if needed. Referrals should be considered for individual and possibly adjunctive family therapy. CBT and interpersonal therapy (IPT) both have evidence for improving depressive symptoms in children and adolescents. CBT includes a focus on building coping skills to change negative thought patterns that predominate in depressive conditions. It also helps identify, label, and verbalize feelings and misperceptions. In therapy, efforts are also made to resolve conflicts between family members and improve communication skills within the family.

Mild to moderate depressive symptoms often improve with psychotherapy alone. When the symptoms of depression are moderate and persistent, or severe, antidepressant medications may be indicated (see Table 7–11). A positive family history of depression increases the risk of early-onset depression in children and adolescents and the chances of a positive response to antidepressant medication. Depression in toddlers and young children is best approached with parent–child relational therapies.

The carefully conducted Treatment of Adolescent Depression Study (TADS) is a major source of evidence for clinic guidelines regarding the treatment of depression in children and adolescents. This study found that CBT combined with fluoxetine led to the best outcomes in the treatment of pediatric depression during the first 12 weeks of treatment. Although our knowledge is still evolving, these findings suggest that when recommending or prescribing an antidepressant, the provider should consider concurrently recommending CBT or IPT. Providers should discuss the options for medication treatment, including which medications have FDA approval for pediatric indications (see Table 7–6). Target symptoms should be carefully monitored for improvement or worsening, and it is important to ask and document the responses about any suicidal thinking and self-injurious behaviors.

▶ Special Considerations Regarding the Use of Antidepressant Medication

There are some special considerations when prescribing the various classes of antidepressant medication. Table 7–11 outlines the distinct differences between some of the most used antidepressant medications.

A. Selective Serotonin Reuptake Inhibitors

Each SSRI has different FDA indications. Providers can choose to treat with an SSRI that has not received FDA approval for a specific indication or age group. Typical considerations for using a medication without FDA approval include the side-effect profile and/or whether another family member has responded to a specific medication. In these instances, providers should inform the patient and family that they are using a medication off-label.

The therapeutic response for SSRIs should be expected 4–6 weeks after a therapeutic dose has been reached although many individuals may experience partial or full benefit earlier. The starting dose for a child younger than 12 years is generally half the starting dose for an adolescent, but young children may eventually need doses similar to adolescents or adults. Pharmacokinetic studies suggest that SSRIs may be metabolized faster in young children, leading to shorter half-lives. SSRIs are usually given once a day, in the morning with breakfast, but lower doses of sertraline should be administered twice daily. Individuals who experience sedation (1 in 10) or find mornings difficult to remember to take their medication may prefer to take the medication at bedtime. Caution should be used in cases of known liver disease, or chronic or severe illness where multiple medications may be prescribed, because SSRIs are metabolized in the liver. In addition, caution should be used when prescribing for an individual with a family history of bipolar disorder, or when the differential diagnosis includes bipolar disorder, because antidepressants can induce manic or hypomanic symptoms.

Adverse effects of SSRIs are often dose related and time limited: GI distress and nausea (can be minimized by taking medication with food), headache, tremulousness, decreased appetite, weight loss, insomnia, sedation (10%), and sexual dysfunction (25%). Irritability, social disinhibition, restlessness, and emotional excitability can occur in approximately 20% of children taking SSRIs, and activation is more likely to occur with preadolescent children. It is important to systematically monitor for side effects. SSRIs other than fluoxetine should be discontinued slowly to minimize withdrawal symptoms including flu-like symptoms, dizziness, headaches, paresthesia, and emotional lability.

All SSRIs inhibit the hepatic microsomal enzyme system. The order of inhibition is fluoxetine > fluvoxamine > paroxetine > sertraline > citalopram > escitalopram. This can lead to higher-than-expected blood levels of concomitant medications. Taking tryptophan while on an SSRI may result in serotonergic syndrome of psychomotor agitation and GI distress. A potentially fatal interaction that clinically resembles neuroleptic malignant syndrome (NMS) may occur when SSRIs are administered concomitantly with monoamine oxidase inhibitors (MAOIs). Fluoxetine has the longest half-life of the SSRIs and should not be initiated within 14 days of the discontinuation of an MAOI, or an MAOI initiated within at least 5 weeks of the discontinuation of fluoxetine. One should be cautious of prescribing SSRIs in conjunction with ibuprofen and other nonsteroidal anti-inflammatory drugs (NSAIDs) for concerns of GI or other bleeding.

B. Serotonin Norepinephrine Reuptake Inhibitors

Serotonin norepinephrine reuptake inhibitors (SNRIs), which include venlafaxine, duloxetine, desvenlafaxine, and milnacipran, are antidepressants that primarily inhibit reuptake of serotonin and norepinephrine. Desvenlafaxine is the major active metabolite of the antidepressant venlafaxine. It is approved for the treatment of major depression in adults. Contraindications for this class of medication include hypertension, which is typically dose related. SNRIs also can increase heart rate. The most common adverse effects are nausea, nervousness, and sweating. SNRIs should be discontinued slowly to minimize withdrawal symptoms, including flu-like symptoms, dizziness, headaches, paresthesia, and emotional lability. The treatment of resistant depression study in adolescents (TORDIA) compared switching adolescents with depression who had not responded to initial treatment with an SSRI to another SSRI, venlafaxine, or medication plus placebo. Response rates were best for the combination (therapy plus medication) arm but did not differ between the two medications arms. However, the patients treated with venlafaxine experienced more skin problems and elevated blood pressure and heart rate. Duloxetine has been associated with severe skin reactions such as erythema multiforme and Stevens-Johnson syndrome, and venlafaxine has been associated with interstitial lung disease and eosinophilic pneumonia and increased suicidal ideation.

C. Other Antidepressants

Bupropion is an antidepressant that inhibits uptake of norepinephrine and dopamine approved for treatment of major depression in adults. Like the SSRIs, bupropion has very few anticholinergic or cardiotoxic effects. The medication has three different formulations, and consideration for use is based on tolerability and compliance. Bupropion can interfere with sleep, so dosing earlier in the day is paramount to adherence and decreasing side effects. Contraindications of this medication include history of seizure disorder or bulimia nervosa. The most common adverse effects include psychomotor activation (agitation or restlessness), headache, GI distress, nausea, anorexia with weight loss, insomnia, tremulousness, precipitation of mania, and induction of seizures with doses above 450 mg/day.

Mirtazapine is an α_2-antagonist that enhances central noradrenergic and serotonergic activity approved for the treatment of major depression in adults. Mirtazapine should not be given in combination with MAOIs. Very rare side effects are acute liver failure (1 case per 250,000–300,000), neutropenia, and agranulocytosis. More common adverse effects include dry mouth, increased appetite, constipation, weight gain, and increased sedation.

TCAs are an older class of antidepressants, which include imipramine, desipramine, clomipramine, nortriptyline, and amitriptyline. The lack of demonstrated efficacy, high-risk side-effect profile, and potential for lethality with overdose have led steering committees and professional organizations to recommend that primary care providers not prescribe TCAs for depression in children and adolescents. Providers should not be confused by FDA approval of imipramine and desipramine for enuresis in children aged 6 years and older.

▶ Other Considerations

The risk of suicide is the most significant side effect associated with depressive episodes. In addition, adolescents with depression are at higher risk for substance misuse and engaging in self-injurious behaviors such as cutting or burning themselves (without suicidal intent). School performance usually suffers during a depressive episode, as children are unable to concentrate or motivate themselves to complete homework or projects. The irritability, isolation, and withdrawal that often result from the depressive episode can lead to loss of peer relationships and tense dynamics within the family. Refer to section on identifying and addressing suicide risk for additional information.

Depression often coexists with other mental illnesses such as ADHD, ODD, conduct disorder, anxiety disorders, eating disorders, and substance abuse disorders. Medically ill patients also have an increased incidence of depression. Every child and adolescent with depressed mood should be asked directly about suicidal ideation, physical and sexual abuse, and substance use. Depressed adolescents should also be screened for hypothyroidism.

In 2005, the FDA issued a "black box warning" regarding suicidal thinking and behavior for all antidepressants prescribed for children and adolescents. Data from 24 short-term trials of 4–16 weeks that included the use of antidepressants for major depressive disorder or OCD found the risk of suicidal thinking and behavior during the first few months of treatment was 4%, twice the placebo risk of 2% and there was indication in original combined analysis that paroxetine had a higher risk for suicidal thoughts and behaviors. No suicides occurred in these trials. Subsequent meta-analysis estimated this risk to be lower. Although children face an initial

increased risk of suicidal thinking and behaviors during the first few months of treatment, there is now substantial evidence that antidepressant treatment, over time, is protective against suicide. Best practice is to educate the patient and family regarding both the risks and benefits of antidepressant treatment and monitor carefully for any increase in suicidal ideation or self-injurious urges, as well as improvement in target symptoms of depression, especially in the first 4 weeks and subsequent 3 months after beginning their use.

▶ Prognosis

A comprehensive treatment intervention, including psychoeducation for the family, individual and family psychotherapy, medication assessment, and evaluation of school and home environments, often leads to complete remission of depressive symptoms over a 1- to 2-month period. If medications are started and proven effective, they should be continued for 6–12 months after remission of symptoms to prevent relapse. Early-onset depression (before age 15) is associated with increased risk of recurrent episodes and the potential need for longer-term treatment with antidepressants. Education of the family and child/or adolescent will help them identify depressive symptoms sooner and decrease the severity of future episodes with earlier interventions. Some studies suggest that up to 30% of preadolescents with major depression manifest bipolar disorder at 2-year follow-up. Psychotic symptoms during depression, early-onset depression, and family history of bipolar disorder all increase the risk for bipolar disorder. It is important to reassess the child or adolescent with depressive symptoms regularly for at least 6 months and to maintain awareness of the depressive episode in caring for this child in the future.

2. Disruptive Mood Dysregulation Disorder

ESSENTIALS OF DIAGNOSIS & TYPICAL FEATURES

▶ Persistent irritability and severe behavioral outbursts at least three times a week for 1 year or more.

▶ The mood in between these symptoms is persistently negative (ie, irritable, angry, or sad), which is observable by others.

▶ The tantrums and negative moods are present in at least two settings.

▶ Onset of illness prior to 10 years old.

▶ Chronological or developmental age of at least 6 years old.

▶ A disruption in functioning in more than one setting (eg, home, school, and/or socially).

General Considerations

The prevalence is estimated to be 2%–5% and may decrease from childhood to adolescence. Early studies suggest males are at increased risk for this disorder. Prior to adding this diagnosis to DSM-5, many of these chronically irritable children would have been diagnosed with some variation of bipolar mood disorder; however, evidence from studies of the family history, functional brain studies, and developmental progression suggests that these children are different from individuals with bipolar disorder.

Identification & Diagnosis

Children with DMDD experience severe tantrums in addition to chronic irritability in at least 2 settings. The tantrums must be inconsistent with the developmental age of the child. DMDD cannot be given to individuals older than 18 or younger than 6. Onset must occur by age 10 years. In cases where symptoms overlap between DMDD and ODD; DMDD supersedes ODD. Children who have experienced a manic or hypomanic episode cannot be given this diagnosis. Tantrums that occur only in relation to anxiety-provoking situations or when routines are interrupted suggest a diagnosis of anxiety, autism spectrum disorder, or OCD, and do not meet criteria for DMDD.

Treatment

Psychoeducation can help families engage and remain in treatment when they are often desperate for rapid improvement. These children can be challenging to parent and therapy that includes a parenting component is highly recommended. Identifying and treating comorbid conditions is also vital, especially given the high rates of comorbidity for these patients. Medication trials for this relatively new diagnosis are few but suggest methylphenidate may be effective in reducing symptoms (open-label trial), and the addition of citalopram to methylphenidate treatment may further reduce temper tantrum severity (randomized placebo-controlled trial). Providers may be tempted to try antipsychotics but, given the side-effect profile and lack of evidence, are encouraged to exhaust the above recommendations first.

Other Considerations

The differential diagnosis for DMDD is similar to other mood disorders. Patients with suspected DMDD should be screened for ADHD, anxiety, trauma, learning or communication difficulties, and significant interpersonal and relational deficits. Those with DMDD are at a higher risk than the general population to develop major depressive disorder and anxiety disorders as adults.

Children with DMDD have low frustration tolerance and may misread neutral social cues as threatening. They often function poorly in school and have impaired relations with peers and family. Parents or caregivers of these children are often distressed, and these families tend to seek mental health treatment. Many parents will decrease the demands and limits placed on these children to avoid tantrums. This can include withdrawing their children from developmentally appropriate health promoting activities. Children with DMDD often have dangerous behaviors that lead to psychiatric hospitalization.

2. Bipolar & Related Disorders

ESSENTIALS OF DIAGNOSIS & TYPICAL FEATURES

► Periods of abnormally and persistently elevated, expansive, or irritable mood, and heightened levels of energy and activity.
► Associated symptoms: grandiosity, diminished need for sleep, pressured speech, racing thoughts, impaired judgment.
► Manic symptoms last at least 1 week.
► Not caused by prescribed or illicit drugs.
► Depressive symptoms are commonly reported first.

General Considerations

Onset of bipolar disorder before puberty is uncommon; however, symptoms often begin to develop and may be initially diagnosed as ADHD or disruptive behavior disorders. The lifetime prevalence of bipolar disorder in middle to late adolescence is still low, at 1%–2%, yet it is important to be vigilant as at least 20% of adults with bipolar disorder experience the onset of symptoms before age 20.

Identification & Diagnosis

In about 70% of patients with bipolar disorder, the first symptoms are primarily those of depression. In the remainder, mania, hypomania, or mixed states dominate the presentation. Patients with mania display a variable pattern of elevated, expansive, or irritable mood along with rapid speech, high energy levels, increase in goal-directed activity, difficulty sustaining concentration, and a decreased need for sleep often including lack of fatigue the following day. The child or adolescent may also exhibit hypersexual behavior. It is critical to rule out abuse. Patients with bipolar disorder often do not acknowledge any problem with their mood or behavior, but the change from baseline is notable to others. The clinical picture can be quite dramatic, with florid psychotic symptoms of delusions and hallucinations accompanying extreme hyperactivity and impulsivity. Hypomanic episodes, characteristic of bipolar II disorder, are lower-intensity manic episodes that do not cause social impairment and do not typically last as long as manic episodes. Although common, the co-occurrence of depression with bipolar I disorder is not a diagnostic requirement, while it is for bipolar II disorder. Cyclothymic disorder is diagnosed when the child or adolescent has 1 year of hypomanic symptoms alternating with depressive symptoms that do not meet criteria for a major depressive or hypomanic episode. Symptoms must be interpreted within a developmental context and differentiated from the normal moods and mood changes that occur in childhood and adolescence. Note that other specified bipolar and related disorder criteria describe youth who have hypomania but have not met full criteria for depression, or youth with shorter duration of manic symptoms (2–3 days).

The Mania Rating Scale (Child, CMRS, Youth YMRS, and Parent P-YMRS) can be useful as an additional tool to help patients and families describe moods, but providers should keep in mind that these are not specific. Parent reports of symptoms are typically more diagnostically helpful than patient or teacher reports.

Treatment

It is recommended that primary care providers refer all patients with suspected bipolar mood disorder to a mental health provider for diagnostic clarification and treatment. In situations where bipolar mood disorder is evident, a referral to a psychiatrist is recommended. In cases of severe impairment, hospitalization is required to maintain safety and initiate treatment. Other levels of care that may be appropriate with less severe presentations include day treatment, intensive outpatient therapy (two to three times per week), in home therapy, or routine outpatient therapy. Once stabilization is achieved, it is reasonable for a primary care provider to offer medication management preferably with ongoing access to a child and adolescent psychiatrist if symptoms worsen.

Pediatricians should reinforce the need for ongoing treatments, provide additional psychoeducation, health maintenance, and surveillance for associated problems such as substance misuse, sexually transmitted diseases, and encouraging other supports such as a 504 plan or IEP if indicated.

Psychotherapy and medication are the mainstay of treatment. Medications are chosen based on current symptoms, side effects, family preference, and differ by polarity of symptoms (depression vs mania). The best evidence for treatment for mania is with second-generation antipsychotics, followed by lithium. Nonresponders may require a combination of medications. Lithium, risperidone, aripiprazole, quetiapine, asenapine, and olanzapine have been approved by the FDA for the treatment of acute and mixed manic episodes in adolescents. Other mood stabilizers, lamotrigine, carbamazepine, and valproate are less effective. Lithium and aripiprazole are approved for preventing recurrence.

Patients with bipolar disorder experience depressive symptoms that can be challenging to treat. It is generally recommended that patients should be on a mood stabilizer. At least one mood stabilizer is approved for pediatric bipolar depression (lurasidone). Patients with bipolar disorder who experience a mild depression should receive therapy and other interventions prior to considering adding an antidepressant (refer to depression section) to a second-generation antipsychotic or other mood stabilizer. Choices for additional antidepressants, if the patient fails monotherapy, are like those for depression (see section on depression).

Therapy for children and adolescents with bipolar disorder generally includes psychoeducation, and there is evidence that psychoeducation alone may have some benefit. More recent studies with youth who met criteria for bipolar I and II disorders found family-focused therapy (FFT) to be effective with outcomes related to bipolar depression and mania. Youth at risk for bipolar disorder, based on parent diagnosis, experienced improved outcomes related to hypomania symptoms. Components of this therapy include (1) psychoeducational activities such as monitoring symptoms, recognizing triggers, and the importance of continuing medications, and (2) improving family communication with a focus on problem solving skills, appropriate expression of emotion, and developing and maintaining routines. Other therapies with some evidence include CBT, DBT, interpersonal and social rhythm therapy, and other family therapies.

Other Considerations

Physical or sexual abuse and exposure to domestic violence can also cause children to be moody, labile, hyperactive, and aggressive. PTSD should be considered by reviewing the history of traumatic life events in children with these symptoms. DMDD, ADHD, ODD, and conduct disorder can be difficult to differentiate from bipolar and related disorders. The timing of onset of symptoms, severity and chronicity of irritability, and relation of oppositional or conduct behaviors to mood symptoms can help with this differentiation. For adolescents who are misusing substances, it is important to differentiate if mood symptoms of bipolar are "driving" the substance misuse or substance misuse is leading to mood symptoms. Individuals with manic psychosis may resemble those with schizophrenia or schizoaffective disorder. Psychotic symptoms associated with bipolar disorder should clear with resolution of the mood symptoms, which should also be prominent. Patients with mood lability may have a developing personality disorder. Many patients with bipolar disorder experience a worsening of anxiety with mood episodes. Further complicating this diagnostic difficulty is the relatively high likelihood of comorbid disorders for youth with bipolar disorder. Providers should not miss medical causes of symptoms such as hyperthyroidism, head trauma, and rare presentations of tumors. This is especially relevant if the change in personality has been relatively sudden or is accompanied by other neurologic changes.

Prognosis

The chance of recovery from the mood episode of a bipolar illness that results in diagnosis (index episode) is high (80%), but many youth will experience a recurrence (60%) most likely in the same polarity (depression or mania) as the index episode and are likely to be symptomatic 60% of the time. Early onset, low socioeconomic status, comorbid illness, and family history of mood disorders all are risk factors for worse outcomes. Children and adolescents diagnosed with cyclothymia are at risk of developing bipolar I or II disorder, and youth with bipolar I or II disorder may also change diagnostic categories over time.

Children and adolescents with bipolar illness are at risk for poorer academic, social, legal, and health outcomes. The poor judgment associated with manic episodes predisposes individuals to dangerous, impulsive, and sometimes criminal activity. Legal difficulties can arise from impulsive acts, such as excessive spending and acts of vandalism, theft, or aggression, that are associated with grandiose thoughts. Affective disorders are associated with a 30-fold greater incidence of suicide. Substance misuse and associated risks also may lead to poor outcomes.

DISRUPTIVE, IMPULSE-CONTROL, & CONDUCT DISORDERS

1. Oppositional Defiant Disorder

> ### ESSENTIALS OF DIAGNOSIS & TYPICAL FEATURES
>
> ▶ A pattern of negativistic, hostile, and defiant behavior lasting at least 6 months.
> ▶ Loses temper, argues with adults, defies rules.
> ▶ Blames others for their own mistakes and misbehavior.
> ▶ Angry, easily annoyed, vindictive.
> ▶ Does not meet criteria for conduct disorder.

General Considerations

ODD is more common in families where caregiver, family-level, and/or environmental dysfunction (eg, substance misuse, parental psychopathology, significant psychosocial stress) is present. It is also more prevalent in children with a history of multiple changes in primary caregivers, inconsistent, harsh, or neglectful parenting, abuse, exposure to violence, or serious caregiver relational discord.

Identification & Diagnosis

ODD is usually evident before 8 years of age and may be an antecedent to the development of conduct disorder. The symptoms usually first emerge at home but then extend to school and peer relationships. The disruptive behaviors of ODD are generally less severe than those associated with conduct disorder and do not include hurting individuals or animals, destruction of property, or theft.

Treatment

Interventions include careful assessment of the psychosocial situation and recommendations to support parenting skills and optimal caregiver functioning. Assessment for comorbid psychiatric diagnoses such as learning disabilities, depression, and ADHD should be pursued, and appropriate interventions recommended.

2. Conduct Disorder

> ### ESSENTIALS OF DIAGNOSIS & TYPICAL FEATURES
>
> ▶ A persistent pattern of behavior that includes the following:
>   • Defiance of authority.
>   • Violating the rights of others or societal norms.
>   • Aggressive behavior toward people, animals, or property.

General Considerations

Disorders of conduct affect approximately 9% of males and 2% of females younger than 18 years. This is a very heterogeneous population, and overlap occurs with ADHD, substance misuse, learning disabilities, neuropsychiatric disorders, mood disorders, and family dysfunction. Many of these individuals come from homes where domestic violence, child abuse, substance misuse, shifting parental figures, and poverty are environmental risk factors. Although social learning partly explains this correlation, the genetic heritability of aggressive conduct and antisocial behaviors is currently under investigation.

Identification & Diagnosis

The prototypical child with conduct disorder is a boy with a turbulent home life and academic difficulties. Defiance of authority, fighting, tantrums, running away, school failure, and destruction of property are common symptoms. With increasing age, fire-setting and theft may occur, followed in adolescence by truancy, vandalism, and substance misuse.

Sexual promiscuity, sexual perpetration, and other criminal behaviors may also develop. Hyperactive, aggressive, and uncooperative behavior patterns in the preschool and early school years tend to predict conduct disorder in adolescence with a high degree of accuracy, especially when ADHD goes untreated. A history of reactive attachment disorder is an additional childhood risk factor. The risk for conduct disorder increases with inconsistent and severe parental disciplinary techniques, parental alcoholism, and parental antisocial behavior.

Treatment

Effective treatment can be complicated by the psychosocial problems often found in the lives of children and adolescents with conduct disorders. These problems may also interfere with achieving compliance with treatment recommendations. Multisystemic therapy (MST) can be an effective intervention. MST is an intensive home-based model of care that seeks to stabilize and improve the home environment while strengthening the support system and coping skills of the individual and family.

Identification of learning disabilities and placement in an optimal school environment is critical. Any associated neurologic and psychiatric disorders should be addressed. Juvenile justice system involvement is common in cases where conduct disorder behaviors lead to illegal activities, theft, or assault.

Medications such as mood stabilizers, antipsychotics, stimulants, and antidepressants have all been studied in youth with conduct disorders, yet none has been found to be consistently effective. Each patient suspected of conduct disorder should be screened for a history of trauma and other common psychiatric disorders before medication initiation. Providers should use caution when prescribing various medications off-label for disruptive behavior. Early involvement in programs, such as Big Brothers, Big Sisters, scouts, and team sports, in which consistent adult mentors and role models interact with youth, decreases the chances that the youth will develop antisocial personality disorder.

Other Considerations

Young people with conduct disorders, especially those with more violent histories, have an increased incidence of neurologic signs and symptoms, seizures, psychotic symptoms, mood disorders, ADHD, and learning disabilities. Efforts should be made to identify these associated disorders because they may require specific therapeutic interventions. Conduct disorder is best conceptualized as a final common pathway emerging from a variety of underlying psychosocial, genetic, environmental, and neuropsychiatric conditions.

Prognosis

The prognosis is based on the ability of the child's support system to mount an effective treatment intervention

consistently over time. The prognosis is generally worse for children in whom the disorder presents before age 10 years; those who display a diversity of antisocial behaviors across multiple settings; and those who are raised in an environment characterized by parental antisocial behavior, alcoholism or other substance misuse, and conflict. Nearly one-half of individuals with a childhood diagnosis of conduct disorder develop antisocial personality disorder as adults. The diagnosis of conduct disorder is based on behaviors; antisocial personality disorder includes a pervasive history of these behaviors beginning at age 15, and current markers of sociopathy such as willful deceit, lack of remorse, and manipulation in individuals greater than 18.

SOMATIC SYMPTOM & RELATED DISORDERS

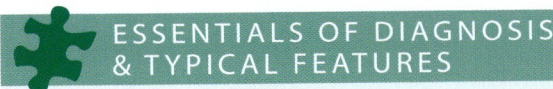

ESSENTIALS OF DIAGNOSIS & TYPICAL FEATURES

► Medically unexplained symptoms are no longer required for these disorders other than conversion disorder. Most disorders in this category are characterized by focus on symptoms within a medical setting.

► Distress and/or functional impairment are present in somatic symptom disorder while functional impairment is more common in conversion disorder.

General Considerations

The category of somatic symptoms and related disorders includes somatic symptom disorder, illness anxiety disorder, conversion disorder (functional neurologic symptom disorder), psychological factors affecting other medical conditions, factitious disorder, and factitious disorder imposed by another (Table 7–15).

Patients with these disorders are commonly encountered in primary care and can be conceptualized as suffering; differences in presentation are likely related to cultural, contextual factors, individual experiences such as trauma, and individual differences such as pain sensitivity. Families and cultures that value physical suffering while devaluing or ignoring psychological distress reinforce the development of these disorders. Family members who are ill, physically disabled, or suffer from any of these disorders can serve as models for children. More extreme parental dysfunction can manifest as factitious disorder imposed on another with the child as the victim.

Identification & Diagnosis

Somatic symptom disorder often presents in school age children and adolescents with the somatic symptom of headaches

Table 7–15. Somatoform disorders in children and adolescents.

Disorder	Major Clinical Manifestations
Somatic symptom disorder, factitious disorder, other specified somatic symptom and related disorder, unspecified somatic symptom and related disorder	A somatic symptom or symptoms cause significant distress, worry, and concern, and may take up considerable time and energy.
Conversion disorder (functional neurologic symptom disorder)	Symptom onset follows psychologically stressful event; symptoms express unconscious feelings and result in secondary gain.
Illness anxiety disorder	Somatic symptoms if present are mild. Focus is on fear of having or developing an illness leading to maladaptive behaviors.
Psychological factors affecting other medical conditions	Psychological or behavioral factors negatively impact a medical illness.
Factitious disorder or factitious disorder imposed on another	Deliberate false presentation of oneself or another (or causing in oneself or another) signs or symptoms of a physical or psychological problem.

or GI distress. Conversion symptoms involve alterations in voluntary motor or sensory function and are often more transient in pediatric patients than adults. Common symptoms include unusual sensory phenomena, paralysis, and movement or seizure-like disorders. A conversion symptom is thought to be an expression of underlying psychological conflict. The specific symptom may be symbolically determined by the underlying conflict and may resolve the dilemma created by the underlying wish or fear (eg, a seemingly paralyzed child need not fear expressing his or her underlying rage or aggressive retaliatory impulses).

Children with conversion disorder may be surprisingly unconcerned about the substantial disability deriving from their symptoms. Symptoms include unusual sensory phenomena, paralysis, vomiting, abdominal pain, intractable headaches, and movement or seizure-like disorders. For both somatic symptom disorder and conversion disorder, the physical symptoms often begin with a stressful event at school, with peers or within the family such as serious illness, a death, or family discord.

▶ **Treatment**

Medical providers are often the first to see the patient and identify these disorders. Many of these patients can be treated within the pediatric primary care setting, utilizing the relationship between the pediatric provider and the family to maximize outcomes. For those who need referral to other settings, ongoing care by the pediatrician can help ensure families engage in other indicated treatments.

In most cases, conversion symptoms resolve quickly when the child and family are reassured that the symptom is a way of reacting to stress. The child is encouraged to continue with normal daily activities, knowing that the symptoms will abate when the stress is resolved. Treatment of conversion disorders includes acknowledging the symptom rather than responding with noninvasive interventions such as physical therapy while continuing to encourage normalization of the symptoms. If the symptom does not resolve with reassurance, further investigation by a mental health professional is indicated. Comorbid diagnoses such as depression and anxiety disorders should be addressed, and treatment with psychopharmacologic agents may be helpful.

Somatic symptom disorder patients may respond to the same treatment. If the family structure or the patient cannot tolerate psychological approaches, somatic symptom patients may respond to regular, short, scheduled medical appointments to address the complaints at hand. In this way they do not need to precipitate emergencies to elicit medical attention. The medical provider should avoid invasive procedures unless clearly indicated and offer sincere concern and reassurance. The provider should also avoid telling the patient "It's all in your head" and should not abandon or avoid the patient, as somatic symptom disorder patients, and their parents, are at great risk of seeking multiple alternative treatment providers and potentially unnecessary treatments. Many parents worry about their child developing or having a serious illness. These families may also benefit from the above approach, in conjunction with encouragement for the pediatric patient to engage in health promoting activities such as involvement in sports.

Treatment for patients who are suffering from psychological factors impacting illness should be targeted to the underlying problem, such as treatment of anxious avoidance, motivational interviewing to target substance abuse, or adherence problems.

Health care providers who suspect factitious disorder imposed on another may need to involve a specialist to confirm the diagnosis. Communication between providers is critical to helping these patients. Child protective services and legal counsel may also need to be alerted. Although parents who are perpetrating factitious disorder imposed on another can appear concerned about the well-being of their child, studies have found child victims' mental health and well-being improved when they were removed from extreme perpetrating caregivers.

▶ **Other Considerations**

Somatic symptoms are often associated with anxiety and depressive disorders. Occasionally, children experiencing psychosis have somatic preoccupations and even somatic delusions.

Children with conversion disorder may have some secondary gain associated with their symptoms. Several reports have pointed to the increased association of conversion disorder with sexual overstimulation or sexual abuse. As with other emotional and behavioral problems, health care providers should always screen for physical and sexual abuse.

► Prognosis

Prognosis is dependent on family factors, age, and disorder. Parents who support the view that symptoms can be related to stress can help patients engage in appropriate treatments. Younger patients with conversion symptoms have better prognosis than older patients with somatic symptom disorder. Patients who have had the disorder for a longer period may be less responsive to treatment. Psychiatric consultation can be helpful and is indicated for severely incapacitated patients.

PSYCHOTIC DISORDERS

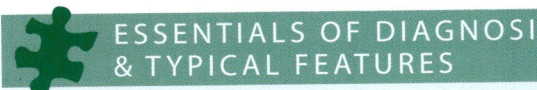

ESSENTIALS OF DIAGNOSIS & TYPICAL FEATURES

- ► Delusional thoughts.
- ► Disorganized speech (rambling or illogical speech patterns).
- ► Disorganized or bizarre behavior.
- ► Hallucinations (auditory, visual, tactile, olfactory).
- ► Paranoia, ideas of reference (belief that random occurrences in the world directly relate to oneself).
- ► Negative symptoms (ie, flat affect, avolition, alogia).

► General Considerations

The prevalence of schizophrenia is about 1 per 10,000 with onset typically between the middle to late teens and early 30s. Symptoms usually begin after puberty, although a full "psychotic break" may not occur until the young adult years. Childhood onset (before puberty) of psychotic symptoms due to schizophrenia is rare and usually indicates a more severe form of the spectrum of schizophrenic disorders. Childhood-onset schizophrenia is more likely to be found in boys.

Schizophrenia has a strong genetic component. Other psychotic disorders that may be encountered in childhood or adolescence include schizoaffective disorder and unspecified psychosis. Unspecified psychosis may be used as a differential diagnosis when psychotic symptoms are present, but the cluster of symptoms is not consistent with a schizophrenia diagnosis.

► Identification & Diagnosis

Children and adolescents display many of the symptoms of adult schizophrenia. Hallucinations or delusions, bizarre and morbid thought content, and rambling and illogical speech are typical. Affected individuals tend to withdraw into an internal world of fantasy and may then equate fantasy with external reality. They generally have difficulty with schoolwork and with family and peer relationships. Adolescents may experience a prodromal period of depression prior to the onset of psychotic symptoms. Most individuals with childhood-onset schizophrenia have had nonspecific psychiatric symptoms or symptoms of delayed development for months or years prior to the onset of their overtly psychotic symptoms.

Obtaining a family history of mental illness is critical when assessing children and adolescents with psychotic symptoms. Psychological testing, particularly the use of projective measures that involve presenting ambiguous stimuli, for example, the Rorschach, is often helpful in identifying or ruling out psychotic thought processes. Psychotic symptoms in children younger than 8 years must be differentiated from manifestations of normal vivid fantasy life or abuse-related symptoms. Children with psychotic disorders often have learning and attention disabilities, in addition to disorganized thoughts, delusions, and hallucinations. In adolescents experiencing psychosis, mania is differentiated by high levels of energy, excitement, and irritability. Any child or adolescent exhibiting new psychotic symptoms requires a medical evaluation consisting of physical and neurologic examinations that include consideration of magnetic resonance imaging and electroencephalogram, drug screening, and metabolic screening for endocrinopathies, Wilson disease, and delirium. Sudden onset of symptoms with rapid decline can be indicative of autoimmune encephalitis, especially when accompanied by motor symptoms or rapid change in cognition.

► Treatment

The treatment of childhood and adolescent schizophrenia focuses on four main areas: (1) decreasing active psychotic symptoms, (2) supporting development of social and cognitive skills, (3) reducing the risk of relapse of psychotic symptoms, and (4) providing support and education to parents and family members. Antipsychotic medications are the primary psychopharmacologic intervention. In addition, a supportive, reality-oriented focus in relationships can help to reduce hallucinations, delusions, and frightening thoughts. In situations where psychosis is evident, a referral to a psychiatrist is recommended. In cases of severe impairment, hospitalization is required to maintain safety and initiate treatment. A special school or day treatment environment may be necessary, depending on the child's or adolescent's ability to tolerate the school day and classroom activities. Support for the family emphasizes the importance of clear, focused communication and an emotionally calm climate in preventing recurrences of overtly psychotic symptoms.

Special Considerations Regarding the Use of Antipsychotic Medication

While it is expected that a psychiatrist will initiate treatment, primary care providers undoubtedly treat children on antipsychotics and should become familiar with management of potential common and severe side effects of this class of medication. The "atypical or second-generation antipsychotics" differ from conventional antipsychotics in their receptor specificity and effect on serotonin receptors. Conventional antipsychotics are associated with a higher incidence of movement disorders and extrapyramidal symptoms due to their wider effect on dopamine receptors. The atypical antipsychotics have a better side-effect profile for most individuals and comparable efficacy for the treatment of psychotic symptoms and aggression, making them the preferred medications. The information that follows primarily focuses on safe use of atypical antipsychotics.

Common adverse effects of the atypical antipsychotics are cognitive slowing, sedation, orthostasis, dystonia, and weight gain. Most side effects tend to be dose related. Less frequent, but important, side effects are development of type 2 diabetes and change in lipid and cholesterol profile. The risk-benefit ratio of the medication for the target symptom should be carefully considered and reviewed with the parent or guardian. Providers should obtain baseline height, weight, and waist circumference; observe and examine for tremors and other abnormal involuntary movements; and establish baseline values for hemoglobin A_{1C} (HbA_{1C}), complete blood count (CBC), liver function tests (LFTs), and lipid profile. Antipsychotics can cause QT prolongation leading to ventricular arrhythmias. Therefore, it is important to obtain an ECG if there is a history of cardiac disease or arrhythmia. Medications that affect the cytochrome P-450 isoenzyme pathway (including SSRIs) may increase the neuroleptic plasma concentration and increase risk of QTc prolongation.

Table 7–16 presents the currently recommended monitoring calendar. Baseline and ongoing evaluations of significant markers are considered standard clinical practice. Other side effects include irregular menses, gynecomastia, and galactorrhea due to increased prolactin, sexual dysfunction, photosensitivity, rashes, lowered seizure threshold, hepatic dysfunction, and blood dyscrasias.

Additional troublesome side effects of antipsychotics include dystonia, akathisia (characterized by an urge to be in constant motion and difficulty sitting still), pseudo-parkinsonism, and tardive dyskinesia (TD). These side effects typically occur in a stepwise fashion and are also dose related. The first three are reversible and typically relieved by anticholinergic agents, such as benztropine (Cogentin) and diphenhydramine, or β-blockers, specifically for akathisia.

Table 7–16. Health monitoring and antipsychotics.

Baseline	After Initiation			Thereafter[a]		
	4 wk	8 wk	12 wk	Quarterly	Annually	q5y
Personal/family history					✓	
Weight (BMI)	✓	✓	✓	✓		
Waist circumference					✓	
BP			✓		✓	
Fasting blood sugar			✓		✓	
Fasting lipid profile			✓			✓

[a]More frequent assessments may be warranted based on clinical status.

The risk of TD is small in patients on atypical antipsychotics and those on conventional antipsychotics for less than 6 months. There are two FDA-approved medications for TD (ie, valbenazine and deutetrabenazine); however, the recommendation is to either lower the dose of the offending agent or switch to an alternative. Withdrawal dyskinesias are reversible movement disorders that appear following withdrawal of neuroleptic medications. Dyskinetic movements develop within 1–4 weeks after withdrawal of the drug and may persist for months.

A severe side effect of antipsychotics is NMS. NMS is a very rare medical emergency primarily associated with conventional antipsychotics, although it has also been reported with atypical antipsychotics. It is manifested by severe muscular rigidity, mental status changes, fever, autonomic lability, and myoglobinemia. NMS can occur without muscle rigidity in patients taking atypical antipsychotics and should be considered in the differential diagnosis of any patient on antipsychotics who presents with high fever and altered mental status. Mortality rates as high as 30% have been reported. Treatment includes immediate medical assessment and withdrawal of the neuroleptic and may require transfer to an intensive care unit.

In cases of significant weight gain or abnormal laboratory values, patients should either be switched to an agent with a decreased risk for these adverse events or should receive specific treatments for the adverse events when discontinuation of the offending agent is not possible. In general, a child and adolescent psychiatrist should evaluate children with psychosis, initiate treatment, and refer to the pediatrician once symptoms are adequately controlled.

Antipsychotics are also used for acute mania and as adjuncts to antidepressants in the treatment of psychotic depression with delusions or hallucinations. Antipsychotics may also be used cautiously in refractory PTSD, in refractory OCD, and in individuals with markedly aggressive behavioral problems unresponsive to other interventions. In some instances, they may be useful for body image distortion and irrational fears about food and weight gain associated with anorexia nervosa.

Prognosis

Schizophrenia is a chronic disorder with exacerbations and remissions of psychotic symptoms. Generally, earlier onset (prior to age 13 years), poor premorbid functioning (oddness or eccentricity), and predominance of negative symptoms (withdrawal, apathy, or flat affect) over positive symptoms (hallucinations or paranoia) predict more severe disability. Later age of onset, normal social and school functioning prior to onset, and predominance of positive symptoms are associated with better outcomes and life adjustment to the illness.

OTHER PSYCHIATRIC CONDITIONS

Dissociative Disorders occur most frequently in the aftermath of traumatic experiences, can be challenging to diagnose, and are best handled by referral to a specialist. Refer to DSM-5-TR™.

Several psychiatric conditions are covered elsewhere in this book. Refer to the following chapters for detailed discussion:

- ADHD: see Chapter 3.
- Autism and pervasive developmental disorders: see Chapter 3.
- Enuresis and encopresis: see Chapter 3.
- Eating disorders: see Chapter 6.
- Intellectual disability/mental retardation: see Chapter 3.
- Substance abuse: see Chapter 5.
- Sleep disorders: see Chapter 3.
- Tourette syndrome and tic disorders: see Chapter 25.

REFERENCES

Anxiety

Anxiety and Depression Association of America: https://adaa.org/.
Blossom JB, Jungbluth N, Dillon-Naftolin E, French W: Treatment for anxiety disorders in the pediatric primary care setting. Child Adolesc Psychiatr Clin N Am 2023; 32:601–611. doi: 10.1016/j.chc.2023.02.003 [PMID: 37201970].
Nicotra CM, Strawn J: Advances in pharmacotherapy for pediatric anxiety disorders. Child Adolesc Psychiatr Clin N Am 2023;32:573–587. doi: 10.1016/j.chc.2023.02.006 [PMID: 37201968].

Attention-Deficit/Hyperactivity Disorder

AAP Practice Parameter: https://publications.aap.org/pediatrics/article/144/4/e20192528/81590/Clinical-Practice-Guideline-for-the-Diagnosis. Accessed July 6, 2023.
American Academy of Pediatrics: Implementing the key action statements: an algorithm and explanation for process of care for the evaluation, diagnosis, treatment, and monitoring of ADHD in children and adolescents. https://publications.aap.org/toolkits/book/337/chapter-abstract/5731242/The-Algorithm?redirectedFrom=fulltext.
Cortese S et al: Comparative efficacy and tolerability of medications for attention-deficit hyperactivity disorder in children, adolescents, and adults: a systematic review and network meta-analysis. Lancet Psychiatry 2018;5(9):727–738. doi: 10.10/16/S2215-0366(18)30269-4 [PMID: 30097390].
Fay TB, Alpert MA: Cardiovascular effects of drugs used to treat attention-deficit/hyperactivity disorder: part 1: epidemiology, pharmacology, and impact on hemodynamics and ventricular repolarization. Cardiol Rev 2019;27(3):113–121. doi:10.1097/CRD.0000000000000233 [PMID: 30365404].
Fay TB, Alpert MA: Cardiovascular effects of drugs used to treat attention-deficit/hyperactivity disorder: part 2: impact on cardiovascular events and recommendations for evaluation and monitoring. Cardiol Rev 2019;27(4):173–178. doi:10.1097/CRD.0000000000000234 [PMID: 30531411].
FDA press release regarding Trigeminal Nerve Stimulation System: https://www.fda.gov/news-events/press-announcements/fda-permits-marketing-first-medical-device-treatment-adhd.
Goode AP et al: Nonpharmacologic treatments for attention-deficit/hyperactivity disorder: a systematic review. Pediatrics 2018;141(6). doi:10.1542/peds.2018-0094 [PMID: 29848556].
Medication guide with pictures of medications, drug class, time of action and other useful information: https://www.adhdmedicationguide.com.
Wolraich ML et al; Subcommittee on Children and Adolescents With Attention-Deficit/Hyperactive Disorder: Clinical practice guideline for the diagnosis, evaluation, and treatment of attention-deficit/hyperactivity disorder in children and adolescents. Pediatrics 2019;144(4):e20192528 [PMID: 32111626].
Riddle M: New findings from the preschoolers with attention-deficit/hyperactivity disorder treatment study (PATS). J Child Adolesc Psychopharmacol 2007;17(5):543–546.

Bipolar Disorder

Brickman HM, Fristad MA: Psychosocial treatments for bipolar disorder in children and adolescents. Annu Rev Clin Psychol 2022;18:291–327. doi: 10.1146/annurev-clinpsy-072220-021237 [PMID: 35216522].
Shain BN; Committee on Adolescence: Collaborative role of the pediatrician in the diagnosis and management of bipolar disorder in adolescents. Pediatrics 2012;130(6):e1725–e1742. doi:10.1542/peds.2012-2756 [PMID: 23184107].
Stepanova E, Findling RL: Psychopharmacology of bipolar disorders in children and adolescents. 2017;64(6) 1209–1222 [PMID: 29173781].

COVID-19

American Academy of Pediatrics. AAP-AACAP-CHA declaration of a national emergency in child and adolescent mental health. October 19, 2021. https://www.aap.org/en/advocacy/child-and-adolescent-healthy-mental-development/aap-aacap-cha-declaration-of-a-national-emergency-in-child-and-adolescent-mental-health/. Accessed October 21, 2021.

American Academy of Pediatrics. Interim Guidance on supporting the emotional and behavioral health needs of children, adolescents, and families during the COVID-19 pandemic. Published September 10, 2022. https://www.aap.org/en/pages/2019-novel-coronavirus-covid-19-infections/clinicalguidance/interim-guidance-on-supporting-the-emotional-and-behavioral-health-needs-of-children-adolescents-and-families-during-the-covid19-pandemic/. Accessed March 13, 2023.

Centers for Disease Control and Prevention. New CDC data illuminate youth mental health threats during the COVID-19 pandemic. Press release. Published March 31, 2022. https://www.cdc.gov/media/releases/2022/p0331-youth-mental-health-covid-19.html. Accessed March 13, 2023.

Racine N, McArthur BA, Cooke JE, Eirich R, Zhu J, Madigan S: Global prevalence of depressive and anxiety symptoms in children and adolescents during COVID-19: a meta-analysis. JAMA Pediatr 2021;175(11):1142–1150. doi:10.1001/jamapediatrics.2021.2482 [PMID: 34369987].

Depression

Brent D et al: Switching to another SSRI or to venlafaxine with or without cognitive behavioral therapy for adolescents with SSRI-resistant depression: the TORDIA randomized controlled trial. JAMA 2008;299(8):901–913. doi: 299/8/901[pii]10.1001/jama.299.8.901 [PMID: 18314433].

Cheung AH, Zuckerbrot RA, Jensen PS, Laraque D, Stein REK; GLAD-PC Steering Group: Guidelines for Adolescent Depression in Primary Care (GLAD-PC): part II. Treatment and ongoing management. Pediatrics 2018;141(3):e20174082. doi: 10.1542/peds.2017-4082 [PMID: 29483201].

Depression Resource Center. American Academy of Child & Adolescent Psychiatry: https://www.aacap.org/AACAP/Families_and_Youth/Resource_Centers/Depression_Resource_Center/Depression_Resource_Center.aspx.

Guidelines for Adolescent Depression in Primary Care (GLAD-PC) Toolkit: The REACH Institute. http://www.gladpc.org.

Kodish I, Richardson L, Schlesinger A: Collaborative and integrated care for adolescent depression. Child Adolesc Psychiatr Clin N Am 2019;28(3):315–325. doi:10.1016/j.chc.2019.02.003 [PMID: 31076110].

March J et al: Treatments for Adolescents with Depression Study (TADS) Team. Fluoxetine, cognitive-behavioral therapy, and their combination for adolescents with depression: Treatment for Adolescents With Depression Study (TADS) randomized controlled trial. JAMA 2004;292(7):807–820. doi:10.1001/jama.292.7.807 [PMID: 15315995].

Zuckerbrot RA et al: Guidelines for Adolescent Depression in Primary Care (GLAD-PC): Part I. Practice preparation, identification, assessment, and initial management. Pediatrics 2018;141(3). doi:10.1542/peds.2017-4081 [PMID: 29483200].

Integrated Collaborative Care

Asarnow JR, Rozenman M, Wiblin J, Zeltzer L: Integrated medical-behavioral care compared with usual primary care for child and adolescent behavioral health: a meta-analysis. JAMA Pediatr 2015;169(10):929–937. doi: 10.1001/jamapediatrics.2015.1141 [PMID: 26259143].

Kolko DJ, Campo J, Kilbourne AM, Hart J, Sakolsky D, Wisniewski S: Collaborative care outcomes for pediatric behavioral health problems: a cluster randomized trial. Pediatrics 2014;133(4):e981–e982 [PMID: 24664093].

Meadows T, Valleley R, Haack MK, Thorson R, Evans J: Physician "costs" in providing behavioral health in primary care. Clin Pediatr 2011;50(5):447–455 [PMID: 21196418].

Minkovitz CS et al: A practice-based intervention to enhance quality of care in the first three years of life: results from the Healthy Steps for Young Children Program. JAMA 2003;290(23):3081–3091 [PMID: 14679271].

Pediatric Integrated Care Resource Center; American Academy of Child and Adolescent Psychiatry. http://integratedcareforkids.org.

Talmi A, Stafford B, Buchholz M: Providing perinatal mental health services in pediatric primary care. Zero to Three 2009;29(5):10–16.

Wissow LS, van Ginneken N, Chandra J, Rahman A: Integrating children's mental health into primary care. Pediatr Clin North Am 2016;63(1):97–113. doi: 10.1016/j.pcl.2015.08.005 [PMID: 26613691].

Miscellaneous

AACAP Facts for Families Disruptive Mood Dysregulation Disorder: https://www.aacap.org/AACAP/Families_and_Youth/Facts_for_Families/FFF-Guide/Disruptive-Mood-Dysregulation-Disorder-_DMDD_-110.aspx. Accessed June 21, 2021.

Adverse Childhood Experiences (ACEs). Centers for Disease Control and Prevention. Violence Prevention: https://www.cdc.gov/violenceprevention/aces/index.html

American Psychiatric Association: Diagnostic and Statistical Manual of Mental Disorders. 5th ed. Washington, DC: American Psychiatric Association; 2013.

Bright Futures: /https://www.brightfutures.org.

Costello EJ: Early detection and prevention of mental health problems: developmental epidemiology and systems of support. J Clin Child Adolesc Psychol 5(6):710–717. doi: org/10.1080/15374416.2016.1236728 [PMID: 27858462].

Roberts RE, Roberts CR, Xing Y: Prevalence of youth-reported DSM-IV psychiatric disorders among African, European, and Mexican American adolescents. J Am Acad Child Adolesc Psychiatry 2006;45(11):1329–1337. doi: 10.1097/01.chi.0000235076.25038.81 [PMID: 17075355].

The Center of Excellence for Infant and Early Childhood Mental Health Consultation (IECMHC). U.S. Department of Health & Human Services. Substance Abuse and Mental Health Services Administration: https://www.samhsa.gov/iecmhc.

Zero to Three: https://www.zerotothree.org.

Obsessive-Compulsive Disorder

Franklin ME et al: Cognitive behavior therapy augmentation of pharmacotherapy in pediatric obsessive-compulsive disorder: the Pediatric OCD Treatment Study II (POTS II) randomized controlled trial. JAMA 2011;306(11):1224–1232 [PMID: 21934055].

International OCD Foundation: https://iocdf.org/.

Pediatric OCD Treatment Study (POST) Team: Cognitive-behavior therapy, sertraline, and their combination for children and adolescents with obsessive-compulsive disorder: the Pediatric OCD Treatment Study (POTS) randomized controlled trial. JAMA 2004;292(16):1969–1976 [PMID: 15507582].

Practice parameter for the assessment and treatment of children and adolescents with obsessive-compulsive disorder. J Am Acad Child Adolesc Psychiatry 2012;51(1):98–113. doi: 10.1016/ja.jaac.2011.09.019 [PMID: 22176943].

Oppositional Defiant Disorder & Conduct Disorder

Byrd AL, Loeber R, Pardini DA: Understanding desisting and persisting forms of delinquency: the unique contributions of disruptive behavior disorders and interpersonal callousness. J Child Psychol Psychiatry 2012;53(4):371–380. doi:10.1111/j.1469-7610.2011.02504.x [PMID: 22176342].

Facts for Families: Disruptive Mood Dysregulation Disorder. American Academy of Child and Adolescent Psychiatry: http://www.aacap.org/App_Themes/AACAP/Docs/facts_for_families/110_disruptive_mood_dysregulation_disorder.pdf.

Viding E, McCrory EJ: Understanding the development of psychopathy: progress and challenges. Psychol Med 2018;48(4):566–577. doi:10.1017/S0033291717002847 [PMID: 29032773].

Posttraumatic Stress Disorder

Cohen JA et al; AACAP Work Group on Quality Issues: Practice parameter for the assessment and treatment of children and adolescents with posttraumatic stress disorder. J Am Acad Child Adolesc Psychiatry 2010;49(4):414–430 [PMID: 20410735].

Cohen JA, Mannarino AP: Trauma-focused cognitive behavior therapy for traumatized children and families. Child Adolesc Psychiatri Clin N Am 2015;24(3):557–570. doi:10.1016/j.chc.2015.02.005 [PMID: 26092739].

Keeshin BR, Strawn JR: Psychological and pharmacologic treatment of youth with posttraumatic stress disorder: an evidence-based review. Child Adolesc Psychiatr Clin N Am 2014;23(2):399–411, x. doi:10.1016/j.chc.2013.12.002 [PMID: 24656587].

Ross DA, Arbuckle MR, Travis MJ, Dwyer JB, van Schalkwyk GI, Ressler KJ: An integrated neuroscience perspective on formulation and treatment planning for posttraumatic stress disorder: an educational review. JAMA Psychiatry 2017;74(4):407–415. doi:10.1001/jamapsychiatry.2016.3325 [PMID: 28273291].

Schizophrenia

Fusar-Poli P, McGorry PD, Kane JM: Improving outcomes of first-episode psychosis: an overview. World Psychiatry 2017;16(3):251–265. doi: 10.1002/wps.20446 [PMID: 28941089].

Haddad PM, Correll CU: The acute efficacy of antipsychotics in schizophrenia: a review of recent meta-analyses. Ther Adv Psychopharmacol 2018;8(11):303–318. doi:10.1177/2045125318781475 [PMID: 30344997].

McClellan J, Stock S; American Academy of Child and Adolescent Psychiatry Committee on Quality Issues: Practice parameter for the assessment and treatment of children and adolescents with schizophrenia. J Am Acad Child Adolesc Psychiatry 2013;52(9):976–990. doi: 10.1016/j.jaac.2013.02.008 [PMID: 23972700].

Sikich L et al: Double-blind comparison of first- and second-generation antipsychotics in early-onset schizophrenia and schizo-affective disorder: findings from the treatment of early-onset schizophrenia spectrum disorders (TEOSS) study. Am J Psychiatry 2008;165(11):1420–1431. doi: appi.ajp.2008.08050756 [PMID: 18794207].

Somatic Disorders

Doss JL, Plioplys S: Pediatric psychogenic nonepileptic seizures: a concise review. Child Adolesc Psychiatr Clin N Am 2018;27(1):53–61. doi:10.1016/j.chc.2017.08.007 [PMID: 29157502].

Herzlinger M, Cerezo C: Functional abdominal pain and related syndromes. Child Adolesc Psychiatr Clin N Am 2018;27(1):15–26. doi:10.1016/j.chc.2017.08.006 [PMID: 29157499].

Suicide

American Foundation for Suicide Prevention: https://afsp.org. Accessed June 21, 2021.

Blades CA, Stritzke WGK, Page AC, Brown JD. The benefits and risks of asking research participants about suicide: a meta-analysis of the impact of exposure to suicide-related content. Clin Psychol Rev 2018;64:1–12. doi:10.1016/j.cpr.2018.07.001 [PMID: 30014862].

Brent DA et al; The Treatment of Adolescent Suicide Attempters study (TASA): Predictors of suicidal events in an open treatment trial. J Am Acad Child Adolesc Psychiatry 2009;48(10):987–996. doi: 10.1097/CHI.0b013e3181b5dbe4 [PMID: 19730274].

Centers for Disease Control and Prevention. WISQARS—Web-based Injury Statistics Query and Reporting System. Accessed March 23, 2023. https://www.cdc.gov/injury/wisqars/index.html

Centers for Disease Control and Prevention. Suicide Data and Statistics. https://www.cdc.gov/suicide/suicide-data-statistics.html. Published January 23, 2023. Accessed March 7, 2023.

Cha CB, Franz PJ, M Guzman E, Glenn CR, Kleiman EM, Nock MK: Annual research review: suicide among youth—epidemiology, (potential) etiology, and treatment. J Child Psychol Psychiatry 2018;59(4):460–482. doi: 10.1111/jcpp.12831 [PMID: 29090457].

Greydanus D, Patel D, Pratt H: Suicide risk in adolescents with chronic illness: implications for primary care and specialty pediatric practice: a review. Dev Med Child Neurol 2010;52(12):1083–1087. doi: 10.1111/j.1469-8749.2010.03771.x [PMID: 20813018].

https://www.nimh.nih.gov/about/director/messages/2020/addressing-the-crisis-of-black-youth-suicide.

Jed Foundation: https://www.jedfoundation.org/.

National Center for the Prevention of Youth Suicide. American Association of Suicidology: https://suicidology.org/2019/09/05/national-center-for-the-prevention-of-youth-suicide-aims-to-engage-youth-in-efforts/

Safe2Tell Colorado: https://safe2tell.org. Accessed June 21, 2021.

Suicide Awareness Voices of Education: https://save.org/

Suicide Prevention Resource Center: http://www.sprc.org.

Suicide Resources: Centers for Disease Control and Prevention. Violence Prevention. https://www.cdc.gov/violenceprevention/suicide/resources.html.

The Columbia Lighthouse Project: https://cssr.columbia.edu. Accessed June 21, 2021.

The Jed Foundation: https://www.jedfoundation.org/ Accessed June 21, 2021. https://www.watsoncoleman.house.gov/uploadedfiles/full_taskforce_report.pdf.

The Trevor Project. 2022 National Survey on LGBTQ Youth Mental Health http://www.thetrevorproject.org/survey-2022/. Published 2022. Accessed March 7, 2023.

Wilcox HC, Wyman PA: Suicide prevention strategies for improving population health. Child Adolesc Psychiatr Clin N Am 2016;25(2):219–233. doi:10.1016/j.chc.2015.12.003 [PMID: 26980125].

Zalsman G et al: Suicide prevention strategies revisited: 10-year systematic review. Lancet Psychiatry 2016;3(7):646–659. doi: 10.1016/S2215-0366(16)30030-X [PMID: 27289303].

Violence

Age-Related Reactions to a Traumatic Event. The National Child Traumatic Stress Network: https://www.nctsn.org/sites/default/files/resources//age_related_reactions_to_traumatic_events.pdf.

Massachusetts Child Psychiatry Access Project: http://www.mcpap.com/.

School Shootings and Other Traumatic Events: How to Talk to Students: http://www.nea.org.

Sood AB, Berkowitz SJ: Prevention of youth violence: a public health approach. Child Adolesc Psychiatr Clin N Am 2016;25(2):243–256. doi:10.1016/j.chc.2015.11.004 [PMID: 26980127].

Talking to Your Children About the Recent Spate of School Shootings. American Psychological Association: https://www.apa.org/topics/violence/school-shooting.

Child Abuse & Neglect

C. Rashaan Ford, MD

Antonia Chiesa, MD

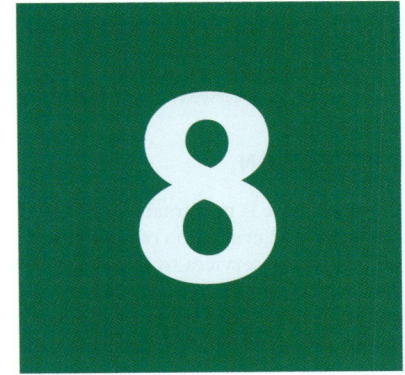

INTRODUCTION

ESSENTIALS OF DIAGNOSIS & TYPICAL FEATURES

► Forms of maltreatment:
- Physical abuse
- Sexual abuse
- Emotional abuse and neglect
- Physical neglect
- Medical care neglect
- Medical child abuse (Munchausen syndrome by proxy)

► Common historical features in child physical abuse cases:
- Implausible mechanism provided for an injury
- Discrepant, evolving, or absent history
- Delay in seeking care
- Event or behavior by a child that triggers a loss of control by the caregiver
- History of abuse in the caregiver's childhood
- Inappropriate affect of the caregiver
- Pattern of increasing severity or number of injuries if no intervention
- Social or physical isolation of the child or the caregiver
- Stress or crisis in the family or the caregiver
- Unrealistic expectations of caregiver for the child

In 2021, an estimated 4 million referrals were made to child protective service agencies, involving the alleged maltreatment of approximately 7.2 million children.

Children 3 years of age and younger have the highest rates of maltreatment. The total number of children confirmed as maltreated by child protective services was estimated to be 600,000 in 2021, yielding an abuse victimization rate of 8.1 per 1000 American children. Neglect is the most common form of maltreatment and was substantiated in 76% of cases, while 16% of cases involved physical abuse and 10.1% involved sexual abuse.

There were 1820 victims of fatal child abuse in 2021 from 50 states, resulting in a rate of 2.46 child abuse deaths per 100,000 children. The rate of African-American child fatalities was about 2.9 times greater than that of White and Hispanic children, a notable public health disparity.

Substance use disorders, poverty and economic strains, parental capacity and skills, and domestic violence are cited as the most common presenting problems in abusive families. Almost a third of substantiated maltreatment cases include domestic violence as a caregiver risk factor. Abuse and neglect of children are best considered in an ecological perspective, which recognizes the individual, family, social, and psychological influences that come together to contribute to the problem. This chapter focuses on the knowledge necessary for the recognition, intervention, and follow-up of the more common forms of child maltreatment and highlights the role of pediatric professionals in prevention. As childhood adversity, including maltreatment, has been shown to have serious implications for life-long health and well-being, the delivery of trauma informed behavioral health treatment is now a standard of care.

Ammerman S, Ryan S, Adelman WP; the Committee on Substance Abuse, the Committee on Adolescence: The impact of marijuana policies on youth: clinical, research, and legal update. Pediatrics 2015;135(3): e769–e785 [PMID: 25624385].

Jacob G, van den Heuvel M, Jama N, Moore AM, Ford-Jones L, Wong PD: Adverse childhood experiences: basics for the paediatrician. Paediatr Child Health 2019;24(1):30–37 [PMID: 30792598].

U.S. Department of Health And Human Services: Administration for Children, Youth, And Families. Child Maltreatment 2019. Https://Www.Acf.Hhs.Gov/Cb/Report/Child-Maltreatment-2021. Accessed March 9, 2023.

PREVENTION

Physical abuse is preventable in many cases. Extensive experience with an evaluation of high-risk families has shown that home visiting services to families at risk can prevent abuse and neglect of children. These services can be provided by public health nurses or trained paraprofessionals, although better outcomes data are available describing public health nurse intervention. Parent education and primary care providers' anticipatory guidance are also helpful, with attention to handling situations that stress parents (eg, colic, crying behavior, and toilet training), age-appropriate discipline, and general education about child developmental issues. Prevention of abusive injuries perpetrated by nonparent caregivers (eg, babysitters, nannies, and unrelated adults in the home) may be addressed by education and counseling of caregivers about safe childcare arrangements and choosing nonviolent life partners. Hospital-based prevention programs that teach parents about the dangers of shaking an infant and how to respond to a crying infant have demonstrated some positive results; however, no one effort has been shown to be completely effective.

The prevention of sexual abuse is more difficult. Most efforts in this area involve teaching children to protect themselves and their "private parts" from harm. The age of toilet training is a suitable time to provide anticipatory guidance to encourage parents to begin this discussion. The most rational approach is to place the burden of responsibility of prevention on the adults who supervise the child and the medical providers rather than on the children themselves. Programs designed to train adults on how to prevent and respond to concerns of child sexual abuse are a crucial resource for youth-serving organizations. Knowing the parents' own history of any victimization is important, as the ability to engage in this anticipatory guidance discussion with a provider and their child may be affected by that history. Promoting internet and social media safety and limiting exposure to sexualized materials and media should be part of this anticipatory guidance.

Efforts to prevent emotional abuse of children have been undertaken through extensive media campaigns. No data are available to assess the effectiveness of this approach. The primary care provider can promote positive, nurturing, and nonviolent behavior in parents. The message that they are role models for a child's behavior is important. Screening for domestic violence during discussions on discipline and home safety can be effective in identifying parents and children at risk. With natural disasters such as the coronavirus disease-19 (COVID-19) pandemic, factors such as parental job loss have been shown to be a predictor of psychological and emotional maltreatment of children. Issues of crime and safety within a community, the educational system, and even the economy may indirectly affect family functioning and can influence a family's capacity to parent and care for a child

American Academy of Pediatrics: HealthyChildren.org: http://www.healthychildren.org. Accessed May 25, 2021.

Bair-Merritt MH: Intimate partner violence. Pediatr Rev 2010 Apr;31(4):145–150; quiz 150.10.1542/pir.31-4-145 [PMID: 20360408].

Barr RG et al: Eight-year outcome of implementation of abusive head trauma prevention. Child Abuse Negl 2018;84:106–114 [PMID: 30077049].

Dubowitz H, Lane WG, Semiatin JN, Magder LS, Venepally M, Jans M: The safe environment for every kid model: impact on pediatric primary care professionals. Pediatrics 2011;127: e962–e970 [PMID: 21444590].

Duffee JH, Mendelsohn AL, Kuo AA, Legano LA, Earls MF; Council on Community Pediatrics; Council on Early Childhood; Committee on Child Abuse and Neglect: Early childhood home visiting. Pediatrics 2017;140(3): e20172150 [PMID: 28847981].

CLINICAL FINDINGS

Child maltreatment may occur either within or outside the family. The proportion of intrafamilial to extrafamilial cases varies with the type of abuse as well as the gender and age of the child. Each of the following conditions may exist as separate or concurrent diagnoses.

Recognition of any form of abuse and neglect of children can occur only if child abuse is considered in the differential diagnosis of the child's presenting medical condition. The advent of electronic medical records can make documenting concerns and patterns of maltreatment more accessible for all care team members. The approach to the family should be supportive, nonaccusatory, and empathetic. The individual who brings the child in for care may not have any involvement in the abuse. Approximately one-third of child abuse incidents occur in extrafamilial settings. Nevertheless, implicit biases, the assumption that the presenting caregiver is "nice and appropriate," combined with the failure to consider the possibility of abuse, can be costly and even fatal. Raising the possibility that a child has been abused is not the same as accusing the caregiver of being the abuser. If the family or presenting caregiver is not involved in the child's maltreatment, they may welcome an explanation for the child's symptoms and the subsequent necessary report and investigation.

In all cases of abuse and neglect, a detailed psychosocial history is important because psychosocial factors may indicate risk for or confirm child maltreatment. This history should include information on who lives or visits regularly in the home, other caregivers, domestic violence, substance abuse, and prior family history of physical or sexual abuse. Inquiring about any previous involvement with social services or law enforcement can help to determine risk.

Physical Abuse

The most common manifestations of physical abuse include bruises, burns, fractures, head trauma, and abdominal injuries. A small but considerable number of unexpected pediatric deaths, particularly in infants and very young children (eg, sudden unexpected infant death), are related to physical abuse.

A. History

The medical diagnosis of physical abuse is based on the presence of a discrepant history, in which the history offered by the caregiver is not consistent with the clinical findings. The discrepancy may exist because the history is absent, partial, changing over time, or simply illogical or improbable. A careful past medical, birth, and family history should also be obtained to assess for any other medical condition that might affect the clinical presentation. The presence of a discrepant history should prompt a request for consultation with a multidisciplinary child abuse pediatrics team or a report to the child protective services agency. This agency is mandated by state law to investigate reports of suspected child abuse and neglect. Investigation by social services and law enforcement officers, as well as a home visit, may be required to sort out the circumstances of the child's injuries.

B. Physical Findings

The findings on examination of physically abused children may include abrasions, alopecia (from hair pulling), bites (Figure 8–1), bruises, burns, dental trauma, fractures, lacerations, ligature marks, or scars. Injuries may be in multiple stages of healing. Primary care providers often play the most

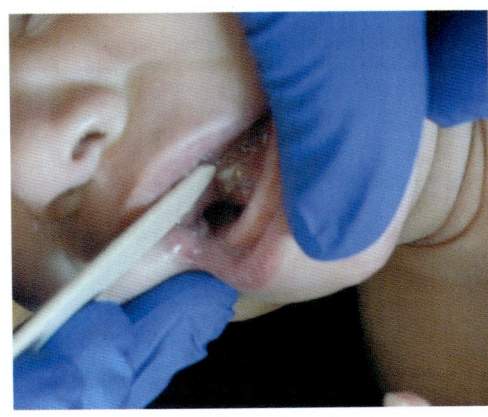

▲ **Figure 8–2.** Frenulum injury.

important role in the recognition of sentinel injuries in children, minor injuries such as frenulum tears (Figure 8–2), subconjunctival hemorrhages (Figure 8–3), or bruising which may be the first sign of child physical abuse before the abuse escalates. Bruises in physically abused children are sometimes patterned (eg, belt marks, looped cord marks, or grab or pinch marks) and are typically found over the soft tissue areas of the body. Toddlers or older children typically sustain accidental bruises over bony prominences such as shins and elbows. Any unexplained bruise in an infant not developmentally mobile should be viewed with concern. Of note, the dating of bruises is not reliable and should be approached cautiously. (Child abuse emergencies are listed in Table 8–1.) Lacerations of the frenulum or tongue and bruising of the lips may be associated with force feeding or blunt force trauma. The mnemonic TEN-4_FACESp (bruising to the torso, ear [Figure 8–4], or neck, frenulum injury, angle of jaw, cheeks [fleshy], eyelids, subconjunctival hemorrhage, and patterned

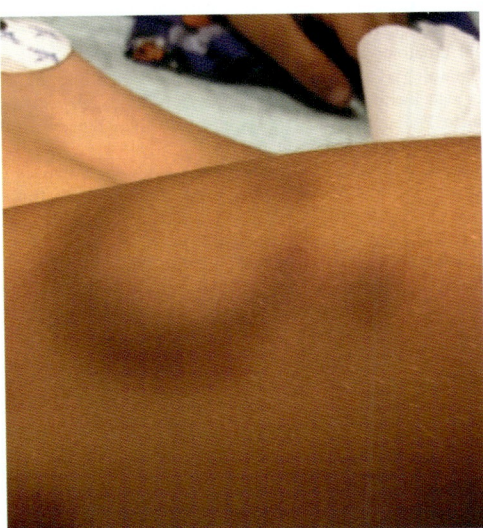

▲ **Figure 8–1.** Bite mark bruising.

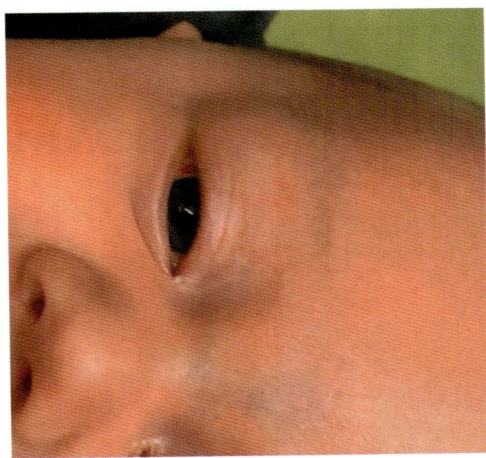

▲ **Figure 8–3.** Subconjunctival hemorrhage.

Table 8–1. Potential child abuse medical emergencies.

Any infant with bruises (especially head, facial, or abdominal), burns, or fractures

Any infant or child younger than 2 y with a history of suspected "shaken baby" head trauma or other inflicted head injury

Any child who has sustained suspicious or known inflicted abdominal trauma

Any child with burns in stocking or glove distribution or in other unusual patterns, burns to the genitalia, and any unexplained burn injury

Any child with disclosure or sign of sexual assault within 48–72 h after the alleged event if the possibility of acute injury is present or if forensic evidence exists

bruising on a child 4 years or younger, and bruising anywhere on a child 4 months and younger) provides an effective screening tool to improve recognition of potentially abused children. Pathognomonic burn patterns include stocking or glove distribution; immersion burns of the buttocks, sometimes with a "doughnut hole" area of sparing; and branding burns such as with cigarettes or hot objects (eg, grill, curling iron, or lighter). The absence of splash marks or a pattern consistent with spillage may be helpful in differentiating accidental from nonaccidental scald burns.

Head and abdominal trauma may present with signs and symptoms consistent with those injuries. Abusive head trauma (eg, shaken baby syndrome) and abdominal injuries may have no visible findings on examination. Symptoms can be subtle and may mimic other conditions such as gastroenteritis. Studies have documented that cases of inflicted head injury will be missed when practitioners fail to consider the diagnosis. A pediatric ophthalmologist should be consulted in cases of suspected abusive head trauma when there is abnormal diagnostic imaging of the head. The finding of retinal hemorrhages in an infant without an appropriate medical condition (eg, leukemia, congenital infection, or clotting disorder) should raise concern about possible

inflicted head trauma. Retinal hemorrhages are not commonly seen after cardiopulmonary resuscitation in either infants or children.

C. Radiologic and Laboratory Findings

Certain radiologic findings are strong indicators of physical abuse. Examples are metaphyseal ("corner" or "bucket handle") fractures of the long bones in infants, spiral fracture of the extremities in nonambulatory infants, rib fractures, spinous process fractures, and fractures in multiple stages of healing. Skeletal surveys in children aged 2 years or younger should be performed when a suspicious injury is diagnosed. Computed tomography or magnetic resonance imaging findings of subdural hemorrhage in infants—in the absence of a clear accidental history—are highly correlated with abusive head trauma. Abdominal computed tomography is the preferred test in suspected abdominal trauma. Any infant or young child with suspected abuse-related head or abdominal trauma should be evaluated immediately by an emergency and/or trauma surgery medical provider.

Coagulation studies and a complete blood cell count with platelets are useful in children who present with multiple or severe bruises. Hepatic transaminases (ALT [alanine aminotransferase] and AST [aspartate aminotransferase]) should be used to screen for abdominal injury, and transaminase levels greater than 80 IU/L should prompt definitive testing for internal injury. Coagulopathy conditions may confuse the diagnostic picture but can be excluded with a careful history, examination, laboratory screens, and hematologic consultation, if necessary.

American Academy of Pediatrics: *Visual Diagnosis of Child Abuse.* 4th ed. American Academy of Pediatrics; 2016 [USB flash drive].

Anderst J, Carpenter SL, Abshire TC, Killough E; AAP Section on Hematology/Oncology, the American Society of Pediatric Hematology/Oncology, the AAP Council on Child Abuse and Neglect. Evaluation for Bleeding Disorders in Suspected Child Abuse. Pediatrics 2022 Oct 1;150(4):e2022059276. doi: 10.1542/peds.2022-059276 [PMID: 36180615].

Christian CW, Block R; American Academy of Pediatrics Committee on Child Abuse and Neglect: Abusive head trauma in infants and children. Pediatrics 2009;123(5):1409–1411 [PMID: 19403508]. Reaffirmed March, 2013.

Flaherty EG, Perez-Rossello JM, Levine MA, Hennrikus WL; American Academy of Pediatrics Committee on Child Abuse and Neglect; Section on Radiology; Section on Endocrinology; Section on Orthopaedics; Society for Pediatric Radiology: Evaluating children with fractures for child physical abuse. Pediatrics 2013;131:4 [PMID: 24470642].

Hymel KP; American Academy of Pediatrics Committee on Child Abuse and Neglect; National Association of Medical Examiners: Distinguishing sudden infant death syndrome from child abuse fatalities. Pediatrics 2006;118:421 [PMID: 16818592]. Reaffirmed March, 2013.

Kempe AM et al: Patterns of skeletal fractures in child abuse: systematic review. BMJ 2008;337:a1518 [PMID: 18832412].

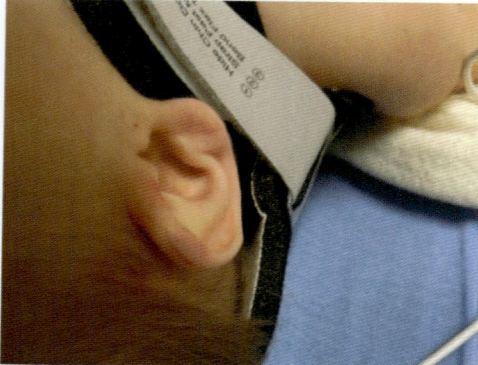

▲ **Figure 8–4.** Ear bruising.

Pierce MC et al: Validation of a clinical decision rule to predict abuse in young children based on bruising characteristics. JAMA Netw Open 2021 Apr 1;4(4):e215832 [PMID: 33852003].

Sheets LK, Leach ME, Koszewski IJ, Lessmeier AM, Nugent M, Simpson P: Sentinel injuries in infants evaluated for child physical abuse. Pediatrics 2013;131(4):701–707 [PMID: 23478861].

Sexual Abuse

Sexual abuse is defined as the engaging of dependent, developmentally immature children in sexual activities that they do not fully comprehend and to which they cannot give consent, or activities that violate the laws and taboos of a society. It includes all forms of incest, sexual assault or rape, and pedophilia, and may involve fondling, oral-genital-anal contact, all forms of intercourse or penetration, exhibitionism, voyeurism, exploitation, prostitution, and the involvement of children in the production of pornography. Over the past decade, there has been a small downward trend nationally in rates of child sexual abuse; however, the exploitation and enticement of children via the Internet and social media and human trafficking cases have gained increases in recognition.

A. History

Sexual abuse may come to the clinician's attention in different ways: (1) The child may be brought in for routine care or for an acute problem, and sexual abuse may be suspected by the medical professional as a result of the history or the physical examination. (2) The parent or caregiver, suspecting that the child may have been sexually abused, may bring the child to the health care provider, and request an examination to rule in or rule out abuse. (3) The child may be referred by child protective services or the police for an evidentiary examination following either disclosure of sexual abuse by the child or an allegation of abuse by a parent or third party. Table 8–2 lists the common presentations of child sexual abuse. Certain high-risk behaviors should prompt recognition of possible human trafficking, including substance misuse, runaway activity, multiple sexual partners, law enforcement history, or presenting to care without identification. If suspected, this should be addressed confidentially with the patient. It should be emphasized that except for acute trauma, certain sexually transmitted infections (STIs), or forensic laboratory evidence, none of these presentations is specific. The presentations listed should arouse suspicion of the possibility of sexual abuse and lead the practitioner to ask the appropriate questions in a compassionate and nonaccusatory manner. Asking the young child nonleading, age-appropriate questions is important and is often best handled by the most experienced interviewer after a report is made. Community agency protocols may exist for child advocacy centers that help in the investigation of these reports. Concerns expressed about sexual abuse in the context of divorce and custody disputes should be handled in the same manner, with the same

Table 8–2. Presentations of sexual abuse.

General or direct statements about sexual abuse
Sexualized knowledge, play, or behavior in developmentally immature children
Sexual abuse of other children by the victim
Behavioral changes
  Sleep disturbances (eg, nightmares and night terrors)
  Appetite disturbances (eg, anorexia, bulimia)
  Depression, social withdrawal, anxiety
  Aggression, temper tantrums, impulsiveness
  Neurotic or conduct disorders, phobias or avoidant behaviors
  Guilt, low self-esteem, mistrust, feelings of helplessness
  Hysterical or conversion reactions
  Suicidal, runaway threats or behavior
  Excessive masturbation
Medical conditions
  Recurrent abdominal pain or frequent somatic complaints
  Genital, anal, or urethral trauma
  Recurrent complaints of genital or anal pain, discharge, bleeding
  Enuresis or encopresis
  Sexually transmitted infections
  Pregnancy
Promiscuity or prostitution, sexual dysfunction, fear of intimacy
School problems or truancy
Substance abuse

objective, nonjudgmental documentation. The American Academy of Pediatrics has published guidelines for the evaluation of child sexual abuse as well as others relating to child maltreatment.

B. Physical Findings

The genital and anal findings of sexually abused children, as well as the normal developmental changes and variations in prepubertal female hymens, have been described in journal articles and visual diagnosis guides. To maintain a sense of comfort and routine for the patient, the genital examination should be conducted in the context of a full body checkup. For nonsexually active, prepubertal girls, an internal speculum examination is rarely necessary unless there is suspicion of internal injury, and in those cases it is advised to perform the examination under anesthesia and with the assistance of the gynecology team. The external female genital structures can be well visualized using labial separation and traction with the child in the supine frog leg or knee-chest position. Most victims of sexual abuse exhibit no physical findings. The reasons for this include delay in disclosure by the child, abuse that may not cause physical trauma (eg, fondling, oral-genital contact, or exploitation by pornographic photography), or rapid healing of minor injuries such as labial, hymenal, or anal abrasions, contusions, or lacerations. Nonspecific abnormalities of the genital and rectal regions such as erythema, rashes, and irritation may not suggest sexual abuse in the absence of a corroborating history, disclosure, or behavioral changes.

Certain STIs should strongly suggest sexual abuse in prepubertal children. *Neisseria gonorrhoeae* infection or syphilis beyond the perinatal period is diagnostic of sexual abuse. *Chlamydia trachomatis*, herpes simplex virus, trichomoniasis, and human papillomavirus are all sexually transmitted, although the course of these potentially perinatally acquired infections may be protracted. Herpes simplex can be transmitted by other means; however, the presence of an infection should prompt a careful assessment for sexual abuse. Risk is higher in children older than five with isolated herpetic genital lesions. In the case of human papillomavirus, an initial appearance of venereal warts beyond the toddler age should prompt a discussion regarding concerns of sexual abuse. Human papillomavirus is a ubiquitous virus and can be spread innocently by caregivers with hand lesions. Finally, sexual abuse must be considered with the diagnosis of *C trachomatis* or human immunodeficiency virus (HIV) infections when other modes of transmission (eg, transfusion or perinatal acquisition) have been ruled out. Postexposure prophylaxis medications for HIV in cases of acute sexual assault should be considered only after assessment of risk of transmission and consultation with an infectious disease expert.

Nucleic acid amplification tests (NAATs) have been used with increasing frequency for screening of STIs in sexual abuse victims, including for children younger than 12 years. For prepubertal children, NAATs can be used for vaginal specimens or urine from girls. If a NAAT is positive, a second confirmatory NAAT test that analyzes an alternate target of the genetic material in the sample or a standard culture is needed. For boys and for extragenital specimens, culture is still the preferred method. Finally, the Centers for Disease Control and Prevention and the AAP Redbook list guidelines for the screening and treatment of STIs in the context of sexual abuse.

C. Examination, Evaluation, and Management

The forensic evaluation of sexually abused children should be performed in a setting that prevents further emotional distress. All the components of a forensic evidence collection kit may not be indicated in the setting of child sexual abuse (as opposed to adult rape cases); the clinical history and exposure risk should guide what specimens are collected. The forensic evidence collection kit guides the practitioner through a stepwise collection of evidence and cultures. This should occur in an emergency department or clinic where chain of custody for specimens can be ensured. The most experienced examiner (pediatrician, APP, nurse examiner, or child advocacy center) is preferable. If the history indicates that the adolescent may have had contact with the ejaculate of a perpetrator within 120 hours, a cervical examination to look for semen or its markers (eg, acid phosphatase) should be performed according to established protocols.

Prior to any speculum examination of an assault victim, it is important to consider the child's physiologic and emotional maturation, and whether the child has been sexually active or had a speculum examination in the past. More important, if there is a history of possible sexual abuse of any child within the past several days, and the child reports a physical complaint or a physical sign is observed (eg, genital or anal bleeding or discharge), the child should be examined for evidence of trauma. Colposcopy may be critical for determining the extent of the trauma, and photodocumentation may be helpful in providing documentation for the legal system.

STI screening should include testing for *N gonorrhoeae* and *C trachomatis*, and vaginal secretions evaluated for *Trichomonas*. These infections and bacterial vaginosis are the most frequently diagnosed infections among older girls who have been sexually assaulted. RPR, hepatitis B, and HIV serology should be drawn at baseline and 6 weeks, 3 months, and 6 months after last contact. Pregnancy testing should be done as indicated.

Acute sexual assault cases that involve trauma or transmission of body fluid should have STI prophylaxis. Using adult doses of ceftriaxone (500 mg IM in a single dose), metronidazole (2 g orally in a single dose), and azithromycin (1 g orally in a single dose) should be offered when older or adolescent patients present for evaluation. (Pediatric treatment and dosing are calculated by weight and can be found in standard references.) Hepatitis B vaccination should be administered to all patients, and hepatitis B immunoglobulin should be given if the perpetrator is known to be infected with hepatitis B. No effective prophylaxis is available for hepatitis C. Evaluating the perpetrator for an STI, if possible, can help determine risk exposure and guide prophylaxis. HIV prophylaxis (Biktarvy 50-200-25 mg for patients weighing ≥ 25 kg; Biktarvy 30-120-15 mg for patients weighing 14–25 kg should be considered in certain circumstances (see Chapter 44). For postpubertal girls, contraception should be given if the sexual assault occurred within 120 hours.

Although it is often difficult for persons to complete recommended follow-up examinations weeks after an assault, primary care providers may play a crucial and trusted role in follow-up, as such examinations are essential to detect new infections, complete immunization with hepatitis B vaccination if needed, and continue psychological support.

Adams JA et al: Updated guidelines for the medical assessment and care of children who may have been sexually abused. J Pediatr Adolesc Gynecol 2016 Apr;29(2):81–87 [PMID: 26220352].

Centers for Disease Control and Prevention: Sexually Transmitted Diseases Treatment Guidelines 2015: http://www.cdc.gov/std/tg2015. Accessed May 8, 2021.

Chiesa A, Goldson E: Child sexual abuse. Pediatr Rev 2017;38(3):105–118 [PMID: 28250071].

Girardet RG et al: HIV post-exposure prophylaxis in children and adolescents presenting for reported sexual assault. Child Abuse Negl 2009;33:173 [PMID: 19324415].

Greenbaum VJ, Dodd M, McCracken C: A short screening tool to identify victims of child sex trafficking in the health care setting. Pediatr Emerg Care 2018 Jan;34(1):33–37 [PMID: 26599463].

Noll JG, Shenk CE: Teen birth rates in sexually abused and neglected females. Pediatrics 2013;131:e1181–e1187 [PMID: 23530173].

Thackeray et al: Forensic evidence collection and DNA identification in acute child sexual assault. Pediatrics 2011;128:227–232 [PMID: 21788217].

Emotional Abuse & Neglect

Emotional or psychological abuse has been defined as the rejection, ignoring, criticizing, isolation, or terrorizing of children, all of which have the effect of eroding their self-esteem. The most common form is verbal abuse or denigration. Children who witness domestic violence should be considered emotionally abused, as a growing body of literature has shown the negative effects of intimate partner violence on child development.

The most common feature of emotional neglect is the absence of normal parent-child attachment and a subsequent inability to recognize and respond to an infant's or child's needs. A common manifestation of emotional neglect in infancy is nutritional (nonorganic) growth faltering. Emotionally neglectful parents appear to have an inability to recognize the physical or emotional states of their children. For example, an emotionally neglectful parent may ignore an infant's cry if the cry is perceived incorrectly as an expression of anger. This misinterpretation leads to inadequate nutrition and failure to thrive.

Emotional abuse may cause nonspecific symptoms in children. Loss of self-esteem or self-confidence, sleep disturbances, somatic symptoms (eg, headaches and stomach aches), hypervigilance, or avoidant or phobic behaviors (eg, school refusal or running away) may be presenting complaints. These complaints may also be seen in children who experience domestic violence. Emotional abuse can occur in the home or day care, school, sports team, or other settings.

Physical Neglect & Growth Faltering

Physical neglect is the failure to provide the necessary food, clothing, and shelter and a safe environment in which children can grow and develop. Although often associated with poverty, physical neglect involves a more serious problem than just lack of resources. There is often a component of emotional neglect and either a failure or an inability, intentionally or otherwise, to recognize and respond to the needs of the child.

A. History

Given that neglect is the most common form of abuse, providers should be proactive in their approach to recognition and treatment. Physical neglect—which must be differentiated from the deprivations of poverty of other social determinants of health—will be present even after adequate social resources have been provided to families in need. The clinician must evaluate the psychosocial history, family dynamics, social determinants of health, and parental mental health when neglect is a consideration and is in a unique position to intervene when warning signs first emerge. A careful social services evaluation of the home and entire family may be required. The primary care provider must work closely with a social service agency and explain the known medical information to help guide their investigation and decision-making.

The history offered in cases of growth faltering (failure to thrive) is often discrepant with the physical findings. Infants who have experienced a significant deceleration in growth may not be receiving adequate amounts or appropriate types of food despite the dietary history provided. Medical conditions causing poor growth in infancy and early childhood can be ruled out with a detailed history and physical examination with minimal laboratory tests. A psychosocial history may reveal maternal depression, family chaos or dysfunction, or other previously unknown social risk factors (eg, substance misuse, violence, poverty, or psychiatric illness). Hospitalization of the severely malnourished patient is sometimes required, but most cases are managed on an outpatient basis.

B. Physical Findings

Approach to assessment, physical examination findings, and diagnostic evaluation of infants and children with nonorganic growth faltering are discussed in detail in Chapter 11. Screening for other injuries may be helpful if concurrent physical abuse is suspected. Placement in a setting in which the child can be fed and monitored can be a useful diagnostic approach. Hospital or out of home placement may occur at the recommendation of social services.

Medical Care Neglect

Medical care neglect is failure to provide the needed treatment to infants or children with life-threatening illness or other serious or chronic medical conditions. This diagnosis should be considered when caregivers have a clear understanding of the child's condition and the consequences of not providing the recommended treatment, and the provider has tried to address barriers to care.

Medical Child Abuse

Previously referred to as Munchausen syndrome by proxy, medical child abuse is the preferred term for a unusual clinical scenario in which a caregiver seeks inappropriate and unnecessary medical care for a child. Often, the caregiver either simulates or creates the symptoms or signs of illness in a child. However, the use of the term medical child abuse emphasizes harm caused to the child as opposed to the psychopathology or motivation of the caregiver. Cases can be complicated, and a detailed review of all medical documentation and a multidisciplinary approach is required. Fatal cases have been reported.

A. History

The child can present with a long list of medical problems or often bizarre, recurrent complaints. Repetitive visits, persistent doctor shopping, and enforced invalidism (eg, not accepting that the child is healthy and reinforcing that the child is somehow ill) are also described in the original definition of Munchausen syndrome by proxy.

B. Physical Findings

Children may present with the signs and symptoms of whatever illness is factitiously produced or simulated. More often, they are reported to be ill and have a normal clinical appearance. Among the most common reported presentations are recurrent apnea, dehydration from induced vomiting or diarrhea, sepsis when contaminants are injected into a child, change in mental status, fever, gastrointestinal bleeding, and seizures.

C. Radiologic and Laboratory Findings

Recurrent polymicrobial sepsis (especially in children with indwelling catheters), recurrent apnea, chronic dehydration of unknown cause, or other highly unusual unexplained laboratory findings should raise the suspicion of medical child abuse. Toxicological testing may also be useful.

Flaherty EG, MacMillan HL; American Academy of Pediatrics; Committee on Child Abuse and Neglect: Caregiver-fabricated illness in a child: a manifestation of child maltreatment. Pediatrics 2013;32:3 [PMID: 23979088].

Hibbard R: Clinical report: psychological maltreatment. Pediatrics 2012 Oct;130(2):372–378.

Hymel KP; American Academy of Pediatrics; Committee on Child Abuse and Neglect: When is lack of supervision neglect? Pediatrics 2006; 118:1296 [PMID:16951030].

Larson-Nath C, Biank VF: Clinical review of failure to thrive in pediatric patients. Pediatr Ann 2016;45(2);e46–e49 [PMID: 26878182].

Roesler T, Jenny C: *Medical Child Abuse: Beyond Munchausen Syndrome by Proxy*. American Academy of Pediatrics; 2009.

DIFFERENTIAL DIAGNOSIS

The differential diagnosis for abuse and neglect may be straightforward. It can also be more elusive as in the case of multiple injuries that may raise concern for an underlying medical condition or in situations where complex, but non-specific behavior changes or physical symptoms reflect the emotional impact of maltreatment.

The differential diagnosis of all forms of physical abuse can be considered in the context of a detailed trauma history, family medical history, radiographic findings, and laboratory testing. The diagnosis of osteogenesis imperfecta or other collagen or bone disorders, for example, may be considered in the child with skin and joint findings or multiple fractures with or without the classic radiographic presentation and is best made in consultation with a geneticist, an orthopedic surgeon, and a radiologist. Trauma—accidental or inflicted—leads the differential diagnosis list for subdural hematomas. Coagulopathy; disorders of copper, amino acid, or organic acid metabolism (eg, Menkes syndrome and glutaric acidemia type 1); chronic or previous central nervous system infection; birth trauma; or congenital central nervous system malformation (eg, arteriovenous malformations or cerebrospinal fluid collections) may need to be ruled out in some cases. It should be recognized, however, that children with these rare disorders can also be victims of abuse or neglect.

There are medical conditions that may be misdiagnosed as sexual abuse. When abnormal physical examination findings are noted, knowledge of these conditions is imperative to avoid misinterpretation. The differential diagnosis includes vulvovaginitis, lichen sclerosus, dermatitis, labial adhesions, congenital urethral or vulvar disorders, Crohn disease, and accidental straddle injuries to the labia. In most circumstances, these can be ruled out by careful history and examination.

TREATMENT

A. Management

Physical abuse injuries, STIs, and medical sequelae of neglect should be treated immediately. Children with growth faltering related to emotional and physical neglect may need to be placed in a setting for which they can be safely cared. Likewise, the child in danger of recurrent abuse or neglect needs to be placed in a safe environment. Studies show that the likelihood of abuse in a sibling of an abused child is significantly increased, so diagnostic screening for all siblings of an abused child should be performed. Psychosocial vulnerabilities are common; therefore, a multidisciplinary approach that supports family engagement is helpful. Cooperation and coordination with clinical social work and mental health colleagues is crucial. Given the developmental and emotional implications, prompt referral to mental health resources for any patient with a history of child abuse or neglect is crucial, although not every child with a history of maltreatment will need long-term mental health treatment. There are also effective interventions for improving parenting and attachment problems that are common in child maltreatment cases. Pediatricians should be aware of community partners and resources to help families in need of services.

B. Reporting

In the United States, clinicians and many other professionals who come in contact with or care for children are mandated reporters. If abuse or neglect is suspected, a report must be made to the local or state agency designated to investigate such matters. In most cases, this will be the child protective services agency. Law enforcement agencies may also receive such reports. The purpose of the report is to permit professionals to gather the information needed to determine whether the child's environment (eg, home, school, day care setting, or foster home) is safe. Recent studies document physician barriers to reporting, but providers should be mindful that good faith and non-biased reporting is a legal requirement for any suspicion of abuse. Failure to report concerns may have legal ramifications for the provider or serious health and safety consequences for the patient. Many hospitals and communities make child protection teams or consultants available when there are questions about the diagnosis and management in a child abuse case. A listing of child abuse pediatric consultants is available from the American Academy of Pediatrics.

Finally, communication with social services, case management, and careful follow-up by primary care providers are crucial to ensuring ongoing safety of child.

Flaherty E, Legano L, Idzerda S; Council on Child Abuse and Neglect: Ongoing pediatric health care for the child who has been maltreated. Pediatrics 2019;143(3):e20190284 [PMID: 30886109].

Garner AS et al; Committee on Psychosocial Aspects of Child and Family Health; Committee on Early Childhood, Adoption, and Dependent Care; Section on Developmental and Behavioral Pediatrics: Early childhood adversity, toxic stress, and the role of the pediatrician: translating developmental science into lifelong health. Pediatrics 2012;129;e224–e231 [PMID: 22201148].

Mankad K, Sidpra J, Oates AJ, Calder A, Offiah AC, Choudhary A: Sibling screening in suspected abusive head trauma: a proposed guideline. Pediatr Radiol 2021 May;51(6):872–875 [PMID: 33999232].

National Child Traumatic Stress Network: http://www.nctsn.org/. Accessed June 24, 2019.

Sege R et al: To report or not to report: examination of the initial primary care management of suspicious childhood injuries. Acad Pediatr 2011;11(6):460–466 [PMID: 21996468].

Sege RD, Amaya-Jackson L; American Academy of Pediatrics Committee on Child Abuse and Neglect, Council on Foster Care, Adoption and Kinship Care; American Academy of Child and Adolescent Psychiatry Committee on Child Maltreatment and Violence; National Center for Child Traumatic Stress: Clinical considerations related to the behavioral manifestations of child maltreatment. Pediatrics 2017;139(4):e20170100 [PMID: 28320870].

PROGNOSIS

Depending on the extent of injury resulting from physical or sexual abuse, the prognosis for complete recovery varies. Serious physical abuse that involves head injury, multisystem trauma, severe burns, or abdominal trauma carries significant morbidity and mortality risk. Hospitalized children with a diagnosis of child abuse or neglect have longer stays and are more likely to die. Long-term medical and developmental consequences are common. For example, children who suffer brain damage related to abusive head injury can have significant neurologic impairment, such as cerebral palsy, vision problems, epilepsy, microcephaly, and learning disorders. Other injuries like minor bruises or burns, fractures, and even injuries resulting from penetrating genital trauma can heal well and with no sequelae.

The emotional and psychological outcomes for child victims are often the most detrimental. Research demonstrates that there are clear neurobiologic effects of child maltreatment and other types of early childhood toxic stress. Physiologic changes to the brain can adversely affect the mental and physical health development of children for decades. Adverse childhood experiences (ACEs) have been associated with chronic adult health problems, suicide, alcoholism and drug abuse, anxiety and depression, violence, and early death. Despite the potential consequences, the effects of maltreatment can be mitigated. There are effective, evidence-based interventions for child maltreatment. Some children may need extra help addressing emotional regulation, coping skills, and rebuilding trust. The primary care provider plays an important role in assuring appropriate medical and mental health care for maltreated children and families, and in advocating for victims across the child and young adult lifespan.

Centers for Disease Control and Prevention: Adverse Childhood Experiences Study. http://www.cdc.gov/violenceprevention/acestudy. Accessed June 24, 2019.

Child Welfare Information Gateway: Long-Term Consequences of Child Abuse and Neglect. https://www.childwelfare.gov/pubpdfs/long_term_consequences.pdf. Accessed June 24, 2019.

Office of the Administration for Children and Families: Within Our Reach: A National Strategy to Reduce Child Abuse Fatalities. https://www.acf.hhs.gov/cb/resrouce/cecanf-final-report. Accessed June 24, 2019.

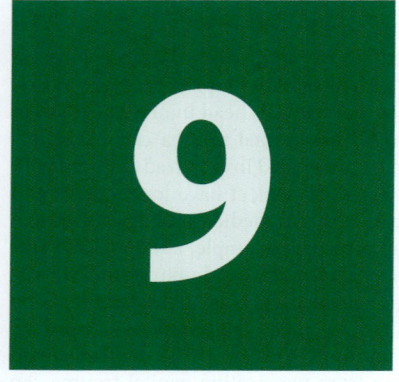

Ambulatory & Office Pediatrics

Meghan Treitz, MD

Daniel Nicklas, MD

David Fox, MD

INTRODUCTION

Pediatric ambulatory outpatient services provide children and adolescents with preventive health care and acute and chronic care management services and consultations.

The development of a physician-patient-parent relationship is crucially important if the patient and parent are to effectively confide their concerns. This relationship develops over time, with regular visits, and is facilitated by the continuity of clinicians and other staff members. A successful relationship occurs when patients and/or parents experience advice as valid and effective. Anticipatory guidance should be age-appropriate and timely to be most helpful. Important skills include choosing vocabulary that communicates understanding and competence, demonstrating commitment of time and attention to the concern, and showing respect for areas that the patient or parent does not wish to address (assuming that there are no concerns relating to physical or sexual abuse or neglect). Parents and patients expect that their concerns will be managed confidentially, and that the clinician understands and sympathizes with those concerns. The effective physician-patient-parent relationship is one of the most satisfying aspects of ambulatory pediatrics.

PEDIATRIC HISTORY

A unique feature of pediatrics is that the history represents an amalgam of parents' objective reporting of facts (eg, fever for 4 days), parents' subjective interpretation of their child's symptoms (eg, infant's crying interpreted by parents as abdominal pain), and for older children their own history of events. Parents and patients may provide a specific and detailed history, or a vague history that necessitates more focused probing. Parents may or may not be able to distinguish whether symptoms are caused by organic illness or a psychological concern. Understanding the family and its hopes for and concerns about the child can help in the process of distinguishing organic, emotional, and/or behavioral conditions, thus minimizing unnecessary testing and intervention.

Although the parents' concerns need to be understood, it is essential also to obtain as much of the history as possible directly from the patient. Direct histories provide firsthand information and give the child a sense of agency over their situation.

Obtaining a comprehensive pediatric history is time consuming. Many offices provide questionnaires for parents to complete before the clinician sees the child. Data from questionnaires allow the provider to address problems in detail while more quickly reviewing areas that are not of concern. Developmental and mental health screening saves provider time and can yield critical information. However, failure to review and assimilate this information prior to the interview may cause a parent or patient to feel that the time and effort have been wasted.

Elements of the history that will be useful over time should be readily accessible in the medical record, including demographic data, a problem list, chronic medications, immunizations, allergies, and previous hospitalizations.

The components of a comprehensive pediatric history are listed in Table 9–1. The information should, ideally, be obtained at the first office visit. Items 8 and 9, and a focused review of systems (ROS), should be addressed at each acute or chronic care visit. The entire list should be reviewed and augmented with relevant updates at each health supervision visit.

PEDIATRIC PHYSICAL EXAMINATION

During the pediatric physical examination, time must be taken to allow the patient to become familiar with the examiner. Interactions and instructions help the child understand what is occurring and what is expected. A gentle, friendly manner and a quiet voice help establish a setting that yields a nonthreatening physical examination. The examiner should take into consideration the need for a quiet child, the extent

Table 9–1. Components of the pediatric historical database.[a]

1. Demographic data	Patient's legal name and preferred name and preferred pronouns, date of birth, social security number, sex, race, parents' names (first and last), siblings' names, and payment mechanism.
2. Problem list	Major or significant problems, including dates of onset and resolution.
3. Allergies	Triggering allergen, nature of the reaction, treatment needed, and date allergy was diagnosed.
4. Chronic medications	Name, concentration, dose, and frequency of chronically used medications.
5. Birth history	Maternal health during pregnancy such as bleeding, infections, smoking, alcohol and any medications, complications of pregnancy; duration of labor; form of delivery; and labor complications. Infant's birth weight, gestational age, Apgar scores, and problems in the neonatal period.
6. Screening procedures	Results of newborn screening, vision and hearing screening, any health screen, or screening laboratory tests. (Developmental screening results are maintained in the development section; see item 14.)
7. Immunizations	Type(s) of vaccine, date administered, vaccine manufacturer and lot number, and name and title of the person administering the vaccine; injection site, previous reaction and contraindications (eg, immunodeficiency or an evolving neurologic problem), date on vaccine information statement (VIS), and date VIS was provided.
8. Reasons for visit	The patient's or parents' concerns, stated in their own words, serve as the focus for the visit.
9. Present illness	A concise chronologic summary of the problems necessitating a visit, including the duration, progression, exacerbating factors, ameliorating interventions, and associations.
10. Medical history	A statement regarding the child's functionality and general well-being, including a summary record of significant illnesses, injuries, hospitalizations, and procedures.
11. Diet	Eating patterns, relative amounts of carbohydrates, fat, and protein in the diet, type and quantity of milk. Inquiry about intake of fast food, candy, and sugar sweetened beverages.
12. Family history	Information about the illnesses of relatives, preferably in the form of a family tree.
13. Social history	Family constellation, relationships, parents' educational background, religious and cultural preference, and the role of the child in the family; socioeconomic profile of the family to identify resources available to the child, access to services that may be needed, and anticipated stressors.
14. Development	(1) Attainment of developmental milestones (including developmental testing results); (2) social habits and milestones (toilet habits, play, major activities, sleep patterns, discipline, peer relationships); (3) school progress and documentation of specific achievements and grades.
15. Sexual history	Sex education, sexual development, sexual secondary characteristics, sexual attraction and gender expression, sexually transmitted diseases, pubertal onset, and birth control measures.
16. ROS, review of systems	Common symptoms in each major body system.

[a]The components of this table should be included in a child's medical record and structured to allow easy review and modification. The practice name and address should appear on all pages.

of trust established, and the possibility of an emotional response when deciding the order in which the child's organ systems are examined. Unpleasant procedures (eg, otoscopic examination in young children, genitourinary [GU] examination in older children) should be deferred until the end of the examination. The examination should proceed efficiently and systematically.

Because young children may fear the examination and become fussy, simple inspection is important. For example, the examiner can observe the child's respiratory rate and work of breathing from across the room (often by having a parent lift the child's shirt) before moving near the child for the remainder of the examination. Observation will also provide the examiner with an opportunity to assess development and parent-child interactions.

Clothing should be removed slowly and gently to avoid threatening the child. A parent or the child is usually the best person to do this. Modesty should always be respected, and gowns or drapes should be provided. Examinations of adolescents should be chaperoned whenever a pelvic examination or a stressful or painful procedure is performed.

Examination tables are convenient, but a parent's lap is a comfortable location for a young child. For most purposes, an adequate examination can be conducted on a "table" formed by the parent's and examiner's legs as they sit facing each other.

Although a thorough physical examination is important at every age, certain components of the examination may change based on the age of the patient. An astute clinician can detect signs of important clinical conditions in an asymptomatic child. In infancy, for example, physical examination can reveal the presence of craniosynostosis, congenital heart disease, or developmental dysplasia of the hip. Similarly, examination of a toddler may reveal pallor suggestive of iron-deficiency anemia, or strabismus. The routine examination of an older child or adolescent may reveal scoliosis or acanthosis nigricans (a finding associated with insulin resistance).

HEALTH SUPERVISION VISITS

Pediatric primary care providers follow periodicity schedules that delineate the frequency of well child visits and the recommended screenings and assessments that should be completed from the prenatal visit through age 21. The American Academy of Pediatrics and Bright Futures (supported by the US Department of Health and Human Services and the Maternal and Child Health Bureau have developed comprehensive health supervision guidelines that include recommendations for measurements, sensory screening, developmental/social/behavioral/mental health, physical examination, procedures, and oral health. The current version of the table can be accessed at https://downloads.aap.org/AAP/PDF/periodicity_schedule.pdf. In areas where evidence-based information is lacking, expert opinion has been used as the basis for these plans. The *Bright Futures Guidelines* emphasizes working collaboratively with families, recognizing the need for attention toward children with medical complexity, gaining cultural competence, and addressing complementary and alternative care, as well as integrating mental health care into the primary care setting. Practitioners should remember that guidelines are not meant to be rigid; services should be individualized according to the child's needs. The AAP publishes Health Supervision Guidelines for Children with Down Syndrome that includes the additional items that should be performed for well visits in this population.

During health supervision visits, the practitioner should review child development and acute and chronic problems, conduct a complete physical examination, order appropriate screening tests, and anticipate future developments. New historical information should be elicited through an interval history. Development should be assessed by parental report and clinician observation. In addition, systematic use of formal parent-directed screening tools, such as the Ages and Stages Questionnaire (ASQ) or the Parents' Evaluation of Developmental Status (PEDS), is recommended. Growth parameters should be carefully recorded, and weight, length/height, head circumference (up to age 3), and body mass index (BMI) (for > 2 years) should be plotted and evaluated using established growth charts. Vision and hearing should be assessed subjectively at each visit, with objective assessments at intervals beginning after the child is old enough to cooperate with the screening test, usually starting at 4 years of age.

Because less than 4% of asymptomatic children have physical findings on routine health maintenance visits, a major portion of the health supervision visit is devoted to anticipatory guidance. This portion of the visit enables the health care provider to address behavioral and developmental concerns, injury prevention, nutritional issues, and school problems; and other age-appropriate issues that will arise before the next well-child visit.

American Academy of Pediatrics Periodicity Schedule: https://www.aap.org/periodicityschedule. Accessed July 11, 2024.

Bright Futures Resources: https://brightfutures.aap.org/Pages/default.aspx. Accessed July 6, 2023.

Bull MJ; Committee on Genetics: Health supervision for children with Down syndrome. Pediatrics 2011;128(2)393–406, reaffirmed 2016 [PMID: 21788214]. https://pediatrics.aappublications.org/content/128/2/393. Accessed July 6, 2023.

Hagan JF, Shaw JS, Duncan PM (eds): *Bright Futures: Guidelines for Health Supervision of Infants, Children, and Adolescents.* 4th ed. Elk Grove Village, IL: American Academy of Pediatrics; 2017.

DEVELOPMENTAL & BEHAVIORAL ASSESSMENT

Addressing developmental and behavioral problems is one of the central features of pediatric primary care. The term *developmental delay* refers to the circumstance in which a child has not demonstrated a developmental skill (such as walking independently) by an age at which the vast majority of normally developing children have accomplished this task. Developmental delays are quite common: approximately 18% of children younger than 18 years either have developmental delays or have conditions that place them at risk of developmental delays.

Pediatric practitioners are in a unique position to assess the development of their patients. This developmental assessment should ideally take the form of *developmental surveillance*, in which a skilled individual monitors development in multiple domains (gross motor, fine motor, language, and personal or social) over time as part of providing routine care. Developmental surveillance includes several key elements: listening to parent concerns, obtaining a developmental history, making careful observations during office visits, periodically screening all infants and children for delays using screening tools with validity evidence, recognizing conditions and circumstances that place children at increased risk of delays, and referring children who fail screening tests for further evaluation and intervention.

The prompt recognition of children with developmental delays is important for several reasons. Children with delays can be referred for a wide range of developmental therapies, such as those provided by physical, speech or language, and/or educational therapists. Children with delays, regardless of the cause, make better developmental progress if they receive appropriate developmental therapies than if they do not. Many infants and toddlers younger than 3 years with delays are eligible to receive a range of therapies and other services, often provided in the home, at no cost to families. Children aged 3 years and older with delays are eligible for developmental services through the local school system.

Several parent and physician-administered developmental screening tools are available and should be utilized to more efficiently incorporate this process in the busy well-child care visit. The PEDS, ASQ, and the Child Development Inventories (CDI) are screening tests that rely on parent report. Other screening tools, such as the Denver II screening test, the Early Language Milestone Scale (see Chapter 3, Figure 3–1), and the Bayley Infant Neurodevelopmental Screener, involve the direct observation of a child's skills by a care provider. All developmental screening tests have their strengths and weaknesses. For example, whereas the Denver II has relatively high sensitivity for detecting possible developmental delays, the specificity is poorer, and this may lead to the over referral of normal children for further developmental testing.

In addition to general developmental screening, autism-specific screens (such as the Modified Checklist for Autism in Toddlers [MCHAT]) should be administered at the 18- and 24-month health supervision visits.

The Survey of Well-being of Young Children (SWYC) is a newer tool that includes developmental milestones, emotional/behavioral domains, autism screening (at appropriate ages), and family context.

Regardless of the approach taken to developmental screening, there are a number of important considerations: (1) The range of normal childhood development is broad, and therefore a child with a single missing skill in a single developmental area is less likely to have a significant developmental problem than a child showing multiple delays in several developmental areas (eg, gross motor and language delays); (2) continuity of care is important because development is best assessed over time; (3) it is beneficial to routinely use formal screening tests to assess development; (4) if developmental delays are detected in primary care, these patients need referral for developmentally focused therapies and close follow-up; and (5) parents appreciate when attention is paid to their child's development and generally react positively to referrals for appropriate developmental therapies.

Age-based expectations for normal development are presented in Chapter 3, as well as a discussion of the recommended medical and neurodevelopmental evaluation of a child with a suspected developmental disorder.

In addition to developmental issues, pediatric providers are an important source of information and counseling for parents regarding a broad range of behavioral issues. The nature of the behavioral problems, of course, varies with the child's age. Some common issues raised by parents are discussed in detail in Chapter 3. Behavioral issues in adolescents are discussed in Chapter 4.

Links to Commonly Used Screening Instruments and Tools (Bright Futures) from AAP: https://publications.aap.org/toolkits/resources/15625/?autologincheck=redirected. Accessed May 1, 2023.

Lipkin PH, Macias MM: Promoting optimal development: identifying infants and young children with developmental disorders through developmental surveillance and screening. Pediatrics 2020;145(1):e20193449 [PMID: 31843861].
Talmi A et al: Improving developmental screening documentation and referral completion. Pediatrics 2014 Oct;134(4): e1181–e1188. doi: 10.1542/peds.2012-1151 [Epub 2014 Sep 1] [PMID: 25180272].

GROWTH PARAMETERS

Monitoring appropriate growth is pivotal in ambulatory pediatric practice. Height, weight, and head circumference are carefully measured at each well-child examination and plotted on age- and sex-specific growth charts. The Centers for Disease Control and Prevention (CDC) recommends use of the World Health Organization (WHO) growth standards to monitor growth for infants and children ages 0–2 in the United States. The WHO standards are based on an international sample of 8500 babies who were predominantly breast-fed for at least 4 months, still nursing at 1 year and living in nonsmoking households. Diagnosis-specific growth charts are available for infants born preterm and infants with Down syndrome, as well as Prader-Willi, Williams syndrome, Turner syndrome, Marfan syndrome, and others, though there are limitations to their use (see references).

To ensure accurate weight measurements for longitudinal comparisons, infants should be undressed completely, and young children should be wearing underpants only. Recumbent length is plotted on the chart until approximately 2 years of age. When the child is old enough to be measured upright, height should be plotted on the charts for ages 2–20 years. Routine measurements of head circumference may cease if circumferential head growth has been steady for the first 2 years of life. However, if a central nervous system (CNS) problem exists or develops, or if the child has growth deficiency, this measurement continues to be useful. Tracking the growth velocity for each of these parameters allows early recognition of deviations from normal.

It is useful to note that in the first year of life, it is common for height and weight measurements to cross over a percentile line. After approximately 18 months, most healthy children tend to follow the curve within one growth channel.

Determination of whether a child's weight falls within a healthy range relies on growth charts. For children younger than 2 years, the weight-for-length chart is used. For children 2–18 years, a BMI chart is used, which is a measure that correlates with adiposity- and obesity-related comorbidities. The BMI is calculated as the weight (in kilograms) divided by the squared height (in meters). The BMI is useful for determining obesity (BMI $\geq$ 95th percentile for age) and overweight (BMI between 85th and 95th percentiles), as well as underweight status (BMI $\leq$ 5th percentile for age). It must be emphasized that "eyeballing" overweight or underweight is frequently inaccurate and should not substitute for careful evaluation of the data on growth charts.

CDC and WHO growth charts: http://www.cdc.gov/growthcharts/. Accessed May 6, 2023.

CDC's Growth Charts for Children With Special Needs (module): http://depts.washington.edu/growth/cshcn/text/page1a.htm. Accessed May 6, 2023.

Growth Charts for specific conditions compiled by the University of Washington: http://depts.washington.edu/nutrpeds/fug/growth/specialty.htm. Accessed May 6, 2023.

Grummer-Strawn LM et al: Use of World Health Organization and CDC growth charts for children aged 0–59 months in the United States. MMWR Recomm Rep 2010;59(RR-9):115 [PMID: 20829749].

US Preventive Services Task Force: Screening for obesity in children and adolescents: US Preventive Services Task Force recommendation statement. JAMA 2017;317(23):2417–2426 [PMID: 28632874].

BLOOD PRESSURE

Blood pressure screening at well-child visits starts at age 3 years. There are some conditions that warrant blood pressure monitoring at an earlier age:

- History of preterm birth, very low birth weight, or other neonatal complication requiring intensive care
- Congenital heart disease (repaired or nonrepaired)
- Recurrent urinary tract infections (UTIs), hematuria, or proteinuria
- Known renal disease or urologic malformations
- Family history of congenital renal disease
- Solid organ transplant
- Malignancy or bone marrow transplant
- Treatment with drugs known to raise blood pressure (steroids, oral contraceptives)
- Other conditions associated with hypertension (neurofibromatosis, tuberous sclerosis, etc.)
- Evidence of elevated intracranial pressure

Accurate determination of blood pressure requires proper equipment (stethoscope, manometer and inflation cuff, or an automated system) and a cooperative, seated subject in a quiet room. Although automated blood pressure instruments are widely available and easy to use, blood pressure readings from these devices are typically 5 mm Hg higher for diastolic and 10 mm Hg higher for systolic blood pressure compared with auscultatory techniques. Therefore, the diagnosis of hypertension should not be made based on automated readings alone. Additionally, blood pressure varies by the height and weight of the individual. Consequently, hypertension is diagnosed as a systolic or diastolic blood pressure greater than the 95th percentile based on the age and height percentiles of the patient using charts from the AAP Clinical Practice Guidelines (see references).

The width of the inflatable portion of the cuff should be 40%–50% of the circumference of the limb. Overweight children need a larger cuff size to avoid a falsely elevated blood pressure reading. Cuffs that are too narrow will overestimate and those that are too wide will underestimate the true blood pressure. Hypertension should not be diagnosed based on readings at one visit, but rather three separate occasions of documented hypertension. Repeated measurements at different visits over time should be tracked using flowcharts in an electronic medical record or equivalent in a paper chart.

Children with repeated blood pressure readings from the 90th to the 95th percentile may be classified as having elevated blood pressure. Children with blood pressures greater than between the 95th and 99th percentile plus 12 mm of Hg are classified as stage 1 hypertension, and those greater than the 99th percentile plus 12 mm of Hg are termed stage 2 hypertension.

Patients with elevated blood pressure should receive lifestyle recommendations at each visit (diet, exercise, and weight management) and have blood pressure rechecked in 6 months. If blood pressures remain elevated at three time points, the patient will need diagnostic evaluation and possible subspecialty referral, generally to nephrology or a multidisciplinary clinic. See Chapter 24 for details.

Flynn JT et al: Clinical practice guideline for screening and management of high blood pressure in children and adolescents. Pediatrics 2017;140(3):e20171904. doi: org/10.1542/peds.2017-1904 [PMID: 28827377].

Hypertension Quality Improvement Resources and Tools from the AAP: https://www.aap.org/en-us/professional-resources/quality-improvement/quality-improvement-resources-and-tools/Pages/hypertension.aspx. Accessed July 6, 2021.

VISION & HEARING SCREENING

Examination of the eyes and an assessment of vision should be performed at every health supervision visit. Eye problems are relatively common in children: refractive errors (including myopia, hyperopia, and astigmatism), amblyopia (loss of visual acuity from cortical suppression of the vision of the eye), and/or strabismus (misalignment of the eyes) occur in 5%–10% of preschoolers. Assessment of vision should include visual inspection of the eyes and eyelids, alignment of eyes, and visual acuity.

Starting at birth, the movement and alignment of the eyes should be assessed, and the pupils and red reflexes examined. The red reflex, performed on each pupil individually and then on both eyes simultaneously, is used to detect eye opacities (eg, cataracts or corneal clouding) and retinal abnormalities (eg, retinal detachment or retinoblastoma). By 3 months of age, an infant should be able to track or visually follow a moving object, with both eyes.

Starting after age 3 years, formal testing of visual acuity should be done if possible. This can be performed in the office with a variety of tests, including the tumbling E chart or picture tests such as Allen cards. In these tests, each eye is tested separately, with the contralateral eye completely covered. Credit is given for any line on which the child gets 2 or less letters or pictures incorrect. Children who are unable to cooperate should be retested, ideally within 6 months, and those who cannot cooperate with repeated attempts should be referred to an ophthalmologist. Any two-line discrepancy between the two eyes, even within the passing range (eg, 20/20 in one eye, 20/30 in the other in a child aged $\geq$ 6 years) should be referred to an ophthalmologist.

Throughout childhood, clinicians should screen for undetected strabismus (ie, ocular misalignment). The corneal light reflex test can be used starting at 3 months and the cover test can be used beginning at 6 months to assess for strabismus. The corneal light reflex test, the cover test, and visual acuity test are described further in Chapter 16.

Recommendations for vision screening and indications for referral are listed in Table 9–2. Referral to an ophthalmologist is also recommended for preterm infants for evaluation of retinopathy of prematurity (ROP), as well as children with a family history of amblyopia, strabismus, retinoblastoma, or retinal degeneration. Children with Down syndrome should

be referred to an ophthalmologist at 6 months of age given their increased risk for refractive error, strabismus, and cataracts.

Approximately 3 in every 1000 newborns have moderate, severe, or profound hearing loss. Hearing loss, if undetected, can lead to substantial impairments in speech, language, and cognitive development. Early detection and intervention of hearing loss leads to better outcomes for children. Thus, universal hearing screening is provided to newborns in most parts of the United States. Hearing in infants is assessed using either evoked otoacoustic emissions or auditory brainstem-evoked responses. Because universal newborn hearing screening is sometimes associated with false-positive test results, confirmatory audiology testing is required for abnormal tests.

Informal behavioral testing of hearing, such as observing an infant's response to a shaken rattle, may be unreliable. In fact, parental concerns about hearing are of greater predictive value than the results of informal tests, and such concerns should be taken seriously. Prior to age 4, children should be referred to an audiologist for testing if a concern arises. Conventional screening audiometry, in which a child raises her hand when a sound is heard, can be performed starting at age 4. Each ear should be tested at 500, 1000, 2000, and 4000 Hz for ages 4–10 with the addition of 6000 and 8000 during adolescence. Patients are referred at threshold levels of greater than 20 dB at any of these frequencies. Any evidence of hearing loss should be substantiated by repeated testing, and if still abnormal, a referral for a formal hearing evaluation should be made.

The AAP periodicity schedule recommends routine hearing screening at 4, 5, 6, 8, and 10 years of age and several times during adolescence. Children with any risk factors for hearing loss should be closely followed and receive more frequent screening. Several inherited or acquired conditions increase the risk of hearing loss. Sometimes hearing loss can be mistaken for inattention, and so hearing screening should be part of workup for attention problems. Additional details regarding hearing assessment are provided in Chapter 18.

Table 9–2. Recommended vision screening in the primary care office.

Test	Age for Screening	Indication(s) for Referral
Inspection of eyes and lids	All	
Red reflex	Birth until child can read eye chart	Abnormal red reflex, asymmetry of the red reflexes, or partially obscured red reflex
Assessment of fixation and following	Starting at 2 mo	Poor fixation/following by 3 mo
Corneal light reflex for assessing strabismus	3 mo to 5 y	Asymmetry of light reflex (in relation to iris and pupil)
Cover testing for assessing strabismus	6 mo to 5 y	Presence of refixation movement
Fundoscopic examination	Starting at 3 y	
Preliterate eye chart testing	Starting at 3–4 y	Unable to pass 20/40 for ages 3–5 or 20/30 for 6 and older; also refer if there is a difference of two or more lines between the eyes

AAP Committee on Practice and Ambulatory Medicine, Section on Ophthalmology, American Association of Certified Orthoptists; American Association for Pediatric Ophthalmology and Strabismus; American Academy of Ophthalmology: Visual system assessment in infants, children, and young adults by pediatricians. Pediatrics 2016;137(1):28–30, reaffirmed 2021 [PMID: 29756730].

Harlor AD, Bower C; American Academy of Pediatrics Committee on Practice and Ambulatory Medicine, Section of Otolaryngology: Hearing assessment in infants and children: recommendations beyond neonatal screening. Pediatrics 2009;124(4):1252–1263 [PMID: 19786460].

Loh AR, Chiang MF: Pediatric vision screening. Pediatr Rev 2018 May;225–234 [PMID: 29716965].

Resources for Early Hearing Detection and Intervention: https://www.aap.org/en-us/advocacy-and-policy/aap-health-initiatives/PEHDIC/Pages/Early-Hearing-Detection-and-Intervention.aspx. Accessed April 21, 2023.

Newborn Screening

Newborn screening involves population-wide testing for metabolic and genetic diseases. It has become an essential component in a public health program that screens millions of newborns every year. Blood samples are collected by heel stick from newborns before hospital discharge, and results are usually available within 1 week. Some states routinely repeat blood testing after 7 days of life, while others recommend it if the child is discharged in less than 24 hours. The state-to-state variation seen in newborn screen panels has begun to diminish as a result of national recommendations. Current guidelines for a uniform screening panel recommend screening for 37 core conditions with another 26 detectable through differential diagnosis. Most states have adopted these guidelines.

Infants with a positive screening result should receive close follow-up, with additional confirmatory studies performed at a center with experience in doing these tests. Screening tests are usually accurate, but the sensitivity and specificity of a particular screening test must be carefully considered. If symptoms of a disease are present despite a negative result on a screening test, the infant should be tested further. Newborn screening has benefited thousands of infants and their families, preventing and diminishing the morbidity of many diseases. At the same time, the emotional cost of false-positive screening is a continuing challenge. Parents report high levels of stress during the evaluation process. Recommendations for useful resources, given the variability of information on the internet, and prompt clinical services can help reduce this distress.

Calonge N et al; Advisory Committee on Heritable Disorders in Newborns and Children: Committee report: method for evaluating conditions nominated for population-based screening of newborns and children. Genet Med 2010 Mar;12(3):153–159 [PMID: 20154628].

National Newborn Screening by State: https://newbornscreening.hrsa.gov/your-state#c. Accessed May 6, 2023.

Recommended Uniform Screening Panel: https://www.hrsa.gov/advisory-committees/heritable-disorders/rusp. Accessed May 6, 2023.

Lead Screening

The developing infant and child are at risk of lead poisoning or toxicity because of their propensity to place objects in the mouth and their efficient absorption of this metal. Children with lead toxicity are typically asymptomatic. High blood levels (> 70 mcg/dL) can cause severe health problems such as seizures and coma. Numerous neuropsychological deficits have been associated with lead exposure. Even blood lead levels less than 10 mcg/dL have been correlated with lower intelligence quotients. The primary source of lead exposure in this country remains lead-based paint, even though most of its uses have been banned since 1977. Other common sources of lead include water pumped through lead pipes and imported items such as clay pots. Lead levels have declined nationally from a mean of 16 mcg/dL in 1976 to less than 2 mcg/dL in 2008. However, considerable variation in lead levels exists in different regions of the United States, and many children at risk of lead toxicity are not currently screened. Despite the wide variation in the prevalence of lead toxicity, the CDC recommends universal lead screening for children at ages 1 and 2 and targeted screening for older children living in communities with a high percentage of old housing (> 27% of houses built before 1950) or a high percentage of children with elevated blood lead levels (> 12% of children with levels > 10 mcg/dL). Children enrolled in Medicaid are required to be screened at 12 and 24 months.

Communities with inadequate data regarding local blood lead levels should also undergo universal screening. Caregivers of children between 6 months and 6 years of age may be interviewed by questionnaire about environmental risk factors for lead exposure (Table 9–3), although the data to support the use of this screening are inconclusive. If risk factors are present, a blood lead level should be obtained. An elevated capillary (fingerstick) blood sample should always be confirmed by a venous sample. There is no safe level of lead in a child's blood, and in 2021 the CDC lowered the reference level to 3.5 mcg/dL. This level should be used to identify children at risk in order to initiate public health actions. The recommended actions can be viewed on the CDC website (see references).

The cognitive development of children with confirmed high blood levels should be evaluated and attempts made to identify the environmental source. Local public health

Table 9–3. Elements of a lead-risk questionnaire.

Recommended questions
1. Does your child live in or regularly visit a house built before 1950? This could include a day care center, preschool, the home of a baby sitter or relative.
2. Does your child live in or regularly visit a house built before 1978 with recent, ongoing, or planned renovation or remodeling?
3. Does your child have a sister or brother, housemate, or playmate being followed for an elevated lead level?

Questions that may be considered by region or locality
1. Does your child live with an adult whose job (eg, at a brass/copper foundry, firing range, automotive or boat repair shop, or furniture refinishing shop) or hobby (eg, electronics, fishing, stained-glass making, pottery making) involves exposure to lead?
2. Does your child live near a work or industrial site (eg, smelter, battery recycling plant) that involves the use of lead?
3. Does your child use pottery or ingest medications that are suspected of having a high lead content?
4. Does your child have exposure to old, nonbrand-type toys or burning lead-painted wood?
5. Does your child play on an athletic field with artificial turf?

centers or poison control centers can often aid in evaluating the patient's home. Concurrent iron deficiency should be treated if present. Chelation of lead is indicated for levels of 45 mcg/dL and higher and is urgently required for levels above 70 mcg/dL. All families should receive education to decrease the risk of lead exposure. With any elevated lead level, rescreening should be performed at recommended intervals.

American Academy of Pediatrics Council on Environmental Health: Prevention of Childhood Lead Toxicity. Pediatrics 2005;116(4):1036–1046 [PMID: 16199720].
Centers for Disease Control and Prevention: Childhood Lead Poisoning Prevention. https://www.cdc.gov/nceh/lead/default.htm. Accessed May 10, 2023.
Lead fact sheet (English and Spanish): https://www.cdc.gov/nceh/lead/docs/lead-levels-in-children-fact-sheet-508.pdf. Accessed July 6, 2021.
Markowitz M: Lead poisoning: an update. Pediatr Rev 2021;42(6):304–313 [PMID: 34074717].

Iron Deficiency

Iron deficiency is the most common nutritional deficiency in the United States. Severe iron deficiency causes anemia, behavioral problems, and cognitive effects, but recent evidence suggests that even iron deficiency without anemia may cause behavioral and cognitive difficulties. Some effects, such as the development of abnormal sleep cycles, may persist even if iron deficiency is corrected in infancy.

Risk factors for iron deficiency include preterm or low-birth-weight birth, multiple pregnancy, iron deficiency in the mother, exclusive breast-feeding, use of nonfortified formula or cow's milk before age 12 months, and an infant diet that is low in iron-containing foods. Infants and children with chronic illness, restricted diet, or extensive blood loss (such as gastrointestinal bleeding or injury) are at risk for iron deficiency.

Primary prevention of iron deficiency should be achieved through dietary means, including feeding ground up meats and iron-containing cereals by age 6 months, avoiding low-iron formula during infancy, and limiting cow's milk to 24 oz per day in children aged 1–5 years.

Universal screening for anemia should occur at approximately 12 months of age by obtaining a complete blood count (CBC) without differential, hemoglobin, or hematocrit. Premature and low-birth-weight infants may need testing before 6 months of age.

A full CBC to look at mean corpuscular volume (MCV) can aid in the evaluation. Serum ferritin, recommended by the WHO, is a useful test to evaluate iron deficiency, as it can also pick up iron deficiency in the absence of anemia and provides more specificity in detecting iron deficiency. Because ferritin is an acute-phase reactant and can be falsely reassuring in the presence of inflammation, infection, or malignancy, some experts recommend obtaining a concurrent C-reactive protein (CRP) for accurate interpretation of the ferritin level. Elevated lead levels can cause iron-deficiency anemia and should be explored as a cause for at-risk infants and children.

Management of iron deficiency with or without anemia includes treatment doses of 3–6 mg/kg body weight of *elemental* iron.

Baker RD et al; American Academy of Pediatrics; Committee on Nutrition: Diagnosis and prevention and iron-deficiency anemia in infants and young children (0–3 years of age). Pediatrics 2010;126:1040 [PMID: 20923825].
Greer FR, Baker RD: Early childhood chronic iron deficiency and later cognitive function: the conundrum continues. Pediatrics. 2022 Dec 1;150(6):e2022058591. doi: 10.1542/peds.2022-058591 [PMID: 36412053].
Oatley H et al: Screening for iron deficiency in early childhood using serum ferritin in the primary care setting. Pediatrics 2018 Dec;142(6) [PMID: 30487142].

Hypercholesterolemia & Hyperlipidemia

Cardiovascular disease is the leading cause of death in the United States, and research has documented that the atherosclerotic process begins in childhood. Genetic factors, diet, and physical activity all play a role in the disease process. Nonfasting lipid screening is recommended universally for children between the ages of 9 and 11 and 17 and 21. Fasting lipid screening is recommended between the ages of 2 and 8, and ages 12 and 16 if risk factors are present. Diet and weight management strategies are the primary interventions. However, consideration of pharmacotherapy should be made for severe dyslipidemia (LDL ≥ 190 mg/dL that persists after 6 months of diet modification or LDL > 160 mg/dL for moderate- and at-risk patients). The target for treatment is LDL less than 130 mg/dl.

Daniels SR: Guidelines for Screening, Prevention, Diagnosis and Treatment of Dyslipidemia in Children and Adolescents. [Updated 2020 Jan 18]. In: Feingold KR et al (eds): *Endotext [Internet]*. South Dartmouth, MA: MDText.com, Inc.; 2000. https://www.ncbi.nlm.nih.gov/books/NBK395579/.
Kubo T et al: Usefulness of non-fasting lipid parameters in children. J Pediatr Endocrinol Metab 2017;30(1):77–83 [PMID: 27977407].
Stewart J et al: Hyperlipidemia. Pediatr Rev 2020;41(8):393–402 AND Addendum to "Hyperlipidemia" Pediatr Rev 2021;42(10):579–580 [PMID: 32737252].

Tuberculosis

According to the CDC, 8916 cases of tuberculosis (TB) were reported in the United States in 2019 (2.7 per 100,000 people). TB testing can be performed by a skin test or a blood test. The Mantoux test (five tuberculin units of purified protein derivative) is the only recommended skin test. The interferon-gamma release assays (IGRAs) are blood tests that can be useful for patients who have been immunized with bacille Calmette-Guerin (BCG) or for patients who may have difficulty returning for a second appointment to look for skin reaction. See Chapter 42 for additional information on tuberculosis.

Targeted screening for latent TB for high-risk individuals is the recommended approach based on available evidence. The following screening questions have been validated to determine high-risk status:

1. Was your child born outside the United States? If yes, this question would be followed by: Where was your child born? If the child was born in Africa, Asia, Latin America, or Eastern Europe, a TB testing should be performed.

2. Has your child traveled outside the United States? If yes, this question would be followed by: Where did the child travel, with whom did the child stay, and how long did the child travel? If the child stayed with friends or family members in Africa, Asia, Latin America, or Eastern Europe for more than 1 week cumulatively, TB testing should be performed.

3. Has your child been exposed to anyone with TB disease? If yes, this question should be followed by questions to determine if the person had TB disease or latent TB infection (LTBI), when the exposure occurred, and what the nature of the contact was. If confirmed that the child has been exposed to someone with suspected or known TB disease, TB testing should be performed. If it is determined that a child had contact with a person with TB disease, notify the local health department per local reporting guidelines.

4. Does your child have close contact with a person who has a positive TB test? If yes, go to question 3.

American Academy of Pediatrics: Tuberculosis. In: David W. Kimberlin MD, FAAP, ed. 2021. Red Book: 2021-2024 Report of the Committee on Infectious Diseases - 32nd Ed. Printed in the United States of America. American Academy of Pediatrics. Holmberg PJ: Tuberculosis in Children. Pediatr Rev 2019;40(4): 168-178.

Screening of Adolescent Patients

Adolescents may present with chief complaints that are not the true concern for the visit. Repeating the question "Is there anything else you would like to discuss?" should be considered. Since suicide is a leading cause of morbidity and mortality in this age group, screening with the Pediatric Symptom Checklist for Youth or other validated tools that are age-appropriate is recommended (https://www.brightfutures.org/mentalhealth/pdf/professionals/ped_sympton_chklst.pdf).

Testing adolescents for blood cholesterol, TB, and HIV should be offered based on high-risk criteria outlined in this chapter and in Chapter 41. Female patients should have a screening hematocrit once after the onset of menses. During routine visits, adolescents should be questioned sensitively about risk factors (eg, multiple partners; early onset of sexual activity, including sexual abuse) and symptoms (eg, genital discharge, infectious lesions, pelvic pain) of sexually transmitted infections (STIs). Because STIs are often not symptomatic, urine polymerase chain reaction (PCR) for gonorrhea and chlamydia and screening tests for trichomoniasis should be considered. Current guidelines recommend that the first Papanicolaou (Pap) test should be performed at age 21 years, regardless of onset of sexual activity. A complete pelvic examination should be performed when evaluating lower abdominal pain in an adolescent.

See Chapter 4 for additional details on adolescent preventive services.

American Academy of Pediatrics Bright Futures Medical Screening Reference Table: https://downloads.aap.org/AAP/PDF/Bright%20Futures/MSRTable_AdolVisits_BF4.pdf?_ga=2.165897533.2085857802.1683391591-1957068794.1683391590. Accessed May 6, 2023.
Centers for Disease Control and Prevention: National Center for HIV, Viral Hepatitis; STD, and TB Prevention: Tuberculosis Surveillance Reports. http://www.cdc.gov/nchhstp/default.htm. Accessed May 6, 2023.

ANTICIPATORY GUIDANCE

An essential part of the health supervision visit is anticipatory guidance. During this counseling, the clinician directs the parent's or the older child's attention to issues that may arise in the future. Guidance must be appropriate to age, focus on concerns expressed by the parent and patient, and address issues in depth rather than run through several issues superficially. Both oral and printed materials are used. When selecting written materials, providers should be sensitive to issues of literacy and primary language spoken by the family members. Areas of concern include diet, injury prevention, developmental and behavioral issues, and health promotion.

Smoking Cessation

The deleterious effects of second-hand smoke (SHS) on children's health are well documented, and the AAP has highlighted the importance of tobacco screening and counseling at each pediatric visit. One-third of children live in a home with an adult smoker. The *Ask*, *Advise*, and *Refer* methodology has been shown to be a feasible approach to smoking cessation. Ask families if there is a smoker at home, advise the family about the benefit of cessation for the child, and refer to a formal cessation program if the family member is ready to quit.

Injury Prevention

For children and adolescents aged 1–19 years, unintentional injuries are the number one cause of death. In every age category, male patients are at higher risk than female patients for unintentional injury.

Injury prevention counseling is an important component of each health supervision visit and can be reinforced during all visits. Counseling should focus on problems that are frequent and age appropriate. Passive strategies of prevention should be emphasized because these are more effective than active strategies; for example, placing chemicals out of reach in high, locked cupboards to prevent poisoning will be more effective than instructing parents to watch their children closely.

Informational handouts about home safety, such as *The Injury Prevention Program* (TIPP; available from the AAP), can be provided in the waiting room. Advice can then be tailored to the specific needs of each family, with reinforcement from age-specific TIPP handouts.

A. Motor Vehicle Injuries

The primary cause of death of children in the United States is motor vehicle injuries. In 2020, 38% of children aged 12 years or younger who were killed in motor vehicle accidents were unrestrained.

The type and positioning of safety seats can be confusing. While car seat and booster seat laws differ by state, a recent AAP policy statement describes the best practice recommendations. All infants and toddlers should ride in a rear-facing car safety seat until 2 years of age or until they reach the weight and height limits for convertible car safety seats (usually 35–40 pounds). Infants may ride in infant-only seats (which often have a carrying handle and snap into a base that is secured in the car) until they reach the height and weight limit for that seat, and then transition to a convertible car seat. Once a child reaches 2 years of age (or younger than 2 if outgrown the weight and height limit of a convertible car seat), he or she can ride in a forward-facing car safety seat with a harness. The safest scenario is for a child to remain in a car safety seat with a harness as long as possible. Once a child reaches the weight or height limits of a forward-facing seat, he or she may be transitioned to a belt-positioning booster until the vehicle's lap-and-shoulder belt fits properly (child can sit with his back against the vehicle seat, bend his knees at the edge of the seat, have the belt positioned in the center of the shoulder and across the chest, and have the lap belt touching the thighs). These criteria are generally met once a child reaches a height of 4 ft 9 in and is between the ages of 8 and 12 years. All children younger than 13 years should be restrained in the rear seats of the vehicle.

Unfortunately, restraint use shows a decreasing trend with advancing age: children from 1 to 8 years of age use restraints over 90% of the time, but those 8–12 years of age use restraints less than 85% of the time. African American and Hispanic children use child safety seats less often than white children.

The use of portable electronic devices increases the risk of motor vehicle accidents. Using a cell phone while driving is associated with a threefold increase in motor vehicle accidents. Texting while driving poses an even greater danger. All should avoid these risks and adults should model safe practices.

B. Recreational Injuries: Bicycling, Skiing, and Snowboarding Injuries

Bicycle accidents are a primary cause of sports-related head injuries in children and adolescents, with 26,000 emergency department visits attributed to this each year. Pediatrics providers should recommend that children, adolescents, and their adult caregivers should wear properly fitting helmets specific to the sport (bicycling, skiing/snowboarding, ice skating, and equestrian sports) and advise that helmets be replaced if involved in an accident. Community-based interventions, especially those that provide free helmets, have been shown to increase observed bike helmet wearing. While there is no federal law mandating bicycle helmets, 21 states have passed legislation requiring bicycle helmets.

Snow sports, such as skiing and snowboarding, have high rates of head injury. Traumatic brain injuries are the leading cause of death for pediatric age skiers. Studies have shown a decrease in head injuries associated with helmet use.

C. Firearm Injuries and Violence Prevention

As of 2020, firearms are the leading cause of death in children ages 1–19 years in the United States, with the increasing numbers of gun-related deaths by suicide and homicide. It is estimated that one-third of children in the United States live in a home with a firearm. Counseling parents about firearm storage can reduce the risk of death and injury and should thus be an integral component of primary care pediatrics. The most effective way to prevent firearm injuries is to remove guns from the home. Families who keep firearms at home should lock them in a cabinet or drawer and store ammunition in a separate locked location.

D. Drowning and Near Drowning

Drowning is the leading cause of injury-related death in children ages 1–4 years and the second leading cause of injury-related death in children ages 5–19 years. An estimated 8700 children younger than 20 years old were taken to a hospital emergency department for a drowning event in 2017, with nearly 1000 deaths. Children younger than 1 year are most likely to drown in the bathtub. Buckets filled with water also present a risk of drowning to the older infant or toddler. For children aged 1–4 years, drowning or near drowning occurs most often in swimming pools; and for school-aged children and teens, drowning occurs most often in large bodies of water (eg, swimming pools or open water). Parents should be cautioned that inflatable swimming devices are not a substitution for approved live vests or close supervision and can give a false sense of security.

All children should be taught to swim, and recreational swimming should always be supervised. Home pools must be fenced securely, and parents should know how to perform cardiopulmonary resuscitation. A phone should be available near the swimming area. Because drowning is a leading cause of death by injury in children, the AAP has produced a Drowning Prevention "toolkit" for pediatric providers and families (see references).

E. Fire and Burn Injuries

Fires and burns are the leading cause of injury-related deaths in the home. Categories of burn injury include smoke inhalation; flame contact; scalding, and electrical, chemical, and ultraviolet burns. Scalding is the most common type of burn in children. Most scalds involve foods and beverages, but nearly one-fourth of scalds are with tap water, and for that reason it is recommended that hot water heaters be set to a maximum of 120°F. Most fire-related deaths result from smoke inhalation. Smoke detectors can prevent 85% of the injuries and deaths caused by fires in the home. Families should discuss a fire plan with children and practice emergency evacuation from the home.

Sunburn is a common thermal injury and often is not recognized because symptoms of excessive sun exposure usually do not begin until after the skin has been damaged. Repeated sunburn and excessive sun exposure are associated with skin cancers. Prevention of sunburn is best achieved by sun avoidance, particularly during the midday hours of 10 AM to 4 PM. A sunscreen with a minimum sun protection factor (SPF) of 30 that protects against both UVA and UVB rays should be used on sunny and cloudy days to help protect against sunburn. Hats, sunglasses, and long-sleeved swim shirts are also important aspects of safe sun exposure. The safety of sunscreen is not established for infants younger than 6 months; thus, sun avoidance, appropriate clothing, and hats are recommended for this age group. In extreme circumstances in which shade is not available, a minimal amount of sunscreen can be applied to small areas, including the face and back of the hands.

F. Choking

Choking is a leading cause of injury and death in young children. Choking hazards include food and small objects. Children younger than 3 are particularly at risk because they do not have fully coordinated chewing and swallowing, and they are more apt to put small objects in their mouth. Foods that are commonly associated with choking include hot dogs, hard candy, nuts, popcorn, raw vegetables, and chunks of meat, fruit, or cheese. Common nonfood items that pose a risk for choking include coins, latex balloons, button batteries, marbles, small toys, and small toy parts. Parents and caregivers should be trained in CPR and choking first aid.

American Academy of Pediatrics: Drowning Prevention Toolkit: https://www.aap.org/en-us/about-the-aap/aap-press-room/campaigns/drowning-prevention/Pages/default.aspx. Accessed May 1, 2023.

American Academy of Pediatrics: Gun Safety and Injury Prevention Resources. https://www.aap.org/en/patient-care/gun-safety-and-injury-prevention/. Accessed May 1, 2023.

American Academy of Pediatrics, Committee on Injury, Violence, and Poison Prevention: Prevention of choking among children. Pediatrics 2010;125:601 [PMID: 20176668].

Bunik et al: The ONE step initiative: quality improvement in a pediatric clinic for secondhand smoke reduction. Pediatrics 2013 Aug;132(2):e502–e511 [PMID: 23858424].

Centers for Disease Control and Prevention (CDC): Child Passenger Safety. https://www.cdc.gov/transportationsafety/child_passenger_safety/cps-factsheet.html. Accessed May 10, 2023.

Centers for Disease Control and Prevention (CDC): WISQARS (Web-based Injury Statistics Query and Reporting System): www.cdc.gov/injury/wisqars/index.html. Accessed May 10, 2023.

Denny SA; American Academy of Pediatrics; Committee on Injury, Violence, and Poison Prevention: prevention of drowning. Pediatrics 2019;143e20190850 [PMID: 30877146].

Durbin DR: Child passenger safety. Pediatrics 2018;142(5): e20182461 [PMID: 30166367].

Lee LK et al: Firearm-related injuries and deaths in children and youth: injury prevention and harm reduction. Pediatrics 2022;150(6) [PMID: 36207776].

Lee LK et al: Helmet use in preventing head injuries in bicycling, snow sports, and other recreational activities and sports. Pediatrics 2022;150(3):e2022058878 [PMID: 35965276].

NUTRITION COUNSELING

Screening for nutritional problems and guidance for age-appropriate dietary choices should be part of every health supervision visit. Overnutrition, undernutrition, and eating disorders can be detected by a careful analysis of dietary and activity patterns interpreted in the context of a child's growth pattern.

Human milk feeding is the preferred method for infant feeding for the first year of life. Pediatricians should assist mother-infant dyads with latch and help manage breast-feeding difficulties in the early newborn period. For exclusively and partially breast-fed infants, vitamin D supplementation should be given. Iron-fortified formula should be used in situations when breast-feeding is contraindicated such as HIV, active untreated TB, galactosemia, and certain medications. As noted in Chapter 11, the positive benefits of continued breast-feeding and breast milk by mothers who have used illicit drugs should be balanced in individual cases against the risk of transmission of such drugs to the infant via the milk. After the first year, breast-feeding may continue or whole cow's milk can be given because of continued rapid growth and high-energy needs. After 2 years of life, milk with 2% fat or lower may be offered. Baby foods and appropriately prepared table foods should be introduced between 4 and

6 months of age and self-feeding with finger foods encouraged by 7–8 months of age.

When obtaining a dietary history, it is helpful to assess the following: who purchases and prepares food, who feeds the child, whether meals and snacks occur at consistent times and in a consistent setting, whether children are allowed to snack or "graze" between meals, the types and portion sizes of food and drinks provided, the frequency of eating meals in restaurants or eating take-out food, and whether the child eats while watching television.

For children 2 years of age and older, a prudent diet consists of diverse food sources, encourages high-fiber foods (eg, fruits, vegetables, grain products), and limits sodium and fat intake. Since obesity is increasingly prevalent, processed foods, sugar-sweetened drinks or soda, and candy should be avoided or limited. National programs such as 5210 and Choose My Plate are evidence-supported references that providers can use. Parents should be gently reminded that they are modeling for a lifetime of eating behaviors in their children, both in terms of the types of foods they provide and the structure of meals (ie, the importance of the family eating together). For additional information on nutritional guidelines, undernutrition, and obesity, see Chapter 11; for eating disorders, see Chapter 6; and for adolescent obesity, see Chapter 4.

Women, Infants, and Children (WIC) food packages reflect the recommendations above and include provision of more fruits and vegetables, whole grains, yogurt and soy products, low-fat milk, and limitations on juice. Breast-feeding mothers receive more food as part of their package, less formula supplementation, and breast-fed infants receive baby food meats as a first food (because of more iron and zinc).

American Academy of Pediatrics Section on Breastfeeding Policy Statement: Breastfeeding and the use of human milk. Pediatrics 2012;129:e841 [PMID: 22371471].
Hampl S et al: American Academy of Pediatrics clinical practice guideline for the prevention, assessment, and treatment of children and adolescents with obesity. Pediatrics 2023;151(2):e2022060640 [PMID: 36622115].
WIC Food Packages: https://www.fns.usda.gov/wic/wic-food-packages. Accessed May 10, 2023.

COUNSELING ABOUT TELEVISION & OTHER MEDIA

Screen time and social media have a significant influence on children and adolescents. The average child in the United States watches approximately 3–5 hours of television per day, and this does not include time spent watching movies, playing video games, playing on computers or tablets, accessing the Internet, or using cell phones. Considering these other forms of media, current estimates are around 7.5 hours of media exposure per day for average 8- to 18-year-olds.

Having a television set in the bedroom increases daily media exposure and is also associated with sleep disturbances. According to the Kaiser Family Foundation, over 70% of 8- to 19-year-olds have a television in their bedrooms.

Watching television may have both positive and negative effects. Programs directed toward early childhood may increase knowledge and imagination and may also teach empathy and acceptance of diversity. However, excessive television viewing of programs with inappropriate content has been shown to have negative effects with respect to violence, sexuality, substance abuse, nutrition, social skills, and body self-image. More recent data suggest that excessive viewing in childhood may have a long-lasting negative effect on cognitive development and academic achievement. Clinicians should assess media exposure in their patients and offer parents concrete advice. Screen time for all media, including television, movies, DVDs, video games, computer activities, computers, tablets, the internet, and cell phones, should be limited. The AAP recommends that children less than 18- to 24-months-old should not have any screen time (unless it is video chatting), and that children 2–5 years be limited to 1-hour total screen time each day. The television should not be on during mealtimes, at night, or naptimes. Parents should themselves watch sensibly, monitor the program content to which their children are exposed, watch programs and discuss interesting content with children, remove television sets from all bedrooms, and encourage alternative activities. Parents should be advised that research consistently shows that exposure to media violence correlates with childhood aggression.

Social networking sites are becoming increasingly popular, and clinicians need to encourage parents to monitor participation and be aware of potential problems with cyberbullying, "Facebook depression," sexting, and exposure to inappropriate content on sites such as YouTube. Free family media use plans are available through the AAP (www.HealthyChildren.org/MediaUsePlan).

Chassiakos Y, Radesky J, Christakis D, Moreno M, Cross C: Children and adolescents and digital media. Pediatrics 2016;138(5):e20162593. doi: 10.1542/peds.2016-2593 [PMID: 27940795].
Hill D et al: Media and young minds. Pediatrics 2016;138(5):e20162591 [PMID: 27940793].
Radesky J, Christakis D: Increased screen time: implications for early childhood development and behavior. Pediatr Clin North Am 2016;63(5):827–839 [PMID: 27565361].

IMMUNIZATIONS

A child's immunization status should be assessed at every visit and every opportunity should be taken to vaccinate. Even though parents may keep an immunization record, it is critical that providers also keep an accurate record of a child's immunizations. This information should be written in a prominent location in the paper or electronic chart or kept in an immunization registry.

Despite high overall national immunization coverage levels, areas of under immunization continue to exist in the United States. An understanding of true contraindications (vs "false contraindications") and a "no missed opportunities" approach to immunization delivery has been shown to successfully increase immunization levels. Therefore, it is important that clinicians screen records and administer required immunizations at all types of visits, not just well child visits, and administer all needed vaccinations simultaneously. Additionally, clinicians should operate reminder or recall systems, in which parents of underimmunized children are prompted by mail, telephone, and text messages (particularly with adolescents) to visit the clinic for immunization. The assessment of clinic-wide immunization levels and feedback of these data to providers have also been shown to increase immunization rates.

Parent refusal of immunizations is an issue in some communities. It is useful for the provider to direct parents toward reliable sources to help them make an informed decision. A wealth of information for parents and providers about immunizations is available at the National Immunization Program's website (www.cdc.gov/vaccines). The vaccine schedule is also easily available online (www.cdc.gov/vaccines/schedules).

Hamborsky J, Kroger A; Centers for Disease Control and Prevention; Public Health Foundation: *Epidemiology and Prevention of Vaccine-Preventable Diseases*, E-Book: The Pink Book; 2015. https://www.cdc.gov/vaccines/pubs/pinkbook/index.html. Accessed May 6, 2023.

Kroger A, Bahta L, Long S, Sanchez P. General Best Practice Guidelines for Immunization. Best Practices Guidance of the Advisory Committee on Immunization Practices (ACIP).

Other Types of General Pediatric Service

ACUTE-CARE VISITS

Acute-care visits account for 30% or more of the general pediatrician's office visits. Office personnel should determine the reason for the visit and whether it is an emergent situation, obtain a brief synopsis of the child's symptoms, carefully document vital signs, and list known drug allergies. The clinician should document the events related to the presenting problem. The record should include supporting physical examination data and a diagnosis. Treatments and follow-up instructions must be recorded, including when to return to the office if the problem is not ameliorated. Immunization status should be screened. Depending on the severity of illness, this may also be an opportunity for age-appropriate health maintenance screenings and anticipatory guidance.

PRENATAL VISITS

Ideally, a couple's first trip to a physician's office should take place before the birth of their baby. A prenatal visit goes a long way toward establishing trust and enables a pediatric provider to learn about a family's expectations, concerns, and fears regarding the anticipated birth.

In addition to helping establish a relationship between parents and pediatric providers, the prenatal visit can be used to gather information about the parents and the pregnancy, provide information and advice, and identify high-risk situations. A range of information can be provided to parents regarding feeding choices and the benefits of breast-feeding; injury prevention, including sleeping position and the appropriate use of car seats; and techniques for managing colic. Potential high-risk situations that may be identified include mental health issues in the parents, a history of domestic violence, or maternal medical problems that may affect the infant. A prenatal visit also allows the pediatric provider to counsel about expectations in the newborn period. If the infant develops a problem during the newborn period, parents know who and when to call for assistance.

Yogman MD et al: The prenatal visit. Pediatrics 2018;142(1): e20181218 [PMID: 29941679].

SPORTS PHYSICALS

A preparticipation physical examination (PPE) is a recommended part of every routine well-child and adolescent care visit. Physicians should be recommending exercise and activity to every child, not just those participating in organized sports. Laws regarding frequency of PPE vary by state. Refer to the section Preparticipation Physical Evaluation in Chapter 27 for details of this visit, which should follow the same guidelines when done in the primary care office. The AAP has a toolkit with detailed information and forms that can streamline the PPE visit.

A few specific conditions bear mentioning during the counseling phase of the sports participation, including the risks and danger of concussions and performance-enhancing drugs. A list of medical conditions that may affect sports participation can be found in the references. Appropriate protective equipment should be encouraged.

American Academy of Pediatrics Preparticipation Exam toolkit: https://www.aap.org/en/patient-care/preparticipation-physical-evaluation/. Assessed May 10, 2023.

Miller SM: The sports preparticipation evaluation. Pediatr Rev 2019;40(3):108–128 [PMID: 30824496].

Rice SG; American Academy of Pediatrics Council on Sports Medicine and Fitness: Medical conditions affecting sports participation. Pediatrics 2008;121(4):841–848. doi: org/10.1542/peds.2008-0080 [PMID: 18381550].

CHRONIC DISEASE MANAGEMENT

Chronic disease in pediatrics is defined as illness that has been present for more than 3 months. Around 25% children and 35% adolescents have illnesses that meet the definition of a chronic illness. The most common chronic conditions in pediatric practice include asthma, obesity or overweight, attention-deficit/hyperactivity disorder (ADHD), and allergic diseases, but also include congenital anomalies and other conditions. Many patients with chronic conditions are cared for only by a primary care provider. However, when subspecialist care is required, the primary care provider plays an integral part of the care to deal with the complexity of these conditions, which also includes understanding the child's growth and development, routine health promotion and anticipatory guidance, evaluating for social issues, advocating for children and their families, and care coordination.

The goal of chronic disease management is to optimize quality of life while minimizing the side effects of treatment interventions. Problem lists should be used to document chronic diagnoses and monitor associated medications. The child and family's emotional responses to chronic illness should be addressed, and referrals to counselors should be offered if needed. Nutrition and the management of medical devices (eg, catheters, gastrostomy tubes) may need to be addressed, and care coordinated with appropriate specialists.

Blanco MA et al: Caring for medically complex children in the outpatient setting. Adv Pediatr 2021;68:89–102 [PMID: 34243861].
White PH et al: Supporting the health care transition from adolescence to adulthood in the medical home. Pediatrics 2018;142(5):e20182587 [PMID: 30705144].

MEDICAL HOME

The medical home is a concept in which children and their families have an identified, easily accessible primary care provider or group of primary care providers within an office. The AAP has identified seven characteristics of a medical home. The medical home must be (1) accessible, meaning that it must be within the child's community, physically accessible, and all insurances accepted; (2) family centered, with mutual responsibility and decision-making between the patient or family and medical provider, and the family is recognized as an expert of the child; (3) continuous, (ie, the same medical professionals provide the continuity of care); (4) comprehensive, with provisions made such that ambulatory and inpatient care are available 24 hours per day, 7 days a week, for 52 weeks of the year; (5) coordinated, with a plan of care developed by the physician and family that is communicated to other providers and agencies as needed; (6) compassionate, meaning that concern is expressed and efforts are made to understand the patient's and family's perspective; and (7) culturally effective, in that the cultural background of the patient and family is respected and incorporated into care, and services are provided in the family's primary language or through a trained medical interpreter.

All children should have a medical home, but it is particularly crucial for children with special health care needs or those with one or more chronic health conditions expected to last more than a year. A primary care provider through a medical home should be available for children to assist families with the coordination of consultant recommendations and development of a care plan to implement recommendations.

American Academy of Pediatrics: The medical home. Pediatrics 2002;110:184 [PMID: 12093969].
Medical Home Resources from the American Academy of Pediatrics: https://www.aap.org/en-us/professional-resources/practice-transformation/medicalhome/Pages/home.aspx. Accessed April 25, 2023.

MENTAL & BEHAVIORAL HEALTH

Parents frequently consult their pediatrician on a large variety of parenting and behavioral health issues. Common topics on which the pediatrician must be comfortable counseling include discipline, temper tantrums, toilet training, biting, and sleep problems.

In addition, there are mental health issues that pediatricians will commonly address in the primary care setting, including ADHD, anxiety, depression, school problems, or family stressors (such as separation, divorce, or remarriage). After assessing the situation, the primary care physician must decide whether the child's and family's needs are within his or her area of expertise or whether referral to another professional such as a psychologist or an education specialist would be appropriate.

The pediatrician should know the warning signs of childhood depression, anxiety, and bipolar disorder, and have a low threshold for referral of these concerns to the appropriate mental health professional. Ideally, mental health services not provided by the clinician are available in the same setting where physical health services are obtained.

Integrated Mental & Behavioral Health in the Primary Care Setting

In the United States, approximately 20% of school-age children suffer from a diagnosable emotional impairment. Prevalence is higher for children living in poor socioeconomic circumstances. About 75% of all children with psychiatric disturbances are seen in primary care settings, and half of all pediatric office visits involve behavioral, psychosocial, or educational concerns.

Child and family concerns routinely manifest in the context of visits with pediatric primary care providers. Parents are most likely to turn to their primary health care provider for information regarding parenting and child development than to another specialist. However, many pediatric providers in community settings do not feel equipped to address the growing mental health and behavioral needs of the populations they serve due to lack of training and perceived lack of support from mental health providers and systems.

Studies have shown that improved detection of mental health conditions is best done when there is a true partnership between clinical providers and families. A small number of clinic settings have moved forward with providing integrated behavior, development, and mental health training for physicians. The HealthySteps Program includes training for pediatric providers on delivering enhanced developmental services in pediatric primary care settings. Families participating in HealthySteps received more developmental services, were more satisfied with the quality of care provided, were more likely to attend well-child visits, receive vaccinations on time and were less likely to use severe discipline techniques with their children. Participation in the program also increased the likelihood that mothers at risk for depression would discuss their symptoms with someone in the pediatric setting.

American Academy of Pediatrics, Committee on Psychosocial Aspects of Child and Family Health and Task Force on Mental Health: The future of pediatrics: mental health competencies for pediatric primary care. Pediatrics 2009 Jul;124:410–421 [PMID: 19564328].

Asarnow J, Rozenman M, Wiblin J, Zeltzer L: Integrated medical-behavioral care compared with usual primary care for child and adolescent behavioral health: a meta-analysis. JAMA Pediatr 2015;169(10):929–937 [PMID: 26259143].

TELEPHONE MANAGEMENT & WEB-BASED INFORMATION

Providing appropriate, efficient, and timely clinical advice over the telephone is a critical element of pediatric primary care in the office setting. An estimated 20%–30% of all clinical care delivered by general pediatric offices is provided by telephone. Telephone calls to and from patients occur both during regular office hours and after the office has closed. The personnel and systems in place to handle office hours versus before- and after-hours calls may differ. In either circumstance, several principles are important: (1) advice is given only by clinicians or other staff with formal medical education (eg, nurse, medical assistant), (2) staff is given additional training in providing telephone care, (3) documentation is made of all pertinent information from calls, (4) standardized guidelines covering the most common pediatric symptoms are used, and (5) a physician is always available to handle urgent or difficult calls.

During routine office hours, approximately 20%–25% of all telephone calls to pediatric offices involve clinical matters. Many of these calls, however, are routine in nature, and an experienced nurse within the office can screen calls and provide appropriate advice by telephone. Calls from inexperienced

or anxious parents about simple concerns should be answered with understanding and respect. Parents who call with an emergency should be told to hang up and call 911. Other types of calls received during office hours should be promptly transferred to a physician or advanced practice provider: (1) calls regarding hospitalized patients, (2) calls from other medical professionals, and (3) calls from parents who demand to speak with a physician. When in doubt about the diagnosis or necessary treatment, nurses giving telephone advice should err on the side of having the patient seen in the office.

After-hours telephone answering services are available to many clinicians. Pediatric call centers, although not available in all communities, have benefits. Calls are managed using standardized guidelines, the call centers are typically staffed by nurses with abundant pediatric experience, the calls are well documented, and call centers often perform ongoing quality assurance. Extensive research on pediatric call centers has revealed a high degree of appropriate referrals to emergency departments, safety in terms of outcomes, parent satisfaction with the process, and savings to the health care system.

In general, after-hours pediatric telephone calls tend to be more serious than calls made during regular office hours. Deciding the disposition (which patients need to be seen, where they need to be seen, and how urgently), is the most important aspect of these after-hours telephone encounters. Several factors influence this final patient disposition: (1) the age of the patient, (2) the duration and type of symptom, (3) the presence of any underlying chronic condition, (4) whether the child appears "very sick" to the caller, and (5) the anxiety level of the caller. Once all the pertinent medical information is gathered, a decision is made about whether the child should be seen immediately (by ambulance vs car), seen in the Emergency Department or an urgent care setting or in the office later (today vs tomorrow), or whether the illness can be safely cared for at home. At the end of the call, it should be confirmed that parents understand and feel comfortable with the plan for their child.

The internet has become a common tool used in pediatric office settings. Information about the practice and providers, the care of common minor problems, scheduling of appointments, insurance issues, prescription refills, and laboratory test results are often available using the web. Pertinent health information, with appropriate permissions and authority, can often be provided via the electronic medical record to other locations such as hospitals and pharmacies. A well-functioning website is now a crucial service of pediatric practice.

ADVOCACY & COMMUNITY PEDIATRICS

Community pediatrics is "a perspective that enlarges the pediatrician's focus from one child to all children in the community." Pediatricians have historically been very involved in supporting and developing services for vulnerable children in their communities. As a group, pediatricians recognize that communities are integral determinants of a child's health and that the synthesis of public health and personal health principles and practices is important in the practice of community pediatrics.

Advocacy refers to the act of representing or pleading a cause on behalf of another. Pediatricians and other providers who care for children have a responsibility to be a voice for a population who cannot vote or advocate for themselves very effectively. Advocacy can be broken down into three categories: individual (patient-based), community, and legislative (policy-based).

Pediatricians in practice frequently engage in one-on-one advocacy, which may take the form of writing a letter of medical necessity or referring children and families to valuable services and resources. Pediatricians must be familiar with programs in the community. For example, children with special health care needs may be eligible for services typically funded through state health departments and through programs such as those provided based on the Individuals With Disabilities Education Act (IDEA). A variety of community-based immunization programs can provide access to needed immunizations for eligible children. Food and nutrition programs such as the federally funded WIC program provide sources of food at no cost to eligible families. Finally, subsidized preschool and childcare services such as the federally funded Head Start program provide preschool programs for qualifying children.

Community advocacy goes beyond the walls of the office or hospital. Pediatricians can become involved with local organizations that help children in the community. Pediatricians and other child advocates can work with community partners to address issues that influence child health. Community advocacy might focus on a particular condition (such as obesity) or environmental factors (such as exposure to violence) or improving health prevention (such as promoting programs to incorporate oral health into well-child visits). Finally, pediatricians can learn about issues that affect children and work to affect change at a local, state, or national level. Physician advocates may write or call their legislators, educate the public and disseminate information by writing letters or opinion pieces, provide expert testimony for legislative committees, or even help draft laws.

Camero K et al: Community advocacy in pediatric practice: perspectives from the field. Pediatr Clin N Am 2023;70:43–51 [PMID: 36402470].
Chamberlain LJ et al: Making advocacy part of your job: working for children in any practice setting. Pediatr Clin N Am 2023;70:25–34 [PMID: 36402468].
Earnest MA et al: Physician Advocacy: what is it and why do we do it? Acad Med 2010;85:63 [PMID: 20042825].

TOXIC STRESS

Chronic or significant stressors can have a tremendous impact on children, as well as increase their risk for medical, social, and substance abuse problems later in life. The Adverse Childhood Experiences (ACE) study showed a strongly positive relationship between childhood trauma [abuse (emotional/physical/sexual), household challenges (domestic violence, substance abuse, mental illness, parental separation/divorce, incarcerated family member), and neglect (emotional/physical)] with life-long medical and social problems. When a child experiences chronic stressors, but does not have buffering relationships, toxic stress occurs. Primary care pediatric providers can help families build resiliency by encouraging caregivers to take care of themselves and teaching them how to spend nurturing time with their children. Trauma-informed care is medical care with a focus on acknowledging and responding to the effects of trauma on children, families, and caregivers, which can improve patient/family engagement and health outcomes.

American Academy of Pediatrics Trauma-informed care resources: https://www.aap.org/en/patient-care/trauma-informed-care/. Accessed May 12, 2023.
Felitti VJ: Relationship of childhood abuse and household dysfunction to many of the leading causes of death in adults: the Adverse Childhood Experiences (ACE) study. Am J Prev Med 1998:14:245 [PMID: 9635069].
Forkey H et al: Trauma-informed care. Pediatrics. 2021;148(2): e2021052580 [PMID: 34312292].

COMMON GENERAL PEDIATRIC ISSUES

Ear Pain

Ear pain is common in children. While many parents are concerned for "ear infections" (acute otitis media) which prompts their visit, there are many causes for ear pain, including otitis externa ("swimmers ear"), sinus pressure, cerumen impaction, trauma to ear canal or tympanic membrane (often from use of a cotton-tipped swab), and dental pain that radiates to the ear. A thorough history and physical examination are needed to arrive at a correct diagnosis. See Chapter 18 for additional information on diagnosis and treatment of acute otitis media, otitis media with effusion, acute otitis externa, and cerumen impaction.

While ear pain is a common complaint, the general pediatrician will note that an infant tugging on his ears who has no other symptoms of illness has likely just discovered their ears and are playing with them as a result. Anticipatory guidance around all ear complaints should include discouraging use of any foreign objects, including cotton tip swabs, in the ear canal.

Fever

When evaluating a child with fever, one should elicit information about the duration of fever, how the temperature was taken, the maximum height of fever documented at home, all associated symptoms, any chronic medical conditions, any medications taken, medication allergies, fluid intake, urine output, exposures and travel, and any additional features of the illness that concern the parents (Table 9–4). In the office, temperature, heart rate, respiratory rate, and blood pressure should be documented, as well as oxygen saturation if the child has any increased work of breathing. A complete physical examination, including a neurologic examination, should then be performed, with attention paid to the child's degree of toxicity and hydration status. A well-appearing, well-hydrated child with evidence of a routine viral infection can be safely sent home with symptomatic treatment and careful return precautions.

Special consideration is given for evaluation and management of febrile infants under 60 days of life because of the possibility of serious disease, including sepsis. Treatment guidelines are stratified by infant age. Refer to local clinical guidelines or the AAP's Clinical Practice Guideline: Evaluation and Management of well-appearing febrile infants 8–60 days old for complete diagnostic and management algorithms.

While fever can be an isolated symptom in the first 24 hours of common childhood illnesses, children who present with fever but without any symptoms or signs of a focal infection beyond 48 hours are often a diagnostic and management challenge. When fever lasts for 8 days without an obvious source, it is defined as a fever of unknown origin (FUO) and the possible differential diagnosis becomes broad and requires a stepwise approach.

Fever phobia is a term that describes parents' anxious response to the fevers that all children experience. In one study, 91% of caregivers thought that a fever could cause harmful effects. Around 7% of parents thought that if they did not treat the fever, it would keep going higher. Parents need to be reassured that fevers lower than 41.7°C do not cause brain damage. They should be counseled that fever is helpful, as it is the body's way of fighting infection. Parents should be educated that, although fevers can occasionally cause seizures—in which case their child needs to be seen—febrile seizures are generally harmless and likewise do not cause brain damage.

Several safe and effective medications are available for the treatment of fever. Acetaminophen is indicated in children older than 2 months who have fever of 39°C or are uncomfortable. Acetaminophen is given in a dosage of 15 mg/kg of body weight per dose and can be given every 4 hours. The other widely used antipyretic is ibuprofen, which can be used in children 6 months and older. Ibuprofen is given in a dosage of 10 mg/kg of body weight per dose and can be given every 6 hours. Ibuprofen and acetaminophen are similar in safety and their ability to reduce fever. Aspirin should not be used for treating fever in any child or adolescent, because of its association with the development of Reye syndrome (particularly during infections with varicella and influenza). With all antipyretics, parents should be counseled to be very careful with dosing and frequency of administration as poisoning can be dangerous. Alternating acetaminophen and ibuprofen is not recommended.

Sore Throat

While viral pharyngitis is the most common cause of sore throat, strep pharyngitis is spread commonly among school aged children. Coxsackie virus and herpangina are seen frequently, especially in toddlers and preschoolers. (See Chapter 18 for details.)

Supportive care for sore throat may involve cold fluids (including popsicles) or warm fluids (warmed herbal tea, apple juice, broth) depending on child's preferences, a teaspoon of honey if the child is older than 12 months. Additional options for older children include saltwater gargles and sucking on hard candies.

Table 9–4. Guidelines for evaluating children with fever.

See immediately if:
1. Child is < age 3 mo with fever > 38°C.
2. Fever is > 40.6°C.
3. Child is crying inconsolably or whimpering.
4. Child is crying when moved or even touched.
5. Child is difficult to awaken.
6. Child's neck is stiff.
7. Purple spots or dots are present on the skin.
8. Child's breathing is difficult and not better after nasal passages are cleared.
9. Child is drooling saliva and is unable to swallow anything.
10. A convulsion has occurred.
11. Child has sickle cell disease, splenectomy, human immunodeficiency virus (HIV), chemotherapy, organ transplant, chronic steroids.
12. Child acts or looks "very sick".

See within 24 h if:
1. Child is 3–6 mo old (unless fever occurs within 48 h after a diphtheria-tetanus-pertussis vaccination and infant has no other serious symptoms).
2. Fever exceeds 40°C (especially if child is < age 3 y).
3. Burning or pain occurs with urination.
4. Fever has been present for > 24 h without an obvious cause or identified site of infection.
5. Fever has subsided for > 24 h and then returned.
6. Fever has been present > 72 h.

Respiratory Infections

Respiratory infections are a seasonal occurrence in pediatrics. Most infectious coughs are viral in nature, associated with upper respiratory infections, and do not require antibiotics. Lower respiratory infections, including viral infections (bronchiolitis or viral pneumonitis) and bacterial pneumonia must be considered. See Chapter 19.

Concerned parents will often bring a child with the common cold to clinic for evaluation. It is important to provide parents with actionable items as well as reassurance. While cough and cold medications are contraindicated in children less than 6 years old due to the potential for serious side effects, symptoms can be managed with supportive measures: drinking plenty of fluids, a teaspoon of honey for cough or sore throat if the child is 12 months or older, use of saline nose drops, and nasal suctioning (with bulb suction or nasal aspirator). Parents should be advised that children often have upwards of eight colds per year, often concentrated in the winter months creating a perception that their child is "always sick."

Dysuria

UTIs are seen in pediatrics from early infancy through adolescence and beyond. Symptoms can vary based on the age of the child. In infants, fever may be the only symptom. See Chapter 24 for details about diagnosis and management of UTI. Vulvovaginitis is common in prepubescent girls with a history of dysuria and examination notable for vulvar erythema. Families should be advised on proper hygiene (wiping front-to-back), wearing cotton underwear, and avoiding soap on the sensitive genital skin (including bubble baths). Sitz baths and petroleum jelly can provide comfort.

In the medical home, providers should be cognizant about following recommendations for imaging following UTI (see Chapter 24), particularly when following up a child diagnosed with UTI in another setting.

Growth Deficiency

Growth faltering or growth deficiency—formerly termed failure to thrive—is deceleration of growth velocity, resulting in crossing two major percentile lines on the growth chart. The diagnosis also is warranted if a child younger than 6 months has not grown for 2 consecutive months or if a child older than 6 months has not grown for 3 consecutive months. Growth deficiency occurs in about 8% of children. The history and physical examination will identify the cause of growth reduction in most cases (Table 9–5). Acceptable weight gain varies by age

Table 9–5. Components of initial evaluation for growth deficiency.

Birth history: newborn screening result; rule out intrauterine growth retardation, anoxia, congenital infections
Feeding and nutrition: difficulty sucking, chewing, swallowing
Feeding patterns: intake of formula, milk, juice, solids
Stooling and voiding of urine: diarrhea, constipation, vomiting, poor urine stream
Growth pattern: several points on the growth chart are crucial
Recurrent infections
Hospitalizations
Human immunodeficiency virus (HIV) risk factors
Developmental history
Social and family factors: family composition, financial status, supports, stresses; heritable diseases, heights and weights of relatives
Review of system

(Table 9–6). Refer to the section on pediatric undernutrition in Chapter 11 for information on assessment and management of this issue.

It is important for the primary care pediatrician to understand that just because an infant crosses a growth percentile does not mean an infant necessarily has a problem. Infants can cross growth curves normally, either "lagging down" or "shooting up." This crossing of growth percentiles is usually normal if it meets the following criteria: change in body weight and length are symmetrical, the size of the infant parallels the midparental weight and stature, the development remains normal, and a new growth curve is subsequently established, usually around 15 months of age; this also can be seen in the exclusively breast-fed infants at 4–6 months. WHO growth curves are now the standard and are based on children from various countries who were exclusively or primarily breast-fed in the first 4 months of life.

Table 9–6. Acceptable weight gain by age.

Age (mo)	Weight Gain (g/day)
Birth to 3	20–30
3–6	15–20
6–9	10–15
9–12	6–11
12–18	5–8
18–24	3–7

REFERENCES

Antoon JW et al: Pediatric fever of unknown origin. Pediatr Rev 2015;36(9):380–391 [PMID: 26330472].

Barker SJ: Honey for acute cough in children. Paediatr Child Health 2016;21(4):199–200 [PMID: 27429573].

Jackson EC: Urinary tract infections in children: knowledge update and salute to the future. Pediatr Rev 2015;36(4):153–166 [PMID: 25834219].

Pantell RH et al: Clinical practice guideline: evaluation and management of well-appearing febrile infants 8-60 days old. Pediatrics 2021;148(2):e2021052228 [PMID: 34281996].

Schmitt BD: *My Child Is Sick: Expert Advice for Managing Common Illnesses and Injuries*. 3rd ed. American Academy of Pediatrics; 2022.

Smith SM et al: Over-the-counter (OTC) medication for children and adults in community settings. Cochrane Database Syst Rev 2014;11:CD001831 [PMID: 25420096].

Tang MN et al: Failure to thrive or growth faltering: medical, developmental/behavioral, nutritional, and social dimensions. Pediatr Rev 2021;42(11):590–603 [PMID: 34725219].

Web Resources

American Academy of Pediatrics: http://www.aap.org. Accessed May 6, 2023.

Bright Futures National Health Promotion Initiative: http://www.brightfutures.org. Accessed June 29, 2019.

Centers for Disease Control and Prevention (vaccines and immunizations home page): http://www.cdc.gov/vaccines. Accessed May 6, 2023.

National Information Center for Children and Youth With Disabilities: https://www.parentcenterhub.org/. Accessed May 6, 2023.

Immunization

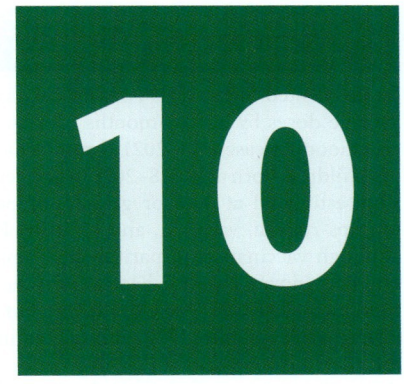

Joshua T. B. Williams, MD

Jessica R. Cataldi, MD, MSCS

Matthew F. Daley, MD

Sean T. O'Leary, MD, MPH

Immunization is one of the greatest public health achievements of modern times. Largely due to immunization, the annual incidences of diphtheria, paralytic poliomyelitis, measles, mumps, rubella, and *Haemophilus influenzae* type b (Hib) in the United States have fallen by more than 99% compared with the average annual incidences of these diseases in the 20th century. Invasive pneumococcal disease in children younger than 5 years has declined steeply since routine pneumococcal vaccination began in 2000. Similarly, rotavirus vaccination is associated with substantial declines in hospitalizations and emergency department visits for diarrheal illnesses in young children. Childhood immunization has also led, through herd immunity, to significant decreases in several infectious illnesses in adults, including pneumococcal, rotavirus, and varicella disease. The coronavirus disease 2019 (COVID-19) pandemic disrupted health care delivery and was associated with declines in routine vaccination for infants, children, and adolescents; efforts to regain these coverage losses are ongoing.

Every year, approximately 3.6 million children are born in the United States, and successful immunization of each birth cohort requires the concerted effort of parents, health care providers, public health officials, and vaccine manufacturers. Modern vaccines have a high degree of safety, serious adverse events following vaccination are rare, and vaccination benefits strongly outweigh these rare risks.

This chapter starts with general principles regarding immunization and the recommended pediatric and adolescent vaccination schedules, followed by a discussion of vaccine safety. Each recommended vaccine is then discussed. Vaccines given in special circumstances are discussed in the final section. Commonly used acronyms (eg, Centers for Disease Control and Prevention [CDC]) in this and other vaccine-related publications are defined with their first use in the text.

Because the immunization field is rapidly changing, it is important for health care providers to seek the most up-to-date information available. The recommendations outlined are current but will change as technology evolves and our understanding of the epidemiology of vaccine-preventable diseases changes. Several useful sources for regularly updated information about immunization are the following:

1. The Centers for Disease Control and Prevention (CDC). It maintains a website with extensive vaccine-related resources, including recommendations of the Advisory Committee on Immunization Practices (ACIP), vaccination schedules, Vaccine Information Statements (VISs), and detailed information for the public and providers. Available at: www.cdc.gov/vaccines.

2. CDC Contact Center. The CDC-INFO contact center provides services to the public and health care professionals regarding a variety of health-related issues, including immunizations. Available at: www.cdc.gov/cdc-info, or by phone at 1-800-232-4636 (English and Spanish).

3. *The Red Book: Report of the Committee on Infectious Diseases.* Published at 3-year intervals by the American Academy of Pediatrics (AAP). A revised *Red Book* was published in 2024. Updates are published in the journal *Pediatrics* and can also be accessed at redbook.solutions.aap.org/.

4. Immunize.org. This nonprofit organization creates and distributes educational materials for the public and health care providers. All materials are provided free of charge and can be accessed at www.vaccineinformation.org (for the public) or www.immunize.org (for health care providers).

5. The Vaccine Education Center at Children's Hospital of Philadelphia. Contains extensive vaccine-related materials, including regarding vaccine safety and vaccine ingredients. Available at: www.chop.edu/centers-programs/vaccine-education-center.

STANDARDS FOR PEDIATRIC IMMUNIZATION PRACTICES

In the United States, every infant requires over two dozen vaccine doses by age 18 months to be protected against 15 childhood diseases. By 2021, immunization coverage rates for children born in 2018–2019 who were aged 24 months were estimated at 90% or greater for poliovirus, measles-mumps-rubella, varicella, and hepatitis B (HepB) vaccines, although vaccination disparities were observed by race and ethnicity, poverty status, health insurance status, and Metropolitan Statistical Area residence. For children entering kindergarten in 2021–2022, immunization coverage dropped for a second consecutive year to 94% for state-required vaccines. The CDC recommends the following specific proven strategies to increase vaccination coverage rates: (1) assessing and providing feedback on practice/provider immunization rates; (2) keeping accurate immunization records; (3) recommending vaccination to parents with evidence-based communication techniques, and reinforcing when to return for vaccination; (4) sending reminder messages to parents; (5) sending reminder messages to providers; (6) reducing missed opportunities to vaccinate; (7) reducing barriers to vaccination within the practice; and (8) improving access to the Vaccines for Children (VFC) program.

The National Childhood Vaccine Injury Act of 1986 requires that for each vaccine covered under the Vaccine Injury Compensation Program, parents should be advised about the risks and benefits of vaccination in a standard manner, using VIS forms produced by CDC. Each time a Vaccine Injury Compensation Program–covered vaccine is administered, the current version of the VIS must be provided to the nonminor patient or legal guardian. Required vaccination documentation in the medical record includes the vaccine manufacturer, lot number, administration date, and expiration date. The VIS version and date and site and route of administration should also be recorded.

Needles used for vaccination should be sterile and disposable to minimize contamination. A 70% solution of alcohol is appropriate for disinfecting the stopper of the vaccine container and the skin at the injection site. A 5% topical emulsion of lidocaine-prilocaine applied to the site of vaccination for 30–60 minutes prior to the injection minimizes pain, especially when multiple vaccines are administered. Ethyl chloride spray can also be used as a rapid topical anesthetic. This can be especially helpful for children very fearful of needles and those who may otherwise need some restraint to be safely vaccinated. A separate syringe and needle should be used for each vaccine.

Compliance with the manufacturer's recommendations for route and site of administration of injectable vaccines are critical for safety and efficacy. With few exceptions (eg, rotavirus vaccines, Bacillus Calmette-Guérin [BCG] vaccine), all vaccines are given either intramuscularly or subcutaneously. All vaccines containing an adjuvant must be administered intramuscularly to avoid local irritation or granuloma formation. Intramuscular injections are given at a 90-degree angle to the skin, using a needle that is sufficiently long to reach the muscle tissue, but not so long as to injure underlying nerves, blood vessels, or bones. The anterolateral thigh is the preferred site of vaccination in newborns and children up to 2 years of age, and the deltoid muscle is the preferred site for children aged 3–18 years, although the anterolateral thigh is an acceptable site. Needle length and location should be ⅝ in. in newborn infants (thigh), 1 in. in infants 1- to 12-month-olds (thigh), 1–1½ in. in 1- to 18-year-olds (thigh), and ⅝–1 in. in 1- to 18-year-olds (deltoid). Subcutaneous injections should be administered at a 45-degree angle into the anterolateral aspect of the thigh (for infants < 12 months) or the upper outer triceps area (for children aged ≥ 12 months) using a 23- or 25-gauge, ⅝-in needle. Pulling back on the syringe prior to vaccine injection (aspiration) is not recommended. If multiple vaccines are to be administered in a single limb, they should be spaced an inch apart.

Many combinations of vaccines can be administered simultaneously without increasing the risk of adverse effects or compromising immune response. Depending on the combination vaccine used, children may receive an "extra" dose of HepB or Hib; these additional doses are not harmful. Inactivated vaccines can be given simultaneously with, or at any time after, a different vaccine. Injectable or intranasal live-virus vaccines (eg, measles-mumps-rubella [MMR], varicella [VAR], or live attenuated influenza vaccine [LAIV]), if not administered on the same day, should be given at least 4 weeks apart. If an immunoglobulin (Ig) or blood product has been administered, live-virus vaccination should be delayed 3–11 months to avoid interference with the immune response. The interval depends on the product given (details can be found at: www.cdc.gov/vaccines/hcp/acip-recs/general-recs/timing.html#t-05).

With the large number of vaccine preparations available, interchangeability of vaccines is an issue. All brands of HepB and Hepatitis A (HepA) vaccines are interchangeable. Haemophilus influenza type b (Hib) vaccine preparations dictate either a three-dose or four-dose series, according to the preparation. For vaccines containing acellular pertussis antigens, it is recommended that the same brand be used, but when the brand is unknown or the same brand is unavailable, any vaccine with diphtheria and tetanus toxoids and acellular pertussis should be used to continue vaccination. Exceptions to this rule are the serogroup B meningococcal (MenB) vaccines, which are not interchangeable under any circumstance. Extending recommended intervals between vaccinations does not alter final antibody titers, and lapsed schedules do not require restarting the series.

The numerous vaccines and other immunologic products used in routine practice vary in the storage temperatures required. Most vaccines should never be subjected to freezing temperatures (measles-mumps-rubella-varicella [MMRV] and VAR, which should be stored frozen, are exceptions).

Product package inserts should be consulted for detailed information on vaccine storage conditions and shelf life.

Vaccines very rarely (about one case per million doses) cause acute anaphylactic-type reactions. All vaccine providers should have the equipment, medications, staff, established protocols, and training to manage emergencies that may occur following vaccination.

CDC: General best practice guidelines for immunization. Best practices guidance of the Advisory Committee on Immunization Practices (ACIP). https://www.cdc.gov/vaccines/hcp/acip-recs/general-recs/.
CDC: Vaccination coverage by age 24 months among children born during 2018 and 2019—National Immunization Survey-Child, United States, 2019–2021. MMWR Morb Mortal Wkly Rep 2020; 72(2):33–38 [PMID: 36634013].
CDC: Vaccination coverage with selected vaccines and exemption rates among children in kindergarten—United States, 2021-22 School Year. MMWR Morb Mortal Wkly Rep 2023;72(2):26–32 [PMID: 36634005].
McNeil MM et al: Risk of anaphylaxis after vaccination in children and adults. J Allergy Clin Immunol 2016;137:868 [PMID: 26452420].

ROUTINE CHILDHOOD & ADOLESCENT IMMUNIZATION SCHEDULES

Each year, the CDC recommends immunization schedules for children and adolescents, which are an important guide for vaccination providers. Vaccines in the schedules are roughly ordered by the age at which the vaccines are first given. Table 10–1 is the 2024 schedule of routine immunizations for normal infants, children, and adolescents from birth through 18 years of age. Table 10–2 is the 2024 schedule for persons aged 4 months through 18 years who start vaccination late or are more than 1 month behind the routine immunization schedule. Annually updated immunization schedules are available at www.cdc.gov/vaccines.

Combination vaccines address the problem of large numbers of injections during a clinic visit. Currently available combination vaccines include MMR, MMRV, and various combinations of Hib, HepB, inactivated polio vaccine (IPV), and DTaP, including DTaP-HepB-IPV, DTaP-IPV-Hib, and DTaP-IPV-Hib-HepB. Separate vaccines should not be combined into one syringe by the provider unless approved by the Food and Drug Administration (FDA) because this could decrease the efficacy of vaccine components.

VACCINE SAFETY

Vaccine Safety Monitoring

The United States has a sophisticated, multifaceted system to monitor the safety of licensed vaccines. The Vaccine Adverse Event Reporting System (VAERS), the Vaccine Safety Datalink (VSD), the Biologics Effectiveness and Safety (BEST) Initiative, and the Clinical Immunization Safety Assessment (CISA) system each provide distinct contributions to monitoring vaccine safety. VAERS is a national passive surveillance system administered jointly by the FDA and CDC to accept reports from health care providers and the public about possible vaccine-related adverse events. Reports of adverse events possibly related to vaccination can be made via the Internet (vaers.hhs.gov) or by telephone (1-800-822-7967). As a passive surveillance system, VAERS is subject to limitations, including underreporting, overreporting, the reporting of events that are temporally but not causally related to vaccination, the lack of denominator data, and the lack of a comparison group. The VSD and BEST, in comparison, are active surveillance systems with continuous safety monitoring of vaccines in defined patient populations. The CISA system is designed to develop protocols for the evaluation, diagnosis, and treatment of adverse events following immunization.

Vaccine Contraindications & Precautions

All vaccines have certain contraindications and precautions that guide their administration. A contraindication indicates that the potential vaccine recipient is at increased risk of a serious adverse event. In the setting of precautions, the benefits and risks of vaccination must be carefully weighed prior to a decision regarding vaccination. Precautions are often temporary, in which case vaccination can resume once the precaution no longer applies. Contraindications and precautions are listed with each vaccine in this chapter. Additional detailed information is available from the CDC (www.cdc.gov/vaccines), in the AAP's *Red Book*, and in vaccine package inserts.

Dudley MZ et al: The state of vaccine safety science: systematic reviews of the evidence. Lancet Infect Dis 2020;20:e80 [PMID: 32278359].
Gidengil C et al: Safety of vaccines used for routine immunization in the United States: an updated systematic review and meta-analysis. Vaccine 2021;39:3696 [PMID: 34049735].

VACCINATION IN SPECIAL CIRCUMSTANCES

Minor Acute Illnesses

Minor acute illnesses, with or without low-grade fever, are not contraindications to vaccination, because there is no evidence that vaccination under these conditions increases the rate of adverse effects or decreases efficacy. A moderate to severe febrile illness may be a reason to postpone vaccination. Routine physical examination and temperature assessment are not necessary before vaccinating healthy infants and children.

Table 10–1. Recommended Child and Adolescent Immunization Schedule for ages 18 years or younger, United States, 2024.

These recommendations must be read with the notes that follow. For those who fall behind or start late, provide catch-up vaccination at the earliest opportunity as indicated by the green bars. To determine minimum intervals between doses, see the catch-up schedule (Table 2).

Vaccine and other immunizing agents	Birth	1 mo	2 mos	4 mos	6 mos	9 mos	12 mos	15 mos	18 mos	19–23 mos	2–3 yrs	4–6 yrs	7–10 yrs	11–12 yrs	13–15 yrs	16 yrs	17–18 yrs
Respiratory syncytial virus (RSV-mAb [Nirsevimab])		1 dose depending on maternal RSV vaccination status, See Notes				1 dose (8 through 19 months), See Notes											See Notes
Hepatitis B (HepB)	1st dose	◀── 2nd dose ──▶			◀─────── 3rd dose ───────▶												
Rotavirus (RV): RV1 (2-dose series), RV5 (3-dose series)			1st dose	2nd dose	See Notes												
Diphtheria, tetanus, acellular pertussis (DTaP <7 yrs)			1st dose	2nd dose	3rd dose		◀── 4th dose ──▶					5th dose					
Haemophilus influenzae type b (Hib)			1st dose	2nd dose	See Notes		3rd or 4th dose, See Notes										
Pneumococcal conjugate (PCV15, PCV20)			1st dose	2nd dose	3rd dose		◀── 4th dose ──▶										
Inactivated poliovirus (IPV <18 yrs)			1st dose	2nd dose	◀─────── 3rd dose ───────▶							4th dose					
COVID-19 (1vCOV-mRNA, 1vCOV-aPS)							1 or more doses of updated (2023–2024 Formula) vaccine (See Notes)										
Influenza (IIV4)							Annual vaccination 1 or 2 doses							Annual vaccination 1 dose only			
Influenza (LAIV4)											Annual vaccination 1 or 2 doses			Annual vaccination 1 dose only			
Measles, mumps, rubella (MMR)					See Notes		◀── 1st dose ──▶					2nd dose					
Varicella (VAR)					See Notes		◀── 1st dose ──▶					2nd dose					
Hepatitis A (HepA)					See Notes		2-dose series, See Notes										
Tetanus, diphtheria, acellular pertussis (Tdap ≥7 yrs)														1 dose			
Human papillomavirus (HPV)														See Notes			
Meningococcal (MenACWY-CRM ≥2 mos, MenACWY-TT ≥2 years)														1st dose		2nd dose	
Meningococcal B (MenB-4C, MenB-FHbp)														See Notes			
Respiratory syncytial virus vaccine (RSV [Abrysvo])														Seasonal administration during pregnancy, See Notes			
Dengue (DEN4CYD; 9–16 yrs)														Seropositive in endemic dengue areas (See Notes)			
Mpox																	

Legend:
- Range of recommended ages for all children
- Range of recommended ages for catch-up vaccination
- Range of recommended ages for certain high-risk groups
- Recommended vaccination can begin in this age group
- Recommended vaccination based on shared clinical decision-making
- No recommendation/not applicable

Reproduced from Centers for Disease Control (CDC) https://www.cdc.gov/vaccines/schedules/hcp/imz/child-adolescent.html.

Table 10–2. Recommended Catch-up Immunization Schedule for Children and Adolescents Who Start Late or Who Are More than 1 Month Behind, United States, 2024.

The table below provides catch-up schedules and minimum intervals between doses for children whose vaccinations have been delayed. A vaccine series does not need to be restarted, regardless of the time that has elapsed between doses. Use the section appropriate for the child's age. **Always use this table in conjunction with Table 1 and the Notes that follow.**

Vaccine	Minimum Age for Dose 1	Minimum Interval Between Doses			
		Dose 1 to Dose 2	Dose 2 to Dose 3	Dose 3 to Dose 4	Dose 4 to Dose 5
Children age 4 months through 6 years					
Hepatitis B	Birth	4 weeks	**8 weeks** *and* **at least 16 weeks after first dose** minimum age for the final dose is 24 weeks		
Rotavirus	6 weeks Maximum age for first dose is 14 weeks, 6 days.	4 weeks	**4 weeks** maximum age for final dose is 8 months, 0 days.		
Diphtheria, tetanus, and acellular pertussis	6 weeks	4 weeks	4 weeks	6 months	**6 months** A fifth dose is not necessary if the fourth dose was administered at age 4 years or older *and* at least 6 months after dose 3
Haemophilus influenzae type b	6 weeks	**No further doses needed** if first dose was administered at age 15 months or older. **4 weeks** if first dose was administered before the 1st birthday. **8 weeks (as final dose)** if first dose was administered at age 12 through 14 months.	**No further doses needed** if previous dose was administered at age 15 months or older **4 weeks** if current age is younger than 12 months *and* first dose was administered at younger than age 7 months *and* at least 1 previous dose was PRP-T (ActHIB®, Pentacel®, Hiberix®, Vaxelis®) or unknown **8 weeks** *and* **age 12 through 59 months (as final dose)** if current age is younger than 12 months *and* first dose was administered at age 7 through 11 months; **OR** if current age is 12 through 59 months *and* first dose was administered before the 1st birthday *and* second dose was administered at younger than age 15 months; **OR** if both doses were PedvaxHIB® and were administered before the 1st birthday	**8 weeks (as final dose)** This dose only necessary for children age 12 through 59 months who received 3 doses before the 1st birthday.	
Pneumococcal conjugate	6 weeks	**No further doses needed** for healthy children if first dose was administered at age 24 months or older **4 weeks** if first dose was administered before the 1st birthday **8 weeks (as final dose for healthy children)** if first dose was administered at the 1st birthday or after	**No further doses needed** for healthy children if previous dose was administered at age 24 months or older **4 weeks** if current age is younger than 12 months *and* previous dose was administered at <7 months old **8 weeks (as final dose for healthy children)** if previous dose was administered between 7–11 months (wait until at least 12 months old); **OR** if current age is 12 months or older *and* at least 1 dose was administered before age 12 months	**8 weeks (as final dose)** This dose is only necessary for children age 12 through 59 months regardless of risk, or age 60 through 71 months with any risk, who received 3 doses before age 12 months.	
Inactivated poliovirus	6 weeks	4 weeks	**4 weeks** if current age is <4 years **6 months (as final dose)** if current age is 4 years or older	**6 months (minimum age 4 years for final dose)**	
Measles, mumps, rubella	12 months	4 weeks			
Varicella	12 months	3 months			
Hepatitis A	12 months	6 months			
Meningococcal ACWY	2 months MenACWY-CRM 2 years MenACWY-TT	8 weeks	See Notes	See Notes	
Children and adolescents age 7 through 18 years					
Meningococcal ACWY	Not applicable (N/A)	8 weeks			
Tetanus, diphtheria; tetanus, diphtheria, and acellular pertussis	7 years	4 weeks	**4 weeks** if first dose of DTaP/DT was administered before the 1st birthday **6 months (as final dose)** if first dose of DTaP/DT or Tdap/Td was administered at or after the 1st birthday	**6 months** if first dose of DTaP/DT was administered before the 1st birthday	
Human papillomavirus	9 years	**Routine dosing intervals are recommended.**			
Hepatitis A	N/A	6 months			
Hepatitis B	N/A	4 weeks	**8 weeks** *and* **at least 16 weeks after first dose**		
Inactivated poliovirus	N/A	4 weeks	**6 months** A fourth dose is not necessary if the third dose was administered at age 4 years or older *and* at least 6 months after the previous dose.	A fourth dose of IPV is indicated if all previous doses were administered at <4 years **OR** if the third dose was administered <6 months after the second dose.	
Measles, mumps, rubella	N/A	4 weeks			
Varicella	N/A	**3 months** if younger than age 13 years. **4 weeks** if age 13 years or older			
Dengue	9 years	6 months	6 months		

For vaccination recommendations for persons ages 19 years or older, see the Recommended Adult Immunization Schedule, 2024.

Additional information

- For calculating intervals between doses, 4 weeks = 28 days. Intervals of ≥4 months are determined by calendar months.
- Within a number range (e.g., 12–18), a dash (–) should be read as "through."
- Vaccine doses administered ≤4 days before the minimum age or interval are considered valid. Doses of any vaccine administered ≥5 days earlier than the minimum age or minimum interval should not be counted as valid and should be repeated as age-appropriate. **The repeat dose should be spaced after the invalid dose by the recommended minimum interval.** For further details, see Table 3-2, Recommended and minimum ages and intervals between vaccine doses, in *General Best Practice Guidelines for Immunization*.
- Information on travel vaccination requirements and recommendations is available at https://www.cdc.gov/travel/.
- For vaccination of persons with immunodeficiencies, see Table 8-1, Vaccination of persons with primary and secondary immunodeficiencies, in *General Best Practice Guidelines for Immunization*, Immunization in Special Clinical Circumstances (In: Kimberlin DW, Barnett ED, Lynfield Ruth, Sawyer MH, eds. Red Book: 2021–2024 Report of the Committee on Infectious Diseases. 32nd ed. Itasca, IL: American Academy of Pediatrics; 2021:72–86).
- For information about vaccination in the setting of a vaccine-preventable disease outbreak, contact your state or local health department.
- The National Vaccine Injury Compensation Program (VICP) is a no-fault alternative to the traditional legal system for resolving vaccine injury claims. All vaccines included in the child and adolescent vaccine schedule are covered by VICP except for dengue, PPSV23, RSV, Mpox and COVID-19 vaccines. Mpox and COVID-19 vaccines that are covered by the Countermeasures Injury Compensation Program (CICP). For more information, see www.hrsa.gov/vaccinecompensation or www.hrsa.gov/cicp.

Covid-19 vaccination
(Minimum age: 6 months [Moderna and Pfizer-BioNTech COVID-19 vaccines], 12 years [Novavax COVID-19 Vaccine])

Routine vaccination

Age 6 months–4 years
- Unvaccinated:
  ○ 2-dose series of updated (2023–2024 Formula) Moderna at 0, 4–8 weeks
  ○ 3-dose series of updated (2023–2024 Formula) Pfizer-BioNTech at 0, 3–8, 11–16 weeks
- Previously vaccinated* with 1 dose of any Moderna: 1 dose of updated (2023–2024 Formula) Moderna 4–8 weeks after the most recent dose.
- Previously vaccinated* with 2 or more doses of any Moderna: 1 dose of updated (2023–2024 Formula) Moderna at least 8 weeks after the most recent dose.
- Previously vaccinated* with 1 dose of any Pfizer-BioNTech: 2-dose series of updated (2023–2024 Formula) Pfizer-BioNTech at 0, 8 weeks (minimum interval between previous Pfizer-BioNTech and dose 1: 3–8 weeks).
- Previously vaccinated* with 2 or more doses of any Pfizer-BioNTech: 1 dose of updated (2023–2024 Formula) Pfizer-BioNTech at least 8 weeks after the most recent dose.

Age 5–11 years
- Unvaccinated: 1 dose of updated (2023–2024 Formula) Moderna or Pfizer-BioNTech vaccine.
- Previously vaccinated* with 1 or more doses of Moderna or Pfizer-BioNTech: 1 dose of updated (2023–2024 Formula) Moderna or Pfizer-BioNTech at least 8 weeks after the most recent dose.

Age 12–18 years
- Unvaccinated:
  ○ 1 dose of updated (2023–2024 Formula) Moderna or Pfizer-BioNTech vaccine
  ○ 2-dose series of updated (2023–2024 Formula) Novavax at 0, 3–8 weeks
- Previously vaccinated* with any COVID-19 vaccine(s): 1 dose of any updated (2023–2024 Formula) COVID-19 vaccine at least 8 weeks after the most recent dose.
- *Note: Previously vaccinated is defined as having received any Original monovalent or bivalent COVID-19 vaccine (Janssen, Moderna, Novavax, Pfizer-BioNTech) prior to the updated 2023–2024 formulation.

There is no preferential recommendation for the use of one COVID-19 vaccine over another-when more than one recommended age-appropriate vaccine is available.

Administer an age-appropriate COVID-19 vaccine product for each dose. For information about transition from age 4 years to age 5 years or age 11 years to age 12 years during COVID-19 vaccination series, see Tables 1 and 2 at www.cdc.gov/vaccines/covid-19/clinical-considerations/interim-considerations-us.html#covid-vaccines.

Current COVID-19 schedule and dosage formulation available at www.cdc.gov/covidschedule. For more information on Emergency Use Authorization (EUA) indications for COVID-19 vaccines, see www.fda.gov/emergency-preparedness-and-response/coronavirus-disease-2019-covid-19/covid-19-vaccines

Special situations
Persons who are moderately or severely immunocompromised**

Age 6 months–4 years
- Unvaccinated:
  ○ 3-dose series of updated (2023–2024 Formula) Moderna at 0, 4, 8 weeks
  ○ 3-dose series of updated (2023–2024 Formula) Pfizer-BioNTech at 0, 3, 11 weeks.
- Previously vaccinated* with 1 dose of any Moderna: 2-dose series of updated (2023–2024 Formula) Moderna at 0, 4 weeks (minimum interval between previous Moderna and dose 1: 4 weeks).
- Previously vaccinated* with 2 doses of any Moderna: 1 dose of updated (2023–2024 Formula) Moderna at least 4 weeks after the most recent dose.
- Previously vaccinated* with 3 or more doses of any Moderna: 1 dose of updated (2023–2024 Formula) Moderna at least 8 weeks after the most recent dose.
- Previously vaccinated* with 1 dose of any Pfizer-BioNTech: 2-dose series of updated (2023–2024 Formula) Pfizer-BioNTech at 0, 8 weeks (minimum interval between previous Pfizer-BioNTech and dose 1: 3 weeks).
- Previously vaccinated* with 2 or more doses of any Pfizer-BioNTech: 1 dose of updated (2023–2024 Formula) Pfizer-BioNTech at least 8 weeks after the most recent dose.

Age 5–11 years
- Unvaccinated:
  ○ 3-dose series of updated (2023–2024 Formula) Moderna at 0, 4, 8 weeks
  ○ 3-dose series updated (2023–2024 Formula) Pfizer-BioNTech at 0, 3, 7 weeks.
- Previously vaccinated* with 1 dose of any Moderna: 2-dose series of updated (2023–2024 Formula) Moderna at 0, 4 weeks (minimum interval between previous Moderna and dose 1: 4 weeks).
- Previously vaccinated* with 2 doses of any Moderna: 1 dose of updated (2023–2024 Formula) Moderna at least 4 weeks after the most recent dose.
- Previously vaccinated* with 3 or more doses of any Moderna: 1 dose of updated (2023–2024 Formula) Moderna or Pfizer-BioNTech at least 8 weeks after the most recent dose.

Age 12–18 years
• Unvaccinated:
  ○ 3-dose series of updated (2023–2024 Formula) Moderna at 0, 4, 8 weeks
  ○ 3-dose series of updated (2023–2024 Formula) Pfizer-BioNTech at 0, 3, 7 weeks
  ○ 2-dose series of updated (2023–2024 Formula) Novavax at 0, 3 weeks
• Previously vaccinated* with 1 dose of any Moderna: 2-dose series of updated (2023–2024 Formula) Moderna at 0, 4 weeks (minimum interval between previous Moderna dose and dose 1: 4 weeks).
• Previously vaccinated* with 2 doses of any Moderna: 1 dose of updated (2023–2024 Formula) Moderna at least 4 weeks after the most recent dose.
• Previously vaccinated* with 1 dose of any Pfizer- BioNTech: 2-dose series of updated (2023–2024 Formula) Pfizer-BioNTech at 0, 4 weeks (minimum interval between previous Pfizer-BioNTech dose and dose 1: 3 weeks).
• Previously vaccinated* with 2 doses of any Pfizer- BioNTech: 1 dose of updated (2023–2024 Formula) Pfizer-BioNTech at least 4 weeks after the most recent dose.
• Previously vaccinated* with 3 or more doses of any Moderna or Pfizer-BioNTech: 1 dose of any updated (2023–2024 Formula) COVID-19 vaccine at least 8 weeks after the most recent dose.
• Previously vaccinated* with 1 or more doses of Janssen or Novavax or with or without dose(s) of any Original monovalent or bivalent COVID-19 vaccine: 1 dose of any updated (2023–2024 Formula) COVID-19 vaccine at least 8 weeks after the most recent dose.

There is no preferential recommendation for the use of one COVID-19 vaccine over another when more than one recommended age-appropriate vaccine is available.

Administer an age-appropriate COVID-19 vaccine product for each dose. For information about transition from age 4 years to age 5 years or age 11 years to age 12 years during COVID-19 vaccination series, see Tables 1 and 2 at www.cdc.gov/vaccines/covid-19/clinical-considerations/interim-considerations-us.html#covid-vaccines.

Current COVID-19 schedule and dosage formulation available at www.cdc.gov/covidschedule. For more information on Emergency Use Authorization (EUA) indications for COVID-19 vaccines, see www.fda.gov/emergency-preparedness-and-response/coronavirus-disease-2019-covid-19/covid-19-vaccines

*Note: Previously vaccinated is defined as having received any Original monovalent or bivalent COVID-19 vaccine (Janssen, Moderna, Novavax, Pfizer-BioNTech) prior to the updated 2023–2024 formulation.

**Note: Persons who are moderately or severely immunocompromised have the option to receive one additional dose of updated (2023–2024 Formula) COVID-19 vaccine at least 2 months following the last recommended updated (2023–2024 Formula) COVID-19 vaccine dose. Further additional updated (2023–2024 Formula) COVID-19 vaccine dose(s) may be administered, informed by the clinical judgement of a healthcare provider and personal preference and circumstances. Any further additional doses should be administered at least 2 months after the last updated (2023–2024 Formula) COVID-19 vaccine dose. Moderately or severely immunocompromised children 6 months–4 years of age should receive homologous updated (2023–2024 Formula) mRNA vaccine dose(s) if they receive additional doses.

Contraindications and Precautions
For contraindications and precautions to COVID-19 vaccination, see Appendix.

Dengue vaccination
(minimum age: 9 years)

Routine vaccination
• Age 9–16 years living in dengue endemic areas AND have laboratory confirmation of previous dengue infection-3-dose series administered at 0, 6, and 12 months
• Endemic areas include Puerto Rico, American Samoa, US Virgin Islands, Federated States of Micronesia, Republic of Marshall Islands, and the Republic of Palau. For updated guidance on dengue endemic areas and pre-vaccination laboratory testing see www.cdc.gov/mmwr/volumes/70/rr/rr7006a1.htm?s_cid=rr7006a1_w and www.cdc.gov/dengue/vaccine/hcp/index.html
• Dengue vaccine should not be administered to children traveling to or visiting endemic dengue areas.

Diphtheria, tetanus, and pertussis (DTaP) vaccination (minimum age: 6 weeks [4 years for Kinrix® or Quadracel®])

Routine vaccination
• 5-dose series at age 2, 4, 6, 15–18 months, 4–6 years
- Prospectively: Dose 4 may be administered as early as age 12 months if at least 6 months have elapsed since dose 3.
- Retrospectively: A 4th dose that was inadvertently administered as early as age 12 months may be counted if at least 4 months have elapsed since dose 3.

Catch-up vaccination
• Dose 5 is not necessary if dose 4 was administered at age 4 years or older and at least 6 months after dose 3.
• For other catch-up guidance, see Table 10-2.

Special situations
• Wound management in children less than age 7 years with history of 3 or more doses of tetanus-toxoid-containing vaccine: For all wounds except clean and minor wounds, administer DTaP if more than 5 years since last dose of tetanus-toxoid-containing vaccine. For detailed information, see www.cdc.gov/mmwr/volumes/67/rr/rr6702a1.htm

Haemophilus influenzae type b vaccination
(minimum age: 6 weeks)

Routine vaccination
• ActHIB®, Hiberix®, Pentacel®, or Vaxelis®: 4-dose series (3 dose primary series at age 2, 4, and 6 months, followed by a booster dose* at age 12–15 months)
- *Vaxelis® is not recommended for use as a booster dose. A different Hib-containing vaccine should be used for the booster dose.
• PedvaxHIB®: 3-dose series (2-dose primary series at age 2 and 4 months, followed by a booster dose at age 12–15 months)

Catch-up vaccination
• Dose 1 at age 7–11 months: Administer dose 2 at least 4 weeks later and dose 3 (final dose) at age 12–15 months or 8 weeks after dose 2 (whichever is later).
• Dose 1 at age 12–14 months: Administer dose 2 (final dose) at least 8 weeks after dose 1
• Dose 1 before age 12 months and dose 2 before age 15 months: Administer dose 3 (final dose) at least 8 weeks after dose 2.
• 2 doses of PedvaxHIB® before age 12 months: Administer dose 3 (final dose) at 12–59 months and at least 8 weeks after dose 2.
• 1 dose administered at age 15 months or older: No further doses needed
• Unvaccinated at age 15–59 months: Administer 1 dose.
• Previously unvaccinated children age 60 months or older who are not considered high risk: Do not require catch-up vaccination

For other catch-up guidance, see Table 2. Vaxelis® can be used for catch-up vaccination in children less than age 5 years. Follow the catch-up schedule even if Vaxelis® is used for one or more doses. For detailed information on use of Vaxelis® see www.cdc.gov/mmwr/volumes/69/wr/mm6905a5.htm.

Special situations
• Chemotherapy or radiation treatment:
Age 12–59 months
- Unvaccinated or only 1 dose before age 12 months: 2 doses, 8 weeks apart

- 2 or more doses before age 12 months: 1 dose at least 8 weeks after previous dose

Doses administered within 14 days of starting therapy or during therapy should be repeated at least 3 months after therapy completion.

- Hematopoietic stem cell transplant (HSCT):
  - 3-dose series 4 weeks apart starting 6 to 12 months after successful transplant, regardless of Hib vaccination history
- Anatomic or functional asplenia (including sickle cell disease):

Age 12–59 months
- Unvaccinated or only 1 dose before age 12 months: 2 doses, 8 weeks apart
- 2 or more doses before age 12 months: 1 dose at least 8 weeks after previous dose

Unvaccinated* persons age 5 years or older
- 1 dose

- Elective splenectomy:

Unvaccinated* persons age 15 months or older
- 1 dose (preferably at least 14 days before procedure)

- HIV infection:

Age 12–59 months
- Unvaccinated or only 1 dose before age 12 months: 2 doses, 8 weeks apart
- 2 or more doses before age 12 months: 1 dose at least 8 weeks after previous dose

Unvaccinated* persons age 5–18 years
- 1 dose

- Immunoglobulin deficiency, early component complement deficiency:

Age 12–59 months
- Unvaccinated or only 1 dose before age 12 months: 2 doses, 8 weeks apart
- 2 or more doses before age 12 months: 1 dose at least 8 weeks after previous dose

*Unvaccinated = Less than routine series (through age 14 months) OR no doses (age 15 months or older)

Hepatitis A vaccination
(minimum age: 12 months for routine vaccination)

Routine vaccination
- 2-dose series (minimum interval: 6 months) at age 12–23 months

Catch-up vaccination
- Unvaccinated persons through age 18 years should complete a 2-dose series (minimum interval: 6 months).
- Persons who previously received 1 dose at age 12 months or older should receive dose 2 at least 6 months after dose 1.
- Adolescents age 18 years or older may receive the combined HepA and HepB vaccine, Twinrix®, as a 3-dose series (0, 1, and 6 months) or 4-dose series (3 doses at 0, 7, and 21–30 days, followed by a booster dose at 12 months).

International travel
- Persons traveling to or working in countries with high or intermediate endemic hepatitis A (www.cdc.gov/travel/):
  - Infants age 6–11 months: 1 dose before departure; revaccinate with 2 doses, separated by at least 6 months, between age 12–23 months.
  - Unvaccinated age 12 months or older: Administer dose 1 as soon as travel is considered.

Hepatitis B vaccination
(minimum age: birth)

Birth dose (monovalent HepB vaccine only)
- Mother is HBsAg-negative:
  - All medically stable infants ≥2,000 grams: 1 dose within 24 hours of birth
  - Infants <2,000 grams: Administer 1 dose at chronological age 1 month or hospital discharge (whichever is earlier and even if weight is still <2,000 grams).
- Mother is HBsAg-positive:
  - Administer HepB vaccine and hepatitis B immune globulin (HBIG) (in separate limbs) within 12 hours of birth, regardless of birth weight. For infants <2,000 grams, administer 3 additional doses of vaccine (total of 4 doses) beginning at age 1 month.
  - Final (3rd or 4th) dose: administer at age 6 months (minimum age 24 weeks)
  - Test for HBsAg and anti-HBs at age 9–12 months. If HepB series is delayed, test 1–2 months after final dose. Do not test before age 9 months.
- Mother's HBsAg status is unknown: if other evidence suggestive of maternal hepatitis B infection exists (e.g., presence of HBV DNA, HBeAg-positive, or mother known to have chronic hepatitis B infection), manage infant as if mother is HBsAg-positive.
  - Administer HepB vaccine within 12 hours of birth, regardless of birth weight.
  - For infants <2,000 grams, administer HBIG in addition to HepB vaccine (in separate limbs) within 12 hours of birth. Administer 3 additional doses of vaccine (total of 4 doses) beginning at age 1 month.
  - Final (3rd or 4th) dose: administer at age 6 months (minimum age 24 weeks)
  - Determine mother's HBsAg status as soon as possible. Test for HBsAg and anti-HBs at age 9–12 months. If HepB series is delayed, test 1–2 months after final dose. Do not test before age 9 months.

Routine series
- 3-dose series at age 0, 1–2, 6–18 months (use monovalent HepB vaccine for doses administered before age 6 weeks)
- Infants who did not receive a birth dose should begin the series as soon as feasible (see Table 10-2).
- Administration of 4 doses is permitted when a combination vaccine containing HepB is used after the birth dose.
- Minimum age for the final (3rd or 4th) dose: 24 weeks
- Minimum intervals: dose 1 to dose 2: 4 weeks/dose 2 to dose 3: 8 weeks/dose 1 to dose 3: 16 weeks (when 4 doses are administered, substitute "dose 4" for "dose 3" in these calculations)

Catch-up vaccination
- Unvaccinated persons should complete a 3-dose series at 0, 1–2, 6 months.
- Adolescents age 11–15 years may use an alternative 2-dose schedule with at least 4 months between doses (adult formulation Recombivax HB® only).
- Adolescents age 18 years or older may receive a 2-dose series of HepB (Heplisav-B®) at least 4 weeks apart.
- Adolescents age 18 years or older may receive the combined HepA and HepB vaccine, Twinrix®, as a 3-dose series (0, 1, and 6 months) or 4-dose series (3 doses at 0, 7, and 21–30 days, followed by a booster dose at 12 months).
- For other catch-up guidance, see Table 10-2.

Special situations
Revaccination is not generally recommended for persons with a normal immune status who were vaccinated as infants, children, adolescents, or adults.
- Post-vaccination serology testing and revaccination (if anti-HBs < 10mIU/mL) is recommended for certain populations, including:
  - Infants born to HBsAg-positive mothers
  - Hemodialysis patients
  - Other immunocompromised persons-For detailed revaccination recommendations, see www.cdc.gov/vaccines/hcp/acip-recs/vacc-specific/hepb.html.

Note: Heplisav-B and PreHevbrio are not recommended in pregnancy due to lack of safety data in pregnant persons.

Human papillomavirus vaccination
(minimum age: 9 years)

Routine and catch-up vaccination
- HPV vaccination routinely recommended at age 11–12 years (can start at age 9 years) and catch-up HPV vaccination recommended for all persons through age 18 years if not adequately vaccinated

• 2- or 3-dose series depending on age at initial vaccination:
- Age 9–14 years at initial vaccination: 2-dose series at 0, 6–12 months (minimum interval: 5 months; repeat dose if administered too soon)
- Age 15 years or older at initial vaccination: 3-dose series at 0, 1–2 months, 6 months (minimum intervals: dose 1 to dose 2: 4 weeks / dose 2 to dose 3: 12 weeks / dose 1 to dose 3: 5 months; repeat dose if administered too soon)
• Interrupted schedules: If vaccination schedule is interrupted, the series does not need to be restarted.
• No additional dose recommended when any HPV vaccine series has been completed using the recommended dosing intervals.

Special situations
• Immunocompromising conditions, including HIV infection: 3-dose series, even for those who initiate vaccination at age 9 through 14 years.
• History of sexual abuse or assault: Start at age 9 years.
• Pregnancy: Pregnancy testing not needed before vaccination; HPV vaccination not recommended until after pregnancy; no intervention needed if vaccinated while pregnant

Influenza vaccination
(minimum age: 6 months [IIV], 2 years [LAIV], 18 years [recombinant influenza vaccine, RIV4])

Routine vaccination
• Use any influenza vaccine appropriate for age and health status annually:
- 2 doses, separated by at least 4 weeks, for children age 6 months–8 years who have received fewer than 2 influenza vaccine doses before July 1, 2023, or whose influenza vaccination history is unknown (administer dose 2 even if the child turns 9 between receipt of dose 1 and dose 2)
- 1 dose for children age 6 months–8 years who have received at least 2 influenza vaccine doses before July 1, 2023
- 1 dose for all persons age 9 years or older
• For the 2023-2024 season, see www.cdc.gov/mmwr/volumes/72/rr/rr7202a1.htm.
• For the 2024–25 season, see the 2024–25 ACIP influenza vaccine recommendations.

Special situations
• Egg allergy, hives only: Any influenza vaccine appropriate for age and health status annually
• Egg allergy with symptoms other than hives (e.g., angioedema, respiratory distress) or required epinephrine or another emergency medical intervention: see Appendix listing contraindications and precautions

• Severe allergic reaction (e.g., anaphylaxis) to a vaccine component or a previous dose of any influenza vaccine: see Appendix listing contraindications and precautions

Measles, mumps, and rubella vaccination
(minimum age: 12 months for routine vaccination)

Routine vaccination
• 2-dose series at age 12–15 months, age 4–6 years
• MMR or MMRV may be administered
Note: For dose 1 in children age 12–47 months, it is recommended to administer MMR and varicella vaccines separately. MMRV may be used if parents or caregivers express a preference.

Catch-up vaccination
• Unvaccinated children and adolescents: 2-dose series at least 4 weeks apart
• The maximum age for use of MMRV is 12 years.
• Minimum interval between MMRV doses: 3 months

Special situations
International travel
• Infants age 6–11 months: 1 dose before departure; revaccinate with 2-dose series at age 12–15 months (12 months for children in high-risk areas) and dose 2 as early as 4 weeks later.
• Unvaccinated children age 12 months or older: 2-dose series at least 4 weeks apart before departure

Meningococcal serogroup A,C,W,Y vaccination
(minimum age: 2 months [MenACWY-CRM, Menveo], 2 years [MenACWY-TT, MenQuadfi], 10 years [MenACWY-TT/MenB-FHbp, Penbraya])

Routine vaccination
• 2-dose series at age 11–12 years; 16 years

Catch-up vaccination
• Age 13–15 years: 1 dose now and booster at age 16–18 years (minimum interval: 8 weeks)
• Age 16–18 years: 1 dose

Special situations
Anatomic or functional asplenia (including sickle cell disease), HIV infection, persistent complement component deficiency, complement inhibitor (e.g., eculizumab, ravulizumab) use:
• Menveo
- Dose 1 at age 2 months: 4-dose series (additional 3 doses at age 4, 6 and 12 months)
- Dose 1 at age 3–6 months: 3- or 4- dose series (dose 2 [and dose 3 if applicable] at least 8 weeks after previous dose until a dose is received at age 7 months or older, followed by an additional dose at least 12 weeks later and after age 12 months)

- Dose 1 at age 7–23 months: 2-dose series (dose 2 at least 12 weeks after dose 1 and after age 12 months)
- Dose 1 at age 24 months or older: 2-dose series at least 8 weeks apart
• MenQuadfi®
- Dose 1 at age 24 months or older: 2-dose series at least 8 weeks apart
Travel in countries with hyperendemic or epidemic meningococcal disease, including countries in the African meningitis belt or during the Hajj (www.cdc.gov/travel/):
• Children less than age 24 months:
- Menveo® (age 2–23 months)
  • Dose 1 at age 2 months: 4-dose series (additional 3 doses at age 4,6 and 12 months)
  • Dose 1 at age 3–6 months: 3- or 4-dose series (dose 2 [and dose 3 if applicable] at least 8 weeks after previous dose until a dose is received at age 7 months or older, followed by an additional dose at least 12 weeks later and after age 12 months)
  • Dose 1 at age 7–23 months: 2-dose series (dose 2 at least 12 weeks after dose 1 and after age 12 months)
- Menactra® (age 9–23 months)
  • 2-dose series (dose 2 at least 12 weeks after dose 1; dose 2 may be administered as early as 8 weeks after dose 1 in travelers)
• Children age 2 years or older: 1 dose Menveo® or MenQuadfi®

First-year college students who live in residential housing (if not previously vaccinated at age 16 years or older) or military recruits:
• 1 dose Menveo® or MenQuadfi®
Adolescent vaccination of children who received MenACWY prior to age 10 years:
• Children for whom boosters are recommended because of an ongoing increased risk of meningococcal disease (e.g., those with complement deficiency, HIV, or asplenia): Follow the booster schedule for persons at increased risk.
• Children for whom boosters are not recommended (e.g., a healthy child who received a single dose for travel to a country where meningococcal disease is endemic): Administer MenACWY according to the recommended adolescent schedule with dose 1 at age 11–12 years and dose 2 at age 16 years.
Note: For MenACWY booster dose recommendations for groups listed under "Special situations" and in an outbreak setting and additional meningococcal vaccination information, see www.cdc.gov/mmwr/volumes/69/rr/rr6909a1.htm.

Children age 10 years or older may receive a single dose of Penbraya as an alternative to separate administration of MenACWY and MenB when both vaccines would be given on the same clinic day (see "Meningococcal serogroup B vaccination" section below for more information)

Meningococcal serogroup B vaccination
(minimum age: 10 years [MenB-4C, Bexsero®; MenB-FHbp, Trumenba®; MenACWY-TT/MenB-FHbp, Penbraya™])

For additional information on shared clinical decision-making for MenB, see www.cdc.gov/vaccines/hcp/admin/downloads/isd-job-aid-scdm-mening-b-shared-clinical-decision-making.pdf.

Shared clinical decision-making
Adolescents not at increased risk age 16–23 years (preferred age 16–18 years) based on shared clinical decision-making:
- Bexsero®: 2-dose series at least 1 month apart
- Trumenba®: 2-dose series at least 6 months apart; if dose 2 is administered earlier than 6 months, administer a 3rd dose at least 4 months after dose 2.

Special situations
Anatomic or functional asplenia (including sickle cell disease), persistent complement component deficiency, complement inhibitor (e.g., eculizumab, ravulizumab) use:
• Bexsero®: 2-dose series at least 1 month apart
• Trumenba®: 3-dose series at 0, 1–2, 6 months

Note: Bexsero® and Trumenba® are not interchangeable; the same product should be used for all doses in a series.

For MenB booster dose recommendations for groups listed under "Special situations" and in an outbreak setting and additional meningococcal vaccination information, see www.cdc.gov/mmwr/volumes/69/rr/rr6909a1.htm.

Children age 10 years or older may receive a dose of Penbraya™ as an alternative to separate administration of MenACWY and MenB when both vaccines would be given on the same clinic day. For age-eligible children not at increased risk, if Penbraya™ is used for dose 1 MenB, MenB-FHbp (Trumenba) should be administered for dose 2 MenB. For age-eligible children at increased risk of meningococcal disease, Penbraya™ may be used for additional MenACWY and MenB doses (including booster doses) if both would be given on the same clinic day and at least 6 months have elapsed since most recent Penbraya™ dose

Mpox vaccination
(minimum age: 18 years [Jynneos®])

Special situations
• Age 18 years and at risk for Mpox infection: 2-dose series, 28 days apart.
  ○ Risk factors for Mpox infection include:
    ▪ Persons who are gay, bisexual, and other MSM, transgender or nonbinary people who in the past 6 months have had:
    ▪ A new diagnosis of at least 1 sexually transmitted disease
    ▪ More than 1 sex partner
    ▪ Sex at a commercial sex venue
    ▪ Sex in association with a large public event in a geographic area where Mpox transmission is occurring
    ▪ Persons who are sexual partners of the persons described above
    ▪ Persons who anticipate experiencing any of the situations described above
• Pregnancy: There is currently no ACIP recommendation for Jynneos use in pregnancy due to lack of safety data in pregnant. Pregnant persons with any risk factor described above may receive Jynneos.

For detailed information, see: www.cdc.gov/vaccines/acip/meetings/downloads/slides-2023-10-25-26/04-MPOX-Rao-508.pdf

Contraindications and Precautions
For contraindications and precautions to Mpox vaccination, see Mpox Appendix.

Pneumococcal vaccination
(minimum age: 6 weeks [PCV15], [PCV20], 2 years [PPSV23])

Routine vaccination with PCV
• 4-dose series at age 2, 4, 6, 12–15 months

Catch-up vaccination with PCV
• Healthy children ages 2–4 years with any incomplete* PCV series: 1 dose PCV
• For other catch-up guidance, see Table 10-2.

Note: For children without risk conditions, PCV20 is not indicated if they have received 4 doses of PCV13 or PCV15 or another age appropriate complete PCV series.

Special situations
Children and adolescents with cerebrospinal fluid leak; chronic heart disease; chronic kidney disease (excluding maintenance dialysis and nephrotic syndrome); chronic liver disease; chronic lung disease (including moderate persistent or severe persistent asthma); cochlear implant; or diabetes mellitus:

Age 2–5 years
• Any incomplete* PCV series with:
  ○ 3 PCV doses: 1 dose PCV (at least 8 weeks after the most recent PCV dose)
  ○ Less than 3 PCV doses: 2 doses PCV (at least 8 weeks after the most recent dose and administered at least 8 weeks apart)
• Completed recommended PCV series but have not received PPSV23
  ○ Previously received at least 1 dose of PCV20: no further PCV or PPSV23 doses needed
  ○ Not previously received PCV20: administer 1 dose PCV20 OR 1 dose PPSV23 administer at least 8 weeks after the most recent PCV dose.

Age 6–18 years
• Not previously received any dose of PCV13, PCV15, or PCV20: administer 1 dose of PCV15 or PCV20. If PCV15 is used and no previous receipt of PPSV23, administer 1 dose of PPSV23 at least 8 weeks after the PCV15 dose.**
• Received PCV before age 6 years but have not received PPSV23
  ○ Previously received at least 1 dose of PCV20: no further PCV or PPSV23 doses needed
  ○ Not previously received PCV20: administer 1 dose PCV20 OR 1 dose PPSV23 at least 8 weeks after the most recent PCV dose. If PPSV23 is used, administer either PCV20 or dose 2 PPSV23 at least 5 years after dose 1 PPSV23.
• Received PCV13 only at or after age 6 years: administer 1 dose PCV20 OR 1 dose PPSV23 at least 8 weeks after the most recent PCV13 dose.
• Received 1 dose PCV13 and 1 dose PPSV23 at or after age 6 years: no further doses of any PCV or PPSV23 indicated.

Children and adolescents on maintenance dialysis, or with immunocompromising conditions such as nephrotic syndrome; congenital or acquired asplenia or splenic dysfunction; congenital or acquired immunodeficiencies; diseases and conditions treated with immunosuppressive drugs or radiation therapy, including malignant neoplasms, leukemias, lymphomas, Hodgkin disease, and solid organ transplant; HIV infection; or sickle cell disease or other hemoglobinopathies:

Age 2–5 years
• Any incomplete* PCV series:
  ○ 3 PCV doses: 1 dose PCV (at least 8 weeks after the most recent PCV dose)

o Less than 3 PCV doses: 2 doses PCV (at least 8 weeks after the most recent dose and administered at least 8 weeks apart)

• Completed recommended PCV series but have not received PPSV23

o Previously received at least 1 dose of PCV20: no further PCV or PPSV23 doses needed

o Not previously received PCV20: administer 1 dose PCV20 OR 1 dose PPSV23 at least 8 weeks after the most recent PCV. If PPSV23 is used, administer 1 dose of PCV20 or dose 2 PPSV23 at least 5 years after dose 1 PPSV23.

Age 6-18 years

• Not previously received any dose of PCV13, PCV15, or PCV20: administer 1 dose of PCV15 or 1 dose of PCV20. If PCV15 is used and no previous receipt of PPSV23, administer 1 dose of PPSV23 at least 8 weeks after the PCV15 dose.**

• Received PCV before age 6 years but have not received PPSV23

o Previously received at least 1 dose of PCV or PPSV23: no additional dose of PCV or PPSV23

o Not previously received PCV20: administer 1 dose PCV20 OR 1 dose PPSV23 at least 8 weeks after the most recent PCV dose. If PPSV23 is used, administer either PCV20 or dose 2 PPSV23 at least 5 years after dose 1 PPSV23.

o Received PCV13 only at or after age 6 years: administer 1 dose PCV20 OR 1 dose PPSV23 at least 8 weeks after the most recent PCV13 dose. If PPSV23 is used, administer 1 dose of PCV20 or dose 2 PPSV23 at least 5 years after dose 1 PPSV23.

o Received 1 dose PCV13 and 1 dose PPSV23 at or after age 6 years: administer 1 dose PCV20 OR 1 dose PPSV23 at least 8 weeks after the most recent PCV13 dose and at least 5 years after dose 1 PPSV23

*Incomplete series = Not having received all doses in either the recommended series or an age-appropriate catch-up series. See Table 2 in ACIP pneumococcal recommendations at stacks.cdc.gov/view/cdc/133252

**When both PCV15 and PPSV23 are indicated, administer all doses of PCV15 first. PCV15 and PPSV23 should not be administered during the same visit.

Contraindications and Precautions

For guidance on determining which pneumococcal vaccines a patient needs and when, please refer to the mobile app, which can be downloaded here: www.cdc.gov/vaccines/vpd/pneumo/hcp/pneumoapp.html

For contraindications and precautions to Pneumococcal conjugate (PCV), see PCV Appendix and Pneumococcal polysaccharide (PPSV23), see PPSV23 Appendix (https://

www.cdc.gov/vaccines/schedules/hcp/imz/child-schedule-notes.html#appendix-PPSV23).

Poliovirus vaccination
(minimum age: 6 weeks)

Routine vaccination

• 4-dose series at ages 2, 4, 6-18 months, 4-6 years; administer the final dose on or after age 4 years and at least 6 months after the previous dose.

• 4 or more doses of IPV can be administered before age 4 years when a combination vaccine containing IPV is used. However, a dose is still recommended on or after age 4 years and at least 6 months after the previous dose.

Catch-up vaccination

• In the first 6 months of life, use minimum ages and intervals only for travel to a polio-endemic region or during an outbreak.

• IPV is not routinely recommended for U.S. residents age 18 years or older.

Series containing oral polio vaccine (OPV), either mixed OPV-IPV or OPV-only series:

• Total number of doses needed to complete the series is the same as that recommended for the U.S. IPV schedule. See www.cdc.gov/mmwr/volumes/66/wr/mm6601a6.htm?s_%20cid=mm6601a6_w.

• Only trivalent OPV (tOPV) counts toward the U.S. vaccination requirements.

- Doses of OPV administered before April 1, 2016, should be counted (unless specifically noted as administered during a campaign).

- Doses of OPV administered on or after April 1, 2016, should not be counted.

- For guidance to assess doses documented as "OPV", see www.cdc.gov/mmwr/volumes/66/wr/mm6606a7.htm?s_cid=mm6606a7_w.

• For other catch-up guidance, see Table 2.

Respiratory syncytial virus immunization
(minimum age: birth [Nirsevimab, RSV-mAB (Beyfortus™)])

Routine vaccination

• Infants born October – March in most of the continental United States*

o Mother did not receive RSV vaccine OR mother's RSV vaccination status is unknown: administer 1 dose nirsevimab within 1 week of birth in hospital or outpatient setting

o Mother received RSV vaccine less than 14 days prior to delivery: administer 1 dose nirsevimab within 1 week of birth in hospital or outpatient setting

o Mother received RSV vaccine at least 14 days prior to delivery: nirsevimab not needed but can be considered in rare circumstances at the discretion of healthcare providers (see special populations and situations at cdc.gov/vaccines/vpd/rsv/hcp/child-faqs.html)

• Infants born April–September in most of the continental United States*

o Mother did not receive RSV vaccine OR mother's RSV vaccination status is unknown: administer 1 dose nirsevimab shortly before start of RSV season*

o Mother received RSV vaccine less than 14 days prior to delivery: administer 1 dose nirsevimab shortly before start of RSV season*

o Mother received RSV vaccine at least 14 days prior to delivery: nirsevimab not needed but can be considered in rare circumstances at the discretion of healthcare providers (see special populations and situations at cdc.gov/vaccines/vpd/rsv/hcp/child-faqs.html)

Infants with prolonged birth hospitalization** (e.g., for prematurity) discharged October through March should be immunized shortly before or promptly after discharge.

Special situations

• Ages 8-19 months with chronic lung disease of prematurity requiring medical support (e.g., chronic corticosteroid therapy, diuretic therapy, or supplemental oxygen) any time during the 6-month period before the start of the second RSV season; severe immunocompromise; cystic fibrosis with either weight for length <10th percentile or manifestation of severe lung disease (e.g., previous hospitalization for pulmonary exacerbation in the first year of life or abnormalities on chest imaging that persist when stable)**:

o 1 dose nirsevimab shortly before start of second RSV season*

• Ages 8-19 months who are American Indian or Alaska Native:

o 1 dose nirsevimab shortly before start of second RSV season*

• Age-eligible and undergoing cardiac surgery with cardiopulmonary bypass**: 1 additional dose of nirsevimab after surgery. For additional details see special populations and situations at www.cdc.gov/vaccines/vpd/rsv/hcp/child-faqs.html

*Note: While the timing of the onset and duration of RSV season may vary, nirsevimab may be administered October through March in most of the continental United States. Providers in jurisdictions with RSV seasonality that differs from most of the continental United States (e.g., Alaska, jurisdiction with tropical climate) should follow guidance from public health authorities (e.g., CDC, health departments) or regional medical centers on timing of

Rotavirus vaccination
(minimum age: 6 weeks)

Routine vaccination
- Rotarix®: 2-dose series at age 2 and 4 months
- RotaTeq®: 3-dose series at age 2, 4, and 6 months
- If any dose in the series is either RotaTeq® or unknown, default to 3-dose series.

Catch-up vaccination
- Do not start the series on or after age 15 weeks, 0 days.
- The maximum age for the final dose is 8 months, 0 days.
- For other catch-up guidance, see Table 10-2.

Tetanus, diphtheria, and pertussis (Tdap) vaccination
(minimum age: 11 years for routine vaccination, 7 years for catch-up vaccination)

Routine vaccination
- Adolescents age 11–12 years: 1 dose Tdap
- Pregnancy: 1 dose Tdap during each pregnancy, preferably in early part of gestational weeks 27–36.
- Note: Tdap may be administered regardless of the interval since the last tetanus- and diphtheria-toxoid-containing vaccine.

Catch-up vaccination
- Adolescents age 13–18 years who have not received Tdap: 1 dose Tdap, then Td or Tdap booster every 10 years
- Persons age 7–18 years not fully vaccinated* with DTaP: 1 dose Tdap as part of the catch-up series (preferably the first dose); if additional doses are needed, use Td or Tdap.
- Tdap administered at age 7–10 years:
  - Children age 7–9 years who receive Tdap should receive the routine Tdap dose at age 11–12 years.
  - Children age 10 years who receive Tdap do not need the routine Tdap dose at age 11–12 years.
- DTaP inadvertently administered on or after age 7 years:
  - Children age 7–9 years: DTaP may count as part of catch-up series. Administer routine Tdap dose at age 11–12 years.
  - Children age 10–18 years: Count dose of DTaP as the adolescent Tdap booster.
- For other catch-up guidance, see Table 10-2.

Special situations
- Wound management in persons age 7 years or older with history of 3 or more doses of tetanus-toxoid-containing vaccine: For clean and minor wounds, administer Tdap or Td if more than 10 years since last dose of tetanus-toxoid-containing vaccine; for all other wounds, administer Tdap or Td if more than 5 years since last dose of tetanus-toxoid-containing vaccine. Tdap is preferred for persons age 11 years or older who have not previously received Tdap or whose Tdap history is unknown. If a tetanus-toxoid-containing vaccine is indicated for a pregnant adolescent, use Tdap.
- For detailed information, see www.cdc.gov/mmwr/volumes/69/wr/mm6903a5.htm.

*Fully vaccinated = 5 valid doses of DTaP OR 4 valid doses of DTaP if dose 4 was administered at age 4 years or older

Varicella vaccination
(minimum age: 12 months)

Routine vaccination
- 2-dose series at age 12–15 months, 4–6 years
- VAR or MMRV may be administered*
- Dose 2 may be administered as early as 3 months after dose 1 (a dose inadvertently administered after at least 4 weeks may be counted as valid)

*Note: For dose 1 in children age 12–47 months, it is recommended to administer MMR and varicella vaccines separately. MMRV may be used if parents or caregivers express a preference.

Catch-up vaccination
- Ensure persons age 7–18 years without evidence of immunity (see MMWR at www.cdc.gov/mmwr/pdf/rr/rr5604.pdf) have a 2-dose series:
  - Age 7–12 years: routine interval: 3 months (a dose inadvertently administered after at least 4 weeks may be counted as valid)
  - Age 13 years and older: routine interval: 4–8 weeks (minimum interval: 4 weeks)
  - The maximum age for use of MMRV is 12 years.

---

administration based on local RSV seasonality. Although optimal timing of administration is just before the start of the RSV season, nirsevimab may also be administered during the RSV season to infants and children who are age-eligible.

**Note: Nirsevimab can be administered to children who are eligible to receive palivizumab. Children who have received nirsevimab should not receive palivizumab for the same RSV season.

For further guidance, see www.cdc.gov/mmwr/volumes/72/wr/mm7234a4.htm and www.cdc.gov/vaccines/vpd/rsv/hcp/ child-faqs.html

Contraindications and precautions
For contraindications and precautions to RSV monoclonal antibody (RSV-mAb), see RSV monoclonal antibody Appendix.

Respiratory syncytial virus vaccination
(RSV [Abrysvo™])

Routine vaccination
- Pregnant at 32 weeks 0 days through 36 weeks and 6 days gestation from September through January in most of the continental United States*: 1 dose RSV vaccine (Abrysvo™). Administer RSV vaccine regardless of previous RSV infection.
  - Either maternal RSV vaccination or infant immunization with nirsevimab (RSV monoclonal antibody) is recommended to prevent respiratory syncytial virus lower respiratory tract infection in infants.
- All other pregnant persons: RSV vaccine not recommended.

There is currently no ACIP recommendation for RSV vaccination in subsequent pregnancies. no data are available to inform whether additional doses are needed in later pregnancies.

*Note: Providers in jurisdictions with RSV seasonality that differs from most of the continental United States (e.g., Alaska, jurisdiction with tropical climate) should follow guidance from public health authorities (e.g., CDC, health departments) or regional medical centers on timing of administration based on local RSV seasonality.

Contraindications and Precautions
For contraindications and precautions to Respiratory syncytial virus vaccine (RSV), see RSV Appendix.

Children With Chronic Illnesses

Most chronic diseases are not contraindications to vaccination; in fact, children with chronic diseases may be at greater risk of complications from vaccine-preventable diseases, such as influenza and pneumococcal infections. Premature infants are a good example. They should be immunized according to their chronological, not gestational, age. Vaccine doses should not be reduced for preterm or low-birth-weight infants. One exception is children with progressive central nervous system disorders. Vaccination with DTaP should be deferred until the neurologic condition has been clarified and/or is stable.

Immunodeficient Children

Congenitally immunodeficient children should not be immunized with live-virus vaccines (oral polio vaccine [OPV, not available in the United States], rotavirus, MMR, VAR, MMRV, yellow fever, or LAIV) or live-bacteria vaccines (BCG or live typhoid fever vaccine). Depending on the nature of the immunodeficiency, other vaccines are safe but may fail to evoke an immune response. Children with cancer and children receiving high-dose corticosteroids or other immunosuppressive agents should not be vaccinated with live vaccines. This contraindication does not apply if the malignancy is in remission and chemotherapy has not been administered for at least 90 days. Live-virus vaccines may also be administered to previously healthy children receiving low to moderate doses of corticosteroids (defined as up to 2 mg/kg/day of prednisone or prednisone equivalent, with a 20 mg/day maximum) for less than 14 days; children without other immunodeficiency receiving short-acting alternate-day corticosteroids; children being maintained on physiologic corticosteroid therapy; and children receiving only topical, inhaled, or intra-articular corticosteroids.

Contraindication of live-pathogen vaccines also applies to children with human immunodeficiency virus (HIV) infection who are severely immunosuppressed. Those who receive MMR should have at least 15% CD4 cells, a CD4 lymphocyte count equivalent to CDC immunologic class 2, and be asymptomatic from their HIV. MMR for these children is routinely recommended at 12 months of age and after at least 3 months on antiretroviral therapy. VAR vaccination is also recommended for HIV-infected children with CD4 cells preserved or recovered as listed earlier. MMR and VAR are not contraindicated in household contacts of immunocompromised children. HIV-infected children who were vaccinated before their HIV was treated should be reimmunized to ensure adequate protection. The recommended immunization schedule for immunocompromised children is available at https://www.cdc.gov/vaccines/schedules/hcp/imz/child-indications.html.

Allergic or Hypersensitive Children

Severe hypersensitivity reactions are rare following vaccination (1.53 cases per 1 million doses). They are generally attributable to a trace component of the vaccine other than to the antigen; for example, MMR, IPV, and VAR contain microgram quantities of neomycin, and IPV also contains trace amounts of streptomycin and polymyxin B. Children with known anaphylactic responses to these antibiotics should not be given these vaccines. Trace quantities of egg antigens may be present in both inactivated and live influenza and yellow fever vaccines. Guidelines for influenza vaccination in children with egg allergies have recently changed. The trace amounts of egg protein are generally considered below the threshold needed to induce an allergic reaction and there has been no increased risk of anaphylaxis documented in children with severe egg allergies. Therefore, children with severe egg allergy can be vaccinated with influenza vaccine with no special precautions beyond those for any other vaccine. Some vaccines (MMR, MMRV, and VAR) contain gelatin. For any persons with a history of anaphylactic reaction to gelatin or any component contained in a vaccine, the vaccine package insert should be reviewed, and additional consultation sought, such as from a pediatric allergist. Some tips and rubber plungers of vaccine syringes contain latex. These vaccines should not be administered to individuals with a history of severe anaphylactic allergy to latex but may be administered to people with less severe allergies. Thimerosal has been an organic mercurial compound used as a preservative in vaccines since the 1930s. While there is no evidence that thimerosal has caused serious allergic reactions or autism, all routinely recommended vaccines for infants have been manufactured without thimerosal since mid-2001. Thimerosal-free formulations of injectable influenza vaccine are available, and LAIV does not contain thimerosal.

Other Special Circumstances

Detailed recommendations for preterm low-birth-weight infants; pediatric transplant recipients; Alaskan Natives/American Indians; children in residential institutions or military communities; or refugees, new immigrants, or travelers are available from the CDC (at http://www.cdc.gov/vaccines) and from the AAP's *Red Book*.

CDC general recommendations on immunization: https://www.cdc.gov/vaccines/hcp/acip-recs/general-recs/index.html. Accessed March 10, 2023.
Kelso JM: Administering influenza vaccine to egg-allergic persons. Expert Rev Vaccines 2014;13:1049 [PMID: 24962036].

COMMUNICATING WITH PARENTS ABOUT VACCINES

Most parents in the United States choose to vaccinate their children. In children born in 2018–2019, 0.9% received no vaccines by age 24 months. However, parental concern about vaccines is common. While there are myriad reasons given for not vaccinating, several themes recur. Some parents do not believe their children are at risk for vaccine-preventable diseases. Other parents do not believe that certain vaccine-preventable diseases, such as varicella and pertussis, are particularly serious. There are also widespread concerns about the safety of vaccines, usually based on misinformation. Health care providers have a critically important role in discussing the known risks and benefits of vaccination with parents, as they are consistently shown to be the most trusted source of vaccine information for parents.

AAP, CDC, and others have developed resources to guide providers on how best to communicate with parents about vaccines and how to address specific vaccine concerns. A presumptive recommendation ("We have three shots to do today") is likely more effective than a participatory approach ("Have you thought about the shots he is due for today?"). For parents who resist or have questions about vaccines, some will agree to be vaccinated after simply receiving the necessary knowledge. For many, however, simply correcting misinformation is not enough, and may increase resistance to vaccination. For these parents, it is best to avoid arguments or rebuttals. Motivational interviewing has shown promise as an effective communication technique for both childhood and adolescent vaccines. Other promising techniques include pivoting away from discussions of vaccine side effects to emphasize the importance of the vaccine for disease prevention, personal recommendations ("I vaccinate my own children according to the recommended schedule"), promotion of social norms ("Almost all of our patients are fully vaccinated"), or highlighting circumstances that increase risk ("These infectious diseases are just a plane flight away.").

Parents with questions may be directed to trusted websites, such as those of the AAP (https://healthychildren.org), CDC (www.cdc.gov/vaccines), Immunize.org, formerly the Immunization Action Coalition (www.immunize.org), and Vaccinate Your Family (https://vaccinateyourfamily.org/).

Edwards KM et al; American Academy of Pediatrics: Committee on Infectious Diseases; the Committee on Practice and Ambulatory Medicine: Countering vaccine hesitancy. Pediatrics 2016;138 [PMID: 27573088].
https://www.cdc.gov/vaccines/hcp/conversations/index.html. Accessed March 10, 2023.
https://www.aap.org/en/patient-care/immunizations/communicating-with-families-and-promoting-vaccine-confidence/. Accessed March 10, 2023.

HEPATITIS B VACCINATION

Hepatitis B (HepB) virus is a partially double-stranded DNA virus, a member of the *Hepadnaviridae* family of viruses, and a major cause of cirrhosis and hepatocellular carcinoma worldwide. HepB infection occurs when blood, semen, or other body fluid containing the virus enters the body of a nonimmune person. This can occur through perinatal exposure; by needle- or razor-sharing; or by contact with an infected person's bodily fluids. Reported cases of acute HepB have declined dramatically in the United States, largely attributable to vaccination. Based on recent surveillance data, the incidence of acute HepB has declined by almost 90% since 1985 and, after remaining stable from 2011 to 2019, declined again in 2020. Declines noted in 2020 may be related to the COVID-19 pandemic, with fewer people seeking health care or getting tested. Regardless, HepB disparities are significant, with newly reported chronic HepB cases among Asian and Pacific Islander persons (17.6 cases per 100,000 people) nearly 12 times the rate among non-Hispanic white persons.

Success in reducing HepB in the United States is due, in large part, to a comprehensive HepB prevention strategy initiated in 1991. The four central elements of this approach are (1) immunization of all infants beginning at birth; (2) routine screening of all pregnant women for HepB infection, and provision of HepB immunoglobulin (HBIg) to all infants born to infected mothers; (3) routine vaccination of previously unvaccinated children and adolescents; and (4) vaccination of adults at increased risk of HepB infection. The estimated proportion of US children receiving a birth dose of HepB vaccine has increased steadily from 2014 to 2019, reaching 80% for children born from 2018 to 2019. These efforts have contributed to the greatest declines in new cases of HepB among children younger than 15 years, in whom rates have decreased by 98% since 1985.

While high immunization rates have been achieved in young children (93% of children born in 2018 and 2019 were fully immunized at age 24 months), there has been less success in identifying HepB-infected mothers and at immunizing high-risk adults. Of the estimated 23,000 mothers who deliver each year who are hepatitis B surface antigen (HBsAg) positive, only 9000 are identified through prenatal screening. While there is an average of 90 cases of perinatally acquired HepB infection reported to the CDC every year, the actual number of perinatal cases is estimated to be 10–20 times higher. This indicates a significant missed opportunity for prevention in exposed infants, given that administration of HepB vaccine in conjunction with HBIg is 95% effective at preventing mother-to-infant transmission of the virus. Further, many hospitals do not routinely offer HepB to all newborns, despite AAP and ACIP recommendations for universal newborn HepB vaccination.

All pregnant women should be routinely screened for HBsAg. Infants born to HBsAg-positive mothers should receive both HepB and HBIg immediately after birth. Infants for whom the maternal HBsAg status is unknown should receive vaccine (but not HBIg) within 12 hours of birth. In such circumstances, the mother's HBsAg status should be determined as soon as possible during her hospitalization and the infant given HBIg if the mother is HBsAg positive. For all infants, the HepB immunization series should be started at birth, with the first dose given prior to 24 hours of age. The only exception is for children with a weight less than 2000 g; they should receive 1 dose at chronological age 1 month or hospital discharge (whichever is earlier, even if weight is < 2000 g).

Routine immunization with three doses of HepB is recommended for all infants and all previously unvaccinated children aged 0–18 years. A two-dose schedule is available for adolescents. Screening for markers of past infection before vaccinating is not indicated for children and adolescents but may be considered for high-risk adults. Because HepB vaccines consist of an inactivated subunit of the virus, they are not contraindicated in immunosuppressed individuals or pregnant women.

▶ **Vaccines Available**

1. HepB vaccine (Recombivax HB, Merck) contains recombinant HepB only.
2. HepB vaccine (Engerix-B, GlaxoSmithKline) contains recombinant HepB only.
3. DTaP-HepB-IPV (Pediarix, GlaxoSmithKline) contains vaccines against diphtheria, tetanus, pertussis, HepB, and poliovirus.

4. HepB vaccine (Heplisav-B, Dynavax Technologies) contains recombinant HepB only, with an adjuvant; approved for adults 18 years and older.
5. DTaP-IPV-Hib-HepB (Vaxelis, Merck) contains DTaP, IPV, Hib, and HepB vaccines.

Only the noncombination vaccines (Recombivax HB and Engerix-B) can be given between birth and 6 weeks of age. Any single or combination vaccine listed above can be used to complete the HepB vaccination series, including the hexavalent combination vaccine (Vaxelis, Merck). A combination vaccine against hepatitis A (HepA) and hepatitis B (Twinrix, GlaxoSmithKline) is available, but is only licensed in the United States for persons 18 years and older.

▶ **Dosage & Schedule of Administration**

HepB is recommended for all infants and children in the United States. Table 10–3 presents the vaccination schedule for newborn infants, dependent on maternal HBsAg status. Infants born to mothers with positive or unknown HBsAg status should receive HepB vaccine within 12 hours of birth.

Table 10–3. Hepatitis B vaccine schedules for newborn infants ≥ 2000 g, by maternal hepatitis B surface antigen (HBsAg) status.[a]

Maternal HBsAg Status	Single Antigen Vaccine		Single Antigen Followed by Combination Vaccine	
	Dose	Age	Dose	Age
Positive[b]	1[c]	Birth (≤ 12 h)	1[c]	Birth (≤ 12 h)
	HBIg[d]	Birth (≤ 12 h)	HBIg	Birth (≤ 12 h)
	2	1–2 mo	2	2 mo
			3	4 mo
	3[e]	6 mo	4[e]	6 mo
Unknown[f]	1[c]	Birth (≤ 12 h)	1[c]	Birth (≤ 12 h)
	2	1–2 mo	2	2 mo
			3	4 mo
	3[e]	6 mo	4[e]	6 mo
Negative	1[c]	Birth (< 24 h)	1[c]	Birth (< 24 h)
	2	1–2 mo	2	2 mo
			3	4 mo
	3[e]	6–18 mo	4[e]	6 mo

[a]See text for vaccination of preterm infants weighing less than 2000 g.
[b]Infants born to HBsAg-positive mothers should be tested at 9–12 months after completion of the immunization series for anti-HBs and HBsAg.
[c]Pediarix should not be administered before age 6 weeks.
[d]Hepatitis B immune globulin (HBIg) should be administered intramuscularly in a separate anatomic site from vaccine.
[e]The final dose in the vaccine series should not be administered before age 24 weeks (164 days).
[f]Mothers should have blood drawn and tested for HBsAg as soon as possible after admission for delivery; if the mother is found to be HBsAg-positive, the infant should receive HBIg as soon as possible, but no later than age 7 days.
Reproduced from Schillie S, Vellozzi C, Reingold A, et al. Prevention of Hepatitis B Virus Infection in the United States: Recommendations of the Advisory Committee on Immunization Practices. MMWR Recomm Rep. 2018 Jan 12;67(1):1-31.

Infants born to HBsAg-negative mothers should receive the vaccine prior to 24 hours of age.

For children younger than 11 years not previously immunized, three intramuscular doses of HepB are needed. Adolescents aged 11–15 years have two options: the standard pediatric three-dose schedule or two doses of adult Recombivax HB (1.0 mL dose), with the second dose administered 4–6 months after the first dose. Certain patients may have reduced immune response to HepB vaccination, including preterm infants weighing less than 2000 g at birth, the elderly, immunosuppressed patients, and those receiving dialysis. Infants whose mothers are HBsAg-positive or with unknown HBsAg status should receive both HepB and HBIg within 12 hours of birth. Pediatric hemodialysis patients and immunocompromised persons may require larger doses or an increased number of doses, with dose amounts and schedules available in the most recent CDC HepB recommendations (see references).

▶ Contraindications & Precautions

HepB should not be given to persons with a serious allergic reaction to yeast or to any vaccine components. Individuals with a history of serious adverse events, such as anaphylaxis, after receiving HepB should not receive additional doses. Vaccination is not contraindicated in persons with a history of Guillain-Barré syndrome (GBS), multiple sclerosis, autoimmune disease, other chronic conditions, or in pregnancy.

▶ Adverse Effects

The overall rate of adverse events following vaccination is low. Those reported are minor, including fever (1%–6%) and pain at the injection site (3%–29%). There is no evidence of an association between vaccination and sudden infant death syndrome, multiple sclerosis, autoimmune disease, or chronic fatigue syndrome.

▶ Postexposure Prophylaxis

Postexposure prophylaxis is indicated for unvaccinated persons with perinatal, sexual, household, percutaneous, or mucosal exposure to HepB virus. When prophylaxis is indicated, unvaccinated individuals should receive HBIg (0.06 mL/kg) and the first dose of HepB at a separate anatomic site. Sexual and household contacts of someone with chronic (as opposed to acute) infection should receive HepB only. All vaccinated persons not previously tested for antibody should be tested for anti-HBs after exposure to HepB. If antibody levels are adequate (≥ 10 mIU/mL), no treatment is necessary. If levels are inadequate (< 10 mIU/mL) and the exposure was to HBsAg-positive blood, HBIg and vaccination are required. For nonvaccinated individuals with percutaneous or mucosal exposure to blood, HepB should be given, and HBIg considered depending on the HBsAg status of the person who was the source of the blood exposure.

▶ Antibody Preparations

HBIg is prepared from HIV-negative and hepatitis C virus–negative donors with high titers of HBsAg. The process used to prepare this product inactivates or eliminates any undetected HIV and hepatitis C virus.

American Academy of Pediatrics, Committee on Infectious Diseases: Elimination of perinatal hepatitis B: providing the first vaccine dose within 24 hours of birth. Pediatrics 2017;140(3):e20171870 [PMID: 28847980].

CDC: Hepatitis B Surveillance 2020. https://www.cdc.gov/hepatitis/statistics/2020surveillance/hepatitis-b.htm. Accessed February 17, 2023.

Schillie S et al: Prevention of hepatitis B virus infection in the United States: recommendations of the Advisory Committee on Immunization Practices. MMWR Recomm Rep 2018;67(RR-1):1 [PMID: 29939980].

ROTAVIRUS VACCINATION

Rotavirus, a genus of double-stranded RNA viruses, is the leading cause of hospitalization and death from acute gastroenteritis in young children worldwide. It is spread through fecal-oral transmission, contact with contaminated surfaces, and by eating contaminated foods. The burden of rotavirus is particularly severe in the developing world, where as many as 215,000 children die each year from rotavirus-associated dehydration and other complications. While deaths from rotavirus were uncommon in the United States (20–60 deaths per year) prior to the introduction of rotavirus vaccine, rotavirus infections caused substantial morbidity nationally with an estimated 2.7 million diarrheal illnesses, 410,000 office visits, and 55,000–70,000 hospitalizations each year.

Rotavirus vaccination has been routinely recommended in the United States since 2006. Two rotavirus vaccines are currently available, a pentavalent rotavirus vaccine (RV5; RotaTeq) and a monovalent rotavirus vaccine (RV1; Rotarix). Hospitalizations and outpatient visits for rotavirus disease have fallen significantly among vaccinated infants in the United States, and disease has also declined among unimmunized older children and adults, reflecting herd protection.

Rotavirus vaccination has also reduced morbidity and mortality from rotavirus disease worldwide. While effectiveness of rotavirus vaccines is somewhat lower in developing countries, disease burden is so high that the public health impact of rotavirus vaccination is substantial in developing countries that have introduced these vaccines. Extensive efforts are underway to develop more effective, lower cost, heat-stable rotavirus vaccines for use in the developing world.

RV5 and RV1 are known to cause intussusception, although rarely. Intussusception risk has been estimated at 1 excess case per 20,000–100,000 vaccinated infants. At this level of risk, the benefits of vaccination against rotavirus disease continue to greatly outweigh the risks in the United States and globally.

Vaccines Available

1. RV5 (Rotateq, Merck) is a pentavalent, live, oral, human-bovine reassortant rotavirus vaccine. The vaccine is a liquid, does not require any reconstitution, and does not contain any preservatives. The dosing tube is latex-free.
2. RV1 (Rotarix, GlaxoSmithKline) is a monovalent, live, oral, attenuated human rotavirus vaccine. The vaccine needs to be reconstituted with 1 mL of diluent using a prefilled oral applicator. The vaccine does not contain any preservatives. The oral applicator contains latex.

Dosage & Schedule of Administration

Either RV5 or RV1 can be used to prevent rotavirus gastroenteritis. RV5 should be administered orally, as a three-dose series, at 2, 4, and 6 months of age. RV1 should be administered orally, as a two-dose series, at 2 and 4 months of age. For both rotavirus vaccines, the minimum age for dose 1 is 6 weeks, and the maximum age for dose 1 is 14 weeks and 6 days. The vaccination series should not be started at 15 weeks of age or older because of the lack of safety data around administering dose 1 to older infants. The minimum interval between doses is 4 weeks. All doses should be administered by 8 months and 0 days of age. While the ACIP recommends that the vaccine series be completed with the same product (RV5 or RV1) used for the initial dose, if this is not possible, providers should complete the series with whichever product is available.

Either rotavirus vaccine can be given simultaneously with all other recommended infant vaccines. No restrictions are placed on infant breast or formula feeding before or after receiving rotavirus vaccine. Infants readily swallow the vaccine in most circumstances; however, if an infant spits up or vomits after a dose is administered, the dose should not be readministered; the infant can receive the remaining doses at the normal intervals.

Contraindications & Precautions

Rotavirus vaccine should not be given to infants with a severe hypersensitivity to any components of the vaccine, to infants who had a serious allergic reaction to a previous dose of the vaccine, or to infants with a history of intussusception from any cause. RV1 should not be given to infants with a severe latex allergy. Both vaccines are contraindicated in infants with severe combined immunodeficiency (SCID). RV vaccines should be avoided in infants whose mother received a biologic response modifier (eg, etanercept) during pregnancy. Vaccination should be deferred in infants with acute moderate or severe gastroenteritis. Limited data suggest that rotavirus vaccination is safe and effective in premature infants. Small trials in Africa demonstrated that RV1 and

RV5 were well tolerated and immunogenic in HIV-infected children. However, vaccine safety and efficacy in infants with immunocompromising conditions, preexisting chronic gastrointestinal conditions (eg, Hirschsprung disease or short-gut syndrome), or a prior episode of intussusception has not been established. Clinicians should weigh the potential risks and benefits of vaccination in such circumstances. Infants living in households with pregnant women or immunocompromised persons can be vaccinated.

One special consideration is vaccination of hospitalized infants who are approaching the upper age limit (14 weeks 6 days) for starting the RV series. Due to concerns over nosocomial spread and potential shedding, the ACIP recommends that hospitalized infants who are eligible to receive RV vaccines wait to receive their first vaccine at or after hospital discharge. However, several US institutions and other countries, such as Australia, routinely allow administration of RV to hospitalized infants. Recent studies evaluating nosocomial spread of RV after vaccination in neonatal intensive care units or other hospital settings have not shown clinically significant disease transmission or side effects in medically stable children. As the window to initiate vaccination closes at age 15 weeks, vaccination of hospitalized children may become standard in future years as additional safety data on this practice accrues.

Adverse Effects

In addition to the slightly increased risk of intussusception, in prelicensure trials RV5 was associated with a very small but statistically significant increased risk of vomiting and diarrhea, and RV1 with a similarly small but significant increased risk of cough or runny nose.

Cortese MM, Parashar UD; CDC: Prevention of rotavirus gastroenteritis among infants and children: recommendations of the Advisory Committee on Immunization Practices (ACIP). MMWR Recomm Rep 2009;58(RR-2):1 [PMID: 19194371].

Lo Vecchio A et al: Rotavirus immunization: global coverage and local barriers for implementation. Vaccine 2017;35:1637 [PMID: 28216189].

Pahud B, Pallotto EK: Rotavirus immunization for hospitalized infants: are we there yet? Pediatrics 2018;141:e20173499 [PMID: 29212882].

Tate JE et al: Intussusception rates before and after the introduction of rotavirus vaccine. Pediatrics 2016;138:e20161082 [PMID: 27558938].

DIPHTHERIA-TETANUS-ACELLULAR PERTUSSIS VACCINATION

Diphtheria, tetanus, and pertussis vaccines have been given in a combined vaccine for many decades and have dramatically reduced each of these diseases. The efficacy with antigens in the combined vaccine is similar to that with antigens in single component vaccines. DTP vaccines containing whole-cell pertussis antigens are used widely in the world but have been entirely replaced in the United States with DTaP vaccines, which contain purified, inactivated components of the pertussis bacterium.

Diphtheria is caused by a gram-positive bacillus, *Corynebacterium diphtheriae*. It is a toxin-mediated disease, with diphtheria toxin causing local tissue destruction, as in pharyngeal and tonsillar diphtheria, as well as systemic disease, particularly myocarditis and neuritis. The overall case fatality rate is between 5% and 10%, with higher death rates in persons younger than 5 years or older than 40 years. The clinical efficacy of diphtheria vaccine is estimated to be greater than 95%. Since 2004, largely because of successful vaccination programs, only a few cases of diphtheria have been reported in the United States each year.

The anaerobic gram-positive rod *Clostridium tetani* causes tetanus, usually through infection of a contaminated wound. When *C tetani* colonizes devitalized tissue, the exotoxin tetanospasmin is disseminated to inhibitory motor neurons, resulting in generalized rigidity and spasms of skeletal muscles. Tetanus-prone wounds include (1) puncture wounds, including those acquired due to body piercing, tattooing, and intravenous drug abuse; (2) animal bites; (3) lacerations and abrasions; and (4) wounds resulting from nonsterile neonatal delivery and umbilical cord care (neonatal tetanus). In persons who have completed the primary vaccination series and have received a booster dose within the past 10 years, vaccination is virtually 100% protective. In 2019, 26 cases of tetanus were reported in the United States.

Pertussis is also primarily a toxin-mediated disease caused by *Bordetella pertussis*, which is called "whooping cough" because of the high-pitched inspiratory whoop that can follow intense paroxysms of cough. Pertussis complications include death, often from associated pneumonia, seizures, and encephalopathy. Pertussis incidence in the United States declined dramatically between the 1940s and 1980s, but beginning in the early 1980s, incidence has been slowly increasing, with adolescents and adults accounting for a greater proportion of reported cases. Reasons for increased incidence include improved detection of cases with better laboratory testing methodology (polymerase chain reaction), increased recognition of cases in adolescents and adults, and waning protection from prior infection or from childhood vaccination with only acellular pertussis vaccines. Infants younger than 6 months have the highest rate of pertussis infection (78 cases per 100,000); greater than 90% of pertussis deaths occur in neonates and infants younger than 3 months.

In 2019, 18,617 cases of pertussis were reported in the United States despite widespread underreporting with many localized outbreaks necessitating enhanced vaccination programs. A single booster dose of a different formulation, Tdap, is now recommended for all adolescents and adults, and pregnant women with each pregnancy. Tdap can also be used at age 7–9 years in children behind on vaccination. Providing a booster dose of pertussis-containing vaccine may prevent adolescent and adult pertussis cases, and it also has the potential to reduce the spread of pertussis to infants, who are most susceptible to pertussis complications.

▶ Vaccines Available

A. Diphtheria, Tetanus, and Acellular Pertussis Combinations

1. DTaP (Daptacel, Sanofi; Infanrix, GlaxoSmithKline) contains tetanus toxoid, diphtheria toxoid, and acellular pertussis vaccine. DTaP is licensed for ages 6 weeks through 6 years and can be used for doses 1–5.

2. Tdap (Boostrix, GlaxoSmithKline) is a tetanus-reduced dose diphtheria-acellular pertussis vaccine formulated for persons 10 years of age and older, including adults and the elderly.

3. Tdap (Adacel, Sanofi) is a tetanus-diphtheria-acellular pertussis vaccine approved for persons 11–64 years of age.

B. DTaP Combined With Other Vaccines

1. DTaP-HepB-IPV (Pediarix, GlaxoSmithKline) contains DTaP combined with poliovirus and HepB vaccines. It is approved for the first three doses of the DTaP and IPV series, given at 2, 4, and 6 months of age. Although it is approved for use through age 6 years, it is not licensed for booster doses. It cannot be used, for example, as the fourth dose of DTaP (typically given at 15–18 months of age).

2. DTaP-IPV-Hib (Pentacel, Sanofi) contains DTaP, IPV, and Hib vaccines. The Hib component is Hib capsular polysaccharide bound to tetanus toxoid. This vaccine is approved for use as doses 1–4 of the DTaP series among children 6 weeks to 4 years of age. It is typically given at 2, 4, 6, and 15–18 months of age, and should not be used as the fifth dose in the DTaP series.

3. DTaP-IPV (Kinrix, GlaxoSmithKline; also Quadracel, Sanofi) contains DTaP and IPV vaccines. The vaccine is licensed for children 4–6 years of age, for use as the fifth dose of the DTaP vaccine series and the fourth dose of the IPV series.

4. DTaP-IPV-Hib-HepB (Vaxelis, Merck) contains DTaP, IPV, Hib, and HepB vaccines. Approved for use as a three-dose series at 2, 4, and 6 months of age; not approved for use at 4–6 years of age as the final booster dose of IPV.

C. Diphtheria and Tetanus Combinations

1. DT (generic, Sanofi) contains tetanus toxoid and diphtheria toxoid to be used only in children younger than 7 years with a contraindication to pertussis vaccination.

2. Td (Tenivac, Sanofi; generic, Massachusetts Biological Labs) contains tetanus toxoid and a reduced quantity of diphtheria toxoid; typically used for adults requiring tetanus prophylaxis.

D. Tetanus Only

TT (generic, Sanofi) contains tetanus toxoid only and can be used for adults or children. However, the use of this single-antigen vaccine is generally not recommended because of the need for periodic boosting for both diphtheria and tetanus; it is available only on the international market.

▶ Dosage & Schedule of Administration

Although several different vaccines are available, a few general considerations can guide their use in specific circumstances. DTaP (alone or combined with other vaccines) is used for infants and children between 6 weeks and 6 years of age. Children 7–10 years of age not fully immunized against pertussis (meaning those who have not received five prior doses of DTaP, or four doses of DTaP if the fourth dose was given on or after the fourth birthday), who have no contraindications to pertussis immunization, should receive a single dose of Tdap for pertussis protection. For adolescents and adults, a single dose of Tdap is used, followed by booster doses of Td every 10 years; a detailed description of Tdap use is provided later in this chapter.

The primary series of DTaP vaccination should consist of four doses, given at 2, 4, 6, and 15–18 months of age. The fourth dose may be given as early as 12 months of age if 6 months have elapsed since the third dose. Giving the fourth dose between 12 and 15 months of age is indicated if the provider thinks the child is unlikely to return for a clinic visit between 15 and 18 months of age. Children should receive a fifth dose of DTaP at 4–6 years of age. However, a fifth dose of DTaP is not needed if the fourth dose was given after the child's fourth birthday. The same brand of DTaP should be used for all doses if feasible.

▶ Contraindications & Precautions

DTaP vaccines should not be used in individuals who have had an anaphylactic-type reaction to a previous vaccine dose or to a vaccine component. DTaP should not be given to children who developed encephalopathy, not attributable to another identified cause, within 7 days of a previous dose of DTaP or DTP. DTaP vaccination should also be deferred in individuals with progressive neurologic disorders, such as infantile spasms, uncontrolled epilepsy, or progressive encephalopathy, until their neurologic status is clarified and stabilized.

Precautions to DTaP vaccination include high fever ($\geq 40.5°F$), persistent inconsolable crying, or shock-like state within 48 hours of a previous dose of DTP or DTaP; seizures within 3 days of a previous dose of DTP or DTaP; GBS less than 6 weeks after a previous tetanus-containing vaccine; or incident moderate or severe acute illness with or without a fever.

▶ Adverse Effects

Local reactions, fever, and other mild systemic effects occur with acellular pertussis vaccines at one-fourth to two-thirds the frequency noted following whole-cell DTP vaccination. Moderate to severe systemic effects, including fever of 40.5°C, persistent inconsolable crying lasting 3 hours or more, and hypotonic-hyporesponsive episodes, are *much* less frequent than with whole-cell DTP. These are without sequelae. Severe neurologic effects have not been temporally associated with DTaP vaccines in use in the United States. Data are limited regarding differences in reactogenicity among currently licensed DTaP vaccines. More severe local reactions at injection sites appear to occur with increasing dose number (including swelling of the thigh or entire upper arm) after receipt of the fourth and fifth doses for all currently licensed DTaP vaccines.

▶ Diphtheria Antibody Preparations

Diphtheria antitoxin is manufactured in horses. Sensitivity to diphtheria antitoxin must be tested before it is given. Dosage depends on the size and location of the diphtheritic membrane and an estimate of the patient's level of intoxication. Consultation on the use of diphtheria antitoxin is available from the CDC's National Center for Immunization and Respiratory Diseases. Diphtheria antitoxin is not commercially available in the United States and must be obtained from the CDC.

▶ Tetanus Antibody Preparations

Human tetanus immune globulin (TIg) is indicated in the management of tetanus-prone wounds in individuals who have had an uncertain number or fewer than three tetanus immunizations. Persons fully immunized with at least three doses do not require TIg, regardless of the nature of their wounds (Table 10–4). The optimal dose of TIg has not been established, but some experts recommend 500 IU, which appears to be as effective and causing less discomfort, as a single dose of 3000–6000 units with part of the dose infiltrated around the wound.

http://www.cdc.gov/vaccines/pubs/pinkbook/dip.html. Accessed February 17, 2023.

http://www.cdc.gov/vaccines/pubs/pinkbook/pert.html. Accessed February 17, 2023.

http://www.cdc.gov/vaccines/pubs/pinkbook/tetanus.html. Accessed February 17, 2023.

Annual statistics from the Nationally Notifiable Infectious Diseases and Conditions Tables, United States. https://wonder.cdc.gov/nndss/nndss_annual_tables_menu.asp. Accessed February 17, 2023.

Table 10–4. Guide to tetanus prophylaxis in routine wound management.

History of Adsorbed Tetanus Toxoid (Doses)	Clean, Minor Wounds		All Other Wounds[a]	
	DTaP, Tdap, or Td[b]	TIG[c]	DTaP, Tdap, or Td[b]	TIG[c]
< 3 or unknown	Yes	No	Yes	Yes
≥ 3	No if < 10 y since last tetanus-containing vaccine dose	No	No[d] if < 5 y since last tetanus-containing vaccine dose	No
	Yes if ≥ 10 y since last tetanus-containing vaccine dose	No	Yes if ≥ 5 y since last tetanus-containing vaccine dose	No

Tdap indicates booster tetanus toxoid, reduced diphtheria toxoid, and acellular pertussis vaccine; DTaP, diphtheria and tetanus toxoids and acellular pertussis vaccine; Td, adult-type diphtheria and tetanus toxoids vaccine; TIG, tetanus immune globulin (human).
[a]Such as, but not limited to, wounds contaminated with dirt, feces, soil, and saliva; puncture wounds; avulsions; and wounds resulting from missiles, crushing, burns, and frostbite.
[b]DTaP is used for children younger than 7 years. Tdap is preferred over Td for underimmunized children 7 years and older who have not received Tdap previously.
[c]Immune globulin intravenous should be used when TIG is not available.
[d]More frequent boosters are not needed and can accentuate adverse effects.
Reproduced from Centers for Disease Control and Prevention (CDC).

HAEMOPHILUS INFLUENZAE TYPE B VACCINATION

H influenzae type b (Hib) causes a wide spectrum of serious illnesses, particularly in young children, including meningitis, epiglottitis, pneumonia, septic arthritis, and cellulitis. Hib is surrounded by a polysaccharide capsule (polyribosylribitol phosphate [PRP]) that contributes to virulence. Antibodies to this polysaccharide capsule confer immunity to the disease. When Hib polysaccharide is chemically bonded (conjugated) to certain protein carriers, the conjugate vaccine induces T-cell–dependent immune memory that is highly effective in young children. Importantly, polysaccharide-protein conjugate vaccines also prevent carriage of the bacterium, limiting spread from asymptomatic carriers to others in the community. All Hib vaccines are polysaccharide-protein conjugates.

Bacterial serotyping is required to differentiate infections caused by Hib from those caused by other encapsulated and nonencapsulated *H influenzae* strains. In the early 1980s, roughly 20,000 cases of invasive Hib disease occurred each year in the United States. Because of the introduction of protein conjugate Hib vaccines, only 18 cases of invasive Hib disease occurred in children younger than 5 years in 2019.

▶ Vaccines Available

Five vaccines against Hib disease are available in the United States; three are Hib-only vaccines, and two are combination vaccines. Each vaccine contains Hib polysaccharide conjugated to a protein carrier, but different protein carriers are used. The Hib conjugate vaccine that uses a meningococcal outer membrane protein carrier is abbreviated PRP-OMP. PRP-T vaccine uses a tetanus toxoid carrier.

▶ Hib-Only Vaccines

1. Hib (PedvaxHIB, Merck, uses PRP-OMP), for use at 2, 4, and 12–15 months of age.
2. Hib (ActHIB, Sanofi, uses PRP-T), for use at 2, 4, 6, and 12–15 months of age.
3. Hib (Hiberix, GlaxoSmithKline, uses PRP-T), for use at 2, 4, 6, and 12–15 months of age.

▶ Hib Combined With Other Vaccines

1. DTaP-IPV-Hib (Pentacel, Sanofi, uses PRP-T) contains DTaP, IPV, and Hib vaccines. This vaccine is approved for use in children 6 weeks to 4 years of age and administered at 2, 4, 6, and 15–18 months of age.
2. DTaP-IPV-Hib-HepB (Vaxelis, Merck, uses PRP-OMP) contains DTaP, IPV, Hib, and HepB vaccines. Approved for use as a three-dose series at 2, 4, and 6 months of age; not approved for use at 12–15 months of age as the final booster dose of Hib.

▶ Dosage & Schedule of Administration

Hib vaccination is recommended for all infants in the United States. The recommended interval between doses in the primary series is 8 weeks, but a minimal interval of 4 weeks is permitted. For infants who missed the primary vaccination series, a catch-up schedule is used (see Table 10–2). Hib vaccine is not generally recommended for children aged 5 years or older.

Contraindications & Precautions

Hib vaccine should not be given to anyone who has had a severe allergic reaction to a prior Hib vaccine dose or to any vaccine components. Hib vaccine should not be given to infants before 6 weeks of age.

Adverse Effects

Adverse reactions following Hib vaccination are uncommon. Between 5% and 30% of vaccine recipients experience swelling, redness, or pain at the vaccination site. Systemic reactions such as fever and irritability are rare.

Annual statistics from the Nationally Notifiable Infectious Diseases and Conditions Tables, United States. https://wonder.cdc.gov/nndss/nndss_annual_tables_menu.asp. Accessed February 17, 2023.

Briere EC: Food and Drug Administration approval for use of Hiberix as a 3-dose primary *Haemophilus influenzae* type b (Hib) vaccination series. MMWR Morb Mortal Wkly Rep 2016;65:418 [PMID: 27124887].

Briere EC, Rubin L, Moro PL, Cohn A, Clark T, Messonnier N; Division of Bacterial Diseases; National Center for Immunization and Respiratory Diseases; CDC: Prevention and control of *Haemophilus influenzae* type b disease: recommendations of the Advisory Committee on Immunization Practices (ACIP). MMWR Recomm Rep 2014;63(RR-01):1 [PMID: 24572654].

Centers for Disease Control and Prevention (Vaccines & Preventable Diseases: Hib): https://www.cdc.gov/vaccines/vpd/hib/hcp/index.html. Accessed February 17, 2023

PNEUMOCOCCAL VACCINATION

Before the routine use of pneumococcal conjugate vaccines in infants, *Streptococcus pneumoniae* (pneumococcus) was the leading cause of invasive bacterial disease in children. Pneumococcus remains a leading cause of febrile bacteremia, bacterial sepsis, meningitis, and pneumonia in children and adults in the United States and worldwide. It is also a common cause of otitis media and sinusitis. Over 90 serotypes of pneumococcus have been identified, and immunity to the capsular polysaccharide antigen of one serotype does not confer immunity to other serotypes.

A seven-valent pneumococcal conjugate vaccine (PCV7) was first licensed in the United States in 2000. Routine use of PCV7 led to a dramatic decrease in pneumococcal disease overall, however, disease caused by pneumococcal serotypes not included in PCV7 increased. In 2010, a 13-valent pneumococcal conjugate vaccine (PCV13) was licensed for use in the United States. This vaccine contains the serotypes in PCV7 and an additional six pneumococcal serotypes, with the capsular polysaccharide antigens of each serotype individually conjugated to a nontoxic diphtheria cross-reactive material (CRM) carrier protein. In 2022, a 15-valent pneumococcal conjugate vaccine (PCV 15) was licensed and recommended for use in children 6 months and older to be used interchangeably with PCV13.

Subsequently, in September of 2023, the CDC published updated guidelines for the use of a 20-valent pneumococcal conjugate vaccine (PCV20) for children. Currently, the CDC recommends use of PCV 20 as an option to the use of PCV15 in the following scenarios: (1) routine vaccination of children aged 2-23 months, (2) catch-up vaccination for healthy children aged 24-59 months who have not received age-appropriate doses; and children aged 24-71 months with underlying medical conditions at increased risk for pneumococcal disease who have not yet received age-appropriate doses. PCV13 is no longer recommended for routine immunizations. Recommendations were also updated for children 2-18 years with any risk conditions.

In addition to PCV15 and PCV20, a 23-valent pneumococcal nonconjugated polysaccharide vaccine (PPSV23) is available in the United States, but its use in children is limited to those with certain chronic medical conditions. However, it does not produce a long-lasting immune response and does not reduce nasopharyngeal carriage. While all children and adults are at risk of pneumococcal disease, certain children are at particularly high risk and need enhanced protection against pneumococcal disease including the use of PPSV23 in addition to PCV15 or PCV20. Table 10–5 details the indications for administration of additional doses of PCV15 and PCV20 and PPSV23 in children aged 6–18 years (i.e., following the completion of a primary series with PCV15 or PCV20 or in children who received 1 or fewer doses of PCV15 or PCV20).

Since the introduction of PCV13, the incidence of invasive pneumococcal disease has decreased dramatically among children younger than 5 years and decreased by more than 50% among older adults, largely due to indirect effects of vaccination among children.

Vaccines Available

1. PCV13 (Prevnar13, Pfizer), for use in children 6 weeks of age and older and for adults.
2. PCV15 (Vaxneuvance, Merck), for use in children 6 weeks of age and older and for adults.
3. PCV20 (Prevnar20, Pfizer), for use in children 6 weeks of age and older and for adults.
4. PPSV23 (Pneumovax23, Merck), for use in children 2 years of age and older and for adults.

Dosage & Schedule of Administration

PCV15 and PCV20 are given as a 0.5-mL intramuscular dose. PPSV23 is given as a 0.5-mL dose by either the intramuscular or subcutaneous route.

PCV15 and PCV20 are routinely recommended for infants at 2, 4, 6, and 12–15 months of age. Healthy children

Table 10–5. Medical conditions or other indications for administration of PCV15[a] or PCV20[a] and indications for PPSV23[b] administration and revaccination for children aged 6–18 years.[c] (Note: PCV15 or PCV20 recommended for all children 2–59 months of age; this table lists additional vaccination recommendations after completion of the primary series).

Risk Group	Underlying Medical Condition	PCV15/20 Recommended	PPSV23 Recommended	PPSV23 Revaccination 5 Years After First Dose
Immunocompetent children	Chronic heart disease[d]		√	
	Chronic kidney disease (excluding maintenance dialysis / nephrotic syndrome)		√	
	Chronic liver disease		√	
	Chronic lung disease[e]		√	
	Diabetes mellitus		√	
	Cerebrospinal fluid leaks	√	√	
	Cochlear implants	√	√	
Children with immunocompromising conditions	Maintenance dialysis or nephrotic syndrome	√	√	√
	Sickle cell disease/other hemoglobinopathies	√	√	√
	Congenital or acquired asplenia, or splenic dysfunction	√	√	√
	Congenital or acquired immunodeficiencies[f]	√	√	√
	Human immunodeficiency virus infection	√	√	√
	Diseases and conditions treated with immunosuppressive drugs or radiation therapy[g]	√	√	√
	Solid organ transplant	√	√	√

[a]15-valent or 20-valent pneumococcal conjugate vaccine.
[b]23-valent pneumococcal polysaccharide vaccine.
[c]Children aged 2–5 years with chronic conditions (eg, heart disease or diabetes), immunocompromising conditions (eg, human immunodeficiency virus), functional or anatomic asplenia (including sickle cell disease), cerebrospinal fluid leaks, or cochlear implants, and who have not previously been vaccinated are recommended to receive PCV15 or PCV20.
[d]Including cyanotic congenital heart disease, congestive heart failure, and cardiomyopathies.
[e]Including chronic obstructive pulmonary disease, emphysema, and moderate persistent or severe persistent asthma.
[f]Including B- (humoral) or T-lymphocyte deficiency, complement deficiencies (particularly C1, C2, C3, and C4 deficiencies), and phagocytic disorders (excluding chronic granulomatous disease).
[g]Including malignant neoplasms, leukemias, lymphomas, and Hodgkin disease.
Reproduced from Centers for Disease Control and Prevention (CDC): Use of 15-valent pneumococcal conjugate vaccine among U.S. children: updated recommendations of the Advisory Committee on Immunization Practices—United States, 2022. *MMWR Morb Mortal Wkly Rep* 2022 Sep 16;71(37):1174–1181.

24–59 months of age who are unvaccinated or did not complete the four-dose PCV series should receive a single dose of PCV15 or PCV20. Children 24–71 months of age at high risk of pneumococcal disease (see Table 10–5) should receive two doses of PCV15 or PCV20 (if they previously received fewer than three doses) or one dose of PCV15 or PCV20 (if they previously received three doses). High-risk children 24–71 months of age should also receive a dose of PPSV23, at least 8 weeks after their final dose of PCV15 or PCV20. If not previously vaccinated against pneumococcus, most high-risk children 6–18 years of age should receive one dose of PCV15, followed at least 8 weeks later by PPSV23, with PPSV23 repeated 5 years later for some conditions. Alternatively, children high-risk children 6-18 years of age who are not previously vaccinated may receive 1 dose of PCV20 with no additional doses of any pneumococcal vaccine indicated thereafter. Updated and detailed schedule information is available at the CDC (at http://www.cdc.gov/vaccines) and AAP (https://publications.aap.org/redbook), including guidance regarding situations in which children have begun their pneumococcal vaccination series with PCV13 and are now continuing with PCV15 or PCV20.

Both PCV15/20 and PPSV23 are recommended in most high-risk children because while PPSV23 is less immunogenic than PCV15/20, PPSV23 covers additional serotypes that may cause disease. Table 10–5 also includes the indications for revaccination with PPSV23.

Contraindications & Precautions

For both PCV15/20 and PPSV23, vaccination is contraindicated in individuals who suffered a severe allergic reaction such as anaphylaxis after a previous vaccine dose or to a vaccine component. PPSV23 should not be given together with a pneumococcal conjugate vaccine (i.e., PCV15 or PCV20) but can be administered concurrently with other childhood vaccines. MenACWY-D (Menactra [Sanofi Paseur]) should not be administered concomitantly or within 4 weeks of PCV15 or PCV 20 administration in order to avoid potential interference with the immune response to either pneumococcal conjugate vaccine.

Adverse Effects

The most common adverse effects associated with PCV15 and PCV20 administration are fever, injection site reactions, irritability, and increased or decreased sleep. With PPSV23, 30%–50% of vaccine recipients develop pain and redness at the injection site. Fewer than 1% develop systemic side effects such as fever and myalgia. Anaphylaxis is rare. PPSV23 appears to be safe and immunogenic during pregnancy, although safety data are lacking regarding vaccination during the first trimester of pregnancy.

CDC: Use of 13-valent pneumococcal conjugate vaccine and 23-valent pneumococcal polysaccharide vaccine among children aged 6–18 years with immunocompromising conditions: recommendations of the Advisory Committee on Immunization Practices (ACIP). MMWR 2013;62:521 [PMID: 23803961].

CDC: Use of 15-Valent Pneumococcal Conjugate Vaccine Among U.S. Children: Updated Recommendations of the Advisory Committee on Immunization Practices - United States, 2022. MMWR Recomm Rep 2022;71(37) [PMID: 36107786]

CDC: ACIP updates: Recommendations for use of 20-valent pneumococcal conjugate vaccine in children – United States, 2023. MMWR Morb Mort Wkly Rep. 2023;72(39):1072.

Wasserman M et al: Twenty-year public health impact of 7- and 13-valent pneumococcal conjugate vaccines in US children. Emerg Infect Dis 2021;27:1627 [PMID: 34013855].

POLIOMYELITIS VACCINATION

Polioviruses are highly infectious, spread primarily by fecal-oral and oral-oral routes, and cause acute flaccid paralysis via destruction of motor neurons. There are three polio serotypes; immunity to one serotype does not confer immunity to the others. Poliomyelitis can be prevented by vaccination. Type 2 poliovirus was declared eradicated in 2015, and type 3 poliovirus was declared eradicated in 2019. Polio eradication has not been achieved, but polio worldwide has decreased from ~350,000 cases annually in the prevaccination era to fewer than 30 wild-type polio cases detected in 2022. Afghanistan and Pakistan are the remaining endemic countries for wild-type polio. Two different types of poliovirus vaccines are used globally: an injectable inactivated polio vaccine (IPV) and an OPV. Only IPV is available for use in the United States.

Attenuated vaccine strains used in OPV can rarely mutate into pathogenic strains and cause polio disease. Referred to as circulating vaccine-derived poliovirus, this phenomenon further complicates eradication efforts. There has been a recent resurgence of vaccine-derived poliovirus outbreaks, particularly in parts of Africa, with 1856 paralytic cVDPV cases reported globally from January 2020 to April 2022, primarily as a result of interruptions of vaccination campaigns during the COVID-19 pandemic. In July 2022, a case of paralytic polio was identified in an unvaccinated young adult in New York state in an area with low vaccination coverage. Continued efforts at polio control will be needed, including use of IPV in all countries currently using OPV, and the development of novel OPV vaccines specifically designed to prevent reversion to pathogenic strains. For updates on the worldwide polio eradication program, go to www.polioeradication.org.

Vaccines Available

1. IPV (IPOL, Sanofi) is given intramuscularly or subcutaneously.
2. DTaP-HepB-IPV (Pediarix, GlaxoSmithKline) contains DTaP, HepB, and IPV vaccines. Approved for use at 2, 4, and 6 months of age; not approved for use at 4–6 years of age as the final booster dose of IPV; given intramuscularly.
3. DTaP-IPV-Hib (Pentacel, Sanofi) contains DTaP, IPV, and Hib vaccines. Approved for use at 2, 4, 6, and 15–18 months of age; not approved for use at 4–6 years of age as the final booster dose of IPV; given intramuscularly.
4. DTaP-IPV-Hib-HepB (Vaxelis, Merck) contains DTaP, IPV, Hib, and HepB vaccines. Approved for use as a three-dose series at 2, 4, and 6 months of age; not approved for use at 4–6 years of age as the final booster dose of IPV; given intramuscularly.
5. DTaP-IPV (Kinrix, GlaxoSmithKline) contains DTaP and IPV vaccines. Licensed for children 4–6 years of age, for use as a final booster dose of IPV; given intramuscularly.

Dosage & Schedule of Administration

In the United States, all children without contraindications should receive an IPV-containing vaccine at 2, 4, 6–18 months, and 4–6 years of age. A dose of IPV should be given at 4 years of age or older, regardless of the number of prior doses of IPV. Completely immunized adult visitors to areas of continuing wild-type poliovirus circulation should receive a booster dose of IPV. Unimmunized or incompletely immunized adults and children should receive two (preferably three) doses of IPV prior to travel.

Contraindications & Precautions

IPV vaccination is contraindicated in individuals who suffered a severe allergic reaction such as anaphylaxis after a previous vaccine dose or to a vaccine component. IPV vaccination should be deferred during moderate or severe acute illness with or without fever. Pregnancy is also a precaution to IPV vaccination. Receipt of previous doses of OPV is not a contraindication to IPV.

Adverse Effects

Minor local reactions, such as pain or redness at the injection site, may occur following IPV vaccination. No serious adverse reactions following IPV vaccination have been described.

Chumakov K et al: Polio eradication at the crossroads. Lancet Glob Health 2021:S2214 [PMID: 34118192].

Kalkowska DA et al: The impact of disruptions caused by the COVID-19 pandemic on global polio eradication. Vaccine 2021:S0264 [PMID: 33962838].

Rachlin et al: Progress toward polio eradication—worldwide, January 2020–April 2022. MMWR Morb Mortal Wkly Rep 2022;71(19) [PMID: 35552352].

INFLUENZA VACCINATION

Influenza viruses comprise four species of RNA viruses from the *Orthomyxoviridae* family, which circulate seasonally in the United States from late fall to early spring. Influenza is primarily transmitted by respiratory droplets. Since 2010, the CDC estimates that between 140,000 and 960,000 hospitalizations and up to 36,000 deaths per year in the United States have been attributable to influenza. Influenza causes significant morbidity in children under age two years and among those with high-risk medical conditions. Disparities in influenza hospitalization and in-hospital deaths are pronounced, especially among Black, Indigenous, and Latino people, and are associated with disparities in influenza vaccination coverage. Notably, influenza A causes global pandemics, such as the 1918 H1N1 and the 2009 H1N1 pandemics.

Each year, recommendations are formulated in the spring regarding the constituents of influenza vaccine for the coming season. Influenza vaccines contain either three strains (ie, trivalent: two influenza A strains and one of two influenza B lineages) or four strains (ie, quadrivalent: two influenza A and two influenza B lineages). The pandemic 2009 H1N1 strain is incorporated into seasonal influenza vaccines. Children at high risk of seasonal influenza-related complications include those with hemoglobinopathies or with chronic cardiac, pulmonary (including asthma), metabolic, renal, and immunosuppressive diseases (including immunosuppression caused by medications or by HIV); and those with any condition (eg, cognitive dysfunction, spinal cord injuries, seizure disorders, or other neuromuscular disorders) that can compromise respiratory function or the handling of respiratory secretions, or that can increase the risk of aspiration. Children and adolescents receiving long-term aspirin therapy are also at risk of influenza-related Reye syndrome. Healthy children aged 6–23 months are at substantially increased risk of influenza-related hospitalizations, and children aged 24–59 months remain at increased risk of influenza-related clinic and emergency department visits and hospitalizations, but less so than younger children.

Annual influenza vaccination is routinely recommended for all persons older than 6 months. Physicians should identify high-risk children in their practices and encourage parents to seek influenza vaccination for their children and themselves as soon as influenza vaccine is available. Influenza prevention will help prevent lower respiratory tract disease or other secondary complications in high-risk groups, thereby decreasing hospitalizations and deaths.

Vaccines Available

Most inactivated influenza vaccine virus is grown in eggs and formalin inactivated; it may contain trace quantities of thimerosal, which is used as a preservative in multidose vials. Only split-virus or purified viral antigens are available in the United States. Fluzone (Sanofi), Afluria (Seqirus), Fluarix (GlaxoSmithKline), and FluLaval (Biomedical Corp of Quebec) are approved for children 6 months and older. A cell-culture–based vaccine Flucelvax (Seqirus) is approved for children 4 years and older. There are several additional influenza vaccines licensed for adults but not for children, including a high-dose vaccine for older adults, a recombinant vaccine, and an adjuvanted vaccine. An intranasal LAIV (FluMist, AstraZeneca) is approved for healthy children and adults aged 2–49 years.

Dosage & Schedule of Administration

A. Inactivated Influenza Virus Vaccine (IIV)

The optimal time to initiate vaccination is as soon as vaccine is available in the early fall. However, providers should continue vaccinating individuals as long as vaccine is available and there is influenza activity in the community. Children younger than 6 months should not be immunized. Two doses administered at least 4 weeks apart are recommended for children younger than 9 years who did not receive two doses in the past. Older children receiving vaccine for the first time require only a single dose. Inactivated vaccine is recommended for all pregnant women and those contemplating pregnancy during the influenza season, as complications from influenza infection are greatly increased in the third trimester and up to 2 weeks postpartum.

Newborns are also protected. Simultaneous administration with other routine vaccines is acceptable.

B. Live Attenuated Influenza Virus Vaccine (LAIV)

The vaccine is supplied in a prefilled single-use sprayer, approximately half of which is sprayed into each nostril. If the patient sneezes during administration, the dose should not be repeated. It can be administered to children with minor illnesses but should not be given if significant nasal congestion is present. Because it is a live vaccine, it should be administered 48 hours after cessation of therapy in children receiving postexposure anti-influenza antiviral drugs, and these should not be given for 2 weeks after vaccination. Two doses are recommended for children younger than 9 years who did not receive two vaccine doses in the past. One dose is recommended for individuals 9–49 years of age.

▶ Contraindications & Precautions

A. Inactivated Influenza Virus Vaccine

Inactivated influenza vaccine is contraindicated in individuals with a severe allergic reaction, such as anaphylaxis, to a previous dose of an inactivated influenza vaccine component. However, guidelines for influenza vaccination in children with egg allergies have recently changed. Previously, only children with hives following exposure to egg could be vaccinated without referral to an allergist for evaluation of vaccination risk. Now, children with more serious allergic reactions to egg, such as angioedema, respiratory symptoms, or anaphylaxis, can receive any licensed, age-appropriate influenza vaccine (ie, IIV or LAIV), in any inpatient or outpatient medical setting, from a health care provider who is able to recognize and manage severe allergic conditions.

B. Live Attenuated Influenza Virus Vaccine

LAIV is contraindicated in individuals with a history of severe allergic reaction to any component of the vaccine, to a previous dose of any influenza vaccine, and in children and adolescents receiving concomitant aspirin or aspirin-containing therapy. LAIV should not be administered to the following persons: (1) children younger than 24 months because an increased risk of hospitalization and wheezing was observed in clinical trials; (2) individuals with asthma or children younger than 5 years with recurrent wheezing unless the potential benefit outweighs the potential risk; (3) pregnant women; and (4) individuals with known or suspected immunodeficiency diseases or immunosuppressed states.

All health care workers, including those with asthma and other underlying health conditions, can administer LAIV. Health care workers who are vaccinated with LAIV can safely provide care to patients within a hospital or clinic, except for severely immunosuppressed patients that require a protected environment (ie, bone marrow transplant patients). In this instance, there should be a 7-day interval between receiving LAIV and care for these patients.

▶ Adverse Effects

A. Inactivated Influenza Virus Vaccine

Injection site reactions are the most common adverse events after inactivated influenza vaccine administration. A small proportion of children will experience some systemic toxicity, consisting of fever, malaise, and myalgias. These symptoms generally begin 6–12 hours after vaccination and may last 24–48 hours. Cases of GBS followed the swine influenza vaccination program in 1976–1977, but careful study by the Institute of Medicine showed no association with that vaccine in children and young adults—nor in any age group that received vaccines in subsequent years.

B. Live Attenuated Influenza Virus Vaccine

The most common adverse reactions include runny nose or nasal congestion in all ages and fever higher than 37.7°C in children 2–6 years of age. These reactions occurred more often with the first dose and were self-limited.

AAP; Committee on Infectious Diseases: Recommendations for prevention and control of influenza in children, 2022–2023. Pediatrics 2022;150(4):e2022059274. [PMID: 36065749].

CDC: Prevention and control of seasonal influenza with vaccines: recommendations of the Advisory Committee on Immunization Practices—United States, 2022–23 Influenza Season. MMWR 2022;71(1):1–28 [PMID: 36006864].

MEASLES, MUMPS, & RUBELLA VACCINATION

Due to an effective vaccination program beginning in 1963, measles was declared eliminated from the United States in 2000. Until 2008, there were only sporadic importations of measles from countries with lower vaccination rates, but since then there have been numerous outbreaks of measles involving viral transmission within the United States, again after initial exposure to imported cases. In 2018–2019, there were numerous outbreaks of measles across the United States, primarily in insular communities, resulting in the most cases in the United States in any year since 1992. As a result of an organized misinformation campaign, the largest of these outbreaks occurred in New York State in orthodox Jewish communities. In outbreaks such as these, most people who developed measles were unvaccinated.

In the United States, after adding mumps vaccine to the childhood schedule in 1977, there was a 99% decline in mumps to fewer than 300 cases each year between 2001 and 2003. However, since then, there have been several large outbreaks, particularly in 2016–2017 when there were over 9000 cases. University outbreaks accounted for half of all outbreaks and 40% of total mumps cases. Many of these outbreaks were in populations that had a high proportion of individuals fully vaccinated with two doses of MMR vaccine. As a result of these large outbreaks, in 2017 ACIP recommended a third dose of a mumps-containing vaccine in persons previously vaccinated with two doses of a mumps-containing vaccine who are identified by public health as at increased risk for mumps because of an outbreak.

The rubella vaccine is primarily intended to prevent the serious consequences of rubella infection in pregnant women: miscarriage, fetal demise, and congenital rubella syndrome. In the United States and elsewhere, the approach has been to vaccinate young children. Over time, this approach has led to most women being rubella immune by the time they reach child-bearing age; herd immunity also reduces transmission to susceptible women. With the use of rubella vaccines, rubella and congenital rubella syndrome were declared eliminated in the United States in 2004. There are now fewer than 10 rubella cases per year, and all cases since 2012 have been infected while living or traveling outside the country.

Despite many reports in the lay press and on the Internet of a link between MMR and autism, there is overwhelming scientific evidence that there is no causal association between the two. There is also no evidence that separation of MMR into its individual component vaccines lessens the risk of any vaccine adverse event, and such practice is not recommended.

▶ Vaccines Available

1. Measles-mumps-rubella (MMR II, Merck): MMR II is a lyophilized preparation of measles, mumps, and rubella vaccines. The measles and mumps portions are prepared using chick embryo tissue cultures, and rubella is grown in human diploid cells. There is no adjuvant and no preservative. It contains small amounts of gelatin, sorbitol, and neomycin. The individual components of MMR II are no longer available.

2. Measles-mumps-rubella (PRIORIX, GlaxoSmithKline): PRIORIX is a preparation of live attenuated measles, mumps, and rubella strains. It contains small amounts of sorbitol and mannitol and may also contain residual amounts of neomycin, ovalbumin, and bovine serum albumin from the manufacturing process. PRIORIX is formulated without preservatives and is administered as subcutaneous injection (the same as M-M-R II)

3. MMRV: A combined live attenuated measles, mumps, rubella, and varicella vaccine (ProQuad, Merck) is licensed for use in children 1–12 years of age. The measles, mumps, and rubella components are identical to MMR II. The varicella component has a higher varicella-zoster virus (VZV) titer than the varicella-only (VAR) vaccine.

▶ Dosage & Schedule of Administration

A. Routine Vaccination

MMR II and PRIORIX can be used interchangeably. Measles, mumps, and rubella vaccinations should be given as MMR or MMRV at 12–15 months and again at 4–6 years of age. Both MMR and MMRV can cause febrile seizures, although uncommonly. Because febrile seizures following MMRV occur at a rate twice that of MMR at the younger age, the ACIP recommends that after a discussion of the benefits and risks of both vaccination options with the parents or caregivers, either MMR or MMRV may be given at 12–15 months of age. MMRV is the preferred vaccine at 4–6 years of age if available; no excess risk of febrile seizures following MMRV vaccination has been observed at 4–6 years of age. A personal or family history of febrile seizures in an infant is considered a precaution for the use of MMRV; and MMR and VAR given separately are preferred. A dose of 0.5 mL should be given subcutaneously. The second dose of MMR or MMRV is recommended at school entry to help prevent school-based measles and mumps outbreaks. Children not reimmunized at school entry should receive their second dose by age 11–12 years. If an infant receives MMR before 12 months of age (such as for travel), two additional doses are required to complete the series, the first after 12 months of age and the second at least 1 month later. Ig interferes with the immune response to the attenuated vaccine strains of MMR and MMRV. Therefore, MMR and MMRV immunization should be deferred by 3–11 months after Ig administration, depending on the type of Ig product received. Consult the AAP's *Red Book* for specific recommendations.

For measles, mumps, and rubella, most persons can be considered immune if they were fully vaccinated at appropriate intervals, or were born before 1957, or if there is laboratory evidence of serologic immunity or disease. However, special considerations apply to health care workers: for those born before 1957, laboratory confirmation of immunity or disease should be performed, and nonimmune health care workers should be vaccinated. A clinical diagnosis of any of these diseases is not acceptable evidence of immunity. For rubella, susceptible pubertal girls and postpubertal women identified by prenatal screening should be immunized after delivery. Whenever rubella vaccination is offered to a woman of childbearing age, pregnancy should be ruled out and the woman advised to prevent conception for 3 months following vaccination. If a pregnant woman is vaccinated or becomes pregnant within 3 weeks of vaccination, she should be counseled regarding the risk to her fetus, although no cases of rubella-vaccine–related fetal anomalies have been reported. The risk of congenital rubella syndrome after wild-type maternal infection in the first trimester of pregnancy is 20%–85%. All susceptible adults in institutional settings (including colleges), day care center personnel, military personnel, and hospital and health care personnel should be immunized.

B. Vaccination of Travelers

People traveling abroad should be immune to measles, mumps, and rubella. Infants 6–11 months of age traveling to high-risk areas should receive one dose of MMR prior to travel followed by either MMR or MMRV at 12–15 months of age (given at least 4 weeks after the initial dose) and either MMR or MMRV at 4–6 years of age to complete the series. Children older than 12 months who are traveling to high-risk areas should receive two doses separated by at least 4 weeks. Children traveling internationally to lower-risk areas should be immunized as soon as possible after their first birthday and complete the series at 4–6 years of age in the usual fashion.

C. Revaccination Under Other Circumstances

Persons entering college and other institutions for education beyond high school, medical personnel beginning employment, and persons traveling abroad should have documentation of immunity to measles and mumps, defined as receipt of two doses of measles vaccine after their first birthday, birth before 1957, or a laboratory documented measles or mumps history.

D. Outbreak Control of Measles

A community outbreak is defined as a single documented case of measles. Control depends on immediate protection of all susceptible persons (defined as persons who have no documented immunity to measles in the affected community). The *Red Book* offers guidance on exposure to measles cases by age, vaccination status, and immunocompromising conditions.

E. Outbreak Control of Mumps

Persons previously vaccinated with two doses of a mumps-containing vaccine who are identified by public health as at increased risk for mumps because of an outbreak should receive a third dose of a mumps-containing vaccine to improve protection against mumps disease and related complications.

▶ Contraindications & Precautions

MMR and MMRV vaccines are contraindicated in pregnant women, women intending to become pregnant within the next 28 days, immunocompromised persons, and persons with an anaphylactic reaction to a prior dose or vaccine component. It is also contraindicated in children receiving high-dose corticosteroid therapy (≥ 2 mg/kg/day, or 20 mg/day total, for longer than 14 days) with the exception of those receiving physiologic replacement doses. In these patients, an interval of 1 month between cessation of steroid therapy and vaccination is sufficient. Leukemic patients who have been in remission and off chemotherapy for at least 3 months can receive MMR and MMRV safely. Persons with HIV infection should receive two doses of MMR vaccine according to the recommended schedule if they do not have evidence of current severe immunosuppression. MMRV is contraindicated in HIV-positive individuals. Children with minor acute illnesses (including febrile illnesses), egg allergy, or a history of tuberculosis should be immunized. MMR and MMRV may be safely administered simultaneously with other routine pediatric immunizations.

▶ Adverse Effects

Between 5% and 15% of individuals receiving MMR become febrile to 39.5°C or higher about 6–12 days following vaccination, lasting approximately 1–2 days, and 5% may develop a transient morbilliform rash. MMR and MMRV vaccines can cause febrile seizures, typically 8–14 days after vaccination; these febrile seizures have not been associated with any long-term complications. Other serious adverse events following vaccination are rare and include anaphylaxis, transient thrombocytopenia (1 per 40,000 vaccine recipients), and arthralgias (more common in adults than children).

▶ Antibody Preparations Against Measles

Ig is effective at preventing measles if given to a nonimmune person within 6 days of exposure to measles. However, the immunity conferred by Ig should be considered temporary. Infants younger than 12 months who have been exposed to measles should receive 0.5 mL/kg of Ig, given intramuscularly (see AAP *Red Book* for detailed recommendations). Pregnant women without evidence of measles immunity and severely immune-compromised persons (regardless of evidence of measles immunity) who are exposed to measles should receive 400 mg/kg of Ig given intravenously. Ig given intramuscularly (0.5 mL/kg, maximum dose, 15 mL) may be given to more immune-competent exposed persons without evidence of immunity, with priority for those with the most intense contact with a case.

Albertson JP et al: Mumps outbreak at a university and recommendation for a third dose of measles-mumps-rubella vaccine—Illinois, 2015–2016. MMWR Morb Mortal Wkly Rep 2016;65:731 [PMID: 27467572].

CDC: Prevention of measles, rubella, congenital rubella syndrome, and mumps, 2013: summary recommendations of the Advisory Committee on Immunization Practices (ACIP). MMWR Recomm Rep 2013;62:1 [PMID: 23760231].

Krow-Lucal et al: Measles, mumps, rubella vaccine (PRIORIX): recommendations of the Advisory Committee on Immunization Practices—United States, 2022. MMWR Recomm Rep 2022;71(46) [PMID: 36395065].

VARICELLA VACCINATION

Prior to a vaccine, there were approximately 4 million cases of VZV infection annually in the United States, mostly in children younger than 10 years, with 11,000 hospitalizations and 100 deaths per year. A live, attenuated varicella vaccine (VAR) was licensed in the United States in 1995, and the incidence, morbidity, mortality, and medical costs associated with varicella infection declined significantly. However, it became apparent that there is "breakthrough" (usually very mild) varicella occurring in about 15% of immunized patients. Outbreaks of wild-type infectious VZV were reported in schools with high one-dose VAR vaccination coverage (96%–100%). Varicella attack rates among these children varied between 11% and 17%, and thus it was concluded that a single VAR dose could not prevent endemic varicella.

A second dose of VAR in children greatly increases the magnitude of the anti-VZV antibody response, which is a correlate of vaccine efficacy. A combination MMRV vaccine has also been shown to be immunologically noninferior to the MMR and VAR components administered separately. MMRV is effective as primary immunization or as a booster administered to children age 4–6 years. The two-dose regimen is almost 100% effective against severe varicella, and the risk of breakthrough varicella is threefold less than the risk with a one-dose regimen. Therefore, ACIP and the AAP recommend two doses of VAR for children older than 12 months and for adolescents and adults without evidence of immunity.

The vaccine is also effective in preventing or modifying VZV severity in susceptible individuals exposed to VZV if used within 3 days (and possibly up to 5 days) of exposure, with an efficacy of 95% for preventing any postexposure disease and 100% for preventing moderate or severe disease. There is no evidence that postexposure prophylaxis increases the risk of vaccine-related adverse events or interferes with development of immunity.

▶ Vaccines Available

1. A cell-free preparation of Oka strain VZV is produced and marketed in the United States as Varivax (Merck). Each dose contains trace amounts of neomycin, fetal bovine serum, and gelatin. There is no preservative.
2. MMRV (measles-mumps-rubella-varicella, ProQuad, Merck) is licensed for use in children 1–12 years of age. MMRV is well tolerated and provides adequate immune response to all of the antigens it contains. In MMRV, the varicella component is present in higher titer than in VAR. Concomitant administration of MMRV with DTaP, Hib, and HepB vaccines is acceptable.

▶ Dosage & Schedule of Administration

Two doses (0.5 mL) of VAR are recommended for immunization of healthy children aged 12 months and older, and for adolescents and adults without evidence of immunity. For children aged 12 months to 12 years, the immunization interval is at least 3 months, and for persons 13 years or older, it is 4 weeks. MMRV is approved only for healthy children aged 12 months to 12 years. A second dose of catch-up vaccination is required for children, adolescents, and adults who previously received one dose of VAR vaccine. All children should have received two doses of VAR before prekindergarten or school. HIV-infected children (≥ 15% CD4+ cells) should receive two doses of the single-antigen vaccine (with at least a 3-month interval between doses).

VAR may be given simultaneously with MMR at separate sites. If not given simultaneously, the interval between administration of VAR and MMR must be greater than 28 days. Simultaneous VAR administration does not appear to affect the immune response to other childhood vaccines. VAR should be delayed 5 months after receiving intravenous immune globulin, blood, or plasma. In addition, persons who received VAR should not be administered an antibody-containing product for at least 2 weeks or an antiviral medication active against varicella for at least 3 weeks. If this occurs, the individual may need to be tested for immunity or revaccinated. After a discussion of the benefits and risks of both vaccination options with the parents or caregivers (see section Adverse Effects), either MMR or MMRV may be given at 12–15 months. MMRV is the preferred vaccine if available at 4–6 years of age.

▶ Contraindications & Precautions

Contraindications to VAR vaccination include a severe allergic reaction after a previous vaccine dose or to a vaccine component. Because VAR and MMRV are live-virus vaccines, they are also contraindicated in children who have acquired treatment-related cellular immunodeficiencies or congenital T-cell abnormalities. The exception to this rule is the recommendation that VAR be administered to HIV-infected children who are not severely immunosuppressed. Household contacts of immunodeficient patients should be immunized. VAR should not be given to pregnant women; however, the presence of a pregnant mother in the household is not a contraindication to immunization of a child within that household. A personal or family history of febrile seizures in an infant is considered a precaution for the use of MMRV; administration of MMR and VAR separately is preferred for the first dose.

▶ Adverse Events

In approximately 20% of vaccinees, minor injection site reactions occur. Additionally, 3%–5% of patients will develop a rash at the injection site, and an additional 3%–5% will develop a sparse varicelliform rash outside of the injection site. These rashes typically consist of two to five lesions and may appear 5–26 days after immunization. The two-dose vaccine regimen is generally well tolerated with a safety profile comparable to that of the one-dose regimen. The incidence of fever and varicelliform rash is lower after the second dose than the first. Although VAR is contraindicated in pregnancy, there have been hundreds of inadvertent administrations of vaccine to pregnant women tracked by the "Pregnancy Registry for Varivax" with no known cases of congenital varicella syndrome or increases in fetal abnormalities.

Studies comparing MMRV to MMR and VAR administered concomitantly showed more systemic adverse events following MMRV (fever 21.5% vs 14.9% and measles-like rash 3% vs 2.1%, respectively). The risk of febrile seizures in children 12–23 months old with the MMRV preparation is twice that of MMR and VAR given separately, resulting in one additional febrile seizure per 2300–2600 children vaccinated with MMRV.

Transmission of vaccine virus from healthy vaccinees to other healthy persons is very rare; has never been documented in the absence of a rash in the index case; and has only resulted in mild disease. Herpes zoster can occur in recipients of VAR in immunocompetent and immunocompromised persons. Many of these cases were found to be caused by unappreciated latent wild-type virus. The age-specific risk of herpes zoster infection is much lower in children following VAR immunization than after natural infection, and it also tends to be milder.

▶ Antibody Preparations

In the event of an exposure to varicella, there are currently two antibody preparations potentially available in the United States for postexposure prophylaxis, VariZIG (Kamada Pharmaceuticals) and intravenous Ig. Exposure is defined as a household contact or playmate contact (> 1 h/day), hospital contact (in the same or contiguous room or ward), or intimate contact with a person with herpes zoster deemed contagious. Susceptibility is defined as the absence of a reliable history of varicella or varicella vaccination. Uncertainty in this designation may be resolved with an appropriate test for anti-VZV antibody. Passive postexposure prophylaxis is indicated for neonates, pregnant women, and immunocompromised patients, including those with cancer or taking immunosuppressive therapies.

VariZIG should be administered as soon as possible after exposure, ideally within 96 hours, but may be given within 10 days postexposure. If VariZIG is not available, it is recommended that intravenous Ig be used in its place. The dose is 400 mg/kg administered once. A subsequent exposure does not require additional prophylaxis if this occurs within 3 weeks of intravenous Ig administration.

AAP Committee on Infectious Diseases: Prevention of varicella: recommendations for use of quadrivalent and monovalent varicella vaccines in children. Pediatrics 2011;128:630 [PMID: 21873692].

CDC: Updated recommendations for use of VariZIG—United States, 2013. MMWR Morb Mortal Wkly Rep 2013;62:574 [PMID: 23863705].
Leung J, Dooling K, Marin M, Anderson TC, Harpaz R: The impact of universal varicella vaccination on herpes zoster incidence in the United States: comparison of birth cohorts preceding and following varicella vaccination program launch. J Infect Dis 2022;21:226(Suppl 4):S470–S477 [PMID: 36265856].

HEPATITIS A VACCINATION

The incidence of hepatitis A (HepA) in the United States had decreased dramatically from an average of 28,000 cases annually in the years prior to availability of a HepA vaccine to 1390 cases reported in 2015. More recently HepA incidence increased to over 12,000 cases reported in 2018 in part related to outbreaks among persons experiencing homelessness or drug use. Widespread outbreaks have continued involving more than 37 states through 2023.

Initial vaccination recommendations for HepA targeted high-risk individuals, primarily adults. However, this targeted approach did not work well, and children, who are more likely than adults to be asymptomatic while infected, often contributed to the spread of HepA. Therefore, since 2006 HepA vaccination has been routinely recommended for children 12–23 months of age. Vaccination has changed the epidemiology of HepA infection, such that most cases now occur in adults, often related to travel or contaminated food.

In addition to routine immunization of children 12–23 months of age, HepA vaccination is indicated for the following groups: (1) unvaccinated children 2–18 years old, (2) international travelers to countries with moderate to high rates of HepA, (3) adolescent and adult males who have sex with men, (4) persons who use injection or noninjection drugs, (5) persons with occupational risk for exposure to HepA, (6) unvaccinated persons who anticipate close contact with an international adoptee from countries with moderate to high rates of HepA, (7) persons experiencing homelessness, (8) persons with HIV, and (9) persons with chronic liver disease.

HepA vaccines are all inactivated and include two single-antigen vaccines and one combination vaccine.

▶ Vaccines Available

1. HepA (Havrix, GlaxoSmithKline), for use in children 12 months of age and older, and adults.
2. HepA (Vaqta, Merck), for use in children 12 months of age and older, and adults.
3. HepA-HepB (Twinrix, GlaxoSmithKline) contains HepA and HepB vaccines. Approved for use in adults 18 years of age and older.

▶ Dosage & Schedule of Administration

The two HepA vaccines given in childhood (Havrix and Vaqta) are given as a two-dose series. The first dose is recommended at 12–23 months of age; the second dose is recommended 6–18 months later. For individuals 12 months through 18 years of age, these vaccines are administered intramuscularly in a dose of 0.5 mL. Adults 19 years of age and older can receive Havrix (two doses of 1.0 mL each, separated by at least 6 months), Vaqta (two doses of 1.0 mL each, separated by at least 6 months), or Twinrix (for adults ≥ 18 years, 1.0 mL per dose, in a three-dose series at 0, 1, and 6 months). If needed, such as for imminent travel, Twinrix can be given on an accelerated four-dose schedule, with doses on days 0, 7, and 21–30, with a booster dose given 12 months after the first dose.

Contraindications & Precautions

HepA vaccine should not be given to anyone with a prior severe allergic reaction, such as anaphylaxis, after a previous vaccine dose or to a vaccine component. Moderate or severe acute illness is a precaution to vaccination. Pregnant people should be vaccinated for the same indications as nonpregnant people; vaccination during pregnancy should be weighed against the risk of HepA infection.

Adverse Effects

Adverse reactions, which are uncommon and mild, consist of pain, swelling, and induration at the injection site, fever, headache, and loss of appetite. There have been no reports of serious adverse events attributed definitively to HepA vaccine.

Postexposure Prophylaxis

Postexposure prophylaxis is recommended for unvaccinated household or sexual contacts of persons with serologically confirmed HepA and for unvaccinated child care staff and attendees in outbreak situations. Postexposure prophylaxis may also be recommended in food-borne outbreaks, depending on the extent and timing of exposure. Postexposure prophylaxis of unimmunized persons should consist of either a single dose of HepA vaccine or Ig (0.1 mL/kg), given as soon as possible after exposure. Ig should be used for children younger than 12 months and anyone for whom vaccination is contraindicated. The efficacy of Ig when given more than 2 weeks after exposure has not been established. For healthy people 12 months through 40 years of age who have not previously completed the two-dose vaccine series, HepA vaccine should be given. For those more than or equal to 40 years of age, Ig may be given in addition to HepA vaccine if there was a high-risk exposure or high risk of complications related to HepA infection. Exposed persons aged more than or equal to 12 months who are immunocompromised or have chronic liver disease should receive both HepA vaccine and Ig. If HepA vaccine and Ig are given at the same time, the vaccine and Ig should be administered at different injection sites.

Preexposure Prophylaxis

Children aged 6–11 months should receive HepA vaccine for preexposure prophylaxis prior to international travel and then receive two additional doses on the age-appropriate schedule. Ig is indicated as preexposure prophylaxis prior to international travel in children younger than 6 months and for travelers more than 6 months of age for whom vaccination is contraindicated. For persons 40 years or older, and those older than 6 months, who are immunocompromised or have chronic liver disease, Ig may be given in addition to HepA vaccine for preexposure prophylaxis prior to travel if there is a high risk for exposure or high risk for complications related to HepA infection. Recommended Ig IM dosages are 0.1 mL/kg in a single intramuscular dose if the duration of exposure is up to 1 month, 0.2 mL/kg for exposure up to 2 months, and 0.2 mL/kg repeated every 2 months for exposure more than 2 months.

CDC (Vaccines & Preventable Diseases: Hepatitis A): https://www.cdc.gov/vaccines/vpd/hepa/hcp/index.html. Accessed February 15, 2023.

Nelson NP et al: Prevention of hepatitis A virus infection in the United States: recommendations of the Advisory Committee on Immunization Practices, 2020. MMWR Recomm Rep 2020;69(No. RR-5):1 [PMID: 32614811].

MENINGOCOCCAL VACCINATION

Infections with *Neisseria meningitidis* cause significant morbidity and mortality, with approximately 350 cases occurring in the United States annually. Even with appropriate treatment, meningococcal disease has an estimated case-fatality rate of 10%–14%, and up to 19% of survivors are left with serious disabilities, including neurologic deficits, hearing loss, and loss of limbs. Six serogroups of meningococcus (A, B, C, W, X, and Y) cause nearly all serious disease worldwide; serogroups B, C, and Y predominate in the United States. Serogroup B is responsible for more than 50% of cases in children younger than 1 year in the United States; it is also responsible for several recent outbreaks on college campuses, although cases outside of the newborn period appear to be generally decreasing.

Vaccination recommendations are somewhat complex because disease rates vary substantially by age and depending on whether a chronic condition increasing meningococcal disease risk is present. The most current vaccination recommendations are available at www.cdc.gov/vaccines/vpd/mening/.

Two quadrivalent meningococcal polysaccharide-protein conjugate vaccines are available (MenACWY; tradenames Menveo and MenQuadfi), providing protection against serogroups A, C, W, and Y. MenACWY vaccination is recommended for all adolescents in the United States.

Three vaccines are available that protect against serogroup B disease (MenB), Bexsero, Penbraya, and Trumenba. For healthy young adults who do not have a chronic health condition predisposing to meningococcal disease, Bexsero and Trumenba are not universally recommended. However, these vaccines may be used with clinical discretion to reduce the risk of serogroup B meningococcal disease. These two vaccines are not interchangeable; the same vaccine product must be used for all doses in the series. Pentavalent meningococcal vaccine (MenABCWY, trade name Penbraya) is recommended as an option for vaccination of people 10 years or older who are getting MenACWY and MenB vaccines at the same visit. If a patient receives MenABCWY vaccine, then Trumenba should be used for additional MenB doses.

Meningococcal disease risk is significantly higher among children traveling to countries with endemic meningococcal disease and those with certain chronic conditions, including anatomic or functional asplenia (including sickle cell disease), HIV infection, complement component deficiencies, or treatment with complement inhibitors (such as eculizumab and ravulizumab). MenACWY vaccination is recommended before adolescence for these children and the vaccination schedule depends on the age of the child, vaccine product and any chronic condition; details are available at https://www.cdc.gov/vaccines/pubs/pinkbook/mening.html.

Children with anatomic or functional asplenia, complement component deficiency and those treated with complement inhibitors are also at increased risk of meningococcal serogroup B disease and should receive Bexsero or Trumenba starting at 10 years of age. Finally, meningococcal disease outbreaks occasionally occur in the United States, and vaccination may be recommended against the serogroups causing the outbreak.

Vaccines Available

1. MenACWY (Menveo, GlaxoSmithKline): contains serogroups A, C, Y, and W capsular polysaccharide, conjugated to CRM_{197}, a nontoxic mutant of diphtheria toxoid. Two-vial presentation licensed for use in persons 2 months through 55 years of age; one-vial presentation for use in persons aged 10–55 years.

2. MenACWY (MenQuadfi, Sanofi Pasteur): contains serogroups A, C, Y, and W capsular polysaccharide, covalently linked to tetanus toxoid; for use in persons 2 years and older.

3. MenB (Trumenba, Pfizer): contains recombinant lipidated factor H–binding protein (fHBP) variants from N meningitidis serogroup B; for use in persons aged 10–25 years.

4. MenB (Bexsero, GlaxoSmithKline): contains recombinant N meningitidis serogroup B proteins neisserial adhesin A (NadA), neisserial heparin-binding antigen (NHBA), fHbp, and outer membrane vesicles (OMV); for use in persons aged 10–25 years.

5. MenABCWY (Penbraya, Pfizer): contains serogropus A, C, W, and Y capsular polysaccharides, conjugated to tetanus toxoid; recombinated fHBP variants from N meningitidis serogroup B; for use in persons aged 10–25 years.

Dosage & Schedule of Administration

MenACWY is given as an intramuscular dose of 0.5 mL. If a dose is inadvertently administered subcutaneously, it does not need to be repeated. MenB is given as an intramuscular dose of 0.5 mL in a prefilled syringe. These vaccines can be given at the same time as other vaccines, at a different anatomic site. Protective antibody levels are typically achieved within 10 days of vaccination. MenACWY should be given at age 11 or 12 years, with a booster dose given at age 16 years. For children at increased risk of meningococcal disease, MenACWY vaccination should be given as early as 2 months of age with schedule dependent on child age, vaccine product, and any chronic condition.

Trumenba may be given as a three-dose series (at 0, 1–2, and 6 months) for those at increased risk or a two-dose series (at 0 and 6 months) for healthy teens. Bexsero is a two-dose series given at least 1 month apart. MenB should be given to persons age 10 years or older at increased risk of serogroup B meningococcal disease (complement deficiencies, taking complement inhibitors, asplenia, microbiologists, or serogroup B outbreaks). MenB may also be given to healthy adolescents and young adults, under shared decision-making between patient, parent/guardian, and health care provider.

Contraindications & Precautions

MenACWY is contraindicated in anyone with a known severe allergic reaction to any component of the vaccine, including to any other meningococcal, diphtheria toxoid-, tetanus toxoid-, or CRM_{197}-containing vaccine. MenACWY can be given to individuals who are immunosuppressed and given during pregnancy if clinically indicated.

Adverse Effects

MenACWY and MenB are generally well tolerated in adolescent patients. Local vaccination reactions among persons 11–18 years old receiving MenACWY or MenB include pain, redness, swelling, or induration at the injection site. The most common solicited complaints among children aged 2–10 years were injection site pain and irritability. More severe systemic reactions after MenACWY or MenB vaccination are less common and include fever, headache, fatigue, malaise, myalgias, or arthralgias.

Mbaeyi SA et al: Meningococcal vaccination: recommendations of the Advisory Committee on Immunization Practices, United States, 2020. MMWR Recomm Rep 2020;69:1 [PMID: 33417592].

TETANUS-REDUCED DIPHTHERIA-ACELLULAR PERTUSSIS VACCINATION (ADOLESCENTS & ADULTS)

Pertussis causes disease in all age groups. Although the burden of disease is highest in infants younger than 12 months, pertussis incidence has been rising in children and adolescents, due in part to waning immunity after administration of acellular pertussis vaccines. Routine vaccination with tetanus-reduced dose diphtheria-acellular pertussis (Tdap) has been recommended since 2006. Adolescent, adult, and elderly immunization not only has the capacity to protect vaccine recipients from pertussis but also should limit spread of pertussis from adults to infants and decrease overall pertussis endemicity.

▶ Vaccines Available

1. Tdap (Boostrix, GlaxoSmithKline) contains tetanus toxoid, diphtheria toxoid, and three acellular pertussis antigens (detoxified pertussis toxin [PT], filamentous hemagglutinin [FHA], and pertactin) and is licensed for use in persons aged 10 years and older.
2. Tdap (Adacel, Sanofi) contains tetanus toxoid, diphtheria toxoid, and five acellular pertussis antigens (PT, FHA, pertactin, and fimbriae types 2 and 3) and is licensed for use in persons aged 11–64 years.

▶ Dosage & Schedule of Administration

Adolescents 11–18 years of age should receive a 0.5-mL dose of Tdap intramuscularly in the deltoid; the preferred age for Tdap immunization is 11–12 years. Adults 19–64 years of age should receive a single dose of Tdap, followed by Td or Tdap booster every 10 years. Adults 65 years of age and older should receive a single dose of Tdap if they have not previously received Tdap and if they anticipate close contact with an infant younger than 12 months. People who are pregnant should receive a Tdap booster with each pregnancy, ideally between 27 and 36 weeks of gestation. Tdap can be administered in this circumstance regardless of the interval since the last tetanus- or diphtheria toxoid–containing vaccine. Tdap and MCV4 should be administered during the same visit if both vaccines are indicated.

▶ Contraindications & Precautions

Contraindications to Tdap include severe allergic reaction to any vaccine component and encephalopathy (eg, coma, prolonged seizures) not attributable to an identifiable cause within 7 days of administration of a vaccine with pertussis components. Precautions for Tdap administration include GBS

occurring within 6 weeks of a previous dose of a tetanus toxoid-containing vaccine, history of Arthus reaction following a previous dose of tetanus or diphtheria toxoid–containing vaccine, a progressive neurologic disorder, uncontrolled epilepsy, or progressive encephalopathy until the condition has stabilized.

▶ Adverse Effects

Pain, redness, or swelling at the injection site are the most frequently reported local adverse events; headache and fatigue are the most frequently reported systemic adverse events.

Cherry JD: The prevention of severe pertussis and pertussis deaths in young infants. Expert Rev Vaccines 2019;18:205 [PMID: 30736722].
Havers FP et al: Use of tetanus toxoid, reduced diphtheria toxoid, and acellular pertussis vaccines: updated recommendations of the Advisory Committee on Immunization Practices—United States, 2019. MMWR Morb Mortal Wkly Rep 2020;69:77 [PMID: 31971933].
Zerbo O et al: Acellular pertussis vaccine effectiveness over time. Pediatrics 2019;144:e20183466 [PMID: 31182549].

HUMAN PAPILLOMAVIRUS VACCINATION

Human papillomavirus (HPV) is the most common sexually transmitted infection in the United States and worldwide. Most of the estimated 14 million persons newly infected every year in the United States have no symptoms. Up to 75% of new infections occur among persons 15–24 years of age. HPV infection is associated with cancers in females and males including anal, cervical, oral, penile, vaginal, and vulvar cancer. Other HPV serotypes, distinct from those that cause cancer, cause genital warts in females and males.

More than 15 years has passed since HPV vaccines were licensed. In that time, substantial positive population-level health impacts have been observed, with large reductions in HPV infections, anogenital wart diagnoses, and cervical intraepithelial neoplasia. Strong herd immunity effects have also been observed, with decreasing HPV prevalence among the unvaccinated as well as the vaccinated.

A nine-valent HPV vaccine (9vHPV; tradename Gardasil 9) is approved for use in the United States for females and males. The vaccine protects against seven cancer-causing HPV types (types 16, 18, 31, 33, 45, 52, and 58), and two genital wart-associated HPV types (types 6 and 11). Two other licensed HPV vaccines, including a bivalent vaccine (tradename Cervarix) and a quadrivalent vaccine (Gardasil), are no longer distributed in the United States.

Routine HPV vaccination is recommended by ACIP for females and males aged 11–12 years and may be given as early as age 9 years. Because there is some evidence of increased uptake when introduced at a younger age, the AAP recommends starting the series between the ages of 9 and 12, at an age that the provider deems optimal for acceptance and completion of the vaccination series. Catch-up vaccination is recommended for females and males aged 13–26 years who were not previously vaccinated or have not completed the full vaccine series. While not universally recommended, vaccination of adults 27–45 years of age not previously vaccinated can be considered. Individuals who test positive for a high-risk HPV type, have an abnormal Pap test, or may have been exposed to HPV are still likely to benefit from HPV vaccination through prevention of other HPV types.

Vaccines Available

1. Nine-valent HPV vaccine (Gardasil 9, Merck), contains HPV-6, 11, 16, 18, 31, 33, 45, 52, and 58 L1 proteins and is licensed for use in persons aged 9–45 years.

Dosage & Schedule of Administration

HPV vaccine is administered intramuscularly as two or three separate 0.5-mL doses depending on age at initial vaccination. For healthy adolescents initiating the series prior to their 15th birthday, two doses separated by 6–12 months are recommended (minimum interval 5 months). Three doses are recommended for those initiating vaccination on or after the 15th birthday and for persons with immunocompromising conditions. For those requiring three doses, the second dose should be administered 1–2 months after the first dose and the third dose 6 months after the first dose. The minimum interval between the first and second doses is 4 weeks; the minimum recommended interval between the second and third doses of vaccine is 12 weeks. HPV vaccine may be administered with other vaccines. If the vaccine schedule is interrupted, the series need not be restarted. There is currently no recommendation for repeat vaccination with 9vHPV for persons who have completed a vaccination series with bivalent or quadrivalent HPV vaccine. Additional information on HPV vaccination recommendations can be found at: www.cdc.gov/vaccines/vpd/hpv/hcp/recommendations.html.

Contraindications & Precautions

HPV vaccine is contraindicated in persons with a history of anaphylaxis to any vaccine component. HPV vaccine is not recommended for use in pregnancy. The vaccine can be administered to persons with minor acute illnesses and to immunocompromised persons.

Adverse Effects

Injection site pain, mild to moderate swelling, and erythema are the most common adverse events reported by vaccine recipients. Fever, nausea, and dizziness have been reported less frequently. As with any vaccination, syncope can occur following HPV vaccination; adolescents should be seated or lying down during and for 15 minutes after vaccination, to prevent injuries from falls should syncope occur.

Meites E et al: Human papillomavirus vaccination for adults: updated recommendations of the Advisory Committee on Immunization Practices. MMWR Morb Mortal Wkly Rep 2019;68:698 [PMID: 31415491].

Rosenblum HG et al: Declines in prevalence of human papillomavirus vaccine-type infection among females after introduction of vaccine—United States, 2003–2018. MMWR Morb Mortal Wkly Rep 2021;70:415 [PMID: 33764964].

Perkins RB et al: Improving HPV vaccination rates: a stepped-wedge randomized trial. Pediatrics 2020;146:e20192737 [PMID: 32540986].

COVID-19 VACCINATION

In the late fall of 2019, a novel, highly contagious and virulent coronavirus, SARS-CoV-2, was detected. COVID, the disease caused by SARS-CoV-2, rapidly spread across the world, resulting in an unprecedented global pandemic. As of April 2023, 760 million cases and 6.9 million deaths have been reported worldwide, counts that greatly underestimate the true burden. People at increased risk of severe illness with COVID-19 include older adults, those with underlying medical conditions, pregnant or recently pregnant people, and racial and ethnic minorities. However, no age group has been spared: As of April 2023, nearly 2000 children and adolescents younger than 18 years in the United States have died from COVID-19.

Given the transmissibility and severity of COVID-19, the limitations of available treatments, and the temporizing nature of nonpharmaceutical measures such as social distancing, vaccination provides the surest path through the pandemic. Several highly effective vaccines against COVID-19 have been authorized for emergency use during this public health emergency or have received full FDA licensure. Initially, three COVID-19 vaccines were available in the United States: two vaccines utilizing messenger RNA (mRNA) technology (Pfizer-BioNTech and Moderna), and one vaccine using adenoviral vector technology (Janssen/Johnson & Johnson). Since the rollout of adult vaccines in 2021, an additional COVID-19 vaccine has been approved by the FDA for use in children (Novavax), and numerous monovalent and bivalent COVID-19 booster vaccines have been approved for use in children 6 months and older.

Pfizer-BioNTech COVID-19 vaccines contain mRNA encoding for a stabilized form of the spike protein of SARS-CoV-2, which is essential to viral attachment and invasion of human cells. After vaccination, the uniquely "packaged" mRNA is taken intracellularly and spike protein is produced by cellular protein synthetic mechanisms, resulting in a robust anti-spike immune response. In a phase II/III clinical trial with more than 43,000 participants, Pfizer-BioNTech COVID-19 vaccine was 95.0% effective at preventing symptomatic lab-confirmed COVID-19.

Moderna COVID-19 vaccines similarly contain mRNA encoding for a stabilized form of spike protein and produces a strong anti-spike immune response. In a phase III clinical trial with more than 30,000 participants, the Moderna COVID-19 vaccine was 94.1% effective at preventing symptomatic lab-confirmed disease.

The Janssen/Johnson & Johnson COVID-19 vaccine uses a human adenoviral vector encoding for a stabilized spike protein. The vector is replication-incompetent so that it infects cells but will not produce more virus. After vaccination, the adenoviral vector infects cells, spike protein is produced and presented to host immune cells to stimulate an anti-spike immune response produced. In a phase III clinical trial enrolling more than 40,000 participants across multiple countries, the vaccine was 74.4% effective in the United States at preventing symptomatic lab-confirmed disease. Janssen/Johnson & Johnson COVID-19 vaccines are not recommended for children.

A fourth COVID-19 vaccine—Novavax—was authorized by the FDA in 2022. It contains a SARS-CoV-2 recombinant spike protein, along with a strong adjuvant to stimulate the immune to response to SARS-CoV-2 spike proteins. The vaccine was found to be 90% effective against mild, moderate, and severe disease in a phase III trial involving 30,000 participants ages 18 and older, and authorization expanded to include adolescents 12–17 based on a pediatric trial.

Vaccine Availability, Dosage, & Schedule of Administration

COVID-19 vaccine availability, dosages, and vaccination schedules are rapidly evolving, with multiple products available for children of all ages that differ by vaccine product. For those with moderate to severe immunocompromise, additional vaccine doses are recommended. Additional booster vaccines may be forthcoming as COVID-19 epidemiology evolves. *Continuously updated information from the CDC about COVID-19 disease is available at https://www.cdc.gov/coronavirus/2019-nCoV/index.html, and the most up-to-date information about current vaccine recommendations is available at https://www.cdc.gov/vaccines/hcp/acip-recs/vacc-specific/covid-19.html.*

Contraindications & Precautions

The currently authorized COVID-19 vaccines should not be administered to individuals with a history of a severe allergic reaction (such as anaphylaxis) to any component of the respective vaccine. Recommendations regarding precautions will evolve. As of March 2023, children who developed myocarditis or pericarditis after a first dose of an mRNA vaccine should defer receiving the second dose. Those with a history of myocarditis or pericarditis prior to COVID-19 vaccination may receive any authorized vaccine. Currently authorized vaccines are not live vaccines and may be safety administered to immunocompromised individuals.

▶ Adverse Effects

At the start of the COVID-19 vaccination program in the United States, very intensive vaccine safety monitoring systems were put in place. Utilizing these systems, several rare and potentially serious vaccine adverse events have been detected following COVID-19 vaccination. Anaphylaxis has been reported following mRNA vaccines, with a reporting rate of approximately 5 cases per 1 million doses administered; symptom onset was typically within 15–30 minutes of vaccination, and cases responded to appropriate treatment. Thrombosis with thrombocytopenia syndrome has been reported following Janssen/Johnson & Johnson vaccination, particularly among women 18–49 years of age; the reporting rate among women of this age was approximately 7 cases per 1 million doses administered. GBS has been reported following Janssen/Johnson & Johnson vaccination; the reporting rate was approximately 8 cases per 1 million doses administered.

Myocarditis and pericarditis have been detected following vaccination with mRNA vaccines, with cases predominantly occurring among adolescent males, with symptom onset typically within 3–4 days, more commonly after the second vaccine dose. The clinical course of myocarditis/pericarditis is typically mild, with complete resolution of symptoms, although affected individuals are being closely followed to assess the risk of any longer-term sequelae. In light of the rarity of these adverse events, it was calculated that the benefit of preventing COVID-19 and its complications far exceeds the risk of any rare complication.

Clinical care considerations for COVID-19 vaccination: https://www.cdc.gov/vaccines/covid-19/clinical-considerations/index.html.
Information related to myocarditis and pericarditis: https://www.cdc.gov/vaccines/covid-19/clinical-considerations/myocarditis.html.
Overview of COVID-19 vaccines: https://www.cdc.gov/vaccines/covid-19/index.html.
Up-to-date information about current vaccine recommendations: https://www.cdc.gov/vaccines/hcp/acip-recs/vacc-specific/covid-19.html.

VACCINATIONS FOR SPECIAL SITUATIONS

RABIES VACCINATION

After symptoms of infection develop, rabies is almost invariably fatal in humans. While sylvan animal and bat rabies in the United States is common, the incidence of human rabies is very low, with fewer than three cases per year. Although dogs represent the most important vector for human rabies worldwide, in the United States because of widespread vaccination of dogs and cats, the most common rabies virus variants responsible for human rabies are bat related. Rabies is also common in skunks, raccoons, and foxes; it is uncommon in rodents.

Human rabies is preventable with appropriate and timely local wound care and postexposure prophylaxis with both passive and active immunization. Immediately after an animal bite, wounds should be flushed and aggressively cleaned with soap and water. If possible, the wound should not be sutured. Passive immunization after high-risk exposure consists of the injection of human rabies immune globulin (RIg) near the wound. Active immunization requires completing a schedule of immunization with one of the two available rabies vaccines licensed in the United States. Postexposure prophylaxis can be controversial, and local public health officials should be consulted before postexposure rabies prophylaxis is started to avoid unnecessary vaccination and to assist in the proper handling of the animal (if confinement or testing of the animal is appropriate). Rabies immunization can be considered for some children traveling to countries where rabies is endemic.

Vaccines Available

1. HDCV (human diploid cell vaccine; IMOVAX, Sanofi Pasteur), approved or all age groups.
2. PCECV (purified chick embryo cell vaccine; RabAvert, Bavarian Nordic), approved for all age groups.

Dosage & Schedule of Administration

These two inactivated rabies vaccines are equally safe and effective for both preexposure and postexposure prophylaxis. For each vaccine, 1 mL is given intramuscularly in the deltoid (for adults and older children) or anterolateral thigh (for infants and young children). The volume of the dose is not reduced for children. Vaccine should not be given in the gluteal region.

Postexposure Prophylaxis

After an individual has possibly been exposed to rabies, decisions about whether to initiate postexposure prophylaxis must be made urgently, in consultation with local public health officials.

1. In previously unvaccinated individuals—After prompt and thorough wound cleansing, an individual exposed to rabies should receive rabies vaccination and RIg. Vaccination is given on the day of exposure (day 0) and on days 3, 7, and 14 following exposure. Immunocompromised individuals should receive an additional dose on day 28. RIg should also be given as soon as possible after exposure, ideally on the day of exposure, in a recommended dose of 20 IU/kg. If anatomically possible, the entire dose of RIg should be infiltrated into and around the wound. Any remaining RIg

should be administered intramuscularly at an anatomic site distant from the location used for rabies vaccination. If RIg was not administered when vaccination was begun, it can be administered up to 7 days after the first dose of vaccine. Postexposure prophylaxis failures have occurred only when deviation from the above protocol occurred (eg, no cleansing of the wound, less than usual amount of RIg, no RIg at the wound site, or vaccination in the gluteal area).

2. In previously vaccinated individuals—RIg should not be administered, and only two doses of vaccine on days 0 and 3 after exposure are needed.

Contraindications & Precautions

Rabies vaccine is contraindicated in persons with a history of anaphylaxis to any vaccine component. The same vaccine (HDCV or PCEC) should be used throughout the vaccination series; however, if severe allergic reactions occur completing the series with the alternate vaccine may be advisable.

Adverse Effects

The rabies vaccines are relatively free of serious reactions. Local reactions at the injection site, such as pain, swelling, induration, or erythema range, are most common. Mild systemic reactions, such as headache, nausea, muscle aches, and dizziness, occur less frequently. An immune complex-like reaction occurs in about 6% of adults 2–21 days after receiving booster doses of rabies vaccine; symptoms may include generalized urticaria, arthralgias, arthritis, and angioedema.

Travelers to countries where rabies is endemic may need immediate postexposure prophylaxis and may have to use locally available vaccines and RIg. In some countries, the only vaccines available may be nerve tissue vaccines derived from the brains of adult animals or suckling mice, and the RIg may be of equine origin. Although adverse reactions to RIg are uncommon and typically mild, nervous tissue rabies vaccines may induce neuroparalytic reactions in 1:200–1:8000 vaccines; this significant risk is another justification for preexposure vaccination prior to travel in areas where exposure to potentially rabid animals is likely.

Antibody Preparations

In the United States, RIg is prepared from the plasma of human volunteers hyperimmunized with rabies vaccine. The recommended dose is 20 IU/kg body weight.

CDC (Rabies information page): https://www.cdc.gov/rabies/medical_care/vaccine.html. Accessed February 16, 2023.
Rao AK et al: Use of a modified preexposure prophylaxis vaccination schedule to prevent human rabies: recommendations of the Advisory Committee on Immunization Practices — United States, 2022. MMWR Morb Mortal Wkly Rep 2022; 71:619–627 [PMID: 35511716].

Rupprecht CE et al: Use of a reduced (4-dose) vaccine schedule for postexposure prophylaxis to prevent human rabies: recommendations of the Advisory Committee on Immunization Practices. MMWR Recomm Rep 2010;59(RR-2):1 [PMID: 20300058].

TYPHOID FEVER VACCINATION

Typhoid fever causes an estimated 11–21 million illnesses and over 200,000 deaths each year worldwide; in the United States an estimated 5700 cases occur (about 350 cases are reported) each year, predominantly related to international travel.

Two vaccines against *Salmonella enterica typhi*, the bacterium that causes typhoid fever, are available in the United States: a live attenuated vaccine given orally (Ty21a) and an inactivated vaccine composed of purified capsular polysaccharide (ViCPS) given parenterally. Both vaccines protect 50%–80% of vaccine recipients. The oral vaccine is commonly used because of its ease of administration. However, noncompliance with the oral vaccine dosing schedule occurs frequently, and correct usage should be stressed or the parenteral ViCPS vaccine used.

Routine typhoid vaccination is recommended only for individuals who are traveling to typhoid-endemic areas or who reside in households with a documented typhoid carrier. Although typhoid fever occurs throughout the world, areas of highest incidence include southern Asia and sub-Saharan Africa. Travelers should be advised that because the typhoid vaccines are not fully protective, and because of the potential for other food- and waterborne illnesses, careful selection of food and drink and appropriate hygiene remain necessary when traveling internationally.

Vaccines Available

1. Parenteral inactivated ViCPS (Typhim Vi, Sanofi Pasteur) is for intramuscular use in people 2 years of age and older.
2. Oral live attenuated Ty21a vaccine (Vivotif, Emergent BioSolutions) is supplied as enteric-coated capsules for use in people 6 years of age and older.

Dosage & Schedule of Administration

ViCPS is administered as a single intramuscular dose (0.5 mL) in the deltoid muscle, with boosters needed every 2 years if exposure continues.

The dose of the oral vaccine (Ty21a) is one capsule every other day for a total of four capsules, taken 1 hour before meals. The capsules should be kept refrigerated and taken with cool liquids. A repeat full course of four capsules is recommended every 5 years if exposure continues. Mefloquine and chloroquine may be given at the same time as the oral vaccine; however, if mefloquine is administered, immunization with Ty21a should be delayed for 24 hours. Proguanil should be administered only if 10 days have lapsed since the last dose of oral vaccine. Oral typhoid vaccine should be given more than 3 days after completing systemic antibiotics.

Contraindications & Precautions

As with all live attenuated vaccines, Ty21a should not be given to immunocompromised patients.

Adverse Reactions

Both the oral and parenteral vaccines are well tolerated, and adverse reactions are uncommon and usually self-limited. The oral vaccine can cause gastroenteritis-like illness, fatigue, and myalgia, whereas the parenteral vaccine can cause injection site pain and swelling, myalgia, and headache.

CDC (Typhoid Fever and Paratyphoid Fever information page): https://www.cdc.gov/typhoid-fever/typhoid-vaccination.html. Accessed February 16, 2023.

Jackson BR et al: Updated recommendations for the use of typhoid vaccine—Advisory Committee on Immunization Practices, United States, 2015. MMWR Morb Mortal Wkly Rep 2015;64:305 [PMID: 25811680].

CHOLERA VACCINATION

Cholera is caused by toxigenic *Vibrio cholera* bacteria of serogroup O1 (> 99% of global cases) or O139. The illness manifests as watery diarrhea that can be severe and rapidly fatal without prompt fluid rehydration. Annually in the United States fewer than 25 cases are reported and most occur among travelers to countries where cholera is endemic or epidemic.

A single-dose, live attenuated monovalent oral vaccine, CVD103-HgR (Vaxchora) is approved by the FDA for use for travelers, age 18–64 years, who are traveling to areas of the world with active cholera transmission. The vaccine has 90% efficacy against severe diarrhea at 10 days after vaccination and 80% efficacy 3 months postvaccination. CVD103-HgR should not be given to patients who have received antibiotics within the preceding 14 days. CVD103-HgR is an oral live attenuated vaccine that can be shed in the stool and potentially transmitted to close contacts. Additional cholera vaccines are available in countries outside the United States. Vaccinated travelers should continue to utilize careful selection of food and drink and use appropriate hygiene when traveling internationally.

Vaccine Available

1. CVD 103-HgR (Vaxchora, Emergent BioSolutions) is a live-attenuated monovalent oral vaccine that is FDA approved in the United States. In December of 2020, the maker of Vaxchora temporarily stopped making and selling it because of the SARS-CoV-2 pandemic. This vaccine may be in limited supply or unavailable.

CDC: Recommendations of the Advisory Committee on Immunization Practices for use of cholera vaccine. MMWR Morb Mortal Wkly Rep 2017;66:482 [PMID: 28493859].

JAPANESE ENCEPHALITIS VACCINATION

Japanese encephalitis (JE) virus is a mosquito-borne flavivirus. Although most infections are asymptomatic, those with neurologic disease suffer high morbidity and mortality. It is endemic in parts of Asia, although the risk to most travelers to Asia is low. Travel to rural areas and extended travel in endemic areas may increase the risk. Travelers to JE-endemic countries should be advised of risks of JE and the importance of measures to reduce mosquito bites. One safe and effective vaccine is available in the United States. Vaccination is not recommended for short-term travelers whose visit will be restricted to urban areas or outside of a well-defined JE transmission season, but vaccination is recommended for travelers who plan to spend more than 1 month in endemic areas during the JE transmission season. Vaccination should be *considered* for short-term travelers to endemic areas during the JE transmission season if they will travel outside of an urban area and their activities will increase the risk of JE exposure (time outdoors in rural/agricultural areas, outdoor recreation activities, sleeping in places without mosquito protection) and should also be considered for travelers to an area with an ongoing JE outbreak.

▶ Vaccines Available & Schedule of Administration

JE-VC (IXIARO, Novartis) is an inactivated Vero cell–derived JE vaccine licensed for use in people 2 months of age and older. It is given intramuscularly in a two-dose series at 0 and 28 days (or 0 and 7–28 days for adults 18–65 years). A booster dose should be given 1 year or more after the primary series if ongoing or repeat exposure to JE virus is expected. The dose for people 3 years or older, each dose is 0.5 mL; if 2–35 months old, each dose is 0.25 mL. Adverse reactions include pain at the injection site, headache, myalgias, and fever. JE vaccination is contraindicated for anyone who has had a severe allergic reaction to a previous vaccine dose or component.

CDC: Infectious diseases related to travel: Japanese encephalitis. CDC Health Information for International Travel, 2020. https://wwwnc.cdc.gov/travel/yellowbook/2020/travel-related-infectious-diseases/japanese-encephalitis. Accessed February 20, 2023.

Hills SL et al: Japanese encephalitis vaccines: recommendations of the Advisory Committee on Immunization Practices (ACIP). MMWR Recomm Rep 2019; 68(RR-1):1 [PMID: 31518342].

TUBERCULOSIS VACCINATION

Approximately one-fourth of the world's population is infected with *Mycobacterium tuberculosis*, and TB disease is a leading cause of death in low- and middle-income nations, killing approximately 1.5 million people annually. In the United States, TB is less common, and most cases occur in persons born abroad or in their close contacts. BCG vaccine consists of live attenuated *Mycobacterium bovis*. BCG is the most widely used vaccine in the world. It can be given any time after birth, sensitizes the vaccinated individual for 5–50 years, and stimulates both B-cell and T-cell immune responses. BCG vaccine reduces the risk of tuberculous meningitis and disseminated TB in pediatric populations by 50%–100% when administered in the first month of life. Efficacy against pulmonary tuberculosis has been variable (0%–80%) depending on the study setting and other factors. BCG is not recommended for use in the United States, nor is it recommended for travel.

▶ Vaccines Available & Schedule of Administration

There is one licensed BCG vaccine in the United States produced by Organon Teknika Corporation (BCG Vaccine). It is administered intradermally. Adverse effects occur in 1%–10% of healthy individuals, including local ulceration, regional lymph node enlargement, and very rarely lupus vulgaris. The live attenuated BCG vaccine is contraindicated in pregnant women and in immunocompromised individuals, because it can cause extensive local adenitis and disseminated or fatal infection.

BCG almost invariably causes its recipients to be tuberculin skin test (TST)-positive (5–7 mm), but the reaction often becomes negative after 3–5 years. An interferon-γ release assay (IGRA) TB test should be negative in such individuals. A positive TST test in a child with a history of BCG vaccination who is being investigated for TB as a case contact should be interpreted as indicating infection with *M tuberculosis*.

CDC (TB information page): https://www.cdc.gov/tb/topic/basics/vaccines.htm. Accessed February 20, 2023.

Roy A et al: Effect of BCG vaccination against *Mycobacterium tuberculosis* infection in children: systematic review and meta-analysis. BMJ 2014;349:g4643. doi:10.1136/bmj.g4643 [PMID: 25097193].

YELLOW FEVER VACCINATION

Yellow fever virus is a mosquito-borne flavivirus that is endemic in sub-Saharan Africa and South America. A live attenuated vaccine against yellow fever is available in the United States but is available only at official yellow fever vaccination locations and should only be given after consultation with travel medicine specialists or public health officials. Immunization against yellow fever is indicated for children 9 months or older traveling to endemic areas. Proof of vaccination against yellow fever may be required for travel to certain countries.

▶ Vaccines Available & Schedule of Administration

YF vaccine (YF-VAX, Sanofi) is made from the 17D yellow fever attenuated virus strain grown in chick embryos. It is given as a subcutaneous injection of 0.5 mL. Immunity following vaccination is long lasting, and booster doses are no longer recommended for most travelers.

Yellow fever vaccine is contraindicated in infants younger than 6 months (due to an increased risk of vaccine-associated encephalitis), in persons with anaphylactic egg allergy, and in immunocompromised individuals or individuals with a history of thymus disease. There is no contraindication to giving other live-virus vaccines simultaneously with yellow fever vaccine.

Adverse reactions are generally mild, consisting of low-grade fever, mild headache, and myalgia. Although very uncommon, several types of severe adverse reactions can occur following vaccination. Serious allergic reactions occur in roughly 1 case per every 55,000 vaccine recipients. The risk of vaccine-associated neurotropic disease within 30 days following vaccination has been estimated to be 1 case per every 125,000 vaccine recipients. The risk of severe multiple organ system failure following vaccination (vaccine-associated viscerotropic disease) has been estimated at 1 case per every 250,000 vaccine recipients. Health care providers should administer yellow fever vaccine only to persons truly at risk of exposure to yellow fever.

CDC (Yellow Fever information page): https://www.cdc.gov/yellowfever/vaccine/index.html. Accessed February 20, 2023.
Reno E et al: Prevention of yellow fever in travellers: an update. Lancet Infect Dis 2020 Jun;20(6):e129 [PMID: 32386609].

PASSIVE PROPHYLAXIS

Immune globulin (Ig) may prevent or modify infection with hepatitis A virus if administered in a dose of 0.02 mL/kg within 14 days after exposure. Measles infection may be prevented or modified in a susceptible person if Ig is given in a dose of 0.5 mL/kg within 6 days after exposure. Pathogen-specific (hyperimmune) preparations of Ig include TIg, HBIg, RIg, CMV Ig (IV), botulism Ig (IV), and varicella-zoster Ig (VariZIG). These are obtained from donors known to have high titers of antibody against the pathogen in question. Ig must be given only by the route (IV or IM) for which it is recommended. The dose varies depending on the clinical indication. Adverse reactions include pain at the injection site, headache, chills, dyspnea, nausea, and anaphylaxis, although all but the first are rare.

▶ Palivizimab and Nirsevimab

Palivizumab (Synagis, MedImmune) is a humanized monoclonal antibody against RSV that is used to prevent RSV infection in high-risk populations with monthly doses during RSV season (Table 10–6). Palivizumab is administered in a dose of 15 mg/kg once a month beginning with the onset of the RSV season and continuing until the end of the season.

Table 10.6. Eligibility criteria for palivizumab prophylaxis of high-risk infants and young children based on AAP policy statement.

- Infants born before 29 wk, 0 days, who are aged < 12 mo at the start of RSV season
- Infants aged < 12 mo with chronic lung disease (CLD) of prematurity, defined as gestational age < 32 wk, 0 days, and requiring > 21% oxygen for at least the first 28 days after birth; for the second year of life in children with a history of CLD, consideration of prophylaxis is recommended only for infants who continue to require medical support (chronic corticosteroids, diuretics, or supplemental oxygen) in the 6 mo prior to the start of RSV season
- Certain children aged < 12 mo with significant congenital heart disease (acyanotic heart disease on medication to control heart failure and will require cardiac surgical procedures, infants with moderate to severe pulmonary hypertension)
- Infants with a neuromuscular disease or congenital anomaly that impairs the ability to clear respiratory secretions
- Infants aged < 24 mo who are profoundly immunocompromised at the start of RSV season
- Infants aged < 24 mo with severe cystic fibrosis (respiratory hospitalizations or weight for length < 10th percentile)

Specific guidance for use in infants and young children at increased risk of hospitalization from RSV is available in the American Academy of Pediatrics' recently re-affirmed policy statement on prophylaxis: https://publications.aap.org/pediatrics/article/134/2/415/33013/Updated-Guidance-for-Palivizumab-Prophylaxis-Among. The maximum number of doses recommended in any one season is five, and palivizumab does not interfere with response to routine childhood vaccinations. Prophylaxis should be discontinued in any child who experiences a breakthrough hospitalization.

Nirsevimab (Beyfortus, Astrazeneca & Sanofi) is a long-acting monoclonal antibody product intended for use in neonates and infants to protect against respiratory syncytial virus (RSV) disease, particularly medically attended disease. Nirsevimab was approved on July 17, 2023 and is preferred over palivizumab because of its convenience, duration, and efficacy. The Advisory Committee on Immunization Practices (ACIP) and American Academy of Pediatrics (AAP) recommend Nirsevimab for:

- Infants aged <8 months born during or entering their first RSV season whose pregnant parent did not receive RSVpreF vaccine, whose pregnant parent's RSVpreF vaccination status is unknown, or who were born <14 days after the pregnant parent's RSVpreF vaccination
- Infants and children 8-19 months of age who are at increased risk of severe RSV disease and entering their second RSV season, including those recommended by the AAP to receive palivizumab (Table 10-6), regardless

of RSV vaccination status of the pregnant parent. This includes:

- Infants and children with chronic lung disease of prematurity who required medical support (chronic corticosteroid therapy, diuretic therapy, or supplemental oxygen) at any time during the 6-month period before the start of the second RSV season.
- Infants and children who are severely immunocompromised.
- Infants and children with cystic fibrosis who have manifestations of severe lung disease (previous hospitalization for pulmonary exacerbation in the first year of life or abnormalities on chest imaging that persist when stable) or have weight-for-length that is less than the 10th percentile.
- American Indian and Alaska Native children.

Providers should consider equity and access to nirsevimab in passive prophylaxis considerations. If nirsevimab is not available or not feasible to administer, high-risk infants who are recommended to receive palivizumab in the first or second year of life should receive palivizumab, as previously recommended, until nirsevimab becomes available. Generally, high-risk infants whose pregnant parent received a recommended RSV vaccine < 14 days prior to delivery do not require palivizumab. The following are considerations regarding palivizumab versus nirsevimab administration for high-risk infants during the same RSV season:

- If nirsevimab is administered, palivizumab should not be administered later that season
- If palivizumab was administered initially for the season and <5 doses were administered, the infant should receive 1 dose of nirsevimab. No further palizivumab doses should be given. There is no minimum interval between the last dose of palivizumab and the sole dose of nirsevimab, and nirsevimab should be administered no later than 30 days after the last palivizumab dose, when possible (palivizumab protection wanes after 30 days).
- If palivizumab was administered in season 1 and the child is eligible for RSV prophylaxis in season 2, the child should receive nirsevimab in season 2 whenever available. If nirsevimab continues to be unavailable, palivizumab should be administered as previously recommended.

While the timing of the onset and the duration of RSV seasons may vary, nirsevimab may be administered from October through the end of March in the continental United States. Clinicians should administer nirsevimab in the first week of life for infants born shortly before or during the RSV season, including during the birth hospitalization. Simultaneous administration of nirsevimab with age-appropriate vaccines is recommended.

AAP Recommendations for the Prevention of RSV Disease in Infants and Children. Updated February 21, 2024. *Red Book Online*. American Academy of Pediatrics. Accessed March 4, 2024.

Brady MT et al.: Policy statement—updated guidance for palivizumab prophylaxis among infants and young children at increased risk of hospitalization for respiratory syncytial virus infection. Pediatrics 2014;134(2):415–420 [PMID: 25070315].

Fleming-Dutra KE, Jones JM, Roper LE, et al. Use of the Pfizer Respiratory Syncytial Virus Vaccine During Pregnancy for the Prevention of Respiratory Syncytial Virus–Associated Lower Respiratory Tract Disease in Infants: Recommendations of the Advisory Committee on Immunization Practices—United States, 2023. MMWR Morb Mortal Wkly Rep. ePub: 6 October 2023.

Jones JM, Fleming-Dutra KE, Prill MM, et al. Use of nirsevimab for the prevention of respiratory syncytial virus disease among infants and young children: recommendations of the Advisory Committee on Immunization Practices – United States, 2023. MMWR Morb Mortal Wkly Rep. 2023;72(34):920-925.

Normal Childhood Nutrition & Its Disorders

Liliane K. Diab, MD

Laura E. Primak, RD, CNSC

Matthew A. Haemer, MD, MPH

The importance of nutrition in medicine transcends the basic need for energy and for preventing deficiencies. Nutrition from preconception and throughout infancy, childhood, and adolescence is not only essential for growth and neurodevelopment, but it also plays a pivotal role in overall wellness, susceptibility to chronic diseases, and adult long-term health. Nutrition is a common foundational requirement across cultures and all ages. The pediatric medical provider is in a unique position to be able to assess nutrition issues acutely and longitudinally, guide families in addressing nutrition needs and concerns, and promote evidence-based nutrition recommendations.

NUTRITIONAL REQUIREMENTS

NUTRITION & GROWTH

The nutrient requirements of children are influenced by growth rates that vary with age and are especially important during early postnatal life (Table 11–1). The period between conception and 2 years of age is referred to as "the critical 1000-day window." Nutrient intake during this time is considered a modifiable factor that can profoundly affect cognitive development, lifelong mental health, as well as impact health risks for obesity, hypertension, and diabetes. Optimizing nutrient provision and healthy intake in infancy/childhood helps provide an early foundation for future growth and development throughout the lifecycle.

DIETARY REFERENCE INTAKE

The dietary reference intakes (DRIs) include four reference values for nutrients and are used to assess and plan the diets of healthy individuals based on their age and gender.

1. **Recommended Dietary Allowance (RDA):** The average daily level of a nutrient intake sufficient to meet the requirements of nearly all (97%–98%) healthy individuals in a specific age and gender group.

2. **Estimated Average Requirement (EAR):** The average daily level of a nutrient intake estimated to satisfy the needs of 50% of healthy individuals in a specific age and gender group.

3. **Adequate Intake (AI):** Established using observational data when evidence is insufficient to develop an RDA

4. **Tolerable Upper Intake Level (UL):** The maximum daily nutrient intake level unlikely to cause adverse health outcomes.

The Acceptable Macronutrient Distribution Range (AMDR) is the calculated range of energy from protein, carbohydrates, and lipids recommended for a healthy diet.

Otten JJ, Hellwig JP, Meyers LD: *DRI, Dietary Reference Intakes: The Essential Guide to Nutrient Requirements.* Washington, DC: National Academies Press; 2006:xiii, 543.

ENERGY

There is no DRI for energy. Estimated energy requirements (EER) are used instead. The significant determinants of energy expenditure are (1) basal metabolism (reflected in resting energy expenditure (REE), (2) physical activity, (3) growth (1 g of new tissue is estimated to require 3–6 kcal/day), and (4) the thermogenic effect of food (hence energy requirements are less when using parenteral nutrition). Suggested guidelines for energy and protein intake for different age groups are given in Table 11–2. Because of the high nutrient requirements for growth and the body composition, the young infant is especially vulnerable to undernutrition. Slowed physical growth is an early and prominent sign of undernutrition in the young infant. The limited fat stores of the very young infant mean that energy reserves are modest. The relatively large size and continued growth of the brain renders the central nervous system (CNS) especially vulnerable to the effects of malnutrition in early postnatal life.

After the first four years, energy requirements expressed on a body weight basis decline progressively. The estimated daily

Table 11–1. Growth rates in infancy.

Age (mo)	g/day
0–3	20–30
3–6	15–20
6–9	10–15
9–12	10
12–18	6
18–24	6

WHO Child Growth Standards based on length/height, weight, and age. Acta Paediatr Suppl 2006;450:76–85.

energy requirement is about 40 kcal/kg/day at the end of adolescence. Approximate daily energy requirements can be calculated by adding 100 kcal/y to the base of 1000 kcal/day at the age of one year. Appetite and growth are reliable indices of caloric needs in most healthy children, but intake also depends to some extent on the energy density of the food offered. Individual energy requirements of healthy infants and children vary considerably, and malnutrition and disease increase the variability. Preterm infant energy requirements can exceed 120 kcal/kg/day, especially during illness or when catch-up growth is desired.

Food and Agricultural Organization: Human energy requirements. Scientific Background Papers from the Joint FAO/WHO/UNU Expert Consultation. Oct. 17–24, 2001. Rome, Italy. Public Health Nutr 2005 Oct;8(7A):929–1228 [PMID: 16277811].

PROTEIN

Protein is the primary functional and structural component of all the cells in the body. The most important defining characteristic of the quality of a protein from a nutritional point of view is its amino acid composition and its digestibility. Amino acids have traditionally been classified as essential and nonessential. A conditionally essential amino acid requires a dietary source when endogenous synthesis cannot meet metabolic demand. The nine essential amino acids are histidine, isoleucine, leucine, lysine, methionine, phenylalanine, threonine, tryptophan, and valine. The quality of a source of dietary protein depends on its essential amino acid composition necessary for the growth, maintenance, and repair of the human body. Proteins from animal sources such as milk, cheese, yogurt, fish, meat, poultry, and eggs provide all essential amino acids and are called "complete proteins." Proteins from vegetarian sources, such as legumes, vegetables, grains, nuts, and seeds, tend to lack one or more of the essential amino acids and are referred to as "incomplete" proteins. Appropriate mixtures of vegetarian proteins are necessary to achieve high protein quality. For example, wheat and rice are low in lysine, and legumes are commonly low in methionine.

The AMDR for protein is 5%–20% of total calories for children 1–3 years old, 10%–30% for children 4–8 years old, and 10%–35% for individuals older than 18 years of age. Data are lacking to establish a UL for protein or amino acids. The mechanisms for removal of excess nitrogen are efficient and moderate excesses of protein are not harmful in healthy individuals, however intake of greater than 3.5 g protein per kilogram of body mass may exceed the renal capacity for nitrogen excretion. Data are limited on amino acid consumption from dietary supplements. We recommend caution when using any single amino acid at a level significantly higher than typically found in food.

Protein requirements per unit of body weight decline rapidly during infancy as growth velocity decreases. The protein content of human milk decreases from 1.4–1.6 g/100 mL in early lactation to 0.8–1.0 g/100 mL at 3–4 months, then to 0.7–0.8 g/100 mL after 6 months, consistent with the expected decline in growth velocity. Recent research suggests that the higher protein content of typical infant formulas (2–2.5 g/100 mL) relative to breast milk is associated with excess weight gain.

Protein requirements increase in the presence of skin or gut losses, burns, trauma, and infection. Requirements also increase during catch-up growth accompanying recovery from malnutrition (~0.2 g of protein per gram of new tissue deposited).

National Academies of Sciences, Engineering, and Medicine. *Dietary Reference Intakes: The Essential Guide to Nutrient Requirements*. Washington, DC: The National Academies Press; 2006.

LIPIDS

Fats are an essential energy source for the body, especially for infants. Fat aids in absorbing the fat-soluble vitamins A, D, E, and K and are needed for myelination of the CNS. Fatty acids esterified into lipids are the major components of fat in the diet. They are classified according to their chain length into short chain fatty acids (< 8 carbon atoms), medium (8–11 carbon atoms), intermediate (12–15 carbon atoms), and long-chain fatty acids (> 16 carbon atoms). They are further classified based on the number, type, and position of the double bonds, of which there may be none (saturated fatty acids), one (monounsaturated fatty acids), or two or more (polyunsaturated fatty acids [PUFA]). There are two isomeric forms of the double bands: *cis* and *trans*. Plant and mammalian cells have only *cis* bonds. *Trans* bonds from food with partially hydrogenated oil are considered harmful.

Unsaturated fatty acids are more readily absorbed than saturated fatty acids except for medium-chain triacylglycerols (MCTs), which contain primarily saturated medium-chain fatty acids. MCTs have high water solubility and are rapidly transported to the liver through portal venous transport. MCTs improve fat absorption in low-birth-weight infants

Table 11–2. Estimated energy and protein needs for pediatric patients.

	Age	Estimated Energy Requirement (EER)[a–c] (kcal/kg/day)	Resting Energy Expenditure (REE)[d] (kcal/kg/day)	Protein:RDA[e] (g/kg/day)	Protein:Hospitalized Patients[f] (g/kg/day)
Preterm < 30 wk		120–140	60–75		3.6–4.5
Infants	0–2 mo	110–130[e]	45–60[e]	1.52*	1.5–2.5
	2–3 mo	102	55	1.52*	1.5–2.5
	4–6 mo	82	55	1.52*	1.5–2.5
	7–12 mo	80	55	1.2–1.5	1.5–2.5
	13–35 mo	82	55	1.05	1.5–2.5
Males	3 y	85	55	1.05	1.5–2.5
	4–5 y	70	45	0.95	1.5–2
	6–7 y	64	40–45	0.95	1.5–2
	8 y	59	40	0.95	1.5
Females	3 y	82	55	1.05	1.5–2.5
	4–5 y	65	45	0.95	1.5–2
	6–7 y	61	40–45	0.95	1.5–2
	8 y	59	55	0.95	1.5
Males	9–11 y	49	30–40	0.95	1.5
	12–13 y	44	30	0.95	1.5
	14–16 y	39	30	0.85	1.5
	17–18 y	37	30	0.85	1.5
	> 18 y	36	30	0.8	1.2–1.5
Females	9–11 y	42	30–40	0.95	1.5
	12–13 y	40	30	0.95	1.5
	14–16 y	33	25	0.85	1.5
	17–18 y	31	25	0.85	1.5
	> 18 y	34	25	0.8	1.2–1.5

[a]Adapted from Dietary Reference Intakes: EER (new DRI/IOM equation) & PA Co-Efficients (sedentary), 2005.
[b]Adapted from ASPEN *Pediatric Nutrition Support Handbook*, 2nd ed, 2015.
[c]Adapted from Texas Children's Hospital *Pediatric Nutrition Support Reference Guide*, 11th ed, 2016.
[d]Adapted from WHO (World Health Organization) Tech Rep Ser 1985;724:1–206.
[e]Adapted from Dietary Reference Intakes: Recommended Dietary Allowance (RDA).
[f]Guidelines for the Provision and Assessment of Nutrition Support Therapy in the Pediatric Critically Ill Patient: Society for Critical Care Medicine and ASPEN, 2017.
Preterm: Proceedings of the Global Neonatal Consensus Symposium: Feeding the Preterm Infant, October 13–15, 2010, Chicago, IL. J Pediatr 2013;162(3 Suppl):S1–116.
*Adequate intake (AI).

(LBWIs) and patients with absorptive defects and chronic inflammatory bowel disease. The caloric density of MCT is 7.6 kcal/g compared to 9 kcal/g for long-chain triglycerides. The potential side effects of MCT administration include diarrhea when given in large quantities; and, if they are the only source of lipids, deficiency of essential fatty acids (EFAs).

EFAs are PUFAs that the human body cannot synthesize. EFAs include (1) omega-6 PUFA: the parent of this series is linoleic acid (18:2ω6), the precursor of arachidonic acid (ARA 20:4ω6), and (2) omega-3 polyunsaturated fatty acid: the parent is alpha linolenic acid (18:3ω3), and leading derivatives are (EPA 20:6ω3) and docosahexaenoic acid (DHA, 22:6ω3). Omega-6 fatty acid deficiency is associated with rough scaly skin dermatitis, growth failure, capillary fragility, increased fragility of erythrocytes, thrombocytopenia, poor wound healing, and susceptibility to infection.* It leads to decreased ARA and increased synthesis of eicosatrienoic acid from oleic acid and is diagnosed by elevated eicosatrienoic acid:ARA (triene:tetraene) ratio. The clinical features of deficiency of omega-3 fatty acids are less well defined, and the eicosatrienoic acid:ARA (triene:tetraene) ratio is normal in isolated omega-3 deficiency.

Human milk lipids are composed of 35%–40% saturated fatty acids, 45%–50% monounsaturated, and 15% PUFAs. The long-chain PUFA profile in human milk is affected by the maternal diet. In the western world, there is an increase in the omega-6:omega-3 ratio, indicating a suboptimal intake of omega-3 associated with higher consumption of omega-6.

The ADMR for fat in the first year of life is based on exclusive breast-feeding in the first 6 months of life and breast-feeding in addition to complimentary food from 6 to 12 months old. The AMDR for total fat is estimated at 20%–35% of calories for adults and children aged four and older and 30%–40% for children ages 1–3 years. The Dietary Guidelines for Americans (DGA) 2020–2025 recommended that saturated fat should not exceed 10% of total calories starting at 2 years of age. The AMDRs for linoleic acid are 5%–10%, and for alpha-linolenic is 0.6%–1.2%.

Dietary Guidelines for Americans 2020–2025: https://dietaryguidelines.gov.
National Academies of Sciences, Engineering, and Medicine: *Dietary Reference Intakes: The Essential Guide to Nutrient Requirements*. Washington, DC: The National Academies Press; 2006. https://doi.org/10.17226/11537.

CARBOHYDRATES

Carbohydrates are converted to glucose in the body and provide a valuable source of energy. The energy density of carbohydrates is 4 kcal/g. Carbohydrates are classified by their number of sugar units: monosaccharides (1 unit/eg, glucose), disaccharides (2 units/eg, lactose), oligosaccharides (3–10 units), and polysaccharides (> 10 units/eg, starch, glycogen). Starchy food that is less processed and slowly absorbed may have a health advantage over simple sugars due to their lower glycemic index (GI). A food's GI is a measurement of the increase in blood glucose 2 hours after its consumption. Foods are ranked on a scale of 0–100, with glucose given a value of 100. The lower a food's GI, the slower blood sugar rises after eating that food. The glycemic load (GL) is the product of the GI and the amount of carbohydrates, thereby accounting for the total glycemic effect of food. Studies suggest a beneficial effect of a low index/load diet in children and adolescents with obesity and a possible preventive effect against type 2 diabetes.

After the first 2 years of life, 50%–60% of energy requirements should be derived from carbohydrates, with no more than 10% from simple sugars as recommended by the World Health Organization (WHO) and the 2020–2025 DGA, or less than 25 g of sugar added to foods per day as recommended by the American Heart Association in 2018. The DGA also recommends avoiding added sugars for children younger than 2 years. These dietary guidelines are, unfortunately, not reflected in the typical diets of North American children, who on average derive 25% of their energy intake from sucrose and less than 20% from complex carbohydrates.

Dietary fiber, as defined by the Institute of Medicine (IOM), comprises nondigestible carbohydrates and lignin that are intrinsic and intact in plants. These substances resist hydrolysis and absorption in the human small intestine.

Dietary fiber can be classified into two main categories: soluble fiber and insoluble fiber. Soluble fiber dissolves in water to form a gel-like substance in the digestive tract. This type of fiber is known for its ability to help lower cholesterol levels and regulate blood sugar levels by slowing down the absorption of glucose. Soluble fiber is found in foods such as oats, barley, legumes, fruits (such as apples and citrus fruits), and vegetables (such as carrots and broccoli).On the other hand, insoluble fiber does not dissolve in water and adds bulk to the stool, helping to promote regular bowel movements and prevent constipation. It also aids in maintaining the health of the digestive system by speeding up the passage of food and waste through the intestines. Insoluble fiber is commonly found in whole grains (such as wheat bran and brown rice), nuts, seeds, and the skins of fruits and vegetables. Many foods contain a combination of both soluble and insoluble fiber, contributing to a balanced and nutritious diet. The DRIs recommend 14 g of fiber per 1000 kcal consumed. The American Academy of Pediatrics (AAP) recommends that children older than 2 years consume in grams per day an amount of fiber equal to 5 plus the age in years. Dietary carbohydrates play an important role in human nutrition and comprise a variety of foods including grains, vegetables, fruits, legumes, and dairy products. Table 11–3 lists examples of some dietary and functional fiber and their health benefits.

Browne NT, Cuda SE: Nutritional and activity recommendations for the child with normal weight, overweight, and obesity with consideration of food insecurity: an Obesity Medical Association (OMA) Clinical Practice Statement 2022 Obesity Pillars 2. Doi: org/10.1016/j.obpill.2022.100012.
Carlson JL et al: Health effects and sources of prebiotic dietary fiber. Curr Dev Nutr 2018;2(3);nzy005. doi:10.1093/cdn/nzy005 [PMID: 30019028].

MAJOR MINERALS

Dietary sources, absorption, metabolism, and deficiency of the major minerals are summarized in Table 11–4. Recommended intakes are provided in Table 11–5.

---

*Adapted from Centers for Disease Control and Prevention: Recommendations for using fluoride to prevent and control dental caries in the United States. Centers for Disease Control and Prevention. *MMWR Recomm Rep* 2001 Aug 17;50(RR-14):1-42.

Table 11–3. Examples of dietary fiber and health benefits.

Fiber	Source	Benefit
Beta-glucans (soluble)	Oat and barley	Prebiotic/may help normalize glucose and cholesterol level.
Cellulose, hemicellulose (insoluble)	Cereal, grains, fruits, veggies	Absorbs water and bulks stool, laxative effect.
Guar gum (soluble)	Seeds	May help normalize glucose and cholesterol level.
Inulin, oligofructose, oligosaccharides, fructooligosaccharides (soluble)	Onions, asparagus, soybeans, leeks, oats, bananas, wheat	May add bulk to stool and have a laxative effect/prebiotic/may help normalize blood glucose. Patients with irritable bowel syndrome can have bloating and upset stomach.
Lignin (insoluble)	Wheat, corn bran, nuts, flaxseed	Laxative effect.
Pectin (soluble)	Apples, berries, fruits	May help normalize blood sugar and cholesterol.
Psyllium (soluble)	Extracted from psyllium seeds	Laxative, may help normalize blood glucose and cholesterol levels.

Source: Harvard School of Public Health.

Table 11–4. Major minerals.

Mineral	Absorption/Metabolism	Deficiency Causes	Deficiency Clinical Features
Calcium *Dietary sources:* dairy products, legumes, broccoli, green leafy vegetables.	20%–30% from diet; 60% from HM. Enhanced by lactose, glucose, protein; impaired by phytate, fiber, oxalate, unabsorbed fat. Absorption is regulated by serum calcitriol, which increases when PTH is secreted in response to low plasma-ionized calcium. PTH also promotes the release of calcium from bone. Renal excretion.	Can occur in preterm infants without adequate supplementation and in lactating adolescents with limited calcium intake or in patients with steatorrhea.	Osteopenia or osteoporosis, tetany.
Phosphorus *Dietary sources:* meats, eggs, dairy products, grains, legumes, and nuts; high in processed foods and sodas.	80% from diet. PTH decreases tubular resorption of phosphorus in kidneys; homeostasis is maintained by GI tract and kidneys.	Rare, but can occur in preterm infants fed unfortified HM (results in osteoporosis and rickets, sometimes hypercalcemia). Also seen in patients with protein-energy malnutrition and may occur with refeeding.	Muscle weakness, bone pain, rhabdomyolysis, osteomalacia, and respiratory insufficiency.
Magnesium *Dietary sources:* vegetables, cereals, nuts.	Kidneys regulate homeostasis by decreasing excretion when intake is low.	Occurs as part of refeeding syndrome with protein-energy malnutrition. Renal disease, malabsorption, or magnesium wasting medications may lead to depletion. May cause secondary hypocalcemia.	Neuromuscular excitability, muscle fasciculation, neurologic abnormalities, ECG changes.
Sodium *Dietary sources:* processed foods, table salt.	Hypo- and hypernatremic dehydration are discussed in Chapter 23. Kidneys are the primary site of homeostatic regulation.	Results from excess losses associated with diarrhea and vomiting.	Anorexia, vomiting, hypotension, and mental apathy. Severe malnutrition, stress, and hypermetabolism may lead to excess intracellular sodium, affecting cellular metabolism.

(Continued)

Table 11–4. Major minerals. (*Continued*)

Mineral	Absorption/Metabolism	Deficiency	
		Causes	**Clinical Features**
Chloride *Dietary sources:* table salt or sea salt, seaweed, and many vegetables.	Homeostasis is closely linked to sodium. Plays an important role in physiologic mechanisms of kidneys and gut.	Can occur in infants fed low chloride containing diets, or in children with cystic fibrosis, vomiting, diarrhea, chronic diuretic therapy, or Bartter syndrome.	Associated with failure to thrive and especially poor head growth; anorexia, lethargy, muscle weakness, vomiting, dehydration, hypovolemia. *Laboratory findings:* may include hypochloremia, hypokalemia, metabolic alkalosis, hyperreninemia.
Potassium *Dietary sources:* nuts, whole grains, meats, fish, beans, fruits and vegetables, especially bananas, orange juice.	Kidneys control potassium homeostasis via the aldosterone renin-angiotensin endocrine system. The amount of total body potassium depends on lean body mass.	Occurs in protein-energy malnutrition (eg, total body depletion + refeeding syndrome) and can cause cardiac failure and sudden death if not treated proactively. With loss of lean body mass, excessive potassium is excreted in urine in any catabolic state. Can also occur during acidosis, from diarrhea, and from diuretic use. Hyperkalemia may result from renal insufficiency.	Muscle weakness, mental confusion, arrhythmias.

ECG, electrocardiogram; GI, gastrointestinal; HM, human milk; PTH, parathyroid hormone.

TRACE ELEMENTS

Trace elements with a recognized role in human nutrition are iron, iodine, zinc, copper, selenium, manganese, molybdenum, chromium, cobalt (as a component of vitamin B$_{12}$), and fluoride. Information on food sources, functions, and deficiencies of the trace elements is summarized in Table 11–6. Supplemental fluoride recommendations are listed in Table 11–7. DRIs of trace elements are summarized in Table 11–5.

Anemia is discussed in Chapter 30. Iron deficiency (ID) is the most prevalent micronutrient deficiency worldwide and can result in neurobehavioral abnormalities that can be irreversible. Early detection of at-risk infants and children with appropriate monitoring and supplementation is essential to mitigate the negative long-term impact of deficiency.

Table 11–5. Summary of dietary reference intakes for selected major minerals and trace elements.

	0–6 mo	7–12 mo	1–3 y	4–8 y	9–13 y	14–18-y Male	14–18-y Female
Calcium (mg/day)	210[a]	270[a]	500[a]	800[a]	1300[a]	1300[a]	1300[a]
Phosphorus (mg/day)	100[a]	275[a]	460[a]	500	1250	1250	1250
Magnesium (mg/day)	30[a]	75[a]	80	130	240	410	360
Iron (mg/day)	0.27[a]	11	7	10	8	11	15
Zinc (mg/day)	2[a]	3	3	5	8	11	9
Iodine (mcg/day)	110[a]	130	90	90	120	150	150
Copper (mcg/day)	200[a]	220[a]	340	440	700	890	890
Selenium (mcg/day)	15[a]	20[a]	20	30	40	55	55

[a]Adequate intakes (AI). All other values represent the Recommended Dietary Allowances (RDAs). Both the RDA and AI may be used as goals for individual intakes.

Table 11–6. Summary of trace elements.

Mineral	Deficiency		Treatment
	Causes	Clinical Features	
Zinc *Dietary sources:* meats, shellfish, legumes, nuts, and whole-grain cereals. *Functions:* component of many enzymes and gene transcription factors; plays critical roles in nucleic acid metabolism, protein synthesis, and gene expression; supports membrane structure and function.	Diets low in available zinc (high phytate), unfortified synthetic diets; malabsorptive diseases (enteritis, celiac disease, cystic fibrosis); excessive losses (chronic diarrhea); inborn errors of zinc metabolism (acrodermatitis enteropathica, mammary gland zinc secretion defect). Inadequate intake in breast-fed infants after age 6 mo. Preterm birth and low birth weight are risk factors.	Mild: impaired growth, poor appetite, impaired immunity. Moderate to severe: mood changes, irritability, lethargy, impaired immune function, increased susceptibility to infection; acro-orificial skin rash, diarrhea, alopecia. Response to zinc supplement is gold standard for diagnosis of deficiency; plasma zinc levels are lowered by acute phase response.	1 mg/kg/day of elemental zinc for 2–3 mo (eg, 4.5 mg/kg/day of zinc sulfate salt), given separately from meals and iron supplements. With acrodermatitis enteropathica, 30–50 mg Zn^{2+}/day (or more) sustains remission.
Copper *Dietary sources:* meats, shellfish, legumes, nuts, and whole-grain cereals. *Functions:* vital component of several oxidative enzymes: cytochrome c oxidase (electron transport chain), cytosolic and mitochondrial superoxide dismutase (free radical defense), lysyl oxidase (cross-linking of elastin and collagen), ferroxidase (oxidation of ferrous storage iron prior to transport to bone marrow).	Generalized malnutrition, prolonged PN without supplemental copper, malabsorption, or prolonged diarrhea. Prematurity is a risk factor.	Osteoporosis, enlargement of costochondral cartilages, cupping and flaring of long bone metaphyses, spontaneous rib fractures. Neutropenia and hypochromic anemia resistant to iron therapy. Defect of copper metabolism (Menkes kinky hair syndrome) results in severe CNS disease. Low plasma levels help to confirm deficiency; levels are normally very low in young infants. Age-matched normal data are necessary for comparison. Plasma levels are raised by acute phase response.	1% copper sulfate solution (2 mg of salt) or 500 mcg/day elemental copper for infants.
Selenium *Dietary sources:* seafood, meats, garlic (geochemical distribution affects levels in foods). *Function:* essential component of glutathione peroxidase.	Inadequate dietary intake; can occur with selenium-deficient PN. Renal disease. Prematurity	Skeletal muscle pain and tenderness, macrocytosis, loss of hair pigment. Keshan disease, an often fatal cardiomyopathy in infants and children in areas of China with Selenium-poor soil.	Minimum recommended selenium content for full-term infant formulas is 1.5 mcg/100 kcal, and for preterm formulas, 1.8 mcg/100 kcal. PN should be supplemented.
Iodine *Dietary source:* iodized salt. Typical fortification provides 225 mcg/5 g. *Functions:* essential component of thyroid hormones; regulates metabolism, growth, and neural development.	Inadequate dietary intake.	Neurologic endemic cretinism (severe mental retardation, deaf mutism, spastic diplegia, and strabismus) occurs with severe deficiency. Myxedematous endemic cretinism occurs in some central African countries where signs of congenital hypothyroidism are present.	Use of iodized salt is effective in preventing goiter. Injections of iodized oil can also be used for prevention.
Fluoride *Function:* incorporated into the hydroxyapatite matrix of dentin.	Inadequate intake (unfluoridated water supply).	Low intake increases incidence of dental caries.	See Table 11–6 for supplementation guidelines. Excess fluoride intake results in fluorosis.

CNS, central nervous system; PN, parenteral nutrition.

Table 11–7. Supplemental fluoride recommendations (mg/day).

Age	Concentration of Fluoride in Drinking Water		
	< 0.3 ppm	0.3–0.6 ppm	> 0.6 ppm
6 mo–3 y	0.25	0	0
3–6 y	0.5	0.25	0
6–16 y	1	0.5	0

Adapted from Centers for Disease Control and Prevention: Recommendations for using fluoride to prevent and control dental caries in the United States. Centers for Disease Control and Prevention. MMWR Recomm Rep 2001 Aug 17;50(RR-14):1–42.

The following list highlights the essential clinical pearls regarding ID:

- ID is a state of insufficient iron to maintain physiologic functions.
- Anemia is a late manifestation of ID.
- Laboratory evaluation of iron status should include a ferritin and inflammatory marker (ferritin is an acute phase reactant and can be falsely elevated even in the presence of a minor viral infection).
- It is estimated that 15%–16% of children have ID without anemia.
- The AAP recommends supplementing the breast-fed infant with iron 1 mg/kg/day starting at 4 months of age until a diet high in iron-rich food is established.
- Premature infants need an iron supplement of 2 mg/kg/day.
- Iron dose for ID without anemia: 3 mg/kg/day given as one daily dose.

Georgieff MK, Krebs NF, Cusick SE: The benefits and risks of iron supplementation in pregnancy and childhood. Annu Rev Nutr 2019 Aug 21;39:121–146. doi: 10.1146/annurev-nutr-082018-124213 [PMID: 31091416].
Schwarzenberg SJ et al; AAP Committee on Nutrition: Advocacy for improving nutrition in the first 1000 days to support childhood development and adult health. Pediatrics 2018;141(2): e20173716 [PMID: 29358479].

VITAMINS

In general, highly restrictive diets (eg, those in which entire food groups are absent) should prompt consideration of vitamin deficiencies. For example, numerous cases of scurvy have been reported in children with autism who have had markedly constrained diets. Figures 11–1 and 11–2 illustrate skin findings in a patient who developed scurvy due to highly restricted diet. Patients with malnutrition and with chronic

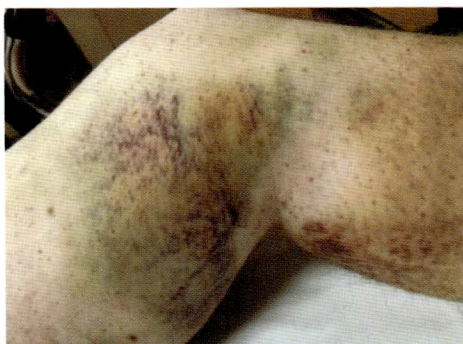

▲ **Figure 11–1.** Scurvy in a 17-year-old with ARFID and restricted eating (pasta, meat, and soda only). **Ecchymoses** on the inner thighs.

illness are also at higher risk for micronutrient deficiencies. Untreated fat-malabsorption syndromes (eg, cystic fibrosis, celiac disease, short gut syndrome), in addition to the physiologic sequelae of bariatric surgery are associated with deficiencies of fat-soluble vitamins. See Table 11–8 for other general circumstances that should prompt assessment for vitamin deficiencies.

Fat-Soluble Vitamins

Because they are insoluble in water, the fat-soluble vitamins require digestion and absorption of dietary fat and a carrier system for transport in the blood. Deficiencies of these vitamins develop more slowly than deficiencies of water-soluble vitamins because the body accumulates stores of the fat-soluble vitamins. Prematurity and some childhood conditions (especially those with fat malabsorption) place children at risk (see Table 11–8). Excessive intake carries potential for toxicity (Table 11–9). A summary of reference intakes is found in Table 11–10. Dietary sources of fat-soluble vitamins,

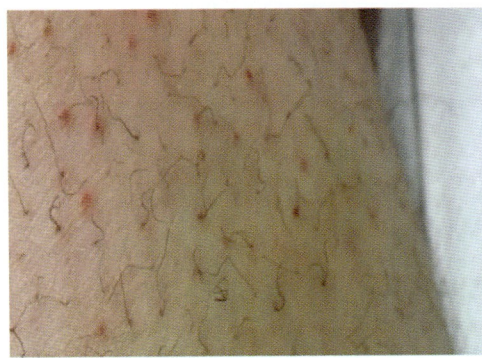

▲ **Figure 11–2.** Cork-screw hair, characteristic of scurvy, which can develop in 30–40 days of a diet deficient of vitamin C.

Table 11–8. Circumstances associated with risk of vitamin deficiencies.

Circumstance	Possible Deficiency
Preterm birth	All vitamins
Severe Malnutrition	B_1, B_2, folate, A
Synthetic diets without adequate fortification (including total parenteral nutrition)	All vitamins
Vitamin-drug interactions	Folate, B_{12}, D, B_6
Fat malabsorption syndromes	Vitamins A, D, E, K
Breast-feeding with malnourished mother and/or limited complementary foods	B_1,[a] folate,[b] B_{12},[c] D,[d] K[e]
Periconceptional	Folate
Severe Obesity	Vitamin D
Bariatric surgery (all types)	B vitamins, Vitamin D
Highly restrictive diet	Vitamin C, B vitamins, vitamin D

[a]Malnourished mother or maternal alcoholism.
[b]Folate-deficient mother.
[c]Vegan mother or maternal pernicious anemia.
[d]Infant not exposed to sunlight and mother's vitamin D status suboptimal.
[e]Prophylaxis omitted.

their absorption/metabolism, and causes and clinical features of deficiency are summarized in Table 11–11. Vitamin deficiency and related diagnostic laboratory findings and treatment are detailed in Table 11–12.

Recent recognition of low levels of 25-OH-vitamin D in a relatively large percentage of the population and the broad range of functions beyond calcium absorption have led many experts including the AAP to recommend a daily intake of at least 400 IU (10 mcg/day) for all infants, including those who are breast-fed, beginning shortly after birth. A recent study illuminated the need for greater attention and adherence to the vitamin D supplementation guidelines, with less than 40% of infants in the United States meeting recommended vitamin D intakes. Nutritional rickets, caused by vitamin D deficiency and/or low calcium intake, is a preventable global health problem for infants, children, and adolescents. Beyond 12 months of age, all children need to meet their nutritional requirement for vitamin D through diet and/or supplementation; the IOM recommends 400–600 IU/day (10–15 mcg/day).

Chang SW, Lee HC: Vitamin D and health—the missing vitamin in humans. [Review]. Pediatr Neonatol 2019 Jun;60(3):237–244. doi: 10.106/j.pedneo.2019.04.007. Epub 2019 Apr 17 [PMID: 31101452].
Simon AE, Ahrens KA: Adherence to vitamin D intake guidelines in the United States. Pediatrics 2020 Jun;145(6):e20193574. doi: 10.1542/peds.2019-3574 [PMID: 32424077].
Soheilipour F, Hamidabad NM: Vitamin D and calcium status among adolescents with morbid obesity undergoing bariatric surgery. Obes Surg 2022 Mar;32(3):738–741. doi: 10.1007/s11695-021-05809-0 [PMID: 34799812].

Table 11–9. Effects of vitamin toxicity.

Pyridoxine
Sensory neuropathy at doses > 500 mg/day
Niacin
Histamine release → cutaneous vasodilation; cardiac arrhythmias; cholestatic jaundice; gastrointestinal disturbance; hyperuricemia; glucose intolerance
Folic acid
May mask B_{12} deficiency, hypersensitivity
Vitamin C
Diarrhea; increased oxalic acid excretion; renal stones
Vitamin A
(> 20,000 IU/day): Vomiting, increased intracranial pressure (pseudotumor cerebri); irritability; headaches; insomnia; emotional lability; dry, desquamating skin; myalgia and arthralgia; abdominal pain; hepatosplenomegaly; cortical thickening of bones of hands and feet
Vitamin D
(> 50,000 IU/day): Hypercalcemia; vomiting; constipation; nephrocalcinosis
Vitamin E
(> 25–100 mg/kg/day intravenously): Necrotizing enterocolitis and liver toxicity (but probably due to polysorbate 80 used as a solubilizer)
Vitamin K
Lipid-soluble vitamin K: Very low order of toxicity
Water-soluble, synthetic vitamin K: Vomiting; porphyrinuria; albuminuria; hemolytic anemia; hemoglobinuria; hyperbilirubinemia (do not give to neonates)

Table 11–10. Summary of dietary reference intakes for select vitamins.

	0–6 mo	7–12 mo	1–3 y	4–8 y	9–13 y	14–18-y Male	14–18-y Female
Thiamin (mg/day)	0.2[a]	0.3[a]	0.5	0.6	0.9	1.2	1.0
Riboflavin (mg/day)	0.3[a]	0.4[a]	0.5[a]	0.6[a]	0.9[a]	1.3[a]	1.0[a]
Pyridoxine (mg/day)	0.1[a]	0.3[a]	0.5	0.6	1.0	1.3	1.2
Niacin (mg/day)	2[a]	4[a]	6	8	12	16	14
Pantothenic acid (mg/day)	1.7[a]	1.8[a]	2[a]	3[a]	4[a]	5[a]	5[a]
Biotin (mcg/day)	5[a]	6[a]	8[a]	12[a]	20[a]	25[a]	25[a]
Folic acid (mcg/day)	65[a]	80[a]	150	200	300	400	400
Cobalamin (mcg/day)	0.4[a]	0.5[a]	0.9	1.2	1.8	2.4	2.4
Vitamin C (mg/day)	40[a]	50[a]	15	25	45	75	65
Vitamin A (mcg/day)	400[a]	500[a]	300	400	600	900	700
Vitamin D (IU/day)	200[a,b]	200[a,b]	200[a,b]	200[a,b]	200[a,b]	200[a,b]	200[a,b]
Vitamin E (mg/day)	4[a]	5[a]	6	7	11	15	15
Vitamin K (mcg/day)	2[a]	2.5[a]	30[a]	55[a]	60[a]	75[a]	75[a]

[a]Adequate Intakes (AI). All other values represent the Recommended Dietary Allowances (RDAs). Both the RDA and AI may be used as goals for individual intakes.
[b]American Academy of Pediatrics in 2008 recommended 400 IU/day vitamin D for infants, children, and adolescents.
Data from National Academy of Sciences, Food and Nutritional Board, Institute of Medicine: *Dietary Reference Intakes, Applications in Dietary Assessment*. Washington, DC: National Academy Press; 2000. http://www.nap.edu.

Table 11–11. Summary of fat-soluble vitamins.

Vitamin	Absorption/Metabolism	Deficiency	
		Causes	Clinical Features
Vitamin A *Dietary sources:* dairy products, eggs, liver, meats, fish oils. Precursor β-carotene is abundant in yellow and green vegetables. *Functions:* has critical role in vision, helping to form photosensitive pigment rhodopsin; modifies differentiation and proliferation of epithelial cells in respiratory tract; and is needed for glycoprotein synthesis.	Retinol is stored in liver and from there is exported, attached to RBP and prealbumin. RBP may be decreased in liver disease or in protein energy malnutrition. Circulating RBP may be increased in renal failure.	Occurs in premature infants, in association with inadequately supplemented PN; protein energy malnutrition (deficiency worsened by measles); dietary insufficiency and fat malabsorption.	Night blindness, xerosis, xerophthalmia, Bitot spots, keratomalacia, ulceration and perforation of cornea, prolapse of lens and iris, and blindness; follicular hyperkeratosis; pruritus; growth retardation; increased susceptibility to infection.
Vitamin K *Dietary sources:* leafy vegetables, fruits, seeds; synthesized by intestinal bacteria. *Functions:* necessary for the maintenance of normal plasma levels of coagulation factors II, VII, IX, and X; essential for maintenance of normal levels of the anticoagulation protein C; essential for osteoblastic activity.	Absorbed in proximal small intestine in micelles with bile salts; circulates with VLDL.	Occurs in newborns, especially those who are breast-fed and who have not received vitamin K prophylaxis at delivery; in fat malabsorption syndromes; and with use of unabsorbed antibiotics and anticoagulant drugs (warfarin).	Bruising or bleeding in GI tract, genitourinary tract, gingiva, lungs, joints, and brain.

(Continued)

Table 11–11. Summary of fat-soluble vitamins. (*Continued*)

Vitamin	Absorption/Metabolism	Deficiency	
		Causes	Clinical Features
Vitamin E *Dietary sources:* vegetable oils, some cereals, dairy, wheat germ, eggs. *Functions:* free-radical scavenger, stops oxidation reactions. Located at specific sites in cell membrane to protect polyunsaturated fatty acids in membrane from peroxidation and thiol groups and nucleic acids; also acts as cell membrane stabilizer; may function in electron transport chain; may modulate chromosomal expression.	Emulsified in intestinal lumen with bile salts; absorbed via passive diffusion; transported by chylomicrons and VLDL.	May occur with preterm birth, cholestatic liver disease, pancreatic insufficiency, abetalipoproteinemia, and short bowel syndrome. Isolated inborn error of vitamin E metabolism. May result from increased consumption during oxidant stress.	Hemolytic anemia; progressive neurologic disorder with loss of deep tendon reflexes, loss of coordination, vibratory and position sensation, nystagmus, weakness, scoliosis, and retinal degeneration.
Vitamin D *Dietary sources:* fortified milk and formulas, egg yolk, fatty fish. *Functions:* calcitriol, the biologically active form of vitamin D, stimulates intestinal absorption of calcium and phosphate, renal reabsorption of filtered calcium, and mobilization of calcium and phosphorus from bone.	Normally obtained primarily from cholecalciferol (D_3) produced by UV radiation of dehydrocholesterol in skin. Ergocalciferol (D_2) is derived from UV irradiation of ergosterol in skin. Vitamin D is transported from skin to liver, attached to a specific carrier protein.	Results from a combination of inadequate sunlight exposure, dark skin pigmentation, and low dietary intake. Breast-fed infants are at risk because of low vitamin D content of human milk. Cow's milk and infant formulas are routinely supplemented with vitamin D. Deficiency also occurs in fat malabsorption syndromes. Hydroxylated vitamin D may be decreased by CYP-450–stimulating drugs, hepatic or renal disease, and inborn errors of metabolism.	Osteomalacia (adults) or rickets (children), in which osteoid with reduced calcification accumulates in bone. *Clinical findings:* craniotabes, rachitic rosary, pigeon breast, bowed legs, delayed eruption of teeth and enamel defects, Harrison groove, scoliosis, kyphosis, dwarfism, painful bones, fractures, anorexia, and weakness. *Radiographic findings:* cupping, fraying, flaring of metaphyses.

CYP, cytochrome P; GI, gastrointestinal; PN, parenteral nutrition; PTH, parathyroid hormone; RBP, retinol-binding protein; UV, ultraviolet; VLDL, very-low-density lipoproteins.

Water-Soluble Vitamins

The risk of toxicity from water-soluble vitamins is not as great as that associated with fat-soluble vitamins because excesses are excreted in the urine. However, deficiencies of these vitamins develop more quickly than fat-soluble vitamins because of limited stores. The clinician should maintain a high index of suspicion for water soluble vitamins deficiencies when managing patients on restricted diets (autism, strict vegan diet), in the setting of malnutrition and morbid obesity, and post bariatric surgery. Table 11–13 summarizes water-soluble vitamins. Table 11–14 provides a quick reference for the assessment of micronutrient deficiencies based on symptoms.

Diab L, Krebs NF: Vitamin excess and deficiency. Pediatr Rev 2018 Apr;39(4):161–179. doi: 10.1542/pir.2016.0068 [PMID: 29610425].

INFANT FEEDING

BREAST-FEEDING

Breast-feeding provides optimal nutrition for the normal infant during the early months of life. The WHO and the AAP recommend exclusive breast-feeding for approximately the first 6 months of life, with continued breast-feeding along with appropriate complementary foods through the first 2 years of life. Numerous immunologic factors in breast milk (including secretory immunoglobulin A [IgA], lysozyme, lactoferrin, bifidus factor, oligosaccharides, and macrophages) provide protection against GI and upper respiratory infections.

In resource limited countries, lack of refrigeration and contaminated water supplies make formula feeding especially hazardous. Although formulas are made to resemble breast milk, they cannot replicate the nutritional or immune

Table 11–12. Evaluation and treatment of deficiencies of fat-soluble vitamins.

Vitamin Deficiency	Diagnostic Laboratory Findings and Treatment		
Vitamin A	*Laboratory findings:* serum retinol < 20 mcg/dL; molar ratio of retinol:RBP < 0.7 is also diagnostic. *Treatment:* xerophthalmia requires 5000–10,000 IU/kg/day for 5 days PO or IM; with fat malabsorption, standard dose is 2500–5000 IU. Toxicity effects are listed in Table 11–8.		
Vitamin K	*Laboratory findings:* assess plasma levels of PIVKA or PT. *Treatment:* Oral: 2.5–5.0 mg/day or IM/IV: 1–2 mg/dose as single dose.		
Vitamin E	*Laboratory findings:* normal serum level is 3–15 mg/mL for children. Ratio of serum vitamin E to total serum lipid is normally ≥ 0.8 mg/g. *Treatment:* large oral doses (up to 100 IU/kg/day) correct deficiency from malabsorption; for abetalipoproteinemia, 100–200 IU/kg/day are needed.		
Vitamin D	*Laboratory findings:* low serum phosphorus and calcium, high alkaline phosphatase, high serum PTH, low 25-OH-cholecalciferol. American Academy of Pediatrics recommends supplementation, as follows: 400 IU/day (10 mcg) for all breast-fed infants, beginning in first 2 mo of life and continuing until infant is receiving ≥ 500 mL/day of vitamin D-fortified formula or cow's milk. Treatment for vitamin D deficiency (if level < 20)		
	Age	**Therapeutic Dose**	**Preventive Dose**
	Infants 0- to 1-year-old	2000 IU (50 mcg) per day or 50,000 IU (1250 mcg) once weekly for 6 wk until blood level is above 30 ng/mL	400–1000 IU/day (10–25 mcg/day)
	Children 1- to 18-year-old	2000 IU (50 mcg) per day or 50,000 IU (1250 mcg) once weekly for 6 wk until blood level is > 30 ng/mL	600–1000 IU/day (15–25 mcg/day)

IM, intramuscular; IV, intravenous; PIVKA, protein-induced vitamin K absence; PO, by mouth; PT, prothrombin time; PTH, parathyroid hormone; RBP, retinol-binding protein.

composition of human milk. Additional differences of physiologic importance continue to be identified. Furthermore, breast-feeding can foster the maternal-child bond.

Breast-feeding is the predominant *initial* mode of feeding young infants in the United States. Unfortunately, breast-feeding rates remain low among several subpopulations, including low-income, minority, and young mothers. Many mothers face obstacles in maintaining lactation once they return to work, and rates of breast-feeding at 6 months are considerably less than the goal of 50%. The use of an electric breast pump can help maintain lactation when mothers and infants are separated for extended periods.

Absolute contraindications to breast-feeding are rare. They include active tuberculosis (in the mother) and galactosemia (in the infant). Breast-feeding is associated with maternal-to-child transmission of human immunodeficiency virus (HIV), but the risk is influenced by duration and pattern of breast-feeding and maternal factors, including immunologic status and presence of mastitis. Complete avoidance of breast-feeding by HIV-infected women is presently the only mechanism to prevent maternal-infant transmission. HIV-infected mothers in developed countries are recommended to refrain from breast-feeding if safe alternatives are available. In developing countries, the use of antiretroviral therapy (ART) and exclusive breast-feeding is encouraged for the first 6 months, with continued breast-feeding up to 24 months with age-appropriate complementary feeding; if ART is not available, avoidance of breast-feeding may be considered. The protection of the child against diarrheal illness and malnutrition may outweigh the risk of HIV transmission via breast milk. In such circumstances, HIV-infected women should be encouraged to exclusively breast-feed for 6 months.

In newborns weighing less than 1750 g, human milk should be fortified to increase protein, calcium, phosphorus, micronutrient content, and caloric density. Breast-fed infants with cystic fibrosis can be breast-fed successfully if exogenous pancreatic enzymes are provided. All infants with cystic fibrosis should receive supplemental vitamins A, D, E, K, and sodium chloride. Those with growth faltering should receive caloric supplementation.

Meek JY, Noble L; Section on Breastfeeding, Policy Statement: Breastfeeding and the use of human milk. Pediatrics 2022 Jul 1;150(1):e2022057988. doi: 10.1542/peds.2022-057988 [PMID: 35921640].

Table 11–13. Summary of water-soluble vitamins.

Vitamin/Population at Risk	Function	Food Source	Deficiency	Laboratory Test / Treatment
Energy-Releasing B Vitamins				
Thiamine (B1) Population at risk: Alcoholism (low intake, defective metabolism) elderly, high carbohydrate diet from unenriched grains or milled rice, anorexia nervosa patients and refeeding after starvation due to insufficient stores to handle increased demand to metabolize carbohydrates. Bariatric surgery.	Thiamin pyrophosphate is a coenzyme in oxidative decarboxylation (pyruvate dehydrogenase, α-ketoglutarate dehydrogenase, and transketolase).	Whole and enriched grains, lean pork, legumes	*"Dry" Beriberi (paralytic or nervous):* peripheral neuropathy, with impairment of sensory, motor, and reflex functions, ophthalmoplegia, vomiting *"Wet" Beriberi:* high output congestive heart failure ± signs of dry beriberi *Cerebral beriberi:* (Wernicke-Korsakoff encephalopathy) ophthalmoplegia, ataxia, mental confusion, memory loss	Thiamine level Treatment dose: 50–100 mg IM or IV
Riboflavin (B2) Rare in the US	Coenzyme of several flavoproteins (eg, flavin mononucleotide [FMN] and flavin adenine dinucleotide [FAD]) involved in oxidative/electron transfer enzyme systems.	Dairy products, meat, poultry, wheat germ, leafy vegetables	Cheilosis; angular stomatitis; glossitis; soreness and burning of lips and mouth; dermatitis of nasolabial fold and genitals; ± ocular signs (photophobia → indistinct vision).	Erythrocyte Glutathione Reductase Activity coefficient (EGRAC increases in deficiency).
Niacin (B3) Deficiency can happen after months of low intake, historically in areas where corn is major source of protein and calories. Also seen in malabsorption and with some meds (isoniazid).	Hydrogen-carrying coenzymes: nicotinamide-adenine dinucleotide (NAD), nicotinamide-adenine dinucleotide phosphate (NADP); decisive role in intermediary metabolism. Pantothenic acid Major component of coenzyme A.	Meats, poultry, fish, legumes, wheat, all foods except fats; synthesized in body from tryptophan.	Pellagra The 4 Ds: Dermatitis, especially on sun-exposed areas; Diarrhea; Dementia; Death Toxicity: High doses can cause peripheral vasodilation and flushing.	Serum niacin.
Biotin Deficiency can be due to suppressed intestinal flora and impaired intestinal absorption; regular intake of raw egg whites.	Component of several carboxylase enzymes involved in fat and carbohydrate metabolism.	Yeast, liver, kidneys, legumes, nuts, egg yolks (synthesized by intestinal bacteria).	Scaly dermatitis; alopecia; irritability; lethargy.	
Hematopoietic B Vitamins				
Folate Population at risk: Breast-fed infants whose mothers are folate-deficient; term infants fed cow's milk or goat's milk; kwashiorkor; chronic overcooking of food sources; malabsorption of folate because of a congenital defect; celiac disease; drugs (phenytoin). Increased requirements: chronic hemolytic anemias, diarrhea, malignancies, extensive skin disease, cirrhosis, pregnancy.	Tetrahydrofolate has essential role in one-carbon transfers. Essential role in purine and pyrimidine synthesis; deficiency → arrest of cell division (especially bone marrow and intestine).	Leafy vegetables (easily destroyed in cooking), fruits, whole grains, wheat germ, beans, nuts	Megaloblastic anemia; neutropenia; growth retardation; delayed maturation of central nervous system in infants; diarrhea (mucosal ulcerations); glossitis; neural tube defects.	*RBC folate* reflects tissue stores. Serum folate reflects recent intake *Elevated homocysteine level.*

Vitamin B$_{12}$ Absorbed in the distal ileum after cleavage of dietary protein and binding to intrinsic factor secreted by gastric parietal cells. Population at risk: 1. Bariatric surgery 2. Vegetarian diet without supplementation 3. Autoimmune conditions associated with antibodies to intrinsic factor 4. Breastfed infant of deficient mothers	Synthesis of methionine with simultaneous synthesis of tetrahydrofolate (reason for megaloblastic anemia in B$_{12}$ deficiency). Adenosyl cobalamin (mitochondria) is coenzyme for mutases and dehydratases.	Eggs, dairy products, liver, meats; none in plants	Megaloblastic anemia; hypersegmented neutrophils; neurologic degeneration: paresthesia, gait problems, depression.	Increased methylmalonic acid level. Increased homocysteine level. Serum B12 levels can be used only as a screen and indicates deficiency if level is < 271 pg/mL. Treatment: IM 1,000ug daily × 2–7 days, followed by either oral/sublingual daily dosing or weekly IM injections based on clinical response.
Other Water-Soluble Vitamins				
Vitamin B$_6$ (Pyridoxine) Use of isoniazid, end stage renal disease, malabsorption such as celiac, genetic conditions, poor diet.	Prosthetic group of transaminases, etc, involved in amino acid interconversions; prostaglandin and heme synthesis; central nervous system function; carbohydrate metabolism; immune development.	Animal products, vegetables, whole grains.	Listlessness; irritability; seizures; anemia; cheilosis; glossitis.	Pyridoxal phosphate Homocysteine.
Vitamin C (Ascorbic acid) Diet lacking fruits and vegetables, increased requirements in wound healing and burn, smokers.	Antioxidant/reducing agent. Collagen synthesis. Enhances iron absorption.	Fruits and vegetables.	Scurvy: Irritability, apathy, pallor; increased susceptibility to infections; hemorrhages under skin, petechiae in mucous membranes, in joints and under periosteum; long bone tenderness; costochondral beading; often presents with refusal to walk secondary to joint pain.	Ascorbic acid level.

Table 11–14. Quick reference for the assessment of micronutrient deficiencies based on symptoms.

Nutrient	Rash/Skin Findings	Mouth Lesions	Neurologic Symptoms	Anemia	Other
Vitamin A	X				Eye findings, blindness
Thiamine B1			X		Beriberi, CHF
Riboflavin B2		X			
Niacin B3	X		X		Pellagra
Pyridoxine B6		X	X	X	
Vitamin B$_{12}$		X	X	X	
Folate		X		X	
Vitamin C	X	X			Bone pain, refusal to walk
Vitamin D					Bone pain, fractures
Vitamin E			X	X	Loss of reflexes
Vitamin K	X	X			
Copper			X	X	Osteopenia, neutropenia
Iron			X	X	
Zinc	X				

Support of Breast-Feeding

In developed countries, health professionals play a significant role in supporting and promoting breast-feeding. Perinatal hospital routines and early pediatric care can have great influence on the successful initiation of breast-feeding by promoting prenatal and postpartum education, frequent mother-baby contact, advice about breast-feeding technique, demand feeding, rooming-in, avoidance of bottle supplements, and early follow-up after delivery. Increasing maternal confidence, family support, adequate maternity leave, and advice about common problems such as sore nipples can foster success. Medical providers can advocate for hospital policies that support breast-feeding.

Very few women are physically unable to nurse their babies, but both maternal and/or infant factors can impact successful initiation of nursing and lactogenesis. Mothers with obesity and/or insulin resistance often have delayed lactogenesis, and thus a potential need for additional breast-feeding support to establish successful lactation should be anticipated. The newborn is generally fed ad libitum every 2–3 hours, with longer intervals (4–5 hours) at night. Thus, a newborn infant nurses at least 8–10 times a day, which should stimulate a generous milk supply. In neonates, a loose stool is often passed with each feeding; stooling frequency decreases by age 3–4 months. Failure to pass several stools a day in the early weeks of breast-feeding and decreased number of wet diapers is always a concern. However, AI is not guaranteed in the presence of regular stooling and voiding. Infants require less volume of milk to maintain hydration than for adequate growth. Expressing milk using an electric breast pump may be indicated if the mother returns to work or if the infant is preterm, cannot suck adequately, or is hospitalized.

Bunik M: The pediatrician's role in encouraging exclusive breast-feeding. [Review] Pediatr Rev 2017 Aug;38(8):353–368. doi: 10.154/pir.2016-0109 [PMID: 28765198].

Technique of Breast-Feeding

Breast-feeding can be started as soon as both mother and baby are stable after delivery, ideally within the first hour. Correct positioning and breast-feeding technique ensure effective nipple stimulation and breast emptying with minimal nipple discomfort.

To nurse while the mother is sitting, the infant should be held at the height of the breast and turned to face the mother so that their abdomens touch. The mother's arms supporting the infant should be held tightly at her side, bringing the baby's head in line with her breast. The breast should be supported by the lower fingers of her free hand, with the nipple compressed between the thumb and index fingers to make it more protractile. When the infant opens its mouth, the mother should quickly insert as much nipple and areola as possible.

The most common cause of poor early weight gain in breast-fed infants is poorly managed mammary engorgement, which rapidly decreases milk supply. Unrelieved engorgement can result from long intervals between feeding, improper infant suckling, a nondemanding infant, sore nipples, maternal or infant illness, nursing from only one breast, and latching difficulties. Poor technique, maternal dehydration, stress, or excessive fatigue can contribute. Some infants may need to wake up to feed at night. Primary lactation failure occurs in less than 5% of women.

A sensible guideline for duration of feeding is 5 minutes per breast at each feeding the first day, 10 minutes on each side at each feeding the second day, and 10–15 minutes per side thereafter. A vigorous infant can obtain most of the available milk in 5–7 minutes, but additional sucking time ensures breast emptying, promotes milk production, and satisfies the infant's sucking urge. The side on which feeding is commenced should be alternated. The mother may break suction gently after nursing by inserting her finger between the baby's gums.

Follow-up

Assessment before discharge should focus on identifying dyads needing additional support. All mother-infant pairs require early follow-up. The second through fourth days postpartum when milk secretion becomes copious is a critical time. Failure to empty the breasts during this time can cause engorgement, which quickly leads to diminished milk production.

Common Problems

Nipple tenderness requires attention to proper positioning of the infant and correct latch-on. Nursing for shorter periods, beginning feedings on the less sore side, air drying the nipples well after nursing, and use of lanolin cream may provide relief. Severe nipple pain and cracking usually indicates improper latch. Temporary pumping may be needed.

The symptoms of mastitis include flu-like symptoms with breast tenderness, firmness, and erythema. Antibiotic therapy covering β-lactamase–producing organisms should be given for 10 days. Analgesics may be necessary, but breastfeeding should be continued. Breast pumping may be helpful adjunctive therapy.

Breast-feeding jaundice is exaggerated physiologic jaundice associated with low intake of breast milk, infrequent stooling, and poor weight gain (see Chapter 2). If possible, the jaundice should be managed by increasing the frequency of nursing and, if necessary, augmenting the infant's sucking with regular breast pumping. Supplemental feedings may be necessary, but care should be taken not to decrease breast milk production further.

Maternal Drug Use

Factors playing a role in the transmission of drugs in breast milk include the route of administration, dosage, molecular weight, pH, and protein binding. Very few drugs are absolutely contraindicated in breast-feeding mothers; these include radioactive compounds, antimetabolites, lithium, diazepam, chloramphenicol, antithyroid drugs, and tetracycline. For up-to-date information, a regional drug center should be consulted.

Maternal use of illicit or recreational drugs may be a contraindication to breast-feeding, but the risks to the infant should be balanced by the benefits of milk and breast-feeding. Expression of milk for a feeding or two after use of a drug is not an acceptable compromise. With the increasing number of states legalizing cannabis, marijuana has become one of the most commonly used drugs during pregnancy and lactation. There is a paucity of clinical data regarding the possible long-term neurobehavioral and developmental effects on the breast-fed infant of a cannabis using mother. Given that cannabis metabolites are detectable in breast milk, for up to 2 or 3 weeks, the AAP and the American College of Obstetricians and Gynecologists recommend counseling lactating mothers to cease use of marijuana and limit any potential secondhand exposure. The breast-fed infants of mothers taking methadone alone as part of a medication-assisted treatment program for opioid addiction have generally not experienced ill effects when the dose is less than 40 mg/day.

United States National Library of Medicine Drugs and Lactation Database (Lactmed): ncbi.nlm.nih.gov/books/NBK501922/.

Wymore E et al: Persistence of D-9-tetrahydrocannabinol in human breast milk. JAMA Pediatr 2021 Jun 1;(6):632–634. doi: 10.1001/jamapediatrics.2020.6098 [PMID: 33683306].

Nutrient Composition

The nutrient composition of human milk is compared to that of cow's milk and formulas in Table 11–15. Outstanding characteristics include (1) lower but highly bioavailable protein content, which is adequate for the normal infant; (2) generous quantity of the EFAs alpha-linolenic acid (an omega-3 fatty acid) and linoleic acid (an omega-6 fatty acid); (3) long-chain PUFAs, of which DHA is thought to be especially important; (4) relatively low sodium and solute load; and (5) lower concentration of highly bioavailable minerals, which are adequate for the needs of normal breast-fed infants for approximately 6 months.

Complementary Feeding

The AAP and WHO recommend the introduction of solid foods in normal infants at about 6 months of age, with continued breast-feeding as mutually desired through 24 months of age or use of an iron fortified infant formula until 1 year of age. Fortified cereals, fruits, vegetables, and meats should complement the breast milk diet. Human milk content of iron and zinc become inadequate to meet infants' needs by 6 months, necessitating food sources of these important

Table 11–15. Composition of human and cow's milk and typical infant formula (per 100 kcal).

Nutrient (unit)	Minimal Level Recommended[a]	Mature Human Milk	Typical Commercial Formula	Cow's Milk (mean)
Protein (g)	1.8[b]	1.3–1.6	2.3	5.1
Fat (g)	3.3[c]	5	5.3	5.7
Carbohydrate (g)	—	10.3	10.8	7.3
Linoleic acid (mg)	300	560	2300	125
Vitamin A (IU)	250	250	300	216
Vitamin D (IU)	40	3	63	3
Vitamin E (IU)	0.7/g linoleic acid	0.3	2	0.1
Vitamin K (mcg)	4	2	9	5
Vitamin C (mg)	8	7.8	8.1	2.3
Thiamin (mcg)	40	25	80	59
Riboflavin (mcg)	60	60	100	252
Niacin (mcg)	250	250	1200	131
Vitamin B_6 (mcg)	15 mcg/g protein intake	15	63	66
Folic acid (mcg)	4	4	10	8
Pantothenic acid (mcg)	300	300	450	489
Vitamin B_{12} (mcg)	0.15	0.15	0.25	0.56
Biotin (mcg)	1.5	1	2.5	3.1
Inositol (mg)	4	20	5.5	20
Choline (mg)	7	13	10	23
Calcium (mg)	5	50	75	186
Phosphorus (mg)	25	25	65	145
Magnesium (mg)	6	6	8	20
Iron (mg)	1	0.1	1.5	0.08
Iodine (mcg)	5	4–9	10	7
Copper (mcg)	60	25–60	80	20
Zinc (mg)	0.5	0.1–0.5	0.65	0.6
Manganese (mcg)	5	1.5	5–160	3
Sodium (mEq)	0.9	1	1.7	3.3
Potassium (mEq)	2.1	2.1	2.7	6
Chloride (mEq)	1.6	1.6	2.3	4.6
Osmolarity (mOsm)	—	11.3	16–18.4	40

[a]Committee on Nutrition, American Academy of Pediatrics.
[b]Protein of nutritional quality equal to casein.
[c]Includes 300 mg of essential fatty acids

nutrients. Pureed meats may be introduced as an early complementary food to meet iron, zinc, and protein needs. Single-ingredient complementary foods are introduced one at a time at 3- to 4-day intervals before a new food is given to assess for allergy or intolerance. Fruit juice is not necessary, and if given should be in a cup, not a bottle, and less than 4 oz/day. Whole cow's milk can be introduced after the first year of life. Non-soy plant-based milks (eg, oat, rice, almond) do not contain a comparable nutrient profile to cow milk and should not be considered an appropriate alternative when planning a toddler's diet.

While breast milk, dairy, soy, legume, and other vegetable sources of protein can provide adequate protein for growth, vegetarian foods are impractical as sources of iron or zinc. A vegetarian diet places older breast-fed infants and toddlers at risk for iron and zinc deficiency because of their high requirements during rapid growth and because animal-based foods are best sources of these nutrients. To meet requirements, infants and toddlers consuming vegetarian diets should be offered fortified foods, including cereals and formula and may also require daily supplementation of iron and zinc. A vegan diet that omits all animal protein sources will require supplementation of vitamin B_{12} as well. Guidance from a pediatric registered dietitian is suggested for families seeking for their infant or toddler to follow a vegetarian or vegan diet to ensure adequate protein, calorie, vitamin, and micronutrient intakes.

Results of large-scale randomized controlled trials have shifted recommended practice around peanut consumption in infancy by the AAP and National Institute of Allergy and Infectious Diseases (NIAID). For infants with severe eczema or egg allergy but without evidence of active peanut sensitization by skin prick test or specific peanut IgE, introduction of 6–7 g/wk of peanut protein served as a puree is recommended to begin at 4–6 months to reduce the risk of peanut allergy. Infants with less severe eczema are recommended to start consuming peanut purees around 6 months. Furthermore, it was the expert opinion of the NIAID panel that infants without risk factors for food allergy should have age-appropriate peanut-containing products introduced into the diet with other purees and solid foods in a manner consistent with familial and cultural norms.

Fleischer DM et al: A consensus approach to the primary prevention of food allergy through nutrition: guidance from the American Academy of Allergy, Asthma, and Immunology; American College of Allergy, Asthma, and Immunology; and the Canadian Society for Allergy and Clinical Immunology. J Allergy Clin Immunol Pract 2021 Jan;9(1):22-43.e4. doi: 10.1016/j.jaip.2020.11.002 [PMID: 33250376].

Merritt RJ et al: NASPGHAN Committee on Nutrition. North American Society for Pediatric Gastroenterology, Hepatology, and Nutrition Position Paper: Plant-based milks. J Pediatr Gastroenterol Nutr 2020 Aug;71(2):276–281. doi: 10.1097/MPG.0000000000002799 [PMID: 32732790].

SPECIAL DIETARY PRODUCTS FOR INFANTS

Table 11–16 offers a comprehensive overview and comparison of various infant formulas.

Soy Protein Formulas

The medical indications for soy formulas are rare: galactosemia and hereditary lactase deficiency. Soy formulas provide an option when a vegetarian diet is preferred. Soy protein formulas are often used in cases of suspected intolerance to cow's milk protein, though cow's milk hydrolysate formulas are preferred because 30% and 40% of infants intolerant to cow's milk protein will also react to soy protein. In contrast to this T-cell–mediated protein intolerance, those infants with less commonly documented IgE-mediated allergy to cow's milk protein do not typically cross-react to soy formula. Soy formula is not considered suitable for use with preterm neonates. Infants with congenital hypothyroidism receiving soy formula require close monitoring of free thyroxine and thyroid-stimulating hormone (TSH) measurements and may need increased hormone replacement to achieve normal thyroid function tests.

Semielemental & Elemental Formulas

Semielemental formulas include protein hydrolysate formulas. The major nitrogen source of most of these products is casein hydrolysate, supplemented with selected amino acids, but partial hydrolysates of whey are also available. These formulas contain an abundance of EFA from vegetable oil; certain brands also provide substantial amounts of MCTs. Elemental formulas are available with free amino acids and varying levels and types of fat components.

Semi-elemental and elemental formulas are invaluable for infants with significant malabsorption syndromes. They are also effective in term infants who cannot tolerate cow's milk and soy protein. The nutrient profiles of these formulas were not developed for the preterm infant and must be used cautiously, with clear indication and close monitoring in this population.

Burris AD et al: Cow's milk protein allergy in term and preterm infants: clinical manifestations, immunologic pathophysiology, and management strategies. Neoreviews 2020 Dec;21(12): e795–e808. doi:10.1542/neo.21-12-e795 [PMID: 33262206].

De Silva D et al: European Academy of Allergy, Clinical Immunology Food Allergy, Anaphylaxis Guidelines Group. Preventing food allergy in infancy and childhood: systematic review of randomised controlled trials. Pediatr Allergy Immunol 2020 Oct;31(7):813–826. doi: 10.1111/pai.13273. Epub 2020 Jun 18 [PMID: 32396244].

Formula Additives

Occasionally, it may be necessary to increase the caloric density of an infant feeding to provide more calories or to restrict

Table 11–16. Major categories of infant formulas.

Category	Examples	Features and Comments
Cow-milk protein	Similac Advance *(48:52 whey:casein ratio)* Similac 24 with iron Enfamil NeuroPro Enfamil Enspire	With lactose
Partially hydrolyzed cow-milk and whey protein	Good Start Gentle *(100% whey)* Similac Total Comfort *(Hydrolyzed protein)* Gentlease Good Start Soothe	Reduced lactose; not hypoallergenic but may prevent atopic disease
Cow-milk protein without lactose	Similac Sensitive *(18:82 whey:casein ratio)*	Lactose free
Soy protein	Similac soy isomil Isomil Prosobee	Lactose free; not for premature infants
Premature (NICU only)	Similac special care *(60:40 20&24 kcal; 50:50 30 kcal whey:casein ratio)* Enfamil Premature	Cow-milk protein, reduced lactose, 40%–50% fat as MCT
Premature transitional (post NICU discharge/not for full-term infant)	NeoSure *(50:50 whey:casein ratio)* EnfaCare	Standard at 22 kcal/oz; cow-milk protein, reduced lactose, 25% fat as MCT
Semielemental/hydrolyzed	Alimentum *(hydrolyzed protein)* Pregestimil *(hydrolyzed protein)* Nutramigen *(hydrolyzed protein)* Gerber extensive HA	Extensively hydrolyzed formula. Contains MCT (Alimentum 33%, Pregestimil 55%, Nutramigen 0%). Hydrolyzed casein, lactose free. Used for protein allergy and malabsorption.
Elemental	EleCare Infant Neocate Infant Puramino Alfamino Infant	Free amino acids and with MCT (EleCare 33%). Used in severe protein allergy or malabsorption.
Fat modified (high MCT)	Enfaport *(60:40 whey:casein ratio)*	30 kcal/oz concentrate; cow-milk protein, lactose free, 83% fat as MCT. Typically used for chylous effusions, lymphatic anomalies, or FA oxidation defects

fluid intake. Concentrating formula to 24–26 kcal/oz is usually well tolerated, delivers an acceptable renal solute load, and increases the density of all the nutrients. Beyond this, individual macronutrient additives (Table 11–17) are usually used to achieve the desired caloric density (up to 30 kcal/oz) based on the infant's needs and underlying condition(s). A pediatric dietitian can provide guidance in formulating calorically dense infant formula feedings. The caloric density of breast milk can be increased by adding infant formula powder or any of the additives used with infant formula. Because of their specialized nutrient composition, human milk fortifiers are generally used only for preterm infants.

Special Formulas

Special formulas are those in which one component, often an amino acid, is reduced in concentration or removed for the dietary management of a specific inborn metabolic disease.

Also included under this heading are formulas designed for specific disease states, such as hepatic failure, pulmonary failure with chronic carbon dioxide retention, and renal failure. Complete information regarding the composition of formulas can be found in reference texts and in the manufacturers' literature.

NUTRITION FOR CHILDREN 2 YEARS & OLDER

Because diet impacts overall health as well as the development of chronic diseases such as diabetes, obesity, and cardiovascular disease, teaching healthy eating behaviors at a young age is an important preventative measure.

Salient features of the DGA for children older than 2 years include the following:

1. Three regular meals per day, ideally eaten together as a family, and one or two healthy snacks.

Table 11–17. Common infant formula additives.

Additive	Kcal/g	Kcal/Tbsp	Kcal/mL	Comments
Dry rice cereal	3.75	15	—	Thickens formula but not breast milk
Benecalorie (Nestle)	7.7	112.5 (2.4 g protein)	7.5	High-calorie liquid supplement; calcium caseinate, high oleic sunflower oil, mono- and di-glycerides (7 g protein/44 mL container)
MCT oil (Mead Johnson)	8.3	116	7.7	Not a source of essential fatty acids
Microlipid (Nestle)	9	68.5	4.5	Safflower oil emulsion with 0.4 g linoleic acid/mL; mixes easily with enteral formulas
Vegetable oil	9	124	8.3	Does not mix well
Beneprotein (Nestle)	3.6	16.7 (4 g protein);	—	Whey protein, soy lecithin (25 kcal/scoop); 1 scoop = 7 g
Duocal (Nutricia)	4.9	42	—	Protein-free mix of hydrolyzed corn starch (60% kcal) and fat (35% MCT)

MCT, medium-chain triglyceride.

2. *A variety of foods*: diet should be nutritionally complete and promote optimal growth and activity.

3. Choose a variety of vegetables of all types, including seasonally fresh vegetables, as well as frozen and canned varieties.

4. Choose a variety of fruits, especially whole fruits. No added sugar canned fruits, or fruits canned in juice or light syrup, as well as dried no-added-sugar fruits and frozen fruits can be healthy choices when fresh fruit is not available.

5. Eat grains, at least half of which are whole grains.

6. Dairy products in moderation, including low fat or fat-free milk, yogurt, cheese and/or lactose free versions and fortified soy beverages and yogurt as alternatives. Encourage plain drinking water for thirst and hydration between meals.

7. Eat a variety of protein foods, including lean meats, poultry, and eggs; seafood, beans, peas, lentils, nuts, seeds, and soy products, with portions appropriate for age.

8. Include healthy oils such as vegetable and olive oils, as well as oils found naturally in foods such as seafood and nuts/seeds. Limit saturated fat to less than 10% of total calories starting at age 2.

9. Limit added sugars to less than 10% of total daily calories per day starting at age 2. This includes sugar sweetened beverages (eg, regular soda, juice drinks, sports drink, and fruit flavored drinks with sugar), as these drinks displace nutrient-dense beverages and foods.

10. Choose foods lower in sodium and minimize the regular consumption of highly processed foods, including canned foods, prepackaged frozen meals, and fast-food items.

Lifestyle counseling for children should also include maintenance of a body mass index (BMI) in the healthy range; regular physical activity, limiting sedentary behaviors; avoidance of smoking; and screening for hypertension starting at age 3 years. Current recommendations from the National Heart Lung and Blood Institute are to routinely screen all children for familial hyperlipidemia using a fasting or non-fasting lipid panel once at age 9–11, and to consider screening children at younger ages who have additional risk factors (obesity, diabetes, family history of early onset cardiovascular disease). The preferred time for screening occurs before puberty, when hormonal changes render lipids unreliable in predicting levels in adulthood.

PICKY EATING

Picky eating can cause considerable distress for parents/caregivers, negatively impact family relationships, and may lead to nutritional inadequacy and weight gain concerns. While there is currently no consensus definition as to what defines picky eating, there are general characteristics to consider. Children with infant feeding issues, premature birth, history of illnesses, as well as those with autism or ADHD may have a higher prevalence of picky eating. As part of normal development, toddlers and young children seek to assert independence and control over their environments. This can manifest in selective behaviors with regard to what and how much to eat. It is important to differentiate between problematic and non-problematic picky eating. Neophobia is often seen in young children with initial refusal to eat or try certain foods. New foods can take 8–10 exposures before acceptance. Children may also exhibit erratic and inconsistent intake, often reflecting a decline in calorie needs/kg and a normal slower rate of growth compared to infancy. These behaviors usually resolve on their own. In the absence of growth faltering and significant dietary restrictions, children are adept at eating what they need over time when they are offered a variety of nourishing choices. Characteristics associated with problematic picky eating include limited total dietary/calorie intake, decreased variety of foods, increased sensory sensitivity to taste, texture, and smell, small range of liked foods, avoidance of mealtimes, disinterest in food and eating, and growth/weight gain concerns.

Addressing picky eating involves a family centered intervention plan, as behaviors of parents/caregivers and the child are intertwined. Allowing the child to graze throughout the day, pressuring or forcing a child to eat, offering rewards for eating, or punishing for failure to eat should be discouraged. Parents/caregivers should be encouraged to establish a structured meal/snack schedule, eat as a family to model desirable behavior, encourage the child to help with food preparation, serve a variety of food choices, and ultimately allow the child to decide how much they choose to eat.

It is important to distinguish between picky eating and avoidant/restrictive food intake disorder (ARFID). ARFID is a relatively new disease diagnosis in *Diagnostic and Statistical Manual of Mental Disorders*, 5th Edition (DSM-5) and International Classification of Diseases, 11th Revision (ICD-11). ARFID can be a diagnostic and therapeutic dilemma for many health professionals. Patients with ARFID have a lack of interest in eating or avoidance of certain foods, which may result in micronutrient deficiencies, weight loss or lack of expected weight gain, dependence on tube feeding, nutritional supplements, and impaired psychosocial functioning. The symptoms cannot be explained by a current medical condition or co-occurring other psychiatric disorders. ARFID can occur in normal weight and overweight children, where energy intake may be maintained but overall diet quality is poor. Nutrient deficiencies commonly observed are B vitamins, vitamin C, vitamin K, vitamin D, zinc, potassium, iron, as well as inadequate protein and calories. Treatment strategies will need to be adapted to age, development, severity of symptoms, and degree of undernutrition. A multidisciplinary team can address increasing calories and nutrient intake with oral nutrition supplements, need for micronutrient supplementation and biochemical assessment/monitoring, temporary use of enteral feedings, and behavior modification/psychological treatments as needed. See the section on Pediatric Malnutrition for additional considerations.

Adolescent Nutrition

Adolescence represents a time of significant change, encompassing physiologic, social, cognitive, and psychological alterations that interplay to impact the nutritional needs of this age group. Globally there is a public health crisis for adolescents, with the prevalence of overweight and obesity rising while simultaneously a high burden of undernutrition, especially in resource-limited countries, remains a major factor

contributing to intergenerational malnutrition (see sections on Malnutrition and Obesity).

Multiple factors impact nutritional adequacy in this age group, including increased independence in food choices, increased influence of peers, decreased vegetable, fruit, and overall fiber intake, increased consumption of processed and energy dense/low nutrient quality foods, and decreased physical activity. Food insecurity remains a major factor for many. Adolescence is also a period where youth are more likely to experiment with fad diets based on the prevalence of dieting culture and body image issues, influenced and reinforced by social medial content.

Pregnancy in undernourished and/or stunted teens presents many risks for the mother and newborn, including small for gestational age births, premature births, anemia in mother and greater risk for infant ID, increased risk for stillbirth, and greater risk of preeclampsia and eclampsia, systemic infections, and maternal mortality. Addressing nutritional needs of this high-risk group is required to break the cycle of intergenerational growth failure and poverty.

Dietary Guidelines for Americans 2020–2025: https://dietaryguielines.gov.

Stewart J et al: Hyperlipidemia. Pediatr Rev 2020 Aug;41(8): 393–402. doi: 10.1542/pir.2019-0053 [PMID: 32737252].

Taylor CM, Emmett PM. Picky eating in children: causes and consequences. Proc Nutr So 2019 May;78(2):161–169. doi: 10.1017/S0029665118002586 [PMID: 30392488].

USDA MyPlate healthing eating guide: https://myplate.gov.

Zimmerman J, Fisher M: Avoidant/restrictive food intake disorder (ARFID). Curr Probl Pediatr Adolesc Health Care 2017 Apr;47(4):95–103. doi: 10.1016/j.cppeds.2017.02.005 [PMID: 28532967].

PEDIATRIC MALNUTRITION

ESSENTIALS OF DIAGNOSIS

► Imbalance between nutrient requirements and intake leading to deficit in energy, protein, micronutrients, or all of the above that may negatively affect growth, development, and other relevant outcomes. It can be illness or non-illness related.

► Wasting is defined as being too thin for height and is commonly seen in periods of acute undernutrition.

► Stunting is defined as being too short for age with length z-score −2 and is more prevalent with chronic undernutrition.

► Most common cause for malnutrition is insufficient caloric intake.

► The most common micronutrient deficiencies associated with malnutrition are iron and zinc.

General Considerations

The causes of pediatric malnutrition are usually multifactorial in origin. In developed countries it is often seen in the setting of acute or chronic illness, with estimates of 25% of hospitalized children experiencing acute malnutrition. However, non-illness–related causes including psychosocial dynamics and feeding issues are prominent as well. In resource limited countries, food scarcity and limited variety interplay with the burden of acute and chronic infections and respiratory/diarrheal diseases leading to high rates of malnutrition globally.

Classification

The severity assessment of undernutrition is essential because it dictates management. To assess malnutrition effectively, it is crucial to evaluate various aspects of growth, including weight gain velocity (Table 11–1), linear growth velocity, weight for length, BMI (Body Mass Index), and head growth. These growth and anthropometric parameters should be measured longitudinally and plotted on the appropriate growth chart for the child's sex, age (corrected if premature), and, if known, on growth charts created for genetic conditions such as trisomy 21 or Turner syndrome.

The AAP and US Centers for Disease Control and Prevention (CDC) recommend the 2006 WHO charts for children up to 2 years of age who are measured supine for length. The CDC 2000 growth charts are recommended for children and adolescents (age 2–20 years) when measured with a standing height. The severity of malnutrition (mild, moderate, or severe) may be determined by plotting the z-score (standard deviation [SD] from the mean) for each of these anthropometric values (Table 11–18).

Infants younger than 6 months are vulnerable to linear growth faltering, and use of weight-for-length alone may underestimate the degree of malnutrition. Weight gain velocity should be strongly considered in this case. Bilateral pitting edema without an alternative explanation (such as heart, liver, or renal disease) is characteristic of **kwashiorkor**. Edema in the setting of malnutrition classifies as **severe malnutrition regardless of weight status** (Figure 11–3).

▶ Approach to the Child With Suspected Undernutrition

The term *failure to thrive* is not preferred as it is not patient centered, lacks specificity, and implies neglect or failure of the care giver. *Growth faltering* is the more widely accepted terminology used to refer to a slower rate of weight gain than expected for age and gender. When growth faltering is identified, a more thorough investigation is essential to determine the degree of undernutrition and plan for treatment options.

1. **Anthropometrics and growth: Assess** severity using multiple growth data points when available. Degree of undernutrition can still be classified when single data points are available for weight, length or height, BMI, and mid-upper arm circumference by assessing z-scores.

2. **Comprehensive history:** Include details of diet intake and feeding patterns (including restrictive intake, grazing feeding pattern, inappropriate foods for age and development, excessive juice, sugar-sweetened beverages, or water intake); past medical history, including birth and developmental history; family history; social history; and review of systems. Assess intake of all food groups.

3. **Physical examination:** Include careful examination of skin (for rashes), mouth, eyes, nails, and hair for signs of micronutrient and protein deficiencies, as well as for abnormal neurologic function (eg, loss of deep tendon reflexes, abnormal strength, and tone), refer to Table 11–14.

4. **Laboratory studies:** Laboratory studies are generally of low yield for diagnosis of growth faltering in the absence of other findings. Typical screening laboratories include a chemistry panel, complete blood count, and iron panel, including ferritin (and marker of inflammation, eg, C-reactive protein [CRP] or erythrocyte sedimentation rate [ESR]). Thyroid function testing is indicated for linear growth faltering. Serology for celiac disease may also be warranted for toddlers, especially with short stature or linear growth faltering.

5. **Assess the risk for refeeding syndrome:** Refeeding syndrome may occur with nutritional rehabilitation. During

Table 11–18. Nutritional status assessment and classification of malnutrition.

Method	No Malnutrition	Mild Malnutrition	Moderate Malnutrition	Severe Malnutrition
Weight for height percent of median	> 90%	80%–89%	70%–79%	< 70%
Weight for height z-score	> −1	−1 to −1.9	−2 to −2.9	< −3
BMI z-score*	> −1	−1 to −1.9	−2 to −2.9	< −3
Length/height z-score*	Not applicable	No data but z-score* < −2 suggest stunting	No data but z score* < −2 suggest stunting	< −3
MUAC for children 6–59 mo old			11.5–12.4 cm	< 11.5 cm

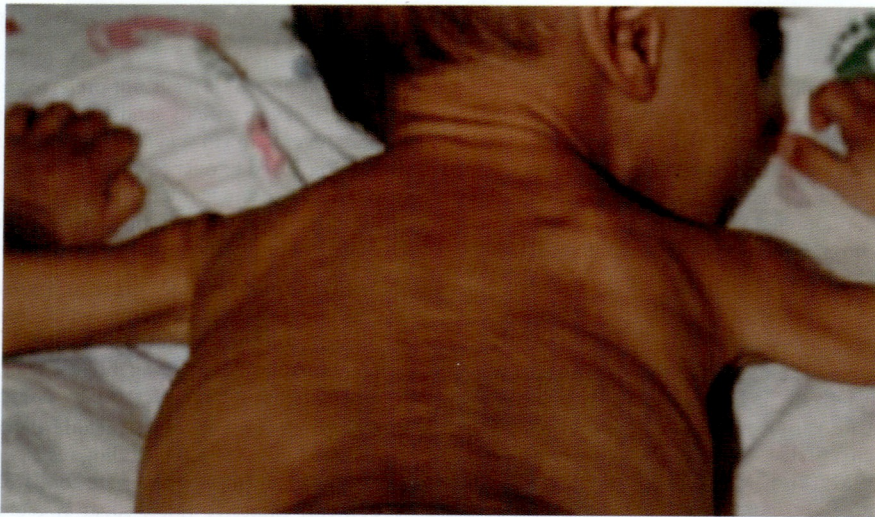

▲ **Figure 11–3.** 1-year-old with severe malnutrition. Note the lack of subcutaneous fat tissue and the profound weakness of the patient who was not able to sit or lift his head up.

refeeding, increased glucose levels lead to increased insulin and decreased glucagon secretion. Insulin stimulates potassium absorption into the cells through the sodium-potassium ATPase symporter, which also transports glucose into the cells. Magnesium and phosphate are also taken up into the cells. Water follows by osmosis. *These processes decrease the serum levels of phosphate, potassium, and magnesium, all of which are depleted prior to refeeding in severe malnutrition.* The clinical features of the refeeding syndrome occur because of the functional deficits of these electrolytes (congestive cardiac failure and cardiac arrhythmia). It is essential to monitor for hypophosphatemia, hypokalemia, hypomagnesemia, and hyperglycemia for the first roughly 3–4 days in which caloric intake is advanced to the goal desired for weight gain during nutritional rehabilitation (until stable). Calorie intake should be increased slowly to avoid metabolic instability. Refer to Table 11–19 for risk factors for refeeding syndrome.

► **Treatment**

Caloric supplementation should start immediately while etiology is investigated. Consultation with a speech therapist for a suck-and-swallow evaluation should be considered if the history suggests difficulty with oral feeds. Hospitalization is indicated for cases of severe and edematous malnutrition due to the risk for refeeding syndrome, as well as for patients with suboptimal response after 2–3 months of outpatient management. Every effort to maintain breast-feeding relationship in breast-fed infants should be made, including lactation support and expressing and fortification of the breastmilk.

Caregiver feeding behaviors are as essential as caloric intake. Parents should be encouraged to be responsive to the infant and toddlers' cues of hunger and satiety and to have a structured schedule with meals and snacks provided every 2–3 hours, ideally eating with other family members. Poor eating is often a learned behavior in response to parenting style and family dynamics. Strong and persistent food refusals that limit overall food intake and variety warrant further investigation (See section on Picky Eating and ARFID). Grazing behavior should be avoided because it interferes with intake at mealtime. The number of calories from oral nutritional supplements should be carefully considered so it does not blunt the child's appetite. However, children with oral motor difficulties may need to consume more calories

Table 11–19. Risk factors for refeeding syndrome.

Patients are at risk for refeeding syndrome if they have one or more of the following:
• Severe malnutrition (marasmus or kwashiorkor)
• Weight loss ≥ 15% in the past 3–6 mo.
• Little or no nutritional intake for > 10 days.
• Low levels of potassium, phosphate, or magnesium before feeding
Patients are at risk for refeeding syndrome if they have two or more of the following:
• Moderate malnutrition
• Weight loss ≥ 10% in the past 3–6 mo
• Little or no nutritional intake for ≥ 5 days
• History of alcohol misuse or drugs, including insulin, chemotherapy, antacids, or diuretics

in a liquid form. Consultation with a pediatric dietitian can be helpful for educating the family. Children whose households are chaotic and children who are abused, neglected, or exposed to poorly controlled mental illness may be described as poor eaters, and may fail to gain. Careful assessment of the social environment of such children is critical, and disposition options may include support services, close medical follow-up visits, counseling, and even foster placement.

The same anthropometric measures used to diagnosis malnutrition should be used to measure progress and recovery from the malnourished state. The target recovery rate of weight gain is 150% of the average rate of weight gain per age. Many children with malnutrition require micronutrient supplementation. This should be guided by assessment of diet adequacy, presence of physical findings, biochemical measures, and severity of malnutrition. For details on the treatment of kwashiorkor, we recommend reviewing the specific guidelines from the WHO, including empiric antibiotics.

American Academy of Pediatrics: Growth faltering in newborns and infants web resource: Aap.org/en/patient-care/newborn-and-infant-nutrition/growth-faltering-in-newborns-and-infants/. Accessed July 24, 2023.

Becker P et al: Consensus Statement of the Academy of Nutrition and Dietetics/American Society for Parenteral and Enteral Nutrition: Indicators recommended for the identification and documentation of pediatric malnutrition (undernutrition). Nutr Clin Pract 2015 Feb;30(1):147–161. doi: 10.1177/0884533614557642 [PMID: 25422273].

Bhutta AZ et al: Severe childhood malnutrition. Nat Rev Dis Primers 2017 Sep 21;3:17067. doi: 10.1038/NRDP.2017.67. Review [PMID: 28933421].

da Silva JSV et al; Parenteral Nutrition Safety and Clinical Practice Committees, American Society for Parenteral and Enteral Nutrition: ASPEN consensus recommendations for refeeding syndrome. Nutr Clin Pract 2020 Apr;35(2):178–195. doi: 10.1002/ncp.10474 [PMID: 32115791].

PEDIATRIC OVERWEIGHT & OBESITY

ESSENTIALS OF DIAGNOSIS & TYPICAL FEATURES

► Excessive rate of weight gain; upward change in BMI percentiles (see also Chapter 3 for obesity in adolescents).

► BMI for age between the 85th and 95th percentiles indicates overweight.

► BMI for age greater than 95th percentile indicates obesity and is associated with increased risk of secondary complications.

► BMI for age greater than 99th percentile, or a BMI that exceeds 120% of the 95th percentile, indicates severe obesity and a higher risk of complications.

► General Considerations

The prevalence of childhood and adolescent obesity has increased rapidly in the United States and many other parts of the world. As of 2018, NHANES data show that 19.3% of 2- to 19-year-olds in the United States have obesity and 6.1% have severe obesity, with even higher rates among minority and economically disadvantaged children. Obesity prevalence increases with age: 13.4% among 2- to 5-year-olds, 20.3% among 6- to 11-year-olds, 21.2% among 12- to 19-year-olds, and 42.4% among all adults. The increasing prevalence of childhood obesity is related to a complex combination of socioeconomic, epigenetic, and biological factors. A significant increase in childhood obesity prevalence occurred during the coronavirus disease-19 (COVID-19) pandemic, affecting minority and economically disadvantaged children most severely.

Childhood obesity, especially when severe, is associated with significant comorbidities. In 2023, the AAP published a comprehensive Clinical Practice Guideline for the Evaluation and Treatment of Children and Adolescents with Obesity including guidance on diagnosis and management of comorbid conditions. See Table 11–20 for a list of complications from childhood obesity.

Hampl SE et al: Clinical practice guideline for the evaluation and treatment of children and adolescents with obesity. Pediatrics 2023 Feb 1;151(2):e2022060640. doi: 10.1542/peds.2022-060640 [PMID: 36622115].

► Clinical Findings

A. Definitions

BMI is the standard measure of obesity in adults and children. BMI is correlated with more accurate but less clinically feasible measures of body fatness and is calculated with readily available information: weight and height (kg/m^2). Routine plotting of the BMI on age- and gender-appropriate charts (http://www.cdc.gov/growthcharts) can identify those with excess weight. BMI between the 85th and 95th percentiles for age and sex identifies those who are overweight; BMI at or above the 95th percentile for age and sex defines obesity and is associated with increased risk of secondary complications. Severe obesity is defined as a BMI for age and sex at or above the 99th percentile. An alternative definition of severe obesity provides a framework for clinicians to better quantify severe obesity in children as class 2 if greater than 120%–140% of the 95th percentile or greater than 35 kg/m^2, or class 3 if greater than 140% of the 95th percentile or greater than 40 kg/m^2 and correspond to the class definitions of obesity in adulthood. The degree of obesity as a percent of the 95th percentile can be tracked on special growth charts created for this purpose. An upward change in BMI percentiles should prompt evaluation and possible treatment. For

Table 11–20. Selected complications of childhood obesity.

System	Condition	Note	Review of Systems
Pulmonary	Obstructive sleep apnea	13%–33% of youth with obesity	Snoring, apnea, poor sleep, nocturnal enuresis, AM headaches, fatigue, poor school performance
	Obesity-hypoventilation syndrome	Severe obesity, restrictive lung disease, may lead to right heart failure	Dyspnea, edema, somnolence
Cardiovascular	Hypertension	3 occasions > 95th percentile on NHLBI tables for gender, age, and height	
	Lipid abnormalities	Total cholesterol 170–199 borderline, > 200 high LDL 110–129 borderline, > 130 high, HDL < 40 low	
		TG > 150 high	Assess for pancreatitis if TG > 400, nausea, vomiting, abdominal pain
GI	NAFLD	10%–25% of youth with obesity; elevated ALT; rule out other liver disease if ALT highly elevated; steatohepatitis may progress to fibrosis, cirrhosis	Commonly asymptomatic; rarely abdominal pain: vague, recurrent
	GERD	Increased abdominal pressure	Abdominal pain: heartburn
	Gallstones	Associated with rapid weight loss	Abdominal pain: right upper or epigastric
	Constipation	Associated with inactivity, r/o encopresis	Abdominal pain: distension, hard infrequent stools, soiling/incontinence
Endocrine	Impaired glucose metabolism	Elevated fasting glucose = 100–125	Acanthosis nigricans
		Impaired glucose tolerance = 2-h OGTT 140–199	
	T2DM	Random glucose > 200 with symptoms; fasting glucose > 126, 2-h OGTT > 200, HgA_{1c} > 6.5	Polyuria and polydipsia, unintentional weight loss
	PCOS	Diagnoses requires two of three: Hyperandrogenism Oligomenorrhea Polycystic ovaries—ultrasound not used in criteria for adolescents; insulin resistance; risk of infertility and endometrial cancer	Oligomenorrhea (< 9 menses/y), hyperandrogenism Hyperandrogenism: hirsutism, acne
	Hypothyroid	Associated with poor linear growth	Asymptomatic until uncompensated: linear growth failure, cold intolerance, decline in school performance, coarse features, thin hair
Neurology/ophthalmology	Pseudotumor cerebri	Papilledema, vision loss possible, consult neuro/ophthalmology	Headaches (severe, recurrent), often worse in AM
Orthopedic	Blount disease	Stress injury to medial tibial growth plate, often painless	Bowed legs, ± knee pain
	SCFE	More likely to progress to bilateral disease in obese	Hip, groin, or knee pain; limp with leg held in external rotation
Dermatology	Acanthosis nigricans	Secondary effect of elevated insulin	Darkening of skin on neck, axillae, groin, ± skin tags
	Intertrigo/furunculosis/panniculitis	Examine skin folds, pannus; bacteria, and/or yeast	Rash/infection in skin folds, inflammatory papules
	Hidradenitis suppurativa	Draining cysts in axillae or groin	Rash/infection in skin folds, blocked glands, recurrent and unrelenting

(Continued)

Table 11–20. Selected complications of childhood obesity. (*Continued*)

System	Condition	Note	Review of Systems
Psychiatric	Depression/anxiety	May lead to worsening obesity if untreated	Full psycho/social review, including mood, school performance, peer and family relationships
	Eating disorder	Assess for binging ± purging behavior	
	History of abuse	Increases risk of severe obesity	

ALT, alanine aminotransferase; GERD, gastroesophageal reflux disease; GI, gastrointestinal; HDL, high-density lipoprotein; HgA$_{1C}$, hemoglobin A$_{1C}$; LDL, low-density lipoprotein; NAFLD, nonalcoholic fatty liver disease; NHLBI, National Heart, Lung, and Blood Institute; OGTT, oral glucose tolerance test; PCOS, polycystic ovarian syndrome; SCFE, slipped capital femoral epiphysis; T2DM, type 2 diabetes mellitus; TG, triglycerides.

children younger than 2 years, weight for length greater than 95th percentile indicates overweight and warrants further assessment of energy intake and feeding behaviors.

B. Risk Factors

There are multiple risk factors for developing obesity, reflecting the complex relationships between genetic and environmental factors. Family history is a strong risk factor. Parental obesity, especially in both parents, strongly increases the odds of a child having obesity in childhood and adulthood.

Risk factors in the home environment offer targets for intervention. Consumption of sugar-sweetened beverages, lack of family meals, large portion sizes, foods prepared outside the home, excess screen time, poor sleep, and lack of activity are all associated with risk of excessive weight gain.

C. Assessment

Early recognition of rapid weight gain or high-risk behaviors is important. Anticipatory guidance or intervention earlier in childhood and before weight gain becomes severe is more likely to be successful than delayed intervention. Routine evaluation at well-child visits should include the following:

1. Measurement of weight and height, calculation of BMI, and plotting on age- and sex-appropriate growth charts (http://www.cdc.gov/growthcharts). Evaluate for upward crossing of BMI percentiles.

2. History regarding diet and activity patterns (Table 11–21); family history, and review of systems. Physical examination should include blood pressure measurement, distribution of adiposity (central vs generalized), though waist circumference standards for age and sex are not available for US children; markers of comorbidities, such as acanthosis nigricans, hirsutism, hepatomegaly, and orthopedic abnormalities; and physical stigmata of genetic syndromes (eg, Prader-Willi syndrome).

3. Laboratory studies are recommended as follows for children beginning by age 10 years or at onset of puberty. Consider testing for comorbid conditions at younger ages when obesity is severe:

   - Overweight with personal or family history of heart disease risk factors—fasting lipid profile, fasting glucose and/or hemoglobin A$_{1C}$, alanine aminotransferase (ALT).
   - Obesity—fasting lipid profile, fasting glucose and/or hemoglobin A$_{1C}$, ALT.
   - Other studies should be guided by findings in the history and physical.
   - When severe obesity is early in onset (typically by age 2–5 years), consider genetic testing for monogenic severe obesity disorders, especially when hyperphagia and/or apparently slowed metabolism is present. Melanocortin pathway agonist therapy has recently been approved by the Food and Drug Administration (FDA) to treat some of these rare disorders.

Table 11–21. Suggested areas for assessment of diet and activity patterns.

Diet
- Portion sizes: adult portions for young children
- Frequency of meals away from home (restaurants or takeout)
- Frequency/amounts of sugar-sweetened beverages (soda, juice drinks)
- Meal and snack pattern: structured vs grazing, skipping meals
- Frequency of eating fruits and vegetables
- Frequency of family meals
- Television viewing while eating

Activity
- Time spent in sedentary activity: television, video games, computer, or smartphone
- Time spent in vigorous activity: organized sports, physical education, free play
- Activities of daily living: walking to school, chores, yard work
- Sleep duration: risk of obesity is increased with inadequate sleep

Clément K et al; Setmelanotide POMC and LEPR Phase 3 Trial Investigators: Efficacy and safety of setmelanotide, an MC4R agonist, in individuals with severe obesity due to LEPR or POMC deficiency: single-arm, open-label, multicentre, phase 3 trials. Lancet Diabetes Endocrinol 2020 Dec;8(12):960–970. Epub 2020 Oct 30 [PMID: 33137293].

Treatment

Treatment should be based on risk factors, including age, severity of obesity, and comorbidities, as well as family history. For children with uncomplicated obesity, the primary goal is to achieve healthy eating and activity patterns, not necessarily to achieve ideal body weight. For children with a secondary complication, improvement of the complication is an important goal. In general, weight goals for children with obesity range from weight maintenance to up to 1 lb/mo weight loss for those younger than 12 years, and up to 2 lb/wk for those older than 12 years. More rapid weight loss should be monitored for pathologic causes that may be associated with nutrient deficiencies and linear growth stunting (Table 11–22).

Treatment focused on behavior changes in the context of family involvement has been associated with sustained weight loss and decreases in BMI. The US Preventive Services Task Force has identified that behavioral interventions most likely to be successful for childhood obesity treatment are intensive, with 26 or more contact hours. Motivational interviewing is a recommended counseling approach for discussions about excess weight gain in children in the primary care setting. This form of counseling uses open-ended questioning and reflective statements to explore and resolve ambivalence toward change and accepts resistance nonjudgmentally.

Clinicians should assess the family's readiness to take action. Providers should engage the family in collaborative decision-making about which behavior change goals will be targeted and what level of intervention will be pursued. Improving dietary habits and activity levels concurrently is desirable for successful weight management. The entire family should adopt healthy eating patterns, with parents modeling healthy food choices, controlling foods brought into the home, and guiding appropriate portion sizes. Enjoyable physical activity should be promoted, and screen time should be limited. The 2023 AAP Clinical Practice Guidelines consensus recommendations emphasize that watchful waiting is not an appropriate approach to childhood obesity and that the best available treatment should be offered. While access may vary, treatment options may include intensive health behavior and lifestyle treatment, anti-obesity pharmacotherapy, and for patients with severe obesity, bariatric surgery.

Pharmacotherapy can be an adjunct to dietary, activity, and behavioral treatment. Orlistat, a lipase inhibitor, combination therapy with phentermine and topiramate, and GLP-1 agonists liraglutide and semaglutide have been FDA approved to treat obesity in patients older than 12 years. Other medications approved for use in adults are used off-label by providers who have expertise in obesity medicine. Bariatric surgery is performed in some centers for adolescents with severe obesity. In carefully selected and closely monitored patients, surgery can result in significant weight loss with a reduction or resolution of comorbidities, including type 2 diabetes, more frequently than in adults undergoing the same surgery.

Inge TH, Ryder JR: The current paradigm of bariatric surgery in adolescents. Nat Rev Gastroenterol Hepatol 2023 Jan;20(1):1–2. doi: 10.1038/s41575-022-00713-8 [PMID: 36447025].

Weghuber D et al; STEP TEENS Investigators: Once-weekly semaglutide in adolescents with obesity. N Engl J Med 2022 Dec 15;387(24):2245–2257. doi: 10.1056/NEJMoa2208601. Epub 2022 Nov 2. [PMID: 36322838].

Table 11–22. Weight management goals.

Age (y)	BMI (%)	Weight Change Goal to Achieve BMI < 85%
2–5	85–94	Maintain weight
	95–98	Maintain weight, or if complications lose 1 lb/mo
	99	Lose 1 lb/mo
6–11	85–94	Maintain weight
	95–98	Lose 1 lb/mo
	99	Lose 2 lb/wk
12–18	85–95	Maintain weight
	95–98	Lose 2 lb/wk
	99	Lose 2 lb/wk

BMI, body mass index; %, percentile for age and sex.

NUTRITION SUPPORT

ENTERAL

Indications

Enteral nutrition support is indicated when a patient cannot adequately meet nutritional needs by oral intake alone and has a functioning GI tract. This method of support can be used for short- and long-term delivery of nutrition. Even when the gut cannot absorb 100% of nutritional needs, some enteral feedings should be attempted. Enteral nutrition, full or partial, has many benefits:

1. Maintaining gut mucosal integrity and supporting the gut microbiome

2. Preserving gut-associated lymphoid tissue
3. Stimulating gut hormones and bile flow

Access Devices

Nasogastric feeding tubes can be used for supplemental enteral feedings, but generally are not used for more than 3 months because of the complications of otitis media and sinusitis. Initiation of nasogastric feeding usually requires a brief hospital stay to ensure tolerance to feedings and to allow for parental instruction in tube placement and feeding administration.

If long-term feeding support is anticipated, a more permanent feeding device, such as a gastrostomy tube, may be considered. Referral to a home care company is necessary for equipment and other services such as nursing visits and dietitian follow-up.

Initiation and advancement of tube feeding:

Table 11–23 suggests appropriate timing for initiation and advancement of drip and bolus feedings, according to a child's age. Clinical status and tolerance to feedings should ultimately guide their advancement.

In medically stable patients, the enteral feeding schedule should be developmentally appropriate (eg, 5–6 small feedings/day for a toddler). When night drip feedings are used in conjunction with daytime feeds, it is suggested that less than 50% of goal calories be delivered at night to maintain a daytime sense of hunger and satiety. This will be especially important once a transition to oral intake begins.

Monitoring

Frequent assessment of anthropometrics, medical status changes, biochemical indices, and tolerance to enteral feeds with documentation of delivered nutrition intake versus goal intake is essential in managing this nutritionally challenging population.

Mehta NM et al: Guidelines for the provision and assessment of nutrition support therapy in the pediatric critically ill patient: Society of Critical Care Medicine and American Society for Parenteral and Enteral Nutrition. J Parenter Enteral Nutr 2017 Jul; 41(5):706–742. doi: 10.1177/0148607117711387. Epub 2017 Jun 2 [PMID: 286868444].

PARENTERAL NUTRITION

Indications

A. Peripheral Parenteral Nutrition (PPN)

PPN is indicated when complete enteral feeding is temporarily impossible or undesirable. Short-term partial intravenous (IV) nutrition via a peripheral vein is a preferred alternative to administration of dextrose and electrolyte solutions alone. Because of the osmolality of the solutions required, it is usually impossible to achieve total calorie and protein needs with parenteral nutrition via a peripheral vein.

B. Total Parenteral Nutrition (TPN)

TPN should be provided only when clearly indicated. Apart from the expense, numerous risks are associated with this method of feeding (see Complications). Even when TPN is indicated, every effort should be made to provide at least a minimum of nutrients enterally to help preserve the integrity of the GI mucosa and of GI function. The primary indication for TPN is the loss of function of the GI tract that prohibits the provision of required nutrients by the enteral route. Important examples include short bowel syndrome, some congenital defects of the GI tract, and preterm birth.

In recent years, several injectable essential nutrients have been in short supply in the US pharmaceutical market. Nutrition support teams should develop clinical guidelines to ensure injectable micronutrients are available for those patients who have the greatest need, for example, preterm infants and children with long-term dependence upon TPN. Policies to promote use of enteral micronutrient preparations

Table 11–23. Guidelines for the initiation and advancement of tube feedings.

| Age | Drip Feeds | | Bolus Feeds | |
	Initiation	Advancement	Initiation (mL)	Advancement
Preterm	1–2 mL/kg/h	5–10 mL/kg q8–12 h over 5–7 day as tolerated	10–20 mL/kg	20–30 mL/kg/day as tolerated
Birth–12 mo	5–10 mL/h	5–10 mL q2–8 h	10–60	20–40 mL q3–4 h
1–6 y	10–15 mL/h	10–15 mL q2–8 h	30–90	30–60 mL q feed
6–14 y	15–20 mL/h	10–20 mL q2–8 h	60–120	60–90 mL q feed
> 14 y	20–30 mL/h	20–30 mL q2–8 h	60–120	60–120 mL q feed

can also help to reduce the reliance on parenteral supplies. National recommendations for the management of IV essential nutrient shortages are available from the American Society for Parenteral and Enteral Nutrition (ASPEN—http://www.nutritioncare.org).

Hardy G et al: Parenteral provision of micronutrients to pediatric patients: an international expert consensus paper. JPEN J Parenter Enteral Nutr 2020 Sept;44 (Suppl 2):S5–S23. doi: 10.1002/jpen.1990 [PMID: 32767589].

Parenteral Product Shortages: https://www.nutritioncare.org/ProductShortages/.

Catheter Selection & Position

An indwelling central venous catheter is preferred for long-term IV nutrition. For periods of up to 3–4 weeks, a percutaneous central venous catheter threaded into the superior vena cava from a peripheral vein can be used. For the infusion of dextrose concentrations higher than 12.5%, the tip of the catheter should be in the superior vena cava.

Complications

A. Mechanical

Mechanical complications include trauma to the adjacent tissues and organs and clotting of the catheter. Addition of heparin (1000 U/L) to the solution is an effective means of preventing this complication.

B. Septic

Septic complications are the most common cause of nonelective catheter removal. Fever over 38°C–38.5°C in a patient with a central catheter should be considered a line infection until proved otherwise. Cultures should be obtained, and IV antibiotics empirically initiated. Removing the catheter may be necessary with certain infections (eg, fungal), and catheter replacement may be deferred until infection is treated.

C. Metabolic

Components of PN solutions, including intravenous lipid emulsions (ILEs), are susceptible to oxidation when exposed to light, resulting in reactive oxygen species production. This oxidative stress can be associated with bronchopulmonary dysplasia, retinopathy of prematurity, necrotizing enterocolitis, and intestinal failure-associated liver disease (IFALD). Based on literature reviews and reports of adverse outcomes in premature infants on PN, expert recommendation is for photoprotection of PN admixtures and ILEs.

The most challenging metabolic complication is cholestasis, particularly common in preterm infants of very low birth weight with prolonged feeding intolerance, infants with congenital gut disorders requiring surgery, such as those with gastroschisis, and infants with short gut syndrome following surgical resections for disorders such as necrotizing enterocolitis. See discussion on IFALD in Chapter 22 for details.

Baskin KM et al: Evidence-based strategies and recommendations for preservation of central venous access in children. J Parenter Enteral Nutr 2019 Apr 21. doi: 10.1002/jpen.1591[PMID: 31006886].

Robinson DT et al: Recommendations for photoprotection of parenteral nutrition for premature infants: an ASPEN position paper. Nutr Clin Pract 2021;36:927–941. doi: org/10.1002/ncp.10747 [PMID: 34472142].

NUTRIENT REQUIREMENTS & DELIVERY

Energy

When patients are fed intravenously, no fat and carbohydrate intakes are unabsorbed, and no energy is used in nutrient absorption. These factors account for at least 7% of energy in the diet of the enterally fed patient. The intravenously fed patient usually expends less energy in physical activity. Average energy requirements may therefore be lower in children fed intravenously, by a total of 10%–15%. Caloric guidelines for the IV feeding of infants and young children are outlined below.

The guidelines are averages, and individuals vary considerably. Especially for critically ill children, use of indirect calorimetry to measure REE is recommended. When this is not feasible, use of the Schofield weight-height equation or WHO equation for determining energy needs without stress factors is recommended, with frequent reassessment of energy needs to avoid unintended overfeeding or underfeeding. Factors that may significantly increase the energy requirement estimates include exposure to cold environment, fever, sepsis, burns, trauma, cardiac or pulmonary disease, and catch-up growth after malnutrition. Patients should be hemodynamically stable prior to any initiation of parenteral nutrition, and then frequently assessed for ability to transition to enteral feedings.

With a few exceptions, such as some cases of respiratory insufficiency, at least 50%–60% of energy requirements are provided as glucose. Up to 40% of calories may be provided by IV fat emulsions in infants and young children. For complex or critically ill infants and children, guidance from practitioners with expertise in nutrition support (registered dietitians, physicians, pharmacists, etc) should be enlisted to formulate macronutrient composition of the infusate.

Dextrose

Dextrose is the main energy source provided by TPN. The energy density of IV dextrose (monohydrate) is 3.4 kcal/g. IV dextrose suppresses gluconeogenesis and can be oxidized directly, especially by the brain, red and white blood cells,

Table 11–24. Pediatric macronutrient guidelines for total parenteral nutrition.

	Dextrose		Amino Acids	Lipids
	mg/kg/min	g/kg/day	g/kg/day	g/kg/day
Age	50%–60% kcal		10%–20% kcal	30%–40% kcal
Preterm	Initial 5–8	Initial 7–11	Initial 1.5–2	Initial 0.5–1
	Max 11–12.5	Max 16–18	Max 3–4	Max 2.5–3.5
Birth–12 mo	Initial 6–8	Initial 9–11	Initial 1.5–2	Initial 1
	Max 11–15	Max 16–21.5	Max 3	Max 2.5–3.5
1–6 y	Initial 6–7	Initial 8–10	Initial 1–1.5	Initial 1
	Max 10–12	Max 14–17	Max 2–2.5	Max 2.5–3.5
> 6 y	Initial 5–7	Initial 8–10	Initial 1	Initial 1
	Max 9	Max 13	Max 1.5–2	Max 3
> 10 y	Initial 4–5	Initial 5–7	Initial 1	Initial 1
	Max 6–7	Max 8–10	Max 1.5–2	Max 2–3
Adolescents	Initial 2–3	Initial 3–4	Initial 1	Initial 0.5–1
	Max 5–6	Max 7–8	Max 1.5–2	Max 2

and wounds. Because of the high osmolality, concentrations of dextrose greater than 10%–12.5% cannot be delivered via a peripheral vein or improperly positioned central line.

Dosing guidelines: The standard initial quantity of dextrose administered will vary by age (Table 11–24). Tolerance to IV dextrose normally increases rapidly due to suppression of hepatic glucose production. Dextrose can be increased by 2.5 g/kg/day, by 2.5%–5%/day, or by 2–3 mg/kg/min/day if there is no glucosuria or hyperglycemia. Standard final infusates for infants via a properly positioned central venous line usually range from 15% to 25% dextrose, though concentrations of up to 30% dextrose may be used at low flow rates. Tolerance to IV dextrose loads is markedly diminished in the preterm neonate, in critically ill patients, and in hypermetabolic states. Hyperglycemia is associated with significant complications especially during the acute phase of critical illness, and IV dextrose dosing may need to be reduced and reassessed daily to promote normoglycemia.

Problems associated with IV dextrose administration include hyperglycemia, hyperosmolality, and glucosuria (often with osmotic diuresis and dehydration). Possible causes of hyperglycemia include the following: (1) inadvertent infusion of higher dextrose rates than ordered and achieving higher glucose concentrations than desired, (2) uneven flow rate, (3) sepsis, (4) persistent glucose production in stress situations (including administration of catecholamines or corticosteroids), and (5) pancreatitis. If these causes have been addressed and severe hyperglycemia persists, the use of insulin may be considered. IV insulin reduces hyperglycemia by suppressing hepatic glucose production

and increasing glucose uptake by muscle and fat tissues. The use of IV insulin also increases the risk of hypoglycemia. Excessive dextrose infusion paired with insulin infusion can exceed mitochondrial oxidation capacity, produce excess reactive oxidation species leading to cell death and local and systemic inflammation. Intensive care management strategies that promote enteral feeding and reduce IV dextrose exposure have improved outcomes for critically ill patients. Hence, insulin should be used cautiously, and enteral feeding is strongly preferred. A standard IV dose is 1 U/4 g of carbohydrate, but much smaller quantities may be adequate and, usually, one starts with 0.2–0.3 U/4 g of carbohydrate.

Hypoglycemia may occur after an abrupt decrease in or cessation of IV glucose. When cyclic IV nutrition is provided, the IV glucose load should be decreased steadily for 1–2 hours prior to discontinuing the infusion. If the central line must be removed, the IV dextrose should be tapered gradually over several hours.

Oxidation rates for infused dextrose decrease with age. It is important to note that the ranges for dextrose administration provided in Table 11–24 are guidelines and that individual patients may require either less or more dextrose. Quantities of dextrose in excess of maximal glucose oxidation rates are used initially to replace depleted glycogen stores; hepatic lipogenesis occurs thereafter. Excess hepatic lipogenesis may lead to a fatty liver (steatosis). Lipogenesis produces carbon dioxide, as does glucose oxidation. Thus, excess dextrose may elevate the $Paco_2$ and aggravate respiratory insufficiency or impede weaning from a respirator.

Lipids

ILEs are an indispensable component of TPN as a noncarbohydrate energy source in an iso-osmolar solution. They provide a source of EFA and aid in the delivery of fat-soluble vitamins. The most used ILE in neonates and pediatrics are 20% lipid emulsions, which provide 2 kcal/mL or 10 kcal/g (9 kcal/g from lipid plus glycerol component). ILEs (Table 11–25) are composed of either single oil-based formulations or composite formulations with two or more oil sources. ILE are often used to provide 30%–40% of calorie needs for infants and up to 30% of calorie needs in older children and teens.

Adverse effects of ILE can include hypertriglyceridemia, fat overload syndrome, and IFALD. These can be minimized by starting with modest quantities, avoiding excessive rates of infusion, and not providing higher doses than recommended for age and clinical condition. Monitoring TGs is standard practice upon initiation and at regular intervals thereafter, especially with prematurity, sepsis, malnutrition, and prolonged TPN/ILE use. If hypertriglyceridemia occurs, it is preferable to maintain enough ILE to provide EFA versus discontinuation if possible. Dextrose load should also be evaluated with hypertriglyceridemia, as increased lipogenesis from excess glucose may be a factor.

IV lipid dosing guidelines: Check serum TGs before starting and after increasing the dose. Commence with 1 g/kg/day, given over 12–20 hours or 24 hours in small preterm infants. Advance by 0.5–1.0 g/kg/day, every 1–2 days, up to goal (see Table 11–24). As a general rule, do not increase the dose if the serum TG level is above 400 mg/dL during infusion or if the level is greater than 250 mg/dL 6–12 hours after cessation of the lipid infusion. Serum TG levels above 400–600 mg/dL may precipitate pancreatitis. In patients for whom normal amounts of IV lipid are contraindicated, 4%–8% of calories as IV lipid should be provided to prevent EFA deficiency.

Lapillonne A et al: ESPGHAN/ESPEN/ESPR/CSPEN guidelines of pediatric parenteral nutrition: lipids. Clin Nutr 2018 Dec; 37(6 Pt. B):2324–2336. doi: 10.1016/j.clin.2018.06.946 Epub 2018 Jun 18 [PMID: 30143306].

Protein

One gram of nitrogen is produced by 6.25 g of protein (1 g of protein contains 16% nitrogen). Caloric density of protein is equal to 4 kcal/g.

A. Protein Requirements

Protein requirements for IV nutrition are generally the same as those for normal oral feeding (see Table 11–2). When PN is provided to critically ill infants and children, the recommendation is for a minimum intake of 1.5 g protein/kg body weight, and optimal intakes may be higher.

B. Intravenous Amino Acid Solutions

Nitrogen requirements can be met by commercially available amino acid solutions. For infants, including preterm infants, the use of TrophAmine (McGaw) is associated with a more normal plasma amino acid profile, superior nitrogen retention, and a lower incidence of cholestasis. TrophAmine contains 60% essential amino acids, is relatively high in branched-chain amino acids, contains taurine, and is compatible with the addition of cysteine within 24–48 hours after administration. The dose of added cysteine is 40 mg/g of TrophAmine. The relatively low pH of TrophAmine enhances solubility of calcium and phosphorus.

C. Dosing Guidelines

Amino acids can be started at 1–2 g/kg/day in most patients (see Table 11–24). In severely malnourished infants, the initial amount should be 1 g/kg/day. In infants of very low birth weight, there is evidence that higher initial amounts of amino acids are tolerated with little indication of protein "toxicity." Larger quantities of amino acids in relation to calories can minimize a negative nitrogen balance even when the infusate is hypocaloric. Amino acid intake can be

Table 11–25. Intravenous lipid emulsions.

Intravenous Lipid Emulsions	Composition	FDA-Approved Neonatal and Pediatric Indications for Use
Intralipid (Baxter Healthcare Corp.)	Soybean oil base	Provide calories and EFA when oral or enteral nutrition is not possible, insufficient, or contraindicated
Nutrilipid (B. Braun Medical, Inc.)	Soybean oil base	Provide calories and EFA when oral or enteral nutrition is not possible, insufficient, or contraindicated
Omegaven (Fresenius-Kabi)	Fish oil base	May be used short term for rescue treatment of IFALD; lower amount of EFA
SMOFlipid (Fresenius-Kabi)	Soybean oil, MCT oil, olive oil, fish oil base	Provide calories and EFA (when recommended amounts/age are provided) when oral or enteral nutrition is not possible, insufficient, or contraindicated

EFA, essential fatty acid; FDA, Food and Drug Administration; IFALD, intestinal failure-associated liver disease; MCT, medium-chain triacylglycerol.

advanced by 0.5–1.0 g/kg/day toward the goal. Normally the final infusate will contain 2%–3% amino acids, depending on the rate of infusion. Concentration should not be advanced beyond 2% in peripheral vein infusates due to osmolality.

D. Monitoring

Monitoring for tolerance of the IV amino acid solutions should include blood urea nitrogen. Serum alkaline phosphatase, γ-glutamyltransferase, and bilirubin should be monitored to detect the onset of cholestatic liver disease.

Joosten K, Verbruggen S: PN Administration in critically ill children in different phases of the stress response. Nutrients 2022 Apr 27;14(9):1819. doi: 10.3390/nu14091819 [PMID: 35565787].

Mehta NM et al: Guidelines for the provision and assessment of nutrition support therapy in the pediatric critically ill patient: society of critical care medicine and American Society for Parenteral and Enteral Nutrition. J Parenter Enteral Nutr 2017 Jul; 41(5):706–742. doi: 10.1177/0148607117711387. Epub 2017 Jun 2 [PMID: 286868444].

Minerals & Electrolytes

A. Calcium, Phosphorus, and Magnesium

Intravenously fed preterm and full-term infants should be given relatively high amounts of calcium and phosphorus. Current recommendations are as follows: calcium, 500–600 mg/L; phosphorus, 400–450 mg/L; and magnesium, 50–70 mg/L. After 1 year of age, the recommendations are as follows: calcium, 200–400 mg/L; phosphorus, 150–300 mg/L; and magnesium, 20–40 mg/L. The ratio of calcium to phosphorous should be 1.3:1.0 by weight or 1:1 by molar ratio. These recommendations are deliberately presented as milligrams per liter of infusate to avoid inadvertent administration of concentrations of calcium and phosphorus that are high enough to precipitate in the tubing. During periods of fluid restriction, care must be taken not to inadvertently increase the concentration of calcium and phosphorus in the infusate. These recommendations assume an average fluid intake of 120–150 mL/kg/day and an infusate of 25 g of amino acid per liter. With lower amino acid concentrations, the concentrations of calcium and phosphorus should be decreased.

B. Electrolytes

Standard recommendations are given in Table 11–26. After chloride requirements are met, the remainder of the anion required to balance the cation should be given as acetate to avoid the possibility of acidosis resulting from excessive chloride. Electrolyte concentrations should be modified based on the flow rate and if indications dictate for the individual patient. If patient is at risk for refeeding syndrome, consult ASPEN consensus guidelines for electrolyte supplementation to avoid serious metabolic complications. Generous quantities of potassium and phosphorus may be needed.

Table 11–26. Electrolyte requirements for parenteral nutrition.

Electrolyte	Preterm Infant (mEq/kg)	Full-Term Infant (mEq/kg)	Child (mEq/kg)	Adolescent (mEq/kg)
Sodium	2–5	2–3	2–3	60–150
Chloride	2–5	2–3	2–3	60–150
Potassium	2–3	2–3	2–3	70–180

da Silva JSV et al: Parenteral Nutrition Safety and Clinical Practice Committees, American Society for Parenteral and Enteral Nutrition. ASPEN consensus recommendations for refeeding syndrome. Nutr Clin Pract 2020 Apr;35(2):178–195. doi: 10.1002/ncp.10474. Epub 2020 Mar 2. Erratum in: Nutr Clin Pract. 2020 Jun;35(3):584–585 [PMID: 32115791].

C. Trace Elements

Trace elements should be provided daily in recommended amounts based on age (Table 11–27) unless an altered dose is necessary based on hepatic or renal function or documented deficiency. Commercially available preparations are available, or micronutrients can be individually dosed. IV zinc requirements may be as high as 400 mcg/kg for preterm infants and can be up to 250 mcg/kg for infants with short bowel syndrome and significant GI losses of zinc. When IV nutrition is supplemental or limited to fewer than 2 weeks, and preexisting nutritional deficiencies are absent, only zinc need routinely be added.

IV copper requirements are relatively low in the young infant because of the presence of hepatic copper stores. These are significant even in the 28-week fetus. Circulating levels of copper and manganese should be monitored in the presence of cholestatic liver disease. If monitoring is not feasible, temporary withdrawal of added copper and manganese is advisable in cholestasis.

Copper and manganese are excreted primarily in the bile, but selenium, chromium, and molybdenum are excreted primarily in the urine. These trace elements, therefore, should be administered with caution in the presence of renal failure.

Vitamins

Three vitamin formulations are available for use in pediatric parenteral nutrition: MVI Pediatric (Hospira), Infuvite Pediatric (Baxter), and the adult formulation MVI-12 (AstraZeneca). It is important to note that MVI-12 contains no vitamin K Detailed content information is available from manufacturers as well as from the Federal Drug Administration (FDA). For dosing considerations during national shortages, recommendations are available from the ASPEN.

Table 11–27. PN trace element daily dosing.

Trace Element	Preterm Neonates (mcg/kg)	Term Neonates (3–10 kg) (mcg/kg)	Children (10-40 kg)	Adolescents (> 40 kg)
Zinc	400	250	50 mcg/kg *max 5000 mcg/day	2–5 mg
Copper	20	20	20 mcg/kg *max 500 mcg/day	200–500 mcg
Manganese	1	1	1 mcg/kg *max 55 mcg/day	40–100 mcg
Chromium	0.05–0.3	0.2	0.2 mcg/kg *max 5 mcg/day	5–15 mcg
Selenium	2	2	2 mcg/kg *max 100 mcg/day	40–60 mcg

It is essential to follow national guidelines in order to prevent deficiencies and use available products appropriately. A dose of 40 IU/kg/day of vitamin D (maximum 400 IU/day) is adequate for both full-term and preterm infants.

ASPEN: *Appropriate Dosing for Parenteral Nutrition: ASPEN Recommendations.* January 2019. http://www.nutritioncare.org/PNDosing.

Federal Drug Administration data sheet, Infuvite Pediatric: https://www.accessdata.fda.gov/drugsatfda_docs/label/2008/021265s015lbl.pdf.
Federal Drug Administration data sheet, M.V.I Pediatric: https://www.accessdata.fda.gov/drugsatfda_docs/label/2017/018920s036lbl.pdf.
Federal Drug Administration data sheet, MVI-12: https://www.accessdata.fda.gov/drugsatfda_docs/label/2004/08809scf052_mvi-12_lbl.pdf.

Table 11–28. Summary of suggested monitoring for parenteral nutrition.

Variables	Acute Stage	Long-Term[b]
Growth	Daily	Weekly
Weight	Weekly	
Length	Weekly	
Head circumference		
Urine		
Glucose (dipstick)	With each void	With changes in intake or status
Specific gravity	Void	
Volume	Daily	
Blood		
Glucose	4 h after changes,[a] then daily × 2 day	Weekly
Na^+, K^+, Cl, CO_2, blood urea nitrogen	Daily for 2 days after changes,[a] then twice weekly	Weekly
Ca^{2+}, Mg^{2+}, P	Initially, then twice weekly	Weekly
Total protein, albumin, bilirubin, aspartate transaminase, and alkaline phosphatase	Initially, then weekly	Every other week
Zinc and copper	Initially according to clinical indications	Monthly
Triglycerides	Initially, 1 day after changes,[a] then weekly	Weekly
Compete blood count	Initially, then twice weekly; according to clinical indications (see text)	Twice weekly

[a]Changes include alterations in concentration or flow rate.
[b]Long-term monitoring can be tapered to monthly or less often, depending on age, diagnosis, and clinical status of patient.

Fluid Requirements

The initial fluid volume and subsequent increments in flow rate are determined by basic fluid requirements, the patient's clinical status, and the extent to which additional fluid administration can be tolerated and may be required to achieve adequate nutrient intake. Calculation of initial fluid volumes to be administered should be based on standard pediatric practice. If replacement fluids are required for ongoing abnormal losses, these should be administered via a separate line.

Monitoring

Vital signs should be checked on each shift. With a central catheter in situ, a fever of greater than 38.5°C requires peripheral and central-line blood cultures, urine culture, complete physical examination, and examination of the IV entry point. Instability of vital signs, elevated white blood cell count with left shift, and glycosuria suggest sepsis. Removal of the central venous catheter should be considered if the patient is toxic or unresponsive to antibiotics.

A. Physical Examination

Monitor especially for hepatomegaly (differential diagnoses include fluid overload, congestive heart failure, steatosis, and hepatitis) and edema (differential diagnoses include fluid overload, congestive heart failure, hypoalbuminemia, and thrombosis of superior vena cava).

B. Intake and Output Record

Calories and volume delivered should be calculated from the previous day's actual intake and output records. The following entries should be noted on flow sheets: IV, enteral, and total fluid (mL/kg/day); dextrose (g/kg/day or mg/kg/min); protein (g/kg/day); lipids (g/kg/day); energy (kcal/kg/day); and percent of energy from enteral nutrition.

C. Growth, Urine, and Blood

Routine monitoring guidelines are given in Table 11–28. These are minimum requirements, except in the very long-term stable patient. Individual variables should be monitored more frequently as indicated, as should additional variables or clinical indications.

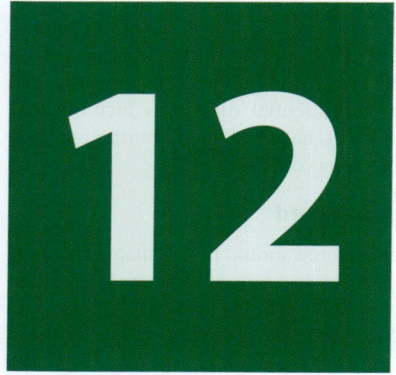

Emergencies & Injuries

Cortney Braund, MD
Laura Rochford, MD

INTRODUCTION TO PEDIATRIC EMERGENCIES & INJURIES

Of the approximately 140 million annual emergency department (ED) visits in the United States, over 30 million (20%) are for pediatric patients. Though the vast majority (97%) of children presenting for ED evaluation are discharged home, nearly 1 million each year require hospital admission in the ED and, sadly, nearly 3000 children die every year in US EDs.

INITIAL APPROACH TO THE ACUTELY ILL INFANT OR CHILD

ESSENTIALS OF DIAGNOSIS & TYPICAL FEATURES

- ▶ Most causes of pediatric cardiac arrest are due to hypoxia from respiratory failure.
- ▶ Hypotension is a *late* finding in pediatric shock; early signs may include tachycardia, capillary refill > 2 seconds, skin mottling, and decreased mental status.

A pediatric patient in serious distress may either present with a known diagnosis or in cardiorespiratory failure of unknown cause. The initial approach must be simple and consistent to rapidly identify and reverse life-threatening conditions. Once stabilized, the provider must then carefully consider the underlying cause, focusing on those that are treatable or reversible. Specific diagnoses can then be made, and targeted therapy initiated.

Pediatric cardiac arrest most commonly results from progressive respiratory deterioration or shock. Unrecognized deterioration may lead to bradycardia, agonal breathing, hypotension, and ultimately asystole. Resulting hypoxic and ischemic insult to the brain and other vital organs make neurologic recovery extremely unlikely, even if the child survives the arrest. When cardiopulmonary arrest does occur, survival is rare and most often associated with significant neurological impairment. Current data reflect a 6% survival rate for out-of-hospital cardiac arrest, 8% for those who receive prehospital intervention, and 27% survival rate for in-hospital arrest. Children who respond to rapid intervention with ventilation and oxygenation alone or to less than 5 minutes of advanced life support are much more likely to survive neurologically intact. In fact, more than 70% of children with respiratory arrest who receive rapid and effective bystander resuscitation survive with good neurologic outcomes. Therefore, it is essential to recognize the child who is at risk for progressing to cardiopulmonary arrest and to provide aggressive intervention before asystole occurs.

Of note, "compressions only" cardiopulmonary resuscitation (CPR) has been touted to encourage bystander CPR for adult out-of-hospital cardiac arrests. In the pediatric population, however, giving rescue breaths as well as chest compressions is still recommended and should be provided for infants and children in cardiac arrest due to the predominance of respiratory causes of arrest.

THE ABCs OF RESUSCITATION

A severely ill child should be rapidly evaluated in a deliberate sequence known as the *ABCs*: *A*irway patency, *B*reathing adequacy, and *C*irculation integrity. Each should be addressed before proceeding to the next step (keeping in mind that a patient in pulseless arrest should have the ABCs addressed simultaneously per PALS [pediatric advanced life support] guidelines).

Age-appropriate equipment (including laryngoscope blade, endotracheal tubes [ETTs], nasogastric or orogastric tubes, intravenous (IV) lines, and an indwelling urinary catheter) and monitors (cardiorespiratory monitor, pulse oximeter, and appropriate blood pressure cuff) should be assembled

Table 12–1. Equipment sizes and estimated weight by age.

Age (y)	Weight (kg)	Laryngeal Mask Airway (LMA) Size	Endotracheal Tube Size (mm)[a,b]	Laryngoscope Blade Size	Chest Tube (Fr)	Foley (Fr)
Premature	1-2.5	1	2.5 (uncuffed only)	0	8	5
Term newborn	3	1	3.0 (uncuffed only)	0-1	10	8
1	10	1.5	3.5–4.0	1	18	8
2	12	2	4.5	1	18	10
3	14	2	4.5	1	20	10
4	16	2	5.0	2	22	10
5	18	2	5.0-5.5	2	24	10
6	20	2-2.5	5.5	2	26	12
7	22	2.5	5.5–6.0	2	26	12
8	24	3	6.0	2	28	14
10	32	4	6.0-6.5	2-3	30	14
Adolescent	50	4	7.0	3	36	14
Adult	70		8.0	3	40	14

[a]Internal diameter.
[b]Decrease tube size by 0.5 mm if using a cuffed tube.

and readily available. See Table 12–1 for endotracheal tube and laryngeal mask airway sizes. After the newborn/neonatal age, cuffed ETTs are preferred, per the 2020 PALS updates, to reduce air leak and reduce need for ETT exchange later. Use a length-based emergency tape for all resuscitation medications and equipment (including ETT sizing). Alternatively, for newborn/neonatal patients, you may refer to Neonatal Resuscitation Program (NRP) guidelines for ETT sizing. For patients over 2 years old, you may use (Age/4) + 3.5 for cuffed ETT size, per PALS. Cuff inflation pressures should always be below 20 cm H_2O.

Airway

In all children, look for evidence of spontaneous breathing. Breath sounds such as stridor, stertor, gurgling, or increased work of breathing without air movement are suggestive of airway obstruction. Significant airway obstruction is associated with altered level of consciousness, including agitation or lethargy.

If concerned for airway compromise, the airway is managed initially by noninvasive means such as oxygen administration, positioning, chin lift, jaw thrust, suctioning, nasal trumpet, or oral airway. Invasive maneuvers, such as endotracheal intubation, supraglottic device (ie, laryngeal mask airway [LMA]), or rarely, cricothyroidotomy, may be required if the noninvasive maneuvers are unsuccessful. The following discussion assumes that basic life support has been instituted.

Knowledge of pediatric anatomy is important for airway management. Children's tongues are large relative to their oral cavities, and the larynx is high and anteriorly located. Infants are obligate nasal breathers; therefore, secretions, blood, or foreign bodies in the nasopharynx can cause significant distress.

1. Place the head in the sniffing position. In the patient without concern for cervical spine injury, the neck should be slightly flexed, and the head extended. This position aligns the oral, pharyngeal, and tracheal planes. In infants and children younger than about 8 years, the relatively large occiput causes significant neck flexion and poor airway positioning. This is relieved by placing a towel roll under the shoulders, thus returning the child to a neutral position (Figure 12–1). In an older child (where the occiput is proportionally less prominent), more head extension is necessary. Avoid hyperextension of the neck, especially in infants.

2. Perform the head tilt/chin lift or jaw thrust maneuver (Figure 12–2). Lift the chin upward while avoiding pressure on the submental triangle or lift the jaw by traction upward on the angle of the jaw. Important: head tilt/chin lift must not be done if cervical spine injury is possible. (See section Approach to the Pediatric Trauma Patient.)

3. Assess airway for foreign material. If a foreign body is of concern, proceed in a stepwise approach. If concern for a partial airway obstruction from a foreign body

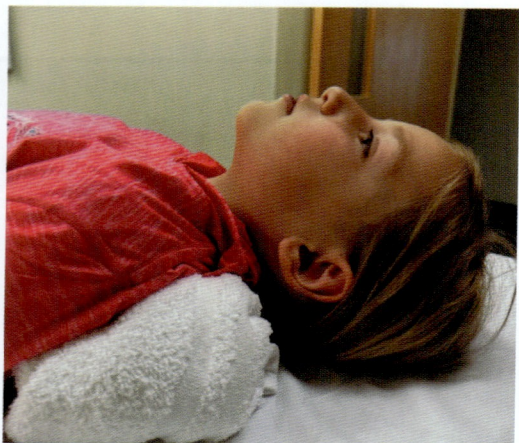

▲ **Figure 12–1.** Correct positioning of the child younger than 8 years for optimal airway alignment: a folded sheet or towel is placed beneath the shoulders to accommodate the occiput and align the oral, pharyngeal, and tracheal airways.

(ie, child is still able to phonate, cough, or cry on their own), allow the child to sit in position of comfort (often upright) and activate emergent airway team (anesthesia or ENT stat) for removal of foreign body in the OR. If the foreign body becomes fully occlusive (indicated by loss of ability to phonate), attempt Heimlich maneuverer or back thrusts per BLS guidelines. If unsuccessful and the patient becomes unresponsive, attempt removal under direct visualization using laryngoscope blade and Magill forceps. Do *not* perform blind finger sweeps. If the preceding maneuvers are unsuccessful, consider intubating and advancing the ETT to push the foreign body into the right mainstem purposefully, then pulling the ETT back to ventilate the left lung. Emergent cricothyrotomy is another option in the setting of "can't intubate/can't ventilate".

4. Assuming no foreign body is suspected, but airway obstruction persists (ie, a post ictal patient), attempt to reposition the head, then proceed with insertion of an airway adjunct, such as the oropharyngeal or naso-pharyngeal airway (Figure 12–3). Such adjuncts may relieve upper airway obstruction due to prolapse of the tongue into the posterior pharynx, the most common cause of airway obstruction in unconscious children. The correct size for an oropharyngeal airway is obtained by measuring from the upper central gumline to the angle of the jaw (Figure 12–4) and should be used only in the unconscious victim. Proper sizing is paramount, as an oropharyngeal airway that is too small will push the tongue further into the airway while one that is too large will obstruct the airway. Nasopharyngeal airways

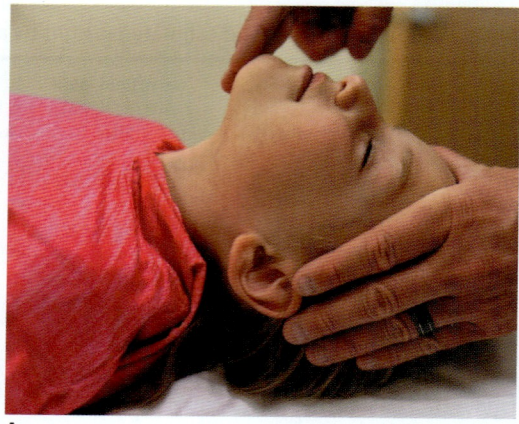

A

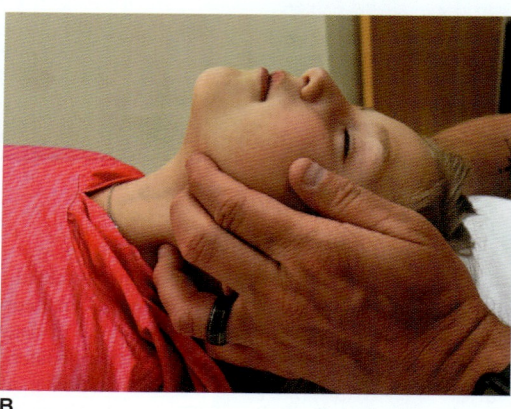

B

▲ **Figure 12–2.** **A:** Opening the airway with the head tilt and chin lift in patients without concern for spinal trauma: gently lift the chin with one hand and push down on the forehead with the other hand. **B:** Opening the airway with jaw thrust in patients with concern for spinal trauma: lift the angles of the mandible; this moves the jaw and tongue forward and opens the airway without bending the neck.

should fit snugly within the nares and should be equal in length to the distance from the nares to the tragus (Figure 12–5). This airway adjunct should be avoided in children with significant injuries to the midface due to the risk of intracranial perforation through a damaged cribriform plate.

Breathing

Assessment of respiratory status begins with inspection. *Look* for adequate and symmetric chest rise and fall, rate, and work of breathing (eg, accessory muscle use, retractions, flaring, and grunting), skin color, and tracheal deviation. Pulse oximetry measurement and end-tidal CO_2 determination are

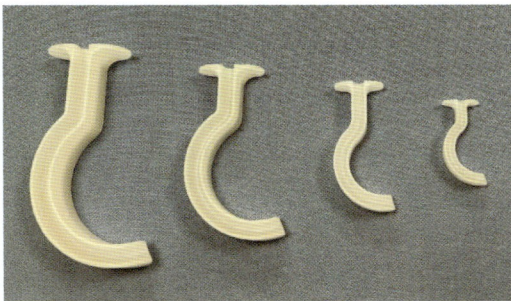

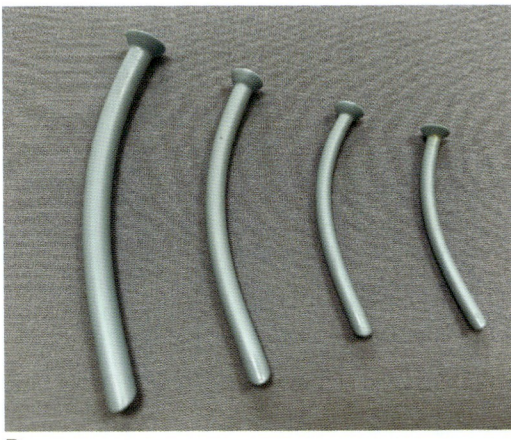

▲ **Figure 12–3. A:** Oropharyngeal airways of various sizes. **B:** Nasopharyngeal airways of different sizes.

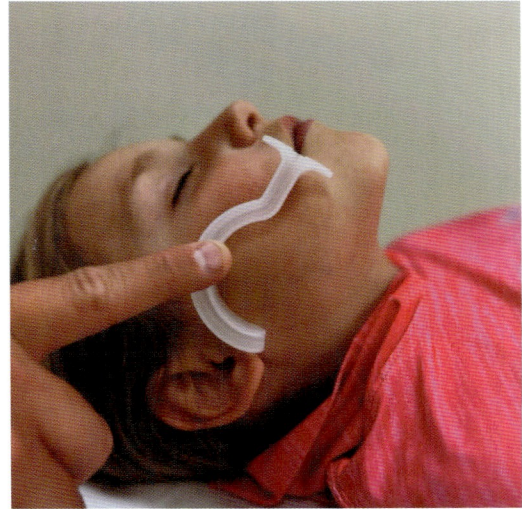

▲ **Figure 12–4.** Size selection for the oropharyngeal airway: hold the airway next to the child's face and estimate proper size by measuring from the upper central gumline to the angle of the jaw.

of aspiration, and a decreased likelihood that return of spontaneous circulation will be achieved during cardiac arrest. If the chest does not rise and fall easily with bagging, reposition the airway and assess for foreign material as previously described. The presence of asymmetrical breath sounds in a child in shock or in severe distress suggests pneumothorax and is an indication for needle thoracostomy. In small

highly desirable. *Listen* for adventitious breath sounds such as wheezing. Auscultate for air entry, symmetry of breath sounds, and rales. *Feel* for subcutaneous crepitus.

If spontaneous breathing is inadequate, initiate positive-pressure ventilation with a bag valve mask (BVM) and 100% oxygen. Assisted ventilations should be coordinated with the patient's efforts if present. Effective ventilation with a BVM is a difficult skill that requires training and practice. To begin, ensure a proper seal by choosing a mask that encompasses the area from the bridge of the nose to the cleft of the chin. Form an E–C clamp around the mask to seal the mask tightly to the child's face. The thumb and index finger form the "C" surrounding the mask, while the middle, ring, and small fingers lift the jaw into the mask (Figure 12–6). Use only enough force and volume to make the chest rise visibly. Two-person ventilation is optimal. When proper technique is used, BVM ventilation is effective in most cases.

Adequacy of BVM ventilation is reflected with appropriate chest rise and auscultation of bilateral air entry. Avoid hyperventilation, as it may lead to barotrauma, increased risk

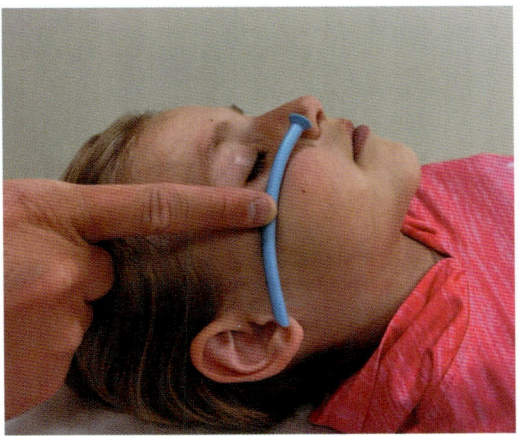

▲ **Figure 12–5.** Size selection for the nasopharyngeal airway: hold the airway next to the child's face and estimate proper size by measuring from the nares to the tragus.

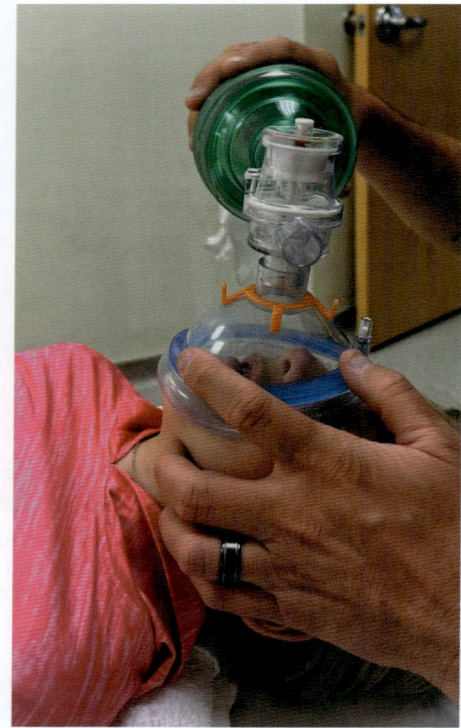

A

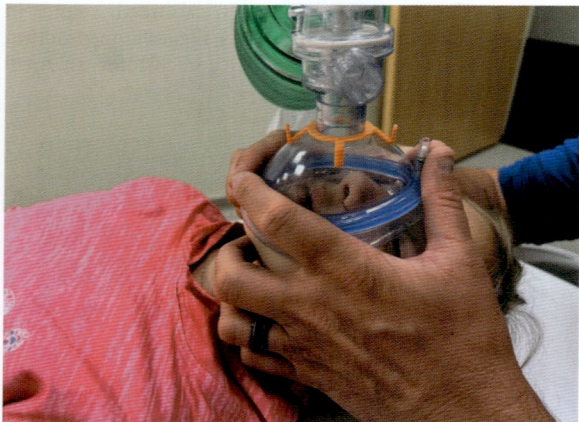

B

▲ **Figure 12–6. A:** Bag-valve-mask ventilation, one-person technique: the thumb and index finger form the "C" surrounding the mask, while the middle, ring, and little fingers lift the jaw into the mask. **B:** Bag-valve-mask ventilation, two-person technique: the first rescuer forms the "C" and "E" clamps with both hands; the second rescuer provides ventilation.

children, the transmission of breath sounds throughout the chest may impair the ability to auscultate the presence of a pneumothorax. *Note:* Effective oxygenation and ventilation are the keys to successful resuscitation.

Cricoid pressure (Sellick maneuver) has not been shown to reduce the risk of aspiration and is no longer recommended by the American Heart Association.

Circulation

The methodical assessment of blood circulation is critical to the diagnosis of shock, defined as the inadequate perfusion of vital organs. Circulation may be assessed in the following ways.

A. Pulses

Check adequacy of peripheral pulses and compare them with central pulses. In the infant, central pulses should be checked at the brachial artery.

B. Heart Rate

Compare with age-specific norms. Tachycardia can be a nonspecific sign of distress; bradycardia for age is a sign of imminent arrest and necessitates aggressive resuscitation.

C. Blood Pressure

It is vital to understand that shock may be present even with normal blood pressure. As intravascular volume falls, peripheral vascular resistance increases. Blood pressure is maintained until there is 35%–40% depletion of blood volume, followed by precipitous and often irreversible deterioration. **Compensated** shock occurs where there is normal blood pressure but signs of decreased organ perfusion. When blood pressure also falls, **decompensated (hypotensive)** shock is present. Hypotension should be immediately recognized and treated. Blood pressure determination should be performed manually using an appropriately sized cuff because automated machines can give erroneous readings in children.

D. Extremities

As shock progresses, extremities become cooler from distally to proximal. A child whose extremities are cool distal to the elbows and knees is in severe shock.

E. Capillary Refill Time

When fingertip pressure is applied to a patient's distal extremity and released, blood should refill the area in less than 2 seconds. A prolonged capillary refill time in the setting of other signs of shock indicates a compensated shock state while flash capillary refill may indicate warm shock. It is important to recognize that capillary refill time is influenced by ambient temperature, limb position, body site, age of the patient, and room lighting.

F. Mental Status

Assess the patient's mental status using Glasgow coma scale (GCS), as hypoxia, hypercapnia, poor cerebral perfusion, or ischemia will result in altered mental status.

G. Skin Color

Skin that is pale, gray, mottled, or ashen may indicate compromised circulatory status.

MANAGEMENT OF SHOCK

IV access is essential but can be difficult to establish in children with shock. Peripheral access, especially via the antecubital veins, can be attempted using short, wide-bore catheters to allow maximal flow rates. Two IVs should be started in severely ill children. The external jugular vein can be a useful site as well. Intraosseous (IO) access is an ideal alternative in any severely ill child (ie, hypotensive, decompensated septic shock, altered mental status) when IV access cannot be established rapidly (within 90 seconds). IO placement should be considered first in patients who present with cardiac arrest or in a severely decompensated state (apneic, unresponsive, in extremis, seizing.) Both manual and automated insertion devices are available for pediatric patients. Evidence suggests that automated devices result in faster, more successful IO placement compared to manual devices. Decisions on more invasive access (ie, central line) should be based on individual expertise, availability of ultrasound for guidance, as well as the urgency of obtaining access. Common sites include the femoral and internal jugular veins. In newborns, the umbilical vein may be cannulated. Arterial access may be indicated for intensive care unit (ICU) level patients needing continuous blood pressure monitoring.

Differentiation of Shock States & Initial Therapy

Management of shock is guided by etiology.

A. Hypovolemic Shock

The most common type of shock in the pediatric population is hypovolemia, leading to decreased preload. Frequent causes include dehydration, diabetic ketoacidosis (DKA), heat illness, and hemorrhage. Normal saline or lactated Ringer solution (isotonic crystalloid) is given as initial therapy in shock and should be initiated even in normotensive patients. There is no advantage to the early administration of colloid (albumin). Give 20 mL/kg (maximum 1 L/bolus) and repeat as necessary, until perfusion normalizes. Reassess after each intervention. Early use of blood products (ie, packed red blood cells ± massive transfusion protocol) is indicated in trauma patients.

B. Distributive Shock

Distributive shock results from vasodilation and subsequent decreased preload. Examples are sepsis, anaphylaxis, and neurogenic shock due to spinal cord injury. Initial therapy is isotonic volume replacement with crystalloid, but pressors may be required if perfusion does not normalize after delivery of two 20-mL/kg boluses of crystalloid (total of 40 mL/kg). Outcomes improve when normal heart rate for age, normalized blood pressure, and a capillary refill in less than 2 seconds are achieved within the first hour of symptom onset. Early identification of septic shock and rapid delivery of goal-directed therapies including fluids, antibiotics, and pressors (as indicated) within the first hour of presentation to the ED can reduce mortality and neurologic morbidity risks twofold. Recently updated recommendations from the American College of Critical Care Medicine stress the importance of aggressively correcting hypotension in the pediatric population. Norepinephrine and epinephrine are preferentially used as pressors for distributive shock.

C. Cardiogenic Shock

Cardiogenic shock can occur as a complication of congenital heart disease (ie, unrecognized ventricular septal defect [VSD], hypoplastic left heart), myocarditis in an otherwise healthy patient, dysrhythmias (eg, prolonged unrecognized supraventricular tachycardia [SVT]), ingestions (eg, clonidine), cardiomyopathy, or as a complication of prolonged shock due to any cause (eg, postcardiac arrest). Signs of cardiogenic shock may be subtle and mimic primary respiratory or primary gastrointestinal (GI) pathologies (eg, nausea, vomiting). Diagnosis may be suggested by any of the following: sustained tachycardia, tachypnea, cyanosis, poor weight gain (in infants), worsened clinical status after intravenous fluid (IVF) bolus, abnormal rhythm, jugular venous distention (JVD), rales, S_3 or S_4, friction rub, narrow pulse pressure, or hepatomegaly. Chest radiographs may show cardiomegaly and/or pulmonary edema, but these are not sensitive indicators. Upon recognition, inotropes (ie, low-dose epinephrine, milrinone), positive pressure (ie, bilevel positive airway pressure [BiPAP]), and possibly afterload reducers may be necessary to sustain blood pressure and improve perfusion. Giving multiple boluses of fluid is deleterious, which is why frequent reassessment and comprehensive monitoring is essential. Bedside ultrasound is useful in rapidly determining if cardiac function is adequate and whether a pericardial effusion is present.

D. Obstructive Shock

Obstructive shock is rare in the pediatric population and involves impaired cardiac output secondary to obstruction of forward flow of blood. Examples include cardiac tamponade, tension pneumothorax, massive pulmonary embolism, congenital cardiac lesion (ie, certain ductal dependent lesions such as critical coarctation of the aorta), or clotting of a Blalock and Taussig (B-T) shunt. Management is directed toward resolution of the obstruction. For instance, in the case of a critical coarctation, management should include emergent prostaglandin to reopen the ductus arteriosus while awaiting surgical repair.

▶ Observation & Further Management

Clinically reassess physiologic response to each fluid bolus to determine additional needs. Serial central venous pressure determinations or a chest radiograph may help determine volume status. Place an indwelling urinary catheter to monitor urine output.

Caution must be exercised with volume replacement if intracranial pressure (ICP) is potentially elevated, as in severe head injury, diabetic ketoacidosis, heart failure, or meningitis. Even in such situations, however, normal intravascular volume must be restored to achieve adequate mean arterial and cerebral perfusion pressure.

SUMMARY OF INITIAL APPROACH TO THE ACUTELY ILL INFANT OR CHILD

Assess the ABCs in sequential fashion and, before assessing the next system, immediately intervene if physiologic derangement is detected. It is essential that each system be reassessed after each intervention to ensure improvement and prevent failure to recognize clinical deterioration.

Agency for Healthcare Research and Quality: https://datatools. ahrq.gov/hcupnet/ Accessed July 16, 2023.
Davis AL et al: American college of critical care medicine clinical practice parameters for hemodynamic support of pediatric and neonatal shock. Critical Care Med 2017;45(6):1061–1093 [PMID: 28509730].
Pediatric Advanced Life Support: Provider Manual. American Heart Association; 2020.
Surviving sepsis campaign international guidelines. Pediatrics 2020;145(5). https://doi.org/10.1542/peds.2020-0629.

EMERGENCY PEDIATRIC DRUGS

Although careful attention to airway and breathing remains the mainstay of pediatric resuscitation, medications are often needed. Rapid delivery to the central circulation, which can be via peripheral IV catheter, is essential. Infuse medications close to the catheter's hub and flush with saline to achieve the most rapid systemic effects. In the rare instance that no IV or IO access is achievable, important emergency resuscitation drugs such as epinephrine, atropine, and naloxone may be given endotracheally (see dosing in Table 12–2). However, the dose, absorption, and effectiveness of drugs given via this route are either unknown or controversial. The use of length-based emergency measuring tapes that contain preprinted drug dosages, equipment sizes, and IV fluid amounts (Broselow tapes) or preprinted resuscitation drug charts is much more accurate than estimation formulas and helps minimize dosing errors. Selected emergency drugs used in pediatrics are summarized in Table 12–2.

▼ APPROACH TO THE PEDIATRIC TRAUMA PATIENT

Unintentional injuries are the leading cause of death for children older than 1 year. Motor-vehicle traffic injuries and falls are the two leading mechanisms of injury. Head and abdominal injuries are particularly common and clinically important. A coordinated team approach to the severely injured child will optimize outcomes. A calm atmosphere in the receiving area will contribute to thoughtful care. To provide optimal multidisciplinary care, regional pediatric trauma centers provide dedicated teams of pediatric specialists in emergency pediatrics, trauma surgery, orthopedics, neurosurgery, and critical care. However, most children with severe injuries are not seen in these centers. Community providers must often provide initial assessment and stabilization of the child with life-threatening injuries before transport to a verified pediatric trauma center.

MECHANISM OF INJURY

Document the time of occurrence, the type of energy transfer (eg, hit by a car, fall from playground), secondary impacts (if the child was thrown by the initial impact), appearance of the child at the scene, interventions performed, and clinical condition during transport. The report of emergency service personnel is invaluable. Forward all this information with the patient to the referral facility if secondary transport occurs.

INITIAL ASSESSMENT & MANAGEMENT

Most children who reach a hospital alive survive to discharge, therefore close attention to cerebral resuscitation and ensuring best neurologic outcomes must be the foremost consideration when treating children with serious injuries. Strict attention to the ABCs (see the previous section) ensures optimal oxygenation, ventilation, and perfusion and, ultimately, cerebral perfusion.

The primary and secondary survey is a method for evaluating and treating injured patients in a systematic way that provides a rapid assessment and stabilization phase, followed by a head-to-toe examination and definitive care phase.

PRIMARY SURVEY

The primary survey is designed to immediately identify and treat all physiologic derangements resulting from trauma. The mnemonic, *ABCDE*, is a simple way to remember the

Table 12–2. Important emergency pediatric drugs.

Drug	Indications	Dosage and Route	Comment
Epinephrine	1. Bradycardia, especially hypoxic-ischemic 2. Hypotension (by infusion) 3. Asystole 4. Fine ventricular fibrillation refractory to initial defibrillation 5. Pulseless electrical activity 6. Anaphylaxis (IM)	*Bradycardia and cardiac arrest:* 0.01 mg/kg of 1:10,000 solution IV/IO: 0.1 mg/kg of 1:1000 solution ET Anaphylaxis: 0.01 mg/kg of 1:1000 solution SC/IM Maximum dose: 0.3 mg. May repeat every 3-5 min. Constant infusion by IV drip: 0.1-1 mcg/kg/min.	Epinephrine is the single most important drug in pediatric resuscitation. Recent pediatric studies have shown no added advantage to high-dose epinephrine in terms of survival to discharge or neurologic outcome. Because other studies have indicated adverse effects, including increased myocardial oxygen consumption during resuscitation and worsened postarrest myocardial dysfunction, high-dose epinephrine is no longer recommended.
Glucose	1. Hypoglycemia 2. Altered mental status (empirical) 3. With insulin, for hyperkalemia	0.5-1 g/kg IV/IO. Continuous infusion may be necessary.	2-4 mL/kg D_{10}W, 1 -2 mL/kg D_{25}W.
Naloxone	1. Opioid overdose 2. Altered mental status (empirical)	0.1 mg/kg IV/IO/ET; maximum single dose, 2 mg. May repeat as necessary.	Side effects are few. A dose of 2 mg may be given in children ≥ 5 years or > 20 kg. Repeat as necessary, or give as constant infusion in opioid overdoses.
Sodium bicarbonate	1. Documented metabolic acidosis 2. Hyperkalemia	1 mEq/kg IV or IO; by arterial blood gas: 0.3 x kg x base deficit. May repeat every 5 min.	Infuse slowly. Sodium bicarbonate will be effective only if the patient is adequately oxygenated, ventilated, and perfused. Some adverse side effects.
Calcium chloride 10%	1. Documented hypocalcemia 2. Calcium channel blocker overdose 3. Hyperkalemia, hypermagnesemia	20 mg/kg slowly IV, preferably centrally, or IO with caution. Maximum single dose 2 g.	Calcium is no longer indicated for asystole. Potent tissue necrosis results if infiltration occurs. Use with caution and infuse slowly.

D_5W would be 10 mL/kg; D_{50}W would be 1 mL/kg; D_{10}W/D_{25}W, 10%/25% glucose in water; ET, endotracheally; IO, intraosseously; IV, intravenously; SC, subcutaneously. D_{50}W is not recommended PIV and use caution with D_{25}. D_{10} is preferred for neonates (newborn–1 month of age).

general steps of the primary survey: *A*irway, with cervical spine control; *B*reathing; *C*irculation, with hemorrhage control; *D*isability (neurologic deficit); *E*xposure (maintain a warm *E*nvironment, undress the patient completely, and *E*xamine).

If the patient is apneic or has agonal breaths, the sequence reverts to the *CAB*s of PALS resuscitation (*c*hest compressions, open the *a*irway, provide two rescue *b*reaths). Please refer to PALS guidelines for further information. Refer to preceding discussion regarding details of the ABC assessment. Modifications in the trauma setting are added as follows:

Airway

Failure to manage the airway appropriately is the most common cause of preventable morbidity and death. Administer 100% high-flow oxygen to all patients. Initially, provide cervical spine protection initially by manual inline immobilization, not traction, until a cervical spine collar can be placed.

Breathing

Most ventilation problems are resolved adequately by the airway maneuvers described earlier and by positive-pressure ventilation. Sources of traumatic pulmonary compromise include pneumothorax, hemothorax, pulmonary contusion, flail chest, and central nervous system (CNS) depression. Asymmetric breath sounds, particularly with concurrent tracheal deviation, cyanosis, or bradycardia, suggest pneumothorax, possibly under tension. To evacuate a tension pneumothorax, insert a large-bore catheter-over-needle assembly attached to a syringe through the second intercostal space in the midclavicular line into the pleural cavity and withdraw air. If a pneumothorax or hemothorax is present (evident by the sound of hissing as the air is evacuated), place a chest tube in the fourth or fifth intercostal space in the anterior axillary line. Connect to water seal. Insertion should be over the rib to avoid the neurovascular bundle that runs below the rib margin. Open pneumothoraces can be treated temporarily by taping petrolatum-impregnated gauze on three sides over the wound, creating a flap valve.

A child with a depressed level of consciousness (GCS score < 9), a need for prolonged ventilation, severe head trauma, or an impending operative intervention requires endotracheal intubation after bag-mask preoxygenation. Orotracheal intubation is the route of choice and is possible while maintaining cervical spine immobilization. Nasotracheal intubation may be possible in children 12 years of age or older who have spontaneous respirations, if not contraindicated by midfacial injury.

Supraglottic devices, such as the LMA, are being used with increasing frequency, in both the prehospital and hospital settings. The device consists of a flexible tube attached to an inflatable rubber mask (Figure 12–7). The LMA is inserted blindly into the hypopharynx and is seated over the larynx, occluding the esophagus. Advantages to its use include ease and speed of insertion, lower potential for airway trauma, and higher first-pass success rates. Patients remain at higher risk for aspiration with LMA use compared with orotracheal intubation; therefore, the LMA should not be used for prolonged, definitive airway management. Newer, second-generation supraglottic devices are available that consist of a noninflatable cuff and fit over the laryngeal inlet. Rarely, if tracheal intubation cannot be accomplished, particularly in the setting of massive facial trauma, cricothyroidotomy may be necessary. Needle cricothyroidotomy using a large-bore

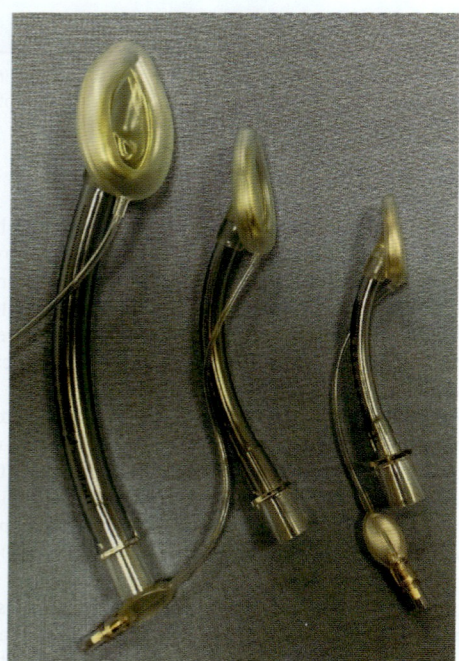

▲ **Figure 12–7.** Laryngeal mask airways of various sizes.

catheter through the cricothyroid membrane is the procedure of choice in patients younger than 12 years in this setting.

Circulation

Evaluation for ongoing external or internal hemorrhage is important in trauma evaluation. Large-bore IV access should be obtained early during the assessment, preferably at two sites. If peripheral access is not readily available, an IO line is established. Determine hematocrit and urinalysis in all patients. Blood type and crossmatch should be obtained in the hypotensive child unresponsive to isotonic fluid boluses or with known hemorrhage. Consider coagulation studies, chemistry panel, liver transaminases, lipase, and toxicologic screening as clinically indicated.

External hemorrhage can be controlled by direct pressure. To avoid damage to adjacent neurovascular structures, avoid placing hemostats on vessels, except in the scalp. Determination of the site of internal hemorrhage can be challenging. Common sites include the chest, abdomen, retroperitoneum, pelvis, and thighs. Bleeding into the intracranial vault rarely causes shock in children except in infants. Evaluation by an experienced clinician with adjunctive computed tomography (CT) or ultrasound will localize the site of internal bleeding.

Suspect cardiac tamponade after penetrating or blunt injuries to the chest if shock, pulseless electrical activity, narrowed pulse pressure, distended neck veins, hepatomegaly, or muffled heart sounds are present. Ultrasound may be diagnostic if readily available. Diagnose and treat with pericardiocentesis and rapid volume infusion.

Treat signs of poor perfusion vigorously: A tachycardic child with a capillary refill time of 3 seconds or more, or other evidence of diminished perfusion, is in *shock* and is sustaining vital organ insults. Recall that hypotension is a late finding. If perfusion does not normalize after initial crystalloid infusion or there are known sources of bleeding, 10 mL/kg of packed red blood cells is infused. Rapid reassessment must follow each bolus. Lack of response or recurring signs of hypovolemia suggest the need for ongoing blood transfusion and possible surgical exploration.

A frequent problem is the brain-injured child who is at risk for intracranial hypertension and who is also hypovolemic. In such cases, circulating volume must be restored to ensure adequate cerebral perfusion; therefore, fluid replacement is required until perfusion normalizes. Thereafter provide maintenance fluids with careful serial reassessments.

Disability-Neurologic Deficit

Assess pupillary size and reaction to light and the level of consciousness. The level of consciousness can be reproducibly characterized by the AVPU (Alert, Voice, Pain, Unresponsive) system (Table 12–3). Pediatric GCS assessments can be done as part of the secondary survey (Table 12–4).

Table 12–3. AVPU system for evaluation of level of consciousness.

A Alert
V Responsive to Voice
P Responsive to Pain
U Unresponsive

Exposure & Environment

Significant injuries can be missed unless the child is completely undressed and examined fully, both anterior and posterior. Any patient transported on a backboard should be removed as soon as possible, as pressure sores may develop on the buttocks and heels of an immobilized patient within hours.

Infants and children cool rapidly due to their high ratio of surface area to body mass. Maintaining normal body temperature is essential as hypo- and hyperthermia can have negative consequences. Hypothermia compromises outcomes except with isolated head injuries; therefore, continuously monitor the body temperature and use warming techniques as necessary. It is important to be mindful in patients with acute brain injuries that hyperthermia can adversely affect outcomes, therefore warming only to maintain normal body temperature in these scenarios.

Monitoring

Cardiopulmonary monitors, pulse oximetry, and end-tidal CO_2 monitors should be put in place immediately. At the completion of the primary survey, additional catheters and airway adjuncts may need to be placed. See Table 12–1 for age/weight-appropriate equipment sizes.

A. Nasogastric or Orogastric Tube

Children's stomachs should be assumed to be full, so a nasogastric tube needs to be placed upon completion of the primary survey. Gastric distention from positive-pressure ventilation increases the chance of vomiting and aspiration. Of note, the nasogastric route should be avoided in patients with significant midface trauma.

B. Urinary Catheter

An indwelling urinary bladder catheter should be considered to monitor urine output. Contraindications are based on the risk of urethral transection; signs include blood at the meatus or in the scrotum or a displaced prostate detected on rectal examination. Urine should be tested for blood. After the initial flow of urine with catheter placement, the urine output should exceed 1 mL/kg/h.

SECONDARY SURVEY

After the Primary Survey and resuscitation phase, a secondary survey consisting of focused history and a head-to-toe examination should be performed to reveal all injuries and determine priorities for definitive care.

History

Obtain a rapid, focused history from the patient (if possible), available family members, or prehospital personnel. The AMPLE mnemonic is frequently used:

- A—Allergies
- M—Medications
- P—Past medical history/pregnancy
- L—Last meal
- E—Events/environment leading to the injury

Table 12–4. Glasgow coma scale.[a]

Eye-opening response	
Spontaneous	4
To speech	3
To pain	2
None	1
Verbal response: Child (*Infant modification*)[b]	
Oriented (*Coos, babbles*)	5
Confused conversation (*Irritable cry, consolable*)	4
Inappropriate words (*Cries to pain*)	3
Incomprehensible sounds (*Moans to pain*)	2
None	1
Best upper limb motor response: Child (*Infant modification*)[b]	
Obeys commands (*Normal movements*)	6
Localizes pain (*Withdraws to touch*)	5
Withdraws to pain	4
Flexion to pain	3
Extension to pain	2
None	1

[a]The appropriate number from each section is added to total between 3 and 15. A score less than 8 usually indicates CNS depression requiring positive-pressure ventilation.
[b]If no modification is listed, the same response applies for both infants and children.

Physical Examination

A. Skin

Search for lacerations, hematomas, burns, swelling, and abrasions, and remove superficial foreign material. Cutaneous findings may indicate underlying pathology (eg, a flank hematoma overlying a renal contusion), although surface signs may be absent even with significant internal injury. Do not remove penetrating foreign objects because vital respiratory components, vascular structures, or organs may be involved and require removal in a controlled environment by a surgeon. Make certain that the child's tetanus immunization status is current. Consider tetanus immune globulin for incompletely immunized children.

B. Head

Evaluate for hemotympanum and for clear or bloody cerebrospinal fluid leak from the nares. The hematoma over the mastoid ("battle sign") and periorbital hematomas ("raccoon eyes") are late signs of basilar skull fracture. Explore wounds, evaluating for foreign bodies and defects in galea or skull. CT scan of the head is an integral part of evaluation for altered level of consciousness, posttraumatic seizure, or focal neurologic findings (see section Head Injury). Pneumococcal vaccine may be considered for basilar skull fractures as a preventive measure for meningitis.

C. Spine

Cervical spine injury must be excluded in all children. This can be done clinically in children older than 4 or 5 years with normal neurologic findings on examination who are able to deny midline neck pain or midline tenderness on palpation of the neck and who have no other painful distracting injuries that might obscure the pain of a cervical spine injury. If radiographs are indicated, a cross-table lateral neck view is obtained initially followed by anteroposterior, odontoid, and, in some cases, oblique views. Normal studies do not exclude significant injury, either bony or ligamentous, or involving the spinal cord itself. Therefore, an obtunded child should be maintained in cervical spine immobilization until the child has awakened and an appropriate neurologic examination can be performed. The entire thoracolumbar spine must be palpated, and areas of pain or tenderness examined by radiography.

D. Chest

Children may sustain significant internal injury without outward signs of trauma. The most common type of injuries sustained from blunt chest trauma is pulmonary contusions which may lead to hypoxemia. Pneumothoraces are detected and decompressed during the primary survey. Hemothoraces can occur with rib fractures or with injury to intercostal vessels, large pulmonary vessels, or lung parenchyma. Tracheobronchial disruption is suggested by large, continued air leak despite chest tube decompression. Myocardial contusions and aortic injuries are unusual in children.

E. Abdomen

Blunt abdominal injury is common in multisystem injuries. Significant injury may exist without cutaneous signs or instability of vital signs. Abdominal pain and tenderness coupled with a linear contusion across the abdomen ("seat belt sign") increases the risk of intra-abdominal injury threefold. Tenderness, guarding, distention, diminished or absent bowel sounds, or poor perfusion mandate immediate evaluation by a pediatric trauma surgeon. Injury to solid viscera frequently can be managed nonoperatively in stable patients; however, intestinal perforation or hypotension necessitates operative treatment. Intra-abdominal injury is highly likely if the aspartate transaminase (AST) is greater than 200 U/L or the alanine transaminase (ALT) greater than 125 U/L; however, elevated levels that are below these thresholds do not exclude significant injury if a significant mechanism has occurred. When measured serially, a hematocrit of less than 30% also may suggest intra-abdominal injury in blunt trauma patients. Coagulation studies are rarely beneficial if no concomitant head injury is present. There is no single test that can reliably predict intra-abdominal injury and therefore laboratory interpretation requires close clinical correlation. Laboratory studies are often most valuable in the nonverbal or obtunded patient, to increase the suspicion for injury and subsequent need for imaging.

Trauma ultrasonography, or the FAST (focused assessment with sonography for trauma), is routinely used in the adult trauma population. The purpose of the four-view examination (Morison pouch, splenorenal pouch, pelvic retrovesical space, and subcostal view of the heart) is to detect free fluid or blood in dependent spaces. In adults, such detection indicates clinically significant injury likely to require surgery. Accuracy and indications in children are much less clear. This examination has a high specificity rate to rule in free abdominal fluid, but low sensitivity to rule out significant intra-abdominal injury. Solid-organ injuries are more frequently missed. Additionally, much of the pediatric trauma management is nonoperative and therefore detection of free fluid by ultrasound in children is less likely to lead to surgery or result in a change in management. At least one recent study showed no change in the rate of pediatric patients eventually undergoing abdominal CT regardless of FAST findings.

F. Pelvis

Pelvic fractures are classically manifested by pain, crepitus, and abnormal motion. Significant blood loss into the pelvis may occur due to vascular injury. Unexplained tachycardia or hypotension should prompt evaluation of the pelvis. Pelvic fracture is a relative contraindication to urethral catheter insertion. A rectal examination is performed to evaluate tone, tenderness, or blood in the stool.

G. Genitourinary System

If urethral transection is suspected, perform a retrograde urethrogram before catheter placement. Diagnostic imaging of the child with hematuria less than 50 red blood cells per high-power field (hpf) often includes CT scan or occasionally, IV urograms. Management of kidney injury is largely nonoperative except for renal pedicle injuries.

H. Extremities

Long bone fractures are common but rarely life threatening. Test for pulses, perfusion, and sensation. Neurovascular compromise requires immediate orthopedic consultation. Treatment of open fractures includes antibiotics, tetanus prophylaxis, and orthopedic consultation.

I. Central Nervous System

Most deaths in children with multisystem trauma are from head injuries, so optimal neurointensive care is important. Significant injuries include diffuse axonal injury; cerebral edema; subdural, subarachnoid, and epidural hematomas; and parenchymal hemorrhages. Spinal cord injuries occur less commonly. Level of consciousness should be assessed serially. A full sensorimotor examination should be performed. Deficits require immediate neurosurgical consultation and should be considered for a patient with a GCS less than 12. Extensor or flexor posturing represents intracranial hypertension until proven otherwise. If accompanied by a fixed, dilated pupil, such posturing indicates that a herniation syndrome is present, and mannitol or 3% hypertonic saline should be given if perfusion is normal (see further discussion in next section). Treatment goals include aggressively treating hypotension to optimize cerebral perfusion, providing supplemental oxygen to keep saturations above 90%, achieving eucapnia (end-tidal CO_2 35–40 mm Hg), avoiding hyperthermia, and minimizing painful stimuli. Early rapid sequence intubation, sedation, and paralysis should be considered. Mild prophylactic hyperventilation is no longer recommended, although brief periods of hyperventilation are still indicated in the setting of acute herniation. Seizure activity warrants exclusion of significant intracranial injury. In the trauma setting, seizures are frequently treated with fosphenytoin or levetiracetam. The use of high-dose corticosteroids for suspected spinal cord injury has not been prospectively evaluated in children and is not considered standard of care. Corticosteroids are not indicated for head trauma.

Centers for Disease Control and Prevention, National Center for Injury Prevention and Control, Division of Unintentional Injury Prevention: https://www.cdc.gov/safechild/child_injury_data.html. Accessed April 30, 2023

Drexel S, Azarow K, Jafri MA: Abdominal trauma evaluation for the pediatric surgeon. Surg Clin North Am 2017 Feb;97(1):59–74 [PMID: 27894432].

Fornari, M, Lawson S: Pediatric blunt abdominal trauma and point-of-care ultrasound. Pediatr Emerg Care 2021 Dec;37(12):624–629 [PMID: 34908375].

Liang et al: The utility of the focused assessment with sonography in trauma examination in pediatric blunt abdominal trauma: a systematic review and meta-analysis. Pediatr Emerg Care 2019 Mar 12 [PMID: 30870341].

HEAD INJURY

Closed-head injuries range in severity from minor asymptomatic trauma without sequelae to fatal injuries. Even after minor closed-head injury, long-term disability and neuropsychiatric sequelae can occur.

ESSENTIALS OF DIAGNOSIS & TYPICAL FEATURES

► Traumatic brain injury (TBI) is the most common injury in children.

► Rapid acceleration-deceleration forces (eg, the shaken infant) as well as direct trauma to the head can result in brain injury.

► Rapid assessment can be made by evaluating mental status with the GCS score and assessing pupillary light response.

► All head injuries require a screening evaluation with symptom inventory and complete neurologic examination.

► Prevention

Wearing helmets while riding wheeled recreational devices, playing contact sports, and participating in snow sports is a simple strategy for preventing head injuries. Over 50% of children fail to wear helmets when riding bicycles; rates are lower with other wheeled devices. Adolescents are less likely to use protective equipment and warrant special attention when discussing helmet use. More stringent helmet use while playing contact sports and return to play recommendations are now in place in child and high school sports programs. Toppled televisions, dressers, and other unsecured furniture can also result in mild to severe head injuries in young children; anticipatory guidance regarding properly securing furniture should be provided to parents.

Clinical Findings

A. Signs and Symptoms

Head injury symptoms are nonspecific and may include headache, dizziness, nausea/vomiting, disorientation, amnesia, slowed thinking, and perseveration. Loss of consciousness is not necessary to diagnose a concussion (see Chapter 27 for more on concussion). Worsening symptoms in the first 24 hours may indicate more severe TBI. Obtain vital signs and assess the child's level of consciousness by the AVPU system (see Table 12–3) or GCS (see Table 12–4), noting irritability or lethargy and pupillary equality, size, and light reaction. Perform a physical examination, including a detailed neurologic examination, being mindful of the mechanism of injury. Cerebrospinal fluid or blood from the ears or nose, hemotympanum, or the later appearance of periorbital hematomas ("raccoon eyes") or "battle sign" (bruising over the mastoid process) imply a basilar skull fracture as discussed previously. Evaluate for associated injuries, paying special attention to the cervical spine. Consider child abuse; injuries observed should be consistent with the history, the child's developmental stage, and the injury mechanism.

B. Imaging Studies

CT may be indicated. However, close observation for a period of time may be appropriate management and reduces the use of CT. A 2009 multicenter investigation of head-injured patients presenting to the ED derived and validated a decision rule for identifying those children at very low risk of clinically important TBIs (Figure 12–8). Plain films are not generally indicated. In infants, a normal neurologic examination does not exclude significant intracranial hemorrhage. Consider imaging if large scalp hematomas or concerns of nonaccidental trauma are present in younger children.

Differential Diagnosis

CNS infection, toxicological ingestions, or other medical causes of altered mental status may present similarly to head injuries which often have no external signs of injury. In young infants when no history is available, one must also consider sepsis and inborn errors of metabolism.

Complications

A. Central Nervous System Infection

Open-head injuries (fractures with overlying lacerations) pose an infection risk due to direct contamination. Basilar skull fractures that involve the cribriform plate or middle ear cavity may allow a portal of entry for *Streptococcus pneumoniae*. Pneumococcal vaccination is considered for such cases.

B. Acute Intracranial Hypertension

Close observation will detect early signs and symptoms of elevated increased ICP. Early recognition is essential to avoid disastrous outcomes. Symptoms include altered mental status, headache, vision changes, vomiting, gait difficulties, and pupillary abnormalities. Papilledema is a cardinal sign of increased ICP. Other signs may include stiff neck, cranial nerve palsies, and hemiparesis. Cushing triad (bradycardia, hypertension, and irregular respirations) is a late and ominous finding. If considering lumbar puncture, consider CT scan prior if there is concern for elevated ICP due to risk of herniation. Lumbar puncture should be deferred in the unstable patient.

1. Treatment—Therapy for elevated ICP must be swift and aggressive. Maintenance of adequate oxygenation, ventilation, and perfusion is paramount. Rapid sequence intubation is often necessary to protect the airway using a sedative and paralytic to decrease the ICP elevation accompanying intubation. Lidocaine is a controversial adjunct pretreatment medication (administered 2–3 minutes prior to RSI attempt) and is thought to blunt increases in ICP during intubation by suppressing cough and gag reflexes and protecting cerebral perfusion. Avoid hypoperfusion and hypoxemia, as both are associated with increased risk of morbidity and mortality. Hyperventilation (goal Pco_2 30–35 mm Hg) is reserved for acute herniation; otherwise, maintain Pco_2 between 35 and 40 mm Hg. Mannitol (0.5–1 g/kg IV), an osmotic diuretic, will reduce brain water during acute herniation. Hypertonic (3%) saline may also be used as a 5-mL/kg bolus doses or 1–2 mL/kg/h infusion. Adjunctive measures to decrease ICP include elevating the head of the bed 30 degrees, maintaining the head in a midline position, and treating hyperpyrexia (fever) and pain. Obtain immediate neurosurgical consultation. Further details about management of intracranial hypertension (cerebral edema) are presented in Chapter 14.

C. Prognosis

For children with mild injuries, concussion symptoms should be followed closely, return to sport only when symptom-free at rest and during exercise without medication use and then followed by a graduated return-to-play protocol. All states now have a concussion law and most require a physician's note to return to play. In addition to sport limitations, patients may require a modified academic schedule and additional academic accommodations, including shorter days, longer testing periods, and less homework. Most children recover fully within 1–2 weeks. Acute symptoms seen in the ED do not correlate with long-term outcome, and therefore it is crucial for all patients to have follow-up management by their primary care physician. Proper management of concussion is critical to reduce the long-term sequelae. Persistent symptoms indicate the need for rehabilitation and/or neuropsychological referral.

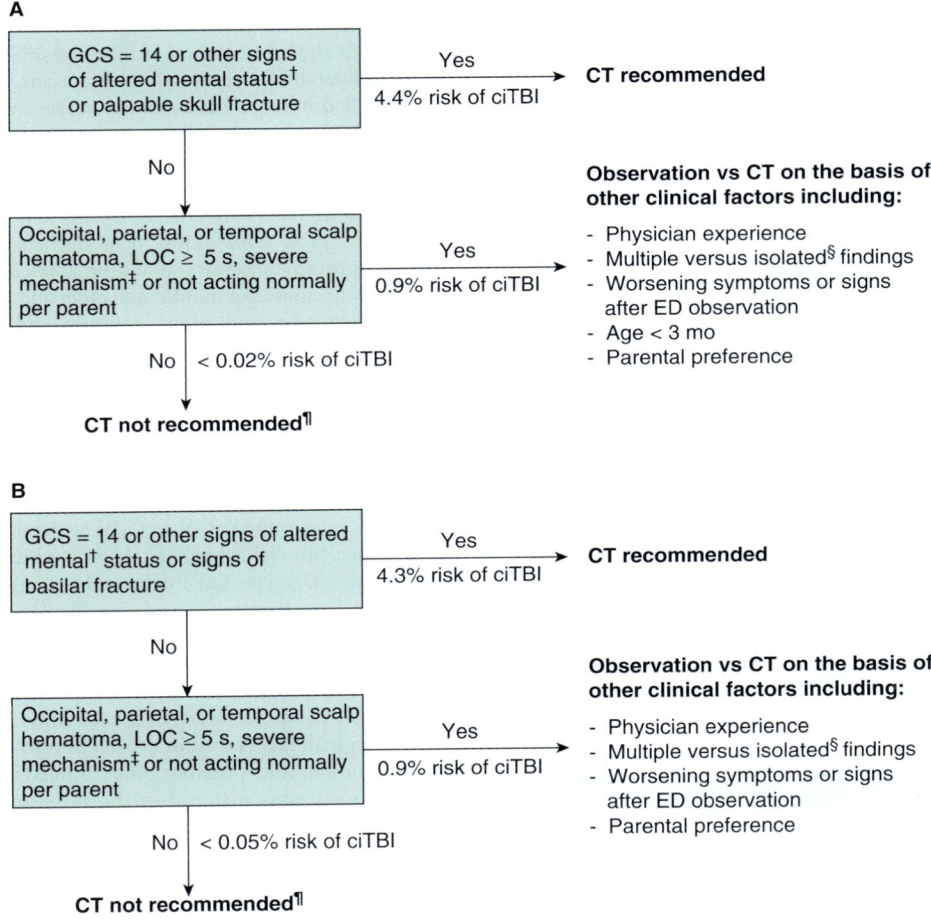

A

GCS = 14 or other signs of altered mental status† or palpable skull fracture
— Yes / 4.4% risk of ciTBI → **CT recommended**

— No ↓

Occipital, parietal, or temporal scalp hematoma, LOC ≥ 5 s, severe mechanism‡ or not acting normally per parent
— Yes / 0.9% risk of ciTBI →

— No / < 0.02% risk of ciTBI ↓

CT not recommended¶

Observation vs CT on the basis of other clinical factors including:

- Physician experience
- Multiple versus isolated§ findings
- Worsening symptoms or signs after ED observation
- Age < 3 mo
- Parental preference

B

GCS = 14 or other signs of altered mental† status or signs of basilar fracture
— Yes / 4.3% risk of ciTBI → **CT recommended**

— No ↓

Occipital, parietal, or temporal scalp hematoma, LOC ≥ 5 s, severe mechanism‡ or not acting normally per parent
— Yes / 0.9% risk of ciTBI →

— No / < 0.05% risk of ciTBI ↓

CT not recommended¶

Observation vs CT on the basis of other clinical factors including:

- Physician experience
- Multiple versus isolated§ findings
- Worsening symptoms or signs after ED observation
- Parental preference

ciTBIa, clinically important traumatic brain injury; CT, computed tomography; ED, emergency department; GCS, Glasgow coma scale; LOC, loss of consciousness.
†Other signs of altered mental status: agitation, somnolence repetitive questioning, or slow response to verbal communication.
‡Severe mechanism of injury: motor vehicle crash with patient ejection, death of another passenger, or rollover; pedestrian or bicyclist without helmet struck by motorized vehicle; falls of more than 3 ft (or more than 5 ft for panel B); or head struck by a high-impact object.
§Patients with certain isolated findings (ie, with no other findings suggestive of traumatic brain injury), such as isolated LOC, isolated headache, isolated vomiting, and certain type of isolated scalp hematomas in infants older than 3 mo, have a risk of ciTBI substantially lower than 1%.
¶Risk of ciTBI exceedingly low, generally lower than risk of CT-induced malignancies. Therefore, CT scans are not indicated for most patients in this group.

▲ **Figure 12–8.** Suggested CT algorithm for children younger than 2 years (**A**) and for those aged 2 years and older (**B**) with GCS scores 14–15 after head trauma. (Reproduced with permission From Kuppermann N et al: Identification of children at very low risk of clinically-important brain injuries after head trauma: a prospective cohort study. Lancet 2009;374(9696):1160–1170.)

The Centers for Disease Control and Prevention's (CDC's) Heads Up program has accessible concussion and return to play information online and is a valuable resource for parents, coaches, and health care providers.

The prognosis for children with moderate to severe injuries depends on many factors, including severity of initial injury, presence of hypoxia or ischemia, development and subsequent management of intracranial hypertension, and associated injuries.

Centers for Disease Control and Prevention, National Center for Injury Prevention and Control, Division of Unintentional Injury Prevention: https://www.cdc.gov/headsup/index.html. Accessed April 30, 2023.

Grubenhoff JA et al: Acute concussion symptom severity and delayed symptom resolution. Pediatrics 2014;134(1):54–62 [PMID: 24958583].

Kuppermann N et al: Identification of children at very low risk of clinically-important brain injuries after head trauma: a prospective cohort study. Lancet 2009;374(9696):1160–1170 [PMID: 19758692].

McCrory P et al: Consensus statement on concussion in sport: the 5th International Conference on Concussion in Sport held in Berlin, October 2016. Br J Sports Med 2017;51:838–847 [PMID: 28446457].

Nigrovic LE et al: The effect of observation on cranial computed tomography utilization for children after blunt head trauma. Pediatrics 2011;127(6):1067–1073 [PMID: 21555498].

Rotter J, Kamat D: Concussion in children. Pediatric Annals 2019;48(4):e182–e185 [PMID: 30986320].

BURNS

THERMAL BURNS

ESSENTIALS OF DIAGNOSIS & TYPICAL FEATURES

- ▶ Burn patterns can distinguish accidental burns from inflicted burns.
- ▶ Burns are categorized into three classes based on skin layer involved: superficial, partial thickness, and full thickness.
- ▶ Burns of the hands, feet, face, eyes, ears, and perineum are always considered to be major burns.

Burns are a common cause of accidental death and disfigurement in children. Common causes include hot water or food, appliances, flames, grills, vehicle-related burns, and curling irons. Burns occur commonly in toddlers—in boys more frequently than in girls. The association with child abuse and the preventable nature of burns constitute an area of major concern in pediatrics.

▶ Prevention

Hot liquids should be placed as far as possible from counter edges and parents/caregivers should take care when holding a child while drinking a hot beverage. While cooking, panhandles should be turned away from stove edge. Water heater thermostats should be turned to less than 120°F (49°C). Irons and electrical cords should be kept out of reach of children. Barriers around fireplaces are crucial. Infants and young children should wear protective clothing including hats when outdoors. Infant approved sunscreen should be applied and reapplied frequently to children 6 months and older and younger infants during extended periods of sun exposure outdoors.

▶ Clinical Findings

A. Signs and Symptoms

Superficial-thickness burns are painful, dry, red, and hypersensitive. Sunburn is an example. Partial-thickness burns are subgrouped as superficial or deep, depending on appearance. Superficial partial-thickness burns are red and often blister. Deep partial-thickness burns are pale, edematous, blanch with pressure, and they display decreased sensitivity to pain. Full-thickness burns affect all epidermal and dermal elements. A full-thickness wound is white or black, dry, depressed, leathery in appearance, and insensate. Deep full-thickness burns are the most severe, extending through all layers of skin as well as into the underlying fascia, muscle, and possibly bone. Singed nasal or facial hair, carbonaceous material in the nose and mouth, and stridor indicate inhalational burns and may herald critical airway obstruction.

Up to 25% of burns in children may be due to child physical abuse. Burn patterns can help distinguish inflicted from accidental causes. Patterns concerning for inflicted burns include symmetric immersion burns with glove and stocking distributions with sharp margins; buttock burns that spare the center and result in a "doughnut appearance"; simultaneous deep burns of the buttocks, perineum, and both feet; burns with clear pattern of the hot object such as an iron or cigarette lighter; and lower extremity burns that spare flexor surfaces. Additionally, if there is delay in seeking care, unknown or unwitnessed cause of burn, or if the burn pattern does not fit the mechanism, consider child abuse.

B. Laboratory Findings

Laboratory evaluation is rarely indicated. With extensive partial- and full-thickness burns, baseline complete blood cell count (CBC), basic metabolic panel, and creatinine kinase are helpful for tracking infectious or renal complications. Consider carbon monoxide poisoning after inhalational injury. If there is an index of suspicion, obtain an arterial blood gas and carboxyhemoglobin level.

C. Imaging Studies

Imaging studies are rarely indicated. Neck x-rays should not delay intubation when inhalational injury is suspected.

Differential Diagnosis

The differential diagnosis of burns is limited when a history is provided. In the preverbal child when no history is available, the primary alternate consideration is cellulitis.

Complications

Superficial- and superficial partial-thickness burns typically heal well. Deep partial- and full-thickness burns are at risk of scarring. Loss of barrier function predisposes to infection. Damage to deeper tissues in full-thickness burns may result in loss of function, contractures, and in the case of circumferential burns, compartment syndrome. Renal failure secondary to myoglobinuria from rhabdomyolysis is also a concern with more severe burns.

Treatment

Burn extent can be classified as major or minor as determined by calculating the percent of body surface area (BSA) affected by partial- or full-thickness burns. Superficial thickness burns are not counted when assessing % BSA. Minor burns are less than 10% BSA for partial-thickness burns, or less than 2% for full-thickness burns. Partial- or full-thickness burns of the hands, feet, face, eyes, ears, and perineum are considered major.

A. Superficial- and Partial-Thickness Burns

These burns generally can be treated in the outpatient setting. Wounds with a potential to cause disfigurement or functional impairment—especially wounds of the face, hands, feet, digits, or perineum—should be referred promptly to a burn surgeon. Analgesia is paramount. After parenteral narcotic administration, initial treatment of partial thickness burns with blisters consists of saline irrigation followed by application of clear antibiotic ointment and a nonadherent dressing (eg, petroleum gauze). Digits should be individually dressed to prevent adhesions. Because of the pain associated with aggressive debridement and the ability to provide an infectious barrier, smaller blisters may be left intact under the dressing. Larger bullae are typically drained and require aggressive pain control or sedation. Protect the wound with a bulky dressing, reexamine within 48 hours and serially thereafter. Treatment at home with cool compresses and optimizing pain control with medications.

B. Full-Thickness, Deep or Extensive Partial-Thickness, and Subdermal Burns

Major burns require attention to the ABCs of trauma management. Early establishment of an artificial airway is critical with oral or nasal burns because of their association with inhalation injuries and critical airway obstruction. If singeing of the oro- or nasopharynx is noted on initial exam, consider early intubation.

Perform a primary survey (see earlier discussion). Consider toxicity from carbon monoxide, cyanide, or other combustion products. Place a nasogastric tube and bladder catheter. The secondary survey identifies associated injuries, including those suggestive of abuse.

Fluid losses can be substantial. Initial fluid resuscitation should restore adequate circulating volume. Subsequent fluid administration must account for increased losses. Fluid needs are based on weight and percentage of BSA with partial- and full-thickness burns. Figure 12–9 shows percentages of BSA by region in infants and children. The Parkland formula for fluid therapy is 4 mL/kg/% BSA burned for the first 24 hours, with half administered in the first 8 hours, in addition to maintenance rates. The use of burn tables improves calculation of appropriate fluids. Goal urine output is 1–2 mL/kg/h.

Children with burns greater than 10% BSA in a circumferential pattern, who are suspicious for abuse, or with burns associated with inhalational injury, explosions, or fractures, should be admitted. Additionally, admission is warranted for adequate pain control in a patient requiring parenteral analgesia. Burns greater than 20% BSA or full thickness burns greater than 2% BSA should be admitted to a children's hospital or burn center. Children with full-thickness burns require immediate hospitalization at a burn center under the care of a burn specialist.

Prognosis

Outcome depends on many factors. Healing occurs with minimal damage to epidermis in superficial burns. In contrast, full-thickness burns will be hard, uneven, and fibrotic unless skin grafting is provided. In general, the greater the surface area and depth of burn injury, the greater the risk of long-term morbidity and mortality.

ELECTRICAL BURNS

Electrical injuries vary from exposure to low-voltage, high-voltage, or lightning strike source. Children electrocuted with household current (low-voltage injury) who are awake and alert at the time of medical evaluation are unlikely to have significant injury. An electrocardiogram (ECG) is not necessary, but a urinalysis should be considered for severe electrical injury as rhabdomyolysis may result. Brief contact with a high-voltage source results in a contact burn and is treated accordingly. Infants and toddlers may bite electric cords, resulting in burns to the commissure of the lips. A late complication is labial artery hemorrhage. If current passes through the body, the pattern of the injury depends on the path of the current. Exposure to high-voltage current

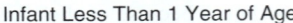

Infant Less Than 1 Year of Age

Name _____ Age _____ Ward _____

1st-degree erythema not to be included.

2nd-degree   3rd-degree

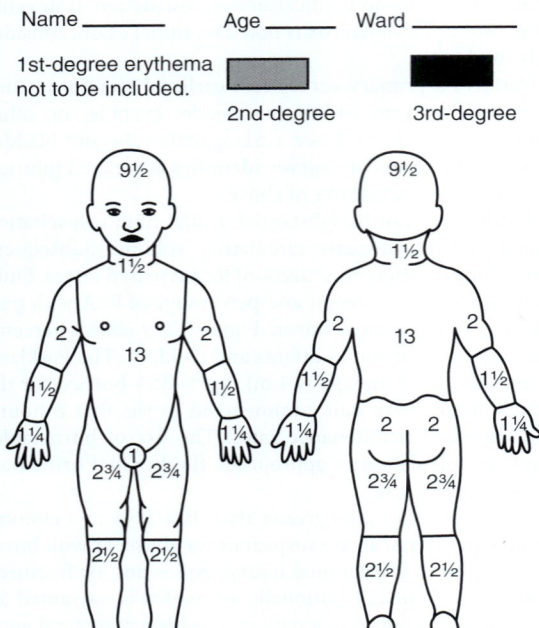

Variations From Adults Distribution in Infants and Children (in Percent).

	New-born	1 Year	5 Years	10 Years
Head	19	17	13	11
Both thighs	11	13	16	17
Both lower legs	10	10	11	12
Neck	2			
Anterior trunk	13			
Posterior trunk	13			
Both upper arms	8	These percentages		
Both lower arms	6	remain constant at		
Both hands	5	all ages		
Both buttocks	5			
Both feet	7			
Genitalia	1			
	100			

▲ **Figure 12–9.** Lund and Browder modification of Berkow scale for estimating extent of burns. (The table under the illustration is compiled from Berkow data.)

often induces a "locking-on" effect due to alternating current causing tetany. Extensive nerve and muscle injury, fractures, cardiac arrhythmias, and dermal burns are possible, and laboratory evaluation and cardiac monitoring should be performed. Lightning strikes are more likely to induce asystole and blast trauma. These patients often have no obvious physical injuries but can present in cardiopulmonary arrest.

Arbuthnot MK, Garcia AV: Early resuscitation and management of severe pediatric burns. Semin Pediatr Surg 2019 Feb;28(1): 73–78 [PMID: 30824139].

Lindford AJ, Lim P, Klass B, Mackey S, Dheansa BS, Gilbert PM: Resuscitation tables: a useful tool in calculating pre-burns unit fluid requirements. Emerg Med J 2009;26(4):245–249 [PMID: 19307382].

Strobel AM, Fey R: Emergency care of pediatric burns. Emerg Med Clin North Am 2018 May;36(2):441–458 [PMID: 29622333].

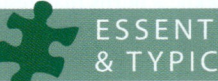

DISORDERS DUE TO EXTREMES OF ENVIRONMENT

HEAT-RELATED ILLNESSES & HEAT STROKE

ESSENTIALS OF DIAGNOSIS & TYPICAL FEATURES

► Heat illness is a spectrum ranging from heat cramps to life-threatening heat stroke.

► A high index of suspicion is required to make the diagnosis given the lack of specific symptoms and a usually normal or only slightly elevated temperature.

▶ Prevention

Avoid exposure to extremes of temperature for extended periods. Plan athletic activities for early morning or late afternoon and evening. Acclimatization, adequate water, shade, and rest periods can prevent heat-related illness.

▶ Clinical Findings

Heat cramps: also called exercise associated muscle cramping, heat cramps are brief, severe cramps of skeletal or abdominal muscles following exertion. Core body temperature is normal or slightly elevated. Electrolyte disturbance is rare and mild: laboratory evaluation is not indicated.

Heat exhaustion includes multiple, vague constitutional symptoms following heat exposure Patients continue to sweat and have varying degrees of sodium and water depletion. Core temperature should be monitored frequently and can range from 101°F to 104°F. Symptoms and signs include weakness, fatigue, headache, disorientation (only mild or quickly resolving), thirst, nausea with or without vomiting, and occasionally muscle cramps without CNS dysfunction. **Heat stroke** is a life-threatening failure of thermoregulation. Diagnosis is based on a rectal temperature above 40°C (> 104°F) with associated altered mental status in a patient after heat exposure. Although lack of sweating is sometimes seen, it is not a necessary criterion for diagnosis. Symptoms are like those of heat exhaustion, but severe CNS dysfunction is a hallmark. Patients may be incoherent or combative. In severe cases, vomiting, shivering, coma, seizures, nuchal rigidity, and posturing may be present. Cellular hypoxia, enzyme dysfunction, and disrupted cell membranes lead to global end-organ derangements and patients may develop rhabdomyolysis, myocardial necrosis, electrolyte abnormalities, acute tubular necrosis and renal failure, hepatic degeneration, acute respiratory distress syndrome (ARDS), and disseminated intravascular coagulation (DIC).

Differential Diagnosis

Viral gastroenteritis, sepsis and other infectious processes, neuroleptic malignant syndrome, malignant hyperthermia, hyponatremia, and anticholinergic poisoning may present similarly.

Treatment

Removal from the offending environment and removal of clothing are the first steps in managing any heat-related illness. **Heat cramps** typically respond to rest and rehydration with electrolyte solutions. Severe cramping and **heat exhaustion** should prompt evaluation of electrolytes to guide IV fluid rehydration.

Heat Stroke Management

1. Address ABCs.
2. Place monitors, including a continuous rectal temperature probe.
3. Initiate active cooling immediately, including: ice packs (neck, groin, and axillae), and a cooling blanket. (***Note:*** cold water submersion, with care to keep the head above water safely, is the gold standard and EMS may initiate this in the field prior to transportation, if the diagnosis is confirmed and possible.) Discontinue active cooling measures once core temperature reaches 38°C to prevent shivering.
4. Administer IV fluids: isotonic crystalloid for hypotension; cooled fluids are acceptable. Consider central venous pressure monitoring.
5. Consider diazepam once the patient starts to shiver, as shivering can interfere with the cooling process.
6. Order laboratory tests: point of care glucose, blood gas, CBC, CMP, CK, UA.
7. Admit to the pediatric ICU.

Prognosis

Full recovery is expected for heat cramps and heat exhaustion. Patients with heat stroke are at risk of end-organ damage. However, even in this critically ill population, most children recover fully with intensive management. Outcome is directly related to duration and elevation of temperature.

HYPOTHERMIA

ESSENTIALS OF DIAGNOSIS & TYPICAL FEATURES

► Hypothermia is defined as a core temperature of less than 35°C.
► Children are at increased risk due to a greater BSA-weight ratio.
► In children, hypothermia is most often associated with water submersion.

Prevention

Given the high association with submersion injuries, children should be carefully monitored around water. Proper use of life vests is critical.

Clinical Findings

A. Signs and Symptoms

Hypothermia is defined as a core temperature of less than 35°C. Peripheral vasoconstriction leads to cool, mottled skin. Shivering increases heat production to two to four times basal levels. As temperature falls, heart rate slows and mental status declines. Severe cases (< 28°C) mimic death: patients are pale or cyanotic, pupils may be fixed and dilated, muscles are rigid, and there may be no palpable pulses. Heart rates as low as 4–6 beats/min may provide adequate perfusion due to lowered metabolic needs in severe hypothermia. Besides cold exposure, disorders that cause incidental hypothermia include sepsis, metabolic derangements, ingestions, CNS disorders, and endocrinopathies. Neonates, trauma victims, intoxicated patients, and the chronically disabled are particularly at risk. With fast-onset hypothermia leading to pulselessness, the metabolic rate is reduced substantially before hypoxemia occurs and these patients can be successfully resuscitated with intact neurologic outcomes. Because of this, death is not pronounced until the patient has been rewarmed (to 32°C–34°C) and remains pulseless despite resuscitative efforts.

B. Laboratory Findings

For moderate to severe hypothermia, standard evaluation includes point of care glucose, blood gas, CBC, comprehensive metabolic panel (CMP), coagulation studies, and toxicology screen. Coagulopathy, hyperglycemia, and acidosis are common. Correction of derangements is accomplished by rewarming and resuscitating the patient.

C. Imaging Studies

Submersion is the most common cause of pediatric hypothermia. Chest x-ray (CXR) should be performed to assess for pulmonary edema and/or aspiration. Other radiographic studies should be performed according to history, with special consideration of possible trauma. ECG may also be considered, which may reveal interval abnormalities, T-wave inversions, and Osborn waves.

► Treatment

A. General Considerations

Management of hypothermia is largely supportive and focuses on rewarming. Continuously monitor core body temperature using a rectal thermometer, or in severe cases, an esophageal probe or a temperature sensing foley (as rectal probes often lag core temperatures). Warmed fluids can be given to ensure adequate preload. Handle patients gently as the hypothermic myocardium is exquisitely prone to arrhythmias. Ventricular fibrillation may occur spontaneously or because of minor handling, or invasive procedures or aggressive compressions. If asystole or ventricular fibrillation is present on the cardiac monitor, perform chest compressions and use standard PALS techniques as indicated. Defibrillation and pharmacologic therapy (eg, epinephrine) are more likely to be successful once core rewarming has occurred. Epinephrine doses may accumulate in the periphery due to vasoconstriction, and one approach for hypothermic patients in cardiac arrest is to limit to two to three doses of code-dose epinephrine. Glucose derangements should be corrected. With severe hypothermia, early consideration of extracorporeal membrane oxygenation (ECMO) is encouraged if available.

B. Rewarming

Rewarming techniques are categorized as passive external, active external, or active core rewarming. Passive rewarming, such as removing wet clothing, covering with blankets, is appropriate only for mild cases (32°C–35°C). Active external rewarming methods are appropriate for moderate to severe hypothermia and include warming lights, heating pads, the use of an electric warming blanket, and warm bath immersion. Be aware of a drop in core temperature after rewarming has begun, which occurs when vasodilation allows cooler peripheral blood to be distributed to the core circulation. This phenomenon is called *afterdrop*.

Active core rewarming techniques supplement active external warming for moderate to severe hypothermia. The techniques include warmed, humidified oxygen, warmed (40°C) crystalloid IV fluids, and warm bladder, peritoneal, and/or pleural lavage. If available, ECMO is the preferred method for rewarming a severely hypothermic patient, as it stabilizes volume, electrolyte disturbances while being safest for the heart.

► Prognosis

Recovery of the hypothermic victim is multifactorial. If associated with submersion injury (see next), CNS anoxic injuries and lung injury play a major role. Mortality rates are high and are related to the presence of underlying disorders and injuries. Children with a core temperature as low as 19°C have survived without neurologic compromise.

SUBMERSION INJURIES

ESSENTIALS OF DIAGNOSIS & TYPICAL FEATURES

► CNS and pulmonary injuries account for major morbidity.
► Child may appear well at presentation, but pulmonary changes can occur up to 6–8 hours later.

► Prevention

The World Health Organization defines *drowning* as the process of experiencing respiratory impairment from submersion/immersion in liquid. The terms *wet* or *dry drowning*, *near-drowning*, and others are no longer used; nonfatal drowning describes survivors. Water hazards are ubiquitous; even toilets, buckets, and washing machines pose a threat. Risk factors include epilepsy, alcohol, and lack of supervision, male sex, and African American race. Prevention strategies include fencing around public and private pools (at least 4 ft high, surrounded on all sides, self-closing/self-latching), the use of life vests, avoiding swimming alone, and adequate supervision (including "touch supervision" for younger children, ie, always keeping swimming children within arm's reach and in sight). Swimming lessons may have a role in a comprehensive prevention strategy, even for children 1–4 years of age.

► Clinical Findings

A. Signs and Symptoms

Depending on the duration of submersion, degree of hypoxia, and presence or absence of cardiac arrest, children may appear clinically dead or completely normal. Major morbidity stems from CNS and pulmonary insult. Cough, nasal flaring, grunting, retractions, wheezes or other lung sounds, and cyanosis can occur. Hypoxia, acidosis, and hypothermia may also be present, and can progress to bradycardia and ultimately cardiac arrest. A child rewarmed to 32°C–34°C but who remains pulseless is unlikely to survive to discharge or will have severe neurologic deficits. Until a determination of brain death can be made, however, aggressive resuscitation should continue in a patient with return of circulation. Cardiovascular changes include myocardial depression and arrhythmias. Later, children may develop ARDS, hypoxic brain injury and increased ICP.

B. Laboratory Findings

Electrolyte alterations are generally negligible for drowning. For drowning resulting in cardiac arrest, obtain glucose, blood gas, lactate, CBC, CMP, and coagulation studies in assessment of end organ damage.

C. Imaging Studies

Chest radiographs may be obtained if the patient is symptomatic to assess for pulmonary edema. Careful attention to cardiac rhythm and obtaining an ECG may be helpful in identifying patients with long QTc. CT of the brain is warranted when the patient is comatose or believed to have suffered prolonged asphyxia or blunt head trauma. Consider cervical spine imaging in patients where diving or intoxication may be involved.

► Treatment

Care is supportive. For children who appear well initially, observe for 6–8 hours on pulse oximetry for evidence of late pulmonary compromise and consider obtaining CXR if hypoxia or any other symptoms develop. Respiratory distress, an abnormal chest radiograph, or hypoxemia require supplemental oxygen, cardiopulmonary monitoring, and admission. For those who present in cardiac arrest, careful adherence to PALS guidelines is warranted, with an emphasis on rewarming if hypothermic, in addition to the following considerations. Early use of ECMO can be beneficial in cold water drowning/cardiac arrest with severe hypothermia. A shockable rhythm is found in less than 5% of drowning patients and is especially relevant in patients with long QTc (who can sometimes have torsades de pointes and subsequent pulseless ventricular tachycardia precipitated by cold water). Among those requiring CPR, up to 86% experience vomiting. Patients who warrant intubation may benefit from a lung protective strategy (including lower tidal volumes, ie, 4 kg–6 mL/kg ideal body weight). Careful fluid management is also warranted, balancing the need for preload and the risk of fluid overload. Less than 0.01% of drowning patients have a cervical spine injury, so routine use of C collar is not indicated unless the history is suggestive of high-risk mechanism.

► Prognosis

Anoxia from laryngospasm or aspiration leads to irreversible CNS damage after only 4–6 minutes. A child must fall through ice or directly into icy water for cerebral metabolism to be slowed sufficiently by hypothermia to provide protection from anoxia. Survival of the drowning victim depends on the duration of anoxia and the degree of lung injury. Children experiencing brief submersion with effective, high-quality resuscitation are likely to recover without sequelae.

AAP: https://www.aap.org/en-us/advocacy-and-policy/aap-health-initiatives/healthy-child-care/Pages/Safety-and-Injury-Prevention.aspx. Accessed June 30, 2019.

Brenner RA et al: Association between swimming lessons and drowning in childhood: a case-control study. Arch Pediatr Adolesc Med 2009;163(3):203–210 [PMID: 19255386].

Denny SA et al: Prevention of drowning. Pediatrics 2021;148(2). https://doi.org/10.1542/peds.2021-052227. Accessed May 1, 2023.

Safety and Injury Prevention: https://www.cdc.gov/earlycare/safety/index.html

Vanden H, Terry L, and Laurie M: Part 12: Cardiac Arrest in Special Situations | Circulation. AHA, https://www.ahajournals.org/doi/full/10.1161/circulationaha.110.971069. Accessed May 1, 2023.

▼ LACERATIONS

ESSENTIALS OF DIAGNOSIS & TYPICAL FEATURES

► The basic objectives of wound management are to stop bleeding, prevent infection, and ensure wound healing that achieves optimal functional and cosmetic outcomes.

► Options for wound closure include staples, sutures, and tissue adhesives.

Lacerations are a common reason to visit an ED. Lacerations can range from minor cuts that require no repair to complex lacerations that may require surgical consultation for adequate repair. The goals of laceration repair are to stop ongoing bleeding, prevent infection, and ensure wound healing that achieves optimal functional and cosmetic outcomes. Technical instruction of laceration repair is beyond this text's scope as we present the basics of laceration wound care.

► Clinical Findings

A. Signs and Symptoms

Lacerations present in a variety of shapes and sizes and occur over all parts of the body. Patients may present immediately after the injury or several days later. Wounds may contain foreign material, involve muscular, vascular, bony, tendon/ligamentous structures, or extend into joint spaces.

Options for wound repair include staples, suture material (both absorbable and nonabsorbable), and tissue adhesives. Tissue adhesives should *never* be used for highly contaminated wounds (eg, bites).

B. Imaging Studies

Imaging is usually not indicated for simple lacerations; however, plain x-rays may be indicated in certain situations. Lacerations caused by penetrating or crush injury may be associated with fractures. Lacerations across joints require specific evaluation for penetration of the joint space. Foreign bodies may be present in wounds and therefore careful attention must be made to assess complete removal when present.

▶ Treatment

Obtain information regarding mechanism and age of the injury. Assess extent of the wound with identification of foreign bodies, neurovascular compromise, tendon/ligament damage, muscle, or joint involvement. Obtain appropriate surgical consultations as needed.

Provide adequate analgesia or anesthesia, using topical or injectable methods prior to wound care. Irrigate the wound using normal saline (tap water is an appropriate alternative) with high pressure (5–8 psi [pounds per square inch]). Debride devitalized tissue, remove foreign material, and then close wound using staples, sutures, or tissue adhesive. Antibiotic ointment may be applied after wound repair. Consider tetanus prophylaxis depending on immunization status. Patients should return as instructed to have suture material removed if needed (Table 12–5).

▶ Prognosis

Functional and aesthetically pleasing cosmetics is generally achieved with initial repair. Complex lacerations may involve multiple visits with surgical service for wound reconstruction.

Table 12–5. Timing of suture removal.

Area of Body	Number of Days
Face	3-4
Neck	5-6
Scalp	6-7
Chest or abdomen	7
Arms and backs of hands	7
Legs and tops of feet	10
Back	10
Palms of hands or soles of feet	14

Harman S et al: Efficacy of pain control with topical lidocaine-epinephrine-tetracaine during laceration repair with tissue adhesive in children: a randomized controlled trial. CMAJ 2013;185(13):E626–E634 [PMID: 23897942].

Navanandan N, Renna-Rodriguez M, DiStefano M: Pearls in pediatric wound management. Clin Pediatr Emerg Med 2017 March;18(1):53–61.

Trott A: *Wounds and Lacerations: Emergency Care and Closure.* 3rd ed. Mosby INC: Philadelphia, PA; 2012.

Weiss EA et al: Water is a safe and effective alternative to sterile normal saline for wound irrigation prior to suturing, a prospective, double-blind, randomized, controlled clinical trial. BMJ Open 2013;16:3(1) [PMID: 23325896].

▼ ANIMAL & HUMAN BITES

Bites account for many visits to the ED. Most fatalities are due to dog bites. Human and cat bites cause the majority of infected bite wounds.

DOG BITES

▶ Clinical Findings

A. Signs and Symptoms

Dogs may cause abrasions, lacerations, and puncture wounds. Larger dogs may tear skin, subcutaneous tissue, and muscle, or even cause fractures. Other signs and symptoms are related to the structures injured.

B. Imaging Studies

Bites caused by large dogs associated with significant crush injury may be associated with fractures. Dislodged teeth may also be present in the wound. Plain x-rays may be indicated.

▶ Treatment

Provide appropriate analgesia or anesthesia before starting wound care. Debride any devitalized tissue and remove foreign matter. Irrigate using normal saline with high pressure (> 5 psi) and volume (> 1 L). Consider tetanus prophylaxis if it has been greater than 5 years since immunization. Rabies risk is low among dogs in developed countries; prophylaxis is rarely indicated. Suture wounds only if necessary for cosmesis as closure increases the risk of infection. Wound closure should be avoided on hands and feet if possible. **Do not use tissue adhesives due to risk of infection.** Bites involving a tendon, joint, periosteum, or associated with fracture require prompt orthopedic surgery consultation.

Pasteurella canis and *Pasteurella multocida*, streptococci, staphylococci, and anaerobes may infect dog bites. Broad-spectrum coverage with amoxicillin and clavulanic acid is first-line therapy. Prophylactic antibiotics do not decrease infection rates in low-risk dog bites, except those involving the hands and feet. Closure should not be performed more than 24 hours after initial injury due to increasing rates of infection.

Complications

Complications of dog bites include scarring, skin infections, CNS infections, septic arthritis, osteomyelitis, endocarditis, sepsis, and posttraumatic stress.

CAT BITES

Clinical Findings

A. Signs and Symptoms

Cat bites typically result in abrasions and puncture wounds. The risk of infection is higher when compared to dog bites as cat bites produce a deeper puncture wound. Within 12 hours, untreated bites may result in cellulitis or, when involving the hand, tenosynovitis, and septic arthritis. Other signs and symptoms are related to the structures injured. Cat scratch disease (CSD) can occur after bites or scratches, especially from kittens. Local findings include a papule, vesicle, or pustule at the site of inoculation. The hallmark of CSD is regional lymphadenitis. See Chapter 42 for a detailed discussion of CSD.

B. Laboratory Findings

Serologic tests for *Bartonella henselae* are available when cat scratch is suspected. C-reactive protein and erythrocyte sedimentation rate may be useful to monitor treatment response in infected cat bites.

Complications

Cellulitis, tenosynovitis, and septic arthritis are important potential complications of cat bites. Systemic illness is rare.

Treatment

Management is like that for dog bites. Provide appropriate analgesia or anesthesia before starting wound care. Debride any devitalized tissue and remove foreign matter. With isolated puncture wounds, high-pressure irrigation is contraindicated as it may force bacteria deeper into the tissue. Avoid chlorhexidine or povidone-iodine. Instead, use large volume water or saline.

Consider tetanus prophylaxis in the under- or unimmunized. As with dogs, rabies risk is low in developed countries and prophylaxis is rarely indicated. Cat bites should *not* be closed except when necessary for cosmesis.

Pasteurella multocida is the most common pathogen. Prophylactic antibiotics are recommended for all cat bites. First-line treatment is amoxicillin and clavulanic acid. Strongly consider surgical consultation and/or admission and parenteral antibiotics for infected wounds on the hands and feet due to higher risk of infection and worsened clinical outcomes.

HUMAN BITES

Most infected human bites occur during fights when a clenched fist strikes bared teeth. Pathogens most commonly include streptococci, staphylococci, anaerobes, and *Eikenella corrodens*. Hand wounds and deep wounds should be treated with antibiotic prophylaxis against *E corrodens* and gram-positive pathogens with a penicillinase-resistant antibiotic (amoxicillin with clavulanic acid). Wound management is the same as for dog bites. Only severe lacerations involving the face should be sutured. Other wounds can be managed by delayed primary closure or healing by secondary intention. A major complication of human bite wounds is infection of the metacarpophalangeal joints. A hand surgeon should evaluate clenched-fist injuries from human bites if extensor tendon injury is identified or joint involvement is suspected.

Halaas GW: Management of foreign bodies in the skin. Am Fam Physician 2007;76(5):683 [PMID: 17894138].
Savu AN, Schoenbrunner AR, Politi R, Janis JE: Practical review of the management of animal bites. Plast Reconstr Surg Glob Open 2021 Sep;9(9):e3778 [PMID: 34522565].

PAIN MANAGEMENT & PROCEDURAL SEDATION

Relief of pain and anxiety is paramount in providing care to pediatric patients and should be assessed and managed. Parenteral agents are effective, safe, and produce few side effects if used judiciously. Intranasal administration of several sedative and narcotic medications is now an accepted route of administration and may omit the need for IV placement. Many agents also have amnestic properties. Refer to Chapter 32 for more information on typical analgesic medications used in pediatric emergency care.

Procedures such as fracture reduction, laceration repair, burn care, sexual assault examinations, abscess incision and drainage, lumbar puncture, and diagnostic procedures such as CT and magnetic resonance imaging may all be performed more effectively and compassionately if effective analgesia, anxiolysis, or sedation is used. The clinician should decide whether procedures will require analgesia, anxiolysis, sedation, or a combination of methods.

Safe and effective sedation requires thorough knowledge of the selected agent and its side effects, suitable monitoring devices, resuscitative medications, equipment, and personnel. The decision to perform procedural sedation and analgesia (PSA) must be patient-oriented and tailored to specific procedural needs, while ensuring the child's safety throughout the procedure. To successfully complete this task, a thorough preprocedural assessment should be completed, including a directed history and physical examination. Risks, benefits, and limitations of the procedure should be discussed with the parent or guardian and informed; verbal consent must be obtained. PSA goals in the ED setting usually involve minimal or moderate sedation. Minimal sedation is a state in which the patient's sensorium is dulled, but he or she is still responsive to verbal stimuli. Moderate sedation is a depression of consciousness in which the child responds to tactile stimuli. In both cases, airway reflexes are preserved. It is important to remember that sedation is a continuum, and the child may drift to deeper, unintended levels of sedation. Ensure appropriate resuscitative equipment and personnel are readily available when providing analgesia, anxiolysis, and sedation.

American Academy of Pediatrics; Coté CJ et al: Guidelines for monitoring and management of pediatric patients before, during, and after sedation for diagnostic and therapeutic procedures. Pediatrics 2019;143(6):e20191000. doi: 10.1542/peds.2019-1000 [PMID: 31138666].

Couloures KG et al: Impact of provider specialty on pediatric procedural sedation complication rates. Pediatrics 2011;127(5):e1154–e1160 [PMID: 21518718].

Hartling L et al: What works and what's safe in pediatric emergency procedural sedation: an overview of reviews. Acad Emerg Med 2016 May;23(5):519–530. doi: 10.1111/acem.12938. Epub 2016 Apr 24. Review [PMID: 26858095].

Ryan PM, Kienstra AJ, Cosgrove P, Vezzetti R, Wilkinson M: Safety and effectiveness of intranasal midazolam and fentanyl use in combination in the pediatric emergency department. Am J Emerg Med 2019 Feb;37(2):237–240. Epub 2018 May 17 [PMID: 30146398].

Pediatric Toxicology

George Sam Wang, MD

Barry H. Rumack, MD

Richard C. Dart, MD, PhD

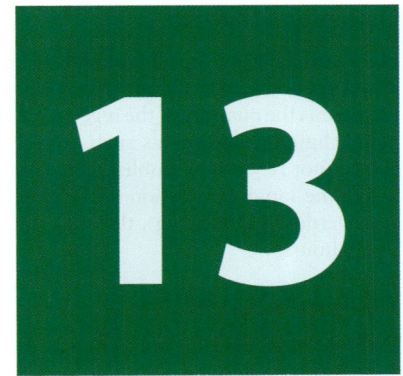

INTRODUCTION

Exposure to toxic substances occurs in children of all ages. Children younger than 6 years are primarily involved in unintentional exposures, with the peak incidence in 2-year-olds. Of the more than 2 million exposures reported by the American Association of Poison Control Centers' National Poison Data System in 2021, almost 60% of exposures occurred in those younger than 20 years: 40% in children aged 5 years and younger, 6% aged 6–12 years, and 9% aged 13–19 years. Fortunately, young children's exposures are typically unintentional and in low dose or volume. They can be exposed to intentional malicious administration through the actions of parents or caregivers and involvement of child abuse specialists is helpful in these cases (see Chapter 8). Recreational drug use and intentional ingestions account for more exposures in the adolescent population. From July 2019 through December 2021, the median monthly overdose deaths among persons aged 10–19 years increased 109%, with 90% of deaths involving opioids. Illicit fentanyl has been responsible for majority of these overdose deaths. Fentanyl is being sold as other prescription pharmaceuticals such as Xanax, Oxycodone (often referred as "M30's"), and Vicodin. Fentanyl has also been found in heroin, methamphetamine, and cocaine. Industrial or manufacturing processes may be associated with homes and farms, and exposures to hazardous substances should be considered in the history.

Pediatric patients also have special considerations pertaining to nonpharmaceutical toxicologic exposures. Their shorter stature places them lower to the ground as well as the fact that many are crawling, and some gas and vapor exposures will gather closer to the ground. They may have a greater inhalational exposure due to their higher minute ventilation. They may not be physically mature enough to remove themselves from exposures. They also have a large body surface area to weight ratio making them vulnerable to topical exposures and hypothermia.

Counterfeit Pills. Drug Fact Sheet, Drug Enforcement Administration. Available at: https://www.dea.gov/sites/default/files/2021-05/Counterfeit%20Pills%20fact%20SHEET-5-13-21-FINAL.pdf. Last accessed 2/21/2023.

Gummin DD et al: 2021 Annual Report of the American Association of Poison Control Centers' National Poison Data System (NPDS): 39th Annual Report. Clin Toxicol (Phila). 2022 Dec;60(12):1381–1643 [PMID: 36602072].

Tanz LJ et al: Drug Overdose Deaths Among Persons Aged 10-19 Years – United States, July 2019-December 2021. MMWR Morb Mortal Wkly Rep. 2022 Dec 16;71(50):1576–1582 [PMID: 36520659].

PHARMACOLOGIC PRINCIPLES OF TOXICOLOGY

In the evaluation of the poisoned patient, it is important to compare the anticipated pharmacologic or toxic effects with the patient's clinical presentation. If the history is that the patient ingested a sedative 30 minutes ago, but the clinical examination reveals dilated pupils, tachycardia, dry mouth, absent bowel sounds, and active hallucinations—clearly anticholinergic toxicity—diagnosis and therapy should proceed accordingly. In addition, standard pharmacokinetics (absorption, distribution, metabolism, and elimination) often cannot be applied in the setting of a large dose, since these parameters have been extrapolated from healthy volunteers receiving therapeutic doses.

Absorption

Depending on the route, absorption rates can vary in general, intravenous/intra-arterial > inhalation > sublingual > intramuscular > subcutaneous (SQ) > intranasal > oral > rectal > dermal. Large overdoses, hypotension, and decreased gut mobility are factors that can delay absorption.

Elimination Half-Life

The $t_{1/2}$ of an agent must be interpreted carefully. Most published $t_{1/2}$ values are for therapeutic dosages. The $t_{1/2}$ may increase as the quantity of the ingested substance increases for many common intoxicants such as salicylates. For example, one cannot rely on the published $t_{1/2}$ for salicylate (2 hours) to assume rapid elimination of the drug. In an acute salicylate overdose (150 mg/kg), the apparent $t_{1/2}$ is prolonged to 24–30 hours.

Volume of Distribution

The volume of distribution (Vd) of a drug is determined by dividing the amount of drug absorbed by the blood level. With aspirin for example, the Vd is 150–170 mL/kg body weight, or 10 L in an average adult. In contrast, digoxin distributes well beyond total body water. Because the calculation produces a volume above body weight, this figure is referred to as an "apparent Vd."

Body Burden

Body burden represents the total amount of drug or toxin within the body and may be useful to determine the dose absorbed from an ingestion. For example, a 20-kg child with an acetaminophen blood level of 200 mcg/mL (200 mg/L) would have a body burden of 4000 mg of acetaminophen. This is ascertained by taking the volume of distribution of 1 L times the weight of the child times the blood level in mg/L. This would be consistent with an overdose history of having consumed eight extra strength 500-mg tablets but would not be consistent with a history of therapeutic administration of 15 mg/kg for four doses. Formula for body burden by patient weight: Dose = Vd*Cp*W, where Vd is the volume of distribution, Cp is the plasma level, and W is the weight in kilograms.

Metabolism & Excretion

The route of excretion or detoxification are usually the liver and kidneys. Disease states impacting liver and kidney function can alter pharmacokinetics. Newborns and toddlers can have low Cytochrome P450 enzyme activity. Methanol, for example, is metabolized to the toxic product, formic acid. This metabolic step may be blocked by the antidote fomepizole or ethanol, and patients with renal failure may not eliminate methanol as readily.

Blood & Urine Concentrations

Care of the poisoned patient should never be guided solely by laboratory measurements. For many recreational drugs, urine assays can detect for several days after acute use. However, detection does not equate to acute intoxication and assays can have false positives and negatives. Blood concentration results often do not return in time to influence acute management. Initial treatment should be directed at symptomatic and supportive care, guided by clinical presentation, followed by more specific therapy based on laboratory determinations. CAUTION: Many laboratories report a normal range. When an overdose has occurred several hours earlier (or later) than expected peak times, the lab may report a level that is within the normal range. It is important to look at the timing as well as signs and symptoms when an overdose is considered.

PREVENTING CHILDHOOD POISONINGS

Inclusion of poison prevention as part of routine well-child care visits should begin at the 6-months. All poison control centers in the United States can be reached by dialing 1-800-222-1222; the call will be automatically routed to the correct regional center.

GENERAL ASSESSMENT OF EXPOSURES AND INGESTIONS

Obtaining Information About the Exposure

Basic information about the exposure from caregivers, patients, and first responders includes the agent and amount of agent ingested, route of exposure, intent, the patient's present condition, and the time elapsed since the exposure. It may be crucial to determine all the kinds of drugs and chemicals in the home. These may include drugs used by family members and their medical histories, dietary or herbal supplements, foreign medications, chemicals associated with the hobbies or occupations of family members, or the purity of the water supply.

Other pertinent information includes the product ingredients, and potential maximum amounts of the drug or chemical involved. If the specific substance is not identified, it is important that the surroundings be searched for possible containers or other clues. Ingredients of commercial products and medications can be obtained from a certified regional poison center. It is important to have the actual container at hand when calling. Safety data sheets (SDSs) can be helpful in providing product ingredients and concentration information. Caution should be used with online resources and information about treatment from toxicity as these can be incorrect or inappropriate.

Address Initial Resuscitation Evaluation

As in all emergencies, the principles of treatment are attention to Pediatric Advance Life Support algorithms in resuscitation: circulation, airway, and breathing. The most important treatment in toxicologic exposures is symptomatic and supportive care, followed by determining specific toxicologic treatment.

Treat Burns & Skin Exposures

Chemical burns may occur following exposure to strongly acidic or strongly alkaline agents should be decontaminated by flooding with sterile saline solution or water. A burn unit should be consulted with significant injury. Emergency department personnel should wear appropriate personal protective equipment (PPE) to prevent secondary exposure and contamination. Ocular exposures can initially be decontaminated at home by placing the child in the shower allowing the water to indirectly flow from the top of the head into the eyes. Otherwise, irrigation with subsequent assessment of pH and signs for ocular injury should be performed in the ED.

OTHER THERAPIES

Prevention of Absorption

A. Emesis and Lavage

These measures are rarely used in pediatric patients and have their own associated risk. They should not be used routinely in the management of ingestion and should be performed only in consultation with a poison center or medical toxicologist.

B. Activated Charcoal (AC)

The routine use of AC has decreased substantially in recent years, especially in unintentional pediatric ingestions where lick, sip, taste ingestions are rarely dangerous. AC can be considered in patients who are awake, alert, and able to drink it voluntarily, but it should not be routinely administered to all poisoned patients. It should never be given to patients with altered sensorium who are unable to protect their airway due to risk of aspiration. It is not recommended in ingestions of heavy metals, hydrocarbons, caustics, and solvent ingestions. The dose of AC is 1–2 g/kg (maximum, 100 g) per dose. Multidose AC may be useful for those agents that slow passage through the gastrointestinal (GI) tract, but repeated doses of sorbitol or saline cathartics must not be given. Repeated doses of cathartics may cause electrolyte imbalances and fluid loss.

C. Catharsis

Cathartics do not improve outcome and should be avoided.

D. Whole Bowel Irrigation (WBI)

WBI uses an orally administered, nonabsorbable hypertonic solution such as CoLyte or GoLYTELY. The effectiveness of this procedure in poisoned patients remains controversial. Preliminary recommendations for the use of WBI include ingestions with sustained-release preparations, mechanical movement of items through the bowel (eg, drug packets, iron tablets, lead foreign bodies), and substances that are poorly absorbed by AC (eg, lithium, iron). Underlying bowel pathology and intestinal obstruction are relative contraindications to its use. Consultation with a certified regional poison center is recommended.

Enhancement of Excretion

Excretion of certain substances can be hastened by urinary alkalinization or hemodialysis (HD) and is reserved for special circumstances.

A. Urinary Alkalinization

Urinary alkalinization should be chosen on the basis of the substance's pK_a, so that ionized drug will be trapped in the tubular lumen and not reabsorbed. Alkaline diuresis is mainly used for salicylate toxicity ($pK_a \sim 3$). Urinary alkalinization is achieved with sodium bicarbonate infusion. It is important to observe for hypokalemia, caused by the shift of potassium intracellularly. If complications such as renal failure or pulmonary edema are present, HD or hemoperfusion may be required.

B. Hemodialysis (HD)

HD is useful in the treatment of some poisons and in the general management of a critically ill patient. Characteristics of drugs amendable to HD include low molecular weight, low-protein binding, and low volume of distribution. Continuous hemofiltration techniques may be used when hypotensive patients may not tolerate traditional HD; however, clearance rates will be slower. HD should be considered part of supportive care if the patient satisfies any of the following criteria:

1. Potentially life-threatening toxicity that is caused by a dializable drug and cannot be treated by conservative means.

2. Renal failure or insufficiency.

3. Marked hyperosmolality or severe acid–base or electrolyte disturbances not responding to therapy.

American Academy of Clinical Toxicology; European Association of Poisons Centers and Clinical Toxicologists: Position statement and practice guidelines on the use of multi-dose activated charcoal in the treatment of acute poisoning. J Toxicol Clin Toxicol 1999;37:731 [PMID: 10584586].

Benson et al: Poison paper update: gastric lavage. Clin Toxicol 2013 Mar;51(3):140–146 [PMID: 23418938].

Chyka PA et al: Position paper: single-dose activated charcoal. American Academy of Clinical Toxicology; European Association of Poison Centres and Clinical Toxicologists. Clin Toxicol (Phila) 2005;43:61 [PMID: 15822758].

Hojer et al: Position paper update: ipecac syrup for gastrointestinal decontamination. Clin Toxicol 2013 Mar;15(3):134–139 [PMID: 23406298].

King et al: Extracorporeal removal of poisons and toxins. Clin J Am Soc Nephrol 2019;14(9):1408–1415 [PMID: 31439539].

Thanacoody R et al: Position paper update: whole bowel irrigation for gastrointestinal decontamination of overdose patients. Clin Toxicol (Phila) 2015 Jan;53(1):5–12 [PMID: 25511637].

The Extracorporeal Treatments in Poisoning Workgroup (EXTRIP): https://www.extrip-workgroup.org/. Accessed January 30, 2023.

MANAGEMENT OF SPECIFIC COMMON SUBSTANCES

ACETAMINOPHEN (PARACETAMOL, APAP)

Overdosage of APAP is common and can produce severe hepatotoxicity. Less than 0.1% of young children develop hepatotoxicity after APAP overdose. In young children, toxicity most commonly results from repeated overdosage arising from confusion about the age-appropriate dose, use of multiple products that contain APAP, or unintentional large volume ingestion.

APAP is normally metabolized in the liver. A small percentage of the drug goes through a pathway leading to a toxic metabolite (NAPQI). Normally, this electrophilic reactant is removed harmlessly by conjugation with glutathione. In overdosage, the supply of glutathione becomes exhausted, and NAPQI may bind covalently to components of liver cells to produce necrosis.

▶ Treatment

Treatment is to administer N-acetylcysteine (NAC). Both oral and intravenous routes of administration are equally efficacious. The blood APAP concentration should be obtained 4 hours after a single acute ingestion or as soon as possible thereafter and plotted on Figure 13–1. NAC is administered to patients whose APAP levels plot above the toxic range on the nomogram. The nomogram is used only for acute ingestion, not repeated supratherapeutic or unknown ingestions. In these situations, consider NAC for patients with a supratherapeutic APAP concentration, or elevated liver transaminitis. NAC is effective even when given more than 24 hours after ingestion, although it is most effective when given within 8 hours post ingestion.

There are now several NAC dosing regimens used in clinical practice. Two of the most common methods of intravenous administration are either the three-bag or the two-bag regimen. The three-bag method consists of a loading dose of 150 mg/kg administered over 15–60 minutes; followed by a second infusion of 50 mg/kg over 4 hours, and then a third infusion of 100 mg/kg over 16 hours. The two-bag regimen administers a similar amount of NAC over the treatment course but involves a slower loading dose that has been associated with lower adverse reactions (nonallergic anaphylactoid reactions) and medication errors. The two-bag method is administered as a 200 mg/kg IV bolus over 4 hours, followed by 100 mg/kg over 16 hours. Patient-tailored therapy is critical when utilizing the IV "20-hour" protocol and those patients who still have APAP measurable and/or elevated aspartate transaminase/alanine transaminase (AST/ALT) may need treatment beyond the 20 hours called for in the product insert.

AST–serum glutamic oxaloacetic transaminase (AST–SGOT), ALT–serum glutamic pyruvic transaminase (ALT–SGPT), serum bilirubin, and plasma prothrombin time should be followed daily. Significant abnormalities of liver function may not peak until 72–96 hours after ingestion. Fomepizole (Antizol, 4-MP) is being experimentally utilized for acetaminophen overdose especially in patients with delay to treatment and following massive ingestion. It is best to consult a poison center.

Akakpo JY, et al: Comparing N-acetylcysteine and 4-methylpyrazole as antidotes for acetaminophen overdose. Arch Toxicol 2022 Feb;96(2):453–465 [PMID: 34978586].

Dart RC, Rumack BH: Patient-tailored acetylcysteine administration. Ann Emerg Med 2007;50:280–281 [PMID: 17418449].

Hoyte C, Dart RC: Transition to two-bag intravenous acetylcysteine for acetaminophen overdose: a poison center's experience. Clin Toxicol (Phila) 2019 Jan 28:1–2 [PMID: 30689437].

Sudanagunta S et al: Comparison of two-bag versus three-bag N-acetylcysteine regimens for pediatric acetaminophen toxicity. Ann Pharmacother 2023 Jan;57(1):36–43 [PMID: 35587124].

ALCOHOL, ETHYL (ETHANOL)

Alcoholic beverages, tinctures, cosmetics, perfumes, mouthwashes, food extracts (vanilla, almond, etc), rubbing alcohol, and hand sanitizers are common sources of alcohol ingestion in children. Alcohol is even available in powdered form for mixing and consumption. In most states, alcohol levels of 50–80 mg/dL are considered compatible with impaired senses, and levels of 80–100 mg/dL are considered evidence of intoxication. (Blood levels cited here are for adults; comparable figures for children are not available.) Children can show a change in sensorium with blood levels as low as 10–20 mg/dL and have higher risk for hypoglycemia than adults; any child displaying such changes should be seen immediately.

Recent erroneous information regarding hand sanitizers has indicated that a "lick" following application on the hand could cause toxicity in children. However, hand sanitizers contain 62% ethanol and toxicity following small ingestion is possible. Potential blood ethanol concentration following consumption of a 62% solution in a 10-kg child is calculated as follows:

1 oz = 30 mL × 62% = 18.6 mL of pure ethanol
18.6 mL × 0.79 (the specific gravity)
= 14.7 g of ethanol, or 14,700 mg

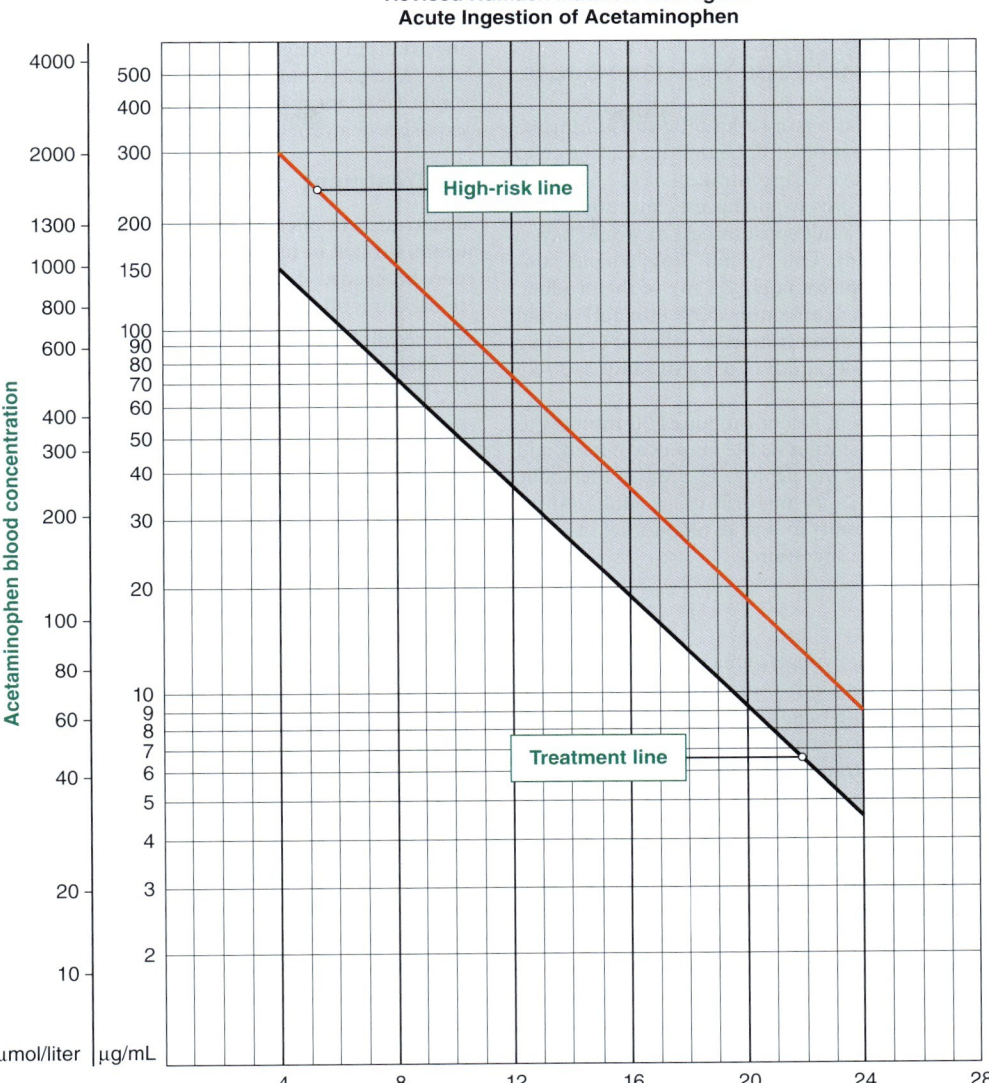

Revised Rumack-Matthew Nomogram
Acute Ingestion of Acetaminophen

High-risk line

Treatment line

Acetaminophen blood concentration

µmol/liter | µg/mL

Hours postingestion

The original Rumack-Matthew nomogram line, derived from patient data, begins at 200 µg/mL at 4 hours after ingestion (Rumack and Matthew 1975). The treatment line (safety line) beginning at 150 µg/mL at 4 hours was derived as 25% lower than the original nomogram line (Rumack et al 1981). A line beginning at 300 µg/mL at 4 hours was derived as 50% greater than the original nomogram line to denote patients and increased risk of developing liver injury (Smilkstein et al, 1988). Acetylcysteine should be initiated if a serum or plasma acetaminophen blood concentration drawn 4 to 24 hours after ingestion falls on or above the treatment line.

▲ **Figure 13–1.** Semilogarithmic plot of plasma acetaminophen levels versus time. (Reproduced with permission from Rumack et al, Acetaminophen Toxicity: Experimental and Clinical Advances. Elsevier; 2024.)

In a 10-kg patient, the total body water distribution (Vd) will be 6 L.

$$14{,}700 \text{ mg} \div 6 \text{ L} = 2450 \text{ mg/L} \rightarrow 2450 \text{ mg/L} \div 10 = 245 \text{ mg/dL}$$

Based on these calculations, a 10-kg child consuming 0.5 oz would have a concentration of 122.5 mg/dL; a 20-kg child consuming 1 oz would have a concentration of 122.5 mg/dL; a 30-kg child consuming 1 oz would have a concentration of 81.7 mg/dL; and a 70-kg adult consuming 1 oz would have a concentration of 35 mg/dL. One "pump" from a hand sanitizer bottle dispenses approximately 2.5 mL of the product. If ingested, this amount (containing 62% ethanol) would create a blood ethanol concentration as follows: (1) 10-kg child: 23.1 mg/dL, (2) 20-kg child: 11.6 mg/dL, and (3) 30-kg child: 7.7 mg/dL.

Complete absorption of alcohol requires 30 minutes to 6 hours, depending on the volume, the presence of food, and the time spent consuming the alcohol. The rate of metabolic degradation is constant (~ 20 mg/dl/h in an adult). Absolute ethanol, 1 mL/kg, results in a peak blood level of about 100 mg/dL in 1 hour after ingestion.

▶ Treatment

Management of sedation, hypoglycemia and acidosis is usually the only measure required. Administer IV dextrose if blood glucose is less than 60 mg/dL. Death is usually caused by CNS depression and subsequent respiratory failure. Secondary evaluation for traumatic injury and coingestants should also be performed.

AMPHETAMINES (STIMULANTS, METHAMPHETAMINE, 3,4-METHYLENEDIOXY-*N*-METHYLAMPHETAMINE)

▶ Clinical Presentation

A. Acute Exposure

Amphetamine, 3,4-methylenedioxy-*N*-methylamphetamine (MDMA), and methamphetamine use is common because of the widespread availability of "diet pills" and the use of "ecstasy," "speed," "crank," "crystal," and "ice" by adolescents. (Care must be taken in the interpretation of slang terms because they have multiple meanings.) Diversion of drugs used for attention-deficit/hyperactivity disorder, such as methylphenidate, is becoming more common. There are also new psychoactive substances (NPS) such as synthetic cannabinoids ("spice, K2") and MPDV or mephedrone ("bath salts, plant food"), which cause effects similar to stimulants.

Symptoms include central nervous system (CNS) stimulation, anxiety, hyperactivity, hyperpyrexia, diaphoresis, hypertension, abdominal cramps, nausea and vomiting, and inability to void urine. MDMA has been associated with hyponatremia and seizures. Severe cases often include rhabdomyolysis and acidosis. Deaths can occur in unintentional ingestions in young children. A toxic psychosis indistinguishable from paranoid schizophrenia may occur. Methamphetamine laboratories in homes are a potential cause of childhood exposure to a variety of hazardous and toxic substances.

▶ Treatment

The treatment of choice are benzodiazepines, such as lorazepam, titrated in increments to effect. Very large total doses may be needed. In cases of extreme agitation or hallucinations, droperidol (0.1 mg/kg per dose) or haloperidol (up to 0.1 mg/kg) parenterally has been used. Hyperthermia should be aggressively controlled, and intubation and paralysis may be required.

Carvalho M et al: Toxicity of amphetamines: an update. Arch Toxicol 2012;86(8):1167–1231 [PMID: 22392347].

Shafi A et al: New psychoactive substances: a review and updates. Ther Adv Psychopharmacol 2020 Dec 17;10:2045125320967197 [PMID: 33414905].

Wang GS, Hoyte C: Novel drugs of abuse. Pediatr Rev 2019 Feb;40(2):71–78 [PMID: 30709973].

ANESTHETICS, LOCAL

Intoxication from local anesthetics may be associated with CNS stimulation, acidosis, delirium, ataxia, shock, seizures, and death. Methemoglobinemia has been reported following local mouth or dental analgesia, typically with benzocaine or prilocaine. It has also been reported with the use of topical anesthetic preparations in infants. The maximum recommended dose for SQ infiltration of lidocaine is 4.5 mg/kg (Table 13–1). Oral teething anesthetic products have been voluntarily recalled due to adverse events.

Local anesthetics used in obstetrics cross the placental barrier and are not efficiently metabolized by the fetal liver. Mepivacaine, lidocaine, and bupivacaine can cause fetal bradycardia, neonatal depression, and death. Unintentional injection of mepivacaine into the head of the fetus during paracervical anesthesia has caused neonatal asphyxia, cyanosis, acidosis, bradycardia, seizures, and death.

▶ Treatment

If the anesthetic has been ingested, mucous membranes should be cleansed carefully, topical applications should be cleaned and irrigated. Oxygen administration is indicated, with assisted ventilation if necessary. Symptomatic methemoglobinemia is treated with 1% methylene blue, 0.2 mL/kg (1–2 mg/kg per dose, IV) over 5–10 minutes. Acidosis and dysrhythmias may be treated with sodium bicarbonate, hypotension with vasopressors, seizures with benzodiazepines, and bradycardia with atropine. In the event of cardiac arrest, 20% lipid (fat) emulsion therapy should be initiated.

Table 13–1. Pharmacologic properties of local anesthetics.

	pK$_a$	Protein Binding (%)	Relative Potency	Duration of Action	Approximate Maximum Allowable Subcutaneous Dose (mg/kg)
Esters					
Chloroprocaine	9.3	Unknown	Intermediate	Short	10
Cocaine	8.7	92	Low	Medium	3
Procaine	9.1	5	Low	Short	10
Tetracaine	8.4	76	High	Long	3
Amides					
Bupivacaine	8.1	95	High	Long	2
Etidocaine	7.9	95	High	Long	4
Lidocaine	7.8	70	Low	Medium	4.5
Mepivacaine	7.9	75	Intermediate	Medium	4.5
Prilocaine	8.0	40	Intermediate	Medium	8
Ropivacaine	8.2	95	Intermediate	Long	3

Reproduced with permission from Nelson et al: *Goldfrank's Toxicologic Emergencies.* 9th ed. New York, NY: McGraw Hill; 2011.

Initial 1.5 mL/kg bolus over 1 minute, followed by 0.25 mL/kg/min for up to 20–30 minutes until spontaneous circulation returns. Repeat bolus can be considered.

Gosselin S et al: Evidence-based recommendations on the use of intravenous lipid emulsion therapy in poisoning. Clin Toxicol (Phila) 2016 Sep 8;1–25 [PMID: 27608281].

Long B et al: Local anesthetic systemic toxicity: a narrative review for emergency clinicians. Am J Emerg Med 2022 Sep;59:42–48 [PMID: 35777259].

McMahon et al: Local anesthetic systemic toxicity in the pediatric patient. Am J Emerg Med 2022 Apr;54:325 e3–325.e6 [PMID: 34742600].

ANTIHISTAMINES & COUGH & COLD PREPARATIONS

Medications included in this area are antihistamine (brompheniramine, chlorpheniramine, diphenhydramine, doxylamine), antitussive (dextromethorphan), expectorant (guaifenesin), and decongestant (pseudoephedrine, phenylephrine). In 2007, manufacturers voluntarily removed preparations intended for use in children younger than 4 years from the market. Most adverse events stem from unintentional ingestions of supratherapeutic doses of antihistamines or dextromethorphan. A high proportion of life-threatening cases are associated with child abuse (sedating a child with medication).

Although antihistamines typically cause CNS depression, children can react paradoxically with excitement, hallucinations, delirium, ataxia, tremors. In overdose settings, seizures followed by CNS depression, respiratory failure, or cardiovascular collapse can occur. A potentially toxic dose is 10–50 mg/kg of the most commonly used antihistamines, but toxic reactions have occurred at much lower doses. Anticholinergic effects such as dry mouth, fixed dilated pupils, flushed face, fever, and hallucinations may be prominent. Dextromethorphan can lead to altered mentation, hallucinations, nystagmus, and serotonin toxicity in large ingestions or when taken with other serotonergic agents. Death may occur with massive overdose.

▶ Treatment

Benzodiazepines, such as lorazepam (0.1 mg/kg IV), can be used to control seizures or agitation. Physostigmine (0.5–2.0 mg IV, slowly administered) dramatically reverses the delirium and agitation of the anticholinergic effects of antihistamines; however, the duration of effect is short, and an infusion may be needed. Hypotension should be treated with normal saline at a dose of 10–20 mg/kg and a vasopressor if necessary. Sodium bicarbonate may be useful for QRS widening and dysrhythmias at a dose of 1–2 mEq/kg, making certain that the arterial pH does not exceed 7.55.

Green JL et al: Safety profile of cough and cold medication use in pediatrics. Pediatrics 2017 Jun;139(6): e20163070. [PMID: 28562262].

Halmo LS et al: Pediatric fatalities associated with over-the-counter cough and cold medications. Pediatrics. 2021 Nov;148(5): e2020049536 [PMID 34607934].

Wang GS et al: A randomized trial comparing physostigmine vs lorazepam for treatment of antimuscarinic (anticholinergic) toxidrome. Clin Toxicol (Phila) 2021 Aug;59(8):698–704 [PMID: 33295809].

BARBITURATES & BENZODIAZEPINES

Barbiturates are rarely used today and have mostly been replaced with benzodiazepines for their use in seizures or for sedation. The toxic effects of barbiturates include confusion, poor coordination, coma, miotic or fixed dilated pupils, and respiratory depression. Ingestion of more than 6 mg/kg of long-acting or 3 mg/kg of short-acting barbiturates is usually toxic. Benzodiazepines typically cause CNS depression and lethargy without hemodynamic compromise in unintentional oral ingestions. Large oral overdoses, coingestants with other sedative/hypnotics, or iatrogenic IV overdose can cause cardiovascular collapse or respiratory depression.

▶ Treatment

Careful, conservative management with emphasis on maintaining a clear airway, adequate ventilation, and control of hypotension is critical. Urinary alkalization and the use of multiple-dose charcoal may decrease the elimination half-life of phenobarbital but have not been shown to alter the clinical course. Flumazenil can be considered if severe CNS depression or respiratory depression develops after benzodiazepine overdose using a dose of 0.01 mg/kg IV (maximum dose of 0.2 mg).

Bachhuber MA et al: Increasing benzodiazepine prescriptions and overdose mortality in the United States, 1996–2013. Am J Public Health 2016 Apr;106(4):686–688 [PMID: 26890165].
Kreshak AA et al: Flumazenil administration in poisoned pediatric patients. Pediatr Emerg Care 2012;28(5):488 [PMID: 22531190].

BELLADONNA ALKALOIDS (ATROPINE, JIMSONWEED, POTATO LEAVES, SCOPOLAMINE, STRAMONIUM)

The effects of anticholinergic (or antimuscarinic) compounds include dry mouth; thirst; decreased sweating with hot, dry, flushed skin; high fever; and tachycardia. The pupils are dilated, and vision is blurred. Speech and swallowing may be impaired. Agitation, delirium, and coma are common. Leukocytosis may occur, confusing the diagnosis.

Atropinism has been caused by normal doses of atropine or homatropine eye drops. Many common plants (such as Datura Stramonium/Jimson Weed), over-the-counter medications (antihistamines and sleep aids), and antipsychotics contain belladonna alkaloids or medications with anticholinergic effects (Photo 1)

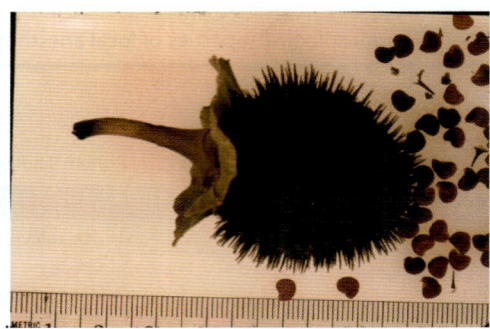

▶ Treatment

Gastric emptying is slowed by anticholinergics; thus, gastric decontamination may be useful even if delayed. If the patient is awake and showing no signs or symptoms, administration of AC can be considered. Benzodiazepines should be administered to control agitation. Bolus dosing should be given in escalating doses, and high doses may be required. Physostigmine (0.5–2.0 mg IV, administered slowly) dramatically reverses the central agitation and delirium, and infusions have been used to sustain the response. Hyperthermia should be aggressively controlled. Catheterization may be needed if the patient cannot void.

Arens AM, Kearney T: Adverse effects of physostigmine. J Med Toxicol 2019 Feb 11 [PMID: 31414401].
Glaststein M et al: Belladonna alkaloid intoxication: the 10-year experience of a large tertiary care pediatric hospital. Am J Ther 2013 Nov;20 [PMID: 24263161].
Wang GS et al: A randomized trial comparing physostigmine vs lorazepam for treatment of antimuscarinic (anticholinergic) toxidrome. Clin Toxicol (Phila) 2020 Dec 9:1–13 [PMID: 33295809].

β-BLOCKERS & CALCIUM CHANNEL BLOCKERS

β-Blockers (BB) and calcium channel blockers (CCB) primarily cause cardiovascular toxicity, bradycardia, hypotension, and various degrees of heart block; cardiac dysrhythmias may develop. Severe toxicity can cause CNS depression (typically due to hemodynamic collapse). Propranolol is associated with seizures and also QRS widening. Hyperglycemia can be seen with CCB toxicity.

▶ Treatment

Initial stabilization with IV fluid resuscitation with isotonic fluids should be initiated. Atropine can be given for symptomatic bradycardia. Calcium at doses of 20 mg/kg and repeated as needed should be administered. Infusions of calcium chloride 10%, 0.2–0.5 mL/kg/h, can be started after initial bolus dosing. Glucagon can be administered; 50–100 mcg/kg (5–10 mg) IV bolus followed by 2–5 mg/h infusion if readily available. Vasopressors such as epinephrine or norepinephrine should be started before persistent hypotension or bradycardia. In patients who are severely poisoned and refractory to these initial measures, high-dose insulin euglycemic therapy (HIET) should be initiated. Doses for HIET begin at 0.5–1 U/kg/h and can be escalated as needed. ECMO can be used in cases of refractory cardiogenic shock. Your regional poison control center or medical toxicologist should be contacted for further details on dosing of this therapy.

Cole et al: High dose insulin for beta-blocker and calcium channel-blocker poisoning. Am J Emerg Med 2018 Oct;36(10): 1817–1824 [PMID: 29452919].

Krenz JR, Kayaked Y: An overview of hyperinsulinemic-euglycemic therapy in calcium channel blocker and β-blocker overdose. Pharmacotherapy 2018 Nov;38(11):1130–1142 [PMID: 30141827].

St-Onge M et al: Experts consensus recommendations for the management of calcium channel blocker poisoning in adults. Crit Care Med 2017 Mar;45(3):e306–e315 [PMID: 27749343].

Upchurch C et al: Extracorporeal membrane oxygenation use in poisoning: a narrative review with clinical recommendations. Clin Toxicol (Phila) 2021 Oct;59(10):877–887 [PMID: 34396873].

CANNABIS (MARIJUANA)

Cannabis is becoming more readily available as most US states have allowed cannabis for medical conditions, and almost half allow recreational cannabis. It is also available for use in multiple forms, including high concentrated products (dabs, butters, waxes), vaporizers, and infused edible products that all can have high concentrations of THC (tetrahydrocannabinol), the most psychoactive component. Cannabidiol (CBD) is another cannabinoid that has gained significant popularity. A pharmaceutical product is FDA approved for the use of refractory seizures in children. However, many unregulated CBD products are being used for many nonapproved conditions. It is not expected to result in significant toxicity in the overdose setting; however, non-FDA-approved products may contain other ingredients, including THC.

Young children who ingest edible products have a degree of sleepiness and ataxia. However, more severe symptoms can develop, including CNS depression, coma, and respiratory depression requiring mechanical ventilation. Symptoms in young children can last over 24 hours. Inhalational use of high-concentrated products can lead to tachycardia, hypertension, agitation, and acute psychosis. Habitual use has led to significant nausea, vomiting, and abdominal pain relieved by hot showers, often labeled "cannabinoid hyperemesis syndrome" (CHS). Symptomatic and supportive care is the mainstay for treatment: supporting cardiorespiratory adverse effects and treating psychosis and agitation with benzodiazepines or antipsychotics. Capsaicin cream and haloperidol have been reported to improve CHS symptoms.

Perisetti A et al: Cannabis hyperemesis syndrome: an update on pathophysiology and management. Ann Gastroenterol 2020 Nov–Dec;33(6):571–578 [PMID: 33162734].

Tweet MS et al: Pediatric edible cannabis exposures and acute toxicity: 2017–2021. Pediatrics 2023 Jan 3: e2022057761 [PMID 36594224].

CARBON MONOXIDE

Carbon monoxide (CO) is a colorless, odorless gas produced from burning various fuels. Onset of symptoms may be more rapid and more severe if the patient lives at a high altitude, has a high respiratory rate (ie, infants), is pregnant, or has myocardial insufficiency or lung disease. Normal blood may contain up to 5% carboxyhemoglobin (10% in smokers). Neonates may have elevated carboxyhemoglobin levels due to breakdown of bilirubin.

Presenting symptoms can include nonspecific symptoms such as headache or flu-like illness. Other effects include confusion, unsteadiness, and coma. Other signs may include improvement of symptoms after leaving the exposed environment. The outcome of severe toxicity may be complete recovery, vegetative state, or any degree of neuropsychiatry injury between these extremes.

▶ Treatment

The biologic half-life of CO on room air is approximately 200–300 minutes; on 100% oxygen, it is 60–90 minutes. Thus, 100% oxygen should be administered immediately. Hyperbaric oxygen (HBO) therapy at 2.0–2.5 atm of oxygen shortens the half-life to 30 minutes but is practically difficult to deploy in a timely manner. The use of HBO therapy for delayed neurologic sequelae can be considered but remains controversial and the primary focus of care should be acute resuscitation and stabilization in consultation with a medical toxicologist. After the level has been reduced to near zero, therapy is aimed at the nonspecific sequelae of anoxia. Evaluation of the source should be performed before the patient is discharged.

Buckley NA et al: Hyperbaric oxygen for carbon monoxide poisoning. Cochrane Database Syst Rev 2011;13(4):CD002041 [PMID: 21491385].

Macnow TE et al: Carbon monoxide poisoning in children: diagnosis and management in the emergency department. Pediatr Emerg Med Pract 2016 Sep;13(9):1–24 [PMID: 27547917].

CAUSTIC INGESTIONS

Both acids and alkalis can burn the skin, mucous membranes, and eyes (Photo 2). Vomiting, dysphagia, airway emergencies, burns, and abdominal pain can occur after ingestion. Respiratory distress may be due to edema of the epiglottis, pulmonary edema resulting from inhalation of fumes, or pneumonia. In severe cases, mediastinitis, intercurrent infections, or shock can occur. Perforation of the esophagus or stomach is rare. Residual lesions include esophageal, gastric, and pyloric strictures (which increases risk for cancer) and scars of the cornea, skin, and oropharynx.

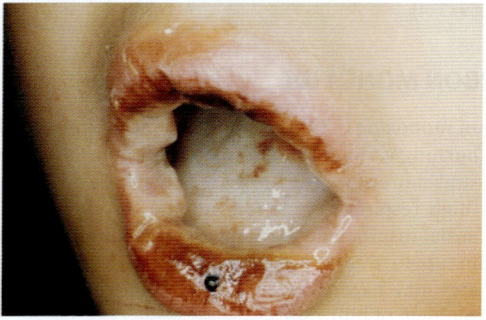

1. Acids (Hydrochloric, Hydrofluoric, Nitric, & Sulfuric Acids; Sodium Bisulfate)

Strong acids are commonly found in metal and toilet bowl cleaners, batteries, and other products, and can lead to coagulative necrosis. Hydrofluoric (HF) acid is a particularly dangerous acid. HF creates a penetrating burn that can last hours or days. Large dermal exposure or small ingestion of HF may produce life-threatening hypocalcemia.

2. Bases (Liquid Clog Removers – such as Crystal Drano, Detergents, Bleach—Examine the Label or Call a Poison Center to Determine Contents)

Alkalis can potentially produce more severe injuries than acids, resulting in liquefactive necrosis. Some substances, such as clog removers, are quite toxic, whereas the chlorinated bleaches (3%–6% solutions of sodium hypochlorite) are usually not toxic in small amounts. Chlorinated bleaches when mixed with a strong acid (toilet bowl cleaners) or ammonia, may produce irritating chlorine or chloramine gas, respectively. These gases can cause mucous membrane irritation or lung injury if inhaled in a closed space (eg, bathroom).

▶ Treatment

Emetics and lavage are contraindicated. Can be diluted with water but take care not to induce emesis by excessive fluid administration. Neutralization should not be attempted. Burned areas of the skin, mucous membranes, or eyes should be washed with copious amounts of warm water. The eye should be irrigated for 20 minutes. Ophthalmologic consultation should be obtained for significant caustic eye injuries. An endotracheal tube may be required due to airway involvement such as laryngeal edema. The absence of oral lesions does not rule out the possibility of laryngeal or esophageal burns. Esophagoscopy should be performed if the patient has

significant burns or difficulty in swallowing, drooling, vomiting, or stridor. Evidence is not conclusive, but corticosteroids may be helpful in significant esophageal burns. Antibiotics may be needed if mediastinitis develops, but they should not be used prophylactically.

HF burns on skin are treated with 10% calcium gluconate gel or calcium gluconate infusion. Ingestion of HF may require large doses of IV calcium or cardiovascular monitoring. Therapy should be guided by calcium levels, the electrocardiogram (ECG), and clinical signs.

Chirica M et al: Caustic ingestion. Lancet 2017;389:2014–2052 [PMID: 28045663].

Usta M et al: High doses of methylprednisolone in the management of caustic esophageal burns. Pediatrics 2014;133(6): E1518–E1524 [PMID: 24864182].

CENTRAL α₂-ADRENERGIC AGONIST

Central α_2-adrenergic agonists are common over-the-counter and prescribed medications. The imidazolines are found in nasal decongestants and eye drops to relieve redness. Clonidine and guanfacine are used to treat attention deficit hyperactivity disorder or hypertension. Dexmedetomidine is an IV central α_2-adrenergic agonist used for sedation. Xylazine is a veterinary tranquilizer that has been found as an adulterant in illicit opioids. These medications exert their effects by decreasing presynaptic release of catecholamines at the α_2-adrenergic receptors in the brain, resulting in decreased sympathetic outflow.

▶ Clinical Findings

Patients can present similar to an opioid toxidrome with miosis, CNS depression, and respiratory depression. Other common effects include bradycardia and hypotension.

▶ Treatment

If the patient becomes obtunded, or has inability to protect their airway, intubation may be indicated. Naloxone has been tried to reverse signs of toxicity with varying success. Symptomatic bradycardia can be treated with IV fluid resuscitation or atropine. Hypotension should be treated initially with IV fluid resuscitation, followed by vasopressors if needed.

Deutsch SA, De Jong AR: Xylazine complicating opioid ingestions in young children. Pediatrics 2023 Jan 1;151(1):e2022058684 [PMID: 36550066].

Seger DL, Loden JK: Naloxone reversal of clonidine toxicity: dose, dose, dose. Clin Toxicol (Phila) 2018 Oct;56(10):873–879 [PMID: 29544366].

Wang et al: Unintentional pediatric exposures to central alpha-2 agonists reported to the National Poison Data System. J Pediatr 2014;164(1):149–152 [PMID: 24094880].

COCAINE

Cocaine is absorbed intranasally, via inhalation or ingestion. Effects are noted almost immediately when the drug is taken intravenously or smoked and are delayed for about an hour when the drug is taken orally or nasally. Cocaine prevents the reuptake of endogenous catecholamines, thereby causing an initial sympathetic discharge, followed by catechol depletion after chronic abuse.

▶ Clinical Findings

A local anesthetic and vasoconstrictor, cocaine is also a potent stimulant to both the CNS and the cardiovascular system. The initial tachycardia, hyperpnea, hypertension, and stimulation of the CNS are often followed by coma, seizures, hypotension, and respiratory depression. In severe cases of overdose, various dysrhythmias may be seen due blockade of sodium channels. If large doses are taken intravenously, myocardial infarction, dysrhythmias, rhabdomyolysis, or hyperthermia may result that can result in death.

Cocaine can be contaminated with levamisole (veterinary anthelmintic), which can lead to systemic vasculitis and agranulocytosis.

▶ Treatment

Cocaine metabolites can be positive in urine for 3–5 days after exposure. For cardiac involvement/chest pain, an ECG is indicated. Signs of myocardial infarction should be treated accordingly, and QRS widening should be treated with sodium bicarbonate. Seizures are treated with IV benzodiazepines. Because cocaine abuse may deplete norepinephrine, an indirect agent such as dopamine may be less effective than a direct agent such as norepinephrine for hypotension. Agitation is best treated with a benzodiazepine.

Heard K et al: Mechanisms of acute cocaine toxicity. Open Pharmacol J 2008;2(9):70–78 [PMID: 19568322].
Vagi SJ: Passive multistate surveillance for neutropenia after use of cocaine or heroin possibly contaminated with levamisole. Ann Emerg Med 2013 Apr;61(4):468–474 [PMID: 23374417].

COSMETICS & RELATED PRODUCTS

Cosmetics and personal care products are the most frequently involved substance in pediatric patients younger than 5 years and third most common in all ages. Most of them do not cause significant toxicity. The relative toxicities of commonly ingested products in this group are listed in Table 13–2.

TRICYCLIC ANTIDEPRESSANTS

Tricyclic antidepressants (TCA) (eg amitriptyline, imipramine) have a very low ratio of toxic to therapeutic doses, and even a moderate overdose (> 1 g) can have serious effects.

Table 13–2. Relative toxicities of cosmetics and similar products.

High toxicity	Low/minimal toxicity
Permanent wave neutralizers (hydrogen peroxide)	Perfume
Moderate toxicity	Deodorants
Fingernail polish (various ingredients)	Bath salts
Fingernail polish remover (acetone, alcohols)	Liquid makeup
Hair tonic (alcohols)	Cleansing cream, lotions

With the transition to SSRI for mood disorder, TCA is less commonly seen as an overdose agent. Diphenhydramine toxicity can have similar symptoms as TCA and is more readily available. Diphenhydramine can cause toxicity in doses greater than 10 mg/kg or 1 g TCA.

Overdosage can cause a progression of illness beginning with sudden onset coma within 1–2 hours of ingestion, followed by seizures, hypotension, and dysrhythmias within hours.

▶ Treatment

After a significant ingestion, decontamination should include administration of AC unless the patient is already symptomatic. Benzodiazepines should be given for seizures.

An ECG should be obtained in all patients. A QRS interval greater than 100 milliseconds specifically identifies patients at risk to develop seizures and 160 milliseconds for dysrhythmias. If dysrhythmias or tachycardia are demonstrated, the patient should be admitted and monitored until free of irregularity for 24 hours. The onset of dysrhythmias is rare beyond 24 hours after ingestion.

Bolus administration of sodium bicarbonate (1–2 mEq/kg) is recommended for all patients with progressive or prolonged QRS and significant dysrhythmias to achieve a pH of 7.5–7.6. If intubated, hyperventilation may be helpful. Lidocaine may be added for treatment of arrhythmias. Lipid-emulsion therapy has been used in the setting of cardiotoxicity.

TCA blocks the reuptake of catecholamines, thereby producing initial hypertension followed by hypotension due to its effect on peripheral α receptors. Vasopressors (such as norepinephrine) are generally effective.

Blaber MS et al: "Lipid rescue" for tricyclic antidepressant cardiotoxicity. J Emerg Med 2012;43(3):465–467 [PMID: 22244291].
Kerr GW et al: Tricyclic antidepressant overdose: a review. Emerg Med J 2001;18:236 [PMID: 11435353].
Palmer RB et al: Adverse events associated with diphenhydramine in children, 2008–2015. Clin Toxicol (Phila) 2020 Feb;58(2):99–106 [PMID: 31062642].

DIGITALIS & OTHER CARDIAC GLYCOSIDES

Acute toxicity with digitalis is typically the result of incorrect dosing, and chronic toxicity is due to unrecognized renal insufficiency or dehydration. In acute overdosage, hyperkalemia is a sign of life-threatening toxicity. Clinical features include nausea, vomiting, diarrhea, headache, delirium, confusion, and occasionally, coma. Cardiac dysrhythmias typically involve bradydysrhythmias, but every type of dysrhythmia has been reported in digitalis intoxication, including atrial fibrillation, paroxysmal atrial tachycardia, and atrial flutter. Transplacental intoxication by digitalis has been reported. Cardiac glycosides, such as yellow oleander and foxglove, can cause digitalis toxicity in large ingestions as well.

Treatment

If patient is awake and alert, consider administering AC. Adequate fluid resuscitation is essential to aid in renal elimination.

The patient must be monitored carefully for ECG changes. Bradycardias have been treated with atropine. Phenytoin, lidocaine, magnesium salts (but not in renal failure), amiodarone, and bretylium have been used to correct arrhythmias.

Definitive treatment is with digoxin immune Fab (ovine). Indications for its use include hypotension or any dysrhythmia, typically ventricular dysrhythmias and progressive bradydysrhythmias, or hyperkalemia (K > 5) in an acute overdose. Elevated T waves indicate high potassium and may be an indication for digoxin immune Fab use. Techniques of determining dosage and indications related to levels, when available, are described in product literature. High doses of digoxin immune Fab may be needed in cardiac glycoside overdose. Extracorporeal treatment is not indicated for digoxin toxicity.

Botelho AFM et al: A review of cardiac glycosides: Structure, toxicokinetics, clinical signs, diagnosis and antineoplastic potential. Toxicon 2019 Feb;158:63–68 [PMID: 30529380].
Mowry JB: Extracorporeal treatment for digoxin poisoning: systematic review and recommendations from the EXTRIP Workgroup. Clin Toxicol (Phila) 2016;54(2):103–114 [PMID: 26795743].
Rajapakse S: Management of yellow oleander poisoning. Clin Toxicol (Phila) 2009;47(3):206–212 [PMID: 19306191].

LOPERAMIDE (IMODIUM) & DIPHENOXYLATE WITH ATROPINE (LOMOTIL)

Ingestions of loperamide up to 0.4 mg/kg can safely be managed at home. There has been a recent rise in loperamide use to self-treat opioid addiction. In overdose setting, it can have opioid-like toxicity and has been associated with cardiac dysrhythmias in both acute overdose and chronic abuse. The FDA recalled Lomotil (diphenoxylate and atropine) for diarrhea in 2017; however, it may be still present in the home.

Diphenoxylate is a synthetic narcotic and can lead to opioid toxicity, and atropine sulfate can lead to anticholinergic toxicity.

Treatment

Naloxone hydrochloride (0.4–2.0 mg IV in children and adults) should be given for signs of respiratory depression. Repeated doses may be required because the duration of action of diphenoxylate is considerably longer than that of naloxone. Dysrhythmias should be treated according to ACLS/PALS.

Eggleston W et al: Loperamide toxicity: recommendations for patient monitoring and management. Clin Toxicol (Phila) 2020 May;58(5):355–359 [PMID: 31684751].
Vakkalanka JP, Charlton NP, Holstege CP: Epidemiologic trends in loperamide abuse and misuse. Ann Emerg Med 2016, Nov 4 [PMID: 27823872].

DISINFECTANTS & DEODORIZERS

1. Naphthalene

Naphthalene and camphor are less commonly found in mothballs, disinfectants, and deodorizers. Naphthalene can be absorbed after ingestion and through the skin and lungs. It is potentially hazardous to store baby clothes in naphthalene because baby oil is an excellent solvent that may increase dermal absorption. Metabolic products of naphthalene may cause methemoglobinemia and severe hemolytic anemia. Other physical findings include vomiting, diarrhea, jaundice, oliguria, anuria, coma, and seizures. Camphor can cause seizures 1–2 hours after ingestion.

Treatment

If the patient is awake and alert, consideration can be given for administering AC. Methemoglobinemia and hemolysis may occur 24–48 hours after ingestion. Life-threatening hemolysis and anemia may require blood transfusions. Seizures from camphor should be treated with benzodiazepines.

2. p-Dichlorobenzene, Phenolic Acids, & Others

Disinfectants and deodorizers containing p-dichlorobenzene or sodium sulfate are now more commonly found in mothballs and much less toxic than those containing naphthalene. They typically cause mucous membrane irritation and GI upset.

Disinfectants containing phenolic acids are highly toxic, especially if they contain a borate ion. Phenol precipitates tissue proteins and can also cause systemic toxicity resulting in respiratory alkalosis followed by metabolic acidosis. Some phenols cause methemoglobinemia. Phenol is readily absorbed topically and from the GI tract, causing local injury, diffuse capillary damage, and, in some cases, methemoglobinemia. Pentachlorophenol, which has been used in terminal rinsing of diapers, has caused infant fatalities by causing metabolic acidosis.

The toxicity of alkalis, quaternary ammonium compounds, pine oil, and halogenated disinfectants varies with the concentration of active ingredients. Wick deodorizers are usually of moderate toxicity. Iodophor disinfectants are the safest. Spray deodorizers are not usually toxic, because a child is not likely to swallow a very large dose.

Signs and symptoms of acute quaternary ammonium compound ingestion include diaphoresis, mucosal irritation, vomiting, diarrhea, cyanosis, hyperactivity, coma, seizures, hypotension, abdominal pain, and pulmonary edema. Acute liver or renal failure may develop later.

▶ **Treatment**

Mainstay to phenol toxicity is symptomatic and supportive care. Anticonvulsants or measures to treat shock may be needed.

Because phenols are absorbed through the skin, exposed areas should be irrigated copiously with water. Undiluted polyethylene glycol may be a useful solvent as well.

Moss MJ et al: An algorithm for identifying mothball composition. Clin Toxicol (Phila) 2017 Sep;55(8):919–921 [PMID: 28541143].
Van Berkel M et al: Survival after acute benzalkonium chloride poisoning. Hum Toxicol 1988;7:191 [PMID: 3378808].
Vearrier D et al: Phenol toxicity following cutaneous exposure to Creolin®: a case report. J Med Toxicol 2015 Jun;11(2):227–231 [PMID: 25326371].

DISK "BUTTON" BATTERIES

Over 60% of disk or button batteries ingested by children are obtained from manufactured household products. These batteries measure between 10 and 25 mm in diameter. Batteries impacted in the esophagus can lead to a significant injury both from leakage of alkaline contents and electrical injury. This is a life-threatening emergency as fatalities have been reported in association with esophageal perforation or aortofistula formation.

When a history of disk battery ingestion is obtained, radiographs of the entire respiratory tract and GI tract should be taken immediately so that the battery can be located, and the proper therapy determined.

▶ **Treatment**

Any concern of or witnessed disk battery ingestion should be referred immediately for evaluation and radiographs. If readily available, 10 mL of honey every 10 minutes for up to 6 doses is recommended en route to hospital evaluation (if the child is > 1 year of age) but should not delay transportation or hospital evaluation. Upon arrival to an ED, sucralfate suspension 10 mL every 10 minutes should

be administered until sedation is given for endoscopy. If the disk battery is located in the esophagus, it must be removed immediately as any prolonged time in the esophagus can cause injury. Consultation with GI or surgical subspecialty is recommended.

Location of the disk battery below the esophagus has been rarely associated with tissue damage. It may take as long as 7 days for spontaneous passage to occur. Lack of movement in the GI tract may not require removal in an asymptomatic patient. Patients less than 5 years of age swallowing button batteries greater than 20 mm in diameter may have difficulties passing through the pylorus.

Asymptomatic patients with known time of ingestion, patients greater than 5 years old, and with disk batteries past the lower esophageal junction may potentially be observed and stools examined for passage of the battery. If the battery has not passed within 7 days or if the patient becomes symptomatic, radiographs should be repeated. If the battery has come apart or appears not to be moving, a purgative, enema, or nonabsorbable intestinal lavage solution should be considered. If these methods are unsuccessful, surgical intervention may be required.

Anfang RR et al: pH-neutralizing esophageal irrigations as a novel mitigation strategy for button battery injury. Laryngoscope 2019 Jan;129(1):49–57 [PMID: 29889306].
Button Battery Ingestion Guideline for Health Care Providers: https://www.rmpdc.org/system/user_files/Documents/Button%20Disc%20Battery%20Guideline%20for%20Management%202018%20Ver%203.pdf. Accessed January 30, 2023.
Sethia R et al: Current management of button battery injuries. Laryngoscope Investig Otolaryngol 2021 Apr 15;6(3):549–563 [PMID: 34195377].

ETHYLENE GLYCOL & METHANOL

Ethylene glycol and methanol are alcohols that can lead to significant toxicity. The primary source of ethylene glycol is antifreeze, whereas methanol is present in windshield wiper fluid. Ethylene glycol causes severe metabolic acidosis and renal failure. Methanol causes metabolic acidosis and blindness. Onset of symptoms with both agents occurs within several hours after ingestion. Rarely, other glycol ethers can cause acidosis, but only in the setting of large ingestions.

▶ **Treatment**

The primary treatment is to block the enzyme alcohol dehydrogenase, which converts both toxic alcohols to their toxic metabolites. This is accomplished with fomepizole (loading dose of 15 mg/kg). Ethanol could be used if fomepizole is unavailable but can lead to CNS depression and hypoglycemia in children. HD is indicated with high concentrations, persistent or severe metabolic acidosis, or end-organ toxicity.

Beauchamp GA et al: Toxic alcohol ingestion: prompt recognition and management in the emergency department. Emerg Med Pract 2016 Sep;18(9):1–20 [PMID: 27538060].

Brent J: Fomepizole for the treatment of pediatric ethylene and diethylene glycol, butoxyethanol, and methanol poisonings. Clin Toxicol (Phila) 2010;48(5):401–406 [PMID: 20586570].

Wang GS et al: Severe poisoning after accidental pediatric ingestion of glycol ethers. Pediatrics 2012;130(4):e1026–e1029 [PMID: 23008459].

γ-HYDROXYBUTYRATE, γ-BUTYROLACTONE, 1,4-BUTANEDIOL, FLUNITRAZEPAM, & KETAMINE

γ-Hydroxybutyrate (GHB), γ-butyrolactone (GBL), and butanediol have become popular drugs of abuse in adolescents and adults. GHB is a CNS depressant that is structurally similar to the inhibitory neurotransmitter γ-aminobutyric acid (GABA). GBL and butanediol are converted in the body to GHB. These drugs cause deep but short-lived coma; the coma often lasts only 1–4 hours. Flunitrazepam (Rohypnol) is a benzodiazepine analog that can lead to somnolence and CNS depression. Ketamine is a dissociative anesthetic that can also cause rapid onset and resolution of altered mental status and CNS depression. Although all of these drugs are often referred to as "date rape" drugs, ethanol is the most commonly used substance in drug-facilitated assault.

Treatment consists of supportive care with close attention to airway and endotracheal intubation if respiratory depression develops. Withdrawal from GHB, GBL, or butanediol is similar to other GABA agonist agents. Treatment is with sedatives such as benzodiazepines.

Schep LJ et al: The clinical toxicology of gamma-hydroxybutyrate, gamma-butyrolactone and 1,4-butanediol. Clin Toxicol (Phila) 2012;50(6):458–470 [PMID: 22746383].

HYDROCARBONS (BENZENE, FUELS, PETROLEUM DISTILLATES, ESSENTIAL OILS)

Ingestion of hydrocarbons cause irritation of mucous membranes, CNS depression, or aspiration pneumonitis. Hydrocarbons with high volatility, low viscosity, and low surface tension have a higher risk of aspiration pneumonitis. Benzene, kerosene, red seal oil furniture polish, and some of the essential oils are very dangerous. A dose exceeding 1 mL/kg is likely to cause CNS depression. A history of coughing or choking, as well as vomiting, suggests aspiration with resulting hydrocarbon pneumonia. Pulmonary edema and hemorrhage, blebs, cardiac dilation, and dysrhythmias can occur following large overdoses. Several weeks may be required for full resolution of hydrocarbon pneumonia.

▶ Treatment

Both emetics and lavage should be avoided. Initial approach in treatment includes observing for CNS depression or respiratory distress. Patients who are asymptomatic with a normal chest x-ray (CXR) after 8 hours are unlikely to develop significant illness; however, patients who develop respiratory symptoms, hypoxia, or CXR changes should be observed.

The usefulness of corticosteroids is debated, and antibiotics should be reserved for patients with infections (pneumonitis can cause fevers and infiltrates). Surfactant therapy for severe hydrocarbon-induced lung injury has been used successfully. Extracorporeal membrane oxygenation has been successful in at least two cases of severe pulmonary disease.

Makrygianni EA et al: Respiratory complications following hydrocarbon aspiration in children. Pediatr Pulmonol 2016 Jun;51(6):560–569 [PMID: 26910771].

Mastropietro SW et al: Early administration of intratracheal surfactant (calfactant) after hydrocarbon aspiration. Pediatrics 2011;127(6):e1600–e1604 [PMID: 21624800].

Sommer C et al. Surfactant for the management of pediatric hydrocarbon ingestion. Am J Emerg Med. 2018 Dec;36(12):2260–2262 [PMID: 30236893].

Tormoehlen LM: Hydrocarbon toxicity: a review. Clin Toxicol (Phila) 2014;52(5):479–489 [PMID: 24911841].

IBUPROFEN

Most exposures in children do not produce symptoms. In one study, for example, children ingesting up to 2.4 g remained asymptomatic. When symptoms occur, the most common are abdominal pain, vomiting, drowsiness, and lethargy. In rare cases, apnea (especially in young children), seizures, metabolic acidosis, hypotension, and coma have occurred.

▶ Treatment

If a child has ingested less than 100 mg/kg, supportive care for GI upset is typically all that is needed. When the ingested amount is more than 400 mg/kg, seizures or CNS depression may occur. There is no specific antidote. Neither alkalization of the urine nor HD is helpful in elimination of ibuprofen. However, HD may be needed to correct acid–base abnormalities.

Cuzzolin L et al: NSAID-induced nephrotoxicity from the fetus to the child. Drug Safety 2001;242:9 [PMID: 11219488].

Marciniak KE et al: Massive ibuprofen overdose requiring extracorporeal membrane oxygenation for cardiovascular support. Pediatr Crit Care Med 2007;8:180–182 [PMID: 17273120].

INSECT STINGS (BEE, WASP, & HORNET)

Insect stings are painful but not usually dangerous; however, death from anaphylaxis may occur. Bee venom has hemolytic, neurotoxic, and histamine-like activities that can on rare occasions cause hemoglobinuria and severe anaphylactoid reactions. Massive envenomation from numerous stings or stings from Africanized bees may cause hemolysis, rhabdomyolysis, and shock leading to multiple-organ failure.

▶ Treatment

The physician should remove the stinger, taking care not to squeeze the attached venom sac. For anaphylaxis, IM epinephrine should be administered. Albuterol, corticosteroids, and antihistamines are useful ancillary drugs but have no immediate effect.

For the more usual stings, cold compresses, acetaminophen, ibuprofen, and antihistamines are sufficient.

> Hughes RL: A fatal case of acute renal failure from envenoming syndrome after massive bee attack: a case report and literature review. Am J Forensic Med Pathol 2019 Mar;40(1):52–57 [PMID: 30531211].

INSECTICIDES

The petroleum distillates or other organic solvents used in these products are often as toxic as the insecticide itself.

1. Organophosphate (Cholinesterase-Inhibiting) Insecticides (eg, Chlorothion, Malathion, Parathion, Phosdrin, TEPP)

The clinical findings are the result of irreversible cholinesterase inhibition, which causes an accumulation of acetylcholine. The onset of symptoms occurs within 12 hours of exposure. Symptoms can include dizziness, headache, blurred vision, miosis, tearing, salivation, nausea, vomiting, diarrhea, shortness of breath, dyspnea, sweating, weakness, muscular twitching, seizures, loss of reflexes and sphincter control, and coma. Red cell cholinesterase levels should be measured as soon as possible, however typically do not return in a timely fashion to influence care. In general, a decrease of red cell cholinesterase to below 25% of normal indicates significant exposure.

Repeated low-grade exposure may result in sudden, acute toxic reactions. This syndrome usually occurs after repeated household spraying rather than agricultural exposure.

Although all organophosphates act by inhibiting cholinesterase activity, they vary greatly in their toxicity. Parathion, for example, is 100 times more toxic than malathion. Toxicity is influenced by the specific compound, type of formulation (liquid or solid), vehicle, and route of absorption (lungs, skin, or GI tract). The timeframe for irreversible inhibition also varies, also called aging.

▶ Treatment

Proper PPE is needed to prevent secondary exposure to health care and emergency personnel. Decontamination of skin, nails, hair, and clothing with soapy water is extremely important. Atropine plus a cholinesterase reactivator, pralidoxime, is an antidote for organophosphate insecticide toxicity. Atropine is used to reverse muscarinic parasympathetic effects such as increased secretions and bradycardia. Appropriate starting dose of atropine is 2–4 mg IV in an adult and 0.05 mg/kg in a child. Severe toxicity may require large quantities of atropine administered over 24 hours or an infusion. Glycopyrrolate can also be used if delirium occurs.

Because atropine antagonizes the muscarinic parasympathetic effects of the organophosphates but does not affect the nicotinic receptor, it does not improve muscular weakness. Although the benefits remain controversial, pralidoxime should also be given immediately in severe cases and repeated every 6–12 hours as needed (25–50 mg/kg diluted to 5% and infused over 5–30 minutes at a rate of no > 500 mg/min).

2. Carbamates (eg, Carbaryl, Sevin, Zectran)

Carbamate insecticides are reversible inhibitors of cholinesterase. The signs and symptoms of intoxication are similar to those associated with organophosphate toxicity but are generally less severe and irreversible cholinesterase inhibition is not observed. Atropine titrated to effect is sufficient treatment.

3. Pyrethrins/Pyrethroids

There are common insecticides that are extracted from the *Chrysanthemum* flower. They usually have no significant toxicity in humans due to rapid hydrolysis. Allergic reaction and asthma-like symptoms can occur. In large overdose coma, and seizures have been reported. Antihistamines, short-acting benzodiazepines, and atropine are helpful as symptomatic treatment.

> Blumberg A et al: Utility of 2-pyridine aldoxime methyl chloride (2-PAM) for acute organophosphate poisoning: a systematic review and meta-analysis. J Med Toxicol 2018 Mar;14(1):91–98 [PMID: 29299760].
> Diaz JH: Chemical and plant-based insect repellents: efficacy, safety, and toxicity. Wilderness Environ Med 2016 Mar;27(1):153–163 [PMID: 26827259].
> King AM et al: Organophosphate and carbamate poisoning. Emerg Med Clin North Am 2015 Feb;33(1):133–151 [PMID: 25455666].

IRON

Overall, significant iron ingestions have continued to decrease in the United States. Iron has many different formulations with varying amounts of elemental iron. Three common formulations include ferrous fumarate (33%), ferrous sulfate (20%), and ferrous gluconate (12%). Doses of more than 20 mg/kg of elemental iron will cause significant symptoms. Five stages of intoxication may occur in iron toxicity: (1) Severe gastroenteritis 30–60 minutes after ingestion and may be associated with shock, acidosis, coagulation defects, and coma; this phase usually lasts 4–6 hours; (2) phase of improvement, lasting 2–12 hours, during which patient looks better; (3) delayed vasoplegic shock 12–48 hours after ingestion; metabolic acidosis, fever, leukocytosis, and coma may also be present; (4) hepatoxicity with hepatic failure; and (5) residual pyloric stenosis, which may develop about 4 weeks after the ingestion.

▶ **Treatment**

GI decontamination is based on clinical assessment. The patient should be referred to a health care facility if symptomatic or if the history indicates toxic amounts (typically > 20 mg/kg of elemental iron).

Shock is treated in the usual manner. Deferoxamine, a specific chelating agent for iron forms a soluble complex that is excreted in the urine. IV deferoxamine chelation therapy should be instituted if the patient has a metabolic acidosis, or if the peak serum iron exceeds 500 mcg/dL at 4–5 hours after ingestion.

Deferoxamine should not be delayed until serum iron levels are available in patients with symptoms consistent of severe toxicity. Intravenous administration should be given at a dosage of 10–15 mg/kg/h. Infusion rates up to 35 mg/kg/h have been used in life-threatening toxicity; however, rapid IV administration can cause hypotension. Generally, it can be stopped after 12–24 hours with resolution of acidosis, declining concentrations, and clinical improvement. The use of deferoxamine for greater than 24 hours has been associated with acute respiratory distress syndrome (ARDS). HD or exchange transfusion can be used to increase the excretion of the dialyzable complex. Urine output should be monitored and urine sediment examined for evidence of renal tubular damage.

Chang TP, Rangan C: Iron poisoning: a literature-based review of epidemiology, diagnosis, and management. Pediatr Emerg Care 2011 Oct;27(10):978–985 [PMID: 21975503].

Leonard JB et al: Iron packaging regulations in the United States and pediatric morbidity: a retrospective cohort study. Clin Pediatr (Phila) 2020 May;59(4–5):375–379 [PMID: 31976760].

LEAD

Lead toxicity occurs insidiously in children younger than 5 years, no detectable lead concentration is considered safe. The most likely sources of lead include flaking leaded paint, artist's paints, fruit tree sprays, solder, brass alloys, home-glazed pottery, fumes from burning batteries, and foreign country remedies. Only paint containing less than 1% lead is safe for interior use (eg, furniture, toys). Repetitive ingestions of small amounts of lead are far more serious than a single massive exposure. Toxic effects are likely to occur if more than 0.5 mg of lead per day is absorbed. In the United States, lead levels continue to decline and are more common abroad, so particular attention should be paid to immigrant and refugee populations or the use of foreign remedies.

Lead toxicity (plumbism) causes vague symptoms, including weakness, irritability, weight loss, vomiting, personality changes, ataxia, constipation, headache, and colicky abdominal pain. Late severe manifestations consist of developmental delays, seizures, and coma associated with increased intracranial pressure, which is a medical emergency.

Blood lead levels are used to assess the severity of exposure. A complete blood count and serum ferritin concentration should be obtained; iron deficiency increases absorption of lead. Glycosuria, proteinuria, hematuria, and aminoaciduria can occur. Abnormal capillary blood lead levels should be repeated with venous samples to rule out laboratory error. A microcytic, hypochromic anemia with basophilic stippling of the red cells and reticulocytosis may be present in plumbism. Stippling of red blood cells is absent in cases involving only recent ingestion.

▶ **Treatment**

Refer to the Centers for Disease Control and Prevention (CDC) guidelines for the most up-to-date recommendations on lead treatment and evaluation. There is no "safe" concentration of lead. Removing the source of exposure is the most important initial treatment to toxicity. Succimer is an orally administered chelator approved for use in children and reported to be as efficacious as calcium edetate. Oral succimer is recommended in asymptomatic children at blood lead levels 45–69 mcg/dL. The initial dose is 10 mg/kg (350 mg/m^2) every 8 hours for 5 days. The same dose is then given every 12 hours for 14 days. At least 2 weeks should elapse between courses. Blood lead levels increase somewhat (ie, rebound) after discontinuation of therapy. Courses of IM dimercaprol/BAL (300–450 mg/m^2/day) and IV calcium sodium edetate/CaNa$_2$EDTA (1000–1500 mg/m^2/day) should be considered in symptomatic children, cases with encephalopathy, or levels over 70 mcg/dL.

Encephalopathy associated with cerebral edema needs to be treated with standard measures. Anticonvulsants may be needed. Iron supplementation should be started. A high-calcium, high-phosphorus diet and large doses of vitamin D may remove lead from the blood by depositing it in the bones. A public health team should evaluate the source of the lead. Necessary corrections should be completed before the child is returned home.

Braun JM et al: Effect of residential lead-hazard interventions on childhood blood lead concentrations and neurobehavioral outcomes: a randomized clinical trial. JAMA Pediatr 2018 Oct 1; 172(10):934–942 [PMID: 30178064].

Childhood Lead Poisoning Prevention Program: Centers for Disease Control and Prevention. https://www.cdc.gov/nceh/lead/default.htm. Accessed January 31, 2023.

Reuben A et al: Association of childhood blood lead levels with cognitive function and socioeconomic status at age 38 years and with IQ change and socioeconomic mobility between childhood and adulthood. JAMA 2017 Mar 28;317(12):1244–1251 [PMID: 28350927].

Rogan WJ et al: Treatment of lead-exposed children trial group: the effect of chelation therapy with succimer on neuropsychological development in children exposed to lead. N Engl J Med 2001;344:1421 [PMID: 11346806].

MAGNETS

Ingestion of multiple small magnets can cause bowel obstructions in children. Recent cases have resulted in warnings and a recall of high-powered magnetic balls by the Consumer Product Safety Commission following intestinal perforation and death in a 20-month-old child. Obstruction may occur following ingestion of as few as two magnets. Radiographs should be obtained, and surgical consultation may be indicated.

Alfonzo MJ et al: Magnetic foreign body ingestions. Pediatr Emerg Care 2016 Oct;32(10):698–702 [PMID: 27749667].

Sola R et al: Magnet foreign body ingestion: rare occurrence but big consequences. J Pediatr Surg 2018 Sep;53(9):1815–1819 [PMID: 28899548].

MARINE ENVENOMATIONS

There are many venomous aquatic marine organisms that can lead to significant envenomations in humans. Cnidaria (jellyfish) are found in on both coasts in the US and are abundant in the water surrounding Australia and Indo-Pacific region. Along their tentacles, they have stinging organelles called *nematocysts*. The venom from the barbs within the nematocysts can cause dermonecrosis, myonecrosis, and rarely more systemic effects such as hemolysis or cardiotoxicity. Systemic effects are more common from *Chironex fleckeri* species of the coasts Australia. Stingrays (*Chondrichthyes*) have a tapered retro-serrated spin in the tail. Common clinical effects include localized trauma, pain, and rarely systemic symptoms may develop (dysrhythmias, seizures, cardiovascular collapse). Lionfish (*Pterois*) is a common fish found in saltwater aquariums (Photo 3). They have venom stored in their dorsal spines. The venom mostly causes localized swelling, erythema and pain. Stonefish can cause similar symptoms, but also lead to more systemic symptoms such as cardiovascular compromise. Blue-ringed Octopus and pufferfish have tetrodotoxin, which blocks neurologic sodium channels which lead to flaccid paralysis.

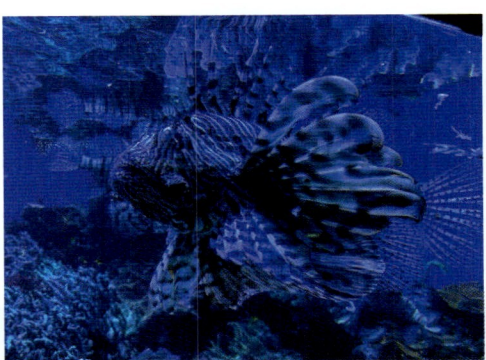

▶ Treatment

In the United States, sea water should be used to remove jellyfish tentacles from the patient. A credit card or seashell may also be used to scrape off tentacles and nematocysts but should not be used if this increases pain. Vinegar, baking soda, and meat tenderizer may increase discharges from the nematocysts from US jellyfish. In contrast, vinegar may be more beneficial in removing jellyfish tentacles in the Indo-Pacific and Australia. For jellyfish, lionfish, and stingrays, hot water immersion can be used to inactivate toxin and for pain control, as they all have heat labile toxins. For stingrays, wounds should be explored for embedded material as they can lead to infection.

American RedCross Scientific Advisory Council Scientific Review – Jellyfish Stings: June 2016. https://www.redcross.org/content/dam/redcross/Health-Safety-Services/scientific-advisory-council/Scientific%20Advisory%20Council%20SCIENTIFIC%20REVIEW%20-%20Jellyfish%20Stings.pdf. Accessed February 2, 2023.

Li L, McGee RG, Isbister G, Webster AC: Interventions for the symptoms and signs resulting from jellyfish stings. Cochrane Database Syst Rev 2013;(12):CD009688 [PMID: 24318773].

Yanagihara AA, Wilcox CL: Cubozoan sting-site seawater rinse, scraping, and ice can increase venom load: upending current first aid recommendations. Toxins (Basel) 2017;9(3):105 [PMID: 28294982].

MUSHROOMS

Toxic mushrooms are often difficult to distinguish from edible varieties. Contact a poison control center to obtain identification assistance. Symptoms vary with the species ingested, time of year, stage of maturity, quantity eaten, and method of preparation. Most mushrooms lead to early GI symptoms and do not lead to significant toxicity; however, some can be fatal and so it is critical to determine from poison center experts what mushroom may have been involved. Drinking alcohol and eating certain mushrooms may cause a reaction like that seen with disulfiram and alcohol. *Psilocybin* mushroom is taken for its hallucinogenic properties. Amanita muscaria (Fly Agaric) can lead to GI symptoms, sedation, hallucinations and delirium (Photo 4). Cooking destroys some toxins but not the deadly one produced by *Amanita phalloides*, which is responsible for 90% of deaths due to mushrooms. Mushroom toxins are absorbed relatively slowly. Onset of symptoms within 2 hours of ingestion suggests muscarinic toxin, whereas a delay of GI symptoms for 6–48 hours after ingestion is concerning for *Amanita* (amanitin). Patients who have ingested *A phalloides* may die of hepatic failure.

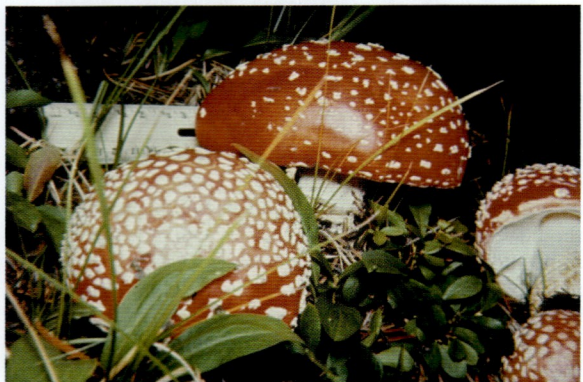

▶ Treatment

Treatment of mushroom toxicity is highly specialized and consultation with a poison center is highly recommended. Try to identify the mushroom if the patient is symptomatic. Local botanical gardens, university departments of botany, and societies of mycologists may be able to help. Supportive care with IV fluid resuscitation may be needed due to emesis and diarrhea. If the patient has muscarinic signs, give atropine, 0.05 mg/kg IM (0.02 mg/kg in toddlers), and repeat as needed (usually every 30 minutes). Agitation and hallucinations from hallucinogenic mushrooms may need benzodiazepines. In the case of *A phalloides*, silibinin, penicillin, biliary drainage, and ultimately liver transplantation have all been used.

North American Mycological Association: Mushroom poisoning syndromes. http://www.namyco.org/toxicology/poison_syndromes.html. Accessed March 3, 2021.
Ye Y et al: Management of *Amanita phalloides* poisoning: a literature review and update. J Crit Care 2018 Aug;46:17–22 [PMID: 29627659].

NITRITES, NITRATES, PENTACHLOROPHENOL, & DINITROPHENOL

Nitrites and nitrates are strong oxidizing agents. Symptoms from significant oxidant stress can include hemolytic anemia, methemoglobinemia, and hemodynamic collapse. Nitrite and nitrate compounds found in the home include amyl nitrite, butyl nitrates, isobutyl nitrates, nitroglycerin, pentaerythritol tetranitrate, sodium nitrite, nitrobenzene, and phenazopyridine. Untreated well water can also be a source. Pentachlorophenol and dinitrophenol (DNP), which are found in wood preservatives, produce methemoglobinemia and severe acidosis because of uncoupling of oxidative phosphorylation. DNP is illicitly sold as a weight loss supplement. Symptoms from methemoglobinemia do not usually occur until 15%–50% of the hemoglobin has been converted to methemoglobin.

▶ Treatment

In the setting of a recent ingestion, consider administering activated charcoal if the patient is awake and alert. Decontaminate affected skin with soap and water. Respiratory and cardiovascular support may be needed. If the blood methemoglobin level exceeds 30%, or if levels cannot be obtained and the patient is symptomatic, give a 1% solution of methylene blue (0.2 mL/kg IV) over 5–10 minutes. Avoid perivascular infiltration because it causes necrosis of the skin and SQ tissues. A dramatic change in the degree of cyanosis should occur. Transfusion is occasionally necessary due to hemolytic crisis from oxidant stress.

Cortazzo JA et al: Methemoglobinemia: a review and recommendations for management. J Cardiothorac Vasc Anesth 2014;28(4): 1055–1059 [PMID: 23953868].
Potts AJ et al: Toxicoepidemiology and predictors of death in 2,4-dinitrophenol (DNP) toxicity. Clin Toxicol (Phila) 2020 Oct 6;1–6 [PMID: 33021407].

OPIOIDS

Opioid-related medical problems may include substance use and addiction, withdrawal in a newborn infant (see Chapter 2), and unintentional overdoses. Opioids can vary in onset of action and duration of action. Fentanyl contamination in heroin and other illicitly sold pharmaceuticals (sold as oxycodone-M30's, Xanax) have increased, contributing to the highest ever overdose death rate. This includes contamination in illicitly sold oxycodone and alprazolam. Many commonly prescribed opioids are not detected in urine drug immunoassays. Detection of semisynthetic and synthetic opioids, such as fentanyl, will require confirmatory testing. Trafficking and the use of benzimidazole opioids, or nitazenes, have been increasing identified in illicitly sold drugs and toxicology cases.

▶ Treatment

A. Overdose

Symptoms of opioid toxicity includes sedation and respiratory depression. In severe toxicity, hypotension, bradycardia, and respiratory arrest can occur. The indication for the administration of naloxone is respiratory depression.

Suggested weight-based dosing for naloxone hydrochloride range from 0.01 to 0.1 mg/kg IV. Alternatively, starting doses from 0.04 to 0.4 mg IV have been recommended using the lowest effective dose without precipitating withdrawal, with escalating doses until a response is seen. Intranasal naloxone (usually 4 mg) has become widely used both in and out of hospital for opioid toxicity due to ease of administration. Return in symptoms can occur after naloxone as duration of action is usually 30–90 minutes. Naloxone infusion can be used for persistent symptoms. Depending on the formulation, some opioid exposures (such as buprenorphine and methadone) may need to be observed for 24 hours due to the duration of action and may need higher doses of naloxone to reverse the symptoms.

B. Opioid Withdrawal

Symptomatic care is the initial goal for opioid withdrawal. Symptoms can include diaphoresis, vomiting, myalgias, diarrhea, tremor, and restlessness. Clonidine, loperamide, ibuprofen, ondansetron and IVF have all been used to control symptoms. Ultimately, mediations for opioid use disorder (buprenorphine, methadone) may be needed control withdrawal symptoms, in conjunction with psychotherapy for the management of opioid use disorder. See Chapter 2 (The Newborn Infant) for information regarding Neonatal Abstinence Syndrome.

Benzimidazole-Opioids. Drug Enforcement Administration: https://www.deadiversion.usdoj.gov/drug_chem_info/benz-imidazole-opioids.pdf. Accessed January 31, 2023.

CHoSEN Collaborative: https://www.chosencollaborative.org/toolkit.html. Accessed January 31, 2023.

Joynt PY, Wang GS: Fentanyl contaminated "M30" pill overdoses in pediatric patients. Am J Emerg Med 2021 Dec;50:811.e3–811.e4 [PMID: 34030905].

Suzuki J, El-Haddad S: A review: fentanyl and non-pharmaceutical fentanyls. Drug Alcohol Depend 2017 Feb 1;171:107–116 [PMID: 28068563].

Tanz LJ et al: Drug overdose deaths among persons aged 10-19 years—United States, July 2019–December 2021. MMWR Morb Mortal Wkly Rep 2022 Dec 16;71(50):1576–1582 [PMID: 36520659].

ORAL ANTIDIABETICS (SULFONYLUREAS, METFORMIN)

Noninsulin hypoglycemic and antidiabetic medications include α-glucosidase inhibitors, biguanides (metformin), dipeptidyl peptidase-4 inhibitors (-gliptins), glucagon-like peptides (-glutide), meglitinides (-glinide), sodium glucose transporter inhibitors (-flovzin), sulfonylureas, and thiazolidinediones (-glitazone). They are all used to treat hyperglycemia in diabetics. Sulfonylureas (acetohexamide, glipizide, glyburide) are the only oral hypoglycemic that actively secretes endogenous insulin and can cause hypoglycemia.

The meglitinides (nateglinide, repaglinide) have scarce reports of hypoglycemia. Biguanides can cause metabolic acidosis and hyperlactatemia in acute large overdose or in conjunction with renal failure.

▶ Treatment

Children with possible exposures to sulfonylureas should be observed for 12–24 hours. The mainstay of treatment is treating hypoglycemia. If the patient is awake and alert, with minimal symptoms, PO glucose can be given. With more severe hypoglycemia or symptomatic, immediate treatment with 0.5–1 g/kg IV dextrose bolus should be administered. With repeated episodes of hypoglycemia, once euglycemia is achieved, octreotide should be given at 1 mcg/kg SC/IV every 6–8 hours as needed for hypoglycemia. Metformin toxicity should be treated supportively and HD may be needed for severe acid–base abnormalities or patients with renal failure.

Glatstein M et al: Octreotide for the treatment of sulfonylurea poisoning. Clin Toxicol (Phila) 2012;50(9):795–804 [PMID: 23046209].

Llamado R et al: Continuous octreotide infusion for sulfonylurea-induced hypoglycemia in a toddler. J Emerg Med 2013 Dec;45(6): e209–e213 [PMID: 23827165].

Wang G et al: Review of biguanide (metformin) toxicity. J Intensive Care Med 2019 Nov–Dec;34(11–12):863–876 [PMID: 30126348].

ANTIPSYCHOTICS (TYPICAL & ATYPICAL)

Typical antipsychotics include butyrophenones (droperidol, haloperidol), and the phenothiazines (promethazine, chlorpromazine, thioridazine). Atypical antipsychotics include benzapines (clozapine, olanzapine, quetiapine) and indoles (risperidone, ziprasidone).

▶ Clinical Findings

A. Extrapyramidal Crisis

Episodes characterized by torticollis, stiffening of the body, spasticity, speech difficulties, catatonia, and inability to communicate although conscious are typical manifestations. Extrapyramidal symptoms (EPS) may represent idiosyncratic reactions impacting dopamine and acetylcholine receptors. EPS are more common with typical antipsychotics (butyrophenones, phenothiazines). EPS in children most often occur after prochlorperazine or after receiving a butyrophenone for psychosis.

B. Overdose

Lethargy and deep prolonged coma are the most common symptoms seen in antipsychotic toxicity. Of the typical antipsychotics, promazine, chlorpromazine, and prochlorperazine are the drugs most likely to cause respiratory depression and precipitous drops in blood pressure. Risperidone and quetiapine are atypical antipsychotics that can cause CNS depression. Clozapine, olanzapine, and quetiapine most commonly cause hypotension and antimuscarinic symptoms. QTc prolongation can occur, most commonly with thioridazine and ziprasidone, however dysrhythmias are rare.

C. Neuroleptic Malignant Syndrome

Neuroleptic malignant syndrome (NMS) is a rare idiosyncratic complication that may be lethal. It is caused by a decrease in central dopaminergic neurotransmission resulting in autonomic dysfunction. It is a syndrome involving mental status change (confusion, coma), motor abnormalities (lead pipe rigidity, clonus), and autonomic dysfunction (tachycardia, hyperpyrexia). Typically, it occurs 1–2 weeks after starting therapy, can occur at therapeutic doses, and may last for several days to weeks.

▶ **Treatment**

Acute extrapyramidal signs can initially be treated with IV administration of diphenhydramine, 1–2 mg/kg (maximum, 50 mg), benztropine mesylate, 1–2 mg IV (1 mg/min), or benzodiazepines. Further doses may be needed.

NMS is treated by discontinuing the drug and treating hyperthermia and agitation aggressively with benzodiazepines and sedation. Hypotension may be treated with standard agents, starting with isotonic saline administration followed by vasopressors. In refractory cases, bromocriptine can be considered, although the evidence for its use is not clear.

Levine M et al: Overdose of atypical antipsychotics: clinical presentation, mechanisms of toxicity and management. CNS Drugs 2012;26(7):601–611 [PMID: 22668123].
Pileggi DJ et al: Neuroleptic malignant syndrome. Ann Pharmacother 2016 Nov;50(11):973–981 [PMID: 27423483].

PLANTS

Some common ornamental, garden, and wild plants are potentially toxic. Only in a few cases will small amounts of a plant cause severe illness or death. Table 13–3 lists common toxic plants, symptoms and signs of toxicity and treatment.

Table 13–3. Poisoning due to plants.[a]

	Symptoms and Signs	Treatment
Arum family: *Caladium, Dieffenbachia,* callally, dumb cane (oxalic acid)	Burning of mucous membranes and airway obstruction secondary to edema caused by calcium oxalate crystals.	Accessible areas should be thoroughly washed. Corticosteroids may relieve airway obstruction
Castor bean plant (ricin—a toxalbumin) Jequirity bean (abrin—a toxalbumin)	*Bean needs to be pulverized. Whole beans do not cause toxicity.* Mucous membrane irritation, nausea, vomiting, bloody diarrhea, blurred vision, circulatory collapse, acute hemolytic anemia, convulsions, uremia.	Symptomatic and supportive care
Foxglove, lily of the valley, and oleander[b]	Nausea, diarrhea, visual disturbances, and -cardiac dysrhythmias.	See treatment for digitalis drugs in text
Jimsonweed: See Belladonna Alkaloids section in text	Anticholinergic toxidrome: mydriasis, dry mouth, tachycardia, and hallucinations.	Benzodiazepines for agitation, physostigmine
Larkspur (ajacine, *Delphinium,* delphinine)	Nausea and vomiting, irritability, muscular paralysis, and central nervous system depression.	Symptomatic and supportive care
Monkshood (aconite)	Numbness of mucous membranes, visual disturbances, tingling, dizziness, tinnitus, hypotension, bradycardia, and convulsions.	Symptomatic and supportive care
Poison hemlock (coniine)	Mydriasis, trembling, dizziness, bradycardia. Central nervous system depression, and muscular paralysis. Death is due to respiratory paralysis.	Symptomatic and supportive care
Rhododendron (grayanotoxin)	Abdominal cramps, vomiting, severe diarrhea, muscular paralysis. Central nervous system and circulatory depression. Hypertension with very large doses.	Symptomatic and supportive care
Water hemlock (cicutoxin).	Nausea, vomiting, abdominal pain. Followed by seizures. Severe ingestions can result in rhabdomyolysis, metabolic acidosis, and renal failure.	Symptomatic and supportive care, benzodiazepines for seizures

[a]Many other plants cause minor irritation but are not likely to cause serious problems unless large amounts are ingested. Data from Lampe KF, McCann MA: *AMA Handbook of Poisonous and Injurious Plants.* American Medical Association; 1985.
[b]Done AK: Ornamental and deadly. Emerg Med 1973;5:255.

Contact your poison control center for assistance with identification and treatment recommendations.

PSYCHOTROPIC DRUGS

Psychotropic drugs include illicit drugs such as lysergic acid diethylamide (LSD) and phencyclidine (PCP). There has been an increase in poison center calls pertaining to adolescent use of LSD in recent years. Increase in young adult use and unintentional pediatric ingestions have been associated with cannabis legalization. There has been a rise in the use and detection of novel psychoactive substances (NPS). These drugs can be new synthetic drugs, or analogs of older recreational drugs.

▶ Clinical Findings

Psychoactive drugs can cause mydriasis, unexplained bizarre behavior, visual and auditory hallucinations, and generalized undifferentiated psychotic behavior. Cannabis products, especially high potency products, can cause tachycardia, anxiety, dysphoria, agitation, and vomiting. In children, cannabis ingestion of edibles can lead to serious symptoms including coma and respiratory depression.

▶ Treatment

Only a small percentage of the persons using drugs come to the attention of physicians; those who do are usually experiencing adverse reactions such as panic states, drug psychoses, homicidal or suicidal thoughts, or respiratory depression.

Even with cooperative patients, an accurate history is difficult to obtain. A drug history is most easily obtained in a quiet spot by a gentle, nonthreatening, honest examiner, and without the parents present. Illicit drugs can be adulterated with one or more other compounds, and the exact dose is usually unknown. Friends may be a useful source of information.

A common drug problem is the "bad trip," which is usually a panic reaction. This is best managed by speaking calmly with the patient and minimizing auditory and visual stimuli. Avoiding drug therapy may help avoid complicating the clinical course. However, benzodiazepines can be used if a sedative effect is required with an aggressive or agitated patient. Antipsychotics may be helpful, although may exacerbate unrecognized toxidromes.

Michienzi AE, Borek HA: Emerging agents of substance use/misuse. Emerg Med Clin North Am 2022 May;40(2):265–281 [PMID: 35461623].

Ng P et al: Adolescent exposures to traditional and novel psychoactive drugs, reported to National Poison Data System (NPDS), 2007–2017. Drug Alcohol Depend 2019 Sep 1;202:1–5 [PMID: 31279256].

Wang GS et al: Common substances of abuse. Pediatr Rev 2018 Aug;39(8):403–414 [PMID: 30068741].

Wang GS et al: Novel drugs of abuse. Pediatr Rev 2019 Feb;40(2):71–78 [PMID: 30709973].

SALICYLATES

The use of child-resistant containers, public education, and more common use of other analgesics and antipyretics have reduced the incidence of acute salicylate toxicity. It is common for people to mistake OTC analgesics (aspirin, nonsteroidal anti-inflammatory drugs [NSAIDs], acetaminophen) in the therapeutic and overdose setting. Oil of wintergreen can contain large amounts of methylsalicylates.

Salicylates uncouple oxidative phosphorylation, leading to increased heat production, excessive sweating, and dehydration. Salicylates interfere with glucose metabolism and may cause hypo- or hyperglycemia. Respiratory center stimulation occurs early which can be evidenced as Kussmaul breathing. The severity of acute intoxication can, in some measure, be judged by serum salicylate levels. High levels are always dangerous irrespective of clinical signs, and low levels may be misleading in chronic cases.

In mild and moderate toxicity, vomiting is a common presenting symptom and patients may complain of tinnitus or hearing loss. Physical examination findings can include fatigue, diaphoresis, and tachypnea with a Kussmaul respiratory pattern. Laboratory findings include a mixed respiratory alkalosis and metabolic acidosis, and ECG may reveal flattened T waves. In severe intoxication (occurring in severe acute ingestion with high salicylate levels and in chronic toxicity with lower levels), respiratory response is unable to overcome the metabolic overdose which may lead to hyperthermia, pulmonary edema, seizures, and death.

Once the urine becomes acidic, less salicylate is excreted. Until this process is reversed, the half-life will remain prolonged, because metabolism contributes little to the removal of salicylate. Chronic severe toxicity may occur as early as 3 days after a regimen of salicylate is begun. Chronic symptoms can be non-specific: vomiting, diarrhea, fatigue, and dehydration.

▶ Treatment

Charcoal binds salicylates well and can be given for acute ingestions in patients with normal mentation. Mild toxicity may require only the administration of oral fluids and confirmation that the salicylate level is falling (< 30 mg/dL). In moderate toxicity, IVF must be administered at a rate of 2–3 mL/kg/h to correct dehydration and produce urine with a pH of greater than 7.0 to promote excretion. Initial IV solutions should be isotonic (D_5W with 150 mEq sodium bicarbonate) and will likely require potassium supplementation.

Patients with renal failure, pulmonary edema, mental status changes, seizures, or concentrations of greater than 100 mg/dL should be considered for HD.

Davis JE: Are one or two dangerous? Methyl salicylate exposure in toddlers. J Emerg Med 2007 Jan;32(1):63–69 [PMID: 17239735].
Juurlink DN et al: Extracorporeal treatment for salicylate poisoning: systematic review and recommendations from the EXTRIP workgroup. Ann Emerg Med 2015 Aug;66(2):165–181 [PMID: 25986310].

SCORPION STINGS

Scorpion stings are common in the southwestern United States. The most common scorpions in the United States are *Vejovis*, *Hadrurus*, *Androctonus*, and *Centruroides* species. Stings by the first three produce edema and pain. Stings by *Centruroides* (the Bark scorpion) are most clinically significant and can cause tingling or burning paresthesia that begin at the site of the sting. In small children, autonomic instability and severe neurologic symptoms can develop including hypersalivation, restlessness, muscular fasciculation, abdominal cramps, opisthotonos, seizures, urinary incontinence, and respiratory failure.

▶ Treatment

Analgesics should be provided for local symptoms. For *Centruroides* stings, sedation with benzodiazepines is the primary therapy. Antivenom is reserved for severe symptoms (recommended dosing of 1–3 vials). In severe cases, the airway may become compromised by secretions and weakness of respiratory muscles and endotracheal intubation may be required. The prognosis is good as long as the patient's airway is managed appropriately, and sedation is achieved.

Boyer LV et al: Antivenom for critically ill children with neurotoxicity from scorpion stings. N Engl J Med 2009; 360:2090–2098 [PMID: 19439743].
Klotz et al: Scorpion stings and antivenom use in Arizona. Am J Med 2021;S0002-9343(21)00106-6 [PMID: 33631163].

SELECTIVE SEROTONIN REUPTAKE INHIBITORS (SSRIs)

Citalopram (Celexa), fluoxetine (Prozac), paroxetine (Paxil), sertraline (Zoloft), and many other agents comprise this class of drugs. Adverse effects in therapeutic dosing include sedation, suicidal thoughts, aggressive behavior, and extrapyramidal effects. Overdose results symptoms due to an increase of serotonin (5-hydroxytryptamine [5-HT]): autonomic instability (hypertension, tachycardia, hyperthermia), altered mental status, and peripheral neurologic findings (myoclonus, clonus, and hyperreflexia). Seizures may occur, and QTc prolongation may be observed, although it is rarely clinically significant due to the tachycardia.

▶ Treatment

The presence of high-grade fever, seizures and high CK may be associated with severe serotonin toxicity. Treatment of agitation and hyperthermia with benzodiazepines is most beneficial. Hypotension may be treated with fluids or norepinephrine. Oral cyproheptadine is an antagonist of serotonin, but evidence for significant benefits of use is limited. Oral doses of 0.25 mg/kg/day divided every 6 hours to a maximum of 12 mg/day may be useful in treating the serotonin syndrome. Adults and older adolescents have been treated with 12 mg initially followed by 2 mg every 2 hours to a maximum of 32 mg/day.

Boyer EW, Shannon M: The serotonin syndrome. N Engl J Med 2005; 352:1112–1120 [PMID: 15784664].
Nguyen H et al: An 11-year retrospective review of cyproheptadine use in serotonin syndrome cases reported to the California Poison Control System. J Clin Pharm Ther 2019 Apr;44(2):327–334 [PMID: 30650197].
Prakash S et al: Fatal serotonin syndrome: a systemic review of 56 cases in the literature. Clin Toxicol (Phila) 2021;59(2):89–100 [PMID: 33196298].

SNAKE BITES

Nearly all envenomous snake bites in the United States are caused by pit vipers (rattlesnakes, water moccasins, and copperheads) (Photo 5). A few are caused by elapids (coral snakes), and occasional bites occur from cobras and other nonindigenous exotic snakes kept as pets. Snake venom is a complex mixture of enzymes, peptides, and proteins that may have predominantly cytotoxic, neurotoxic, hemotoxic, or cardiotoxic effects. Up to 25% of bites by pit vipers do not result in venom injection. US pit viper venom predominantly causes local injury with pain, tissue necrosis, edema, and thrombocytopenia.

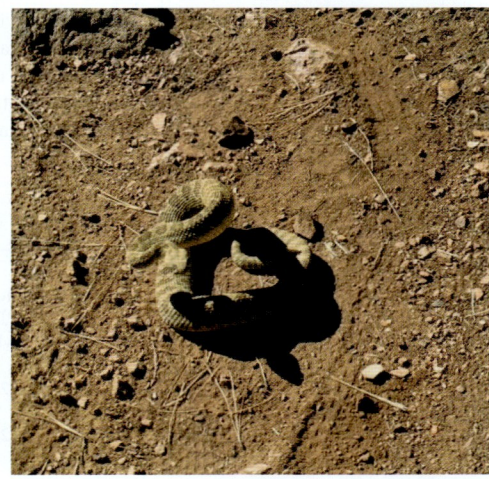

The outcome depends on the size of the child, the degree of envenomation, the type of snake, and the effectiveness of treatment. Swelling and pain occur soon after rattlesnake bite and are a certain indication that envenomation has occurred. During the first few hours, swelling and ecchymosis extend proximally from the bite. The bite can have a double puncture mark surrounded by ecchymosis. Hematemesis, melena, hemoptysis, and other manifestations of coagulopathy rarely develop in severe cases. Respiratory difficulty, anaphylactoid symptoms, and shock may occur. Deaths occur rarely.

Coral snake envenomation causes little local pain, swelling, or necrosis, and systemic reactions are often delayed. The signs of coral snake envenomation include bulbar paralysis, dysphagia, and dysphoria; these signs may appear in 5–10 hours and may be followed by total peripheral paralysis and death in 24 hours.

▶ Treatment

A. Emergency (First Aid) Treatment

The most important first-aid measure is transportation to a medical facility. Splint the affected extremity and minimize the patient's motion. Tourniquets and ice packs are contraindicated. Incision and suction are not useful for either crotalid or elapid snake bite.

B. Definitive Medical Management

Upon arrival at a health care facility, wound should be cleaned and affected extremity elevated. Administer an opioid to control pain. Blood should be drawn for complete blood counts, clotting time and platelet function, and fibrinogen.

Specific antivenom is indicated when signs of progressive envenomation are present. For coral snake bites, an eastern coral snake antivenom (Wyeth Laboratories) is available for patients who develop neurologic symptoms. Patients with pit viper bites should receive polyvalent crotaline antivenom IV (Fab or Fab$_2$) if progressive local injury, coagulopathy, or systemic signs (eg, hypotension, confusion) are present. See package labeling or call your poison center for details of use. Antivenom will halt (not resolve) progression of symptoms and improve hemorrhage, pain, and shock. For coral snake bites, observation is warranted for 12–24 hours to observe for any development of neurologic toxicity. If they do develop (ptosis, respiratory depression), give 3–5 vials of antivenom in 250–500 mL of isotonic saline solution if available, repeat as necessary.

In rare cases, fasciotomy to relieve pressure within muscular compartments is required from pit viper envenomation; recommend measurements of pressures before decision to perform fasciotomy as swelling usually does not involve deep compartments. Antibiotics are not needed unless clinical signs of infection occur. Tetanus status should be updated and early physiotherapy helps improve recovery. Recurrent coagulopathy and thrombocytopenia may occur after discharge, and patients should have follow-up examinations and repeat laboratory values within 1 week after hospital discharge.

Gerardo CJ et al: Coagulation parameters in copperhead compared to other Crotalinae envenomation: secondary analysis of the F(ab')2 versus Fab antivenom trial. Clin Toxicol (Phila) 2017 Feb;55(2):109–114 [PMID: 27806644].

Levine M et al: When it comes to snakebites, kids are little adults: a comparison of adults and children with rattlesnake bites. J Med Toxicol 2020 Oct;16(4):444–451 [PMID: 32394223].

Mascarenas DN et al: Comparison of F(ab')2 and Fab antivenoms in rattlesnake envenomation: first year's post-marketing experience with F(ab')2 in New Mexico. Toxicon 2020 Oct 30;186:42–45 [PMID: 32763251]

Miller AD et al: Recurrent coagulopathy and thrombocytopenia in children treated with crotalidae polyvalent immune fab: a case series. Pediatr Emerg Care 2010 Aug;26(8):576–582 [PMID: 20693856].

SOAPS & DETERGENTS

1. Soaps

Soap is made from salts of fatty acids. Ingestion of soap bars may cause vomiting and diarrhea, but they have a low toxicity.

2. Detergents

Detergents are non-soap synthetic products used for cleaning purposes because of their surfactant properties. Commercial products include granules, powders, and liquids. Dishwasher detergents are very alkaline and can cause caustic burns. Low concentrations of bleaching and antibacterial agents as well as enzymes are found in many preparations. The pure compounds are moderately toxic, but the concentration used is too small to alter the product's toxicity significantly. Occasional primary or allergic irritative phenomena have been noted in persons who frequently use such products and in employees manufacturing these products. Unit dose detergents, or pods, have become popular and have packaging attractive to young children. They are usually a mix of glycol ethers, ethyl alcohol, and surfactant. They typically cause local irritation but can lead to more severe symptoms, including corneal injuries, CNS depression, and respiratory distress if ingested.

A. Cationic Detergents

Cationic detergents are quaternary ammonium salts of amines with acetates, chlorides or bromides. In dilute solutions (0.5%) cause mucosal irritation, but higher concentrations (10%–15%) may cause caustic burns to mucosa.

Common clinical effects include nausea and vomiting. Rarely in large ingestions, cardiovascular collapse, coma, and seizures. As little as 2.25 g of some cationic agents have caused death in an adult. In four cases, 100–400 mg/kg of benzalkonium chloride caused death. Cationic detergents are rapidly inactivated by tissues and ordinary soap. Because of the caustic potential and rapid onset of seizures, emesis is not recommended. Anticonvulsants may be needed.

B. Anionic Detergents

Most common household detergents are anionic (sodium salts of sulphonated long chain alcohols or hydrocarbons). Anionic detergents irritate the skin by removing natural oils. Although ingestion causes diarrhea, intestinal distention, and vomiting, no fatalities have been reported. The only treatment usually required is to discontinue use if skin irritation occurs and replace fluids and electrolytes. Induced vomiting is not indicated following ingestion of automatic dishwasher detergent, because of its alkalinity.

Day et al: Liquid laundry detergent capsules (PODS): a review of their composition and mechanisms of toxicity, and of the circumstances, routes, features, and management of exposures. Clin Toxicol (Phila) 2019 Nov;57(11):1053–1063 [PMID: 31130018]

Sjogren PP et al: Upper aerodigestive injuries from detergent ingestion in children. Laryngoscope 2017 Feb;127(2):509–512 [PMID: 27470579].

SPIDER BITES

Most medically important bites in the United States are caused by the black widow spider (*Latrodectus mactans*) and the North American brown recluse (violin) spider (*Loxosceles reclusa*). Positive identification of the spider is helpful, because many spider bites may mimic those of the brown recluse spider.

1. Black Widow Spider (*Latrodectus*)

The black widow spider is endemic to nearly all areas of the United States. The female has a characteristic black shiny body, and many species have a red hourglass on the ventral surface (Photo 6). The initial bite causes sharp fleeting pain that spreads centripetally. Local and systemic muscular cramping, abdominal pain, periorbital edema, nausea and vomiting, tachycardia, and hypertension are common. Facial swelling may also occur. Systemic signs of black widow spider bite may be confused with other causes of acute abdomen. Although paresthesias, nervousness, and transient muscle spasms may persist for weeks, recovery from the acute phase is generally complete within 2–3 days. Death is extremely rare.

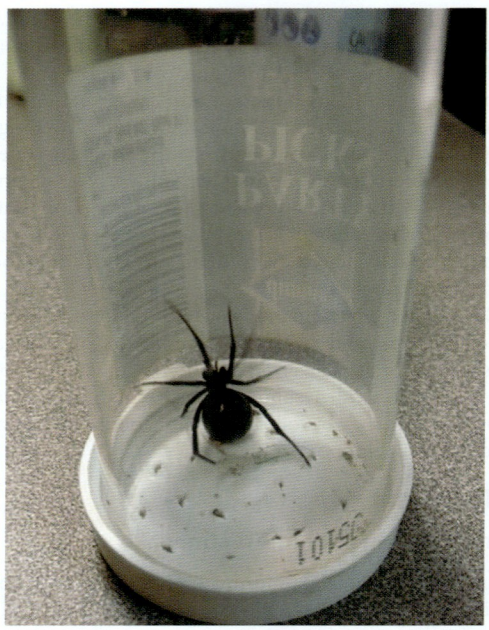

Initial pain control should be achieved with the use of benzodiazepines and opioids. Antivenom has limited availability but is effective in treatment of symptoms and is recommended in severe cases in which the previously mentioned therapies have failed. Because it is a whole IgG horse serum, serum sickness may develop in patients 5–7 days after treatment.

2. Brown Recluse Spider (*Loxosceles*)

The North American brown recluse spider is most commonly found in the central and Midwestern areas of the United States. Its bite characteristically produces a localized reaction with progressively severe pain within 24 hours. The initial bleb on an erythematous ischemic base is replaced by a black eschar within 1 week. This eschar separates in 2–5 weeks, leaving an ulcer that heals slowly. Systemic signs (loxoscelism) include cyanosis, morbilliform rash, fever, chills, malaise, weakness, nausea and vomiting, joint pains, hemolytic reactions with hemoglobinuria, jaundice, and delirium and are more common in children. Deaths are rare although fatal disseminated intravascular coagulation has been reported.

Although of unproved efficacy, the following therapies have been used: dexamethasone, 4 mg IV four times a day, during the acute phase; polymorphonuclear leukocyte inhibitors, such as dapsone or colchicine. Supportive wound care is recommended, with possible reconstruction/debridement with surgical consultation. Plasma exchange has been described for severe hemolysis.

Glatstein M et al: Treatment of pediatric black widow spider envenomation: a national poison center's experience. Am J Emerg Med 2018 Jun;36(6):998–1002 [PMID: 29133072].

Halmo et al: *Latrodectus* facies after *Latrodectus hesperus* envenomation in a pediatric patient. J Emerg Med 2019 Oct;57(4):523–526 [PMID: 31492593].

Said A et al: Successful use of plasma exchange for profound hemolysis in a child with loxoscelism. Pediatrics 2014 Nov;134(5):e1464–e1467 [PMID: 25349320].

VITAMINS

Unintentional ingestion of excessive amounts of vitamins rarely causes significant problems. Rare cases of hypervitaminosis A do occur, however, particularly in patients with poor hepatic or renal function. Chronic doses more than 50,000–100,000 IU are required for toxicity. Hypervitaminosis A can result in increased intracranial pressure, ocular toxicity, and hepatotoxicity. The fluoride contained in many multivitamin preparations is not a realistic hazard, because a 2- or 3-year-old child could eat 100 tablets, containing 1 mg of sodium fluoride per tablet, without experiencing serious symptoms. Iron toxicity has been reported with multivitamin tablets containing iron; most gummy vitamins do not contain iron. Pyridoxine abuse has caused neuropathies; nicotinic acid can result in flushing, and rarely hypotension and hepatotoxicity.

Wooltorton E. Too much of a good thing? Toxic effects of vitamin and mineral supplements. CMAJ 2003 Jul 8;169(1):47–48 [PMID: 12847042].

WARFARIN (COUMADIN) & NOVEL/DIRECT ORAL ANTICOAGULANTS (NOAC)

Warfarin is used as an anticoagulant and rodenticide. Long-acting anticoagulant rodenticides (eg brodifacoum, difenacoum) can cause a more serious toxicologic problem than warfarin as the anticoagulant activity may persist for periods ranging from 6 weeks to several months. However, most unintentional ingestions can be watched at home without further evaluation. If there are concerns for large ingestions, a prothrombin time at 48 hours can determine extent of toxicity. Treatment with vitamin K_1 at high doses may be needed for weeks for long-acting anticoagulant rodenticide toxicity.

Refer to published American College of Chest Physicians guidelines on management of bleeding in patient receiving vitamin K antagonists. With evidence for bleeding, preferred reversal agent is four-factor prothrombin complex concentrated (PCC), followed by fresh frozen plasma (FFP) and recombinant factor 7. Without significant bleeding, oral vitamin K is recommended.

Newer oral anticoagulants have been developed that have direct inhibition to specific clotting factors. Examples include direct Xa inhibitors (apixaban, edoxaban, rivaroxaban), and direct thrombin (IIa) inhibitors (dabigatran). Toxic doses have not been established, but unintentional ingestions do not typically lead to significant toxicity. If available, chromogenic antifactor Xa assay can quantitate direct Xa inhibition, and ecarin clotting time (ECT) or dilute thrombin time (dTT) is the most sensitive coagulation parameter for direct thrombin inhibitors. Idarucizumab and andexanet alfa are now available for the reversal of dabigatran and factor Xa inhibitors, respectively. Their availability and clinical experience in overdose are limited. If not available, activated four-factor PCC, recombinant Factor VII, or FFP should be used to treat potentially life-threatening bleeding.

Gunja N, Coggins A, Bidny S: Management of intentional super warfarin poisoning with long-term vitamin K and brodifacoum levels. Clin Toxicol (Phila) 2011;49(5):385–390 [PMID: 21740137].

Otero J et al: Direct oral anticoagulant reversal in the pediatric emergency department. Pediatr Emerg Care 2022 Nov 1;38(11):621–625 [PMID: 36314863].

Ravel et al: Management of patients on non-vitamin K antagonist oral anticoagulants in the acute care and periprocedural setting: a scientific statement from the American Heart Association. Circulation 2017 Mar 7;135(10):e604–e633 [PMID: 28167634].

Stevens SM et al: Executive summary: antithrombotic therapy for VTE disease: second update of the CHEST guideline and expert panel report. Chest 2021 Dec;160(6):2247–2259 [PMID: 34352279].

Critical Care

Amy C. Clevenger, MD, PhD

Angela S. Czaja, MD, MSc, PhD

Ryan J. Good, MD

Michele Loi, MD

Christopher Ruzas, MD

INTRODUCTION

Critical care medicine is the discipline of caring for patients with acute life-threatening conditions or conditions likely to cause serious harm if not rapidly addressed. This work requires a detailed understanding of human physiology, the pathophysiology of severe illness and injury, the intricate interactions between organ systems and therapies, as well as an understanding of and experience with the rapidly changing technologies available in a modern pediatric intensive care unit (PICU). The science of caring for the critically ill patient continues to advance rapidly as the molecular mediators of illness have become better defined and new therapies are brought into clinical use. Critical care, then, is a highly complex, multidisciplinary field in which optimal patient outcomes require a team-oriented approach, including critical care physicians and nurses; respiratory therapists; pharmacists; consulting specialists; physical, occupational, and recreational therapists; and social services specialists.

MONITORING & TECHNOLOGY

MONITORING

▶ Respiratory Monitoring

Pulse oximetry measures *arterial oxygen saturation* (Sao_2) continuously and noninvasively. However, pulse oximetry readings can be much less accurate in patients with saturations below 80%, poor skin perfusion, or significant movement and can overestimate the Sao_2 in patients with darker skin. In addition, pulse oximetry can be dangerously inaccurate in certain clinical settings such as carbon monoxide poisoning or methemoglobinemia. To directly measure arterial oxygen content, direct arterial blood gas sampling must be performed.

Knowing the partial pressure of oxygen (Pao_2) and inspired oxygen content (Fio_2), gas exchange impairment may be estimated through measures such as the Pao_2/Fio_2 ratio (used in diagnosing acute respiratory distress syndrome [ARDS]) or the *alveolar-arterial oxygen difference* ($A-aDO_2$, or A–a gradient). The A–a gradient is less than 15 mm Hg under normal conditions, widening with diffusion impairment, shunts, and ventilation-perfusion mismatch V/Q mismatch; gradients over 400 mm Hg are strongly associated with mortality. Although calculation of the intrapulmonary shunt fraction (the percentage of pulmonary blood flow that passes through nonventilated areas of the lung) is possible with a pulmonary arterial catheter, the use of the latter has declined significantly over the past decade.

End-tidal CO_2 ($ETco_2$) *monitoring* measures exhaled carbon dioxide (CO_2) noninvasively, allowing for continuous assessment of ventilation. Normally, the $ETco_2$ level closely approximates the alveolar CO_2 level (P_Aco_2), which should equal arterial CO_2 levels ($Paco_2$) because carbon dioxide diffuses freely across the alveolar-capillary barrier. However, $ETco_2$ may not accurately reflect the $Paco_2$ in patients with increased dead space ventilation (tidal volume that does not participate in gas exchange) or severe airway obstruction. $Paco_2$ is directly measured through blood gas analysis. Although venous or capillary samples may be used, these values can be misleading in patients with poor perfusion or difficult blood draws, and thus, arterial samples are the most reliable and accurate.

▶ Cardiovascular Monitoring

Noninvasive blood pressure monitoring may be sufficient for many critically ill children, but for others, *invasive hemodynamic monitoring* for diagnostic and therapeutic reasons may be required. *Arterial catheters* provide continuous arterial blood pressure readings, and the shape of the waveform is helpful in evaluating cardiac output. *Central venous catheters* allow monitoring of central venous pressure (CVP) and central venous oxygen saturation and can provide useful information about relative changes in volume status as therapies are administered. Indirect assessments of global oxygen delivery through laboratory monitoring of arterial pH, lactate, and central venous oxygen saturation can be performed. Normal central venous saturation is 25%–30% lower than arterial oxygen saturation (i.e. 70%–75% in normally saturated patients). If oxygen delivery is inadequate for the needs of the tissues, a greater portion of that oxygen will be consumed and the central venous saturation will be lower than normal. However, some patients (such as those with septic shock) may have an elevated central venous saturation (> 80%) due to impaired oxygen utilization by the tissues. Near-infrared spectroscopy (NIRS) can provide noninvasive assessments of regional tissue oxygenation with transcutaneous probes. Both the absolute value and percent decrease in NIRS values may reflect adequacy of regional tissue oxygen delivery.

Neurologic Monitoring

Critically ill children may have continuous neurologic monitoring with electroencephalography (EEG) and/or an intracranial pressure (ICP) monitor. Continuous EEG identifies clinical and subclinical seizure activity and provides information about general cerebral electrical activity, particularly in sedated and/or brain-injured patients. ICP monitors directly measure ICP, either continuously or intermittently. Fiberoptic ICP monitors can be placed in different intracranial spaces but are most commonly placed within the brain parenchyma. An external ventricular drain (EVD) can also monitor ICP but only intermittently, as drainage needs to be stopped to allow for closed volume pressure monitoring.

TECHNOLOGY

Mechanical Ventilation

The goals of mechanical ventilation are to facilitate the movement of gas into and out of the lungs (ventilation) and to improve oxygen uptake into the bloodstream (oxygenation). Positive-pressure ventilation (PPV) can be delivered either noninvasively or invasively via an artificial airway (endotracheal tube [ETT] or tracheostomy tube).

Noninvasive Ventilation

Noninvasive ventilation (NIV) provides PPV through various interfaces (mouthpiece or nasal; face or helmet mask) and has become an integral tool in the management of both acute and chronic respiratory failure. NIV modes include continuous positive airway pressure (CPAP), bilevel positive airway pressure (BiPAP), or average volume-assured pressure support (AVAPS). CPAP refers to the constant application of airway pressure, whereas BiPAP cycles between a higher inspiratory positive airway pressure (IPAP) and a lower expiratory positive airway pressure (EPAP) with each breath. The additional inspiratory support with BiPAP improves tidal volume and ventilation in patients who are breathing shallowly and can improve oxygenation by providing a higher mean airway pressure (MAP). AVAPS also delivers bilevel support but targets a set tidal volume within an allowable inspiratory pressure range rather than a set inspiratory pressure.

Conventional Mechanical Ventilation

Conventional mechanical ventilators deliver PPV invasively, with specific modes being defined by the pattern of breathing and several variables set by the clinician. Breathing during mechanical ventilation can be classified as spontaneous (controlled by patient) or mandatory (controlled by machine). The breathing pattern provided by the ventilator can be set to one of three configurations: continuous mandatory ventilation (CMV; ventilator determines the size and duration of all breaths), intermittent mandatory ventilation (IMV; ventilator delivers mandatory breaths, but additional spontaneous breaths between and during mandatory breaths are allowed, permitting weaning of ventilator support by reducing the number of mandatory breaths), and continuous spontaneous ventilation (CSV; patient initiates and controls all breaths, but the ventilator can assist those efforts). In addition to the breathing pattern, the settings chosen will determine how breaths should be initiated (trigger variable) and terminated (cycle variable), both of which can be either patient- or time-dependent. They also specify whether the ventilator will deliver a specific tidal volume (volume-controlled modes) or a specific pressure (pressure-controlled modes) and place limits to prevent excessive pressure or volume from being delivered by the ventilator.

As there is a current lack of evidence supporting one mode of ventilation over another, both volume-controlled and pressure-controlled modes are commonly used in PICUs. The most important considerations are understanding potential physiologic effects with a certain mode as applied to a child's respiratory condition and ensuring that appropriate limits are applied to the settings. For example, with pressure-controlled ventilation, high airway pressures may be avoided, limiting barotrauma or worsening lung injury. However, changes in the compliance of the respiratory system will lead to fluctuations in the actual tidal volume delivered to the patient with this mode, risking either inadequate or excessive tidal volumes at times. Volume-controlled ventilation, on the other hand, ensures more reliable delivery of the desired tidal volume and thus better control of ventilation and reduced risk of atelectasis from hypoventilation. However, as changes in lung compliance leads to fluctuations in the peak airway pressure generated by the breath, there is higher risk of barotrauma from excessive airway pressures and difficulties overcoming leaks in the ventilator circuit. In any mode of ventilation, the minimum distending pressure applied to the lung during the respiratory cycle is determined by setting the *positive end-expiratory pressure* (PEEP). PEEP helps prevent the end-expiratory collapse of open lung units, thus preventing atelectasis and intrapulmonary shunting.

High-Frequency Oscillatory Ventilation

High-frequency oscillatory ventilation (HFOV) is an alternative mode of mechanical ventilation in which the ventilator provides very small tidal volumes, at high rates (eg, 5–10 Hz, or 300–600 breaths/min) around a higher MAP. HFOV can achieve and maintain higher MAPs without high peak inspiratory pressures or large tidal volumes, theoretically providing a lung-protective strategy for diffuse lung disease such as ARDS. Disadvantages of HFOV include poor tolerance by patients who are not heavily sedated or paralyzed, risk of cardiovascular compromise due to high MAP, and risk of gas-trapping and barotrauma in patients with highly heterogeneous lung disease or severe obstructive disease. This mode of ventilation has been used successfully in neonates, older pediatric patients, and adults, although recent work has suggested that HFOV may be associated with worse outcomes in adults ARDS. Therefore, while HFOV may still be used in select patients, it may have a more limited role in ARDS.

Extracorporeal Membrane Oxygenation

Extracorporeal membrane oxygenation (ECMO) provides cardiovascular and/or respiratory support when other supportive measures are insufficient to maintain adequate gas exchange or oxygen delivery. ECMO circuits generally consist of a membrane oxygenator, a heater, and a pump. Central venous blood from the patient is directed out of the body, oxygenated, warmed, and returned back to the patient. ECMO can be provided in two major modes: venoarterial (VA) and venovenous (VV). VA ECMO, which requires cannulation of a large central artery and vein, bypasses the lungs and the heart, thus supporting both the cardiovascular and respiratory systems. VV ECMO, provided via either a single cannula into the internal jugular with dual lumens to allow venous drainage and return through the same cannula or separate cannulas for drainage and return in different veins, provides extracorporeal oxygenation and carbon dioxide removal, but the patient's own cardiac output is required to provide systemic oxygen delivery. VV ECMO use has increased over the past 15 years, with the advantage of reduced risk for systemic and cerebral emboli compared to VA ECMO. While VV ECMO is primarily indicated for respiratory failure, patients with moderate hemodynamic compromise can also experience improvements in circulatory status, likely due to improved oxygenation and acid base status and decreased intrathoracic pressures with so-called "rest settings" (ie, reduced mechanical ventilation pressure support and respiratory rates to lessen ventilator-induced lung injury).

ECMO is indicated for patients with potentially reversible cardiovascular and/or respiratory failure. Serious complications such as central nervous system (CNS) injury, hemorrhage, and infection can occur. Determining the optimal time to consider ECMO initiation is one of the most challenging aspects of using this technology. Despite an increase in the complexity of patients placed on ECMO, survival has remained acceptable over the past two decades. According to recent registry data, 60% of pediatric respiratory failure patients who are supported with ECMO survive, and survival rates are even better for ECMO patients with a diagnosis of viral pneumonia (especially due to respiratory syncytial virus) and without significant comorbidities. In both neonatal and adult randomized controlled trials, patients with severe respiratory failure who were referred to an ECMO center for consideration of ECMO had improved survival, even though not all patients were actually placed on ECMO. These results emphasize the importance of early referral to experienced centers if ECMO is to be considered.

Renal Replacement Therapy

Renal replacement therapy should be considered for serious electrolyte disturbances, drug or toxin overdoses, refractory acidosis, or when fluid overload associated with *acute kidney injury* (AKI) is not responsive to fluid restriction and/or diuretic use. Renal replacement modalities include peritoneal dialysis, intermittent hemodialysis, and continuous renal replacement therapy (CRRT), also known as continuous VV hemofiltration either with dialysis (CVVHD; performed with a dialysate to allow solute control) or without dialysis (CVVHF; ultrafiltration alone to control intravascular volume). CRRT involves sending patient venous blood through an extracorporeal filtration circuit and pump to provide slow, continuous fluid removal and/or dialysis. Advantages of CRRT, making it the often-preferred modality for PICU patients, include (1) in hemodynamically labile patients, a slower continuous rate of fluid removal may be better tolerated and more precisely controlled; (2) solute and fluid removal can be regulated separately; and (3) potential for easing of fluid restrictions so that nutrition can be improved. Disadvantages include technical complexity, including anticoagulation of the circuit and the need for central venous access. Retrospective studies and the few available prospective studies have suggested that early initiation of CRRT may be associated with lower mortality when comparing CRRT with other modes of renal replacement during severe pediatric sepsis.

Point-of-Care Ultrasound

Point-of-care ultrasound (POCUS) for procedural guidance has become widespread and, in some cases, standard of care. This technology allows for greater accuracy for procedural interventions and potentially reduced risk of adverse events.

While the strongest evidence base for the benefits exists for central venous catheter placement, POCUS can facilitate other procedures including PIV placement, arterial cannulation, and thoracentesis. POCUS is also increasingly used for diagnostics purposes, including assessment of volume status through measurement of inferior vena cava size and collapsibility, characterization of cardiac function, and evaluation of pleural effusions.

Alibrahim O et al: Mechanical ventilation and respiratory support in the pediatric intensive care unit. Pediatr Clin North Am 2022;69(3):587–605 [PMID: 35667763].

Burton L et al: Point-of-care ultrasound in the pediatric intensive care unit. Front Pediatr 2022;9:830160 [PMID: 35178366].

Cashen K et al: Extracorporeal membrane oxygenation in critically ill children. Pediatr Clin North Am 2022;69(3):425–440 [PMID: 35667755].

de Galasso et al: Dialysis modalities for the management of pediatric acute kidney injury. Pediatr Nephrol 2020;35(5):753–765 [PMID: 30887109].

RESPIRATORY CRITICAL CARE

ACUTE RESPIRATORY FAILURE

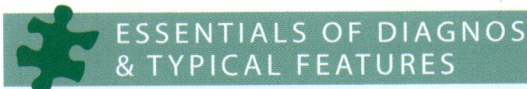

ESSENTIALS OF DIAGNOSIS & TYPICAL FEATURES

▶ Inability to deliver oxygen or remove carbon dioxide.

▶ PaO_2 is low while $PaCO_2$ is normal in hypoxemic respiratory failure (V/Q mismatch, diffusion defects, and intrapulmonary shunt).

▶ PaO_2 is low and $PaCO_2$ is high in hypercapnic respiratory failure (alveolar hypoventilation seen in central nervous system [CNS] dysfunction, oversedation, and neuromuscular disorders).

▶ Noninvasive mechanical ventilation can be an effective treatment for hypercapnic respiratory failure and selected patients with hypoxemic respiratory failure.

▶ Conventional mechanical ventilation should be accomplished within a strategy of "lung-protective" ventilation.

▶ Extracorporeal membrane oxygenation (ECMO) is a viable option for patients failing conventional mechanical ventilation.

▶ Pathogenesis

Acute respiratory failure, defined as the inability of the respiratory system to adequately deliver oxygen or remove carbon dioxide, is a major cause of morbidity and mortality in infants and children. Anatomic and developmental differences place infants and young children at higher risk than older children or adults for respiratory failure. An infant's thoracic cage is more compliant, allowing a greater tendency toward alveolar collapse. The intercostal muscles are poorly developed and unable to achieve the "bucket-handle" motion characteristic of adult breathing, and the diaphragm is shorter and relatively flat with fewer type I muscle fibers, making it less effective and more easily fatigued. The infant's airways are also smaller in caliber resulting in greater resistance to airflow and greater susceptibility to occlusion by mucus plugging and mucosal edema, particularly in the setting of respiratory infections. Alveoli in children are smaller and have less collateral ventilation than adults, again resulting in a greater tendency to collapse and develop atelectasis. Finally, young infants may have a more reactive pulmonary vascular bed, impaired immune system, or residual effects from prematurity, all of which increase the risk of respiratory failure.

Respiratory failure can be due to inadequate oxygenation (hypoxemic respiratory failure) or inadequate ventilation (hypercapnic respiratory failure) or both. Hypoxemic respiratory failure occurs in three situations: (1) *V/Q mismatch*, when blood flows to inadequately ventilated lung or when ventilated areas of the lung are inadequately perfused; (2) *diffusion defects*, caused by thickened alveolar membranes or excessive interstitial fluid at the alveolar-capillary junction; and (3) *intrapulmonary shunt*, when structural anomalies in the lung allow blood to flow through the lung without participating in gas exchange. Hypercapnic respiratory failure results from impaired alveolar ventilation, due to conditions such as increased dead space ventilation (eg, pneumonia, asthma), reduced respiratory drive due to CNS dysfunction or oversedation, or neuromuscular disorders (Table 14–1).

▶ Clinical Findings

The clinical findings in respiratory failure are the result of hypoxemia, hypercapnia, and arterial pH changes. Common features are summarized in Table 14–2. These features may not be clinically obvious, and many are nonspecific. As a result, a strictly clinical assessment of respiratory failure is not always reliable, and clinical findings of respiratory failure should be supplemented by laboratory data such as blood gas analysis.

▶ Modes of Respiratory Support

Patients with severe hypoxemia, hypoventilation, or apnea require immediate assistance with bag and mask ventilation. Although assisted ventilation can generally be maintained for some time with a properly sized mask, gastric distention, emesis leading to aspiration of gastric contents, and inadequate tidal volumes leading to atelectasis are possible complications. For patients with acute respiratory failure, *endotracheal intubation* and initiation of mechanical

Table 14–1. Types of respiratory failure.

Findings	Causes	Examples
Hypoxemic (type I) Pao$_2$ low Paco$_2$ normal	Ventilation-perfusion (V/Q) defect	Positional (supine in bed), acute respiratory distress syndrome (ARDS), atelectasis, pneumonia, pulmonary embolus, bronchopulmonary dysplasia
	Diffusion impairment	Pulmonary edema, ARDS, interstitial pneumonia
	Shunt	Pulmonary arteriovenous malformation, congenital adenomatoid malformation
	Low oxygen content	High-altitude
Hypercapnic (type II) Pao$_2$ low Paco$_2$ high	Hypoventilation	Neuromuscular disease (polio, Guillain-Barré syndrome), head trauma, sedation, chest wall dysfunction (burns), kyphoscoliosis, severe reactive airways

ventilation can be lifesaving. Safe placement of an ETT in infants and children requires experienced personnel and appropriate equipment at the bedside, including a correctly sized mask, Ambu bag, oral airways, ETTs, and appropriate suction catheters. See Chapter 12 for specific steps in preparing for pediatric intubation. Patients with normal airway anatomy may be intubated under intravenous (IV) anesthesia by experienced personnel. The specific agents selected should target sedation, analgesia, and neuromuscular blockade (Table 14–3). Additional details about medications can be found in section Sedation & Analgesia in the PICU. Endotracheal intubation of high-risk patients, such as those with significant upper airway obstruction (eg, patients with croup, epiglottitis, foreign bodies, or subglottic stenosis), mediastinal masses, or suspected or known difficult airways

Table 14–2. Clinical features of respiratory failure.

Respiratory
  Wheezing
  Expiratory grunting
  Decreased or absent breath sounds
  Flaring of alae nasi
  Retractions of chest wall
  Tachypnea, bradypnea, or apnea
  Cyanosis
Neurologic
  Restlessness
  Irritability
  Headache
  Confusion
  Convulsions
  Coma
Cardiac
  Bradycardia or excessive tachycardia
  Hypotension or hypertension
General
  Fatigue
  Sweating

should be approached with extreme caution; minimal sedation should be used, and neuromuscular blocking agents should be strictly avoided unless trained airway specialists decide otherwise.

Appropriately sizing the ETT is important for reducing complications and providing adequate respiratory support. An inappropriately large ETT is a risk factor for subglottic pressure necrosis, potentially leading to scarring and stenosis requiring surgical repair. An inappropriately small ETT can result in excessive air leak around the ETT, making adequate ventilation and oxygenation difficult and impairing the ability to clear secretions effectively. Two useful methods for calculating the correct size of ETT for a child are (1) using a Broselow tape to measure height and determine the corresponding ETT size or (2) in children older than 2 years, choosing a tube size using the formula ETT size = (16 + age in years) ÷ 4. Either cuffed or uncuffed tubes may be used, although a cuffed tube can ensure more effective mechanical ventilation. Assessment of an audible leak (with cuff deflated) at pressures less than 15–20 cm H$_2$O generally indicates acceptable ETT size. If there is insufficient leak, the decision to change the ETT needs to be carefully considered, especially in those with severe lung disease. Approximate proper insertion depth (in cm) as measured at the teeth can be estimated by tripling the size of the ETT. Correct placement of the ETT should be confirmed by auscultation for equal bilateral breath sounds and by detecting carbon dioxide using either a colorimetric filter or quantitative capnography. A chest radiograph is necessary for final assessment of a correctly positioned ETT, which should terminate in the mid-trachea between the thoracic inlet and the carina, at approximately the level of the second thoracic vertebra.

In patients not requiring immediate intubation, several modalities can be used to provide respiratory support, including supplemental oxygen, heated high-flow nasal cannula (HHFNC), and NIV. *Supplemental oxygen* with a nasal cannula or oxygen mask may be adequate to treat patients with mild respiratory insufficiency (Table 14–4). For patients

Table 14–3. Drugs commonly used for controlled endotracheal intubation.

Drug	Class of Agent	Dose	Advantages	Disadvantages
Atropine	Anticholinergic	0.02 mg/kg IV, minimum of 0.1 mg	Prevents bradycardia, dries secretions	Tachycardia, fever; seizures and coma with high doses
Fentanyl	Opioid (sedative)	1–3 mcg/kg IV	Rapid onset, hemodynamic stability	Respiratory depression, chest wall rigidity with rapid administration in neonates
Midazolam	Benzodiazepine (sedative)	0.1–0.2 mg/kg IV	Rapid onset, amnestic	Respiratory depression, hypotension
Etomidate	Anesthetic	0.2–0.4 mg/kg IV	Rapid onset, hemodynamic stability, lowers ICP	Suppresses adrenal function, should not be used in sepsis
Ketamine	Dissociative anesthetic	1–2 mg/kg IV 2–4 mg/kg IM	Rapid onset, bronchodilator, hemodynamic stability	Increases oral and airway secretions; potential myocardial depressant with chronic heart failure
Propofol	Anesthetic	1–2 mg/kg IV	Rapid onset, short-acting	Hypotension, contraindicated with egg or soy allergies
Rocuronium	Nondepolarizing muscle relaxant	1–1.2 mg/kg IV	Rapid onset, suitable for rapid sequence intubation, lasts 30 min	Requires refrigeration; can be reversed with Sugammadex
Succinylcholine	Depolarizing muscle relaxant	1 mg/kg IV	Rapid onset, short-acting	Hyperkalemia, dysrhythmias, cardiac arrest; malignant hyperthermia in susceptible children; contraindicated in chronic myopathies, acute burn or significant crush injuries

ICP, intracranial pressure; IM, intramuscularly; IV, intravenously.

requiring more support, HHFNC can be considered. *HHFNC* devices deliver heated and humidified oxygen mixtures via nasal cannula at flow rates higher than possible with cooler dry air. Depending on the flow rate and size of patient, HHFNC can also generate some amount of positive pressure and potentially improve work of breathing without further escalation of support. Generally, flow rates of 1–2 L/kg/min are considered high flow in infants and children (up to a maximum of 25 L/min), although some studies have utilized up to 60 L/min in adults. HHFNC use has been studied in children with bronchiolitis and appears to be well tolerated. However, if the patient is not improving on HHFNC, additional escalation of respiratory support may be warranted, including initiation of PPV through NIV or via ETT.

The best candidates for NIV are patients with moderate lung disease, patients in the recovery phases of their illness, or

Table 14–4. Supplemental oxygen therapy.

Source	Maximum % O$_2$ Delivered	Range of Rates (L/min)	Advantages	Disadvantages
Nasal cannula	35–40	0.125–4	Easily applied, relatively comfortable	Uncomfortable at higher flow rates, requires open nasal airways, easily dislodged, lower % O$_2$ delivered, nosebleeds
Simple mask	50–60	5–10	Higher % O$_2$, good for mouth breathers	Unsure of delivered % O$_2$
Face tent	40–60	8–10	Higher % O$_2$, good for mouth breathers, less restrictive	Unsure of delivered % O$_2$
Nonrebreathing mask	80–90	5–10	Highest O$_2$ concentration, good for mouth breathers	Unsure of delivered % O$_2$
Oxyhood	90–100	5–10	Stable and accurate O$_2$ concentration	Difficult to maintain temperature, hard to give airway care

Table 14–5. Suggested settings for NIV and conventional MV initiation.

Noninvasive Positive-Pressure Ventilation		
	Starting Settings	**Considerations**
CPAP	6–10 cm H_2O	If inspiratory support required, consider BiPAP or AVAPS
BiPAP	IPAP 12–16 cm H_2O, EPAP 6–8 cm H_2O	Higher IPAP may be needed with significant obstruction, or higher ventilatory support
AVAPS	Targeted TV 8–10 mL/kg, pressure limit range 20–30 cm H_2O, EPAP 6–8 cm H_2O	Adjust pressure limits based on respiratory compliance
Conventional Mechanical Ventilation		
	Starting Settings	**Considerations**
Volume control	Targeted TV 6–8 mL/kg, PEEP 6–8 cm H_2O, respiratory rate 12–20 breaths/min, I-time 0.3	Lower TV and higher PEEP for lung-protective strategies, limiting plateau pressures; permissive hypercapnia if not contraindicated (eg, elevated ICP)
Pressure control	Peak inspiratory pressure 20–30 cm H_2O, PEEP 6–8 cm H_2O, respiratory rate 12–20 breaths/min, I-time 0.3	Adjust PIP for targeted TV, higher PEEP for impaired oxygenation; permissive hypercapnia if not contraindicated (eg, elevated ICP)

AVAPS, average volume assured pressure support; BiPAP, bilevel positive airway pressure; CPAP, continuous positive airway pressure; EPAP, expiratory positive airway pressure; ICP, intracranial pressure; IPAP, inspiratory positive airway pressure; MV, mechanical ventilation; NIV, noninvasive ventilation; PEEP, positive end-expiratory pressure; TV, tidal volume.

those with primarily hypercapnic respiratory failure, such as patients with muscular dystrophies or other forms of neuromuscular weakness. Patients suffering from coma, impaired respiratory drive, an inability to protect their airway, or cardiac or respiratory arrest are not candidates for NIV. Suggested initial NIV settings are listed in Table 14–5 but should be titrated based on the patient's work of breathing and gas exchange. Close respiratory monitoring of patients initiated on NIV is critical, as NIV may mask symptoms of progressive respiratory failure, making eventual intubation more precarious. In patients with severe respiratory failure or those who are not improving with NIV, endotracheal intubation and initiation of mechanical ventilation should not be delayed.

▶ Setting & Adjusting the Ventilator

The overall approach to mechanical ventilation is to optimize gas exchange while minimizing the adverse effects of PPV. The principles of this "lung-protective ventilation strategy" are to safely recruit underinflated lung, sustain lung volume, minimize phasic overdistention, and decrease lung inflammation. To achieve this balance, careful consideration of the patient's respiratory disease process and other organ impairments such as cardiovascular instability or neurologic injury is essential. When initiating mechanical ventilation, the ICU clinician sets the respiratory rate, inspiratory time (I-time), level of PEEP, and either a targeted volume or the peak inspiratory pressure in volume-controlled or pressure-controlled modes, respectively. Ventilated patients require careful *monitoring* for the efficacy of mechanical ventilation, including respiratory rate and activity, chest wall movement, quality

of breath sounds and adequacy of gas exchange, with careful adjustment of settings as needed to optimize both ventilation ($Paco_2$) and oxygenation (Pao_2).

Ventilation is most affected by the delivered minute ventilation (tidal volume multiplied by respiratory rate). Thus, manipulations of the respiratory rate or tidal volume can improve abnormal $Paco_2$ values (hyper- or hypocarbia). Increasing the respiratory rate and/or tidal volume will increase the minute ventilation, which should decrease the $Paco_2$ levels; conversely, decreases in respiratory rate or tidal volume should act in the opposite fashion. When manipulating the respiratory rate, ensuring sufficient exhalation time is important, particularly in patients with significant airway obstruction (eg, asthma). Additionally, for patients with extensive alveolar collapse, ventilation can also improve with strategies to recruit and maintain open previously collapsed lung units through increased PEEP.

Oxygenation is primarily affected by adjustments in the inspired oxygen concentration and the MAP during the respiratory cycle. Increases in inspired oxygen concentration will generally increase arterial oxygenation unless there is significant right-to-left intracardiac or intrapulmonary shunting. Titration to the minimum Fio_2 necessary to achieve adequate oxygenation is important because high concentrations of inspired oxygen (eg, above 60%–65%) may lead to hyperoxic lung injury. Patients requiring high levels of oxygen may need a higher MAP to recruit underinflated lung units not participating in gas exchange and increase the functional residual capacity (FRC). Increases in PEEP, peak inspiratory pressure, and I-time will increase the MAP and may improve arterial oxygenation. However, if increases in MAP lead to decreased cardiac output by decreasing venous return or overdistention of alveoli rather than recruitment of collapsed alveoli, V/Q matching may worsen, resulting in worsened oxygenation. Additional complications of high MAP include gas trapping, CO_2 retention, and barotrauma with resultant air leaks. Finally, if cardiac output diminishes sufficiently to impair oxygen delivery, oxygen delivery to the tissues may be compromised despite an increase in oxygenation. Therefore, careful consideration of respiratory and cardiovascular goals is essential.

General guidelines in setting the ventilator are provided in Table 14–5, with specific principles of mechanical ventilation in ARDS and asthma further discussed in the following text. However, irrespective of ventilator mode or initial settings, the patient should be continually monitored, and adjustments should be made based on underlying pathophysiology, effectiveness of gas exchange, and overall cardiopulmonary status.

► Troubleshooting

Troubleshooting a sudden deterioration in the mechanically ventilated patient should begin with examining the patient. Determine whether the ETT is patent and in the correct position by auscultating for bilateral breath sounds, attempting to pass a suction catheter, assessing for detectable $ETco_2$, and the use of direct laryngoscopy, if necessary. A chest x-ray may also be helpful for ensuring appropriate ETT positioning. If the ETT is patent and correctly positioned, the next step is to determine whether any changes in the physical examination—such as poor or unequal chest rise or absent or unequal breath sounds—suggest atelectasis, bronchospasm, pneumothorax, or pneumonia. Next, determine whether hemodynamic deterioration could be underlying acute respiratory compromise (shock or sepsis). If the problem cannot be readily identified, take the patient off the ventilator and begin manual ventilation by hand-bagging. Hand-bagging can support the patient while the ventilator is checked for malfunction and allow assessment of changes in compliance, informing necessary ventilator adjustments.

► Escalation to Other Modes of Respiratory Support

If a child with acute respiratory failure is unable to maintain effective gas exchange without injurious levels of mechanical ventilation, escalation to other modes of support should be considered, including HFOV or ECMO. If the center does not have ability for ECMO, early referral to a center that does is essential.

► Supportive Care of the Mechanically Ventilated Patient

Patients undergoing mechanical ventilation require meticulous supportive care. Careful attention must be directed toward optimizing patient comfort and decreasing anxiety to reduce ventilator dyssynchrony and impaired gas exchange. Sedating medications are often required (see section Sedation & Analgesia in the PICU). However, oversedation of the ventilated patient may lead to longer durations of ventilation and difficulty weaning from the ventilator; therefore, standardized assessments of sedation level and targeting treatment to the minimum sedation level necessary are important.

For patients with severe respiratory illness, even small physical movements can compromise gas exchange and in such cases, neuromuscular blockade may be needed. Nondepolarizing neuromuscular blocking agents are most commonly used, given as intermittent doses or as continuous infusions. Extra care must be taken to ensure that levels of sedation are adequate, as these medications will mask many of the usual signs of patient discomfort. In addition, ventilator support may need to be increased to compensate for the elimination of patient respiratory effort.

Mechanically ventilated patients can usually be fed enterally with the use of temporary or existing feeding tubes. In patients in whom reflux or emesis is a major concern, transpyloric feeding or parenteral nutrition should be considered. *Ventilator-associated pneumonia* (VAP) is a significant complication of mechanical ventilation, leading to longer ICU stays and increased hospital costs. Preventative measures to reduce the risk of VAP include proper hand washing prior to respiratory care, elevation of the head of the bed to 30 degrees to prevent reflux, frequent turning of the patient, proper oral care, use of closed suction circuits on all ventilated patients and avoidance of breaking the closed suction system, sedation protocols to minimize sedation administration, and daily assessment of extubation readiness.

Mechanical ventilation should be weaned and discontinued as soon as safely possible. Successful extubation requires overall improvement in clinical status, adequate gas exchange, adequate respiratory muscle strength, and ability to protect the airway. Extubation failure rates in mechanically ventilated children have been estimated between 4% and 20%. To assess extubation readiness, a trial of spontaneous breathing may be conducted in which the patient remains intubated and breathes either without assistance (through a T-piece) or with a low level of pressure support (through the ventilator) for a defined period of time, usually 1–2 hours. The patient is observed carefully for signs of rapid shallow breathing or worsened gas exchange during this trial, and, if neither is observed, the patient can generally be safely extubated. In some children, support with NIV after extubation may facilitate the transition from mechanical ventilation.

Faustino EV et al: Accuracy of extubation readiness test in predicting successful extubation in children with acute respiratory failure from lower respiratory tract disease. Crit Care Med 2017;45(1):94–102 [PMID: 27632676].

Lee JH et al: Tracheal intubation practices and safety across international PICUs: a report from National Emergency Airway Registry for Children. Pediatr Crit Care Med 2019;20(1):1–8 [PMID: 30407953].

Nikolla DA et al: Change in frequency of invasive and noninvasive respiratory support in critically ill pediatric subjects. Respir Care 2021;66(8):1247–1253 [PMID: 33947789].

Ricard J et al: Use of nasal high flow oxygen during acute respiratory failure. Intensive Care Med 2020;46(23):2238–2247 [PMID: 32901374].

MAJOR RESPIRATORY DISEASES IN THE PEDIATRIC ICU

ACUTE RESPIRATORY DISTRESS SYNDROME

ESSENTIALS OF DIAGNOSIS & TYPICAL FEATURES

▶ Acute respiratory distress syndrome (ARDS) is a severe form of lung injury characterized by hypoxemia and noncardiogenic pulmonary edema.

▶ ARDS can arise because of either direct pulmonary injury or systemic conditions, such as sepsis.

▶ Lung protective mechanical ventilation and careful fluid management are crucial to good outcomes in ARDS patients.

ARDS is a syndrome of acute respiratory failure characterized by increased pulmonary capillary permeability, resulting in bilateral diffuse alveolar infiltrates on chest radiography, decreased lung compliance, and hypoxemia refractory to supplemental oxygen. Current consensus diagnostic criteria for ARDS in adult patients, known as the Berlin definition, include (1) acute onset, (2) bilateral pulmonary infiltrates on chest radiograph, (3) no clinical evidence of left atrial hypertension, and (4) severe hypoxemia based on the P/F ratio. Pediatric criteria for diagnosing ARDS are similar, but with notable differences including allowing for pulmonary infiltrates to be unilateral, utilizing the oxygenation index (OI, $MAP \times FIO_2 \times 100 \div PaO_2$) as the marker of ARDS severity in mechanically ventilated patients, and broadening the oxygenation criteria to include measures based on pulse oximetry saturations (Table 14–6).

▶ Presentation & Pathophysiology

ARDS may be precipitated by a variety of insults, including coronavirus-19 (COVID-19; Table 14–7). Pneumonia and sepsis account for most ARDS cases in children. Despite the diversity of potential causes, the clinical presentation is remarkably similar in most cases. ARDS can be divided into four clinical phases (Table 14–8). In phase 1, the patient may have dyspnea and tachypnea with a relatively normal PaO_2 and hyperventilation-induced respiratory alkalosis.

During phase 2, hypoxemia worsens, and respiratory distress becomes more clinically apparent, with cyanosis, tachycardia, irritability, and dyspnea. Early radiographic changes include the appearance of confluent alveolar infiltrates initially appearing in dependent lung fields, in a pattern suggestive of pulmonary edema. Pulmonary hypertension, reduced lung compliance, and increased airways resistance are also commonly observed in ARDS. Although chest x-rays show bilateral infiltrates, computed tomography (CT) imaging of adults demonstrates heterogeneous lung involvement: (1) consolidated areas which require high inflation pressures to open, (2) areas that are overinflated, and (3) areas that are

Table 14–6. Diagnostic criteria for ARDS.

Findings	Berlin Definition (Adults)	PALICC Definition (Children)
Timing	Within 1 wk of inciting event	No difference
Origin of pulmonary edema	Not fully explained by left ventricular failure or fluid overload; utilization of echocardiography to exclude elevated left atrial pressures as evidence of cardiac etiology	No difference
Radiographic findings	Bilateral opacities not fully explained by effusion, atelectasis, or pulmonary nodules	Bilateral **OR** unilateral opacities
Hypoxemia	Mild: P/F ≤ 300 mm Hg Moderate: P/F ≤ 200 mm Hg Severe: P/F ≤ 100 mm Hg *Minimum PEEP ≥ 5 cm H$_2$O	Invasive mechanical ventilation - Mild: 4 ≤ OI < 8 (5 ≤ OSI < 7.5) - Moderate: 8 ≤ OI < 16 (7.5 ≤ OSI < 12.3) - Severe: OI ≥ 16 (OSI ≥ 12.3) Noninvasive ventilation: P/F < 300 or S/F < 264

*ARDS, acute respiratory distress syndrome; OI, oxygenation index; OSI, oxygenation saturation index; P/F, PaO$_2$/FIO$_2$ ratio; PALICC, Pediatric Acute Lung Injury Consensus Conference; PEEP, positive end-expiratory pressure; S/F, SpO$_2$/FIO$_2$ ratio.

Table 14–7. Acute respiratory distress syndrome (ARDS) risk factors.

Direct Lung Injury	Indirect Lung Injury

Pneumonia
Aspiration of gastric contents
Inhalation injury (heat or toxin)
Pulmonary contusion
Hydrocarbon ingestion or
   aspiration
Near-drowning
	Sepsis
	Shock
	Burns
	Trauma
	Fat embolism
	Drug overdoses (including
	   aspirin, opioids, barbiturates,
	   tricyclic antidepressants)
	Transfusion of blood products
	Pancreatitis

normally inflated or repetitively opened and collapsed with each breath. Attempts to improve oxygenation by recruiting collapsed dependent lung regions occur at the expense of damaging nondependent regions by hyperinflation. This process, termed *volutrauma*, incites a potent inflammatory response that is capable of worsening nonpulmonary organ dysfunction. Even in normal lungs, ventilation with large tidal volumes and low PEEP levels can produce a lung injury that is indistinguishable from ARDS. This phenomenon is called *ventilator-induced lung injury*. Thus, mechanical injury from PPV is superimposed on the initial insult and is an integral part of the pathogenesis of ARDS.

Phase 3 of ARDS (subacute, 2–10 days after lung injury) is characterized by worsening of hypoxemia with an increasing shunt fraction, as well as a further decrease in lung compliance. Some patients develop an accelerated fibrosing alveolitis. The mechanisms responsible for these changes are unclear. In phase 4 of ARDS (chronic, 10–14 days after lung injury), fibrosis, emphysema, and pulmonary vascular obliteration occur. During this phase, oxygenation generally improves, but the lung becomes more fragile and susceptible to barotrauma. Air leak is common among patients ventilated with high airway pressures at this late stage. Patients have increased dead space and difficulties with ventilation are common. Airway compliance remains low because of ongoing pulmonary fibrosis and insufficient surfactant production. Secondary infections are frequent in the subacute and chronic phases of ARDS and can impact clinical outcomes. Mechanisms responsible for increased susceptibility to infection during this phase are not well understood.

Table 14–8. Pathophysiologic changes of acute respiratory distress syndrome.

Radiography	Symptoms	Laboratory Findings	Pathophysiology
Phase 1 (early changes)			
Normal radiograph	Dyspnea, tachypnea, normal chest examination	Mild pulmonary hypertension, normoxemic or mild hypoxemia, hypercapnia	Neutrophil sequestration, no clear tissue damage
Phase 2 (onset of parenchymal changes)			
Patchy alveolar infiltrates; normal heart size	Dyspnea, tachypnea, cyanosis, tachycardia, coarse rales	Moderate to severe hypoxemia, increasing shunt, decreased lung compliance, pulmonary hypertension, normal wedge pressure	Neutrophil infiltration, vascular congestion, increased lung permeability, pulmonary edema, fibrin strands, platelet clumps, type I epithelial cell damage
Phase 3 (acute respiratory failure with progression, 2–10 days)			
Diffuse alveolar infiltrates; air bronchograms; decreased lung volume; normal heart size	Tachypnea, tachycardia, sepsis syndrome, signs of consolidation, diffuse rhonchi	Worsening shunt fraction, further decrease in compliance, increased minute ventilation, impaired oxygen extraction	Increased interstitial and alveolar inflammatory exudate with neutrophils and mononuclear cells, type II cell proliferation, beginning fibroblast proliferation, thromboembolic occlusion
Phase 4 (pulmonary fibrosis, pneumonia with progression, > 10 days)			
Persistent diffuse infiltrates; superimposed new pneumonic infiltrates; air leak; normal heart size or enlargement due to cor pulmonale	Symptoms as above, recurrent sepsis, evidence of multiorgan system failure	Phase 3 changes persist; recurrent pneumonia, progressive lung restriction, impaired tissue oxygenation, impaired oxygen extraction; multiorgan system failure	Type II cell hyperplasia, interstitial thickening; infiltration of lymphocytes, macrophages, fibroblasts; loculated pneumonia or interstitial fibrosis; medial thickening and remodeling of arterioles

Treatment

Ventilator management of ARDS is directed at protecting vulnerable lung regions from cyclic alveolar collapse at end expiration and protecting nondependent, overinflated lung regions from hyperinflation at end inspiration (open lung, or lung-protective, strategy). The mode of mechanical ventilation is less important than limiting phasic alveolar stretch and stabilizing lung units prone to repetitive end-expiratory collapse. A landmark, multicenter randomized trial of adult ARDS patients demonstrated a ventilation strategy using a 6-mL/kg (ideal body weight) tidal volume had a 22% mortality reduction and less extrapulmonary organ failure compared to one allowing tidal volumes of 12 mL/kg. Although this trial has not been replicated in pediatric patients, application of these same management principles has gained widespread acceptance. The general approach to mechanical ventilation in pediatric ARDS is to limit the tidal volume (ie, 6–8 mL/kg ideal body weight), limit the alveolar plateau pressure (the pressure at end-inspiration) to 25–30 cm H_2O or less, and target a level of PEEP to maintain acceptable oxygen saturations for end-organ perfusion. Targeting 88%–90% oxygen saturation may be reasonable for many patients, especially if it allows for an FIO_2 of 60% or less to minimize injurious hyperoxia. In general, this can be accomplished by incremental increases in PEEP until adequate oxygenation is achieved or until a limiting side effect of the PEEP is reached. Clinicians should minimize the ETT cuff leak (if possible), ensure an appropriate plane of patient sedation, and optimize the ventilation to perfusion relationship by verifying that the patient's intravascular volume status is appropriate. Unless a clear contraindication exists (eg, increased ICP), permissive hypercapnia (ie, accepting elevated $PaCO_2$ with reasonable pH ranges) should be allowed.

Fluid management is an important element of the care of patients with ARDS. Given the increased pulmonary capillary permeability in ARDS, further pulmonary edema accumulation is likely with any elevation in pulmonary hydrostatic pressures. Evidence in adults has shown that a "conservative" fluid strategy targeting lower cardiac filling pressures (CVP < 4 mm Hg) is associated with better oxygenation and a shorter duration of mechanical ventilation compared to a "liberal" fluid strategy targeting a CVP 10–14 mm Hg. Fluid restriction should only be implemented after hemodynamic variables stabilize, however, and volume resuscitation should not be denied to hemodynamically unstable patients with ARDS.

For patients failing these standard approaches of mechanical ventilation and fluid restriction, several alternative or rescue therapies are available. *Prone positioning* is a technique of changing the patient's position in bed from supine to prone, with the goal of improving ventilation of collapsed dependent lung units via postural drainage and improved V/Q matching. This technique can dramatically improve gas exchange in the short term, particularly for patients early during ARDS, but the gains are often not sustained. Clinical trials of prone positioning in adults have shown a survival benefit in those with severe disease, but no pediatric study has shown a clear improvement in mortality or in duration of mechanical ventilation. HFOV has been used successfully for many years in pediatric patients with ARDS; however, studies in adults have shown no benefit or an increase in mortality with HFOV. Based on the ability of *inhaled nitric oxide* (iNO) to reduce pulmonary artery pressure and improve the matching of ventilation with perfusion without producing systemic vasodilation, iNO can be used as a therapy for refractory ARDS. Several multicenter trials of iNO in the treatment of ARDS, both in adults and in children, showed acute improvements in oxygenation in subsets of patients, but no significant improvement in overall survival. As a result, iNO cannot be recommended as a standard therapy for ARDS. *ECMO* has been increasingly used to support pediatric patients with severe ARDS, although the impact on outcomes in pediatric ARDS has not been compared with lung protective ventilation strategies in a prospective randomized trial.

Patients with ARDS require careful cardiorespiratory monitoring to allow for careful titration of mechanical ventilation and assessment of need for escalation. Additionally, renal, hepatic, and GI function should be watched closely because of the prognostic implications of multiorgan dysfunction in ARDS. Finally, as secondary infections are common and contribute to increased mortality rates, surveillance for infection is important by obtaining appropriate cultures and following the temperature curve and white blood cell count.

Outcomes

Reported mortality rates for pediatric ARDS vary depending upon the diagnostic criteria used, presence of coexisting conditions, and the quality and consistency of supportive care provided. In general, mortality rates have improved over time, ranging from 8% to 40%, with immunocompromised patients at higher risk of death. Across all subpopulations of pediatric ARDS patients, non-pulmonary organ failure remains an important cause of mortality. Morbidity and long-term outcomes are less clearly understood. Limited data suggest that some children with severe ARDS can have respiratory symptoms for years after the original insult, highlighting the need for close follow-up of pulmonary function.

ARDS Definition Task Force: Acute respiratory distress syndrome: the Berlin definition. JAMA 2012;307(23):2526–2533 [PMID: 22797452].

Emeriaud G et al: Executive summary of the second international guidelines for the diagnosis and management of pediatric acute respiratory distress syndrome (PALICC-2). Pediatr Crit Care Med 2023;24(2):143–168 [PMID: 36661420].

Killien EY et al: Outcomes of children surviving pediatric acute respiratory distress syndrome: from the pediatric acute lung injury consensus conference. Pediatr Crit Care Med 2023;24:S28–S44 [PMID: 36661434].

Yehya N et al: Definition, incidence and epidemiology of pediatric acute respiratory distress syndrome: from the second Pediatric Acute Lung Injury Consensus Conference. Pediatr Crit Care Med 2023;24(12 Suppl 2): S87–S98 [PMID: 36661438].

SEVERE ASTHMA EXACERBATION

ESSENTIALS OF DIAGNOSIS & TYPICAL FEATURES

► Severe asthma exacerbation (previously known as *status asthmaticus*) is reversible small airway obstruction refractory to sympathomimetic and anti-inflammatory agents that may progress to respiratory failure without prompt and aggressive intervention.

► Dyspnea at rest that interferes with the ability to speak can be an ominous sign.

► Absence of wheezing may be misleading because, to produce a wheezing sound, the patient must take in sufficient air.

► Patients with severe respiratory distress, signs of exhaustion, alterations in consciousness, elevated $Paco_2$, or acidosis should be admitted to the PICU.

Pathogenesis

Life-threatening asthma exacerbations are caused by severe bronchospasm, excessive mucus secretion, inflammation, and edema of the airways (see Chapter 19). Infants and children are at particular risk for respiratory failure from asthma due to several structural and mechanical features of their lungs: less elastic recoil, a more compliant chest wall, thicker airway walls leading to greater peripheral airway resistance for any degree of bronchoconstriction, increased airway reactivity to bronchoconstrictors, and fewer collateral channels of ventilation. Risk factors for severe asthma exacerbation include obesity, lower socioeconomic status, non-Caucasian race, and a prior history of previous ICU admissions or intubations.

Clinical Findings

Patients with severe asthma exacerbations can have a variety of constitutional and cardiorespiratory findings. They often have tachypnea, increased use of accessory muscles, and variable aeration. Diffuse wheezing is usually present, but absence of wheeze may indicate severe obstruction impeding airflow. Dyspnea at rest that interferes with the ability to speak and cyanosis is also an ominous sign. These children may display signs of panic, exhaustion, or an altered level of consciousness. Agitation, drowsiness, or confusion can be signs of elevated $Paco_2$ levels and impending respiratory failure.

These patients generally have elevated heart rates secondary to stress, dehydration, and β-agonist therapy, and may have systolic and/or diastolic hypotension. Diastolic pressures less than 40 mm Hg in conjunction with extreme tachycardia may impair coronary artery filling and predispose to cardiac ischemia, which can present with chest pain and ST changes on electrocardiogram. Pulsus paradoxus (ie, an exaggerated decrease in systolic blood pressure with inspiration) may be observed and can be used as a marker of disease severity and response to treatment.

Laboratory Findings

In addition to continuous pulse oximetry, blood gas measurements should be considered in critically ill patients with status asthmaticus to evaluate gas exchange and acid–base balance. Patients with severe asthma exacerbations typically have increased minute ventilation and should be expected to have a $Paco_2$ less than 40 mm Hg. Normal to elevated $Paco_2$ levels suggest respiratory failure. Desaturation on room air may indicate severely impaired gas exchange and impending respiratory failure but also may occur with initiation of $β_2$-agonist therapy and associated V/Q mismatching. The presence of metabolic acidosis may signify relative dehydration, inadequate cardiac output, or underlying infection, but can also be related to type B lactic acidosis (ie, lactate production not related to tissue hypoxia or hypoperfusion) from $β_2$-agonist therapy.

Patients may demonstrate decreased serum potassium, magnesium, and/or phosphate, especially with prolonged $β_2$-agonist use. Leukocytosis is commonly observed during asthma exacerbations and may be due to infection or to demargination of polymorphonuclear leukocytes as a result of stress or corticosteroid treatment. Measurement of other inflammatory markers can be useful if there is concern for infection.

Chest x-rays should be obtained in patients presenting with severe asthma exacerbations to evaluate for treatable conditions such as pneumonia, foreign-body aspiration, air leak, or a chest mass. Pneumothorax and pneumomediastinum are common complications of severe exacerbations detected with chest radiography. Severe wheezing without a prior history of asthma should raise suspicion for alternative diagnoses such as foreign-body aspiration or congenital anomalies. Electrocardiograms are not routinely recommended but may be indicated to rule out cardiac ischemia, especially in patients with known cardiac disease, extreme tachycardia and low diastolic blood pressure, or complaints of chest pain.

Treatment

The key treatment strategy for severe asthma exacerbation is to reverse the underlying process swiftly and aggressively before respiratory failure requiring endotracheal intubation and mechanical ventilation ensues, given the complications of providing mechanical ventilation to patients with severe airflow obstruction. Children with severe asthma exacerbations require IV access, continuous pulse oximetry, and cardiorespiratory monitoring, as close monitoring of gas exchange, cardiovascular status, and mental status are crucial to assessing response to therapy and determining appropriate interventions.

Because of inadequate minute ventilation and V/Q mismatching, patients with severe asthma exacerbations are almost always hypoxemic and should receive supplemental humidified oxygen immediately to maintain saturations more than 90%. Children with clinical signs of dehydration should receive appropriate fluid resuscitation. The hemodynamic effects of β₂-agonist therapy (eg, peripheral vasodilation, diastolic hypotension) may also require further fluid resuscitation to maintain cardiac output and avoid cardiac ischemia. Antibiotics are generally not recommended for treatment of severe asthma exacerbations unless a coexisting bacterial infection is identified or suspected.

The first-line treatment for rapidly reversing airflow obstruction is administration of inhaled selective short-acting β₂-*agonist* therapy such as albuterol (Table 14–9). The frequency of administration will vary based on the severity of symptoms and the occurrence of adverse side effects. Patients with severe distress and poor inspiratory flow rates may have inadequate delivery of inhaled medications and may require subcutaneous or IV medication. Subcutaneous epinephrine or terbutaline, a relatively specific β₂-agonist, may be used for initial treatment. Side effects of β₂-agonist therapy, including

tachycardia and other arrhythmias as well as diastolic hypotension, are usually more severe with systemic administration. In addition to β₂-agonist therapy, immediate administration of systemic *corticosteroids* to decrease associated inflammation is critical to the early management of life-threatening asthma exacerbations. Because enteral medications may not be tolerated in patients with severe exacerbations, administration of IV or IM steroids should be considered.

For severe exacerbations unresponsive to these initial treatments, additional therapies may be considered despite limited pediatric evidence. *Ipratropium bromide*, an inhaled anticholinergic bronchodilator, is commonly used in the emergency department and is a reasonable intervention in the PICU, despite limited evidence of efficacy. *Magnesium sulfate* has bronchodilatory properties and may also be considered for patients who are unresponsive to early treatment or who have impending respiratory failure. NIV may be used to support patients with severe asthma exacerbations and help avoid the need for intubation and mechanical ventilation. Because of its noninvasive interface, spontaneous breathing and upper airway function are preserved, allowing the patient to provide his/her own airway clearance. Recent adult data demonstrated a lower risk of invasive mechanical ventilation and mortality associated with NIV use during severe asthma exacerbations. Pediatric data are limited to small studies and case series but describe improvements in gas exchange and respiratory effort. Careful titration of inspiratory and expiratory pressures is essential, however, to avoid complications of PPV such as air leak.

Table 14–9. Medical therapies for severe asthma exacerbation.

Medication	Mechanism of Action	Dosing and Administration	Common Side Effects
Albuterol	β₂-Agonist	Inhaled *Intermittent:* 2.5–5 mg every 10–15 min *Continuous:* 10–30 mg/h	Tachycardia, hypotension, hypoxemia, myocardial ischemia
Terbutaline	β₂-Agonist	Intravenous *Loading dose:* 10 mcg/kg *Continuous infusion:* 0.5–5 mcg/kg/min	Tachycardia, hypotension, hypoxemia, myocardial ischemia
Epinephrine	Nonselective adrenergic agonist	Subcutaneous or intramuscular 0.01 mg/kg every 20 min	Tachycardia, hypertension
Corticosteroids	Decrease inflammation	Intravenous, intramuscular, or oral *Dexamethasone:* 0.6 mg/kg daily *Methylprednisolone:* 1–2 mg/kg in two divided doses	Agitation, hypertension, hyperglycemia
Ipratropium bromide	Anticholinergic	Inhaled 250–500 mcg every 8 h	Blurred vision, mydriasis, tachycardia
Magnesium sulfate	Prevents calcium flux into smooth muscle cells	Intravenous 50 mg/kg/dose	Hypotension, flushing
Aminophylline	Prevents degradation of cyclic guanosine monophosphate	Intravenous *Loading dose:* 5.7 mg/kg *Continuous infusion:* 0.5–1 mg/kg/h *Target serum level:* 10 mcg/mL	Narrow therapeutic window, seizures, arrhythmias; routine use not recommended

Heliox-driven albuterol nebulization can also be considered for patients refractory to conventional therapy. Heliox is a mixture of helium and oxygen with lower density than ambient air that can improve airway delivery of albuterol and gas exchange through improved laminar flow. A mixture of at least 60%–70% helium is required to be effective, limiting its use in patients with higher oxygen requirements.

Methylxanthines, such as *theophylline and aminophylline*, may also be considered for the management of severe asthma, although their use remains controversial. The pharmacokinetics of these agents are erratic, and serious side effects such as seizures and cardiac arrhythmias may occur. These concerns, in addition to mixed evidence of benefit, have led to a general recommendation against the routine use of methylxanthines for asthma exacerbations. Nevertheless, they may have a role in individual severe cases. When a methylxanthine is used, close therapeutic drug monitoring is essential and consultation with a pharmacist recommended.

If aggressive management fails to result in significant improvement, endotracheal intubation and *mechanical ventilation* may be necessary. Patients who present with apnea or coma should be intubated immediately. If there is steady deterioration despite maximal medical therapy for asthma, intubation should occur before acute respiratory arrest. The intubation procedure can be dangerous, given the high risk of barotrauma and cardiovascular collapse, and should be performed by the most experienced provider available.

Mechanical ventilation for patients with asthma is difficult because severe airflow obstruction often leads to very high airway pressures, air trapping, and resultant barotrauma. Therefore, the goal of mechanical ventilation is to maintain adequate oxygenation and ventilation with the least amount of barotrauma until other therapies are successful in reversing airflow obstruction. This approach typically means accepting some degree of hypercarbia to avoid complications of aggressive ventilation. Because of the severe inspiratory and expiratory airflow obstruction, these patients will require long inspiratory times to deliver a breath and long expiratory times to avoid air trapping. Either volume- or pressure-targeted modes of ventilation can be used, although volume and pressure limits should be closely monitored. In general, the ventilator rate should be decreased until the expiratory time is long enough to allow emptying prior to the next machine breath. The level of PEEP should be titrated to minimize air trapping from either auto-PEEP or dynamic obstruction. If possible, and when a patient moves toward extubation, a CSV mode is useful, as the patient can control the I-time and flow rate.

These ventilator strategies and the resulting hypercarbia typically are uncomfortable, requiring that patients be heavily sedated. Ketamine is a dissociative anesthetic with bronchodilatory properties that can be used to facilitate intubation and as a sedative infusion for intubated patients. Ketamine can also increase bronchial secretions, which may limit its use in certain patients or require administration of an anticholinergic agent. Barbiturates and morphine should be avoided, as both can increase histamine release and worsen bronchospasm. Many patients will also require neuromuscular blockade initially to optimize ventilation and minimize airway pressures. In intubated patients not responding to these strategies, inhaled anesthetics, such as isoflurane, should be considered. These agents act not only as anesthetics but also cause airway smooth muscle relaxation. Inhalational anesthetics must be used with caution, however, as they can also cause significant hypotension due to vasodilation and myocardial depression. Finally, the use of ECMO has been reported for severe asthma exacerbations and could be considered as a rescue therapy.

▶ **Prognosis**

Severe asthma exacerbations remain among the most common reasons for admission to the PICU and are associated with a mortality rate of 1%–3%, especially in patients with a previous PICU admission. Careful but expedient management can reduce morbidity and mortality. As many as 75% of patients admitted to the PICU with life-threatening asthma flares will be readmitted with a future exacerbation, emphasizing the need for careful outpatient follow-up of this high-risk population.

Abu-Kishk et al: Long-term outcome after pediatric intensive care unit asthma admissions. Allergy Asthma Proc 2016 Nov;37(6):169–175 [PMID: 27931294].
Grunwell JR et al: Geospatial analysis of social determinants of health identifies neighborhood hot spots associated with pediatric intensive care use for life-threatening asthma. J Allergy Clin Immunol Pract 2022;10(4):981–991 [PMID: 34775118].
Smith MA et al: Changes in the use of invasive and noninvasive mechanical ventilation in pediatric asthma: 2009–2019. Ann Am Thorac Soc 2023;20(2):245–253 [PMID: 36315585].

CARDIOVASCULAR CRITICAL CARE

SHOCK

ESSENTIALS OF DIAGNOSIS & TYPICAL FEATURES

▶ Shock is defined as the inadequate delivery of oxygen and nutrients to tissues to meet metabolic needs.

▶ Shock can result from decreased delivery of oxygen, inadequate delivery of oxygen in the face of increased demands, or from impaired utilization of oxygen.

▶ Shock can be categorized as compensated, hypotensive, or irreversible.

▶ Early recognition and intervention are essential to improving patient outcomes from shock.

Pathogenesis

Shock is a syndrome characterized by inadequate oxygen delivery to meet the body's metabolic demands. Shock can complicate multiple different disease processes and can be categorized based on the primary physiologic disturbance: hypovolemic, cardiogenic, obstructive (eg, tamponade, pneumothorax), and distributive (eg, septic shock or vasodilation secondary to anaphylaxis) (see Chapter 12). Dissociative shock (impaired use of oxygen despite adequate delivery) can also occur in situations such as carbon monoxide poisoning. Shock, regardless of underlying etiology, can be best understood as an imbalance between delivery of oxygen to the tissues and consumption of oxygen by the tissues. Metabolic failure may occur as a result of reduced oxygen delivery, increased tissue demand, or impaired oxygen utilization, or combinations of all three conditions. These may result in anaerobic cellular metabolism, hypoxia, lactic acidosis, and, ultimately, irreversible cellular damage.

Oxygen delivery (DO_2) is defined as the product of the *cardiac output* and the *oxygen content of arterial blood* (Cao_2). Cardiac output, in turn, is determined by ventricular stroke volume (SV) and heart rate (HR). SV is influenced by preload, afterload, contractility, and cardiac rhythm. *Preload* can be decreased as a result of hypovolemia due to hemorrhage or dehydration or as a result of vasodilation due to anaphylaxis, medications, or septic shock. Impaired *contractility* can occur with conditions such as cardiomyopathy, myocardial ischemia/reperfusion following a cardiac arrest, postcardiac surgery, multisystem inflammatory syndrome in children (MIS-C) following SARS-CoV-2 infection, and sepsis. *Afterload* can be increased with elevated systemic vascular resistance as seen in late septic shock and cardiac dysfunction. Cardiac dysrhythmias can alter cardiac output and contribute to inadequate oxygen delivery (see Chapter 20).

The oxygen content of arterial blood consists primarily of the oxygen *bound* to hemoglobin and, to a much smaller extent, the oxygen *dissolved* in the blood. Therefore, illnesses that affect the oxygen saturation of hemoglobin (eg, impaired gas exchange) or alter hemoglobin concentration (eg, severe anemia from hemorrhage) can impair oxygen delivery. Abnormal hemoglobins (eg, carboxyhemoglobin and methemoglobin) can also reduce oxygen delivery.

Clinical Findings

The clinical presentation of shock can be categorized into recognizable stages: compensated, hypotensive or decompensated, and irreversible. Patients in *compensated shock* have relatively normal blood pressures, and compensatory mechanisms preserve oxygen delivery. In infants, a compensatory increase in cardiac output is achieved primarily by increases in HR, given the limited ability of infants to increase SV. In older patients, SV and HR both increase to improve cardiac output. Blood pressure remains normal initially because of peripheral vasoconstriction and increased systemic vascular resistance. Decline in blood pressure occur late, defining *hypotensive or decompensated shock*. Patients in hypotensive shock are at risk of developing multiorgan dysfunction syndrome (MODS), which in turn carries a high risk of mortality. In extreme cases, organ damage can progress to the point that restoration of oxygen delivery will not improve organ function, a condition known as *irreversible shock*.

The symptoms and signs of shock may vary by etiology but, in general, result from end-organ dysfunction caused by inadequate oxygen delivery. Because this condition can progress rapidly to serious illness or death, rapid assessment of a child in shock is essential to determining treatment. In patients with impaired cardiac output and peripheral vasoconstriction, the skin will be cool and pale with delayed capillary refill (>3 seconds) and thready pulses. Additionally, the skin may appear gray or ashen, particularly in newborns, and mottled or cyanotic in patients with decreased cardiac output. In contrast, patients with vasodilatory shock (eg, with sepsis) can present with warm skin with brisk capillary refill and bounding pulses. The detection of peripheral edema is a worrisome sign and can indicate severe vascular leak due to sepsis or poor cardiac output with fluid and sodium retention. The skin examination can also provide insight into the diagnosis (eg, presence of a rash such as purpura fulminans may indicate an infectious etiology) or reveal the site and extent of traumatic injury. Cracked, parched lips, and dry mucous membranes may indicate severe volume depletion.

Tachycardia is an important and early sign of shock and is typically apparent well before hypotension. Not all patients can mount an appropriate HR increase, however, and bradycardia in a patient with shock is particularly ominous. Peripheral pulses will weaken first in shock as cardiac output is diverted to the body core. Discrepancy in pulses between lower extremities and upper extremities, particularly in an infant, may indicate a critical coarctation of the aorta with closure of the ductus arteriosus. The presence of a gallop on examination can indicate heart failure, while a pathologic murmur suggests the possibility of congenital heart disease or valvular dysfunction. A rub or faint, distant heart sounds may indicate a pericardial effusion. Rales, hypoxia, and increased work of breathing occur in patients with shock from heart failure or acute lung injury. Severe metabolic acidosis due to shock is often associated with tachypnea and compensatory respiratory alkalosis. Urine output less than 0.5 mL/kg/h in a pediatric patient should be considered abnormally low, reflecting decreased renal blood flow. Hepatomegaly may suggest right heart failure or fluid overload, splenomegaly may suggest an oncologic/infiltrative process, and abdominal distension may suggest gastrointestinal obstruction or perforated viscus as the etiology of shock. The level of consciousness reflects the adequacy of brain cortical perfusion. When brain perfusion is severely impaired, alteration of consciousness occurs. Lack of motor response and failure to cry in response to venipuncture or lumbar puncture is highly concerning. Inadequate perfusion of deeper brain structures can result in loss of sympathetic tone, irregular respirations, and respiratory arrest. The PODIUM collaborative has defined clinical and laboratory criteria to standardize determination of organ dysfunction.

▶ Monitoring & Evaluation

In addition to cardiorespiratory monitoring, laboratory and radiographic studies in the patient with suspected shock should be performed to evaluate the etiology of shock, assess the extent of impaired oxygen delivery, and identify signs of end-organ dysfunction due to inadequate oxygen delivery. Some studies should be performed in all patients with shock and others selected based on category of shock (Table 14–10).

Laboratory indicators of organ dysfunction include evidence of anaerobic metabolism such as acidemia and elevated lactate, increased serum creatinine, and abnormal liver function tests (elevated transaminases or reduced production of clotting factors). Electrolyte abnormalities may be present, including hypo- or hypernatremia, hyperkalemia or hyperphosphatemia (eg, with renal failure), and low ionized calcium levels. Coagulation panels can be used to detect

Table 14–10. Laboratory studies in the setting of shock.

Evaluation for infectious etiology
Sources include blood, urine, tracheal secretions, CSF, wound, pleural fluid, or stool
Stains, cultures, and other microbiologic tests (PCR, immunofluorescent antibody stains) for bacteria, fungus, viruses
Evaluation of organ function
Pulmonary: ABG (evaluate acid–base status, evaluation of oxygen delivery/consumption)
Cardiac: ABG, mixed venous saturation, lactate
Liver: LFTs, coagulation studies
Renal (and hydration status): BUN, creatinine, bicarbonate, serum sodium
Hematology: WBC count with differential, hemoglobin, hematocrit, platelet count
Evaluation for DIC: PT, PTT, fibrinogen, D-dimer
Extent of inflammatory state: CRP, WBC, ESR, procalcitonin, ferritin
Additional studies
Electrolytes
Ionized calcium
Magnesium
Phosphate

ABG, arterial blood gas; ACTH, adrenocorticotropic hormone; BUN, blood urea nitrogen; CRP, C-reactive protein; CSF, cerebrospinal fluid; DIC, disseminated intravascular coagulation; ESR, erythrocyte sedimentation rate; LFTs, liver function tests; PCR, polymerase chain reaction; PT, prothrombin time; PTT, partial thromboplastin time; WBC, white blood cell.

disseminated intravascular coagulation (DIC), particularly in patients with purpura fulminans or petechiae or in those at risk for thrombosis. Laboratory testing for infectious etiologies should be performed in cases of septic shock.

The selection of imaging studies should be guided by the presumed etiology of shock. For patients presenting with shock secondary to trauma, standard trauma protocols to evaluate injury and potential sites of hemorrhage are indicated (see Chapter 12). Chest x-rays can evaluate the extent of airspace disease and presence of pleural effusions or pneumothorax and evaluate for pulmonary edema and cardiomegaly. CT of the chest or abdomen may be indicated to better evaluate sites of infection in septic shock, and echocardiography can provide important information about cardiac anatomy and function.

▶ Treatment of Shock

The approach to treating shock is tailored to the suspected or determined etiology. However, irrespective of the underlying cause, the end result of shock is organ dysfunction, which if untreated can lead to irreversible multiorgan failure and, possibly, death. Therefore, early recognition of shock, coupled with early control of the underlying cause (eg, decompression of tension pneumothorax, surgical control of hemorrhage, or infectious source control) and supportive care, is necessary to minimize end-organ injury and improve survival. *Airway, breathing, and circulation* should be rapidly assessed and appropriately stabilized. Children with pulmonary processes and acute respiratory failure may require intubation and mechanical ventilation. Even with normal lungs or gas exchange, intubation may be indicated for children with altered mental status and inability to protect the airway, poor respiratory effort, or significant hemodynamic instability (to reduce metabolic demand). A temporary intraosseous line should be placed if IV access cannot be rapidly obtained for resuscitation fluids and medications. A central venous catheter should be considered in patients with hemodynamic instability, particularly if they require ongoing resuscitation and infusions of vasoactive medications. Femoral venous access can be simpler and safer for central venous access, but subclavian and internal jugular locations provide more accurate and consistent central venous saturation and pressure monitoring, although with the additional risk of pneumothorax with placement. Ultrasound guidance can improve the rapidity and accuracy of placing central venous lines.

Hemodynamic support can be provided with fluid resuscitation and/or vasoactive infusions. The amount of fluid and choice of vasoactive medication will depend upon the underlying etiology and responsiveness to therapy. Children with cardiogenic shock may have elevated ventricular filling pressures (> 20 mm Hg) and, thus, while increasing preload may augment cardiac output for some patients, many may not tolerate significant fluid administration without further impairment in contractility. In these children, smaller increments of fluid should be administered, if at all, with earlier consideration of vasoactive medication.

For other types of shock, early aggressive fluid resuscitation, targeted to measurable physiologic endpoints of organ perfusion, should be prioritized. Fluid resuscitation should begin with 20 mL/kg increments administered over 5–10 minutes and repeated as necessary. Initial fluid resuscitation should consist of crystalloid (salt solution). Albumin has been shown to be safe in adults and children with septic shock and should be considered when patients have received large volumes of crystalloid and require ongoing resuscitation. Blood and blood products can be used for volume administration in patients with acute bleeding or DIC.

Fluid administration should be titrated to reverse hypotension and achieve normal capillary refill, pulses, level of consciousness, and urine output. Large volumes of fluid for acute stabilization in children with hypovolemic or septic shock may be necessary to restore adequate oxygen delivery and do not necessarily increase the incidence of ARDS or cerebral edema. Patients who do not respond rapidly to 40–60 mL/kg should be monitored in an intensive care setting and considered for vasoactive medication infusion therapy and invasive hemodynamic monitoring. If pulmonary edema or hepatomegaly develops, additional fluid should be avoided and vasoactive medication infusions should be considered, and cardiac function should be evaluated.

Inotropic and vasopressor agents should be considered for patients with refractory shock despite receiving 60 mL/kg of fluid resuscitation or for patients with cardiogenic shock (Table 14–11). Inotropic medications improve cardiac contractility but can increase myocardial oxygen demand and arrhythmia risk; vasopressor medications increase vascular tone and resistance but can increase cardiac afterload. Selection of inotropic or vasopressor therapy should be based on the hemodynamic state and reassessed with changes in clinical course. Several of these medications in diluted forms can be delivered through an intraosseous or peripheral line until stable central access is secured. *Epinephrine* or *norepinephrine* is recommended as first-line vasoactive infusions for treatment of shock in the pediatric population. Generally, epinephrine has a greater net effect on cardiac output due to improvement in contractility, while norepinephrine has a greater net effect on vascular tone and is preferred for vasodilatory shock states. *Vasopressin* may be considered for patients failing catecholamine infusions but has not been clearly shown to improve outcomes. In patients with low cardiac output and high systemic vascular resistance, *milrinone*, a type III phosphodiesterase inhibitor with inotropic and vasodilator activity, can be added to other more potent inotropic agents. However, milrinone has a longer half-life and is less titratable and can have prolonged clearance with renal impairment. Alternatively, *dobutamine* (a selective

β-agonist) may be used to improve myocardial contractility and reduce afterload. As hypocalcemia may contribute to cardiac dysfunction in shock, *calcium* replacement should be given to normalize ionized calcium levels. *Dopamine* (an α- and β-adrenergic agonist) is no longer recommended for adults or children with septic shock due to arrhythmogenic effects in this population. If hemodynamics and oxygen delivery remain inadequate despite adequate fluid resuscitation and vasoactive medication support, ECMO can be considered as a life-saving measure for patients with recoverable causes of shock.

Blood products can be important supportive therapies in patients with shock. *Packed red blood cells* can be administered to improve oxygen-carrying capacity. In hemodynamically stable patients, hemoglobin levels are often maintained over 7 g/dL, while the transfusion threshold can be increased to 10 g/dL in unstable patients. DIC is common in shock, particularly septic shock, due to endothelial damage, formation of microvascular emboli, and consumptive coagulopathy. Thus, a process beginning as increased coagulation leads to a bleeding diathesis. *Platelets* are generally transfused when platelet counts are less than 20,000/μL, or less than 40,000–60,000/μL in a patient with bleeding or requiring surgical intervention. For severe coagulopathies associated with bleeding in the setting of shock, standard treatment includes *fresh frozen plasma* (FFP) or, for fibrinogen replacement, *cryoprecipitate*, with close monitoring of prothrombin time (PT), international normalized ratio (INR), partial thromboplastin time (PTT), and fibrinogen.

SEPSIS

ESSENTIALS OF DIAGNOSIS & TYPICAL FEATURES

▶ Sepsis and septic shock remain major causes of death in children worldwide.

▶ Early recognition and intervention are keys to improving patient outcome.

▶ Systematic approaches to the treatment of sepsis can improve survival.

Sepsis and septic shock remain important causes of morbidity and mortality across the world. The number of organ systems affected by sepsis is a particularly important prognostic factor, with the risk of death rising with the number of organ failures: single organ failure is associated with a mortality rate of 7%–10%, while patients with failure of four organs have a mortality rate of up to 50%. Therefore, careful management of patients with sepsis to minimize organ dysfunction is essential.

Table 14–11. Pharmacologic support of the patient with shock.

Drug	Dose (mcg/kg/ min)	α-Adrenergic Effect[a]	β-Adrenergic Effect[a]	Vasodilator Effect	Actions and Advantages	Disadvantages
Norepinephrine	0.05–1	+++	+++	None	Potent vasoconstric-tor (systemic and pulmonary), increases SVR	Reduced cardiac output if afterload is too high; renal and splanchnic ischemia
Epinephrine	0.05–1	++ to +++ (dose-related)	+++	+ (at lower doses, via β$_2$)	Strong inotrope and chronotrope; increases SVR	Tachycardia, dysrhythmias; can cause myocardial necrosis at high doses
Vasopressin	0.0003–0.008 (U/kg/min)	None	None	None	Potent vasopressor (V1), increases SVR	Coronary ischemia, splanchnic hypoperfu-sion, not well studied in pediatrics
Dopamine	1–20	+ to +++ (dose-related)	+ to ++ (dose-related)	None	Moderate inotrope, wide and safe dosage range, short half-life	Neuroendocrine effects; may increase pulmo-nary artery pressure
Dobutamine	1–10	None	++	+ (via β$_2$)	Moderate inotrope; less chronotropy, fewer dysrhythmias than epinephrine	Marked variation among patients, tachycardia
Milrinone	0.25–0.75	None	None	++	Decreases SVR and PVR; increases cardiac contractility but only mild increase in myocardial O$_2$ consumption	Longer half-life, renal clearance limits use in kidney injury
Nitroprusside	0.05–8	None	None	+++ (arterial and venous vasodila-tion)	Potent vasodilator, decreases SVR and PVR, very short-acting.	Toxic metabolites (thio-cyanates and cyanide); increased intracranial pressure; ventilation-perfusion mismatch; methemoglobinemia

[a]+, small effect; ++, moderate effect; +++, potent effect. PVR, pulmonary vascular resistance; SVR, systemic vascular resistance.

▶ Definition & Pathophysiology

Defining sepsis has been challenging, with earlier definitions of sepsis using overlapping and sometimes confusing terms such as systemic inflammatory response syndrome (SIRS), septic shock, and severe sepsis. In 2016, the adult defini-tions and criteria (Sepsis-3) were revised and simplified into a dichotomy of sepsis or septic shock. Sepsis is defined as "life-threatening organ dysfunction resulting from a dys-regulated host immune response to infection," and septic shock is reserved for the subset of patients with "particularly profound circulatory, cellular, and metabolic abnormalities associated with a greater risk of mortality." Septic shock is identified by persistent requirement of vasoactive medi-cations and a lactate greater or equal to 2 mmol/L despite adequate volume resuscitation. The 2020 Surviving Sepsis

guidelines for children use both prior definitions and the Sepsis-3 definitions in formulating the evidence base for recommendations.

Organ failure associated with sepsis is due to both impaired oxygen delivery and impaired utilization of deliv-ered oxygen. The etiology of impaired oxygen utilization is not well understood but is likely multifactorial, including maldistribution of blood flow in the microcirculation and mitochondrial dysfunction. Recent work has also identified the critical role of the innate immune system, derangements of adaptive immunity, and microvascular thrombi in the pathophysiology of sepsis, contributing to impaired oxy-gen delivery to the tissues, impaired oxygen utilization, and metabolic downregulation, leading to end-organ dysfunc-tion and, ultimately, to death if the process is not reversed.

► Treatment of Sepsis

Standardized treatment guidelines are available from several professional organizations, most prominently the American Heart Association Pediatric Advanced Life Support (PALS) guidelines for initial management of shock in children and the Surviving Sepsis Campaign guidelines for management of sepsis in adults and children. A key principle of both guidelines is that early recognition and treatment of shock and sepsis, preferably stemming from a consistent organized clinical approach, improve outcomes in all age groups.

There are several particular considerations in treating shock when sepsis is the etiology. When selecting medications for intubation, agents that may contribute to adrenal suppression should be avoided. The approach to mechanical ventilation should be similar to that of a lung-protective strategy (ie, limiting inspiratory pressures and maintaining adequate recruitment). Because of low systemic vascular resistance in combination with hypovolemia, children with septic shock may require more fluid resuscitation than with other causes of shock, which should be administered within the first few hours of recognition. Current pediatric guidelines recommend either epinephrine or norepinephrine for first-line therapy of septic shock. Vasopressin infusion can also be considered for catecholamine-refractory septic shock.

If hemodynamics remain inadequate despite aggressive fluid and pressor support, the patient can be considered to have *catecholamine-resistant septic shock*. This condition may be related to critical illness-related corticosteroid insufficiency (CIRCI), a state of impaired adrenal responsiveness that may occur in as many as 30% of critically ill patients. Absolute adrenal insufficiency, characterized by impaired adrenal responsiveness, low-circulating cortisol concentrations, and often associated with adrenal hemorrhage, can be seen in up to 50% of children with catecholamine-resistant septic shock. Although the evidence related to steroid administration and outcomes is conflicting, steroid supplementation can be considered for children with catecholamine-resistant septic shock. Children with fulminant meningococcemia, congenital adrenal hyperplasia, or recent steroid exposure are at the highest risk of absolute adrenal insufficiency and should receive hydrocortisone treatment.

As with other causes of shock, identifying and reversing the cause of sepsis is essential. Empiric *antimicrobials* should be delivered promptly, ideally within *1 hour* of presentation in patients with suspected septic shock. Antibiotics should be chosen according to the most likely cause of infection. While it is highly desirable to obtain cultures prior to initiation of antibiotics to guide the choice and duration of antibiotic coverage, acquisition of cultures should never delay antibiotic administration in patients with suspected sepsis. Early and aggressive control of sources of infection is essential for patients with sepsis and septic shock, including surgical drainage of abscesses or other infected spaces or removal of infected foreign bodies such as vascular catheters.

Bembea MM et al: Pediatric Organ Dysfunction Information Update Mandate (PODIUM) Contemporary Organ Dysfunction Criteria: executive summary. Pediatrics 2022;149:S1–S12 [PMID: 34970673].

Duff JP et al: 2019 American Heart Association focused update on pediatric advanced life support: an update to the American Heart Association guidelines for cardiopulmonary resuscitation and emergency cardiovascular care. Circulation 2019;140(24):e904–e914 [PMID: 31722551].

Rudd KE et al: Global, regional, and national sepsis incidence and mortality, 1990–2017: analysis for the Global Burden of Disease Study. Lancet 2020;395:200–211 [PMID: 31954465].

Surviving Sepsis Campaign website (a good source for information on sepsis including protocols and order bundles for the care of patients with sepsis): https://www.sccm.org/SurvivingSepsis-Campaign/Home. Accessed June 2, 2021.

Weiss SL et al: Surviving sepsis campaign international guidelines for management of septic shock and sepsis-associated organ dysfunction in children: Pediatr Crit Care Med 2020;21(2):e52–e106 [PMID: 32032273].

▼ NEUROCRITICAL CARE

Pediatric neurocritical care is a multidisciplinary field focused on critically ill pediatric patients with neurologic injury due to conditions such as traumatic brain injury (TBI), stroke, status epilepticus, and hypoxic-ischemic brain injury. Neurointensivists work to better understand the distinct pathophysiologic and clinical features of pediatric brain injury, develop and apply new diagnostic and monitoring strategies to better understand brain function and dysfunction in real time, and formulate pediatric-specific management guidelines for common neurocritical care problems.

TRAUMATIC BRAIN INJURY

ESSENTIALS OF DIAGNOSIS & TYPICAL FEATURES

► Traumatic brain injury (TBI) presents in a variety of ways, from alterations in memory or alertness (mild confusion to unresponsiveness), irritability, seizures, and even poor feeding/emesis. TBI should be high on the differential for all patients matching these descriptions.

► Significant alterations in blood flow and/or metabolic state (eg, hypotension, hypoxia, hypoglycemia, hypercapnia, hyperthermia, seizures) can exacerbate brain injury. Timely identification and correction of these factors are essential.

► Early signs and symptoms of intracranial hypertension tend to be nonspecific. The classic Cushing triad of bradycardia, hypertension, and apnea occurs late and is often incomplete.

TBIs can be conceptualized as occurring in two phases. *Primary injury* occurs at the moment that injury disrupts bone, blood vessels, and brain tissue. Prevention through helmets, safety belts, and other injury prevention efforts is the only true means to reduce primary injury. *Secondary injury* is the indirect result of the primary injury and develops minutes to days after the initiating event. Reducing secondary injury is the focus of first responders, emergency medicine doctors, and intensivists. Management of the brain-injured child aims to optimize delivery of oxygen and nutrients (supply) while reducing hypermetabolic states (demand). Therapy focuses on avoidance of factors such hypoxia, hypotension, hypoglycemia, hyperthermia, infection, seizures, and agitation.

▶ Pathogenesis

The skull contains a fixed total volume composed of the brain, cerebrospinal fluid (CSF), and blood. An increase in volume of one component must therefore be offset by a decrease in one of the other components to maintain a constant ICP (Monro-Kellie doctrine). After a brain injury, the volume of any or all these components may increase to an extent that it cannot be compensated by the other components, resulting in increased ICP. *Intracranial hypertension* is defined as an ICP over 20 mm Hg (vs < 15 mm Hg in healthy children) and is associated with increased morbidity and mortality in brain-injured patients. Intracranial hypertension may occur due to other illnesses in addition to TBI (Table 14–12), but in all cases, the pathogenesis of intracranial hypertension can be understood by considering each of the intracranial components.

The uninjured brain occupies about 80% of the volume within the skull, but this volume can increase dramatically after brain injury as a result of cerebral edema. *Cytotoxic edema* is the most common form of cerebral edema seen in the PICU and is the least easily treated. Cytotoxic edema occurs as a result of direct injury to brain cells, often leading to irreversible cell swelling and death. This form of cerebral edema is typical of TBIs as well as hypoxic-ischemic injuries and metabolic disease. *Vasogenic edema* is frequently associated with trauma, tumors, abscesses, and infarct; breakdown of the tight endothelial junctions that make up the blood-brain barrier (BBB) is a hallmark component. As plasma constituents cross the BBB, extracellular water moves into the brain parenchyma. *Hydrostatic edema*, due to transudation of fluid from the capillaries into the parenchyma as a result of elevated cerebral vascular pressures, and *interstitial edema*, which results from obstructed CSF flow and appears in a typical periventricular distribution, are less common. Cerebral edema can be diagnosed by characteristic findings on either CT or magnetic resonance imaging (MRI) of the brain.

CSF occupies an estimated 10% of the intracranial space. Intracranial hypertension due primarily to obstructed CSF flow or increased CSF volume (eg, primary or secondary hydrocephalus) is generally easily diagnosed by CT scan and treated with appropriate drainage and shunting. CSF drainage can be of benefit in managing intracranial hypertension even in the absence of overt hydrocephalus.

Cerebral blood volume comprises the final 10% of the intracranial space and is affected by cerebral blood flow. Changes in cerebral blood flow occur by alterations in cerebral perfusion pressure (CPP) or vascular resistance. *Cerebral perfusion pressure*, defined as mean systemic arterial pressure minus CVP or ICP, whichever is higher, is the driving pressure across the cerebral circulation. Hypotension, which may occur due to hemorrhage from comorbid injuries or as a part of a systemic inflammatory response following TBI, results in decreased CPP. Changes to cerebral vascular resistance generally result from alterations in vascular diameter in response to metabolic demands or vascular pressures, responses termed *autoregulation*. *Metabolic autoregulation* matches cerebral blood flow to tissue demands. High metabolic rates, such as those induced by fever or seizure activity, increase cerebral blood flow by causing vasodilation, which in turn increases cerebral blood volume; lower metabolic rates allow the vessels to constrict, reducing cerebral blood volume. Partial pressure of carbon dioxide is another important determinant, as elevations in blood $Paco_2$ lead to cerebral vasodilation and decreases in $Paco_2$ lead to vasoconstriction. *Pressure autoregulation*, which works to maintain a constant cerebral blood flow despite variable systemic blood pressures, links cerebral blood pressure to cerebral blood flow. Within the autoregulatory range of blood pressure, cerebral vessels

Table 14–12. Pediatric illnesses commonly associated with intracranial hypertension.

Diffuse processes
  Global hypoxia-ischemia
    Near-drowning
    Hanging/other strangulation
    Cardiorespiratory arrest
  Infectious
    Encephalitis
    Meningitis
  Metabolic
    Reye syndrome
    Liver failure
    Inborn errors of metabolism
  Toxic
    Lead intoxication
    Vitamin A overdose
Focal processes
  Trauma
  Stroke
  Infectious
    Abscess
  Mass lesions
    Tumors
    Hematomas

dilate with low systemic blood pressures or constrict with high systemic blood pressures to maintain constant cerebral blood flow. Above the autoregulatory range, cerebral vessels are maximally constricted, and further increases in systemic pressure will result in increased cerebral blood flow and volume; the opposite is true below the autoregulatory range, and cerebral blood flow will fall with further decreases in systemic pressure. It is not unusual to see partial or complete loss of cerebral blood flow autoregulation following TBI. Cerebral blood flow then becomes dependent on systemic blood pressure.

In addition to direct damage from elevated ICP and cerebral edema, secondary injury following trauma may also occur due to cerebral ischemia and/or neuronal excitotoxicity.

▶ Clinical Findings

The clinical presentation of TBI is dependent on the nature, location, and size of affected areas in the brain, as well as the amount of edema and infringement of CSF pathways. Physical deformities such as skull fractures and exposure of the brain parenchyma may or may not be apparent. Clinical presentation can be subtle, such as a headache from a concussion, or more severe, including manifestations of intracranial hypertension (Table 14–13). Often, early signs and symptoms are nonspecific, particularly in young children, requiring that TBI be included in the differential diagnosis for a wide range of clinical presentations.

Initial examination of the patient with TBI should include assessment of airway patency, breathing, and cardiovascular function. Mental status should be evaluated, and the Glasgow coma scale (GCS) score calculated (see Chapter 12). Once stabilized, a more detailed neurologic examination should be performed, including evaluation of cranial nerves, motor and sensory function, and deep tendon reflexes. Repeated neurologic examinations over time are also needed as neurologic function can change rapidly in brain-injured patients. Head imaging (CT or MRI) is beneficial to identify specific intracranial injuries, determine the need for surgical intervention,

Table 14–13. Signs and symptoms of intracranial hypertension in children.

Early
Poor feeding, vomiting
Irritability, lethargy
Seizures
Late
Coma
Decerebrate responses
Cranial nerve palsies
Abnormal respirations/apnea
Bradycardia
Hypertension

monitor the progression of injuries and cerebral edema, and monitor for the development of complications.

▶ Treatment

Initial stabilization should begin with support of the airway, breathing, and circulation, while avoiding further neurologic injury. Cervical spine immobilization should be strongly considered prior to securing the airway to avoid worsening spinal cord injury. If the GCS is less than 8 or if the patient demonstrates apnea, irregular respirations, significant hypoxia, or other signs concerning for intracranial hypertension, the airway should be secured via endotracheal intubation. Care should be taken to avoid hypercapnia, which will further increase ICP. Similarly, sedative agents used in the process of intubation should be chosen carefully, as adequate sedation is important to blunt further elevations in ICP with airway manipulation. Maintenance of systemic blood pressure is also critically important;. studies in both adult and pediatric patients with head injury show that even a single episode of hypotension is associated with marked increase in mortality rates.

Following intubation and support of systemic blood pressure, treatment strategies in children are largely focused on optimizing cerebral blood flow and reducing metabolic demand. Minimizing intracranial hypertension is a critical component of management, and current treatment guidelines for children with TBI recommend ICP monitoring for all patients with GCS of 8 or less. Elevated ICP (ICP > 20 mm Hg) can be treated with medical or mechanical interventions. Medication treatment strategies to reduce ICP rely on *osmotic therapies* such as hypertonic ($\geq$ 3%) saline and mannitol. Hypertonic saline, commonly given in bolus doses of 2–5 mL/kg of 3% saline or as a continuous infusion, encourages intravascular volume expansion and increases serum osmolality, enhancing movement of excess water out of brain cells and interstitium and into blood vessels for removal by the kidneys. Serum sodium and osmolality should be followed closely to avoid severe hypernatremia or severe hypertonicity. Mannitol, given in doses of 0.25–1 g/kg, exerts a rapid rheologic effect, reducing blood viscosity which improves blood flow and subsequent autoregulatory vasoconstriction. Mannitol also exerts a potent osmotic and diuretic effect. While this may further reduce ICP, it can result in hypovolemia and hypotension, which reduces CPP and exacerbates secondary injury. Volume status and systemic blood pressures should therefore be monitored closely, and treatment should reduce these side effects should be promptly administered. Renal failure due to intravascular volume depletion and acute tubular necrosis is a rare side effect associated with serum osmolality greater than 320 mOsm/L.

Controlled ventilation is another important element of treating intracranial hypertension. Normocapnia, with a goal Paco$_2$ between 35 and 40 mm Hg, is the current standard of care. Hyperventilation to Paco$_2$ levels less than

30 mm Hg—in the past a mainstay in the treatment of intra-cranial hypertension—is no longer recommended because it compromises CNS perfusion and exacerbates secondary injury. However, hyperventilation can be considered emergently for short periods for refractory intracranial hypertension while awaiting more definitive therapy.

Mechanical therapies to reduce ICP are aimed at reducing the volume of intracranial contents. Midline positioning and head elevation to 30 degrees can aid in cerebral venous drainage. CSF drainage can be accomplished by placement of an EVD. Timely surgical evacuation of hematomas and other pathologic masses is also a mainstay of TBI treatment.

In some cases, intracranial hypertension is refractory to initial medical, ventilatory, and mechanical therapies. In these circumstances, the 2019 Pediatric Severe Traumatic Brain Injury guidelines suggest three additional measures that may be considered to reduce ICP: decompressive craniectomy (removal of a portion of the skull and opening of the dura), moderate hypothermia (32°C–33°C), and high-dose *barbiturates*. Risks and benefits of these measures must be carefully considered prior to utilization in an individual patient.

Prevention of ischemia and excitotoxicity are important considerations. Hypoxic episodes (Pao$_2$ < 60 mm Hg) after TBI are associated with increased morbidity and mortality. Maintenance of normal ranges for glucose, calcium, magnesium, and phosphorus may be beneficial. Current guidelines also recommend enteral nutrition within 72 hours of injury.

Finally, optimizing oxygen and nutrient delivery to the injured brain should be facilitated by reducing metabolic demands. Aggressive control of fevers (*controlled normothermia*), using antipyretics and surface cooling devices, is warranted, and continuous temperature monitoring helps prevent over- or under-correction. Induced hypothermia lowers cerebral metabolism, cerebral blood flow, and cerebral blood volume, but has not been shown to improve overall outcome in the pediatric population. *Adequate sedation* to reduce episodes of agitation and/or pain can further reduce metabolic demands and ICP, although bolus administration may contribute to systemic hypotension and cerebral hypoperfusion. *Neuromuscular blockade* can also be considered as an effective adjunctive therapy. *Seizures* occur in approximately 30% of patients with severe head injury and result in increased metabolic demand and potential for secondary injury. Continuous EEG should be used in patients with persistent altered mental status or in those requiring heavy sedation. A short course (7 days) of empiric antiepileptic medication is suggested, and seizures noted on EEG should be treated rapidly. Corticosteroids may be of use in reducing vasogenic cerebral edema surrounding tumors and other inflammatory CNS lesions, but they are not recommended in the treatment of TBI.

Complications

Complications are frequent in patients with TBI and should be anticipated. Nosocomial infections are more common in these patients than other critically ill populations and may lead to worse outcomes. Abnormalities of sodium handling such as diabetes insipidus, syndrome of inappropriate secretion of antidiuretic hormone (SIADH), or cerebral salt wasting are also relatively common and require careful monitoring and intervention. In more severe cases, *cerebral infarctions* may occur as a result of ischemia, thrombosis, and progressive edema compromising blood supply. Finally, *cerebral herniation* is a life-threatening medical emergency, often leading to death or serious disability in brain-injured patients. Cushing triad (bradycardia, hypertension, and altered respirations) may be only partially present in these patients.

Prognosis

Many factors affect the prognosis of patients with TBI, especially the inciting event and severity of injury. It is difficult to predict overall outcome during the initial stabilization period, but lack of improvement in neurologic examination after 24–72 hours (peak period for swelling) is associated with worse outcomes. Follow-up studies have demonstrated that "recovery" occurs over time, even months to years.

Inflicted Traumatic Brain Injury

Inflicted traumatic brain injury (iTBI), also referred to as abusive head trauma (AHT), accounts for a significant portion of TBI in infants and young children. Repetitive brain injuries prior to presentation and global hypoxic-ischemic brain damage (as a result of trauma-induced respiratory failure or cardiac arrest) may complicate the pathophysiology. Management of children with iTBI is similar to those with accidental TBI, but additional evaluations should include an ophthalmologic assessment for retinal hemorrhages and a radiologic skeletal survey to identify occult bone fractures. Child advocacy and law enforcement groups should be notified when abuse is suspected. Children with iTBI often have a worse neurologic outcome compared to accidentally injured children.

HYPOXIC-ISCHEMIC ENCEPHALOPATHY

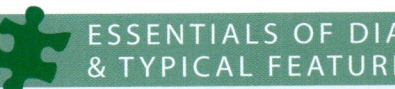

ESSENTIALS OF DIAGNOSIS & TYPICAL FEATURES

► Hypoxic-ischemic encephalopathy should be suspected when altered mental status persists after prolonged hypoxemia or resuscitation from a cardiorespiratory arrest.

Hypoxic-ischemic encephalopathy (HIE) results from global brain hypoxia and ischemia produced by systemic hypoxemia and/or reduced blood flow to the brain. Pediatric HIE is commonly caused by cardiopulmonary arrest due to drowning, hanging or other strangulation, severe respiratory distress, shock, drug overdose/poisoning, nonperfusing arrhythmias, and other insults. Pediatric HIE can be associated with poor neurologic outcome. Like TBI, the extent of brain injury in HIE depends on the duration and severity of the initial inciting event and the development of secondary injury over the minutes to days following re-establishment of cerebral blood flow and oxygen delivery.

Clinical Findings

Signs and symptoms of brain injury secondary to hypoxic-ischemic injury are variable and depend on injury severity and affected brain regions. Manifestations of HIE can include cognitive dysfunction, seizures (clinical and subclinical), status epilepticus, stroke, coma, persistent vegetative state, and irreversible cessation of neurologic function ("brain death").

Treatment

The initial stabilization of a patient with HIE includes airway management, respiratory support, and maintenance of cardiovascular stability. As with TBI, treatment strategies are focused on optimizing cerebral blood flow and mitigating neuronal loss. Blood flow to the brain is dependent on cardiac output, which may be impaired following cardiac arrest and/or injury. Optimization of cardiac function and systemic hemodynamics with fluid resuscitation and inotropic and/or vasopressor agents is necessary to ensure adequate delivery of oxygen and nutrients to the injured brain. Cerebral pressure auto-regulation may also be impaired in children who develop HIE as a result of cardiac arrest. Several studies in adult victims of cardiac arrest suggest that maintaining a higher mean blood pressure may better support the postischemic brain, but the degree of pressure dysregulation and blood pressure targets to optimize cerebral blood flow in the ischemic pediatric brain remain unclear. Intracranial hypertension may develop as a result of cerebral edema, but the utility of ICP monitoring and titration of therapies to a normal ICP in HIE patients has not been clearly defined. Seizures should be aggressively treated, and continuous EEG monitoring is useful for identifying subclinical seizure activity. Similar to TBI, temperature regulation and maintenance of normothermia are essential since the risk of severe disability in patients with HIE increases with fevers. *Therapeutic hypothermia* (target body temperature 33°C–35°C) is a mainstay of treating postcardiac arrest HIE in adults and postanoxic HIE in newborns but published data in the pediatric population do not demonstrate significant benefit.

Prognosis

Accurately predicting outcome in children with HIE is difficult. Out-of-hospital cardiac arrest and/or prolonged cardiopulmonary resuscitation (> 10–15 minutes) are significant risk factors for poor outcome. Other indicators of likely poor outcome include any of the following 24 hours or more after the inciting event: (1) GCS score 3–5; (2) absent pupillary and motor responses; (3) absent spontaneous respiratory effort; (4) bilateral absence of median nerve somatosensory evoked potential; (5) discontinuous, nonreactive, or silent EEG (in the absence of confounding drug administration); and (6) MRI (obtained 72 hours after return of spontaneous circulation) demonstrating watershed, basal ganglia, and brainstem injury. Outcome prediction is enhanced when several assessment modalities are combined; many centers will wait until 48–72 hours after injury for formal prognostication as this reflects the period of peak swelling and other markers of secondary brain injury.

STATUS EPILEPTICUS

ESSENTIALS OF DIAGNOSIS & TYPICAL FEATURES

► Status Epilepticus is defined as a persistent seizure lasting 30 minutes or longer, or several shorter seizures without an intervening return to baseline mental status.

► When a patient without epilepsy presents with status epilepticus, multiple etiologies should be considered, including trauma, stroke, infection, tumors, hypertensive encephalopathy, hyponatremia, and hypoglycemia.

► Comorbid infections in patients with epilepsy can lower their seizure threshold and result in status epilepticus.

► Status epilepticus and its associated treatment can lead to acute cardiorespiratory compromise requiring intervention.

Pathogenesis

Status epilepticus can result from multiple etiologies. In a patient with a prior diagnosis of epilepsy, common infections such as viral respiratory illnesses can lower the seizure threshold enough to result in prolonged seizure activity, as can nonadherence to antiepileptic medications. In patients without a prior diagnosis of epilepsy, the differential diagnosis is broad and includes complex febrile seizure, CNS tumor, TBI, ischemic or hemorrhagic stroke, CNS infection, hypertensive encephalopathy, electrolyte abnormalities (hyponatremia or hypoglycemia), withdrawal to benzodiazepines or alcohol, acute demyelinating encephalomyelitis, previously unrecognized metabolic disorders, autoimmune disorders, and medication ingestion. Regardless of the etiology, the development of status epilepticus occurs due to an imbalance between excitatory and inhibitory neurotransmission, with rhythmic discharges of multiple neurons in a brain region. Left untreated, these discharges can ultimately result in energy failure and long-lasting changes in neurons, including cell death.

Clinical Findings

While seizures and status epilepticus may be focal in nature (involving only one area of the brain and manifesting in a single body part), classic status epilepticus in considered to be generalized tonic-clonic activity with altered mental status, lasting at least 30 minutes. Loss of bladder or bowel continence may occur. Status epilepticus may be associated with profound respiratory abnormalities, apnea, tachycardia, and/or hypertension or hypotension. Because it is a hypermetabolic state, a long postictal period of altered mental status and/or rhabdomyolysis may occur.

Treatment

Resuscitation begins with attention to airway, breathing, and circulation. If a specific etiology for the seizure can be found (eg, hyponatremia), rapid correction of that abnormality (eg, hypertonic saline) usually results in seizure cessation. In the absence of a clear etiology, treatment generally begins with benzodiazepines, most commonly lorazepam 0.1 mg/kg IV, given within the first 5 minutes. This can be repeated, or transition to an alternate agent may be considered. Fosphenytoin 20 mg/kg IV or levetiracetam 20–60 mg/kg in the general pediatric population and phenobarbital 20 mg/kg IV in the neonatal period are common choices. For refractory status epilepticus that persists after these initial agents, next-line therapies may include infusions of midazolam, propofol, ketamine, or a barbiturate. During treatment of refractory status epilepticus, hypoventilation and apnea may occur, and intubation and initiation of mechanical ventilation are often needed. Similarly, antiepileptic-induced hypotension may occur, and support of systemic blood pressure with volume and/or vasopressor medications is recommended.

Brown KL et al: The brain in pediatric critical care: unique aspects of assessment, monitoring, investigations, and follow-up. Intensive Care Med 2022; 48(5):535–547 [PMID: 35445823].

Kochanek P et al: Guidelines for the Management of Pediatric Severe Traumatic Brain Injury, Third Edition: update of the Brain Trauma Foundation Guidelines. Pediatr Crit Care Med 2019;20(3S):S1–S82 [PMID: 30830016].

Smith AE et al: Neuroprognostication in children after cardiac arrest. Pediatr Neurol 2020;108:13–22 [PMID: 32381279].

ACUTE KIDNEY INJURY & RENAL REPLACEMENT THERAPY

Definitions

The kidney is important in maintaining homeostasis for a number of important physiologic processes, including fluid and electrolyte balance, acid–base status, erythropoiesis, and vascular tone. *Acute kidney injury* (AKI) is observed in 10%–40% of the PICU population, most commonly within 24–48 hours of admission. Studies consistently show an independent association between AKI and increased ICU length of stay and mortality.

Pathophysiology

The etiology of AKI in critically ill children is most often multifactorial. Decreased renal perfusion can occur with systemic hypotension from a variety of etiologies or from elevated intra-abdominal pressures reducing local perfusion (eg, abdominal compartment syndrome). In addition to altering hemodynamics, sepsis can lead to disturbances of the renal microvasculature by inflammatory mediators and activation of the coagulation system. Other conditions associated with AKI include hypoxia, pulmonary-renal and hepatorenal syndromes, and toxic metabolic byproducts as in rhabdomyolysis or tumor lysis syndrome. Finally, nephrotoxic medications, most commonly antibiotics (aminoglycosides, vancomycin) and immunosuppressive medications, contribute to as much as 25% of cases of AKI.

Clinical Findings

Critically ill patients with AKI may develop electrolyte abnormalities, severe metabolic acidosis, fluid overload, and hypertension. Although the mechanisms are unclear and likely complex, fluid overload exceeding 10% of body weight has been shown to be an independent risk factor for worse morbidity, including more ventilator days and longer hospital length of stay, and patients overloaded by 20% of their body weight with fluid may have as much as an eightfold increased risk of death. The causal relationship between fluid overload and poor outcome is uncertain, but based on these findings, some experts recommend consideration of renal replacement therapies for patients reaching 10%–20% fluid overload.

Treatment

Management is directed at alleviating potential contributing factors to AKI. Methods to *improve renal perfusion* include maintenance of adequate cardiac output and blood pressure using fluids and/or vasopressor medications, as well as relief of excess intrathoracic and intraabdominal pressures when feasible. *Diuretics* are commonly used to address fluid overload associated with AKI, but these agents have not been shown to improve renal recovery in children and have been associated with an increased risk of death in adults with AKI. *Fluid restriction* can be helpful in managing fluid overload and may be of particular benefit in patients with concomitant lung injury. For patients who fail medical management, renal replacement therapy may be indicated for metabolic and volume control (see Monitoring and Technology). Since treatment of AKI is largely supportive, prevention of AKI through avoidance of dehydration and nephrotoxic medications should also be mainstays of care.

Alobaidi R et al: Association between fluid balance and outcomes in critically ill children: a systematic review and meta-analysis. JAMA Pediatr 2018 Mar 1;172(3):257–268. doi: 10.1001/jamapediatrics.2017.4540 [PMID: 29356810].

Hessey E et al: Renal function follow-up and renal recovery after acute kidney injury in critically ill children. Pediatr Crit Care Med 2017;18(8):733–740 [PMID: 28492401].

Kaddourah A, Basu RK, Bagshaw SM, Goldstein SL; AWARE Investigators: Epidemiology of acute kidney injury in critically ill children and young adults. N Engl J Med 2017 Jan 5;376(1):11–20. doi: 10.1056/NEJMoa1611391 [PMID: 27959707].

Modem V et al: Timing of continuous renal replacement therapy and mortality in critically ill children. Crit Care Med 2014 Apr;42(4):943–953 [PMID: 24231758].

FLUID MANAGEMENT & NUTRITIONAL SUPPORT OF THE CRITICALLY ILL CHILD

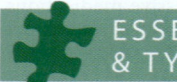

ESSENTIALS OF DIAGNOSIS & TYPICAL FEATURES

▶ Critically ill children are more susceptible to metabolic stress than adults due to lower muscle and fat mass and higher resting energy requirements.

▶ Administration rate and electrolyte composition are important considerations when prescribing IV fluids, and decisions should be tailored to the individual patient.

▶ Early enteral and parenteral feeding may influence morbidity and mortality in critically ill infants and children.

▶ Optimizing nutrition in critically ill children may reduce prolonged nutritional deficiencies, which can last months after an ICU stay.

▶ Fluid Management

Many critically ill children are unable to take oral fluids and food, and, as a result, the ICU provider must carefully consider the needs of the individual patient in prescribing a fluid and nutrition regimen. Standard maintenance IV fluid rate calculations are based on the assumption of a healthy,

normotensive, spontaneously breathing patient. However, the "ideal" amount of fluid to provide a critically ill patient is variable and depends on the underlying condition, current physiologic state, and fluid losses (both measurable and unmeasurable). Total body volume losses may be *increased* by unmeasurable losses (insensible losses) due to fever or tachypnea or by measurable losses from hemorrhage or drainage of fluids (eg, urine). Intravascular volume losses may also occur despite total body fluid overload; for example, inflammatory states can lead to vasodilation and leakage from the vascular space into tissues, producing intravascular hypovolemia. Under these circumstances, fluid administration may need to be increased temporarily. Total body volume losses may be *decreased* by reduced measurable losses (eg, low urine output due to excess antidiuretic hormone secretion) or unmeasurable losses. For example, mechanical ventilators deliver humidified gas, reducing insensible fluid losses from breathing in intubated patients. Under these circumstances, early consideration of fluid restriction and/or diuretic use may be warranted. Electrolyte composition of fluids may also have profound effects on morbidity and mortality in the critically ill patient. For example, hyponatremia has been associated with significant morbidity and mortality in patients at risk of cerebral edema, and isotonic maintenance fluids are recommended. In contrast, patients with chronic kidney disease may benefit from lower sodium content in their IV fluids. Potassium content may need to be increased in IV fluids administered to patients with diabetic ketoacidosis or avoided in patients with acute or chronic renal failure. Therefore, both rate of administration and electrolyte composition are important considerations during selection of IV fluids for each critically ill child.

▶ Nutritional Support

Adequate nutritional support should be provided to the critically ill child as early as possible, as malnutrition is associated with higher rates of infectious and noninfectious complications as well as longer hospital stays and increased hospital costs. In the pediatric ICU, as many as 20% of patients experience either acute or chronic malnutrition, a rate that is largely unchanged over the past 30 years. Malnutrition in PICU patients is typically multifactorial, reflecting increased physiologic and metabolic stresses associated with critical illness (Table 14–14), inaccurate assessments of caloric needs, and/or inadequate delivery of nutrition. The risk of malnutrition is especially high in certain clinical scenarios (Table 14–15) in which specific attention to nutrition is particularly important.

▶ Nutritional Assessment

Early assessment by a pediatric dietitian or nutritionist can be helpful to establish nutritional requirements and identify factors impeding adequate nutrition intake, tolerance, or

Table 14–14. Metabolic responses to severe illness.

Hormone and biological response modifier levels
↑ insulin
↑ glucocorticoids
↑ catecholamines
↑ interleukin-1
↑ tumor necrosis factor
Carbohydrate metabolism
↑ blood glucose
↑ gluconeogenesis
↑ glucose turnover
Glucose intolerance
Fat metabolism
↑ lipid turnover and utilization
Insuppressible lipolysis
ketogenesis
Protein metabolism
↑ muscle protein catabolism
↑ muscle branched-chain amino acid oxidation
↑ serum amino acids
↑ nitrogen losses

Table 14–15. Markers of high risk of malnutrition.

- Underweight (< 5th percentile for age) or overweight (> 85th percentile for age)
- > 10% weight gain or loss during ICU stay
- Failure to consistently meet prescribed caloric goals
- Failure to wean from respiratory support
- Need for muscle relaxants for > 7 days
- Neurologic injury with evidence of dysautonomia
- Oncologic diagnoses
- Burns
- Requiring mechanical ventilation for > 7 days
- Suspected hypermetabolic state (eg, status epilepticus, SIRS) or hypometabolic state (eg, hypothermia, induced coma)
- ICU length of stay > 4 wk

ICU, intensive care unit; SIRS; systemic inflammatory response syndrome.

absorption. The initial caloric needs of the critically ill child can be estimated from calculations of the basal metabolic rate (BMR) or the resting energy expenditure (REE) and applying adjustments to those calculations based on the patient's illness and level of support. Both the BMR and REE calculations represent the energy requirements of a healthy person at rest with a normal temperature and without additional stressors, however, and they can be inaccurate for critically ill children who often manifest significant metabolic instability and hypometabolism, resulting in a higher risk of overfeeding when using calculations alone. Indirect calorimetry (IC) is a more accurate means of directly measuring energy expenditure and determining caloric needs but is more difficult and expensive to perform. Targeted use of IC assessment for identification of patients at highest risk for malnutrition has been suggested (see Table 14–15). IC requires collection of exhaled gases from the patient and can be inaccurate if a significant ETT leak is present, if the F_{IO_2} is more than 60%, or during hemodialysis or CRRT.

▶ Delivery of Nutrition

There are two main methods of nutrient delivery in the severely ill pediatric patient, parenteral and enteral nutrition, each with individual advantages and disadvantages (Table 14–16).

Table 14–16. Methods of delivering nutrition.

	Advantages	Disadvantages

Enteral nutrition	• Associated with fewer infectious complications
	• May be beneficial to maintain gastrointestinal mucosal integrity and motility
	• Low-volume continuous "trophic feeding" generally safe and feasible in all but the most unstable patients
	• Transpyloric feeding may improve tolerance
		• Inadequate mesenteric perfusion in patients with shock requiring vasoactive infusions
		• Complications include:
		  • Vomiting
		  • Diarrhea
		  • Bleeding
		  • Necrotizing enterocolitis
		  • Aspiration events/pneumonia
		  • Mechanical issues (occlusion of tube, errors in placement)

Parenteral nutrition	• Can be used when enteral nutrition cannot be delivered or tolerated
	• Not interrupted by procedures requiring fasting
		• Often requires need of a central venous line to reach full nutrition goals
		• Need for regular metabolic evaluation (glucose, electrolytes, liver function tests, lipase) to adjust parenteral components
		• Complications:
		  • Infection risk with central venous access
		  • Hyperglycemia
		  • Hypertriglyceridemia
		  • Hepatobiliary abnormalities

Regardless of route of nutrition, *monitoring* should include routine physical examination, serial measures of growth (weight, skinfold thickness), serial monitoring of serum electrolyte and mineral concentrations, and repeated measurements of caloric needs when available.

Marino LV et al: Micronutrient status during paediatric critical illness: a scoping review. Clin Nutr 2020; 39(12):3571–3593 [PMID: 32371094].

Mehta NM et al: Guidelines for the provision and assessment of nutrition support therapy in the pediatric critically ill patient: Society of Critical Care Medicine and American Society for Parenteral and Enteral Nutrition. JPEN J Parenter Enteral Nutr 2017 Jul;41(5):706–742 [PMID: 28686844].

SEDATION & ANALGESIA IN THE PICU

ESSENTIALS OF DIAGNOSIS & TYPICAL FEATURES

► Pain control and relief of anxiety are standard of care for all patients in the PICU.

► Sedation and analgesia must be individualized for each patient and reassessed frequently to avoid inadequate or excessive medication.

► Sedative and analgesic medications have unique sets of physiologic effects and side effects, and these agents should only be used with adequate monitoring and support to address potential adverse events.

Children admitted to the PICU often require analgesic and/or anxiolytic medications to reduce overt pain/anxiety or allow them to tolerate therapies (eg, mechanical ventilation, procedures, etc.). When determining which medications to initiate, it is important to distinguish between anxiety and pain, because pharmacologic therapy may be directed at either or both of these symptoms (Table 14–17). Additional considerations in medication selection are the route of administration and the anticipated duration of treatment. For example, children who require more frequent dosing or tighter control of pain/sedation level may benefit from a continuous infusion, whereas patients undergoing a bedside procedure may only require a small number of discrete doses. Potential adverse effects in particular clinical circumstances are another important consideration in sedative and analgesic selection.

► Sedation

Sedative (anxiolytic) medications may be indicated when the goals of treatment are to reduce anxiety, facilitate treatment or procedures, maintain safety during acute confusional states, and diminish physiologic responses to stress

Table 14–17. Commonly used intravenous medications for pain and anxiety control.

Drug	Suggested Starting Dose	Advantages	Disadvantages	Usual Duration of Effect
Morphine	0.1 mg/kg; continuous infusion, 0.05–0.1 mg/kg/h	Pain relief, reversible	Respiratory depression, hypotension, nausea, suppression of gastrointestinal (GI) motility, histamine release	2–4 h
Hydromorphone	0.015 mg/kg; continuous infusion, 1.5–3 mcg/kg/h	Pain relief, reversible	Respiratory depression, histamine release, nausea, suppression of GI motility	2–4 h
Fentanyl	1–2 mcg/kg; continuous infusion, 0.5–2 mcg/kg/h	Excellent pain relief, reversible, short half-life	Respiratory depression, chest wall rigidity, severe nausea and vomiting	30 min
Midazolam	0.1 mg/kg; continuous infusion 0.05–0.2 mg/kg/h	Short half-life, sedation, seizure control	Respiratory depression	20–40 min
Lorazepam	0.1 mg/kg	Longer half-life, sedation, seizure control	Nausea and vomiting, respiratory depression, phlebitis	2–4 h
Diazepam	0.1 mg/kg	Sedation, seizure control, muscle spasm relief	Respiratory depression, jaundice, phlebitis	1–3 h
Dexmedetomidine	0.2–0.7 mcg/kg/h	Sedation without respiratory depression	Bradycardia, hypotension	10 min–2 h

(such as tachycardia, hypertension, or increased ICP). The most commonly used agents in the PICU are benzodiazepines, but multiple other agents may be used in certain clinical scenarios. All sedatives should be carefully titrated to effect to avoid under- or over-sedation and reduce side effects.

A. Benzodiazepines

Benzodiazepines work through the neuroinhibitory transmitter γ-aminobutyric acid (GABA) system, resulting in anxiolysis, sedation, hypnosis, skeletal muscle relaxation, and anticonvulsant effects. Benzodiazepines provide little to no analgesia and thus need to be combined with other medications when pain control is required. Commonly used benzodiazepines in the PICU include midazolam, lorazepam, and diazepam. Each has differing half-lives, resulting in varying durations of effect, and multiple possible routes of administration. *Midazolam* has the shortest half-life and produces excellent retrograde amnesia lasting for 20–40 minutes after a single IV dose. Therefore, it can be used for short-term procedural sedation and anxiolysis with single or intermittent doses or for prolonged sedation as a continuous infusion. *Lorazepam* has a longer half-life than midazolam (or diazepam) and can achieve sedation for as long as 6–8 hours. It has less effect on the cardiovascular and respiratory systems than other benzodiazepines and is commonly used for short-term sedation or initial treatment of seizures. *Diazepam* has a longer half-life than midazolam and is used most commonly to treat muscle spasticity and seizures.

Common side effects after benzodiazepine administration include respiratory depression and cardiovascular compromise, especially if given rapidly or in high doses. In some children, benzodiazepines can cause a paradoxical effect, producing greater agitation than sedation. Additional side effects vary by patient population or by the specific benzodiazepine administered or route chosen. Most benzodiazepines are metabolized in the liver and use should be carefully considered in patients with liver failure, as side effects may be prolonged and/or occur at lower doses. Continuous infusions of lorazepam should be avoided because its preservative, polyethylene glycol, can accumulate in patients with renal insufficiency and produce a metabolic acidosis. A disadvantage of diazepam in the PICU is the long half-life of its intermediary metabolite, nordazepam, which may accumulate and prolong sedative effect.

B. Other Sedative Medications

Ketamine is a phencyclidine derivative that produces a trance-like state of immobility and amnesia known as dissociative anesthesia. Ketamine does not cause significant respiratory depression at nonanesthetic doses, an advantage for the nonintubated patient. Ketamine has direct negative inotropic effects, but these are countered by stimulation of the sympathetic nervous system resulting in an increase in HR, blood pressure, and cardiac output for most patients. These effects may make ketamine a good choice for hemodynamically unstable patients unless there is concern that the patient may be catecholamine depleted, such as in the setting of chronic heart failure. Additionally, ketamine has bronchodilatory properties and, thus, may be useful for children with status asthmaticus. Finally, it has strong analgesic effects and therefore may be used as a single agent for sedation for painful procedures. The main side effects seen with ketamine are increased salivary and tracheobronchial secretions and unpleasant dreams or hallucinations. Atropine or glycopyrrolate may be administered ahead of time to reduce secretions, and concurrent administration of benzodiazepines may reduce the hallucinatory effects. Historical concerns of increased ICP with administration have not been demonstrated in more recent studies. Although most frequently used for short-term sedation, low-dose continuous infusions may be used in selected patients.

Dexmedetomidine is a selective α_2-adrenoreceptor agonist that produces sedation, anxiolysis, and some analgesia with minimal respiratory depression. It allows for the ability to rouse the patient easily if necessary. These advantages have resulted in increasing use in critically ill children for minimally painful procedural sedation as well as sedation to facilitate both invasive and noninvasive mechanical ventilation. The most frequent side effects observed are dose-related bradycardia and hypotension. Dexmedetomidine is primarily used as a short- or long-term continuous infusion. The use of dexmedetomidine may also mitigate the need for increasing doses of opioids and benzodiazepines in patients requiring multiple sedative medications.

Propofol is an anesthetic IV induction agent with strong sedative effects. Its main advantages are a rapid onset and recovery time resulting from its rapid hepatic metabolism. Because propofol has no analgesic properties, an analgesic agent should be concurrently administered for painful procedures. Propofol can cause significant vasodilation, resulting in dose-related hypotension, in addition to dose-dependent respiratory depression. Propofol infusion syndrome is a sudden-onset, profound, and potentially fatal acidosis that may occur with longer-term infusions.

Barbiturates (eg, phenobarbital) can cause direct myocardial and respiratory depression and are, in general, poor choices for standard sedation of critically ill patients.

▶ Analgesia

Opioid and nonopioid analgesics are the mainstay of treatment for acute and chronic pain in the PICU. Although several other medications used for sedation also have analgesic properties, they are uncommonly used for primary treatment of pain.

A. Opioid Analgesics

All opioids provide analgesia, but the dose required to produce adequate analgesia varies significantly between patients. Therefore, the best approach to dosing with opioids is to start with a low dose and titrate to effect, monitoring for side effects. The choice and mode of delivery of agents within this class depends upon the physiologic state of the child and the etiology of pain. In an awake and developmentally capable patient, a patient-controlled analgesia (PCA) approach with an infusion pump may be appropriate. Each of these medications may also be administered intermittently, in which case half-life and tolerability of side effects may be the primary considerations. For many patients in the PICU, a continuous infusion may be the best option. Several IV medications are commonly used as a continuous infusion or by PCA, including fentanyl, morphine, and hydromorphone. For children who have more chronic, less severe pain and who can tolerate oral medications, there are many different options, including hydrocodone, hydromorphone, morphine, methadone, and oxycodone.

The most common side effects of opioids are nausea, pruritus, slowed intestinal motility, miosis, cough suppression, and urinary retention. Opioids can also cause sedation and respiratory depression in higher or more frequent doses. Morphine can cause histamine release leading to pruritus and even hypotension. As opioids are metabolized in the liver, with metabolites excreted in the urine, patients with hepatic or renal impairment may have prolonged responses to administration.

B. Nonopioid Analgesics

Nonopioid analgesics used to treat mild to moderate pain include acetaminophen, aspirin, and other nonsteroidal anti-inflammatory drugs (NSAIDs). Because the effects of these agents can be additive with opiates, a combination of opiate and nonopiate medications can be a very effective approach to pain management in the ICU. *Acetaminophen* is the most commonly used analgesic in pediatrics in the United States and is the drug of choice for mild to moderate pain because of its low toxicity and minimal side-effect profile. With chronic use and higher doses, acetaminophen may cause liver and renal toxicity. *NSAIDs* are reasonable alternatives for the treatment of pain, particularly those conditions associated with inflammation. All NSAIDs carry the risk of gastritis, renal compromise, and bleeding due to inhibition of platelet function, limiting their use in patients with thrombocytopenia, bleeding, and kidney disease. *Ketorolac* is the only IV NSAID currently available. It can be very effective for children who cannot take oral medications or for those who require a faster onset of action. Because of the concerns for more serious renal toxicity with longer-term use, ketorolac is primarily used for shorter-term pain control. *Ibuprofen* and *naproxen* are options for patients who can tolerate oral medications.

▶ Titration of Sedative & Analgesic Dosing, Delirium, & Withdrawal Syndromes

Analgesic and anxiolytic agents have a number of disadvantages in addition to those described above, including short- and long-term cognitive deficits, increased risk of delirium, and withdrawal syndromes. To minimize risk of these unwanted effects, doses of these agents should be titrated multiple times daily to provide the minimum dosage necessary. Several scoring systems are available to assess the level of sedation and analgesia and help guide management decisions. In an awake and verbal patient, a pain scale can be used to determine the level of pain and need for treatment. In a nonverbal patient, this assessment can be more difficult, and scoring systems such as the COMFORT score, State Behavioral Scale (SBS), and Richmond Agitation and Sedation Scale (RASS) can be used. These tools allow for better communication among team members with regard to the goals of treatment and the effectiveness of any changes in medications. When using these measures, however, the provider should also exclude or address physiologic causes of agitation, such as hypoxemia, hypercapnia, or cerebral hypoperfusion caused by low cardiac output.

As with adult patients, critically ill children are at risk for developing *delirium*. Delirium may present with a wide variety of symptoms, commonly grouped as hypoactive, hyperactive, or mixed. Hyperactive delirium is associated with restlessness, agitation, emotional lability, and combativeness. Hypoactive delirium, on the other hand, may be more difficult to recognize; patients may be quiet, withdrawn, and apathetic with decreased responsiveness. PICU delirium scales including the Pediatric Confusion Assessment Method for the ICU (pCAM-ICU) and Cornell Assessment of Pediatric Delirium (CAPD) may help better assess for delirium in the PICU population.

In critically ill children, as in adults, the risk of developing delirium appears to increase with severity of illness, administration of sedative medications such as benzodiazepines, and greater sleep disturbances. Suggested strategies for preventing and treating delirium include reducing sedative exposure, promoting normal circadian rhythms with greater activity during the day and quiet, dark rooms at night, and ensuring the presence of parents and objects familiar to the child. Finally, in more extreme situations, treatment with medications can be considered. Quetiapine is a newer antipsychotic agent that has shown promise in early studies for treating pediatric delirium. Older antipsychotics such as haloperidol are still used at times but their side effect profile warrants caution. Dexmedetomidine may also be an effective medication for treatment of delirium, but this use has not been well studied in the pediatric population.

Withdrawal syndromes are another important aspect of the use of sedative and analgesic agents in the ICU. Long-term administration and high doses of continuous infusions of opioids or benzodiazepines can lead to tolerance and physical dependence. Acute reductions or cessation of these medications can result in withdrawal symptoms such as agitation, tachypnea, tachycardia, sweating, and diarrhea. Gradual tapering of the medication dosage over 7–10 days often effectively prevents withdrawal symptoms. This gradual reduction may be facilitated by transitioning to intermittent dosing of longer half-life agents, such as methadone or lorazepam. While weaning opiates or benzodiazepines, providers should assess twice daily for symptoms of withdrawal. This assessment can be facilitated by symptom scores such as the Withdrawal Assessment Tool-1 (WAT-1). A higher WAT-1 score suggests greater withdrawal symptoms and may indicate a need to slow the weaning plan. Conversely, if the WAT-1 score is consistently low, the patient is likely to tolerate the current pace or, possibly, an accelerated dose reduction.

Curley MA et al: Protocolized sedation vs usual care in pediatric patients mechanically ventilated for acute respiratory failure: a randomized clinical trial. JAMA 2015 Jan 27;313(4):379–389 [PMID: 25602358].
Smith HAB et al: 2022 Society of Critical Care Medicine clinical practice guidelines on prevention and management of pain, agitation, neuromuscular blockade and delirium in critically ill pediatric patients with consideration of the ICU environment and early mobility. Pediatr Crit Care Med 2022;23(2):e74–e110 [PMID: 35119438].

END-OF-LIFE CARE & DEATH IN THE PICU

ESSENTIALS OF DIAGNOSIS & TYPICAL FEATURES

▶ End-of-life discussions in the PICU should include the patient, if possible, and family members as well as the medical team.

▶ PICU providers may assist in defining the limits of care provided, facilitating withdrawal of life support, and providing compassionate palliative care.

▶ The palliative care and ethics teams, if available, may facilitate end-of-life discussions in the PICU.

▶ Withdrawal of life-sustaining therapies should include a plan to treat any pain and discomfort.

▶ Brain death determination requires a systematic and age-appropriate evaluation consistent with institutional policies.

▶ Tissue and organ donation must be considered with every death.

▶ Grief/bereavement support for the family as well as medical team members should be provided following every death in the PICU.

Death in the PICU

In-hospital pediatric deaths occur infrequently. A large proportion of these pediatric deaths occur in the PICU, and pediatric intensivists may be called upon to help define the limits to care provided, assist in the withdrawal of life-sustaining medical therapies (LSMTs), and provide compassionate palliative care. End-of-life discussions may have occurred prior to PICU admission for some children with congenital or chronic diseases. For other children, their PICU stay may be the first time a child or family discusses end-of-life decisions. Regardless of the individual patient's situation, the medical team has a responsibility to facilitate discussions regarding the goals of care in an honest and sensitive manner.

Deaths without any limitations on patient care comprise a small minority (10%–12%) of pediatric ICU deaths. In these circumstances, most recent studies have found greater family satisfaction with the care provided if family members are allowed to witness ongoing resuscitative efforts. The remainder of pediatric deaths is divided between brain death declarations (23%) and decisions to limit or withdraw LSMTs (65%).

Brain Death

Patients with severe neurologic injuries may meet the criteria for a diagnosis of brain death. Brain death is diagnosed by a clinical examination (Table 14–18) based on published guidelines and is recognized as legally equivalent to somatic

Table 14–18. Brain death examination.

- Patient must have normal blood pressure, core temperature > 35°C, normal electrolytes and glucose, and not be receiving sedating medications or muscle relaxants.
- 24-h waiting period suggested following CPR or severe brain injury before first brain death examination.
- Flaccid coma with no evidence of cortical function.
- Absence of brain stem reflexes:
  - Apnea ("apnea test": no respirations seen with $PaCO_2$ > 60 mm Hg and a change in $PaCO_2$ > 20 mm Hg).
  - Fixed dilated pupils with no response to light.
  - Absence of corneal reflexes.
  - Absence of eye movements including spontaneous, oculocephalic (doll's eye), or oculovestibular (cold caloric). Do not perform oculocephalic maneuver if there is potential for cervical spine injury.
  - Absence of gag and cough reflex.
- Examination consistent throughout observation period as documented by two separate clinical examinations by two different attending physicians.
- Recommended observation periods between brain death examinations:
  - 24 h: term newborn to 30 days
  - 12 h: 31–18 years
- Ancillary testing (cerebral angiography, radionuclide scanning, electroencephalography, or transcranial Doppler ultrasonography) recommended if unable to perform cranial nerve examination or apnea testing due to patient instability or injuries.

(cardiopulmonary) death in all 50 US states. The general approach to the diagnosis of brain death is similar in most medical centers, but subtle institutional variations make it imperative for PICU providers to be familiar with their own institutional policies on brain death declaration. Once a patient is declared legally brain dead, further medical support is no longer indicated, although the timing of discontinuation of mechanical life support should be discussed and agreed upon with the patient's family.

Brain death is determined through a complete clinical assessment. First and foremost, the provider must be confident that the patient's condition is irreversible and must exclude any potentially reversible conditions that may produce signs similar to brain death (such as hypotension, hypothermia, or the presence of sedating medications, toxins or electrolyte derangements). The brain death examination is a formal clinical examination directed at demonstrating absence of cortical function (flaccid coma without evidence of response to stimuli) and brainstem function (cranial nerve testing). In order to meet the definition of brain death, guidelines require that qualified physicians document one or two (separated by a period of observation) clinical examinations consistent with brain death (ie, no evidence of brain function). If a patient cannot tolerate some portion of the clinical examination (typically apnea testing) or is very young (especially < 1 year of age), an ancillary test such as EEG or cerebral perfusion scan may provide supporting evidence of brain death. Once a child has been declared brain dead, the time of death is noted as occurring at the completion of the final examination even if the child is still receiving cardiopulmonary support.

▶ Limitation or Withdrawal of Life-Sustaining Medical Therapies

Most patients who die in the pediatric ICU will do so following a decision to limit or withdraw medical support. The discussions leading to these decisions should include the patient (to the extent possible given his/her medical condition and developmental age), family members, and members of the medical team, as well as social workers, child life specialists and chaplains. The primary goals of these discussions should be to (1) communicate information regarding the patient's medical status and anticipated prognosis and (2) clarify the goals of ongoing medical care both in regard to the patient's current status and in the event of an acute decompensation. If the opinion of the medical team is that the patient's condition is likely irreversible, the options for care include (1) continuing current support with escalation as deemed medically reasonable by the health care team, (2) continuing current support but not adding any new therapies, or (3) withdrawal of LSMTs such as mechanical ventilation and/or hemodynamic support. The first two options may include a decision to not initiate cardiopulmonary resuscitation in the event of a respiratory or cardiac arrest (do-not-attempt resuscitation

[DNAR]). The third option presumes a DNAR, but this must be explicitly written in the medical record and communicated to team members.

Discussions with patients and families regarding the decision to limit resuscitation or to withdraw LSMT should be conducted by experienced personnel with the ability to communicate in a clear and compassionate manner and should occur at an appropriate time and place. Cultural needs should be considered prior to major discussions and may include the need for a translator or spiritual guidance. Discussions should begin with a clear statement that the goal is to make decisions in the best interest of the patient and that the health care team will support the patient and family in making reasonable decisions based on that goal. Potential options regarding limitations of care or withdrawal of care should be clearly explained for the decision makers. Withdrawal of LSMT can be considered when the pain and suffering inflicted by prolonging and supporting life outweighs the potential benefit for the individual. If there is no reasonable chance of recovery, the patient has the right to a natural death in a dignified and pain-free manner. The health care team should emphasize that decisions are not irrevocable and that if at any time the family or health care providers wish to reconsider the decision, full medical therapy can be reinstituted until the situation is clarified.

Prior to the withdrawal of LSMT, the patient's family and care team should be prepared for the physiologic process of dying. Key facets of the process to discuss include the possibility of agonal respirations, which can be disturbing to witness for family members and care providers, as well as the unpredictable length of time that the process may require. Additionally, the fact that the patient will ultimately have a cardiopulmonary arrest and a member of the medical team will declare the time of death should be discussed. The family should also be reassured that the patient will be given appropriate doses of medications to treat signs and symptoms of pain or discomfort and that neither they nor the patient will be abandoned by the medical team during this process.

▶ Palliative Care & Bioethics Consultation

Palliative care teams and ethics consultation services are important resources to help the health care team and families address difficult end-of-life decision making. For families of children with congenital or chronic diseases, the palliative care team may have established relationships with the patient and family outside of the acute illness. For patients with new conditions or whose prognosis has changed, the palliative care team may be newly introduced in the PICU. In either case, the palliative care team can bring invaluable support and resources for families during end-of-life discussions. A more comprehensive discussion of palliative care can be found in Chapter 32.

If conflict arises surrounding decisions about limiting medical care, an ethics consultation can aid the process by helping to identify, analyze, and resolve ethical problems. Ethics consultation can independently clarify views and allow the health care team, patient, and family to make decisions that respect patient autonomy and promote maximum benefit and minimal harm to the patient.

▶ Tissue & Organ Donation

Organ transplantation is standard therapy for many pediatric conditions and many children die while awaiting a transplant due to short supply of organs. The gift of organ donation can be a positive outcome for a family from the otherwise tragic loss of their child's life. The 1986 U.S. Federal Required Request Law mandates that all donor-eligible families be approached about potential organ donation. The decision to donate must be made free of coercion, with informed consent, and without financial incentive. State organ-procurement agencies provide support and education to care providers and families to make informed decisions.

To be a solid organ donor, the patient must be declared dead and have no conditions contraindicating donation. The most frequent type of solid organ donor in the PICU is a brain-dead donor. The unmet demand for donor organs has, however, led to the emergence of protocols for procuring solid organs from donors following cardiac death. Donation after cardiac death has been described by different terminology over time, with the most recent nomenclature being Donation after Circulatory Determination of Death (DCDD). In these cases, the patient does not meet brain death criteria but has an irreversible disease process and the family or patient has decided to withdraw life-sustaining therapy and consented to attempted organ donation. In the DCDD process, LSMT is withdrawn, and comfort measures are provided as per usual care. The withdrawal of care may take place in the PICU or the operating room without any surgical staff present, depending upon institutional policy. Once the declaring physician has determined cessation of cardiac function, the patient is observed for an additional short time period for autoresuscitation (the return of cardiac activity without medical intervention). After this waiting period, the patient is declared dead. Upon declaration of death, transplant surgeons are then allowed to enter the room and the organs are immediately harvested for donation. If the patient does not die within a predetermined time limit after discontinuation of LSMT, comfort measures continue but solid-organ donation is abandoned due to long ischemic times with a high probability the organs will not be viable for transplant. Tissue (heart valves, corneas, skin, and bone) can be donated following a "traditional" cardiac death (no pulse or respirations), brain death, or DCDD.

▶ Bereavement & Grief Support

After any pediatric death, bereavement and grief support for families and health care providers are essential components of comprehensive end-of-life care. Families may need information about care of the body after the death, funeral arrangements, and autopsy decisions as well as about educational, spiritual, and other supportive resources available. Members of the medical team may feel their own grief and sense of loss with the death of a patient. These emotions, if not appropriately addressed, can negatively affect their personal and professional lives. Therefore, similar supportive services should be available to health care workers caring for dying children.

Buang SNH et al: Palliative and critical care: their convergence in the pediatric intensive care unit. Front Pediatr 2022;10:907268 [PMID: 35757116].

Kirschen MP et al: Epidemiology of brain death in the pediatric intensive care units in the United States. JAMA Pediatr 2019;173(5):469–476 [PMID: 30882855].

Nakagawa T et al: Guidelines for the determination of brain death in infants and children: an update of the 1987 task force recommendations. Pediatrics 2011;128(3):e720–e740 [PMID: 21873704].

▼ QUALITY IMPROVEMENT INITIATIVES IN THE PICU

Quality improvement and patient safety initiatives in the PICU are essential to providing high quality and reliable care to complex and critically ill pediatric patients. National and local reporting requirements for a number of *hospital-acquired conditions* (HACs) including central line-associated bloodstream infections, catheter-associated urinary tract infections, unplanned extubations, VAPs and venous thromboembolism have led to the development of collaboratives focused on data gathering and sharing of best practices for prevention of those conditions. Improving quality and safety practices relies on creating both a culture of transparency and safe reporting of adverse events and tools or workflows designed to help reduce the likelihood of error. As an example, multipronged efforts to reduce catheter-related bloodstream infections include checklists or bundled tools to ensure strict adherence to sterile procedure during catheter insertion, sterile practice when accessing the catheter during care, reductions in the number of times the catheter is accessed, and removal of catheters at the earliest safe opportunity. Improving communication during handoffs and cardiopulmonary resuscitation quality are two additional initiatives to optimize patient outcomes in the PICU.

Hsu HE et al: Health care-associated infections among critically ill children in the US, 2013–2018. JAMA Pediatr 2020 Dec 1;174(12):1176–1183. doi: 10.1001/jamapediatrics.2020.3223 [PMID: 33017011] [PMCID: PMC7536620].

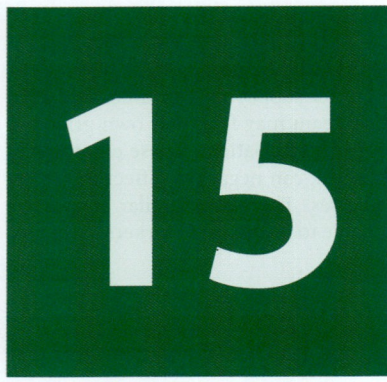

Skin

Lori D. Prok, MD
Carla X. Torres-Zegarra, MD

GENERAL PRINCIPLES

DIAGNOSIS OF SKIN DISORDERS

Examination of the skin requires that the entire surface of the body be palpated and inspected in good light. The onset and duration of each symptom should be recorded, together with a description of the primary lesion and any secondary changes, using the terminology in Table 15–1. In practice, characteristics of skin lesions are described in an order opposite to that shown in Table 15–1. Begin with distribution, then configuration, color, secondary changes, and primary changes. For example, guttate psoriasis could be described as "generalized, discrete, red, or scaly papules." Of note, cutaneous lesions may present differently in patients with varying skin tones, and historically, mainstream dermatology literature and training have not focused on skin of color. The reader is encouraged to explore dermatologic manifestations in a variety of skin colors. An excellent reference is given by Taylor and Kelly, 2016. Several online and social media platforms, including the Instagram account "Brown Skin Matters" offer follower-submitted photographs and other helpful resources.

DISORDERS OF THE SKIN IN NEWBORNS

TRANSIENT DISEASES IN NEWBORNS

1. Milia

Milia are tiny epidermal cysts filled with keratinous material. These 1- to 2-mm white papules occur predominantly on the face in 40% of newborns. Their intraoral counterparts are called *Epstein pearls* and occur in up to 60%–85% of neonates. These cystic structures spontaneously rupture and exfoliate their contents.

2. Sebaceous Gland Hyperplasia

Prominent white to yellow papules at the opening of pilosebaceous follicles without surrounding erythema—especially over the nose—represent overgrowth of sebaceous glands in response to maternal androgens. They occur in more than half of newborns and spontaneously regress in the first few months of life.

3. Neonatal Acne

Inflammatory papules and pustules with occasional comedones predominantly on the face occur in as many as 20% of newborns. Although neonatal acne can be present at birth, it most often occurs between 2 and 4 weeks of age. Spontaneous resolution occurs over a period of 6 months to 1 year. A rare entity that is often confused with neonatal acne is **neonatal cephalic pustulosis**. This is a more monomorphic eruption with red papules and pustules on the head and neck that appears in the first month of life. There is associated neutrophilic inflammation and yeasts of the genus *Malassezia* (*Pityrosporum*). This eruption will resolve spontaneously but responds to topical antiyeast preparations (ie, ketoconazole 2% cream).

4. Harlequin Color Change

A cutaneous vascular phenomenon unique to neonates in the first week of life occurs when the infant (particularly one of low birth weight) is placed on one side. The dependent half develops an erythematous flush with a sharp demarcation at the midline, and the upper half of the body becomes pale. The color change usually subsides within a few seconds after the infant is placed supine but may persist for as long as 20 minutes.

5. Mottling or Cutis Marmorata

A lace-like pattern of bluish, reticular discoloration representing dilated cutaneous vessels appears over the extremities and

Table 15–1. Examination of the skin.

Clinical Appearance	Description and Examples
Primary lesions (first to appear)	
Macule	Any flat circumscribed color change in the skin < 1 cm. Examples: white (vitiligo), brown (junctional nevus), purple (petechia).
Patch	Any flat circumscribed color change in the skin > 1 cm. Examples: white (nevus depigmentosa), brown (café au lait macule), purple (purpura).
Papule	A solid, elevated area < 1 cm in diameter whose top may be pointed, rounded, or flat. Examples: acne, warts, small lesions of psoriasis.
Plaque	A solid, circumscribed area > 1 cm in diameter, usually flat-topped. Example: psoriasis.
Vesicle	A circumscribed, elevated lesion < 1 cm in diameter and containing clear serous fluid. Example: blisters of herpes simplex.
Bulla	A circumscribed, elevated lesion > 1 cm in diameter and containing clear serous fluid. Example: bullous impetigo.
Pustule	A vesicle containing a purulent exudate. Examples: acne, folliculitis.
Nodule	A deep-seated mass with indistinct borders that elevates the overlying epidermis. Examples: tumors, granuloma annulare. If it moves with the skin on palpation, it is intradermal; if the skin moves over the nodule, it is subcutaneous.
Wheal	A circumscribed, flat-topped, firm elevation of skin resulting from tense edema of the papillary dermis. Example: urticaria.
Secondary changes	
Scales	Dry, thin plates of keratinized epidermal cells (stratum corneum). Examples: psoriasis, ichthyosis.
Lichenification	Induration of skin with exaggerated skin lines and a shiny surface resulting from chronic rubbing of the skin. Example: chronic atopic dermatitis.
Erosion and oozing	A moist, circumscribed, slightly depressed area representing a blister base with the roof of the blister removed. Examples: burns, impetigo. Most oral blisters present as erosions.
Crusts	Dried exudate of plasma on the surface of the skin following disruption of the stratum corneum. Examples: impetigo, contact dermatitis.
Fissures	A linear split in the skin extending through the epidermis into the dermis. Example: angular cheilitis.
Scars	A flat, raised, or depressed area of fibrotic replacement of dermis or subcutaneous tissue. Examples: acne scar, burn scar.
Atrophy	Depression of the skin surface caused by thinning of one or more layers of skin. Example: lichen sclerosus.
Color	
	The lesion should be described as white, red, yellow, brown, tan, or blue. Particular attention should be given to the blanching of red lesions. Failure to blanch suggests bleeding into the dermis (petechiae).
Configuration of lesions	
Annular (circular)	Annular nodules represent granuloma annulare; annular scaly papules are more apt to be caused by dermatophyte infections.
Linear (straight lines)	Linear papules represent lichen striatus; linear vesicles, incontinentia pigmenti; linear papules with burrows, scabies.
Grouped	Grouped vesicles occur in herpes simplex or zoster.
Discrete	Discrete lesions are independent of each other.
Distribution	
	Note whether the eruption is generalized, acral (hands, feet, buttocks, face), or localized to a specific skin region.

often the trunk of neonates exposed to lowered room temperature. This feature is transient and usually disappears completely on rewarming. This can be mistaken for the mottling that occurs with sepsis, but the infant will be ill appearing.

6. Erythema Toxicum

Up to 50% of full-term infants develop erythema toxicum. At 24–48 hours of age, blotchy erythematous macules 2–3 cm in diameter appear, most prominently on the chest but also on the back, face, and extremities. These are occasionally present at birth. Onset after 4–5 days of life is rare. The lesions vary in number from a few up to as many as 100. Incidence is much higher in full-term versus premature infants. The macular erythema may fade within 24–48 hours or may progress to formation of urticarial wheals in the center of the macules or, in 10% of cases, pustules. Examination of a Wright-stained smear of the lesion reveals numerous eosinophils. No organisms are seen on Gram stain. These findings may be accompanied by peripheral blood eosinophilia of up to 20%. The lesions fade and disappear within 5–7 days.

7. Transient Neonatal Pustular Melanosis

Transient neonatal pustular melanosis is a pustular eruption in African-America newborns. The pustules rupture leaving a collarette of scale surrounding a macular hyperpigmentation. Unlike erythema toxicum, the pustules contain mostly neutrophils and often involve the palms and soles.

8. Sucking Blisters

Bullae, either intact or as erosions (representing the blister base) without inflammatory borders, may occur over the forearms, wrists, thumbs, or upper lip. These presumably result from vigorous sucking in utero. They can persist in the newborn period but resolve without complications.

9. Miliaria

Obstruction of the eccrine sweat ducts occurs often in neonates and produces one of two clinical scenarios. Superficial obstruction in the stratum corneum causes miliaria crystallina, characterized by tiny (1- to 2-mm), superficial grouped vesicles without erythema over intertriginous areas and adjacent skin (eg, neck, upper chest). More commonly, obstruction of the eccrine duct deeper in the epidermis results in erythematous grouped papules in the same areas and is called miliaria rubra. Rarely, these may progress to pustules. Heat and high humidity predispose the patient to eccrine duct pore closure. Removal to a cooler environment is the treatment of choice.

10. Subcutaneous Fat Necrosis

This entity presents in the first 7 days of life as reddish or purple, sharply circumscribed, firm nodules occurring over the cheeks, buttocks, arms, and thighs. Cold injury is thought to

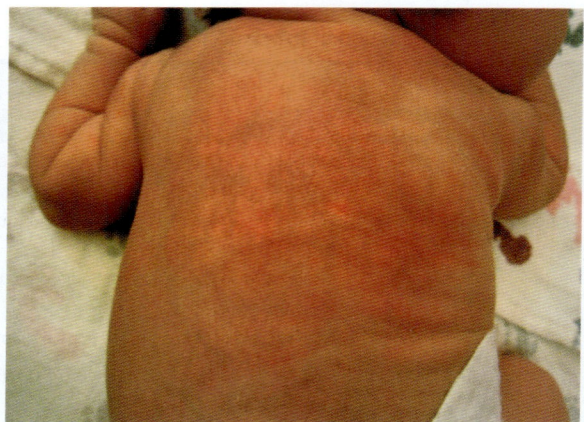

▲ **Figure 15–1.** Subcutaneous fat necrosis on the back of a newborn.

play an important role, and the clinical manifestations have been observed after iatrogenically induced and therapeutic hypothermia. These lesions resolve spontaneously over a period of weeks, although in some instances they may calcify. Affected infants should be screened for hypercalcemia that can develop up to 28 weeks after these skin changes are noted (Figure 15–1).

Rayala BZ, Morell DS: Common skin conditions in children: neonatal skin lesions. FP Essent 2017 Feb;453:11–17 [PMID: 28196316].

Stefanko NS et al: Subcutaneous fat necrosis of the newborn and associated hypercalcemia: a systematic review of the literature. Pediatr Dermatol 2019 Jan;36(1):24–30 [PMID: 30187956].

Taylor SC et al: *Taylor and Kelly's Dermatology for Skin of Color.* 2nd ed. McGraw-Hill; 2016.

PIGMENT CELL BIRTHMARKS, NEVI, & MELANOMA

Birthmarks may involve an overgrowth of one or more of any of the normal components of skin (eg, pigment cells, blood vessels, lymph vessels). A nevus is a hamartoma of highly differentiated cells that retain their normal function.

1. Dermal melanocytosis

A blue-black macule found over the lumbosacral area in 90% of darker-skinned infants is "dermal melanocytosis." The term "Mongolian spot" is no longer considered an appropriate term to be used to describe this condition. These macules or patches are occasionally noted over the shoulders and back and may extend over the buttocks. Histologically, they consist of spindle-shaped pigment cells suspended deep in the dermis. The lesions fade somewhat with time as a result of darkening of the overlying skin, but some traces may persist into adult life. The presence of this cutaneous finding should

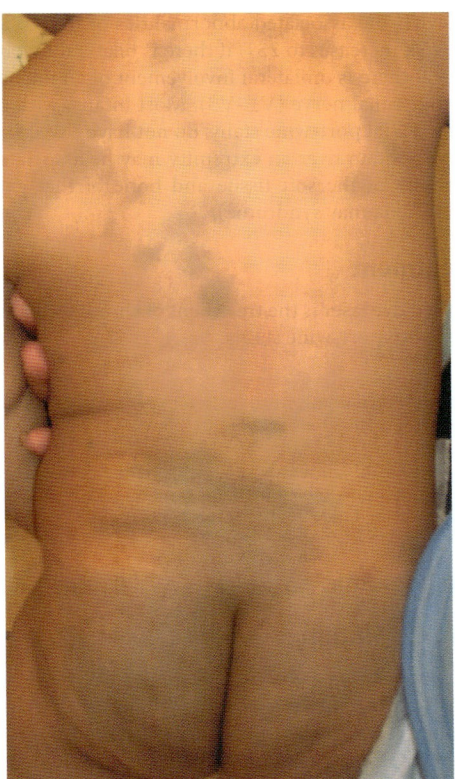

▲ **Figure 15–2.** Dermal melanocytosis of the back and buttocks.

be documented in the newborn physical examination, lest it be mistaken for bruising (Figure 15–2).

2. Café au Lait Macule

A café au lait macule is a light-brown, oval macule (dark brown on brown or black skin) that may be found anywhere on the body. Café au lait spots over 1.5 cm in greatest diameter are found in 10% of white and 22% of black children. These lesions persist throughout life and may increase in number with age. The presence of six or more such lesions with diameter larger than 0.5 cm in a prepuberal child or 1.5 cm in an adolescent or adult is a major diagnostic criterion for neurofibromatosis type 1 (NF-1). Patients with McCune-Albright syndrome (see Chapter 34) have a large, unilateral café au lait macule (Figure 15–3).

3. Spitz Nevus

A Spitz nevus presents as a reddish-brown smooth solitary papule appearing on the face or extremities. Histologically, it consists of epithelioid and spindle-shaped nevomelanocytes that may demonstrate nuclear pleomorphism. Although

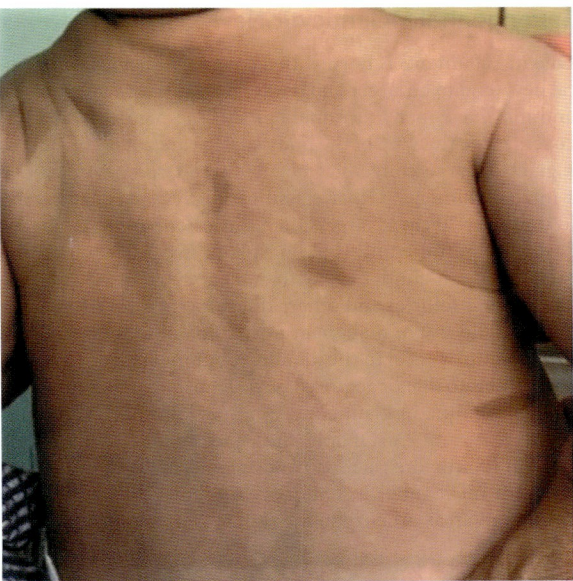

▲ **Figure 15–3.** Café au lait macules on the back.

these lesions can look concerning histologically, they follow a benign clinical course in most cases.

MELANOCYTIC NEVI

1. Common Moles

Well-demarcated, brown to brown-black macules represent junctional nevi. They can appear in the first years of life and increase with age. Histologically, single and nested melanocytes are present at the junction of the epidermis and dermis. Approximately 20% may progress to compound nevi—papular lesions with melanocytes both in junctional and intradermal locations. Intradermal nevi are often lighter in color and can be fleshy and pedunculated. Melanocytes in these lesions are located purely within the dermis. Nevi look dark blue (blue nevi) when they contain more deeply situated spindle-shaped melanocytes in the dermis.

2. Melanoma

Melanoma in prepubertal children is very rare. Pigmented lesions with variegated colors (red, white, blue), notched borders, asymmetrical shape, and very irregular or ulcerated surfaces should prompt suspicion of melanoma. Ulceration and bleeding are advanced signs of melanoma. If melanoma is suspected, wide local excision and pathologic examination should be performed.

3. Congenital Melanocytic Nevi

One in 100 infants is born with a congenital nevus. Congenital nevi tend to be larger and darker brown than acquired nevi and may have many terminal hairs. If the pigmented plaque covers more than 5% of the body surface area, it is considered a giant or large congenital nevus; these large nevi occur in 1 in 20,000 infants. Other classification systems characterize lesions over 20 cm as large. Often the lesions are so large they cover the entire trunk (bathing trunk nevi). Histologically, they are compound nevi with melanocytes often tracking around hair follicles and other adnexal structures deep in the dermis. The risk of malignant melanoma in small congenital nevi is controversial in the literature, but most likely very low, and similar to that of acquired nevi. Transformation to malignant melanoma in giant congenital nevi has been estimated between 1% and 7%. Of note, these melanomas often develop early in life (before puberty) and in a dermal location. Two-thirds of melanomas in children with giant congenital nevi develop in areas other than the skin.

Jahnke MN et al: Care of congenital melanocytic nevi in newborns and infants: Review and management recommendations. Pediatrics 2021 Dec 1;148(6):e2021051536 [PMID: 34845496].
Kalani N et al: Pediatric melanoma: characterizing 256 cases from the Colorado Central Cancer Registry. Pediatr Dermatol 2019 Mar;36(2):219–222 [PMID: 30793788].
LaVigne EA et al: Clinical and dermoscopic changes in common melanocytic nevi in school children: the Framingham school nevus study. Dermatology 2005;211:234 [PMID: 16205068].
Simons EA: Congenital melanocytic nevi in young children: histopathologic features and clinical outcomes. J Am Acad Dermatol 2017;76(5):941–947 [PMID: 28242090].

VASCULAR BIRTHMARKS

1. Capillary Malformations

▶ Clinical Findings

Capillary malformations are an excess of capillaries in localized areas of skin. The degree of excess is variable. The color of these lesions ranges from light red-pink to dark red.

Nevus simplexes are the light red macules found over the nape of the neck, upper eyelids, and glabella of newborns. Fifty percent of infants have such lesions over their necks. Eyelid and glabellar lesions usually fade completely within the first year of life. Lesions that occupy the total central forehead area usually do not fade. Those on the neck persist into adult life.

Port-wine stains are dark red macules appearing anywhere on the body. A bilateral facial port-wine stain or one covering the entire half of the face may be a clue to Sturge-Weber syndrome (SWS), which is characterized by seizures, mental retardation, glaucoma, and hemiplegia (see Chapter 25). The overall risk of a facial port-wine stain having the associated abnormalities of the SWS is 8%, but the risk increases to 25% if there is bilateral involvement of V1 or if there is unilateral involvement of all the branches of the trigeminal nerve (V1–V3). Most infants with smaller, unilateral facial port-wine stains do not have SWS. Similarly, a port-wine stain over an extremity may be associated with hypertrophy of the soft tissue and bone of that extremity (Klippel-Trénaunay syndrome).

▶ Treatment

The pulsed dye laser is the treatment of choice for infants and children with port-wine stains.

Eberson SN et al: A basic introduction to pediatric vascular anomalies. Semin Intervent Radiol 2019 Jun;36(2):149–160 [PMID: 31123389].
Sara Sabeti et al: Consensus statement for the management and treatment of port-wine birthmarks in Sturge-Weber syndrome. JAMA Dermatology 2021 [PMID: 33175124].

2. Hemangioma

▶ Clinical Findings

A red, rubbery vascular plaque or nodule with a characteristic growth pattern is a hemangioma. The lesion is often not present at birth but is represented by a permanent blanched area on the skin that is supplanted at age 2–4 weeks by red papules. Hemangiomas then undergo a rapid growth or "proliferative" phase within the first 5–7 weeks of life, where growth of the lesion is out of proportion to growth of the child. Growth then slows and, at 9–12 months, growth stabilizes or ceases completely, and the lesion slowly involutes over the next several years. Histologically, hemangiomas are benign tumors of capillary endothelial cells. They may be superficial, deep, or mixed. The terms *strawberry* and *cavernous* are misleading and should not be used. The biologic behavior of a hemangioma is the same despite its location. Fifty percent reach maximal regression by age 5 years, 70% by age 7 years, and 90% by age 9 years, leaving redundant skin, hypopigmentation, and telangiectasia. Local complications include superficial and deep ulcerations particularly for hemangiomas involving the lips and diaper area, leading to pain and scarring. Disfigurement can result from large facial infantile hemangiomas, or those involving the nasal tip or ears. There is also potential for functional impairment in periorbital hemangiomas that may block vision.

Large plaque-like facial hemangiomas may be associated with underlying abnormalities, including intracranial and aortic arch vascular abnormalities accompanying a large facial Infantile hemangioma associated with PHACES syndrome (Posterior fossa malformations, Hemangioma, Arterial anomalies, Cardiac anomalies, Eye anomalies, Supraumbilical

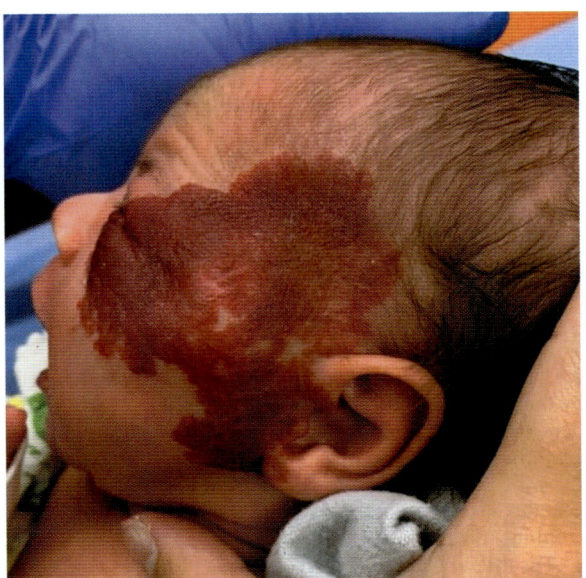

▲ **Figure 15–4.** Facial hemangioma on the face in an infant with PHACES syndrome.

raphe or Sternal pit). Similarly, large sacral hemangiomas may be associated with spinal dysraphism and genitourinary abnormalities as seen in LUMBAR syndrome (Lower body hemangioma and other cutaneous defects, Urogenital anomalies, Myelopathy, Bone deformities, Anorectal malformations, arterial anomalies, Renal anomalies). Rare complications include airway obstruction seen with hemangiomas involving lower face in a "beard distribution." Early intervention and referral to a pediatric dermatologist is recommended for certain hemangiomas based on location and associated risk factors to prevent complications (Figure 15–4).

▶ **Treatment**

Complications that require immediate treatment are (1) visual obstruction (with resulting amblyopia), (2) airway obstruction (hemangiomas of the head and neck ["beard hemangiomas"] may be associated with subglottic hemangiomas), (3) cardiac decompensation (high-output failure), (4) ulceration, and (5) association with underlying anomalies. Historically, the preferred treatment for complicated hemangiomas was systemic prednisolone. Currently, oral propranolol (2 mg/kg/day divided bid) has replaced systemic steroids as the treatment of choice for infantile hemangiomas. Reported side effects are sleep disturbance and acrocyanosis. Hypoglycemia and bradycardia have been described but are rarely seen. Recommendations on pretreatment cardiac evaluation vary between institutions. The topical β-adrenergic receptor antagonist timolol,

administered as a gel-forming solution (GFS), is successful in treating small superficial hemangiomas. If the lesion is ulcerated or bleeding, wound care and pulsed dye laser treatment is indicated to initiate ulcer healing and immediately control pain. The Kasabach-Merritt syndrome, characterized by platelet trapping with consumption coagulopathy, does not occur with solitary cutaneous hemangiomas. It is seen only in association with rare vascular tumors such as kaposiform hemangioendotheliomas and tufted angiomas.

Krowchuk DP et al: Clinical practice guideline for the management of infantile hemangiomas. Pediatrics 2019 Jan;143(1). pii: e20183475 [PMID: 30584062].
Smithson SL: Consensus statement for the treatment of infantile haemangiomas with propranolol. Australas J Dermatol 2017;58(2):155–159 [PMID: 28251611].

3. Lymphatic Malformations

Lymphatic malformations may be superficial or deep. Superficial lymphatic malformations present as fluid-filled vesicles often described as resembling "frog spawn." Deep lymphatic malformations are rubbery, skin-colored nodules occurring most commonly in the head and neck. They often result in grotesque enlargement of soft tissues. Histologically, they can be either macrocystic or microcystic.

▶ **Treatment**

Therapy includes compression garments, sclerotherapy with injection of doxycycline, surgical excision, and most recently sirolimus (mToR inhibitor).

EPIDERMAL BIRTHMARKS

1. Epidermal Nevus

▶ **Clinical Findings**

The majority of these birthmarks present in the first year of life. They are hamartomas of the epidermis that are warty to papillomatous plaques, often in a linear array. They range in color from skin-colored to dirty yellow to brown. Histologically they show a thickened epidermis with hyperkeratosis. The condition of widespread epidermal nevi associated with other developmental anomalies (central nervous system [CNS], eye, and skeletal) is called the epidermal nevus syndrome.

▶ **Treatment**

Treatment once or twice daily with topical calcipotriene or keratolytic may flatten some lesions. Fractionated CO_2 laser can be used to remove hyperkeratotic epidermis. The only definitive cure is surgical excision.

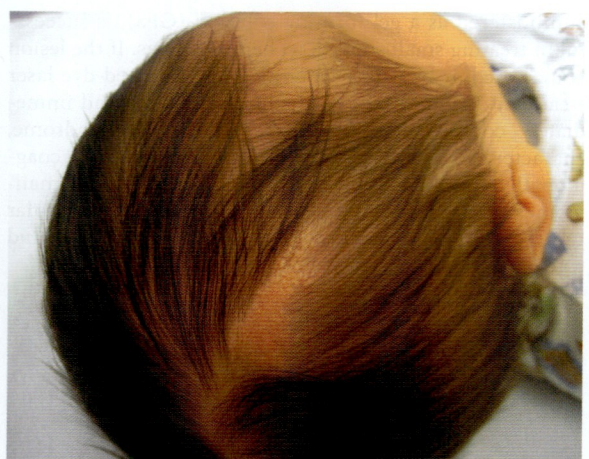

▲ **Figure 15–5.** Nevus sebaceus on the scalp of an infant.

2. Nevus Sebaceus

▶ Clinical Findings

This is a hamartoma of sebaceous glands and underlying apocrine glands that is diagnosed by the appearance at birth of a yellowish, hairless plaque in the scalp or on the face. The lesions can be contiguous with an epidermal nevus on the face, and widespread lesions can constitute part of the epidermal nevus syndrome.

Histologically, nevus sebaceus represents an overabundance of sebaceous glands without hair follicles. At puberty, with androgenic stimulation, the sebaceous cells in the nevus divide, expand their cellular volume, and synthesize sebum, resulting in a warty mass (Figure 15–5).

▶ Treatment

Because it has been estimated that approximately 1% of these lesions will develop secondary epithelial tumors, including basal cell carcinomas, trichoblastomas, and other benign tumors, surgical excision at puberty is recommended by many experts, while ongoing clinical surveillance is favored by others. The majority of the tumors develop in adulthood, although basal cell carcinomas have been reported in childhood and adolescence.

CONNECTIVE TISSUE BIRTHMARKS (JUVENILE ELASTOMA, COLLAGENOMA)

▶ Clinical Findings

Connective tissue nevi are smooth, skin-colored papules 1–10 mm in diameter that are grouped on the trunk. A solitary, larger (5–10 cm) nodule is called a shagreen patch and is histologically indistinguishable from other connective tissue

nevi that show thickened, abundant collagen bundles with or without associated increases of elastic tissue. Although the shagreen patch is a cutaneous clue to tuberous sclerosis (see Chapter 25), the other connective tissue nevi occur as isolated events.

▶ Treatment

These nevi remain throughout life and need no treatment.

HEREDITARY SKIN DISORDERS

1. Ichthyosis

Ichthyosis is a term applied to several diseases characterized by the presence of excessive scales on the skin. These disorders represent a large and heterogeneous group of genetic and acquired defects of cornification of the skin. Classification of these diseases is clinically based, although the underlying genetic causes and pathophysiologic mechanisms responsible continue to be elucidated.

Disorders of keratinization are characterized as syndromic when the phenotype is expressed in the skin and other organs or nonsyndromic when only the skin is affected. Ichthyoses may be inherited or acquired. Inherited disorders are identified by their underlying gene defect if known. Acquired ichthyosis may be associated with malignancy and medications, or a variety of autoimmune, inflammatory, nutritional, metabolic, infectious, and neurologic diseases. These disorders are diagnosed by clinical examination, with supportive findings on skin biopsy (including electron microscopy) and mutation analysis if available.

▶ Treatment

Treatment consists of controlling scaling with ammonium lactate (Lac-Hydrin or AmLactin) 12% or urea cream 10%–40% applied once or twice daily. Daily lubrication and a good dry skin care regimen are essential.

Takeichi T, Akiyama M: Inherited ichthyosis: non-syndromic forms. J Dermatol 2016 Mar;43(3):242–251 [PMID: 26945532].
Yoneda K: Inherited ichthyosis: syndromic forms. J Dermatol 2016 Mar;43(3):252–263 [PMID: 26945533].

2. Epidermolysis Bullosa

This is a group of heritable disorders characterized by skin fragility with blistering. Several subtypes are recognized, based on the ultrastructural level of skin cleavage due to known genetic mutations.

For the severely affected, much of the surface area of the skin may have blisters and erosions, requiring daily wound care and dressings. These children are prone to frequent skin infections, anemia, growth problems, mouth erosions and esophageal strictures, and chronic pain issues. They are also at increased risk of squamous cell carcinoma, a common cause of death in affected patients.

▶ Treatment

Treatment consists of protection of the skin with topical emollients as well as nonstick dressings. The other medical needs and potential complications of the severe forms of epidermolysis bullosa require a multidisciplinary approach. For the less severe types, protecting areas of greatest trauma with padding and dressings as well as intermittent topical or oral antibiotics for superinfection are appropriate treatments. If hands and feet are involved, reducing skin friction with 5% glutaraldehyde every 3 days is helpful.

Fine JD et al: Inherited epidermolysis bullosa: updated recommendations on diagnosis and classification. J Am Acad Dermatol 2014 Jun;70(6):1103–1126 [PMID: 24690439].
Has C et al: Consensus reclassification of inherited epidermolysis bullosa and other disorders with skin fragility. Br J Dermatol 2020 Oct;183(4):614–627 [PMID: 32017015].

▼ COMMON SKIN DISEASES IN INFANTS, CHILDREN, & ADOLESCENTS

ACNE

Acne affects 85% of adolescents. The onset of adolescent acne is between ages 7 and 10 years in 40% of children. The early lesions are usually limited to the face and are primarily closed comedones.

▶ Pathogenesis

The primary event in acne formation is obstruction of the sebaceous follicle and subsequent formation of the microcomedo (not evident clinically). This is the precursor to all future acne lesions. This phenomenon is androgen-dependent in adolescent acne. The four primary factors in the pathogenesis of acne are (1) plugging of the sebaceus follicle, (2) increased sebum production, (3) proliferation of *Cutibacterium acnes* in the obstructed follicle, and (4) inflammation. Many of these factors are influenced by androgens.

Drug-induced acne should be suspected in teenagers if all lesions are in the same stage at the same time and if involvement extends to the lower abdomen, lower back, arms, and legs. Drugs responsible for acne include corticotropin (adrenocorticotropic hormone [ACTH]), glucocorticoids, androgens, hydantoins, and isoniazid, each of which increases plasma testosterone.

▶ Clinical Findings

Open comedones are the predominant clinical lesion in early adolescent acne. The black color is caused by oxidized melanin within the stratum corneum cellular plug. Open comedones do not progress to inflammatory lesions. Closed comedones, or whiteheads, are caused by obstruction just beneath the follicular opening in the neck of the sebaceous follicle, which produces a cystic swelling of the follicular duct directly beneath the epidermis. Most authorities believe that closed comedones are precursors of inflammatory acne lesions (red papules, pustules, nodules, and cysts). In typical adolescent acne, several different types of lesions are present simultaneously. Severe, chronic, inflammatory lesions may rarely occur as interconnecting, draining sinus tracts. Adolescents with cystic acne require prompt medical attention because ruptured cysts and sinus tracts result in severe scar formation.

▶ Differential Diagnosis

Consider rosacea, nevus comedonicus, flat warts, miliaria, molluscum contagiosum, and the angiofibromas of tuberous sclerosis.

▶ Treatment

Different treatment options are listed in Table 15–2. Recent data have indicated that combination therapy that targets multiple pathogenic factors increases the efficacy of treatment and rate of improvement.

A. Topical Keratolytic Agents

Topical keratolytic agents address the plugging of the follicular opening with keratinocytes and include retinoids, benzoyl peroxide, and azelaic acid. The first-line treatment for both comedonal and inflammatory acne is a topical retinoid (tretinoin [retinoic acid], adapalene, and tazarotene). These are the most effective keratolytic agents and have been shown to prevent the microcomedone. These topical agents may be used once daily, or the combination of a retinoid applied to acne-bearing areas of the skin in the evening and a benzoyl peroxide gel or azelaic acid applied in the morning may be used. This regimen will control 80%–85% of cases of adolescent acne.

B. Topical Antibiotics

Topical antibiotics are less effective than systemic antibiotics and at best are equivalent in potency to 250 mg of tetracycline orally once a day. One percent clindamycin phosphate solution is the most efficacious topical antibiotic. Most *C acnes* strains are now resistant to topical erythromycin solutions. Topical antibiotic therapy alone should never be used. Multiple studies have shown a combination of benzoyl peroxide or a retinoid, and a topical antibiotic are more effective than the antibiotic alone. Benzoyl peroxide has been shown to help minimize the development of bacterial resistance at sites of application. The duration of application of topical

Table 15–2. Acne treatment.

Type of Lesion	Treatment
Comedonal acne	One of the following: Tretinoin, 0.025%, 0.05%, or 0.1% cream; 0.01% or 0.025% gel; 0.4% or 0.1% microgel Adapalene, 0.3% gel, 0.1% gel or solution; 0.05% cream
Papular inflammatory acne	One from first grouping, plus one of the following: Benzoyl peroxide, 2.5%, 4%, 5%, 8%, or 10% gel or lotion; 4% or 8% wash Azelaic acid, 15% or 20% cream Clindamycin, 1% lotion, solution, or gel Combination products include benzoyl peroxide-erythromycin (Benzamycin); benzoyl peroxide-clindamycin (Duac, BenzaClin, Acanya); tretinoin-clindamycin (Ziana, Veltin)
Pustular inflammatory acne	One from first grouping, plus one of the following oral antibiotics: Minocycline or doxycycline, 50–100 mg, bid
Nodulocystic acne	Isotretinoin, 1 mg/kg/day, goal dose 120–150 mg/kg total

antimicrobials should be limited unless benzoyl peroxide is used. Several combination products (benzoyl peroxide and clindamycin, tretinoin and clindamycin, adapalene, and benzoyl peroxide) are available, which may simplify the treatment regimen and increase patient compliance.

C. Systemic Antibiotics

Antibiotics that are concentrated in sebum, such as tetracycline, minocycline, and doxycycline, should be reserved for moderate to severe inflammatory acne. The usual dose of tetracycline is 0.5–1.0 g divided twice a day on an empty stomach; minocycline and doxycycline 50–100 mg taken once or twice daily can be taken with food. Oral antibiotics should never be used alone without concurrent retinoid and/or benzoyl peroxide. Recent recommendations are that oral antibiotics should be used for a finite time, and then discontinued as soon as there is improvement in the inflammatory lesions, and for no more than 6 months if no improvement is seen. The tetracycline antibiotics should not be given to children younger than 8 years due to the effect on dentition (staining of teeth). Doxycycline may induce significant photosensitivity, and minocycline can cause bluish-gray dyspigmentation of the skin, vertigo, headaches, and drug-induced lupus. These antibiotics have anti-inflammatory effects in addition to decreasing *C acnes* in the follicle.

D. Oral Retinoids

An oral retinoid, 13-*cis*-retinoic acid (isotretinoin), is the most effective treatment for severe cystic or treatment resistant acne. The precise mechanism of its action is unknown, but apoptosis of sebocytes, decreased sebaceous gland size, decreased sebum production, decreased follicular obstruction, decreased skin bacteria, and general anti-inflammatory activities have been described. The initial dosage is 0.5–1 mg/kg/day. This therapy is reserved for severe nodulocystic acne or acne recalcitrant to aggressive standard therapy. Side effects include dryness and scaling of the skin, dry lips, and, occasionally, dry eyes and dry nose. Fifteen percent of patients may experience some mild achiness with athletic activities. Up to 10% of patients experience mild, reversible hair loss. Elevated liver enzymes and blood lipids have rarely been described. Acute depression and mood changes have been reported, but no definitive relationship to the drug has been proven. Most importantly, isotretinoin is teratogenic. Because of this and other potential side effects, it is not recommended unless strict adherence to the Food and Drug Administration (FDA) guidelines is ensured. The FDA has implemented a registration program (iPLEDGE) that must be used to obtain and/or prescribe isotretinoin.

E. Other Acne Treatments

Hormonal therapy (oral contraceptives) is often an effective option for female patients who have perimenstrual flares of acne or have not responded adequately to conventional therapy. Adolescents with endocrine disorders such as polycystic ovary syndrome also see improvement of their acne with hormonal therapy and spironolactone 50–100 mg PO bid. Oral contraceptives can be added to a conventional therapeutic regimen and should always be used in female patients who are prescribed oral isotretinoin unless absolute contraindications exist. There are growing data regarding the use of light, laser, and photodynamic therapy in acne. However, existing studies are of variable quality, and although there is evidence to suggest that these therapies offer benefit in acne, the evidence is not sufficient to recommend any device as monotherapy in acne.

F. Patient Education and Follow-up Visits

The multifactorial pathogenesis of acne and its role in the treatment plan must be explained to adolescent patients. Good general skin care includes washing the face consistently and using only oil-free, noncomedogenic cosmetics, face creams, and hair sprays. Acne therapy takes 8–12 weeks to produce improvement, and this delay must be stressed to the patient. Realistic expectations should be encouraged in the adolescent patient because no therapy will eradicate all future acne lesions. A written education sheet is useful. Follow-up visits should be made every 3–4 months. An objective method to chart improvement, including photographs, should be documented by the provider because patients' assessment of improvement can be inaccurate.

Bienenfeld A: Oral antibiotic therapy for acne vulgaris: an evidence-based review. Am J Clin Dermatol 2017;18(4):469–490 [PMID: 28255924].

Habeshiam KA et al: Current issues in the treatment of acne vulgaris. Pediatrics 2020 May;145(Suppl 2):S225–S230 [PMID: 32358215].

BACTERIAL INFECTIONS OF THE SKIN

1. Impetigo

Erosions covered by honey-colored crusts are diagnostic of impetigo. Staphylococci and group A streptococci in combination are the pathogens in this disease, which histologically consists of superficial invasion of bacteria into the upper epidermis, forming a subcorneal pustule.

▶ **Treatment**

Impetigo should be treated with an antimicrobial agent effective against *Staphylococcus aureus* and group A streptococci (β-lactamase–resistant penicillins or cephalosporins, clindamycin, amoxicillin–clavulanate) for 7–10 days. Topical mupirocin, polymyxin, gentamycin, and erythromycin are also effective but not recommended in children because of the need to eradicate nasopharyngeal carriage. In severe and recalcitrant cases, skin swab for bacterial culture should be performed prior to initiation of empiric antibiotic therapy.

2. Bullous Impetigo

In bullous impetigo there is, in addition to the usual erosion covered by a honey-colored crust, a border filled with clear fluid. Staphylococci may be isolated from these lesions, and systemic signs of circulating exfoliatin are absent. Bullous impetigo lesions can be found anywhere on the skin, but a common location is the diaper area.

▶ **Treatment**

Treatment with oral antibiotic for 7–10 days is effective. Application of cool compresses to debride crusts is a helpful symptomatic measure.

3. Ecthyma

Ecthyma is a firm, dry crust, surrounded by erythema that exudes purulent material. It represents invasion by group A β-hemolytic streptococci through the epidermis to the superficial dermis, therefore it is often referred as a deeper form of impetigo. This should not be confused with ecthyma gangrenosum. Lesions of ecthyma gangrenosum may be similar in appearance, but they are seen in a severely ill or immuno-compromised patient and are due to systemic dissemination of bacteria, usually *Pseudomonas aeruginosa*, through the bloodstream.

▶ **Treatment**

Treatment is with systemic penicillin.

4. Cellulitis

Cellulitis is characterized by erythematous, hot, tender, ill-defined, edematous plaques accompanied by regional lymphadenopathy. Histologically, this disorder represents invasion of microorganisms into the lower dermis and sometimes beyond, with obstruction of local lymphatics. Group A β-hemolytic streptococci and coagulase-positive staphylococci are the most common causes; pneumococci and *Haemophilus influenzae* (in younger unvaccinated children) are rare causes. Staphylococcal infections are usually more localized and more likely to have a purulent center; streptococcal infections spread more rapidly, but these characteristics cannot be used to specify the infecting agent. An entry site of prior trauma or infection (eg, varicella, dermatophyte) is often present. Septicemia is a potential complication.

▶ **Treatment**

Treatment is with an appropriate systemic antibiotic.

5. Folliculitis

A pustule at a follicular opening represents folliculitis. Deeper follicular infections are called furuncles (single follicle) and carbuncles (multiple follicles). Staphylococci and streptococci are the most frequent pathogens. Lesions are painless and tend to occur in crops, usually on the buttocks and extremities in children. Methicillin-resistant *S aureus* (MRSA) is now an increasing cause of folliculitis and skin abscesses. Cultures of persistent or recurrent folliculitis for MRSA are advisable.

▶ **Treatment**

Treatment consists of measures to remove follicular obstruction—either warm, wet compresses for 24 hours or topical keratolytics such as those used for acne. Topical or oral antistaphylococcal antibiotics may be required.

6. Abscess

An abscess occurs deep in the skin, at the bottom of a follicle or an apocrine gland, and is diagnosed as an erythematous, firm, acutely tender nodule with ill-defined borders. Staphylococci are the most common organisms.

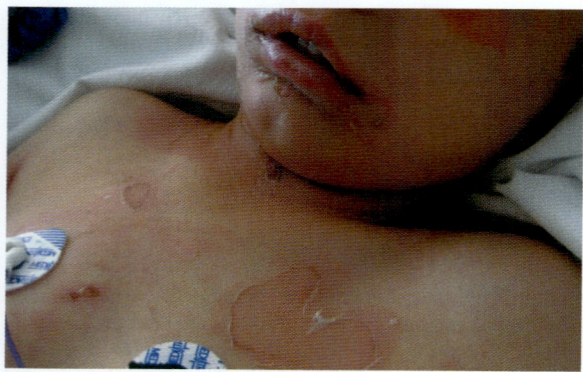

▲ **Figure 15–6.** Characteristic clinical findings in staphylococcal scalded skin syndrome.

▶ Treatment

Recent studies have suggested that incision and drainage alone may be adequate for uncomplicated MRSA skin abscesses in otherwise healthy patients. In more extensive cases adjuvant systemic antibiotics may be required.

7. Scalded Skin Syndrome

This entity consists of the sudden onset of bright red, acutely painful skin, most obvious perorally, periorbitally, and in the flexural areas of the neck, the axillae, the popliteal and antecubital areas, and the groin. The slightest pressure on the skin results in severe pain and separation of the epidermis (positive Nikolsky sign). The disease is caused by a circulating toxin (exfoliatin) elaborated by phage group II staphylococci. Exfoliatin binds to desmoglein-1 resulting in a separation of cells in the granular layer. The causative staphylococci may be isolated from the nasopharynx, an abscess, sinus, blood culture, joint fluid, or other focus of infection, but not from the skin (Figure 15–6).

▶ Treatment

Treatment is with systemic antistaphylococcal drugs.

McNeil JC, Fritz SA: Prevention strategies for recurrent community-associated *Staphylococcus aureus* skin and soft tissue infections. Curr Infect Dis Rep 2019 Mar 11;21(4):12 [PMID: 30859379].
Yamamoto LG: Treatment of skin and soft tissue infections. Pediatr Emerg Care 2017 Jan;33(1):49–55 [PMID: 28045842].

FUNGAL INFECTIONS OF THE SKIN

1. Dermatophyte Infections

Dermatophytes become attached to the superficial layer of the epidermis, nails, and hair, where they proliferate. Fungal infection should be suspected with any red and scaly lesion.

▶ Classification & Clinical Findings

A. Tinea Capitis

Thickened, broken-off hairs with erythema and scaling of underlying scalp are the distinguishing features (Table 15–3). Hairs are broken off at the surface of the scalp, leaving a "black dot" appearance. Diffuse scaling of the scalp and pustules are also seen. A boggy, fluctuant mass on the scalp called a kerion, represents an exaggerated host response to the organism. *Microsporum canis* and *Trichophyton tonsurans* are the cause. Fungal culture should be performed in all cases of suspected tinea capitis.

B. Tinea Corporis

Tinea corporis presents either as annular marginated plaques with a thin scale at the periphery and clear center or as an annular confluent dermatitis. The most common organisms are *Trichophyton mentagrophytes*, *Trichophyton rubrum*, and *M canis*. The diagnosis is made by scraping thin scales from the border of the lesion, dissolving them in 20% potassium hydroxide (KOH), and examining for hyphae (Figure 15–7).

C. Tinea Cruris

Symmetrical, sharply marginated lesions in inguinal areas occur with tinea cruris. The most common organisms are *T rubrum*, *T mentagrophytes*, and *Epidermophyton floccosum*.

D. Tinea Pedis

Tinea pedis presents with red scaly soles, blisters on the instep of the foot, or fissuring between the toes. *T rubrum* and *T mentagrophytes* are the cause.

Table 15–3. Clinical features of tinea capitis.

Most Common Organisms	Clinical Appearance	Microscopic Appearance in KOH
Trichophyton tonsurans (90%)	Hairs broken off 2-3 mm from follicle; "black dot"; diffuse pustule; seborrheic dermatitis-like; no fluorescence	Hyphae and spores within hair
Microsporum canis (10%)	Thickened broken-off hairs that fluoresce yellow-green with Wood lamp	Small spores outside of hair; hyphae within hair

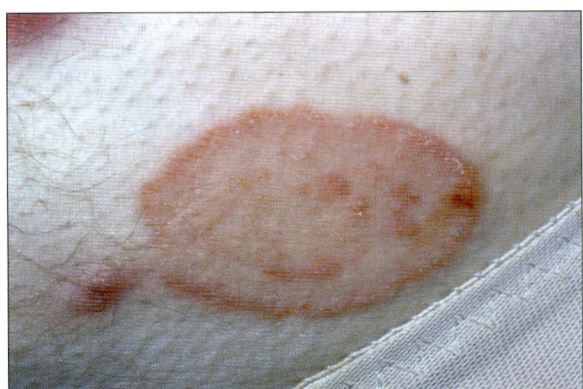

▲ **Figure 15–7.** Tinea corporis.

E. Tinea Unguium (Onychomycosis)

Loosening of the nail plate from the nail bed (onycholysis), giving a yellow discoloration, is the first sign of fungal invasion of the nails. Thickening of the distal nail plate then occurs, followed by scaling and a crumbly appearance of the entire nail plate surface. *T rubrum* is the most common cause. The diagnosis is confirmed by KOH examination and fungal culture. Usually only one or two nails are involved. If every nail is involved, psoriasis, lichen planus, or idiopathic trachyonychia is a more likely diagnosis than fungal infection.

▶ **Treatment**

The treatment of dermatophytosis is quite simple: If hair is involved (ie, scalp infections), systemic therapy is necessary. Griseofulvin and terbinafine are both effective. Terbinafine does not work for *M canis*. Topical antifungal agents do not enter hair or nails in sufficient concentration to clear the infection. The absorption of griseofulvin from the gastrointestinal tract is enhanced by a fatty meal; thus, whole milk or ice cream taken with the medication increases absorption. The dosage of griseofulvin is 20 mg/kg/day divided bid (maximum 500 mg/dose). With hair infections, cultures should be done every 4 weeks, and treatment should be continued for 4 weeks following a negative culture result. The side effects are few, and the drug has been used successfully in the newborn period. Terbinafine dosing is weight dependent: 62.5 mg/day, < 20 kg; 125 mg/day, 20–40 kg; 250 mg/day, > 40 kg. For nails, daily administration of topical ciclopirox 8% (Penlac nail lacquer) can be considered; however, success rates are lower than 20%, terbinafine can be used for 6–12 weeks or pulsed-dose itraconazole (50 mg/twice a day < 20 kg; 100 mg/twice a day, 20–40 kg; 200 mg/twice a day, > 40 kg) given in three 1-week pulses separated by 3 weeks.

Tinea corporis, tinea pedis, and tinea cruris can be treated effectively with topical medication after careful inspection to make certain that the hair and nails are not involved.

Treatment with any of the imidazoles, allylamines, benzylamines, or ciclopirox applied twice daily for 3–4 weeks is recommended.

Chen X et al: Systemic antifungal therapy for tinea capitis in children. Cochrane Database Syst Rev 2016 May 12;(5):CD004685 [PMID: 27169520].

2. Tinea Versicolor

Tinea versicolor is a superficial infection caused by *Malassezia globosa*, a yeast-like fungus. It characteristically causes polycyclic connected hypopigmented macules and very fine scales in areas of sun-induced pigmentation. In winter, the polycyclic macules appear reddish brown. Recurrent infection is common.

▶ **Treatment**

Treatment consists of application of selenium sulfide (Selsun), 2.5% suspension, zinc pyrithione shampoo, or topical antifungals. Selenium sulfide and zinc pyrithione shampoo should be applied to the whole body and left on overnight. Treatment can be repeated again in 1 week and then monthly thereafter. It tends to be somewhat irritating, and the patient should be warned about this difficulty. Topical antifungals are applied twice a day for 1–2 weeks. Fluconazole 400 mg single dose may also be used.

3. *Candida* Infections

▶ **Clinical Findings**

Candida albicans causes diaper dermatitis; thick, white patches on the oral mucosa (thrush); fissures at the angles of the mouth (perleche); and periungual erythema and nail plate abnormalities (chronic paronychia) (see also Chapter 43). *Candida* dermatitis is characterized by sharply defined erythematous patches, sometimes with eroded areas. Pustules, vesicles, or papules may be present as satellite lesions. Similar infections may be found in other moist areas, such as the axillae and neck folds. This infection is more common in children who have recently received antibiotics (Figure 15–8).

▶ **Treatment**

A topical imidazole cream is the drug of first choice for *C albicans* infections. In diaper dermatitis, the cream form can be applied twice a day. In oral thrush, nystatin suspension should be applied directly to the mucosa with the parent's finger or a cotton-tipped applicator. In candidal paronychia, the antifungal agent is applied over the area, covered with occlusive plastic wrapping, and left on overnight after the application is made airtight. Refractory candidiasis will respond to a brief course of oral fluconazole.

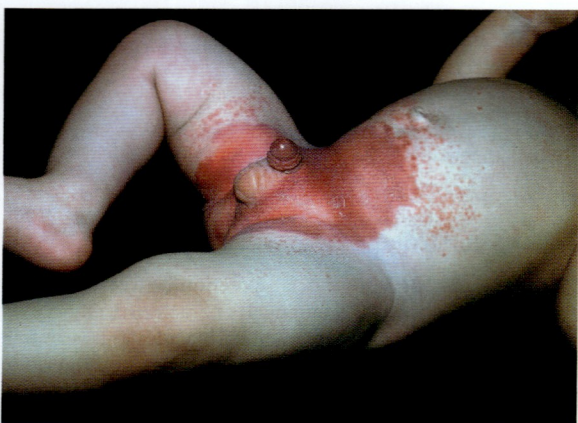

▲ **Figure 15–8.** Candidal diaper dermatitis.

VIRAL INFECTIONS OF THE SKIN

1. Herpes Simplex Infection

▶ Clinical Findings

Painful, grouped vesicles or erosions on a red base suggest herpes simplex (see also Chapter 40). Rapid immunofluorescent tests for herpes simplex virus (HSV) and varicella-zoster virus (VZV) are available. A Tzanck smear is done by scraping a vesicle base with a No. 15 blade, smearing on a glass slide, and staining the epithelial cells with Wright stain. The smear is positive if epidermal multinucleated giant cells are visualized. A positive Tzanck smear indicates herpesvirus infection (HSV or VZV). In infants and children, lesions resulting from herpes simplex type 1 are commonly seen on the gingiva, lips, and face. Involvement of a digit (herpes whitlow) will occur if the child sucks the thumb or fingers. Herpes simplex type 2 lesions are seen on the genitalia and in the mouth in adolescents. Cutaneous dissemination of herpes simplex occurs in patients with atopic dermatitis (eczema herpeticum) and appears clinically as very tender, monomorphic punched-out erosions among the eczematous skin changes. Herpes gladiatorum occurs on the face, lateral neck, and medial arms and is commonly seen in wrestlers and rugby players.

▶ Treatment

The treatment of HSV infections is discussed in Chapter 40.

2. Varicella-Zoster Infection

▶ Clinical Findings

Grouped vesicles in a dermatome, usually on the trunk or face, suggest varicella-zoster reactivation. Zoster in children may not be painful and usually has a mild course. In patients with compromised host resistance, the appearance of an erythematous border around the vesicles is a good prognostic sign. Conversely, large bullae without a tendency to crusting and systemic illness imply a poor host response to the virus. Varicella-zoster and herpes simplex lesions undergo the same series of changes: papule, vesicle, pustule, crust, slightly depressed scar. Lesions of primary varicella appear in crops, and many different stages of lesions are present at the same time (eg, papules), eccentrically placed vesicles on an erythematous base ("dew drop on a rose petal"), erosions, and crusts.

▶ Treatment

The treatment of VZV infections is discussed in Chapter 41.

3. Human Immunodeficiency Virus Infection

▶ Clinical Findings

The average time of onset of skin lesions after perinatally acquired human immunodeficiency virus (HIV) infection is 4 months; after transfusion-acquired infection, it is 11 months (see also Chapter 41). Persistent oral candidiasis and recalcitrant candidal diaper rash are the most frequent cutaneous features of infantile HIV infection. Severe or recurrent herpetic gingivostomatitis, varicella zoster infection, and molluscum contagiosum infection occur. Recurrent staphylococcal pyodermas, tinea of the face, and onychomycosis are also observed. A generalized dermatitis with features of seborrhea (severe cradle cap) is extremely common. In general, persistent, recurrent, or extensive skin infections should make one suspicious of HIV infection.

▶ Treatment

The treatment of HIV infections is discussed in Chapter 46.

VIRUS-INDUCED TUMORS

1. Molluscum Contagiosum

Molluscum contagiosum is a poxvirus that induces the epidermis to proliferate, forming a pale papule. Molluscum contagiosum consists of umbilicated, flesh-colored papules in groups anywhere on the body. They are common in infants and preschool children, as well as sexually active adolescents (Figure 15–9).

▶ Treatment

Treatment for molluscum is usually observational. Other treatments are either immunologic (topical imiquimod, oral cimetidine, intralesional *Candida* antigen injection) or cytodestructive (topical cantharidin, cryotherapy with more than 80%. Liquid nitrogen is painful, user dependent, and can lead to blistering and scarring. Topical salicylic acid may also be used. Large mosaic plantar warts are treated most effectively by applying 40% salicylic acid plaster cut with a scissors to fit the lesion. The adhesive side of the plaster is placed against the lesion and taped securely in place with duct or athletic tape. The plaster and tape should be placed on Monday through Friday. Over the weekend, the patient should soak the skin in warm water for 30 minutes to soften it. Then the white, macerated tissue should be pared with a pumice stone, cuticle scissors, or a nail file. This procedure is repeated every week, and the patient is seen every 4 weeks. Most plantar warts resolve in 6–8 weeks when treated in this way. Vascular pulsed dye lasers are a useful adjunct therapy for the treatment of warts.

For flat warts, a good response to 0.025% tretinoin gel or topical imiquimod cream, applied once daily for 3–4 weeks, has been reported. *C albicans* antigen, 0.3 mL injected every 4–6 weeks intradermally into the lesion for has been effective

Surgical excision, electrosurgery, and nonspecific burning laser surgery should be avoided; these modalities do not have higher cure rates and result in scarring. Cantharidin may cause small warts to become larger and should not be used.

Venereal warts (condylomata acuminata) (see Chapter 44) may be treated with imiquimod, 25% podophyllum resin (podophyllin) in alcohol, or podofilox, a lower concentration of purified podophyllin, which is applied at home. Podophyllin should be painted on the lesions in the practitioner's office and then washed off after 4 hours. Re-treatment in 2–3 weeks may be necessary. Podofilox is applied by the patient once daily, Monday through Thursday, whereas imiquimod is used three times a week on alternating days. Lesions not on the vulvar mucous membrane but on the adjacent skin should be treated as a common wart and frozen.

No wart therapy is immediately and definitively successful. Realistic expectations should be set and appropriate follow-up treatments scheduled.

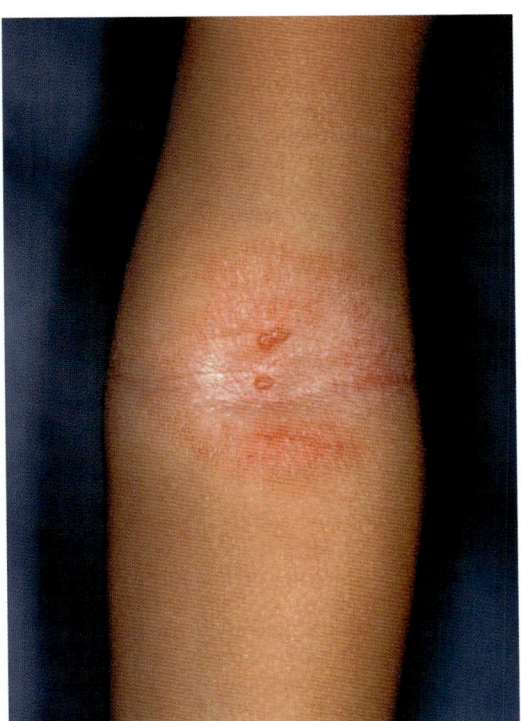

▲ **Figure 15–9.** Molluscum contagiosum with associated "molluscum dermatitis".

liquid nitrogen, and curettage). Destructive therapies can be painful and potentially scarring. Choosing not to treat is an appropriate alternative, depending on patient symptoms. Left untreated, the lesions resolve over months to years.

2. Warts

Warts are skin-colored papules with rough (verrucous) surfaces caused by infection with human papillomavirus (HPV). There are over 200 types of this DNA virus, which induces the epidermal cells to proliferate, thus resulting in the warty growth. Flat warts are smoother and smaller than common warts and are often seen on the face and other sun-exposed areas. Certain types of HPV are associated with certain types of warts (eg, flat warts) or location of warts (eg, genital warts).

▶ Treatment

Thirty percent of warts will clear in 12 months, and 60% will clear in 24 months. As with molluscum, the treatment of warts is also immunologic (topical imiquimod, oral cimetidine, intralesional *Candida* antigen injection, and squaric acid contact therapy) or cytodestructive. 5-fluoruracil applied directly to warts under occlusion for 12 weeks has been approved to be used in children with a success rate of

Gladsio JA et al: 5% 5-Fluorouracil cream for treatment of verruca vulgaris in children. Pediatr Dermatol 2009 May–Jun;26(3): 279–285 [PMID: 19706088].

Park IU, Introcaso C, Dunne EF: Human papillomavirus and genital warts: a review of the evidence for the 2015 Centers for Disease Control and Prevention Sexually Transmitted Diseases Treatment Guidelines. Clin Infect Dis 2015 Dec 15;61 (Suppl 8): S849–S855 [PMID: 26602622].

INSECT INFESTATIONS

1. Scabies

▶ Clinical Findings

Scabies is suggested by linear burrows about the wrists, ankles, finger webs, areolas, anterior axillary folds, genitalia, or face (in infants). Often there are excoriations, honey-colored crusts, and pustules from secondary infection. Identification of the female mite or her eggs and feces is necessary to confirm the diagnosis. Apply mineral oil to a No. 15 blade and scrape an unscratched papule or burrow and examine microscopically to confirm the diagnosis. In a child who is often scratching, scrape under the fingernails. Examine the parents for unscratched burrows.

▶ Treatment

Permethrin 5% is the treatment of choice for scabies. It should be applied as a single overnight application and repeated in 7 days to patient and household contacts. It is recommended that in children younger than 2 years, the application of topical permethrin cream should include the face. In older children and adults, this medication should be applied from the neck down. Oral ivermectin 200 mcg/dose × 1 and repeated in 7 days may be used in resistant cases.

2. Pediculoses (Louse Infestations)

▶ Clinical Findings

The presence of excoriated papules and pustules and a history of severe itching at night suggest infestation with the human body louse. This louse may be discovered in the seams of underwear but not on the body. In the scalp hair, the gelatinous nits of the head louse adhere tightly to the hair shaft. The pubic louse may be found crawling among pubic hairs, or blue-black macules may be found dispersed through the pubic region (maculae cerulea). The pubic louse is often seen on the eyelashes of newborns.

▶ Treatment

Initial treatment of head lice is often instituted by parents with an over-the-counter pyrethrin or permethrin product. These products are not ovicidal, and are more effective if nits are removed manually, by hand or with a lice comb. If head lice are not eradicated after two applications 7 days apart with these products, malathion 0.5% is ovicidal and highly effective but is toxic, if ingested, and flammable. A second application 7–9 days after initial treatment may be necessary. Other ovicidal products include topical ivermectin and spinosad (oral ivermectin is also effective but is not FDA approved for this indication). These ovicidal products do not require manual nit removal. Treatment of pubic lice is similar. Treatment of body lice is clean clothing and washing the infested clothing at high temperature.

3. Papular Urticaria

▶ Clinical Findings

Papular urticaria is characterized by grouped erythematous papules surrounded by an urticarial flare and distributed over the shoulders, upper arms, legs, and buttocks in infants. Although not a true infestation, these lesions represent delayed hypersensitivity reactions to stinging or biting insects. Fleas from dogs and cats are the usual offenders. Less commonly, mosquitoes, lice, scabies, and bird and grass mites are involved. The sensitivity is transient, lasting 4–6 months. Usually, no other family members are affected. It is often difficult for the parents to understand why no one else is affected.

▶ Treatment

The logical therapy is to remove the offending insect, although in most cases it is very difficult to identify the exact cause. Topical corticosteroids and oral antihistamines will control symptoms.

DERMATITIS (ECZEMA)

The terms *dermatitis* and *eczema* are currently used interchangeably in dermatology, although the term *eczema* truly denotes an acute weeping dermatosis. All forms of dermatitis, regardless of cause, may present with acute edema, erythema, and oozing with crusting, mild erythema alone, or lichenification. Lichenification is diagnosed by thickening of the skin with a shiny surface and exaggerated, deepened skin markings. It is the response of the skin to chronic rubbing or scratching.

Although the lesions of the various dermatoses are histologically indistinguishable, clinicians have nonetheless divided the disease group called dermatitis into several categories based on known causes in some cases and differing natural histories in others.

1. Atopic Dermatitis

ESSENTIALS OF DIAGNOSIS & TYPICAL FEATURES

▶ Clinical features of atopic dermatitis:

▶ Essential feature: Pruritus (or parental reporting of itching or rubbing) in the past 12 months, plus at least three of the following:

- History of generalized dry skin in the past 12 months
- Personal history of allergic rhinitis or asthma (or history in first-degree family member if patient is < 4 years old)
- Onset before 2 years of age
- History of skin crease involvement (antecubital or popliteal fossae, front of ankles, neck, periorbital)
- Visible flexural dermatitis (if child is < 4 years, include cheeks or forehead, and extensor surface of limbs)

Pathogenesis

Atopic dermatitis is a polygenic disease with positive and negative modifiers. Atopic dermatitis results from an interaction among susceptibility genes, the host environment, skin barrier defects, pharmacologic abnormalities, and immunologic response. The case for food and inhalant allergens as specific causes of atopic dermatitis is not strong. There is significant evidence that a primary defect in atopic dermatitis is an abnormality in the skin barrier formation due to defects in the filaggrin gene. Not all people with filaggrin abnormalities have atopic dermatitis and not all people with atopic dermatitis have filaggrin abnormalities.

Clinical findings

A. Symptoms and Signs

Most patients go through three clinical phases. In the first, infantile eczema, the dermatitis begins on the cheeks and scalp and frequently expresses itself as oval patches on the trunk, later involving the extensor surfaces of the extremities. The usual age at onset is 2–3 months, and this phase ends at age 18 months to 2 years. Only one-third of all infants with infantile eczema progress to phase 2 childhood or flexural eczema in which the predominant involvement is in the antecubital and popliteal fossae, the neck, the wrists, and sometimes the hands or feet. This phase lasts from age 2 years to adolescence. Only one-third of children with typical flexural eczema progress to adolescent eczema, which is usually manifested by the continuation of chronic flexural eczema along with hand and/or foot dermatitis. Atopic dermatitis is quite unusual after age 30 years.

Differential Diagnosis

All other types of dermatitis must be considered.

A few patients with atopic dermatitis have immunodeficiency with recurrent pyodermas, unusual susceptibility to HSVs, hyperimmunoglobulinemia E, defective neutrophil and monocyte chemotaxis, and impaired T-lymphocyte function (see Chapter 33).

Complications

A faulty epidermal barrier predisposes the patient with atopic dermatitis to dry, itchy skin. Inability to hold water within the stratum corneum results in rapid evaporation of water, shrinking of the stratum corneum, and cracks in the epidermal barrier. Such skin forms an ineffective barrier to the entry of various irritants. Chronic atopic dermatitis is frequently infected secondarily with S aureus or Streptococcus pyogenes. HSV virus may also superinfect atopic dermatitis and severe widespread disease is known as Kaposi's varicelliform eruption or eczema herpeticum. Patients with atopic dermatitis have a deficiency of antimicrobial peptides in their skin, which may account for the susceptibility to recurrent skin infection.

Treatment

Topical Glucocorticoids

Twice-daily application of topical corticosteroids is the mainstay of treatment for all forms of dermatitis (Table 15–4). Topical steroids can also be used under wet dressings. After wet dressings are discontinued, topical steroids should be applied only to areas of active disease. They should not be applied to normal skin to prevent recurrence. Only low-potency steroids (see Table 15–4) are applied to the face or intertriginous areas.

Wet Dressings

By placing the skin in an environment where the humidity is 100% and allowing the moisture to evaporate to 60%, pruritus is relieved. Evaporation of water stimulates cold-dependent nerve fibers in the skin, and this may prevent the transmission of the itching sensation via pain fibers to the CNS. It is also vasoconstrictive, thereby helping to reduce the erythema and also decreasing the inflammatory cellular response.

The simplest form of wet dressing consists of one set of wet underwear (eg, "long johns") worn under dry pajamas. Cotton socks are also useful for hand or foot treatment. The underwear should be soaked in warm (not hot) water and wrung out until no more water can be expressed.

Table 15–4. Topical glucocorticoids.

Glucocorticoid	Concentrations
Low potency[a] = 1–9	
Hydrocortisone	0.5%, 1%, 2.5%
Desonide	0.05%
Moderate potency = 10–99	
Mometasone furoate	0.1%
Hydrocortisone valerate	0.2%
Fluocinolone acetonide	0.025%
Triamcinolone acetonide	0.01%
Amcinonide	0.1%
High potency = 100–499	
Desoximetasone	0.25%
Fluocinonide	0.05%
Halcinonide	0.1%
Super potency = 500–7500	
Betamethasone dipropionate	0.05%
Clobetasol propionate	0.05%

[a]1% hydrocortisone is defined as having a potency of 1.

Dressings can be worn overnight for a few days up to 1 week. When the condition improves, wet dressings are discontinued.

Relief of Itching

If itching is significant, the use of oral antihistamines can be most helpful. A strategy of cetirizine 2.5–10 mg in the morning plus hydroxyzine 1 mg/kg in a single evening dose can be most effective.

A. Acute Stages of Dermatitis

Application of wet dressings and medium-potency topical corticosteroids is the treatment of choice for acute, weeping atopic eczema. The use of wet dressings is outlined at the beginning of this chapter. Superinfection with *S aureus*, *S pyogenes*, and HSV may occur, and appropriate systemic therapy may be necessary. If the expected improvement is not seen, bacterial and HSV cultures should be obtained to identify the possibility of a superinfection.

B. Chronic Stages of Dermatitis

Treatment is aimed at avoiding irritants and restoring moisture to the skin. No soaps or harsh shampoos should be used, and the patient should avoid woolen or any rough clothing. Bathing is minimized to every second or third day. Twice-daily lubrication of the skin is very important.

Nonperfumed creams or lotions are suitable lubricants. Plain petrolatum is an acceptable lubricant, but some people find it too greasy and during hot weather it may also cause considerable sweat retention. Liberal use of a thick moisturizer four to five times daily as a substitute for soap is also satisfactory as a means of lubrication. A bedroom humidifier is often helpful. Topical corticosteroids should be limited to medium strength (see Table 15–4). There is seldom a reason to use super or high-potency corticosteroids in atopic dermatitis. In superinfected atopic dermatitis, systemic antibiotics for 10–14 days are necessary.

Tacrolimus and pimecrolimus ointments are topical calcineurin-inhibitor immunosuppressive agents that are effective in atopic dermatitis. Because of concerns about the development of malignancies when similar medications are administered in high-dose IV forms, tacrolimus and pimecrolimus are usually reserved for children older than 2 years with atopic dermatitis unresponsive to low-potency topical steroids. It has been argued that an increased risk of malignancy has not been seen in immunologically normal individuals using these products. Narrow-band UV-B is recommended for extensive disease, starting with twice-weekly sessions in addition to topical steroids. Numerous immunosuppressive have been successful in controlling severe generalized eczema, including methotrexate, mycophenolate mofetil, azathioprine, or cyclosporine. Dupilumab (Dupixent) is the first biological therapy approved to treat atopic dermatitis in patients 6 months and older with moderate-to-severe atopic

dermatitis that is not well controlled with prescription topical or systemic therapies or who cannot use topical therapies. This antibody blocks IL-4 and IL-13, inhibiting immune system and subsequent inflammation. Several JAK inhibitor medications in oral and topical form have also received recent FDA approved for treatment of atopic dermatitis in patients over age 12. Leukotriene antagonists (used in asthma) are not effective.

Treatment failures in chronic atopic dermatitis are most often the result of noncompliance or nonadherence to a consistent therapy plan. This is a frustrating disease for parent and child. Return to a normal lifestyle for the parent and child is the ultimate goal of therapy.

Barrett M, Luu M: Differential diagnosis of atopic dermatitis. Immunol Allergy Clin North Am 2017 Feb;37(1):11–34 [PMID: 27886900].

Eichenfeld LF et al: Recent developments and advances in atopic dermatitis: a focus on epidemiology, pathophysiology, and treatment in the pediatric setting. Paediatr Drugs 2022 Jul;24(4): 293–305. [PMID: 35698002].

Yang EJ et al: Recent developments in atopic dermatitis. Pediatrics 2018 Oct;142(4). pii: e20181102 [PMID: 30266868].

1. Nummular Eczema

Nummular eczema is characterized by numerous symmetrically distributed coin-shaped patches of dermatitis, principally on the extremities. These may be acute, oozing, and crusted or dry and scaling. The differential diagnosis should include tinea corporis, impetigo, and atopic dermatitis.

▶ Treatment

The same topical measures should be used as for atopic dermatitis, although more potent topical steroids may be necessary.

2. Primary Irritant Contact Dermatitis (Diaper Dermatitis)

Contact dermatitis is of two types: primary irritant and allergic. Primary irritant dermatitis develops within a few hours, reaches peak severity at 24 hours, and then disappears. Allergic contact dermatitis (described in the next section) has a delayed onset of 18 hours, peaks at 48–72 hours, and often lasts as long as 2–3 weeks even if exposure to the offending antigen is discontinued.

Diaper dermatitis, the most common form of primary irritant contact dermatitis seen in pediatric practice, is caused by prolonged contact of the skin with urine and feces, which contain irritating chemicals such as urea and intestinal enzymes.

▶ Clinical Findings

The diagnosis of diaper dermatitis is based erythema and scaling of the skin in the perineal area and the history of prolonged skin contact with urine or feces, with sparing of inguinal folds. This is frequently seen in the "good baby" who sleeps many hours through the night without waking. In 80% of cases of diaper dermatitis lasting more than 3 days, the affected area is colonized with *C albicans* even before appearance of the classic signs of a beefy red, sharply marginated dermatitis with satellite lesions. Streptococcal perianal cellulitis and infantile psoriasis should be included in the differential diagnosis.

▶ Treatment

Treatment consists of changing diapers frequently. The area should only be washed with clean cloth and water following a bowel movement. Because rubber or plastic pants prevent evaporation of the contactant and enhance its penetration into the skin, they should be avoided as much as possible. Air drying is useful. Treatment of long-standing diaper dermatitis should include application of a barrier cream such as zinc oxide with each diaper change and an imidazole cream twice a day.

3. Allergic Contact Dermatitis

▶ Clinical Findings

Plants such as poison ivy, poison sumac, and poison oak cause most cases of allergic contact dermatitis in children. Allergic contact dermatitis has all the features of delayed type (T-lymphocyte–mediated) hypersensitivity. Many substances may cause such a reaction; other than plants, nickel sulfate, potassium dichromate, and neomycin are the most common causes. Nickel is found to some degree in all metals. Nickel allergy is commonly seen on the ears secondary to the wearing of earrings, and near the umbilicus from pants snaps and belt buckles. The true incidence of allergic contact dermatitis in children is unknown. Children often present with acute dermatitis with blister formation, oozing, and crusting. Blisters are often linear and of acute onset.

▶ Treatment

Treatment of contact dermatitis in localized areas is with potent topical corticosteroids. In severe generalized involvement, prednisone, 1–2 mg/kg/day orally for 10–14 days, can be used.

Brown C, Yu J: Pediatric allergic contact dermatitis. Immunol Allergy Clin North Am 2021 Aug;41(3):393–408 [PMID: 34225896].

4. Seborrheic Dermatitis

▶ Clinical Findings

Seborrheic dermatitis is an erythematous scaly dermatitis accompanied by overproduction of sebum occurring in areas rich in sebaceous glands (ie, the face, scalp, and perineum).

This common condition occurs predominantly in the newborn and at puberty, the ages at which hormonal stimulation of sebum production is maximal. Although it is tempting to speculate that overproduction of sebum causes the dermatitis, the exact relationship is unclear.

Seborrheic dermatitis on the scalp in infancy is clinically similar to atopic dermatitis, and the distinction may become clear only after other areas are involved. Psoriasis also occurs in seborrheic areas in older children and should be considered in the differential diagnosis.

▶ Treatment

Seborrheic dermatitis responds well to low-potency topical corticosteroids, antifungal shampoos (ketoconazole 1% or 2%), and antidandruff shampoos. For severe recalcitrant cases, pulse courses of oral itraconazole have been shown to be effective.

5. Dandruff

Dandruff is physiologic scaling or mild seborrhea, in the form of greasy scalp scales. The cause is unknown. Treatment is with medicated dandruff shampoos.

6. Dry Skin Dermatitis (Asteatotic Eczema, Xerosis)

Children who live in arid climates are susceptible to dry skin, characterized by large cracked scales with erythematous borders. The stratum corneum is dependent on environmental humidity for its water, and below 30% environmental humidity the stratum corneum loses water, shrinks, and cracks. These cracks in the epidermal barrier allow irritating substances to enter the skin, predisposing the patient to dermatitis.

▶ Treatment

Treatment consists of increasing the water content of the skin in the immediate external environment. House humidifiers are very useful. Minimize bathing to every second or third day.

Frequent soaping of the skin impairs its water-holding capacity and serves as an irritating alkali, and all soaps should therefore be avoided. Frequent use of emollients (eg, Cetaphil, Eucerin, Vaseline, Vanicream) should be a major part of therapy.

7. Keratosis Pilaris

Follicular papules containing a white inspissated scale characterize keratosis pilaris. Individual lesions are discrete and may be red. They are prominent on the extensor surfaces of the upper arms and thighs and on the buttocks and cheeks. In severe cases, the lesions may be generalized (Figure 15–10).

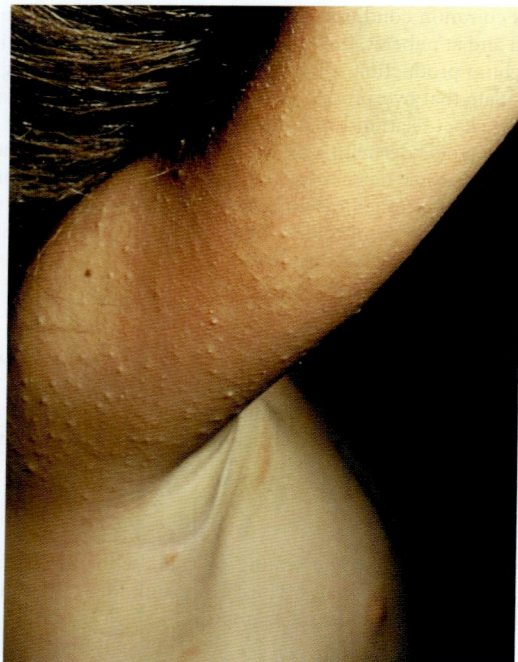

▲ **Figure 15–10.** Keratosis pilaris on the arm.

Treatment

Treatment is with keratolytics such as urea cream, salicylic acid, glycolic acid, or lactic acid, followed by skin hydration.

8. Pityriasis Alba

White, scaly macular areas with indistinct borders are seen over extensor surfaces of extremities and on the cheeks in children with pityriasis alba. Sun tanning exaggerates these lesions. Histologic examination reveals a mild dermatitis. These lesions may be confused with tinea versicolor.

Treatment

Low-potency topical corticosteroids may help decrease any inflammatory component and may lead to faster return of normal pigmentation. Strict sun avoidance and sun protection is also recommended.

COMMON SKIN TUMORS

If the skin moves with the nodule on lateral palpation, the tumor is located within the dermis; if the skin moves over the nodule, it is subcutaneous. Seventy-five percent of lumps in childhood will be either epidermoid cysts (60%) or pilomatricomas (15%).

1. Epidermoid Cysts

Clinical Findings

Epidermoid cysts are the most common type of cutaneous cyst. Other names for epidermoid cysts are epidermal cysts, epidermal inclusion cysts, and "sebaceous" cysts. This last term is a misnomer since they contain neither sebum nor sebaceous glands. Epidermoid cysts can occur anywhere but are most common on the face and upper trunk. They usually arise from and are lined by the stratified squamous epithelium of the follicular infundibulum. Clinically, epidermoid cysts are dermal nodules with a central punctum, representing the follicle associated with the cyst. They can reach several centimeters in diameter. **Dermoid cysts** are areas of sequestration of skin along embryonic fusion lines. They are present at birth and occur most commonly on the lateral eyebrow. When present in the midline nasal dorsum, they develop a superficial pit. Imaging prior to any intervention is recommended in this case to evaluate for intracranial connection (Figure 15–11).

Treatment

Epidermoid cysts can rupture, causing a foreign-body inflammatory reaction, or become infected. Infectious complications should be treated with antibiotics. Definitive treatment of epidermoid and dermoid cysts is surgical excision.

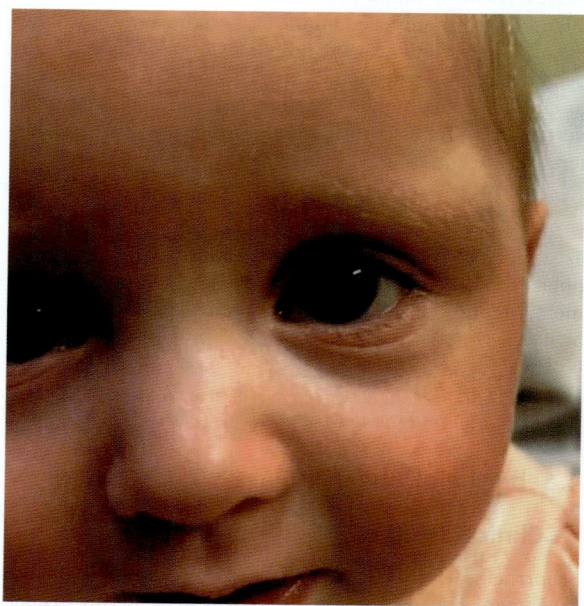

▲ **Figure 15–11.** Dermoid cyst of the left lateral brow.

2. Pilomatricomas

These are benign tumors of the hair matrix. They are most commonly seen on the face and upper trunk. They are firm, multilobuled dermal nodules. Their color varies, flesh colored or blue. The firmness is secondary to calcification of the tumor.

▶ Treatment

Treatment is by surgical excision.

3. Granuloma Annulare

Violaceous circles or semicircles of nontender intradermal nodules found over the lower legs and ankles, the dorsum of the hands and wrists, and the trunk suggest granuloma annulare. Histologically, the disease appears as a central area of tissue death (necrobiosis) surrounded by macrophages and lymphocytes (Figure 15–12).

▶ Treatment

No treatment is necessary. Lesions resolve spontaneously within 1–2 years in most children.

4. Pyogenic Granuloma

These lesions appear over 1–2 weeks at times following skin trauma as a dark red papule with an ulcerated and crusted surface that may bleed easily with minor trauma. Histologically, this represents excessive new vessel formation with or without inflammation (granulation tissue). It should be regarded as an abnormal healing response.

▶ Treatment

Pulsed dye laser, Imiquimod 5% cream and Timolol 0.05% GFS daily have been successful in treating very small lesions. Curettage followed by electrocautery is the treatment of choice for larger or recurrent lesions.

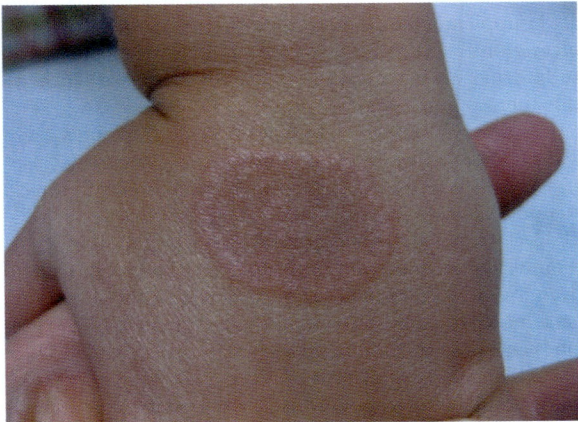

▲ **Figure 15–12.** Granuloma annulare.

5. Keloids

Keloids are scars of delayed onset that continue to grow for up to several years and to progress beyond the initial wound margins. The tendency to develop keloids is inherited. They are often found on the face, earlobes, neck, chest, and back.

▶ Treatment

Treatment includes intralesional injection with triamcinolone acetonide, 20–40 mg/mL, or excision and injection with corticosteroids. For larger keloids, excision followed by postoperative radiotherapy may be indicated.

PAPULOSQUAMOUS ERUPTIONS

Papulosquamous eruptions (Table 15–5) comprise papules or plaques with varying degrees of scale.

1. Pityriasis Rosea

▶ Pathogenesis & Clinical Findings

Pink to red, oval plaques with fine scales that tend to align with their long axis parallel to skin tension lines (eg, "Christmas tree pattern" on the back) are characteristic lesions of pityriasis rosea. The generalized eruption is usually preceded for up to 30 days by a solitary, larger, scaling plaque with central clearing and a scaly border (the herald patch). The herald patch is clinically similar to ringworm and can be confused. In whites, the lesions are primarily on the trunk; in blacks, lesions are primarily on the extremities and may be accentuated in the axillary and inguinal areas (inverse pityriasis rosea).

This disease is common in school-aged children and adolescents and is presumed to be viral in origin. The role of human herpesvirus 7 in the pathogenesis of pityriasis rosea is debated. The condition lasts 6–12 weeks and may be pruritic.

▶ Differential Diagnosis

The major differential diagnosis is secondary syphilis, and a VDRL (Venereal Disease Research Laboratories) test should be done if syphilis is suspected, especially in high-risk patients

Table 15–5. Papulosquamous eruptions in children.

Psoriasis
Pityriasis rosea
Tinea corporis
Lichen planus
Pityriasis lichenoides (acute or chronic)
Dermatomyositis
Lupus erythematosus
Pityriasis rubra pilaris
Secondary syphilis

with palm or sole involvement. Fever and widespread lymph-adenopathy are often found in secondary syphilis. "Pityriasis rosea" lasting more than 12 weeks is likely to be pityriasis lichenoides.

Treatment

Exposure to natural sunlight may help hasten the resolution of lesions. Oral antihistamines and topical steroids can be used for pruritus. Often, no treatment is necessary. Pityriasis rosea that lasts more than 12 weeks should be referred to a dermatologist for evaluation.

2. Psoriasis

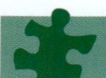

ESSENTIALS OF DIAGNOSIS & TYPICAL FEATURES

▶ Erythematous papules and plaques with thick, white scales.

▶ Elbows, knees, and scalp often affected.

▶ Nail pitting and distal onycholysis.

Pathogenesis

The pathogenesis of psoriasis is complex and incompletely understood. It has immune-mediated inflammation, is a familial condition, and multiple psoriasis susceptibility genes have been identified. There is increased epidermal turnover; psoriatic epidermis has a turnover time of 3–4 days versus 28 days for normal skin. These rapidly proliferating epidermal cells produce excessive stratum corneum, giving rise to thick, opaque scales.

Clinical Findings

Psoriasis is characterized by erythematous papules covered by thick white scales. Guttate (drop like) psoriasis is a common form in children that often follows by 2–3 weeks an episode of streptococcal pharyngitis. The sudden onset of small papules (3–8 mm), seen predominantly over the trunk and quickly covered with thick white scales, is characteristic of guttate psoriasis. Chronic psoriasis is marked by thick, large scaly plaques (5–10 cm) over the elbows, knees, scalp, and other sites of trauma. Pinpoint pits in the nail plate are seen, as well as yellow discoloration of the nail plate resulting from onycholysis. Psoriasis occurs frequently on the scalp, elbows, knees, periumbilical area, ears, sacral area, and genitalia.

Differential Diagnosis

Papulosquamous eruptions that present problems of differential diagnosis are listed in Table 15–5.

Treatment

Topical corticosteroids are the initial treatment of choice. Penetration of topical steroids through the enlarged epidermal barrier in psoriasis requires that more potent preparations be used, for example, fluocinonide 0.05% (Lidex) or clobetasol 0.05% (Temovate) ointment twice daily.

The second line of therapy is topical vitamin D_3 medications such as calcipotriene (Dovonex) or, calcitriol (Vectical), applied twice daily or the combination of a superpotent topical steroid twice daily on weekends and calcipotriene or calcitriol twice daily on weekdays.

Topical retinoids such as tazarotene (0.1%, 0.5% cream, gel) can be used in combination with topical corticosteroids to help restore normal epidermal differentiation and turnover time.

Anthralin therapy is also useful. Anthralin is applied to the skin for a short contact time (eg, 20 minutes once daily) and then washed off with a neutral soap (eg, Dove). This can be used in combination with topical corticosteroids.

Crude coal tar therapy is messy and stains bedclothes. The newer tar gels (Estar, PsoriGel) and one foam product (Scytera) cause less staining and are most efficacious. They are applied twice daily. These preparations are sold over the counter and are not usually covered by insurance plans.

Scalp care using a tar shampoo requires leaving the shampoo on for 5 minutes, washing it off, and then shampooing with commercial shampoo to remove scales. It may be necessary to shampoo daily until scaling is reduced.

More severe cases of psoriasis are best treated by a dermatologist. Narrow band UVB phototherapy and multiple systemic medications and new biologic agents (antibodies, fusion proteins, and recombinant cytokines) are effective in more widespread, severe cases. Methotrexate given at a dose of 0.3–0.6 mg/kg PO weekly is generally well tolerated by patients. Common side effects include nausea, abdominal pain, fatigue, headaches, and anorexia. Folic acid supplementation decreases risk of nausea, mucosal ulcerations, and macrocytic anemia. Live vaccines and sulfa drugs are not recommended while the patient is on this therapy.

Systemic retinoids are given at a dose of 0.5–1 mg/kg/day. They are very effective for erythrodermic and pustular psoriasis and are more efficacious when combined with topical steroids, UV light, methotrexate, or cyclosporine.

Cyclosporine is given at a dose of 3–5 mg/kg/day for 3–4 months and then titrated off. Side effects include renal and liver toxicity, hypertrichosis, and increased risk for future leukemias, lymphomas, and cutaneous carcinomas. Live vaccines and macrolide antibiotics are not recommended while the patient is on this therapy.

Biologics are a growing field in the treatment of childhood psoriasis and are best managed in a consultative dermatology setting.

Menter A et al: Joint American Academy of Dermatology-National Psoriasis Foundation guidelines of care for the management and treatment of psoriasis in pediatric patients. J Am Acad Dermatol 2020 Jan;82(1):161–201 [PMID: 31703821].

Relvas M, Torres T: Pediatric psoriasis. Am J Clin Dermatol 2017 Dec;18(6):797–811 [PMID: 28540590].

HAIR LOSS (ALOPECIA)

Hair loss in children (Table 15–6) imposes great emotional stress on the patient and the parent. A 60% hair loss in a single area is necessary before hair loss can be detected clinically. Examination should begin with the scalp to determine whether inflammation, scale, or infiltrative changes are present. The hair should be gently pulled to see if it is easily removable. Hairs should be examined microscopically for breaking and structural defects and to see whether growing or resting hairs are being shed. Placing removed hairs in mounting fluid (Permount) on a glass microscope slide makes them easy to examine.

Three diseases account for most cases of hair loss in children: alopecia areata, tinea capitis (described earlier in this chapter), and hair pulling.

1. Alopecia Areata

▶ **Clinical Findings**

Complete hair loss in a localized area is called alopecia areata. This is the most common cause of hair loss in children. An immunologic pathogenic mechanism is suspected because dense infiltration of lymphocytes precedes hair loss. Fifty percent of children with alopecia areata completely regrow their hair within 12 months, although as many may have a relapse in the future.

A rare and unusual form of alopecia areata begins at the occiput and proceeds along the hair margins to the frontal scalp. This variety, called *ophiasis*, often eventuates in total scalp hair loss (alopecia totalis). The prognosis for regrowth in ophiasis is poor.

▶ **Treatment**

Superpotent topical steroids, minoxidil (Rogaine), contact therapy, and anthralin are topical treatment options. Systemic corticosteroids given to suppress the inflammatory response will result in hair growth, but the hair may fall out again when the drug is discontinued. Systemic corticosteroids should never be used for a prolonged time period. In children with alopecia totalis, a wig may be helpful. Treatment induced hair growth does not alter risk of recurrence. New therapies including topical and systemic Janus kinase (JAK) inhibitors have obtained recent FDA approval for treatment of alopecia areata in children older than 12.

Barton VR et al. Treatment of pediatric alopecia areata: a systematic review. J Am Acad Dermatol 2022. Jun;86(6):1318-1334. [PMID: 33940103].

2. Hair Pulling

▶ **Clinical Findings**

Traumatic hair pulling causes the hair shafts to be broken off at different lengths, with an ill-defined area of hair loss, petechiae around follicular openings, and a wrinkled hair shaft on microscopic examination. This behavior may be merely habit, an acute reaction to severe stress, trichotillomania, or a sign of another psychiatric disorder. Eyelashes and eyebrows rather than scalp hair may be pulled out.

▶ **Treatment**

If the behavior has a long history, psychiatric evaluation may be helpful. Cutting or oiling the hair to make it slippery is an aid to behavior modification.

REACTIVE ERYTHEMAS

1. Erythema Multiforme

▶ **Clinical Findings**

Erythema multiforme begins with papules that later develop a dark center and then evolve into lesions with central bluish discoloration or blisters and the characteristic target lesions (iris lesions) that have three concentric circles of color change. Erythema multiforme has sometimes been diagnosed in patients with severe mucous membrane involvement, but Stevens-Johnson syndrome is the diagnosis when severe involvement of conjunctiva, oral cavity, and genital mucosa also occur.

Many causes are suspected, particularly concomitant HSV; drugs, especially sulfonamides; and *Mycoplasma* infections.

Table 15–6. Other causes of hair loss in children.

Hair loss with scalp changes
Atrophy:
Lichen planus
Lupus erythematosus
Birthmarks:
Epidermal nevus
Nevus sebaceous
Aplasia cutis congenita
Hair loss with hair shaft defects (hair fails to grow out enough to require haircuts)
Monilethrix—alternating bands of thin and thick areas
Pili annulati—alternating bands of light and dark pigmentation
Pili torti—hair twisted 180 degrees, brittle
Trichorrhexis invaginata (bamboo hair)—intussusception of one hair into another
Trichorrhexis nodosa—nodules with fragmented hair

Recurrent erythema multiforme is usually associated with reactivation of HSV. In erythema multiforme, spontaneous healing occurs in 10–14 days, but Stevens-Johnson syndrome may last 6–8 weeks.

▶ **Treatment**

Treatment is symptomatic in uncomplicated erythema multiforme. Removal of offending drugs is an obvious measure. Oral antihistamines such as cetirizine 5–10 mg every morning and hydroxyzine 1 mg/kg/day at bedtime are useful. Cool compresses and wet dressings will relieve pruritus. Steroids have not been demonstrated to be effective. Chronic acyclovir therapy has been successful in decreasing attacks in patients with herpes-associated recurrent erythema multiforme.

2. Drug Eruptions

Drugs may produce urticarial, morbilliform, scarlatiniform, pustular, bullous, or fixed skin eruptions. Urticaria may appear within minutes after drug administration, but most reactions begin 7–14 days after the drug is first administered. These eruptions may occur in patients who have received these drugs for long periods, and eruptions continue for days after the drug has been discontinued. Drug eruptions with fever, eosinophilia, and systemic symptoms (DRESS syndrome) is most commonly seen with anticonvulsants but may be seen with other drugs. Drugs commonly implicated in skin reactions are listed in Table 15–7.

Table 15–7. Common drug reactions.

Urticaria
Barbiturates
Opioids
Penicillins
Sulfonamides
Morbilliform eruption
Anticonvulsants
Cephalosporins
Penicillins
Sulfonamides
Fixed drug eruption, erythema multiforme, toxic epidermal necrolysis, Stevens-Johnson syndrome
Anticonvulsants
Nonsteroidal anti-inflammatory drugs
Sulfonamides
DRESS syndrome
Anticonvulsants
Photodermatitis
Psoralens
Sulfonamides
Tetracyclines
Thiazides

DRESS syndrome, drug eruptions with fever, eosinophilia, and systemic symptoms.

Heinze A et al: Characteristics of pediatric recurrent erythema multiforme. Pediatr Dermatol 2018 Jan;35(1):97–103 [PMID: 29231254].

MISCELLANEOUS SKIN DISORDERS SEEN IN PEDIATRIC PRACTICE

1. Aphthous Stomatitis

Recurrent erosions on the gums, lips, tongue, palate, and buccal mucosa are often confused with herpes simplex. A smear of the base of such a lesion stained with Wright stain will aid in ruling out herpes simplex by the absence of epithelial multinucleate giant cells. A culture for herpes simplex is also useful in differential diagnostics. The cause remains unknown, but T-cell–mediated cytotoxicity to various viral antigens has been postulated.

TREATMENT

There is no specific therapy for this condition. Rinsing the mouth with liquid antacids provides relief in most patients. Topical corticosteroids in a gel base may provide some relief. In severe cases that interfere with eating, prednisone, 1 mg/kg/day orally for 3–5 days, will suffice to abort an episode. Colchicine, 0.2–0.5 mg/day, sometimes reduces the frequency of attacks.

2. Vitiligo

Vitiligo is characterized clinically by the development of areas of depigmentation. These are often symmetrical and occur mainly on extensor surfaces. The depigmentation results from a destruction of melanocytes. The basis for this destruction is unknown, but immunologically mediated damage is likely and vitiligo sometimes occurs in individuals with autoimmune endocrinopathies.

TREATMENT

Treatment is with potent topical steroids or tacrolimus. Topical calcipotriene has also been used. Narrow-band ultraviolet B radiation (UVB 311 nm) in booth or via handheld device ("excimer" laser) may be used in many cases. The topical JAK inhibitor ruxolitinib was recently FDA approved for treatment of non-segmental vitiligo in patients over age 12. Response to treatment of all types is slow, often requiring many months to years.

Roohaninasab M et al: Therapeutic options and hot topics in vitiligo with special focus on pediatrics' vitiligo: a comprehensive review study. Dermatol Ther 202 1Jan;34(1):e14550 [PMID: 33200859].

Eye

Lauren Mehner, MD, MPH
Jennifer Lee Jung, MD

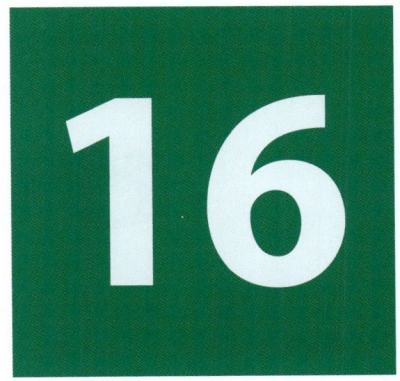

16

INTRODUCTION

Normal vision is a sense that develops during infancy and childhood. Pediatric ophthalmology emphasizes early diagnosis and treatment of pediatric eye diseases to obtain the best possible visual outcome. Eye disease can also be a manifestation of systemic disease.

COMMON NONSPECIFIC SIGNS & SYMPTOMS

Nonspecific signs and symptoms commonly occur as the chief complaint or as an element of the history of a child with eye disease. Five of these findings are described here, along with a sixth—abnormal red reflex.

RED EYE

Redness (injection, hyperemia) of the bulbar conjunctiva or deeper vessels is a common presenting complaint. It may be localized or diffuse. Causes include infection, inflammation (ocular or systemic), allergy, irritation from noxious agents (acidic or alkali exposure), and trauma. Subconjunctival hemorrhage may be traumatic, spontaneous, or associated with hematopoietic disease, vascular anomalies, or inflammatory processes.

TEARING

Tearing in infants is usually due to nasolacrimal obstruction but may also be associated with congenital glaucoma, in which case photophobia and blepharospasm may also be present. Any irritation in the eye can cause tearing including infections, allergy, and dryness.

DISCHARGE

Purulent discharge is usually associated with bacterial conjunctivitis. *Watery discharge* occurs with viral conjunctivitis/keratitis, iritis, and corneal abrasions/foreign bodies. *Mucoid discharge* may be a sign of allergic conjunctivitis or nasolacrimal obstruction. Infants with nasolacrimal duct obstruction (NLDO) commonly have tearing associated with yellow crusts, but their eye remains white and quiet. A mucoid discharge due to allergy typically contains eosinophils, whereas a purulent bacterial discharge contains polymorphonuclear leukocytes.

PAIN & FOREIGN-BODY SENSATION

Pain in or around the eye may be due to foreign bodies, corneal abrasions, lacerations, acute infections of the globe or ocular adnexa, iritis, and elevated eye pressure. Large refractive errors or poor accommodative ability may manifest as headaches and eye strain. Trichiasis (misdirected lashes) and contact lens problems also cause ocular discomfort.

PHOTOPHOBIA

Acute aversion to light may occur with corneal abrasions, foreign bodies, and uveitis. Squinting of one eye in bright light is a common sign of intermittent exotropia (eye drifting). Photophobia is present in infants with glaucoma, albinism, aniridia, and retinal dystrophies such as achromatopsia. Photophobia is common after ocular surgery and after pharmacologic dilation of the pupil.

ABNORMAL RED REFLEX

Checking for an abnormal red reflex is a crucial part of every pediatric examination starting from the newborn period. Abnormal red reflex can be unilateral or bilateral. Any abnormality altering the penetration of light into the retina can result in abnormal red reflex. This includes cloudy corneas, cloudy lens (cataracts), abnormality in the retina itself, and significant refractive errors (nearsightedness, farsightedness, astigmatism). Causes of cloudy corneas include congenital glaucoma, Peter anomaly, infections, and anterior segment

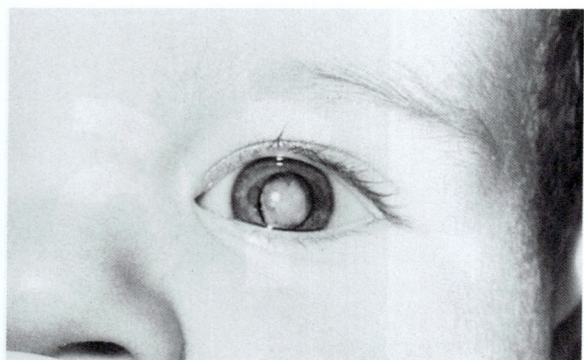

▲ **Figure 16–1.** Leukocoria of the left eye caused by congenital cataract.

dysgenesis. Leukocoria (white pupil) can be caused by cataracts or retinal problems like retinoblastoma (RB), retinal detachment, *Toxocara* infection, and Coats disease (nonhereditary retinal vascular disorder) (Figure 16–1).

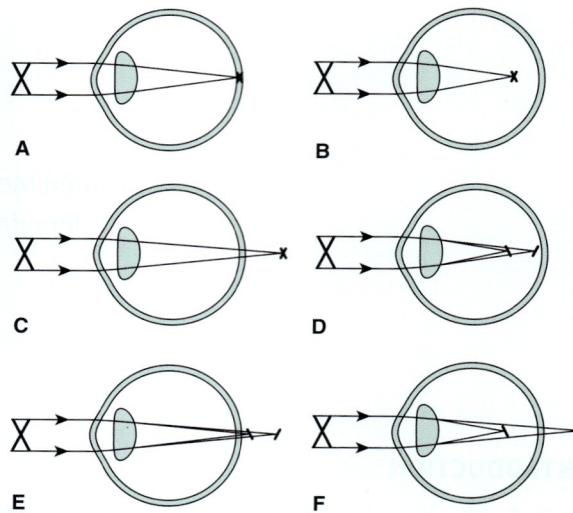

▲ **Figure 16–2.** Different refractive states of the eye. **A:** Emmetropia. Image plane from parallel rays of light falls on retina. **B:** Myopia. Image plane focuses anterior to retina. **C:** Hyperopia. Image plane focuses posterior to retina. **D:** Astigmatism, myopic type. Images in horizontal and vertical planes focus anterior to retina. **E:** Astigmatism, hyperopic type. Images in horizontal and vertical planes focus posterior to retina. **F:** Astigmatism, mixed type. Images in horizontal and vertical planes focus on either side of retina.

REFRACTIVE ERRORS

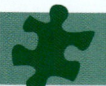
ESSENTIALS OF DIAGNOSIS & TYPICAL FEATURES

▶ Significant refractive errors (myopia, hyperopia, astigmatism, or anisometropia) may cause decreased visual acuity (VA), refractive amblyopia, and strabismus.

▶ Symptoms and signs of uncorrected refractive error include blurred vision, squinting, headaches, fatigue with visual tasks, and failed vision screening.

▶ Pathogenesis

Refractive error refers to the optical state of the eye (Figure 16–2). The shape of the cornea and, to a lesser extent, the shape of the lens and length of the eye play a role in the refractive state of the eye. Children at particular risk for refractive errors requiring correction with glasses include those who are born prematurely; have Down syndrome; have parents with refractive errors; or have certain systemic conditions such as Stickler, Marfan, or Ehlers-Danlos syndrome.

▶ Diagnosis

There are three common refractive errors: myopia, hyperopia, and astigmatism. High refractive errors or inequality of the refractive state between the two eyes (anisometropia) can cause amblyopia (reduced vision caused by conditions affecting normal vision development). The refractive state can be determined by instrument-based screening or by an eye care professional. The use of the autorefractor in children can overestimate the amount of nearsightedness. Cycloplegia is used to fully relax their accommodation, and the process of retinoscopy is used to determine the accurate refractive error in children.

▶ Treatment

Refractive errors in children are most commonly treated with glasses. An eye care professional can determine if the refractive error requires treatment. Contact lenses are prescribed for children with very high or asymmetrical refractive errors and adolescents who do not want to wear glasses. Laser refractive surgery is not indicated for most children.

MYOPIA (NEARSIGHTEDNESS)

For the myopic individual, objects nearby are in focus; those at a distance are blurred. There is a global rise in prevalence of myopia. Onset is typically in elementary school age and often progresses throughout adolescence and young adulthood.

A myopic person may squint to produce a pinhole effect, which improves distance vision. Treatment requires glasses or contact lenses. Daily use of low-dose atropine 0.01% eye drops has been shown to slow myopia progression by approximately 50%. Side effects include minimal pupil dilation and loss of accommodation without reduction in VA.

HYPEROPIA (FARSIGHTEDNESS)

A hyperopic child is able to see clearly both at distance and at near because the child can focus on near objects through the process of accommodation if the hyperopia is not excessive. Large amounts of uncorrected hyperopia can cause esotropia (crossed eyes) as accommodation and convergence are closely linked. Most young children have hyperopic refraction that diminishes with age and does not require glasses.

ASTIGMATISM

When either the cornea or the crystalline lens is not perfectly spherical, an image will not be sharply focused in one plane. Schematically, there will be two planes of focus. This refractive state is described as *astigmatism*. Large amounts of astigmatism can cause amblyopia, and it is treated with glasses or toric contact lenses. Keratoconus is a corneal disorder that results in progressive corneal thinning and irregular astigmatism and requires special attention. It is more commonly seen in children with Down syndrome, atopy, and connective tissue disorders.

OPHTHALMIC EXAMINATION

The ophthalmic examination should be a part of every well-child assessment. A history of poor vision, misalignment of the eyes, failed vision screening, eyelid malposition, abnormal pupil reactivity or shape, and an asymmetric/abnormal red reflex requires referral to an ophthalmologist. Prompt detection and treatment of ocular conditions can prevent a lifetime of visual disability.

From birth to 3 years of age, the ophthalmic examination should include taking a history for ocular problems, vision assessment, inspection of the eyelids and eyes, pupil examination, ocular motility assessment, and red reflex check. Instrument-based screening may be attempted at this age.

The ophthalmic examination of children older than 3 years should include all of the previously mentioned tests and VA testing with eye charts such as HOTV, Snellen, or LEA. Testing of binocular vision, or the use of both eyes at the same time, can be accomplished by various stereoacuity tests. Instrument-based screening can identify children with amblyogenic risk factors and are particularly useful in children with language barriers or cognitive delays. See AAPOS.org for vision screening and referral recommendations.

HISTORY

Elements of the ocular history include onset of the complaint, its duration, laterality, previous treatment, and associated systemic symptoms. If an infectious disease is suspected, ask about possible contact with others having similar findings. The history should include prior ocular disease, perinatal and developmental history, history of allergy, and history of familial ocular disorders.

VISUAL ACUITY

Visual acuity (VA) testing is the most important test of visual function and should be part of every well-child check.

In the sleeping newborn, the presence of lid squeezing to bright light is an adequate response. At age 6 weeks, eye-to-eye contact with slow, following movements is usually present. By age 3 months, the infant should demonstrate fixing and following ocular movements for objects at a distance of 2–3 ft. At age 6 months, interest in movement across the room is the norm. Vision can be recorded for the presence or absence of fixing and following behavior, and whether vision is steady (unsteady when nystagmus is present) and maintained when the other eye is uncovered.

Children who can identify or match objects on a chart can provide direct measurements of their VA. This may be possible in children as young as 3 years. Vision is tested first with both eyes open on large optotypes to ensure that the child understands the test. Then, vision should be tested monocularly, preferably with one eye patched (with tape or occlusive patch) to prevent peeking. Glasses should be worn during vision test.

Currently preferred optotypes are LEA and HOTV symbols. For those who can identify letters, Snellen or Sloan charts are recommended. Most accurate assessment is obtained when using charts with lines of optotypes (letter or symbol) or single optotype with crowding bars around it. Using single optotypes without crowding bars can overestimate VA. Crowding bars surrounding an optotype make individual letters more difficult to identify by an amblyopic eye, thus increasing the sensitivity to detect amblyopia.

"Critical line" screening is an effective method for identifying children with potentially serious vision problems and can be administered more quickly than the "threshold" method of starting at the top and reading down to the smallest discernable line. The "critical line" is the age-dependent line a child is expected to see and pass. This critical line to pass becomes smaller in size as age increases. Most eye charts have four to six optotypes per line. Passing the screening requires the child to correctly answer the majority of the optotypes present on the critical line appropriate for his or her age (Table 16–1).

Children with nystagmus (eye shaking) require special considerations during vision testing. They may have a compensatory head position (head turn or tilt) to achieve their

Table 16–1. "Critical line" vision screening evaluation.

Age (mo)	Critical Line for Vision
36–47	20/50
48–59	20/40
≥ 60	20/30 or 20/32 in some charts

null point (where shakiness is dampened). Because VA can decrease when forced to face straight ahead, these children should be tested in their compensatory head positions. In addition, children with nystagmus often also have "latent nystagmus," which results in worsened shakiness when one eye is covered. For this reason, testing both eyes simultaneously without occlusion gives a better VA measurement than when either eye is tested individually.

Instrument-based screening modalities including photo screeners and autorefractors are used by various volunteer programs, schools, daycare facilities, and physician offices. Instrument screening does not screen directly for amblyopia but rather for amblyogenic factors that include strabismus, media opacities, eyelid ptosis, and refractive errors depending on the device. If the screening results suggest an amblyogenic factor, children are referred to an eye care professional for a complete eye examination. Problems exist with sensitivity and specificity of the instruments and poor follow-up for referrals to eye care professionals. If available, instrument-based screening can be initiated beginning at age 12 months. Once children can read, optotype-based acuity should supplement instrument-based testing.

American Academy of Ophthalmology: Visual screening for Infants and Children—2022. October 2022. https://www.aao.org/education/clinical-statement/vision-screening-infants-children-2022.

Donahue SP, Baker CN: Procedures for the evaluation of the visual system by pediatricians. Pediatrics 2016 Jan;137(1). doi: 10.1542/peds.2015-3597 [PMID: 26644488].

Pineles SL et al: Atropine for the prevention of myopia progression in children: a report by the American Academy of Ophthalmology. Ophthalmology 2017 Dec;124(12):1857–1866. doi: 10.1016/j.ophtha.2017.05.032 [PMID: 28669492].

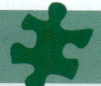

ESSENTIALS OF DIAGNOSIS & TYPICAL FEATURES

▶ Corneal light reflex evaluation (Hirschberg test) is performed by shining a penlight at the patient's eyes, observing the reflections of each cornea, and estimating whether the lights appear to be positioned symmetrically.

▶ Simultaneous examination of both pupils at the same time with a handheld ophthalmoscope is called the *Brückner test*.

Red Reflex Test

An ophthalmoscope is used to check the red reflex of both eyes. The examiner should use the largest diameter of light and have the setting at zero. The room should be darkened for maximal pupil dilation. Both pupils are evaluated with the ophthalmoscope at arm's length from the child with the child looking straight at the light. If the child is looking off to the side, the reflex can be asymmetric. The observed red reflexes should be a light orange-yellow in color in lightly pigmented eyes or a dark red in darkly pigmented brown eyes. A difference in quality of the red reflexes between the two eyes constitutes a positive Brückner test and requires referral to an ophthalmologist. The American Academy of Pediatrics (AAP), American Association for Pediatric Ophthalmology and Strabismus (AAPOS), and the American Academy of Ophthalmology (AAO) policy statements for red reflex testing can be accessed at https://www.aao.org/clinical-statement/procedures-evaluation-of-visual-system-by-pediatri.

EXTERNAL EXAMINATION

A penlight provides good illumination for inspection of the anterior segment of the globe and its adnexa. A slit lamp provides optimal illumination and magnification for an ocular examination.

In cases of suspected foreign body, pulling down on the lower lid provides excellent visualization of the inferior cul-de-sac (palpebral conjunctiva). Visualizing the upper cul-de-sac and superior bulbar conjunctiva is possible by having the patient look down, while the upper lid is lifted up. The upper lid should be everted to evaluate the superior tarsal conjunctiva (Figure 16–3).

When indicated for further evaluation of the cornea, a small amount of fluorescein solution should be instilled into the lower cul-de-sac. A Wood lamp or a blue filter cap placed over a penlight will illuminate the epithelial defects as yellow-green. Disease-specific staining patterns may be observed. For example, herpes simplex lesions of the corneal epithelium produce a dendrite or branchlike pattern. A foreign body lodged beneath the upper lid shows one or more vertical lines of stain on the cornea due to the constant movement of the foreign body over the cornea. Contact lens overwear produces a central staining pattern. A fine, scattered punctate pattern may be a sign of medication toxicity. Punctate erosions of the inferior third of the cornea can be seen with staphylococcal blepharitis or exposure keratitis secondary to incomplete lid closure.

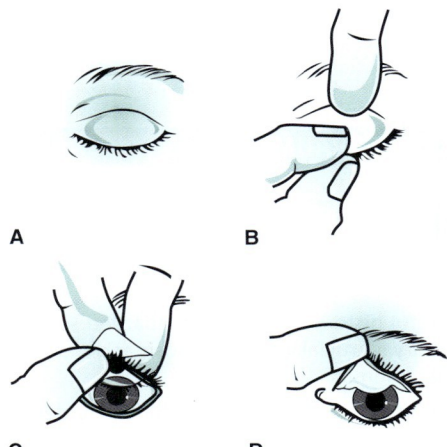

▲ Figure 16–3. Eversion of the upper lid. **A:** The patient looks downward. **B:** The fingers pull the lid down, and an index finger or cotton tip is placed on the upper tarsal border. **C:** The lid is pulled up over the finger. **D:** The lid is everted.

PUPILS

The pupils should be evaluated for reaction to light, regularity of shape, and equality of size as well as for the presence of afferent pupillary defect (APD). This defect, which occurs in optic nerve disease, is evaluated by the swinging flashlight test (see section Diseases of the Optic Nerve). Irregular pupils are associated with iritis, trauma, pupillary membranes, and structural defects such as iris coloboma (see section Iris Coloboma).

Pupils vary in size due to lighting conditions and age. In general, infants have miotic (constricted) pupils. Children have larger pupils than either infants or adults, whereas the elderly have miotic pupils.

Anisocoria, a size difference between the two pupils, may be physiologic if the size difference is within 1 mm. Anisocoria can result when the abnormal pupil is smaller (Horner syndrome) or when it is bigger (third nerve palsy, Adie tonic pupil, trauma, medication). Systemic antihistamines and scopolamine patches can dilate the pupils and interfere with accommodation (focusing).

ALIGNMENT & MOTILITY EVALUATION

Alignment and motility should be tested because amblyopia is associated with strabismus. Ocular motility should be evaluated in the six cardinal positions of gaze (Table 16–2; Figure 16–4).

Alignment can be assessed in several ways. Observation is an educated guess about whether the eyes are properly aligned. Corneal light reflex evaluation (Hirschberg test) is

Table 16–2. Function and innervation of each of the extraocular muscles.

Muscle	Function	Innervation
Medial rectus	Adductor	Oculomotor (third)
Lateral rectus	Abductor	Abducens (sixth)
Inferior rectus	Depressor, adductor, extorter	Oculomotor
Superior rectus	Elevator, adductor, intorter	Oculomotor
Inferior oblique	Elevator, abductor, extorter	Oculomotor
Superior oblique	Depressor, abductor, intorter	Trochlear (fourth)

performed by shining a penlight and checking where the light reflects off each cornea. If the reflection of light is noted temporally on one cornea while in the middle on the other cornea, esotropia (crossed eyes) is suspected (Figure 16–5). Nasal reflection on one cornea of the light suggests exotropia (outward deviation). Pseudostrabismus is the appearance of crossed eyes due to wide nasal bridge and/or prominent epicanthal skin folds that cover the medial portion of the sclera. Despite the false impression of esotropia, they will have symmetric corneal light reflexes.

Cover testing is the most accurate method of alignment evaluation. As the child attends to the target, each eye is alternately covered. A shift in an eye's alignment as it assumes fixation onto the target is a possible indication of strabismus (Figure 16–6). A deviated eye that has very poor vision will not fixate on a target. Consequently, spurious results to cover testing may occur, which can happen with disinterest on the part of the patient, small-angle strabismus, and inexperience in administering cover tests.

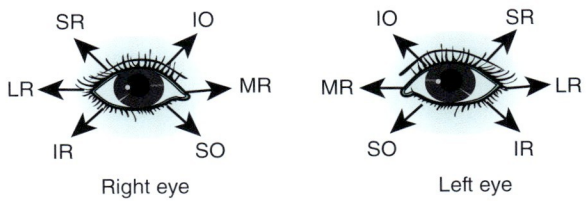

MR = medial rectus LR = lateral rectus
SR = superior rectus IR = inferior rectus
SO = superior oblique IO = inferior oblique

▲ Figure 16–4. Cardinal positions of gaze and muscles primarily tested in those fields of gaze. Arrows indicate position in which each muscle is tested.

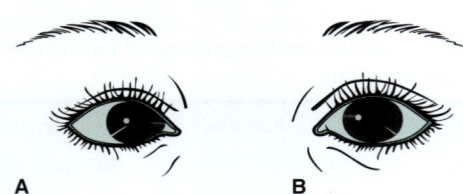

▲ **Figure 16–5. A.** Temporal displacement of light reflection showing esotropia (inward deviation) of the right eye. **B.** Nasal displacement of the reflection would show exotropia (outward deviation) of the left eye.

Intermittent strabismus is a normal finding in infancy. However, if this persists beyond 4 months of age, referral to ophthalmology is necessary.

OPHTHALMOSCOPIC EXAMINATION

A handheld ophthalmoscope allows visualization of the ocular fundus. As the patient's pupil becomes more constricted, viewing the fundus becomes more difficult. Although pupillary dilation can precipitate an attack of closed-angle glaucoma in the predisposed adult, children are very rarely predisposed to angle closure. Exceptions include those with a dislocated lens, past surgery, or an eye previously compromised by a retrolental membrane, such as in ROP. Structures to be observed during ophthalmoscopy include the optic disc, blood vessels, the macular reflex, and retina, as well as the clarity of the vitreous media. By increasing the amount of plus lens dialed into the direct ophthalmoscope, the point of focus moves anteriorly from the retina to the lens and finally to the cornea.

OCULAR TRAUMA

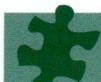

ESSENTIALS OF DIAGNOSIS & TYPICAL FEATURES

▶ A careful history of the events that led to the ocular injury is crucial in the diagnosis and treatment of ocular trauma.

▶ If the extent of the eye injury is difficult to determine or if it is sight threatening, it is best to cover the eye with a shield and refer to ophthalmology urgently.

PREVENTION OF OCULAR INJURIES

Safety/sport goggles or prescription glasses should be used while in laboratories and industrial arts classes, when operating power tools, hammers, nails, and while participating in organized sports. The one-eyed individual should be specifically advised to always wear polycarbonate eyeglasses and goggles for all sports. High-risk activities such as boxing and the martial arts should be avoided by one-eyed children.

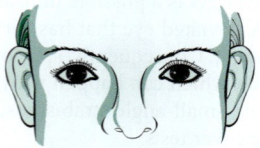

Eyes straight (maintained in position by fusion).

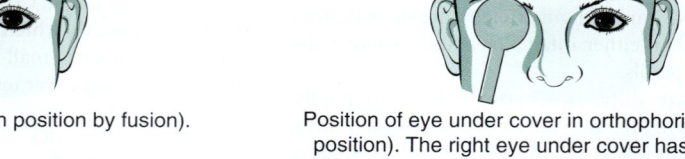

Position of eye under cover in orthophoria (fusion-free position). The right eye under cover has not moved.

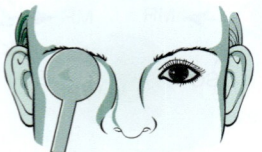

Position of eye under cover in esophoria (fusion-free position). Under cover, the right eye has deviated inward. Upon removal of cover, the right eye will immediately resume its straight-ahead position.

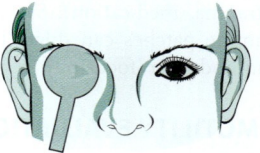

Position of eye under cover in exophoria (fusion-free position). Under cover, the right eye has deviated outward. Upon removal of the cover, the right eye will immediately resume its straight-ahead position.

▲ **Figure 16–6.** Cover testing. The patient is instructed to look at a target at eye level 20 ft away. Note that in the presence of constant strabismus (ie, a tropia rather than a phoria), the deviation will remain when the cover is removed. (Reproduced with permission from Riordan-Eva P, Cunningham ET: *Vaughan & Asbury's General Ophthalmology*, 18th ed. New York, NY: McGraw Hill; 2011.)

CORNEAL ABRASION

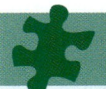

ESSENTIALS OF DIAGNOSIS & TYPICAL FEATURES

► The cornea is one of the most sensitive parts of the body. Corneal abrasion can cause severe ocular pain, tearing, and blepharospasm.

► All corneal abrasion should be evaluated for possible foreign body under eyelids or on the eye surface.

► Pathogenesis

Children often suffer corneal abrasions accidentally while playing with siblings or pets and participating in sports. Contact lens users may develop abrasions due to poorly fitting lenses, overnight wear, and the use of torn or damaged lenses.

► Prevention

Proper contact lens care and parental supervision can prevent activities that can lead to a corneal abrasion.

► Clinical Findings

Corneal abrasions produce sudden and severe eye pain after an inciting event. Decreased vision secondary to pain and tearing are common complaints. Eyelid edema, tearing, injection of the conjunctiva, and poor cooperation with the ocular examination due to pain are common signs. Pain improves with instillation of ophthalmic anesthetic drops and can aid in examination. Fluorescein dye will stain the abrasion bright yellow-green when illuminated with Wood lamp (Figure 16–7). Both upper and lower eyelids should be everted to evaluate for foreign bodies.

► Differential Diagnosis

Ocular or adnexal foreign bodies, corneal ulcer, and corneal laceration.

► Complications

Possible vision loss from corneal infection and scarring.

► Treatment

Topical anesthetic should never be prescribed to patients as it can lead to corneal melting and/or infection. Ophthalmic ointment, such as erythromycin ointment, lubricates the surface of the cornea and helps prevent infections. Patching the affected eye when a large abrasion is present may provide comfort, but it is not advised for corneal abrasions caused by contact lens wear or other potentially contaminated sources. Frequent follow-up is required until healing is complete.

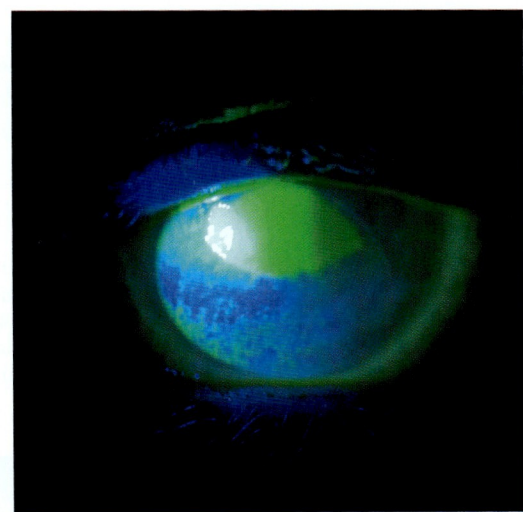

▲ **Figure 16–7.** Fluorescein stain of large inferior corneal abrasion illuminated with Wood lamp.

► Prognosis

Excellent if corneal infection and scarring do not occur.

OCULAR FOREIGN BODIES

ESSENTIALS OF DIAGNOSIS & TYPICAL FEATURES

► Vertical corneal abrasion can be a sign of foreign body under the eyelid, so lid eversion should be performed.

► Prevention

Protective goggles or prescription glasses can help prevent ocular injuries and should be encouraged while participating in sports and activities at risk for eye injuries.

► Clinical Findings

Foreign bodies on the surface of the globe and palpebral conjunctiva usually cause discomfort, tearing, and a red eye. Pain with blinking suggests that the foreign body may be trapped under the eyelid or on the corneal surface.

Magnification with a slit lamp may be needed for inspection. Foreign bodies that lodge on the upper palpebral conjunctiva are best viewed by everting the lid on itself and removing the foreign body with a cotton applicator.

Differential Diagnosis

Corneal abrasion, corneal ulcer, and globe rupture/laceration.

Complications

Pain, infection, and potential vision loss from scarring.

Treatment

When foreign bodies are noted on the bulbar conjunctiva or cornea (Figure 16–8), removal of the foreign body with irrigation or with a cotton applicator after instillation of a topical anesthetic can be attempted. Referral to an ophthalmologist may be necessary if the aforementioned measures fail to remove the foreign body or if a corneal rust ring secondary to a metallic foreign body is present. Patients should be warned that foreign-body sensation may persist for 1–2 days even after removal due to the epithelial defect that occurs after removal. An ophthalmic antibiotic ointment is typically prescribed for several days after foreign-body removal.

Prognosis

Usually excellent with prompt treatment.

INTRAOCULAR FOREIGN BODIES & PERFORATING OCULAR INJURIES

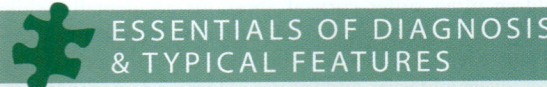

ESSENTIALS OF DIAGNOSIS & TYPICAL FEATURES

► Signs of perforating ocular injuries include irregularly shaped pupil, shallow anterior chamber, hyphema (blood in the anterior chamber), or dark tissue showing through the white sclera (Figure 16–9).

Pathogenesis

Intraocular foreign bodies and penetrating injuries/corneal/scleral laceration (ruptured globes) are most often caused by being in close proximity to high-velocity projectiles such as windshield glass broken during a motor vehicle accident, metal grinding without the use of protective safety goggles, BB gun injury, and sports-related injuries.

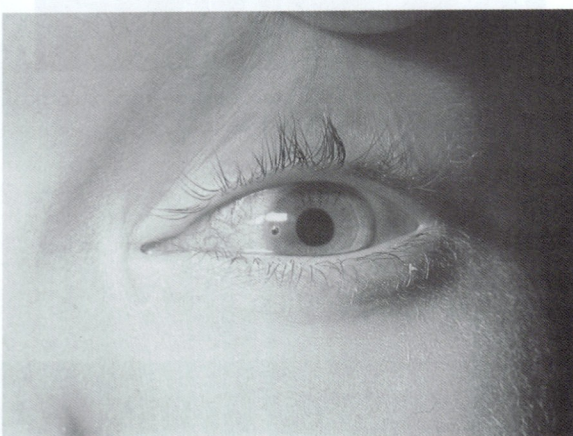

A

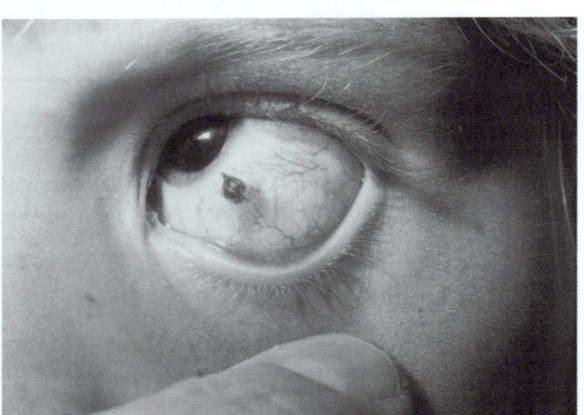

B

▲ **Figure 16–8.** **A:** Corneal foreign body at the nasal edge of the cornea. **B:** Subconjunctival foreign body of graphite.

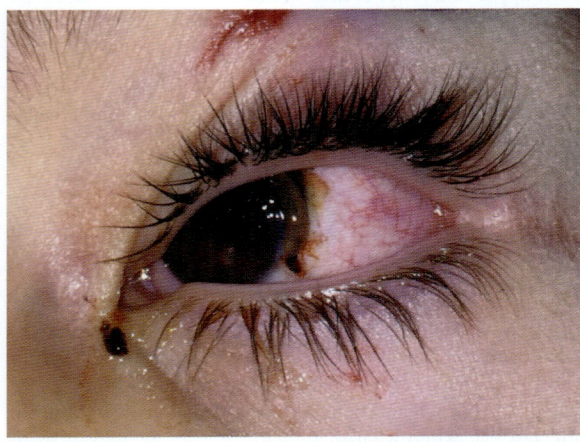

▲ **Figure 16–9.** Corneoscleral laceration with dark uveal tissue expulsed from wound, irregular pupil and hyphema.

Prevention

Use protective eyewear when engaging in activities that may be a risk for ocular injury.

Clinical Findings

Sudden ocular pain with vision loss occurs after an inciting event. Diagnosis may be difficult if obvious signs of globe rupture as stated above are not present.

Computed tomographic (CT) scan is useful in evaluating ocular trauma, including bony injury and intraocular foreign bodies. Nonradiopaque materials such as glass will not be seen on imaging. Magnetic resonance imaging (MRI) must be avoided if a magnetic foreign body is suspected. Ocular ultrasound should not be performed on suspected globe injury.

Differential Diagnosis

Corneal abrasion and superficial foreign body of the eye or eyelids.

Complications

Traumatic cataract, retinal detachment, intraocular infection, loss of vision or eye.

Treatment

In cases of suspected intraocular foreign body or perforation of the globe, it may be best to keep the child at rest, gently shield the eye with a metal shield or cut-down paper cup and keep the extent of examination to a minimum to prevent expulsion of intraocular contents. In this setting, the child should be given nothing by mouth in case eye examination under anesthesia or surgical repair is required. Emergent consultation with ophthalmologist is warranted.

Prognosis

Prognosis depends on the extent of the trauma.

BLUNT ORBITAL TRAUMA

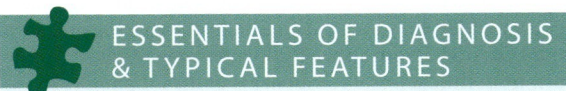

ESSENTIALS OF DIAGNOSIS & TYPICAL FEATURES

► In "white-eyed blowout fracture," injury to the eye and lids may appear minimal except for restriction of eye movements, especially upgaze. It requires emergent surgery.

► In orbital compartment syndrome, the eyelids will be too tight to open with fingers or instruments due to pressure from within the orbit associated with retrobulbar hemorrhage.

Pathogenesis

Blunt trauma to the orbit can lead to orbital fractures. Retrobulbar hemorrhage (bleeding behind the globe within the orbit) can lead to orbital compartment syndrome, which can lead to permanent vision loss.

Prevention

Protective eyewear during athletic activities and adequate supervision of children at home and school.

Clinical Findings

The orbital floor is a common location for a fracture (called a *blowout fracture*). Patients can have double vision, pain with eye movements, and restriction of extraocular movements. *White-eyed blowout fracture* is a greenstick fracture with entrapment of orbital contents within the fracture; the only abnormality on examination may be restricted eye movements, especially upward. Entrapment of orbital contents often stimulates the oculocardiac reflex resulting in bradycardia and emesis. CT scan is helpful in diagnosing the extent of injuries. Consultation with an ophthalmologist is necessary to determine the full spectrum of the injuries.

Orbital compartment syndrome is also an emergency requiring immediate treatment. Patients present with severe eyelid edema and proptosis. Eyelid tightness is due to pressure from within the orbit pushing the eye out. Neuroimaging will show retrobulbar hemorrhage and proptosis. This is distinct from just severe eyelid edema that can be seen in orbital fractures, especially with orbital roof fracture. Although orbital compartment syndrome can still occur, orbital fractures can decompress pressure build up within the orbit.

Treatment

Orbital compartment syndrome requires emergent lateral eyelid canthotomy and cantholysis to decompress the orbit. Treatment should not be delayed to image the orbits. Prompt treatment can prevent permanent vision loss.

Patients with clinical signs of muscle entrapment require urgent surgical repair to avoid permanent ischemic injury to the involved extraocular muscle. Large fractures may need nonurgent repair to prevent enophthalmos (sunken appearance to the orbit). Patients with any orbital fracture must be warned not to blow their nose as it can cause orbital emphysema and worsening proptosis.

Cold compresses or ice packs for brief periods in the first 24 hours after injury may help reduce hemorrhage and swelling.

Prognosis

The prognosis depends on the severity of the blunt trauma, associated ocular injuries, and extent of the orbit fractures.

LACERATIONS

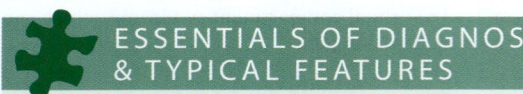

ESSENTIALS OF DIAGNOSIS & TYPICAL FEATURES

▶ Lacerations of the nasal third of the eyelid are at risk for lacrimal system injury.

Pathogenesis

Lacerations of the eyelids and lacrimal system often result from dog bites, car accidents, falls, and fights.

Prevention

Supervision of children at home and at school.

Clinical Findings

Eyelid lacerations may be partial or full thickness in depth. Foreign bodies, such as glass or gravel, may be present depending on the mechanism of the injury.

Differential Diagnosis

Globe injury may be associated with eyelid lacerations as well.

Complications

Poor surgical repair of lacerations of the eyelid margin can result in eyelid malposition, which causes chronic ocular surface irritation and possible corneal scarring.

Treatment

Superficial lacerations away from the lid margins can be repaired by non-ophthalmologists. Lacerations involving the lid margin or canaliculus (Figure 16–10) and those associated with significant tissue loss are best repaired by an ophthalmologist and may require intubation of the nasolacrimal system with silicone tubes.

Prognosis

Prognosis depends on severity of the injury, tissue loss, and adequacy of surgical repair.

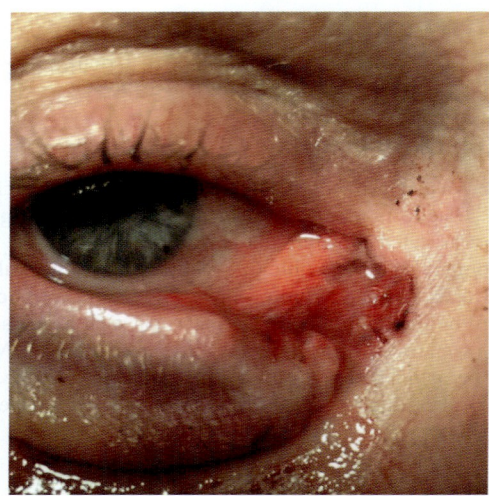

▲ **Figure 16–10.** Laceration involving right lower lid and canaliculus.

BURNS

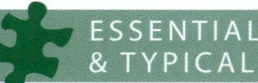

ESSENTIALS OF DIAGNOSIS & TYPICAL FEATURES

▶ For all chemical burns, pH should be checked, and eyes irrigated until pH is close to 7.

▶ In severe burns, the eye may not look red due to perilimbal ischemia.

▶ Alkalis tend to penetrate deeper than acids into ocular tissue and often cause severe injury.

Pathogenesis

Burns of the conjunctiva and cornea may be thermal, radiant, or chemical. Chemical burns with strong acidic and alkaline agents can be blinding and constitute a true ocular emergency. Examples are burns caused by splash injury with cleaning supplies, spilled drain cleaner, and bleach. Radiant energy causes ultraviolet keratitis. Typical examples are welder's burn and burns associated with skiing without goggles in bright sunlight. In addition to thermal and blunt trauma, chemical eye injury can occur from airbag deployment as a result of alkaline burn from the chemical components of the inflation reaction.

Prevention

Protective eyewear when engaging in activities that pose a potential risk for exposure to hazardous chemicals, radiant energy, or when explosive conditions is possible.

Clinical Findings

Superficial thermal burns cause pain, tearing, and injection. Corneal epithelial defects can be diagnosed using fluorescein dye, which will stain areas of the cornea bright fluorescent green where the epithelium is absent. Conjunctiva may be injected diffusely. In severe burns, there is relative lack of redness around the cornea indicative of perilimbal ischemia. Eyelashes may be singed due to thermal burns. The fluorescein dye pattern will show a uniformly stippled appearance of the corneal epithelium in ultraviolet keratitis. It is important to check the pH after any suspected chemical burn injury including airbag deployment.

Differential Diagnosis

Corneal abrasion, foreign body, and traumatic iritis.

Complications

Significant corneal injury, especially if associated with an alkali burn, may lead to scarring and vision loss. Eyelid scarring can result in chronic exposure, dry eye, and entropion or ectropion.

Treatment

Immediate treatment consists of copious irrigation and removal of precipitates as soon as possible after the injury. Irrigation should be continued until the pH is close to 7. Initial stabilization of the injury is initiated by using topical antibiotics. A cycloplegic agent such as cyclopentolate 1% may be added to reduce ciliary spasm that contributes to pain. Topical steroids may also be necessary but should be guided by an ophthalmologist. Ultraviolet keratitis can be extremely painful, and patients often need opioids for pain control. Patients should be referred to an ophthalmologist after immediate first aid has been given.

Prognosis

Prognosis depends on the severity of the injury.

HYPHEMA

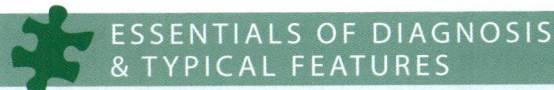

ESSENTIALS OF DIAGNOSIS & TYPICAL FEATURES

▶ Slit-lamp examination or penlight examination may reveal a layer of blood within the anterior chamber.

▶ A hyphema may be microscopic or may fill the entire anterior chamber (Figure 16–11).

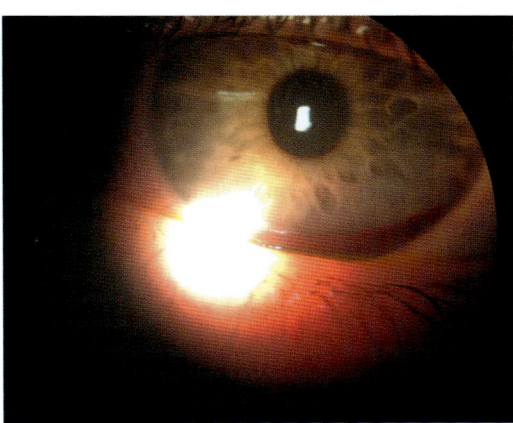

▲ **Figure 16–11.** Hyphema filling approximately 10% of the anterior chamber.

Pathogenesis

Blunt trauma to the globe may cause a hyphema, which is bleeding within the anterior chamber from a ruptured vessel from the iris or in the anterior chamber angle.

Prevention

Protective eyewear and appropriate supervision at home and at school.

Clinical Findings

Blunt trauma severe enough to cause a hyphema may be associated with additional ocular injury, including lens subluxation, cataract, retinal edema or detachment, and ruptured globe. It is important to note the height and color of the hyphema. Most will be layered inferiorly unless patient has been lying down for a long time, in which case it will be dispersed and have a hazy appearance. Sometimes, it can be seen as a clot over the iris. Total hyphema (100%) may appear black or red. A black total hyphema is referred to as "eight-ball hyphema." The black color is suggestive of impaired aqueous circulation and decreased oxygen concentration. This distinction is important because an eight-ball hyphema is more likely to cause pupillary block and secondary angle closure, which is an ophthalmic emergency. In patients with sickle cell anemia or trait, even a small amount of hyphema can lead to significantly elevated intraocular pressure that can result in permanent vision loss. Therefore, all African Americans should have their sickle cell status determined if hyphema is observed. These patients require extra vigilance in diagnosing and treating hyphema.

▶ Differential Diagnosis

Nontraumatic causes of hyphema include juvenile xanthogranuloma and blood dyscrasias.

▶ Complications

Increased intraocular pressure, glaucoma, permanent corneal staining, and vision loss.

▶ Treatment

A shield should be placed over the eye, the head elevated, and ophthalmologic referral made.

▶ Prognosis

The majority of children with isolated traumatic hyphema do well with outpatient treatment, activity restriction, and close follow-up with an ophthalmologist. Prognosis is worse if intraocular pressure is elevated, the patient has sickle cell disease, or if other associated ocular injuries are present.

ABUSIVE HEAD TRAUMA & NONACCIDENTAL TRAUMA

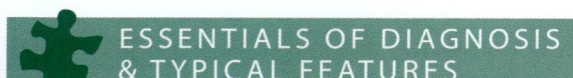

ESSENTIALS OF DIAGNOSIS & TYPICAL FEATURES

▶ Abusive head trauma (AHT), formerly known as *shaken baby syndrome*, is a form of nonaccidental trauma characterized by a constellation of examination findings, including intracranial injury, retinal hemorrhages (RHs), and fractures of long bones or ribs.

▶ The history leading to the diagnosis of AHT is often vague and poorly correlated with the extent of injury.

▶ Pathogenesis

AHT includes shaking as a mechanism of injury, shaking with impact, or impact alone. The most widely accepted theory is that retinal hemorrhages (RHs) occur due to the vitreoretinal traction from accelerating-decelerating forces from shaking alone or combined with impact.

▶ Clinical Findings

Victims may present with irritability, change in mental status, or unexplained seizures. RH can be present in approximately 75% of children with AHT.

Ophthalmic consultation with dilated retinal examination is necessary to document RH, preferably within the first 24 hours and ideally within 72 hours of the acute presentation. If pupillary dilation is not possible due to neurologic checks, one eye can be dilated at a time. Timing is important as intraretinal hemorrhages may resolve rapidly within days, whereas preretinal/subretinal/vitreous hemorrhages can take time. Hemorrhages may be unilateral or bilateral, confined to the posterior pole or involving periphery. Classically, they are multilayered (intraretinal, preretinal, and subretinal), too numerous to count, and diffuse. Traumatic macular retinoschisis (splitting of retinal layers) and folds are very specific for AHT, although they have been reported in severe head crush injuries and fatal accidental traumas. If a blood clot lies over the macula, deprivation amblyopia may occur and may require intraocular surgery by a retinal specialist. Other ocular findings associated with AHT include lid ecchymosis, subconjunctival hemorrhage, hyphema, and optic nerve edema.

▶ Differential Diagnosis

The differential diagnosis of RH includes birth trauma (in < 6 weeks old), sepsis, blood dyscrasia, and severe crush injuries or high-velocity trauma. RH associated with birth trauma is most commonly seen after vacuum-assisted vaginal delivery (> 70%) and least likely after a routine cesarean delivery (< 20%). A team effort between the primary treating physician, neurosurgery, orthopedics, ophthalmology, social services, and law enforcement is crucial in determining the true cause of a patient's injuries.

▶ Complications

Persistent hemorrhages involving the macula can lead to amblyopia. Longitudinal data show that vision can be abnormal in more than 40% of children after AHT. Poor vision can also result from cortical visual impairment in patients with severe neurologic injuries. Children with history of AHT are at higher risk of strabismus, need for strabismus surgeries, and significant refractive error.

▶ Treatment

Management of any systemic injuries is required. Observation by an ophthalmologist for resolution of RH is recommended. Vitreous hemorrhages or large preretinal hemorrhages that do not resolve within several weeks may need surgical treatment by a retinal specialist.

▶ Prognosis

Prognosis depends on the severity of ocular and brain injuries.

Christian CW, Levin AV; Council on Child Abuse and Neglect; section on ophthalmology; AACO; AAPOS; AAO: The eye examination in the evaluation of child abuse. Pediatrics 2018 Aug;142(2):e20181411. doi: 10.1542/peds.2018-1411 [PMID: 30037976].

Weldy E, Shimoda A, Patnaik J, Jung J, Singh J: Long-term visual outcomes following abusive head trauma with retinal hemorrhage. J AAPOS 2019 Dec;23(6):329.e4. doi: 10.1016/j.jaapos.2019.08.276. Epub 2019 Oct 23 [PMID: 3165514].

▼ DISORDERS OF THE OCULAR STRUCTURES

DISEASES OF THE EYELIDS

The eyelids can be affected by various dermatologic, infectious, or inflammatory conditions.

Blepharitis/Blepharokeratoconjunctivitis

ESSENTIALS OF DIAGNOSIS & TYPICAL FEATURES

► Blepharokeratoconjunctivitis (BKC) is a chronic inflammatory disorder of the eyelid and ocular surface that can be sight-threatening.

► Patients with BKC often have chronic, recurrent "pink eye" and frequent chalazia, leading to delay in diagnosis and proper treatment.

► Pathogenesis

Blepharitis is caused by inflammation of the eyelid margin, meibomian gland obstruction, and tear film imbalance. The term *BKC* is used when the conjunctiva and cornea are affected in addition to the lids. Meibomian glands, located in the eyelids, secrete the lipid layer of tear film. Bacterial flora on lid margins secretes enzymes that can further destabilize the tear film. Higher numbers of *Staphylococcus aureus* and *Staphylococcus epidermis* have been cultured in patients with BKC. Refractory cases of BKC can be caused by ocular rosacea or *Demodex* (mite) infestation.

► Prevention

Eyelid hygiene is essential to prevent or control blepharitis. Eyelid scrubs with baby shampoo help decrease the bacterial load on the eyelid margins and lashes. Warm compresses help loosen the secretions of the meibomian glands.

► Clinical Findings

Patients commonly present with concerns of redness, tearing, photophobia, and foreign-body sensation. They may have decreased vision. Diagnosis is clinical with examination findings of the lid margin (thickening, telangiectasia, stye, crusting, collarettes), meibomian gland inspissation, follicular conjunctivitis, and corneal changes (punctate keratitis, corneal opacities, peripheral pannus and vascularization, ulceration, thinning, and scarring). Findings are often bilateral but can be asymmetric. Corneal scarring, if present, is usually peripheral and inferior but can be diffuse and central in severe cases. Vision loss can be from corneal scarring and also from induced astigmatism, leading to amblyopia.

► Differential Diagnosis

Allergic or viral conjunctivitis. Herpes keratitis is the most frequent misdiagnosis. Contrary to BKC, HSV will be unilateral with decreased corneal sensation.

► Complications

Permanent corneal and eyelid margin scarring in severe cases. Amblyopia with vision loss.

► Treatment

It should be emphasized that BKC is a chronic condition with exacerbations and remissions. Treatment is targeted to opening the plugged meibomian glands to clear them of excess bacteria and oily secretions. Hot compresses of the lids with microwavable heat packs and eye masks are essential in melting the glandular debris followed by lid massage to express the glands. Lids should also be scrubbed with baby shampoo daily. When suspecting Demodex, addition of tea tree oil shampoo is helpful. Topical and oral antibiotics can be used to decrease the bacterial burden. These include erythromycin ointment, azithromycin drops, and oral azithromycin. Topical steroids may be required to treat the inflammation and requires close follow-up with an ophthalmologist.

► Prognosis

Generally good with early diagnosis and treatment.

O'Gallagher M, Banteka M, Bunce C, Larkin F, Tuft S, Dahlmann-Noor A: Systemic treatment for blepharokeratoconjunctivitis in children. Cochrane Database Syst Rev 2016 May;30(5):CD011750. doi: 10.1002/14651858.CD011750.pub2 [PMID: 27236587].

O'Gallagher M, Bunce C, Hingorani M, Larkin F, Tuft S, Dahlmann-Noor A: Topical treatments for blepharokeratoconjunctivitis in children. Cochrane Database Syst Rev 2017 Feb 7;2:CD011965. doi: 10.1002/14651858.CD011965.pub2 [PMID: 28170093].

Rousta ST: Pediatric blepharokeratoconjunctivitis: is there a 'right' treatment? Curr Opin Ophthalmol 2017 Sep;28(5):449–453. doi: 10.1097/ICU.0000000000000399 [PMID: 28696955].

Chalazion

ESSENTIALS OF DIAGNOSIS & TYPICAL FEATURES

▶ A chalazion is an aseptic, nontender eyelid nodule.

▶ Patients report slowly enlarging lump with variability in size from day to day.

▶ Pathogenesis

Obstruction of the eyelid meibomian glands with resultant inflammation, fibrosis, and lipogranuloma formation.

▶ Prevention

See section Blepharitis/Blepharokeratoconjunctivitis.

▶ Clinical Findings

Eyelid nodule of variable size and localized erythema of the corresponding palpebral conjunctiva that may be associated with a yellow lipogranuloma (Figure 16–12). It is a nontender, painless lesion.

▶ Differential Diagnosis

Clinical presentation of acute chalazion and internal hordeolum can be difficult to distinguish, but management is the same.

▶ Treatment

See section Blepharitis. Since chalazia are inflammatory and not infectious, antibiotics are not necessary. If incision and curettage are needed because the lesion is slow to resolve, the child will often require a general anesthetic.

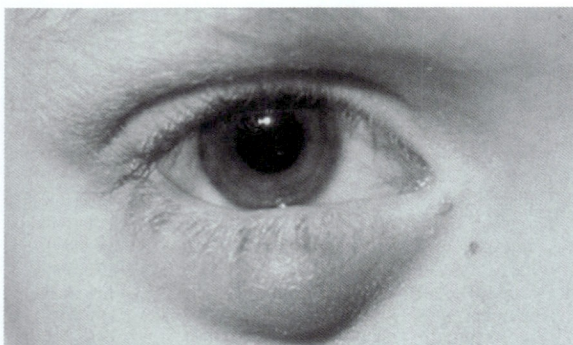

▲ **Figure 16–12.** Chalazion. Right lower lid, external view.

▶ Prognosis

Generally good.

Wu AY, Gervasio KA, Gergoudis KN, Wei C, Oestreicher JH, Harvey JT: Conservative therapy for chalazia: is it really effective? Acta Ophthalmol 2018 Jun;96(4):e503–e509. doi: 10.1111/aos.13675. Epub 2018 Jan 16 [PMID: 29338124].

Hordeolum

ESSENTIALS OF DIAGNOSIS & TYPICAL FEATURES

▶ Hordeolum is a painful red bump on the eyelid caused by an acute bacterial infection of eyelash hair follicle or Meibomian glands.

▶ It is a self-limiting condition lasting 1–2 weeks.

▶ Pathogenesis

Hordeolum is usually caused by *Staphylococcus* infection occurring from stasis of eyelid glands, which normally produce antiseptic secretions. External hordeolum (stye) occurs from blockage of the sebaceous (Zeis) and sweat (Moll) glands, resulting in painful red swollen bump that develops into a pustule. Internal hordeolum is due to blockage of Meibomian glands, and pustules form on the inner side of the eyelids.

▶ Prevention

See section Blepharitis.

▶ Clinical Findings

It presents as painful, red bump on the eyelid with localized erythema. Pustule can be seen on the eyelid margin for external hordeolum or on the palpebral conjunctiva for internal hordeolum (Figure 16–13).

▶ Differential Diagnosis

Periorbital cellulitis, chalazion.

▶ Treatment

Hordeolum generally drain spontaneously without any treatment. Treatments used for chalazia can be helpful (warm compresses, lid massage, lid scrubs). Erythromycin ointment can provide lubrication. Oral antibiotic is rarely indicated unless infection leads to periorbital cellulitis, when systemic antibiotic is necessary. Incision and draining of a persistent lesion can be performed by ophthalmologists.

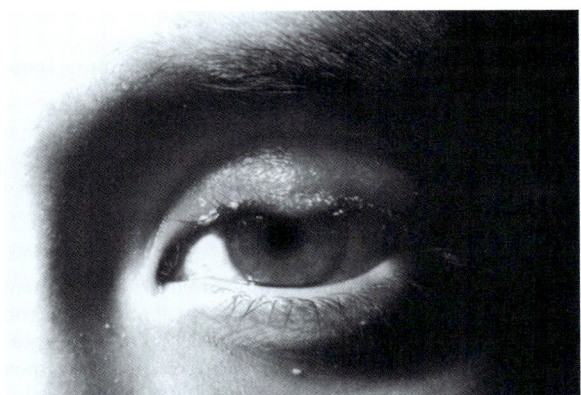

▲ **Figure 16–13.** Hordeolum and blepharitis, left upper lid.

 Prognosis

Generally good.

VIRAL EYELID DISEASE

ESSENTIALS OF DIAGNOSIS & TYPICAL FEATURES

▶ Molluscum contagiosum can cause dome-shaped, shiny nodules with central umbilication on skin, including eyelids. It can cause recurrent ipsilateral conjunctivitis.

▶ Herpes simplex virus (HSV) and herpes zoster usually cause unilateral disease.

▶ Pathogenesis

HSV may involve the conjunctiva and lids at the time of primary herpes simplex infection resulting in blepharoconjunctivitis. Vesicular lesions with an erythematous base occur. Herpes zoster causes a painful vesicular disease in association with a skin eruption in the dermatome of the ophthalmic branch of the trigeminal nerve.

▶ Prevention

Avoid contact with individuals with active HSV infection.

▶ Clinical Findings

A vesicular rash is the most common sign of herpes viral eyelid infection. Fluorescein dye should be administered topically to the affected eye followed by examination with a cobalt blue light to assess for the presence of dendrites. When vesicles are present on the tip of the nose with herpes zoster (Hutchinson sign), ocular involvement, including iritis, is more likely. Eyelid edema in herpes zoster ophthalmicus (HZO) can be severe and mistaken for preseptal cellulitis. Herpes simplex and herpes zoster can be diagnosed and distinguished by polymerase chain reaction (PCR). Molluscum contagiosum lesions are typically umbilicated papules, which may or may not be inflamed. It can cause acute or chronic follicular conjunctivitis.

▶ Differential Diagnosis

Impetigo.

▶ Complications

Conjunctivitis and keratitis (corneal infection).

▶ Treatment

Herpes simplex blepharoconjunctivitis can be treated with systemic acyclovir or valacyclovir. An alternative includes topical ganciclovir 0.15%. Treatment of ophthalmic herpes zoster with systemic nucleoside analogues within 3 days after onset may reduce the morbidity. Molluscum contagiosum lesions may be treated with observation, cautery, or excision.

▶ Prognosis

Generally good unless corneal involvement is present. Recurrence may occur and can involve the cornea, warranting an eye examination every time HSV recurrence is suspected.

MISCELLANEOUS EYELID INFECTIONS

Pediculosis

Pediculosis of the lids (phthiriasis palpebrarum) is caused by *Pthirus pubis*. Nits and adult lice can be seen on the eyelashes when viewed with appropriate magnification. Mechanical removal as well as medical treatment is effective (see Chapter 15). Other bodily areas of involvement must also be treated if involved. Family members and contacts may also be infected.

Papillomavirus

Papillomavirus may infect the lid and conjunctiva. Warts may be recurrent, multiple, and difficult to treat. Treatment modalities include cryotherapy, cautery, carbon dioxide laser, and surgery.

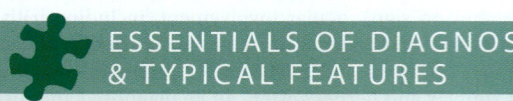

EYELID PTOSIS

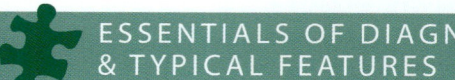

ESSENTIALS OF DIAGNOSIS & TYPICAL FEATURES

▶ Eyelid ptosis is droopy eyelid that may be unilateral or bilateral. Children may have a chin-up position to compensate for the droopiness.

▶ Ptosis can lead to amblyopia from deprivation or from significant astigmatism that is induced by the droopy eyelid.

▶ Pathogenesis

Eyelid ptosis—a droopy upper lid (Figure 16–14)—may be congenital or acquired but is usually congenital in children owing to a defective levator muscle. Other causes of ptosis are myasthenia gravis, lid injuries, third nerve palsy, and Horner syndrome (see section Horner Syndrome). Marcus Gunn jaw-winking phenomenon is a congenital ptosis associated with synkinetic movements of the upper eyelid and muscles of mastication. It is due to an aberrant connection between the motor branches of trigeminal nerve innervating the external pterygoid muscle and the superior branches of oculomotor nerve supplying the levator palpebrae superioris.

▶ Clinical Findings

The upper eyelid is lower than normal, which narrows the vertical dimension of the palpebral fissure. In congenital ptosis, the upper lid crease is poorly defined or absent with poor elevation of lid when looking up due to fibrotic levator muscle. This may be compensated by the use of forehead muscles to lift the brow. It is important to note the extraocular motility and check for anisocoria in any child with ptosis.

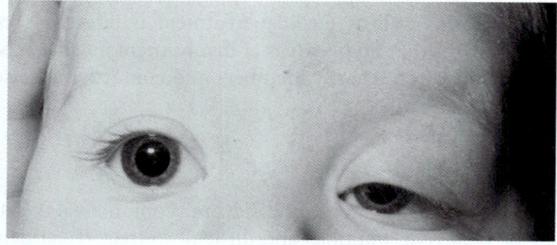

▲ **Figure 16–14.** Congenital ptosis of severe degree, left upper lid.

▶ Differential Diagnosis

Congenital ptosis, traumatic ptosis, neurogenic ptosis (oculomotor nerve palsy), Horner syndrome.

▶ Complications

Amblyopia.

▶ Treatment

Children with ptosis should be monitored for development of amblyopia. They may require correction of refractive error. Surgical correction is indicated for moderate to severe ptosis. Generally, surgery is delayed until preschool age when most of the facial growth has occurred, but it can be considered earlier in the presence of amblyopia or severe chin-up position.

▶ Prognosis

The prognosis depends on the presence of amblyopia and whether it is adequately treated.

HORNER SYNDROME

ESSENTIALS OF DIAGNOSIS & TYPICAL FEATURES

▶ Horner syndrome, which may be congenital or acquired, presents with signs of unequal pupils (anisocoria), eyelid ptosis, and anhidrosis.

▶ Pathogenesis

The syndrome is caused by an abnormality of the sympathetic chain. Most cases of pediatric Horner syndrome are idiopathic or caused by birth trauma. Acquired cases may occur in children who have had cardiothoracic surgery, trauma, neoplasm, or brainstem vascular malformation. Most worrisome is a Horner syndrome caused by neuroblastoma of the sympathetic chain in the apical lung region.

▶ Clinical Findings

Parents may notice unequal pupils or different colored eyes. Penlight examination of the eyes may reveal anisocoria and eyelid ptosis of the affected eye. The affected pupil is smaller in size, and the difference is most pronounced in the dark as the problem lies in poor dilation due to sympathetic dysfunction. Ptosis is usually mild with a well-defined upper lid crease. The whole eye may appear smaller due the smaller palpebral fissure from upper lid ptosis and lower lid elevation

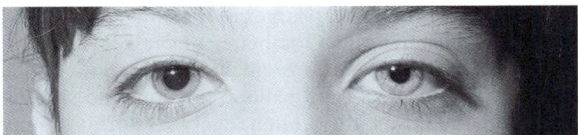

▲ **Figure 16–15.** Congenital Horner syndrome. Ptosis, miosis, and heterochromia. Lighter colored iris is on the affected left side.

(lower lid also has sympathetic innervation). A key finding of *congenital* Horner syndrome is iris heterochromia, with the lighter colored iris on the affected side (Figure 16–15). Anhidrosis can occur in congenital and acquired cases. Of note, not all of the three signs must be present to make the diagnosis.

Pharmacologic assessment of the pupils with topical cocaine and hydroxyamphetamine will help determine whether Horner syndrome is due to a preganglionic or postganglionic lesion of the sympathetic chain, but these drugs are difficult to obtain in a clinical setting. The use of apraclonidine may be more practical, but its use is limited in pediatric population as it can lead to lethargy and bradycardia. Physical examination, including palpation of the neck and abdomen for masses, should be performed. The need for an extensive evaluation for neuroblastoma (urinary catecholamine test, MRI of the brain, neck, chest, abdomen, and abdominal ultrasound) in children with isolated Horner syndrome remains controversial as many studies show that isolated Horner syndrome is an unlikely sign of "occult" neuroblastoma, and sedation and gadolinium involved in MRI are not without risk. Further evaluation of children with Horner syndrome is recommended for suspicious cases without a history of trauma, surgery, or pneumonia, in the presence of other signs or symptoms of neuroblastoma.

▶ Differential Diagnosis

Congenital or neurogenic ptosis and physiologic anisocoria.

▶ Complications

Prognosis depends on the etiology. Ptosis associated with Horner syndrome is usually mild and rarely results in amblyopia.

▶ Treatment

Management of any underlying disease is required. The ptosis and vision should be monitored by an ophthalmologist.

▶ Prognosis

Prognosis depends on the etiology. The vision is usually normal.

Ben SA, Ash S, Luckman J, Toledano H, Goldeberg-Cohen N: Likelihood of diagnosing neuroblastoma in isolated Horner syndrome. J Neuroophthalmol 2019;39(3):308–312. doi: 10.1097/WNO.0000000000000764 [PMID: 30801444].

Graef S, Chiu HH, Wan MJ: The risk of a serious etiology in pediatric Horner syndrome: indications for a workup and which investigations to perform. J AAPOS 2020 Jun;24(3):143.e1–143.e6. doi: 10.1016/j.jaapos.2020.02.012. Epub 2020 Jun 6 [PMID: 32522708].

EYELID TICS

Eyelid tics may occur as a transient phenomenon lasting several days to months. Although a tic may be an isolated finding in an otherwise healthy child, it may also occur in children with multiple tics, attention-deficit/hyperactivity disorder, or Tourette syndrome. Caffeine consumption may cause or exacerbate eyelid tics. If the disorder is a short-lived annoyance, no treatment is needed.

▼ DISORDERS OF THE NASOLACRIMAL SYSTEM

NASOLACRIMAL DUCT OBSTRUCTION

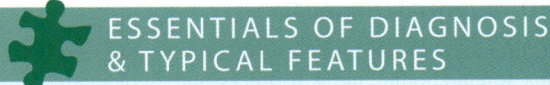

ESSENTIALS OF DIAGNOSIS & TYPICAL FEATURES

► Nasolacrimal duct obstruction (NLDO) occurs in up to 20% of infants aged < 1 year.

► Most cases (> 90%) clear spontaneously during the first year.

▶ Pathogenesis

Congenital NLDO occurs from mechanical obstruction located distally at the valve of Hasner. Nasolacrimal obstruction is more commonly seen in individuals with craniofacial abnormalities or Down syndrome.

▶ Prevention

Not applicable.

▶ Clinical Findings

NLDO can be unilateral, bilateral, and asymmetric in severity. Signs and symptoms include tearing (epiphora) or mucoid discharge from the affected eye(s), especially in the morning (Figure 16–16). The conjunctiva is usually white and quiet, distinguishing it from infectious conjunctivitis. The eyelid skin can become irritated from constant wetness or dabbing.

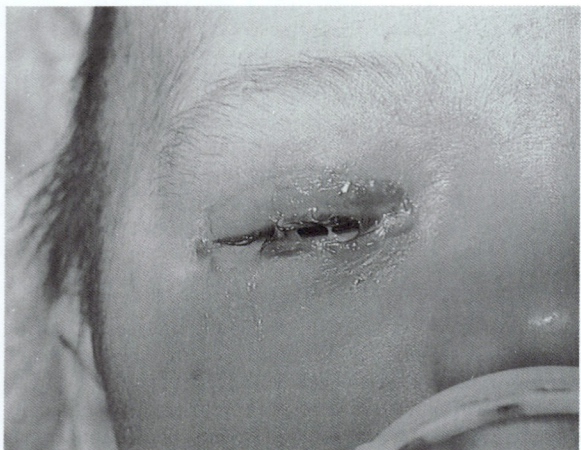

▲ **Figure 16–16.** Nasolacrimal obstruction, right eye. Mattering on upper and lower lids.

Fluorescein dye disappearance test can evaluate the clearance of dye from the tear meniscus in both eyes over a 5-minute period.

Differential Diagnosis

The differential diagnosis of tearing includes congenital glaucoma, foreign bodies, nasal disorders, and, in older children, allergies. Light sensitivity and blepharospasm suggest possible congenital glaucoma and warrant an urgent ophthalmic referral.

Complications

Dacryocystitis, orbital cellulitis, and higher prevalence of anisometropic amblyopia have been demonstrated in children with congenital NLDO.

Treatment

Massage over the nasolacrimal sac may empty debris from the nasolacrimal sac and clear the obstruction, although the efficacy of massage in clearing nasolacrimal obstruction is debated. The use of topical antibiotics/ointment should be reserved only for concurrent signs of conjunctivitis or dacryocystitis as there is no evidence that it affects resolution of NLDO and can also promote overgrowth of resistant flora that can cause chronic NLD infection.

The mainstay of surgical treatment is probing, which has 75%–80% success rate. Probing is recommended for children older than 12 months due to high rate of spontaneous resolution. Review of published reports supports the efficacy and safety of both in-office and facility-based (under general anesthesia) surgeries for unilateral NLDO. Probing of bilateral NLDO is better under general anesthesia. Additional procedures include infraction of the inferior nasal turbinate and balloon dilation, and silicone tube intubation. Much less often, dacryocystorhinostomy (DCR) is required.

Prognosis

Generally good with surgical treatment.

Morrison DG et al: Office-or Facility-based probing for congenital nasolacrimal duct obstruction: a report by the AAO. Ophthalmology 2021 Jun;128(6):920–927. doi:10.1016/j.ophtha.2020/10.028. Epub 2020 Dec 24 [PMID: 33358412].
Vagge A et al: Congenital nasolacrimal duct obstruction (CNLDO): a review. Diseases 2018 Dec;6(4):96. doi: 10.3390/diseases6040096 [PMID: 30360371].

CONGENITAL DACRYOCYSTOCELE

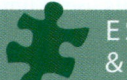 ESSENTIALS OF DIAGNOSIS & TYPICAL FEATURES

▶ Congenital dacryocystocele (CDC) presents as a bluish mass located below the medial canthus.

▶ This entity is different from regular congenital NLD obstruction and is associated with high rates of acute dacryocystitis and intranasal cysts and warrants urgent ophthalmology and ENT referral.

Pathogenesis

CDC is thought to result from obstructions proximal and distal to the nasolacrimal sac.

Clinical Findings

CDC presents in the neonatal period with the majority within the first 10 days of life. It is most often a unilateral (80%) bluish mass lesion, which may or may not be compressible, and can displace the medial canthus superiorly (Figure 16–17). Not all patients have associated epiphora/discharge. More than one-half can be associated with intranasal cysts that can cause grunting sounds, respiratory distress, and feeding difficulties. Therefore, nasal endoscopic examination should be performed in all cases of CDC. Infection (dacryocystitis) can develop in up to 85%, usually in the first 1–2 weeks of life and can progress to orbital cellulitis and sepsis. Typically, CDCs are isolated and not associated with systemic syndromes.

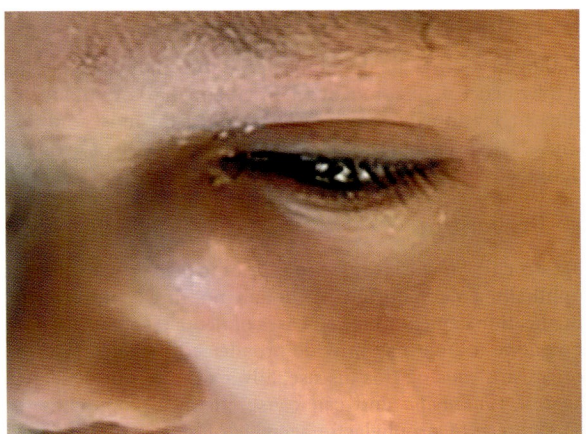

▲ **Figure 16–17.** Congenital dacryocystocele on the left side. Raised, bluish discolored mass of enlarged nasolacrimal sac. Note superiorly displaced medial canthus.

Differential Diagnosis

Eyelid hemangioma, encephalocele, and meningoencephalocele (these are usually located above the medial canthus).

Complications

Dacryocystitis, orbital cellulitis, sepsis, respiratory distress, feeding difficulties.

Treatment

All patients with CDC should be referred to an ophthalmologist urgently due to the high risk of infection and possible need for surgical intervention. Consultation with an ENT specialist is recommended to aid in the diagnosis and treatment of an associated intranasal cyst. In the meantime, parents can perform massage as long as there are no signs of respiratory distress. Nasolacrimal duct probing and endoscopic marsupialization of the intranasal cyst under general anesthesia are often required, but in certain cases, debridement of the intranasal cyst alone may resolve the problem. For treatment of dacryocystitis, hospital admission and the use of systemic antibiotics are advised prior to probing to monitor respiratory status and reduce the rate of probing-induced bacteremia.

Prognosis

Generally good.

Singh S, Ali MJ: Congenital dacryocystocele: a major review. Ophthalmic Plast Reconstr Surg 2019;35:309–317. doi: 10.1097/IOP.0000000000001297 [PMID: 30601463].

DACRYOCYSTITIS

ESSENTIALS OF DIAGNOSIS & TYPICAL FEATURES

▶ Dacryocystitis is an infection of the nasolacrimal sac that causes erythema and edema over the nasolacrimal sac.

▶ Pathogenesis

Acute dacryocystitis is most commonly caused by *S aureus, Streptococcus pneumoniae*, and *Haemophilus* species, in order of frequency. Rare cases of fungal or viral infections have been reported. Congenital NLDO is the most common risk factor for acute dacryocystitis in children. Pediatric acute dacryocystitis can be categorized into four groups that are managed differently: acute dacryocystitis in neonates with dacryocystocele, dacryocystitis with periorbital cellulitis, dacryocystitis post facial trauma, and dacryocystitis associated with orbital abscess.

▶ Prevention

Treatment of NLDO.

▶ Clinical Findings

Acute dacryocystitis presents with inflammation, swelling, tenderness, and pain over the lacrimal sac (located inferior to the medial canthal tendon). Fever may be present. The infection may point externally (Figure 16–18). A purulent discharge within the lacrimal sac may reflux with sac pressure.

Chronic dacryocystitis and recurrent episodes of low-grade dacryocystitis are caused by nasolacrimal obstruction.

▶ Differential Diagnosis

Infected mucocele.

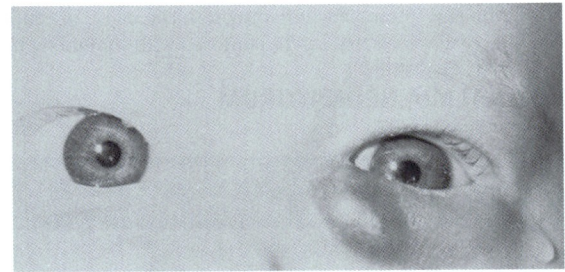

▲ **Figure 16–18.** Acute dacryocystitis in an 11-week-old infant.

Complications

Preseptal cellulitis, orbital cellulitis, and sepsis.

Treatment

Management of acute dacryocystitis depends on the category. All acute types will require systemic antibiotics. Approximately 30% of cases resolve with outpatient treatment, and 56% without early surgical intervention. However, hospital admission is recommended for younger patients and those with dacryocystitis associated with dacryocystocele as they may require probing with marsupialization of intranasal cysts. Dacryocystitis with periorbital cellulitis may need probing after the acute episode. Those that occur from facial trauma often require DCR with stents. Those complicated by orbital abscess require simultaneous abscess drainage with probing and stent placement.

Warm compresses are beneficial to help express discharge from the lacrimal sac.

Prognosis

Generally good.

Alaboudi A, Al-Shaikh OA, Fatani D, Alsuhaibani AH: Acute dacryocystitis in pediatric patients and frequency of nasolacrimal duct patency. Orbit 2021 Feb;40(1):18–23. doi:101080/0167683 0.2020.1717548. Epub 2020 Jan 29 [PMID: 31994430].

Prat D, Magoon K, Karen R, Katowitz JA, Katowitz WR: Management of pediatric acute dacryocystitis. Ophthalmic Plast Reconstr Surg 2021 Sep–Oct;37(5):482–487. doi: 10.1097/IOP.0000000000001932 [PMID: 33782322].

DISEASES OF THE CONJUNCTIVA

Conjunctivitis may be infectious, allergic, or associated with systemic disease. In conjunctivitis, the eye becomes red as a result of blood vessel dilation. Edema can accumulate leading to *chemosis*, a boggy appearance of conjunctiva. When eyelids are everted, there can be a papillary or follicular reaction of the palpebral conjunctiva. In *papillary* reaction, the palpebral conjunctiva has a cobblestoning appearance with large nodules with central vessel core. *Follicular* reaction causes dome-shaped, gel-like nodules surrounded at their base by vessels.

Trauma and intraocular inflammation can cause injection of conjunctival vessels that can be confused with conjunctivitis.

OPHTHALMIA NEONATORUM

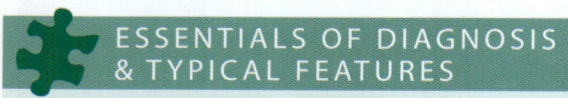

ESSENTIALS OF DIAGNOSIS & TYPICAL FEATURES

▶ Ophthalmia neonatorum (conjunctivitis in the newborn) occurs during the first month of life.

Pathogenesis

Pathogenesis may be due to bacterial infection (gonococcal, staphylococcal, pneumococcal, or chlamydial) or viral infection. In developed countries, *Chlamydia* is the most common cause. Herpes simplex is a rare but serious cause of neonatal conjunctivitis.

Prevention

Treatment of maternal infections prior to delivery can prevent ophthalmia neonatorum. Although no single prophylactic medication can eliminate all cases of neonatal conjunctivitis, povidone-iodine may provide broader coverage against the organisms causing this disease. Silver nitrate is not effective against *Chlamydia* and can cause chemical conjunctivitis. The choice of prophylactic agent is often dictated by local epidemiology and cost considerations, but erythromycin ophthalmic ointment is most routinely administered immediately after birth to help prevent ophthalmia neonatorum.

Clinical Findings

Ophthalmia neonatorum is characterized by redness, discharge, and swelling of the lids and conjunctiva (Figure 16–19). *Neisseria gonorrhoeae* causes severe purulence with pseudomembrane formation and can rapidly lead to corneal perforation. Gram staining of discharge, cultures and PCR amplification for *Chlamydia trachomatis*, *N gonorrhoeae*, and HSV aid will provide an etiologic diagnosis.

Differential Diagnosis

Chemical/toxic conjunctivitis, viral conjunctivitis, and bacterial conjunctivitis.

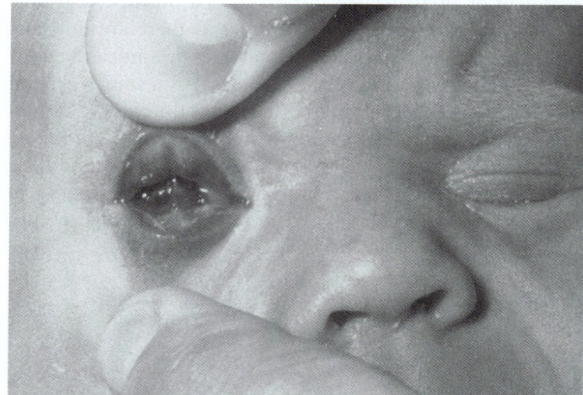

▲ **Figure 16–19.** Ophthalmia neonatorum due to *Chlamydia trachomatis* infection in a 2-week-old infant. Note marked lid and conjunctival inflammation.

Table 16–3. Features and treatment of ophthalmia neonatorum.

Cause	Typical Onset	Features	Topical Treatment	Systemic Treatment
Chlamydia	5–14 days after birth	Mucoid discharge	Erythromycin 4 times daily × 14 days	Erythromycin or azithromycin
Gonorrhea	2–4 days after birth	Hyperpurulent discharge, corneal perforation	Saline lavage, erythromycin	Ceftriaxone or cefotaxime
HSV	4–21 days after birth	Mucoid discharge, corneal involvement	Ganciclovir gel	Acyclovir
Chemical	1 day after birth	Redness, lid swelling	Lubricants	

► Complications

Chlamydia can cause a delayed-onset pneumonitis. Gonococcal infections can cause blindness through corneal perforation and can cause sepsis.

► Treatment

Treatment for ophthalmia neonatorum is shown in Table 16–3. Parents should be examined and receive treatment when a sexually associated pathogen is present. They need close monitoring by an ophthalmologist due to the risk of corneal involvement that can lead to permanent vision loss.

► Prognosis

Prognosis depends on the infectious agent as well as the rapidity of treatment.

BACTERIAL CONJUNCTIVITIS

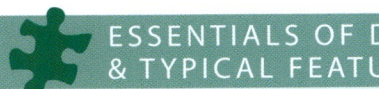

ESSENTIALS OF DIAGNOSIS & TYPICAL FEATURES

► In general, bacterial conjunctivitis is accompanied by a significant purulent discharge.

► Pathogenesis

Common bacterial causes of conjunctivitis in children include *Haemophilus* species, *S pneumoniae*, *Moraxella catarrhalis*, and *S aureus*.

► Prevention

Handwashing and contact precautions.

► Clinical Findings

Presence of significant discharge helps distinguish bacterial from viral conjunctivitis. Regional lymphadenopathy is not a common finding in bacterial conjunctivitis except in cases of oculoglandular syndrome due to *S aureus*, group A β-hemolytic streptococci, *Mycobacterium tuberculosis* or atypical mycobacteria, *Francisella tularensis*, and *Bartonella henselae*. *Chlamydia* serotypes A and C cause trachoma with severe follicular reaction of tarsal conjunctiva that can lead to scarring (Arlt's line), limbal follicles (Herbert pits), and eventual cicatrization of the cornea. Chlamydial D through K causes inclusion conjunctivitis, a unilateral chronic follicular form seen in sexually active adolescents.

► Differential Diagnosis

Viral, allergic, traumatic, or chemical/toxic conjunctivitis.

► Complications

Bacterial conjunctivitis is usually self-limited unless caused by *C trachomatis*, *N gonorrhoeae*, and *N meningitidis*, which may have systemic manifestations and can lead to ocular complications without treatment.

► Treatment

If conjunctivitis is not associated with systemic illness, topical antibiotics such as polymyxin/trimethoprim sulfate or fluoroquinolones may be helpful in hastening the resolution of symptoms. Using a delayed treatment strategy (waiting 3 days for spontaneous improvement) before the use of antibiotics may prevent unnecessary medication. Systemic therapy in addition to topical treatment is recommended for conjunctivitis associated with *C trachomatis*, *N gonorrhoeae*, and *N meningitidis*.

► Prognosis

Generally good.

Alfonso SA, Fawley JD, Alexa Lu X: Conjunctivitis. Prim Care 2015 Sep;42(3):325–345. doi: 10.1016/j.pop.2015.05.001 [PMID: 26319341].

Chen FV, Chang TC, Cavuoto KM: Patient demographic and microbiology trends in bacterial conjunctivitis in children. J AAPOS 2018;22:66–67 [PMID: 29247795].

VIRAL CONJUNCTIVITIS

ESSENTIALS OF DIAGNOSIS & TYPICAL FEATURES

▶ Children with viral conjunctivitis usually present with injection of the conjunctiva of one or both eyes and watery ocular discharge.

▶ Pathogenesis

Adenovirus infection is often associated with pharyngitis, a follicular reaction of the palpebral conjunctiva, and preauricular adenopathy (pharyngoconjunctival fever). Epidemics of adenoviral keratoconjunctivitis occur. Less commonly, acute hemorrhagic conjunctivitis due to Coxsackievirus or enterovirus can present with extensive subconjunctival hemorrhage and injection. Other causes include measles, Zika virus, HSV, and varicella-zoster virus (VZV).

▶ Prevention

Handwashing and contact precautions.

▶ Clinical Findings

Watery discharge associated with conjunctival injection of one or both eyes. Significant eyelid edema can occur. Enlarged preauricular lymph nodes can be present. A vesicular rash involving the eyelids or face suggests HSV or herpes zoster (unilateral).

▶ Differential Diagnosis

Bacterial, allergic, traumatic, or chemical/toxic conjunctivitis.

▶ Complications

Generally, viral conjunctivitis is self-limited. Cornea involvement in epidemic keratoconjunctivitis may prolong the course of disease. Herpes conjunctivitis may be associated with keratitis or retinal involvement.

▶ Treatment

Treatment of adenovirus conjunctivitis is supportive. Children with presumed adenoviral keratoconjunctivitis are considered contagious 10–21 days from the day of onset or as long as the eyes are red. They should stay out of school and group activities until redness and tearing resolve. Strict handwashing precautions are recommended. In severe cases with cornea involvement, a short course of topical steroids can improve the symptoms. However, steroids can also prolong the duration of disease. Steroids should only be used when it is certain that HSV is not the cause.

Herpes conjunctivitis can be treated with topical or oral antivirals (see section Viral Keratitis).

▶ Prognosis

Generally good.

ALLERGIC CONJUNCTIVITIS

ESSENTIALS OF DIAGNOSIS & TYPICAL FEATURES

▶ Itching associated with redness, tearing, and papillary reaction of palpebral conjunctiva.
▶ Commonly seen with allergic rhinitis and asthma.

▶ Prevention

Decreased exposure to allergens.

▶ Clinical Findings

The history of itchy, watery, and red eyes is essential in making the diagnosis of allergic conjunctivitis. Allergic "shiners" or dark circles under eyes can be present. Atopic keratoconjunctivitis (AKC) can cause year-round symptoms. Vernal keratoconjunctivitis (VKC), which is similar to AKC but occurs more often in the spring and summer (75%), is associated with intense tearing, itching, and a stringy discharge. VKC is more common in males, usually in the first decade of life, and may present with giant cobblestone papillae (Figure 16–20) on the tarsal conjunctiva, Horner-Trantas

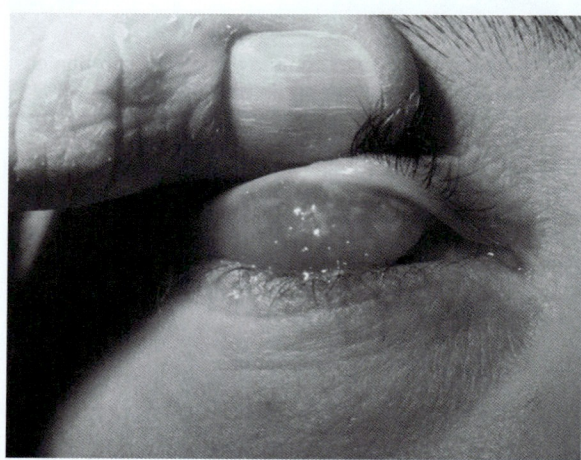

▲ **Figure 16–20.** Vernal conjunctivitis. Cobblestone papillae in superior tarsal conjunctiva.

Table 16–4. Common over-the-counter ocular allergy medications.

Generic Name	Brand Name	Side Effects	Dosage
Mast cell stabilizer			
Lodoxamide tromethamine 0.1%	Alomide	Transient burning or stinging	1 drop 4 times daily—taper
Nedocromil	Alocril	Bitter tasting, nasal congestion (10%)	1 drop 1–2 times daily
Pemirolast potassium	Alamast	Burning, nasal congestion (10%)	
Antihistamines			
Levocabastine HCL 0.05%	Livostin	Headache, burning	1 drop 1–4 times daily
H1–Antihistamines/Mast cell stabilizer combination			
Olopatadine	Patanol, Pataday, Pazeo	Headache, burning or stinging	1 drop 1–2 times daily
Ketotifen	Zyrtec Eye, Claritin Eye, Zaditor, Alaway	Redness, rhinitis	1 drop 3 times daily
Azelastine	Optivar	Burning, bitter taste	1 drop 2 times daily
Alcaftadine	Lastacaft	Burning, stinging	1–2 drops daily
Nonsteroidal anti-inflammatory			
Ketorolac tromethamine 0.5%	Acular	Transient burning or stinging	1 drop 4 times daily
Vasoconstrictor			
Naphazoline HCl 0.1%	AK-Con, Naphcon, Opcon, Vasocon	Mydriasis, increased redness, irritation, discomfort, punctate keratitis, increased intraocular pressure, dizziness, headache, nausea, nervousness, hypertension, weakness, cardiac effects, hyperglycemia, rebound redness	Varies by preparation

dots (white accumulation of degenerated eosinophils and epithelial cells at corneal limbus), phlyctenules (nodular inflammation on conjunctiva or cornea), and even sterile corneal ulcers (shield ulcers) due to rubbing of the giant papillae against the corneal surface. Contact lens wear may induce a giant papillary conjunctivitis that appears similar to the palpebral form of vernal conjunctivitis.

▶ Treatment

Topical ophthalmic solutions that combine both an antihistamine and mast cell stabilizer are very effective at treating allergic conjunctivitis. Table 16–4 lists the various combinations available for treatment of allergic conjunctivitis. Corticosteroids should be used with caution because their extended use causes glaucoma or cataracts and requires close follow-up with an ophthalmologist. Topical antibiotics are used to prevent secondary infections in those with shield ulcers. Systemic antihistamines and limitation of exposure to allergens may help reduce symptoms and are important part of the treatment, especially for AKC.

▶ Prognosis

Generally good but inadequate treatment and poor follow-up can result in corneal scarring and permanently decreased vision.

MUCOCUTANEOUS DISEASES

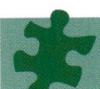
ESSENTIALS OF DIAGNOSIS & TYPICAL FEATURES

▶ Stevens-Johnson syndrome (SJS) and toxic epidermal necrolysis (TEN) are systemic conditions that often affect the eyes, as well as the skin, oral, and genitourinary mucosa.

▶ Ocular involvement may result in permanent conjunctival scarring, eyelid malposition, severe dry eye syndrome, and permanent vision loss. Early intervention is key to preventing ocular complications.

▶ Pathogenesis

SJS/TEN is a spectrum of serious delayed-type hypersensitivity reaction to drugs and viruses. A separate pattern of mucocutaneous eruptions associated with *Mycoplasma pneumoniae* infection, called mycoplasma-induced rash and mucositis (MIRM), has been described. These mucocutaneous conditions can have ocular involvement with potentially permanent and serious ocular complications.

Clinical Findings

Eye involvement can vary in severity from self-limited mild conjunctivitis to sloughing of the entire mucosal surface. Intense inflammation can lead to formation of pseudomembrane, frank membrane, and corneal ulceration. Conjunctival ulceration can result in fusion of bulbar and palpebral conjunctival surfaces in the fornix leading to permanent symblepharon (adhesions between conjunctiva), ankyloblepharon (adhesions between eyelids), and lid malposition. The extent of epithelial cell loss of ocular surface is visualized with fluorescein staining. Patients require daily examinations by ophthalmologists. The severity of ocular involvement may not correlate with systemic skin and mucocutaneous manifestations.

Differential Diagnosis

Viral or bacterial conjunctivitis until the diagnosis of SJS/TEN is apparent.

Complications

Severe ocular involvement can result in permanent scarring of the conjunctiva leading to eyelid malposition, trichiasis (misdirected eyelashes), and vision loss and blindness from chronic ocular irritation and extreme tear film deficiency.

Treatment

Management of acute ocular SJS/TEN/MIRM involves controlling the intense ocular surface inflammation. Treatment of the underlying disease includes discontinuation of offending medications and the use of appropriate antimicrobials as necessary. Aggressive ophthalmic treatment should be initiated as soon as possible, including the use of lubrication, topical corticosteroids, topical cyclosporine, and topical antibiotics. Extensive sloughing requires urgent amniotic membrane transplants to the lid margins and conjunctiva within the first weeks of illness in order to prevent chronic ocular complications.

Prognosis

Prognosis depends on the severity of the underlying condition. Visual prognosis can be excellent with early medical and surgical treatment.

Gregory DG: New grading system and treatment guidelines for the acute ocular manifestations of Stevens-Johnson syndrome. Ophthalmology 2016 Aug;123(8):1653–1658. doi: 10.1016/j.ophtha.2016.04.041 [PMID: 27297404].

DISORDERS OF THE IRIS

IRIS COLOBOMA

> ## ESSENTIALS OF DIAGNOSIS & TYPICAL FEATURES
>
> ► Iris coloboma is a developmental defect due to incomplete closure of the anterior embryonal fissure.
> ► Iris coloboma may occur as an isolated defect or in association with various chromosomal abnormalities and syndromes.

Clinical Findings

Penlight examination of the pupils reveals a keyhole shape to the pupil rather than the normal round configuration (Figure 16–21). A dilated examination by an ophthalmologist is necessary to determine if the coloboma involves additional structures of the eye including the optic nerve, retina, and choroid, in which case vision can be affected. A genetic evaluation is usually recommended due to the high rate of associated genetic syndromes.

Differential Diagnosis

Anterior segment dysgenesis, aniridia, and previous iris trauma.

Complications

Low vision and rarely a secondary retinal detachment from chorioretinal coloboma.

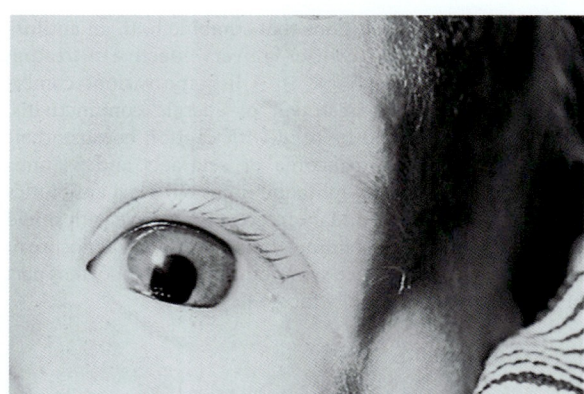

▲ **Figure 16–21.** Iris coloboma located inferiorly.

Treatment

Patients with coloboma should be monitored by an ophthalmologist for signs of amblyopia, significant refractive errors, and strabismus.

Prognosis

The prognosis depends on whether there are other ocular structures involved. Vision is guarded if a large retinal coloboma is present.

ANIRIDIA

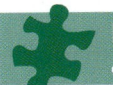

ESSENTIALS OF DIAGNOSIS & TYPICAL FEATURES

► Aniridia is a bilateral congenital disorder that affects all ocular tissue but most notably results in iris hypoplasia (Figure 16–22).

Pathogenesis

Aniridia can occur in isolation without systemic involvement, due to PAX6 gene mutation, or as part of the Wilms tumor-aniridia-genitourinary anomalies-retardation (WAGR) syndrome. One-third of the sporadic cases are associated with WAGR syndrome.

Clinical Findings

Aniridia involves all ocular tissue and can manifest as iris hypoplasia, keratopathy, glaucoma, cataract, optic nerve hypoplasia (ONH), and foveal hypoplasia. If foveal hypoplasia is present, nystagmus is usually apparent by 6 weeks of age due to poor vision. Slit-lamp or penlight examinations reveal little to no visible iris (see Figure 16–22). Photophobia may be present. Glaucoma, cataracts, and keratopathy usually develop with time in teenage years or adulthood.

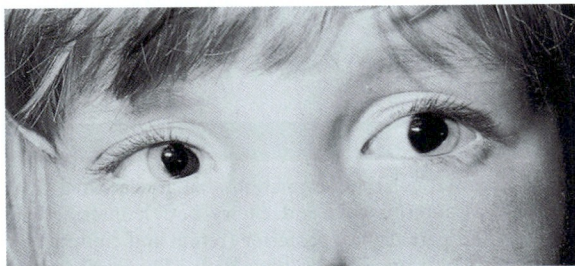

▲ **Figure 16–22.** Bilateral aniridia. Iris remnants present temporally in each eye.

Differential Diagnosis

Microphthalmia, iris coloboma, and previous iris trauma.

Complications

Low vision, cataracts, glaucoma, and keratopathy.

Treatment

An ophthalmologist should evaluate and treat refractive error as well as monitor for signs of cataracts and glaucoma. Abdominal ultrasonography is indicated in the sporadic form of aniridia to diagnose Wilms tumor. Referral to genetics is recommended unless there is clear family history of autosomal dominant aniridia.

Prognosis

Patients tend to have low vision.

ALBINISM

ESSENTIALS OF DIAGNOSIS & TYPICAL FEATURES

► Oculocutaneous albinism (OCA) is a heterogenous group of autosomal recessive disorders causing reduced or absent pigmentation of hair, skin, and eyes. Ocular albinism (OA) is an X-linked recessive disorder where hypopigmentation is limited to eyes only.

Pathogenesis

OCA is most often due to a defect in tyrosine conversion affecting pigment production. There are at least four types of OCA for which the clinical spectrum can vary from complete lack of pigmentation in OCA1A to milder forms where pigments can accumulate over time. OA, which represents 10% of all albinism, is due to a mutation in the *GPR143* gene whose protein product controls the number and size of melanosomes.

Clinical Findings

Iris, skin, and hair color vary with the type of albinism. Iris transillumination defects can be seen, characterized by abnormal transmission of light through an iris with decreased pigment. The iris can appear to be pink in color as the red fundus shows through the hypopigmented iris. This may require slit-lamp examination with retroillumination to detect focal areas of transillumination. Affected individuals usually have poor vision and nystagmus due to foveal hypoplasia. Other ocular abnormalities include abnormal optic pathway projections, strabismus, and poor stereoacuity.

Differential Diagnosis

Albinism may be associated with other systemic manifestations. In Hermansky-Pudlak syndrome, OCA is associated with a platelet abnormality causing bleeding issues. Chédiak-Higashi syndrome is characterized by neutrophil defects, recurrent infections, and OCA. Other conditions associated with albinism are Waardenburg, Prader-Willi, and Angelman syndromes.

Complications

Low vision, strabismus, high refractive errors, and visual field (VF) abnormalities.

Treatment

Children with albinism should be evaluated by a pediatric ophthalmologist to optimize their visual function. Vision teachers in schools and ophthalmic specialists trained in treating low-vision patients can improve the patient's ability to perform activities of daily living and function within society.

Prognosis

Vision is subnormal in most individuals.

MISCELLANEOUS IRIS CONDITIONS

Heterochromia, or a difference in iris color, can occur in congenital Horner syndrome, after iritis, or with tumors and nevi of the iris. Lisch nodules, which occur in type 1 neurofibromatosis, usually become apparent by age 8 years. When seen on slit-lamp examination, Lisch nodules are 1–2 mm in diameter and often beige in color. They do not affect vision. Iris xanthogranuloma occurring with juvenile xanthogranuloma can cause hyphema and glaucoma. Patients with juvenile xanthogranuloma should be evaluated by an ophthalmologist for ocular involvement.

GLAUCOMA

ESSENTIALS OF DIAGNOSIS & TYPICAL FEATURES

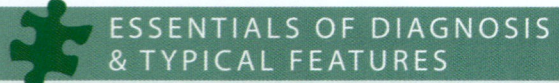

- ▶ Pediatric glaucoma can be congenital or acquired, unilateral or bilateral.
- ▶ The classic triad of symptoms in primary congenital glaucoma (PCG) includes epiphora, photophobia, and blepharospasm.

Clinical Findings

Primary signs of PCG are buphthalmos and corneal clouding. Buphthalmos occurs from elevated eye pressure that leads to enlargement of the globe due to low scleral rigidity of an infant eye. Horizontal breaks in Descemet's membrane called Haab's striae can be visible in the cornea. Unlike in adults, optic nerve cupping may be reversible in children with lowering of eye pressure. In general, a red, inflamed eye is not typical of PCG.

Sudden eye pain, redness, corneal clouding, and vision loss suggest possible pupillary block or angle-closure glaucoma. Urgent referral to an ophthalmologist is indicated. Genetic evaluation should be completed if other systemic abnormalities are noted.

Glaucoma also occurs with ocular and systemic syndromes such as aniridia, anterior segment dysgenesis, Sturge-Weber syndrome, the oculocerebrorenal syndrome of Lowe, Weill-Marchesani syndrome, and the Pierre Robin syndrome. Glaucoma can be secondary to trauma, uveitis, lens dislocation, intraocular tumor, and retinal disorders.

Differential Diagnosis

Buphthalmos is glaucoma until proven otherwise. NLDO can cause tearing, but not the other signs of blepharospasm and photophobia.

Treatment

Treatment depends on the cause, but surgery is often indicated. Topical medications have limited success in pediatric glaucoma but can be used as temporizing measures until the time of surgery. Treatment of refractive error and amblyopia is essential.

Prognosis

In general, the prognosis is guarded although excellent results can be seen. Patients may require multiple surgeries to achieve adequate eye pressure control.

Yu Chan JY, Choy BN, Ng AL, Shum JW: Review on the management of primary congenital glaucoma. J Curr Glaucoma Pract 2015 Sep–Dec;9(3):92–99. doi: 10.5005/jp-journals-10008-1192 [PMID: 26997844].

UVEITIS

Uveitis is intraocular inflammation that is classified anatomically as anterior (iris and ciliary body), intermediate (vitreous and pars plana), posterior (retina and choroid), or panuveitis. The course of uveitis is defined as acute, recurrent, and chronic (lasting more than 3 months). Most pediatric uveitides are idiopathic but can be due to systemic inflammatory conditions, infection, or as part of a masquerade syndrome.

ANTERIOR UVEITIS/IRIDOCYCLITIS/IRITIS

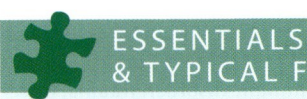

ESSENTIALS OF DIAGNOSIS & TYPICAL FEATURES

▶ Anterior uveitis (also called iritis or iridocyclitis) often presents with redness, photophobia, and blurred vision.

▶ The exception is in children with juvenile idiopathic arthritis (JIA) who are asymptomatic with white eyes and good vision despite severe uveitis resulting in ocular complications.

▶ Etiology

The most commonly diagnosed anterior uveitis in childhood is traumatic iritis, which is an acute anterior uveitis following blunt eye trauma. Uveitis is one of the most frequent and severe extra-articular manifestations of JIA so children with JIA should be screened according to a schedule recommended by the AAP (http://www.aap.org). Uveitis may precede arthritis in 3%–7%. Those with positive ANA and age 6 years or younger at diagnosis or duration 4 years or shorter are at highest risk for chronic anterior uveitis and should be screened by an ophthalmologist every 3 months. Patients with JIA-ERA (enthesitis-related arthritis) and/or positive HLA-B27 are predisposed to acute or recurrent anterior uveitis, which is usually unilateral, episodic, and characterized by acute symptoms. Uveitis is less commonly associated with inflammatory bowel disease (IBD) or psoriatic arthritis (2%–7%). Less common causes of uveitis in children include tubulointerstitial nephritis and uveitis (TINU) and early-onset sarcoidosis/Blau syndrome.

▶ Clinical Findings

Redness, photophobia, pain, and blurred vision usually accompany anterior uveitis with the exception of JIA. Slit-lamp examination reveals anterior chamber cells and protein flare (fogginess) in active anterior uveitis. Cells and protein flare can cause the iris to adhere to the lens capsule resulting in an irregular shaped pupil from posterior synechiae. Cells can settle and form a white layer, called hypopyon, within the anterior chamber. Severe anterior uveitis can also result in posterior involvement (vitritis, optic nerve edema, macular edema).

Band keratopathy, which is a sign of longstanding uveitis, are calcium deposits on the cornea that start in nasal and temporal cornea and encroach centrally. Both uveitis itself and treatment with steroids cause cataract formation.

▶ Differential Diagnosis

Trauma, infection, autoimmune disorders, medications, and masquerade syndromes such as RB, leukemia, and juvenile xanthogranuloma.

▶ Complications

Majority of children with uveitis develop complications (as high as 86% by 3 years after diagnosis). Cataract and glaucoma can develop due to severe inflammation but also due to corticosteroid treatment. Other complications include band keratopathy, cyclitic membranes, optic nerve and retinal edema, and permanent decreased vision.

▶ Treatment

Corticosteroids are the first-line treatment for acute and chronic uveitis. Cycloplegic agents help release and prevent iris adhesion to the lens and also reduce ciliary muscle spasm that causes photophobia and eye pain. Depending on the etiology, systemic immunosuppressive agents may be needed. Methotrexate is the most commonly used systemic therapy for children. Other options include anti–tumor necrosis factor-α (anti-TNFα) agents and T-cell inhibitors for refractory cases.

▶ Prognosis

Prognosis depends on the severity of ocular inflammation and development of complications.

Angeles-Han et al: 2019 American College of Rheumatology/ Arthritis Foundation Guideline for the Screening, Monitoring, and Treatment of Juvenile Idiopathic Arthritis-Associated Uveitis. Arthritis Care Res 2019 June;71(6):703–716 [PMID: 31021540].

INTERMEDIATE UVEITIS

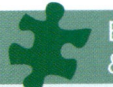

ESSENTIALS OF DIAGNOSIS & TYPICAL FEATURES

▶ Patients with pars planitis may complain of floaters and decreased vision.

▶ Clinical Findings

Intermediate uveitis, which accounts for 5%–27% of pediatric uveitis, is inflammation of the vitreous body, peripheral retina, and/or pars plana. The term "pars planitis" is a particular subset (85%–95%) of intermediate uveitis associated with characteristic snowbank and snowball formation in the absence of an infectious or systemic disease.

Pars planitis has a bimodal age distribution and affects both children (5–15 years) and adults (20–40 years). It is most commonly bilateral and can be asymmetric. Pars planitis may "burn out" after 5–15 years.

Most common clinical symptoms are blurry vision and floaters. Less commonly, patients can have red eye, photophobia, or pain. Some are asymptomatic and are diagnosed incidentally on routine eye examination. A dilated examination is crucial to identifying vitritis and inflammation along the pars plana (snowballs and snowbanking).

Differential Diagnosis

Intermediate uveitis is most often idiopathic but can be associated with systemic disease such as MS and sarcoidosis. Infectious causes include toxoplasmosis and Lyme disease.

Complications

The most common cause of decreased vision is from macular edema. Other ocular complications include cataract, optic nerve edema, and glaucoma.

Treatment

Treatment is corticosteroids as first line, but many may need systemic immunosuppression. Vitrectomy by a retinal surgeon or cryotherapy may be needed in refractory cases.

Prognosis

Prognosis depends on the severity of the disease and secondary complications. Younger children often have worse prognosis due to delayed detection and development of amblyopia.

Chauhan K, Tripathy K. Pars Planitis. [Updated 2023 Aug 25]. In: StatPearls [Internet]. Treasure Island (FL): StatPearls Publishing; 2024 Jan. Available from: https://www.ncbi.nlm.nih.gov/books/NBK436019/.

POSTERIOR UVEITIS

ESSENTIALS OF DIAGNOSIS & TYPICAL FEATURES

► Children with ocular toxoplasmosis may complain of blurred vision and have a white retinal lesion that appears like a "headlight in the fog" owing to the overlying vitritis.

Clinical Findings

The terms *choroiditis*, *retinitis*, and *retinochoroiditis* denote the tissue layers primarily involved in posterior uveitis. Fundus examination by an ophthalmologist and serologic testing are used to identify or rule out the causes of posterior uveitis. Most common cause of posterior chorioretinitis in children is infection (TORCH, HSV, CMV, toxoplasmosis, *Toxocara canis*).

Differential Diagnosis

Posterior uveitis due to autoimmune disorder, trauma, infection, malignancy, or idiopathic etiology.

Complications

Permanent vision loss due to retinal scarring and detachment.

Treatment

Congenital toxoplasmosis infections are treated with systemic antimicrobials (see Chapter 43). Reactivated toxoplasmosis with vision-threatening lesions also requires treatment. Treatment of acute retinal necrosis includes antiviral medication, corticosteroids, and prophylactic laser. Treatment of toxocariasis includes periocular corticosteroid injections and vitrectomy. The benefit of anthelminthic medications, such as albendazole, thiabendazole, and mebendazole, is not well established, as they can worsen the inflammatory response as the larvae die.

Prognosis

The prognosis for vision depends on the severity of retinal and systemic involvement.

Chan NSW, Choi J, Cheung CMG: Pediatric uveitis. Asia-Pac J Ophthalmol 2018 May–Jun;7(3):192–199 [PMID: 29682916].

▼ DISORDERS OF THE CORNEA

CLOUDY CORNEA

ESSENTIALS OF DIAGNOSIS & TYPICAL FEATURES

► Corneal clouding can be caused by developmental abnormalities, metabolic disorders, trauma, and infection.

Clinical Findings

The cornea may have a white, hazy appearance on penlight examination. Findings can be unilateral or bilateral. The red reflex may be decreased or absent.

► Differential Diagnosis

Corneal clouding, tearing, blepharospasm, and photophobia in a newborn are signs of congenital glaucoma until proven otherwise. Peters anomaly and sclerocornea are congenital malformations of the anterior segment of the eye that can be unilateral or bilateral. Direct trauma to the cornea during a forceps delivery can result in corneal haze, scarring, and significant amblyopia. Systemic abnormalities, such as developmental delay and liver or kidney failure, associated with cloudy cornea, suggest metabolic disorders such as mucopolysaccharidoses, Wilson disease, and cystinosis. Corneal infiltrates occur with viral infections, staphylococcal lid disease, and corneal dystrophies. Interstitial keratitis is a manifestation of congenital syphilis.

A complete ocular evaluation by an ophthalmologist is required and should be completed urgently when congenital glaucoma is suspected.

► Complications

Amblyopia.

► Treatment

Treatment depends on the underlying condition. Surgical treatment of glaucoma and possible corneal transplantation or keratoprosthesis may be required.

► Prognosis

Prognosis depends on the amount of corneal involvement and response to surgical treatment. Corneal transplants have a very high frequency of rejection and subsequently a poor prognosis in children.

Fecarotta CM, Huang WW: Pediatric genetic disease of the cornea. J Pediatr Genet Dec 2014;3(4):195–207. doi: 10.3233/PGE-14102 [PMID: 27625877].

VIRAL KERATITIS

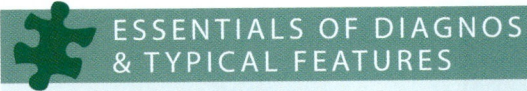

ESSENTIALS OF DIAGNOSIS & TYPICAL FEATURES

- ► A dendritic or branch-like pattern can be seen with fluorescein staining in herpetic keratitis.
- ► Children with HSV keratitis may not complain of eye pain due to decreased corneal sensation.

► Clinical Findings

In the anterior segment, HSV can present as blepharoconjunctivitis, keratitis (epithelial, stromal, or endothelial), and keratouveitis. Most often, children present with recurrent unilateral red eye with tearing, photophobia, and decreased vision. In epithelial keratitis, fluorescein administration will reveal areas of staining when viewed with a blue light. The pattern of epithelium staining may be dendritic and irregular, or round if a geographic ulcer is present. In stromal keratitis, there is corneal haze, scarring, and neovascularization, usually without epithelial fluorescein staining. Stromal keratitis is more commonly seen in children than in adults due to increased inflammatory response. Recurrence is more common in children, especially with stromal keratitis. Up to 75% of children with herpes keratitis develop damage to the corneal nerves leading to decreased corneal sensation and complications associated with neurotrophic cornea. Bilateral disease in adults has been associated with atopy and immune suppression, but this relationship remains unclear in children.

HZO is more commonly seen in adults but can present in children. It occurs with reactivation of VZV involving the ophthalmic branch of the trigeminal nerve and can affect the ocular structures anywhere from the conjunctiva to the optic nerve. In the cornea, punctate keratitis and pseudodendrites represent swollen, poorly adherent epithelial cells having a "stuck on" appearance. In contrast to HSV dendrites, these pseudodendrites lack terminal bulbs and dichotomous branching and stain poorly with fluorescein.

Adenovirus can cause bilateral epidemic keratoconjunctivitis with corneal subepithelial infiltrates (see section Viral Conjunctivitis). Adenovirus conjunctivitis may progress to keratitis 1–2 weeks after onset. Vision may be decreased.

► Differential Diagnosis

BKC and allergic conjunctivitis.

► Treatment

Oral acyclovir is a well-tolerated and effective treatment for children with HSV infection. Topical treatment can also be helpful in refractory cases of acyclovir-resistant strains of HSV. For acute HZO, oral antiviral medication can be helpful when started within 72 hours of onset of disease. Topical antivirals for HZO are controversial. Topical steroids are used for the treatment of stromal keratitis with close monitoring by an ophthalmologist. Long-term prophylactic oral acyclovir is frequently used in children with stromal keratitis or those with recurrence and continued for at least 1 year after the last recurrence.

In adenovirus keratoconjunctivitis, no treatment is necessary as it is most often self-limiting. However, judicious use of topical steroids can help decrease the symptoms (see section Viral Conjunctivitis).

► Prognosis

Recurrence of herpetic keratitis is common in children. Recurrence with corneal involvement can occur as epithelial (dendritic) keratitis or stromal (deeper in cornea) keratitis. Permanent vision loss due to scarring and amblyopia is common in children with HSV keratitis, occurring in more than 50% of affected children.

Vadoothker S, Andrews L, Jeng BH, Levin MR: Management of herpes simplex virus keratitis in the pediatric population. Pediatr Infect Dis J 2018 Sep;37(9):949–951. doi: 10.1097/INF.0000000000002114 [PMID: 29794647].

CORNEAL ULCERS

ESSENTIALS OF DIAGNOSIS & TYPICAL FEATURES

► Acute pain, decreased vision, injection, a white corneal infiltrate or ulcer (Figure 16–23), and hypopyon (pus in the anterior chamber) may be present.

▶ Pathogenesis

Most common risk of infectious keratitis and corneal ulcer is contact lens use, especially with extended wear, overnight use, orthokeratology, and using tap water for cleaning. Common pathogens are *Pseudomonas aeruginosa*, **staphylococci**, and *Acanthamoeba*. In children younger than 3 years, ocular trauma is a common cause of infectious corneal ulcers.

▶ Clinical Findings

Patients present with acute pain, photophobia, redness, and decreased vision. On examination, they have a white spot on the cornea with overlying epithelial defect that stains with fluorescein (see Figure 16–23). Other examination findings include corneal thinning, anterior chamber inflammation, and hypopyon. *Acanthamoeba* keratitis can cause unilateral or bilateral rapidly progressing ulcers with pain that seems out of proportion to examination findings.

▶ Differential Diagnosis

Viral keratitis, corneal abrasion, and penetrating foreign body.

▶ Complications

Corneal perforation and corneal scarring.

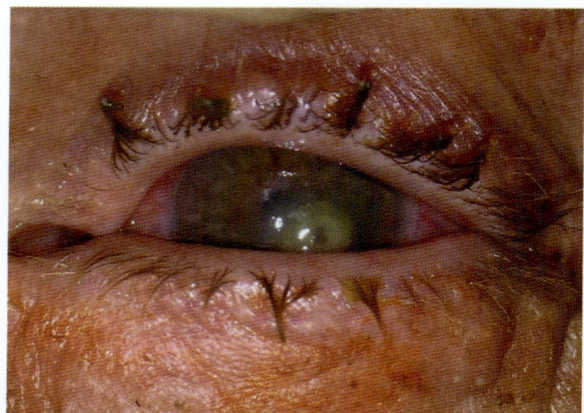

▲ **Figure 16–23.** Corneal ulcer. Note white infiltrate located on inferior cornea.

▶ Treatment

Treatment of corneal ulcers requires special expertise, and urgent referral to an ophthalmologist is necessary. It is helpful for patients to bring their contact lens and case, which can be used for culture.

▶ Prognosis

Prognosis depends on how large the ulcer is and whether the central cornea is involved.

DISORDERS OF THE LENS

Lens disorders involve abnormality of clarity or position. Lens opacification (Figure 16–24) can affect vision depending on its density, size, and position. Visual potential is also influenced by age at onset and the success of amblyopia treatment.

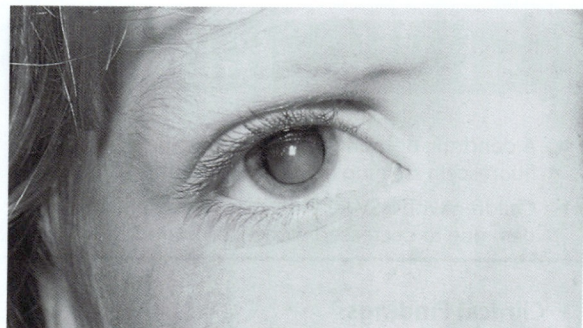

▲ **Figure 16–24.** Cataract causing leukocoria.

CATARACTS

ESSENTIALS OF DIAGNOSIS & TYPICAL FEATURES

► Absence or asymmetry of a red reflex, leukocoria, poor fixation, strabismus, or nystagmus may be due to a cataract, which requires an urgent referral to an ophthalmologist.

Etiology

Cataracts in children may be unilateral or bilateral, may exist as isolated defects, or may be accompanied by other ocular disorders or systemic disease. Systemic associations include syndromes such as Down and Lowe syndromes and metabolic disorders like galactosemia, Wilson disease, diabetes, and hypocalcemia. Genetic mutation is a common cause; inheritance pattern is most often autosomal dominant, although autosomal recessive or X-linked forms occur. Thus, it is important to ask about family history of early cataracts. The majority of non-syndromic bilateral congenital cataracts have no identifiable cause. If there is no family history of bilateral cataracts, laboratory investigation for infectious, genetic, and metabolic causes of bilateral congenital cataracts is indicated. Infectious etiologies, evaluated by TORCH titers, are less common in the United States. In contrast, unilateral cataracts are usually isolated, developmental, not inherited, and rarely associated with a systemic disease. Other causes include trauma, uveitis, and tumor.

Differential Diagnosis

Cloudy cornea, intraocular tumor, and retinal detachment.

Complications

Pediatric cataracts are frequently associated with deprivation amblyopia.

Treatment

Early diagnosis and treatment are necessary to prevent deprivation amblyopia in children younger than 9 years. Cataracts that are visually significant require removal. Visually significant unilateral cataracts in infants are removed prior to 6 weeks of age and bilateral cataracts within 8 weeks of age to reduce the risk of deprivation amblyopia. Rehabilitation of the vision will require the correction of refractive errors and amblyopia treatment. Contact lenses, glasses, bifocals, and artificial intraocular lenses are used to correct refractive errors after cataract extraction. Concomitant treatment of associated amblyopia, glaucoma, and the underlying systemic disease is indicated.

Prognosis

The ultimate VA depends on the age when the cataract developed and was removed, whether it was unilateral or bilateral, whether it was associated with glaucoma, and compliance with amblyopia treatment.

DISLOCATED LENSES/ECTOPIA LENTIS

ESSENTIALS OF DIAGNOSIS & TYPICAL FEATURES

► Most common cause of ectopia lentis is trauma, but if trauma was minor, evaluation for underlying diseases that predispose to ectopia lentis should be considered.

Etiology

Marfan syndrome, homocystinuria, Weill-Marchesani syndrome, sulfite oxidase deficiency, hyperlysinemia, syphilis, Ehlers-Danlos syndrome, and trauma.

Clinical Findings

In dislocation, lens may be free-floating in the vitreous, anterior chamber, or lie on the retina. Subluxation, which is more common, refers to partial displacement, and the edge of the lens can be seen through the pupil when shining a light or with a slit-lamp examination. Refraction often reveals significant astigmatism. A complete ophthalmic evaluation, as well as genetic and metabolic evaluation, may be warranted.

Complications

Ectopia lentis can cause decreased vision and amblyopia due to induced refractive errors. Another ophthalmologic concern is pupillary block glaucoma, in which a malpositioned unstable lens blocks the normal flow of aqueous humor from the ciliary body (posterior to the pupil), where it is produced, into the trabecular meshwork (anterior to the pupil).

Treatment

Surgical lensectomy may be required if vision is not improved significantly with glasses or contact lenses. Underlying metabolic and/or genetic disorders require a multidisciplinary approach.

Prognosis

Prognosis depends on the severity of the lens dislocation and need for lensectomy.

DISORDERS OF THE RETINA

RETINAL HEMORRHAGES IN THE NEWBORN

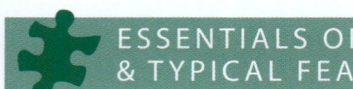

ESSENTIALS OF DIAGNOSIS & TYPICAL FEATURES

▶ RHs associated with birth most often resolves by 6 weeks of life.

Clinical Findings

Birth-related RHs can occur in approximately 25% of newborns. RHs are more commonly seen after spontaneous vaginal delivery with higher rates up to 50% after vacuum- or forceps-assisted deliveries. RHs are less common after cesarean sections but still occur (5%). Most RHs from birth resolve by 6 weeks. Examination of the retina of an otherwise healthy full term newborn infant is not indicated.

Differential Diagnosis

See section Abusive Head Trauma & Nonaccidental Trauma.

Treatment

Observation is indicated since RHs of the newborn usually disappear by 6 weeks of life.

Prognosis

Excellent.

RETINOPATHY OF PREMATURITY

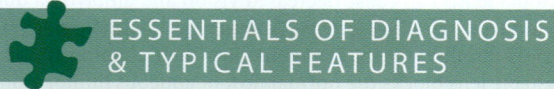

ESSENTIALS OF DIAGNOSIS & TYPICAL FEATURES

▶ Retinopathy of prematurity (ROP) screening examinations are recommended for infants with:
  • Birth weight ≤ 1500 g or
  • Gestational age ≤ 30 weeks or
  • Select infants with an unstable clinical course who may not meet the above criteria

Pathogenesis

Normal retinovascular development in humans starts in utero from the optic nerve and wraps around to the front of the eye to reach completion around 40 weeks gestation. Premature infants are at risk for developing abnormal peripheral retinal vascularization, which may lead to retinal detachment and blindness. In utero, the retina is in a state of physiologic hypoxia resulting in elevated vascular endothelial growth factor (VEGF) that facilitates retinal angiogenesis. After birth, premature infants are exposed to hyperoxia from both atmospheric and supplemental oxygen, which slows down vascularization with vasoconstriction and obliteration (phase 1 ROP). This eventually leads to peripheral retinal hypoxia which drives increased production of VEGF. In addition, a relative nutritional deficiency occurs in premature infants resulting in decreased serum IGF1, a vital regulator of VEGF. Unregulated VEGF leads to phase 2 of ROP characterized by abnormal proliferation of vessels that grow into the vitreous rather than on the retina.

Prevention

The risk of vision loss from ROP can be reduced by timely screening of premature infants by an ophthalmologist.

Clinical Findings

The Cryotherapy for Retinopathy of Prematurity (CRYO-ROP) study outlined a standard nomenclature to describe the progression and severity of ROP (Table 16–5). Since retinal blood vessels emanate from the optic nerve and do not fully cover the developing retina until term, the optic nerve is used as the central landmark. The most immature zone of the retina, zone I, is the most posterior concentric imaginary circle around the optic nerve. The nasal peripheral area is zone II, and temporal periphery is zone III. The stages of the abnormal vessels are numbered from zero (simply incomplete vascularization) through stage 5.

Table 16–5. Stages of retinopathy of prematurity.

Stage I	Demarcation line or border dividing the vascular from the avascular retina.
Stage II	Ridge. Line of stage I acquires volume and rises above the surface retina to become a ridge.
Stage III	Ridge with extraretinal fibrovascular proliferation.
Stage IV	Subtotal retinal detachment.
Stage V	Total retinal detachment.

Initial examinations are performed 4 weeks after delivery or at 31 weeks for those with GA 26 weeks or less. The frequency of follow-up examinations depends on the findings and the risk factors for developing ROP. Most infants are evaluated every 1–3 weeks, depending on the severity of ROP. ROP often persist beyond original due date. Examinations can be discontinued when the retinas are fully vascularized. Complete retinal vascularization may be prolonged in infants with moderate to severe ROP.

Complications

Low vision and retinal detachment.

Treatment

Treatment of ROP is indicated when there is type I ROP (zone I ROP with any stage and plus disease [severe vessel dilation and tortuosity], zone I ROP stage III without plus disease, zone II ROP with stage II or III and plus disease) as defined by the Early Treatment Retinopathy of Prematurity (ETROP) study. Treatment includes laser photocoagulation and, in certain cases, anti-VEGF intravitreal injections. Surgical treatment for a retinal detachment involves scleral buckling or a lens-sparing vitrectomy by a vitreoretinal specialist.

Prognosis

Most cases of ROP do not progress to retinal detachment and require no treatment. However, ROP remains a leading cause of blindness in children. Premature infants, especially those who had ROP, are at a higher risk of developing strabismus, amblyopia, and refractive error than the average child.

Fierson WM; American Academy of Pediatrics Section on Ophthalmology; American Academy of Ophthalmology; American Association for Pediatric Ophthalmology and Strabismus; American Association of Certified Orthoptists: Screening examination of premature infants for retinopathy of prematurity. Pediatrics 2018;142(6). pii: e20183061 [PMID: 30824604].

RETINOBLASTOMA

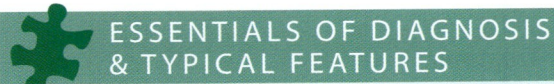

ESSENTIALS OF DIAGNOSIS & TYPICAL FEATURES

▶ Retinoblastoma (RB) is the most common primary intraocular malignancy of childhood, with an incidence estimated between 1 in 14,000–18,000 live births, and 8000 new cases each year globally.

▶ 90% of tumors are diagnosed before age 5 years.
▶ A complete review of RB can be found in Chapter 31 Neoplastic Disease.

RETINAL DETACHMENT

ESSENTIALS OF DIAGNOSIS & TYPICAL FEATURES

▶ A retinal detachment may present as an abnormal or absent red reflex.
▶ Older children may complain of decreased vision, flashes, floaters, or VF defects.

Pathogenesis

Common causes are trauma, ocular anomalies, and history of ocular surgery. The most common inherited cause of childhood retinal detachment is Stickler syndrome, a genetic connective tissue disorder. Other risk factors include high myopia, ROP, and Marfan syndrome.

Clinical Findings

Symptoms of detachment are floaters, flashing lights lasting seconds, and loss of VF; however, children often cannot appreciate or verbalize their symptoms. Self-injurious behavior is associated with high rates of retinal detachment and traumatic cataracts.

Differential Diagnosis

Intraocular tumor.

Complications

Vision loss, strabismus.

Treatment

Treatment of retinal detachment is surgical. Examination under anesthesia with prophylactic cryotherapy or laser photocoagulation is recommended for all patients with Stickler syndrome.

Prognosis

Prognosis depends on the location and duration of the detachment.

DIABETIC RETINOPATHY

ESSENTIALS OF DIAGNOSIS & TYPICAL FEATURES

► Diabetic retinopathy (DR) is a specific microvascular complication of diabetes mellitus. Patients with type 1 diabetes are at higher risk of developing severe proliferative retinopathy leading to visual loss than are those with type 2 diabetes.

▶ Prevention & Detection

Risk factors for developing DR include longer duration of disease and poor glycemic control. The screening guidelines differ among different medical societies. The AAP recommends that children older than 9 years should be examined by an ophthalmologist within 3–5 years after the onset of type 1 diabetes. Based on research in adults with type 2 diabetes, screening examination is recommended at initial diagnosis and annually thereafter for children with type 2 diabetes.

▶ Clinical Findings

Acute onset of diabetes may be accompanied by sudden blurred vision due to shift in refractive error and/or cataract formation. DR can range in severity from mild, moderate, or severe non-proliferative retinopathy to proliferative retinopathy that can lead to tractional retinal detachment. Macula edema may occur with any retinopathy. Vision-threatening DR is less common in children.

▶ Complications

Vision loss due to vitreous hemorrhage, macular edema, neovascular glaucoma, cataracts, and/or retinal detachment.

▶ Treatment

Good glycemic control is essential to decrease the risk and severity of DR. Severe proliferative DR requires pan-retinal laser photocoagulation, intravitreal anti-VEGF medication, or vitreoretinal surgery (or combination). Most children with DR do not require treatment until adulthood.

▶ Prognosis

Prognosis depends on the severity of the retinopathy and associated complications.

Geloneck MM, Forbes BJ, Shaffer J, Ying GS, Binenbaum G: Ocular complications in children with diabetes mellitus. Ophthalmology 2015 Dec;122(12):2457–2464. doi: 10.1016/j.ophtha.2015.07.010 [PMID: 26341461].

Wang SY, Andrews CA, Herman WH, Gardner TW, Stein JD: Incidence and risk factors for developing diabetic retinopathy among youths with type 1 or type 2 diabetes throughout the United States. Ophthalmology 2016 Nov 30. doi: 10.1016/j.ophtha.2016.10.031 [PMID: 27914837].

DISEASES OF THE OPTIC NERVE

OPTIC NEUROPATHY

ESSENTIALS OF DIAGNOSIS & TYPICAL FEATURES

► Poor optic nerve function may result in decreased central or peripheral vision, decreased color vision, strabismus, and nystagmus.

▶ Clinical Findings

Optic nerve disorders can be due to congenital malformation, malignancy, inflammation, infection, infiltration, medication toxicity, metabolic or genetic disorders, ischemia, and trauma. Optic nerve function is evaluated by checking VA, color vision, pupillary response, and VFs.

The swinging flashlight test is used to assess the relative function of each optic nerve. It is performed by shining a light alternately in front of each pupil to check for an APD. Normal pupil should constrict when the light is shined directly into it and also when the light is shined into the fellow eye (consensual pupil constriction). An abnormal response in the affected eye is pupillary dilation when the light is directed into that eye after having been shown in the other eye with its healthy optic nerve. Hippus—rhythmic dilating and constricting movements of the pupil—can be confused with an APD. Patients with bilateral optic nerve dysfunction may not show an APD but have bilaterally sluggishly reactive pupils.

The optic nerve is evaluated as to size, shape, color, and vascularity. Anatomic anomalies of the optic nerve include colobomatous defects, optic nerve pits, and hypoplasia.

▶ Treatment

Management of the underlying condition resulting in the optic neuropathy is necessary.

▶ Prognosis

Prognosis depends on the severity of optic neuropathy and the underlying disease.

OPTIC NERVE HYPOPLASIA

ESSENTIALS OF DIAGNOSIS & TYPICAL FEATURES

▶ Optic nerve hypoplasia (ONH), regardless of laterality or neuroanatomic abnormalities, is an independent risk factor for hypothalamic-pituitary dysfunction, which occurs in 60%–80%.

▶ Neuroimaging of the brain and endocrine consultation should be performed in all patients with ONH.

Pathogenesis

ONH is a complex congenital disorder, involving a spectrum of anatomic malformations and clinical manifestations ranging from isolated hypoplasia of one or both optic nerves to extensive brain malformations, hypothalamic-pituitary dysfunction, and neurocognitive disability. ONH is considered as part of the septo-optic dysplasia or de Morsier syndrome due to the co-occurrence of hypothalamic-pituitary dysfunction and absent septum pellucidum. Absent septum pellucidum has no prognostic significance. Growth hormone abnormality is the most common endocrine dysfunction in children with ONH. Most cases of ONH are nonhereditary.

To date, the most consistently found risk factors for ONH are young maternal age and primiparity although the mechanism by which these lead to ONH development still needs to be elucidated.

Clinical Findings

Visual function with ONH ranges from functional vision to complete blindness. Vision impairment is nonprogressive. If only one eye is involved, the child usually presents with strabismus (usually esotropia). If both eyes are affected, nystagmus is usually the presenting sign. Visual signs often may not develop until children are at least 3 months of age. Systemic signs of congenital hypopituitarism may present earlier with signs, including prolonged hyperbilirubinemia, transient or permanent hypoglycemia, or poor linear growth.

Ophthalmoscopy is performed to directly visualize the optic nerves and to determine the severity of the hypoplasia. In ONH, optic nerves can be smaller than average to nearly absent. Vessels are often abnormal in caliber. Classic "double-ring sign" refers to the circular hypo- or hyperpigmented ring (scleral canal) seen around the small optic nerve.

Treatment

ONH is an incurable congenital disorder. Sensory amblyopia and significant refractive errors should be treated by an ophthalmologist. Strabismus surgery may be necessary in certain patients. Endocrine abnormalities should be managed as necessary. A referral to a teacher for the visually impaired is a beneficial adjunct to children with ONH at any age to help optimize vision.

Prognosis

Severe bilateral ONH may result in blindness.

Ryabets-Lienhard A, Stewart C, Borchert M, Geffner ME: The optic nerve hypoplasia spectrum: review of the literature and clinical guidelines. Adv Pediatr 2016 Aug;63(1):127–146. doi: 10.1016/j.yapd.2016.04.009 [PMID: 27426898].

PAPILLEDEMA

ESSENTIALS OF DIAGNOSIS & TYPICAL FEATURES

▶ Optic nerve edema is abnormal swelling of the optic nerves. Causes include elevated intracranial pressure (ICP), infection, inflammation, ischemia, and infiltrative causes.

▶ *Papilledema* is a specific term used for optic nerve edema caused by elevated ICP.

Pathogenesis

In papilledema, ICP can be elevated primarily (idiopathic intracranial hypertension [IIH]/pseudotumor cerebri) or secondarily as a direct result of an identifiable condition. Secondary causes include intracranial mass, structural abnormalities (Chiari malformation, obstructive hydrocephalus), vascular causes (cerebral venous sinus thrombosis, hypertensive emergency), or medication induced. Most common medications associated with papilledema are tetracycline antibiotics, vitamin A derivatives, growth hormone supplementation, and corticosteroid use or withdrawal.

IIH is a poorly understood primary cause of intracranial hypertension with normal brain parenchyma and cerebrospinal constituents. In children, IIH is divided into prepubertal and pubertal groups. In the pubertal group, female gender and obesity are associated with IIH, similar to adults.

Not every patient with elevated ICP develops papilledema. It is speculated that transmission of ICP to the optic nerve sheath results in axoplasmic flow stasis leading to papilledema. There may be anatomic variations in the optic canal that provide protective effects in some individuals. In addition, optic nerves with atrophy may not swell even in the setting of severely elevated ICP.

Clinical Findings

Acute rise in ICP can result in headaches, tinnitus, nausea, vomiting, and vision changes (transient visual obscurations). Patients can develop diplopia from sixth nerve (CN VI) palsy that occurs when elevated ICP leads to a downward displacement of the brainstem that stretches CN VI as it crosses over the petrous ridge and enters Dorello's canal. CN VI palsy associated with elevated ICP is more commonly seen in children compared to adults. Photophobia is also a unique symptom of elevated ICP seen in children. Gradual rise in ICP may not cause obvious symptoms. For IIH, symptoms tend to be less obvious in younger patients. Optic nerve edema may be an incidental finding in a routine eye examination in young children.

Direct visualization of the optic nerve by ophthalmoscopy reveals an elevated disc with indistinct margins, dilated and tortuous vessels that may be obscured by the edema around the disc margin, and central hyperemia of the nerve head. Hemorrhages may be present in more severe cases. Optic nerve changes are often bilateral but can be asymmetric.

When optic nerve edema is noted, it is important to search for the cause. MRI of the brain with and without contrast is the preferred method of neuroimaging. MRV is recommended in atypical cases to rule out venous sinus thrombosis. In IIH, characteristic MRI findings are empty sella turcica, decreased pituitary gland size, optic nerve tortuosity, perioptic subarachnoid space enlargement, posterior globe flattening, and intraocular protrusion of the optic nerve head. These findings are not direct causes of elevated ICP but associated findings that may be seen in IIH patients. When a mass or structural abnormality is ruled out with neuroimaging, obtaining a lumbar puncture (LP) for opening pressure and CSF analysis may be necessary. Elevated ICP in children 18 years and younger is greater than 25 cm H_2O in nonobese, nonsedated children, and greater than 28 cm H_2O for all others.

Other ancillary modalities for evaluation include optic coherence tomography, which may show thickened retinal nerve fiber layer, and VF tests, which most commonly show an enlarged blind spot.

Differential Diagnosis

Pseudopapilledema is a normal variant of the optic disc in which the disc appears elevated, with indistinct margins and a normal vascular pattern. Pseudopapilledema sometimes occurs in hyperopic individuals. Optic disc drusen, which are acellular deposits that calcify over time, is commonly misdiagnosed as papilledema. Optic nerve edema can also be caused by infections and inflammation.

Treatment

Treatment of papilledema depends on the cause. Cessation of inciting agents may be adequate in medication-related papilledema. Anticoagulation and antibiotics may be needed for cerebral venous sinus thrombosis. For IIH, medications that are commonly used include acetazolamide, topiramate, and furosemide. For obese individuals with IIH, weight loss and healthy diet can be significantly helpful. When conservative treatment fails, or there are concerns for optic nerve compression, options such as ventriculoperitoneal or lumbo-peritoneal shunts and optic nerve sheath fenestration may be necessary.

Complications

Optic atrophy and vision loss.

Prognosis

Prognosis depends on the underlying etiology, duration, and control of the increased ICP.

Aylward SC, Way AL: Pediatric intracranial hypertension: a current literature review. Curr Pain Headache Rep 2018 Feb 13;22(2):14. doi: 10.1007/s11916-018-0665-9 [PMID: 29441432].

Phillips PH, Sheldon CA: Pediatric pseudotumor cerebri syndrome. J Neuroophthalmol 2017 Sep;37(Suppl 1):S33–S40 [PMID: 28806347].

Sheldon CA: Pediatric idiopathic intracranial hypertension: age, gender, and anthropometric features at diagnosis in a large, retrospective, multisite cohort. Ophthalmology 2016 Nov;123(11):2424–2431. doi: 10.1016/j.ophtha.2016.08.004 [PMID: 27692528].

OPTIC NEURITIS

ESSENTIALS OF DIAGNOSIS & TYPICAL FEATURES

▶ Compared to adults, optic neuritis (ON) in children is more often bilateral, more often associated with papillitis (up to 69% vs 33% in adults), more often present after a preceding viral illness, less often associated with painful eye movements, but with more severe visual deficit.

Pathogenesis

ON in children is a heterogenous disorder that may occur as an isolated event (ie, postinfectious, idiopathic) or as a component of a generalized inflammatory CNS disease or an underlying rheumatologic condition such as systemic lupus erythematosus. Inflammatory CNS diseases that can present with ON include acute disseminated encephalomyelitis (ADEM), multiple sclerosis (MS), and neuromyelitis optica (NMO).

Clinical Findings

Cardinal features of ON are decreased VA, abnormal color vision (notably red color desaturation), pain with eye movements, and VF deficits. APD will be present in unilateral cases. Symptoms may present over hours to days. Anterior ON results in optic nerve edema (papillitis). Patients with posterior ON may have normal appearing nerves on examination despite signs of optic nerve dysfunction and abnormal MRI findings.

Diagnostic workup includes LP, MRI, serum autoimmune and rheumatologic studies, and complete ophthalmic examination. MRI of the brain/orbits with and without contrast may show thickening of the optic nerves on T1-weighted imaging, bright T2 signal along the optic nerve or chiasm, and post-gadolinium enhancement. Up to 36% of children who present with ON are eventually diagnosed with MS clinically or radiologically. Likelihood is higher in children with white matter lesions in MRI of the brain and cerebrospinal fluid (CSF) oligoclonal bands (present in 80% of children with MS vs 15% in monophasic ON). Normal MRI at the time of ON conveys a low likelihood of MS.

Severe bilateral ON with severe vision loss, poor response to steroids, signs of hypothalamic/brainstem symptoms, or the presence of longitudinally extensive lesions of the optic nerve and spinal cord should prompt evaluation of serum aquaporin-4 (AQP4) IgG (NMO IgG). A positive test for AQP4-IgG supports the diagnosis of NMO.

ON is also now known to be the predominant phenotype of MOG-Ab positive-associated disease, a more recently described non-MS subgroup of CNS demyelination characterized by presence of serum myelin oligodendrocyte glycoprotein antibodies (MOG-Ab). MOG seropositivity is also found in some patients with ADEM and some NMO spectrum disorder patients who lack serologic evidence of AQP4-IgG.

Differential Diagnosis

Papilledema, infection, and neoplasm.

Complications

Decreased vision, color vision, peripheral vision, and contrast sensitivity. ON may be the first manifestation of relapsing disease that can result in ocular and systemic disability.

Treatment

No clinical trials have been performed for pediatric ON. Clinical practice follows evidence from the optic neuritis treatment trial (ONTT) where recovery after IV steroids followed by oral steroids was more rapid than after placebo or oral steroids alone. Although treatment may not change the medical outcome, recovery of visual symptoms can be shortened from 7 to 2 weeks, which may prevent psychosocial challenges faced by children, including the need to make up schoolwork and other sequelae from visual limitations. Plasma exchange (PLEX) or intravenous immunoglobulin therapy may be considered for refractory cases.

Prognosis

Prognosis depends on the underlying disease process. Despite the severe vision deficit at presentation, the majority have good visual recovery.

Gise RA, Heidary G: Update on pediatric optic neuritis. Curr Neurol Neurosci Rep 2020 Mar 3;20(3):4. doi: 10.1007/s11910-020-1024-x [PMID: 32124097].

OPTIC ATROPHY

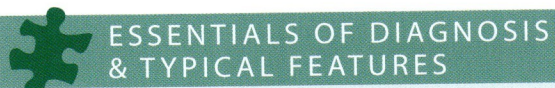

ESSENTIALS OF DIAGNOSIS & TYPICAL FEATURES

► Optic atrophy is the pathologic endpoint of numerous diseases that result in intrinsic and extrinsic insults to optic nerves.

Clinical Findings

Most common causes of optic atrophy are tumors, warranting a timely evaluation and diagnosis. Perinatal events such as intraventricular hemorrhage or periventricular white matter changes in premature infants are emerging as a common cause of optic atrophy. Other causes include structural intracranial abnormalities (craniosynostosis, hydrocephalus), post-papilledema or papillitis, toxins, ischemia, and inherited causes (autosomal dominant, autosomal recessive, X-linked, and mitochondrial). Neuroimaging is helpful for delineating CNS abnormalities.

Direct examination of the optic nerve by ophthalmoscopy reveals an optic nerve head with a cream or white color and possibly cupping. Vessels may appear attenuated. Patients may not complain of decreased vision but often have low vision on examination. Nystagmus can be present if optic atrophy was acquired as an infant.

Complications

Vision loss, decreased peripheral vision or central scotoma, and contrast sensitivity.

Treatment

There is no treatment to reverse optic atrophy.

Prognosis

Prognosis depends on the severity of the optic nerve atrophy and associated neurologic deficits.

DISEASES OF THE ORBIT

PRESEPTAL & ORBITAL CELLULITIS

ESSENTIALS OF DIAGNOSIS & TYPICAL FEATURES

▶ Significant eyelid edema, pain with eye movements, blurred or double vision, and proptosis (bulging of eye) suggest orbital cellulitis.

Pathogenesis

The fascia of the eyelids joins with the fibrous orbital septum to isolate the orbit from the lids. The orbital septum helps decrease the risk of an eyelid infection extending into the orbit. Infections arising anterior to the orbital septum are termed *preseptal*. Infection involving structures posterior to the septum (eye itself, muscles and fat around eye, and optic nerve) is called orbital cellulitis and may result in serious complications, such as a subperiosteal abscess, cavernous sinus thrombosis, cerebral abscess, meningitis, septicemia, and optic neuropathy.

Preseptal (periorbital) cellulitis can arise from a local exogenous source such as an abrasion or insect bite of the eyelid, may spread from other infections (hordeolum, dacryocystitis), or result after hematogenous spread from respiratory infection or otitis media. *S aureus* and *S pyogenes* are the most common pathogens cultured from external sources. Preseptal cellulitis can progress to orbital cellulitis.

Orbital cellulitis most commonly arises from paranasal sinus infection (most commonly ethmoid sinusitis). The pathogenic agents are those of acute or chronic sinusitis—respiratory flora and anaerobes. In addition to the normal culprits of preseptal cellulitis, *Streptococcus anginosus* is an emerging cause of orbital cellulitis and often causes a more serious infection with increased frequency of intracranial or spinal abscesses that may require neurosurgical intervention.

Rhino-orbital-cerebral mucormycosis is an uncommon but devastating infection that can lead to blindness and death in children with immunosuppression and poorly controlled diabetes.

Clinical Findings

Children with preseptal cellulitis present with red and swollen eyelids, pain, and mild fever. The vision, eye movements, and eye itself are normal. Culture should be obtained if there is an obvious site of infection on the skin.

Orbital cellulitis presents with orbital signs, which are proptosis, eye movement restriction, decreased vision, and an APD. The eye often appears red and chemotic. CT with contrast helps establish the extent of the infection within the orbit and sinuses and evaluate for subperiosteal abscess.

Differential Diagnosis

Severe conjunctivitis can cause (often bilateral) eyelid swelling and redness that can mimic preseptal/orbital cellulitis. Other masquerading diseases are primary or metastatic neoplasm of the orbit, orbital pseudotumor (idiopathic orbital inflammation), and orbital foreign body with secondary infection.

Complications

Orbital cellulitis can result in permanent vision loss due to compressive optic neuropathy. Proptosis can cause corneal exposure, dryness, and scarring. Cavernous sinus thrombosis, intracranial extension, blindness, and death can result from severe orbital cellulitis.

Treatment

Most preseptal cellulitis can be managed as an outpatient with oral antibiotics with strict counseling on returning for clinical worsening. Initial therapy for orbital cellulitis infection is with broad-spectrum systemic antibiotics, which may be later narrowed based on culture findings and clinical improvement. Treatment may require surgical drainage for subperiosteal abscess and drainage of infected sinuses, which is a crucial part of the therapy. Surgery is indicated for decreased vision attributable to orbital cellulitis, failure to improve clinically after 24–48 hours of IV antibiotics, or demonstration of worsened abscess on repeat CT. Patients with proptosis, eye movement restriction, elevated eye pressure, and age greater than 9 years are significantly more likely to require surgical intervention.

Prognosis

Most patients do well with timely treatment.

Williams KJ, Allen RC: Paediatric orbital and periorbital infections. Curr Opin Ophthalmol 2019 Sep;30(5):349–355 [PMID: 31261188].

CRANIOFACIAL ANOMALIES

ESSENTIALS OF DIAGNOSIS & TYPICAL FEATURES

▶ Children with syndromic or nonsyndromic cranio-synostosis should be examined by an ophthalmologist at the time of diagnosis and before and after craniofacial surgery.

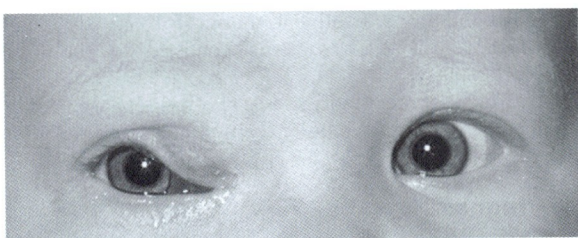

▲ **Figure 16–25.** Right upper-lid hemangioma causing ptosis.

▶ Clinical Findings

Ocular abnormalities associated with craniofacial abnormalities involving the orbits include visual impairment, proptosis, corneal exposure, hypertelorism (widely spaced orbits), strabismus, amblyopia, papilledema, refractive errors, optic atrophy, and high prevalence of NLDO. In nonsyndromic craniosynostosis patients, annual eye examination until age 7–9 is recommended. In syndromic craniosynostosis patients, biannual examinations until age 7–9 and yearly thereafter is recommended.

▶ Treatment

Orbital and ocular abnormalities associated with craniofacial anomalies often require a multispecialty approach. Management may require orbital and strabismus surgery. Ophthalmologists also treat amblyopia, refractive errors, and corneal exposure when present.

Ganesh A et al: An update of ophthalmic management in craniosynostosis. J AAPOS 2019 Apr; 23(2):66–76 [PMID: 30928366].

ORBITAL TUMORS

ESSENTIALS OF DIAGNOSIS & TYPICAL FEATURES

▶ The most common benign tumor of infancy is capillary hemangioma, arising in the first few weeks of life and exhibiting a characteristic sequence of growth and spontaneous involution (Figure 16–26).

▶ The most common primary malignant tumor of the orbit is rhabdomyosarcoma.

▶ Clinical Findings

Capillary hemangiomas may be located superficially in the lid or deep in the orbit and can cause ptosis (Figure 16–25), refractive errors, and amblyopia. Deeper lesions may cause proptosis.

Orbital dermoid cysts are benign congenital orbital choristomas that vary in size and are usually found temporally at the brow and orbital rim or supranasally. These lesions are firm, well encapsulated, and mobile. Rupture of the cyst causes a severe inflammatory reaction.

Lymphangioma occurring in the orbit is typically poorly encapsulated, increases in size with upper respiratory infection, and is susceptible to hemorrhage. Other benign tumors of the orbit are varix, plexiform neurofibroma, teratoma, and tumors arising from bone, connective tissue, and neural tissue.

Orbital rhabdomyosarcoma (see Chapter 31) grows rapidly and displaces the globe. The average age at onset is 6–7 years. The tumor is often initially mistaken for orbital swelling due to insignificant trauma or can mimic orbital cellulitis.

Tumors metastatic to the orbit also occur; neuroblastoma is most common. The patient may exhibit proptosis, orbital ecchymosis (raccoon eyes), Horner syndrome, or opsoclonus (dancing eyes). Ewing sarcoma, leukemia, Burkitt lymphoma, and Langerhans cell histiocytosis may involve the orbit.

Examination of vision, eye movements, eyelids, and orbits often reveals amblyopia, eyelid malposition, strabismus, and proptosis. Neuroimaging with CT or MRI is required to delineate the location and size of orbital tumors.

▶ Differential Diagnosis

Orbital pseudotumor (idiopathic orbital inflammation) and orbital cellulitis.

▶ Treatment

Topical and systemic β-blockers have shown success in treating capillary hemangiomas. Treatment is indicated if the lesion is large enough to cause amblyopia. Induced astigmatism or amblyopia (or both) are treated with glasses and patching, respectively. Treatment of orbital dermoids is by excision.

Treatment modalities for rhabdomyosarcoma include radiation, chemotherapy, and surgery. With expeditious diagnosis and proper treatment, the survival rate of patients with orbital rhabdomyosarcoma confined to the orbit approaches 90%.

Treatment of metastatic disease requires management by an oncologist and may require chemotherapy and radiation therapy.

Prognosis

Prognosis depends on the underlying disease.

NYSTAGMUS

ESSENTIALS OF DIAGNOSIS & TYPICAL FEATURES

▶ Nystagmus is an involuntary rhythmic oscillation of eyes. It may be unilateral or bilateral or be gaze dependent.

▶ Nystagmus can be caused by poor vision. Reduced VA can also occur from nystagmus due to excessive motion of images on the retina.

Pathogenesis

Nystagmus can be grouped into infantile nystagmus, which usually appears in the first 3–6 months of life, and acquired nystagmus, which appears later in life. Infantile nystagmus can be idiopathic, associated with retinal diseases (ie. retinal dystrophy), due to low vision (ie, ONH, foveal hypoplasia), or due to visual deprivation early in life (ie, cataracts). Foveal hypoplasia can be isolated or be associated with aniridia, albinism, and achromatopsia.

Nystagmus can also occur with normal ocular structures and seemingly normal CNS development. Infantile nystagmus syndrome, also known as congenital motor nystagmus, is an ocular disorder of unknown etiology that presents at birth or early infancy. Positive family history may be present. Latent nystagmus occurs when one eye is occluded and can be seen in patients with strabismus. Acquired nystagmus can result from neurologic disorders, vestibular dysfunction, and drug toxicity.

Clinical Findings

When characterizing nystagmus, the examiner can note the laterality (unilateral, bilateral, asymmetric), plane (horizontal, vertical, torsional), conjugacy, amplitude, and frequency of nystagmus.

Nystagmus due to low vision or foveal hypoplasia may exhibit a slow "roving" nystagmus. Infantile nystagmus syndrome is characterized by horizontal, uniplanar nystagmus that increases in intensity with fixation and decreases in intensity with convergence and at a null point (gaze where shakiness is the least). Children may have an abnormal head posture to hold their gaze at the null point. They may have crossing (esotropia) due to nystagmus blockage syndrome, since nystagmus is dampened by convergence. Children with infantile nystagmus do not complain of oscillopsia (perception of oscillations in vision). See-saw nystagmus is associated with a suprasellar mass (ie, craniopharyngioma).

Spasmus nutans, in which a rapid, shimmering, asymmetric nystagmus occurs often with head bobbing and torticollis, is a benign disorder that resolves with time. Clinically, nystagmus of spasmus nutans is indistinguishable from nystagmus due to optic pathway glioma. MRI of brain/orbits, with and without contrast, is necessary to determine if the cause of the nystagmus is due to a CNS disease.

Neurologic disease should be suspected, and neuroimaging performed in acquired nystagmus and when nystagmus is unilateral or asymmetrical. An electroretinogram may be required to rule out retinal pathology as the cause of nystagmus if neuroimaging is normal.

Differential Diagnosis

Opsoclonus (chaotic bilateral eye movements) and voluntary eye movements (cannot be prolonged).

Treatment

Therapy is directed at managing the underlying ocular or CNS disease. An ophthalmologist can optimize vision by correcting significant refractive errors and strabismus. The range of vision varies depending on the cause of the nystagmus. Some patients may benefit from extraocular muscle surgery and contact lenses.

Prognosis

Most affected individuals have subnormal vision, but spasmus nutans usually improves with time.

AMBLYOPIA

ESSENTIALS OF DIAGNOSIS & TYPICAL FEATURES

▶ Amblyopia is decreased vision in one or both eyes resulting from abnormal or inadequate stimulation of the visual system during the critical early period of visual development.

▶ Amblyopia is defined as a difference of best-corrected VA of two lines or more on an acuity chart between the two eyes.

Pathogenesis

Amblyopia is classified according to its cause. Unilateral amblyopia has two main causes: strabismus (misalignment of the eyes resulting in abnormal binocular interaction and decreased vision of the nondominant eye) and anisometropia (difference in refractive error between two eyes resulting in poor visual input in one eye). Bilateral amblyopia can result from high refractive errors (high hyperopia, myopia, or astigmatism). Deprivation amblyopia due to organic causes such as cataracts, corneal opacities, lid ptosis, or vitreous hemorrhage is least common but most difficult to treat. Children can have combined or mixed mechanism amblyopia as well.

Normal binocular development leads to progressive refinement of monocular VA, stereoacuity (3D vision), and fusion of images from both eyes. The critical early period for vision development is thought to end around 8 years of age. Individuals with amblyopia may have not only decreased VA but also decreased contrast sensitivity, stereoacuity, and fixation stability, and increased vulnerability to "crowding," difficulty identifying shapes surrounded by visual "clutter."

Prevention

Vision screening and referral to an eye care professional if amblyopia is suspected.

Clinical Findings

Screening for amblyopia should be a component of periodic well-child examinations. The single best screening technique to discover amblyopia is obtaining VA in each eye. In preverbal children unable to respond to VA assessment, amblyogenic factors are sought, including strabismus, media opacities, unequal Brückner reflexes (pupillary red reflexes), and a family history suggestive of strabismus, amblyopia, or ocular disease occurring in childhood (see section Ophthalmic Examination).

Treatment

The earlier treatment is begun, the better will be the chance of improving VA. Treatment is continued until amblyopia resolves or until at least 8–9 years of age. Amblyogenic factors such as refractive errors are addressed. Because of the extreme sensitivity of the visual nervous system in infants, congenital cataracts and media opacities must be diagnosed and treated within the first few weeks of life. Visual rehabilitation and amblyopia treatment must then be started to foster visual development.

After eradicating amblyogenic factors, the mainstay of treatment is to increase stimulation of the amblyopic eye by part-time occlusion (patching) of the amblyopic eye. Other treatment modalities include "fogging" the sound eye with

cycloplegic drops (atropine) and Luminopia™, which is an FDA-approved binocular therapy for amblyopia.

Prognosis

Prognosis depends on the compliance with treatment and the cause of amblyopia.

STRABISMUS

ESSENTIALS OF DIAGNOSIS & TYPICAL FEATURES

▶ Strabismus is misalignment of the eyes.

▶ Its prevalence in childhood is about 2%–3%.

▶ Strabismus is categorized by the direction of the deviation (esotropia, exotropia, hypertropia, hypotropia) and its frequency (constant or intermittent).

▶ Strabismus and amblyopia are related but different entities. Strabismus can often cause unilateral amblyopia.

ESOTROPIA (CROSSED EYES)

ESSENTIALS OF DIAGNOSIS & TYPICAL FEATURES

▶ Pseudoesotropia can result from prominent epicanthal folds and wide nose bridges that give the appearance of crossed eyes when they are actually straight.

▶ Esotropia is deviation of the eyes toward the nose or eye crossing.

Pathogenesis

Primary infantile esotropia (also known as congenital esotropia) has its onset in the first year of life. The deviation of the eyes toward the nose is large and obvious. The most frequent type of acquired esotropia is the accommodative type (Figure 16–26). Onset is usually between ages 2 and 5 years. The deviation is variable in magnitude and constancy and is often accompanied by amblyopia. Refractive accommodative esotropia is associated with a high hyperopic refraction. In another type, the deviation is worse with near than with distant vision (high AC/A accommodative esotropia). This type of esodeviation is usually associated with lower refractive errors.

Esotropia can be associated with certain syndromes. In Möbius syndrome (congenital facial diplegia), a sixth nerve

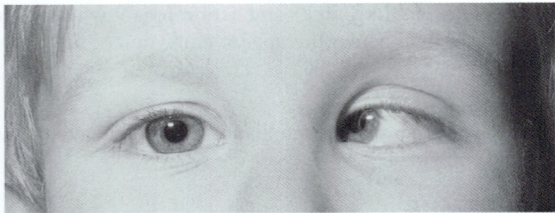

A

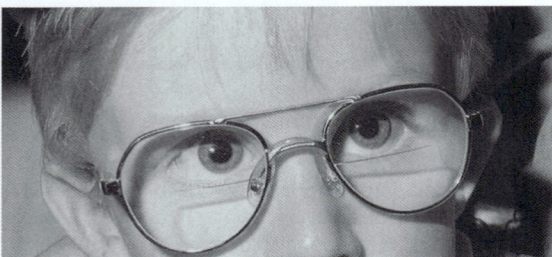

B

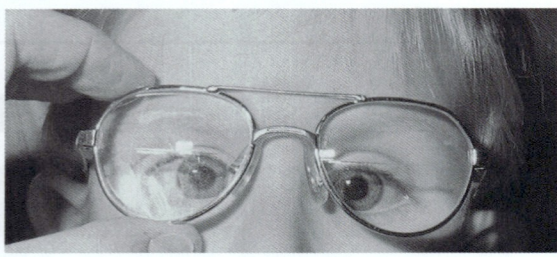

C

▲ **Figure 16–26.** Accommodative esotropia. **A:** Without glasses, esotropia; **B:** With glasses, well aligned at distance; **C:** At near with bifocal correction.

palsy causing esotropia is associated with palsies of the VII and XII cranial nerves and limb deformities. Duane syndrome can affect the medial or lateral rectus muscles (or both). It may be an isolated defect or may be associated with a multitude of systemic defects (eg, Goldenhar syndrome). Duane syndrome is often misdiagnosed as a sixth (abducens) nerve palsy. The left eye is involved more commonly, but both eyes can be involved. Girls are affected more frequently.

After age 5 years, any esotropia of recent onset should arouse suspicion of CNS disease. Intracranial masses, hydrocephalus, demyelinating diseases, and IIH are causes of abducens palsy, where patients may present with esotropia and diplopia. Papilledema is often, but not invariably, present with increased ICP.

Besides the vulnerability of the abducens nerve to increased ICP, it is susceptible to infection and inflammation. Otitis media and Gradenigo syndrome (inflammatory disease of the petrous bone) can cause sixth nerve palsy. Less commonly, migraine and diabetes mellitus are considerations in children with sixth nerve palsy.

▶ **Clinical Findings**

Observation of the reflection of a penlight on the cornea, the corneal light reflex, is an accurate means of determining if the eyes are straight. This is a good way to differentiate true esotropia from pseudostrabismus. If strabismus is present, the corneal light reflex will not be centered in one or both eyes. Observation of eye movements may reveal restriction of eye movements in certain positions of gaze. Children with unilateral paretic or restrictive causes of esotropia may develop face turns toward the affected eye to maintain binocularity. The face turn is an attempt to maintain binocularity away from the field of action of the paretic muscle. Alternate cover testing of the eyes while the child is fixating on a near and/or distant target will reveal refixation movements in the opposite direction of the deviation. Motility, cycloplegic refraction, and a dilated funduscopic examination by an ophthalmologist are necessary to determine the etiology of esotropia. Some children require imaging studies and neurologic consultation.

▶ **Complications**

Amblyopia and poor stereoacuity/depth perception.

▶ **Treatment**

Surgery is the mainstay of treatment for primary infantile esotropia. Surgery is typically performed between 6 months and 2 years of age to obtain optimal results.

Management of accommodative esotropia includes glasses with or without bifocals, amblyopia treatment, and, in some cases, surgery.

Underlying neurologic disease should be referred to the appropriate specialists for further management.

▶ **Prognosis**

Usually good.

EXOTROPIA (WALL-EYED, DRIFTING OF EYES)

 ESSENTIALS OF DIAGNOSIS & TYPICAL FEATURES

▶ Exotropia is a type of strabismus in which the eyes are divergent (Figure 16–27).
▶ Exotropia may be intermittent or constant.

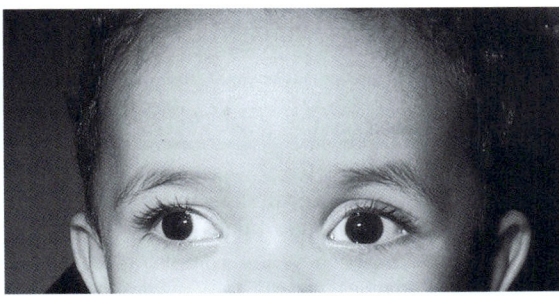

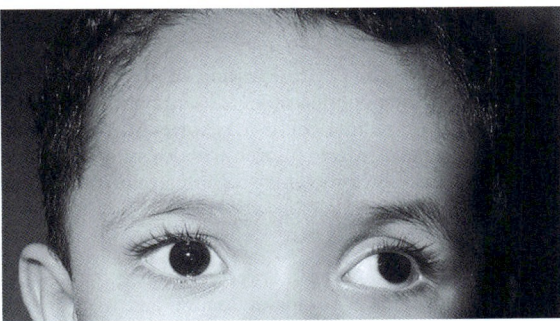

▲ **Figure 16–27.** Exotropia. **A:** Fixation with left eye. **B:** Fixation with right eye.

▶ Clinical Findings

The deviation of the eyes toward the ears most often begins intermittently and usually after age 2 years. Congenital (infantile) exotropia is rare in an otherwise healthy infant. Early-onset exotropia may occur in infants and children with severe neurologic problems. All children with constant, congenital exotropia require CNS neuroimaging. Referral to an ophthalmologist is indicated.

Evaluation of the corneal light reflex reveals the penlight's reflection in the deviated eye is displaced nasally. Cover uncover test or alternate cover test will reveal refixation eye movements inward (toward the nose) when exotropia is present.

Convergence insufficiency is a special type of exotropia where the deviation is larger at near compared to distance. They have poor convergence (ability to converge or cross their eyes when looking at a near target). Common symptoms include asthenopia, binocular diplopia, or visual blur with near visual tasks.

▶ Complications

Poor stereoacuity/depth perception. Amblyopia is less commonly seen in exotropia compared to esotropia but can occur in monocular or poorly controlled exotropia.

▶ Treatment

Treatment of exotropia includes observation, glasses, and/ or surgery. Indications for surgery of intermittent exotropia include poor control of deviation, large angle deviation, and worsening stereoacuity. Convergence insufficiency is the only type of strabismus with scientific evidence that orthoptic exercises can improve symptoms and signs. Classic exercise is pencil push-ups, which can be performed at home or in the office. There are other computer-based exercises that can help reduce the symptoms of convergence insufficiency. Vision exercises or therapy for all other types of strabismus are not endorsed by pediatric ophthalmologists due to the lack of scientific evidence.

▶ Prognosis

Generally good.

UNEXPLAINED DECREASED VISION IN INFANTS & CHILDREN

ESSENTIALS OF DIAGNOSIS & TYPICAL FEATURES

▶ Cortical/cerebral visual impairment (CVI) is visual impairment that is not fully explainable by eye examination findings and deemed to be due to neurologic injury.

▶ Pathogenesis

Occult causes of poor vision and blindness in children may be due to hereditary retinal dystrophies such as Leber congenital amaurosis and optic nerve abnormalities, including ONH and atrophy.

CVI is characterized by bilateral VA or VF loss in the presence of a normal eye examination or greater than expected vision loss based on the degree of ocular pathology. The term *cortical visual impairment* was first applied as an umbrella term to describe impairments of visual processes like VA, contrast sensitivity, and VFs. But since injuries can involve more than the outer cortex of the brain, the term *cerebral visual impairment* (CVI) was later adopted. CVI can occur from generalized cerebral damage or from insults in the postgeniculate visual pathway (dorsal and/or ventral pathways). Hypoxic-ischemic injury is the most common cause of CVI. Other causes include trauma, intracranial hemorrhage, periventricular leukomalacia, infections, metabolic/genetic disorders, in utero drug exposures, structural brain abnormalities, and seizures.

Functional vision loss describes acute subjective vision loss in children without organic cause. Acute stress may bring on these symptoms.

Clinical Findings

Patients with CVI may have poor eye contact, fail to fixate and follow a visual target, or be unresponsive to visual threat. These neurobehavioral characteristics can fluctuate due to medical and environmental factors. Wandering or roving eye movements and nystagmus are common. Eye poking can be seen in some infants with low vision. Children with CVI often have difficulties with complex visual input due to crowding effect.

Referral to an ophthalmologist is indicated to determine the etiology of the low vision. Diagnostic tests such as an electroretinogram and visual evoked response may be required. Imaging studies of the brain, genetics, and neurology consultations may be useful.

Patients with functional vision loss often have a normal eye examination, including normal eye structures and lack of APD but have abnormalities just in the subjective portions (VA, VF). Some may have an overlay of functional vision loss on their pre-existing eye conditions. A thorough examination is required to rule out organic causes before diagnosis of functional vision loss is made.

Differential Diagnosis

Delayed visual maturation (temporary dysfunction of higher cortical centers; symptoms improve with time), vision loss due to an ocular disease.

Treatment

Vision rehabilitation specialists (low vision optometrist, teachers for visually impaired) and support groups are helpful for patients with CVI. Goal is to maximize their vision. Patients with functional vision loss often do well with support and reassurance.

Prognosis

Generally poor for vision for CVI patients.

Chang MY, Borcert MS: Advances in the evaluation and management of cortical/cerebral visual impairment in children. Surv Ophthalmol 2020 Nov–Dec;65(6):708–724 [PMID: 32199940].

LEARNING DISABILITIES & DYSLEXIA

ESSENTIALS OF DIAGNOSIS & TYPICAL FEATURES

▶ Learning disabilities and dyslexia result in poor reading comprehension and writing.

▶ Children often have vague complaints of ocular fatigue, headaches, and difficulty reading.

Clinical Findings

Evaluation of the child with learning disabilities and dyslexia should include ophthalmologic examination to identify any ocular disorders that could cause or contribute to poor school performance. Most children with learning difficulties have no demonstrable problems on ophthalmic examination.

Treatment

A multidisciplinary approach is recommended by the AAP, the AAPOS, and the AAO for evaluating and treating children with learning disabilities. According to the joint AAP report, there is no scientific evidence to support the claims that visual training, muscle exercises, ocular pursuit-and-tracking exercises, behavioral/perceptual vision therapy, "training" glasses, prisms, and colored lenses and filters are effective treatments for learning disabilities, dyslexia, and strabismus. There is no evidence that children who participate in vision therapy are more responsive to educational instruction than children who do not participate.

Handler SM, Fierson WM; Section on Ophthalmology; Council on Children With Disabilities; American Academy of Ophthalmology; American Association for Pediatric Ophthalmology and Strabismus; American Association of Certified Orthoptists: Learning disabilities, dyslexia, and vision. Pediatrics 2011;127(3):e818–e856 [PMID: 21357342].
Rucker JC, Phillips PH: Efferent vision therapy. J Neuroophthalmol 2017 Jan 4;1–7. doi: 10.1097/WNO.0000000000000480 [PMID: 28059865].

Web Resources

American Academy of Ophthalmology: www.aao.org.
American Association of Pediatric Ophthalmology and Strabismus: www.aapos.org.
EyeWiki—American Academy of Ophthalmology: https://eyewiki.org/Main_Page.

Oral Medicine & Dentistry

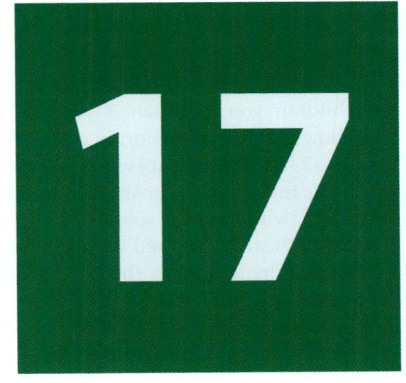

Anne R. Wilson, DDS, MS

Abidin Hakan Tuncer, DDS, DMD, MPH, FSCD

Chaitanya P. Puranik, BDS, MS, MDentSci, PhD

Katherine L. Chin, DDS, MS

PEDIATRIC ORAL HEALTH

Concept of the Dental Home

Establishing a dental home, by age 1 year or when the first tooth erupts, provides a vital foundation for oral health promotion and prevention of oral disease, such as early childhood caries (ECC). The American Academy of Pediatric Dentistry describes the dental home as "the ongoing relationship between the dentist and the patient, inclusive of all aspects of oral health care delivered in a comprehensive, continuously accessible, coordinated, and family-centered way." The dental home involves ongoing interactions among patients, parents, dentists, dental professionals, and nondental professionals, which increases awareness of factors influencing oral health.

Achieving optimal oral health care as part of a dental home requires a general dentist knowledgeable about pediatric oral health or a pediatric dentist as a specialist for children and complex oral health needs. Together, the dentist and primary caregiver can develop a comprehensive preventive program based on disease susceptibility. Similar to preventive guidance as part of a medical home, a preventive oral health plan for children provides anticipatory guidance on age-appropriate measures. This includes oral hygiene practices, importance of fluoride, dietary guidance, dental trauma prevention, and benefits of a dental home. Addressing risk factors for ECC is a vital component of anticipatory guidance during routine visits to medical and dental providers.

Prenatal & Perinatal Factors & Infant Oral Health Care

During the prenatal and perinatal periods, medical care providers should provide preventive information to mothers about the potential consequences of their oral health, which may impact their own health and pregnancies. Pregnancy-related gingivitis commonly occurs and, if untreated, may result in periodontal disease. Also, a mother's and/or primary caregiver's oral health knowledge, behaviors, and attitudes have an influence on the oral health trajectory of children.

During the postnatal period, oral health promotion provides an opportunity for caregivers to establish the foundation for preventive oral health. This enables caregivers to (1) develop oral health goals, (2) their role in reaching these goals, and (3) learn and maintain optimal preventive oral health behaviors. Typically, pediatricians encounter newborns and infants at an earlier age than dental providers, providing an opportunity for early oral health promotion to address risk factors associated with ECC. Pediatricians are encouraged to incorporate caries-risk assessment and anticipatory guidance focused on oral health in their practice.

Caries-risk assessment estimates the likelihood of developing disease based on the complex interaction of risk factors at multiple levels. Caries-risk assessment forms are available to physicians and other nondental health care providers through the American Academy of Pediatric Dentistry and American Academy of Pediatrics. By 6 months of age, every infant should have a caries-risk assessment performed by a pediatric health care provider. Since the risk of caries increases with age, anticipatory guidance by pediatricians and nondental health care providers is recommended beyond age 3 years as part of routine pediatric care.

Mouradian WE et al: Addressing disparities in children's oral health: a dental-medical partnership to train family practice residents. Dent Educ 2003 Aug;67(8):886–895 [PMID: 12959162].

Sanchez OM, Childers NK: Anticipatory guidance in infant oral health: rationale and recommendations. Am Fam Physician 2000 Jan 1;61(1):115–120, 123–124 [PMID: 10643953].

Watt RG: From victim blaming to upstream action: tackling the social determinants of oral health inequalities. Community Dent Oral Epidemiol 2007;35(1):1–11 [PMID: 17244132].

ORAL EXAMINATION OF CHILDREN

Examination Positioning

For children younger than 3 years, a knee-to-knee position allows oral examination in a safe and comfortable way (Figure 17–1). The parent is instructed to sit facing the provider. The infant is then positioned on the parent's lap facing the parent, with each leg wrapped around the parent's waist. The child's head is lowered onto a pillow on the provider's lap for examination, with the parent instructed to stabilize the child's arms and legs with their hands and elbows. Crying during examination is a normal response in healthy children and allows better visualization of the oral cavity. For older, more cooperative children, oral examination is performed in a dental chair.

Extraoral Examination

Extraoral examination includes assessing overall facial symmetry and facial proportions by dividing in equal thirds. The length of each facial third is usually equal or similar. Extraoral findings such as muscle strain over the chin may reflect a skeletal or orthodontic problem. Submandibular glands and lymph nodes should be palpated to identify enlargement or pain. Temporomandibular joint (TMJ) examination determines range of motion and deviation while opening or closing the jaw, and crepitations or clicking during movement that may indicate underlying joint pathology.

Intraoral Examination

The newborn's mouth is lined with an intact, smooth, and moist mucosa (Figure 17–2). The alveolar ridges are continuous and relatively smooth. The sagittal and vertical maxillomandibular relationships are different at birth, with an anterior open bite before the onset of tooth eruption.

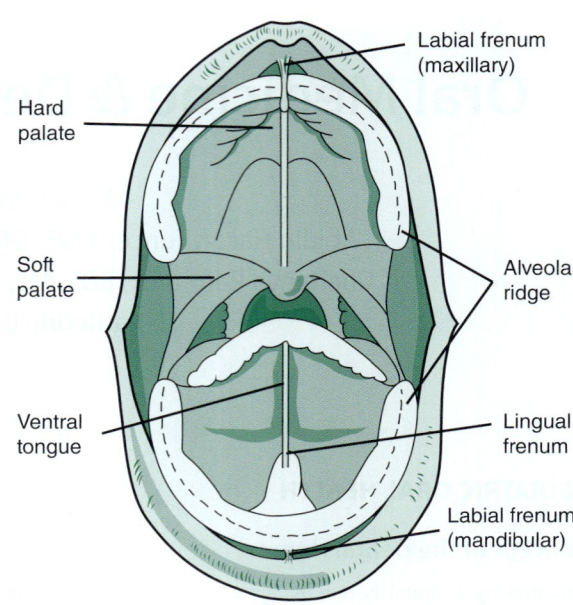

▲ **Figure 17–2.** Normal anatomy of the newborn mouth.

The mouth is more triangularly shaped, and the oral cavity is small and filled by the tongue.

Frena

Maxillary and mandibular frena are located in the anterior midline region (Figure 17–3), and accessory frena are often present posteriorly. A more prominent midline maxillary

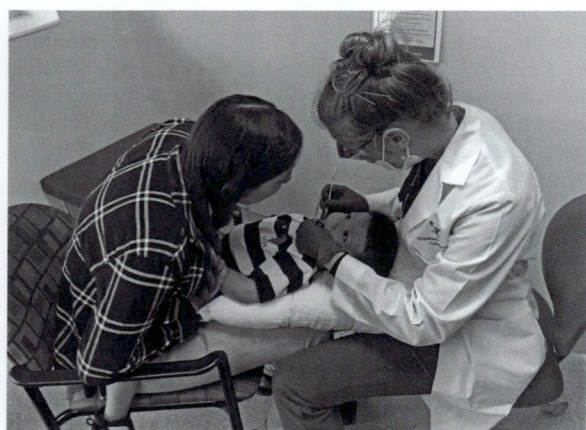

▲ **Figure 17–1.** Knee-to-knee position.

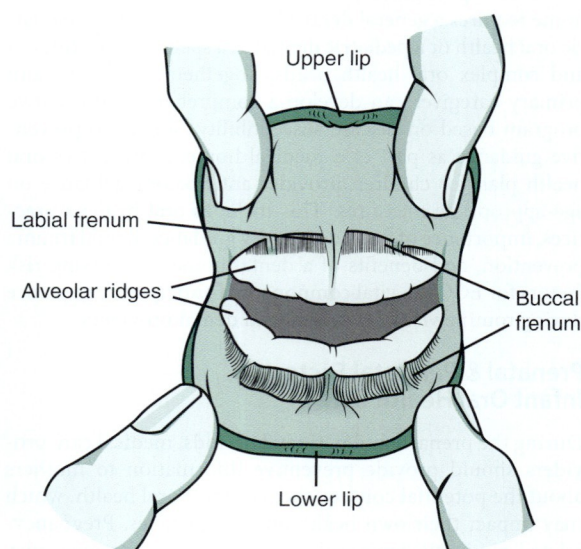

▲ **Figure 17–3.** The frena.

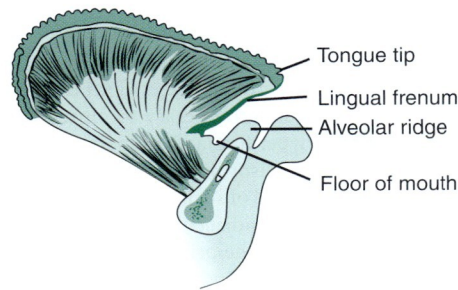

- Tongue tip
- Lingual frenum
- Alveolar ridge
- Floor of mouth

▲ **Figure 17–4.** Normal position of lingual frenum.

labial frenum is observed in 25% of children and diminishes in size and recedes apically with normal development and dental eruption.

The tongue is connected to the floor of the mouth by the lingual frenum (Figures 17–4 and 17–5), whereas the upper lip is connected to gingiva above the upper central incisors by the maxillary frenum. With ankyloglossia, the frenal attachment extends up to the tip of the tongue or high up on the alveolar ridge (see Figure 17–5) and may restrict movement. Ankyloglossia typically does not inhibit normal growth and development, but can cause feeding problems, such as difficulty latching or pain during nursing. Other signs of a tight frenum attachment involving the tongue or lip include a heart-shaped or bifid appearance of the tongue with restricted protrusive movements or blanching of the lip when everted towards the nose. In most cases breastfeeding will improve with frenotomy of the lingual frenum shortly after birth. In contrast, frenotomy of the maxillary frenum is rarely indicated as there is no evidence this reduces breast-feeding difficulties.

Soft Tissue Variations

The most common soft tissue pathology in newborns are neonatal cysts, including Bohn's nodules, Epstein pearls, and dental lamina cysts. Bohn's nodules are located on the buccal and lingual aspects of the alveolar ridges. Epstein pearls along the mid-palatal raphe, and dental lamina cysts are found on the alveolar mucosa. These cysts are 1–3 mm round, smooth,

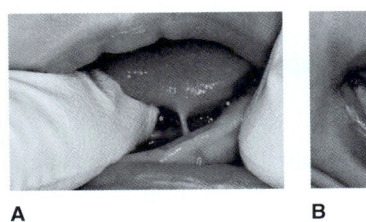

A

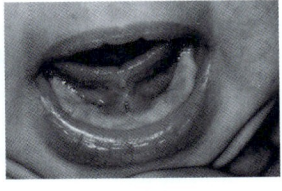

B

▲ **Figure 17–5.** Ankyloglossia (tongue-tie) in a 6-week-old, before **(A)** and after **(B)** lingual frenectomy.

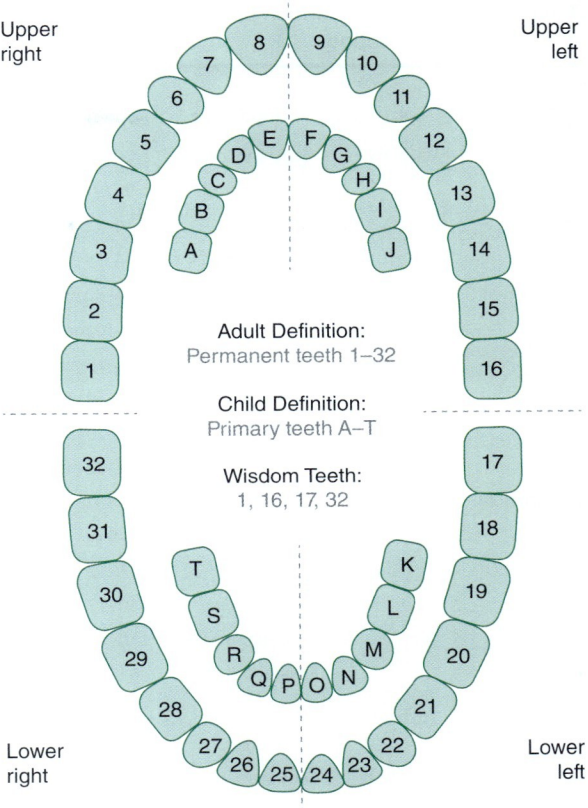

Upper right

Upper left

Adult Definition:
Permanent teeth 1–32

Child Definition:
Primary teeth A–T

Wisdom Teeth:
1, 16, 17, 32

Lower right

Lower left

▲ **Figure 17–6.** Universal numbering system for primary and permanent dentition.

nontender white, gray, or yellow nodules that are self-limiting and typically resolve by 3 months of age.

Intraoral Hard Tissue

The development of alveolar bone is evident with the formation of tooth buds and later eruption of the primary teeth and permanent teeth. Alveolar bone encases the developing tooth buds and supports the teeth through periodontal ligament attachments.

Hard tissue formation of the primary teeth begins at approximately 14 weeks in utero, with all 20 primary teeth calcified to varying degrees and traces of enamel of first permanent molars present at birth. Primary teeth generally begin eruption around 7 months of age but may appear as early as 3–4 months or as late as 12–16 months of age as shown in the table of the estimated eruption periods for the primary and permanent dentition. Once the patient has a complete set of permanent teeth (excluding third molars), they are considered to have adolescent dentition (Table 17–1).

Table 17–1. Estimated eruption periods for the primary and permanent dentition.

Dentition	Arch	Tooth Type	Estimated Eruption
Primary	Maxillary	Central incisor	8–12 mo
		Lateral incisor	9–14 mo
		Canine	16–22 mo
		First molar	14–19 mo
		Second molar	24–30 mo
	Mandibular	Central incisor	6–10 mo
		Lateral incisor	10–16 mo
		Canine	16–24 mo
		First molar	14–20 mo
		Second molar	24–32 mo
Permanent	Maxillary	Central incisor	7–8 y
		Lateral incisor	8–9 y
		Canine	11–12 y
		First premolar	10–12 y
		Second premolar	10–12 y
		First molar	6–7 y
		Second molar	12–13 y
		Third molar	17–20 y
	Mandibular	Central incisor	5–7 y
		Lateral incisor	6–8 y
		Canine	9–10 y
		First premolar	10–11 y
		Second premolar	11–12 y
		First molar	5–6 y
		Second molar	12–13 y
		Third molar	17–20 y

Tooth Numbering Systems

Tooth numbering systems enable clinicians to communicate unequivocally about a patient's dentition. In the United States, the Universal Numbering System (Figure 17–6) assigns the uppercase letters A–T for primary teeth and numbers 1–32 for permanent teeth. The initial designation begins on the upper right, most posterior tooth and continues along the upper teeth to the left side. The count then drops to the lower, most posterior tooth on the left side and continues along the bottom teeth ending on the lower right side.

Hard Tissue Variations

Potential variations in dental hard tissues involve the number and size of primary and permanent teeth. An extra tooth or teeth are referred to as supernumerary tooth/teeth and the condition is known as hyperdontia. If a supernumerary tooth occurs in the maxillary incisor midline area, it is referred to as mesiodentes. The removal of such a tooth is recommended when hindering eruption of adjacent permanent incisors.

Tooth agenesis is rare in the primary dentition and more prevalent in the permanent dentition. The most frequently missing permanent teeth are the third molars, followed by mandibular second premolars and maxillary lateral incisors. Tooth agenesis is caused by several independent defective genes, which can act alone or in combination with other genes. It can occur as an isolated problem but is common with cleft lip/cleft palate or as part of the phenotype of over 200 syndromes, including ectodermal dysplasia.

Minor variations in the size of teeth are common. Macrodontia refers to abnormally large teeth and microdontia is the term for teeth that are smaller than the expected size. Apart from the number and shape of the teeth, there may be abnormalities in the overall formation of the hard tissue structures such as enamel and dentin (amelogenesis imperfecta or dentinogenesis imperfecta, respectively).

Eruption Symptoms

Many symptoms are attributed to tooth eruption or teething. However, temporal association with fever, upper respiratory infection, or systemic illness is coincidental rather than related to dental eruption. Medical evaluation for diagnosing other sources is recommended.

Common therapies for teething pain in children include application of over-the-counter teething gels or liquids containing benzocaine, which in rare circumstances can cause methemoglobinemia. While "natural" benzocaine-free formulations are available, systemic analgesics such as acetaminophen or ibuprofen are safe and effective. Chewing on a teething object can be beneficial, if only for distraction purposes.

Eruption cysts/hematomas of the alveolar mucosa overlying an erupting tooth may occur as an asymptomatic localized red to purple, round, raised, and smooth lesion. Treatment is rarely needed as these resolve with tooth eruption.

Pathologies of Tooth Eruption

▶ Natal Teeth

On rare occasions (1:3000), natal teeth are present at birth and neonatal teeth erupt within the first month of life. These are most commonly (85%) primary mandibular incisors and normal teeth with 10% as supernumerary teeth. Although the preferred approach is to leave the tooth in place, natal teeth that are hypermobile, or of inferior structural quality should be extracted. Other potential indications for removing natal teeth include nursing difficulties and sharp incisal edges causing laceration of the infant's ventral tongue surface.

Delayed Eruption

Premature loss of a primary tooth can either delay or accelerate eruption of the successor permanent tooth. Accelerated eruption occurs when the primary tooth is removed within 6–9 months of its normal exfoliation, but loss of the primary tooth more than 1 year before expected exfoliation typically delays eruption of its successor. Loss of a primary tooth often causes adjacent teeth to tip or drift into the resulting space, leading to space loss for the successor permanent tooth. Placement of a space maintainer can prevent such space loss.

Ectopic Eruption

Insufficient space in the dental arch may cause permanent teeth to erupt ectopically. Permanent mandibular incisors erupt from the lingual and over-retention of the primary predecessors can result in a "double row of teeth." If the primary tooth remains firmly in place, extraction is indicated.

Impaction

Impaction occurs when a permanent tooth is prevented from erupting. Although crowding is a frequent reason, over-retained primary or supernumerary teeth are other causes. The teeth most often affected in the developing dentition are the maxillary incisors and canines. Often, correct alignment occurs with early extraction of the preceding or adjacent primary teeth. If this approach is ineffective, surgical exposure of the impacted tooth and orthodontic treatment are indicated.

Dean JA, Avery DR, McDonald RE: *McDonald and Avery's Dentistry for the Child and Adolescent.* 10th ed. Maryland Heights, MO: Mosby Elsevier, 2016.

DENTAL CARIES

Dental caries is the most common chronic disease of childhood and the most prevalent unmet health need of US children. Largely a disease of poverty, dental caries primarily affects children and adolescents in disadvantaged families impacted by negative social determinants leading to adverse health outcomes.

Early Childhood Caries

Early childhood caries (ECC) is a virulent and rapidly progressive form of caries in a child younger than 6 years that is defined as one or more decayed (d), missing (m), or filled (f) primary tooth surfaces (s) designated as the *dmfs* score. Severe ECC (S-ECC) is defined as any smooth-surface caries in a child younger than 3 years, and from 3 to 5 years a *dmfs* score of 1 or more in maxillary front teeth or a total *dmfs* score of 4 or higher. This is associated with an increased risk for hospitalization, emergency department visits, and school absences due to pain and infection. Chronic oral disease can impact growth and diminishes quality of life.

Pathogenesis

Development of dental caries involves interaction of biologic factors: (1) the host oral environment; (2) cariogenic dietary substrate; (3) cariogenic microorganisms; and (4) cumulative exposure to fermentable carbohydrates and acid exposure duration. The most studied oral microorganism implicated in dental caries of infants and children is *Streptococcus mutans* (MS). Host and environmental factors contribute to acquiring and establishing commensal oral microbiota. Exposure to the maternal oral microbiome occurs prenatally and colonization continues perinatally and postnatally. Factors associated with infants' and children's microbiota include eruption of teeth, oral hygiene habits and free-sugar consumption, exposure to antibiotics, maternal smoking, and oral health status of the caregiver.

Dental plaque is an adherent biofilm harboring acidogenic bacteria in proximity to enamel. As bacteria metabolize fermentable carbohydrates, production of lactic acid solubilizes calcium phosphate in tooth enamel. Demineralization of dental enamel occurs below pH 5.5. Saliva and its buffering capacity are important modifiers of demineralization. Demineralization of enamel and dentin can be halted or even reversed by redeposition of calcium, phosphate, and fluoride from saliva.

Caries Prevention

Prevention of dental caries necessitates restoration of the delicate balance between pathologic factors and protective influences. The most studied protective influences include fluoride, sugar substitutes (xylitol), and frequency of brushing. Among these, only fluoride from topical and systemic sources (food, beverages, drinking water, and oral care products) has demonstrated a consistent protective effect.

Dietary Guidelines

Since dental caries requires prolonged exposure to fermentable carbohydrates, recommended dietary practices for young children include giving only water in the bottle at bedtime, weaning from the bottle between 12 and 18 months of age, and encouraging drinking from an uncovered cup (instead of a no-spill training cup). Sugar-containing carbonated beverages, 100% juice, and powdered beverages should be avoided.

Dietary counseling should be in accordance with the World Health Organization (WHO) recommendations to maintain free-sugar consumption at less than 10% of total daily energy intake and preferably below 5% of the total energy intake. Foods considered to be protective against caries are high in fat, protein, and minerals, such as milk and cheese, which contain calcium and phosphate.

Oral Hygiene

Soon after birth, caregivers should clean intra-oral mucosal surfaces daily using a moist, soft cloth. Once teeth erupt, oral hygiene is initiated as formation of dental caries has been associated with biofilm accumulation on tooth surfaces. Due to a lack of manual dexterity in children younger than 8 years, caregivers should supervise children's oral hygiene and floss their children's teeth in areas with contact between teeth. Removal of biofilm from tooth surfaces without concomitant use of fluoridated toothpaste is less effective in caries reduction. Caregivers should be instructed regarding the appropriate amount of fluoridated toothpaste at each brushing; "smear or rice-sized amount" (age < 3 years) or "pea-sized" amount (ages 3–6 years) of toothpaste. The benefits of fluoride-containing toothpaste can be extended by brushing teeth twice daily and either avoiding or rinsing minimally after brushing. Caregivers should be advised to initiate the use of fluoridated toothpaste upon eruption of the primary dentition. Nonfluoridated toothpaste is not recommended.

Fluoride

Fluoride is a one of the most effective means of caries prevention through both topical and systemic mechanisms of action. By both routes of administration, fluoride can improve the dentin and enamel of erupted and unerupted teeth. Topical application inhibits bacterial metabolism by interfering with enzyme activity, inhibits demineralization, and enhances remineralization.

Systemic benefits are achieved by oral ingestion from sources such as fluoridated drinking water, beverages, infant formulas, and prepared food. Initiation of community water fluoridation in the 1950s has been associated with significant reductions in dental caries. The U.S. Department of Health and Human Services has specified a level of 0.7 ppm fluoride in community water supplies to balance the benefits of preventing dental caries while minimizing the risk for developmental enamel defects from excess systemic fluoride or fluorosis.

Fluoride supplements also help reduce dental caries prevalence and should be considered for children who are at high caries risk and without access to fluoridated community water. This will depend on age and other fluoride sources. A child's total exposure to all sources of fluoride must be thoroughly evaluated before supplements are prescribed to avoid enamel fluorosis. Infants receiving concentrated formula as the main source of nutrition are at increased risk for enamel fluorosis in the permanent dentition if fluoride-containing formulas are reconstituted with fluoridated water.

A. Fluoride Varnish for High-Risk Populations

Well-child visits with physicians allows for application of fluoride varnish among children at risk for dental caries (ICD-10-CM Diagnosis Code Z29.3: Encounter for Prophylactic Fluoride Administration). The varnish's adherent resin base provides extended fluoride contact with the tooth surface without systemic absorption. Post-treatment guidelines include avoiding brushing, flossing, and crunchy foods for at least 4 hours and up to 24 hours for optimal adherence and topical absorption of fluoride into enamel.

Treatment of Caries

Caries is clinically diagnosed by visual and tactile oral examination supplemented by radiographs, which detect caries on the surfaces between teeth. Dental caries initially can present on visible enamel surfaces as a white, chalky-appearing area along the gingival margin or on approximated tooth surfaces. Pediatricians may observe early disease referred to as non-cavitated lesions, which provides the opportunity for highlighting areas of concern with caregivers. Continuation of disease results in enamel loss and cavitated areas that may feature light to deep brown spots or cavities.

In the initial stages of decay with loss of tooth structure, removal of carious tooth structure and restoration can repair the tooth. As decay progresses into the pulp, inflammation and pain may develop. Once the pulp becomes necrotic, a periapical abscess develops (Figure 17–7), which usually causes severe pain, fever, and swelling. Pediatricians may

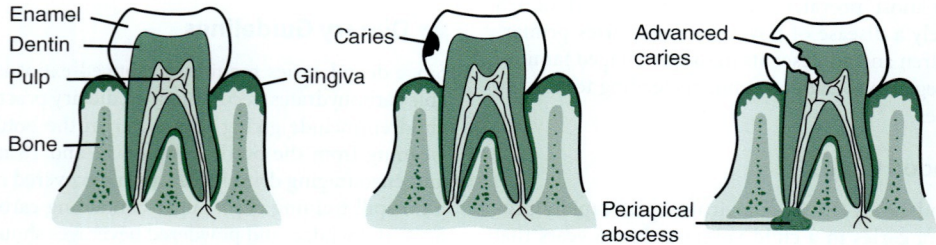

▲ **Figure 17–7.** Tooth anatomy and progression of caries.

encounter clinical signs of an abscess including localized gingival inflammation, fistula or parulis formation, mobility, and intraoral swelling. Antibiotics are indicated in advanced infections featuring systemic sequelae such as fever and extraoral swelling. However, definitive resolution requires dental extraction or root canal therapy.

Silver diamine fluoride has been utilized to slow or arrest caries progression in select patients. Use may be considered in circumstances where the risk of morbidity or mortality under sedation or general anesthesia outweighs the benefit of definitive restorations and for patients with special management considerations unable to tolerate definitive restorative care in clinical settings. Application produces a permanent black discoloration of carious defects.

Achembong LN, Kranz AM, Rozier RG: Office-based preventive dental program and statewide trends in dental caries. Pediatrics 2014 Apr;133(4):e827–e834 [PMID: 24685954].

Guideline: *Sugars Intake for Adults and Children*. Geneva, Switzerland: World Health Organization; 2015. https://www.ncbi.nlm.nih.gov/books/NBK285537/.

Riggs E et al: Interventions with pregnant women, new mothers, and other primary caregivers for preventing early childhood caries. Cochrane Database Syst Rev 2019 Nov 20;2019(11):CD012155. doi: 10.1002/14651858.CD012155.pub2 [PMID: 31745970].

Rozier RG et al: Evidence-based clinical recommendations on the prescription of dietary fluoride supplements for caries prevention: a report of the American Dental Association Council on Scientific Affairs. J Am Dent Assoc 2010 Dec;141(12):1480–1489 [PMID: 21158195].

US Preventive Services Task Force; Davidson KW et al: Screening and interventions to prevent dental caries in children younger than 5 years: US Preventive Services Task Force Recommendation Statement. JAMA 2021 Dec 7;326(21):2172–2178. doi: 10.1001/jama.2021.20007 [PMID: 34874412].

PERIODONTAL DISEASE

Periodontal diseases are a group of conditions affecting a tooth's supporting structures: bone, gingiva, and periodontal ligament (Figure 17–8). Plaque and bacterial accumulation in the gingival margin cause a localized inflammation of the gingival tissue adjacent to a tooth. This initial phase, called dental biofilm-induced gingivitis, is found almost universally in children and adolescents. This affects about half of the population by 5 years of age and reaches a prevalence of nearly 100% at puberty. Nonmicrobial gingivitis is associated with genetic, inflammatory, immune, metabolic, and endocrine factors and exacerbated by inconsistent oral hygiene. Gingivitis is reversible and generally improves with removal of microbial biofilm and consistent oral hygiene.

Periodontitis, the subsequent phase, is characterized by irreversible loss of the periodontal attachment and destruction of alveolar bone due to gingival inflammation. Periodontitis is staged based on the severity and complexity of the management and grading depends on the progression and treatment response. Abnormalities in neutrophil function such as chemotaxis, phagocytosis, and antibacterial activity increase the risk of periodontitis. *Actinobacillus actinomycetemcomitans* in combination with *Bacteroides* species are implicated in this disease process. Periodontitis is most easily arrested in the initial stages before deep pockets develop with gradual loss of attachment. Treatment consists of combined surgical and nonsurgical mechanical debridement and antibiotic therapy.

Medical conditions, hormonal alterations with puberty, certain medications, and malnutrition can intensify the inflammatory response to microbial biofilm. Periodontitis in children is a manifestation of systemic diseases and predisposing factors including genetics, immune response, dental tissue anatomy, and oral health behaviors.

Periodontal diseases of children and adolescents. Pediatr Dent 2016;38(6):388–396 [PMID: 27931482].

Treatment of plaque-induced gingivitis, chronic periodontitis, and other clinical conditions. Pediatr Dent 2016;38(6):403–411 [PMID: 27931484].

DENTAL EMERGENCIES

▶ Orofacial Trauma

Orofacial trauma includes abrasions or lacerations of the lips, gingiva, tongue, or oral mucosa and frena, and may involve damage to the teeth. Lacerations should be cleansed, inspected for foreign bodies, and sutured if necessary. Radiographs of lacerations of the tongue, lips, or cheeks are indicated when missing embedded tooth fragments or other foreign bodies are suspected as palpation alone is often inadequate. All patients with facial trauma should be evaluated for jaw fractures. Blows to the chin are among the most common childhood orofacial traumas and are a leading cause of condylar fracture, which should be suspected if significant pain or deviation occurs with mouth opening.

Tooth-related trauma affects the dental hard tissues and pulp, the alveolar process, and the periodontal tissues. The range of dental injuries involves root, crown, and alveolar fractures; concussion, subluxation, intrusive, extrusive, and lateral luxations; and avulsion. Figure 17–9 demonstrates

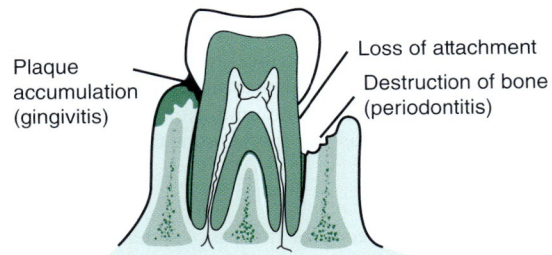

Plaque accumulation (gingivitis)

Loss of attachment

Destruction of bone (periodontitis)

▲ **Figure 17–8.** Periodontal disease.

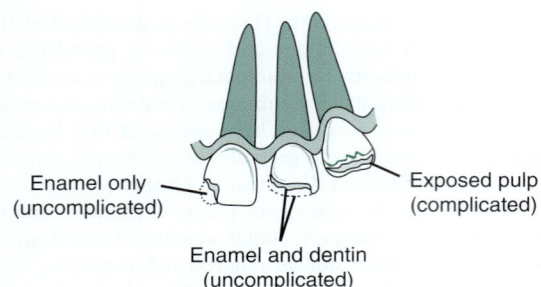

▲ Figure 17–9. Patterns of crown fractures.

different degrees of tooth fractures, and Figure 17–10 shows the types of luxation injuries.

Primary Teeth

The most common injuries in the primary dentition are luxation injuries, with the greatest incidence of trauma occurring between 2 and 3 years of age. Treatment recommendations are primarily to assess the risk of damage to the developing permanent tooth that is lingual to the apex of the primary tooth root. Parents should be advised of potential permanent tooth complications such as enamel hypocalcification, dilacerations (severe angular distortions of the crown or root of a tooth), ectopic eruption, or impaction caused by intrusion injuries of the primary maxillary anterior teeth. Parents should be informed that an avulsed primary tooth is not replanted as risk of infection and damage to the permanent tooth successor outweighs the aesthetic benefit of having the primary tooth in place.

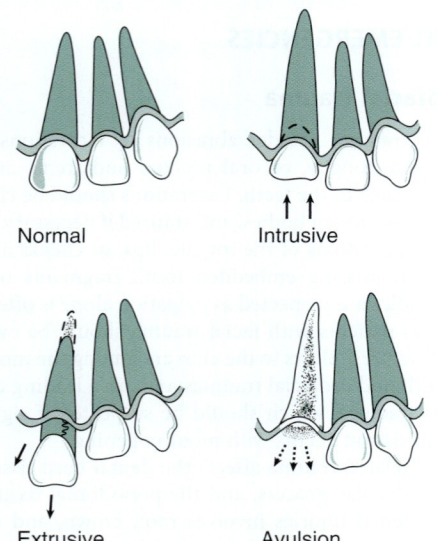

▲ Figure 17–10. Patterns of luxation injuries.

Permanent Teeth

The most common injury in the permanent dentition is crown fracture occurring secondary to falls, motor vehicle accidents, other traumatic events, and sports. Treatment is aimed at preserving the health of the pulp, the tooth's inner anatomy consisting of connective and neurovascular tissue. Intrusions of permanent teeth are managed with repositioning unless the tooth is immature and has incomplete root formation, the intrusion is minor (less than 3 mm), or there is no reeruption after a few weeks. Laterally and extrusively luxated teeth are repositioned and splinted for up to 2 weeks. Splints should stabilize the tooth in correct position while allowing physiologic movement of the tooth.

An avulsed permanent tooth should be replanted into its socket as soon as possible at or near the accident scene after gentle rinsing with clean water, provided that the child is immunocompetent and without certain types of severe cardiac disease requiring antibiotic prophylaxis. The patient must seek emergency dental care immediately thereafter. Hank's balanced salt solution (HBSS) maintains the pH and osmotic balance of periodontal ligament cells which surround the tooth root and is the best storage and transport medium for avulsed teeth that are to be replanted. The next best storage mediums in decreasing order are milk, saline, saliva (buccal vestibule), or water. Because the prognosis for viability worsens rapidly as time outside the mouth increases, the commercially available Food and Drug Administration (FDA)–approved Save-a-Tooth kit containing HBSS should be part of first-aid kits in school and sports facilities.

Alveolar Fracture

Severe injuries can result in a fractured alveolus. The alveolar ridge and teeth within the fractured segment often move together when palpated and result in a disturbance in occlusion. Fractures should be evaluated radiographically to determine their extent and involvement with the remaining teeth.

Home Care, Follow-up, & Prevention

Outcome is improved with adherence to home care instructions and dental follow-up visits. Excellent oral hygiene and rinsing with 0.12% chlorhexidine gluconate solution for 1–2 weeks reduces the presence of bacteria in the affected areas and promotes healing. A soft diet for 1–2 weeks and prevention of further injury is critical to healing. Additionally, for infants pacifier use should be avoided. Following healing, prevention of future dental trauma should be encouraged through mouthguard use for sports prone to injuries.

Antibiotic Usage

There is limited evidence for the use of systemic antibiotics for dental injuries; however, antibiotic prescription remains at the discretion of the clinician as traumatic dental injuries frequently occur in unclean environments and are often accompanied by soft tissue lacerations, maxillofacial trauma, and affect medically compromised patients. For avulsion injuries, amoxicillin or penicillin is the antibiotic of choice for the first week after replantation. Tetracycline or doxycycline are effective alternatives for penicillin-allergic children. Notable side effects of the tetracyclines are staining of permanent teeth, thus long courses (longer than 21 days for doxycycline) are not given to children younger than 8 years if an alternative exists. However, a single course of a doxycycline, which causes less tooth discoloration than tetracycline, can be safely used in all age groups.

Odontogenic Infections

Odontogenic infections can result from carious lesions, restorations approximating the pulp tissue, periodontal complications, and dental trauma. If left untreated, pain, a dental abscess, and facial cellulitis can result. Serious complications such as dehydration from difficulties with eating or drinking, cavernous sinus thrombosis, and Ludwig's angina can develop. Prompt intervention and removal of the odontogenic source of infection is indicated to avoid adverse sequelae and antibiotics recommended with systemic progression. Topical medications are of limited value for pain relief, but acetaminophen or ibuprofen can help relieve pain.

Alveolar Abscess

When left untreated, pulpal infection can progress through bone and periosteum to produce an alveolar abscess. In its acute form, the abscess presents as a painful and diffuse infection of the gingival soft tissues that requires immediate attention. Treatment includes root canal therapy or extraction for the drainage of pus and pain relief. A chronic alveolar abscess (or parulis) is a localized smaller swelling confined to the gingival tissue associated with the infected tooth that does not represent an urgent situation. Antibiotic therapy is not warranted as the pus is draining through a fistula tract and may give the patient a false sense of curing the disease. Definitive treatment of the abscess requires completely removing the source of infection by either root canal therapy or extraction of the offending tooth.

Facial Cellulitis

Facial cellulitis results if the odontogenic infection invades the facial spaces. Elevated temperature, lethargy, difficulty swallowing, and difficulty breathing are signs of serious infections. Swelling of the midface—especially the bridge of the nose and the lower eyelid—should be urgently evaluated as a potential dental infection. Eliminating the source of the odontogenic infection by either root canal therapy or extraction of the offending tooth is required. Antibiotic administration is also essential to accelerate resolution of

the cellulitis. Occasionally root canal therapy or extraction is delayed for several days while antibiotics are administered orally or intravenously (for hospitalized patients) so that the infection can be properly drained. The first-line antibiotic of choice is penicillin and secondarily clindamycin or ampicillin-sulbactam (Unasyn). Hospitalization is a prudent choice for younger children with severe facial cellulitis especially if other systemic signs and symptoms are present or if there is concern for compliance.

Bourguignon C et al: International association of Dental Traumatology guidelines for the management of traumatic dental injuries: 1. Fractures and luxations. Dent Traumatol 2020;36(4):314–330 [PMID: 32475015].
Day PF et al: International association of dental traumatology guidelines for the management of traumatic dental injuries: 3. Injuries in the primary dentition. Dent Traumatol 2020;36(4):343–359 [PMID: 32458553].
Fouad AF et al: International association of dental traumatology guidelines for the management of traumatic dental injuries: 2. Avulsion of permanent teeth. Dent Traumatol 2020;36(4):331–342 [PMID: 32460393].

SPECIAL PATIENT POPULATIONS

Oral Conditions

Children with special health care needs (C-SHCN) may have dental and/or oral soft tissues anomalies as a manifestation of a systemic condition or secondary to medical interventions. Hypodontia and delayed eruption are oral manifestations of certain disorders such as trisomy 21. Osteogenesis imperfecta can be associated with dentinogenesis imperfecta—a defect affecting the dentin of primary and permanent teeth. Chemotherapy and radiation therapy can have immediate and long-term oral effects. Immediate effects include xerostomia, particularly from salivary gland exposure to radiation, mucositis, and severe pain due to atrophy of the oral mucosa, and predisposition to various fungal and bacterial infections. Long-term effects include microdontia, hypocalcification, short and blunted roots, and delayed tooth eruption. Hematopoietic stem cell transplantation patients are at risk for oral fungal and herpes simplex virus infections during the initial engraftment and reconstitution period. Allogeneic transplants predispose a child to oral graft-versus-host disease, which can cause ulcerations, erosive lesions, or whitish reticulations affecting various oral soft tissues.

Preventive Measures

Dental caries affects C-SHCN relative to their medical condition. Long-term use of medications that contain sucrose or induce xerostomia is associated with increased caries risk. Frequent consumption of supplemental nutrition drinks high in carbohydrates significantly increases the risk for dental caries. Simple preventive steps such as rinsing with fluoridated water or mouth rinse, and/or tooth brushing with fluoridated toothpaste after each medication or supplemental nutrition intake can lower caries risk. The prescription of sugar-free alternatives for medications is recommended.

For some C-SHCN, frequent vomiting or gastroesophageal reflux disease (GERD) can weaken the enamel of teeth and increase caries risk due to acidic exposure. For patients with such concerns, rinsing with fluoridated water or mouth rinse after a vomiting episode is recommended. Toothbrushing immediately afterwards should be avoided due to abrasive effects of toothbrushing on the weakened enamel surfaces.

The susceptibility of C-SHCN to periodontal diseases increases with difficulty in performing oral hygiene due to oral aversions, limited mouth opening, or erratic body movements. Parents may perceive brushing their child's teeth as unnecessary when not taking food by mouth. However, gastric-tube–fed children typically exhibit increased calculus buildup due to the lack of mechanical stimulation of the gingival tissues associated with oral feedings, increasing risk for periodontal disease.

▶ Preventive Measures for the Oncology Patient

It is imperative that a dentist knowledgeable about pediatric oncology evaluates children with cancer soon after diagnosis. The aims are to (1) develop a dental treatment plan in collaboration with the oncologist prior to cancer therapy, (2) inform the patient and caregivers about the importance of good oral hygiene, and (3) remove all existing and potential sources of dental infection (eg, abscessed teeth, extensive caries) before the child becomes neutropenic from chemotherapy. Failure to do so can result in consequences, such as an abscess due to undiagnosed caries, which can compromise oncology management.

Preventive strategies aimed at reducing oral complications from oncology therapy include a noncariogenic diet, fluoride therapy, mucositis prevention through meticulous oral hygiene, and patient/parent education. In children receiving radiation therapy, customized fluoride applicators and artificial saliva in combination with regular follow-up visits minimizes rapid and extensive destruction of teeth due to xerostomia.

▶ Dental Treatment Considerations

Indications for Antibiotic Prophylaxis

Certain dental procedures including tooth brushing result in transient bacteremia. Patients at increased risk for bacteremia-induced infections require prophylactic antibiotic coverage prior to invasive dental procedures. Indications include children with cardiac conditions such as a history of infective endocarditis, repaired congenital heart disease with residual defects or valvular regurgitation and unrepaired cyanotic congenital heart disease, prosthetic cardiac valves or material, and cardiac transplant with valvulopathy. For nonvalvular devices such as indwelling vascular catheters and cardiovascular implantable electronic devices, antibiotic coverage is not indicated after placement. Hydrocephalus shunts with vascular access (ie, ventriculocardiac, ventriculovenous) require antibiotic prophylaxis to minimize risk for infection from dental procedures, whereas the nonvascular type (ie, ventriculoperitoneal, ventriculoatrial) does not. Current guidelines reflect antibiotic premedication for a smaller subset of patients due to risk of developing drug-resistant bacteria and adverse reactions to antibiotics.

Antibiotic prophylaxis is not indicated for dental patients with pins, plates, screws, or other orthopedic hardware not within a synovial joint. Likewise, patients with total joint replacements do not routinely require antibiotic prophylaxis. If unsure of risk, consultation with the orthopedic surgeon is indicated.

For immunocompromised patients, the absolute neutrophil count (ANC) is important because of the risk for systemic sepsis from dental procedures. For neutrophil levels above 2000/mm^3, antibiotic prophylaxis is not indicated. Between 1000 and 2000/mm^3, prophylaxis is subject to the clinical judgment of the dentist, the patient's health status, and planned procedures. Both the dentist and physician should discuss the need for antibiotic prophylaxis in these unique circumstances.

Management of Bleeding Disorders

Oral surgical procedures on any child with a bleeding disorder require a coordinated approach between the child's hematologist and dentist. Patients with mild bleeding disorders (eg, mild von Willebrand disease) can be treated in ambulatory dental settings with local hemostatic measures such as topical hemostatic agents (eg, Gelfoam, thrombin). Patients with severe coagulation disorders (eg, severe hemophilia A and/or factor VIII antibodies) requiring dental surgery should be managed in hospital settings in consultation with a hematologist. Intraoperatively, topical hemostatic agents within tooth sockets and suturing immediately following extractions reduces bleeding complications.

For patients receiving anticoagulation therapy, dosage reduction before dental surgery is generally not recommended as the risk of embolism outweighs the risk for bleeding complications. In these instances, the dentist should consult with the hematologist to obtain the most recent international normalized ratio (INR) and discuss the appropriate anticoagulation level at which a dental procedure can occur. The administration of a "bridging agent" such as enoxaparin in preparation for the planned dental procedure reduces postoperative bleeding concerns while minimizing embolic complications.

Patients undergoing chemotherapy and/or hematopoietic stem cell transplantation are also at risk for intra-oral bleeding. Elective dental care should be deferred when the platelet count is less than 60,000/μL. Typically, platelet counts greater than 60,000/μL do not require additional measures for dental procedures, while lower levels require supportive measures and pre- and postoperative platelet transfusions.

PDQ® Supportive and Palliative Care Editorial Board. PDQ Oral Complications of Chemotherapy and Head/Neck Radiation. Bethesda, MD: National Cancer Institute. https://www.cancer.gov/about-cancer/treatment/side-effects/mouth-throat/oral-complications-hp-pdq. Accessed May 3, 2023.

Schiffer CA et al: Platelet transfusion for patients with cancer: American Society of Clinical Oncology Clinical Practice Guideline Update. J Clin Oncol 2018;36(3):283–299 [PMID: 29182495].

Wilson WR et al: Prevention of viridans group streptococcal infective endocarditis: a scientific statement from the American Heart Association. Circulation 2021;143(20):e963–e978. https://www.ahajournals.org/doi/pdf/10.1161/CIR.0000000000000969. Accessed May 03, 2023.

ORTHODONTIC REFERRAL

The pediatric dentist is involved in the timely detection of orthodontic concerns in the mixed or permanent dentition and facilitates appropriate referral to an orthodontist for correction of the malocclusion to promote normal growth development of jaws and teeth. For any child with a cleft palate or other craniofacial growth disorder, referral is indicated when maxillary permanent incisors erupt, and alveolar bone grafting is contemplated.

Proffit WR, Sarver DM, Ackerman JL: Orthodontic diagnosis: the problem-oriented approach. In: Proffit WR, Fields HW, Sarver DM (eds): Contemporary Orthodontics. 5th ed. St. Louis, MO: Mosby; 2012:150–219.

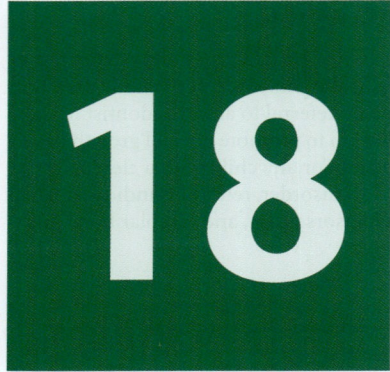

18

Ear, Nose, & Throat

Patricia J. Yoon, MD
Melissa A. Scholes, MD
Brian W. Herrmann, MD

THE EAR

INFECTIONS OF THE EAR

1. Acute Otitis Externa

ESSENTIALS OF DIAGNOSIS & TYPICAL FEATURES

► Rapid onset of symptoms within the past 3 days.
► Symptoms of ear canal inflammation, including otalgia, itching, or fullness, with or without hearing loss or jaw pain.
► Tenderness on movement of the tragus or pinna is a classic finding.

► Differential Diagnosis

Acute or chronic otitis media with eardrum rupture, furunculosis of the ear canal, herpes zoster oticus, mastoiditis, referred temporomandibular joint pain, and chronic otitis externa (OE).

► Pathogenesis

OE is a cellulitis of the soft tissues of the external auditory canal (EAC), which can extend to surrounding structures such as the pinna, tragus, and lymph nodes. Humidity, heat, and moisture in the ear are known to contribute to the development of OE; thus, it is more common in the summer months and in humid climates. It more often occurs in children and young adults and is responsible for more than 500,000 emergency room visits per year.

Cerumen serves as a hydrophobic protective barrier to the underlying skin and its acidic pH inhibits bacterial and fungal growth. Trauma to the ear canal skin from things such as cotton swabs, fingernails, or earbuds, can break the skin-cerumen barrier, which is the first step in developing OE. Dermatologic conditions such as atopic dermatitis can also predispose one to OE. The most common organisms causing OE are *Staphylococcus aureus*, *Staphylococcus epidermidis*, and *Pseudomonas aeruginosa*. However, anaerobic bacteria are also seen. Fungal infection occurs in 2%–10% of patients, usually following treatment for a bacterial OE.

► Clinical Findings

Symptoms include acute onset of pain, aural fullness, decreased hearing, and itching in the ear. Symptoms tend to peak within 3 days. Manipulation of the pinna or tragus causes considerable pain that is usually out of proportion to examination. Discharge may be present and be clear or purulent and may also cause secondary eczema of the auricle. The EAC is typically swollen and narrowed, and the patient may resist any attempt to insert an otoscope. Debris is often present in the canal, and it may be difficult to visualize the tympanic membrane (TM). However, it is important to determine the status of the eardrum to rule out secondary OE caused by middle ear drainage that may need to be managed differently.

► Complications

If untreated, cellulitis of neck and face may result. Immunocompromised individuals or uncontrolled diabetics can develop malignant OE, which is a spread of the infection to the skull base with resultant osteomyelitis. This is a life-threatening condition and should be evaluated emergently if suspected.

► Treatment

Management of OE includes pain control, removal of debris from the canal, topical antimicrobial therapy, and avoidance of causative factors. Cultures are not routinely sent on initial presentation as most cases will resolve with these primary interventions. Fluoroquinolone eardrops alone are first-line therapy for OE in the absence of systemic symptoms; however, combination drops that also contain a steroid, such as ciprofloxacin with dexamethasone, can hasten recovery by addressing the edema and inflammatory response as well. The topical therapy chosen must be non-ototoxic in case a perforation or patent tube is present; if the TM cannot be visualized, a perforation should be presumed to exist. If the ear canal is too edematous to allow entry of the eardrops, a Pope ear wick (expandable sponge) should be placed to ensure antibiotic delivery. If symptoms persist after 48–72 hours, the patient should be reassessed to confirm diagnosis and exclude other causes for their symptoms. If drainage persists despite therapy, cultures should be sent. Oral antibiotics are indicated for any signs of invasive infection, such as fever, cellulitis of the face or auricle, or tender periauricular or cervical lymphadenopathy. In such cases, in addition to ototopical therapy, cultures of the ear canal discharge should be sent, and an antistaphylococcal antibiotic prescribed while awaiting culture results. The ear should be kept dry until the infection has cleared. Patients can have difficulty applying drops to the affected ear canal, which may cause prolonged symptoms and treatment failures. If this is suspected, thoroughly explain and demonstrate the application of the topical therapy as outlined in the Clinical Practice Guideline on Acute Otitis Externa.

American Academy of Family Physicians: Acute otitis externa [clinical practice guideline]; 2019. https://www.aafp.org/family-physician/patient-care/clinical-recommendations/all-clinical-recommendations/acute-otitis-externa.html. Accessed January 3, 2023.
Rosenfeld RM et al: Clinical practice guideline: acute otitis externa executive summary. Otolaryngol Head Neck Surg 2014 Nov; 150(2):161–168 [PMID: 24492208].

Web Resources

Goguen LA: External otitis: pathogenesis, clinical features and diagnosis. https://www.uptodate.com/contents/external-otitis-pathogenesis-clinical-features-and-diagnosis?search=external%20otitis&source=search_result&selectedTitle=2~30&usage_type=default&display_rank=2. Last updated: July 12, 2022. Accessed July 5, 2023.
Jackson EA, Geer K. Acute otitis externa: rapid evidence review. Am Fam Physician 2023 Feb;107(2):145–151 [PMID: 36791445].
Waitzman AA et al: Otitis Externa. Updated April 7, 2022. http://emedicine.medscape.com/article/994550-overview. Accessed July 5, 2023.

2. Acute Otitis Media

Acute otitis media (AOM) is the most common reason antibiotics are prescribed for children in the United States. It is an acute infection of the middle ear space associated with inflammation, effusion, or, if a patent tympanostomy tube or perforation is present, otorrhea (ear drainage).

ESSENTIALS OF DIAGNOSIS & TYPICAL FEATURES

▶ Moderate to severe bulging of the TM or new otorrhea not associated with OE.

▶ Mild bulging of the TM and less than 48 hours of otalgia (ear-holding, tugging, or rubbing in a nonverbal child) or intense erythema of the TM.

▶ Middle ear effusion (MEE), proven by pneumatic otoscopy or tympanometry, must be present.

▶ Differential Diagnosis

Otitis media with effusion (OME), OE, bullous myringitis, acute mastoiditis, dental or TMJ pain, acute viral pharyngitis, and middle ear mass.

▶ Clinical Findings

Two findings are critical in establishing a diagnosis of AOM: a bulging TM and MEE. The presence of MEE is best determined by visual examination and either pneumatic otoscopy or tympanometry (Figure 18–1). To distinguish AOM from OME, signs and symptoms of middle ear inflammation and acute infection must be present. Otoscopic findings specific for AOM include a bulging TM, impaired visibility of ossicular landmarks, yellow or white effusion (pus), an opacified and inflamed eardrum, and occasionally squamous exudate or bullae on the eardrum.

A. Pathophysiology and Predisposing Factors

1. Eustachian tube dysfunction (ETD)—The Eustachian tube regulates middle ear pressure and allows for drainage of the middle ear. The ciliated respiratory epithelium of the Eustachian tube also defends against pathogens by producing lysozyme and mucus, which helps rid the ear of microorganisms. It must periodically open to prevent the development of negative pressure and effusion in the middle ear space. If the Eustachian tube does not work properly, negative pressure leads to transudation of cellular fluid into the middle ear, as well as influx of fluids and pathogens from the nasopharynx and adenoids. The transudate then becomes infected by the pathogens present, creating infection in the middle ear space. The Eustachian tube of infants and young children is more prone to dysfunction because it is shorter, more compliant, and more horizontal than in adults. The Eustachian tube reaches its adult configuration by the age of 7 years. Children with craniofacial differences, such as those with trisomy 21 or

Right tympanic membrane

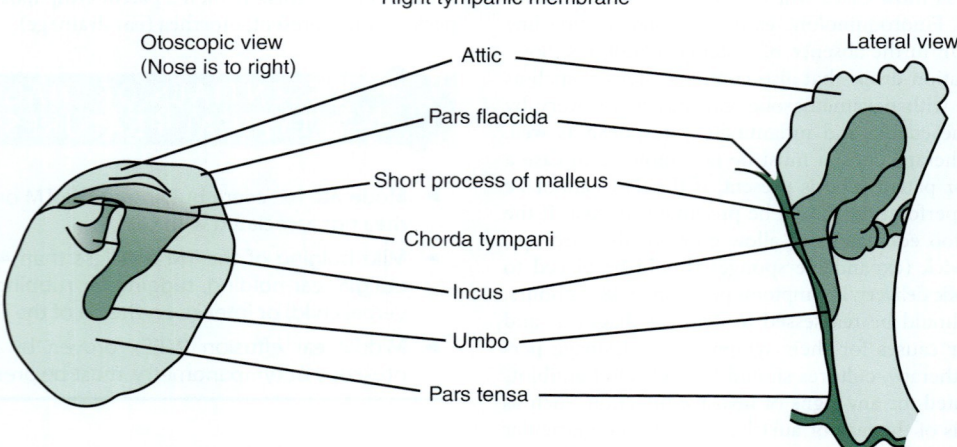

▲ **Figure 18–1.** Tympanic membrane.

cleft palate, may be particularly susceptible to ETD because of abnormal anatomy of the Eustachian tube.

2. Bacterial colonization—Nasopharyngeal colonization with *Streptococcus pneumoniae, Haemophilus influenzae,* or *Moraxella catarrhalis* increases the risk of AOM, whereas colonization with normal flora such as viridans streptococci may prevent AOM by inhibiting growth of these pathogens.

3. Viral upper respiratory infections (URIs)—URIs impair Eustachian tube function by causing adenoid hypertrophy and edema of the Eustachian tube itself. Viral infections also inhibit the antibacterial properties of mucus and mucociliary clearance.

4. Smoke exposure—Passive smoke increases the risk of persistent MEE by enhancing colonization, prolonging the inflammatory response, and impeding drainage of the middle ear through the Eustachian tube. For infants aged 12–18 months, cigarette exposure is associated with an 11% per pack increase in the duration of MEE.

5. Impaired host immune defenses—Immunocompromised children such as those with selective IgA deficiency usually experience recurrent AOM, rhinosinusitis, and pneumonia. However, most children who experience recurrent or persistent otitis only have selective impairments of immune defenses against specific otitis pathogens.

6. Bottle feeding—Bottle feeding especially with bottle propping in the crib or car seat increases the risk of AOM because of aspiration of contaminated secretions into the middle ear space. Breast-feeding reduces the incidence of acute respiratory infections and provides immunoglobulin A (IgA) antibodies that reduce colonization with otitis pathogens.

7. Season—The incidence of AOM correlates with the activity of respiratory viruses, accounting for the annual surge in otitis media cases during the winter months in temperate climates.

8. Daycare attendance—Children exposed to large groups of children have more respiratory infections and OM. The increased number of children in day care over the past three decades has undoubtedly played a major role in the increase in AOM.

9. Genetic susceptibility—Genetics is thought to play a role in 40%–70% of ear infections. Most of the genes responsible regulate immunity. However, environmental and pathogen-related causes also play a role. The role of genetics in AOM is an area of active research.

10. Age—Children ages 1–3 years are at greatest risk for AOM and 70% of all children experience one or more episodes of AOM before their second birthday.

B. Microbiology of Acute Otitis Media

Bacterial or viral pathogens can be detected in up to 96% of middle ear fluid samples from patients with AOM. Peak activity of respiratory syncytial virus, metapneumovirus, and influenza A corresponds with increased visits for AOM and 71% of middle ear aspirates from children undergoing ear tube surgery for recurrent OM contain viruses. Polybacterial infections are seen in up to 55% of cases, with bacterial and viral coinfections occurring in up to 70%. *S pneumoniae* and *H influenzae* account for 35%–40% and 30%–35% of isolates, respectively. With widespread use of the pneumococcal conjugate vaccine starting in 2000, the incidence of AOM caused by *H influenzae* rose while that of the *S pneumoniae* vaccine

Table 18–1. Microbiology of acute otitis media (AOM).

Organism	Percentage of AOM Cases
S pneumoniae	35–40
H influenzae	30–35
M catarrhalis	15–25
S pyogenes	4

serotypes declined. However, there has been an increase in disease caused by S pneumoniae serotypes not covered by the vaccine, as well as S aureus. The third most common pathogen cited is M catarrhalis, which causes 15%–25% of AOM cases in the United States (Table 18–1). The fourth most common organism in AOM is Streptococcus pyogenes, which is found more frequently in school-aged children than in infants. S pyogenes and S pneumoniae are the predominant causes of mastoiditis.

Drug-resistant S pneumoniae is a common pathogen in AOM and strains may be resistant to only one drug class (eg, penicillins or macrolides) or to multiple classes. Children with resistant strains tend to be younger and to have had more unresponsive infections. History of antibiotic treatment in the preceding 3 months increases the risk of harboring resistant pathogens.

C. Examination Techniques and Procedures

1. Pneumatic otoscopy—AOM is often overdiagnosed, leading to inappropriate antibiotic therapy, unnecessary surgical referrals, and significant associated costs. Contributing to errors in diagnosis is the temptation to accept the diagnosis without removing enough cerumen to adequately visualize the TM, and the mistaken belief that a red TM establishes the diagnosis. Redness of the TM is often a vascular flush caused by fever or crying.

A pneumatic otoscope with a rubber suction bulb and tube is used to assess TM mobility. When used correctly, pneumatic otoscopy can improve diagnostic ability by 15%–25%. The largest possible speculum should be used to provide an airtight seal and maximize the field of view. When the rubber bulb is gently squeezed, the TM should move freely with a snapping motion; if fluid is present in the middle ear space, the mobility of the TM will be absent or resemble a fluid wave. The ability to assess mobility is compromised by failure to achieve an adequate seal with the otoscope and poor visualization of the TM.

2. Cerumen removal—In order to adequately visualize the TM, cerumen (ear wax) removal is an essential skill for anyone who cares for children. Please refer to section Ear Canal Foreign Body & Cerumen Impaction.

3. Tympanometry—Tympanometry can be helpful in assessing middle ear status, particularly when pneumatic otoscopy

is inconclusive or difficult to perform. Tympanometry can reveal the presence or absence of an MEE but cannot differentiate between acutely infected fluid (AOM) and a chronic effusion (also referred to as OME).

Tympanometry measures TM compliance and displays it in graphic form. It also measures the volume of the ear canal, which can help differentiate between an intact and perforated TM.

Standard 226-Hz tympanometry is not reliable in infants younger than 6 months. A high-frequency (1000 Hz) probe is used in this age group.

Tympanograms can be classified into four major patterns, as shown in Figure 18–2. The pattern shown in Figure 18–2A, characterized by maximum compliance at normal atmospheric pressure, indicates a normal TM, good Eustachian tube function, and absence of effusion. Figure 18–2B identifies a nonmobile TM with normal volume, which indicates MEE. Figure 18–2C indicates an intact, mobile TM with excessively negative middle ear pressure (> –150 daPa), indicative of poor Eustachian tube function. Figure 18–2D shows a flat tracing with a large middle ear volume, indicative of a patent tube or TM perforation.

► Treatment

A. Pain Management

Pain is the primary symptom of AOM, and the 2013 clinical practice guidelines emphasize the importance of addressing this symptom. As it may take 1–3 days before antibiotic therapy leads to a reduction in pain, ibuprofen or acetaminophen should be administered as needed to relieve discomfort. Topical analgesics have a very short duration, and studies do not support efficacy in children younger than 5 years.

B. The Observation Option

The choice to observe an episode of AOM and not treat with antibiotics is an option in otherwise healthy children with mild to moderate otitis media without other underlying conditions such as cleft palate, craniofacial abnormalities, immune deficiencies, cochlear implants, or tympanostomy tubes. The decision should be made in conjunction with the parents, and a mechanism must be in place to provide antibiotic therapy if there is worsening of symptoms or lack of improvement within 48–72 hours. A Safety-Net Antibiotic Prescription (SNAP) given to parents with instructions to be filled only if symptoms do not resolve lowered overall antibiotic use in a large pediatric practice-based research network. The American Academy of Pediatrics clinical practice guidelines include age, presence of otorrhea, severity of symptoms, and laterality as criteria for antibiotic treatment versus observation (Table 18–2).

C. Antibiotic Therapy

Antibiotics have been shown to shorten the duration of AOM and prevent complications. Some have advocated observation

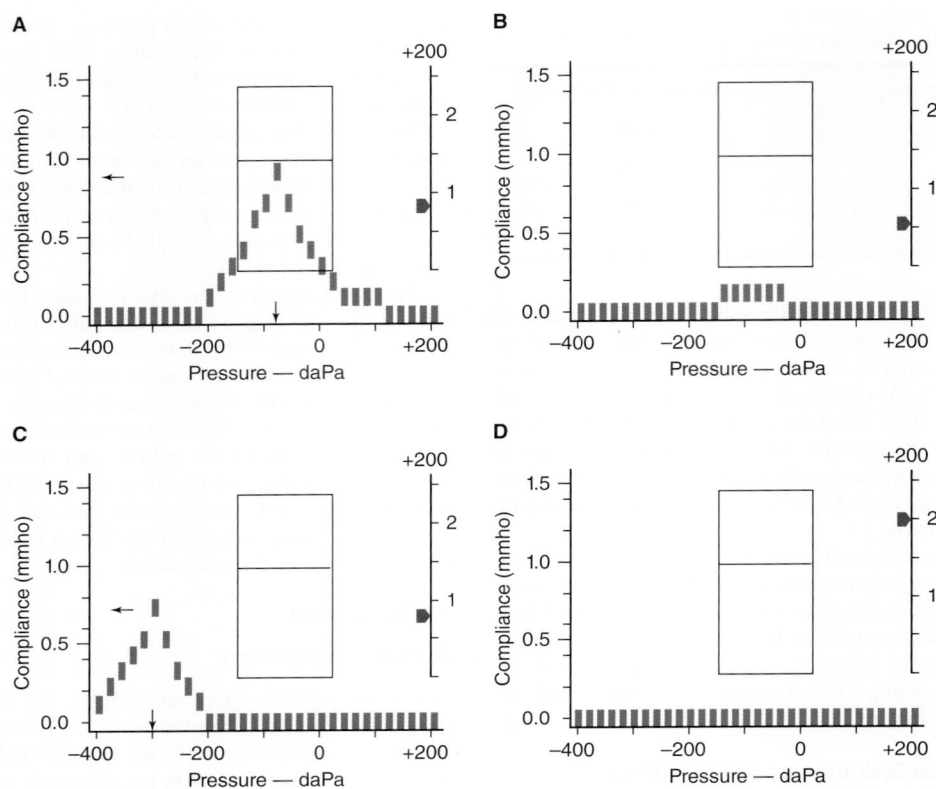

▲ **Figure 18–2.** Four types of tympanograms obtained with Welch-Allyn MicroTymp 2. **A:** Normal middle ear. **B:** Otitis media with effusion or AOM. **C:** Negative middle ear pressure due to ETD. **D:** Patent tympanostomy tube or perforation in the TM. Same as B except for a very large middle ear volume.

in healthy, older children; however, studies have demonstrated that the use of antibiotics improves patient outcomes in early and late stages of AOM. High-dose amoxicillin remains the first-line antibiotic for treating AOM, even with a high prevalence of drug-resistant *S pneumoniae*, because data show that isolates of the bacteria remain susceptible to the drug 83%–87% of the time.

Amoxicillin-clavulanate enhanced strength (ES), with 90 mg/kg/day of amoxicillin dosing (14:1 ratio of amoxicillin:

Table 18–2. Recommendations for initial management of uncomplicated AOM.[a]

Age	Otorrhea With AOM[a]	Unilateral or Bilateral AOM[a] With Severe Symptoms[b]	Bilateral AOM[a] Without Otorrhea	Unilateral AOM[a] Without Otorrhea
6 mo to 2 y	Antibiotic therapy	Antibiotic therapy	Antibiotic therapy	Antibiotic therapy or additional observation
≥ 2 y	Antibiotic therapy	Antibiotic therapy	Antibiotic therapy or additional observation	Antibiotic therapy or additional observation[c]

[a]Applies only to children with well-documented AOM and a high certainty of diagnosis.
[b]A toxic-appearing child, persistent otalgia for more than 48 hours, temperature > 39°C (102.2°F) in the past 48 hours, or if there is uncertain access to follow-up after the visit.
[c]This plan of initial management provides an opportunity for shared decision-making with the child's family for those categories appropriate for initial observation. If observation is offered, a mechanism must be in place to ensure follow-up and begin antibiotics if the child worsens or fails to improve within 48–72 hours of AOM onset.

clavulanate), is an appropriate choice when a child has had amoxicillin in the last 30 days or is clinically failing after 48–72 hours on amoxicillin (Table 18–3) or has concomitant conjunctivitis. Purulent conjunctivitis is often caused by nontypeable *H influenzae*. The regular strength formulations of amoxicillin-clavulanate (7:1 ratio) should not be doubled in dosage to achieve 90 mg/kg/day of amoxicillin, because the increased amount of clavulanate will cause diarrhea.

Three oral cephalosporins (cefuroxime, cefpodoxime, and cefdinir) are more β-lactamase–stable and are alternative choices in children who develop a papular rash with amoxicillin (see Table 18–3). Of these, cefdinir suspension is most palatable; the other two have a bitter aftertaste which is difficult to conceal.

A second-line antibiotic is indicated when a child experiences symptomatic infection within 1 month of finishing amoxicillin; however, repeated use of high-dose amoxicillin is indicated if more than 4 weeks have passed without symptoms. Macrolides are not recommended as second-line agents because *S pneumoniae* is resistant in approximately 30% of respiratory isolates, and because virtually all strains of *H influenzae* have an intrinsic macrolide efflux pump, which pumps the antibiotic out of the bacterial cell. However, if there is a history of type 1 hypersensitivity reaction, macrolides may be used.

Reasons for failure to eradicate a sensitive pathogen include drug noncompliance, poor drug absorption, or vomiting of the drug. If a child remains symptomatic for longer than 3 days while taking a second-line agent, a tympanocentesis is useful to identify the causative pathogen. If a highly resistant pneumococcus is found or if tympanocentesis is not feasible, intramuscular ceftriaxone at 50 mg/kg/dose for 3 consecutive days is recommended. If a child has experienced a severe reaction, such as anaphylaxis, to amoxicillin, cephalosporins should not be substituted. Otherwise, the risk of cross-sensitivity is less than 0.1%. Multidrug-resistant *S pneumoniae* poses a treatment dilemma and newer antibiotics, such as fluoroquinolones or linezolid, may need to be used. However, these drugs are not approved by the US Food and Drug Administration (FDA) for the treatment of AOM in children.

In patients with tympanostomy tubes with uncomplicated acute otorrhea, ototopical antibiotics (fluoroquinolone eardrops) are first-line therapy. The eardrops serve two purposes: (1) They treat the infection and (2) they physically "rinse" drainage from the tube which helps prevent plugging of the tube. Oral antibiotics are not indicated in the absence of systemic symptoms.

If a TM perforation has occurred with otorrhea then topical antibiotics are recommended as first-line agents due to the

Table 18–3. Antibiotic therapies for AOM.

A. Initial Immediate or Delayed Antibiotic Treatment	
First-Line Treatment	**Alternative Treatments (if Penicillin-Allergic)**
Amoxicillin (80–90 mg/kg/day in two divided doses) • For children aged < 2 y or children of all ages with severe symptoms, treat for 10 days. • Age 2–6 y with mild-moderate symptoms, treat for 7 days. • Age > 6 y with mild-moderate symptoms, treat for 5 days. or Amoxicillin-clavulanate (90 mg/kg/day or amoxicillin, with 6.4 mg/kg/day of clavulanate in two divided doses) • For patients who have received amoxicillin in the previous 30 days or who have otitis-conjunctivitis syndrome	Cefdinir (14/mg/kg/day in one or two doses) Cefuroxime (30 mg/kg/day divided BID) Cefpodoxime (10 mg/kg/day in two divided doses) Ceftriaxone (50 mg IM or IV per day for 1 or 3 days) • If unable to take oral medications For children with severe penicillin allergies (IgE-mediated events) or known cephalosporin allergy: • Trimethoprim-sulfamethoxazole • Macrolides • Clindamycin (30–40 mg/kg/day, divided TID)
B. Antibiotic Treatment After 48–72 h of Failure of Initial Antibiotic	
First-Line Treatment	**Alternative Treatment**
Amoxicillin-clavulanate (90 mg/kg/day or amoxicillin, with 6.4 mg/kg/day of clavulanate in two divided doses) • For patients who have received amoxicillin in the previous 30 days or who have otitis-conjunctivitis syndrome. or Ceftriaxone (50 mg IM or IV per day for 3 days)	Ceftriaxone (50 mg IM or IV per day for 3 days) Clindamycin (30–40 mg/kg/day, divided TID) with or without a third-generation cephalosporin Consider tympanocentesis Consult specialist
C. Recurrence > 4 wk After Initial Episode	
1. A new pathogen is likely, so restart first-line therapy. 2. Be sure diagnosis is not OME, which may be observed for 3–6 mo without treatment.	

ability to provide high concentrations of antibiotic directly to the middle ear. Topical fluoroquinolone otic drops (ofloxacin and ciprofloxacin) with or without steroids are considered safe for administration into the middle ear. If there is a large amount of debris or drainage in the ear canal, the canal may need to be suctioned first to allow drops to gain access to the middle ear.

D. Tympanocentesis

Tympanocentesis is performed by placing a needle through the TM and aspirating the middle ear fluid. The fluid is sent for culture and sensitivity. Indications for tympanocentesis are (1) AOM in an immunocompromised patient, (2) research studies, (3) evaluation for presumed sepsis or meningitis, such as in a neonate, (4) unresponsive otitis media despite courses of two appropriate antibiotics, and (5) acute mastoiditis or other suppurative complications.

E. Prevention of Acute Otitis Media

1. Antibiotic prophylaxis—Strongly discouraged due to poor efficacy and concern for antibiotic resistance.

2. Possible lifestyle modifications—Parental education plays a major role in decreasing AOM.

- Smoking is a risk factor both for URI and AOM. Primary care physicians should provide information on smoking cessation programs and measures.

- Breast-feeding protects children from AOM. Clinicians should encourage exclusive breastfeeding for 6 months or longer.

- Bottle-propping in the crib should be avoided. It increases AOM risk due to the reflux of milk into the Eustachian tubes.

- Pacifiers are controversial. There may be a protective effect of pacifiers against SIDS, but they may increase risk of AOM. Currently, the recommendation from the American Academy of Family Physicians is to wean pacifiers after 6 months of age to reduce the risk of AOM.

- Day care is a risk factor for AOM, but working parents may have few alternatives. Possible alternatives include care by relatives or childcare in a setting with fewer children.

3. Surgery—Tympanostomy tubes are effective in the treatment of recurrent AOM as well as OME.

4. Immunologic evaluation and allergy testing—While immunoglobulin subclass deficiencies may be more common in children with recurrent AOM, there is no practical immune therapy available. More serious immunodeficiencies, such as selective IgA deficiency, should be considered in children who suffer from a combination of recurrent AOM, rhinosinusitis, and pneumonia. In the school-aged child or preschooler with an atopic background, skin testing may be beneficial in identifying allergens that can predispose to AOM.

5. Vaccines—The pneumococcal conjugate and influenza vaccines are recommended. The seven-valent pneumococcal conjugate vaccine (PCV7) was introduced in the United States in 2000, and the 13-valent pneumococcal conjugate vaccine (PCV13) in 2010. The transition from PCV7 to PCV13 has resulted in a decline of otitis media among children younger than 2 years due to decreased risk of both the first and subsequent episodes of otitis media.

Barenkamp SJ et al: Panel 4: report of the microbiology panel. Otolaryngol Head Neck Surg 2017 April;156(4 Suppl):S51–S62 [PMID: 28372529].

Donaldson JD: Acute otitis media. Emedicine. Updated December 27, 2021. https://emedicine.medscape.com/article/859316-overview.

Lieberthal AS et al: The diagnosis and management of acute otitis media. Pediatrics 2013;131:e964–e999 [PMID: 23439909].

Rosenfeld RM et al: Executive summary of clinical practice guideline on tympanostomy tubes in children (update). Otolaryngol Head Neck Surg 2022 Feb;166(2):189–206. doi: 10.1177/01945998211065661 [PMID: 35138976].

Schilder AG et al: Panel 7: otitis media and complications. Otolaryngol Head Neck Surg 2017;156(4s):S88–S105 [PMID: 28372534].

Wald ER: Acute otitis media in children: clinical manifestations and diagnosis. Up to Date. Updated April 22, 2022.

Wiese AD et al: Changes in otitis media episodes and pressure equalization tube insertions among young children following introduction of the 13-valent pneumococcal conjugate vaccine: a birth-cohort based study. Clin Infect Dis 2019 Nov 27;69(12):2162–2169. doi: 10.1093/cid/ciz142 [PMID: 30770533].

3. Otitis Media With Effusion

ESSENTIALS OF DIAGNOSIS & TYPICAL FEATURES

- ► MEE with decreased TM mobility on examination, confirmed by pneumatic otoscopy or tympanometry.
- ► No signs or symptoms of acute inflammation.
- ► OME should *not* be treated with antibiotics, intranasal or systemic steroids, antihistamines, or decongestants.

► Clinical Findings

OME is the presence of fluid in the middle ear space without signs or symptoms of acute inflammation. This is common, with 90% of children having one episode of OME by age 5. On examination, the TM may be opacified and thickened and the middle ear fluid can be clear, amber-colored, or opaque. Pneumatic otoscopy can confirm the presence of a MEE. If the pneumatic otoscopy examination is uncertain, tympanometry should be performed to confirm presence of middle ear fluid.

Children with OME can develop AOM if the middle ear fluid should become infected. After AOM, fluid can remain in the ear for several weeks, with 25% of patients having a persistent MEE at 3 months after treatment. It is important to distinguish OME from AOM because the former does not benefit from treatment with antibiotics. OME can be associated with hearing loss, balance issues, ear discomfort, behavioral concerns, and reduced quality of life.

▶ Management

An audiology evaluation should be performed after approximately 3 months of continuous bilateral effusion in most children. However, children who are at risk of language delay due to socioeconomic circumstances, craniofacial anomalies, autism, ADHD, or other risk factors should undergo a hearing evaluation at the time that OME is diagnosed. Children with hearing loss or speech delay should be referred to an otolaryngologist for possible tympanostomy tube placement. Antibiotics, antihistamines, and steroids have not been shown to be useful in the treatment of OME.

In uncomplicated cases, OME is observed for 3 months prior to consideration for tympanostomy tube placement. Longer periods of observation may be acceptable in children with normal or very mild hearing loss on audiogram, no risk factors for speech and language issues, and no structural changes to the TM. These children should be followed every 3–6 months until the effusions clear or problems develop. Indications for tympanostomy tubes include hearing loss greater than 40 dB, TM retraction pockets, ossicular erosion, adhesive atelectasis, and cholesteatoma. In children older than 4, adenoidectomy may be recommended with ear tubes as studies show this can reduce failure rate and need for additional surgeries.

▶ Prognosis & Sequelae

Prognosis is variable based on age of presentation. Infants who are very young at the time of first otitis media are more likely to need surgical intervention. Other factors that decrease the likelihood of resolution are onset of OME in the summer or fall, history of prior tympanostomy tubes, presence of adenoids, and hearing loss greater than 30 dB.

Rosenfeld RM et al: Clinical practice guideline: otitis media with effusion executive summary (update). Otolaryngol Head Neck Surg 2016 Feb;154(2):201–214. doi: 10.1177/019459981562440 7.26833645 [PMID: 26833645].
Rosenfeld RM et al: Executive summary of clinical practice guideline on tympanostomy tubes in children (update). Otolaryngol Head Neck Surg 2022 Feb;166(2):189–206. doi: 10.1177/01945998211065661 [PMID: 35138976].

4. Complications of Otitis Media

A. Changes of the Tympanic Membrane

Tympanosclerosis is an acquired disorder of calcification and scarring of the TM and middle ear structures secondary to inflammation. If tympanosclerosis involves the ossicles, a conductive hearing loss may result. The term *myringosclerosis* applies to calcification of the TM only and is a common sequela of OME and AOM. Myringosclerosis may also develop at the site of a previous tympanostomy tube; tympanosclerosis is not a common sequela of tube placement. Myringosclerosis rarely causes hearing loss unless the entire TM is involved ("porcelain eardrum").

The appearance of a small defect or invagination of the pars tensa or pars flaccida of the TM suggests a retraction pocket. Retraction pockets occur when chronic inflammation and negative pressure in the middle ear space produce atrophy and atelectasis of the TM.

Continued inflammation can cause adhesions to form between the retracted TM and the ossicles. This condition, referred to as *adhesive otitis*, predisposes one to formation of a cholesteatoma or fixation and erosion of the ossicles.

B. Cholesteatoma

A greasy-looking or pearly white mass seen in a retraction pocket or perforation behind the eardrum suggests a cholesteatoma (Figure 18–3). If infection is superimposed, serous or purulent drainage will be seen and the middle ear cavity may contain granulation tissue or even polyps. Persistent, recurrent, or foul-smelling otorrhea following appropriate medical management should make one suspect a cholesteatoma and prompt an ENT (Ear-Nose-Throat/Otolaryngology) referral.

C. Tympanic Membrane Perforation

Occasionally, an episode of AOM may result in rupture of the TM. Discharge from the ear is seen, and often there is rapid relief of pain. Perforations due to AOM usually heal

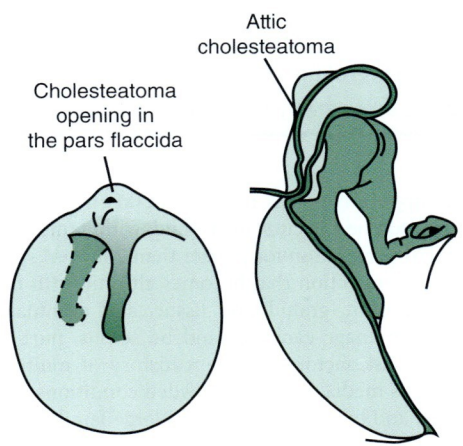

▲ **Figure 18–3.** Attic cholesteatoma, formed from an in-drawing of an attic retraction pocket.

Cholesteatoma opening in the pars flaccida

Attic cholesteatoma

spontaneously within a couple of weeks. Ototopical antibiotics are recommended for a 10- to 14-day course and patients should be referred to an otolaryngologist 2–3 weeks after the rupture for examination and hearing evaluation.

When perforations fail to heal, surgical repair may be needed. TM repair is generally delayed until the child is older and Eustachian tube function has improved. Repair of the eardrum (tympanoplasty) is generally deferred until around 7 years of age, which is approximately when the Eustachian tube reaches adult orientation.

In the presence of a perforation, water activities should be limited to surface swimming, preferably with the use of an ear plug.

D. Facial Nerve Paralysis

The facial nerve traverses the middle ear as it courses through the temporal bone to its exit at the stylomastoid foramen. Normally, the facial nerve is completely encased in bone, but occasionally bony dehiscence in the middle ear is present, exposing the nerve to infection and making it susceptible to inflammation during an episode of AOM. The acute onset of a facial nerve paralysis should not be deemed idiopathic Bell palsy until all other causes have been excluded. If middle ear fluid is present, prompt myringotomy and tube placement are indicated. Computed tomography (CT) is indicated if a cholesteatoma or mastoiditis is suspected.

E. Chronic Suppurative Otitis Media

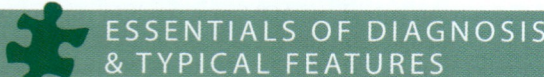

ESSENTIALS OF DIAGNOSIS & TYPICAL FEATURES

▶ Ongoing purulent ear drainage from the middle ear through either a perforation of the eardrum or a tympanostomy tube.

▶ Hearing loss of the affected ear is common.

▶ May be associated with cholesteatoma.

Chronic suppurative otitis media (CSOM) is present when persistent otorrhea occurs in a child with tympanostomy tubes or TM perforation for greater than 2–6 weeks. It starts with an acute infection that becomes chronic with mucosal edema, ulceration, granulation tissue, and eventual polyp formation. Drainage can vary and be serous, purulent, or cheese-like. Risk factors include a history of multiple episodes of otitis media, living in crowded conditions, day care attendance, and being a member of a large family. The most common associated bacteria is *P aeruginosa*, followed by *S aureus*, *Proteus* species, *Klebsiella pneumoniae*, and diphtheroids. Polymicrobial infections are seen in 5%–10% of cases.

Visualization of the TM, meticulous cleaning with culture of the drainage, and appropriate antimicrobial therapy, usually topical, are the keys to management. Ototopicals with steroids are felt to be superior to steroid-free ototopicals, especially when granulation tissue is present.

Occasionally, CSOM may be a sign of cholesteatoma or other disease process such as foreign body, neoplasm, Langerhans cell histiocytosis, tuberculosis, granulomatosis, fungal infection, or petrositis. If CSOM is not responsive to culture-directed treatment, imaging and biopsy may be needed to rule out other possibilities. Patients with facial palsy, vertigo, or other CNS signs should be referred immediately to an otolaryngologist.

Web Resources

Rosario DC, Mendez MD: Chronic suppurative otitis. 2023 Jan 31. In: StatPearls [Internet]. Treasure Island, FL: StatPearls Publishing; 2023 Jan– [PMID: 32119479].

Varughese D: Chronic suppurative otitis media. http://emedicine.medscape.com/article/859501-overview. Updated June 19, 2023. Accessed July 6, 2023.

F. Labyrinthitis

Suppurative infections of the middle ear can spread into the membranous labyrinth of the inner ear. Symptoms include vertigo, hearing loss, and fevers. The child often appears extremely toxic. Intravenous antibiotic therapy is used, and intravenous steroids may also be used to help decrease inflammation. Sequelae can be serious, including a condition known as *labyrinthitis ossificans*, or bony obliteration of the inner ear, including the cochlea, leading to profound hearing loss.

G. Mastoiditis

ESSENTIALS OF DIAGNOSIS & TYPICAL FEATURES

▶ AOM is almost always present.

▶ Postauricular pain and erythema.

▶ Ear protrusion (late finding).

▶ Pathogenesis

Mastoiditis occurs when infection spreads from the middle ear space to the mastoid portion of the temporal bone, which lies just behind the ear and contains air-filled spaces. Mastoiditis can range in severity from inflammation of the mastoid periosteum to bony destruction of the mastoid air cells (coalescent mastoiditis) with abscess development.

Mastoiditis can occur in any age group, but more than 60% of the patients are younger than 2 years. Many children do not have a prior history of recurrent AOM.

Clinical Findings

A. Symptoms and Signs

Patients with mastoiditis usually have postauricular pain, fever, and an outwardly displaced pinna. On examination, the mastoid area often appears indurated and red and with disease progression, it may become swollen and fluctuant. The earliest finding is severe tenderness on mastoid palpation. AOM is almost always present. Late findings include a pinna that is pushed forward by postauricular swelling and an ear canal that is narrowed due to pressure on the posterosuperior wall from the mastoid abscess. In infants younger than 1 year, swelling occurs superior to the ear and pushes the pinna downward rather than outward.

B. Imaging Studies

The best way to determine the extent of disease is by CT scan. Early mastoiditis is radiographically indistinguishable from AOM, with both showing opacification but no destruction of the mastoid air cells. With progression of mastoiditis, coalescence of the mastoid air cells is seen with bone destruction. Mastoiditis is a clinical diagnosis, based on pain as well as physical examination findings.

C. Microbiology

The most common pathogens are *S pneumoniae* followed by *H influenzae* and *S pyogenes*. Rarely, gram-negative bacilli and anaerobes are isolated. In the preantibiotic era, up to 20% of patients with AOM developed mastoiditis requiring mastoidectomy. Antibiotics decrease the incidence and morbidity of acute mastoiditis. However, acute mastoiditis still occurs in children who are treated with antibiotics for an acute ear infection. In the Netherlands, where only 31% of AOM patients receive antibiotics, the incidence of acute mastoiditis is 4.2 per 100,000 person-years. In the United States, where more than 96% of patients with AOM receive antibiotics, the incidence of acute mastoiditis is 2 per 100,000 person-years. Despite the routine use of antibiotics, the incidence of acute mastoiditis has been rising in some cities. The pattern change may be secondary to the emergence of resistant *S pneumoniae*.

Differential Diagnosis

Lymphadenitis, parotitis, trauma, tumor, histiocytosis, OE, and furuncle.

Complications

Meningitis can be a complication of acute mastoiditis and should be suspected when a child has associated high fever,

stiff neck, severe headache, or other meningeal signs. Lumbar puncture should be performed for diagnosis after imaging. Brain abscess occurs in 2% of mastoiditis patients and may be associated with persistent headaches, recurring fever, or changes in sensorium. Facial palsy, sigmoid sinus thrombosis, epidural abscess, cavernous sinus thrombosis, and thrombophlebitis may also be encountered.

Treatment

Intravenous antibiotic treatment alone may be successful if there is no evidence of coalescence or abscess on CT. However, if there is no improvement within 24–48 hours, surgical intervention should be undertaken. Minimal surgical management starts with tympanostomy tube insertion, during which cultures are taken. If a subperiosteal abscess is present, incision and drainage is also performed, with or without a cortical mastoidectomy. Intracranial extension requires complete mastoidectomy with decompression of the involved area.

Antibiotic therapy (intravenous and topical ear drops) is instituted along with surgical management and relies on culture-directed antibiotic therapy for 2–3 weeks. An antibiotic regimen should be chosen which is able to cross the blood-brain barrier. After significant clinical improvement is achieved with parenteral therapy, oral antibiotics are begun and should be continued for 2–3 weeks. A patent tympanostomy tube must also be maintained with the continued use of otic drops until drainage abates.

Prognosis

Prognosis for full recovery is good. Children that develop acute mastoiditis with abscess as their first ear infection are not necessarily prone to recurrent otitis media.

Anne S et al: Medical versus surgical treatment of pediatric acute mastoiditis: a systematic review. Laryngoscope 2019 Mar; 129(3):754–760 [PMID: 30284265].
Chesney J et al: What is the best practice for acute mastoiditis in children? Laryngoscope 2014 May;124(5):1057–1058 [PMID: 23852990].

ACUTE TRAUMA TO THE MIDDLE EAR

Head injuries, a blow to the ear canal, sudden impact with water, blast injuries, or the insertion of pointed objects into the ear canal can lead to perforation of the TM, ossicular chain disruption, facial nerve injury, hearing loss, vertigo, and hematoma of the middle ear. One study reports that 50% of serious penetrating wounds of the TM are due to the parental use of a cotton swab.

If there is facial paralysis, severe vertigo, or subjective hearing loss after ear trauma, urgent otolaryngology consultation is warranted. Middle ear trauma can lead to a perilymphatic fistula which is a breach of the inner ear that causes sensorineural (nerve) hearing loss and vertigo. This hearing loss can be prevented or reversed with emergent surgery. Facial nerve injury in the setting of middle ear trauma also often needs to be addressed emergently with possible facial nerve decompression. Other sequelae of middle ear trauma may be treated with observation. Blood collecting in the middle ear space may cause a conductive hearing loss that will resolve with time. Antibiotics are not necessary unless signs of infection appear. The patient needs to be followed with audiometry or by an otolaryngologist until hearing has returned to normal, which is expected within 6–8 weeks. If the conductive hearing loss does not resolve, there may be injuries to the ossicular chain. CT scan may be needed to evaluate the middle ear structures in this case.

Traumatic TM perforations should be referred to an otolaryngologist for examination and hearing evaluation. Spontaneous healing may occur within 6 months of the perforation. In the acute setting, antibiotic eardrops are often recommended to provide a moist environment that is thought to speed healing.

EAR CANAL FOREIGN BODY & CERUMEN IMPACTION

Foreign bodies of the ear canal, both intentional (placement by patient or other person) and/or accidental (eg, insect, playground mulch), are common in childhood. Cerumen can also be obstructive, acting like a foreign body. These objects can be removed if they are easy to visualize and there is appropriate instrumentation. Factors that may make them difficult to remove include size of foreign body, particularly when large enough to obscure the TM, rounded or globular objects, and objects deep in the ear canal adjacent to the TM. If these conditions exist or you are unable to remove the object on the first attempt, an ENT referral is often necessary for resolution. Vegetable matter should never be irrigated as it can swell and become more difficult to remove. An emergency condition exists if the foreign body is a disk-type battery. An electric current is generated in the moist canal, and a severe burn can occur in less than 4 hours. If the TM cannot be visualized, assume a perforation and avoid irrigation or ototoxic medications.

Cerumen impaction is common in children and using cotton swabs or other devices in the ear canal predisposes to the problem. Not only do these objects block the natural outflow of cerumen, but they can also increase cerumen production from irritation. Cerumen impaction should be removed if it is symptomatic or obstructs visualization of the TM. Education on the proper techniques of ear cleaning (such as only cleaning the external meatus) is important to avoid impactions. Explaining to parents that cerumen production is normal and protective of the ear canal skin can help reinforce proper ear care.

Oyama LC: Foreign bodies of the ear, nose and throat. Emerg Med Clin North Am 2019 Feb;37(1):121–130 [PMID: 30454775].
Schwartz SR: Clinical practice guideline (update). Otolaryngol Head Neck Surg 2017 Jan;156(1 Suppl):S1–S29. doi: 10.1177/0194599816671491.28045591 [PMID: 28045632].
Sharpe SJ, Rochette LM, Smith GA: Pediatric battery-related emergency department visits in the United States, 1990–2009. Pediatrics 2012 Jun;129(6):1111–1117 [PMID: 22585763].

AURICULAR HEMATOMA

Trauma to the outer ear can result in formation of a hematoma between the perichondrium and cartilage of the pinna. This is different from a bruise, which does not change the ear shape and where the blood is in the soft tissue outside of the perichondral layer. A hematoma appears as a boggy purple swelling of the cartilaginous auricle, and the normal folds of the ear are obscured. If untreated, neocartilage is deposited after 7–10 days resulting in "cauliflower ear." To prevent this cosmetic deformity, physicians should urgently refer patients to an otolaryngologist for drainage and application of a pressure dressing.

CONGENITAL EAR MALFORMATIONS

The external ear and EAC start to develop at 3 weeks gestation. Variable anomalies can present depending on timing of abnormal development. **Atresia** is failure of the ear canal to form. This results in conductive hearing loss and should be evaluated within the first 3 months of life by an audiologist and otolaryngologist. **Microtia** is the term used for an external ear that is small, collapsed, or only has an earlobe present. Usually there is a deficiency of cartilage and tissue. **Anotia** refers to an absent external ear. Often, there is an associated atresia with microtia and anotia. Reconstruction of the auricle usually occurs around ages 6–8 years and requires introduction of additional tissue or implants.

Malformations of the auricle can occur that are not due to a deficiency of tissue. This can range from ears that lack the proper folds and therefore protrude from the skull (**prominotia**) to ears that are folded over due to lack of cartilage stiffness or in utero positioning. Taping of the ears into correct anatomic position is very effective if performed in the first 72–96 hours of life. Tape is applied over a molding of wax or plastic and continued for at least 2 weeks. If this window of opportunity is missed or taping is unsuccessful, surgical correction, called an "otoplasty," can be performed at school age.

An ear is considered "low-set" if the upper pole is below eyebrow level. This condition is often associated with other congenital anomalies, and in these patients a genetics evaluation should be considered.

Preauricular tags, ectopic cartilage, fistulas, and cysts require surgical correction primarily for cosmetic reasons. Since the inner ear forms in conjunction with the outer ear children with ear malformations should have their hearing tested. Renal ultrasound should be considered, as external ear anomalies can also be associated with renal anomalies, as both structures form during the same period of embryogenesis. Most preauricular pits are asymptomatic but may become infected and require antibiotic treatment and possible surgical management.

Anstadt EE et al: Neonatal ear molding: timing and technique. Pediatrics 2016 Mar;137(3):e20152831 [PMID: 26908661].

Bly et al: Microtia reconstruction. Facial Plast Surg Clin North Am 2016 Nov;24(4):577–591 [PMID: 27712823].

IDENTIFICATION & MANAGEMENT OF HEARING LOSS

Hearing loss is classified as being conductive, sensorineural, or mixed in nature. Conductive hearing loss occurs when sound transmission is blocked somewhere between the opening of the external ear and the cochlear hair cells. The most common cause of conductive hearing loss in children is fluid in the middle ear. Sensorineural hearing loss (SNHL) is due to a defect in the neural transmission of sound, arising from a defect in the cochlear hair cells or the auditory nerve. Mixed hearing loss is characterized by elements of both conductive and sensorineural loss.

Hearing is measured in decibels (dB). The threshold, or 0 dB, refers to the level at which a sound is perceived in normal subjects 50% of the time. Hearing is considered normal if thresholds are within 20 dB of normal. In children, severity of hearing loss is commonly graded as follows: 20–40 dB mild, 41–55 dB moderate, 56–70 dB moderately severe, 71–90 dB severe, and > 90 dB profound.

Hearing loss can significantly impair a child's ability to communicate and hinder academic, social, and emotional development. Studies suggest that periods of auditory deprivation have enduring effects on auditory processing, even after normal hearing is restored. Even a unilateral hearing loss may be associated with difficulties in school and behavioral issues. Early identification and management of any hearing loss is therefore critical.

Conductive Hearing Loss

The most common cause of childhood conductive hearing loss is otitis media and related conditions such as MEE and ETD. Other causes may include EAC atresia or stenosis, TM perforation, cerumen impaction, cholesteatoma, and middle ear abnormalities, such as ossicular fixation or discontinuity. Often, a conductive loss may be corrected with surgery.

MEE may be serous, mucoid, or purulent, as in AOM. Effusions are generally associated with a mild conductive loss that normalizes once the effusion is gone. The American Academy of Pediatrics recommends that hearing and language skills be assessed in children who have recurrent AOM or MEE lasting longer than 3 months.

Sensorineural Hearing Loss

SNHL arises due to a defect in the cochlear hair cells or the auditory nerve (cranial nerve VIII). The loss may be congenital (present at birth) or acquired. In both the congenital and acquired categories, the hearing loss may be either hereditary (due to a genetic mutation) or nonhereditary. It is estimated that SNHL affects 2–3 out of every 1000 newborns, making this the most common congenital sensory deficit. The incidence is thought to be considerably higher in the neonatal intensive care unit population. Well-recognized risk factors for SNHL in neonates include a family history of childhood SNHL, birthweight less than 1500 g, low Apgar scores (0–4 at 1 minute or 0–6 at 5 minutes), craniofacial anomalies, hypoxia, in utero infections (eg, TORCH syndrome), hyperbilirubinemia requiring exchange transfusion, and mechanical ventilation for more than 5 days.

A. Congenital Hearing Loss

Approximately 50% of congenital hearing loss is nonhereditary. Examples include loss due to infection, teratogenic drugs, and perinatal injuries. The other 50% is attributed to genetic factors. Among children with hereditary hearing loss, approximately one-third of cases are thought to be due to a known syndrome, while the other two-thirds are considered nonsyndromic.

Syndromic hearing loss is associated with malformations of the external ear or other organs, or with medical problems involving other organ systems. Over 660 genetic syndromes that include hearing loss have been described. Although not all syndromes are physically apparent, patients being evaluated for hearing loss should be checked for features commonly associated with these syndromes. These include ear and branchial cleft anomalies (such as pits and tags), ocular abnormalities, white forelock, café au lait spots, and craniofacial anomalies. Some of the more frequently mentioned syndromes associated with congenital hearing loss include the following: Waardenburg, branchio-oto-renal, Usher, Pendred, Jervell and Lange-Nielsen, and Alport.

Over 70% of hereditary hearing loss is nonsyndromic (ie, there are no associated visible abnormalities or related medical problems). The most common known mutation associated with nonsyndromic hearing loss is in the *GJB2* gene, which encodes the protein Connexin 26. The *GJB2* mutation has a carrier rate of about 3% in the general population. Most nonsyndromic hearing loss, including that due to the *GJB2* mutation, is autosomal recessive.

B. Acquired Hearing Loss

Hereditary hearing loss may be delayed in onset, as in Alport syndrome and most autosomal dominant types of nonsyndromic loss. Vulnerability to aminoglycoside-induced hearing loss has also been linked to a mitochondrial gene defect.

Nongenetic etiologies for delayed-onset SNHL include exposure to ototoxic medications, meningitis, autoimmune or neoplastic conditions, noise exposure, and trauma. Infections such as syphilis or Lyme disease have been associated with hearing loss. Hearing loss associated with congenital cytomegalovirus (CMV) infection may be present at birth or may have a delayed onset. The loss is progressive in approximately half of all patients with congenital CMV-associated hearing loss. Other risk factors for delayed-onset, progressive loss include a history of persistent pulmonary hypertension and extracorporeal membrane oxygenation therapy.

C. Congenital CMV Infection and Hearing Loss

Congenital CMV (cCMV)–associated hearing loss can be congenital, but it is more often acquired. It deserves special mention as it is believed to be the most common cause of nongenetic hearing loss in the US pediatric population. cCMV-associated hearing loss can present at birth or have a delayed onset as long as several years. An estimated 0.5%–1% of all newborns are infected in utero by CMV. While some manifest severe symptoms at birth such as petechiae, hyperbilirubinemia, hepatosplenomegaly, seizures, neurologic deficits, and retinitis, 90–95% of newborns with cCMV infection are completely asymptomatic. Thirty to fifty percent of symptomatic and 8%–12% of asymptomatic infants will go on to develop SNHL in early childhood. Congenital CMV infection can only be confirmed in the newborn period, so given that most newborns are asymptomatic during this period, it has been very difficult to accurately determine the percentage of SNHL attributable to cCMV. Currently there is no universal screening for cCMV in the United States, but some centers are now performing targeted screening on newborns who fail newborn hearing screening. There is no consensus on the management of cCMV but trials of valganciclovir have shown promise in the treatment of cCMV hearing loss.

Identification of Hearing Loss

A. Newborn Hearing Screening

Prior to the institution of universal newborn screening, the average age at identification of hearing loss was 30 months. In 1993, a National Institutes of Health Consensus Panel recommended that all newborns be screened for hearing loss prior to hospital discharge. Today, all 50 states and the District of Columbia have Early Hearing Detection and Intervention (EHDI) laws or screening programs. As of 2019, over 98% of newborns in the United States were screened. The EHDI goal is identification and confirmation of hearing loss by 3 months of age and appropriate intervention by the age of 6 months. As subjective testing is not reliable in infants, objective, physiologic methods are used for screening. Auditory brainstem response and otoacoustic emission testing are the two commonly used modalities.

B. Audiologic Evaluation of Infants and Children

A parent's report of an infant's behavior cannot be relied upon for identification of hearing loss, as a deaf infant's behavior can appear normal and easily mislead parents and professionals. Deaf infants are often visually alert and able to actively scan the environment which may be mistaken for an appropriate response to sound. In children, signs of hearing loss include inconsistent response to sounds, not following directions, speech and language delays, and turning the volume up on televisions. Any child who fails a hearing screening or is suspected to have hearing loss should be referred for formal audiometric testing by an audiologist who is knowledgeable about testing pediatric patients.

Audiometry subjectively evaluates hearing. There are several different methods used, and the choice of method is primarily based on patient age. Objective testing methods such as auditory brainstem response and otoacoustic emission testing are used if a child cannot be reliably tested using subjective methods.

In addition to infants who fall into the high-risk categories for SNHL as outlined earlier, hearing should be tested and followed more closely in children with a history of developmental delay, bacterial meningitis, ototoxic medication exposure, neurodegenerative disorders, or a history of infection such as mumps or measles. Children with bacterial meningitis should be referred immediately to an otolaryngologist, as cochlear ossification can necessitate urgent cochlear implantation. Even if a newborn screening was passed, all infants who fall into a high-risk category for progressive or delayed-onset hearing loss, such as in utero CMV exposure, should be referred for regular audiologic monitoring for the first 3 years and at appropriate intervals thereafter to avoid a missed diagnosis.

MANAGEMENT OF HEARING LOSS

While identification of hearing loss is the critical first step, it is largely meaningless without appropriate follow-up and management. Prompt and appropriate intervention can minimize the potential lifelong detrimental effects that hearing loss can have on language, academic, emotional and social development, and hearing-related quality of life. Optimal management requires a multidisciplinary approach. The team may include audiologists, otolaryngologists, speech-language pathologists, early intervention specialists, deaf-hard of hearing educational specialists, and family counselors.

Any child with confirmed hearing loss should be referred to an otolaryngologist for further evaluation and possible medical and/or surgical management. Etiologic workup can include radiographic imaging and/or laboratory tests and should be tailored to each individual patient's history, examination, and audiometric results. Within the past decade, major advances have made comprehensive genetic testing for hearing loss widely available.

The medical management of hearing loss depends upon type and severity. Conductive hearing loss is sometimes fixable if the point at which sound transmission is compromised can be corrected. For example, hearing loss due to effusions usually normalizes once the fluid has cleared, whether by natural means or by placement of tympanostomy tubes. As of yet, SNHL is not reversible. Most sensorineural loss is managed with amplification. Cochlear implantation is an option for many children when amplification is no longer beneficial. It is FDA approved down to the age of 9 months. Unlike hearing aids, cochlear implants do not amplify sound but directly stimulate the cochlea with electrical impulses. Although most children who receive cochlear implants have bilateral hearing loss, they can be helpful in select children with unilateral hearing losses as well.

When hearing loss is diagnosed, it is unknown if it will remain stable, or if it will fluctuate or worsen. Therefore, children with hearing loss should receive ongoing audiologic monitoring, as well as periodic assessments of global development and functional performance.

The Individuals with Disabilities Education Act 2004 (IDEA 2004) is a US law mandating free access to individualized educational opportunities with qualified instructors for children with disabilities, including hearing loss. Part C provides early intervention for children up to age 3 years. Audiologists play a key role in the transition from diagnosis to intervention, as they are required to initiate a referral to their state's Part C program within 7 days of a new confirmed permanent hearing loss diagnosis. An Individualized Family Service Plan (IFSP) is developed and may enlist the services of audiologists, speech-language pathologists, and other related professionals. The IFSP is family-centered, and family support services are often available. Between the ages of 3 and 21 years, children are covered under Part B of IDEA 2004. Part B is managed through the local school systems' special education programs. Under Part B, an Individualized Education Plan (IEP) is developed with a goal of maximizing a child's academic success.

PREVENTION

Appropriate care may treat or prevent certain conditions causing hearing loss. Aminoglycosides and diuretics, particularly in combination, are potentially ototoxic and should be used judiciously and monitored carefully. Given the association of a mitochondrial gene defect with aminoglycoside ototoxicity, use should be avoided, when possible, in patients with a family history of aminoglycoside-related hearing loss. Reduction of repeated exposure to loud noises may prevent high-frequency hearing loss associated with acoustic trauma. Any patient with sudden-onset SNHL should be seen by an otolaryngologist immediately, as in some cases, steroid therapy may reverse the loss if initiated right away.

Web Resources

Congenital CMV and Hearing Loss: https://www.cdc.gov/cmv/hearing-loss.html?CDC_AA_refVal=https%3A%2F%2Fwww.cdc.gov%2Fcmv%2Ffact-sheets%2Fhearing-loss.html. Updated April 28, 2020. Accessed July 4, 2023.

Data and statistics about hearing loss in children: Updated July 21, 2022. https://www.cdc.gov/ncbddd/hearingloss/data.html. Accessed July 4, 2023.

NCHAM: Newborn hearing & infant hearing—early hearing detection and intervention resources and information. http://www.infanthearing.org/screening/. Updated June 15, 2023. Accessed July 4, 2023.

OtoSCOPE Genetic Hearing Loss Testing v.9: https://morl.lab.uiowa.edu/clinical-diagnostic-services/hearing-loss-otoscope®/otoscope®-genetic-hearing-loss-testing-v9. Accessed July 4, 2023.

Shearer AE, Hildebrand MS, Schaefer AM, Smith RJH: Genetic hearing loss overview. http://www.ncbi.nlm.nih.gov/books/NBK1434/. Updated June 29, 2023. Accessed July 4, 2023.

THE NOSE & PARANASAL SINUSES

ACUTE VIRAL RHINITIS

The common cold (viral URI) is the most common pediatric infectious disease, and the incidence is higher in early childhood than in any other period of life (Common Cold; see also Chapter 40). Children younger than 5 years typically have 6–12 colds per year. Approximately 30%–40% are caused by rhinoviruses, of which there are over 100 subtypes. Other culprits include adenoviruses, coronaviruses, enteroviruses, influenza and parainfluenza viruses, and respiratory syncytial virus. Since so many viruses can cause a cold, development of a vaccine has thus far not been successful.

ESSENTIALS OF DIAGNOSIS & TYPICAL FEATURES

- ► Clear or mucoid rhinorrhea, nasal congestion, and sore throat.
- ► Possible fever, particularly in younger children (under 5–6 years).
- ► Possible hoarseness and/or cough.
- ► Symptoms resolve by 7–10 days, but cough and hoarseness can linger for several weeks afterward.

► Differential Diagnosis

Rhinosinusitis (acute or chronic), allergic rhinitis, nonallergic rhinitis, influenza, pneumonia, gastroesophageal reflux disease, asthma, and bronchitis.

Clinical Findings

The patient usually experiences a sudden onset of sore throat followed by clear or mucoid rhinorrhea, nasal congestion, and sneezing. Cough or fever may develop. Although fever is not a prominent feature in older children and adults, in the first 5 or 6 years of life it can be as high as 40.6°C without superinfection. The nose, throat, and TMs may appear red and inflamed. The average duration of symptoms is about 1 week; however, a mild cough may persist for several weeks following resolution of other symptoms. Nasal secretions tend to become thicker and more purulent after day 2 of infection due to shedding of epithelial cells and influx of neutrophils. This discoloration should not be assumed to be a sign of bacterial rhinosinusitis, unless it persists beyond 10–14 days, by which time the patient should normally be experiencing significant symptomatic improvement.

Treatment

Treatment for the common cold is symptomatic (Figure 18–4). Because colds are viral infections, antibiotics are not helpful. Acetaminophen or ibuprofen can relieve fever and pain.

Humidification may provide relief for congestion and cough. Nasal saline drops and bulb suctioning may be used for an infant or child unable to blow his or her nose.

Available scientific data suggest that over-the-counter cold and cough medications are not effective in children and may have serious adverse effects. Use in children under 4 years is not recommended. Antihistamines have not proven effective in relieving cold symptoms in children; in rhinoviral colds, increased levels of histamine are not observed. Oral decongestants may provide symptomatic relief in adults but have not been well studied in children. Studies have shown that most cough medicines are no better than placebo and the use of narcotic antitussives is discouraged, as these may be associated with respiratory depression. There is no convincing evidence that naturopathic or alternative therapies are effective in children.

Only time cures the common cold. Education and reassurance may be the most important "therapy" for parents. They should be informed about the expected nature and duration of symptoms, efficacy and potential side effects of medications, and the signs and symptoms of complications of the common cold, such as bacterial rhinosinusitis, bronchiolitis, or pneumonia.

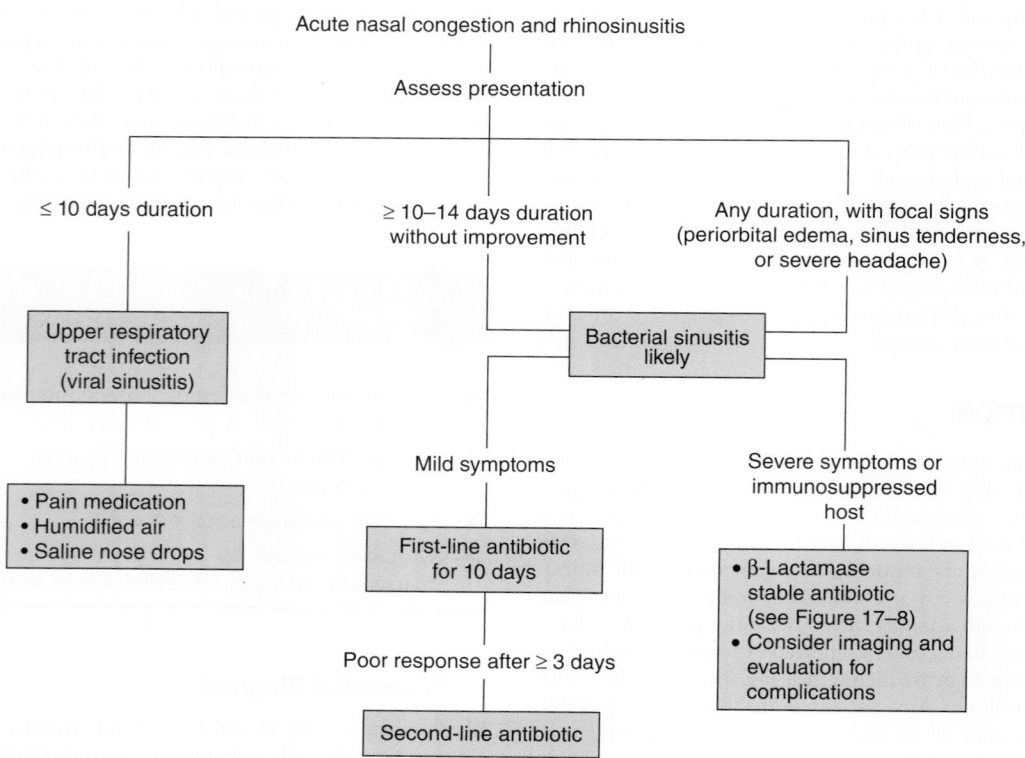

▲ **Figure 18–4.** Algorithm for acute nasal congestion and rhinosinusitis.

Kenealy T, Arroll B: Antibiotics for the common cold and acute purulent rhinitis. Cochrane Database Syst Rev 2013 Jun 4;6: CD000247. doi: 10.1002/14651858.CD000247.pub3 [PMID: 23733381].

Web Resources

US Food and Drug Administration: Should you give your kids medicine for coughs and colds? Updated January 5, 2023: https://www.fda.gov/consumers/consumer-updates/when-give-kids-medicine-coughs-and-colds. Accessed July 4, 2023.

RHINOSINUSITIS

The use of the term *rhinosinusitis* has replaced sinusitis. Rhinosinusitis acknowledges that the nasal and sinus mucosa are involved in similar and concurrent inflammatory processes.

1. Acute Bacterial Rhinosinusitis

Acute bacterial rhinosinusitis (ABRS) is a bacterial infection of the paranasal sinuses, which lasts less than 30 days and the symptoms resolve completely. It is almost always preceded by a cold; it is estimated that 6%–9% of viral URIs are complicated by the development of ABRS. Other predisposing conditions include allergies and trauma. The diagnosis of ABRS is made when a cold does not improve by 10–14 days or worsens after 5–7 days. The maxillary and ethmoid sinuses are most involved; these sinuses are present at birth. Other sinuses may be involved in older children. The sphenoid sinuses typically form by age 5 years, and the frontal sinuses by 7–8 years. Frontal sinusitis is unusual before age 10 years.

ESSENTIALS OF DIAGNOSIS & TYPICAL FEATURES

- ▶ URI symptoms are not improving 10 or more days beyond onset, or symptoms worsen within 10 days after an initial period of improvement.
- ▶ Symptoms may include nasal congestion, nasal drainage, postnasal drainage, facial pain, headache, and fever.
- ▶ Symptoms resolve completely within 30 days.

▶ Pathogenesis

Situations which lead to inflammation of sinonasal mucosa and obstruction of sinus drainage underlie the development of rhinosinusitis. A combination of anatomic, mucosal, microbial, and immune factors is involved. Both viral and bacterial infections play integral roles in the pathogenesis. Viral URIs may cause sinus mucosal injury and swelling, resulting in sinus outflow obstruction and alteration of the normal mucociliary clearance of the sinuses. The bacterial pathogens that commonly cause acute rhinosinusitis are *S pneumoniae, H influenzae* (nontypeable), *M catarrhalis*, and β-hemolytic streptococci.

▶ Clinical Findings

The onset of symptoms in ABRS may be gradual or sudden and commonly include nasal drainage, nasal congestion, facial pressure or pain, postnasal drainage, hyposmia or anosmia, fever, cough, fatigue, maxillary dental pain, and ear pressure or fullness. The physical examination is rarely helpful in making the diagnosis, as the findings are essentially the same as those in a child with an uncomplicated cold.

In complicated or immunocompromised patients, sinus aspiration and culture by an otolaryngologist should be considered to facilitate culture-directed antibiotic therapy. Nasal, nasopharyngeal or throat cultures should not be used, as there is poor correlation between the organisms found in these and sinus aspirates. If the patient is hospitalized because of rhinosinusitis-related complications, blood cultures should also be obtained.

Imaging of the sinuses during acute illness is not recommended unless evaluating for possible complications or for patients with persistent symptoms that do not respond to medical therapy. As with the physical examination, the radiographic findings of ABRS, such as sinus opacification, fluid, and mucosal thickening, are indistinguishable from those seen in the common cold.

▶ Complications

Complications of ABRS occur when infection spreads to adjacent structures like the eye and the brain. *S aureus* (including methicillin-resistant *S aureus*) is frequently implicated in complicated ABRS, as well as *Streptococcus anginosus* (*milleri*), which has been found to be a particularly virulent organism.

Orbital complications are the most common. These complications usually begin as a preseptal cellulitis but can progress to postseptal cellulitis, subperiosteal abscess, orbital abscess, and cavernous sinus thrombosis. Associated signs and symptoms include eyelid edema, restricted extraocular movements, proptosis, chemosis, and altered visual acuity (see Chapter 16).

The most common complication of frontal sinusitis is osteitis of the frontal bone, also known as Pott's puffy tumor. Intracranial extension of infection can lead to meningitis and to epidural, subdural, and brain abscesses. Frequently, children with complicated rhinosinusitis have no prior history of sinus infection.

▶ Treatment

For children with cold symptoms that are not improving by 10 days, observation for up to 3 more days or antibiotic therapy may be chosen, depending upon individual circumstances, such as ability to follow-up and treat with antibiotics if needed. For children with uncomplicated ABRS who have worsening or severe symptoms (fever of at least 39°C and purulent nasal drainage for at least 3 consecutive days), antibiotic therapy is recommended. Antibiotics are generally thought to decrease duration and severity of symptoms.

First-line antibiotic therapy should be amoxicillin or amoxicillin-clavulanate. Cefuroxime, cefpodoxime, and cefdinir are recommended for patients with a non–type I hypersensitivity to penicillin, and in most cases may be safely used in patients with an anaphylactoid reaction, as recent studies seem to indicate almost no risk of a serious reaction to second- and third-generation cephalosporins among these patients. Other agents which may be used, particularly in more severe cases where resistant *S pneumoniae* and *H influenzae* are suspected, include clindamycin, linezolid, and quinolone antibiotics. Due to high resistance of *S pneumoniae* and *H influenzae*, the use of trimethoprim-sulfamethoxazole and azithromycin is not advised.

Duration of therapy should be for 7 days after symptoms have resolved.

Failure to improve after 48–72 hours of antibiotic therapy suggests a resistant organism or potential complication. Second-line therapies should be initiated at this point, or, if the patient is already on amoxicillin-clavulanate or a cephalosporin, intravenous antibiotic therapy should be considered. Imaging and referral for sinus aspiration should be strongly considered as well.

Patients who are toxic, or who have evidence of invasive infection or CNS complications, should be hospitalized immediately. Intravenous therapy with nafcillin or clindamycin plus a third-generation cephalosporin such as ceftriaxone should be initiated until culture results become available.

Decongestants, antihistamines, and nasal saline irrigations are frequently used in acute rhinosinusitis to promote drainage. To date, there are no methodologically sound studies supporting their efficacy in children. If used, topical nasal decongestants, such as oxymetazoline or phenylephrine sprays, should not be used for more than 3 days due to risk of rebound edema. Patients with underlying allergic rhinitis may benefit from intranasal cromolyn or corticosteroid nasal spray.

Shaikh N, Wald ER: Decongestants, antihistamines and nasal irrigation for acute sinusitis in children. Cochrane Database Syst Rev 2014 Oct 27;(10):CD007909 [PMID: 25347280].

Wald ER et al: Clinical practice guideline for the diagnosis and management of acute bacterial sinusitis in children aged 1 to 18 years. Pediatrics 2013;134:e262–e280 [PMID: 23796742].

2. Recurrent or Chronic Rhinosinusitis

Recurrent rhinosinusitis occurs when episodes of ABRS clear for at least 10 days but recur at least four times per year. Chronic rhinosinusitis (CRS) is diagnosed when the child

has not cleared the infection in 90 days but has not developed acute complications. Both symptoms and physical findings are required to support the diagnosis, and CT scan may be a useful in making the diagnosis. Although recent meta-analysis evaluations have resulted in recommendations for ABRS, there is a paucity of data for the treatment of recurrent or CRS. Important factors to consider include allergies, anatomic variations, and disorders in host immunity. Mucosal inflammation leading to obstruction is most often caused by allergic rhinitis and occasionally by nonallergic rhinitis. There is a great deal of evidence that allergic rhinitis, rhinosinusitis, and asthma are all manifestations of a systemic inflammatory response. Gastroesophageal reflux has also been implicated in CRS. Less commonly, CRS is caused by anatomic variations, such as septal deviation, polyp, or foreign body.

Allergic nasal polyps are unusual in children younger than 10 years and should prompt a workup for cystic fibrosis. In cases of chronic or recurrent pyogenic pansinusitis, poor host resistance (eg, an immune defect, primary ciliary dyskinesia, or cystic fibrosis)—though rare—must be ruled out by immunoglobulin studies, electron microscopy studies of respiratory cilia, nasal nitric oxide measurements if available, a sweat chloride test, and genetic testing (see Chapter 19). Anaerobic and staphylococcal organisms are often responsible for CRS. Evaluation by an allergist and an otolaryngologist may be useful in determining the underlying causes.

▶ Treatment

A. Medical Therapy

Antibiotic therapy for CRS is similar to that used for ABRS, but the duration is longer, typically 3–4 weeks. Antimicrobial choice should include drugs effective against staphylococcal organisms. Regular use of nasal saline irrigations and intranasal steroid sprays have been shown to be helpful in the reduction of symptoms of CRS.

B. Surgical Therapy

The mainstay of treatment for pediatric CRS is medical management, with appropriate antibiotic therapy and treatment of comorbid conditions such as allergic rhinitis and asthma. Only a small percentage of children will warrant surgical management.

1. Antral lavage—Antral lavage, generally regarded as a diagnostic procedure, may have some therapeutic value. An aspirate or a sample from the maxillary sinus is retrieved under anesthesia. The maxillary sinus is then irrigated. In the very young child, this may be the only procedure performed.

2. Adenoidectomy—Adenoidectomy is thought to be effective in 50%–75% of children with CRS, up to the age of 12 years. The adenoids serve as a reservoir of pathogenic bacteria and may also interfere with mucociliary clearance and drainage. Biofilms have been reported in the adenoids of children with

CRS and may explain the resistance of these infections to standard antibiotic therapy.

3. Balloon catheter dilation—This method of opening the sinus ostia is safe and less invasive than endoscopic sinus surgery, but its efficacy as superior to adenoidectomy and/or sinus lavage has not clearly been established.

4. Endoscopic sinus surgery—Endoscopic sinus surgery in children was controversial because of concerns regarding facial growth. However, recent studies have not supported this concern. Endoscopic sinus surgery is reported to be effective in over 80% of cases and may be indicated if adenoidectomy or balloon dilation is not effective.

5. External drainage—External drainage procedures are not commonly performed and are reserved for complications arising from ethmoid and frontal sinusitis.

Brietzke SE et al: Clinical consensus statement: pediatric chronic rhinosinusitis. Otolaryngol Head Neck Surg 2014;151(4): 542–553 [PMID: 25274375].

Orlandi RR et al: International consensus statement on allergy and rhinology: rhinosinusitis. Int Forum Allergy Rhinol 2016 Feb 6; (Suppl 1):S22–S209 [PMID: 26889651].

Sedaghat AR et al: Does balloon catheter sinuplasty have a role in the surgical management of pediatric sinus disease? Laryngoscope 2011; 121(10):2053–2054 [PMID: 21952904].

CHOANAL ATRESIA

Choanal atresia occurs in approximately 1 in 7000 live births. The female-male ratio is 2:1, as is the unilateral-bilateral ratio. Bilateral atresia results in severe respiratory distress at birth and requires immediate placement of an oral airway or intubation, and otolaryngology consultation for surgical treatment. Unilateral atresia usually appears later as a unilateral chronic nasal discharge that may be mistaken for CRS. Diagnosis may be suspected if a 6F catheter cannot be passed through the nose and is confirmed by axial CT scan. Approximately 50% of patients with bilateral choanal atresia have CHARGE association (**C**oloboma, **H**eart disease, **A**tresia of the choanae, **R**etarded growth and retarded development or CNS anomalies, **G**enital hypoplasia, and **E**ar anomalies or deafness) (see Chapter 37) or other congenital anomalies.

RECURRENT RHINITIS

Recurrent rhinitis is frequently seen in pediatrics. The child is brought in with the chief complaint of having "one cold after another," "constant colds," or "always being sick." Approximately, two-thirds of these children have recurrent colds; the rest have either allergic rhinitis or recurrent rhinosinusitis.

1. Allergic Rhinitis

Allergic rhinitis is a chronic disorder of the upper airway which is induced by IgE-mediated inflammation secondary to allergen exposure. It is more common in children than in adults and affects up to 40% of children in the United States. It significantly affects quality of life, interfering with physical and social activities, concentration, school performance, and sleep. Allergic rhinitis can contribute to the development of rhinosinusitis, otitis media, and asthma. Symptoms may include nasal congestion, sneezing, rhinorrhea, and itchy nose, palate, throat, and eyes. On physical examination, the nasal turbinates are swollen and may be red or pale pink-purple. Several classes of medications have proven effective in treating allergic rhinitis, including intranasal corticosteroids, oral and intranasal antihistamines, leukotriene antagonists, and decongestants. Ipratropium nasal spray may also be used as an adjunctive therapy. Nasal saline rinses are helpful to wash away allergens. Recent studies have indicated that the use of intranasal steroid sprays may not only decrease the impairment caused by allergic rhinitis symptoms but also help prevent progression to more severe disease and decrease the risk of related comorbidities such as asthma and sleep-disordered breathing. Intranasal steroids can be used in children as young as 2 years.

2. Nonallergic Rhinitis

Nonallergic rhinitis also causes rhinorrhea and nasal congestion, but does not seem to involve an immunologic reaction. Its mechanism is not well understood. Triggers can include sudden changes in environmental temperature, air pollution, and other irritants such as tobacco smoke. Medications can also be associated with nonallergic rhinitis. Nasal decongestant sprays, when used for long periods of time, can cause *rhinitis medicamentosa*, which is a rebound nasal congestion and can be very difficult to treat. Oral decongestants, nasal saline, nasal corticosteroids, antihistamines, and ipratropium spray have all been shown to offer symptomatic relief.

Rachelefsky G, Farrar JR: A control model to evaluate pharmacotherapy for allergic rhinitis in children. JAMA Pediatr 2013; 167(4):380–386 [PMID: 23440263].

Web Resources

American Academy of Allergy, Asthma, and Immunology: Hay Fever/Rhinitis: https://www.aaaai.org/Conditions-Treatments/Allergies/Hay-Fever-Rhinitis. Accessed July 8, 2023.

EPISTAXIS

The nose is a highly vascular structure. In most cases, epistaxis (nosebleed) arises from the anterior nasal septum (Kiesselbach area). It is often due to dryness, nose rubbing, nose blowing, or nose picking. Examination of the anterior septum usually reveals a red, raw surface with fresh clots or old crusts. Presence of telangiectasias, hemangiomas, or varicosities should also be noted. If a patient has been using a nasal corticosteroid spray, check the patient's technique to make sure he or she is not directing the spray toward the septum. If proper technique does not reduce the nosebleeds, the spray should be discontinued.

In fewer than 5% of cases, epistaxis is caused by a bleeding disorder such as von Willebrand disease. A hematologic workup is warranted if any of the following is present: family history of a bleeding disorder; medical history of easy bleeding, particularly with circumcision or dental work; spontaneous bleeding at any site; bleeding that lasts for more than 30 minutes or blood that will not clot with direct pressure by the physician; onset before age 2 years; or a drop in hematocrit due to epistaxis.

Juvenile nasopharyngeal angiofibroma (JNA) is a benign, but often aggressive, tumor that tends to bleed and may present as recurrent epistaxis (45%–60%). JNA is only seen in males; females with JNA should undergo karyotyping. CT and magnetic resonance imaging (MRI) are diagnostic.

▶ **Treatment**

The patient should sit up and lean forward so as not to swallow blood. Swallowed blood may cause nausea and hematemesis. The nasal cavity should be cleared of clots by gentle blowing. The soft part of the nose below the nasal bones is pinched and held firmly enough to prevent arterial blood flow, with pressure over the bleeding site (anterior septum) being maintained for 5 minutes. For persistent bleeding, a one-time only application of oxymetazoline into the nasal cavity may be helpful. If bleeding continues, the bleeding site needs to be visualized. A small piece of gelatin sponge (Gelfoam) or collagen sponge (Surgicel) can be inserted over the bleeding site and held in place.

Friability of the nasal vessels is often due to dryness and can be decreased by increasing nasal moisture. This can be accomplished by daily application of a water-based ointment, such as a nasal saline gel, to the nose. A pea-sized amount is placed just inside the nose and spread by gently squeezing the nostrils. Twice-daily nasal saline irrigation and humidifier use may also be helpful. Aspirin and ibuprofen should be avoided, as should nose picking and vigorous nose blowing. Otolaryngology referral is indicated for refractory cases. Cautery of the nasal vessels is reserved for treatment failures.

NASAL INFECTION

A nasal furuncle is an infection of a hair follicle in the anterior nares. Hair plucking or nose picking can provide a route of entry. The most common organism is S aureus. A furuncle presents as an exquisitely tender, firm, red lump in the anterior nares. Treatment includes antibiotic therapy and drainage. Keflex and dicloxacillin are appropriate antibiotic choices, but in areas of high methicillin-resistant S aureus (MRSA) prevalence, clindamycin or trimethoprim-sulfamethoxazole are recommended. The lesion should be gently incised and drained as soon as it points with a sterile needle. Topical

antibiotic ointment may be of additional value. Because this lesion is in the drainage area of the cavernous sinus, the patient should be followed closely until healing is complete. Parents should be advised never to pick or squeeze a furuncle in this location—and neither should the physician. Associated cellulitis or spread requires hospitalization for administration of intravenous antibiotics.

A nasal septal abscess is usually the result of nasal trauma or a nasal furuncle. Examination reveals fluctuant gray septal swelling, which is usually bilateral. The possible complications are the same as for nasal septal hematoma (see following discussion). In addition, spread of the infection to the CNS is possible. Treatment consists of immediate hospitalization, incision and drainage by an otolaryngologist, and intravenous antibiotic therapy.

NASAL TRAUMA

Rarely, newborn infants present with subluxation of the septal cartilage. In this disorder, the top of the nose deviates to one side, the inferior septal border deviates to the other side, the columella leans, and the nasal tip is unstable. This must be distinguished from the more common transient flattening of the nose caused by the birth process. These subluxations may sometimes be reduced in the nursery, but more difficult cases are done under sedation.

After nasal trauma, it is essential to examine the inside of the nose in order to rule out hematoma of the septum, which can quickly lead to septal necrosis, causing permanent nasal deformity. The diagnosis is confirmed by the abrupt onset of nasal obstruction following trauma and the presence of a boggy, widened nasal septum. A normal nasal septum is only 2–4 mm thick. A cotton swab can be used to palpate the septum. This warrants immediate otolaryngology referral for drainage and packing.

Most blows to the nose result in epistaxis without fracture. A persistent nosebleed after trauma, crepitus, instability of the nasal bones, and external deformity of the nose indicate fracture. Septal injury cannot be ruled out by radiography and can only be ruled out by careful intranasal examination. Patients with suspected nasal fractures should be referred to an otolaryngologist for definitive therapy. Since the nasal bones begin healing immediately, the child must be seen by an otolaryngologist within 48–72 hours of the injury to allow time to arrange for fracture reduction before the bones become immobile.

FOREIGN BODIES IN THE NOSE

If this diagnosis is delayed, unilateral foul-smelling rhinorrhea, halitosis, bleeding, or nasal obstruction often result.

There are many ways to remove nasal foreign bodies. The obvious first maneuver is vigorous nose blowing if the child is old enough. This is usually not possible under the age of 4 years. A parent or caregiver may also try positive pressure by gently blowing in the mouth while occluding the unaffected nostril. If these are not successful, instrumentation is necessary. This requires nasal decongestion, good lighting, and physical restraint. Topical tetracaine or lidocaine may be used for anesthesia in young children, and topical phenylephrine or oxymetazoline are used for decongestion. With the child is properly restrained, most nasal foreign bodies can be removed using a pair of alligator forceps or right-angle instrument through an operating head otoscope. If the object seems unlikely to be removed on the first attempt, is wedged in, or is quite large, the patient should be referred to an otolaryngologist rather than worsening the situation through futile attempts. Irrigation is not recommended due to risk of aspiration.

High-risk foreign bodies include button batteries, disc magnets (one in each nostril), and superabsorbent polymer beads. These can all cause necrosis and destruction of nasal tissues and must be removed immediately; these constitute a foreign body emergency.

Olfactory Disorders

Children with olfactory disorders either have a decrease in their ability to smell or alterations in how odors are perceived. Anosmia is the complete inability to detect odors. Hyposmia is a reduced sense of smell. Parosmia is a distortion in how an odor is perceived. Phantosmia is the sensation of an odor that is not present.

Olfactory disorders can be temporary or permanent. There are three basic causes:

- Physical blockage of the nasal passages—eg, nasal polyps or tumors. Movement of air to the olfactory receptor cells that sit high in the nasal cavity is blocked by such lesions.

- Inflammation and irritation of the nasal passages—eg, viral infections, sinusitis, allergies, smoke exposure.

- Brain or nerve damage—eg, brain tumors, chemical nerve damage, diabetes, medications, malnutrition, head trauma.

In rare cases, children may have congenital anosmia due to absent or hypoplastic olfactory bulbs. This can be determined on high-resolution MRI. Congenital anosmia may be an isolated finding, but it can also be caused by genetic disorders such as Kallmann syndrome (hypogonadism).

An altered sense of smell and taste is a common symptom of SARS-CoV-2 (coronavirus disease-19 [COVID-19]) infection. Most recover over the course of several weeks. For those who do not, olfactory training, with repeated exposure to known odorants, may be helpful. To date, there are no medications that have proven effective in the treatment of post-COVID olfactory and taste dysfunction.

Watson DLB et al: Altered smell and taste: anosmia, parosmia and the impact of long COVID-19. PLoS One 2021;16(9):e0256998 [PMID: 34559820]

THE THROAT & ORAL CAVITY

ACUTE STOMATITIS

Stomatitis is inflammation in the oral cavity and can arise from infection, autoimmune disorders, drug reactions, and chemoradiation. Acute episodes are often painful and limit oral intake.

1. Recurrent Aphthous Stomatitis

Aphthous ulcers, or canker sores, are small painful ulcers (3–10 mm) usually found on the inner aspect of the lips, gingiva, or tongue. Typically lasting 1–2 weeks, there is usually no associated fever or cervical adenopathy. These may reoccur throughout life, with infectious or autoimmune causes suspected. Treatment is symptomatic with acetaminophen or ibuprofen and temporary choice of a bland diet. A topical corticosteroid, such as triamcinolone dental paste or a swish and spit regimen of dexamethasone solution, may also reduce symptomatic duration and intensity. A Cochrane review was unable to promote a single systemic treatment for those unresponsive to local therapy.

Less common causes of recurrent oral ulcers include Behçet disease, familial Mediterranean fever, and PFAPA syndrome (**P**eriodic **F**ever, **A**phthous stomatitis, **P**haryngitis, and cervical **A**denopathy). Behçet disease requires two of the following: genital ulcers, uveitis, and erythema nodosum–like lesions. Patients with Mediterranean fever usually have a positive family history, serosal involvement, and recurrent fever. PFAPA typically begins before the age of 5 years, continues through adolescence, and then spontaneously resolves. Fever and other symptoms recur at regular intervals. Episodes last approximately 5 days and are not associated with other URI symptoms or illnesses. Steroids may shorten episodes but do not prevent recurrence. PFAPA has been shown to resolve with prolonged cimetidine use and adenotonsillectomy.

Brocklehurst P et al: Systemic interventions for recurrent aphthous stomatitis (mouth ulcers). Cochrane Database Syst Rev 2012 Sep 12;(9):CD005411 [PMID: 22972085].
Manthiram K et al: Physician's perspectives on the diagnosis and management of periodic fever, aphthous stomatitis, pharyngitis, and cervical adenitis (PFAPA) syndrome. Rheumatol Int 2017 Jun;37(6):883–889. doi: 10.1007/s00296-017-3688-3 [PMID: 28271158].

2. Herpes Simplex Gingivostomatitis (See Chapter 40)

Herpes simplex virus 1 (HSV-1) is more often associated with oral ulcerations than HSV-2. HSV transmission is almost always through direct contact, and the virus migrates to reside in the trigeminal ganglion. Reactivation from a dormant state can arise from a variety of stimuli, leading to symptomatic ulcerated lesions of the lips and oral cavity.

3. Thrush (See Chapter 43)

Candida is normally found in the oral flora of 60% of the population. In infants it presents as white plaques with an erythematous base that typically involves the buccal mucosa and dorsal tongue. Spread to the pharynx and larynx causes odynophagia and can be seen in older children using inhaled steroids and those with compromised immune systems. The breast-feeding mother-infant dyad require simultaneous treatment—the mother with oral Diflucan and the infant with a one-time application of Gentian Violet or a course of Nystatin suspension.

4. Traumatic Oral Ulcers

Mechanical trauma most commonly occurs on the buccal mucosa secondary to biting by the molars. Thermal trauma, from very hot foods, can also cause ulcerative lesions. Chemical ulcers can be produced by mucosal contact with aspirin or other caustic agents. Oral ulcers can occur with leukemia or on a recurrent basis with cyclic neutropenia. Unexplained oral ulcers, burns, or trauma should raise suspicion for the possibility of nonaccidental trauma or abuse in younger children.

PHARYNGITIS

Figure 18–5 is an algorithm for the management of a sore throat.

1. Acute Viral Pharyngitis

Over 90% of sore throats and fever in children are due to viral infections. The findings seldom point toward any viral agent, but four types of viral pharyngitis are sufficiently distinctive to warrant the following discussion.

► Clinical Findings

A. Infectious Mononucleosis

Findings include exudative tonsillitis, generalized cervical adenitis and fever, usually in patients older than 5 years. A palpable spleen or axillary adenopathy increases the likelihood of the diagnosis. The presence of more than 10% atypical lymphocytes on a peripheral blood smear or a positive mononucleosis spot test supports the diagnosis, although these tests are often falsely negative in children younger than 5 years. Epstein-Barr virus serology showing an elevated IgM-capsid antibody is definitive. Amoxicillin is contraindicated in patients suspected of having mononucleosis because the drug often precipitates a rash.

B. Herpangina

Herpangina ulcers are classically 3 mm in size, surrounded by a halo and are found on the anterior tonsillar pillars, soft palate, and uvula; the anterior mouth and tonsils are spared. Herpangina is caused by the Coxsackie A group of viruses.

Polymerase chain reaction testing is available, but not typically indicated, as this is a self-limited illness.

C. Hand, Foot, and Mouth Disease

This entity is caused by several enteroviruses, one of which (enterovirus 71) can rarely cause encephalitis. Ulcers occur anywhere in the mouth. Vesicles, pustules, or papules may be found on the palms, soles, interdigital areas, and buttocks. In younger children, lesions may be seen on the distal extremities and even the face.

D. Pharyngoconjunctival Fever

This disorder is caused by an adenovirus and often is epidemic. Exudative tonsillitis, conjunctivitis, lymphadenopathy, and fever are the main findings. Treatment is symptomatic.

2. Acute Bacterial Pharyngitis

ESSENTIALS OF DIAGNOSIS & TYPICAL FEATURES

► Sore throat
► At least one of the following:
  • Cervical lymphadenopathy (lymph nodes tender or > 2 cm)
  • Tonsillar exudates
  • Positive group A β-hemolytic *Streptococcus* culture
  • Fever > 38.3°C

► Differential Diagnosis

Viral pharyngitis, infectious mononucleosis, bacterial pharyngitis other than streptococcal, diphtheria, and peritonsillar abscess.

Approximately 20%–30% of children with pharyngitis have a group A streptococcal (GAS) infection. It is most common in children between 5 and 15 years in the winter or early spring. Less common causes of bacterial pharyngitis include *Mycoplasma pneumoniae*, *Chlamydia pneumoniae*, groups C and G streptococci, and *Arcanobacterium hemolyticum*. Of the five, *M pneumoniae* is by far the most common and may cause over one-third of all pharyngitis cases in adolescents and adults.

► Clinical Findings

Sudden onset of sore throat, fever, tender cervical adenopathy, palatal petechiae, a beefy-red uvula, and a tonsillar exudate suggest streptococcal infection. Other symptoms may include headache, stomachache, nausea, and vomiting. The only way to make a definitive diagnosis is by throat culture

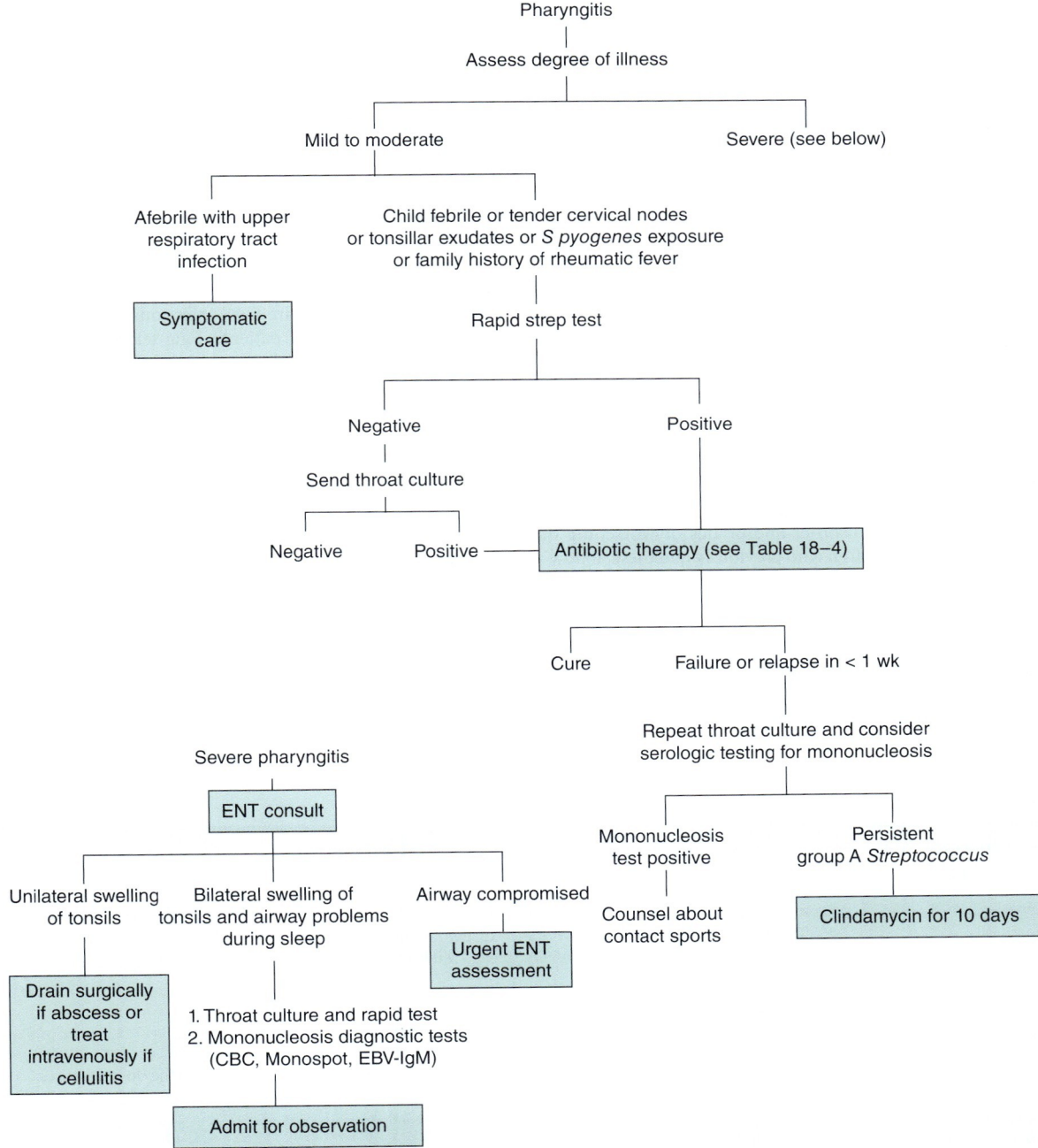

▲ **Figure 18–5.** Algorithm for pharyngitis. CBC, complete blood count; EBV, Epstein-Barr virus; ENT, ear, nose, and throat; IgM, immunoglobulin M.

or rapid antigen test. Rapid antigen tests are very specific but have a sensitivity of only 85%–95%. Therefore, a positive test indicates *S pyogenes* infection, but a negative result requires confirmation by performing a culture. Diagnosis is important because untreated streptococcal pharyngitis can result in acute rheumatic fever, glomerulonephritis, and suppurative complications (eg, cervical adenitis, peritonsillar abscess, otitis media, cellulitis, and septicemia). The presence of conjunctivitis, cough, hoarseness, symptoms of URI, anterior stomatitis, ulcerative lesions, viral rash, and diarrhea should raise suspicion of a viral etiology.

Occasionally, a child with GAS infection develops scarlet fever within 24–48 hours after the onset of symptoms. Scarlet fever is a diffuse, finely papular, erythematous eruption producing a bright red discoloration of the skin, which blanches on pressure. The rash is more intense in the skin creases. The tongue has a strawberry appearance.

A controversial but possible complication of streptococcal infections is Pediatric Autoimmune Neuropsychiatric Disorders Associated with *Streptococcus* (PANDAS). PANDAS is a relatively newly recognized condition. It describes a subset of pediatric patients who experience a sudden onset of obsessive-compulsive disorder and/or tics or worsening of such symptoms in children who previously had these, following a strep infection.

Web Resources

National Institute of Mental Health: PANDAS—Questions and Answers: https://www.nimh.nih.gov/health/publications/pandas/. Updated 2019. Accessed July 4, 2023.

▶ Treatment

Suspected or proven GAS infection should be treated with penicillin (oral or intramuscular) or amoxicillin as outlined in Table 18–4. For patients allergic to penicillin, alternative treatments include cephalexin, azithromycin, and clindamycin. Tetracyclines, sulfonamides (including trimethoprim-sulfamethoxazole), and quinolones should not be used for treating GAS infections.

Repeat culture after treatment is not recommended and is indicated only for those who remain symptomatic, have a recurrence of symptoms, or have had rheumatic fever. Of note, children who have had rheumatic fever are at a high risk of recurrence if future GAS infections are inadequately treated. In this group of patients, long-term antibiotic prophylaxis is recommended, sometimes life-long in patients with residual rheumatic heart disease (see Chapter 20).

In general, the carrier state is harmless, self-limited (2–6 months), and not contagious. An attempt to eradicate the carrier state is warranted only if the patient or another family member has frequent streptococcal infections or if a family member or patient has a history of rheumatic fever or glomerulonephritis. If eradication is chosen, a course of clindamycin for 10 days or rifampin for 5 days should be used.

In the past, daily penicillin prophylaxis was occasionally recommended; however, because of concerns about the development of drug resistance, tonsillectomy is now preferred for patients with recurrent streptococcal tonsillitis. Otolaryngologists' decision for tonsillectomy is guided by Paradise criteria: seven tonsillitis episodes in single year, five

Table 18–4. Treatment of group A streptococcal pharyngitis.[a]

Treatment of acute group A strep pharyngitis		
Antibiotic	**Dose**	**Notes**
Penicillin	Penicillin V 250 mg 2–3 times per day for 10 days if < 27 kg; 500 mg 2–3 times per day for 10 days if > 27 kg; Benzathine Penicillin 600,000 units IM single dose if < 27 kg; 1.2 million units IM single dose if > 27 kg	Resistance to penicillin, amoxicillin, and first-generation cephalosporins has not been reported. Each is equally effective if compliance is ensured.
Amoxicillin	50 mg/kg/day once daily for 10 days (max 1200 mg)	
Cephalexin	25–50 mg/kg/day in 2 divided doses for 10 days	
Clindamycin	20 mg/kg/day in 3 divided doses for 10 days'	Rare resistance reported in the United States.
Azithromycin	12 mg/kg once daily for 5 days (max 500 mg/day)	Some resistance reported in the United States.
Eradication of carrier state		
Clindamycin	20 mg/kg/day in 3 divided doses for 10 days	Most effective.
Cephalexin	25–50 mg/kg/day in 2 divided doses for 10 days	Also effective.
Penicillin + Rifampin	See above penicillin doses; Rifampin 20 mg/kg/day twice daily for final 4 days	

[a]Tetracyclines, sulfonamides (including trimethoprim-sulfamethoxazole), and quinolones should not be used for treating GAS infections.

episodes per year for 2 consecutive years, or three episodes each year for at least 3 years.

Wessels MR: Clinical practice. Streptococcal pharyngitis. N Engl J Med 2011;364(7):648–655 [PMID: 21323542].

PERITONSILLAR CELLULITIS OR ABSCESS (QUINSY)

ESSENTIALS OF DIAGNOSIS & TYPICAL FEATURES

► Severe sore throat.
► Unilateral tonsillar swelling.
► Deviation of the uvula.
► Trismus (limited mouth opening).

Tonsillar infection extending to the surrounding tissues is called *peritonsillar cellulitis*. If untreated, necrosis occurs, with peritonsillar abscess formation. The most common pathogen is β-hemolytic *Streptococcus*, but others include group D *Streptococcus*, *S pneumoniae*, and anaerobes. A severe sore throat and high fever is usually present, and the process is almost always unilateral. The tonsil bulges medially, and the anterior tonsillar pillar is prominent. The soft palate and uvula on the involved side are edematous and displaced toward the uninvolved side. As the infection progresses, trismus, ear pain, dysphagia, and drooling may occur. The most serious complication of untreated peritonsillar abscess is a lateral pharyngeal abscess, which can progress to jugular vein thrombosis and septic thrombi to the lungs (Lemierre syndrome).

While peritonsillar cellulitis will often respond to parenteral antibiotics (penicillin, cephalosporin, or clindamycin), an abscess within the peritonsillar space will usually require drainage. Failure to respond to therapy during the first 12–24 hours indicates a high probability of abscess formation and need for otolaryngology consultation. A peritonsillar abscess may be needle aspirated or formally incised and drained. The risk of bilateral and/or recurrent peritonsillar abscess is low (7%–10%), so tonsillectomy is not usually indicated for a single incident.

RETROPHARYNGEAL ABSCESS

Retropharyngeal lymph nodes drain the oropharynx, nasopharynx, and paranasal sinuses. Infections of these nodes are most often due to β-hemolytic streptococci and *S aureus*. The diagnosis of retropharyngeal abscess should be suspected in a child with fever, respiratory symptoms, and restriction in neck range of motion, particularly with extension.

Dysphagia, drooling, dyspnea, and gurgling respirations may also be present. This occurs most commonly during the first 2 years of life. After this age, the most common cause of retropharyngeal abscess is penetrating injury of the posterior pharyngeal wall.

Prominent swelling on one side of the posterior pharyngeal wall is characteristic. Swelling usually stops at the midline because a medial raphe divides the prevertebral space. Although nonspecific, lateral neck x-ray may demonstrate retropharyngeal tissues wider than the C4 vertebral body; CT scan with contrast can distinguish between soft tissue swelling versus abscess.

Although a retropharyngeal abscess is a surgical emergency, frequently it cannot be distinguished from retropharyngeal adenitis. Immediate hospitalization and intravenous antimicrobial therapy with a semisynthetic penicillin or clindamycin is the first step for most cases. In most instances, a period of 12–24 hours of antimicrobial therapy will help differentiate the two entities. In the child with adenitis, fever will decrease and oral intake will improve. A child with retropharyngeal abscess will typically not improve. A surgeon should incise and drain the abscess under general anesthesia to prevent its extension. Immediate surgical drainage is indicated if there is concern for airway compromise.

LUDWIG ANGINA

Ludwig angina is a rapidly progressive cellulitis of both submandibular spaces that pushes the tongue posteriorly against the pharyngeal wall, causing life threatening airway obstruction. Symptoms include fever and tender swelling of the tongue and floor of the mouth. Most often arising from an odontogenic source, this infection is unusual in infants and children. Group A strep is the most common culprit. Treatment consists of high-dose intravenous clindamycin or ampicillin plus nafcillin until culture and sensitivities are available. Treatment for airway obstruction in patients with Ludwig angina has transitioned through the years from tracheotomy to intensive care unit monitoring and intubation. An otolaryngologist should be consulted for airway evaluation and management, and to perform a drainage procedure if needed.

ACUTE CERVICAL ADENITIS

Local infections of the ear, nose, and throat can involve a regional lymph node and cause abscess formation. The typical case involves a unilateral, solitary, anterior cervical node. About 70% of these cases are due to β-hemolytic streptococcal infection, 20% to staphylococci (including MRSA), and the remainder to viruses, atypical mycobacteria, and *Bartonella henselae*.

The initial evaluation of cervical adenitis should generally include a rapid GAS test, and a complete blood count with differential looking for atypical lymphocytes. A purified protein derivative skin test, looking for nontuberculous mycobacteria, should also be considered. If multiple enlarged nodes are found, a rapid mononucleosis test is useful. Early treatment with antibiotics prevents many cases of adenitis from progressing to suppuration. However, once abscess formation occurs, antibiotic therapy alone is often insufficient and a drainage procedure may be necessary. Because of the increase in community-acquired MRSA, it is a prudent to send a specimen for culture and sensitivity.

Cat-scratch disease, caused by *B henselae*, causes indolent ("cold") adenopathy. The diagnosis is supported if a primary papule is found at the scratch site on the face. In over 90% of patients, there is a history of contact with kittens. The node is usually only mildly tender but may, over a month or more, suppurate and drain. About one-third of children have fever and malaise; rarely neurologic sequelae and prolonged fever occur. Cat-scratch disease can be diagnosed by serologic testing, but testing is not always confirmatory. If blood is to be drawn, one should wait 2–8 weeks after onset of symptoms. Because most enlarged lymph nodes infected with *B henselae* spontaneously regress within 1–3 months, the benefit of antibiotics is controversial. In a placebo-controlled trial, azithromycin for 5 days caused a more rapid decrease in node size. Other drugs likely to be effective include rifampin, trimethoprim-sulfamethoxazole, erythromycin, clarithromycin, doxycycline, ciprofloxacin, and gentamicin (some of these antibiotics may be contraindicated depending on patient age).

Cervical lymphadenitis can also be caused by nontuberculous mycobacterial species or *Mycobacterium avium* complex. Mycobacterial disease is unilateral and may involve several matted nodes. A characteristic violaceous appearance may develop over a prolonged period of time without systemic signs or much local pain. Atypical mycobacterial infections are often associated with positive purified protein derivative skin test reactions less than 10 mm in diameter, and a second-strength (250-test-unit) purified protein derivative skin test is virtually always positive.

Lawrence R, Bateman N: Controversies in the management of deep neck space infection in children: an evidence-based review. Clin Otolaryngol 2017 Feb;42(1):156–163. doi: 10.1111/coa.12692. Epub 2016 Jun 30 [PMID: 27288654].

▶ Differential Diagnosis

A. Neoplasms and Cervical Nodes

Malignant tumors usually are not suspected until adenopathy persists despite antibiotic treatment. Classically, malignant lymph nodes are painless, nontender, and of firm consistency. They may be fixed to underlying tissues. They may occur as a single node, as unilateral nodes in a chain, bilateral cervical nodes, or as generalized adenopathy. Common malignancies that may manifest in the neck include lymphoma, rhabdomyosarcoma, and thyroid carcinoma.

B. Imitators of Adenitis

Several structures in the neck can become infected and resemble a lymph node. The first three masses are of congenital origin.

1. Thyroglossal duct cyst—These are midline, usually near the level of the hyoid bone. Thyroglossal duct cysts move upward when the tongue is protruded or with swallowing. Occasionally, a thyroglossal duct cyst may have a sinus tract with an opening just lateral to the midline. When infected, these can become acutely swollen and inflamed.

2. Branchial cleft cyst—These masses are found along the anterior border of the sternocleidomastoid muscle and are smooth and fluctuant. Sometimes a branchial cleft cyst may be attached to the overlying skin by a small dimple or a draining sinus tract. When infected, they can become a tender mass 3–5 cm in diameter.

3. Lymphatic malformation—Most lymphatic cysts are located in the posterior triangle just above the clavicle. These are soft and compressible and can be transilluminated. Over 60% are noted at birth; the remaining malformations usually become apparent by the age of 2 years. If large enough, they can compromise the patient's ability to swallow and breathe.

4. Parotitis—Parotitis is commonly mistaken for cervical adenitis. The parotid salivary gland crosses the angle of the jaw. Parotitis may be bacterial or viral and may occur unilaterally or bilaterally. Mumps was once the most common cause of viral parotitis, but because of routine vaccinations, parainfluenza is the primary viral cause in the United States. An amylase level will be elevated in parotitis.

5. Ranula—A ranula is a saliva filled cyst in the floor of mouth caused by obstruction of the sublingual salivary gland. A "plunging" ranula extends down through the mylohyoid muscle and can present as a neck mass.

6. Sternocleidomastoid muscle hematoma—Also known as *fibromatosis colli*, these are noted at age 2–4 weeks. On examination, the mass is found to be part of the muscle body and not movable. An associated torticollis usually confirms the diagnosis. A neck ultrasound can help confirm the diagnosis. Treatment involves physical therapy, with range of motion exercises.

TONSILLECTOMY & ADENOIDECTOMY

Tonsillectomy

A tonsillectomy, with or without adenoidectomy, is most often performed for either hypertrophy or recurrent infections. The most common indication for adenotonsillectomy is adenotonsillar hypertrophy associated with an obstructive breathing pattern during sleep (see Chapter 19). Adenotonsillar hypertrophy may also cause other problems such as dysphagia or dental malocclusion.

Recurrent tonsillitis is the second most common reason for tonsillectomy. Tonsillitis is considered "recurrent" when a child has seven or more documented infections in 1 year, five per year for 2 years, or three per year for 3 years. For an infection to be considered clinically significant, there must be a sore throat and at least one of the following clinical features: cervical lymphadenopathy (tender lymph nodes or > 2 cm), OR tonsillar exudate, OR positive culture for group A β-hemolytic *Streptococcus*, OR temperature greater than 38.3°C.

Tonsillectomy is reasonable with fewer infections if the child has missed multiple school days due to infection, has a complicated course, or under other circumstances such as recurrent peritonsillar abscess, persistent streptococcal carrier state, or multiple antibiotic allergies. Unless neoplasm is suspected, tonsil asymmetry is not an indication.

Another indication for tonsillectomy is PFAPA syndrome (see section Recurrent Aphthous Stomatitis), in which fever recurs predictably, typically every 4–8 weeks. Tonsillectomy has been shown to be an effective treatment.

Ingram DG, Friedman NR: Toward adenotonsillectomy in children: a review for the general pediatrician. JAMA Pediatr 2015 Dec;169(12):1155–1161. doi: 10.1001/jamapediatrics.2015.2016. Review [PMID: 26436644].
Mitchell RB et al: Clinical practice guideline: tonsillectomy in children (update). Otolaryngol Head Neck Surg 2019 Feb;160(1 Suppl): S1–S42. doi: 10.1177/0194599818801757 [PMID: 30798778].

Web Resources

American Academy of Otolaryngology/Head and Neck Surgery–Clinical indicators: tonsillectomy, adenoidectomy, adenotonsillectomy in childhood. https://www.entnet.org/resource/clinical-indicators-tonsillectomy-adenoidectomy-adenotonsillectomy-in-childhood/. Updated April 23, 2021. Accessed July 8, 2023.

Adenoidectomy

The adenoid is composed of lymphoid tissue in the nasopharynx and is a part of the Waldeyer ring of lymphoid tissue, which also includes the palatine and lingual tonsils. Enlarged adenoids, with or without infection, can obstruct the nose, alter normal orofacial growth, and interfere with speech, swallowing, and Eustachian tube function. Children who are persistent mouth breathers can develop dental malocclusion and "adenoid facies," where the face appears "pinched" and the maxilla narrowed because the molding pressures of the orbicularis oris and buccinator muscles are unopposed by the tongue. The adenoid can also harbor biofilms, which have been associated with CRS and otitis media.

Indications for adenoidectomy with or without tonsillectomy include upper airway obstruction, orofacial conditions such as mandibular growth abnormalities and dental malocclusion, speech abnormalities, persistent MEE, recurrent otitis media, and CRS.

Complications of Tonsillectomy & Adenoidectomy

The mortality rate associated with tonsillectomy and adenoidectomy is reported to approximate that of general anesthesia alone. The rate of hemorrhage varies between 0.1% and 8.1%, depending on the definition of hemorrhage; the rate of postoperative transfusion is 0.04%. Other potential complications include permanently hypernasal speech (< 0.01%) and, more rarely, nasopharyngeal stenosis, atlantoaxial subluxation, mandibular condyle fracture, and psychological trauma.

Contraindications to Tonsillectomy & Adenoidectomy

A. Palatal Abnormalities

Adenoid tissue should not be removed completely in a child with a cleft palate or submucous cleft palate because of the risk of velopharyngeal incompetence which may cause hypernasal speech and nasal regurgitation. If needed, a partial adenoidectomy can be performed in at-risk children. A bifid uvula can be a sign of a palatal abnormality.

B. Bleeding Disorder

When suspected, bleeding disorders must be diagnosed and treated prior to surgery.

C. Acute Tonsillitis

An elective tonsillectomy and adenoidectomy can usually be postponed until acute tonsillitis is resolved. Urgent tonsillectomy may occasionally be required for tonsillitis unresponsive to medical therapy.

DISORDERS OF THE LIPS

1. Labial Sucking Tubercle

A young infant may present with a small callus in the mid-upper lip. The cause is likely strong sucking in utero but can persist into early infancy. It usually is asymptomatic and disappears after cup feeding is initiated.

2. Cheilitis

Dry, cracked, scaling lips are usually caused by sun or wind exposure. Contact dermatitis from mouthpieces or various woodwind or brass instruments has also been reported. Licking the lips exacerbates cheilitis. Liberal use of lip balm gives excellent results.

3. Inclusion Cyst

Inclusion or mucous retention cysts are due to obstruction of mucous glands or other mucous membrane structures, such as minor salivary glands. In the newborn, they occur on the hard palate or gums and are called *Epstein pearls*. These resolve spontaneously in 1–2 months. In older children, inclusion cysts usually occur on the palate, uvula, or tonsillar pillars. They appear as taut yellow sacs varying in size from 2 to 10 mm. Inclusion cysts that do not resolve spontaneously may undergo incision and drainage. Occasionally, a mucous cyst on the lower lip (mucocele) will require excision for cosmetic reasons.

DISORDERS OF THE TONGUE

1. Geographic Tongue (Benign Migratory Glossitis)

This condition of unknown etiology occurs in 1%–2% of the population with no age, sex, or racial predilection. It is characterized by irregularly shaped patches on the tongue that are devoid of papillae and surrounded by parakeratotic reddish borders. The pattern changes as alternating regeneration and desquamation occurs. The lesions are generally asymptomatic and require no treatment.

2. Fissured Tongue (Scrotal Tongue)

This condition is marked by numerous irregular fissures on the dorsum of the tongue. It occurs in approximately 1% of the population and is usually a dominant trait. It is also frequently seen in children with trisomy 21.

3. Coated Tongue (Furry Tongue)

The tongue becomes coated if mastication is impaired and the patient is limited to a liquid or soft diet. Mouth breathing, fever, or dehydration can accentuate the process. This process is usually self-limited and resolves with return of normal dietary patterns.

4. Macroglossia

Tongue hypertrophy and protrusion may be due to trisomy 21, Beckwith-Wiedemann syndrome, glycogen storage diseases, cretinism, mucopolysaccharidoses, lymphangioma, or hemangioma. Tongue reduction procedures should be considered in otherwise healthy subjects if macroglossia affects airway patency.

HALITOSIS

Bad breath is usually due to acute stomatitis, pharyngitis, rhinosinusitis, nasal foreign body, or dental hygiene problems. In older children and adolescents, halitosis can be a manifestation of CRS, gastric bezoar, bronchiectasis, or lung abscess. The presence of orthodontic devices or dentures can cause halitosis if good dental hygiene is not maintained. Halitosis can also be caused by decaying food particles embedded in cryptic tonsils. Mouthwashes and chewable breath fresheners give limited improvement. Treatment of the underlying cause is indicated, and a dental referral may be in order.

SALIVARY GLAND DISORDERS

1. Parotitis

A first episode of parotitis may safely be considered to be of viral origin, unless fluctuance is present. Mumps was the leading cause until adoption of vaccination; now the leading viruses are parainfluenza and Epstein-Barr virus. HIV infection should be considered if the child is known to be at risk.

2. Suppurative Parotitis

Suppurative parotitis occurs chiefly in newborns and debilitated elderly patients. The parotid gland is swollen, tender, and often erythematous, usually unilaterally. The diagnosis is made by expression of purulent material from Stensen duct. The material should be cultured. Fever and leukocytosis may be present. Treatment includes antibiotic therapy, sialogogues, and warm compresses to the parotid region. *S aureus* is the most common causative organism.

3. Juvenile Recurrent Parotitis

Some children experience recurrent nonsuppurative parotid inflammation with swelling or pain and fever. Juvenile recurrent parotitis (JRP) is most prevalent between the ages of 3 and 6 years, and it generally decreases by adolescence. The cause is unknown, but possible etiologic factors include ductal anomaly, autoimmune, allergy, and genetic. It usually occurs unilaterally. Treatment includes analgesics and some recommend an antistaphylococcal antibiotic for prophylaxis of bacterial infection and quicker resolution. Endoscopy and irrigation of Stensen duct is being performed more frequently, not only to confirm diagnosis but also to provide treatment.

4. Tumors of the Parotid Gland

Mixed tumors, hemangiomas, sarcoidosis, and leukemia can manifest in the parotid gland as a hard or persistent mass. A cystic mass or multiple cystic masses may represent an HIV infection. Workup may require consultation with oncology, infectious disease, hematology, and otolaryngology.

5. Ranula

A ranula is a retention cyst of a sublingual salivary gland. It occurs on the floor of the mouth to one side of the lingual frenulum. It is thin walled and can appear bluish. Referral is indicated to an otolaryngologist for surgical management.

CONGENITAL ORAL MALFORMATIONS

1. Tongue-Tie (Ankyloglossia)

A short lingual frenulum can hinder protrusion and elevation of the tongue. Dimpling of the midline tongue tip is noted with tongue movement. Ankyloglossia can cause feeding difficulties in the neonate, speech problems, and dental problems. If the tongue cannot protrude past the teeth or alveolar ridge or move between the gums and cheek, referral to an otolaryngologist is indicated. A frenulectomy should be performed in the neonatal period if the infant is having difficulty breast-feeding, specifically inefficient milk transfer or persistent pain in the mother. Early treatment is favored because it can easily be performed in clinic. When an infant is even a few months old, general anesthesia is required for the procedure to be performed safely. Lip tie concerns have become more common as breast-feeding initiation is increasing but there is little evidence that this has any effect on nursing, or that surgical lysis of the lip frenum has any real benefits.

O'Shea JE et al: Frenotomy for tongue-tie in newborn infants. Cochrane Database Syst Rev 2017 Mar 11;3:CD011065. doi: 10.1002/14651858.CD011065.pub2 [PMID: 28284020].

2. Torus Palatini

Torus palatini are hard, midline, palate masses which form at suture lines of the bone. They are usually asymptomatic and require no therapy, but they can be surgically reduced if necessary.

3. Cleft Lip & Cleft Palate

A. Submucous Cleft Palate

A bifid uvula is present in 3% of healthy children (see Chapter 37). However, a close association exists between bifid uvula and submucous cleft palate. A submucous cleft can be diagnosed by noting a translucent zone in the middle of the soft palate (zona pellucida). Palpation of the hard palate reveals absence of the posterior bony protrusion. Affected children have a 40% risk of developing persistent MEE. They are at risk for velopharyngeal incompetence, or an inability to close the palate against the posterior pharyngeal wall, resulting in hypernasal speech and nasal regurgitation of food. Children with submucous cleft palate causing abnormal speech or significant nasal regurgitation of food should be referred for possible surgical repair.

B. High-Arched Palate

A high-arched palate is usually a genetic trait of no consequence. It also occurs in children who are chronic mouth breathers and in premature infants who undergo prolonged oral intubation. Some rare causes of high-arched palate are congenital disorders such as Marfan syndrome, Treacher Collins syndrome, and Ehlers-Danlos syndrome. Orthodontic treatment of a high-arched palate can be an effective treatment for childhood OSA.

C. Pierre Robin Sequence

This group of congenital malformations is characterized by the triad of micrognathia, glossoptosis (posterior tongue displacement), and airway obstruction, usually associated with cleft palate. Affected children often present as emergencies in the newborn period because of infringement on the airway by the tongue and also because of feeding difficulties. The main objective of early management is to prevent asphyxia until the mandible becomes large enough to accommodate the tongue. In some cases, this can be achieved by positioning strategies, side-lying or prone when sleeping. Other airway manipulations such as a nasal trumpet may be necessary. Tongue lip adhesion is considered by some surgeons. Mandibular distraction osteogenesis may be performed in the neonatal period to avoid tracheotomy. Rarely, a tracheotomy is required, often in combination with a gastric feeding tube. Cleft palate repair is deferred until 10–12 months of age. These children benefit from multidisciplinary cleft and craniofacial care for ongoing management involving feeding, airway, and speech issues.

Gómez OJ et al: Pierre robin sequence: an evidence-based treatment proposal. J Craniofac Surg 2018 Mar;29(2):332–338. doi: 10.1097/SCS.0000000000004178 [PMID: 29215441].

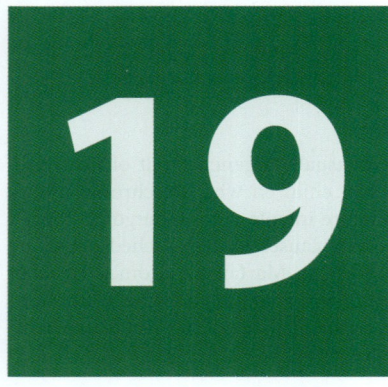

Respiratory Tract & Mediastinum

Paul Stillwell, MD

Emily M. DeBoer, MD

Jordana Hoppe, MD

Paul Houin, MD

Respiratory Tract

Pulmonary diseases account for almost 50% of deaths in children younger than 1 year and about 20% of all hospitalizations of children younger than 15 years. Approximately 7% of children have a chronic respiratory disorder. Understanding the pathophysiology of many pediatric pulmonary diseases is enhanced by an appreciation of the normal growth and development of the lung.

GROWTH & DEVELOPMENT

Normal fetal lung development progresses through five stages (embryonic, pseudoglandular, canalicular, saccular, alveolar) with considerable overlap in the timing of each stage. Interruption of the sequence leads to significant neonatal pulmonary difficulties that may be lifelong. The normal human term newborn infant does not have a full complement of alveoli at birth, usually 100–150 million; this will increase with normal growth to the adult number of 300–600 million alveoli. Infants born prematurely may have difficulty transitioning from fetal life to air breathing due to incomplete alveolarization. This may be accentuated by additional stresses such as higher altitude, suboptimal nutrition, poor air quality, or infections.

Schittney JC: Development of the lung. Cell Tissue Res 2017;367: 427–444. doi: 10.1007/s00441-016-2545-0 [PMID: 28144783].

DIAGNOSTIC AIDS

PHYSICAL EXAMINATION OF THE RESPIRATORY TRACT

The complete pulmonary examination includes inspection, palpation, auscultation, and percussion. *Inspection* of respiratory rate and work of breathing is critical to the detection of pulmonary disease. Tachypnea, decreased sensorium, inconsolability, increased respiratory effort, retraction, poor color, and reduced movement suggest hypoxemia. *Palpation* of tracheal position, symmetry of chest wall movement, and vibration with vocalization can help in identifying intrathoracic abnormalities. A shift in tracheal position from midline suggests pneumothorax or significant unilateral atelectasis. Tactile vibrations (fremitus) may change with consolidation or air in the pleural space. *Auscultation* should assess the intensity and symmetry of breath sounds and the presence of abnormal sounds such as fine or coarse crackles, wheezing, or rhonchi. Wheezing or prolonged expiration suggests intrathoracic airways obstruction. Knowing the lung anatomy helps identify the location of the pathology (Figure 19–1). *Percussion* may identify tympanic or dull sounds that can help define an effusion or pneumothorax but can be challenging in young children.

Acute findings such as cyanosis and altered mental status or chronic signs of respiratory insufficiency including growth failure and digital clubbing suggest pulmonary disease. Evidence of cor pulmonale (loud pulmonic component of the second heart sound, hepatomegaly, elevated neck veins, and, rarely, peripheral edema) signifies pulmonary hypertension and may accompany advanced lung disease.

Respiratory disorders can be secondary to disease in other systems. It is therefore important to look for other conditions such as fever, metabolic acidosis, congenital heart disease, neuromuscular disease, obesity, immunodeficiency, or autoimmune disease.

Bohadana A, Izbicki G, Kraman SS: Fundamentals of lung auscultation. N Engl J Med 2014;370:744–751 [PMID: 24552321].
Zimmerman B, Williams D: Lung sounds. Stat Pearls. https://www.ncbi.nlm.nih.gov/books/NBK537253/. Updated August 29, 2022.

PULMONARY FUNCTION TESTS

Pulmonary function tests (PFTs) objectively measure lung function. They are useful to measure lung health, disease progression or improvement, and evaluate response to

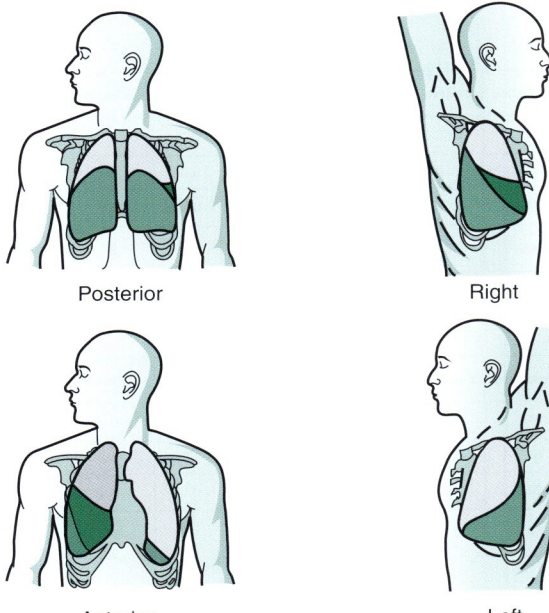

Posterior

Right

Anterior

Left

▲ **Figure 19–1.** Projections of the pulmonary lobes on the chest surface. The upper lobes are white, the right-middle lobe is the darker color, and the lower lobes are the lighter color.

therapy. Serial lung function measurements are often more informative than a single determination, especially in growing children. Patient cooperation and consistent effort is essential for almost all standard PFTs. Most children aged 5 and older can perform pulmonary function testing. Younger children may be able to produce reliable results with coaching and visual incentives. Children with cystic fibrosis (CF), asthma, and other chronic lung conditions should perform PFTs routinely as early as they can cooperate. Spirometric values include forced vital capacity (FVC), which is the total volume of air that is exhaled; forced expiratory volume in 1 second (FEV_1); the ratio of the FEV_1/FVC; forced expiratory flow at the middle of the vital capacity (FEF_{25-75}); and peak expiratory flow rate (PEFR). Reference equations are now available from age 4 to 80 years with the lower limit of normal defined by a z-score of −1.64 in all values. Commonly seen obstructive lung processes include asthma, bronchopulmonary dysplasia (BPD), and CF. Common restrictive lung diseases include chest wall or spine deformities, muscle weakness, and interstitial lung diseases (ILDs). (See Figures 19–2 for spirometry examples.) Confirmation of restrictive lung physiology requires lung volume measurements: total lung capacity, residual volume, and functional residual capacity. Other sophisticated PFTs such as diffusing

capacity, oscillometry, and lung clearance index require special equipment and expertise.

PEFR (the maximal flow recorded during an FVC maneuver) can be assessed by handheld devices. These devices are not as well calibrated as spirometers, and the PEFR measurement can vary greatly with patient effort, so they are not good substitutes for actual spirometry. However, peak flow monitoring can be helpful in a patient with asthma that is difficult to control or has poor perception of symptoms.

Stanojevic S et al: ERS/ATS technical standard on interpretive strategies for routine lung function tests. Eur Respir J 2022; 60:2101499 [PMID: 34949706].

ASSESSMENT OF OXYGENATION & VENTILATION

Arterial blood gas measurements describe the acid–base balance, oxygenation, and ventilation status in the body. Blood gas measurements can categorize acid–base disturbances as respiratory, metabolic, or mixed as well as acute or chronic. Blood gas measurements are affected by abnormalities of ventilation/perfusion ($\dot{V}/\dot{Q}$) matching, respiratory control, ventilation, and respiratory mechanics. In pediatrics, hypoxemia most commonly results from $\dot{V}/\dot{Q}$ mismatch. Common pediatric diseases associated with hypoxemia due to $\dot{V}/\dot{Q}$ mismatch include acute asthma, CF, pneumonia, bronchiolitis, and BPD. Other causes of hypoxemia include hypoventilation, shunts (physiologic and anatomic), and diffusion barriers. Hypercapnia (elevated partial pressure of arterial carbon dioxide [$PaCO_2$]) results from hypoventilation. Causes include decreased central respiratory drive, respiratory muscle weakness, and low-tidal-volume breathing as seen in restrictive lung or chest wall diseases. Hypercapnia can also occur when severe $\dot{V}/\dot{Q}$ mismatch is present, which may occur with severe CF or BPD. Table 19–1 shows normal values for arterial pH, PaO_2, and $PaCO_2$ at sea level and at 5000 ft (approximately the elevation of Denver, Colorado).

Venous blood gas analysis or capillary blood gas analysis can be useful for the assessment of PCO_2 and pH, but not PO_2 or saturation. Noninvasive assessment of oxygenation can be achieved with pulse oximetry (SpO_2). Values of SpO_2 are reliable as low as 80%. Reliability is reduced with poor arterial pulsation (eg, with hypothermia, hypotension, or vasoconstriction). Carbon monoxide bound to hemoglobin results in falsely high SpO_2 readings. Exhaled or end-tidal CO_2 monitoring is most accurate in patients without significant lung disease but can be a noninvasive way to estimate arterial CO_2 content and monitor alveolar ventilation. Monitoring of exhaled or end-tidal CO_2 is commonly used during polysomnogram (PSG), mechanical ventilation, and anesthesia. Transcutaneous PCO_2 monitoring is also feasible but may be less reliable than transcutaneous PO_2 monitoring.

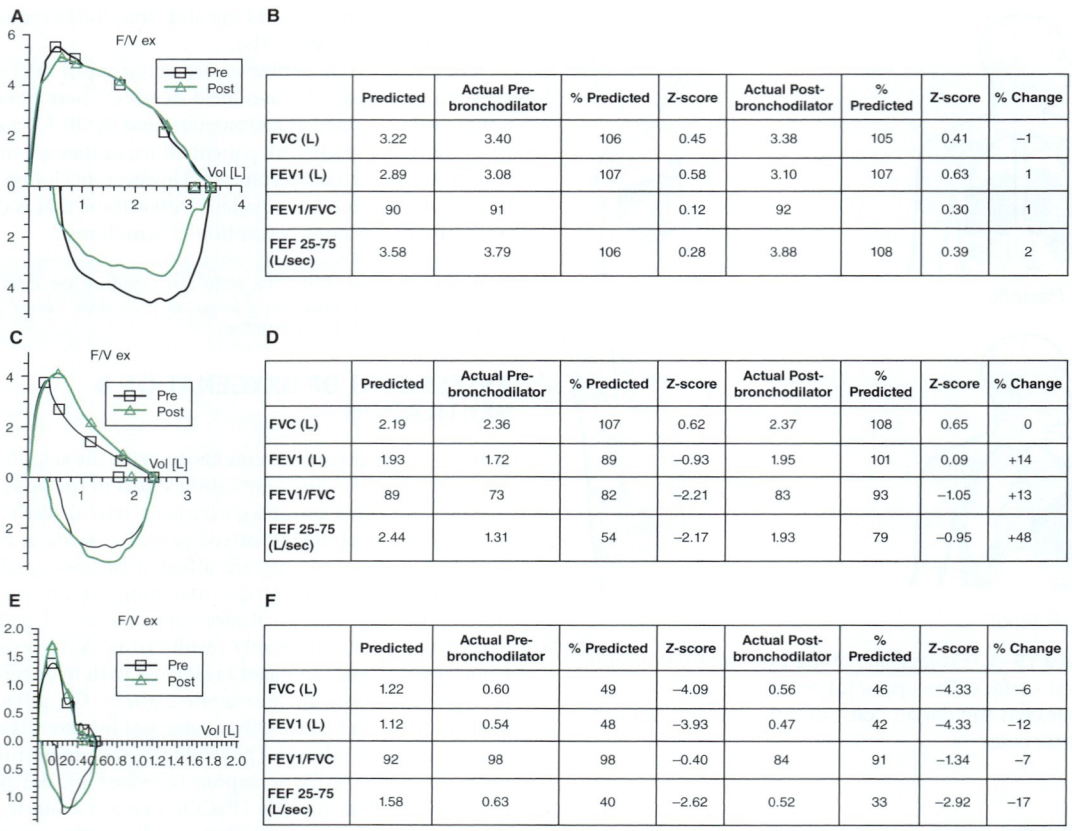

A: Normal spirometry, pre- and postbronchodilator Flow Volume Curve.

B

	Predicted	Actual Pre-bronchodilator	% Predicted	Z-score	Actual Post-bronchodilator	% Predicted	Z-score	% Change
FVC (L)	3.22	3.40	106	0.45	3.38	105	0.41	−1
FEV1 (L)	2.89	3.08	107	0.58	3.10	107	0.63	1
FEV1/FVC	90	91		0.12	92		0.30	1
FEF 25-75 (L/sec)	3.58	3.79	106	0.28	3.88	108	0.39	2

D

	Predicted	Actual Pre-bronchodilator	% Predicted	Z-score	Actual Post-bronchodilator	% Predicted	Z-score	% Change
FVC (L)	2.19	2.36	107	0.62	2.37	108	0.65	0
FEV1 (L)	1.93	1.72	89	−0.93	1.95	101	0.09	+14
FEV1/FVC	89	73	82	−2.21	83	93	−1.05	+13
FEF 25-75 (L/sec)	2.44	1.31	54	−2.17	1.93	79	−0.95	+48

F

	Predicted	Actual Pre-bronchodilator	% Predicted	Z-score	Actual Post-bronchodilator	% Predicted	Z-score	% Change
FVC (L)	1.22	0.60	49	−4.09	0.56	46	−4.33	−6
FEV1 (L)	1.12	0.54	48	−3.93	0.47	42	−4.33	−12
FEV1/FVC	92	98	98	−0.40	84	91	−1.34	−7
FEF 25-75 (L/sec)	1.58	0.63	40	−2.62	0.52	33	−2.92	−17

▲ **Figure 19–2.** **A:** Normal spirometry, pre- and postbronchodilator Flow Volume Curve. The vertical axis represents flow rate, and the horizontal axis represents volume. **B:** Normal Spirometry, typical pre- and postbronchodilator volumes and flow rates. FVC = forced vital capacity; FEV_1 = forced expiratory volume in 1 second; FEV_1/FVC is the ratio of the two measured values. FEF25–75 = forced expiratory flow between 25% and 75% of the FVC. L = liters; L/s = liters/second. Predicted = expected value based on age, sex, height, and ethnicity. Actual prebronchodilator = value measured prior to administration of a short acting bronchodilator. % predicted = ratio of the measured value to the predicted value. Z-score = Standard deviation number from the mean predicted value. Actual postbronchodilator = measure value after administration of a short-acting bronchodilator. % change = change from pre- to post-bronchodilator. **C:** Reversible airflow obstruction spirometry, pre- and postbronchodilator flow volume curve. **D:** Reversible airflow obstruction, typical pre- and postbronchodilator volumes and flow rates. **E:** Restrictive pattern spirometry, pre- and postbronchodilator flow volume curve. Restriction was confirmed by measuring the lung volumes by helium dilution (not shown). **F:** Restrictive pattern spirometry, typical pre- and postbronchodilator volumes and flow rates.

Table 19–1. Normal arterial blood gas values on room air.

	pH	Pao_2 (mm Hg)	$Paco_2$ (mm Hg)
Sea level	7.38–7.42	85–95	36–42
5000 ft	7.36–7.40	65–75	35–40

$Paco_2$, partial pressure of arterial carbon dioxide; Pao_2, partial pressure of arterial oxygen; Sao_2, percent hemoglobin saturation.

Ammaddeo A, Fauroux B: Oxygen and carbon dioxide monitoring during sleep. Paediatr Respir Rev 2016;20:42–44. doi: 10.1016/j.prrv.2015.11.009 [PMID: 26724141].

Berend K, de Vries APJ, Gans ROB: Physiological approach to assessment of acid-base disturbances. N Engl J Med 2014;371:1434–1445 [PMID: 25295502].

Fouzas S, Priftis KN, Anthracopoulos MB: Pulse oximetry in pediatric practice. Pediatrics 2011;128:740 [PMID: 21930554].

DIAGNOSIS OF RESPIRATORY TRACT INFECTIONS

Respiratory tract infections may be caused by bacteria, viruses, atypical bacteria (eg, *Mycoplasma pneumoniae* and *Chlamydia pneumoniae*), *Mycobacterium tuberculosis*, nontuberculous *Mycobacterium*, or fungi (eg, *Aspergillus* and *Pneumocystis jirovecii*). The type of infection suspected, and appropriate diagnostic tests vary depending on factors such as the age of the child, underlying lung disease, immune function, and geographic region. Sources of respiratory tract secretions for diagnostic testing include nasopharyngeal and oropharyngeal swabs, expectorated and induced sputum, tracheal aspirates, direct lung or pleural fluid sampling, bronchoalveolar lavage (BAL) fluid, and gastric aspirates. Spontaneously expectorated sputum is the least invasive way to collect a sample, though it is rarely available or satisfactory from patients younger than 6 years. Sputum induction, performed by inhaling aerosolized hypertonic saline, is a relatively safe, noninvasive means of obtaining lower airway secretions. Tracheal aspirates can be obtained easily from patients with endotracheal or tracheostomy tubes. Cultures of the respiratory tract are commonly used to identify airway pathogens, but molecular diagnostic tests, based on polymerase chain reaction (PCR) amplification and detection of nucleic acid from microbes, are increasingly utilized and are often more rapid and sensitive. Blood and urine samples also may be used for serologic and antigen testing. Because of the coronavirus disease-19 (COVID-19) pandemic, rapid antigen tests to detect Sars-CoV-2 infections have become a common point of care testing option.

Hayden MK, et al. Infectious Diseases Society of America Guidelines on the Diagnosis of COVID-19: Antigen Testing. Infectious Diseases Society of America 2022; Version 2.0.0. Available at https://www.idsociety.org/practice-guideline/covid-19-guideline-antigen testing/ [PMID: 36702617].
Rueda et al: Etiology and challenges of diagnostic testing of community-acquired pneumonia in children and adolescents. BMC Pediatr 2022;22:169 [PMID: 35361166].

IMAGING OF THE RESPIRATORY TRACT

The plain chest radiograph (CXR) remains the foundation for investigating the pediatric thorax. Both frontal (posterior-anterior) and lateral views should be obtained if feasible. The radiograph is useful for evaluating chest wall, heart size and shape, mediastinum, diaphragm, airways, and lung parenchyma. When pleural fluid is suspected, lateral decubitus radiographs may help determine the extent and mobility of the fluid. Lung ultrasound is a point of care test for effusion and complicated pneumonia. When a foreign body is suspected, forced expiratory radiographs may show focal air trapping and shift of the mediastinum to the contralateral side. Lateral neck radiographs can be useful in assessing the size of adenoids and tonsils and in differentiating croup from epiglottitis, the latter being associated with the "thumbprint" sign.

Fluoroscopic studies, including upper gastrointestinal (UGI) series, esophagram, or videofluoroscopic swallow studies (VFSS), are indicated for detection of esophageal compression or swallowing dysfunction in patients with dysphagia, tracheoesophageal fistula, vascular rings and slings, or unexplained cough/respiratory symptoms. Fluoroscopy or ultrasound of the diaphragm can detect paralysis by demonstrating paradoxical movement of the involved hemidiaphragm.

Chest CT is recommended for evaluation of congenital lung lesions, pleural disease (eg, effusion or recurrent pneumothorax), complicated pneumonia, mediastinal disorders (eg, lymphadenopathy), diffuse lung disease (DLD), and bronchiectasis. The addition of contrast helps evaluate masses, nodules, and vasculature. Magnetic resonance imaging (MRI) is also useful for defining vascular and bronchial anatomy. Concerns about radiation exposure in children led to the *Image Gently* campaign, an initiative of the Alliance for Radiation Safety in Pediatric Imaging, dedicated to increasing awareness of the need for radiation protection for children.

Don S et al: Image gently campaign back to basics initiative: ten steps to help manage radiation dose in pediatric digital radiography. AJR Am J Roentgenol 2013;200(5):W431–W436 [PMID: 23617510].
Image Gently Campaign: http://www.imagegently.org/.
Schneebaum et al: Use and yield of chest computed tomography in the diagnostic evaluation of pediatric lung disease. Pediatrics 2009;124:472–479 [PMID: 19620200].

LARYNGOSCOPY & BRONCHOSCOPY

Direct visualization of airway anatomy can be useful for diagnosis or for therapeutic maneuvers. Nasopharyngoscopy or laryngoscopy is used to evaluate the upper airway while the patient is awake. Flexible or rigid bronchoscopy is used to evaluate both the upper and lower airways while the patient is sedated with general anesthesia. Indications for laryngoscopy include hoarseness, stridor, symptoms of obstructive sleep apnea (OSA), and inducible laryngeal obstruction (ILO). Indications for bronchoscopy include wheezing, suspected foreign body, suspected or known tracheoesophageal fistula, recurrent pneumonia, persistent atelectasis, chronic cough, and hemoptysis.

Rigid and flexible bronchoscopes have individual advantages, and for some patients, both should be used sequentially under the same anesthesia. The rigid, open tube instruments have the best optics for visualization of laryngeal cleft, subglottic stenosis, or other structural abnormality and allow surgical intervention to be easily achieved, such as removal of a foreign body. Flexible laryngoscopes and bronchoscopes are of a smaller caliber, and therefore do not stent the airway open during the procedure. Dynamic airway collapse is better evaluated by flexible bronchoscopy, and distal airways can be evaluated better with the flexible scope than with the rigid scope. BAL, a sterile water washing of the distal airway and alveoli, is performed during most diagnostic flexible bronchoscopies. BAL is useful to sample the alveolar space for infection, inflammation, or hemorrhage. Although removal of foreign bodies has been achieved with the flexible bronchoscope, the standard of care in most institutions is to remove foreign bodies via the rigid bronchoscope.

A flexible bronchoscope can also be used to assess placement and patency of an endotracheal tube or to perform awake tracheoscopy (visualizing the distal airways through a tracheostomy tube). In fiberoptic endoscopic evaluation of swallowing (FEES), a laryngoscope is used to visualize the larynx while the patient swallows liquids or food that has been dyed blue or green.

Therapeutic flexible bronchoscopy is performed to suction thick secretions and remove clots or can be combined with interventional procedures including laser or cryotherapy. Transbronchial biopsy in children is limited mainly to rejection in lung transplant patients and may have a role in diagnosing sarcoidosis, but there is low diagnostic yield in most other conditions. Endobronchial ultrasound-guided transbronchial needle aspiration (EBUS-TBNA) has been reported to be useful for evaluation of infection. Video-assisted thoracoscopic lung surgery (VATS) provides a more substantial specimen for pathologic assessment.

Giraldo-Cadavid LF et al: Accuracy of endoscopic and videofluoroscopic evaluations of swallowing for oropharyngeal dysphagia. Laryngoscope 2017 Sep;127(9):2002–2010 [PMID: 27859291].

Nicholai T: The role of rigid and flexible bronchoscopy in children. Paediatr Respir Rev 2011;12:190–195 [PMID: 21722848].

Piccione J et al: Pediatric advanced diagnostic and interventional bronchoscopy. Semin Pediatr Surg 2021;30(3):1501065 [PMID: 34172210].

GENERAL THERAPY FOR PEDIATRIC LUNG DISEASES

OXYGEN THERAPY

Supplemental oxygen (O_2) therapy is used to relieve hypoxemia. The benefits of oxygen may include reducing the work of breathing, reducing respiratory symptoms, relaxing the pulmonary vasculature, and improving feeding tolerance. Patients breathing spontaneously can receive supplemental O_2 via nasal cannula, head hood, or face mask (including simple, rebreathing, nonrebreathing, or Venturi masks). The goal of O_2 therapy is to achieve a PaO_2 of 65–90 mm Hg (at sea level) or SpO_2 above 90%. Lower PaO_2 or SpO_2 levels may be acceptable in certain situations, particularly cyanotic congenital heart disease. The actual O_2 concentration achieved by nasal cannula or mask depends on the flow rate, the type of mask used, and the patient's size. Small changes

in flow rate during O_2 administration by nasal cannula can lead to substantial changes in inspired oxygen concentration in young infants. The amount of oxygen required to correct hypoxemia may vary with activity; for example, an infant with chronic lung disease who uses 0.25 L/min may need more with sleep, activity, or feeding.

Head hood O_2 delivery is not often used if the patient can use a nasal cannula, which allows more mobility. Even at high flow rates, O_2 by nasal cannula rarely delivers inspired oxygen concentrations greater than 40%–45%. In contrast, partial rebreathing and nonrebreathing masks or head hoods can achieve inspired oxygen concentrations as high as 90%–100%. Heated humidified high-flow nasal cannula oxygen delivery allows a much higher high flow rate and is used with increasing frequency when standard low flow supplemental O_2 is not meeting SpO_2 goals.

Levy SD et al: High-flow oxygen therapy and other inhaled therapies in intensive care units. Lancet 2016;387:1867–1878 [PMID: 27203510].

Luo et al: Efficacy of high-flow nasal cannula vs standard oxygen therapy or nasal continuous positive airway pressure in children with respiratory distress: a meta-analysis. J Pediatr 2019;215: 199–208 [PMID: 31570155].

Rahimi S: New guidelines for home oxygen therapy in children. Lancet Respir Med 2019;7(4):301–302. doi: 10.1016/S2213-2600(19)30076-1 [PMID: 30857991].

Walsh BK, Smallwood CD: Pediatric oxygen therapy: a review and update. Respir Care 2017;62(6):645–661. doi: 10.4187/respcare.05245 [PMID: 28546370].

INHALATION OF MEDICATIONS

Inhaled medications are a therapeutic mainstay for pediatric respiratory conditions and are routinely used in patients with CF, BPD, and asthma, as well as in acute illnesses such as infectious laryngotracheobronchitis and bronchiolitis (Table 19–2). Short-acting β-agonists and anticholinergics provide acute bronchodilatation, whereas inhaled corticosteroids and cromones provide anti-inflammatory effects. Nebulized antibiotics have documented benefit in CF and nebulized mucolytic medications (eg, rhDNAse and hypertonic saline) are used in CF and other conditions with impaired secretion control such as non-CF bronchiectasis.

The medications can be delivered by pressurized metered dose inhaler (pMDI), breath activated pMDI, dry powder inhaler (DPI), or compressed air-driven wet nebulization. Careful attention to delivery technique is critical to optimize medication delivery to the airways. A valved holding chamber or similar spacer should be used with pMDI use, and this technique has been shown to be effective in infants as young as 4 months. A face-mask interface is recommended for both pMDI and wet nebulization in infants and toddlers; a simple mouthpiece suffices for older children who can form a seal around the mouthpiece. Delivery technique should be assessed and reviewed at each clinical visit.

Table 19–2. Common uses for inhaled medications in pediatric respiratory illness.

Disease Process	Short-Acting Bronchodilator	Anticholinergic Bronchodilator	Inhaled Steroid	Other
Asthma	Acute relief and prior to exercise to prevent exercise-induced bronchospasm	Acute relief	Chronic use for control of inflammation	Inhaled corticosteroid + long-acting bronchodilator for control
Bronchopulmonary dysplasia	Acute relief	Acute relief	Chronic use for control of inflammation if bronchial reactivity is present	
Cystic fibrosis	Prior to airway clearance	Limited data	Chronic use for control of inflammation if bronchial reactivity is present	Mucolytics and inhaled antibiotics
Infectious laryngotracheo-bronchitis (croup)	Acute relief (racemic epinephrine)		Acute relief (nebulized steroid)	
Bronchiolitis (acute infectious)	Acute relief. May have limited benefit.		Ongoing investigation of inhaled epinephrine and hypertonic saline	Recent interest in inhaled epinephrine and hypertonic saline

Lavorini F, Janson C, Braido F, Stratelis G, Lokke A: What to consider before prescribing inhaled medications: a pragmatic approach for evaluating the current inhaler landscape. Ther Adv Respir Dis 2019;13:1–28. doi: 10.1177/1753466619884532 [PMID: 31805823].

Restreppo MI, Keyt H, Reyes LF: Aerosolized antibiotics. Respir Care 2015;60:762–773 [PMID: 26070573].

AIRWAY CLEARANCE THERAPY

Airway clearance is the mobilization and expulsion of airway secretions or debris. Innate airway clearance comprises mucociliary clearance and cough. Airway clearance therapies intend to reproduce or augment these functions. Currently available airway clearance techniques include manual percussion or chest physiotherapy, postural drainage, forced expiratory technique (huff cough), autogenic drainage, positive expiratory pressure with handheld devices, intermittent positive pressure breathing, high-frequency chest wall oscillation or compression, intrapulmonary percussive ventilation, and manual or mechanical insufflation-exsufflation. All the above except insufflation-exsufflation techniques have been used in CF, bronchiectasis, and tracheobronchomalacia due to impaired mucociliary function. Often, therapies are combined (eg, high-frequency chest wall compression plus huff cough) to maximize the effect. Insufflation-exsufflation (commonly called cough assist) is used when cough force is weakened as in neuromuscular diseases, neurologic injury, or prolonged immobility. The decision about which technique to use should be based on the patient's underlying airway clearance impairment, age, preference, and ability to participate. Bronchodilators or mucolytic medications may be given prior to or during airway clearance therapy. If prescribed, inhaled corticosteroids and inhaled antibiotics should be given after airway clearance therapy so that the airways are first cleared of secretions, allowing the medications to maximally penetrate the lung. Airway clearance has not been shown to be beneficial for patients with acute respiratory illnesses such as pneumonia, bronchiolitis, and asthma. Contraindications to airway clearance therapy include retained foreign body, hemoptysis, untreated pneumothorax, chest trauma, recent airway or open chest surgery, and concerns for increased intracranial pressure. Daily exercise is an important adjunctive therapy for airway clearance and overall lung health.

McIlwaine M et al: Personalizing airway clearance in chronic lung disease. Eur Respir Rev 2017;26:143 [PMID: 28223396].

AVOIDANCE OF ENVIRONMENTAL HAZARDS

Environmental insults can aggravate existing lung diseases, impair pulmonary function, and cause lung disease in children. Outdoor air pollution (ozone and particulates), indoor pollution, diesel exhaust, and household fungi are examples. Environmental tobacco smoke dramatically increases childhood pulmonary morbidity. There is increasing evidence that secondhand exposure to other tobacco products, such as e-cigarettes, is harmful. Smoking family members should be counseled to quit smoking and do everything possible to minimize environmental smoke exposure to the people around them, both secondhand (smoking inhaled directly by child in the room) and thirdhand (smoke inhaled from family member's clothes) exposures. Homes with mold should have remediation, particularly if children with lung disease are in residence. Ozone exposure can be limited by avoiding outdoor activities during the height of daily ozone levels. Recent data show that improvements in air quality reduce lung function impairments in children. Pet exposure and infestations such as cockroaches or mice may be a significant trigger in children who have asthma and allergies to pets or pests.

Bozier et al: The evolving landscape of e-cigarettes: a systematic review of recent evidence. Chest 2020;157:1362–1390 [PMID: 32006591].

Jenssen et al: Protecting children and adolescents from tobacco and nicotine. Pediatrics 2023;151(5):e2023061805 [PMID: 37066689].

Pfeffer PE, Mudway IS, Grigg J: Air pollution and asthma: mechanism of harm and considerations for clinical interventions. Chest 2021;159(4):1346–1355. doi: org/10.1016/j.chest.2020.10.053 [PMID: 33461908].

Tiotiu AI et al: Impact of air pollution on asthma outcomes. Int J Environ Res Public Health 2020;17(17):6212. doi: 10.3390/ijerph17176212 [PMID: 32867076].

Urman R, Garcia E, Berhane K, McConnell R, Gauderman WJ, Gilliland F: The potential effects of policy-driven air pollution interventions on childhood lung development. Am J Respir Crit Care Med 2020;201(4):438–444. doi: 10.1164/rccm.201903-0670OC [PMID: 31644884].

▼ DISORDERS OF AIRFLOW OBSTRUCTION

Airflow obstruction can be extrathoracic (superior to the thoracic inlet, eg, nose, mouth, pharynx, and larynx) or intrathoracic (inferior to the thoracic inlet, eg, trachea, bronchi, and terminal bronchioles). Extrathoracic or upper airway obstruction disrupts the inspiratory phase of respiration producing stridor or "noisy breathing." The differential of upper airway obstruction includes congenital abnormalities, viral infections including croup, and foreign-body aspiration. Intrathoracic or small airway obstruction disrupts the expiratory phase of respiration producing wheezing and prolongation of the expiratory phase. The differential for small airway obstruction includes infection, airway compression (eg, lymphadenopathy), and chronic lung diseases causing airway inflammation such as disorders of mucociliary clearance, dysphagia with aspiration, and asthma.

After assessing whether the obstruction is extrathoracic or intrathoracic, the next challenge is to determine if the obstruction is fixed or variable. Variable obstructions are typically due to dynamic changes in airway caliber between inspiration and exhalation that occurs with laryngomalacia, tracheomalacia, or bronchomalacia producing a central monophonic wheeze. Asthma causes obstruction distally with exhalation and produces a polyphonic or musical wheeze originating from many small airways. Unlike variable obstructions, fixed obstructions are consistent through the breathing cycle. Fixed obstructions are often associated with anatomic abnormalities such as airway stenosis or external compression that may be amenable to surgical correction (Table 19–3).

The onset and progression of the obstruction can provide important clues as to etiology and help determine the urgency of evaluation and management. Obstructions due to dynamic airway collapse (malacia) often improve with age, whereas fixed obstructions may worsen over time or fail to improve with age. Acute onset extrathoracic obstruction is often infectious. Clinical indications that the obstruction is severe include high-pitched stridor or wheezing, biphasic stridor, drooling or dysphagia, poor-intensity breath sounds, severe retractions, and pallor or cyanosis.

Helpful diagnostic studies in the evaluation of upper airway obstruction include chest and lateral neck radiographs and laryngoscopy and/or bronchoscopy. Patients with symptoms of OSA should have a PSG (see section Sleep-Disordered Breathing). Patients who have symptoms of severe chronic obstruction should have an electrocardiogram (ECG) and/or echocardiography (echo) to evaluate for right ventricular hypertrophy and pulmonary hypertension.

Table 19–3. Classification and causes of upper airway obstruction.

Fixed, Extrathoracic, Not Acute	Fixed, Extrathoracic, Acute	Fixed Intrathoracic, Intrinsic	Fixed, Intrathoracic, Extrinsic
Vocal cord paralysis	Infectious laryngotracheobronchitis	Tracheal stenosis	Tumor (compressing the airways)
Laryngeal atresia/web	Epiglottitis	Complete tracheal rings	Vascular ring or sling
Laryngocele/cyst	Bacterial tracheitis	Foreign-body aspiration	Bronchogenic cyst
Laryngeal papillomas	Anaphylaxis	Endobronchial tumor	Congenital pulmonary airway malformation
Subglottic hemangioma	Angioneurotic edema		Esophageal duplication
Tracheal web	Foreign-body aspiration		Congenital lobar overdistention

Diagnostic studies for intrathoracic obstruction may include CXRs, computed tomography (CT), sweat test, PFTs, and bronchoscopy. In older children, flow volume loops created during PFT maneuvers can differentiate fixed from variable airflow obstruction and may identify the site of obstruction. Children with asthma may show improvement in airflow obstruction after administration of albuterol. Treatment should be directed at relieving airway obstruction and correcting the underlying condition if possible.

UPPER AIRWAY OBSTRUCTION

LARYNGOMALACIA

ESSENTIALS OF DIAGNOSIS & TYPICAL FEATURES

▶ Presentation from birth or within the first few weeks of life.

▶ Intermittent, high-pitched, inspiratory stridor.

▶ Moderate to severe symptoms require visualization of the airway.

Laryngomalacia is a congenital disorder in which the cartilaginous support for the supraglottic structures is underdeveloped. It is the most common cause of variable extrathoracic airway obstruction and manifests as **intermittent stridor** in infants, usually within the first 6 weeks of life. Stridor is generally worse in the supine position, with increased activity or crying, with upper respiratory infections, and during feeding. Typically, the condition is benign and resolves by the time the child is 1 year of age, but occasionally signs can be more severe or persist beyond 2 years of age. In mildly affected patients without stridor at rest or retractions, diagnosis is based on history and treatment is not usually needed. In children with severe or atypical symptoms, awake laryngoscopy is performed to confirm inspiratory collapse of an omega-shaped epiglottis with tight aryepiglottic folds. Surgical supraglottoplasty may be recommended in those children with severe stridor, retractions, OSA, and increased work of breathing or those with feeding difficulties or failure to thrive.

Thompson DM et al: Laryngomalacia: factors that influence disease severity and outcomes of management. Curr Opin Otolaryngol Head Neck Surg 2010;18(6):564 [PMID: 20962644].

Thorne MC, Garetz SL: Laryngomalacia: review and summary of current clinical practice in 2015. Paediatr Respir Rev 2016;17:3–8 [PMID: 25802018].

OTHER CAUSES OF CONGENITAL UPPER AIRWAY OBSTRUCTION

Other congenital lesions of the larynx usually present as fixed extrathoracic obstruction and are best evaluated by laryngoscopy and rigid bronchoscopy.

- Laryngeal atresia, also known as complete high airway obstruction syndrome (CHAOS), presents at birth with severe respiratory distress and is often fatal or requires a fetal EXIT (ex utero intrapartum treatment) with immediate tracheostomy.

- Laryngeal web, representing fusion of the anterior portion of the true vocal cords, is associated with hoarseness, aphonia, and stridor at birth and severe cases require intervention.

- Laryngeal cysts are superficial and are generally fluid filled. Laryngoceles communicate with the interior of the larynx and may be either air- or fluid-filled. Both require surgery or laser therapy.

- Subglottic hemangiomas are a rare cause of upper airway obstruction in infants and are associated with cutaneous vascular lesions of the skin in 50%–60% of patients. Although vascular malformations regress spontaneously, airway obstruction requires intervention. Medical management options include propranolol, systemic steroids, or intralesional steroids. Surgical intervention with laser ablation is usually successful. Tracheostomy is rarely required.

- Laryngeal cleft from failure of posterior cricoid fusion is an abnormality of the extrathoracic airway but rarely causes obstruction. Instead, patients may present with dysphagia and aspiration. Children with type 1 laryngeal cleft (at the level of the vocal cords) may or may not aspirate on a VFSS while children with types 2 and 3 clefts almost always do. All types of clefts may result in recurrent or chronic pneumonia and failure to thrive. The diagnosis is made by rigid laryngoscopy/bronchoscopy with attention to spreading the posterior glottic structures apart and assessing for the absence of tissue above the vocal folds. The decision to correct type 1 clefts should be made after multidisciplinary consideration of the pulmonary complications and other comorbidities. Repair of type 1 clefts may be addressed surgically or with an injection laryngoplasty. More severe clefts require surgical repair and may require tracheostomy. Normal swallow function without aspiration may not return for months, even after repair.

- Subglottic stenosis can be congenital or acquired (see acquired disorders of the extrathoracic airway).

Huoh KC, Rosbe KW: Infantile hemangiomas of the head and neck. Pediatr Clin North Am 2013;60(4):937–949 [PMID: 23905829].

Rutter MJ: Congenital laryngeal anomalies. Braz J Otorhinolaryngol 2014 Dec 80(6):533–539 [PMID: 25457074].

INFECTIOUS UPPER AIRWAY OBSTRUCTION

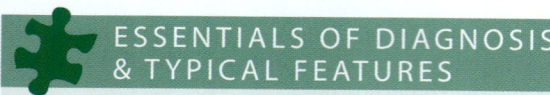

ESSENTIALS OF DIAGNOSIS & TYPICAL FEATURES

▶ New-onset stridor in the setting of an upper respiratory illness or fever.

Acute stridor is the main symptom of croup (viral laryngotracheobronchitis). The differential diagnosis of acute stridor includes epiglottitis, bacterial tracheitis, spasmodic croup, angioedema, laryngeal or esophageal foreign body, retropharyngeal or peritonsillar abscess, or occult presentation of congenital upper airway obstruction. These diagnoses should be considered when symptoms are atypical, or children are critically ill.

1. Croup

Croup generally affects young children 6 months to 5 years of age in the fall and early winter and is most often caused by *parainfluenza virus* serotypes. However, many other viral organisms as well as *M pneumoniae* can cause croup. Edema in the subglottic space accounts for the predominant signs of upper airway obstruction although inflammation of the entire airway is often present.

▶ Clinical Findings

A. Symptoms and Signs

Usually, a prodrome of upper respiratory tract symptoms is followed by a barking cough, laryngitis, and stridor. Fever is usually absent. Patients with mild disease may have stridor when agitated. As obstruction worsens, stridor occurs at rest, accompanied in severe cases by retractions, air hunger, cyanosis, and hypoxemia.

B. Imaging

Anteroposterior and lateral neck radiographs are not routinely indicated for patients with classic presentation of croup. Radiographs are indicated to evaluate for other causes in an atypical presentation or critically ill patient. In croup, a neck radiograph shows subglottic narrowing (the steeple sign) without the irregularities seen in tracheitis and a normal epiglottis. A severely ill patient should never be left unattended in the imaging suite.

▶ Treatment

Treatment of croup is based on the symptoms. Mild croup, signified by a barking cough and no stridor at rest, requires supportive therapy with oral hydration. Dexamethasone or inhaled steroid may be prescribed (see below). Conversely, patients with stridor at rest require active intervention. Oxygen should be administered to patients with oxygen desaturation. Nebulized racemic epinephrine (0.5 mL of 2.25% solution diluted in sterile saline) is commonly used because it has a rapid onset of action within 10–30 minutes, is effective in alleviating symptoms, and decreases the need for intubation.

The efficacy of glucocorticoids in croup is firmly established. Dexamethasone, 0.6 mg/kg intramuscularly as one dose, improves symptoms, reduces the duration of hospitalizations and frequency of intubations, and permits earlier discharge from the emergency department. Oral dexamethasone (0.15 mg/kg) may be equally effective for mild to moderate croup. Prednisolone is not inferior to dexamethasone in equivalent doses, and inhaled budesonide (2–4 mg) can improve symptoms and decrease hospital stay. The use of heliox, a mixture of helium and oxygen, improves turbulent airflow but is not superior to nebulized medication. Heliox use is limited to normoxic children because of its low fractional concentration of inspired oxygen.

If symptoms resolve within 3–4 hours of glucocorticoids and nebulized epinephrine, patients can safely be discharged. If, however, recurrent nebulized epinephrine treatments are required or if respiratory distress persists, patients require hospitalization for close observation, supportive care, and repeated steroid dosing or nebulization treatments as needed. In patients with impending respiratory failure, an airway must be established. Intubation with an endotracheal tube of slightly smaller diameter than would ordinarily be used is reasonably safe. Extubation should be accomplished within 2–3 days to minimize the risk of laryngeal injury. Other underlying causes should be considered in hospitalized patients with persistent symptoms over 3–4 days despite treatment, more severe cases requiring intubation or recurrent episodes.

▶ Prognosis

Most children with croup have an uneventful course and improve within a few days. Some evidence suggests that patients with a history of croup associated with wheezing may have airway hyperreactivity. It is not always clear if the hyperreactivity was present prior to the croup episode or if the viral infection causing croup altered airway function.

Petrocheilou A et al: Viral croup: diagnosis and a treatment algorithm. Ped Pulm 2014;49(5):421 [PMID: 24596395].

Tyler A et al: Variation in inpatient croup management and outcomes. Pediatrics 2017;139(4):e20163582. doi: 10.1542/peds.2016-3582 [PMID: 28292873].

2. Epiglottitis

Epiglottitis is rare in countries with immunization programs that include the *Haemophilus influenzae* conjugate vaccine. If disease occurs, it is likely to be associated with *H influenzae* in unimmunized children, or another organism such as non-typeable *H influenzae*, *Neisseria meningitidis*, or *Streptococcus* species in immunized populations.

► Clinical Findings

A. Symptoms and Signs

The classic presentation is a sudden onset of high fever, dysphagia, drooling, muffled voice, inspiratory retractions, cyanosis, and soft stridor. Patients often sit in the so-called sniffing position, with the neck hyperextended and the chin stretched forward, which gives them the best airway possible under the circumstances. Progression to total airway obstruction may occur and result in respiratory arrest. The definitive diagnosis is made by direct inspection of the epiglottis, a procedure that should be done by an experienced airway specialist under controlled conditions (typically in the operating room during intubation). The typical findings are a cherry-red and swollen epiglottis and swollen arytenoids.

B. Imaging

Diagnostically, lateral neck radiographs may be helpful in demonstrating a classic "thumbprint" sign caused by the swollen epiglottis. Obtaining radiographs, however, may delay important airway intervention.

► Treatment

Once the diagnosis of epiglottitis is made, endotracheal intubation should be performed by an experienced clinician. Most anesthesiologists prefer general anesthesia (but not muscle relaxants) to facilitate intubation. After an airway is established, cultures of the blood and epiglottis should be obtained, and the patient should be started on appropriate intravenous antibiotics to cover *H influenzae* and *Streptococcus* species (ceftriaxone sodium or an equivalent cephalosporin). Extubation can usually be accomplished in 24–48 hours, when direct inspection shows a significant reduction in the size of the epiglottis. Intravenous antibiotics should be continued for 2–3 days, followed by oral antibiotics to complete a 10-day course.

► Prognosis

Prompt recognition and appropriate treatment usually results in rapid resolution of swelling and inflammation. Recurrence is unusual.

Guardiani E et al: Supraglottitis in the era following widespread immunization against *Haemophilus influenzae* type b: evolving principles in diagnosis and management. Laryngoscope 2010;120(11):2183 [PMID: 20925091].

Tibballs J et al: Symptoms and signs differentiating croup and epiglottitis. J Paediatr Child Health 2011;47(3):77 [PMID: 21091577].

3. Bacterial Tracheitis

Acute bacterial tracheitis (pseudomembranous croup) is a severe life-threatening form of laryngotracheobronchitis. As the management of severe viral croup has been improved with the use of dexamethasone, and vaccination has decreased the incidence of epiglottitis, tracheitis is relatively more common as a cause of a pediatric airway emergency requiring admission to the pediatric intensive care unit. This diagnosis must be high in the differential when a patient presents with severe upper airway obstruction and fever. The organism most often isolated is *Staphylococcus aureus*, but organisms such as *H influenzae*, group A *Streptococcus pyogenes*, *Neisseria* species, *Moraxella catarrhalis*, and others have been reported. Viral co-infections including influenza are common. The disease probably represents localized mucosal invasion of bacteria in patients with primary viral croup, resulting in edema, purulent secretions, and pseudo membranes. Chronic tracheitis can cause cough or other symptoms of upper airway obstruction in children with tracheostomies (a nidus for infection) or impaired proximal airway clearance like tracheomalacia. Chronic tracheitis typically presents in an outpatient setting with a more indolent and less severe clinical syndrome than acute bacterial tracheitis.

► Clinical Findings

A. Symptoms and Signs

The early clinical picture is like viral croup; however, instead of gradual improvement, patients develop higher fever, toxicity, and progressive severe upper airway obstruction unresponsive to standard croup therapy. The incidence of sudden respiratory arrest or progressive respiratory failure is high, requiring airway intervention. Findings of toxic shock and acute respiratory distress syndrome may also be seen.

B. Laboratory Findings and Imaging

The white cell count is usually elevated with a left shift. Cultures of tracheal secretions usually demonstrate one of the causative organisms, but blood cultures are often negative. Lateral neck radiographs show a normal epiglottis but severe subglottic and tracheal narrowing with an irregular contour of the proximal tracheal mucosa. Endoscopy showing a normal epiglottis and the presence of copious purulent tracheal secretions and membranes confirms the diagnosis.

► Treatment

Most patients with bacterial tracheitis will be intubated because the incidence of respiratory arrest or progressive respiratory failure is high. Patients may require direct visualization and debridement of the airway in a controlled environment. Patients may also require intensive care for humidification and frequent suctioning to prevent endotracheal tube obstruction by purulent tracheal secretions.

Intravenous antibiotics are indicated to cover *S aureus*, *H influenzae*, and the other organisms. Glucocorticoid therapy may be helpful. Thick secretions persist for several days, usually resulting in longer periods of intubation for bacterial tracheitis than for epiglottitis or croup. Despite the severity of this illness, the reported mortality rate is very low if it is recognized and treated promptly.

Dawood FS et al: Complications and associated bacterial coinfections among children hospitalized with seasonal or pandemic influenza, United States, 2003–2010. J Infect Dis 2014;209(5):686 [PMID: 23986545].

Tebruegge M et al: Bacterial tracheitis: a multi-centre perspective. Scand J Infect Dis 2009;41(8):548–557 [PMID: 19401934].

VOCAL FOLD IMMOBILITY

ESSENTIALS OF DIAGNOSIS & TYPICAL FEATURES

► Hoarseness or stridor.
► May present with difficulty swallowing.

Unilateral or bilateral vocal fold (cord) weakness or paralysis may be congenital; or more commonly, may result from injury to the recurrent laryngeal nerve. Patients may present with varying degrees of hoarseness, dysphagia, or high-pitched stridor. If partial function is preserved (paresis), the adductor muscles tend to move better than the abductors, with a resultant high-pitched inspiratory stridor and normal voice. Risk factors for acquired paresis/paralysis include difficult delivery (especially face presentation), neck and thoracic surgery (eg, ductal ligation or repair of tracheoesophageal fistula), trauma, mediastinal masses, and central nervous system disease (eg, Arnold-Chiari malformation). The differential diagnosis includes damage to the tissue of the vocal fold from traumatic intubation. Unilateral cord paralysis is more likely to occur on the left because the left recurrent laryngeal nerve takes a longer course inferiorly near major thoracic structures. With bilateral vocal cord paralysis, the closer to midline the cords are positioned, the greater the airway obstruction; the more lateral the cords are positioned, the greater the tendency to aspirate and experience hoarseness or aphonia.

Airway intervention (tracheostomy) is rarely indicated in unilateral paralysis but is often necessary for bilateral paralysis. Clinically, paralysis can be assessed by direct visualization of vocal fold function with laryngoscopy or more invasively by recording the electrical activity of the muscles (electromyography). Electromyogram recordings can differentiate vocal fold paralysis from arytenoid dislocation, which has prognostic value. Recovery is related to the severity of nerve injury and the potential for healing.

King EF, Blumin JH: Vocal cord paralysis in children. Curr Opin Otolaryngol Head Neck Surg 2009;17(6):483 [PMID: 19730263].

INDUCIBLE LARYNGEAL OBSTRUCTION

ESSENTIALS OF DIAGNOSIS & TYPICAL FEATURES

► Acute stridor with exercise or anxiety.
► Diagnosis based on clinical suspicion or exercise laryngoscopy.

Inducible laryngeal obstruction (ILO) is a group of disorders previously called vocal cord dysfunction (VCD) that can present in older children and teenagers as acute shortness of breath and noisy breathing when the glottis or supraglottis inappropriately narrows during exercise. Relaxation of the laryngeal structures will resolve the symptoms, but patients may receive asthma therapy inappropriately because the appearance can mimic an acute asthma exacerbation. ILO is important to diagnose because it will not resolve with asthma therapy and can prevent children from having a healthy lifestyle that includes exercise. ILO can be distinguished from asthma because asthma is typically associated with expiratory wheezing usually heard through a stethoscope whereas the noisy breathing with an ILO exacerbation is often audible on inspiration (though some patients may describe their symptoms as wheezing), usually lack cough symptoms, and can sometimes feel discomfort at the neck base. Diagnosis can be made with a classic history and high clinical suspicion, but a laryngoscopy performed during symptoms showing inappropriate laryngeal narrowing is the gold standard method. Treatment includes pursed lip breathing to allow laryngeal relaxation and can be taught by a speech language pathologist or other experienced clinician. Treatment by a multidisciplinary team including a psychologist may be needed. Symptoms may recur during times of increased stress.

Olin JT et al: Inducible laryngeal obstruction during exercise. Phys Sportsmed 2015;43(1):14 [PMID: 25644598].

SUBGLOTTIC STENOSIS

ESSENTIALS OF DIAGNOSIS & TYPICAL FEATURES

► Chronic or recurrent stridor.
► History of airway trauma is common in acquired subglottic stenosis.

Subglottic stenosis may be congenital, or more commonly may result from endotracheal intubation. Neonates and infants are particularly vulnerable to subglottic injury from intubation. The subglottis is the narrowest part of an infant's airway, and the cricoid cartilage, which supports the subglottis, is the only cartilage that completely encircles the airway. This area is therefore susceptible to injury when an endotracheal tube is inserted. The clinical presentation may vary from asymptomatic to severe upper airway obstruction. Subglottic stenosis should be suspected in children who repeatedly fail extubation or children with multiple, prolonged, or severe episodes of croup. Diagnosis is made by direct visualization of the subglottic space with bronchoscopy and maneuvers to size the airway. Tracheostomy is often required when airway compromise is severe. Laryngotracheal reconstruction, in which a cartilage graft from another source (eg, rib) is used to expand the airway, has become the standard procedure for severe subglottic stenosis in children. In mild cases, balloon dilation of the subglottis is a less invasive alternative.

Jefferson ND, Cohen AP, Rutter MJ: Subglottic stenosis. Semin Pediatr Surg Jun 2016;25(3):138–143 [PMID: 27301599].

CONGENITAL INTRATHORACIC AIRWAY OBSTRUCTION

Children with disorders of the intrathoracic airway often present with expiratory sounds such as wheeze, recurrent cough, and/or recurrent pneumonia due to retained secretions. Congenital disorders of intrathoracic airway obstruction can present acutely or with recurrent symptoms of lower airway obstruction. The differential diagnosis for intrathoracic airway obstruction includes tracheobronchomalacia, extrinsic compression from a vascular ring or sling, and congenital anomalies such as bronchogenic cysts.

TRACHEOBRONCHOMALACIA

ESSENTIALS OF DIAGNOSIS & TYPICAL FEATURES

▶ Chronic monophonic wheeze with or without a barking cough.
▶ Respiratory symptoms do not respond to bronchodilators.

▶ Pathogenesis

Tracheomalacia or bronchomalacia exists when the cartilaginous framework of the airway is inadequate to maintain normal airway patency. Airway collapse is dynamic and can lead to partial or complete airway obstruction. Because infant airway cartilage is normally soft, infants have some degree of dynamic collapse of the central airway. Congenital or innate abnormalities of the trachealis or tracheal cartilage are associated with developmental syndromes and other congenital abnormalities such as esophageal atresia with tracheoesophageal fistula or extrinsic compression from a vascular ring. Acquired tracheomalacia has been associated with long-term ventilation of preterm infants due to delayed cartilaginous development with or without direct positive pressure. Other acquired causes include severe tracheobronchitis, surgical repair of airway anomalies such as complete tracheal rings, extrinsic airway compression due to tumors, abscess or cysts, and compression as seen in congenital heart disease with associated ventricular hypertrophy or vascular anomalies.

▶ Clinical Findings

Coarse and recurrent wheezing, cough, or stridor that do not respond to bronchodilators are common findings. Preterm infants with tracheal or bronchomalacia may have hypoxemia that requires continuous nasal cannula or positive pressure ventilation. Symptoms classically present insidiously over the first few months of life and can increase with agitation, excitement, activity, or upper respiratory tract infections. Diagnosis can be made by bronchoscopy or combined inspiratory/expiratory imaging modalities like CT or MRI.

▶ Treatment

Observation is usually indicated for mild symptoms, which generally improve over time with growth. Coexisting lesions such as tracheoesophageal fistulas and vascular rings need primary repair. In severe cases of tracheomalacia, surgical intervention (eg, posterior tracheopexy, aortopexy, or stents) or chronic ventilation (noninvasive or invasive) may be indicated. Unfortunately, tracheostomy without mechanical ventilation is rarely satisfactory because airway collapse continues to exist below the tip of the artificial airway. In children with tracheomalacia, protracted bronchitis due to retained secretions may contribute to chronic cough. Treatment with antibiotics is often effective but may need to be repeated if the malacia and airway obstruction does not resolve.

▶ Prognosis

Tracheobronchomalacia symptom resolution depends on the severity and extent of the malacia and any underlying illness in the child. Children with mild malacia without other underlying lung disease or neuromuscular disease may have at least partial resolution by the time they are 3–4 years old.

Fraga JC, Jennings RW, Kim PC: Pediatric tracheomalacia. Semin Pediatr Surg 2016;25(3):156–164 [PMID: 27301602].

Goyal V, Masters IB, Chang AB: Interventions for primary (intrinsic) tracheomalacia in children. Cochrane Database Syst Rev 2012;CD005304 [PMID: 23076914].

VASCULAR RINGS & SLINGS

ESSENTIALS OF DIAGNOSIS & TYPICAL FEATURES

▶ Characterized by chronic barking cough, wheeze.

▶ Diagnosed with an UGI fluoroscopy series showing esophageal compression.

The most common vascular anomaly to compress the trachea or esophagus is a vascular ring. A vascular ring can be formed by a double aortic arch or a right aortic arch with left ligamentum arteriosum or a patent ductus arteriosus. The pulmonary sling is created when the left pulmonary artery branches off the right pulmonary artery. Other common vascular anomalies that can cause tracheal compression include a left-sided origin of the brachiocephalic artery and a right-sided origin of the left carotid artery. The pulmonary sling may compress the trachea but can also compress the right upper lobe bronchus or the right mainstem takeoff. A pulmonary sling is associated with long segment tracheal stenosis 50% of the time.

▶ Clinical Findings

Symptoms of chronic airway obstruction (eg, stridor, coarse wheezing, and croupy cough) are often worse in the supine position. Respiratory compromise is most severe with double aortic arch and may lead to apnea, respiratory arrest, or even death. Esophageal compression may result in feeding difficulties. UGI fluoroscopy series showing esophageal compression is the mainstay of diagnosis in all but anomalous innominate or carotid artery. CXRs and echos may miss abnormalities. Airway compression can best be assessed by bronchoscopy, and anatomy can be further defined by angiography, chest CT with contrast, or magnetic resonance angiography.

▶ Treatment

Patients with significant symptoms require surgical correction, especially those with double aortic arch. Symptoms usually improve following correction, but patients may have persistent but milder symptoms of airway obstruction with associated tracheomalacia.

Backer CL et al: Vascular rings. Semin Pediatr Surg 2016;25(3): 165–175 [PMID: 27301603].

McLaren CA, Elliott MJ, Roebuck DJ: Vascular compression of the airway in children. Paediatr Respir Rev 2008;9(2):85–94 [PMID: 18513668].

BRONCHOGENIC CYSTS

ESSENTIALS OF DIAGNOSIS & TYPICAL FEATURES

▶ Can present with symptoms of airway compression, infection, or chest pain.

▶ Chest radiograph (CXR) may show a spherical lesion along the airway.

Bronchogenic cysts generally occur in the middle mediastinum (see section Mediastinal Masses) near the carina and adjacent to the major bronchi but can be found elsewhere in the lung. They range in size from 2 to 10 cm. Cyst walls are thin and may contain air, pus, mucus, or blood. Cysts develop from abnormal lung budding of the primitive foregut and can occur in conjunction with other congenital pulmonary malformations such as pulmonary sequestration or lobar emphysema.

▶ Clinical Findings

A. Symptoms and Signs

Bronchogenic cysts can present acutely with respiratory distress in early childhood due to airway compression or with symptoms of infection. Other patients present with chronic symptoms such as chest pain, chronic wheezing, cough, intermittent tachypnea, recurrent pneumonia, or recurrent stridor, depending on the location and size of the cysts and the degree of airway compression. Still other patients remain asymptomatic until adulthood. However, all asymptomatic cysts will eventually become symptomatic; chest pain is the most common presenting complaint. The physical examination is often normal.

B. Laboratory Findings and Imaging Studies

CXRs can show air trapping and hyperinflation of the affected lobes or a spherical lesion with or without an air-fluid level. However, smaller lesions may not be seen on CXRs. CT scan is the preferred imaging study and can differentiate solid versus cystic mediastinal masses and define the cyst's relationship to the airways and the rest of the lung. Fluoroscopy can help determine whether the lesion communicates with the gastrointestinal tract. MRI and ultrasound are other imaging modalities used.

▶ Treatment

Treatment is surgical resection. Resection should be performed as soon as the cyst is detected to avoid future complications including infection. Postoperatively, vigorous pulmonary physiotherapy is required to prevent complications (atelectasis or infection of the lung distal to the site of resection of the cyst).

Chowdhury MM, Chakraboty S: Imaging of congenital lung mal-formations. Semin Pediatr Surg 2015;24(4):168–175 [PMID: 26051049].

Durell J, Lajhoo K: Congenital cystic lesions of the lung. Early Human Dev 2014;90(12):935–939 [PMID: 25448785].

FOREIGN-BODY ASPIRATION & CHOKING

ESSENTIALS OF DIAGNOSIS & TYPICAL FEATURES

► Sudden onset of coughing or respiratory distress.

► Choking or difficulty vocalizing.

► Asymmetrical physical findings of decreased breath sounds or localized wheezing.

► Asymmetrical radiographic findings, especially with forced expiratory view.

Aspiration of a foreign body into the respiratory tract is a significant cause of accidental death each year. The foreign body can lodge anywhere along the respiratory tract. Typically, the foreign body lodges in the supraglottic airway, triggering protective reflexes that result in laryngospasm. Small objects such as coins may pass through the glottis and obstruct the trachea. Signs at the time of aspiration can include coughing, choking, or wheezing. Children 6 months to 3 years are at the highest risk. Onset is generally abrupt, with a history of the child running with food in the mouth or playing with seeds, small coins, or toys. The history may also suggest that an older sibling or child may have fed age-inappropriate foods (eg, nuts and seeds, corn/popcorn, hard candy, carrot slices, or hot dogs) to the younger child.

The diagnosis of choking is established by acute onset with *inability* to vocalize or cough and cyanosis with marked distress (complete obstruction), or with drooling, stridor, and *ability* to vocalize (partial obstruction). Without treatment, progressive cyanosis, loss of consciousness, seizures, bradycardia, and cardiopulmonary arrest can follow.

If a foreign body is in the lower respiratory tract, the acute cough or wheezing may diminish over time only to recur later as chronic cough or persistent localized or monophonic wheezing, asymmetrical breath sounds on chest examination, or recurrent pneumonia in one location. Foreign-body aspiration should be suspected in these children.

Laboratory Findings & Imaging Studies

Acute choking is an emergency that requires immediate treatment without laboratory or imaging studies. Without a witnessed choking event, a high index of suspicion is needed to identify lower airway foreign bodies. Inspiratory and forced expiratory (obtained by manually compressing the abdomen during expiration) CXRs should be obtained if foreign-body aspiration is suspected. Forced expiratory radiographs may show unilateral hyperinflation; but may be normal. If obstruction of a distal airway is complete, atelectasis and related volume loss will be the major radiologic findings. Rigid or flexible bronchoscopy is the gold standard for diagnosis of foreign-body aspiration, but rigid bronchoscopy is the preferred treatment for removal of a foreign body. Virtual bronchoscopy (using 3D rendering with CT) and CT are alternative approaches for detecting a foreign body.

► Treatment

Prevention is paramount. Pediatricians should counsel parents and caregivers regarding age-specific safe foods. Small toys and latex balloons should have age-appropriate choking warnings on their labels. In the event of acute upper airway obstruction due to foreign-body aspiration, emergency treatment depends on the amount of obstruction. If partial obstruction is present, the choking subject should be allowed to use his or her own cough reflex to remove the foreign body. If the obstruction increases or the airway is *completely obstructed*, acute intervention is required and Red Cross recommendations for choking in a child should be followed (see Reference below).

Blind finger sweeps *should not* be performed in infants or children because the finger may push the foreign body further into the airway. The airway should be opened by jaw thrust, and if the foreign body can be directly visualized, careful removal with the fingers or instruments should be attempted. Patients with persistent apnea and inability to achieve adequate ventilation may require emergency intubation, tracheotomy, or needle cricothyrotomy, depending on the setting and the rescuer's skills. If a child of any age becomes unresponsive, cardiopulmonary resuscitation (CPR) is recommended. Chest compressions may help to dislodge the foreign body.

In children with known or suspected lower airway foreign bodies, removal is most successfully performed using rigid bronchoscopy under general anesthesia. Following the removal of the foreign body, β-adrenergic nebulization treatments followed by chest physiotherapy are recommended to help clear related mucus or treat bronchospasm. Flexible bronchoscopy may be adjunct treatment for foreign bodies that are very distal. Failure to identify and remove a foreign body in the lower respiratory tract can result in bronchiectasis or lung abscess from chronic airway obstruction. This risk justifies an aggressive approach to suspected foreign bodies.

Green SS: Ingested and aspirated foreign bodies. Pediatr Rev 2015; 6(10):430–436 [PMID: 26330203].

https://www.redcross.org/take-a-class/first-aid/performing-first-aid/child-baby-first-aid.

CONGENITAL MALFORMATIONS OF THE LUNG PARENCHYMA

PULMONARY AGENESIS & HYPOPLASIA

> ### ESSENTIALS OF DIAGNOSIS & TYPICAL FEATURES
>
> ▶ Pulmonary aplasia is not compatible with life.
>
> ▶ Pulmonary hypoplasia is due to incomplete development.
>
> ▶ Pulmonary hypoplasia often leads to prolonged oxygen requirement and increased oxygen need with illness and activity. Other symptoms vary by degree of hypoplasia.

In unilateral pulmonary agenesis (complete absence of one lung), the trachea continues into a main bronchus and often has complete tracheal rings. Unilateral pulmonary agenesis can be isolated in 24% of reported cases but is usually associated with other anomalies: cardiovascular (40%), vertebral or rib fusion (30%), gastrointestinal (20%), tracheal stenosis (20%), or genitourinary (14%). Two-year survival is estimated at 62% and right agenesis, tracheal stenosis and gastrointestinal anomalies were associated with increased mortality.

Pulmonary hypoplasia is incomplete development of one or both lungs, characterized by a reduction in alveolar number and airway branches, decreasing the surface area for gas exchange. Pulmonary hypoplasia results from premature disruption of lung development. Causes include decreased amniotic fluid production (ie, with renal agenesis), premature loss of amniotic fluid through prolonged premature rupture of membranes, decreased blood flow to the early fetal developing lungs, chromosomal abnormalities, or possibly a primary mesodermal defect affecting multiple organ systems leading to structural immaturity. Chest cage abnormalities, intrathoracic masses, diaphragmatic hernia or elevation, fetal hydrops, severe musculoskeletal disorders, and cardiac lesions may also result in hypoplastic lungs. Infants with advanced BPD can have pulmonary hypoplasia, and thus, postnatal factors may play important roles as well.

▶ Clinical Findings

A. Symptoms and Signs

The clinical presentation is highly variable and related to the severity of hypoplasia. Some newborns present with perinatal stress, severe acute respiratory distress, pneumothorax, and persistent pulmonary hypertension secondary to primary pulmonary hypoplasia. Children with lesser degrees of hypoplasia may present with chronic cough, chronic hypoxemia, tachypnea, wheezing, and recurrent pneumonia.

B. Laboratory Findings and Imaging Studies

Prenatal diagnosis can be made on ultrasound or fetal MRI. CXRs show variable degrees of volume loss in a small hemithorax with mediastinal shift. Pulmonary agenesis can be associated with tracheal deviation, mediastinal shift, and remaining lung herniating into the side of the absent lung. Chest CT scan shows heterogeneous air trapping and atelectasis and better delineates simplification of alveoli, airways, and pulmonary vasculature if the CXR is not definitive. V/Q scans, angiography, and bronchoscopy can demonstrate decreased pulmonary vascularity or premature blunting of airways associated with the maldeveloped lung tissue. Arterial blood gas can help define the degree of hypoxemia and acute and chronic hypoventilation secondary to pulmonary hypoplasia.

▶ Treatment & Prognosis

Treatment and diagnosis are determined by the severity of underlying medical problems, the extent of the hypoplasia and the degree of pulmonary hypertension and usually includes supporting the child with oxygen, and noninvasive or invasive ventilation if needed.

Cotton CM: Pulmonary hypoplasia. Semin Fetal Neonatal Med 2017;22(4):250–255 [PMID: 28709949].

Fukuoka et al: Clinical outcomes of pulmonary agenesis: a systematic review of the literature. Pediatr Pulmonol 2022;57:3060–3068 [PMID: 36069476].

CONGENITAL PULMONARY AIRWAY MALFORMATION

> ### ESSENTIALS OF DIAGNOSIS & TYPICAL FEATURES
>
> ▶ May be diagnosed prenatally by ultrasound.
>
> ▶ Newborns generally present with respiratory distress and evidence of a space-occupying density on chest x-ray.

Congenital pulmonary airway malformations (CPAMs), previously known as congenital cystic adenomatoid malformations, though rare, are the most common congenital lung lesion. They are unilateral space-occupying masses that can appear to be solid or cystic. Histopathology varies based on type of CPAM and may show an increase in terminal

Table 19–4. Types of congenital pulmonary airway malformations.

CPAM Type	Epidemiology (%)	Pathologic Characteristics	Presentation	Prognosis and Treatment
Type 0	1–3	Firm with small cysts and made of irregular bronchial tissue. Often involving entire lung.	Not compatible with life.	Not compatible with life.
Type 1	60–70 of cases	Single or multiple large cysts; rarely bilateral.	Prenatal diagnosis may occur when cysts are large. In the newborn period, respiratory distress will be seen if large cysts expand causing compression of the adjacent lung or mediastinal shift. Smaller cysts may present with recurrent pneumonia later.	Resection leads to symptom resolution.
Type 2	15–20	Bulky, firm masses with small cysts in one lobe.	Often presents with associated nonpulmonary anomalies.	Resection.
Type 3	5–10	Bulky, solid appearance. Small cysts. This CPAM is often large involving one whole lobe or multiple lobes. Frequent mediastinal shift.	Infants present in the newborn period with severe respiratory distress.	50% survival due to the association with cardiac compression and fetal hydrops in large. Infants may be stillborn. Treatment: pre- and postnatal resection.
Type 4	< 10	Large, thin-walled cysts in the periphery of the whole lung or isolated to one lobe.	Newborns present with severe respiratory distress.	Resection.

CPAM, congenital pulmonary airway malformation.

respiratory structures that form intercommunicating cysts of various sizes that are lined by cuboidal or ciliated pseudostratified columnar epithelium. Air passages appear malformed and tend to lack cartilage.

Right and left lungs are involved with equal frequency. These lesions originate in the first 5–22 weeks of gestation during the embryonic period of lung development. They are categorized into five types based on size and number of cysts (Table 19–4).

▶ Clinical Findings

A. Symptoms and Signs

CPAMs are usually identified on routine prenatal ultrasound. In children, 86% are identified by age 5. Presenting symptoms include respiratory distress with hypoxemia, tachypnea, grunting, recurrent pulmonary infection, and possible acute respiratory failure. With type 3 lesions, dullness to percussion may be present. Older patients can present with a spontaneous pneumothorax, cough, fever, failure to thrive, or rarely hemoptysis.

B. Imaging Studies and Differential Diagnosis

CXR findings are usually cystic or mass-like but differ by the type of lesion (see Table 19–4). CT scan without contrast is often helpful in characterizing CPAMs. CPAMs have no systemic blood supply; thus, CT angiography can help differentiate CPAMs from pulmonary sequestrations. Placement of a radiopaque feeding tube into the stomach helps in the differentiation from diaphragmatic hernia.

▶ Treatment

Surgical resection is often required because of potential complications such as hydrops, cardiac compression, risk of infection, and air trapping from poor mucus clearance. Segmental resection is not indicated because smaller cysts may expand after removal of the more obviously affected area. Of note, some prenatal CPAMs have been shown to spontaneously resolve. There is concern that type 4 CPAMs may have the potential to develop into pleural pulmonary blastoma (PBB), a malignant cystic lung tumor, but this is currently controversial and not proven. Because it is difficult to differentiate CPAMs from PBB, surgical removal is recommended. Intrauterine surgery and EXIT (procedures for congenital malformations have become more prevalent at tertiary centers for higher risk patients.

Baird R, Puligandla PS, Laberge JM: Congenital lung malformations: informing best practice. Semin Pediatr Surg 2014;23(5): 270–277 [PMID: 25459011].

David M, Lamas-Pinheiro R, Henriques-Coelho T: Prenatal and postnatal management of congenital pulmonary airway malformation. Neonatology 2016;110(2):101–115 [PMID: 27070354].

Wall J, Coates A: prenatal imaging and postnatal presentation, diagnosis, and management of congenital lung malformations. Curr Opin Pediatr 2014;26(3):315–319 [PMID: 24739492].

PULMONARY SEQUESTRATION

ESSENTIALS OF DIAGNOSIS & TYPICAL FEATURES

► Congenital lung malformation with a systemic artery blood supply usually found in a lower lobe.

► Presents with recurrent pneumonia, chronic cough, or incidentally.

► Diagnosed postnatally by chest CT angiography.

Pulmonary sequestration is the second most common congenital lung abnormality (after CPAM) and originates during the embryonic period of lung development. Sequestrations are characterized by nonfunctional pulmonary tissue that does not communicate with the tracheobronchial tree and receives or delivers its blood supply from one or more anomalous systemic circulation vessels. Sequestrations are classified as either extralobar or intralobar based on whether the sequestration has its own pleural lining.

Intralobar type is more common than extralobar, comprising 75% of the cases of sequestration. Intralobar sequestration (ILS) is an isolated segment of lung within the normal pleural investment that often receives blood from the aorta or one of its arterial branches. Intralobar sequestration is usually found within the lower lobes (98%), 55% are found on the left side, and it is rarely associated with other congenital anomalies (< 2%).

Extralobar sequestration (ELS) has its own distinct pleural lining with blood supplied from the systemic circulation (more typical), from pulmonary vessels, or from both. In contrast to ILS, venous drainage is usually through the systemic or portal venous system. Pathologically, ELS appears as a 0.5–12 cm solitary thoracic lesion near the diaphragm, more commonly on the left, representing 65% of the cases. Abdominal sites are rare but can occur. ELSs are more commonly seen in syndromes with over 50% of patients having other congenital disorders.

► Clinical Findings

Postnatal clinical presentation of ILS includes chronic cough, wheezing, recurrent pneumonias, or rarely with hemoptysis. ELSs are more commonly found incidentally without obvious symptoms.

► Imaging & Treatment

Pulmonary sequestrations can be detected by prenatal ultrasound; doppler may allow for distinction between intralobar and extralobar malformations based on blood supply. CT angiography or magnetic resonance angiography are the best modalities to identify the anomalous systemic arterial supply to the lung, with CT better delineating the surrounding lung tissue. Treatment is surgical resection.

Baird R, Puligandla PS, LaBerge JM: Congenital lung malformations: informing best practice. Semin Pediatr Surg 2014;23(5):270–277 [PMID: 25459011].

Wall J, Coates A: Prenatal imaging and postnatal presentation, diagnosis, and management of congenital lung malformations. Curr Opin Pediatr 2014;26(3):315–319 [PMID: 24739492].

CONGENITAL LOBAR OVERINFLATION

ESSENTIALS OF DIAGNOSIS & TYPICAL FEATURES

► Presents in the first year of life but may be diagnosed prenatally.

► Overinflation of the affected lobe (usually left upper or right middle lobes) on imaging.

Patients with congenital lobar overinflation (CLO), also known as congenital lobar emphysema (CLE), have hyperinflation of the affected lung lobe which can cause respiratory distress. Although the cause of CLO is not well understood, on biopsy some lesions show abnormal orientation or distribution of the bronchial cartilage that is thought to cause bronchial obstruction, leading to a partial ball-valve effect and resultant air trapping of the affected lobe. Males are more commonly affected.

► Clinical Findings

A. Symptoms and Signs

CLO presents most commonly with neonatal respiratory distress or progressive respiratory impairment during the first year of life. Clinical features include respiratory distress, hypoxemia, tachypnea, wheezing, and cough. Breath sounds are reduced on the affected side, perhaps with hyperresonance to percussion, mediastinal displacement and bulging of the chest wall. The mild or intermittent nature of the symptoms in older children or young adults results in delayed diagnosis.

B. Imaging Studies and Differential Diagnosis

Radiologic findings include overdistension of the affected lobe with wide separation of bronchovascular markings, collapse of adjacent lung, shift of the mediastinum away from the affected side, and a depressed diaphragm on the affected side. The most common site of involvement is the left upper lobe (42%) or right middle lobe (35%). The radiographic diagnosis may be confusing in the newborn because of retention of alveolar fluid in the affected lobe causing the appearance of a homogeneous density. Usually, CLO is detected on CXR, but chest CT and bronchoscopy are often used to evaluate for other disorders such as external airway compression (artery, lymphadenopathy, bronchogenic cyst) or internal airway obstruction (mass, mucus plug or foreign body). The differential diagnosis of CLO includes pneumothorax, pneumatocele, atelectasis with compensatory hyperinflation, diaphragmatic hernia, and congenital cystic adenomatoid malformation.

Treatment

When respiratory distress is severe, a segmental or complete lobectomy is usually required. Less symptomatic and older children may do equally well with or without lobectomy.

Seear M et al: A review of congenital lung malformations with a simplified classification system for clinical and research use. Pediatr Surg Int 2017;33(6):657–664 [PMID: 2820492].
Wall J, Coates A: Prenatal imaging and postnatal presentation, diagnosis, and management of congenital lung malformations. Curr Opin Pediatr 2014;26(3):315–319 [PMID: 24739492].

BRONCHOPULMONARY DYSPLASIA (NEONATAL CHRONIC LUNG DISEASE)

ESSENTIALS OF DIAGNOSIS & TYPICAL FEATURES

▶ Respiratory distress after preterm birth.

▶ Required oxygen therapy or positive pressure ventilation at 36 weeks' gestational age or 28 days of life.

▶ Persistent respiratory abnormalities, including physical signs and radiographic findings.

Bronchopulmonary dysplasia (BPD) remains one of the most significant sequelae of acute respiratory distress in the neonatal intensive care unit, with an incidence as high as 68% for infants born at 22–28 weeks' gestation. In addition to preterm infants, full-term newborns with disorders such as meconium aspiration, congenital diaphragmatic hernia, and persistent pulmonary hypertension also can develop BPD. BPD is diagnosed if an infant needs oxygen postnatally for at least 28 days. The severity of BPD assessed at 36 weeks post menstrual age predicts long-term respiratory serious morbidity and mortality (Table 19–5).

Table 19–5. NICHD classification of BPD severity based on respiratory support at 36 weeks postmenstrual age.

BPD Grade	Respiratory Support
I (mild)	< 2 L/min nasal cannula
II (moderate)	> 2 L/min nasal cannula OR Nasal CPAP or NIV
III (severe)	Invasive ventilation

BPD, bronchopulmonary dysplasia; CPAP, continuous positive airway pressure; NIV, noninvasive ventilation.
Data from Jensen EA, et al: The diagnosis of bronchopulmonary dysplasia in very preterm infant. Am J Respir Crit Care Med 2019 Sep 15; 200(6):751–759.

The pathologic findings and clinical course of BPD have changed over time due to technological advances (artificial surfactant, antenatal steroids) and improved ventilatory strategies. Preterm infants born at less than 28 weeks gestation that have received antenatal steroids and surfactant at birth now are termed to have "new BPD" characterized more by simplified (fewer) alveoli, early inflammation, and hypercellularity followed by healing with fibrosis that leads to impaired gas exchange, exercise intolerance, and pulmonary hypertension, but often are able to avoid the severe scarring, stiff lung damage that occurs from prolonged barotrauma from ventilation that is now termed "old BPD."

The mechanisms that cause BPD are unclear, but current studies suggest that structural immaturity of the alveolar-capillary network, surfactant deficiency, atelectasis, and pulmonary edema cause impaired gas exchange that requires mechanical ventilation and supplemental oxygen, which may result in further injury from barotrauma and oxidative stress. Infants can develop aggressive, fibroproliferative pathologic lesions as well as physiologic abnormalities (increased airway resistance) and biochemical markers of lung injury that may predict BPD during the first weeks of life. Ongoing injuries may further contribute to ventilator and oxygen dependence.

Clinical Findings

A. Signs and Symptoms

BPD clinical course ranges from an oxygen requirement that gradually resolves over a few months to more severe disease requiring chronic mechanical ventilation with tracheostomy during early childhood. In general, patients show slow, steady improvements in oxygen or ventilator requirements over time. If not complicated by significant neurologic injury, patients with severe BPD may be able to wean slowly off chronic invasive ventilation (if required) between 2 and 5 years of age, with outliers. Some patients with BPD may also have significant tracheobronchomalacia that can present with desaturation spells that may lead to apnea, bradycardia, and ventilator dyssynchrony. Infants with BPD are at risk of developing pulmonary hypertension because of simplified arterial structure in the parenchyma, and even mild hypoxemia can cause significant elevations of pulmonary arterial pressure.

B. Imaging Studies and Procedures

Flexible bronchoscopy can evaluate for structural lesions (subglottic stenosis, vocal cord paralysis, tracheal or bronchial stenosis, tracheobronchomalacia, or airway granulomas). Video fluoroscopic swallow study can assess for chronic oral microaspiration that is more common with prematurity. High-resolution chest CT or lung biopsy can evaluate for ILD if severity of BPD is out of proportion to gestational age. Echo can evaluate for PDA or pulmonary hypertension. Cardiac catheterization may be necessary if significant pulmonary hypertension is present to evaluate for left heart diastolic dysfunction or pulmonary vein stenosis.

▶ Differential Diagnosis

The differential diagnosis of BPD includes meconium aspiration syndrome, congenital infection (eg, with cytomegalovirus or *Ureaplasma*), CPAM, recurrent aspiration, pulmonary lymphangiectasia, total anomalous pulmonary venous return, overhydration, and childhood ILD.

▶ Treatment

Prenatal maternal systemic steroids, surfactant therapy at birth, and adequate lung recruitment in premature infants decreases BPD risk, mechanical ventilation requirement, and mortality. After birth, short systemic steroid courses can aid in weaning respiratory support, but recurrent or prolonged systemic steroid courses have been associated with an increased incidence of cerebral palsy. Inhaled corticosteroids and β-adrenergic agonists do not decrease the incidence of BPD, but there may be some benefit to infants who have airway hyperreactivity. Chronic or intermittent diuretic therapy improves acute lung function and is commonly used if pulmonary edema is present, but the impact on long-term outcomes is unclear. Diuretics can have adverse effects, including volume contraction, electrolyte imbalances, and nephrocalcinosis; thus, long-term use is usually avoided if possible. If a patient has pulmonary hypertension, the arterial oxygen saturation should be kept above 93% to minimize irreversible pulmonary vascular remodeling with fibrosis.

Routine vaccinations including the influenza vaccine are recommended. Immune prophylaxis of RSV reduces the morbidity of bronchiolitis in infants with BPD. In children older than 2 years with BPD, pneumococcal polysaccharide 23-valent vaccine is recommended in addition to standard pneumococcal vaccination.

▶ Prognosis

Surfactant replacement therapy has had a markedly beneficial effect on reducing morbidity and mortality from BPD.

The incidence of BPD and chronic lung disease due to preterm birth is increasing due to increased survival of extremely preterm infants. The long-term outlook for most survivors is favorable, although follow-up studies suggest that lung function may be altered for life. As smaller, more immature infants survive, chronic lung disease has been associated with increasing abnormal neurodevelopmental outcomes. The incidence of cerebral palsy, hearing/visual impairment, and developmental delays also is increased in infants with BPD, as are feeding abnormalities, behavioral difficulties, and increased irritability.

Gilfillan M, Bhandari A, Bhandari V: Diagnosis and management of bronchopulmonary dysplasia. BMJ 2021 Oct 20;375:n1974. doi: 10.1136/bmj.n1974 [PMID: 34670756].

Jensen et al: The diagnosis of bronchopulmonary dysplasia in very preterm infant. Am J Respir Crit Care Med 2019 Sep 15;200(6): 751–759 [PMID: 30995069].

▼ DIFFUSE LUNG DISEASES

CHILDHOOD INTERSTITIAL LUNG DISEASE SYNDROME

ESSENTIALS OF DIAGNOSIS & TYPICAL FEATURES

▶ Diverse group of rare pulmonary disorders

▶ Can involve the airways, alveoli, and/or interstitium.

▶ Presentation: At least three of the following:

  • Respiratory symptoms: tachypnea, retractions, cough, wheeze, dyspnea

  • Respiratory signs: Inspiratory rales, wheezing, decreased breath sounds, digital clubbing, weight loss

  • Hypoxemia breathing ambient air

  • Abnormality on chest imaging: chest CT scan or plain CXR

▶ Diagnosis: First exclude more common pulmonary diseases that can have similar presentations: CF, BPD, primary ciliary dyskinesia (PCD), aspiration, etc.

▶ Lung biopsy and/or genetic studies often required for precise diagnosis.

Childhood **I**nterstitial and diffuse **L**ung **D**isease (chILD) syndrome is a constellation of signs and symptoms but not a specific diagnosis (Table 19–6). Once recognized, a more specific diagnosis should be pursued. More common pulmonary diseases that can present similarly to chILD should be excluded first, including CF, cardiac disease, asthma, acute or chronic infection, immunodeficiency, thoracic

Table 19–6. Classification of diffuse lung diseases in infancy and childhood.

Developmental disorders	Acinar dysplasia Congenital alveolar dysplasia Alveolar capillary dysplasia with misalignment of pulmonary veins (FOXF1)
Growth abnormalities	Pulmonary hypoplasia Chronic neonatal lung disease/bronchopulmonary dysplasia (BPD) Related to chromosomal defects (eg, Down syndrome) Related to congenital heart disease with normal chromosomes
Specific conditions with undefined etiology	Pulmonary interstitial glycogenosis (PIG) Neuroendocrine cell hyperplasia of infancy (NEHI)
Disorders of surfactant metabolism	Surfactant protein B deficiency (SFTPB) Surfactant protein B deficiency (SFTPC) ABCA3 transporter deficiency NKX2-1 (also TTF-1) Pulmonary alveolar proteinosis (CSF2RB/CSF2RA)
Disorders in a normal host	Bronchiolitis obliterans Cryptogenic organizing pneumonia Hypersensitivity pneumonitis (HP) Chronic aspiration syndromes Eosinophilic pneumonia Toxic inhalations
Associated with systemic or rheumatological diseases	Storage diseases Sarcoidosis Langerhans cell histiocytosis Malignant infiltrates Alveolar hemorrhage syndromes (COPA) Vasculitis (GPA, GBM, EGPA) Tuberous sclerosis with lymphangioleiomyomatosis
Immunocompromised host	Opportunistic infections Drug toxicities Idiopathic diffuse alveolar damage (DAH) Lymphoid hyperplasia and lymphoid interstitial pneumonitis (LIP) Lymphoproliferative disease
Lymphatic disorders	Lymphangiectasis Lymphangiomatosis

Data from Kurland G et al: An official American Thoracic Society clinical practice guideline: classification, evaluation, and management of childhood interstitial lung disease in infancy. Am J Respir Crit Care Med 2013 Aug 1;188(3):376–394 and Dishop MK: Diagnostic pathology of diffuse lung disease in children. Pediatr Allergy Immunol Pulmonol 2010 Mar;23(1):69–85.

cage abnormality, chronic lung disease of prematurity, and aspiration.

Clinical Findings

A. Symptoms and Signs

ChILD can present in infants and young children with respiratory failure and inability to wean supplemental O_2 or alternatively, with cough, exercise intolerance, clubbing, dyspnea, tachypnea, retractions, hypoxemia, barrel chest, and failure to thrive. Crackles are common on chest auscultation.

B. Laboratory Findings

The initial evaluation may include spirometry, lung volumes, diffusing capacity, complete blood count with WBC differential, inflammatory markers, and comprehensive metabolic panel. Both an ECG and echo should be obtained. Other pertinent studies might include immunologic assessment, and biologic markers of collagen vascular disease. Genetic panels are improving and can lead to diagnosis without invasive testing.

C. Imaging Studies

CXRs are normal in up to 10%–15% of patients, but CT scans are almost always abnormal and can be diagnostic.

D. Special Tests

Pulmonary function testing is typically abnormal in chILD. Depending on the specific disease, PFTs may show (1) a restrictive pattern of decreased lung volumes, compliance, and diffusing capacity; (2) an obstructive pattern with hyperinflation and little bronchodilator response; or (3) a mixed obstructive-restrictive pattern. The 6-minute walk test often demonstrates desaturation and reduced distance capacity. Exercise-induced or nocturnal hypoxemia may be the earliest physiologic abnormality in chILD.

Bronchoscopy can exclude anatomic abnormalities and one should obtain BAL for microbiologic and cytologic testing, though it is seldom diagnostic alone. Lung biopsy is often required for a definitive diagnosis, and video-assisted thoracoscopic lung biopsies are preferred rather than transbronchial biopsy.

Differential Diagnosis

Many disorders have similar presentations: CF, cardiac disease, asthma, acute and chronic infection, immunodeficiency, thoracic cage abnormality, chronic lung disease of prematurity, and aspiration.

Complications

Complications from chILD include delays in school, failure to thrive, respiratory failure, and pulmonary hypertension. Mortality and morbidity can be significant and varies by specific diagnosis. Treatment for these diseases also can have significant side effects.

Treatment

The mainstays of treatment include supplemental O_2 and nutritional support. Corticosteroids are used for many chILD diagnoses. Most treatments for chILD are disease specific and based on expert opinion, case reports, and small case series. Patients with severe disease may need noninvasive respiratory support. All patients should be evaluated for comorbidities such as pulmonary hypertension, aspiration, failure to thrive, sleep apnea, and hypoxemia. All vaccines should be provided, including annual influenza vaccine, palivizumab in infancy, and pneumococcal polysaccharide vaccine. Nutritional and respiratory support should be provided to encourage optimal growth and development. Environmental irritant exposure (recreational and occupational) should be avoided. Children with chILD should be evaluated and cared for by an experienced multidisciplinary team. Lung transplantation may be an option for patients with progressive respiratory failure. The chILD Family Foundation can provide further supportive resources for families (http://www.childfoundation.us).

Prognosis

Prognosis varies by chILD diagnosis from mild disease to progressive respiratory failure and death.

Liang T, Vargas SO, Lee EY: Childhood interstitial (diffuse) lung disease: pattern recognition approach to diagnosis in infants. Am J Radiol 2019;212:958–967. doi: org/10.2214/AJR.18.20696 [PMID: 30835521].

Nathan N, Berdah L, Delestrain C, Sileo C, Clement A: Interstitial lung diseases in children. Presse Med 2020;49:1–12. doi: org/10.1016/j.lpm.2019.06.007 [PMID: 32563946].

HYPERSENSITIVITY PNEUMONITIS

ESSENTIALS OF DIAGNOSIS & TYPICAL FEATURES

► Dyspnea on exertion, cough, weight loss, hypoxemia, and fever.
► History of exposure to an inhaled organic particle (birds) or low-molecular-weight chemicals.

Hypersensitivity pneumonitis (HP), or extrinsic allergic alveolitis, is a T-cell–mediated response triggered by an environmental exposure. Both acute and chronic forms may occur. In children, the most common antigen(s) are birds (eg, pigeons, parakeets, parrots, or doves); this is also known as "bird fancier's lung." However, a multitude of other antigens have been documented to cause HP, including moldy hay, compost, logs,

tree bark, sawdust, or aerosols from humidifiers or hot tubs. A high level of suspicion and a thorough environmental exposure history are required to find the diagnosis.

Clinical Findings

A. Symptoms and Signs

Episodic cough and fever can occur following acute exposures. Chronic exposure results in weight loss, fatigue, hypoxemia, and dyspnea. Physical examination findings include crackles, loud cardiac P2 if pulmonary hypertension has developed, and clubbing with chronic HP.

B. Laboratory Findings and Imaging Studies

Acute exposure may cause polymorphonuclear leukocytosis with eosinophilia and airway obstruction or restriction on lung function testing. Chronic HP results in a restrictive pattern.

Chest CT is often diagnostic (with typical exposure, signs, and symptoms) showing small centrilobular nodules, ground-glass opacities, and air-trapping. Chronic HP may progress to pulmonary fibrosis. CXR findings are variable and may include normal lung fields, airspace opacification, and linear nodular or reticulonodular opacities. The cell counts on BAL typically show lymphocytosis. Lung biopsy reveals bronchiolocentric interstitial lymphocytic inflammation, nonnecrotizing, poorly formed interstitial granulomas, and intra-alveolar foci of organizing pneumonia Serum precipitins (precipitating immunoglobin G [IgG] antibodies) to the triggering antigen are less helpful for diagnosis because current tests are not significantly sensitive or specific.

Differential Diagnosis

Patients with acute symptoms may appear to have asthma. Patients with chronic symptoms must be differentiated from other DLDs.

Complications

Prolonged exposure to offending antigens may result in pulmonary hypertension due to chronic hypoxemia, irreversible restrictive lung disease, and pulmonary fibrosis.

Treatment & Prognosis

The primary goal is complete elimination of exposure to the offending antigen. Corticosteroids treatment is often successful at stopping or reversing HP. With early diagnosis and avoidance of offending antigens, the prognosis is excellent.

Vasakova M, Selman M, Morell F, Sterclova M, Molina-Molina M, Raghu G: Hypersensitivity pneumonitis: current concepts of pathogenesis and potential targets for treatment. Am J Respir Crit Care Med 2019;200(3):301–308. doi: 10.1164/rccm.201903-0541PP [PMID: 31150272].

BRONCHIOLITIS OBLITERANS

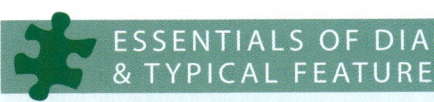

ESSENTIALS OF DIAGNOSIS & TYPICAL FEATURES

▶ Persistent symptoms of airway obstruction (dyspnea on exertion, severe, irreversible airflow obstruction) 8 weeks after the resolution of a lower respiratory tract infection.

▶ Chest CT scan with mosaic pattern of hyperinflation, vascular attenuation, and perhaps bronchiectasis.

Bronchiolitis obliterans (BO) is a rare chronic obstructive lung disease characterized by the scarring of bronchioles from a variety of different insults that have the common final pathway of obliterating the small airway lumen. The most common etiology in children is postinfectious, following a lower airway tract infection with adenovirus, although influenza, rubeola, *Bordetella*, and *Mycoplasma* are also implicated. Other causes include connective tissue diseases, chronic aspiration, Stevens-Johnson syndrome, post transplantation (lung or bone marrow), and inhalational injury. Many cases of BO are idiopathic. Mechanical ventilation for severe adenoviral respiratory infection is a strong risk factor for development of BO.

▶ Clinical Findings

A. Symptoms and Signs

BO usually presents with dyspnea, coughing, and exercise intolerance. On examination they may have expiratory wheezing and eventually an overinflated chest. Sequelae of BO include persistent airway obstruction, recurrent wheezing, bronchiectasis, chronic atelectasis, recurrent pneumonia, and unilateral hyperlucent lung syndrome.

B. Laboratory Findings and Imaging Studies

CXR abnormalities include heterogeneous air trapping and airway wall thickening. Classic findings on chest CT include a mosaic perfusion pattern, vascular attenuation, and central bronchiectasis. Pulmonary function testing showing airway obstruction unresponsive to bronchodilators. CT and PFT may be diagnostic in patients with the appropriate clinical history. Lung biopsy is necessary only in cases where clinical history and/or CT scan are not classic. Transbronchial biopsy can miss the pathology due to its nonuniform distribution. Pathologic findings include airway scarring (eg, with fibrin) with partial or complete obstruction of bronchioles.

▶ Differential Diagnosis

Asthma with remodeling, CF, and BPD must be considered in children with persistent airway obstruction.

▶ Treatment

Supportive care with supplemental oxygen for hypoxemia, routine vaccination, avoidance of environmental irritant exposure, exercise, and nutritional support should be provided. Ongoing airway damage due to problems such as aspiration should be prevented. Inhaled bronchodilators (β-agonists and anticholinergic) may reverse airway obstruction if the disease has a reactive component. Systemic corticosteroids may help reverse the obstruction or prevent ongoing damage; these can be given orally or with monthly intravenous doses (intravenous doses may decrease systemic side effects). Azithromycin is beneficial in BO syndrome after lung transplantation and in patients with bronchiectasis but has been associated with leukemia recurrence after bone marrow transplant thus should be avoided in this condition. Fluticasone, azithromycin, and montelukast have been used to treat BO after hematopoietic stem cell transplantation. Lung transplant may be an option for patients with severe, progressive disease. If bronchiectasis is present, airway clearance and early antibiotics with respiratory illnesses (ie, to treat endobronchitis) are helpful.

▶ Prognosis

Prognosis depends in part on the underlying cause as well as the age of onset. Postinfectious BO tends to be nonprogressive with low mortality and the possibility of slow improvement. Conversely, post transplantation or Stevens-Johnson syndrome–related BO may have a rapidly progressive course leading to death or need for lung transplantation.

Colom AJ, Teper AM: Post-infectious bronchiolitis obliterans. Pediatr Pulmonol 2019;54:212–219. doi: 10.1002/ppul.24221 [PMID: 30548423].

Kavaliunaite E, Aurora P: Diagnosing and managing bronchiolitis obliterans in children. Expert Rev Respir Med 2019;13(5):481–488. doi: 10.1080/17476348.2019.1586537 [PMID: 30798629].

DYSPHAGIA WITH ASPIRATION PNEUMONITIS (OR PNEUMONIA)

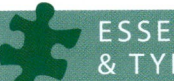

ESSENTIALS OF DIAGNOSIS & TYPICAL FEATURES

▶ History of recurrent aspiration or an aspiration event.

▶ New-onset respiratory distress, oxygen requirement, or fever in a child with known aspiration or after a witnessed aspiration event.

▶ Focal findings on physical examination.

Children with intellectual delay or neurodevelopmental disorders and extreme preterm birth are at increased risk of

Table 19–7. Risk factors for aspiration pneumonia.

Anatomic abnormalities (laryngeal cleft, tracheoesophageal fistula, vocal cord paralysis)
Delayed maturation (genetic disorder or prematurity with hypotonia)
Static encephalopathy
CNS malformation, mass, or traumatic brain injury
Neuromuscular disorders
Seizures
Depressed sensorium (medications)
Near-drowning
Iatrogenic (anesthesia, nasogastric or tracheostomy tubes)
Gastrointestinal disease (reflux, achalasia, or obstruction)

CNS, central nervous system.
Data from Kurland G et al: An official American Thoracic Society clinical practice guideline: classification, evaluation, and management of childhood interstitial lung disease in infancy. Am J Respir Crit Care Med 2013 Aug 1;188(3):376–394 and Dishop MK: Diagnostic pathology of diffuse lung disease in children. Pediatr Allergy Immunol Pulmonol 2010 Mar;23(1):69–85.

dysphagia with chronic aspiration pneumonitis or acute aspiration pneumonia, but it may occur in neurologically normal children as well (Table 19–7). An acute aspiration event may lead to typical pneumonia syndrome with fever, asymmetrical auscultation findings, and asymmetric imaging findings. Chronic aspiration pneumonitis is more indolent and can cause chronic respiratory symptoms of "rattling," cough or wheezing, chronic chest infiltrates, bronchiectasis, or failure to thrive. Pneumonitis is worsened by gram-negative anaerobes and other bacteria present in the mouth.

▶ Clinical Findings

A. Symptoms and Signs

Acute onset of fever, cough, respiratory distress, or hypoxemia in a patient at risk suggests acute aspiration pneumonia. Chest physical findings, such as rales, rhonchi, or decreased breath sounds, may initially be limited to the lung region into which aspiration occurred. Although any region may be affected, the right side—especially the right upper lobe in the supine patient—is commonly affected. In patients with chronic aspiration, "chest rattling" is often described by parents. Generalized rales and wheezing may also be present.

B. Laboratory Findings and Imaging Studies

CXR abnormalities can vary widely. They may reveal lobar consolidation or atelectasis and focal or generalized alveolar or interstitial infiltrates. Complications such as empyema or lung abscess may complicate acute aspiration pneumonia. In some patients with chronic aspiration, perihilar infiltrates with or without bronchiectasis may be seen. If there is clinical concern, chest CT can better delineate these complications.

In patients with chronic aspiration pneumonitis, attempts should be made to evaluate dysphagia and modify the diet. VFSS is typically performed to evaluate swallowing function. Fiberoptic endoscopic examination of swallowing (FEES) is done at specialty centers to directly visualize the larynx during swallowing via laryngoscope. Radionuclide studies have low sensitivity to diagnosis aspiration. Although biomarkers such as lipid-laden macrophages obtained from BAL samples have low sensitivity and specificity, BAL may be considered to diagnose bacterial infection (see section Diagnosis of Respiratory Tract Infections). Anatomic abnormalities such as laryngeal cleft can be evaluated by rigid laryngoscopy/bronchoscopy. Tracheoesophageal fistula is rare and can be difficult to diagnose: UGI fluoroscopy series, rigid or flexible bronchoscopy, or esophageal endoscopy may aid in diagnosis. The role of esophageal disease, gastroesophageal reflux, and impaired esophageal motility in chronic aspiration may warrant evaluation by a gastroenterologist or multidisciplinary aerodigestive team.

▶ Differential Diagnosis

In the acutely ill patient, bacterial and viral pneumonias should be considered. In the chronically ill patient, the differential diagnosis may include disorders causing recurrent pneumonia (eg, immunodeficiencies, ciliary dysfunction, or foreign body), chronic wheezing, or interstitial lung disorders (see the next section), depending on the presentation.

▶ Treatment

Aspiration pneumonia leads to chemical pneumonitis, and supportive treatment is recommended. Antimicrobial therapy for patients who are acutely ill from aspiration pneumonia includes coverage for anaerobic organisms. In general, clindamycin is appropriate initial coverage.

Treatment of dysphagia may include surgical correction of anatomic abnormalities, paced swallowing systems/bottles, thickening of liquids taken by mouth, and feeding and swallowing therapy. Improved oral hygiene, inhaled corticosteroids, and chest physiotherapy may decrease symptoms of aspiration pneumonitis. In patients with compromise of the central nervous system or significant neuromuscular disorders, exclusive feeding by gastrostomy may be required. Because of the widespread causes and consequences of chronic aspiration, multidisciplinary aerodigestive management is often recommended.

Durvasula VS, O'Neill AC, Richter GT: Oropharyngeal dysphagia in children: mechanism, source, and management. Otolaryngol Clin North Am 2014;47(5):691 [PMID: 25213278].

DISORDERS OF THE PULMONARY CIRCULATION

HEMOPTYSIS

ESSENTIALS OF DIAGNOSIS & TYPICAL FEATURES

▶ Coughing up blood or tasting blood after coughing.

▶ New-onset cough, respiratory distress, hypoxemia, or opacity on chest imaging.

Hemoptysis is the expectoration of blood or bloody secretions. Determining the source can be challenging since it may originate in the lower airways and parenchyma, the upper airway and sinuses, or the upper GI tract. The severity can be mild as might occur with viral tracheobronchitis or very large volume as might occur with severe bronchiectasis. The most common pulmonary causes are infections and retained foreign body aspiration; the range of possible causes are listed in the Table 19–8.

The lungs have two sources of blood supply: the pulmonary arteries and the bronchial arteries. The pulmonary artery system is a low-pressure, high-volume system whereas the bronchial artery system is a high-pressure (systemic), low-volume system. As such, large volume hemoptysis usually arises from the bronchial arteries associated with neovascularization caused by chronic inflammation in severe bronchiectasis. The alveolar capillary surface area of the lungs is enormous so considerable bleeding can occur with diffuse alveolar hemorrhage, even from this low-pressure system.

▶ Clinical Findings

A. Symptoms and Signs

Hemoptysis can occur with diseases where hemoptysis might be expected, such as in an adolescent patient with progressive bronchiectasis or in situations where it is not suspected, as

Table 19–8. Pulmonary causes for hemoptysis in children (partial list).

Infections	Systemic vasculitides
Foreign-body aspiration	Pulmonary/airway tumors
Bronchiectasis	Trauma
Congenital airway malformations	Idiopathic/iatrogenic
Congenital heart defects	Toxic inhalations
Pulmonary vascular abnormalities	Factitious
Generalized coagulopathy/thrombosis	

the presenting sign of systemic vasculitis. The presentation depends on whether the bleeding is acute or chronic, small or large volume, and associated symptoms related to the underlying etiology. Symptoms may be mild such as cough and congestion or severe with fever and hemodynamic collapse. Similarly, the signs can vary from nearly normal to cyanosis, pallor, crackles, and impending respiratory failure. Pulmonary hemorrhage may present without hemoptysis in children younger than 5 or 6 years because they may not be able to expectorate the blood.

Estimating the volume of hemoptysis is quite difficult and of uncertain benefit, while estimating the rate of blood loss might be more helpful in determining the severity.

B. Laboratory Findings and Imaging Studies

The patient with illness severe enough to warrant further assessment should undergo a complete blood count with white blood cell count differential, a comprehensive metabolic panel, inflammatory markers, and coagulation studies. Initial imaging includes a CXR and often a chest CT angiogram. The CT angiogram can detect a pulmonary embolism (PE) as well as assess the airways and parenchyma. Flexible bronchoscopy can be considered to localize a bleeding source or identify a specific infectious agent, but this should be done cautiously in a hemodynamically unstable patient and is unlikely to be useful with massive hemoptysis due to the field of view being obscured by the blood. Hemosiderin laden macrophages obtained during the BAL indicate chronic bleeding. Metagenomic next-generation sequencing panels are an excellent test for infectious etiologies. Additional laboratory investigation is directed by the differential diagnosis and might include biomarkers for infections, rheumatologic diseases, systemic vasculitidies, hematologic abnormalities, or malignancy. Echo can help assess cardiac structure and function and look for indications of pulmonary hypertension. Cardiac catheterization may be indicated to identify more obscure vascular abnormalities causing hemoptysis. Lung biopsy often helps establish or confirm the specific cause of the hemorrhage and is particularly useful with pulmonary capillaritis.

▶ Differential Diagnosis

The list of possible pulmonary etiologies of pulmonary hemorrhage is quite broad and diverse (see Table 19–8). Common nonpulmonary sources such as epistaxis and hematemesis need to be evaluated and excluded. A wide variety of specialists, in addition to pulmonologists, are often needed to establish the diagnosis and formulate the most appropriate management plan.

▶ Treatment

Initial management should focus on stabilizing the patient while assessing the severity. For patients with large volume hemoptysis, this is often achieved in the intensive care unit. Supportive treatment may include supplemental O₂, IV fluids, and assisted ventilation. Specific treatment is aimed at the presumed underlying etiology and may include antibiotics for infections and corticosteroids for inflammatory conditions. For hemoptysis related to collagen vascular diseases, disease-modifying drugs are commonly administered along with corticosteroids. Bronchial artery embolization is effective for bleeding related to bronchiectasis. Tranexamic acid, given intravenously, orally, or by nebulization, can be a useful treatment to stop the bleeding regardless of the underlying etiology.

Prognosis

The prognosis for almost all causes of pediatric hemoptysis is favorable with prompt discovery of etiology and a comprehensive multidisciplinary team approach. Chronic, recurrent hemorrhage may lead to pulmonary fibrosis if not prevented early in the course of disease. The outcome for hemorrhage associated with systemic diseases may be related to the damage in other organ systems, particularly the kidney.

Al-Samkari H et al: Antifibrinolytic agents for hemoptysis management in adults with cystic fibrosis. Chest 2019,155(6):1226–1233. doi: org/10.1016/j.chest.2019.02.010 [PMID: 30790551].

Davidson K, Shojaee S: Managing massive hemoptysis. Chest 2020;157(1):77–88. doi: org/10.1016/j.chest.2019.07.012 [PMID: 31374211].

Marquis KM et al: CT for evaluation of hemoptysis. Radiographics 2021;41:742–761. doi: 10.1148/rg.2021200150 [PMID: 33939537].

Shnayder R, Needleman JP: Hemoptysis. Pediatr Rev 2018;39(6): 319–321 [PMID: 29858301].

PULMONARY EMBOLISM

ESSENTIALS OF DIAGNOSIS & TYPICAL FEATURES

► Acute onset chest pain, dyspnea, and tachypnea.
► Known risk factors for thrombosis.
► Pulmonary artery obstruction on CT angiogram.

The incidence of pulmonary embolism (PE) in children is increasing along with an increasing incidence of chronic conditions that predispose patients to thrombosis. Therefore, pediatric providers should have a heightened awareness of this possibility when evaluating children with new onset chest pain, shortness of breath, and tachypnea. Traditional risks for thrombosis are vascular injury, blood flow stasis, and hypercoagulability (Virchow triad), and the most common source of PE is deep venous thrombosis (DVT). Most children who have PE have at least one risk factor for DVT including oral contraceptives, chronic indwelling venous lines, obesity, thrombophilia, congenital heart disease, septicemia, cancer, autoimmune disease, or immobility.

Clinical Findings

A. Symptoms and Signs

The most common symptoms of PE include chest pain, dyspnea, and tachypnea, although in children, these symptoms may be subtle and obscured by underlying conditions. Other symptoms and signs may include cough, hypoxemia, hemoptysis, tachycardia, fever, and syncope. Abnormal findings on physical examination are nonspecific but may include tachypnea, crackles, augmented P2, and evidence of DVT.

B. Laboratory Findings and Imaging Studies

Prediction scores for PE in adults have not been validated in children. Initial laboratory studies should include a CBC with WBC differential, coagulation studies, fibrinogen, and D-dimer, brain natriuretic protein (BNP), lactate and troponin. CT angiograms have supplanted ventilation perfusion scans as the imaging of choice for PE. Doppler ultrasound examination of the extremities is useful for assessing DVT. Echos may help evaluate central pulmonary arterial or atrial thrombosis, paradoxical septal motion, flattened interventricular septum and depressed RV function as well as pulmonary hypertension. If a PE is detected, additional evaluation for acquired or genetic risks for thrombophilia should be obtained (deficits in protein C, protein S, antithrombin III; factor V Leiden variants; elevated homocysteine; anti-phospholipid antibodies).

Treatment

The initial treatment should focus on stabilizing the patient and providing supportive care that might include supplemental O₂, IV fluids, and pain management. Anticoagulation is commonly initiated with low-molecular-weight heparin and/or thrombolysis. For massive, life-threatening PE, thrombectomy may be an option. Options for longer-term anticoagulation include vitamin K antagonists (eg, warfarin) or direct anticoagulants (eg, rivaroxaban, apixaban, dabigatran). Initial treatment should be for at least 3–4 months and is usually supervised by a hematology specialist.

Maggio A et al: Pulmonary embolism in children, a real challenge for the pediatrician: a case report and review of the literature. Acta Biomed 2022 (Suppl);93:e2022055. doi: 10.23750/abm.v93iS3.13070 [PMID: 35666119].

Ross C et al: Acute management of high-risk and intermediate-risk pulmonary embolism in children: a review. Chest 2022; 161(3):791–802. doi: 10.1016/j.chest.2021.09.019 [PMID: 34587483].

PULMONARY EDEMA

ESSENTIALS OF DIAGNOSIS & TYPICAL FEATURES

► Dyspnea, tachypnea, and hypoxemia.
► Inspiratory crackles on examination.
► Evidence of pulmonary edema on chest imaging.

► Pathogenesis

Pulmonary edema is the accumulation of fluid in the alveolar space that is normally occupied by air. The preservation of the alveolar space is a balance between the forces that push fluid out of the vascular space and keep fluids in the vascular space. Tight epithelial and endothelial junctions help prevent fluid leakage out of the vessels and into the interstitial and alveolar spaces. Increased intravascular pulmonary capillary pressures, loss of plasma oncotic proteins, decreased pericapillary extravascular pressures, and loss of vascular integrity can lead to pulmonary edema. Fluid overload, obstruction of lymphatic flow, or obstructed venous drainage can also contribute to pulmonary edema. In children, the most common causes of pulmonary edema include congenital heart disease and increased vascular permeability which occurs with pediatric acute respiratory distress syndrome.

► Clinical Findings

A. Symptoms and Signs

Children with pulmonary edema commonly have increased work of breathing due to decreased lung compliance, leading to retractions and tachypnea. Inspiratory crackles are common, and infants with extensive edema may also wheeze.

B. Imaging Studies

While CXR is not very sensitive to the degree of pulmonary edema, common abnormalities include increased interstitial markings and engorged pulmonary vessels. If the underlying cause is from cardiac dysfunction, cardiomegaly may be present. Pleural effusions may also be seen.

► Treatment

Initial treatment should focus on supportive care with supplemental O_2 and assisted ventilation if indicated. Diuretics and restoring appropriate fluid balance are likely beneficial. Inotropes can improve cardiac performance if there is poor myocardial function. Airway positive pressure may help stop the influx of fluid into the alveoli but is unlikely to push fluid back into the vascular space. If serum albumin is low,

nutritional support improving the albumin level may also decrease the edema. For patients with pulmonary edema associated with renal failure, dialysis is beneficial.

Matthay MA et al: Acute respiratory distress syndrome. Nature Rev Dis Primers 2019;5(1):18. doi: org/10.1038/s41572-019-0069-0 [PMID: 30872586].
O'Brodovich H: Pulmonary edema in infants and children. Curr Opin Pediatr 2005;17:381–384. doi: 10.1097/01.mop.0000159780.42572.6c [PMID: 15891430].

▼ PULMONARY LYMPHATIC DISORDERS

CONGENITAL PULMONARY LYMPHANGIECTASIA

ESSENTIALS OF DIAGNOSIS & TYPICAL FEATURES

► Respiratory distress and oxygen requirement at birth.
► Nonimmune fetal hydrops, chylothorax, and Noonan syndrome.
► Milky pleural fluid with high triglycerides and lymphocytes.
► Diagnosed by chest CT or dynamic contrast-enhanced magnetic resonance lymphangiogram or lung biopsy.

Congenital pulmonary lymphangiectasia is a rare anomaly of the lymphatic system in the lungs. It can be isolated or diffuse and limited to the chest or generalized in other organ systems, most notably the GI tract. The lymphatic channels are dilated, tortuous, and may be muscularized. Most cases are associated with a genetic syndrome, most commonly Noonan, Down, and Turner syndromes. Associated congenital heart defects are common and include total anomalous venous return and hypoplastic left heart syndrome. Diffuse congenital lymphangiectasis is often fatal.

► Clinical Findings

Congenital pulmonary lymphangiectasia generally presents as severe respiratory distress at birth. Occasionally symptoms start after the first few months of life and infrequently they begin later in childhood. Chylothorax and diffuse interstitial markings are common on CXR. Chest CT findings include extensive septal and peribronchovascular thickening and ground glass opacities. Associated pulmonary hypoplasia is common.

► Treatment

Pulmonary lymphangiectasia is very challenging to treat and best done at a tertiary center with multidisciplinary team experience. Respiratory support with oxygen, positive pressure, or mechanical ventilation may be necessary and if excessive pleural effusion is present, chest tube drainage may be needed. Nutritional support with medium-chain triglycerides is preferred enterally to reduce lymphatic flow. Investigational therapeutics such as octreotide or sirolimus often are tried, but studies have not definitively proved their benefit. Other interventions to consider are pleurodesis, ligation of the thoracic duct, and endolymphatic embolization.

Prognosis

Once considered a uniformly fatal disease, survival has been increasing with advanced neonatal care, earlier recognition, and advanced interventional options. Limited pulmonary lymphangiectasis has better survival than diffuse disease, and generalized disease often has less severe pulmonary involvement. If there is associated congenital heart disease, that severity may determine the child's outcome.

ACQUIRED LYMPHATIC OBSTRUCTION

The pulmonary lymphatics can become obstructed following surgery for congenital heart disease, most notably after the Fontan procedure. The pulmonary lymph flow abnormally moves from the thoracic duct toward the pulmonary parenchyma, known as pulmonary lymphatic perfusion syndrome. Embolic obliteration of the abnormal lymph channels by a percutaneous approach is a promising therapeutic option.

Lam CZ et al: Diagnosis of secondary pulmonary lymphangiectasia in congenital heart disease: a novel role for chest ultrasound and prognostic implications. Pediatr Radiol 2017;47:1441–1451. doi: 10.1007/s00247-017-3892-z [PMID: 28631156].

Nakano TA et al: How we approach pediatric congenital chylous effusions and ascites. Pediatr Blood Cancer 2022;69(Suppl 3): e29246. doi: 10.1002/pbc.29246 [PMID: 36070215].

LOWER RESPIRATORY TRACT INFECTIONS

BRONCHIOLITIS

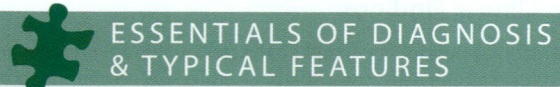

ESSENTIALS OF DIAGNOSIS & TYPICAL FEATURES

- ► Upper respiratory infection prodrome (fever, rhinorrhea), and cough.
- ► Wheezing or rales, tachypnea, retractions, hypoxemia.
- ► Irritability, poor feeding.

Acute viral bronchiolitis is the most common diagnosis responsible for hospitalization at children's hospitals after the neonatal period. Respiratory syncytial virus (RSV) is the most identified viral etiology although other viruses can cause the same clinical scenario, including human metapneumovirus (HMPV), rhinovirus (RV), adenovirus, parainfluenza virus, influenza, and coronaviruses, including the novel corona virus SARS-CoV-2 (COVID-19). Almost all children will have experienced an infection with RSV by the age of 2 years, whether it be a common cold, tracheobronchitis, bronchiolitis, or pneumonia.

Clinical Findings

A. Symptoms and Signs

Bronchiolitis is a clinical diagnosis based on the history of a prodromal upper respiratory tract infection (fever and rhinorrhea) progressing to cough, wheezing, tachypnea, and respiratory distress. Bronchiolitis occurs primarily in infants and toddlers less than 2 years of age. Approximately 1%–3% of the infants with bronchiolitis will require hospitalization due to hypoxemia and/or tachypnea. The most severe infections tend to occur at an early age (< 10 weeks), in infants with: prematurity (< 37 weeks' gestation) with or without chronic lung disease, hemodynamically significant heart disease, neurologic deficits, smoke exposure in the home, poor nutrition, or less than 2 months of breastfeeding. Severe bronchiolitis also occurs more frequently in patients who identify as member of indigenous populations and those in disadvantaged socioeconomic conditions. In temperate climates, bronchiolitis clusters in the winter months with less seasonal variation identified in tropical climates. Patients with bronchiolitis typically have tachypnea, retractions, prolongation of the expiratory phase, crackles, and/or wheezing on examination.

B. Laboratory Findings and Imaging Studies

Although a CXR is not needed for diagnosis, the typical features of bronchiolitis include increased peribronchial markings, over inflation, and subsegmental atelectasis. Because serious bacterial infections associated with bronchiolitis are rare, blood cultures, complete blood counts, and blood gases are not indicated unless the patient is being evaluated for sepsis or acute respiratory failure.

Differential Diagnosis

Children who experience more than one episode of bronchiolitis should be evaluated for asthma or other confounding respiratory condition that predisposes them to recurrent coughing and wheezing.

Treatment

Management of bronchiolitis is mainly supportive by ensuring satisfactory oxygenation, hydration, and suctioning upper airway secretions. Supplemental O_2 by nasal canula usually suffices although the use of heated humidified high-flow O_2

may support oxygenation and limit the escalation of care for patients with hypoxemia refractory to low-flow O_2 by nasal canula. Positive airway pressure delivered in the intensive care unit is beneficial to support oxygenation when less intense support fails, although some children require intubation and mechanical ventilation.

The routine use of inhaled bronchodilators for bronchiolitis is discouraged by most guidelines, citing lack of improvement in oxygenation and duration of hospitalization. Similarly, the use of corticosteroids (usually dexamethasone or prednisolone) has not demonstrated improved clinical outcomes. Studies combining nebulized epinephrine and dexamethasone have suggested potential small benefit. Additional studies are underway. Nebulized hypertonic saline is also under investigation as a potential aid in reducing the secretion burden. Antibiotics have not shown a benefit but are commonly given due to the challenges of interpreting CXRs and concerns for sepsis in young infants.

Prevention

Palivizumab is a monoclonal antibody directed against RSV that may be given prophylactically to high-risk infants, particularly ex-premature babies, that can reduce hospitalization and intensive care use. Palivizumab requires several monthly administrations just prior to the anticipated RSV season, whereas a newer monoclonal antibody, nirsevimab, requires only one infusion per season and its use is pending further evaluation. Maternal vaccination is a newer means of preventing RSV lower respiratory tract infections in newborns.

Prognosis

The outcome for almost all infants and toddlers following acute bronchiolitis is favorable with complete recovery expected, usually by 7–14 days after initial symptoms arise. Children who are severely ill enough to be hospitalized may be at increased risk for asthma following their acute bronchiolitis, particularly if infected with either RV or RSV.

Dalziel SR et al: Bronchiolitis. Lancet 2022;400:392–406. doi: 10.1016/S0140-6736(22)01016-9 [PMID: 35785792].

COMMUNITY ACQUIRED BACTERIAL PNEUMONIA

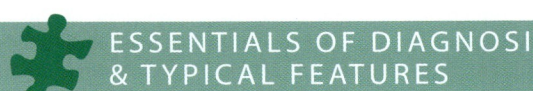

ESSENTIALS OF DIAGNOSIS & TYPICAL FEATURES

▶ Fever, cough, dyspnea.
▶ Focal crackles or decreased breath sounds.
▶ CXR abnormalities (opacities, hilar adenopathy, pleural effusion).

Community-acquired pneumonia (CAP) is a world-wide problem and is the leading cause of childhood mortality in some underserved areas of the world. Next-generation metagenomic sequencing techniques have improved the identification of specific etiologies of CAP, although 20% are nondiagnostic. Viral infection or co-viral infections are the predominant cause of CAP in children with only slight geographic and socioeconomic variation.

In a recent large study in the United States, RSV is the most identified pathogen in children younger than 4 years with RV and HMPV also prominent in this age range. *M pneumoniae* increases in prevalence in the 5- to 9-year age range and predominates along with RV in the 10- to 17-year age range. Documented bacterial infection with *Streptococcus pneumoniae* (3%–4%), *S aureus* (1%), and *S pyogenes* (1%) was both infrequently identified and relatively constant across all childhood age groups.

Clinical Findings

A. Symptoms and Signs

The incidence of CAP is highest in children younger than 2 years and decreases over the remainder of childhood. The symptoms are universal regardless of the etiology and include cough, fever, loss of appetite, tachypnea, respiratory distress, and shortness of breath. Chest auscultation reveals adventitious breath sounds with diffuse or localized crackles and/or wheezing or diminished or absent breath sounds if segmental opacification or pleural effusion is present.

B. Laboratory Findings and Imaging Studies

Guidelines developed by the World Health Organization (WHO) and the British Thoracic Society for diagnosis and management of CAP in children suggest CXR is not necessary for the diagnosis of pneumonia, and managing young children based on solely on tachypnea and respiratory distress as pneumonia has helped reduce mortality in underserved parts of the world. In well-resourced parts of the world, it is common to obtain a CXR to assess the presence or absence of an abnormality that may identify CAP or another disease process. However, CXR findings correlate poorly with the type of organism causing the infection. While it is reasonable to diagnose CAP without a CXR in a mildly ill outpatient based on clinical features alone, more severely ill patients referred for inpatient care should have a CXR (preferably two views) obtained. CXR findings may provide useful information regarding subsequent interventions, such as thoracentesis or chest tube insertion and serve as a baseline if the patient deteriorates.

White blood cell counts and differential counts, C-reactive protein, procalcitonin, and other lab tests are elevated in CAP but lack sensitivity or specificity in identifying bacterial versus viral causes. Blood cultures are rarely positive with CAP unless it is complicated, but even with parapneumonic effusions the blood cultures are positive 30% or less often.

Sputum cultures may be helpful in older children capable of providing a satisfactory sample. Invasive diagnostic procedures should be undertaken in critically ill patients when other means do not adequately identify the cause (see section Diagnosis of Respiratory Tract Infections). PCR technology has improved the ability to detect a wide variety of viral infections but is not indicated in the evaluation of CAP unless the results change management.

► Treatment

Children with CAP or suspected CAP are often treated with antibiotics while recognizing these are mostly viral infections. *S pneumoniae* is the most common bacterial cause of CAP (except in the teenage years), therefore, the initial antibiotic of choice for CAP is amoxicillin for outpatients and ampicillin for inpatients. Antibiotic duration is typically 5–7 days and is adjusted for severity of illness and response to therapy. *M pneumoniae* is the most common organism causing pneumonia in adolescents, therefore initial therapy in this population often is a macrolide antibiotic (such as azithromycin) or a combination of a macrolide and amoxicillin, even though treatment for *M pneumoniae* may not hasten recovery. For children with documented or suspected influenza pneumonia, therapy with an antiviral such as oseltamivir, zanamivir, peramivir, or baloxavir marboxil is recommended.

► Prevention

Childhood pneumonia can be prevented by administering all the recommended childhood vaccines that include coverage against *H influenzae*, *Bordetella pertussis*, *S pneumoniae*, and measles. Annual influenza immunization is recommended for children older than 6 months just prior to the anticipated influenza season.

► Prognosis

The outcome for CAP in children is usually favorable with complete recovery. While mortality in underserved communities is high, it is low in developed countries: estimated to be 1% or less. The CXR is expected to return to normal but may lag the improvement seen clinically. Patients with an excellent clinical recovery from a simple CAP do not require a follow up CXR, but this should be considered if CAP is complicated or recurrent to prove resolution.

Jain S et al: Community-acquired pneumonia requiring hospitalization among U.S. children. N Engl J Med 2015;372:835–845. doi: 10.1056/NEJMoa1405870 [PMID: 25714161].

Messinger AI, Kupfer O, Hurst A, Parker S: Management of pediatric community-acquired bacterial pneumonia. Pediatr Rev 2017;38(9):394–409 [PMID: 28864731].

Zar HJ, Andronikou S, Nicol M: Advances in the diagnosis of pneumonia in children. BMJ 2017;358:j2739. doi: 10.1136/bmj.j2739 [PMID: 28747379].

COMMUNITY-ACQUIRED PNEUMONIA COMPLICATIONS

ESSENTIALS OF DIAGNOSIS & TYPICAL FEATURES

- ► Parapneumonic effusions, empyemas, necrotizing pneumonias, and lung abscesses can complicate pneumonias.
- ► Clinical symptoms, CXRs not improving despite appropriate antibiotic therapy.
- ► Respiratory distress and chest pain.
- ► Persistent fever.
- ► Focal decreased breath sounds.

Pneumonia in childhood is considered complicated if there is a parapneumonic effusion, empyema, lung abscess (necrotizing pneumonia), or if the patient develops acute respiratory failure. These complications are not common but do occur in about 3%–10% of children with CAP and are often preceded by a viral illness. A lung abscess may form during recovery from severe pneumonia or after an aspiration event. If the lung abscess follows an aspiration event, the organisms are commonly anaerobic, and the clinical features can be less dramatic with lower grade fevers and less respiratory distress.

The most identified organism for effusions, empyema and necrotizing pneumonia is *S pneumoniae*, but *S aureus* (both methicillin sensitive and methicillin resistant) can also be the causative organism and should be considered if not responding to appropriate therapy. Less common causative organisms include *H pneumoniae*, *M pneumoniae*, and *Pseudomonas aeruginosa*. Certain clues in the patient's history might indicate that the pneumonia is from an organism less common than viruses or bacteria. For example, *M tuberculosis* should be considered for a patient exposed to a family member with active tuberculosis, one who has travelled to or born from an area where tuberculosis is prevalent, or someone who has been exposed to institutionalized individuals or migrant farm workers. A detailed travel history might uncover a visit to an area of endemic fungal infection such as *Histoplasmosis capsulatum*, *Coccidioidomycosis immitis*, *Blastomycosis dermatitidis*, or *Cryptococcus gattii*. Endemic fungal pneumonias can be a challenge to diagnose and often require a degree of suspicion and the combination of antibody and antigen detection methods in addition to cultures and stains of infected tissues.

▶ Clinical Findings

A. Symptoms and Signs

Pneumonia complications all present similarly with the presence of ongoing respiratory distress, persistent fevers, considerable or progressive radiographic abnormality, and suboptimal response to antibiotic therapy. Many of these children are critically ill and require intensive care unit management. The presence of a pleural effusion or empyema should be suspected in patients with progressive or worsening symptoms despite antibiotic treatment who have decreased intensity breath sounds and dullness to percussion, which is often unilateral.

B. Laboratory and Imaging Studies

Pleural effusions on CXR show blunting of the costophrenic angle and may show a meniscus sign of fluid rising apically on the lateral chest wall (Figure 19–3). Ultrasound can help determine if the fluid is free flowing or loculated and help direct a thoracentesis needle, which if positive for bacteria would suggest an empyema. Loculations indicate a complex effusion or possible empyema. Necrotizing pneumonias and lung abscesses reveal necrotic areas (air-fluid level within a thick-walled cavity) of lung parenchyma on CXR and chest CT and often can be accompanied by effusion or pneumothoraces (Figure 19–4). White blood counts and inflammatory markers (CRP, procalcitonin) may be used in parallel with clinical assessments to track improvement with antibiotic treatment. Bronchoscopy with BAL and sputum cultures can be helpful for determining the causative organism.

▶ Treatment

Small parapneumonic effusions may not need intervention, but larger effusions should be sampled for specific

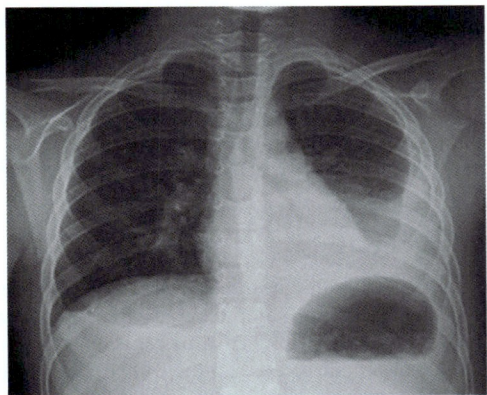

▲ **Figure 19–3.** Chest radiograph demonstrating a left lower lobe opacification with a left pleural effusion in a 9-year-old. No organism was identified despite culturing the pleural fluid.

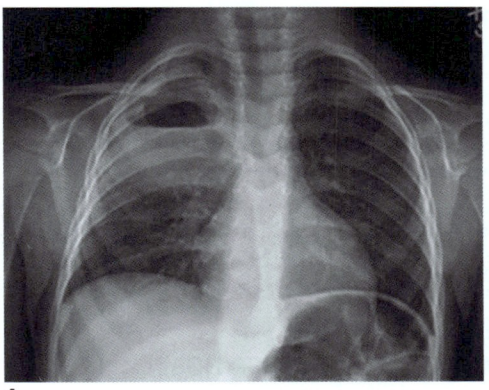

A

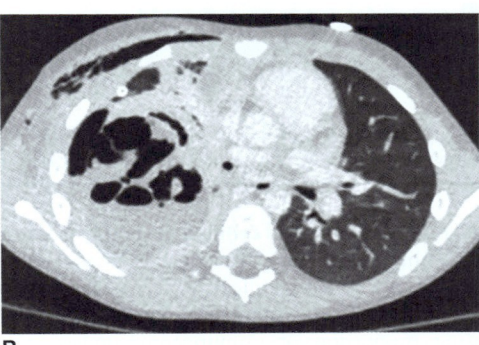

B

▲ **Figure 19–4.** **A:** Chest radiograph demonstrating a thick-walled cavity in the right upper lobe with an air fluid level in a 3-year-old. No organism was identified. **B:** Chest CT scan demonstrating extensive opacification of the right hemithorax with multiple cavitary parenchymal lesions indicating necrotizing pneumonia in a 6-year-old due to *Streptococcus pneumoniae.*

organisms and drained with a chest tube. Complex effusions and empyemas may need more aggressive intervention such as intra-pleural fibrinolytic agents or video-assisted thoracoscopic surgery (VATS). Most patients will return to normal functionally and radiographically over the course of several weeks. Necrotizing pneumonias usually respond to typical systemic antibiotics once the causative organism is appropriately treated but will typically require serial inflammatory markers (CRPs) and clinical monitoring to determine duration of therapy, often lasting weeks.

▶ Prevention

The introduction of the pneumococcal conjugate vaccine (PCV) against *S pneumoniae* has led to a significant reduction in hospitalizations and complicated pneumococcal pneumonias, with recently expanded coverage in 2022 to new vaccines PCV 15 and PCV20 beyond the previous 13 serotypes.

Prognosis

The long-term outlook with pleural effusions is favorable after several weeks. Recovery from a lung abscess is expected, often after several weeks to months. A pneumatocele is a thin walled cavitary structure that may occur after pneumonia has resolved, after trauma, or with hydrocarbon aspiration.

de Benedictis FM, Kerem E, Chang AB, Colin AA, Zar HJ, Bush A: Complicated pneumonia in children. Lancet 2020;396:786–798 [PMID: 32919518].

PNEUMONIA IN THE IMMUNOCOMPROMISED HOST

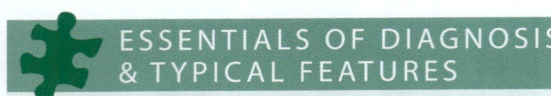

ESSENTIALS OF DIAGNOSIS & TYPICAL FEATURES

▶ The nature of the immunocompromised state may help predict etiology of pulmonary infection.

Patients may have impaired immune responses because of a primary immunodeficiency, from certain disease processes, or iatrogenically from treatment of an underlying disease. Children who have undergone an organ transplant are an increasing proportion of immunocompromised patients. Infectious causes of new pulmonary opacities can occur from typical organisms that infect immunocompetent patients as well as opportunistic organisms that do not infect immunocompetent patients. The type of immunodeficiency can be a clue to which particular or class of organisms is causal. Identifying the specific organism (s) is critical to selecting the best antibiotic regimen.

Bronchoscopy with BAL is often successful at identifying the organism, though less invasive and more commonly performed methods include blood and urine cultures, respiratory pathogen panel nasal swabs, and antigen or antibody measurements. Lung biopsy, performed primarily with VATS, can enhance the diagnostic yield both for infections and noninfectious explanations for the pulmonary opacities, when less invasive testing is unrevealing.

Immunocompromised patients with new pulmonary opacities tend to be quite complex and noninfectious etiologies should be considered in the differential diagnosis, including pulmonary edema, aspiration, venous thromboembolism with PE, lymphoproliferative disease, and reactivation of a latent chronic infection. Complications of therapy for the primary disease process can mimic infections and occur often in patients undergoing hematopoietic stem cell transplantation. These include pulmonary hemorrhage, BO, cryptogenic organizing pneumonia, idiopathic pneumonia syndrome, drug reactions, and radiation injury. Extension of the primary disease process might also be responsible for the new opacities, such as metastatic disease or leukemic infiltrates.

Azoulay E et al: Diagnosis of severe respiratory infections in immunocompromised patients. Intensive Care Med 2020;46:298–314. doi: 10.1007/s00134-019-04906-5 [PMID: 32034433].
Cheng G-S et al: Immunocompromised host pneumonia: definitions and diagnostic criteria. An official American Thoracic Society Workshop Report. Ann Am Thorac Soc 2023;20(3): 341–353. doi: 10.1513/AnnalsATS.202212-1019ST [PMID: 36856712].

DISORDERS OF MUCOCILIARY CLEARANCE

Mucociliary clearance is the primary defense mechanism for the lung. Inhaled particles including microbial pathogens are entrapped in mucus on the airway surface, then cleared by the coordinated action of cilia. The volume and composition of airway surface liquid influence the efficiency of ciliary function and mucus clearance. Mucus that cannot be cleared normally can obstruct the airways. If mucociliary clearance is abnormal, bacteria that are not cleared can cause a vicious cycle of infection, inflammation, and increased mucus production that ultimately leads to airway damage (bronchiectasis). The two main genetic diseases of mucociliary clearance involve disorders of ion transport (CF) and disorders in ciliary function (PCD).

CYSTIC FIBROSIS

ESSENTIALS OF DIAGNOSIS & TYPICAL FEATURES

▶ Greasy, bulky, malodorous stools; failure to thrive, recurrent respiratory infections, digital clubbing.
▶ Bronchiectasis on chest imaging.
▶ Diagnosis with sweat chloride > 60 mmol/L and/or two disease-causing mutations in CFTR gene.

Pathogenesis

Cystic fibrosis (CF), an autosomal recessive disease, results in a syndrome of chronic sinopulmonary infections, malabsorption, and nutritional abnormalities. It is one of the most common lethal genetic diseases in the United States, with an incidence of approximately 1:3000 among Caucasians and 1:9200 in the US Hispanic population and is less common in all other racial and ethnic groups. Although abnormalities occur in the hepatic, gastrointestinal, and male reproductive systems, lung disease is the major cause of morbidity and mortality. Most individuals with CF develop obstructive lung disease associated with chronic infection that leads to progressive loss of pulmonary function.

The cause of CF is a defect in a single gene on chromosome 7 that encodes an epithelial chloride channel called the CF transmembrane conductance regulator (CFTR) protein. The most common mutation is F508del, although approximately 1800 other disease-causing mutations have been identified. Gene mutations lead to absence or defects in CFTR, altering salt and water movement across cell membranes, resulting in abnormally thick secretions in various organs and critically altering host defense in the lung.

▶ Clinical Findings

A. Symptoms and Signs

All states in the United States and many other countries now perform newborn screening for CF by measuring immunoreactive trypsinogen (IRT), a pancreatic enzyme, in blood with or without concurrent DNA testing. Most infants with CF have elevated IRT in the newborn period, although false negative results are possible. In newborns with a positive newborn screen, the diagnosis of CF must be confirmed by sweat testing and/or mutation analysis (https://www.cff.org/intro-cf/newborn-screening-cf). Newborn screening is not diagnostic and false negative values can occur. Therefore, any child presenting with symptoms consistent with CF should undergo a diagnostic sweat test, regardless of newborn screen results.

Approximately 15% of newborns with CF are born with meconium ileus, a severe intestinal obstruction resulting from inspissation of tenacious meconium in the terminal ileum. Meconium ileus is virtually diagnostic of CF, so the infant should be treated presumptively as having CF until a sweat test or genotyping can be obtained. Importantly, meconium ileus can be associated with falsely negative newborn screening (low IRT) and therefore further diagnostic testing is always indicated, regardless of newborn screening results.

Beginning in infancy, failure to thrive can be a common presentation due to malabsorption from exocrine pancreatic insufficiency, failure of the pancreas to produce sufficient enzymes to digest fats and protein. Children with pancreatic insufficiency fail to gain weight despite having a good appetite, and typically have frequent, bulky, foul-smelling, oily stools. Pancreatic insufficiency occurs in about 85% of persons with CF. (Chapter 22 describes gastrointestinal and hepatobiliary manifestations of CF.) Infants with undiagnosed CF may also present with hypoproteinemia (and subsequent edema), anemia, and deficiency of the fat-soluble vitamins A, D, E, and K, because of ongoing steatorrhea.

CF should also be considered in children who present with severe dehydration and hypochloremic alkalosis, bronchiectasis, nasal polyps, chronic sinusitis, rectal prolapse, or unexplained pancreatitis or cirrhosis. Respiratory symptoms can include productive cough, wheezing, recurrent pneumonia, progressive obstructive airways disease, exercise intolerance, dyspnea, or hemoptysis. Chronic airway infection with bacteria, including *S aureus* and *H influenzae*, often begins in the first few months of life, even in asymptomatic infants. Eventually, *P aeruginosa* and other gram-negative opportunistic bacteria become the predominant pathogens. Chronic infection leads to airflow obstruction and progressive airway and lung destruction resulting in bronchiectasis and compromised lung function.

Episodic increases in respiratory symptoms are generically termed pulmonary exacerbations. Clinically, an exacerbation manifests by increased cough and sputum production, decreased exercise tolerance, malaise, weight loss, and a decrease in measures of lung function. Treatment for pulmonary exacerbations generally consists of antibiotics and augmented airway clearance.

B. Laboratory Findings and Imaging Studies

The diagnosis of CF is made by a sweat chloride concentration greater than 60 mmol/L following an abnormal newborn screen or when obtained for clinical symptoms or family history of CF. Sweat testing should be performed at a CF Foundation–accredited laboratory. A diagnosis can also be confirmed by genotyping that reveals two disease-causing CFTR mutations (www.cftr2.org).

Intermediate sweat chloride values of 30–60 may be associated with "mild" CFTR mutations that result in residual functioning CFTR protein. Patients with residual CFTR function typically have adequate pancreatic exocrine function but may develop lung disease. CFTR-related metabolic syndrome (CRMS), diagnosed based on elevated IRT on newborn screen but sweat test less than 60 mmol/L and up to two CFTR mutations, at least one of which is not considered disease-causing, appears to have an even milder disease phenotype. The natural history of this condition is unclear; it is possible that these children may eventually be diagnosed with CF based on increases in sweat chloride and/or in rarer circumstances the development of clinical symptoms. Recent guidelines have suggested that if a child does not meet criteria for a diagnosis of CF after a comprehensive evaluation at age 6, discharge from the CF specialist can be considered with monitoring for symptoms by the family and primary care provider.

▶ Treatment

Individuals with CF should be followed at a CF Foundation–accredited CF care center (http://www.cff.org) in addition to a primary care provider. Care at a CF care center is provided by a multidisciplinary team including pulmonologists and advanced practice providers trained in CF care, nurses, respiratory therapists, dietitians, social workers, psychologists, physical therapists, and pharmacists.

The cornerstone of gastrointestinal treatment is pancreatic enzyme supplementation combined with a high-calorie, high-protein, and high-fat diet. Persons with pancreatic insufficient CF are required to take pancreatic enzyme immediately prior to meals and snacks. Daily multivitamins that contain vitamins A, D, E, and K are also prescribed. Caloric supplements are often added to the diet to optimize growth. Daily salt supplementation also is required to prevent dehydration and hyponatremia, especially during hot weather.

Airway clearance therapy and aggressive antibiotic use form the mainstays of treatment for CF lung disease. Respiratory treatments typically include recombinant human dornase alfa and inhaled hypertonic saline to thin airway mucus for those with chronic *Pseudomonas* infection, inhaled anti-pseudomonal antibiotics (tobramycin or aztreonam), and oral azithromycin are recommended. These therapies have been shown to maintain lung function and reduce the need for hospitalizations and intravenous antibiotics. Early detection of *P aeruginosa* and treatment with inhaled tobramycin can often eradicate the bacteria and delay chronic infection. Bronchodilators and anti-inflammatory therapies are also frequently used in those with airway reactivity.

The development of protein-rescue therapies which directly target the underlying defects in CFTR (termed CFTR modulators) have made significant impacts on the lives of patients with CF. The first treatment that directly works to correct the function of the defective CF protein was approved in 2012. Currently there are four FDA-approved CFTR modulators for people with certain CFTR mutations: ivacaftor, lumacaftor/ivacaftor, tezacaftor/ivacaftor, and elexacaftor/tezacaftor/ivacaftor. These medications will eventually be available to about 90% of the CF population based on genotype. Addition of these modulators to treatment regimens significantly improves lung function and body mass index and reduces exacerbations. These findings have been even more profound with the approval of the highly effective CFTR modulator, elexacaftor/tezacaftor/ivacaftor, which is expected to have significant long-term impacts on lung function, quality of life, and life expectancy. For the remaining 10% of people with CF who do not qualify for CFTR modulators based on genotype, alternate approaches including restoring the CFTR protein or fixing/replacing the CFTR gene will be needed. (https://www.cff.org/research-clinical-trials/path-cure-many-routes-one-mission).

▶ Prognosis

A few decades ago, CF was fatal in early childhood. Now the median life expectancy is approximately 50 years. With the addition of highly effective CFTR modulators, life expectancy is anticipated to increase. Lung transplantation may be performed in those with end-stage lung disease.

Barben J et al: Updated guidance on the management of children with cystic fibrosis transmembrane conductance regulator-related metabolic syndrome/cystic fibrosis screen positive, inconclusive diagnosis (CRMS/CFSPID). J Cyst Fibrosi 2020; Online ahead of print [PMID: 33257262].

Goralski JL, et al. Phase 3 Open-Label Clinical Trial of Elexacaftor/Tezacaftor/Ivacaftor in Children Aged 2-5 Years with Cystic Fibrosis and at Least One F508del Allele. Am J Respir Crit Care Med. 2023 Jul 1;208(1):59-67 [PMID: 36921081].

Middleton PG et al: Elexacaftor-tezacaftor-ivacaftor for cystic fibrosis with a single Phe508del allele. N Engl J Med 2019 Nov 7; 381(19):1809–1819.

Ramsey BW et al: A CFTR potentiator in patients with cystic fibrosis and the G551D mutation. N Engl J Med 2011;365(18): 1663–1672 [PMID: 22047557].

Rosenfeld M, Sontag MK, Ren CL: Cystic fibrosis diagnosis and newborn screening. Pediatr Clin North Am 2016;63(4):599–615 [PMID: 27469178].

PRIMARY CILIARY DYSKINESIA

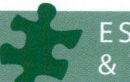

ESSENTIALS OF DIAGNOSIS & TYPICAL FEATURES

► Unexplained neonatal respiratory distress in a term infant.

► Daily year-round cough and nasal congestion.

► Recurrent otitis media with effusions and conductive hearing loss.

► Situs inversus in approximately 50% of cases.

► Diagnosis confirmed by ciliary ultrastructure abnormality on electron microscopy and/or disease-causing mutations in PCD genes.

► Low nasal nitric oxide measurements are suggestive but not diagnostic for PCD.

Primary ciliary dyskinesia (PCD) is a rare, genetic disorder (usually inherited in an autosomal recessive fashion) of impaired mucociliary clearance leading to chronic otosinopulmonary disease. It is believed to occur in approximately 1 in 15,000 births. Approximately half of patients with PCD have situs abnormalities, and men are usually infertile. The triad of situs inversus totalis, bronchiectasis, and chronic sinusitis is known as Kartagener syndrome.

▶ Clinical Findings

A. Symptoms and Signs

Upper and lower respiratory tract manifestations are cardinal features of PCD. Most children with PCD present in the newborn period with respiratory distress (commonly misdiagnosed as neonatal pneumonia or transient tachypnea of the newborn) and often require supplemental oxygen. Upper respiratory tract problems include chronic year-round nasal drainage that begins in the first weeks of life, chronic sinusitis, nasal polyps, and chronic serous otitis media. Conductive hearing loss with chronic middle ear effusion is common. If myringotomy tubes are placed, chronic otorrhea often ensues. Lower respiratory tract features include chronic year-round productive cough, chronic and recurrent bronchitis, and recurrent pneumonia. Patients with PCD are at risk of developing obstructive lung disease and bronchiectasis. Situs inversus totalis occurs in approximately 50% of patients with PCD.

Nonrespiratory ciliopathies that have been associated with PCD include heterotaxy, congenital heart disease, kidney disease, retinitis pigmentosa, and biliary atresia.

B. Laboratory Findings and Imaging Studies

The diagnosis of PCD currently requires a compatible clinical phenotype with at least two of four key clinical features: (1) unexplained neonatal respiratory distress in term infant, (2) year-round daily cough, (3) year-round daily nasal congestion, and (4) organ laterality defect. To confirm the diagnosis of PCD, biallelic pathogenic mutations in PCD-associated genes and/or ultrastructural defects of the cilia by electron microscopy (EM) are also required. Low nasal nitric oxide in combination with a compatible clinical history is suggestive of, but not diagnostic for PCD. Extended genetic testing (> 40 genes on commercially available panels) is emerging as the test of choice but ciliary biopsy may still be necessary to make the diagnosis if genetic testing is normal or inconclusive. Cilia samples may be obtained from either the upper airways (nasal passage) or lower airways (trachea) for EM testing. Significant expertise is required to produce high-quality EM of cilia, and to distinguish primary (genetic) defects from secondary (acquired) defects in ciliary ultrastructure. Multiple different defects in EM can occur including abnormalities in the outer dynein arms, inner dynein arms, radial spokes, and the central apparatus. Some patients with PCD can also have normal EM ultrastructure. There is a strong correlation between genetic mutations and the subsequent ultrastructure abnormalities. Ciliary beat frequency and motion analysis via high-speed videomicroscopy is also used for diagnosis in some settings.

▶ Treatment

At present, no specific therapies are available to correct ciliary dysfunction in PCD. Treatment is largely not evidence-based, and most recommendations are extrapolated from CF and other suppurative lung diseases. Respiratory management includes routine pulmonary monitoring (lung function testing, respiratory cultures, chest imaging), airway clearance by combinations of physiotherapy and physical exercise, and aggressive treatment of upper and lower airways infections.

The first multicenter randomized controlled trial in PCD suggested a benefit of azithromycin maintenance therapy in the reduced the frequency of respiratory exacerbations.

▶ Prognosis

The progression of lung disease in PCD is quite variable. Importantly, persons with PCD are at risk for chronic obstructive lung disease with bronchiectasis. With monitoring and aggressive treatment during times of illness, most individuals with PCD should experience a normal or near-normal life span.

Davis SD et al: Primary ciliary dyskinesia: longitudinal study of lung disease by ultrastructure defect and genotype. Am J Respir Crit Care Med 2019 Jan 15;199(2):190–198 [PMID: 30067075].

Horani A, Ferkol TW: Understanding primary ciliary dyskinesia and other ciliopathies. J Pediatr 2021;230:15–22 [PMID: 33242470].

Kobbernagel HE et al: Efficacy and safety of azithromycin maintenance therapy in primary ciliary dyskinesia (BESTCILIA): a multicentre, double-blind, randomised, placebo-controlled phase 3 trial. Lancet Respir Med 2020 May;8(5):493–505 [PMID: 32380069].

Shapiro AJ et al: Diagnosis of primary ciliary dyskinesia: an official American Thoracic Society clinical practice guideline. Am J Respir Crit Care Med 2018 Jun 15;197(12):e24–e39 [PMID: 29905515].

BRONCHIECTASIS

ESSENTIALS OF DIAGNOSIS & TYPICAL FEATURES

- ▶ Chronic cough with sputum production.
- ▶ Rhonchi or wheezes (or both) on chest auscultation.
- ▶ Diagnosis is confirmed by high-resolution chest CT scan.

▶ Pathogenesis

Bronchiectasis is the permanent dilation of bronchi resulting from airway obstruction by retained mucus secretions or inflammation in response to chronic or repeated infection. It occurs either after an illness (severe pneumonia or foreign-body aspiration) or as a manifestation of an underlying systemic disorder leading to chronic airway inflammation and injury (CF, PCD, chronic aspiration, or immunodeficiency).

▶ Clinical Findings

A. Symptoms and Signs

Persons with bronchiectasis will typically have chronic cough and purulent sputum production. Recurrent respiratory infections and dyspnea on exertion are also common. Hemoptysis occurs less frequently in children than in adults with bronchiectasis. On physical examination, digital clubbing may be seen. Rales, rhonchi, and decreased air entry are often noted during auscultation over the bronchiectatic areas.

B. Laboratory Findings and Imaging Studies

The most common bacteria detected in cultures from the lower respiratory tract include *S pneumoniae, S aureus*, nontypeable *H influenzae*, and *P aeruginosa*. Nontuberculous mycobacterial species may also be detected in patients with bronchiectasis.

Although CXRs may be abnormal, bronchiectasis is diagnosed and defined by high-resolution chest CT. CT imaging reveals the type of bronchiectasis (cylindrical, varicose, cystic) as well as the extent and distribution within the lungs. Airflow obstruction and air trapping is often seen on pulmonary function testing. Airflow obstruction is often fixed (not reversible with bronchodilator use) in bronchiectasis but bronchodilator responsiveness testing should be performed as some patients may benefit.

▶ Differential Diagnosis

The differential diagnosis of bronchiectasis is broad and includes postinfectious etiologies (bacteria, viral, and atypical pathogens), genetic causes (CF, PCD), primary or secondary immunodeficiencies, aspiration, congenital malformations, surfactant deficiencies, collagen-vascular conditions, and allergic bronchopulmonary aspergillosis. The clinical history and physical examination findings can provide important clues as to the underlying etiology and guide the diagnostic testing.

▶ Treatment

The mainstay of treatment for bronchiectasis is airway clearance which has been shown to improve sputum expectoration, measures of lung function, and quality of life. Exercise has also been shown to be beneficial in adults with bronchiectasis but has not been extensively studied in children. Much of the pharmacologic treatments for bronchiectasis have been derived from treatment of CF. Chronic antibiotic use, anti-inflammatory therapy, hyperosmolar agents (hypertonic saline), inhaled corticosteroids, and bronchodilators have not proven effective for non-CF bronchiectasis overall, although individual patients may benefit. However, a large study in adults with idiopathic bronchiectasis concluded that those who received dornase alpha twice a day had more frequent exacerbations, hospitalizations, and lower lung function compared to placebo; thus, dornase alpha is not indicated in adult idiopathic bronchiectasis. Chronic azithromycin has been shown to reduce exacerbations in adults with non-CF bronchiectasis. Whether these results translate to children with idiopathic bronchiectasis is not known. Antibiotics during

pulmonary exacerbations are an important component of bronchiectasis treatment. A multicenter, three-arm, double-dummy, double-blind, randomized placebo-controlled trial in children with non-CF bronchiectasis compared treatment with amoxicillin-clavulanic acid, azithromycin, and placebo to assess the primary outcome of exacerbation resolution at day 14. Oral amoxicillin-clavulanic acid was superior to placebo for exacerbation resolution and duration and is recommended as first-line treatment for mild-moderate exacerbations of bronchiectasis.

Surgical removal of a localized area of lung affected with severe bronchiectasis is considered when the response to medical therapy is poor. Other indications for surgery include repeated hemoptysis and recurrent pneumonia in one area. If bronchiectasis is widespread, surgical resection offers little advantage.

▶ Prognosis

The prognosis depends on the underlying cause and severity of bronchiectasis, the extent of lung involvement, and the response to medical management. Good pulmonary hygiene and avoidance of infectious complications in the involved areas of lung may reverse cylindrical bronchiectasis.

Chang AB, Bush A, Grimwood K: Bronchiectasis in children: diagnosis and treatment. Lancet 2018 Sep 8;392(10150):866–879 [PMID: 30215382].

Goyal V, Chang AB: Bronchiectasis in childhood. Clin Chest Med 2022;43(1):71–88 [PMID: 35236563].

Goyal V et al: Efficacy of oral amoxicillin-clavulanate or azithromycin for non-severe respiratory exacerbations in children with bronchiectasis (BEST-1): a multicenter, three-arm, double-blind, randomized placebo-controlled trial. Lancet 2018 Oct 6; 392(10154):1197–1206 [PMID: 30241722].

Wong C et al: Azithromycin for prevention of exacerbations in non-cystic fibrosis bronchiectasis (EMBRACE): a randomised, double-blind, placebo-controlled trial. Lancet 2012 Aug 18; 380(9842):660–667 [PMID: 22901887].

▼ DISORDERS OF THE CHEST WALL

SCOLIOSIS

ESSENTIALS OF DIAGNOSIS & TYPICAL FEATURES

▶ Scoliosis is a lateral curve of the spine.

▶ Scoliosis is diagnosed based on physical examination and radiologic studies.

▶ Pectus carinatum is a protrusion of the sternum while pectus excavatum is an anterior depression of the chest wall.

Scoliosis is defined as lateral curvature of the spine and is categorized as idiopathic, congenital, syndromic, or neuromuscular. No pulmonary impairment is typically seen with a thoracic curvature of less than 35 degrees. Most cases of idiopathic scoliosis occur in adolescent girls and are corrected before significant pulmonary impairment occurs. Congenital scoliosis of severe degree or with other major abnormalities carries a more guarded prognosis. Patients with progressive neuromuscular disease, such as Duchenne muscular dystrophy, can be at risk for respiratory failure due to severe scoliosis and restrictive lung disease. Severe scoliosis can also lead to impaired lung function and, if uncorrected, possible death from cor pulmonale. (See also Chapter 26.) Small studies indicate that surgical correction of neuromuscular scoliosis should lead to improved quality of life, although pulmonary function may not improve.

Kan et al: Is impaired lung function related to spinal deformities in patients with adolescent idiopathic scoliosis? A systemic review and meta-analysis—SOSORT 2019 award paper. Eur Spine J 2023; 32(1):118–139 [PMID: 36509885].

Kempen et al: Pulmonary function in children and adolescents with untreated idiopathic scoliosis: a systemic review with meta-regression analysis. Spine J 2022;22(7):1178–1190 [PMID: 34963629].

PECTUS EXCAVATUM & PECTUS CARINATUM

Pectus excavatum is anterior depression of the chest wall that may be symmetrical or asymmetrical with respect to the midline. Pectus carinatum is a protrusion of the upper or lower (more common) portion of the sternum, more commonly seen in males. The effects of pectus excavatum and pectus carinatum on cardiopulmonary function are both controversial. While subjective exertional dyspnea has been reported in pectus excavatum and may improve with repair, objective cardiopulmonary function or pulmonary function testing shows inconsistent postoperative results. Therefore, the decision to repair either deformity may be based on cosmetic or psychological considerations, as studies have consistently shown significant improvement in psychological outcomes after surgical repair. Timing of repair is critical and based on growth plate maturation. Pectus excavatum may be associated with congenital heart disease, PCD, and neuromuscular disorders. Pectus carinatum may be associated with systemic diseases such as the mucopolysaccharidoses and congenital heart disease.

Buziashvili D et al: An evidence-based approach to management of pectus excavatum and carinatum. Ann Plast Surg 2019 Mar;82(3):352–358. doi: 10.1097/SAP.0000000000001654 [PMID: 30383585].

Jaroszewski DE et al: Cardiopulmonary function in thoracic wall deformities: what do we really know? Eur J Pediatr Surg 2018;28(4):327–346 [PMID: 30103240].

NEUROMUSCULAR DISORDERS & LUNG DISEASE

ESSENTIALS OF DIAGNOSIS & TYPICAL FEATURES

▶ Neuromuscular disease is associated with impaired cough, sleep-disordered breathing (SDB), and restrictive lung disease in children.

Neuromuscular disorders have multiple etiologies and include weakness of the diaphragm, intercostal muscles, and pharyngeal muscles that inhibit normal breathing (see Chapter 25).

▶ Symptoms & Signs

Neuromuscular weakness leads to weak cough and poor mucus clearance, aspiration and infection, persistent atelectasis, hypoventilation, and respiratory failure in severe cases. Scoliosis, which frequently accompanies neuromuscular disorders, may further compromise respiratory function. The age that respiratory symptoms present for children with progressive or acquired neuromuscular disease depends on the underlying neuromuscular defect and severity. Typical examination findings in children at increased risk for pulmonary disease are a weak cough, decreased air exchange, crackles, and dullness to percussion. The child also may have symptoms of sleep-related hypoventilation or OSA. Positional changes in chest movement and paradoxical thoracoabdominal movement during quiet breathing are indications of respiratory insufficiency. Signs of cor pulmonale may be evident in advanced cases.

▶ Imaging Studies

CXRs generally show small lung volumes, abnormal rib orientation and generalized osteopenia of disuse. If chronic aspiration is present, increased interstitial infiltrates and areas of atelectasis or consolidation may be present. If recurrent pneumonias or dysphagia are present a video fluoroscopic swallow study is warranted. Arterial blood gases demonstrate hypoxemia in the early stages and compensated respiratory acidosis in the late stages. PFTs should be followed over time because abnormalities of decreased vital capacity, decreased inspiratory and/or expiratory pressure, and decreased peak cough flow can worsen over time.

▶ Treatment & Prognosis

Treatment is supportive and includes vigorous airway clearance focused on assisted cough maneuvers, noninvasive ventilation (if worsening vital capacity or hypoventilation), and antibiotics with infection. Supplemental oxygen may correct hypoxemia but does not correct the mechanical defect leading to hypoxemia. Depending on the diagnosis, routine PSG may be indicated to identify hypoventilation before it becomes clinically apparent. Consideration of bilevel positive airway pressure and mechanical airway clearance support, like mechanical in-exsufflation, should be introduced before respiratory failure is present. Because of risk of malignant hyperthermia and difficulty extubating, expert consultation prior to any anesthesia is required.

Many neuromuscular conditions progress to respiratory failure and death. The decision to intubate and ventilate is a difficult one; it should be made only when there is real hope that deterioration, though acute, is potentially reversible or when chronic ventilation is desired. Chronic mechanical ventilation using either noninvasive or invasive techniques is being used more frequently in patients with chronic respiratory insufficiency. New therapies in spinal muscular atrophy, including gene replacement and antisense oligonucleotides, are changing the landscape of this disease.

Antonaci L, Pera MC, Mercuri E: New therapies for spinal muscular atrophy: where we stand and what is next. Eur J Pediatr 2023 Apr 17. doi: 10.1007/s00431-023-04883-8. Epub ahead of print [PMID: 37067602].
Sheehan DW et al: Respiratory management of the patient with Duchenne muscular dystrophy. Pediatrics 2018 Oct;142(Suppl 2): S62–S71 [PMID: 30275250].

DISORDERS OF THE PLEURA & PLEURAL CAVITY

The *parietal* pleura covers the inner surface of the chest wall. The *visceral* pleura covers the outer surface of the lungs. Disease processes can lead to accumulation of air or fluid or both in the pleural space. Pleural effusions are classified as transudates or exudates based on the characteristics of the fluid. Transudates occur when there is imbalance between hydrostatic and oncotic pressure, so that fluid filtration exceeds reabsorption (eg, congestive heart failure). Exudates form because of inflammation of the pleural surface leading to increased capillary permeability (eg, parapneumonic effusions). Other pleural effusions include chylothorax and hemothorax.

Thoracentesis helps characterize the fluid and can provide a definitive diagnosis. Recovered fluid is considered an exudate when Light's criteria are present (pleural fluid–serum protein ratio > 0.5, a pleural fluid–serum LDH ratio > 0.6, or a pleural fluid lactate dehydrogenase (LDH) level greater than two-thirds the upper limit for normal serum LDH). Important additional studies on pleural fluid include cell count; pH and glucose; Gram stain, acid-fast and fungal stains; aerobic and anaerobic cultures; and counterimmunoelectrophoresis for specific organisms. Cytologic examination of pleural fluid should be performed to rule out leukemia or other neoplasm.

Wilcox M et al: Does this patient have an exudative pleural effusion? The rational clinical examination systematic review. JAMA 2014;311(23):2422–2431 [PMID: 24938565].

HEMOTHORAX

ESSENTIALS OF DIAGNOSIS & TYPICAL FEATURES

► Sudden-onset shortness of breath.
► Thoracocentesis reveals blood in the pleural space.

Accumulation of blood in the pleural space can be caused by surgical or accidental trauma, coagulation defects, and pleural or pulmonary tumors. A hemothorax is defined as a parapneumonic effusion when the hematocrit of the fluid is more than 50% of the peripheral blood. Hemopneumothorax may be caused by trauma. Symptoms are related to blood loss and compression of underlying lung parenchyma. There is some risk of secondary infection, resulting in empyema.

► Treatment

Drainage of a hemothorax is required when significant compromise of pulmonary function is present, as with hemopneumothorax. In uncomplicated cases, observation is indicated because blood is readily absorbed spontaneously from the pleural space.

VATS has been used successfully in the management of hemothorax. Chest CT scan is helpful to select patients who may require surgery, as identification of blood and the volume of blood may be more predictive by this method than by CXR.

Broderick SR: Hemothorax: etiology, diagnosis, and management. Thorac Surg Clin. 2013 Feb;23(1):89–96, vi-vii. doi: 10.1016/j. thorsurg.2012.10.003 [PMID: 23206720].

CHYLOTHORAX

ESSENTIALS OF DIAGNOSIS & TYPICAL FEATURES

► Respiratory distress with evidence of fluid in the pleural space on chest imaging.
► Thoracocentesis reveals milky fluid that is high in triglycerides and lymphocytes.

Accumulation of chyle, a fluid of intestinal origin containing fat digestion products (mostly lipids), in the pleural space usually results from accidental or surgical trauma to the thoracic duct. The most common cause of a pleural effusion in the first few days of life is chylothorax due to congenital abnormalities of the lymph vessels or secondary to birth trauma. Abnormalities of lymph vessels are seen in several congenital syndromes such as Down syndrome and Noonan syndrome. In an older child, a chylothorax can be due to laceration or obstruction of the thoracic duct due to trauma or any surgery involving the chest wall (cardiac surgery, scoliosis repair, etc), obstruction of the vessels due to a benign or malignant mass or lymphadenopathy, a granulomatous infection such as tuberculosis, or increased venous pressure due to obstruction or left ventricular failure. Symptoms of chylothorax are related to the amount of fluid accumulation and the degree of compromise of underlying pulmonary parenchyma. Thoracentesis reveals typical milky fluid (unless the patient has been fasting) containing chiefly T lymphocytes.

▶ Treatment

Treatment should be conservative because many chylothoraces resolve spontaneously. Oral feedings with medium-chain triglycerides reduce lymphatic flow through the thoracic duct. Somatostatin or the long-acting somatostatin analogue, octreotide, is a viable therapeutic option. Drainage of chylous effusions should be performed only for those patients with respiratory compromise because the fluid often rapidly reaccumulates. Repeated or continuous drainage may lead to protein malnutrition and T-cell depletion, rendering the patient relatively immunocompromised. If reaccumulation of fluid persists, surgical ligation of the thoracic duct or sclerosis of the pleural space can be attempted, although the results may be less than satisfactory.

Rocha et al: Chylothorax in the neonate—a stepwise approach algorithm. Pediatr Pulmonol 2021;56(10):3093–3105 [PMID: 34324269].
Tutor JD: Chylothorax in infants and children. Pediatrics 2014; 133(4):722–733 [PMID: 24685960].

PNEUMOTHORAX & RELATED AIR LEAK SYNDROMES

ESSENTIALS OF DIAGNOSIS & TYPICAL FEATURES

▶ Sudden-onset shortness of breath.
▶ Focal area of absent breath sounds on chest auscultation.
▶ Shift of the trachea away from the area with absent breath sounds.

Pneumothorax can occur spontaneously in newborns and in older children or, more commonly, because of birth trauma, positive pressure ventilation, underlying obstructive or restrictive lung disease, or rupture of a congenital or acquired lung cyst. Pneumothorax can also occur as an acute complication of tracheostomy. Air is forced from the alveolar spaces into the interstitial spaces of the lung. Migration to the visceral pleura ultimately leads to rupture into the pleural space. Associated conditions include pneumomediastinum, pneumopericardium, pneumoperitoneum, and subcutaneous emphysema. These conditions are more commonly associated with dissection of air into the interstitial spaces of the lung with retrograde dissection along the bronchovascular bundles toward the hilum.

▶ Clinical Findings

A. Symptoms and Signs

The clinical spectrum can vary from asymptomatic to severe respiratory distress. Associated symptoms include cyanosis, chest pain, and dyspnea. Physical examination may reveal decreased breath sounds and hyperresonance to percussion on the affected side with tracheal deviation. When pneumothorax is under tension, cardiac function may be compromised, resulting in hypotension or narrowing of the pulse pressure. Pneumopericardium is a life-threatening condition that presents with muffled heart tones and shock. Pneumomediastinum rarely causes complications other than chest pain.

B. Imaging Studies

CXRs demonstrate the presence of free air in the pleural space. When the pneumothorax is large and under tension, compressive atelectasis of the underlying lung and shift of the mediastinum to the contralateral side may be observed. Cross-table lateral and lateral decubitus radiographs can aid in the diagnosis of free air. Pneumopericardium is identified by the presence of air surrounding the heart, whereas in patients with pneumomediastinum, the heart and mediastinal structures may be outlined with air, but the air does not involve the diaphragmatic cardiac border. Chest CT may identify subtle pleural disease (eg, blebs) in recurrent pneumothoraces. Esophagram can identify if esophageal tear is present in the setting of a pneumomediastinum.

▶ Differential Diagnosis

Acute deterioration of a patient on a ventilator can be caused by tension pneumothorax, obstruction or dislodgment of the endotracheal tube, or ventilator failure. Radiographically, pneumothorax must be distinguished from diaphragmatic hernia, lung cysts, congenital lobar emphysema, and CPAM.

▶ Treatment

Small (< 15%) or asymptomatic pneumothoraces usually do not require treatment and can be managed with close observation. Larger or symptomatic pneumothoraces require drainage. Needle aspiration should be used to relieve tension acutely, followed by chest tube or pigtail catheter placement. Inhalation of 100% oxygen through a nonrebreather to wash out blood nitrogen can be tried but it is controversial whether this procedure is truly beneficial. Pneumopericardium requires immediate identification, and if clinically symptomatic, needle aspiration to prevent death, followed by pericardial tube placement. In older patients with recurrent spontaneous pneumothorax, sclerosing and pleurodesis procedures are sometimes required.

Dotson K, Johnson LH: Pediatric spontaneous pneumothorax. Pediatr Emerg Care 2012;28(7):715–720 [PMID: 22766594].
Johnson NN, Toledo A, Endom EE: Pneumothorax, pneumomediastinum, and pulmonary embolism. Pediatr Clin North Am 2010;57(6):1357–1383 [PMID: 21111122].
Wilson et al: An evidence-based review of primary spontaneous pneumothorax in the adolescent population. J Am Coll Emerg Physicians Open 2021;2(3):e12449 [PMID: 34179877].

MEDIASTINUM

MEDIASTINAL MASSES

ESSENTIALS OF DIAGNOSIS & TYPICAL FEATURES

► Presentation varies depending on the location of the mass.

► Most mediastinal masses are discovered on routine chest x-rays.

Delineation of mediastinal compartments aids in the differential diagnosis of mediastinal masses. Figure 19–5 shows the anatomical borders of the three mediastinal compartments and respective typical mediastinal masses: prevascular (anterior), visceral (middle), and paravertebral (posterior) described by the International Thymic Malignancy Interest Group (ITMIG) classification. In some series, more than 50% of mediastinal tumors occur in the posterior mediastinum and are mainly neurogenic tumors or enterogenous cysts. Most neurogenic tumors in children younger than 4 years are malignant (neuroblastoma or neuroganglioblastoma), whereas a benign ganglioneuroma is the most common histologic type in older children. In the middle and anterior mediastinum, lymphoma and leukemia are the primary concerns. Definitive diagnosis in most instances relies on surgical excision or biopsy for histologic examination.

▶ Clinical Findings

A. Symptoms and Signs

Children with mediastinal masses may present because of symptoms produced by pressure on the esophagus (difficulty swallowing), airways (cough, wheeze, or localized persistent or recurrent infection), nerves (vocal cord paralysis and hoarse voice), or mediastinal vessels (head and neck venous dilation from superior vena cava [SVC] syndrome). Other masses may be discovered incidentally on CXR. Superior mediastinal syndrome presents like SVC syndrome but includes tracheal compression. Hemoptysis can also occur but is an unusual presenting symptom.

B. Laboratory Findings and Imaging Studies

The mass is initially defined by frontal and lateral CXRs together with chest CT scans or MRI. A barium esophagram may help define the extent of a mass. Other studies that may be required include angiography (to define the blood supply to large tumors), echo, ultrasound of the chest, fungal and mycobacterial skin tests, CBC, uric acid, LDH, and urinary catecholamine assays. MRI or myelography may be necessary in children suspected of having a neurogenic tumor in the posterior mediastinum. Mediastinal masses, particularly anterior masses, can cause life-threatening airway compromise in the supine position and during sedation; thus, any sedation or anesthesia should be avoided if possible and performed cautiously.

▶ Treatment & Prognosis

The appropriate therapy and the response to therapy depend on the cause of the mediastinal mass.

Sreedher et al: Pediatric mediastinal masses. Pediatr Radiol 2022;52:1935–1947 [PMID: 35674800].
Vo et al: Imaging evaluation of the pediatric mediastinum: new International Thymic Malignancy Interest Group classification system for children. Pediatr Radiol 2022;52(10):1948–1962 [PMID: 35476071].

SLEEP-DISORDERED BREATHING

ESSENTIALS OF DIAGNOSIS & TYPICAL FEATURES

► Obstructive sleep apnea (OSA) presents with habitual snoring, apnea, or labored respirations.

► Central sleep apnea or periodic breathing may cause subtle pauses in breathing.

► Sleep studies are used to diagnose sleep apnea and guide treatment.

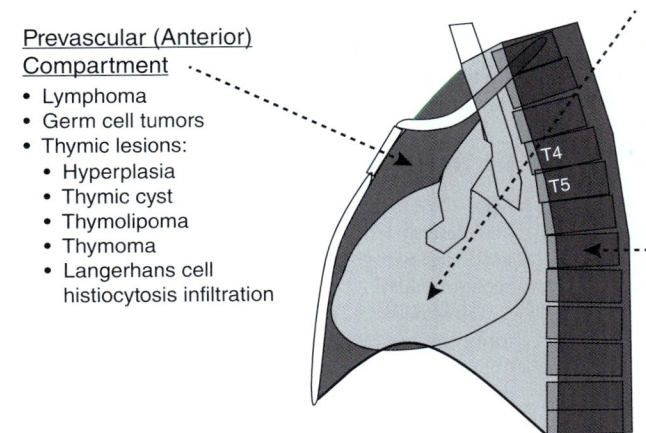

Prevascular (Anterior) Compartment
- Lymphoma
- Germ cell tumors
- Thymic lesions:
  - Hyperplasia
  - Thymic cyst
  - Thymolipoma
  - Thymoma
  - Langerhans cell histiocytosis infiltration

Visceral (Middle) Compartment
- Lymph nodal disease (neoplastic, metastatic)
- Infections (tuberculosis, histoplasmosis)
- Mediastinal fibrosis
- Bronchogenic cyst
- Esophageal duplication cyst
- Tumors of trachea, esophagus, heart, pericardium and great vessels

Paravertebral (Posterior) Mediastinum
- Neurogenic sympathetic ganglion-related tumors
- Nerve sheath tumors
- Paraganglioma
- Extramedullary hematopoiesis
- Discitis or osteomyelitis abscesses

▲ **Figure 19–5.** Mediastinal areas and correlating typical masses.

Sleep-disordered breathing (SDB) is any abnormal respiratory pattern during sleep, which may include noisy breathing, mouth breathing, and/or pauses in breathing that may be obstructive, central, or mixed in etiology. SDB includes obstructive disorders of primary snoring and OSA and central disorders of periodic breathing, central sleep apnea, and hypoventilation syndromes. SDB can decrease children's daytime concentration, impair their growth, cause cardiovascular complications, and systemic inflammation. SDB is a broad clinical diagnosis, but PSG is necessary to determine the specific underlying disorder. Sleep apnea is cessation of breathing and is classified as obstructive (airflow stops despite persistence of respiratory effort) or central (the lack of breathing effort). Hypopnea is decreased (but not absent) airflow and respiratory effort for at least two respiratory cycles with associated oxygen desaturation or arousal.

PRIMARY SNORING & OBSTRUCTIVE SLEEP APNEA

Obstructive sleep apnea (OSA) occurs in approximately 2% of otherwise healthy children. The incidence of OSA is increased in obesity, craniofacial abnormalities, neuromuscular diseases, genetic syndromes (trisomy 21, sickle cell disease, mucopolysaccharidosis), or the use of medications such as hypnotics, sedatives, or anticonvulsants.

▶ Clinical Findings

A. Symptoms and Signs

OSA should be considered with typical nighttime and daytime symptoms:

1. Nighttime symptoms: habitual snoring (more than three times per week) with gasping, pauses, or labored breathing. Other associated symptoms can include night terrors, sleep walking, secondary enuresis, or morning headaches.
2. Daytime symptoms: somnolence, attention deficit, hyperactivity, emotional lability, temperamental behavior, poor weight gain, poor school performance, and recurrent falling asleep in school. Other signs include daytime mouth breathing or dysphagia.

In children, airway obstruction is often associated with nasal congestion, atopy, and adenotonsillar hypertrophy. Tonsillar hypertrophy is most common between the ages of 2 and 7 years. Obesity is widely recognized as an etiologic component in adult OSA and is increasingly recognized in pediatric OSA.

B. Diagnostic Studies: Polysomnogram and Airway Evaluation

AAP's childhood OSA syndrome clinical practice guideline and American Academy of Sleep Medicine (AASM) have similar recommendations, emphasizing that primary care physicians should screen all children for snoring. If the child exhibits additional signs and symptoms of SDB, referral for a PSG is recommended. Referral to an otolaryngologist or sleep specialist is also an option.

The gold standard for diagnosis of OSA is a PSG because overnight oximetry studies can miss obstructive events and history and clinical examination findings do not always correlate with presence or severity of OSA.

The criteria for diagnosing OSA differ between children and adults, and normative values for children are still being

Table 19–9. Comparison of OSA severity in children and adults based on obstructive AHI.

OSA Severity	Obstructive AHI (Children)	Obstructive AHI (Adult)
None	0	0–5
Mild	1–5	5–15
Moderate	5–10	15–30
Severe	> 10	> 30

OSA, Obstructive sleep apnea; AHI, Apnea-Hypopnea Index (events of apnea and hypopnea per hour during polysomnogram).

established, but current suggestions of severity of OSA is shown in Table 19–9.

PSG is recommended for children if the need for surgery is uncertain or if there is discordance between tonsillar size and SDB symptom severity.

If a PSG indicates OSA in a child without tonsillar hypertrophy, an evaluation of the upper airway by awake flexible laryngoscopy should be performed to look for other possible sites of obstruction, including turbinate hypertrophy, adenoid hypertrophy, base of tongue or lingual tonsil hypertrophy, and possible laryngomalacia. The adenoid can also be assessed with a lateral neck x-ray. MRI and drug-induced sleep endoscopy (DISE) in the operating room can also detect sites of upper airway obstruction.

Differential Diagnosis

Periodic limb movement disorders, narcolepsy, circadian rhythm disorders, and behavioral insomnia may mimic the daytime symptoms of OSA.

Treatment

Mild OSA has been shown to improve with nasal steroids and leukotriene inhibitors. If leukotriene inhibitors are used, following for any signs of sadness or depression is recommended.

Most pediatric otolaryngologists perform adenotonsillectomy (AT) in healthy patients with obstructive SDB without obtaining a PSG if there are significant nighttime symptoms and/or daytime symptoms and enlarged tonsils.

Figure 19–6 is an algorithm for management of SDB complaints in an otherwise healthy child. The pathway relies on clinical symptoms and tonsil size. The most commonly used grading scale for tonsil size ranges from 0 to 4. Grade 0 describes prior tonsillectomy; grade 1 tonsils are small and contained within the tonsillar fossa; grade 4 tonsils are so large they may touch ("kissing"). Although the pathway states that an asymptomatic child with markedly enlarged tonsils (4+) should undergo PSG, a period of observation or trial of conservative management is reasonable. Educating the parents about the risks of SDB and what to look for is paramount.

A landmark randomized prospective study on AT outcomes (CHAT Study) demonstrated overall success at 79%. Children with persistent SDB symptoms after AT, more

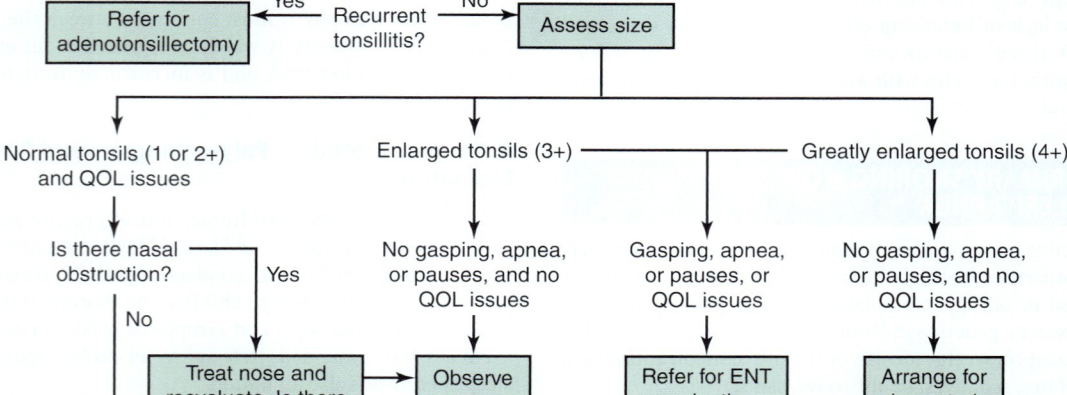

▲ **Figure 19–6.** Algorithm for evaluation of snoring in an otherwise healthy child.

severe OSA, obesity, or other comorbidities should have a postoperative PSG. When OSA persists or AT is contraindicated/refused/delayed, treatment with continuous or bilevel positive airway pressure may be considered.

Regardless of the underlying etiology of SDB, maintaining a healthy weight, addressing abnormal dentition (with the use of orthodontics, such as oral appliances or rapid maxillary expanders), and treating other related pulmonary conditions such as nasal obstruction, allergic rhinitis, and asthma are cornerstones of OSA management.

PERIODIC BREATHING & CENTRAL SLEEP APNEA

Central sleep apnea (CSA) is most common in infants and children, particularly at higher elevations. CSA is a pause in breathing without respiratory effort and may occur in a pattern of alternating apnea and tachypnea known as periodic breathing. Healthy children have been shown to have central apneas lasting 25 seconds without clear consequences. These central respiratory events may be relevant if they occur frequently or are associated with gas exchange abnormalities or sleep fragmentation and then should prompt a thorough evaluation by a pediatric sleep specialist. Supplemental oxygen is often used to reduce oxygen desaturation that can accompany CSA and stabilize the respiratory pattern.

Alsubie HS, BaHammam AS: Obstructive sleep apnoea: children are not little adults. Paediatr Respir Rev 2017 Jan;21:72–79. doi: 10.1016/j.prrv.2016.02.003 [PMID: 27262609].

Marcus CL et al; Childhood Adenotonsillectomy Trial (CHAT): A randomized trial of adenotonsillectomy for childhood sleep apnea. N Engl J Med 2013 Jun 20;368(25):2366–2376 [PMID: 22926173].

BRIEF RESOLVED UNEXPLAINED EVENTS (FORMERLY APPARENT LIFE-THREATENING EVENTS)

ESSENTIALS OF DIAGNOSIS & TYPICAL FEATURES

► Acute, unexpected change in breathing, appearance, and behavior that leads the frightened observer to fear that the infant has died.

► Infants are characterized as low versus high risk to facilitate evaluation and management.

In 2016, the AAP suggested renaming apparent life-threatening events (ALTE) to brief resolved unexplained events (BRUE).

BRUEs are specific to infants younger than 1 year who are observed to have apnea or irregular breathing, cyanosis, or pallor (not redness), marked change in muscle tone (either hypotonia/limpness or hypertonia), or decreased responsiveness that lasts less than 1 minute (more often < 20–30 seconds) and returns to baseline with subsequent reassuring history and physical examination by a clinician. After a BRUE diagnosis, the infant is determined to be either low or high risk, which will determine what, if any, further evaluation is needed. Infants with a BRUE are considered high risk if they are younger than 60 days, born at less than 32 weeks' gestation, received CPR at the time of the event, or have had a prior BRUE.

Immaturity likely plays a major role in the pathogenesis of BRUEs. Classic studies on the nervous system, reflexes, or responses to apnea or gastroesophageal reflux during sleep in infants and immature animals show profound cardiovascular changes during stimulation of the vagus nerve, whereas adults are not affected.

The relationship between BRUE and future risk of SIDS or sudden unexpected infant death (SUID) is not clear, as BRUE infants tend to be younger. See section Sudden Unexpected Infant Death & Sudden Infant Death Syndrome for more detail.

Differential Diagnosis

A careful history, especially gestational age, is the most helpful to determine whether further studies are needed. A study evaluating swallowing in patients with BRUE found that dysphagia and aspiration was the most common abnormality in evaluation of these patients. Table 19–10 classifies disorders that may present as higher-risk BRUEs.

Laboratory Findings & Imaging Studies

Patients with low-risk BRUEs may not need inpatient observation or further testing. One may consider respiratory viral infection including pertussis testing, ECG, brief pulse oximetry, and/or serial observations based on history, examination, or suspicion, but other blood work, lumbar puncture, imaging, acid-suppression therapy, etc are generally discouraged as they provoke unwarranted worry and stress in both patients and caregivers.

Patients with high-risk BRUE, however, should undergo more thorough evaluation for potential underlying etiologies (see Table 19–10), where clinical suspicion prioritizes the appropriate workup. In these cases, patients may be hospitalized for observation to reduce stress on the family and perform diagnostic testing based on the history and physical examination. Laboratory evaluation might include a complete blood count, blood culture with urinalysis, and urine culture for evidence of infection. Serum electrolytes can help evaluate for metabolic disorders, tissue death from hypoxemia, dehydration, ingestions, or chronic hypoventilation.

Table 19–10. Potential causes of brief resolved unexplained events (BRUEs).

Infectious	Viral: respiratory syncytial virus and other respiratory *viruses* Bacterial: sepsis, pertussis, *Chlamydia*
Gastrointestinal	Gastroesophageal reflux with or without obstructive apnea
Respiratory	Airway abnormality; vascular rings, pulmonary slings, tracheomalacia Pneumonia
Neurologic	Seizure disorder Central nervous system infection: meningitis, encephalitis Vasovagal response Leigh encephalopathy Brain tumor
Cardiovascular	Congenital malformation Dysrhythmias Cardiomyopathy
Nonaccidental trauma	Physical abuse Drug overdose Factitious disorder imposed by another (FDIA)
No definable cause	Apnea of infancy

Arterial blood gas studies assess oxygenation and acid–base status. Continuous pulse oximetry in the hospital can assess any changes during eating, sleeping, or screaming.

CXRs can show infiltrates from acute infection or chronic aspiration and evaluate cardiac size from congenital heart disease. ECG is helpful to rule out cardiac dysrhythmias, and echo may be indicated if there is suspicion of congenital heart disease. If history suggests airway obstruction, the airway should be examined either by laryngoscopy, flexible bronchoscopy, or radiographically by CT. VFSS or FEES should be considered to evaluate for dysphagia and aspiration. Upper GI fluoroscopy can evaluate for vascular ring and tracheoesophageal fistula if history is concerning. Infants with reflux and repeated episodes of apnea may benefit from evaluation by a multidisciplinary aerodigestive team.

Depending on the discretion of the clinician, PSG can be useful in detecting abnormalities of cardiorespiratory function, sleep state, oxygen saturation, carbon dioxide retention, and seizure activity. With repeated episodes, apnea, or loss of consciousness, a 24-hour EEG monitoring may be helpful in detecting a seizure disorder.

▶ Treatment

Therapy is directed at the underlying cause if one is found. For both low and high-risk BRUEs, caregivers should be provided with education to reduce modifiable risk factors.

undergo CPR training. Home monitoring has been used in the past, but the efficacy of monitoring has not been demonstrated in controlled trials.

SUDDEN UNEXPECTED INFANT DEATH & SUDDEN INFANT DEATH SYNDROME

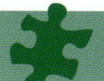

ESSENTIALS OF DIAGNOSIS & TYPICAL FEATURES

▶ Sudden, unexpected death of an infant or child, including accidental suffocation.

Sudden infant death syndrome (SIDS) is defined as the sudden death of an infant younger than 1 year that remains unexplained after a thorough case investigation, including performance of a complete autopsy, examination of the death scene, and review of the clinical history. The postmortem examination is an important feature of the definition because approximately 20% of cases of sudden death can be explained by autopsy findings. After the "Back to Sleep" campaign began in the United States in 1994, the incidence of SIDS declined from approximately 2 per 1000 to 0.5 per 1000 live births. The incidence of SIDS has not changed significantly since 1999.

Sudden unexpected infant death (SUID), defined as any sudden and unexpected infant death, whether explained (such as accidental suffocation or strangulation) or unexplained (such as SIDS) has gained favor as the preferred term to refer to infant deaths that were previously classified as SIDS. SIDS is neither a true diagnosis nor a syndrome and labeling an infant death as SIDS tends to give parents a false sense that the cause of their child's death is known and understood. SUID also includes deaths due to infection, ingestions, metabolic diseases, cardiac arrhythmias, and trauma. Recent evidence shows that the incidence of accidental suffocation and strangulation in bed is increasing due to unsafe sleep surfaces and environments.

▶ Epidemiology & Pathogenesis

Like SIDS, SUID deaths peak between ages 2 and 4 months. Most deaths occur at night, while the infant and the caregiver are sleeping. In fact, the only unifying features of all cases are age and sleep. SUID is more common among socioeconomically disadvantaged populations. Other risk factors include preterm birth, low birth weight, recent infection, young maternal age, high maternal parity, maternal tobacco or drug use, and crowded living conditions. Most of these risk factors are associated with a two to threefold increased incidence but are not specific enough to be useful in predicting which infants will die unexpectedly. Recent immunization is not a risk factor.

Mechanisms of death in SUID are unknown, but maldevelopment or delayed maturation of the brainstem, which is responsible for arousal from sleep, remains the predominant theory. A history of mild symptoms of upper respiratory infection before death is not uncommon.

▶ Treatment/Prevention

Parents should be educated on how to avoid modifiable SUID risk factors, especially in infants at increased risk such as former preterm infants, children exposed to cigarette smoke environmentally or prior to birth, and infants in poor socioeconomic areas (see above).

SIDS AAP Task Force Recommendations:

- Always place a baby on its back to sleep (this includes a baby with reflux).
- Infants should sleep in the parents' room, close to the parents' bed but on a separate surface designed for infants at least for the first 6 months.
- Soft objects and loose bedding, including blankets, nonfitted sheets, stuffed animals, or wedge positioners, should be kept away from the infant's sleep area to reduce the risk of suffocation.

- Zip up wearable blankets are preferred to blankets to keep the infant warm.
- Avoid overheating, overwrapping, and covering the face and head.
- Breast-feeding is recommended.
- Consider offering a pacifier at naptime and bedtime.
- Avoid exposure to cigarette smoke during pregnancy and after birth.
- Car seats, swings, and baby slings should not be used for sleep because the infant's head can fall forward or to the side, compromising the airway.
- Avoid the use of bed rails which increase the risk of suffocation and entrapment.
- Health care professionals, hospital staff, and childcare providers should endorse and model infant safe sleep recommendations from birth.

AAP Task Force on Sudden Infant Death Syndrome: SIDS and other sleep-related infant deaths: updated 2016 recommendations for a safe infant sleeping environment. Pediatrics 2016;138(5):e20162938 [PMID: 27940804].

Tieder JS et al: Brief resolved unexplained events (formerly apparent life-threatening events) and evaluation of lower-risk infants. Pediatrics 2016 May;137(5) [PMID: 27244835].

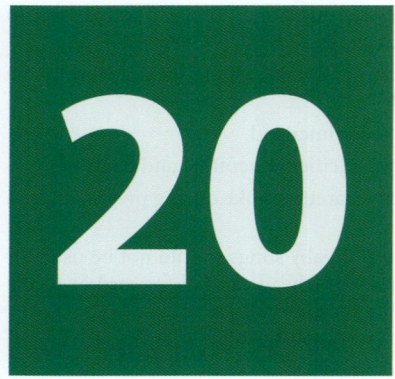

Cardiovascular Diseases

John S. Kim, MD

Dale Burkett, MD

Roni Jacobsen, MD

Johannes Von Alvensleben, MD

INTRODUCTION

Eight in 1000 infants are born with a congenital heart defect. Advances in medical and surgical care allow more than 90% of such children to enter adulthood. Familial and acquired heart diseases, such as Kawasaki disease (KD), viral myocarditis, cardiomyopathies, and rheumatic heart disease, are also a significant cause of morbidity and mortality in children. Pediatric cardiac care includes not only the diagnosis and treatment of congenital and acquired heart disease, but also the prevention of risk factors for adult cardiovascular disease—obesity, smoking, and hyperlipidemia.

◥ DIAGNOSTIC EVALUATION

HISTORY

▶ Signs and Symptoms

Symptoms related to congenital heart defects primarily vary according to the alteration in pulmonary blood flow (Table 20–1). The presence of other cardiovascular symptoms such as palpitations and chest pain should be determined by history in the older child, paying particular attention to the timing (at rest or activity-related), onset, and termination (gradual vs sudden), as well as precipitating and relieving factors.

PHYSICAL EXAMINATION

General

The examination begins with a visual assessment of mental status, signs of distress, perfusion, and skin color. Documentation of heart rate, respiratory rate, blood pressure (in all four extremities), and oxygen saturation is essential. Many congenital cardiac defects occur as part of a genetic syndrome (Table 20–2), and complete assessment includes evaluation of dysmorphic features that may be clues to the associated cardiac defect.

Cardiovascular Examination

A. Inspection and Palpation

Chest conformation should be noted in the supine position. A precordial bulge indicates cardiomegaly. Palpation may reveal increased precordial activity, right ventricular (RV) lift, or left-sided heave; a diffuse point of maximal impulse; or a precordial thrill caused by a grade IV/VI or greater murmur. The thrill of aortic stenosis is found in the suprasternal notch. In patients with severe pulmonary hypertension (PH), a palpable pulmonary closure (P_2) is frequently noted at the upper left sternal border.

B. Auscultation

1. Heart sounds—The first heart sound (S_1) is the sound of atrioventricular (AV) valve closure between the atria and ventricles (mitral and tricuspid valves) and is best heard at the lower left sternal border. Although S_1 has multiple components, only one of these, M_1 (closure of the mitral valve), is usually audible.

The second heart sound (S_2) is the sound of semilunar valve closure between the ventricles and the major arteries (aortic and pulmonary valves). It is best heard at the upper left sternal border. S_2 has two component sounds, A_2 and P_2 (aortic and pulmonic valve closure). Splitting of S_2 varies with respiration, widening with inspiration and narrowing with expiration. Abnormal splitting of S_2 may be an indication of cardiac disease (Table 20–3). A prominent or loud P_2 is associated with PH.

The third heart sound (S_3), if present, is the sound of rapid left ventricular (LV) filling. It occurs in early diastole, after S_2, and is medium- to low-pitched. In healthy children, S_3 diminishes or disappears when going from supine to sitting or standing. A pathologic S_3 is often heard in the presence of

Table 20–1. Symptoms of increased and decreased pulmonary blood flow.

Decreased Pulmonary Blood Flow	Increased Pulmonary Blood Flow
Infant/toddler	
Cyanosis	Tachypnea with activity/feeds
Squatting	Diaphoresis
Loss of consciousness	Poor weight gain
Older child	
Dizziness	Exercise intolerance
Syncope	Dyspnea on exertion, diaphoresis

Table 20–2. Cardiac defects in common syndromes.

Genetic Syndrome	Commonly Associated Cardiac Defect
Down syndrome	AVSD
Turner syndrome	Bicuspid aortic valve, coarctation, dilated aortic root, hypertension
Noonan syndrome	Dysplastic pulmonic valve, HCM
Williams-Beuren syndrome	Supravalvular aortic stenosis, PPS, coronary ostial stenosis
Marfan syndrome	MVP, MR, dilated aortic root
Fetal alcohol syndrome	VSD, ASD
Maternal rubella	PDA, PPS
Loeys-Dietz syndrome	Aneurysmal PDA, dilated aortic root, tortuous arteries throughout the body

ASD, atrial septal defect; AVSD, atrioventricular septal defect; HCM, hypertrophic cardiomyopathy; MR, mitral regurgitation; MVP, mitral valve prolapse; PDA, patent ductus arteriosus; PPS, peripheral pulmonary stenosis; VSD, ventricular septal defect.

Table 20–3. Abnormal splitting of S_2.

Causes of wide split S_2
RV volume overload: ASD, anomalous pulmonary venous return, PI
RV pressure overload: Pulmonary valve stenosis
Delayed RV conduction: RBBB
Causes of narrow split or single S_2
Pulmonary hypertension
Single semilunar valve (aortic atresia, pulmonary atresia, truncus arteriosus)

ASD, atrial septal defect; PI, pulmonic insufficiency; RBBB, right bundle branch block; RV, right ventricle.

poor cardiac function, significant mitral regurgitation, or a large left-to-right shunt. The fourth heart sound (S_4), if present, is associated with atrial contraction into a noncompliant ventricle, as in hypertrophic or restrictive cardiomyopathy or from other causes of diastolic dysfunction, and has a low pitch similar to that of S_3. It occurs just prior to S_1 and is not normally audible.

Ejection clicks are characterized by a short, high-pitched sound and are usually related to dilated great vessels or valve abnormalities. They are heard during ventricular systole, between S1 and S2, and are classified as early, mid, or late. Early ejection clicks at the mid-left sternal border are from the pulmonic valve. Aortic clicks are typically best heard at the right upper sternal border. In contrast to aortic clicks, pulmonic clicks vary with respiration, becoming louder during inspiration. A mid to late ejection click at the apex is most typically caused by mitral valve prolapse (MVP).

2. Murmurs—A heart murmur is the most common cardiovascular finding leading to a cardiology referral. Innocent or functional heart murmurs are common; 40%–45% of children have an innocent murmur at some time during childhood.

A. CHARACTERISTICS—All murmurs should be described based on the following characteristics:

(1) Intensity—Grade I describes a soft murmur heard with difficulty; grade II, soft but easily heard; grade III, loud but without a thrill; grade IV, loud and associated with a precordial thrill; grade V, loud, with a thrill, and audible with the edge of the stethoscope; grade VI, very loud and audible with the stethoscope off the chest.

(2) Quality—Harsh, musical, or rough; high, medium, or low in pitch.

(3) Relationship to cardiac cycle and duration—Systolic ejection (immediately following S_1 with a crescendo/decrescendo change in intensity), pansystolic/holosystolic (onset concurrent with S_1, lasting throughout most of systole and of constant intensity), diastolic, or continuous. The timing of the murmur provides valuable clues as to the underlying pathology (Table 20–4).

(4) Location and radiation—Where the murmur is best heard and where the sound extends.

(5) Variation with position—Audible changes in murmur when the patient is supine, sitting, standing, or squatting.

B. INNOCENT MURMURS—The six most common innocent murmurs of childhood are as follows:

(1) Newborn murmur—Heard in the first few days of life, this murmur is at the lower left sternal border, without significant radiation. It is a soft I–II/VI, low-pitch, short, early systolic murmur that often subsides when mild pressure is applied to the abdomen. It usually disappears by age 2–3 weeks.

(2) Peripheral pulmonary artery stenosis (PPS)—This murmur, often heard in newborns, is caused by increased flow through normal branching of the pulmonary artery

Table 20–4. Pathologic murmurs.

Systolic Ejection	Pansystolic	Diastolic	Continuous
Semilunar valve stenosis	VSD	Semilunar valve regurgitation	PDA
ASD	AV valve regurgitation		AVM
Aortic coarctation		AV valve stenosis	Aortopulmonary collaterals

ASD, atrial septal defect; AV, atrioventricular; AVM, arteriovenous malformation; PDA, patent ductus arteriosus; VSD, ventricular septal defect.

(PA). It is heard with equal intensity at the upper left sternal border, at the back, and in one or both axillae. It is a I–II/VI, short, high-pitched, early systolic ejection murmur and usually disappears by 6 months of age.

(3) *Still's murmur*—This is the most common innocent murmur of early childhood. It is typically heard between 2 and 7 years of age. It is the loudest midway between the apex and the lower left sternal border. Still's murmur is a I-III/VI, musical or vibratory, short, early systolic murmur. It is loudest when the patient is supine and diminishes or disappears with sitting the patient up or with exercise. It can be louder while febrile.

(4) *Pulmonary ejection murmur*—This is the most common innocent murmur in older children and adults. It is heard from age 3 years onward. It is a I-II/VI, soft, low-pitch systolic ejection murmur, at the upper left sternal border. The murmur is louder when the patient is supine or when cardiac output is increased. Unlike the pulmonary flow murmur associated with an atrial septal defect (ASD), there is normal splitting of A_2 and P_2.

(5) *Venous hum*—A venous hum is usually heard after age 2 years. It is a I-II/VI, continuous, low-to-medium pitch musical hum located in the right infraclavicular area and may be accentuated in diastole and with inspiration. It is best heard in the sitting position. Turning the child's neck, placing the child supine, and compressing the jugular vein obliterate the venous hum. The venous hum is caused by turbulence at the confluence of the subclavian and jugular veins.

(6) *Innominate or carotid bruit*—This murmur is more common in the older child and adolescents. It is heard in the right supraclavicular area. It is a II-III/VI, somewhat harsh, long systolic ejection murmur. The bruit can be accentuated by light pressure on the carotid artery and must be differentiated from all types of aortic stenosis. The characteristic findings of aortic stenosis are outlined in more detail later in this chapter.

When innocent murmurs are found in a child, the physician should assure the parents that these are normal heart sounds of the developing child and that they do not represent heart disease.

Extracardiac Examination

A. Arterial Pulse Rate and Rhythm

Cardiac rate and rhythm vary greatly during infancy and childhood, so multiple determinations should be made. This is particularly important for infants (Table 20–5) whose heart rates vary with activity. The rhythm may be regular, or there may be a normal phasic variation with respiration (sinus arrhythmia).

B. Arterial Pulse Quality and Amplitude

A bounding pulse is characteristic of patent ductus arteriosus (PDA), aortic regurgitation, arteriovenous malformation, or any condition with a low diastolic pressure (fever, anemia, or septic shock). Narrow or thready pulses occur in patients with conditions reducing cardiac output such as decompensated heart failure (HF), pericardial tamponade, or severe aortic stenosis. Blood pressure fluctuation greater than 10 mm Hg with respiration is referred to as pulsus paradoxus and can be a sign of pericardial tamponade. The pulses of the upper and lower extremities should be compared. The femoral pulse should be palpable and equal in amplitude and simultaneous with the brachial pulse. A femoral pulse that is absent or weak, or that is delayed in comparison with brachial pulse, suggests coarctation of the aorta.

C. Arterial Blood Pressure

Blood pressures should be obtained in the upper and lower extremities. Systolic pressure in the lower extremities should be greater than or equal to that in the upper extremities. The cuff must cover the same relative area of the arm and leg. Measurements should be repeated several times. A lower blood pressure in the lower extremities suggests coarctation of the aorta.

Table 20–5. Resting heart rates.

Age	Low	High
< 1 mo	80	160
1–3 mo	80	200
2–24 mo	70	120
2–10 y	60	90
11–18 y	40	90

D. Cyanosis of the Extremities

Cyanosis results from an increased concentration of deoxygenated hemoglobin (> 4–5 g/dL) in the blood. Visible cyanosis also accompanies low cardiac output, hypothermia, and systemic venous congestion, even in the presence of adequate oxygenation. Cyanosis should be judged by the color of the mucous membranes (lips, gums, tongue). Bluish discoloration surrounding the mouth (acrocyanosis) does not correlate with cyanosis.

E. Clubbing of the Fingers and Toes

Clubbing is often associated with severe cyanotic congenital heart disease (CHD). It usually appears after age 1 year. Hypoxemia with cyanosis is the most common cause, but clubbing also occurs in patients with endocarditis, chronic liver disease, inflammatory bowel diseases, chronic pulmonary disease, and lung abscess. Digital clubbing may also be a benign genetic variant.

F. Edema

Edema of dependent areas (lower extremities in the older child and the face and sacrum in the younger child) is characteristic of elevated right heart pressure, which may be seen with tricuspid valve pathology or HF.

G. Abdomen

Hepatomegaly is the cardinal sign of right HF in the infant and child. Left HF can ultimately lead to right HF, and therefore hepatomegaly may also be seen in the child with pulmonary edema from lesions causing left-to-right shunting (pulmonary overcirculation) or left HF. Splenomegaly may be present in patients with long-standing HF and is also a characteristic of infective endocarditis (IE). Ascites is another feature of chronic right HF. Examination of the abdomen may reveal shifting dullness or a fluid wave.

Kostopoulou E, Dimitriou G, Karatza A: Cardiac murmurs in children: a challenge for the primary care physician. Curr Pediatr Rev 2019 Mar 20 [PMID: 30907325].
Sumski CA et al: Evaluating chest pain and heart murmurs in pediatric and adolescent patients. Pediatr Clin North Am 2020;67(5): 783–799 [PMID: 32888681].

ELECTROCARDIOGRAPHY

The electrocardiogram or electrocardiography (ECG) is essential for the evaluation of the cardiovascular system. The heart rate should first be determined, then the cardiac rhythm, and then the axis. Finally, assessment of chamber enlargement, cardiac intervals, and ST segments should be performed.

Age-Related Variations

ECG evolves with age. The heart rate decreases and intervals increase with age. Right ventricle (RV) dominance in the newborn changes to left ventricle (LV) dominance in the older infant, child, and adult.

Electrocardiographic Interpretation

Figure 20–1 defines the events recorded by the ECG.

A. Rate

The heart rate varies markedly with age, activity, and state of emotional and physical well-being (see Table 20–5).

B. Rhythm

Sinus rhythm should always be present in healthy children and is defined by ECG findings of (1) P wave before every QRS, (2) QRS after every P wave, (3) regular P-to-P intervals, and (4) regular R-to-R intervals. Extra heartbeats representing premature atrial and ventricular contractions (PAC and PVC) are common during childhood, with atrial ectopy predominating in infants and ventricular ectopy during adolescence. Isolated premature beats in patients with normal heart structure and function are usually benign.

C. Axis

1. P-wave axis—The P wave is generated from atrial contraction, typically originating from the sinus node in the high right atrium (RA). The impulse proceeds leftward and inferiorly, thus leading to a positive deflection in all left-sided and inferior leads (II, III, and aVF) and negative in lead aVR.

2. QRS axis—The net voltage should be positive in leads I and aVF in children with a normal axis. In infants and young children, RV dominance may persist, leading to a negative deflection in lead I. Several congenital cardiac lesions are associated with alterations in the normal QRS axis (Table 20–6).

D. P Wave

In the pediatric patient, the amplitude of the P wave is normally no greater than 3 mm (three small boxes) and the duration no more than 0.08 second (two small boxes). The P wave is best seen in leads II and V_1.

E. PR Interval

The PR interval is measured from the beginning of the P wave to the beginning of the QRS complex. It represents the time it takes to conduct the signal from the sinus node to, and through, the AV node. It increases with age and with slower rates. The PR interval ranges from a minimum of 0.10 second in infants to a maximum of 0.18 second in older children with slow rates. Rheumatic heart disease, digitalis, β-blockers, and calcium channel blockers can prolong the PR interval.

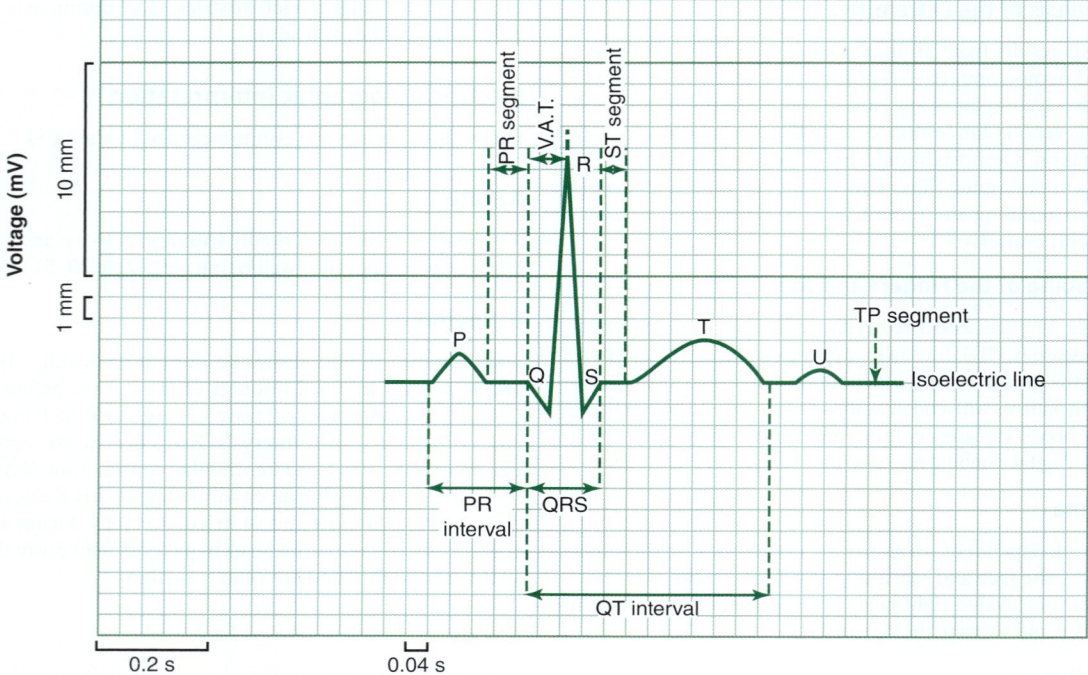

▲ **Figure 20–1.** Complexes and intervals of the electrocardiogram.

F. QRS Complex

This represents ventricular depolarization, and its amplitude and direction of force (axis) reveal the relative ventricular mass in hypertrophy, hypoplasia, and infarction. Abnormal ventricular conduction (eg, left bundle branch block [LBBB] or right bundle branch block [RBBB]) is also revealed.

G. QT Interval

This interval is measured from the beginning of the QRS complex to the end of the T wave. The QT duration may be prolonged as a primary condition or secondarily due to drugs or electrolyte imbalances (Table 20–7). The normal

QT duration is rate-related and must be corrected using the Bazett formula:

$$QTc = \frac{QT\ interval\ (s)}{\sqrt{R-R\ interval\ (s)}}$$

The normal QTc is less than or equal to 0.44 second.

Table 20–6. QRS axis deviation.

Right-Axis Deviation	Left-Axis Deviation
Tetralogy of Fallot	Atrioventricular septal defect
Transposition of the great arteries	Pulmonary atresia with intact ventricular septum
Total anomalous pulmonary venous return	Tricuspid atresia
Atrial septal defect	

Table 20–7. Causes of QT prolongation.[a]

Cardiac medications
Antiarrhythmics: class IA (quinidine, procainamide, disopyramide) class III (amiodarone, sotalol)
Inotropic agents: dobutamine, dopamine, epinephrine, isoproterenol
Noncardiac medications
Antibiotics/antivirals: azithromycin, clarithromycin, levofloxacin, amantadine
Antiemetics: droperidol, ondansetron, promethazine, tropisetron, amisulpride, granisetron, dolasetron
Antipsychotics: risperidone, thioridazine, lithium, haloperidol, prochlorperazine
Sedatives: chloral hydrate, methadone
Other: albuterol, levalbuterol, ondansetron, phenytoin, pseudoephedrine
Electrolyte disturbances: hypokalemia, hypomagnesemia, hypocalcemia

[a]Partial list only.

H. ST Segment

This segment, lying between the end of the QRS complex and the beginning of the T wave, is affected by drugs, electrolyte imbalances, or myocardial injury.

I. T Wave

The T wave represents myocardial repolarization and is altered by electrolytes, myocardial hypertrophy, and ischemia.

O'Connor M, McDaniel N, Brady WJ: The pediatric electrocardiogram. Part I: age-related interpretation. Am J Emerg Med 2008 May;26(4):506–512 [PMID: 18416018].

CHEST RADIOGRAPH

Evaluation of the chest radiograph for cardiac disease should focus on (1) position of the heart, (2) position of the abdominal viscera, (3) cardiac size, (4) cardiac configuration, and (5) character of the pulmonary vasculature. Standard posteroanterior and left lateral chest radiographs are used (Figure 20–2).

Cardiac position is either levocardia (apex of the heart pointing leftward), dextrocardia (apex of the heart pointing rightward), or mesocardia (midline heart). The position of the liver and stomach bubble is either in the normal position (abdominal situs solitus), mirror image inverted (abdominal situs inversus), or variable with midline liver (abdominal situs ambiguous). The heart appears relatively large in normal newborns at least in part due to a prominent thymic shadow. The heart size should be less than 50% of the chest diameter in children older than 1 year. The cardiac configuration on chest radiograph may provide useful diagnostic information (Table 20–8). Some congenital cardiac lesions have a characteristic radiographic appearance that suggests the diagnosis but should not be viewed as conclusive (Table 20–9).

Pulmonary vasculature should be assessed for increased or decreased pulmonary blood flow, which may suggest a possible congenital cardiac diagnosis, particularly in the cyanotic infant (Table 20–10).

Table 20–8. Radiographic changes with cardiac chamber enlargement.

Chamber Enlarged	Change in Cardiac Silhouette on Anteroposterior Film
Right ventricle	Apex of the heart is tipped upward
Left ventricle	Apex of the heart is tipped downward
Left atrium	Double shadow behind cardiac silhouette
	Increase in subcarinal angle
Right atrium	Prominence of right atrial border of the heart

Laya BF et al: The accuracy of chest radiographs in the detection of congenital heart disease and in the diagnosis of specific congenital cardiac lesions. Pediatr Radiol 2006;36:677–681 [PMID: 16547698].

Dextrocardia

Dextrocardia is a radiographic term used when the apex of the heart is pointing rightward. In situs inversus totalis, dextrocardia occurs with reversal of position of all other important organs of the chest and abdomen (eg, liver, lungs, and spleen), and the heart is usually structurally normal. When dextrocardia occurs with the other organs normally located (situs solitus), the heart usually has severe defects. There are other abnormal spatial relationships between the heart and other organs that fall into the realm of heterotaxy syndrome, defined as the existence of two or more abnormal organ relationships. Abnormalities include right isomerism (asplenia syndrome, with duplication of right-sided structures), left isomerism (polysplenia, with duplication of left-sided structures), or indeterminate visceroatrial situs (situs ambiguous). In virtually all cases of situs ambiguous, CHD is present.

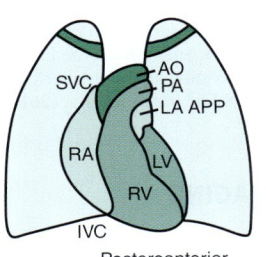 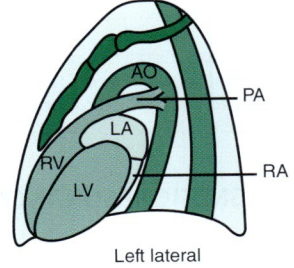

Posteroanterior / Left lateral

▲ **Figure 20–2.** Position of cardiovascular structures in principal radiograph views. AO, aorta; IVC, inferior vena cava; LA, left atrium; LA APP, left atrial appendage; LV, left ventricle; PA, pulmonary artery; RA, right atrium; RV, right ventricle; SVC, superior vena cava.

Table 20–9. Lesion-specific chest radiographic findings.

Diagnosis	Chest Radiograph Appearance
Transposition of the great arteries	Egg on a string
Tetralogy of Fallot	Boot-shaped heart
Unobstructed total anomalous pulmonary venous drainage	Snowman
Obstructed total anomalous pulmonary venous drainage	Small heart with congested lungs
Coarctation	Figure 3 sign + rib notching

Table 20–10. Alterations in pulmonary blood flow in cyanotic cardiac lesions.

Increased Pulmonary Blood Flow	Decreased Pulmonary Blood Flow
Total anomalous pulmonary venous return	Pulmonic stenosis
Tricuspid atresia with large ventricular septal defect	Tricuspid atresia/restrictive ventricular septal defect
Transposition of the great arteries	Tetralogy of Fallot
Truncus arteriosus	Pulmonary atresia with intact ventricular septum

ECHOCARDIOGRAPHY

Echocardiography, a fundamental tool of pediatric cardiology, is performed by placing the ultrasound transducer on areas of the chest and can define cardiac anatomy, blood flow, intracardiac pressures, and ventricular function. M-mode echocardiography generates an image based on the structures visualized along a single line and is typically used to assess ventricular function. Complex intracardiac anatomy and spatial relationships can be described with two-dimensional imaging (Figure 20–3), making possible the accurate diagnosis of CHD.

Doppler ultrasound is used to assess the direction and velocity of blood flow or tissue motion, providing information about intracardiac blood flow and pressure gradients. Three-dimensional echocardiography, tissue Doppler, strain, and strain rate imaging are newer modalities that provide more sophisticated assessment of ventricular function.

Transesophageal echocardiography uses a probe inserted into the esophagus, requiring general anesthesia in infants and children. It is primarily used to guide interventional procedures and surgical repair of CHD but may be of benefit in cases where patients have poor transthoracic windows.

Fetal echocardiography plays an important role in the prenatal diagnosis of CHD. A fetal echocardiogram is recommended if the fetus is considered high risk for CHD or if there is suspicion for fetal arrhythmias based on the obstetric fetal ultrasound. In utero management of fetal arrhythmias and postdelivery planning for the fetus with CHD results in improved outcomes for this challenging group of patients.

Donofrio MT et al: Diagnosis and treatment of fetal cardiac disease: a scientific statement from the American Heart Association. Circulation 2014 May 27;129(21):2183–2242 [PMID: 24763516].

Puchalski MD et al: Guidelines for performing a comprehensive transesophageal echocardiographic examination in children and all patients with congenital heart disease: recommendations from the American Society of Echocardiography. J Am Soc Echocardiogr 2019 Feb;32(2):173–215 [PMID: 30579694].

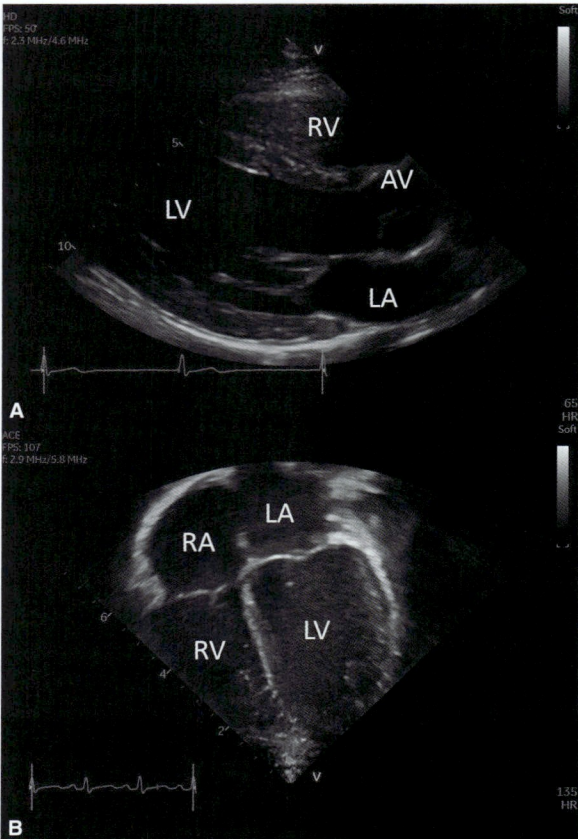

▲ **Figure 20–3.** Two-dimensional echocardiography, from parasternal long-axis (A) and apical four-chamber (B) planes. The images demonstrate the aortic valve (AV), left atrium (LA), left ventricle (LV), right atrium (RA), and right ventricle (RV).

Simpson J et al: Three-dimensional echocardiography in congenital heart disease: an expert consensus document from the European Association of Cardiovascular Imaging and the American Society of Echocardiography. J Am Soc Echocardiogr 2017 Jan;30(1):1–27 [PMID: 27838227].

MAGNETIC RESONANCE IMAGING

Magnetic resonance imaging (MRI) of the heart, which provides dynamic evaluation of structure and blood flow through the heart and thoracic great vessels, is valuable for evaluation and follow-up of acquired and congenital heart disease. Cardiac MRI can quantify valve regurgitation, ventricular function, chamber size, and wall thickness. It is especially useful to characterize RV size and function as this chamber is often difficult to image comprehensively by echocardiography. Because MRI allows computer manipulation of images of the heart and great vessels, three-dimensional MRI is an ideal noninvasive way of obtaining accurate reconstructions of the heart. General anesthesia is often required to facilitate cardiac MRI performance in children younger than 8 years.

Fratz S et al: Guidelines and protocols for cardiovascular magnetic resonance in children and adults with congenital heart disease. J Cardiovasc Magn Reson 2013;15(1):51 [PMID: 23763839].

CARDIOPULMONARY STRESS TESTING

Cardiopulmonary exercise (or stress) testing (CPET) provides objective measurements in children with acquired and congenital heart disease to ascertain limitations, develop exercise programs, and assess effects of medical or surgical therapies. Bicycle ergometers or treadmills can be used in children as young as 7 years. The addition of a metabolic cart enables differentiation of exercise impairment secondary to cardiac or pulmonary limitation or deconditioning. Stress testing is also employed in children with structurally normal hearts who have complaints of exercise-induced symptoms to rule out cardiac or pulmonary pathology. Significant stress ischemia or dysrhythmias warrant physical restrictions or appropriate therapy. Children with poor performance due to suboptimal conditioning benefit from a planned exercise program.

Miliaresis C et al: Cardiopulmonary stress testing in children and adults with congenital heart disease. Cardiol Rev 2014 Nov–Dec;22(6):275–280 [PMID: 25162333].

ARTERIAL BLOOD GASES & PULSE OXIMETRY

Quantifying the partial arterial oxygen pressure (Pa_{O_2}) or O_2 saturation (Sa_{O_2}) during the administration of 100% oxygen—the so-called hyperoxia test—is the most useful method of distinguishing hypoxemia produced primarily by heart disease or by lung disease. In cyanotic heart disease, hypoxemia is caused by shunting of deoxygenated blood to the systemic circulation and, thus, when compared to values obtained while breathing room air, the Sa_{O_2} and Pa_{O_2} increase very little when oxygen is administered. However, in a patient with hypoxemia caused by lung disease, the Sa_{O_2} and Pa_{O_2} usually increase significantly when oxygen is administered. Table 20–11 illustrates the respective responses in patients during the hyperoxia test.

In 2010, the US Department of Health and Human Services (HHS) recommended newborn screening for critical CHD with pulse oximetry screening at 24–48 hours of age. Both the American Academy of Pediatrics (AAP) and American Heart Association (AHA) endorsed this recommendation in 2012.

Table 20–11. Examples of responses to 100% oxygen in lung disease and heart disease.

	Lung Disease		Heart Disease	
	Room Air	100% Fi$_{O_2}$	Room Air	100% Fi$_{O_2}$
Color	Blue → Pink		Blue → Blue	
Oximetry (Sa$_{O_2}$)	60% → 99%		60% → 62%	
Pa$_{O_2}$ (mm Hg)	35 → 120		35 → 38	

Fi$_{O_2}$, fraction of inspired oxygen; Pa$_{O_2}$, partial arterial oxygen pressure; Sa$_{O_2}$, oxygen saturation.
Data from Mahle WT et al: Role of pulse oximetry in examining newborns for congenital heart disease: a scientific statement from the AHA and AAP. Pediatrics 2009 Aug;124(2):823–836.

Martin GR et al: Updated strategies for pulse oximetry screening for critical congenital heart disease. Pediatrics 2020 Jul;146(1):Epub 2020 Jun 4 [PMID: 32499387].

CARDIAC CATHETERIZATION & ANGIOCARDIOGRAPHY

Cardiac catheterization is an invasive method to evaluate anatomic and physiologic conditions in congenital or acquired heart disease. Management decisions may be made based on oximetric, hemodynamic, or angiographic data obtained during catheterization. In an increasing number of cases, intervention may be performed via catheterization that may palliate, or even cure, a congenital heart defect without open heart surgery.

Cardiac Catheterization Data

Figure 20–4 shows oxygen saturation (in percent) and pressure (in millimeters of mercury) values obtained at cardiac catheterization from the chambers and surrounding blood vessels. These values represent the normal range for a school-age child.

A. Oximetry, Shunts, and Cardiac Output

Measurement of oxygen saturation throughout the heart and surrounding blood vessels can provide a wealth of information about a patient's physiology. The difference between systemic saturation (in the aorta) and mixed venous saturation (usually in the superior vena cava [SVC]) is generally inversely proportional to the overall cardiac output. An *increase* in saturation across the *right* side of the heart (anywhere between SVC and PAs) represents a left-to-right shunt with mixing of oxygenated blood with venous blood. Conversely, a *fall* in saturation across the *left* heart, between the pulmonary veins and the aorta, is abnormal and represents

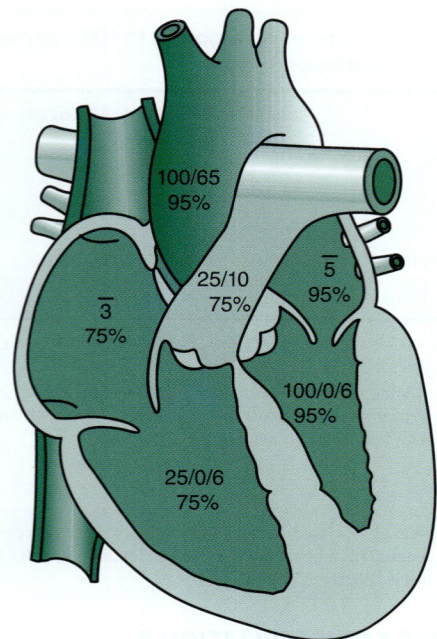

▲ **Figure 20–4.** Pressures (mm Hg) and oxygen saturation (%) obtained by cardiac catheterization in a healthy child. 3, mean pressure of 3 mm Hg in the right atrium; 5, mean pressure of 5 mm Hg in the left atrium. Pressures in the ventricles are described as systolic/diastolic/end diastolic.

addition of deoxygenated blood to oxygenated blood—a right-to-left shunt.

B. Pressures

Pressures should be determined in all chambers and major vessels entered. Systolic pressure in the RV should be equal to the systolic pressure in the PA, just as systolic pressure in the LV should be equal to that of the aorta. The mean pressure in the atria should be nearly equal to the end-diastolic pressure of the ventricles. If a gradient in pressure exists, an obstruction is present, and the severity of the gradient is one criterion for the necessity of intervention.

C. Vascular Resistance

In addition to pressure and flow, vascular resistance can be calculated to further understand cardiac physiology. Resistance is related to pressure and flow as described in the below equation:

$$\text{Resistance} = \frac{\text{Pressure}}{\text{Flow}}$$

To calculate pulmonary vascular resistance (PVR), the pressure drop from the PAs to the left atrium (LA) is divided by pulmonary blood flow (Qp). Patients with pulmonary vascular or heart disease may have elevated PVR, which can adversely impact circulation and heart function. Cardiac catheterization can be performed to evaluate the effects of pharmacologic therapy. An example is monitoring changes in PVR during the administration of nitric oxide or prostacyclin in a child with primary PH.

Angiography

In the past, angiography (injection of contrast via a catheter) was a mainstay for initial diagnosis of CHD. It is still used for diagnostic purposes and is frequently used to plan interventions or evaluate postsurgical anatomy that is poorly seen by noninvasive methods. Cardiac function can be observed, and anatomic abnormalities may be easily identified. Three-dimensional reconstruction can be used to generate images for anatomically accurate 3D printed models.

Interventional Cardiac Catheterization

Interventional cardiac catheterization procedures are performed to occlude lesions such as a PDA, ASD, or ventricular septal defect (VSD). Obstruction of heart valves can be relieved with balloon valvuloplasty. Intervention for vascular obstruction can be accomplished with angioplasty or stent placement. Devices are now available to allow patients to undergo replacement of failing heart valves without open heart surgery. With the improvement in noninvasive imaging, fewer diagnostic cardiac catheterization studies are performed today. The number of interventional procedures, however, is on the rise. Risks of cardiac catheterization are very low for elective studies in older children (< 1%) but are higher in distressed or small patients.

Backes CH et al: Low weight as an independent risk factor for adverse events during cardiac catheterization of infants. Catheter Cardiovasc Interv 2013 Nov 1;82(5):786–794 [PMID: 23436647].

PERINATAL & NEONATAL CIRCULATION

At birth, two events affect the cardiovascular and pulmonary system: (1) the umbilical cord is clamped and (2) breathing commences. As a result, marked changes in the circulation occur. During fetal life, the placenta offers low resistance to blood flow. In contrast, the pulmonary arterioles are markedly constricted and there is high resistance to blood flow in the lungs. Therefore, the majority of blood entering the right side of the heart travels from the RA into the LA across the foramen ovale (right-to-left shunt). In addition, most of the blood that makes its way into the RV and then PAs will flow from the PA into the aorta through the ductus arteriosus (right-to-left shunt). Subsequently, pulmonary blood flow accounts for only 7%–10% of the combined in utero ventricular output.

At birth, as breathing commences, the Po_2 of the small pulmonary arterioles increases, resulting in a decrease in PVR and a dramatic increase in pulmonary blood flow (PBF). Increased oxygen tension, lung distention, and production of nitric oxide as well as prostacyclin all play major roles in the fall in PVR at birth. Conversely, clamping the umbilical cord produces an immediate increase in resistance to flow in the systemic circulation. The PVR falls below that of the systemic circuit, resulting in a reversal in direction of blood flow across the ductus arteriosus, further augmenting PBF.

Functional closure of the ductus arteriosus begins shortly after birth. During the first hour after birth, a small right-to-left shunt is present (as in utero). However, after 1 hour left-to-right shunting predominates. In most cases, right-to-left shunting disappears completely by 8 hours. Although flow through the ductus arteriosus is usually minimal by 5 days of life, the vessel does not close anatomically for 7–14 days.

In fetal life, the foramen ovale serves as a one-way valve shunting blood from the inferior vena cava (IVC) through the RA into the LA. At birth, because of the changes in the pulmonary and systemic vascular resistance and the increase in the quantity of blood returning from the pulmonary veins to the LA, the left atrial pressure rises above that of the RA. This functionally closes the flap of the foramen ovale, preventing flow of blood across the septum. The foramen ovale remains probe patent in 10%–15% of adults.

Persistent pulmonary hypertension of the newborn (PPHN) is a clinical syndrome of full-term infants in which the neonate develops tachypnea and hypoxemia due to persistently elevated PVR during the first 8 hours after birth. These infants have massive right-to-left ductal and/or foramen shunting for 3–7 days because of high PVR. Progressive hypoxemia and acidosis will cause early death unless the pulmonary resistance can be lowered. Increased alveolar Po_2 with hyperventilation, alkalosis, paralysis, surfactant administration, high-frequency ventilation, and cardiac inotropes can usually reverse this process. Treatment with inhaled nitric oxide selectively dilates pulmonary vasculature, produces a sustained improvement in oxygenation, and has resulted in improved outcomes.

In the normal newborn, PVR and pulmonary arterial pressure continue to fall during the first weeks of life due to demuscularization of the pulmonary arterioles. Adult levels of pulmonary resistance and pressure are normally achieved by 4–6 weeks of age. It is at this time typically that signs of pulmonary overcirculation associated with left-to-right shunt lesions such as VSD or (AVSD) appear.

Rudolph AM: The fetal circulation and congenital heart disease. Arch Dis Child Fetal Neonatal Ed 2010;95(2):F132–F136 [PMID: 19321508].

HEART FAILURE

Heart failure (HF) is the clinical condition in which the heart fails to meet the circulatory and metabolic needs of the body. Right and left HF can result from volume or pressure overload of the respective ventricle or an intrinsic abnormality of the ventricular myocardium. Causes of RV volume overload include an ASD, pulmonary valve insufficiency, or anomalous pulmonary venous return. LV volume overload occurs with any left-to-right shunting lesion (eg, VSD, PDA), aortic valve insufficiency, or a systemic arteriovenous malformation. Causes of RV pressure overload include PH, valvar pulmonary stenosis, or severe branch PA stenosis. LV pressure overload results from left heart obstructive lesions such as aortic stenosis or coarctation of the aorta. Abnormalities of the RV myocardium that can result in right HF include Ebstein anomaly and arrhythmogenic RV dysplasia (genetic disorder in which the RV myocardium is replaced by fat). Abnormalities of the LV myocardium are more common and include dilated cardiomyopathy (DCM), myocarditis, or hypertrophic cardiomyopathy (HCM). As a result of elevated LA pressure and impaired relaxation of the LV, left HF can lead to right HF.

HF due to acquired conditions such as myocarditis can occur at any age. Other causes of HF in infants include AVSD, coronary artery anomalies, and chronic arrhythmias. Metabolic, mitochondrial, and neuromuscular disorders can be associated with cardiomyopathy at a variety of ages. Children with HF may present with irritability, diaphoresis with feeds, fatigue, exercise intolerance, or evidence of pulmonary congestion (see Table 20–1).

Treatment of Heart Failure

The treatment of HF should be directed toward the underlying cause as well as the symptoms. Regardless of the etiology, neurohormonal activation occurs early when ventricular systolic dysfunction is present. Plasma catecholamine (norepinephrine) levels increase, causing tachycardia, diaphoresis, and activation of the renin-angiotensin system (which, in turn, results in peripheral vasoconstriction and salt and water retention). Therapies are aimed at improving cardiac performance by targeting the three determinants of cardiac performance: (1) preload, (2) afterload, and (3) contractility.

Inpatient Management of Heart Failure

Patients with cardiac decompensation may require hospitalization for initiation or augmentation of HF therapy.

A. Inotropic and Mechanical Support

1. Afterload reduction and systemic vasodilatation

A. MILRINONE—This phosphodiesterase-3 inhibitor potentiates calcium delivery to the myocardium, thereby improving cardiac inotropy. Milrinone is an inodilator; that is it has systemic and pulmonary vasodilatory effects in addition to causing a dose-dependent increase in cardiac contractility. Thus, milrinone is an effective agent in both right and left HF. The usual intravenous infusion dosage range is 0.25–0.75 mcg/kg/min.

B. NITRATES—Nitroprusside is a nitric oxide donor that induces arterial and venous vasodilatation. Venous vasodilatation allows for increased capacitance, reduction of venous preload, and reduction of right atrial pressure. Arterial vasodilatation reduces LV afterload but can also cause hypotension. A common adverse effect is reflex tachycardia. Nitroglycerin exerts similar effects with increased venous selectivity and is also used to improve coronary blood flow in settings of myocardial infarction or coronary underperfusion following congenital heart surgery. The usual intravenous infusion dosage range for nitroprusside and nitroglycerin is 0.25–3 mcg/kg/min.

2. Enhancement of contractility

Table 20–12 outlines intravenous inotropic agents used to augment cardiac output and their effects on heart rate and systemic vascular resistance. The choice of drug will depend in part on the cause of HF. Norepinephrine would not be utilized alone due to its mild effect on contractility and cardiac output and more profound effect of increasing systemic vascular resistance, and, thus, afterload.

A. EPINEPHRINE—Also known as adrenaline, this catecholamine is a potent stimulator of α_1-, β_1-, and β_2-adrenergic receptors resulting in systemic vasoconstriction, cardiac stimulation, and bronchodilatation. Epinephrine demonstrates dose-dependent effects on the vasculature, with vasodilatation at low doses via β_2 receptors and vasoconstriction at high doses via α_1-receptor activation. The β_1 effects induce both increased inotropy and chronotropy (heart rate). Other non-HF indications for epinephrine include anaphylaxis, bronchoconstriction, shock, bradycardia, and pulseless cardiac arrest.

B. DOPAMINE—This naturally occurring catecholamine increases myocardial contractility primarily via stimulation of adrenergic and dopaminergic receptors. Renal dopamine receptor activation improves renal perfusion.

C. DOBUTAMINE—This synthetic catecholamine increases myocardial contractility secondary to cardiac-specific β-adrenergic activation and produces little peripheral vasoconstriction. Dobutamine does not usually cause marked tachycardia, which is a distinct advantage. However, the drug does not selectively improve renal perfusion like dopamine does.

3. Mechanical circulatory support—Mechanical support is indicated in children with severe, refractory myocardial failure secondary to cardiomyopathy, myocarditis, or following cardiac surgery. Mechanical support is used for a limited time while cardiac function improves or as a bridge to cardiac transplantation.

A. Extracorporeal MEMBRANE OXYGENATION (ECMO)—ECMO is a temporary means of providing gas exchange and hemodynamic support to patients with cardiac or pulmonary failure refractory to conventional therapy (Figure 20–5).

Blood is withdrawn from the patient by a pump via a cannula positioned at the SVC or RA and passes through a membrane oxygenator (to exchange both oxygen and carbon dioxide). Oxygenated blood is then delivered back to the patient through a cannula in the aorta (via the common carotid artery). Systemic anticoagulation is needed to prevent clot formation in the circuit. Risks are significant and include

Table 20–12. Intravenous inotropic agents.

Drug	Dose	Renal Perfusion	Heart Rate	Cardiac Output	SVR
Dopamine	2–5 mcg/kg/min 5–15 15–20 (usual dose for HF 2–10 mcg/kg/min)	↑ via vasodilatation ↑/↓ depending on balance of ↑ cardiac index and ↑ SVR ↓ via vasoconstriction	0 ↑ ↑	0 ↑ ↑	0 ↑↓ ↑
Dobutamine	2–20 mcg/kg/min (usual dose for HF 2–10 mcg/kg/min)	↑ via ↑ cardiac index	Mild ↑	↑	↓
Epinephrine	0.05–2 mcg/kg/min	↑ at low dose via vasodilatation ↓ at high dose via vasoconstriction	↑	↑	↓ at low dose ↑ at high dose
Norepinephrine	0.05–2 mcg/kg/min	↓	0	Very mild ↑	↑↑
Isoproterenol	0.05–5 mcg/kg/min	0	↑↑	↑	↓↓

HF, heart failure; SVR, systemic vascular resistance.

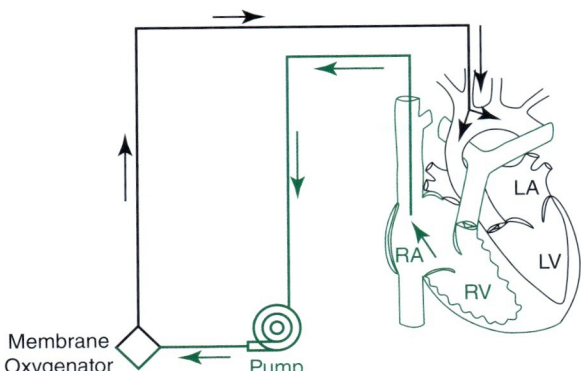

▲ **Figure 20–5.** Extracorporeal membrane oxygenation (ECMO). Deoxygenated blood is pulled from the right atrium (RA) via a pump and passes through a membrane oxygenator before being delivered back to the patient through a cannula in the aorta. LA, left atrium; LV, left ventricle; RA, right atrium; RV, right ventricle.

severe bleeding, infection, end organ injury (kidneys, in particular), stroke, and patient or circuit thrombosis.

B. Ventricular assist device (VAD)—A VAD allows for less invasive hemodynamic support than ECMO. A cannula is usually positioned in the apex of the ventricle and blood is withdrawn from the ventricle using a battery-operated pump implanted in the mediastinum. Blood is returned to the patient through a separate cannula positioned in the aorta or PA, depending on the ventricle being supported. One or both ventricles can be supported. A VAD carries lower risk of circuit thrombosis than ECMO, but risks of infection, patient thrombosis, and bleeding complications remain.

Outpatient Management of Heart Failure

A. Medications

1. Afterload-reducing agents—Oral afterload-reducing agents improve cardiac output by decreasing systemic vascular resistance and, thus, afterload on the LV. Angiotensin-converting enzyme (ACE) inhibitors (captopril, enalapril, and lisinopril) are a first-line therapy in children with HF requiring long-term treatment. These agents reduce LV afterload by blocking angiotensin II–mediated systemic vasoconstriction.

2. β-Blockade—The neurohumoral response to HF includes excessive circulating catecholamines due to activation of the sympathetic nervous system. Although beneficial acutely, this compensatory response over time produces myocardial fibrosis, myocyte hypertrophy, and myocyte apoptosis that contribute to the progression of HF. β-Blockers (eg, carvedilol and metoprolol) antagonize this sympathetic activation and

may offset these deleterious effects. Although clearly beneficial in adults with HF, β-blocker therapy in children with HF does not demonstrate any significant improvement compared to placebo. β-blockers may still be useful adjunctive therapy in some children who are taking ACE inhibitors and have refractory HF requiring additional afterload reduction. Side effects of β-blockers include bradycardia, hypotension, and worsening HF in some patients.

3. Diuretics—Diuretic therapy is often necessary in HF to maintain the euvolemic state and control symptoms related to pulmonary or hepatic congestion caused by sodium and water retention (caused by renin-angiotensin system activation).

A. Furosemide—This loop diuretic inhibits sodium-chloride-potassium cotransport and reabsorption at the loop of Henle. Loop diuretics induce potassium and chloride excretion, producing hypochloremic metabolic alkalosis and hypokalemia, requiring that electrolyte levels be monitored.

B. Thiazides—Thiazide diuretics inhibit sodium-chloride reabsorption at the distal convoluted tubule and are used to complement loop diuretics in severe cases of HF.

C. Spironolactone—Spironolactone is an aldosterone inhibitor used frequently in conjunction with other diuretics for its potassium-sparing effect (often helps avoid the need for potassium supplementation). Though not proven in children, the aldosterone inhibitory effect of spironolactone has benefit in adults with HF separate from its diuretic effect, as aldosterone is associated with the development of fibrosis, sodium retention, and vascular dysfunction.

4. Digitalis—Digitalis is a cardiac glycoside with a positive inotropic effect on the heart and an associated decrease in systemic vascular resistance. The preparation used in clinical practice is digoxin. Large studies in adult patients with HF have not demonstrated decreased mortality of HF with digoxin use, but treatment is associated with reduced hospitalization rates for HF exacerbations. No controlled studies exist in children.

A. Digitalis toxicity—Ventricular dysrhythmia and heart block are characteristic of digoxin toxicity, and any dysrhythmia occurring during digoxin therapy should be attributed to the drug until proven otherwise. Serum digoxin level should be obtained if digoxin toxicity is suspected.

B. Digitalis poisoning—Digoxin poisoning, which most commonly occurs in toddlers who have taken an adult family member's medication, is an acute emergency. The child's stomach should be emptied immediately. Toxicity may induce high grade heart block, for which atropine or temporary pacing may be needed. Digoxin immune Fab can be used to reverse potentially life-threatening intoxication.

Kirk R et al: The International Society of Heart and Lung Transplantation Guidelines for the management of pediatric heart failure: executive summary. J Heart Lung Transplant 2014 Sep;33(9):888–909 [PMID: 25110323].

CARDIAC TRANSPLANTATION

Cardiac transplantation is an effective therapeutic modality for infants and children with end-stage heart disease. Indications for transplantation include (1) progressive HF despite maximal medical therapy; (2) complex CHD that is not amenable to surgical repair or palliation or for which the surgical palliative approach has an equal or higher risk of mortality compared with transplantation; and (3) malignant arrhythmias unresponsive to medical or catheter ablative therapy. Approximately 300–400 pediatric cardiac transplants are performed annually in the U.S., of which 30% are performed in infants. The current estimated graft half-life for children undergoing cardiac transplantation in infancy is over 19 years, and the overall pediatric heart transplant graft half-life is approximately 14 years.

Careful evaluation of the recipient and the donor is performed prior to cardiac transplantation. Assessment of the recipient's PVR is critical, as irreversible and severe PH is a risk factor for post-transplant right HF and early death. End-organ function of the recipient may also influence post-transplant outcome. Donor-related factors that can have an impact on outcome include cardiac function, amount of inotropic support needed, active infection (HIV and hepatitis B and C are considered contraindications to donation for pediatric transplantation in most cases), donor size, and ischemia time prior to transplantation.

Immunosuppression

The ideal post-transplant immunosuppressive regimen allows the immune system to continue to recognize and respond to foreign antigens in a productive manner while avoiding graft rejection. Although there are many different regimens, calcineurin inhibitors (eg, cyclosporine and tacrolimus) remain the mainstay of maintenance immunosuppression in pediatric heart transplantation. Double-drug therapy is often necessary and includes the addition of antimetabolite or antiproliferative medications such as azathioprine, mycophenolate mofetil, or sirolimus. Because of the significant adverse side effects of long-term corticosteroid use, chronic steroid therapy is avoided.

Graft Rejection

Despite advances in immunosuppression, graft rejection remains the leading cause of death in the first 3 years after heart transplantation. Because graft rejection can present in the absence of clinical symptomatology, monitoring for and diagnosing rejection in a timely fashion can be difficult.

Screening regimens include serial physical examination, ECG, echocardiography, and cardiac catheterization with endomyocardial biopsy.

▶ Rejection Surveillance

A. Symptoms and Signs

Acute graft rejection may not cause symptoms in the early stages. With progression, patients may develop signs of HF. There is 50% mortality within 1 year for those suffering an episode of rejection associated with hemodynamic compromise; therefore, early detection is critical.

B. Imaging

In an actively rejecting patient, chest radiography may show cardiomegaly, pulmonary edema, and/or pleural effusions.

C. Electrocardiography

Abnormalities in conduction, reduced QRS voltages, and arrhythmias can occur in graft rejection.

D. Echocardiography

Echocardiography is a useful tool for rejection surveillance. Changes in ventricular compliance and function may initially be subtle but are progressive with increasing duration of rejection. A new pericardial effusion or worsening valvular insufficiency may also indicate rejection.

E. Cardiac Catheterization and Endomyocardial Biopsy

Hemodynamic assessment including ventricular filling pressures, cardiac output, and oxygen consumption can be performed via cardiac catheterization. The endomyocardial biopsy is useful in diagnosing acute graft rejection, but not all episodes of symptomatic rejection result in a positive biopsy result. The appearance of infiltrating lymphocytes with myocellular damage on the biopsy is the hallmark of cell-mediated graft rejection and is helpful if present. The diagnosis of antibody-mediated rejection is challenging, but is based on a combination of clinical symptoms, evidence of complement deposition on endomyocardial biopsy, and new or increasing antibody production (typically anti-human lymphocyte antigen [HLA] antibodies) in the circulation.

▶ Treatment of Graft Rejection

The goal of graft rejection treatment is to reverse the immunologic inflammatory cascade. High-dose corticosteroids are the first line treatment. Frequently, additional therapy with antithymocyte biologic preparations such as antithymocyte globulin (a rabbit-based polyclonal antibody) is needed to reverse rejection. Antibody- and T-cell–mediated rejections are treated similarly, but plasmapheresis and IVIG are added to the treatment regimen of antibody-mediated rejection. Most rejection episodes can be treated effectively if diagnosed promptly. Graft function usually returns to its baseline state, although severe rejection episodes can result in chronic graft failure, graft loss, and death.

Course & Prognosis

The quality of life of pediatric heart transplant recipients is usually quite good. The risk of infection is low after the immediate post-transplant period despite chronic immunosuppression. Nonadherence with lifetime immunosuppression is a significant challenge, especially in adolescent patients. Several recent studies have identified nonadherence as the leading cause of late death. Post-transplant lymphoproliferative disorder, a syndrome related to Epstein-Barr virus infection, can result in a Burkitt-like lymphoma that usually responds to a reduction in immunosuppression but occasionally must be treated with chemotherapy and can be fatal. The overwhelming majority of children are not physically limited and do not require restrictions.

The most common cause of late graft loss is transplant coronary artery disease, known as cardiac allograft vasculopathy (CAV). CAV results from intimal proliferation within the lumen of the coronary arteries that can ultimately result in complete luminal occlusion. These lesions are diffuse and are usually not amenable to bypass grafting, angioplasty, or stent placement. The etiology of these lesions has an immune basis, but the specific pathogenesis is not known, making targeted therapy challenging.

Canter CE et al: Indications for heart transplantation in pediatric heart disease: a scientific statement from the American Heart Association Council on Cardiovascular Disease in the Young; the Councils on Clinical Cardiology, Cardiovascular Nursing, and Cardiovascular Surgery and Anesthesia; and the Quality of Care and Outcomes Research Interdisciplinary Working Group. Circulation 2007 Feb 6;115(5):658–676 [PMID: 17261651].

GENETIC BASIS OF CONGENITAL HEART DISEASE

The importance of genetics as a cause of CHD is becoming more evident, in addition to the impact of maternal exposures (eg, maternal diabetes, alcohol consumption, progesterone use, viral infection, and other teratogens associated with an increased incidence of cardiac malformations). Microdeletion in the long arm of chromosome 22 (22q11) results in DiGeorge syndrome, which is associated with truncus arteriosus, tetralogy of Fallot (ToF), or interrupted aortic arch. Alagille, Noonan, Holt-Oram, and Williams syndromes and trisomies 13, 18, and 21 are all commonly associated with congenital heart lesions. Understanding these associations and further targeted study investigating the genetic basis of other cardiac lesions will offer opportunities for early diagnosis, potential gene therapy, and recurrence risk counseling.

Pierpont ME et al: Genetic basis for congenital heart defects: revisited: a scientific statement from the American Heart Association. Circulation 2018;138: e653–e711 [PMID: 30571578].

ACYANOTIC CONGENITAL HEART DISEASE

DEFECTS IN SEPTATION

1. Atrial Septal Defect

ESSENTIALS OF DIAGNOSIS & TYPICAL FEATURES

► Fixed, widely split S_2, RV heave.
► Grade I–III/VI systolic ejection murmur at the pulmonary area.
► Large shunts cause a diastolic flow murmur at the lower left sternal border (increased flow across the tricuspid valve).
► Frequently asymptomatic.

General Considerations

Atrial septal defect (ASD) is an opening in the atrial septum permitting the shunting of blood between the atria. There are three major types: ostium secundum, ostium primum, and sinus venosus. Ostium secundum is the most common type and represents an embryologic deficiency in atrial septal development. Ostium primum defect is associated with AVSDs. The sinus venosus is intimately related to the right pulmonary veins and, therefore, a sinus venosus defect is associated with abnormal pulmonary venous return.

Ostium secundum ASD is two times more common in females than in males and occurs in 10% of patients with CHD. The defect is most often sporadic but may be familial or have a genetic basis (Holt-Oram syndrome). If unrepaired after the third decade, atrial arrhythmias or PH may develop due to the excessive pulmonary blood flow (PBF). Irreversible PH results in cyanosis as atrial septal shunting becomes right-to-left; ultimately, right HF can occur and is a life-limiting process (Eisenmenger syndrome).

Clinical Findings

A. Symptoms and Signs

Most infants and children with an ASD have no symptoms. Older children and adults can present with exercise intolerance, easy fatigability, or, rarely, HF. The direction of flow across the ASD is determined by the compliance of the ventricles. Because the RV is normally more compliant, shunting across the ASD is left-to-right as blood follows the path of least resistance. Therefore, cyanosis does not occur unless reduced RV compliance occurs (due to dysfunction, usually as a result of PH), leading to reversal of the shunt across the defect.

Peripheral pulses are normal and equal. The heart is usually hyperactive, with an RV heave felt best at the mid-to-lower left sternal border. S_2 at the pulmonary area is widely split and often fixed. In the absence of associated PH, the pulmonary component is normal in intensity. A grade I–III/VI ejection-type systolic murmur, caused by increased flow across the pulmonic valve rather than flow across the ASD, is heard best at the left sternal border in the second intercostal space. A mid-diastolic murmur is often heard in the fourth intercostal space at the left sternal border, caused by increased flow across the tricuspid valve during diastole. The presence of this murmur suggests high flow across the ASD.

B. Imaging

Chest radiography may show cardiac enlargement. The main PA may be dilated, and pulmonary vascular markings increased in large defects owing to increased PBF.

C. Electrocardiography

ECG shows right axis deviation. In the right precordial leads, an rSr' pattern (narrow QRS complex with a small R wave, followed by a deeper S wave, and another small R wave seen in V_1 and/or V_2) is usually present.

D. Echocardiography

Echocardiography shows a dilated RA and RV. Direct visualization of the location of the ASD by two-dimensional echocardiography and demonstration of a left-to-right shunt through the defect by color-flow Doppler confirm the diagnosis; this has eliminated the need for cardiac catheterization prior to surgical or catheter closure of the defect. Assessment of all pulmonary veins should be made to rule out associated anomalous pulmonary venous return.

E. Cardiac Catheterization

Although cardiac catheterization is rarely needed for diagnostic purposes, transcatheter closure of an ostium secundum ASD is now the preferred method of treatment. If catheterization is performed, oximetry shows a significant step-up in oxygen saturation from the SVC to the RA. The PA pressure (PAP) and PVR are usually normal. The ratio of pulmonary-to-systemic blood flow may vary from 1.5:1 to 4:1.

▶ Treatment

Surgical or catheterization closure is generally recommended for symptomatic children with a large ASD and associated

right heart dilatation. In the asymptomatic child with a large hemodynamically significant defect, closure is performed electively at age 1–3 years. In the asymptomatic child with a small defect of no hemodynamic significance, continued observation is recommended to allow time for spontaneous closure; however, elective closure can be considered later in the first decade of life. Most ostium secundum defects are amenable to nonoperative device closure via cardiac catheterization. The mortality for surgical closure for all ASD types is less than 1%. When closure is performed by age 3 years, late complications of RV dysfunction, PH, and dysrhythmias are avoided.

▶ Course & Prognosis

Patients usually tolerate an ASD well in the first two decades of life, and the defect often goes unnoticed until middle or late adulthood. PH and reversal of the shunt are rare late complications. IE is uncommon. Spontaneous closure occurs, most frequently in children with a small and hemodynamically insignificant defect less than 4 mm in diameter; therefore, outpatient observation is recommended. Exercise tolerance in surgically corrected children is generally normal and restriction of physical activity is unnecessary.

Silvestry FE et al: Guidelines for the echocardiographic assessment of atrial septal defect and patent foramen ovale: from the American Society of Echocardiography and Society for Cardiac Angiography and Interventions. J Am Soc Echocardiogr 2015 Aug;28(8):910–958. doi: 10.1016/j.echo.2015.05.015 [PMID: 26239900].

2. Ventricular Septal Defect

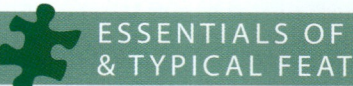

ESSENTIALS OF DIAGNOSIS & TYPICAL FEATURES

▶ Holosystolic murmur at lower left sternal border with RV heave.

▶ Presentation and course depend on size of defect and PVR.

▶ Clinical features include failure to thrive, tachypnea, and diaphoresis with feeds.

▶ General Considerations

Ventricular septal defects (VSDs) accounts for about 30% of all CHD and generally follow one of four courses:

A. Small, Hemodynamically Insignificant Ventricular Septal Defects

Between 80% and 85% of VSDs are small (< 3 mm in diameter) at birth and will close spontaneously. In general, small defects in the muscular interventricular septum will close sooner than those in the membranous septum. Fifty percent of small VSDs will close by age 2 years and 90% by age 6 years, with most of the remaining closing during the school years. In most cases, small VSDs do not require surgical closure.

B. Moderate-Sized Ventricular Septal Defects

Asymptomatic patients with moderate-sized VSDs (3–5 mm in diameter) account for 3%–5% of children with VSDs. In general, these children do not have clear indicators for surgical closure. If the patient is asymptomatic and without evidence of PH, these defects can be followed serially as some close spontaneously over time.

C. Large Ventricular Septal Defects With Normal Pulmonary Vascular Resistance

These defects are usually 6–10 mm in diameter. Unless they become markedly smaller within a few months after birth, they often require surgery. Many infants with large VSDs and normal PVR develop symptoms of failure to thrive, tachypnea, diaphoresis with feeds by age 3–6 months and require correction at that time. Surgery before age 2 years in patients with large VSDs essentially eliminates the risk of PH.

D. Large Ventricular Septal Defects With Pulmonary Vascular Obstructive Disease

The direction of flow across a VSD is determined by the resistance in the systemic and pulmonary vasculature, explaining why flow is usually left-to-right. With large VSDs, ventricular pressures are equalized, resulting in increased PAP. In addition to the increased PAP, shear stress caused by increased PBF causes increased resistance over time. The multicenter National History Study indicates that almost all cases of irreversible PH can be prevented by surgical repair of a large VSD before age 2 years.

▶ Clinical Findings

A. Symptoms and Signs

Patients with small or moderate VSDs usually have no cardiovascular symptoms. Patients with large left-to-right shunts are usually ill early in infancy with frequent respiratory infections, failure to thrive, dyspnea, diaphoresis, and fatigue. Older children may experience exercise intolerance. Over time, with a persistent large left-to-right shunt the pulmonary vascular bed undergoes structural changes, leading to increased PVR and reversal of the shunt from left-to-right to right-to-left (Eisenmenger syndrome) and cyanosis develops.

1. Small left-to-right shunt—No lifts or heaves are present. The first sound at the apex is normal, and the second sound at the pulmonary area is split physiologically. A grade II–IV/VI, medium- to high-pitched, harsh pansystolic murmur is heard best at the left sternal border in the third and fourth intercostal spaces. The murmur radiates over the entire precordium. No diastolic murmurs are heard.

2. Moderate left-to-right shunt—Slight prominence of the precordium with moderate LV heave is evident. A systolic thrill may be palpable at the lower left sternal border between the third and fourth intercostal spaces. The second sound at the pulmonary area is most often split but may be single. A grade III–IV/VI, harsh pansystolic murmur is heard best at the lower left sternal border in the fourth intercostal space. A mitral diastolic flow murmur indicates that PBF and pulmonary venous return are significantly increased by the large shunt.

3. Large ventricular septal defects with pulmonary hypertension—The precordium is prominent, and the sternum bulges. Both LV and RV heaves are palpable. S_2 is palpable in the pulmonary area. A thrill may be present at the lower left sternal border. S_2 is usually single or narrowly split, with accentuation of the pulmonary component. The murmur ranges from grade I to IV/VI and is usually harsh and pansystolic. Occasionally, when the defect is large or ventricular pressures are equalized, a murmur is difficult to hear. A diastolic flow murmur may be heard, depending on the size of the shunt.

B. Imaging

In patients with small shunts, the chest radiograph may be normal. Patients with large shunts have significant cardiac enlargement involving the LV, RV, and LA. The main PA segment may be dilated, and pulmonary vascular markings are increased.

C. Electrocardiography

ECG is normal in small left-to-right shunts. Left ventricular hypertrophy (LVH) usually occurs in patients with large left-to-right shunts and normal PVR. Signs of RVH, in addition to LVH, become evident in patients with PH. Pure right ventricular hypertrophy (RVH) is present in patients with more severe PH induced by long-standing left-to-right shunt (Eisenmenger syndrome).

D. Echocardiography

Two-dimensional and color-flow echocardiography demonstrate the size of a VSD and identify its anatomic location. Doppler can estimate the pressure difference between the ventricles and, thus, identify the presence of PH.

E. Cardiac Catheterization and Angiocardiography

The ability to describe the VSD anatomy and estimate the PAP by echocardiography allows for the majority of isolated defects to be repaired without cardiac catheterization and angiocardiography. Catheterization for hemodynamic assessment is indicated in those patients with signs of PH.

Treatment

A. Medical Management

Patients who develop symptoms can be managed with anti-congestive treatment, particularly diuretics and systemic afterload reduction, prior to surgery or if it is expected that the defect will close spontaneously.

B. Surgical Treatment

Patients with cardiomegaly, poor growth, poor exercise tolerance, or other clinical abnormalities who have a significant shunt typically undergo surgical repair using a synthetic or pericardial patch at age 3–12 months. As a result, Eisenmenger syndrome has been virtually eliminated. The surgical mortality rate for VSD closure is below 2%.

Transcatheter closure of muscular VSDs is also an option. However, catheter device closure of perimembranous VSDs can be associated with a high incidence of heart block and is therefore less commonly performed.

Course & Prognosis

Significant late dysrhythmias are uncommon after surgical or device closure (spontaneously closed defects result in no apparent sequelae). Functional exercise capacity is usually normal (both in cases of intervention and spontaneous closure), and physical restrictions are unnecessary. Adults with corrected defects have normal quality of life.

Jortveit J et al: Mortality and complications in 3495 children with isolated ventricular septal defects. Arch Dis Child 2016 Sep;101(9):808–813. doi: 10.1136/archdischild-2015-310154 [PMID: 27091847].

Sondheimer HM, Rahimi-Alangi K: Current management of ventricular septal defect. Cardiol Young 2006;16(Suppl 3):131–135 [PMID: 17378052].

3. Atrioventricular Septal Defect

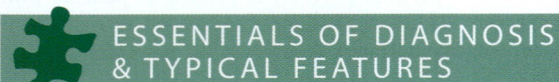

ESSENTIALS OF DIAGNOSIS & TYPICAL FEATURES

▶ Often no murmur in neonates.
▶ Loud pulmonary component of S_2.
▶ Common in infants with Down syndrome.
▶ ECG with extreme left-axis deviation.

General Considerations

Atrioventricular septal defect (AVSD) results from incomplete fusion of the embryonic endocardial cushions that help form the "crux" of the heart (lower portion of the atrial septum,

membranous portion of the ventricular septum, and septal leaflets of the tricuspid and mitral valves). AVSD accounts for about 4% of all CHD. Sixty percent of children with Down syndrome have CHD, and of these, 40% have an AVSD.

AVSDs are defined as partial or complete. In complete AVSD, both atrial and ventricular components of the septal defect are present and the left- and right-sided AV valves share a common ring or orifice. In the partial form of AVSD, there is a primum ASD without a ventricular defect component and there are two separate AV valve orifices (usually with a cleft in the left-sided AV valve). The physiology of the defect is determined by the presence and degree of ventricular shunt. Partial AVSD with an ostium primum ASD behaves like an isolated ASD, with variable amounts of regurgitation through the cleft in the left AV valve. Complete AVSD causes large left-to-right shunts at both the ventricular and atrial levels with variable degrees of AV valve regurgitation. If there is increased PVR, the shunts may be bidirectional. Bidirectional shunting is more common in Down syndrome or in older children who have not undergone repair.

Clinical Findings

A. Symptoms and Signs

The partial form may produce symptoms similar to ostium secundum ASD. Patients with complete AVSD usually have symptoms such as failure to thrive, tachypnea, diaphoresis with feeding, or recurrent bouts of pneumonia.

In the neonate with the complete AVSD, the murmur may be inaudible due ventricular pressures that are equivalent to the relatively equal systemic and pulmonary vascular resistance. After 4–6 weeks, as PVR drops, a nonspecific systolic murmur develops. The murmur is usually not as harsh as that of an isolated VSD. There is both right- and left-sided cardiac chamber enlargement. S_2 is loud, and a pronounced diastolic flow murmur may be heard at the apex and the lower left sternal border.

If severe PH is present, there is usually dominant RV enlargement. S_2 is palpable at the pulmonary area, and no thrill is felt. A nonspecific short systolic murmur is heard at the lower left sternal border. No diastolic flow murmurs are heard. If a right-to-left shunt is present, cyanosis will be evident.

B. Imaging

Cardiac enlargement is always present and pulmonary vascular markings are increased in the complete form. Often, only the right heart size may be increased in partial AVSD, although a severe mitral valve cleft can rarely lead to left heart enlargement as well.

C. Electrocardiography

In all forms of AVSD, there is extreme left-axis deviation (QRS axis of −30° to −90°) and, therefore, the ECG is an important diagnostic tool. First-degree heart block occurs in over 50% of patients with AVSD. Right, left, or combined ventricular hypertrophy is present depending on the defect and the presence or absence of PH.

D. Echocardiography

The anatomy can be well visualized by two-dimensional echocardiography, the diagnostic test of choice. The size of the atrial and ventricular components of the defect can be measured and AV valve regurgitation can be detected. The LV outflow tract is elongated (gooseneck appearance), which produces systemic outflow obstruction in some patients.

E. Cardiac Catheterization and Angiocardiography

Cardiac catheterization is not routinely used to evaluate AVSD but may be used to assess PAPs and resistance in the older infant with Down syndrome, as this patient group is predisposed to early-onset PH. Increased oxygen saturation in the RV or the RA identifies the level of the shunt.

▶ Treatment

Spontaneous closure of AVSD does not occur, and therefore, surgery is required. In partial AVSD, surgery carries a low mortality rate (1%–2%), but patients require follow-up because of late-occurring LV outflow tract obstruction and mitral valve dysfunction. Complete AVSD carries a higher mortality rate. Complete correction in the first year of life, prior to the onset of irreversible PH, is obligatory.

Colen T, Smallhorn JF: Three-dimensional echocardiography for the assessment of atrioventricular valves in congenital heart disease: past, present and future. Semin Thorac Cardiovasc Surg Pediatr Card Surg Annu 2015;18(1):62–71. doi: 10.1053/j.pcsu.2015.01.003 [PMID: 25939845].

Craig B: Atrioventricular septal defect: from fetus to adult. Heart 2006;92:1879–1885 [PMID: 17105897].

PATENT (PERSISTENT) DUCTUS ARTERIOSUS

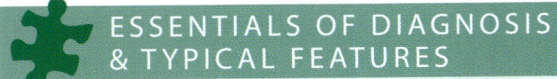

ESSENTIALS OF DIAGNOSIS & TYPICAL FEATURES

▶ Presentation and course depends on size of the ductus arteriosus and the PVR.

▶ Left-to-right shunt occurs if PVR is normal.

▶ Continuous machinery-type murmur.

▶ Bounding peripheral pulses if patent ductus arteriosus (PDA) is large.

▶ Clinical features of a large ductus are failure to thrive, tachypnea, and diaphoresis with feeds.

▶ General Considerations

Patent ductus arteriosus (PDA) is the persistence of the normal fetal vessel joining the PA to the aorta. It closes spontaneously in normal term infants at 1–5 days of age. PDA accounts for 10% of all CHD. The incidence of PDA is higher in infants born at altitudes over 10,000 ft, and it occurs twice as often in females as in males. The frequency of PDA in preterm infants ranges from 20% to 60%. The defect may occur as an isolated abnormality or with associated lesions (commonly coarctation of the aorta and VSD). Patency of the ductus arteriosus may be necessary in some patients with CHD (eg, hypoplastic left heart syndrome or pulmonary atresia). Continuous intravenous infusion of prostaglandin E_1 (PGE_1), a product of arachidonic acid metabolism, can be used to maintain ductal patency.

▶ Clinical Findings

A. Symptoms and Signs

The clinical findings and course depend on the size of the shunt and the severity of PH.

1. Moderate to large patent ductus arteriosus—Pulses are bounding, and pulse pressure is widened due to diastolic run-off through the PDA. S_1 is normal and S_2 is usually narrowly split. In large shunts, S_2 may have a paradoxical split (eg, S_2 narrows on inspiration and widens on expiration) caused by volume overload of the LV and prolonged ejection of blood from this chamber. A characteristic rough machinery murmur, maximal at the second left intercostal space, is present in the absence of other associated CHD. It begins shortly after S_1, rises to a peak at S_2, and passes through the S_2 into diastole, where it becomes a decrescendo murmur and fades before S_1. The murmur tends to radiate well to the anterior lung fields but relatively poorly to the posterior lung fields. A diastolic flow murmur is often heard at the apex.

2. Patent ductus arteriosus with associated pulmonary hypertension—Flow across the PDA is diminished due to increased PVR. S_2 is single and accentuated, and no significant heart murmur is present. The pulses are normal rather than bounding.

B. Imaging

In an isolated PDA, the appearance of the chest radiograph depends on the size of the shunt. If the shunt is small, the heart is not enlarged. If the shunt is large, LA and LV enlargement may be seen. Increased pulmonary vascular markings may be seen in association with increased PBF. The aorta and the main PA segment may also be prominent.

C. Electrocardiography

ECG may be normal or may show LVH, depending on the size of the shunt. In patients with PH caused by increased blood flow, biventricular hypertrophy usually is evident. If PH is associated with PDA, pure RVH is present.

D. Echocardiography

Echocardiography provides direct visualization of the PDA and confirms the direction and degree of shunting. High-velocity left-to-right flow suggests normal PVR, and as PVR drops during the neonatal period, higher velocity left-to-right shunting is usually seen. If PVR becomes elevated and greater than systemic resistance, flow across the PDA will be right-to-left. Associated cardiac lesions and ductal-dependent pulmonary or systemic blood flow must be recognized by echocardiography, as closure of a PDA in this setting would be contraindicated.

E. Cardiac Catheterization and Angiocardiography

PDA closure in the catheterization laboratory with a vascular device is now routine in all but the smallest of neonates and infants.

▶ Treatment

Presence of a symptomatic PDA is common in preterm infants. Indomethacin, a prostaglandin synthesis inhibitor, is often used to close the PDA in premature infants but does not close the PDA of full-term infants or older children. The success of indomethacin therapy is as high as 90% in premature infants with a birth weight greater than 1200 g, but it is less successful in smaller infants. If indomethacin is not effective and the PDA remains hemodynamically significant, surgical ligation should be performed. Alternative medical treatment with acetaminophen has been tried in patients who have contraindications to indomethacin.

Device occlusion in the catheterization laboratory is ideally performed for a symptomatic PDA with normal PAP after the child has reached 5 kg. Surgical closure is indicated when the PDA is large, and the patient is too small for catheter device closure. Patients with large left-to-right shunts require repair by age 1 year to prevent the development of progressive PH.

Caution must be given to closing a PDA in patients with PH and right-to-left shunting across the PDA, as this could result in RV failure. Patients with PH not reactive to inhaled nitric oxide testing should not undergo PDA closure. These patients are made worse by closure because the flow through the PDA allows preserved RV function and maintains cardiac output to the systemic circulation. These patients can be managed with pulmonary vasodilator therapy but eventually may require heart-lung transplant in severe cases.

▶ Course & Prognosis

Spontaneous closure of a PDA may occur up to age 1 year but is rare beyond 1 year. Because endocarditis is a potential complication, some cardiologists recommend percutaneous device closure if the defect persists beyond age 1, even if it is small. Patients with an unrepaired, isolated PDA and small-to-moderate shunts usually do well clinically; however, in the third or fourth decade of life, symptoms of easy fatigability, dyspnea on exertion, and exercise intolerance appear in those patients who develop PH and/or HF. Percutaneous closure can be done later in life if there has not been development of severe PH. For those with severe and irreversible PH, prognosis is not good and heart-lung transplant may be needed.

Lam JY, Lopushinsky SR, MaI W, Dicke F, Brindle ME: Treatment options for pediatric patent ductus arteriosus: systematic review and meta-analysis. Chest 2015 Sep;148(3):784–793. doi: 10.1378/chest.14-2997 [PMID: 25835756].

RIGHT-SIDED OBSTRUCTIVE LESIONS

1. Pulmonary Valve Stenosis

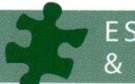

ESSENTIALS OF DIAGNOSIS & TYPICAL FEATURES

▶ Mild or moderate stenosis can be asymptomatic.

▶ Cyanosis and a high incidence of right-sided HF in ductal-dependent lesions.

▶ RV lift with systolic ejection click heard at the third left intercostal space.

▶ S_2 widely split with soft to inaudible P_2; grade I–VI/VI systolic ejection murmur, maximal at the pulmonary area.

▶ Dilated PA on chest radiography.

▶ General Considerations

Pulmonic valve stenosis (PS) accounts for 10% of all CHD. The pulmonary valve annulus is usually small, with poststenotic dilatation of the main PA. Obstruction to PBF across the pulmonary valve causes an increase in RV pressure. Because of the increased RV strain, severe RVH and eventual right-sided HF can occur.

When obstruction is severe and the ventricular septum is intact, a right-to-left shunt will often occur at the atrial level through a patent foramen ovale (PFO). In neonates with severe obstruction and minimal antegrade blood flow (critical PS), left-to-right flow through the PDA is essential, making PGE$_1$ infusion critical at the time of birth.

▶ Clinical Findings

A. Symptoms and Signs

Patients with mild or moderate valvular PS are acyanotic, asymptomatic, and usually well developed and well nourished.

Pulses are normal. The precordium may be prominent, often with palpable RV heave. A systolic thrill is often auscultated in the pulmonary area. A prominent ejection click of pulmonary origin is heard at the third left intercostal space. The click varies with respiration, being more prominent during expiration than inspiration. In mild valvar pulmonary stenosis, S_2 is normal, while in moderate PS, S_2 is more widely split and the pulmonary component is softer. A rough systolic ejection murmur is best heard at the second left interspace and radiates to the back.

Patients with severe valvular obstruction may develop cyanosis early. In severe stenosis, the pulmonary ejection click tends to merge with S_1 and S_2 is single because the pulmonary component cannot be heard. The systolic murmur is usually short.

B. Imaging

The heart size is normal. Poststenotic dilatation of the main PA and the left PA is often evident on chest radiography.

C. Electrocardiography

ECG is usually normal with mild PS. In severe PS, RVH with an RV strain pattern (deep inversion of the T wave) occurs in the right precordial leads (V_{3R}, V_1, V_2). RA enlargement may be present. Right axis deviation occurs in moderate and severe stenosis.

D. Echocardiography

The diagnosis often is made by physical examination, but echocardiography confirms the diagnosis, defines the anatomy, and can identify any associated lesions. Thickened leaflets are seen on the pulmonary valve, with reduced valve leaflet excursion. The transvalvular pressure gradient can be estimated accurately by Doppler, which provides an estimate of RV pressure and can assist in determining the appropriate time to intervene.

E. Cardiac Catheterization and Angiocardiography

Catheterization is reserved for therapeutic balloon valvuloplasty. In severe cases with associated RV dysfunction, a right-to-left shunt at the atrial level is indicated by a lower LA saturation than pulmonary vein saturation. PAP is normal. The gradient across the pulmonary valve varies from 10 to 200 mm Hg. In severe cases, the right atrial pressure is elevated. Angiocardiography in the RV shows a thick pulmonary valve with a narrow opening producing a jet of contrast into the PA. Infundibular (RV outflow tract) hypertrophy may be present and may contribute to obstruction of PBF.

▶ Treatment

Treatment of valvular PS is recommended for children with RV systolic pressure greater than two-thirds of systemic pressure. Immediate correction is indicated for patients with RV pressure equal to or greater than LV pressure. Percutaneous balloon valvuloplasty is the procedure of choice, as it is as effective as surgery in relieving obstruction and causes less valve insufficiency. Surgery is required when balloon pulmonic valvuloplasty is unsuccessful.

▶ Course & Prognosis

Patients with mild PS live normal lives. Even those with moderate stenosis are rarely symptomatic, whereas those with severe valvular obstruction may develop cyanosis in infancy.

After balloon pulmonary valvuloplasty or surgery, most patients have good exercise capacity unless they have significant valvar pulmonary insufficiency (PI), a frequent side effect of intervention). Limitation of physical activity is unwarranted. The quality of life of adults with successfully treated PS and minimal PI is normal. Severe PI can lead to progressive RV dilatation and dysfunction, which may limit exercise capacity and precipitate ventricular arrhythmias and/or right HF in adulthood. Patients with severe PI may benefit from replacement of the pulmonic valve, for which transcatheter valve replacement is becoming more common.

Harrild DM et al: Long-term pulmonary regurgitation following balloon valvuloplasty for pulmonary stenosis risk factors and relationship to exercise capacity and ventricular volume and function. J Am Coll Cardiol 2010 Mar 9;55(10):1041–1047 [PMID: 20202522].

2. Subvalvular Pulmonary Stenosis

Isolated infundibular (subvalvular) PS is rare. It typically is found in combination with other lesions, such as ToF. Infundibular hypertrophy that is associated with a small perimembranous VSD may lead to a "double-chambered RV" characterized by obstruction between the inflow and outflow portion of the RV. The clinical picture is identical to that of pulmonic valve stenosis. Intervention, if indicated, is always surgical because this condition does not improve with balloon catheter dilation.

3. Supravalvular Pulmonary Stenosis

Supravalvular PS is a relatively rare condition defined by narrowing of the main PA. The clinical picture may be identical to valvular PS, although the murmur is maximal in the first intercostal space at the left sternal border and in the suprasternal notch. No ejection click is audible, as the valve itself is not involved. The murmur radiates toward the neck and over the lung fields. William syndrome is associated with supravalvular and PA branch stenosis, as well as supravalvular aortic stenosis. In severe supravalvular PS, surgical treatment is indicated.

4. Pulmonary Artery Branch Stenosis

In pulmonary artery branch stenosis (PABS), there are multiple narrowings of the branches of the PAs, sometimes extending into the vessels in the periphery of the lungs. Systolic murmurs may be heard over both lung fields, anteriorly and posteriorly, radiating to the axilla. Mild, nonpathologic peripheral pulmonary stenosis (PPS) produces a murmur in infancy that resolves by 6 months of age (described above, with other innocent murmurs). William, Alagille, and congenital rubella syndromes are commonly associated with severe forms of PABS. Surgery is often unsuccessful, as areas of stenoses near and beyond the hilum of the lungs are not surgically accessible. Transcatheter balloon angioplasty and even stent placement can treat this condition with moderate success. In some instances, the stenoses improve spontaneously with age.

5. Ebstein Malformation of the Tricuspid Valve

In Ebstein malformation of the tricuspid valve, the septal leaflet of the tricuspid valve is displaced toward the apex of the heart and is attached to the endocardium of the RV rather than at the tricuspid annulus. As a result, a large portion of the RV functions physiologically as part of the RA. This "atrialized" portion of the RV is thin-walled and does not contribute to RV output. The volume of the RV below the displaced tricuspid valve, representing the functioning RV, is diminished. In utero exposure to lithium increases the risk of developing Ebstein malformation.

▶ Clinical Findings

A. Symptoms and Signs

The clinical picture of Ebstein malformation varies with the degree of displacement of the tricuspid valve. In the most extreme form, the septal leaflet is markedly displaced into the RV outflow tract, causing obstruction of antegrade flow into the PA. In such severe cases, the majority of the ventricle is "atrialized" and there is very little functioning RV. The degree of TR may be so severe that forward (antegrade) flow out the RV outflow tract is further diminished, leading to a right-to-left atrial level shunt (across the PFO) and cyanosis. At the opposite extreme, when antegrade PBF is adequate, symptoms may not develop until adulthood when tachyarrhythmias (due to right atrial dilatation or reentrant electrical pathways) occur. These older patients typically have less displacement of the septal leaflet of the tricuspid valve and therefore more functional RV tissue.

B. Imaging

Chest radiography shows cardiomegaly with prominence of the right heart border. The extent of cardiomegaly depends on the degree of tricuspid valve insufficiency and the presence and size of the atrial level shunt. Massive cardiomegaly with a "wall-to-wall heart" (the heart shadow extends laterally across the entire chest cavity) occurs with severe tricuspid valve displacement and/or a restrictive atrial level defect.

C. Electrocardiography

ECG may be normal but usually shows right atrial enlargement and RBBB. There is an association between Ebstein anomaly and Wolff-Parkinson-White (WPW) syndrome, in which case a delta wave is present (short PR with a slurred upstroke of the QRS).

D. Echocardiography

Echocardiography is necessary to confirm the diagnosis and may aid in predicting outcome. Degree of tricuspid valve displacement, size of the RA, and presence of associated atrial level shunt all affect outcome.

▶ Course & Prognosis

In cyanotic neonates, PGE_1 is used to maintain PBF via the PDA until PVR decreases, facilitating antegrade PA flow. If the neonate remains significantly cyanotic, surgical intervention is required. The type of surgical repair depends on the severity of the disease. For example, to decrease the amount of tricuspid regurgitation (TR), surgery may involve atrial plication and tricuspid valve repair. The success of the procedure is highly variable. Late arrhythmias are common due to preexisting atrial dilatation. Postoperative exercise tolerance improves but remains lower than age-related norms. If a significant Ebstein malformation is not treated, atrial tachyarrhythmias frequently begin during adolescence and the enlarged atrialized RV could impede LV function.

Ramcharan TKW et al: Ebstein's anomaly: from fetus to adult-literature review and pathway for patient care. Pediatr Cardiol 2022 Oct;43(7):1409–1428 [PMID: 35460366].

LEFT-SIDED LESIONS

1. Coarctation of the Aorta

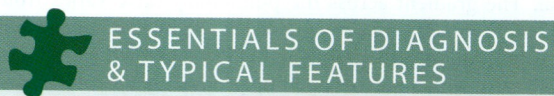

ESSENTIALS OF DIAGNOSIS & TYPICAL FEATURES

► Absent or diminished femoral pulses.
► Upper-to-lower extremity systolic blood pressure gradient.
► Blowing systolic murmur in the back or left axilla.

General Considerations

Coarctation is a narrowing in the aorta, usually in the proximal descending aorta at the insertion of the ductus arteriosus, near the takeoff of the left subclavian artery (which is usually proximal to the obstruction). Coarctation accounts for 7% of all CHD and has a male predominance (1.5:1); many affected females have Turner syndrome (45, XO). Coarctation is associated with bicuspid aortic valve in up to 85% of cases and intracerebral berry aneurysms later in life in 10% of cases.

Clinical Findings

A. Symptoms and Signs

The cardinal physical findings are decreased or absent femoral pulses and a blood pressure gradient between the arms and legs. Normally, blood pressure in the legs is at least that of the arms, and typically higher. This is reversed in coarctation, with upper extremity blood pressure often greater than 15 mm Hg above that of lower extremities; the gradient may be diminished in the setting of significant LV dysfunction or collateralization. Lower extremity pulses may be normal until the PDA closes (ductal patency ensures flow to the descending aorta distal to the coarctation).

Approximately 40% of children with aortic coarctation present as neonates, often with acute LV dysfunction, cardiogenic shock, and lactic acidosis from impaired tissue perfusion when the PDA closes. The remaining 60% of children with coarctation often have no symptoms in infancy, presenting insidiously with systemic hypertension, claudication, or failure to thrive. A systolic or continuous murmur may be present in the left back or left axilla, in addition to possible findings associated with a bicuspid aortic valve, if present. Measurement of blood pressure in all four extremities is key to diagnosis.

B. Imaging

Infants with coarctation and associated LV dysfunction often have marked cardiac enlargement and pulmonary venous congestion on chest radiograph. Older children may have normal LV size but demonstrate a "figure 3" sign (prominent aorta proximal to the coarctation, indentation at the level of the coarctation, and postcoarctation dilatation) or inferior notching of the ribs due to significant collateralization of intercostal arteries bypassing the obstruction. Computed tomography (CT) and MRI are occasionally utilized to provide three-dimensional imaging of the aorta, especially with complex coarctation and extensive aortic hypoplasia.

C. Electrocardiography

ECG in infants with aortic coarctation is often normal, with dominant RV forces, as the RV serves as the systemic ventricle during fetal life. ECGs in older children often demonstrate LVH.

D. Echocardiography

Echocardiography can directly visualize the coarctation and assess ventricular size and function. Color-flow Doppler demonstrates turbulent flow at the coarctation. Development of a coarctation cannot be excluded in the presence of a PDA, as coarctation can occur as PDA closure constricts aortic tissue. Other left heart obstruction lesions, such as bicuspid aortic valve or mitral stenosis, may be present.

E. Cardiac Catheterization and Angiocardiography

Cardiac catheterization and angiocardiography are rarely performed for diagnosis in infants or children with coarctation but are used if transcatheter intervention is planned.

Treatment

Infants with coarctation of the aorta may present in extremis, and the primary resuscitative measure is high dose PGE_1 infusion (0.05–0.1 mcg/kg/min) to reopen the ductus arteriosus and relax ductal tissue in the aorta. PGE_1 infusion may result in apnea, requiring respiratory support. Inotropic support is frequently needed. Once stabilized, the infant should undergo corrective surgery. Palliative neonatal balloon angioplasty is rarely performed in those with substantial cardiac dysfunction. In older children, balloon angioplasty of the coarctation can be the definitive treatment; stent angioplasty may be appropriate if the implanted stent can be expanded to an adult size.

Recurrent coarctation, the primary complication of both surgery and balloon angioplasty, is more common after initial angioplasty intervention. Recurrent coarctation is typically treatable in the catheterization laboratory with angioplasty and possible stent placement.

Course & Prognosis

Children who survive the neonatal period without HF do well through childhood and adolescence. Systemic hypertension is common, even after successful coarctation repair, especially in those repaired after age 5 years. Infective endarteritis is rare before adolescence but can occur in both repaired and unrepaired coarctation. Exercise testing is mandatory prior to participation in competitive athletic activities.

Feltes TF et al: Indications for cardiac catheterization and intervention in pediatric cardiac disease: a scientific statement from the American Heart Association. Circulation 2011 Jun 7;123(22):2607–2652. doi: 10.1161/CIR.0b013e31821b1f10 [PMID: 21536996].

Meadows J, Minahan M, McElhinney DB, McEnaney K, Ringel R: Intermediate outcomes in the prospective, multicenter coarctation of the Aorta Stent Trial (COAST). Circulation 2015 May 12;131(19):1656–1664. doi: 10.1161/CIRCULATIONAHA.114.013937 [PMID: 25869198].

2. Aortic Stenosis

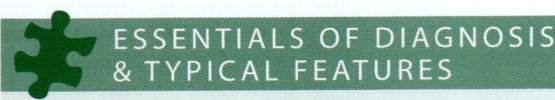

ESSENTIALS OF DIAGNOSIS & TYPICAL FEATURES

► Harsh systolic ejection murmur at the upper right sternal border with radiation to the neck.
► Thrill in suprasternal notch and carotid arteries.
► Systolic click at the apex.
► Dilatation of the ascending aorta on chest radiograph.

General Considerations

Aortic stenosis, accounting for 3%–8% of CHD, is defined as obstruction to outflow from the LV at or near the aortic valve, producing a systolic pressure gradient greater than 10 mm Hg. Three isolated anatomic variants of aortic stenosis exist (at, below, or above the valve), though multiple levels of obstruction commonly occur.

A. Valvular Aortic Stenosis (60%–75%)

Valvular aortic stenosis has a male predominance (as high as 5:1) and is typically associated with a bicuspid or unicuspid aortic valve. A bicuspid aortic valve, present in 1.3% of the population, is composed of only two leaflets or, more commonly, three leaflets with complete or partial fusion of two of the leaflets. A unicuspid aortic valve has fusion of all three leaflets. Leaflet fusion typically results in reduced leaflet mobility and potential obstruction to flow.

B. Subvalvular Aortic Stenosis (10%–20%)

Subvalvular aortic stenosis, also with a male predominance (2–3:1), is associated with a discrete membrane or muscular narrowing in the LV outflow tract that typically develops postnatally. The aortic valve is often structurally normal. Membranes are often attached to the anterior leaflet of the mitral valve. Subaortic membranes are typically progressive and are often associated with other left heart obstructive lesions and perimembranous VSDs.

C. Supravalvular Aortic Stenosis (8%–14%)

Supravalvular aortic stenosis involves narrowing of the ascending aorta, typically just above the aortic sinuses. This is usually associated with an elastin defect, such as in William syndrome (also associated with supravalvular pulmonary stenosis).

Clinical Findings

A. Symptoms and Signs

Isolated valvular aortic stenosis seldom causes symptoms in infancy, though severe congenital aortic valve stenosis can

be associated with significant LV outflow obstruction, dysfunction, and cardiogenic shock and requires a PDA to supply systemic cardiac output ("critical" aortic stenosis). Most patients with aortic stenosis who do not present in infancy have no symptoms, and, except in the most severe cases, do well until the third to fifth decades of life. Some patients have mild exercise intolerance. Infrequently, significant symptoms (eg, exertional chest pain, dizziness, syncope) manifest in the first decade. Sudden death is uncommon but may occur in all forms of aortic stenosis, with the greatest risk in patients with subvalvular obstruction.

Physical findings vary depending on the level of obstruction:

1. Valvular aortic stenosis—If the stenosis is severe, pulses are diminished with a slow upstroke. Palpation reveals an LV thrust at the apex and, possibly, a systolic thrill at the suprasternal notch and over the carotid arteries with moderate or severe stenosis. An aortic ejection click, associated with valve opening, may be heard at the apex, distinct from S_1 and without respiratory variation. A loud, harsh, medium-to-high-pitched ejection-type systolic murmur is present at the right upper sternal border, radiating to the suprasternal notch and carotids; the frequency and intensity of the murmur correlates with stenosis severity.

2. Discrete membranous subvalvular aortic stenosis—The findings are the same as those of valvular aortic stenosis, except that an ejection click is absent. The murmur is located lower on the left sternal border, in the third and fourth intercostal spaces. Associated aortic insufficiency, a common sequela of subaortic stenosis, may produce a high-pitch diastolic decrescendo murmur.

3. Supravalvular aortic stenosis—The harsh systolic murmur is best heard in the suprasternal notch (with possible thrill) and carotids but is well transmitted over the aortic area. There may be a difference in pulses and blood pressure between the right and left arms, with more prominent pulse and higher pressure in the right arm due to the streaming of high velocity blood flow ejected from the LV across the area of stenosis (the Coanda effect).

B. Imaging

In most cases, the heart is not enlarged. The LV, however, may be slightly prominent. In valvular aortic stenosis, poststenotic dilatation of the ascending aorta is common.

C. Electrocardiography

Patients with mild aortic stenosis have a normal ECG. LVH and LV strain may be present with more severe obstruction. Progressive LVH on serial ECG can indicate significant obstruction. LV strain is one indication for intervention.

D. Echocardiography

Echocardiography can be used to reliably diagnose and follow all forms of aortic stenosis. Two-dimensional images and color Doppler can visualize the affected area, and the mean gradient estimated by spectral Doppler approximates the transvalvular gradient measured by cardiac catheterization.

E. Cardiac Catheterization and Angiocardiography

Catheterization demonstrates the pressure gradient from LV to aorta and the anatomic level at which the gradient exists. Catheterization should be considered when echocardiography demonstrates severe valvular aortic stenosis (mean gradient > 40 mm Hg, peak gradient > 70 mm Hg) and in patients with critical aortic stenosis or decreased LV function, regardless of gradient.

▶ Treatment

PGE$_1$ infusion is necessary in critical aortic stenosis until surgical or percutaneous therapy can be performed. Percutaneous balloon valvuloplasty is usually the standard initial treatment for patients with valvular aortic stenosis, though it is typically ineffective for significant annular hypoplasia or subvalvular and supravalvular stenosis. Surgery should be considered in patients with a high residual resting gradient despite balloon valvuloplasty or in the presence of coexisting aortic insufficiency. In many cases, the gradient cannot be significantly diminished by valvuloplasty without producing aortic insufficiency, and patients who develop significant aortic insufficiency require surgical intervention to repair or replace the valve. Surgical options include a mechanical aortic valve replacement in older children or a Ross procedure (translocating the patient's pulmonary valve to the aortic position and placing an RV-to-PA conduit) in infants and children.

Discrete subvalvular aortic stenosis is surgically resected, often at lower gradients than valvular stenosis to prevent progressive damage to the aortic valve by turbulent flow (which may produce valvular aortic insufficiency). Unfortunately, simple resection is followed by recurrence in up to 20%; additional muscle resection lowers this risk of recurrence but is associated with potential heart block or iatrogenic VSD creation.

Supravalvar aortic stenosis requiring repair is usually addressed with surgical patch augmentation of the affected area. Recurrent stenosis is common, as is new stenosis development beyond repair sites.

▶ Course & Prognosis

All forms of LV outflow tract obstruction tend to be progressive. Despite this, with the exception of those with critical aortic stenosis in infancy, patients are usually asymptomatic. Symptoms such as angina, syncope, or HF are rare but imply serious disease. Children often have normal exercise capacity with less-than-moderate stenosis. Children with mild stenosis and normal exercise stress tests may safely participate in vigorous physical activity, including nonisometric competitive sports. Those with moderate stenosis may have restrictions based on symptoms and exercise testing. Children with severe aortic stenosis are predisposed to ventricular dysrhythmias and should refrain from vigorous activity and all isometric exercise.

Otto CM et al: 2020 AHA/ACC guideline for the management of patients with valvular heart disease: a report of the American College of Cardiology/American Heart Association Joint Committee on Clinical Practice Guidelines. Circulation 2021 Feb 2; 143(5):e72–e227 [PMID: 33332150].

Soulatges C et al: Long-term results of balloon valvuloplasty as primary treatment for congenital aortic valve stenosis: a 20-year review. Pediatr Cardiol 2015 Aug;36(6):1145–1152. doi: 10.1007/s00246-015-1134-4 [PMID: 25788411].

3. Mitral Valve Prolapse

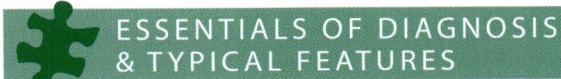

ESSENTIALS OF DIAGNOSIS & TYPICAL FEATURES

- ▶ Midsystolic click.
- ▶ Late systolic "whooping" or "honking" murmur.
- ▶ Typical symptoms include chest pain, palpitations, and dizziness.
- ▶ Often overdiagnosed on routine cardiac ultrasound.

▶ General Considerations

In this condition, as the mitral valve closes during systole, it moves superiorly (prolapses) into the LA. MVP occurs in about 2% of thin female adolescents, a minority of whom have concomitant mitral valve regurgitation (MR). Although MVP is usually an isolated lesion, it can occur in association with connective tissue disorders such as Marfan, Loeys-Dietz, and Ehlers-Danlos syndromes.

▶ Clinical Findings

A. Symptoms and Signs

Most patients with MVP are asymptomatic. Chest pain, palpitations, and dizziness may be reported, but it is unclear whether these symptoms are more common in patients with MVP than in the normal population. Chest pain on exertion is rare and should be assessed with CPET. Significant dysrhythmias have been reported, including premature ventricular contractions and nonsustained ventricular tachycardia. If significant MR is present, atrial arrhythmias may also occur. Standard auscultation technique must be modified to diagnose MVP. A midsystolic click (with or without a systolic murmur) is elicited best in the standing position and is the hallmark of this entity. Conversely, maneuvers that increase LV volume, such as squatting or handgrip exercise, will cause delay or obliteration of the click-murmur complex. The systolic click usually is heard at the apex but may be audible at the left sternal border. A late, short systolic murmur after the click implies MR, which is much less common than isolated MVP. This murmur is not holosystolic, in contrast to rheumatic MR.

B. Imaging

Chest radiograph is generally normal and is not usually indicated in this condition. In the rare case of significant MR, the LA may be enlarged.

C. Electrocardiography

ECG is usually normal but diffuse flattening or inversion of T waves may occur in the precordium.

D. Echocardiography

Echocardiography assesses the degree of prolapse and the presence and degree of regurgitation. Significant superior/posterior systolic movement of the mitral valve leaflets into the LA side of the mitral annulus is diagnostic.

E. Other Testing

Invasive procedures are rarely indicated. Holter monitoring or event recorders may be useful in establishing the presence of ventricular dysrhythmias in patients with palpitations.

▶ Treatment & Prognosis

Propranolol may be effective in treatment of coexisting ventricular arrhythmias. Prophylaxis for infectious endocarditis is not indicated. The natural course of this condition is not well defined. Twenty years of observation indicate that isolated MVP in childhood is usually a benign entity. Surgery for MR is rarely needed.

Delling FN, Vasan RS: Epidemiology and pathophysiology of mitral valve prolapse: new insights into disease progression, genetics, and molecular basis. Circulation 2014 May 27;129(21):2158–2170 [PMID: 24867995].

Otto CM et al: 2020 ACC/AHA guideline for the management of patients with valvular heart disease. A report of the American college of cardiology/American Heart Association Joint Committee on Clinical Practice Guidelines. Circulation 2021;145(5):e35 [PMID: 33332149].

4. Other Congenital Left Heart Valvular Lesions

A. Congenital Mitral Stenosis

Congenital mitral stenosis is a rare disorder in which the valve leaflets are thickened and/or fused, resulting in obstruction to flow into the LV. In many cases, the subvalve apparatus (papillary muscles and chordae tendineae) is also abnormal. When mitral stenosis occurs with other left-sided obstructive lesions, such as subaortic stenosis and coarctation of the aorta, the complex is called Shone syndrome. Most patients develop congestive symptoms early in life with tachypnea, dyspnea, and failure to thrive. Physical examination reveals an accentuated S_1 and a loud pulmonary closure sound. No opening snap is heard. In most cases, a presystolic crescendo murmur is heard at the apex. Occasionally, only a mid-diastolic murmur can be heard. ECG shows right-axis deviation, biatrial enlargement, and RVH. Chest radiography reveals LA enlargement and pulmonary venous congestion. Echocardiography shows abnormal mitral valve structures with reduced leaflet excursion and LA enlargement. Cardiac catheterization reveals an elevated pulmonary capillary wedge pressure and PH, owing to the elevated LA pressure.

Mitral valve repair or mitral valve replacement may be performed, even in young infants. Mitral valve repair is the preferred surgical option, as valve replacement can have a poor outcome, particularly in infants.

B. Cor Triatriatum

Cor triatriatum is a rare abnormality in which the pulmonary veins join in a confluence that is not completely incorporated into the LA. The pulmonary vein confluence communicates with the LA through an opening of variable size that may be obstructed. Patients can present in a similar way to those with mitral stenosis. Clinical findings depend on the degree of obstruction of pulmonary venous flow into the LA. If the communication between the confluence and the LA is small and restrictive to flow, symptoms develop early in life. Echocardiography reveals a linear density in the LA with a pressure gradient present between the pulmonary venous chamber and the true LA. Cardiac catheterization may be needed if the diagnosis is in doubt. High pulmonary wedge pressure and low LA pressure (with the catheter passed through the foramen ovale into the true LA) support the diagnosis. Angiocardiography identifies the pulmonary vein confluence and the anatomic LAs. Coexisting mitral valve abnormalities may be noted, including a supravalvular mitral ring or a dysplastic mitral valve. Surgical repair is always required for cor triatriatum in the presence of an obstructive membrane. Long-term results are good.

Otto CM et al: 2020 AHA/ACC guideline for the management of patients with valvular heart disease: a report of the American College of Cardiology/American Heart Association Joint Committee on Clinical Practice Guidelines. Circulation 2021 Feb 2; 143 (5):e72–e227 [PMID: 33332150].

DISEASES OF THE AORTA

Patients with isolated bicuspid aortic valve and those with Marfan, Loeys-Dietz, Turner, and type IV Ehlers-Danlos syndromes are at risk for progressive aortic dilatation and dissection those.

1. Bicuspid Aortic Valve

Patients with a bicuspid aortic valve have an increased incidence of aortic dilatation and consequent dissection, regardless of the presence of valvular aortic stenosis. Histologic examination demonstrates cystic medial degeneration of the aortic wall, similar to that seen in patients with Marfan syndrome. Patients with an isolated bicuspid aortic valve require regular follow-up to monitor for aortic dilatation, even in the absence of aortic insufficiency or stenosis. Significant aortic dilatation requiring surgical intervention typically does not occur until adulthood.

2. Marfan & Loeys-Dietz Syndromes

Marfan syndrome is an autosomal dominant disorder of the connective tissue caused by a mutation in the fibrillin-1 gene. Spontaneous mutations account for 25%–30% of cases, and thus, negative family history does not rule out Marfan syndrome. Patients are diagnosed by the Ghent criteria (https://www.marfan.org/dx/rules), requiring a minimum of major involvement of two body systems (cardiovascular, ocular, musculoskeletal, pulmonary, or integumentary) plus involvement of a third body system or a positive family history. Cardiac manifestations (which may be present at birth) include aortic dilatation and MVP. Patients with Marfan syndrome are at risk for aortic dissection and are restricted from competitive contact sports and isometric activities. β-Blockers (eg, atenolol), ACE inhibitors, or angiotensin receptor blockers (eg, losartan) are used to lower blood pressure and slow the rate of aortic dilatation. Elective surgical intervention is performed in adolescent and adult patients when the aortic root dimension reaches 50 mm or if there is rapidly progressive aortic root dilatation exceeding 1 cm in 1 year. The ratio of actual-to-expected aortic root dimension is used to determine the need for surgery in the young child. Surgical options include replacement of the dilated aortic root with a composite valve graft (Bentall technique) or sparing of the patient's own aortic valve and replacement of the dilated aortic root with a Dacron tube graft (David procedure). Young age at diagnosis was previously thought to confer a poor prognosis; however, early diagnosis with close follow-up and early medical therapy has more recently been associated with favorable outcomes. Ventricular dysrhythmias may contribute to the mortality in Marfan syndrome.

Loeys-Dietz syndrome is an autosomal dominant disorder of the connective tissue caused by a mutation in the transforming growth factor β (TGFβ) receptor. Loeys-Dietz syndrome is associated with musculoskeletal, skin, and cardiovascular abnormalities, and many patients with Loeys-Dietz were previously thought to have Marfan syndrome. Cardiovascular involvement includes mitral and tricuspid valve prolapse, aneurysms of the PDA, and aortic and PA dilatation. Dissection and aneurysm formation of arteries throughout the body can occur, including in the brachiocephalic arteries.

3. Turner Syndrome

Turner syndrome is caused by spontaneous monosomy of the X chromosome and is associated with cardiovascular abnormalities in approximately 25% of patients. The most commonly associated CHD is coarctation of the aorta with bicuspid aortic valve. As a consequence, patients are at risk for aortic dissection, typically during adulthood. Additional risk factors for aortic dissection that may be present include hypertension (regardless of cause) and coarctation of the aorta. Rare reports of aortic dissection in adult Turner syndrome patients in the absence of any risk factors may suggest the presence of vasculopathy associated with this syndrome. Patients with Turner syndrome require routine cardiology follow-up from adolescence (even in the absence of prior CHD) to monitor for this potentially lethal complication.

Loeys BL et al: The revised Ghent nosology for the Marfan syndrome. J Med Genet 2010;47:476–485 [PMID: 20591885].
Otto CM et al: 2020 AHA/ACC guideline for the management of patients with valvular heart disease: a report of the American College of Cardiology/American Heart Association Joint Committee on Clinical Practice Guidelines. Circulation 2021 Feb 2; 143 (5):e72–e227 [PMID: 33332150].

CORONARY ARTERY ABNORMALITIES

Several anomalies involve the origin, course, and distribution of the coronary arteries. Abnormal origin or course of the coronary arteries is often asymptomatic and can go undetected. However, in some instances these children are at risk for sudden death. The most common congenital coronary artery abnormality in infants is anomalous origin of the left coronary artery from the pulmonary artery (ALCAPA).

Anomalous Origin of the Left Coronary Artery From the Pulmonary Artery

In this condition, the left coronary artery (LCA) arises from the PA rather than the aorta. In neonates, whose PAP is high, perfusion of the left coronary artery may be adequate and the infant may be asymptomatic. By age 2 months, the PAP falls, causing a progressive decrease in myocardial perfusion provided by the anomalous LCA. Ischemia and infarction of the LV results. Immediate surgery is indicated to reimplant the anomalous LCA and restore myocardial perfusion.

▶ Clinical Findings

A. Symptoms and Signs

Neonates appear healthy with relatively normal growth and development until PAP decreases. Presentation may be subtle, with nonspecific complaints of fussiness or intermittent colic, which may be attacks of intestinal angina. Other symptoms may include pallor, wheezing, and sweating, especially during or after feeding. Presentation may be fulminant at age 2–4 months, with sudden, severe HF due to LV dysfunction and associated MR. On physical examination, infants are usually well developed and well nourished. Pulses are typically weak but equal. A prominent left precordial bulge is present. A gallop and/or holosystolic murmur of MR is sometimes present, though frequently auscultation alone reveals no obvious abnormalities.

B. Imaging

Chest radiography may show cardiac enlargement (due to LA enlargement) and pulmonary venous congestion if LV function has been compromised. Cardiac CT with angiography can help evaluate the coronary arteries if not well defined by echocardiography.

C. Electrocardiography

ECG reveals T-wave inversion in leads I, aVL, and the precordial leads V_4–V_7. Deep and wide Q waves are present in leads I, aVL, and sometimes in V_4–V_6. Deep Q waves in these inferolateral leads is a pathognomonic sign for ALCAPA. These ECG findings of myocardial infarction are similar to those in adults.

D. Echocardiography

The diagnosis can be made with echocardiography by visualizing a single large right coronary artery (RCA) arising from the aorta and the anomalous LCA arising from the main PA. Flow reversal in the LCA (heading *toward* the PA, rather than away from the aorta) confirms the diagnosis. LV dysfunction, echo-bright (ischemic) papillary muscles, and MR are commonly seen.

E. Cardiac Catheterization and Angiocardiography

Angiogram of the aorta will fail to show the origin of the LCA. A large RCA fills directly from the aorta, and contrast flows from the RCA system via collaterals into the LCA and finally into the PA. Angiogram of the RV or main PA may show the origin of the anomalous LCA. Rarely, a left-to-right shunt may be detected as oxygenated blood passes through the collateral system, without delivering oxygen to the myocardium, and into the PA.

▶ Treatment & Prognosis

The prognosis of ALCAPA depends in part on the clinical appearance of the patient at presentation. Medical management with diuretics and afterload reduction can help stabilize a critically ill patient, but surgical intervention should not be delayed. Surgery involves reimplantation of the anomalous LCA onto the aorta. The mitral valve may have to be replaced, depending on the degree of injury to the papillary muscles and associated MR. Although a life-threatening problem,

cardiac function nearly always recovers if the infant survives the surgery and postoperative period.

Frommelt P et al: Recommendations for multimodality assessment of congenital coronary anomalies: a guide from the American Society of Echocardiography: developed in collaboration with the Society for Cardiovascular Angiography and Interventions, Japanese Society of Echocardiography, and Society for Cardiovascular Magnetic Resonance. J Am Soc Echocardiogr 2020 Mar;33(3):259–294 [PMID: 32143778].

Neumann A et al: Long-term results after repair of anomalous origin of left coronary artery from the pulmonary artery: Takeuchi repair versus coronary transfer. Eur J Cardiothorac Surg 2017 Feb 1;51(2):308–315. doi: 10.1093/ejcts/ezw268 [PMID: 28186291].

CYANOTIC CONGENITAL HEART DISEASE

TETRALOGY OF FALLOT

ESSENTIALS OF DIAGNOSIS & TYPICAL FEATURES

► Hypoxemic spells during infancy.
► Boot-shaped cardiac silhouette on chest radiograph.
► Systolic ejection murmur at the upper left sternal border.

▶ General Considerations

In tetralogy of Fallot (ToF), anterior deviation of the subpulmonary outflow septum causes narrowing of the RV outflow tract (RVOT). This deviation also results in a VSD, and the aorta then overrides the crest of the ventricular septum. The RV hypertrophies, not because of pulmonary stenosis, but because it is pumping against systemic resistance across a (usually) large VSD. ToF is the most common cyanotic cardiac lesion and accounts for 10% of all CHD.

Obstruction of the RVOT causes a right-to-left shunt across the VSD, resulting in arterial desaturation. The greater the obstruction and the lower the systemic vascular resistance, the greater is the right-to-left shunt. ToF is associated with 22q11 deletion or DiGeorge syndrome in as many as 15% of affected children.

▶ Clinical Findings

A. Symptoms and Signs

Clinical findings vary with the degree of RVOT obstruction. Patients with mild obstruction are minimally or not cyanotic. Those with severe obstruction are deeply cyanotic from birth.

Few children are asymptomatic. In those with significant RVOT obstruction, many have cyanosis at birth, and nearly all have progressive cyanosis by age 4 months. Growth and development are not typically delayed, but easy fatigability and dyspnea on exertion are common. Though less common with early treatment, the fingers and toes show variable clubbing depending on age and severity of untreated cyanosis.

Cyanotic spells, also called "Tet spells" are one of the hallmarks of severe ToF. These spells can occur spontaneously and at any time, but in infants occur most commonly with crying or feeding, while in older children they can occur with exercise. They are characterized by (1) sudden onset of cyanosis or deepening of cyanosis; (2) dyspnea; (3) alterations in consciousness, from irritability to syncope; and (4) decrease in or disappearance of the systolic murmur (as RVOT becomes completely obstructed). These episodes most commonly start at age 4–6 months. Cyanotic spells are treated acutely by administration of oxygen and placing the patient in the knee-to-chest position (to increase systemic vascular resistance). Sedating medications can be helpful, but morphine should be administered cautiously due to its vasodilatory effect. β -Blocker therapy may reduce the RVOT obstruction through its negative inotropic action. Chronic oral prophylaxis of cyanotic spells with β-blockers may be useful to delay surgery, but the onset of Tet spells usually prompts surgical intervention. In fact, in the current era, elective surgical repair generally occurs around the age of 3 months to avoid the development of Tet spells. With earlier diagnosis and treatment, squatting that was historically seen in older children with ToF to increase systemic vascular resistance and force blood through the pulmonary circuit, thus warding off cyanotic spells, is rarely seen.

On examination, an RV lift is palpable. S_2 is predominantly aortic and single. A grade II–IV/VI, rough, systolic ejection murmur is present at the left sternal border in the third intercostal space and radiates well to the back.

B. Laboratory Findings

Older infants or children typically develop polycythemia due to chronic arterial desaturation.

C. Imaging

Chest radiography show a normal-size heart. The RV is hypertrophied, often shown by an upturning of the apex (boot-shaped heart). The main PA silhouette is usually concave due arterial hypoplasia, and pulmonary vascular markings are usually decreased.

D. Electrocardiography

The QRS axis is rightward, ranging from +90 to +180 degrees. The P waves are usually normal. RVH is always present, but RV strain patterns are rare.

E. Echocardiography

Two-dimensional imaging is diagnostic, revealing RV hypertrophy, overriding of the aorta, and a large subaortic VSD. Obstruction at the level of the RVOT and pulmonary valve can be identified.

F. Cardiac Catheterization and Angiocardiography

If a catheterization is done, it reveals a right-to-left shunt across the VSD in most cases. The RV pressure is equalized to the LV if the VSD is large. The PAP (beyond the RVOT obstruction) is invariably low. Pressure gradients may be noted at the pulmonary valvular level, the infundibular level, or both. RV angiography reveals RVOT obstruction and a right-to-left shunt at the VSD. The major indications for cardiac catheterization are to establish coronary artery and distal PA anatomy if not able to be clearly defined by echocardiography.

▶ **Treatment**

A. Palliative Treatment

Most centers currently advocate complete repair of ToF during the neonatal or infant period. However, some centers prefer palliative treatment for small neonates in whom complete correction is deemed risky. Palliation (without complete repair) consists of the surgical insertion of a GoreTex shunt from the subclavian artery to the ipsilateral PA [modified Blalock-Taussig-Thomas (BTT) shunt] to replace the ductus arteriosus (which is ligated and divided) or stenting of the ductus via catheterization. This secures a source of PBF and may allow for growth of the hypoplastic PAs prior to complete surgical correction. The BTT shunt was previously known as the Blalock-Taussig shunt in recognition of Dr. Helen Taussig who identified the problem of inadequate PBF in "blue babies" and Dr. Alfred Blalock who first performed the shunt procedure; however, credit for development of the technique is now given to Dr. Blalock's Black laboratory technician, Vivien Thomas, who was awarded an honorary doctorate by Johns Hopkins University in 1976.

B. Total Correction

Complete surgical repair of ToF is performed at ages ranging from birth to 2 years, depending on the patient's anatomy and degree of cyanosis. The current surgical trend is toward earlier repair for symptomatic infants. During surgery, the VSD is closed and the obstruction to RVOT removed. Although a valve-sparing procedure is preferred, in many cases, a transannular patch is placed across the RVOT and pulmonary valve. When a transannular patch repair is done, the patient has PI that is usually well tolerated for years. However, pulmonary valve replacement is eventually necessary once symptoms (usually exercise intolerance) and RV dilatation occur. Surgical mortality is low.

▶ Course & Prognosis

Infants with severe ToF can be deeply cyanotic at birth and, thus, require early surgery. Complete repair of ToF before age 2 years usually produces a good result. Depending on the extent of the repair required, patients frequently require additional surgery 10–15 years after their initial repair for replacement of the pulmonary valve. Transcatheter pulmonary valve replacement is now performed in some adolescents and young adults with a history of ToF, avoiding the need for open heart surgery. Patients with ToF are at risk for sudden death due to ventricular dysrhythmias. A competent pulmonary valve without a dilated RV appears to diminish arrhythmias and enhance exercise performance.

Valente AM et al: Multimodality imaging guidelines for patients with repaired tetralogy of Fallot: a report from the American Society of Echocardiography: developed in collaboration with the Society for Cardiovascular Magnetic Resonance and the Society for Pediatric Radiology. J Am Soc Echocardiogr 2014 Feb;27(2):111–141 [PMID: 24468055].

PULMONARY ATRESIA WITH VENTRICULAR SEPTAL DEFECT

ESSENTIALS OF DIAGNOSIS & TYPICAL FEATURES

▶ Symptoms depend on the amount of pulmonary blood flow.

▶ Pulmonary blood flow occurs via PDA and/or aortopulmonary collaterals.

▶ May require surgical palliation prior to delayed complete reparative surgery.

Complete atresia of the pulmonary valve, in association with a VSD, is an extreme form of ToF. Because there is no antegrade flow from the RV to the PA, PBF must be derived from a PDA or from major aortopulmonary collateral arteries (MAPCAs). Symptoms depend on the amount of PBF. If PBF is adequate, patients may be stable. If PBF is inadequate, severe hypoxemia occurs and newborns will require PGE_1 infusion to maintain the PDA; however, if the MAPCAs alone are sufficient, the ductus may not contribute significantly to PBF and PGE_1 may be discontinued. Once stabilized, palliation with a BTT shunt or complete repair is undertaken. The decision to perform palliation or complete repair in a newborn is dependent on surgical expertise and preference in combination with PA anatomy. The goal of the shunt is to augment PBF and encourage vascular growth, with complete surgical correction planned several months later. In children

with MAPCAs, relocation of the MAPCAs is performed so that they are connected to the PA (unifocalization) to complete the repair.

Echocardiography is usually diagnostic. Cardiac catheterization and angiocardiography or cardiac MRI can confirm the source(s) of PBF and document size of the distal PAs.

Glatz AC et al: Comparison between patent ductus arteriosus stent and modified Blalock-Taussig shunt as palliation for infants with ductal-dependent pulmonary blood flow: insights from the congenital catheterization research collaborative. Circulation 2018;137(6):589–601 [PMID: 29042354].

PULMONARY ATRESIA WITH INTACT VENTRICULAR SEPTUM

ESSENTIALS OF DIAGNOSIS & TYPICAL FEATURES

▶ Different lesion from pulmonary atresia with VSD.

▶ Cyanosis at birth.

▶ Pulmonary blood flow is ductal dependent and aortopulmonary collateral arteries are rare.

▶ RV-dependent coronary arteries are sometimes present.

▶ General Considerations

Although pulmonary atresia with intact ventricular septum (PA/IVS) sounds as if it might be related to pulmonary atresia with VSD, it is a distinct cardiac condition. As the name suggests, the pulmonary valve is atretic. The pulmonic annulus usually has a small diaphragm consisting of fused valve cusps. There is no VSD. The main PA segment is usually present but usually hypoplastic. There is variable reduction in RV size, a variable that determines the success of two-ventricle surgical repair. Newborns with severe RV hypoplasia that is inadequate in size to support cardiac output may require single ventricle palliation. After birth, the PBF is provided by the PDA. MAPCAs are usually not present, in contrast to pulmonary atresia with VSD. PGE_1 infusion after birth is needed to maintain ductal patency.

▶ Clinical Findings

A. Symptoms and Signs

Neonates are usually cyanotic and become more so as the PDA closes. A blowing systolic murmur may be heard at the pulmonary area due to ductal-dependent PBF. A holosystolic murmur is often heard at the lower left sternal border, as TR is the only egress of blood that enters the RV. A PFO or ASD is essential for decompression of the right side of the heart.

B. Imaging

The heart size varies depending on the degree of TR. With severe TR, RA enlargement may be massive, and the cardiac silhouette may fill the chest on radiograph. In patients with associated tricuspid valve and/or RV hypoplasia, most of the systemic venous return travels right-to-left across the ASD, and so the heart size can be normal.

C. Electrocardiography

ECG reveals a left axis for age (45–90 degrees) in the frontal plane. LV forces dominate the ECG, and there is a paucity of RV forces, particularly with a hypoplastic RV. Findings of RA enlargement are usually striking.

D. Echocardiography

Echocardiography shows atresia of the pulmonary valve with varying degrees of RV and tricuspid valve hypoplasia. Patency of an intra-atrial communication and PDA are verified by echocardiography.

E. Cardiac Catheterization and Angiocardiography

RV pressure often exceeds the systemic pressure. Angiogram of the RV will reveal no filling of the PA. A Rashkind balloon atrial septostomy may be required to open the existing communication across the atrial septum, if inadequate. Some newborns with PA/IVS may have fistulous connections between the RV cavity and the coronary arteries. These connections can persist due to the high pressure generated in the RV and can result in reversal of coronary flow (from the RV). Such RV-dependent coronary circulation can result in myocardial ischemia due to inadequate coronary perfusion. Precise coronary angiography is required to evaluate the coronary anatomy. If the RV is adequate in size and coronary circulation is not RV-dependent, an eventual two-ventricle repair can be planned. The pulmonary valve plate may be perforated and dilated during cardiac catheterization to allow antegrade flow from the RV to the PA and thus encourage RV cavity growth.

Treatment & Prognosis

As in all ductal-dependent lesions, PGE_1 is used to stabilize the patient and maintain the PDA until catheter intervention or surgery can be performed. Surgery is usually undertaken in the first week of life. If the RV is hypoplastic, RV-dependent coronary circulation is present, or the pulmonic valve cannot be opened successfully during cardiac catheterization, a BTT shunt or PDA stenting is performed to establish PBF. Later in infancy, a communication between the RV and PA can be created to stimulate RV cavity growth. If RV hypoplasia precludes two-ventricular repair (and coronary blood flow is normal), an approach similar to that taken for a single ventricle pathway best serves these children (see section Hypoplastic Left Heart Syndrome). Children with significant coronary artery abnormalities are considered for cardiac transplantation because they are at risk for myocardial ischemia and sudden death.

Glatz AC et al: Comparison between patent ductus arteriosus stent and modified Blalock-Taussig shunt as palliation for infants with ductal-dependent pulmonary blood flow: insights from the Congenital Catheterization Research Collaborative. Circulation 2018;137(6)589–601 [PMID: 29042354].

Lowenthal A et al: Prenatal tricuspid valve size as a predictor of postnatal outcome in patients with severe pulmonary stenosis or pulmonary atresia with intact ventricular septum. Fetal Diagn Ther 2014;35(2):101–107 [PMID: 24457468].

Schneider AW et al: More than 25 years of experience in managing pulmonary atresia with intact ventricular septum. Ann Thorac Surg 2014 Nov;98(5):1680–1686 [PMID: 25149048].

TRICUSPID ATRESIA

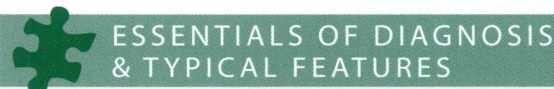

ESSENTIALS OF DIAGNOSIS & TYPICAL FEATURES

► Marked cyanosis present from birth.

► ECG with left-axis deviation, right atrial enlargement, and LVH.

► General Considerations

In tricuspid atresia, there is complete atresia of the tricuspid valve with no direct communication between the RA and the RV. There are two types of tricuspid atresia based on the relationship of the great arteries (normally related or malposed great arteries). The entire systemic venous return must flow through the atrial septum (ASD or PFO) to reach the LA. The LA thus receives both the systemic venous return and the pulmonary venous return. Complete mixing occurs in the LA, resulting in variable degrees of arterial desaturation. Because there is no flow to the RV, development of the RV depends on the presence of left-to-right shunt across a VSD. Severe hypoplasia of the RV occurs when there is no VSD or when the VSD is small.

► Clinical Findings

A. Symptoms and Signs

Symptoms usually develop in early infancy with cyanosis present at birth. Growth and development are poor, and the infant usually exhibits exhaustion during feedings, tachypnea, and dyspnea. Patients with increased PBF may develop HF with less prominent cyanosis. The degree of PBF is most dependent on PVR; those patients with low PVR will have increased PBF. A murmur from a VSD is usually present and heard best at the lower left sternal border.

B. Imaging

The heart is slightly to markedly enlarged. The main PA segment is usually small or absent. The size of the RA is moderately to massively enlarged, depending on the size of the communication at the atrial level. The pulmonary vascular markings are usually decreased but may be increased if pulmonary blood flow is not restricted by the VSD or pulmonary stenosis.

C. Electrocardiography

ECG shows marked left-axis deviation. The P waves are tall and peaked, indicative of RA hypertrophy. LVH or LV dominance is found in almost all cases. RV forces on the ECG are usually low or absent.

D. Echocardiography

Two-dimensional and color-flow Doppler echocardiography is diagnostic and shows absence of the tricuspid valve, the relationship between the great arteries, anatomy of the VSD, presence of an ASD or PFO, and size of the PAs.

E. Cardiac Catheterization and Angiocardiography

Catheterization reveals a right-to-left shunt at the atrial level. Because of mixing in the LA, oxygen saturations in the LV, RV, PA, and aorta are identical to those in the LA. RA pressure is increased if the ASD is restrictive. A balloon atrial septostomy is performed if a restrictive PFO or ASD is present.

▶ Treatment & Prognosis

In infants with unrestricted PBF, conventional anticongestive therapy with diuretics and afterload reduction should be given until the infant begins to outgrow the VSD. Sometimes, a PA band is needed if there is no restriction to PBF to protect the pulmonary bed from excessive flow and development of pulmonary vascular disease.

Staged palliation of tricuspid atresia is the usual approach. In infants with diminished PBF, PGE_1 is given until an aortopulmonary shunt (BTT shunt or ductal stent) can be performed. A Glenn procedure (SVC to PA anastomosis) is done (with takedown of the aortopulmonary shunt, if present) at 4–6 months of life, when saturations begin to fall, and completion of the Fontan procedure (redirection of IVC and SVC to PA) is performed when the child reaches around 15 kg.

The long-term prognosis for children treated by the Fontan procedure is unknown, although patients now are living into their late 20s and early 30s. In the short term, the best results for the Fontan procedure occur in children with low PAPs prior to open-heart surgery.

Wald RM et al: Outcome after prenatal diagnosis of tricuspid atresia: a multicenter experience. Am Heart J 2007;153:772–778 [PMID:17452152].

HYPOPLASTIC LEFT HEART SYNDROME

ESSENTIALS OF DIAGNOSIS & TYPICAL FEATURES

► Minimal cyanosis at birth.
► Minimal auscultatory findings.
► Rapid onset of shock with ductal closure.

▶ General Considerations

Hypoplastic left heart syndrome (HLHS) is caused by obstruction of either inflow to or outflow from the LV. The syndrome occurs in 1.4%–3.8% of infants with CHD. Stenosis or atresia of the mitral and aortic valves is the rule. In the neonate, survival depends on a PDA through which right-to-left flow into the systemic circulation is needed for organ blood flow (and, potentially, for blood flow to the heart itself, via the coronary arteries). Neonates with HLHS are usually initially stable, but they deteriorate rapidly as the ductus closes in the first week of life. Untreated, death is common in the first week of life. Rarely, the ductus remains patent and infants may survive for weeks to months without PGE_1 therapy.

The diagnosis is often made prenatally by fetal echocardiography. Prenatal diagnosis aids in counseling for the expectant parents and planning for delivery of the infant at or near a center with experience in treating HLHS.

▶ Clinical Findings

A. Symptoms and Signs

Neonates with HLHS appear stable at birth because the ductus is patent. They deteriorate rapidly as the ductus closes, with shock and acidosis secondary to inadequate systemic perfusion.

B. Imaging

Chest radiography on the first day of life may be relatively unremarkable. Later, chest radiographs can demonstrate cardiac enlargement with severe pulmonary venous congestion if the PDA has begun closing or if the baby has been placed on supplemental oxygen that increases PBF.

C. Electrocardiography

ECG shows right-axis deviation, RA enlargement, and RVH with a relative paucity of LV forces.

D. Echocardiography

Echocardiography is diagnostic. A hypoplastic aorta and LV with atretic or stenotic mitral and aortic valves are diagnostic. Color-flow Doppler imaging shows right-to-left flow via the PDA to the aorta, often with retrograde flow in the ascending aorta to the coronary arteries.

▶ Treatment & Prognosis

Initiation of PGE$_1$ is essential as systemic circulation depends on a PDA. Later management depends on balancing pulmonary and systemic blood flow, both of which depend on the RV. In the first weeks of life the PVR falls, favoring pulmonary overcirculation and systemic underperfusion, and therapy is directed at encouraging systemic blood flow. Despite hypoxemia and cyanosis, supplemental oxygen is avoided as this will decrease pulmonary resistance and lead to further increases in PBF. Adequate perfusion can usually be obtained by keeping systemic O$_2$ saturation between 65% and 80%, or more accurately, a PO$_2$ of 40 mm Hg.

Staged surgical palliation is the most common management approach. A Norwood procedure, in which the relatively normal main PA is transected and connected to the small ascending aorta, is performed. The entire aortic arch must be reconstructed due to its small size. Then, either a BTT shunt (from the brachiocephalic artery to the PA) or a Sano shunt (from the RV to the PA) must be created to restore PBF. Children who have a Norwood procedure will later require a Glenn anastomosis (SVC to PA connection with takedown of the systemic-pulmonary shunt) followed by a Fontan (IVC to PA connection, completing the systemic venous bypass of the heart) at ages 6 months and 2–3 years, respectively. Despite advances in surgical technique and postoperative care, HLHS remains one of the most challenging lesions in pediatric cardiology, with 1-year survival as low as 70% (although exceeding 95% at some centers).

Heart transplantation is also a treatment option for newborns with HLHS but is currently typically performed only in infants who are considered poor Norwood candidates. Heart transplantation is more commonly utilized in the event of a failed surgical palliation or if the systemic RV fails (often in adolescence or young adulthood).

Some centers offer a "hybrid" approach that is a collaboration between surgeons and interventional cardiologists. In the hybrid procedure, the chest is opened surgically, and bands are placed around the branches of the PA to limit PBF. Next, a stent is placed in the PDA by the interventionalist to maintain systemic output. In the "comprehensive stage 2," the PA bands and ductal stent are taken down, the aortic arch is reconstructed, and the SVC is surgically connected to the PA (Glenn shunt). Overall survival outcomes are comparable to those undergoing the Norwood Stage 1 palliation; however, long-term outcome data are not yet available.

Alsoufi B et al: Results of heart transplantation following failed staged palliation of hypoplastic left heart syndrome and related single ventricle anomalies. Eur J Cardiothorac Surg 2015 Nov;48(5):792–798 [PMID: 25602055].

Oster ME et al: Association of interstage home monitoring with mortality, readmissions, and weight gain: a multicenter study from the National Pediatric Cardiology Quality Improvement Collaborative. Circulation 2015 Aug 11;132(6):502–508 [PMID: 26260497].

Sananes R et al: Six-year neurodevelopmental outcomes for children with single-ventricle physiology. Pediatrics 2021 Feb;147(2):e2020014589 [PMID: 33441486].

TRANSPOSITION OF THE GREAT ARTERIES

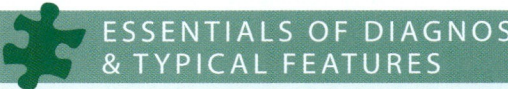

ESSENTIALS OF DIAGNOSIS & TYPICAL FEATURES

- ▶ Cyanotic newborn without respiratory distress.
- ▶ More common in males.

▶ General Considerations

Transposition of the great arteries (TGA) is the second most common cyanotic CHD, accounting for 5% of all cases of CHD. The male-to-female ratio is 3:1. It is caused by an embryologic abnormality in the spiral division of the arterial trunk in which the aorta arises from the RV and the PA from the LV. Patients may also have an associated VSD. Left unrepaired, TGA is associated with a high incidence of early PH. Because pulmonary and systemic circulations are in parallel, survival is impossible without mixing between the two circuits. The most effective mixing occurs at the atrial level via either a PFO or ASD. Some mixing can also occur at the level of the ductus or VSD, if present, but an adequate interatrial communication is needed to prevent severe cyanosis.

▶ Clinical Findings

A. Symptoms and Signs

Neonates are often cyanotic but without respiratory distress or a significant murmur. Infants with a large VSD may be less cyanotic, and they usually have a prominent murmur. The findings on cardiovascular examination depend on the associated intracardiac defects.

B. Imaging

The chest radiograph usually demonstrates an "egg on a string" appearance because the aorta is directly anterior to the main PA, resulting in narrowing of the upper mediastinum.

C. Electrocardiography

Because the newborn ECG normally has RV predominance, the ECG in TGA will frequently look normal.

D. Echocardiography

Echocardiography is diagnostic. Associated defects, such as a VSD, RV or LV outflow tract obstruction, or coarctation, should be evaluated. The atrial septum should be closely examined for any restriction. The coronary anatomy is variable and must be defined prior to surgery.

E. Cardiac Catheterization and Angiocardiography

A Rashkind balloon atrial septostomy is frequently performed if the interatrial communication does not allow for adequate mixing of blood.

▶ Treatment

Early corrective surgery is recommended. The arterial switch operation (ASO) is performed at 4–7 days of life and has replaced the previously performed atrial switch procedures (Mustard and Senning operations). The great arteries are transected above the level of the valves and switched, while the coronaries are separately reimplanted. Large VSDs, if present, are repaired and the ASD is closed. Operative survival after the ASO is greater than 95% in major centers.

Cohen MS: Multimodality imaging guidelines of patients with transposition of the great arteries: a report from the American Society of Echocardiography developed in collaboration with the Society for Cardiovascular Magnetic Resonance and the Society of Cardiovascular Computed Tomography. J Am Soc Echocardiogr 2016 Jul;29(7):571–621. doi: 10.1016/j.echo.2016.04.002 [PMID: 27372954].

Fricke TA et al: Arterial switch operation: operative approach and outcomes. Ann Thorac Surg. 2019;107(1):302–310 [PMID: 30009809].

1. Congenitally Corrected Transposition of the Great Arteries

Congenitally corrected transposition of the great arteries (ccTGA) is a relatively uncommon CHD. In ccTGA, there is discordance between both connections from the atria to ventricles and ventricles to the arteries (ie, the RA drains to a morphologic LV, which supports the PA; conversely, the LA drains to a morphologic RV, which supports the aorta). Commonly associated lesions are VSD and pulmonary stenosis. Patients may present with neonatal cyanosis, HF later in life, or be asymptomatic, depending on the associated lesions. In the absence of associated lesions, patients with ccTGA are often undiagnosed until adulthood.

Previously, surgical repair was directed at VSD closure and relief of pulmonary outflow tract obstruction—a technique that maintained the RV as the systemic ventricle with outflow to the aorta. It is now recognized that these patients have a reduced life span due to systemic RV failure; thus, the double-switch procedure has been advocated. An atrial switch (Mustard or Senning technique) is performed, in which pulmonary and systemic venous blood are baffled such that they drain into the contralateral ventricle (systemic venous return drains into the RV and pulmonary venous return drains into the LV). In addition, an ASO then restores the morphologic LV to its position as systemic ventricle.

Patients with ccTGA have an increased incidence of complete heart block with an estimated risk of 1% per year and an overall frequency of 50%.

Marathe SP et al: Contemporary outcomes of the double switch operation for congenitally corrected transposition of the great arteries. J Thorac Cardiovasc Surg 2022;164(6)1980–1990 [PMID: 35688715].

2. Double-Outlet Right Ventricle

In this uncommon malformation, both great arteries arise from the RV and a VSD allows blood to exit the LV. Presenting symptoms depend on the relationship of the VSD to the semilunar valves. In the absence of outflow obstruction, a large left-to-right shunt exists, and the clinical picture resembles that of a large VSD. If pulmonary stenosis is present, the physiology is similar to ToF. Early primary correction is the goal. LV flow is directed to the aorta across the VSD (closing the VSD), and an RV to PA conduit is placed if there is restriction to PBF. If the aorta is far from the VSD, an arterial switch may be necessary. Echocardiography is usually sufficient to make the diagnosis and determine the orientation of the great arteries and their relationship to the VSD.

Mahle WT et al: Anatomy, echocardiography, and surgical approach to double outlet right ventricle. Cardiol Young 2008; 18(Suppl 3):39–51 [PMID: 19094378].

Pushparajah K et al: A systematic three-dimensional echocardiographic approach to assist surgical planning in double outlet right ventricle. Echocardiography 2013 Feb;30(2):234–238. doi: 10.1111/echo.12037 [PMID: 23167820].

TOTAL ANOMALOUS PULMONARY VENOUS RETURN

ESSENTIALS OF DIAGNOSIS & TYPICAL FEATURES

► Abnormal pulmonary venous connection leading to cyanosis.

► Occurs with or without a murmur and may have accentuated P_2.

► Right atrial enlargement and RVH.

General Considerations

This malformation accounts for 2% of all CHD. Instead of the pulmonary veins draining into the LA, the veins empty into a confluence that usually is located behind the LA. However, the confluence is not connected to the LA and, instead, the pulmonary venous blood drains into the systemic venous system. Therefore, there is complete mixing of the systemic and pulmonary venous blood at the level of the RA. The presentation of a patient with total anomalous pulmonary venous return (TAPVR) depends on the route of drainage into the systemic circulation and whether or not this drainage route is obstructed.

The malformation is classified as either intra-, supra-, or infracardiac. Intracardiac TAPVR occurs when the pulmonary venous confluence drains directly into the heart, usually via the coronary sinus into the RA (rarely draining directly into the RA). Supracardiac (or supradiaphragmatic) TAPVR is most common and defined as a confluence that drains into the right SVC, brachiocephalic vein, or persistent left SVC. In infracardiac (or infradiaphragmatic) TAPVR, the confluence drains into the IVC (most commonly via the portal venous system and occasionally to the ductus venosus).

Infracardiac TAPVR is very frequently obstructed and makes this lesion a potential surgical emergency. Supracardiac TAPVR is less commonly obstructed. Rarely, the pulmonary venous confluence drains to more than one location, called mixed TAPVR. Because the entire venous drainage from the body returns to the RA, an obligatory right-to-left shunt occurs at the level of the atrial septum.

Clinical Findings

A. Unobstructed Pulmonary Venous Return

Patients with unobstructed TAPVR and a large atrial communication tend to have increased PBF and typically present with cardiomegaly and HF (rather than severe cyanosis). Hypoxemia with saturations in the high 80s or low 90s are common. Most patients have elevated PAP owing to elevated PBF.

1. Symptoms and signs—Patients may have mild cyanosis and tachypnea in the neonatal period and early infancy. An RV heave is palpable, and P_2 is increased. A systolic and diastolic murmur may be heard due to increased flow across the pulmonary and tricuspid valves, respectively.

2. Imaging—Chest radiography reveals cardiomegaly involving the right heart and PA. Pulmonary vascular markings are increased.

3. Electrocardiography—ECG shows right axis deviation and varying degrees of RA enlargement and RVH.

4. Echocardiography—Demonstration by echocardiography of a discrete anomalous chamber posterior to the LA

(receiving the pulmonary veins) and an obligatory right-to-left atrial level shunt is diagnostic.

B. With Obstructed Pulmonary Venous Return

Most patients with infracardiac TAPVR and a minority of patients with supracardiac TAPVR have obstructed drainage. The pulmonary venous return is usually obstructed at the level of the ascending or descending vein that connects the confluence to the systemic venous system. Obstruction can be caused from extravascular structures (eg, the diaphragm or airways) or by inherent stenosis within the ascending or descending vein.

1. Symptoms and signs—Infants usually present shortly after birth with cyanosis and respiratory distress. Cardiac examination discloses a striking RV impulse. S_2 is markedly accentuated and single. Although there is often no murmur, sometimes, a systolic murmur is heard over the pulmonary area with radiation over the lung fields. Diastolic murmurs are uncommon.

2. Imaging—Chest radiography demonstrates a small cardiac silhouette and pulmonary venous congestion with associated air bronchograms. The radiographic appearance may lead to an erroneous diagnosis of severe lung disease. In less severe cases, the heart size may be normal with mild pulmonary venous congestion.

3. Electrocardiography—The ECG shows right axis deviation, RA enlargement, and RVH.

4. Echocardiography—Echocardiography shows a small LA and LV, a dilated right heart with findings suggestive of high RV pressure, and an obligatory right-to-left atrial level shunt. Drainage from the pulmonary venous confluence can be traced to a draining vertical vein either cephalad or caudal in supra- or infracardiac TAPVR, respectively.

5. Cardiac catheterization and angiocardiography—If echocardiography is not definitive, cardiac catheterization or CT angiography demonstrates the site of entry of anomalous venous drainage.

Treatment

Surgery is always required for TAPVR. If pulmonary venous return is obstructed, surgery must be performed immediately; obstructed TAPVR represents one of the few surgical emergencies in CHD. If pulmonary venous drainage is not obstructed and atrial septal flow is not restricted, surgical repair can be scheduled nonemergently.

Course & Prognosis

Most children undergoing TAPVR repair experience surgery without complication. However, some surgical survivors develop late stenosis of the pulmonary veins. Pulmonary vein stenosis is an intractable condition that is difficult to treat either with interventional catheterization or surgery and has a poor prognosis, with a risk of postprocedural restenosis.

Marino BS et al: Neurodevelopmental outcomes in children with congenital heart disease: evaluation and management: a scientific statement from the American Heart Association. Circulation 2012 Aug 28;126(9):1143–1172. doi: 10.1161/CIR.0b013e318265ee8a [PMID: 22851541].

Seale AN et al: Total anomalous pulmonary venous connection: outcome of postoperative pulmonary venous obstruction. J Thorac Cardiovasc Surg 2013 May;145(5):1255–1262 [PMID: 22892140].

TRUNCUS ARTERIOSUS

ESSENTIALS OF DIAGNOSIS & TYPICAL FEATURES

▶ Early HF with or without cyanosis.
▶ Systolic ejection click.

▶ General Considerations

Truncus arteriosus accounts for less than 1% of CHD. A single great artery arises from the heart, giving rise to the systemic, pulmonary, and coronary circulations. Truncus arteriosus develops embryologically as a result of failure of the division of the common arterial trunk into the aorta and the PA. A VSD is nearly always present (only rare cases of truncus arteriosus without VSD have been reported). The number of truncus valve leaflets varies from one to six, and the valve may be insufficient or stenotic.

Truncus arteriosus is divided into subtypes by the anatomy of the pulmonary circulation. A single main PA may arise from the base of the trunk and gives rise to branch PAs (type 1). Alternatively, the PAs may arise separately from the common trunk, either in close association with one another (type 2) or widely separated (type 3). This lesion can occur in association with an interrupted aortic arch.

In patients with truncus arteriosus, blood from both ventricles leaves the heart through a single outflow. Thus, oxygen saturation in the PA is equal to that in the systemic arteries. The degree of hypoxemia and cyanosis depends on the ratio of pulmonary to systemic blood flow, which is determined by the balance of systemic and pulmonary vascular resistances.

▶ Clinical Findings

A. Symptoms and Signs

Elevated PBF characterizes most patients with truncus arteriosus. These patients are usually minimally cyanotic and

present in HF. Physical examination reveals a hyperactive precordium. A loud holosystolic murmur with systolic thrill is common at the lower left sternal border. A loud early systolic ejection click is common. S_2 is single and accentuated. A diastolic flow murmur can often be heard at the apex due to increased pulmonary venous return crossing the mitral valve. An additional diastolic murmur of truncus valve insufficiency may be present.

B. Imaging

Chest radiography reveals cardiomegaly, absence of the main PA segment, and a large aorta. The pulmonary vascular markings vary with the degree of pulmonary blood flow.

C. Electrocardiography

The axis is usually normal. RVH or combined ventricular hypertrophy is common.

D. Echocardiography

Echocardiography is diagnostic and demonstrates ventricular septal override of a single great artery (similar to ToF, but no second great artery arises directly from the heart). The origin of the PAs and the degree of truncal valve abnormality can be defined. Color-flow Doppler can aid in the description of pulmonary flow. Echocardiography is critical in identifying associated lesions such as the presence of an interrupted aortic arch which will impact surgical planning.

E. Angiocardiography

Cardiac catheterization is not routinely performed but may be of value in older infants in whom pulmonary vascular disease must be ruled out. The single most important angiogram would be from the truncus root, which will demonstrate both the origin of the PAs and the amount of truncus insufficiency.

▶ Treatment

Anticongestive therapy is needed for patients with increased PBF and HF. Surgery is always required in this condition. Because of HF and the risk of development of pulmonary vascular disease, surgery is usually performed in the neonatal period or in early infancy. The VSD is closed to allow LV egress to the truncus valve. The pulmonary artery (type 1) or arteries (types 2–3) are separated from the truncus and a valved conduit is fashioned from the RV to the PAs.

▶ Course & Prognosis

Children with a good surgical result generally do well. Patients with dysplasia or dysfunction of the truncus valve (which becomes the "neoaortic" valve) may eventually require surgical repair or replacement of this valve. In addition, similar to patients with ToF, patients eventually outgrow the RV-to-PA conduit placed in infancy and require revision of the conduit in later childhood.

O'Byrne ML et al: Morbidity in children and adolescents after surgical correction of truncus arteriosus communis. Am Heart J 2013 Sep;166(3):512–518. doi: 10.1016/j.ahj.2013.05.023 [PMID: 24016501].

ACQUIRED HEART DISEASE

RHEUMATIC FEVER

ESSENTIALS OF DIAGNOSIS & TYPICAL FEATURES

► Preceding group A β-hemolytic streptococcal infection.

► Diagnosis of initial acute rheumatic fever requires two major or one major plus two minor manifestations.

► Diagnosis of recurrent acute rheumatic fever requires two major or one major and two minor or three minor manifestations.

► Major criteria include carditis, arthritis, chorea, erythema marginatum, and subcutaneous nodules.

► Minor criteria include polyarthralgia or monoarthralgia, fever ≥ 38.5°C, elevated inflammatory markers, and prolonged PR interval on ECG.

Rheumatic fever remains a major cause of morbidity and mortality in developing countries that suffer from poverty, overcrowding, and poor access to health care. Even in developed countries, rheumatic fever has not been entirely eradicated. The overall incidence in the United States is less than 1 per 100,000. Group A β-hemolytic streptococcal infection of the upper respiratory tract is the essential trigger in predisposed individuals. The latest attempts to define host susceptibility implicate immune response genes that are present in approximately 15% of the population. The immune response triggered by infection of the pharynx with group A streptococci consists of (1) sensitization of B lymphocytes by streptococcal antigens, (2) formation of antistreptococcal antibody, (3) formation of immune complexes that cross-react with cardiac sarcolemma antigens, and (4) myocardial and valvular inflammatory responses.

The peak age of risk in the United States is 5–15 years. The disease is slightly more common in girls and in African Americans.

► Clinical Findings

Two major or one major and two minor manifestations (plus supporting evidence of streptococcal infection) based on the

Table 20–13. Jones criteria (modified) for diagnosis of rheumatic fever.

Major manifestations
Carditis
Polyarthritis
Sydenham chorea
Erythema marginatum
Subcutaneous nodules
Minor manifestations
Clinical
Previous rheumatic fever or rheumatic heart disease
Polyarthralgia
Fever
Laboratory
Acute phase reaction: elevated erythrocyte sedimentation rate, C-reactive protein, leukocytosis
Prolonged PR interval
Plus
Supporting evidence of preceding streptococcal infection, ie, increased titers of antistreptolysin O or other streptococcus antibodies, positive throat culture for group A *Streptococcus*

modified Jones criteria are needed for the diagnosis of acute rheumatic fever (Table 20–13). Except in cases of rheumatic fever manifesting solely as Sydenham chorea or long-standing carditis, there should be clear evidence of a streptococcal infection such as scarlet fever, a positive throat culture for group A β-hemolytic streptococcus, or increased antistreptolysin O or other streptococcal antibody titers. The antistreptolysin O titer is significantly higher in rheumatic fever than in uncomplicated streptococcal infections.

A. Carditis

Carditis is the most serious consequence of rheumatic fever and varies from minimal to life-threatening HF. The term *carditis* implies pancardiac inflammation, but it may be limited to valves, myocardium, or pericardium. Valvulitis is frequently seen, with the mitral valve most commonly affected. MR is the most common valvular residua of acute rheumatic carditis. Mitral stenosis after acute rheumatic fever is rarely encountered until 5–10 years after the first episode, and, therefore, is much more commonly seen in adults than in children. The aortic valve is the second most common valve affected and is involved more often in males and in African Americans. Aortic insufficiency is occasionally encountered as the sole valvular manifestation of rheumatic carditis. In one large study, the shortest length of time observed for a patient to develop dominant aortic stenosis secondary to rheumatic heart disease was 20 years, so dominant aortic stenosis of rheumatic origin is not seen in pediatric patients.

B. Polyarthritis

Arthritis most commonly involves the large joints (knees, hips, wrists, elbows, and shoulders) and is typically migratory.

Joint swelling and associated limitation of movement should be present. Polyarthritis is a common major criterion, occurring in 80% of patients. Arthralgia alone is not a major criterion.

C. Sydenham Chorea

Sydenham chorea is characterized by involuntary and purposeless movements and is often associated with emotional lability. These symptoms become progressively worse and may be accompanied by ataxia and slurring of speech. Muscular weakness becomes apparent following the onset of the involuntary movements. Chorea is self-limiting, although it may last up to 3 months. Chorea may not be apparent for months to years after an acute streptococcal infection.

D. Erythema Marginatum

A macular, serpiginous, erythematous rash with a sharply demarcated border is present primarily on the trunk and the extremities, usually sparing the face.

E. Subcutaneous Nodules

Subcutaneous nodules usually occur only in severe cases. The nodules vary from 1 mL to 2 cm in diameter, are nontender and freely movable under the skin, and most commonly occur over the joints, scalp, and spinal column.

▶ Treatment & Prophylaxis

A. Treatment of the Acute Episode

1. Anti-infective therapy—Eradication of the streptococcal infection is essential. Long-acting benzathine penicillin is the drug of choice. Depending on the age and weight of the patient, a single intramuscular injection of 0.6–1.2 million units is effective; alternatively, penicillin V (250–500 mg orally two to three times a day for 10 days) or amoxicillin (50 mg/kg up to a maximum 1 g once daily for 10 days) may be used. Narrow-spectrum cephalosporins, clindamycin, azithromycin, or clarithromycin are used in those allergic to penicillin.

2. Anti-inflammatory agents

A. ASPIRIN—Aspirin, 30–60 mg/kg/day, is given in four divided doses. This dose is usually sufficient to affect dramatic relief of arthritis and fever. Higher doses carry a greater risk of side effects, and there are no proven short- or long-term benefits of high doses that produce salicylate blood levels of 20–30 mg/dL. The duration of therapy is tailored to meet the needs of the patient, but 2–6 weeks of therapy with reduction in dose toward the end of the course is usually sufficient. Other nonsteroidal anti-inflammatory drugs (NSAIDs) used because of concerns about Reye syndrome are less effective than aspirin. Influenza vaccination should be strongly recommended for patients receiving aspirin and their household contacts.

B. CORTICOSTEROIDS—There is no clear evidence to support the use of corticosteroids, but they are occasionally used for those with severe carditis.

3. Therapy in heart failure—Treatment for HF is based on symptoms and severity of valve involvement and cardiac dysfunction (see section Heart Failure).

4. Bed rest and ambulation—Bed rest is not required in most cases. Activity level should be commensurate with symptoms, and children should be allowed to self-limit their activity level while affected. Most acute episodes of rheumatic fever are managed on an outpatient basis.

B. Treatment After the Acute Rheumatic Fever Episode

1. Prevention—Prevention of future group A streptococcal infections is critical, as patients who have had rheumatic fever are at greater risk of rheumatic fever recurrence if future group A streptococcal infections are inadequately treated. Follow-up visits are essential to reinforce the necessity for prophylaxis., with regular intramuscular long-acting benzathine penicillin injections preferred to oral medication due to better adherence. Long-term (possibly lifelong) prophylaxis is recommended for patients with residual rheumatic heart disease. More commonly, with no or transient cardiac involvement, 5–10 years of therapy or discontinuance in early adulthood (age 21) (whichever is longer) is an effective approach.

The following preventive regimens are in current use:

A. PENICILLIN G BENZATHINE—600,000 units for less than 27 kg or 1.2 million units for more than 27 kg intramuscularly every 4 weeks is the drug of choice.

B. PENICILLIN V—250 mg orally twice daily is much less effective than intramuscular penicillin benzathine G (5.5 vs 0.4 streptococcal infections per 100 patient-years).

C. SULFADIAZINE—500 mg for less than 27 kg and 1 g for more than 27 kg, once daily. Blood dyscrasias and lesser effectiveness in reducing streptococcal infections make this drug less satisfactory than penicillin benzathine G; however, it is the recommended regimen for penicillin-allergic patients.

D. ERYTHROMYCIN—250 mg orally twice daily may be given to patients who are allergic to both penicillin and sulfonamides. Azithromycin or clarithromycin may also be used.

2. Residual valvular damage—The mitral and aortic valves are most commonly affected by rheumatic fever; the severity of carditis is quite variable. In the most severe cases, cardiac failure or the need for a valve replacement can occur in the acute setting. In less severe cases, valve abnormalities can persist, requiring lifelong medical management and eventual valve replacement. Other patients fully recover without residual cardiac sequelae.

Although antibiotic prophylaxis to protect against endocarditis used to be recommended for those with residual valvular abnormalities, the 2007 revised criteria for prevention of IE recommended routine prophylaxis against endocarditis only if a prosthetic valve is in place.

Kumar RK et al: Contemporary diagnosis and management of rheumatic heart disease: implications for closing the gap: a scientific statement from the American Heart Association. Circulation 2020 Nov 17;142(20):e337–e357 [PMID: 33073615].

KAWASAKI DISEASE

ESSENTIALS OF DIAGNOSIS & TYPICAL FEATURES

► At least 5 days of fever + four of the five following diagnostic criteria:
  • Conjunctival injection without exudate
  • Mucous membrane changes (lips/tongue/pharynx)
  • Peripheral extremity changes (hand/foot erythema and/or swelling)
  • Polymorphous generalized rash
  • Unilateral enlarged cervical lymph node (> 1.5 cm)

► Exclusion of other causes of these findings

► Dilated coronary arteries seen with echocardiogram can help with diagnosis in incomplete Kawasaki disease (KD) that does not fulfill diagnostic criteria.

Kawasaki disease (KD) was first described in Japan in 1967 and was initially called mucocutaneous lymph node syndrome. The cause is unclear, and there is no specific diagnostic test. KD is the leading cause of acquired heart disease in children in the United States. Eighty percent of patients are younger than 5 years (median age at diagnosis is 2 years), and the male-to-female ratio is 1.5:1. Diagnostic criteria are fever for more than 5 days and at least four of the following features: (1) bilateral, painless, nonexudative conjunctivitis with limbic sparing; (2) lip or oral cavity changes (eg, lip cracking and fissuring, strawberry tongue, and inflammation of the oral mucosa); (3) cervical lymphadenopathy greater than or equal to 1.5 cm in diameter and usually unilateral; (4) polymorphous exanthema; and (5) extremity changes (redness and swelling of the hands and feet with subsequent desquamation). In the presence of more than four principal clinical criteria, the diagnosis can be made with fewer than 5 days

Table 20–14. Noncardiac manifestations of Kawasaki disease.

System	Associated Signs and Symptoms
Gastrointestinal	Vomiting, diarrhea, gallbladder hydrops, elevated transaminases
Blood	Elevated ESR or CRP, leukocytosis, hypoalbuminemia, mild anemia in acute phase and thrombocytosis in subacute phase (usually second to third week of illness)
Renal	Sterile pyuria, proteinuria
Respiratory	Cough, hoarseness, infiltrate on chest radiograph
Joint	Arthralgia and arthritis
Neurologic	Mononuclear pleocytosis of cerebrospinal fluid, irritability, facial palsy

CRP, C-reactive protein; ESR, erythrocyte sedimentation rate.

of fever. Clinical features not part of the diagnostic criteria, but frequently associated with KD, are shown in Table 20–14.

The potential for cardiovascular complications is the most serious aspect of KD. Complications during the acute illness include myocarditis, pericarditis, valvular heart disease (usually mitral or aortic regurgitation), and coronary arteritis. Patients with fever for at least 5 days, but fewer than four of the diagnostic features can be diagnosed with incomplete KD, especially if they have coronary artery abnormalities detected by echocardiography. Comprehensive recommendations regarding the evaluation for children with suspected incomplete KD were outlined in a 2017 Statement by the AHA (see reference at the end of this section).

Coronary artery lesions range from mild transient dilatation of a coronary artery to large aneurysms. Aneurysms rarely form before day 10 of illness. Untreated patients have a 15%–25% risk of developing coronary aneurysms. Those at greatest risk for aneurysm formation are males, young infants (< 6 months), and those not treated with intravenous immunoglobulin (IVIG). Most coronary artery aneurysms resolve within 5 years of diagnosis; however, as aneurysms resolve, associated obstruction or stenosis (19% of all aneurysms) may develop, which may result in coronary ischemia. Giant aneurysms (> 8 mm) are less likely to resolve, and nearly 50% eventually become stenotic. Acute thrombosis of an aneurysm can occur, resulting in myocardial infarction that is fatal in approximately 20% of such cases.

► Treatment

Immediate management of KD includes IVIG and high-dose aspirin. This therapy is effective in decreasing the incidence of coronary artery dilatation and aneurysm formation. The currently recommended regimen is 2 g/kg of IVIG administered over 10–12 hours and 80–100 mg/kg/day (some centers use 30–50 mg/kg/day) of aspirin in four divided doses. The duration of high-dose aspirin is institution dependent; many centers reduce the dose once the patient is afebrile for 48–72 hours, while others continue through 5 afebrile days or day 14 of the illness. Once high-dose aspirin is discontinued, low-dose aspirin (3–5 mg/kg/day) is given through the subacute phase of the illness (6–8 weeks) or until coronary artery abnormalities resolve. If fever recurs within 48–72 hours of the initial treatment course and no other source of the fever is detected, a second dose of IVIG is often recommended; however, the effectiveness of this approach has not been clearly demonstrated. Dual therapy with IVIG and another anti-inflammatory agent (either corticosteroids or infliximab) is sometimes used, as it has been shown to reduce inflammation faster and decrease length of hospital stay. Dual therapy has also been demonstrated to be effective in reducing coronary artery dilatation in patients presenting with coronary artery dilatation or aneurysms on their initial echocardiogram. Corticosteroids or other anti-inflammatory therapy (eg, infliximab) should, therefore, be considered for patients with cardiac involvement seen on initial echocardiogram and in those with persistent fever despite one or two infusions of IVIG. Follow-up and long-term management of patients with treated KD depends on the degree of coronary involvement (Table 20–15).

Friedman KG et al: Primary adjunctive corticosteroid therapy is associated with improved outcomes for patients with Kawasaki disease with coronary artery aneurysms at diagnosis. Arch Dis Child 2021 Mar;106(3):247–252 [PMID: 32943389].

Jone PN et al: Infliximab plus intravenous immunoglobulin (IVIG) versus IVIG alone as initial therapy in children with Kawasaki disease presenting with coronary artery lesions: is dual therapy more effective? Pediatr Infect Dis J 2018 Oct;37(10):976–980 [PMID: 29461447].

McCrindle BW et al: Diagnosis, treatment, and long-term management of Kawasaki disease: a scientific statement for health professionals from the American Heart Association [review]. Circulation 2017 Apr 25;135(17):e927–e999. doi: 10 1161/CIR 0000000000000484. Epub 2017 Mar 29 [PMID: 28356445].

INFECTIVE ENDOCARDITIS

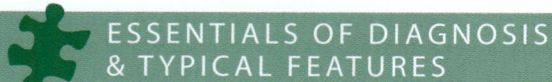

ESSENTIALS OF DIAGNOSIS & TYPICAL FEATURES

▶ Fever and positive blood culture.

▶ Intracardiac oscillating mass, abscess, or new valve regurgitation on echocardiogram.

▶ Elevated erythrocyte sedimentation rate and/or C-reactive protein.

Table 20–15. Long-term management in Kawasaki disease.

Risk Level	Definition	Management Guidelines
I	No coronary artery changes at any stage of the illness	No ASA is needed beyond the subacute phase (6–8 wk). No follow-up beyond the first year.
II	Coronary dilation only (Z-score[a] 2–2.5)	Same as above or clinical follow-up every 2–5 y if persistent coronary dilation.
III	Small coronary aneurysms (Z-score > 2.5 to < 5)	ASA until abnormality resolves. Assess at 6 mo and every 2–3 y thereafter with ECG and echo if < 7 y and every other-year stress testing if > 7 y.
IV	Medium aneurysms (Z-score > 5 to < 10 and absolute dimension < 8 mm)	Long-term ASA ± clopidogrel. Annual follow-up with ECG, echo, and stress testing.
V	Large and giant aneurysms (Z-score > 10 or absolute dimension > 8 mm) or coronary artery obstruction	Long-term ASA ± clopidogrel ± warfarin ± calcium channel blocker to reduce myocardial oxygen consumption. Echo and ECG every 6 mo. Stress testing and Holter examination annually.

ASA, acetyl salicylic acid; ECG, electrocardiogram; echo, echocardiogram.
[a]Coronary artery size assessments are based on standard deviation (Z-score) compared to the normal population.

General Considerations

Bacterial or fungal infection of the endocardium of the heart is rare and usually occurs in the setting of a preexisting abnormality of the heart or great arteries. It may occur in a normal heart during septicemia or as a consequence of infected indwelling central catheters. The frequency of infective endocarditis (IE) appears to be increasing for several reasons: (1) increased survival in children with CHD, (2) greater use of central venous catheters, and (3) increased use of prosthetic material and valves. Pediatric patients without preexisting heart disease are also at increasing risk for IE because of (1) increased survival rates for children with immune deficiencies, (2) long-term use of indwelling lines in ill newborns and patients with chronic diseases, and (3) increased intravenous drug abuse.

Patients at greatest risk are children with unrepaired or palliated cyanotic heart disease (especially in the presence of an aorta to pulmonary shunt), those with implanted prosthetic material, and patients who have had a prior episode of IE. Common organisms causing IE are viridans streptococci (30%–40% of cases), *Staphylococcus aureus* (25%–30%), and fungi (about 5%).

Clinical Findings

A. History

Most patients with IE have a history of heart disease. There may or may not be an antecedent infection or surgical procedure (cardiac surgery, tooth extraction, tonsillectomy). Transient bacteremia occurs frequently during normal daily activities such as flossing or brushing teeth, using a toothpick, and even when chewing food. Although dental and nonsterile surgical procedures also can result in transient bacteremias, these episodes are much less frequent for a given individual. This may explain why a clear inciting event is often not identified in association with IE and also underlies recent changes in guidelines for antibiotic prophylaxis to prevent IE.

B. Symptoms, Signs, and Laboratory Findings

Although IE can present in a fulminant fashion with cardiovascular collapse, often it presents in an indolent manner with fever, malaise, and weight loss. Joint pain and vomiting are less common. On examination, there may be a new or changing murmur, splenomegaly, and hepatomegaly. Classic findings of Osler nodes (tender nodules, usually on the pulp of the fingers), Janeway lesions (nontender hemorrhagic macules on palms and soles), splinter hemorrhages, and Roth spots (retinal hemorrhage) are uncommonly noted in children. Laboratory findings include multiple positive blood cultures, elevated erythrocyte sedimentation rate and/or C-reactive protein, and hematuria. Transthoracic echocardiography can identify large vegetations in some patients, but transesophageal imaging has better sensitivity and may be necessary if the diagnosis remains in question.

Prevention

The 2017 AHA guidelines include revised criteria for patients requiring prophylaxis for IE (Table 20–16). Only the high-risk

Table 20–16. Conditions requiring antibiotic prophylaxis for the prevention of infective endocarditis (IE).

Prosthetic cardiac valves
Prior episode of IE
Congenital heart disease (CHD)
Palliated cyanotic CHD
For 6 months post procedure if CHD repair involves implanted
prosthetic material
Repair of CHD with residual defect bordered by prosthetic material
Cardiac transplant with valvulopathy

patients listed require antibiotic prophylaxis before dental work (tooth extraction or cleaning) and procedures involving the respiratory tract or infected skin or musculoskeletal structures. IE prophylaxis is not recommended for gastrointestinal or genitourinary procedures, body piercing, or tattooing.

Recommended prophylaxis is 50 mg/kg of oral amoxicillin for patients less than 40 kg and 2000 mg for those more than 40 kg. This dose is to be given 1 hour prior to procedure. If the patient is allergic to amoxicillin, alternative prophylactic antibiotic recommendations are included in the guidelines.

Treatment

In general, appropriate antibiotic therapy should be initiated as soon as IE is suspected after several large volume blood cultures have been obtained via separate venipunctures. Therapy can be tailored once the pathogen and its susceptibilities are defined. Vancomycin or a β-lactam antibiotic, with or without gentamicin, for a 6-week course is the most common regimen. If HF occurs and progresses in the face of adequate antibiotic therapy, surgical excision of the infected area and prosthetic valve replacement must be considered.

Course & Prognosis

Factors associated with a poor outcome are delayed diagnosis, presence of prosthetic material, IE associated with cardiac surgery, and infection with *S aureus*. Mortality for bacterial IE in children ranges from 10% to 25%, with fungal IE having a mortality exceeding 50%.

Baltimore RS et al: Infective endocarditis in childhood: 2015 update: a scientific statement from the American Heart Association. Circulation 2015 Oct 13;132(15):1487–1515. doi: 10.1161/CIR.0000000000000298 [PMID: 26373317].

Dixon G et al: Infective endocarditis in children: an update. Curr Opin Infect Dis 2017 Jun;30(3):257–267 [PMID: 28319472].

Otto CM et al: 2020 ACC/AHA guideline for the management of patients with valvular heart disease. A report of the American college of cardiology/American Heart Association Joint Committee on Clinical Practice Guidelines. Circulation 2021; 145(5):e35 [PMID: 33332149].

PERICARDITIS

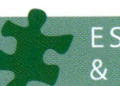

ESSENTIALS OF DIAGNOSIS & TYPICAL FEATURES

- ▶ Chest pain made worse by deep inspiration and decreased by leaning forward.
- ▶ Fever and tachycardia.
- ▶ Shortness of breath.
- ▶ Pericardial friction rub.
- ▶ ECG with elevated ST segments.

General Considerations

Pericarditis is an inflammation of the pericardium. The most common cause of pericarditis in children is a viral infection (eg, coxsackievirus, mumps, Epstein-Barr, adenovirus, influenza, and human immunodeficiency virus [HIV]). Purulent pericarditis results from bacterial infection (eg, pneumococci, streptococci, staphylococci, and *Haemophilus influenzae*) and is less common but potentially life threatening. In some cases, pericardial disease occurs in association with a generalized process such as rheumatic fever, rheumatoid arthritis, uremia, systemic lupus erythematosus, malignancy, or tuberculosis. Pericarditis after cardiac surgery (postpericardiotomy syndrome) is most commonly seen after surgical closure of an ASD. Postpericardiotomy syndrome appears to be autoimmune in nature, with high titers of anti-heart antibody and evidence of acute or reactivated viral illness. The syndrome is often self-limited and responds well to short courses of NSAIDs or corticosteroids.

Clinical Findings

A. Symptoms and Signs

Childhood pericarditis usually presents with sharp, stabbing mid-chest, shoulder, and neck pain made worse by deep inspiration or coughing, but decreased by sitting up and leaning forward. Shortness of breath is common. Physical findings depend on the presence of fluid accumulation in the pericardial space (effusion). In the absence of significant effusion, a characteristic scratchy, high-pitched friction rub may be heard on auscultation. If the effusion is large, heart sounds are distant and muffled and a friction rub may not be present. In the absence of cardiac tamponade, peripheral venous and arterial pulses are normal.

Cardiac tamponade occurs in association with a large effusion or one that has rapidly accumulated. Tamponade is characterized by jugular venous distention, tachycardia, hepatomegaly, peripheral edema, and pulsus paradoxus (characterized by a drop in systolic blood pressure > 10 mm Hg during inspiration). Decreased cardiac filling and subsequent decrease in cardiac output result in the potential for cardiovascular collapse.

B. Imaging

In pericarditis with a significant pericardial effusion, the cardiac silhouette is enlarged. The cardiac silhouette can appear normal if the effusion is small.

C. Electrocardiography

ST segments are commonly elevated in acute pericarditis and PR segment depression may be present. Low voltages or electrical alternans (alteration in QRS amplitude between beats) can be seen with large pericardial effusions.

D. Echocardiography

Serial echocardiography allows a direct, noninvasive estimate of the volume of pericardial fluid and its change over time. Cardiac tamponade is associated with compression of the atria or respiratory alteration of ventricular inflow demonstrated by Doppler imaging.

Diagnosis and Treatment

Diagnostic pericardiocentesis should be considered if the underlying cause is unclear or identification of the pathogen is necessary for targeted therapy. Treatment depends on the cause of pericarditis and the size of the associated effusion. Viral pericarditis is usually self-limited, and symptoms can improve with NSAIDs. Purulent pericarditis requires immediate evacuation of the fluid and appropriate antimicrobial therapy. Cardiac tamponade from any cause must be treated by immediate removal of the fluid, usually via pericardiocentesis. Diuretics should be avoided in the patient with cardiac tamponade because they reduce ventricular preload and can exacerbate the degree of cardiac decompensation.

Prognosis

Prognosis depends to a great extent on the cause of pericardial disease. Constrictive pericarditis can develop following infectious pericarditis (especially if bacterial or tuberculous) and can be difficult to manage.

Adler Y et al: 2015 ESC guidelines for the diagnosis and management of pericardial diseases: the Task Force for the Diagnosis and Management of Pericardial Diseases of the European Society of Cardiology (ESC) endorsed by: The European Association for Cardio-Thoracic Surgery (EACTS). Eur Heart J 2015 Nov 7;36(42):2921–2964. doi: 10.1093/eurheartj/ehv318 [PMID: 26320112].

Avula S et al: Management of acute pericarditis. Curr Opin Cardiol 2023;38(4):364–368 [PMID: 37115909].

CARDIOMYOPATHY

ESSENTIALS OF DIAGNOSIS & TYPICAL FEATURES

- ▶ Failure to thrive, poor appetite, abdominal pain, and/or vomiting.
- ▶ Exercise intolerance, diaphoresis, tachycardia.
- ▶ Tachypnea, cough, orthopnea, and/or shortness of breath.
- ▶ Hepatomegaly, edema, and rales.
- ▶ Fainting or aborted sudden death event.
- ▶ Diagnosis based on echocardiographic findings.

There are five classified forms of cardiomyopathy in children: (1) dilated, (2) hypertrophic, (3) restrictive, (4) arrhythmogenic right ventricular dysplasia (ARVD), and (5) LV noncompaction. Discussion will be limited to the first three, most common forms.

1. Dilated Cardiomyopathy

Dilated cardiomyopathy (DCM) is the most frequent form of childhood cardiomyopathy and occurs with an annual incidence of 4–8 cases per 100,000 population in the United States and Europe. Although usually idiopathic, identifiable causes of DCM include viral myocarditis, untreated tachyarrhythmias, left heart obstructive lesions, congenital abnormalities of the coronary arteries, medication toxicity (eg, anthracycline), and genetic (eg, dystrophin gene defects, sarcomeric mutations) and metabolic diseases (inborn errors of fatty acid oxidation and mitochondrial oxidative phosphorylation defects). Genetic causes are being discovered at an increasing rate, and commercial testing is now available for some of the more common associated gene defects.

▶ Clinical Findings

A. Signs and Symptoms

As myocardial function fails and the heart dilates, cardiac output falls and affected children develop decreased exercise tolerance, failure to thrive, diaphoresis, and tachypnea. As the heart continues to deteriorate, congestive signs such as hepatomegaly and rales develop, and a prominent gallop can be appreciated on examination. The initial diagnosis in a previously healthy child can be difficult, as presenting symptoms can resemble a viral respiratory infection, pneumonia, or asthma.

B. Imaging

Chest radiography shows generalized cardiomegaly with or without pulmonary edema.

C. Electrocardiography

Sinus tachycardia with ST-segment changes is commonly seen on ECG. Criteria for RVH and LVH may also be met, and the QT interval may be prolonged. Evaluation for the presence of supraventricular arrhythmias is critical, as this is one of the few treatable and reversible causes of DCM in children.

D. Echocardiography

The echocardiogram shows LV and LA enlargement with decreased LV-shortening fraction and ejection fraction. The calculated end-diastolic and end-systolic dimensions are increased, and MR is commonly seen. A careful evaluation for evidence of structural abnormalities (especially coronary artery anomalies or left heart obstructive lesions) must be performed.

E. Other Testing

Cardiac catheterization is useful to evaluate hemodynamic status and coronary artery anatomy. Endomyocardial biopsies can aid in diagnosis. Biopsy specimens may show inflammation consistent with acute myocarditis, abnormal myocyte architecture, and/or myocardial fibrosis. Electron microscopy may reveal evidence of mitochondrial or other metabolic disorders. Polymerase chain reaction (PCR) testing may be performed on biopsied specimens to detect viral genome products indicative of infectious myocarditis. CPET is useful for measuring response to medical therapy and as an objective assessment of the cardiac limitations on exercise.

▶ Treatment & Prognosis

Outpatient management of pediatric DCM usually entails combinations of afterload-reducing agents and diuretics (see section Heart Failure). Antithrombotic may be necessary to prevent thrombus formation in the dilated and poorly contractile cardiac chambers. Arrhythmias are more common in dilated hearts and antiarrhythmic therapy is sometimes necessary. Therapy of the underlying cause of cardiomyopathy is always indicated if possible. Unfortunately, despite complete evaluation, greater than 70% of DCM remains idiopathic. If medical management is unsuccessful, cardiac transplantation is considered.

2. Hypertrophic Cardiomyopathy

The most common cause of hypertrophic cardiomyopathy (HCM) is familial HCM, which is found in 1 in 500 individuals. HCM is the leading cause of sudden cardiac death (SCD) in young persons. It most commonly presents in an older child, adolescent, or adult, although it may occur in neonates. Causes of nonfamilial HCM in neonates and young children include glycogen storage disease, Noonan syndrome (including related syndromes such as LEOPARD and Costello syndrome), Friedreich ataxia, maternal gestational diabetes, mitochondrial disorders, and other metabolic disorders.

A. Familial Hypertrophic Cardiomyopathy

Familial HCM is most commonly caused by a mutation in one of the genes that encode proteins of the cardiac sarcomere (β-myosin heavy chain, cardiac troponin T or I, α-tropomyosin, and myosin-binding protein C).

1. Clinical findings—Patients may be asymptomatic despite having significant hypertrophy or may present with symptoms of inadequate coronary perfusion or HF such as angina, syncope, palpitations, or exercise intolerance. Patients may experience SCD as their initial presentation, often precipitated by sporting activities. Although the cardiac examination may be normal on presentation, some patients develop a left precordial bulge with a diffuse point of maximal impulse. An LV heave or an S_4 gallop may be present. If outflow tract obstruction exists, a systolic ejection murmur will be audible. A murmur may not be audible at rest but may be provoked with exercise or positional maneuvers that decrease LV volume (standing), thereby increasing the outflow tract obstruction.

A. Echocardiography—The diagnosis of HCM is usually made by echocardiography, and in most familial cases demonstrates asymmetrical septal hypertrophy, in contrast to concentric hypertrophy that is more commonly seen in young patients with metabolic or other nonfamilial causes. Systolic anterior motion of the mitral valve leaflet may occur and contribute to LV outflow tract obstruction. The mitral valve leaflet may become distorted and result in MR. LV outflow tract obstruction may be present at rest or provoked with monitored exercise. Systolic function is most often hypercontractile in young children but may deteriorate over time, resulting in poor contractility and LV dilatation. Diastolic function is almost always abnormal.

B. Electrocardiography—The ECG may be normal but more typically demonstrates deep Q waves in the inferolateral leads (II, III, aVF, V_5, and V_6) secondary to the increased mass of the hypertrophied septum. ST-segment abnormalities may be seen in the same leads. Age-dependent criteria for LVH and LA enlargement are often met.

C. Other testing—CPET is valuable to evaluate for provocable LV outflow tract obstruction, ischemia, and arrhythmias, and to determine prognosis. Extreme LVH and a blunted blood pressure response to exercise have both been associated with increased mortality in children. Cardiac MRI can be useful for defining areas of myocardial fibrosis or scarring. Patients are at risk for myocardial ischemia, possibly as a result of systolic compression of the intramyocardial coronary arteries along the interventricular septum, myocardial bridging of epicardial coronary arteries (coronaries running within the heart muscles), or an imbalance of coronary artery supply and demand due to the presence of massive myocardial hypertrophy.

D. Cardiac catheterization—Cardiac catheterization may be performed in patients with HCM who have angina, syncope, resuscitated sudden death, or a worrisome stress test. Hemodynamic findings include elevated LA pressure secondary to impaired diastolic filling. If midcavitary LV outflow tract obstruction is present, an associated pressure gradient will be evident. Angiography demonstrates midcavitary LV obliteration during systole. Although uncommonly done currently, myocardial biopsy demonstrates myofiber disarray.

2. Treatment and prognosis—Treatment varies depending on symptoms and phenotype. Affected patients are restricted from competitive athletics and isometric exercise due to associated risk of SCD. Patients with resting or latent LV outflow tract obstruction may be treated with β-blockers, verapamil, or disopyramide with variable success in alleviating obstruction. Patients with severe symptoms despite medical therapy and an

LV outflow tract gradient may require additional intervention. Surgical myectomy with resection of part of the hypertrophied septum has been used in symptomatic patients with good results. At the time of myectomy, the mitral valve may require repair or replacement in patients with a long history of systolic anterior motion of the mitral valve. Ethanol ablation of the myocardium, in which a coronary septal artery branch is selectively infiltrated with ethanol to induce a small targeted myocardial infarction, reduce septal size, and improve obstruction, is used in adults with HCM and LV outflow tract obstruction. The long-term effects of this procedure are unknown, and it is not commonly employed in children.

Risk stratification with respect to SCD is important in HCM. Consideration for placement of internal defibrillators in adult patients are based on the known risk factors for SCD: severe hypertrophy (> 3 cm septal thickness in adults), documented ventricular arrhythmias, syncope, abnormal blood pressure response to exercise, resuscitated sudden death, or a strong family history of HCM with associated sudden death. The criteria for defibrillator placement in children are not as well defined.

B. Glycogen Storage Disease of the Heart

There are at least 10 types of glycogen storage disease. The type that primarily involves the heart is Pompe disease (GSD IIa) in which acid maltase, necessary for hydrolysis of the outer branches of glycogen, is absent. There is marked deposition of glycogen within the myocardium. Affected infants are well at birth, but symptoms of growth and developmental delay, feeding problems, and cardiac failure occur by the sixth month of life. Physical examination reveals generalized muscular weakness, a large tongue, and cardiomegaly without significant heart murmurs. Chest radiography reveals cardiomegaly with or without pulmonary edema. The ECG shows a short PR interval and LVH with ST depression and T-wave inversion over the left precordial leads. Echocardiography shows severe concentric LVH. Although historically children with Pompe disease usually died before age 1 year, recent enzyme replacement clinical trials have shown some promise in reversing hypertrophy and preserving cardiac function. Death may be sudden or result from progressive HF.

3. Restrictive Cardiomyopathy

Restrictive cardiomyopathy is a rare entity in the pediatric population, accounting for less than 5% of all cases of cardiomyopathy. It is usually idiopathic but can be familial or secondary to an infiltrative process (eg, amyloidosis).

▶ Clinical Findings

Patients present with signs of congestive HF due to restriction to ventricular relaxation and associated diastolic dysfunction (with preserved systolic function). The LV is more severely affected than the RV, but the RV is also affected in most cases, resulting in signs and symptoms consistent with biventricular congestion. Patients often present with exercise intolerance, fatigue, chest pain, and orthopnea. Physical examination is remarkable for a prominent S_4 and jugular venous distention.

A. Electrocardiography

ECG demonstrates marked right and left atrial enlargement with normal ventricular voltages. ST-T–wave abnormalities including a prolonged QTc interval may be present.

B. Echocardiography

The diagnosis is confirmed by echocardiography demonstrating normally sized ventricles, normal systolic function, and massively dilated atria. Cardiac MRI is useful in ruling out pericardial abnormalities (restrictive or constrictive pericarditis) and infiltrative disorders.

Treatment & Prognosis

Anticongestive therapy is used for symptomatic relief. The risk of SCD and propensity for rapid progression of irreversible PH warrant close follow-up with early consideration of cardiac transplantation.

Bozkurt B et al: Current diagnostic and treatment strategies for specific dilated cardiomyopathies: a scientific statement from the American Heart Association. 2016;134(23):e579–e646 [PMID: 27832612].

Chen LR et al: Reversal of cardiac dysfunction after enzyme replacement in patients with infantile-onset Pompe disease. J Pediatr 2009 Aug;155(2):271–275, e272 [PMID: 19486996].

Moak JP et al: Long-term follow-up of children and adolescents diagnosed with hypertrophic cardiomyopathy: risk factors for adverse arrhythmic events. Pediatr Cardiol 2011;32(8):1096–1105 [PMID: 21487794].

MYOCARDITIS

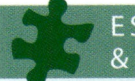

ESSENTIALS OF DIAGNOSIS & TYPICAL FEATURES

► Often occurs in association with a viral infection.

► Signs and symptoms of cardiomyopathy.

► Echocardiogram demonstrates a poorly functioning ventricle with varying degrees of ventricular dilatation.

► May see diffusely low voltages on ECG.

► Elevated inflammatory markers may be present (eg, ESR, CRP).

► Cardiac MRI is an evolving diagnostic tool.

► Endomyocardial biopsy may demonstrate lymphocytic infiltrate and viral PCR positivity.

The most common viral causes of myocarditis are adenoviruses, coxsackie viruses, echoviruses, parvovirus, cytomegalovirus, influenza A virus, and, more recently, severe acute respiratory syndrome coronavirus 2 (SARS-CoV-2). HIV can also cause myocarditis. The ability to identify the causative pathogen has been enhanced by PCR technology, which amplifies identifiable segments of the viral genome from the myocardium of affected children.

Clinical Findings

A. Symptoms and Signs

There are two major clinical patterns. In the first, sudden-onset HF occurs in an infant or child who was previously healthy. This malignant form of the disease is usually secondary to overwhelming viremia with tissue invasion in multiple organ systems, including the heart. The second pattern is characterized by gradual onset of cardiac symptoms, and there may be a history of upper respiratory tract infection or gastroenteritis in the previous month. This more insidious form may have a late postinfectious or autoimmune component. Acute/malignant and gradual/insidious presentations occur at any age.

Signs of HF are variable, but in a decompensated patient with fulminant myocarditis, they include signs of poor systemic perfusion; rapid, weak, and thready pulses; and breathlessness. In those with a more subacute presentation, signs include increased work of breathing, orthopnea, difficulty with feeding in infants, exercise intolerance, and edema of the face and extremities. The patient is usually tachycardic and heart sounds may be muffled and distant; an S_3 or S_4 gallop (or both) are common. Murmurs are usually absent, although a murmur of tricuspid or mitral regurgitation may be heard. Moist rales are usually present at the lung bases. The liver is enlarged and frequently tender.

B. Imaging

Cardiomegaly and pulmonary edema are seen on radiography.

C. Electrocardiography

ECG findings are variable. Classically, there is diffusely low-voltage QRS in all leads with ST-segment depression and inversion of T waves in leads I, III, and aVF. Dysrhythmias, ectopy, and conduction disturbances are common.

D. Echocardiography

Echocardiography demonstrates four-chamber dilatation with poor ventricular function with AV valve regurgitation. A pericardial effusion may be present. Patients with a more acute presentation may have less ventricular dilatation than those with a longer history of HF-related symptoms.

E. Myocardial Biopsy

An endomyocardial biopsy may be helpful in the diagnosis of viral myocarditis. An inflammatory infiltrate with myocyte damage can be seen with hematoxylin and eosin staining. Viral PCR testing of the biopsy specimen may yield a positive result in 30%–40% of patients suspected to have myocarditis.

F. Cardiac MRI

Cardiac MRI is increasing in use as a potential diagnostic modality for myocarditis. Abnormalities suggestive of myocardial edema or inflammation and global relative enhancement (evidence of capillary leak) are evident in acute myocarditis. This imaging method requires general anesthesia in infants and young children, which is associated with significant risk in those with HF and must be a consideration when ordering this test.

▶ Treatment

The inpatient cardiac support measures outlined previously (section Heart Failure) are used in the treatment of these patients. The use of digitalis in a rapidly deteriorating child with myocarditis is dangerous and should be undertaken with great caution, as it may cause ventricular dysrhythmias. Administration of immunomodulating medications such as corticosteroids is controversial. Subsequent to the successful use of IVIG in children with KD, there have been several trials of IVIG in presumed viral myocarditis; however, the therapeutic value of IVIG remains unconfirmed. Initiation of mechanical circulatory support in those with fulminant or severe myocarditis is a therapeutic option as a bridge to transplantation or recovery.

▶ Prognosis

The prognosis is determined by the age at onset, severity of presentation, and the response to therapy. Children presenting with fulminant myocarditis and severe hemodynamic compromise have a 75% early mortality. Those at highest risk for a poor outcome are those presenting in the first year of life. Complete recovery is possible, although some patients who recover clinically have persistent LV dysfunction and require ongoing medical therapy for HF. Children with myocarditis whose ventricular function fails to return to normal may be candidates for cardiac transplantation if they remain symptomatic or suffer growth failure despite maximal medical management. It is possible that subclinical myocarditis in childhood is the pathophysiologic basis for some of the "idiopathic" DCMs that present later in life.

Kawakami R et al: Pathological evidence for SARS-CoV-2 as a cause of myocarditis: JACC review topic of the week. J Am Coll Cardiol 2021 Jan 26;77(3):314–325 [PMID: 33478655].

Law YM et al: Diagnosis and management of myocarditis in children: a scientific statement from the American Heart Association. Circulation 2021;144(6):e123–e135 [PMID: 34229446].

PULMONARY HYPERTENSION

ESSENTIALS OF DIAGNOSIS & TYPICAL FEATURES

► Often subtle, with symptoms of dyspnea, fatigue, chest pain, and syncope.

► Loud pulmonary component of S_2; ECG with RVH.

► Rare, progressive, and often fatal disease without treatment.

▶ General Considerations

Five categories of disorders, with each group sharing similar hemodynamic, pathologic, and management features, are recognized to cause PH: pulmonary arterial hypertension (PAH; group 1); PH due to left heart disease (group 2); PH due to chronic lung disease and/or hypoxia (group 3); chronic thromboembolic PH (group 4); and PH due to multifactorial mechanisms (group 5). PAH (group 1) is a disorder of the pulmonary arterial tree and is defined as a sustained mean PAP 20 mm Hg or greater with a mean pulmonary capillary wedge pressure 15 mm Hg or less and PVR more than 3 indexed Wood units. The etiology of PH in children is very different from adults, with a predominance of idiopathic or CHD-associated PAH (both included in group 1). The incidence of idiopathic and CHD-associated PAH is 1–2 persons per million. Although the outcome for pediatric PH is improving due to the advent of new therapies, prognosis remains guarded, with only 74% survival at 5 years. Familial PH occurs in 6%–12% of affected individuals. When a clear familial association is known, the disease shows evidence of genetic anticipation, presenting at younger ages in subsequent generations.

▶ Clinical Findings

A. Symptoms and Signs

The clinical picture varies with the severity of PH, and usually early symptoms are subtle, delaying the diagnosis. Initial symptoms may be dyspnea, palpitations, or chest pain, often brought on by strenuous exercise. Syncope may be the first symptom, which generally implies severe disease. As the disease progresses, patients have signs of low cardiac output and right HF. Right HF may be manifested by hepatomegaly, peripheral edema, and an S_3 gallop on examination.

Murmurs of pulmonary and TR may be present, and the pulmonary component of S_2 is usually pronounced.

B. Imaging

The chest radiograph most often reveals a prominent main PA and RV enlargement.

C. Electrocardiography

ECG usually shows RVH with an upright T wave in V_1 (when it should be negative in young children). Evidence of right axis deviation and RA enlargement may also be present.

D. Echocardiography

The echocardiogram is an essential tool for diagnosing PH and excluding CHD as a cause. It frequently shows RV hypertrophy and dilatation. In the absence of other structural disease, tricuspid and PI velocity can be used to estimate PA pressures. Other, more nuanced, echocardiographic measures can be used in the evaluation of PH.

E. Cardiac Catheterization and Angiocardiography

Cardiac catheterization is the best method for determining the severity of disease. The procedure is performed to rule out cardiac (eg, restrictive cardiomyopathy) or vascular (eg, pulmonary vein stenosis) causes of PH, determine the severity of disease, and define treatment strategies. The reactivity of the pulmonary vascular bed to short-acting vasodilator agents (oxygen, inhaled nitric oxide, or prostacyclin) can be assessed and used to determine treatment options. Angiography may show a decrease in the number of small PAs with tortuous vessels.

F. Other Evaluation Modalities

Cardiac MRI can be used to evaluate RV function, PA architecture, and hemodynamics, as well as thromboembolic phenomena. CPET can assess disease severity. More simply, a 6-minute walk test, in which distance walked and perceived level of exertion are measured, has a strong independent association with mortality in late disease.

▶ Treatment

The goal of therapy is to reduce PAP, increase cardiac output, and improve quality of life. Patients responsive to pulmonary vasodilator therapy at catheterization are given calcium channel blockers, such as nifedipine or diltiazem. Patients unresponsive to vasodilators initially receive one of three classes of drugs: prostanoids (such as epoprostenol), endothelin receptor antagonists (such as bosentan), or phosphodiesterase-5 inhibitors (such as tadalafil). These agents have distinct mechanisms of action that can reduce PAP.

Antithrombotic therapy is commonly used to prevent thromboembolic events.

Humbert M: 2022 ESC/ERS guidelines for the diagnosis and treatment of pulmonary hypertension: developed by the task force for the diagnosis and treatment of pulmonary hypertension of the European Society of Cardiology (ESC) and the European Respiratory Society (ERS). Eur Heart J 2022;43(38):3618–3731 [PMID: 36821743].

Ivy DD et al: Pediatric pulmonary hypertension. J Am Coll Cardiol 2013 Dec 24;62(25 Suppl):D11726 [PMID: 24355636].

Pulmonary Hypertension Association: www.phassociation.org/.

▼ DISORDERS OF RATE & RHYTHM

Cardiac rhythm abnormalities can occur in two different patient populations: (1) healthy children with structurally normal hearts who have an intrinsic abnormality of the electrical conduction system and (2) at risk children with CHD. In the latter population, changes in cardiac muscle cells associated with a chronic state of altered cardiac hemodynamics and any operative procedures with surgical suture lines/scars place the patients at higher risk for arrhythmias.

The evaluation and treatment of cardiac rhythm disorders have advanced significantly over the last several decades. Arguably, the most significant advancements in the last few years have continued in the area of the genetic basis of rhythm disorders such as long QT syndrome (LQTS). Treatment for cardiac rhythm abnormalities includes clinical monitoring with no intervention, antiarrhythmic medications, invasive electrophysiology study and ablation procedures, pacemakers, and automated implanted cardioverter/defibrillators.

Deal BJ et al: Arrhythmic complications associated with the treatment of patients with congenital cardiac disease: consensus definitions from the Multi-Societal Database Committee for Pediatric and Congenital Heart Disease. Cardiol Young 2008 Dec;18(Suppl 2):202–205 [PMID: 19063792].

DISORDERS OF THE SINUS NODE

▶ Sinus Arrhythmia

Typically, the sinus rate varies with the respiratory cycle (heart rate increases with inspiration and decreases with exhalation), while P-QRS-T intervals remain unchanged. This phasic variation in heart rate is referred to as sinus arrhythmia and may occur with respiratory distress, but it is most often a normal finding in healthy children. In isolation, it never requires treatment; however, it may occur with sinus node or autonomic nervous system dysfunction.

▶ Sinus Bradycardia

Sinus bradycardia is defined based on heart rate values below the normal limit for age (neonates to 6 years, 60 beats/min;

7–11 years, 45 beats/min; > 12 years, 40 beats/min). Physiologic sinus bradycardia is often seen in athletic children. Causes of pathologic sinus bradycardia include hypoxia, central nervous system damage, eating disorders, and medication side effects. Symptomatic bradycardia (syncope, low cardiac output, or exercise intolerance) requires treatment (atropine, isoproterenol, or cardiac pacing).

▶ Sinus Tachycardia

The heart rate normally accelerates in response to stress such as exercise, anxiety, fever, hypovolemia, anemia, or HF. Although sinus tachycardia in the normal heart is well tolerated, symptomatic tachycardia with impaired cardiac output warrants evaluation for CHD, cardiomyopathy, or true tachyarrhythmias. The first evaluation should be with a 12-lead ECG. Treatment may be indicated to correct the underlying cause of sinus tachycardia.

▶ Sinus Node Dysfunction

Sinus node dysfunction is a clinical syndrome of inadequate sinus nodal function and rate. It is defined as one or more of the following: severe sinus bradycardia, sinus pause or arrest, chronotropic incompetence (inability of the heart rate to increase with activity or other demands), or combined bradyarrhythmias and tachyarrhythmias. The abnormality may be due to a true anatomic defect of the sinus node or its surrounding tissue or it may reflect an abnormality of autonomic input. It is a common late finding after repair of CHD, but it is also seen in normal hearts, in unoperated CHD, and in acquired heart diseases. Symptoms usually manifest between 2 and 17 years of age and consist of episodes of presyncope, syncope, palpitations, pallor, or exercise intolerance.

Evaluation of sinus node dysfunction may involve the following a baseline ECG, ambulatory ECG monitoring, and/or an exercise stress test. Treatment for sinus node dysfunction with a permanently implanted pacemaker is indicated only in symptomatic patients.

PREMATURE BEATS

Atrial Premature Beats

Atrial premature beats or premature atrial contractions (PACs) are triggered by an ectopic focus in the atrium. They are one of the most common types of premature beats and occur frequently during the fetal and newborn periods. The premature beat may be conducted to the ventricle and therefore followed by a QRS complex, or it may be nonconducted, as the beat has occurred so early that the AV node is still refractory (Figure 20–6). A brief pause usually occurs until the next normal sinus beat occurs. As an isolated finding, atrial premature beats are benign and require no treatment.

Junctional Premature Beats

Junctional premature beats arise in the AV node or the bundle of His. They induce a normal QRS complex with no preceding P wave. Junctional premature beats are usually benign and require no specific therapy.

Ventricular Premature Beats

Ventricular premature beats or premature ventricular contractions (PVCs) are relatively common, occurring in 1%–2% of patients with normal hearts. They are characterized by an early beat with a wide QRS complex, without a preceding P wave, and with a full compensatory pause following this early beat. PVCs originating from a single ectopic focus all have the same configuration, while those of multifocal origin show varying configurations. The consecutive occurrence of two PVCs is referred to as a ventricular couplet and of three or more as ventricular tachycardia. Most PVCs in otherwise normal patients are usually benign. However, frequent PVCs may result in decreased ventricular function, a phenomenon known as PVC-induced cardiomyopathy. The exact frequency of PVCs necessary to cause a cardiomyopathy is incompletely understood but is most commonly greater than 20% of the total daily beats.

Patients with frequent PVCs are usually evaluated with tests such as a 24-hour ambulatory ECG or with exercise testing to rule out concerning arrhythmias. An echocardiogram may be performed to evaluate ventricular function. The significance of PVCs can also be evaluated by having the patient exercise. As the heart rate increases, benign PVCs usually disappear. If exercise results in an increase or coupling of contractions, underlying disease may be present. Multifocal PVCs are always abnormal and may be more dangerous. They may be associated with drug overdose (tricyclic antidepressants or digoxin toxicity), electrolyte imbalance, myocarditis, or hypoxia. Treatment is directed at correcting the underlying disorder.

SUPRAVENTRICULAR TACHYCARDIA

Supraventricular tachycardia (SVT) is a term used to describe any rapid rhythm originating from the atrium, the AV node, or an accessory pathway. These tachycardias are rapid and narrow complex. They may occur in an otherwise healthy child or may be associated with either congenital or acquired heart disease (cardiomyopathies and myocarditis). The mode of presentation depends on the rate, the presence of underlying cardiac structural or functional abnormalities, coexisting illness, and patient age. An otherwise healthy child with SVT may complain of intermittent periods of rapid heartbeat. An infant with SVT may have poor feeding and increased fatigue (manifesting as less awake time). Incessant tachycardia, even if fairly slow (120–150 beats/min), may cause myocardial dysfunction and HF if left untreated. In children with preexisting

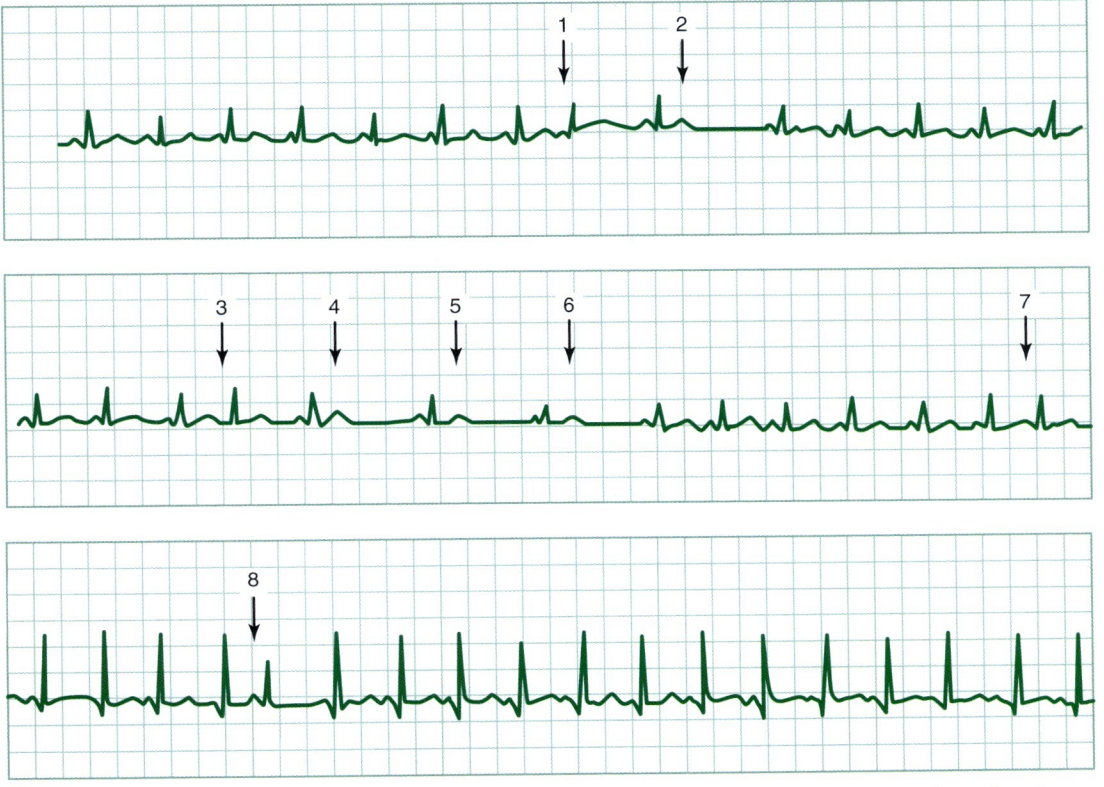

▲ **Figure 20–6.** Lead II rhythm strip with premature atrial contractions. Beats 1, 3, 7, and 8 are conducted to the ventricles, whereas beats 2, 4, 5, and 6 are not.

HF or an underlying systemic disease such as anemia or sepsis, SVT may result in decreased heart function and further signs of hemodynamic instability much more rapidly than in a healthy child.

The mechanisms of tachycardia are generally divided into reentrant and automatic mechanisms and can be described by the location of tachycardia origination (Table 20–17).

Reentrant tachycardias represent approximately 80% of pediatric arrhythmias. They have the following characteristics: they initiate abruptly, they have a fixed rate, they have little variation with fever or internal catecholamines, and they terminate abruptly. They can be terminated with return to sinus rhythm with maneuvers such as vagal maneuvers, administration of adenosine, pacing maneuvers, or direct current (DC) cardioversion. Reentrant tachycardia mechanisms involve electrical conduction traveling down one pathway and then back up another, creating a sustained repetitive circular loop. The circuit can be confined to the atrium (*atrial flutter* in a normal heart or *intra-atrial reentrant tachycardia* in a patient with CHD) (Figure 20–7). It may be confined within the AV node (*AV nodal reentrant tachycardia*),

or it may encompass an accessory connection between atria and ventricle (*accessory pathway–mediated tachycardia*). If, during tachycardia, the electrical impulse travels antegrade (from atria to ventricles) through the AV node and retrograde (from ventricle to atria) back up the accessory pathway, orthodromic reciprocating tachycardia is present. If, instead, the impulse travels antegrade through the accessory pathway and retrograde up through the AV node, antidromic reciprocating tachycardia is present. This latter tachycardia would present as a wide complex tachycardia.

WPW syndrome is a subclass of reentrant tachycardia in which, during sinus rhythm, the impulse travels antegrade down the accessory connection, bypassing the AV node and creating ventricular preexcitation (early eccentric activation of the ventricle with a short PR interval and slurred upstroke of the QRS, a delta wave) (Figure 20–8). Most patients with WPW have otherwise structurally normal hearts. However, WPW has been noted to occur with increased frequency in association with tricuspid atresia, Ebstein anomaly of the tricuspid valve, HCM, and ccTGA. Different from other causes of tachycardia described above in which the arrhythmia is

Table 20–17. Mechanisms of supraventricular tachycardia.

Site of Origination	Automatic Mechanisms	Reentrant Mechanisms
Sinus node	Sinus tachycardia	Sinoatrial node reentry
Atrium	Ectopic atrial tachycardia Multifocal atrial tachycardia	Atrial flutter Intra-atrial reentrant tachycardia Atrial fibrillation
Atrioventricular node	Junctional ectopic tachycardia	Atrioventricular nodal reentrant tachycardia (AVNRT)
Accessory pathways		Concealed accessory pathways Wolff-Parkinson-White (WPW) syndrome Permanent form of junctional reciprocating tachycardia (PJRT) Mahaim fiber tachycardia

postoperative atrial flutter. In this tachycardia, electrically isolated corridors of atrial myocardium act as pathways for sustained reentrant circuits of electrical activity. These tachycardias are chronic, medically refractory, and clinically incapacitating.

The *automatic tachycardias* represent approximately 20% of childhood arrhythmias. The characteristics of automatic arrhythmias include gradual onset, rate variability, variations in rate with fever or increasing internal catecholamines, and gradual offset. Maneuvers such as vagal maneuvers, adenosine, and attempt pacing can alter the rhythm temporarily, but they do not result in termination of the rhythm and return to sinus rhythm as would be seen in reentrant tachycardias. Automatic tachycardias are usually under autonomic influence and can be episodic or incessant. When they are incessant, they are usually associated with HF and a clinical picture of DCM. Automatic tachycardias are created when a focus of cardiac tissue develops an abnormally fast spontaneous rate of depolarization. For ectopic atrial tachycardia, the ECG demonstrates a normal QRS complex preceded by an abnormal P wave (Figure 20–9). Junctional ectopic tachycardia does not have a P wave preceding the QRS waves and may be associated with AV dissociation or 1:1 retrograde conduction.

Cohen MI et al: PACES/HRS expert consensus statement on the management of the asymptomatic young patient with a Wolff-Parkinson-White (WPW, ventricular preexcitation) electrocardiographic pattern: developed in partnership between the Pediatric and Congenital Electrophysiology Society (PACES) and the Heart Rhythm Society (HRS). Heart Rhythm 2012; 9(6):1006–1024 [PMID: 22579340].

▶ Clinical Findings

A. Symptoms and Signs

The presentation of SVT varies with age. Infants tend to have signs of poor perfusion with onset of tachycardia and may

not life threatening, there have been rare cases of sudden collapse from WPW syndrome. The mechanism of this sudden event is the development of atrial fibrillation, conducting down a rapid accessory pathway to the ventricle leading to ventricular fibrillation and sudden death. For this reason, most centers recommend that even asymptomatic patients with WPW undergo an invasive procedure to assess the conduction properties of the WPW accessory pathway.

Improved surgical survival for patients with CHD has created a new, increasingly prevalent, chronic reentrant arrhythmia that is similar to atrial flutter in a normal heart. These arrhythmias have been referred to as intra-atrial reentrant tachycardia, incisional tachycardia, macro-reentry, or

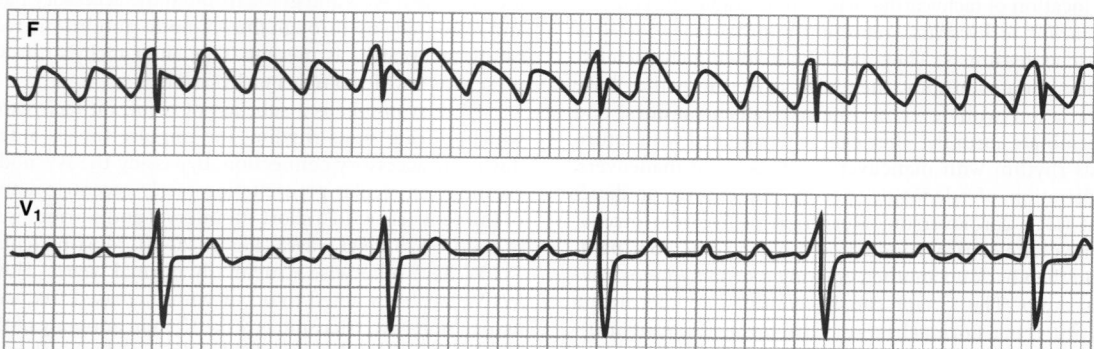

▲ **Figure 20–7.** Leads aVF (F) and V$_1$ showing atrial flutter with "sawtooth" atrial flutter waves.

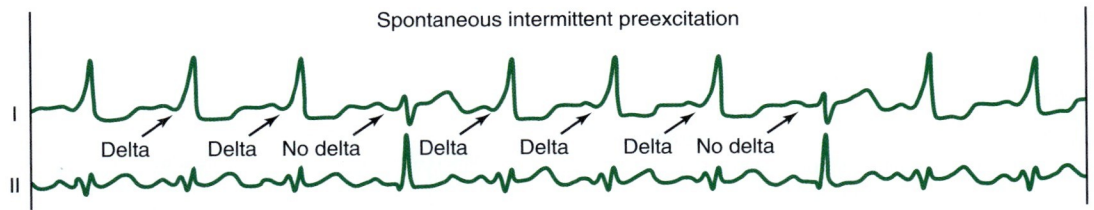

▲ Figure 20–8. Leads I and II with spontaneous intermittent ventricular preexcitation (Wolff-Parkinson-White syndrome).

become irritable. With long duration of tachycardia, symptoms of HF develop. Older children complain of dizziness, palpitations, fatigue, and chest pain; HF is less common than in infants. Heart rates range from 240–300 beats/min in infants to 150–180 beats/min in the teenager.

B. Imaging

Chest radiography is normal during the early course of tachycardia and therefore is usually not obtained. If HF is present, the heart is enlarged and pulmonary edema is evident.

C. Electrocardiography

ECG is the most important tool in the diagnosis of SVT and to define the precise tachycardia mechanism. Findings include a heart rate that is rapid and out of proportion to the patient's physical status. For reentrant mechanisms, the rhythm would be extremely regular with little variability. For automatic mechanisms, the rate would vary or rhythm may be irregular. The QRS complex is usually narrow and appears the same as during normal sinus rhythm. However, the QRS complex is occasionally widened (SVT with aberrant ventricular conduction), in which case the condition may be difficult to differentiate from ventricular tachycardia. The presence of P waves and their association with the QRS are important in determining tachycardia mechanism. With automatic tachycardias, there is often a 1:1 or 2:1 atrial:ventricular relationship with P waves preceding the QRS. With reentrant tachycardias, such as accessory pathway–mediated tachycardias, a small retrograde P wave can often be seen just after the QRS.

▶ Treatment

A. Acute Treatment

During initial episodes of SVT, patients require close monitoring. Acidosis and electrolyte abnormalities should be corrected. The following acute treatments are effective in terminating tachycardia only for patients with reentrant SVT. Acute treatment for automatic SVT is aimed at rate control, usually with a β-blocker.

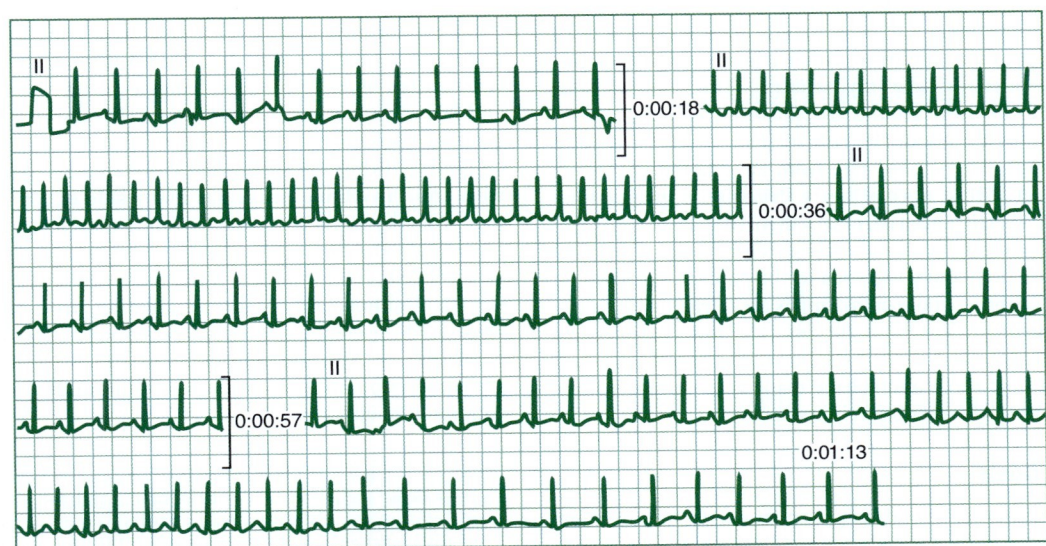

▲ Figure 20–9. Lead II rhythm strip of ectopic atrial tachycardia. The tracing demonstrates a variable rate with a maximum of 260 beats/min, an abnormal P wave, and a gradual termination.

1. Vagal maneuvers—Placing an ice bag on the nasal bridge (for infants) or a Valsalva maneuver (older children) will increase parasympathetic tone and terminate some reentrant tachycardias.

2. Adenosine—Adenosine (0.1–0.2 mg/kg by rapid intravenous bolus) transiently blocks AV conduction and terminates tachycardias that incorporate the AV node or may aid in the diagnosis of arrhythmias confined to the atrium by causing a pause in ventricular conduction and allowing identification of multiple P waves. Heart transplant recipients should not be administered adenosine due to an exaggerated response that results in prolonged block of AV conduction.

3. Direct current cardioversion—Synchronized DC cardioversion (0.5–2 J/kg) should be used immediately when a patient presents in cardiovascular collapse. This will convert a reentrant mechanism to sinus. Automatic tachycardia will not respond to cardioversion.

B. Chronic Treatment

Once the patient has been diagnosed with SVT and the mechanism has been evaluated, long-term treatment options can be considered. Options include monitoring clinically for tachycardia recurrences, medical management with antiarrhythmic medications, or an invasive electrophysiology study and ablation procedure. In infancy and early childhood, antiarrhythmic medications such as digoxin and β-blockers are the mainstay of therapy.

Tachycardias, both automatic and reentrant, can be more definitively addressed with an invasive electrophysiology study and ablation procedure. This is a nonsurgical transvascular catheter technique that desiccates an arrhythmia focus or accessory pathway and permanently cures an arrhythmia. Ablation catheters can utilize either a heat source (radiofrequency) or a cool source (cryoablation). The latter has been reported to be safer around the normal conduction pathway and thus decreases the risk of inadvertent damage to the AV node. The success rate from an ablation procedure in a patient with a normal heart structure is greater than 90%, with a recurrence risk of less than 10%. In patients less than 15 kg, the risks of procedural complications or failed ablation are potentially higher, and the procedure should be reserved for those whose arrhythmias are refractory to medical management. The high success rate, low complication and recurrence rates, and elimination of the need for chronic antiarrhythmic medications have made ablation procedures the primary treatment option in most cases.

▶ Prognosis

SVT in infants and children generally carries an excellent prognosis. It can be treated with medical management and, eventually, with potentially curative ablation procedures. There are, however, rare cases of incessant SVT leading to

HF, and SCD can occur from atrial fibrillation in the presence of WPW. Therefore, all patients with complaints of rapid heartbeats or other symptoms that raise concern for tachyarrhythmia should be referred for evaluation.

Friedman RA: NASPE Expert Consensus Conference: Radiofrequency catheter ablation in children with and without congenital heart disease. Report of the writing committee. North American Society of Pacing and Electrophysiology. Pacing Clin Electrophysiol 2002;25(6):1000–1017 [PMID: 12137336].

VENTRICULAR TACHYCARDIA

Ventricular tachycardia (three or more consecutive PVCs) is uncommon in childhood (Figure 20–10). It is usually associated with underlying abnormalities of the myocardium (myocarditis, cardiomyopathy, myocardial tumors, or postoperative CHD), hypoxia, electrolyte imbalance, or drug toxicity. On occasion, it can be secondary to a primary electrical abnormality in an otherwise normal heart. Sustained ventricular tachycardia can be an unstable situation, and if left untreated, can degenerate into ventricular fibrillation and SCD.

Ventricular tachycardia must be differentiated from accelerated idioventricular rhythm. The latter is a sustained tachycardia occurring in neonates with normal hearts, with a ventricular rate within 10% of the preceding sinus rate. This is a self-limiting arrhythmia that requires no treatment. Because of the consequences of sustained ventricular tachycardia, however, a symptomatic patient with a wide complex tachycardia should be considered to have ventricular tachycardia until proven otherwise.

Acute termination of ventricular tachycardia involves restoration of the normal myocardium when possible (correction of electrolyte imbalance, drug toxicity, etc) and DC cardioversion (1–4 J/kg), cardioversion with lidocaine (1 mg/kg), or administration of amiodarone (5 mg/kg load). Chronic suppression of ventricular arrhythmias with antiarrhythmic drugs has many side effects (including proarrhythmia and death), and, therefore, must be initiated in the hospital under the direction of a pediatric cardiologist. If the etiology of the tachycardia is a primary electrical abnormality, catheter ablation procedures can be offered in select patients as a potentially curative treatment option. Ablation for ventricular tachycardia in the pediatric population is much less commonly performed compared to ablation for SVT.

Al-Khatib SM et al: 2017 AHA/ACC/HRS guideline for management of patients with ventricular arrhythmias and the prevention of sudden cardiac death: a report of the American College of Cardiology/American Heart Association Task Force on Clinical Practice Guidelines and the Heart Rhythm Society. Circulation 2018;138(13):e272–e391 [PMID: 29084731].

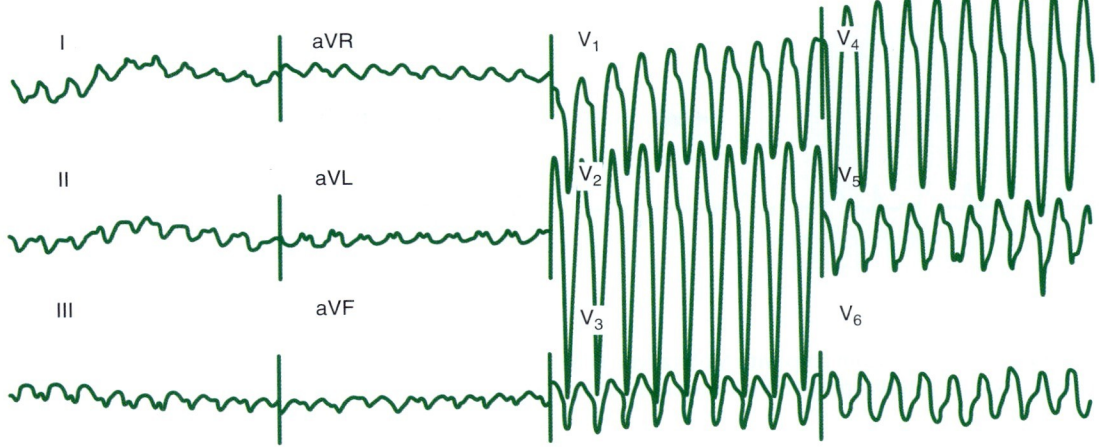

▲ **Figure 20–10.** Twelve-lead ECG from a child with imipramine toxicity and ventricular tachycardia.

LONG QT SYNDROME

Long QT syndrome (LQTS) is a malignant disorder of cardiac conduction in which cardiac repolarization is prolonged (QTc measurement on ECG). This predisposes the patient to sudden episodes of syncope, seizures, or SCD due to a pause-dependent initiation of torsade de pointes, a multifocal ventricular tachycardia. LQTS can be acquired or congenital. Acquired LQTS resulting from altered ventricular repolarization can occur secondary to myocardial toxins, ischemia, or inflammation and predisposes to ventricular arrhythmias. Numerous medications can also cause QT prolongation (see Table 20–7). Congenital LQTS is inherited in an autosomal dominant (more common) or recessive pattern, or it may occur spontaneously. The Jervell and Lange-Nielsen syndrome is also associated with a recessive inheritance pattern and characterized by bilateral sensorineural hearing loss with QTc greater than 500 milliseconds resulting in torsade de pointes. Congenital LQTS is caused by a defect in one of several genes that code for potassium or sodium channels in cardiac myocytes. Different mutations result in discrete subtypes with differing presentations and associations: SCD occurs most commonly during exercise with LQT1; auditory and emotional stimuli are provocative in LQT2; the risk of SCD is greatest with LQT3, in which SCD occurs during sleep. The genetic and phenotypic heterogeneity contributes to the difficulty in diagnosing and managing patients with congenital LQTS. The wide range of QTc values in both unaffected and affected individuals, as well as age-related variation, also confounds the diagnosis. Although a QTc of greater than 460 milliseconds is a reasonable threshold, most individuals in this range are not affected.

Evaluation includes an ECG (demonstrating QTc prolongation), 24-hour ambulatory ECG, and, possibly, an exercise test. A genetic test for the primary genes that cause LQTS is commercially available and is most helpful for identifying affected individuals in a family with LQTS. Unfortunately, this test cannot completely rule out LQTS due to a 25% false-negative rate. The mainstay of treatment for LQTS has been exercise restriction, treatment with β-blockade, and, possibly, placement of an internal cardioverter/defibrillator. Additional therapies specific to particular gene defects are anticipated.

Ackerman MJ et al: HRS/EHRA expert consensus statement on the state of genetic testing for the channelopathies and cardiomyopathies this document was developed as a partnership between the Heart Rhythm Society (HRS) and the European Heart Rhythm Association (EHRA). Heart Rhythm 2011 Aug;8(8):1308–1339. doi: 10.1016/j.hrthm.2011.05.020 [PMID: 21787999].

Kirsh JA: Finding the proverbial "needle in a haystack": identifying presymptomatic individuals with long QT syndrome. Heart Rhythm 2013;10(2):239–240 [PMID: 23219703].

SUDDEN CARDIAC DEATH

Sudden cardiac death (SCD) can be defined as biologic death resulting from abrupt, unexpected cardiovascular collapse from which an individual does not recover. The precise incidence of SCD in young persons is unknown, though an estimated 4000–8000 children in the United States die from SCD annually, compared to more than 300,000 older individuals. SCD in athletic, competitive young persons is rare, with the risk in a high school male athlete of less than 1 in 100,000 patient-years; the risk in female athletes is even lower. The causes of SCD vary with age. In infants (≤ 1 year), approximately one-half of cases may have coronary anomalies, and, in the other half, no structural cause is found. The latter group, described as having "sudden infant death syndrome" (SIDS),

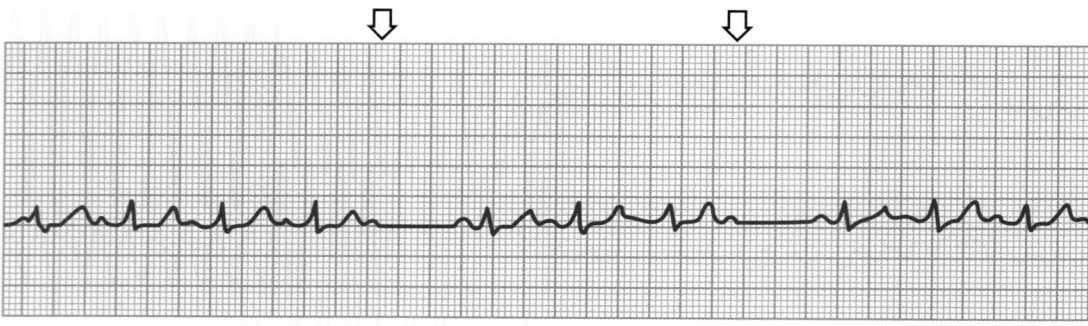

▲ **Figure 20–11.** Lead I rhythm strip with Mobitz type I (Wenckebach) second-degree heart block. There is progressive lengthening of the PR interval prior to the nonconducted P wave (*arrows*).

may have a genetic cardiac ion channel mutation, and up to one-third of SIDS cases are thought to be caused by congenital LQTS. Beyond infancy and into adulthood, the most frequent causes are HCM, myocarditis, primary electrical disturbances, coronary artery abnormalities, and preexisting structural CHD.

As many of causes of SCD are genetic, it is necessary to investigate cases by conducting detailed family histories, assessing for seizures, syncope, or early sudden death. Family members should be examined with an arrhythmia screen consisting of a physical examination, ECG, and echocardiography to detect arrhythmias or cardiomyopathies. Depending on the history, cardiac MRI, signal-averaged ECG, and genetic screening may be helpful.

Emery MS et al: Sudden cardiac death in Aahletes. JACC Heart Fail 2018;6(1):30–40 [PMID: 29284578].

DISORDERS OF ATRIOVENTRICULAR CONDUCTION

▶ General Considerations

The AV node is the electrical connection between the atrium and the ventricles. AV blocks involve a slowing or disruption of this connection.

First-Degree Atrioventricular Block

First-degree AV block is an ECG diagnosis of prolongation of the PR interval. The block does not, in itself, cause problems. It may be associated with structural CHD, namely AVSD and ccTGA, and with diseases such as rheumatic carditis.

Second-Degree Atrioventricular Block

Mobitz type I (Wenckebach) AV block is recognized by progressive prolongation of the PR interval until there is no QRS following a P wave (Figure 20–11). Mobitz type I block

occurs in normal hearts at rest and is usually benign. In Mobitz type II block, there is no progressive lengthening of the PR interval before the dropped beat (Figure 20–12). Mobitz type II block is frequently associated with organic heart disease, and a complete evaluation is necessary.

Complete Atrioventricular Block

In complete AV block, there is no electrical communication between the atria and ventricles. Ventricular rates are much slower than atrial rates and can range from 40–80 beats/min. The most common presentation of complete AV block is a congenital block occurring in a fetus or infant with an otherwise normal heart born who has passively acquired maternal systemic lupus erythematosus-associated antibodies; therefore, it is recommended to screen the mother of an affected infant even if the mother has no symptoms of collagen vascular disease. Congenital complete AV block is also associated with some forms of CHD (AVSD and ccTGA). Acquired complete AV block may be secondary to acute myocarditis, drug toxicity, electrolyte imbalance, hypoxia, and cardiac surgery.

▶ Clinical Findings

The primary finding in children with complete AV block is a significantly low heart rate for age. The diagnosis is often made prenatally when fetal bradycardia is documented. A fetal echocardiogram demonstrates an atrial contraction rate that is higher than the ventricular contraction rate, with no relationship to each other. If the heart rate is sufficiently low, there will be low cardiac output, decreased cardiac function, and development of hydrops fetalis. Postnatal adaptation largely depends on the heart rate; infants with heart rates less than 55 beats/min are at significantly greater risk for low cardiac output, HF, and death. In symptomatic patients, chest radiography can reveal an enlarged heart, and pulmonary edema may be present.

Complete AV block can also occur in older patients. Patients may be asymptomatic or may present with

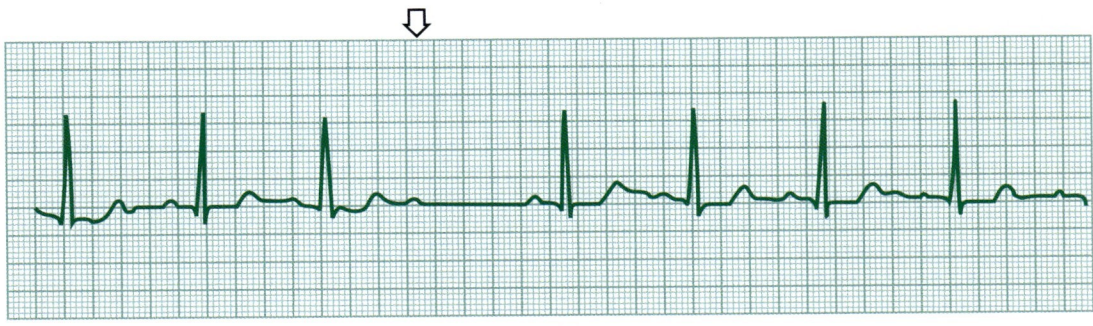

Lead III

▲ **Figure 20–12.** Lead III rhythm strip with Mobitz type II second-degree heart block. There is a consistent PR interval with occasional loss of AV conduction (*arrow*).

presyncope, syncope, or fatigue. Complete cardiac evaluation, including ECG, echocardiography, and Holter monitoring, is necessary to assess the patient for ventricular dysfunction and to relate any symptoms to concurrent arrhythmias.

▶ **Treatment**

When diagnosis of complete AV block is made in a fetus, treatment depends on gestational age, ventricular rate, and presence or absence of hydrops. Some centers have advocated the administration of steroids, IVIG, and/or β-adrenergic stimulation treatment of the mother in some instances, but emergent delivery is sometimes warranted. Postnatal treatment for neonates or older children includes temporary support with infusions of isoproterenol, temporary transvenous pacing, or a temporary transcutaneous pacemaker. The relationship of complete congenital AV block to auto-antibody production and cardiomyopathy is the basis for the consideration of immune modulation (with steroids and IVIG) in both the pregnant mother and the newborn. If neonatal complete AV block persists, long-term treatment involves the placement of a permanent pacemaker.

Baruteau AE et al: Congenital and childhood atrioventricular blocks: pathophysiology and contemporary management. Eur J Pediatr 2016;175(9):1235–1248 [PMID: 27351174].

Trucco SM et al: Use of intravenous gamma globulin and corticosteroids in the treatment of maternal autoantibody-mediated cardiomyopathy. J Am Coll Cardiol 2011 Feb 8:57(6):715–723 [PMID: 21292131].

▼ SYNCOPE (FAINTING)

INTRODUCTION

Syncope is defined as the transient loss of consciousness and postural tone resulting from an abrupt, temporary decrease in cerebral blood flow. It is one of the most common referrals to pediatric cardiology. There is an estimated 30% lifetime risk. Most episodes are self-limited and benign and are known as "simple fainting," vasovagal syncope, or neurocardiogenic syncope. While the pathophysiologic mechanisms are heterogenous and not completely understood, it is thought to reflect a disruption of heart rate and blood pressure control by the autonomic nervous system, resulting in hypotension or bradycardia. Even benign vasovagal syncope, if recurrent, can interfere with and cause a major impact on lifestyle. Rarely, syncope can be the first warning sign of a serious condition such as arrhythmia, CHD, or noncardiac disease.

▶ **Clinical Findings**

The most common initiating event of vasovagal/neuro-cardiogenic syncope is prolonged or rapid assumption of an upright position that results in gravitationally mediated venous pooling in the lower extremities and central hypovolemia, leading to decreased venous return and stroke volume. Alternatively, an emotional or physical stress (pain or fright) or a reflex mechanism related to swallowing or micturition creates a sympathetic response characterized by tachycardia and vasoconstriction followed by a parasympathetic response characterized by bradycardia or asystole, peripheral vasodilation, and decrease in systemic blood pressure and venous return. The result is a short period of loss of consciousness, (< 1–2 minutes). When the patient becomes supine, there is rapid return to baseline behavior. Bowel or bladder incontinence is uncommon, and although seizures rarely occur, myoclonic "jerks" are common. A prodrome consisting of nausea, epigastric pain, clammy sensation, pallor, dizziness, light-headedness, tunnel vision, and weakness is very characteristic of vasovagal/neurocardiogenic syncope. If the prodrome is of sufficient duration, patients may learn to recognize it and lie down to prevent complete loss of consciousness. Some patients with profound bradycardia or asystole may have little to no warning and will typically require additional evaluation to confirm the diagnosis.

Diagnosis

Given that there are many possible causes of syncope, a carefully planned approach is preferred to avoid an involved and expensive diagnostic evaluation. Patient history, family history, physical examination, and an ECG are fundamental and direct the remainder of the evaluation. Important historical details include age (syncope is rare before 10 years of age except for breathing holding syncope); state of hydration; environmental conditions (ambient temperature); activity or body position immediately prior to the syncope episode; frequency and duration of episodes; and any aura, prodrome, or specific symptoms prior to the episode. Witnesses should provide details regarding the patient's condition prior to syncope, duration of loss of consciousness, any injuries or seizure-like movements, loss of bowel or bladder function, heart rate during episode, and duration and nature of recovery. Medication history (prescription and over the counter supplements) is critical and may point to proarrhythmic potential. Pertinent positives of the past medical history include neurologic disorders, traumatic brain injury, and neurosurgical interventions.

It is not uncommon to elicit a history of multiple family members who experienced syncope during adolescence that subsequently resolved. However, if the family history is positive for recurrent syncope, it is important to consider familial disorders such as cardiomyopathy, LQTS, PH, exertional syncope, or primary arrhythmia. Additionally, families should be asked about sudden unexplained death in children or young adults (drownings, single car accidents, SCD, and SIDS), seizures, and congenital deafness.

On physical examination, the general condition should be noted, with particular emphasis on hydration, nutritional status (evidence of eating disorders), and manifestations of thyroid disease. Orthostatic vital signs should be obtained, but care must be taken to follow a strict protocol to avoid false positives. Orthostatic hypotension is defined as a decrease in systolic blood pressure of 20 mm Hg or a decrease in diastolic blood pressure of 10 mm Hg after 3 minutes of standing when compared with blood pressure in the supine or sitting position. Pulse strength, rate, and any differences between upper and lower extremities should be noted. The presence of heart murmurs suggesting anatomic disease should prompt an echocardiogram. Finally, a phenotype of inherited connective tissue disorders (ie, Marfan syndrome) should be considered.

An ECG should be obtained, particularly if syncope is recurrent or occurs with exercise. All patients with exertional syncope, even those with positive orthostatic vital signs, should undergo additional evaluation with an echocardiogram and exercise stress testing. Echocardiograms are necessary to examine for cardiomyopathy, myocarditis, anomalous coronary arteries, and PH. An exercise test may be helpful to identify arrhythmogenic causes of syncope. Tilt table testing is less commonly performed as a positive test is not required for the diagnosis of vasovagal syncope.

Treatment

Maintaining adequate hydration is the mainstay of treatment of vasovagal syncope. While choosing a fluid volume goal is acceptable, having patients target clear urine at least five times per day ensures appropriate intake. Increased dietary salt intake may also aid in maintaining intravascular volume. Counterregulatory maneuvers such as leg pumping, leg crossing, and squatting can ameliorate presyncopal symptoms and frequently avoids complete loss of consciousness. Finally, regular aerobic exercise can improve the vascular tone of the lower extremities. Medications can be useful although are rarely necessary if adequate hydration is established.

Shen WK et al: 2017 ACC/AHA/HRS guideline for the evaluation and management of patients with syncope: a report of the American College of Cardiology/American Heart Association Task Force on Clinical Practice Guidelines and the Heart Rhythm Society. Circulation 2017;136(5):e60–e122 [PMID: 28280231].

CHEST PAIN

ESSENTIALS OF DIAGNOSIS & TYPICAL FEATURES

► Location, severity, intensity, and modulating factors help with diagnosis.

► Often musculoskeletal in origin or due to gastroesophageal reflux.

► Cardiac etiologies are rare and can be associated with pain on exertion.

Overview

Chest pain is a common pediatric complaint, accounting for 3–6 in 1000 emergency and urgent care visits, with median age of 12–13 years and a male predominance (1–1.6:1). Although children with chest pain are commonly referred for cardiac evaluation, chest pain in children is uncommonly cardiac in origin, with a cardiac etiology found in only 2%–5% of emergency department visits and 3%–7% of cardiology clinic visits.

Detailed history and physical examination should guide the appropriate workup of chest pain. The location, duration, intensity, frequency, and radiation of the pain should be documented, as well as associated symptoms and any possible worsening or alleviating factors. The presence of triggering events preceding the pain should be explored. Chest pain during or immediately following exertion should lead to a more elaborate evaluation for a cardiac disorder. Associated symptoms should be evaluated, including syncope, palpitations, nausea/vomiting, shortness of breath, cough, or wheezing. Relation of pain to meals should be investigated. Detailed social history may reveal psychosocial stressors or exposures such as smoking or drug abuse. On physical examination, attention should focus on the following: vital signs; general appearance of the child; the chest wall morphology and musculature; cardiac, pulmonary, and abdominal examination findings; and quality of peripheral pulses. If pain can be reproduced by direct palpation of the chest wall, it is almost always musculoskeletal in origin.

Etiology

Chest pain is typically noncardiac and may be due to a multitude of conditions. Musculoskeletal etiologies are the most common identifiable cause of chest pain and include costochondritis, muscular strain, skeletal abnormality, and trauma. Costochondritis accounts for 26%–41% of all chest pain cases; it is caused by inflammation of the costochondral joints and is reproducible on examination. Respiratory causes include reactive airway disease, pneumonia, pleuritis, and pneumothorax. Gastrointestinal causes of chest pain include gastroesophageal reflux, esophagitis, gastritis, foreign-body ingestion, hiatal hernia, cholecystitis, and referred abdominal pain. Hematologic and oncologic conditions include pulmonary embolism, sickle cell anemia, and tumors. Psychological conditions are more common in adolescents than younger children and include stress, anxiety, panic attacks, somatoform disorder, and depression. On occasion, no identifiable cause is found (idiopathic chest pain), despite sometimes extensive evaluations.

Cardiac disease is itself an infrequent cause of chest pain; however, if misdiagnosed, it may be life threatening. Although chest pain is commonly associated with myocardial ischemia in adults, this association is rare in children. When chest pain is associated with ischemia in the pediatric population, it is often related to substance abuse causing coronary vasospasm or as a consequence of coronary abnormalities caused by prior KD. A history of KD with coronary artery involvement increases the risk of future myocardial infarction secondary to thrombosis of coronary aneurysms. Abnormal origins of the coronary arteries can also be associated with chest pain and SCD due to impaired myocardial blood flow, particularly with exertion. Arrhythmias, including SVT, atrial flutter, and ectopic atrial tachycardia, ventricular tachycardia, complete heart block, or simple ectopy, including PACs or PVCs, can also elicit chest pain, and young children may simply describe the palpitations associated with an arrhythmia as pain. Structural lesions that can cause chest pain include aortic or pulmonary stenosis. Finally, acquired cardiac conditions that can cause chest pain include DCM, myocarditis, pericarditis, rheumatic carditis, and aortic dissection.

Evaluation

In most cases, sophisticated testing is not required. However, if a cardiac origin is suspected, a pediatric cardiologist should be consulted. Evaluation in these instances may include an ECG, chest radiograph, echocardiogram, or ambulatory arrhythmia monitor. In a 10-year study of 3700 patients evaluated for chest pain in a pediatric cardiology clinic, the vast majority of patients had suggestive symptoms (eg, exertional chest pain), concerning family or medical history, abnormal examination, or abnormal ECG. Forty percent of patients underwent echocardiography; incidental cardiac findings (unrelated to chest pain) were found in 4% of patients and a positive finding potentially related to the complaint of chest pain was found in only 0.3% of patients. Rhythm monitors were positive in only 0.4% of patients, most of whom had complaints of palpitations. An exercise stress test was not additive to making a diagnosis. Ultimately, only 1% of patients were found to have a cardiac etiology and there were no SCDs. Children were more likely to die from suicide, confirming that depression and anxiety are potential serious causes of chest pain.

Friedman KG et al: Chest pain and syncope in children: a practical approach to diagnosis of cardiac disease. J Pediatr 2013; 163(3):896–901 [PMID: 23769502].

Sumski CA et al: Evaluating chest pain and heart murmurs in pediatric and adolescent patients. Pediatr Clin North Am 2020; 67(5):783–799 [PMID: 32888681]

▼ PREVENTIVE CARDIOLOGY

HYPERTENSION

Blood pressure should be determined at every pediatric visit beginning at 3 years of age. Since blood pressure is being monitored more carefully, systemic hypertension is more widely recognized as a pediatric problem, now with a prevalence of approximately 3%. Blood pressure must be obtained when the child is relaxed, and an appropriately sized cuff must be used with the sphygmomanometer. The widest cuff that fits between the axilla and the antecubital fossa should be used (covering 60%–75% of the upper arm). The pressure coinciding with the onset (K_1) and the loss (K_5) of the Korotkoff sounds determines the systolic and diastolic blood pressures, respectively. Pediatric standards for blood pressure have been published based on age, gender, and height. Normal blood pressure is defined as less than 90th percentile and less than 120/80; prehypertension, greater than or equal to 90th percentile or greater than or equal to 120/80 and less than 95th percentile; stage 1 hypertension, greater than or equal to 95th percentile and less than 99th percentile + 5 mm Hg; and stage 2 hypertension, greater than or equal to 99th percentile + 5 mm Hg. If a properly measured blood pressure meets or exceeds the 95th percentile, the measurement should be repeated on at least 3 separate occasions over a 2- to 4-week interval. Ambulatory blood pressure monitoring (ABPM) has also become an important diagnostic tool in the evaluation of hypertension in the pediatric and adolescent population. ABPM should be performed for at least 24 hours, with at least 40 total readings during both waking and sleeping hours. In assessing ABPM data, in addition to describing blood pressure values outside the normal range, the percentage of readings that are above the target threshold is useful. If the blood pressure is persistently elevated, a search for the cause should be undertaken. Although most hypertension in children is primary, particularly given the increased incidence of overweight and obese children, the incidence of treatable causes is higher in children than in adults. Causes of secondary hypertension include coarctation of the aorta, renal artery stenosis, chronic renal disease, pheochromocytoma, and medication side effects (eg, steroids).

If a secondary cause is not identified, therapeutic lifestyle change with diet and exercise is the first-line therapy for both prehypertension and hypertension. The main classes of antihypertensive agents used as first-line therapy in children are the same as in adults, including angiotensin converting enzyme inhibitors, angiotensin receptor blockers, calcium channel blockers, and diuretics. The initial agent is usually chosen based on preference and experience of the prescribing provider. β-Blockers and diuretics are safe to use but are often avoided as first-line agents due to concerns about anticipated side effects. Maximizing monotherapy prior to introducing a second agent remains an official guideline.

Flynn JT et al: Ambulatory blood pressure monitoring in children and adolescents: 2022 update: a scientific statement from the American Heart Association. Hypertension 2022;79(7):e114–e124 [PMID: 35603599].

Flynn JT et al: Clinical practice guideline for screening and management of high blood pressure in children and adolescents. Pediatrics 2017;140(3):e20171904 [PMID: 28827377].

Patel SS et al: Ambulatory blood pressure monitoring in pediatrics. Curr Hypertens Rep 2019 Jul 26;21(9):71 [PMID: 31350605].

ATHEROSCLEROSIS & DYSLIPIDEMIAS

Coronary artery disease remains the leading cause of death in the U.S. However, the age-adjusted incidence of death from ischemic heart disease has been decreasing in recent decades as a result of improved diet, decreased smoking, awareness and treatment of hypertension, and increased physical activity.

Serum lipid concentrations in childhood usually remain constant through early adolescence. Abnormal lipid concentrations are relatively common, affecting approximately 1 in 5 adolescents. Lipid disorders are less common, with severe hypercholesterolemia (LDL ≥ 190 mg/dL [≥ 4.9 mmol/L]) only affecting approximately 1 in 250; when present, however, they frequently occur in association with obesity and other risk factors that contribute to increased rates of cardiovascular and metabolic morbidity and mortality. Abnormalities in the lipid profile appearing early in childhood correlate with higher risk for coronary artery disease in adulthood. Low-density lipoprotein (LDL) is atherogenic, while its counterpart, high-density lipoprotein (HDL) has been identified as an anti-atherogenic factor.

Routine lipid screening of children remains controversial. It is reasonable to check a fasting or nonfasting lipoprotein profile in children as early as 2 years old who have a family history of early cardiovascular disease (< 55 years old in men, < 65 years old in women) or significant hypercholesterolemia (total cholesterol > 240 mg/dL) to detect familial hypercholesterolemia (FH) or other rare forms of hypercholesterolemia. AHA guidelines recommend universal pediatric lipid screening at 9–11 years old and then at ages 17–21 years because total cholesterol and LDL-C levels decrease 10%–20% during puberty. Checking a fasting lipid panel is particularly indicated in children and adolescents with obesity or metabolic risk factors (high blood sugar, low HDL, high triglycerides, high blood pressure, large waist circumference).

When children have LDL levels greater than 130 mg/dL on two successive tests, lifestyle therapy including dietary counseling and regular physical activity is indicated. Dietary modification, alone, may decrease cholesterol levels by 5%–20%. If the patient is unresponsive to lifestyle therapy after 3–6 months and at extreme risk (eg, LDL-C ≥ 190 mg/mL, ≥ 160 mg/dL with clinical presentation of FH, HDL < 35 mg/dL, or a history of cardiovascular disease in a first-degree relative at < 40 years of age), drug therapy may be indicated to decrease atherosclerotic cardiovascular disease risk. Statins are the more commonly used agents in the pediatric population and can be started as early as 8–10 years old. Cholestyramine, a bile acid sequestrant (BAS), can be given to children with FH as early as 6 years old, while colesevelam (a BAS) can be used in children 10 years or older. However, these latter agents are rarely used due to poor adherence. Ezetimibe, a cholesterol absorption inhibitor, can be combined with statins to lower LDL-C in children 10 years or older with FH. Niacin is useful for treatment of hypertriglyceridemia.

Grundy SM et al: AHA/ACC/AACVPR/AAPA/ABC/ACPM/ADA/AGS/APhA/ASPC/NLA/PCNA guideline on the management of blood cholesterol: a report of the American College of Cardiology/American Heart Association Task Force on Clinical Practice Guidelines. Circulation 2019 Jun 18;139(25):e1082–e1143. doi: 10.1161/CIR.0000000000000625. Epub 2018 Nov 10. Erratum in: Circulation. 2019 Jun 18;139(25):e1182–e1186 [PMID: 30586774].

Gastrointestinal Tract

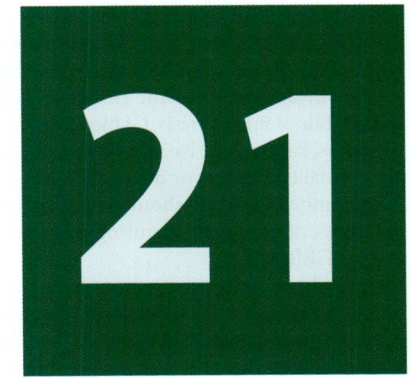

21

David Brumbaugh, MD

Glenn T. Furuta, MD

Edward J. Hoffenberg, MD

Gregory E. Kobak, MD

Robert E. Kramer, MD

Nathalie Nguyen, MD

Seth Septer, DO

Mary Shull, MD

Jason Soden, MD

Thomas Walker, MD

DISORDERS OF THE ESOPHAGUS

GASTROESOPHAGEAL REFLUX & GERD

ESSENTIALS OF DIAGNOSIS & TYPICAL FEATURES

▶ Key definitions:
  - **Gastroesophageal reflux (GER)** refers to uncomplicated recurrent spitting and vomiting in healthy children that resolves spontaneously.
  - **Gastroesophageal reflux disease (GERD)** is present when reflux causes secondary symptoms or complications.
  - **Esophageal manifestations of GERD** include symptoms (heartburn, regurgitation) and mucosal complications (esophagitis, stricture, Barrett esophagus) primarily related to acid exposure in the upper gastrointestinal (GI) tract, primarily the esophagus itself.
  - **Extraesophageal manifestations of GERD** include a myriad of clinical disorders that may be linked to reflux, including upper and lower airway symptoms and findings, as well as dental erosions. In most settings, objective confirmation of extraesophageal reflux complications is challenging.

▶ Clinical Findings

A. Infants With Gastroesophageal Reflux

Gastroesophageal (GE) reflux is common in young infants and is a physiologic event. Frequent postprandial regurgitation, ranging from effortless to forceful, is the most common GI symptom in infants. Infant GER is usually benign, and it is expected to resolve by 12–18 months of life.

Reflux of gastric contents into the esophagus occurs during spontaneous relaxations of the lower esophageal sphincter (LES) that are unaccompanied by swallowing. Factors promoting reflux in infants include small stomach capacity, frequent large-volume feedings, short esophageal length, supine positioning, and slow swallowing response to the flow of refluxed material up the esophagus. Infants' individual responses to the stimulus of reflux, particularly the maturity of their self-settling skills, are important factors determining the severity of reflux-related symptoms. Symptoms such as failure to thrive, food refusal, pain behavior, GI bleeding, upper or lower airway–associated respiratory symptoms, or Sandifer syndrome in infants suggest gastroesophageal reflux disease (GERD).

B. Older Children With Reflux

Older children with GERD complain of adult-type symptoms such as regurgitation into the mouth, heartburn, and dysphagia. Esophagitis can occur as a complication of GERD and requires endoscopy with biopsy for diagnostic confirmation. Children with asthma, cystic fibrosis, developmental delay/spasticity, hiatal hernia (HH), and repaired esophageal atresia—tracheoesophageal fistulas are at increased risk of GERD and esophagitis.

C. Extraesophageal Manifestations of Reflux Disease

Upper airway symptoms (hoarseness, sinusitis, laryngeal erythema, and edema), events of apnea and/or cyanosis, lower airway symptoms (asthma, recurrent pneumonia, recurrent cough), dental erosions, and Sandifer syndrome have all been linked to GERD, although proof of cause-and-effect relationship is challenging.

D. Diagnostic Studies

History and physical examination alone should help differentiate infants with benign, recurrent vomiting (physiologic GER) from those who have red flags for GERD or other underlying primary conditions that may present with recurrent emesis at this age. Warning signs that warrant further investigation in the infant with recurrent vomiting include bile-stained emesis, GI bleeding, onset of vomiting after 6 months, failure to thrive, diarrhea, fever, hepatosplenomegaly, abdominal tenderness or distension, or neurologic changes.

An upper GI series should be considered when anatomic etiologies of recurrent vomiting are considered but is not a test for GERD.

In older children with heartburn or frequent regurgitation, a limited trial of acid-suppressant therapy may be both diagnostic and therapeutic. If a child has symptoms requiring ongoing acid suppressant therapy, or if symptoms fail to improve with empiric therapy, consider referral to a pediatric gastroenterologist to assist in evaluation of complicated GERD, or other diagnoses including eosinophilic esophagitis (EoE).

Esophagoscopy and mucosal biopsies are useful to evaluate for mucosal injury secondary to GERD (Barrett esophagus, stricture, erosive esophagitis), or to evaluate for other diagnoses. Endoscopic evaluation is not requisite for the evaluation of all infants and children with suspected GERD.

Intraluminal impedance and pH monitoring (pH impedance probe) may be indicated to quantify reflux, and to evaluate for objective evidence of symptom associations with regards to atypical reflux presentations. pH impedance studies may have diagnostic yield in evaluating for respiratory or atypical complications of reflux disease, or in evaluating for breakthrough reflux symptoms while a patient is on acid-suppressant therapy.

Pediatric patients with predominant airway and/or pulmonary presentations that are suspected to be GERD-related may benefit from multi-specialty aerodigestive evaluation to include input from feeding specialists, pulmonology, and otolaryngology.

▶ Treatment & Prognosis

Reflux resolves spontaneously in 85% of affected infants by 12 months of age, coincident with developing an erect posture and initiation of solid feedings. Until then, regurgitation volume may be reduced by offering small feedings at frequent intervals and by thickening feedings with rice cereal (2–3 tsp/oz of formula). In infants with unexplained crying or fussy behavior, no evidence supports the empiric use of acid suppression.

In infants with suspected GERD, empiric acid suppression may not be appropriate without careful attention to potential factors leading to symptoms and/or objective testing. Acid suppression may be used to treat suspected esophageal or extraesophageal complications of acid reflux in older infants and children. Because the presentation of milk protein intolerance may be clinically indistinguishable

from GERD in infants, a trial of maternal dairy elimination (breast fed infants) or formula modification (formula fed infants) may be warranted. Pharmacologic options include histamine-2 (H2)–receptor antagonists or proton pump inhibitors (PPIs). PPI therapy has been shown to significantly heal both esophageal mucosal injury and symptoms from GERD within 8–12 weeks. Potential risk factors associated with long-term PPI therapy include risk for infection (pneumonia, *Clostridium difficile*–associated diarrhea), and an increased risk for osteoporosis has been demonstrated in adults. Although there are no standardized recommendations regarding prophylaxis or surveillance for these complications in pediatric patients on long-term PPI therapy, one should consider weaning or discontinuing treatment if it is no longer required. There is no sufficient evidence to support the routine use of prokinetic agents for treatment of pediatric GERD.

Spontaneous resolution is less likely in older children with GERD and those with underlying neurodevelopmental disorders. Episodic symptoms may be controlled with the intermittent use of acid blockers and those with persistent symptoms may require chronic acid suppression. Complications of reflux esophagitis or chronic GERD include feeding dysfunction, esophageal stricture, and anemia (Figure 21–1). Barrett esophagus, a precancerous condition, is very uncommon in children, but it may occur in patients with an underlying primary diagnosis that offers high risk for GERD.

Anti-reflux surgery (Nissen fundoplication) may be considered in a child with GERD who (1) fails medical therapy; (2) is dependent on persistent, aggressive medical therapy; (3) is symptomatic and nonadherent to medical therapy; or (4) has persistent, severe respiratory complications of

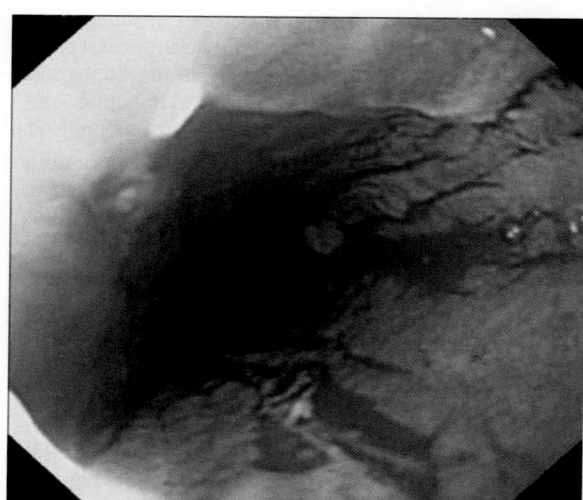

▲ **Figure 21–1.** Esophagitis associated with GERD. Mucosa is erythematous with loss of vascular pattern.

GERD or other life-threatening complications of GERD. Potential complications after antireflux surgery include dumping syndrome, gas bloat syndrome, persistent retching or gagging, or wrap failure.

Gulati IK, Jadcherla SR: Gastroesophageal reflux disease in the neonatal intensive care unit infant: who needs to be treated and what approach is beneficial? Pediatr Clin North Am 2019 Apr;66(2):461–473. doi: 10.1016/j.Pcl.2018.12.012. Epub 2019 Feb 1 [PMID: 30819348].

Mousa H, Hassan M: Gastroesophageal reflux disease. Pediatr Clin North Am 2017 jun;64(3):487–505 [PMID: 28502434].

Rosen R. Gastroesophageal reflux treatment in infancy through young adulthood. Am J Gastroenterol. 2023 Mar 1;118(3):452–458. doi: 10.14309/ajg.0000000000002160. Epub 2022 Dec 24. [PMID: 36717189].

Rosen R et al: Pediatric gastroesophageal reflux clinical practice guidelines: joint recommendations of The North American Society for Pediatric Gastroenterology, Hepatology, and Nutrition and The European Society for Pediatric Gastroenterology, Hepatology, and Nutrition. J Pediatr Gastroenterol Nutr 2018 Mar;66(3):516–554. doi: 10.1097/mpg.0000000000001889 [PMID: 29470322].

EOSINOPHILIC ESOPHAGITIS

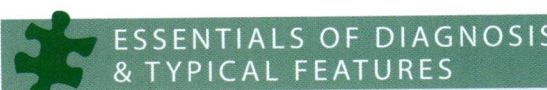

ESSENTIALS OF DIAGNOSIS & TYPICAL FEATURES

▶ Dysphagia, feeding difficulties, esophageal food impaction, and heartburn are common symptoms.

▶ Must rule out other causes for esophageal eosinophilia before assigning diagnosis of EoE.

▶ Esophageal food impaction and esophageal stricture are two most common complications.

▶ Swallowed topical steroids, PPIs, diet elimination and biologics are effective treatments.

Clinical Findings

A. Symptoms and Signs

Eosinophilic esophagitis (EoE) is an increasingly recognized disease that occurs in all ages, but more frequently affects boys. Common initial presentations in young children include feeding difficulties, reflux, abdominal pain, vomiting, and regurgitation. Children may develop compensatory behaviors including careful and lengthy chewing, prolonged mealtimes, washing food down with liquid or avoiding highly textured foods (breads, meats, rice, potatoes). A family or personal history of atopy, asthma, dysphagia, esophageal dilation, or food impaction is often present.

B. Laboratory Findings

Laboratory findings are not helpful in making the diagnosis. Use of a barium coated pill with upper GI series or esophagram can illuminate functional or motility abnormalities if the study shows delayed passage of the barium tablet. Narrow caliber esophagus or focal strictures on upper GI series are also suggestive (Figure 21–2).

Differential Diagnosis

The most common differential diagnoses are GERD with esophagitis, congenital esophageal stricture, and *Candida* esophagitis.

Diagnosis

The diagnosis of EoE is based on clinical symptoms of esophageal dysfunction and histologic findings in esophageal mucosal biopsies (> 15 eosinophils per high-power field), therefore endoscopy is required for diagnosis. Other causes of esophageal eosinophilia, in particular, GERD, must be ruled out.

Treatment

Dietary exclusion of offending allergens (elemental diet, allergy testing directed diets, or empiric elimination diets) is effective treatment, but adherence in older children can be difficult. PPIs and topical corticosteroids are effective drugs for treatment of EoE. Topical corticosteroids are puffed in the mouth and swallowed from a metered dose pulmonary inhaler; this method of administration is different from how

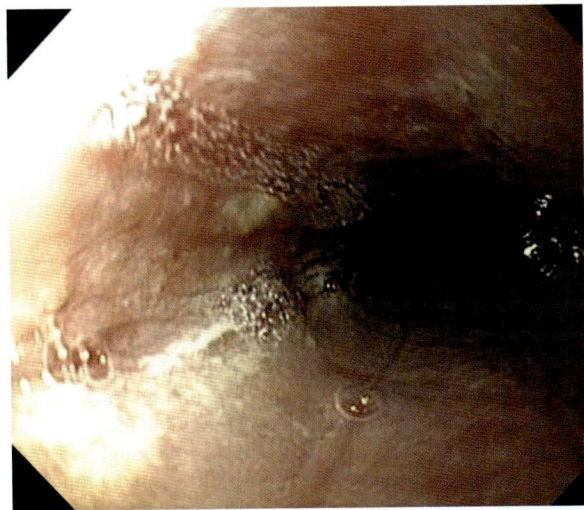

▲ **Figure 21–2.** Esophagitis associated with EoE. Mucosa contains linear folds, white exudate, and has loss of vascular pattern.

topical steroids are administered for the treatment of asthma. Patients should not rinse their mouth or eat for 30 minutes to maximize effectiveness. Diet elimination, topical corticosteroids and PPI have been the mainstays of treatment however, new biologics have been developed. Dupilumab, a monoclonal antibody that blocks the receptor for interleukin-4 and interleukin-13, important cytokines in the pathogenesis of the disease, was the first biologic approved for EoE.

Dellon ES et al: Dupilumab in adults and adolescents with eosinophilic esophagitis. N Engl J Med 2022 Dec 22;387(25):2317–2330. doi: 10.1056/NEJMoa2205982 [PMID: 36546624].

Furuta GT, Katzka DA: Eosinophilic esophagitis. N Engl J Med 2015 Oct 22;373(17):1640–1648 [PMID: 26488694].

Hirano I, Furuta GT: approaches and challenges to management of pediatric and adult patients with eosinophilic esophagitis. Gastroenterology. 2020 Mar;158(4):840–851. [PMID: 31836530].

Nguyen N et al:. Role of pill esophagram to identify pediatric patients with eosinophilic esophagitis amenable to therapeutic dilation. J Pediatr Gastroenterol Nutr 2020 Oct;71(4):530–532 [PMID: 32960542].

Ruffner MA, Spergel JM: Pediatric eosinophilic esophagitis: updates for the primary care setting. Curr Opin Pediatr 2018 Dec;30(6):829–836 [PMID: 3023937].

ACHALASIA OF THE ESOPHAGUS

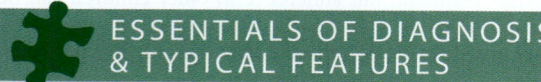

ESSENTIALS OF DIAGNOSIS & TYPICAL FEATURES

► Disorder of esophageal motility causing increased tone and failure of relaxation of LES.

► Rare in children younger than 5

► Presenting symptoms include emesis, dysphagia, and weight loss.

► Barium esophagram with "beaking" at GE junction and tertiary contractions of esophageal wall.

► High-resolution manometry is gold standard for diagnosis.

A. Symptoms and Signs

Pediatric achalasia has an incidence of 0.11 per 100,000, with less than 5% of achalasia occurring in patients younger than 15 years. Presenting symptoms are emesis (84.6%), dysphagia (69.2%), weight loss (46.0%), and chronic cough (46.1%). Patients may eat slowly, regurgitate undigested food, and often require large amounts of fluid when ingesting solid food. Achalasia may present in conjunction with adrenal insufficiency and alacrima as part of 3A syndrome, also known as Allgrove syndrome.

B. Diagnostic Testing

A barium esophagram shows a dilated esophagus with a tapered "beak" at the LES and irregular tertiary contractions, indicative of disordered esophageal peristalsis. Use of timed barium esophagram correlates with manometry in identifying delayed esophageal emptying in children. Esophageal manometry shows high resting pressure and failure of relaxation of the LES after swallowing and abnormal esophageal peristalsis. Use of high-resolution manometry has become the standard in diagnosis and the Chicago classification into types I (classic, no contractility), II (pan-esophageal pressurization) and III (spastic contractions), have been used to indicate prognosis. Clinically, the Eckhardt score has been used to grade symptom severity and outcome of treatment, based on four domains of dysphagia, chest pain, regurgitation and weight loss. Use of functional luminal imaging probe (FLIP) balloons can discriminate lower distensibility and diameter of the esophagogastric junction (EGJ) in pediatric achalasia patients and subsequently be used to perform LES dilation. Biopsies of the EGJ have also demonstrated both lymphocytic inflammation and mast cell degranulation in patients with achalasia.

C. Differential Diagnosis

Congenital or peptic stricture, webs, and masses of the esophagus may mimic achalasia. EoE commonly presents with similar symptoms of dysphagia and food impaction. Cricopharyngeal achalasia is a rare cause of dysphagia in children, but it shares clinical features. Intestinal pseudo-obstruction, multiple endocrine neoplasia type 2b, systemic amyloidosis, and post-vagotomy syndrome cause similar esophageal dysmotility. Teenage girls may be suspected of having an eating disorder. Chagas disease is an acquired achalasia caused by *Trypanosoma cruzi*, where neuronal nitric oxide synthase (nNOS) and ganglion cells are diminished or absent in the muscular layers of the LES.

► Treatment & Prognosis

The primary treatments for pediatric achalasia are Heller myotomy (HM), endoscopic dilation (ED), and most recently, peroral endoscopic myotomy (POEM). Metanalysis of HM and ED success show rates of 78% and 45%, respectively, with similar complication rates. Prospective randomized trials comparing these modalities in children are lacking, but meta-analysis of 14 POEM studies involving more than 400 pediatric patients showed a success rate of 88% with an adverse event rate of 12.9% and a 26.3% rate of erosive esophagitis. Considering that achalasia patients carry a 50× increased risk for esophageal cancer 20–25 years after diagnosis, primarily related to GERD, assessment of risk-benefit ratio of POEM versus HM and ED modalities is particularly critical in the pediatric population. HM typically offers the advantage of being performed in conjunction with fundoplication, helping mitigate the risk of subsequent GERD. Though conventional ED may be falling out of favor compared to these other modalities, increased use of FLIP during endoscopy offers utility in simultaneous diagnosis and intervention during the same procedure, as well as to objectively measure outcomes after POEM and HM.

Howk AA, Clifton MS, Garza JM, Durham MM: Impedance planimetry (Endoflip) assisted laparoscopic esophagomyotomy in pediatric population. J Pediatr Surg 2022 Dec;57(12): 1000–1004. Epub 2022 May 10 [PMID: 35659759].

Nabi Z, Talukdar R, Chavan R, Basha J, Reddy DN: Outcomes of per-oral endoscopic myotomy in children: a systematic review and meta-analysis. Dysphagia 2022 Dec;37(6):1468–1481. Epub 2022 Jan 29 [PMID: 35092485].

Provenzano L et al: Laparoscopic Heller-Dor is a persistently effective treatment for achalasia even in pediatric patients: a 25-year experience at a single tertiary center. Eur J Pediatr Surg 2023 Dec;33(6):493–498 [PMID: 36720247].

CAUSTIC BURNS OF THE ESOPHAGUS

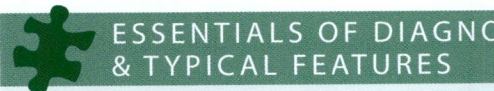

ESSENTIALS OF DIAGNOSIS & TYPICAL FEATURES

▶ Reported history of ingestion, with or without evidence of oropharyngeal injury.

▶ Painful swallowing, drooling, and food refusal typical of esophageal injury.

▶ Endoscopic evaluation of severity and extent of injury at 24–48 hours post-ingestion.

▶ Significant risk for development of esophageal strictures, especially in second- and third-degree lesions.

▶ Clinical Findings

A. Symptoms and Signs

Ingestion of caustic solids or liquids (pH < 2 or pH > 12) produces esophageal lesions ranging from superficial inflammation to deep necrosis with ulceration, perforation, mediastinitis, or peritonitis. Metanalysis encompassing more than 11,000 ingestions indicates a slight male predominance and a mean age of ingestion of 2.78 years. Acidic substances typically have a sour taste and therefore lead to limited injury because of the small volume ingested, causing superficial coagulative necrosis with eschar formation. Conversely, the more benign taste of alkali ingestions may allow for larger volume ingestions and subsequent liquefactive necrosis that can lead to deeper mucosal penetration. Ingestions of liquid detergent capsules or pods have become more common, accidentally in younger children, and intentionally in teenagers. They may cause more respiratory compromise

and neurologic impairment than esophageal injury, as their pH tends to range from 7 to 9. The lips, mouth, and airway should be examined in suspected caustic ingestion, although up to 12% of children without oral lesions can have significant esophageal injury.

B. Imaging Studies

Esophagoscopy is often performed; however, timing is important as endoscopy may not indicate the true severity of injury if it is performed too early (< 24–48 hours) and may increase the risk of perforation if it is performed too late (> 72 hours) due to formation of granulation tissue. Grading of esophageal lesions via the Zargar classification into first degree (superficial injury, erythema only), second degree (transmucosal with erythema, ulceration, and sloughing), and third degree (transmural with circumferential sloughing and deep mucosal ulceration) can help predict prognosis. Circumferential lesions carry the highest risk of stricture formation. If dilation is felt to be necessary, it should not be performed in the acute phase of injury. Plain radiographs of the chest and abdomen may be performed if there is clinical suspicion of perforation. Contrast studies of the esophagus should be performed when endoscopic evaluation is not available, though they are unlikely to detect grades 1 and 2 lesions.

▶ Treatment & Prognosis

Clinical observation is always prudent, as it is often difficult to predict the severity of esophageal injury at presentation. A large study of more than 1500 pediatric ingestions across 40 institutions showed a stricture rate of 11%. Vomiting should not be induced, and administration of buffering agents should be avoided to prevent an exothermic reaction in the stomach. Use of high-dose (1 g/1.73 m^2) methylprednisone for the first 3 days after ingestion significantly decreases the occurrence of esophageal strictures. Broad-spectrum antibiotic coverage with third-generation cephalosporins may be considered to decrease stricture formation by preventing bacterial colonization into necrotic tissue. Acid-blockade is often used to decrease additional injury from acid reflux. A prospective study of 60 children with grade IIb esophageal injury treated with sucralfate 80 mg/kg every 2 hours for 3 days after injury showed a significant reduction in the incidence of strictures.

In cases where caustic stricture develops, ED is the mainstay of therapy. Intralesional injection of corticosteroids can be used to help open strictures in cases where the endoscope is unable to pass, or where repeated dilations alone fail to produce a sustained response. In refractory cases, fully covered, self-expanding, removable esophageal stents, now available in pediatric sizes, may offer additional benefit as a definitive treatment or as abridge to surgical therapy. Topical mitomycin-C in conjunction with dilation has been effective in treatment of refractory caustic strictures of the esophagus. Surgical replacement of the esophagus by colonic interposition or gastric tube may be needed for long strictures. Patients with history of caustic esophageal injury are estimated to have as much as a 1000-fold increased risk for esophageal carcinoma, though no formal surveillance guidelines have been established.

Akhijahani RF et al: Effectiveness of sucralfate in preventing esophageal stricture in children after ingestion of caustic agents. Eur J Pediatr 2023 Jun;182(6):2591–2596. Epub ahead of print [PMID: 36935468].

Flor MM, Ribeiro IB, DE Moura DTH, Marques SB, Bernardo WM, DE Moura EGH: Efficacy of endoscopic topical mitomycin C application in caustic esophageal strictures in the pediatric population: a systematic review and meta-analysis of randomized controlled trials. Arq Gastroenterol 2021 Apr–Jun;58(2):253–261 [PMID: 34231663].

Patterson KN, Beyene TJ, Gil LA, Minneci PC, Deans KJ, Halaweish I: Procedural and surgical interventions for esophageal stricture secondary to caustic ingestion in children. J Pediatr Surg 2023 Sep;58(9):1631–1639. [PMID: 36878759].

FOREIGN BODIES IN THE ALIMENTARY TRACT

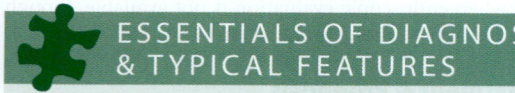

ESSENTIALS OF DIAGNOSIS & TYPICAL FEATURES

▶ Dysphagia, odynophagia, drooling, regurgitation, and chest/abdominal pain are typical symptoms of esophageal foreign body (EFB).

▶ EFBs should be removed within 24 hours of ingestion.

▶ Esophageal button batteries must be removed emergently because of their ability to cause lethal injury.

▶ Most foreign bodies in the stomach will pass spontaneously.

▶ Clinical Findings

Pediatric foreign-body ingestions (FBIs) are common. The rate of children presenting to emergency departments with FBIs has increased in the last two decades in the United States. FBIs are responsible for more than 2400 hospital admissions per year in the United States. The majority (80%–90%) of foreign bodies pass spontaneously with only 10%–20% requiring endoscopic or surgical management. Recent tracking data comparing rates of ED presentation for FBI in children pre- and post-COVID-19 (coronavirus disease 2019) pandemic in the United States showed a disturbing trend toward more frequent and severe FBI events. The most common presenting symptoms of FBI are dysphagia, odynophagia, drooling,

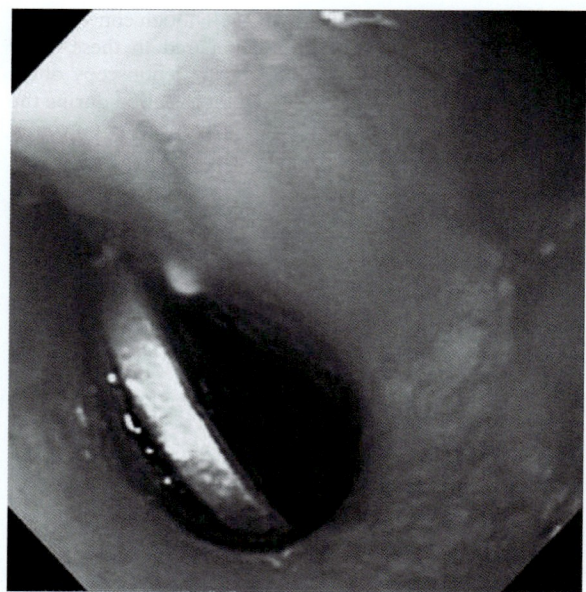

▲ **Figure 21–3.** Foreign body in esophagus. Coin is lodged in the esophageal lumen.

regurgitation, and chest or abdominal pain, but patients may be completely asymptomatic. Cough may become prominent for FBI retained in the esophagus for more than 1 week, especially in toddlers even without a witnessed ingestion.

Coins are the most common FBI in children (Figure 21–3) and tend to lodge in narrowed areas—vallecula, thoracic inlet, GE junction, pylorus, ligament of Treitz, and ileocecal junction, or at the site of congenital or acquired intestinal stenoses. Evaluations to detect FBI start with plain radiographs, but nonradiopaque objects, such as plastic toys, may not appear on standard radiography. If there is clinical concern for a retained EFB that is nonradiopaque, a contrast esophagram is a useful test, though this may delay or increase the risk of anesthesia as endoscopy may not be performed until the contrast has passed the upper GI tract. Point-of-care ultrasound, high-definition radiographs, and computed tomography (CT) scan have been proposed as having utility in early and accurate diagnosis of FBI.

▶ Treatment & Prognosis

Most FBIs can be removed from the esophagus or stomach by flexible endoscopy. During removal of an EFB, the increased risk of airway aspiration supports endotracheal intubation. EFBs should be removed within 24 hours to avoid injury or erosion. The urgency of removal of EFB is dictated by the severity of patient symptoms and the ability to swallow oral secretions.

Esophageal button batteries are especially concerning and should be removed emergently. Button battery ingestion (BBI) may cause an electrical thermal injury in as little as 2 hours and may be complicated by aortoesophageal fistula, tracheo-esophageal fistula, esophageal perforation, esophageal stricture, vocal cord paralysis, discitis, and even death. Although most gastric BBI will pass uneventfully, greater attention is required for larger batteries (> 20 mm) in younger children (< 5 years of age), as there is greater risk for significant injury. Recent multicenter data have shown up to 25% of gastric BBI are symptomatic at presentation and 60% of those undergoing endoscopy showed signs of gastric injury, including perforation. Significant injury and death due to BBI have increased in recent years with the production of larger, higher-voltage lithium batteries. A scoring system has been proposed to predict severe outcomes in pediatric BBI, with 88% probability if all three risk factors of esophageal location on imaging, battery 20 mm or greater, and clinical symptoms are found at presentation.

Esophageal food impaction should always raise the question of underlying esophagitis, especially EoE. Esophageal food impaction is a common presenting symptom in children with EoE and esophageal biopsies should be obtained at the time of food bolus removal or later if it is not felt to be safe at time of removal.

Smooth foreign bodies in the stomach, such as marbles or coins, may be monitored without attempting removal for up to several weeks if the child is asymptomatic. Screws and nails are examples of objects with a blunt end that is heavier than the sharp end and will generally pass without incident. In contrast, double-sided sharp objects that are weighted equally on each end, such as fish bones and wooden toothpicks, should be removed as they can migrate through the wall of the GI tract into other organs. A large retrospective study of sharp and pointed FBI in children demonstrated the need for endoscopic removal in 13.6%, with the remainder passing uneventfully. Objects longer than 5 cm may be unable to pass the ligament of Treitz and should be removed.

Multiple magnets, or a single magnet if ingested along with a metallic object, should be removed due to the risk of fistula or erosion of mucosal tissue trapped between two adherent foreign bodies. Rare earth metal magnets, or neodymium magnets, are very powerful small magnets sold in bulk and may cause bowel obstruction, perforation, or fistula necessitating surgical intervention in up to 43%. Ingestion of multiple magnets should lead to immediate endoscopic removal if technically feasible. If not, their migration through the GI tract should be followed radiographically until they have passed. Ingestion of superabsorbent polymers that expand upon contact with an aqueous environment may result in bowel obstruction when ingested by children.

The use of balanced electrolyte lavage solutions containing polyethylene glycol may help the passage of small, smooth foreign bodies lodged in the intestine. Lavage is especially useful in hastening the passage of foreign bodies that may contain an absorbable toxic material such as a heavy metal.

Neal JT, Monuteaux MC, Porter JJ, Hudgins JD: The effect of COVID-19 stay-at-home orders on the rate of pediatric foreign body ingestions. J Emerg Med 2022 Dec;63(6):729–737. Epub 2022 Sep 14 [PMID: 36289021].
Quitadamo P et al: Sharp-pointed foreign body ingestion in pediatric age. J Pediatr Gastroenterol Nutr 2023 Feb 1;76(2):213–217. Epub 2022 Nov 8 [PMID: 36346952].
Scalise PN et al:. Pediatric button battery ingestion: a single center experience and risk score to predict severe outcomes. J Pediatr Surg 2023 Apr;58(4):613–618. Epub 2022 Dec 22 [PMID: 36646540].

DISORDERS OF THE STOMACH & DUODENUM

HIATAL & PARAESOPHAGEAL HERNIA

Hiatal hernias (HHs) are classified into four types, encompassing both sliding HH and paraesophageal HH. Type I is a sliding HH, in which the GE junction and a portion of the proximal stomach is displaced above the diaphragmatic hiatus. Sliding HHs are common, with data showing a prevalence of nearly 21% of all EGDs performed and a correlation between HHs and clinical symptoms of heartburn and regurgitation in children older than 48 months. Paraesophageal HH's encompass types II, III, and IV of HHs, in which the esophagus and GE junction are in their normal anatomic position, but the gastric cardia is herniated through the diaphragmatic hiatus. In studies of HH, type I accounted for 50.9% of hernias, while II–IV combined accounted for 42.8%. Most HHs are acquired, with congenital paraesophageal hernias being rare in childhood. Patients may present with recurrent pulmonary infections, vomiting, anemia, failure to thrive, or dysphagia. HHs can be associated with linear ulcerations, called Cameron lesions, in the portion of the stomach compressed by the thoracic diaphragm, leading to blood loss and iron deficiency anemia. The most common cause of acquired paraesophageal hernia is previous fundoplication surgery, though they have also been described following blunt abdominal trauma and EA/TEF repair. Following fundoplication, the degree of circumferential surgical dissection of the esophageal hiatus is the most important risk factor for HH. Acquired HH may also occur as a complication of congenital diaphragmatic hernia (CDH) repair in more than 10% of patients, with rates largely determined by type of repair and surgical patch used. Neurologic impairment has been associated with HH, in as many as 22.7%. Risk factors include duration of impairment, presence of wasting, tube feeding, and history of aspiration pneumonia.

Radiographic studies typically reveal a cystic mass in the posterior mediastinum or a dilated esophagus. The diagnosis is typically made with an upper GI series or a CT scan of the chest and abdomen, though diagnosis via ultrasound in the prenatal period has been reported. The presence of a ring in the lower esophagus on upper GI has been found to be associated with HH in 96% of children and should increase the index of suspicion. Treatment in symptomatic cases is generally surgical, with laparoscopic repair being used more commonly. Use of robotic-assisted surgery for HH repair in adults is gaining favor and has been reported in children as small as 20 kg. Other than an increase in residual reflux scores for type I patients, outcomes are not significantly different between types I and II–IV. Fundoplication is generally indicated at the time of repair, as rates of significant GERD requiring surgical intervention have been reported as high as 60%.

Zahn KB et al: Longitudinal follow-up with radiologic screening for recurrence and secondary hiatal hernia in neonates with open repair of congenital diaphragmatic hernia—a large prospective, observational cohort study at one referral center. Front Pediatr 2021 Dec 17;9:796478 [PMID: 34976900].

Zheng J, Zhao J, Jiang H, Zhang L: Clinical application of da Vinci robotic-assisted surgery for esophageal hiatal hernia in children. Asian J Surg 2022 Jan;45(1):510–511. Epub 2021 Nov 23 [PMID: 34836760].

PYLORIC STENOSIS

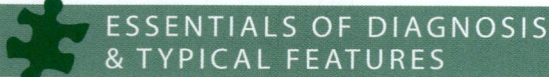

ESSENTIALS OF DIAGNOSIS & TYPICAL FEATURES

► Postnatal muscular hypertrophy of the pylorus.
► Progressive gastric outlet obstruction, nonbilious vomiting, dehydration, and alkalosis in infants younger than 12 weeks.
► Upper GI contrast radiographs or abdominal ultrasound are diagnostic.

The cause of postnatal pyloric muscular hypertrophy with gastric outlet obstruction is unknown. The incidence is 1–8 per 1000 births, with a 4:1 male predominance. Recent studies suggest that erythromycin in the neonatal period is associated with a higher incidence of pyloric stenosis.

▶ Clinical Findings

A. Symptoms and Signs

Projectile postprandial vomiting usually begins between 2 and 4 weeks of age but may start as late as 12 weeks. Vomiting starts at birth in about 10% of cases, and onset of symptoms may be delayed in preterm infants. Vomitus is rarely bilious but may be blood streaked. The upper abdomen may be distended after feeding, and prominent gastric peristaltic waves from left to right may be seen. An oval mass called an "olive" can be felt on deep palpation in the right upper abdomen in a small percentage of infants with pyloric stenosis, especially after vomiting.

B. Laboratory Findings

Hypochloremic alkalosis with potassium depletion is the classic metabolic findings, though low chloride may be seen in as few as 23% and alkalosis in 14.4%. These findings may not be as common in younger infants and their absence should not dissuade from the diagnosis in the appropriate clinical setting. Dehydration causes elevated hemoglobin and hematocrit. Mild unconjugated bilirubinemia occurs in 2%–5% of cases.

C. Imaging

Ultrasonography shows a hypoechoic muscle ring greater than 4 mm thickness with a hyperdense center and a pyloric channel length greater than 15 mm. A barium upper GI series reveals retention of contrast in the stomach and a long narrow pyloric channel with a double track of barium. The hypertrophied muscle mass produces typical semilunar filling defects in the antrum. Infants presenting younger than 21 days may not fulfill these classic ultrasonographic criteria and may require clinical judgment to interpret "borderline" measures of pyloric muscle thickness.

▶ Treatment & Prognosis

Pyloromyotomy is the treatment of choice and consists of incision down to the mucosa along the pyloric length. Treatment of dehydration and electrolyte imbalance is mandatory before surgical treatment, even if it takes 24–48 hours. Patients often vomit postoperatively as a consequence of gastritis, esophagitis, or associated GE reflux.

El-Gohary Y et al: Pyloric stenosis: an enigma more than a century after the first successful treatment. Pediatr Surg Int 2018 Jan;34(1):21–27 [PMID: 29030700].

Vinycomb TI et al: Presentation and outcomes in hypertrophic pyloric stenosis: an 11-year review. J Paediatr Child Health 2019 Oct;55(10):1183–1187 [PMID: 30677197].

GASTRIC & DUODENAL ULCER

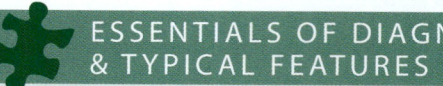

ESSENTIALS OF DIAGNOSIS & TYPICAL FEATURES

► Localized erosions of gastric or duodenal mucosa.
► Pain, vomiting, and bleeding are the most common symptoms.
► Underlying severe illness, *Helicobacter pylori* infection, and nonsteroidal anti-inflammatory drugs (NSAIDs) are the most common causes.

- Eosinophilic GI disease is emerging as an important novel etiology of gastric and duodenal ulcer.
- Successful eradication of *H pylori* infection requires knowledge of regional antimicrobial resistance patterns.
- Diagnosis by endoscopy.

General Considerations

Gastric and duodenal ulcers occur at any age. In the United States, most childhood gastric and duodenal ulcers are associated with underlying illness, toxins, or drugs such as NSAIDs that cause breakdown in mucosal defenses.

Worldwide, the most common cause of gastric and duodenal ulcers is mucosal infection with the bacterium *H pylori*. The prevalence of *H pylori* infection varies greatly by country and increases with poor sanitation, crowded living conditions, and family exposure. Infection is thought to be acquired in childhood, but only in a small percentage of infected persons will infection lead to nodular gastritis, peptic ulcer, or in the case of long-standing infection, gastric lymphoid tumors and gastric adenocarcinoma. In contrast to ulcers secondary to *H pylori*, non–*H pylori* ulcers tend to present at a younger age and are more likely to recur. In a large study of over 1000 children undergoing endoscopy, 5.4% had ulcers, with 47% of these due to *H pylori*, 16.5% related to NSAIDs, and 35.8% unrelated to either *H pylori* or NSAIDs. Recent evidence suggests that the prevalence of non–*H pylori* peptic ulcers is increasing.

Illnesses predisposing to secondary ulcers include central nervous system (CNS) disease, burns, sepsis, multiorgan system failure, chronic lung disease, Crohn disease (CrD), cirrhosis, and rheumatoid arthritis. The most common drugs causing secondary ulcers are aspirin, alcohol, and NSAIDs. NSAID use may lead to ulcers throughout the GI tract but most often clinically relevant in the stomach and duodenum. Severe ulcerative lesions in full-term neonates have been found to be associated with maternal antacid use in the last month of pregnancy.

Clinical Findings

A. Symptoms and Signs

In children younger than 6 years, vomiting and upper GI bleeding are the most common symptoms. Older children are more likely to complain of epigastric abdominal pain. Ulcers in the pyloric channel may cause gastric outlet obstruction. Chronic blood loss may cause iron-deficiency anemia. Deep penetration of the ulcer may erode into a mucosal arteriole and cause acute hemorrhage. Penetrating duodenal ulcers (especially common during cancer chemotherapy, immunosuppression, and in the intensive care setting) may perforate the duodenal wall, resulting in peritonitis or abscess.

B. Diagnostic Studies

Upper GI endoscopy is the most accurate diagnostic examination. The typical endoscopic appearance of an ulcer is a white exudative base with erythematous margins (Figure 21–4). Histopathologic assessment of biopsies obtained at endoscopy provides the opportunity to distinguish between different causes of ulcer disease, including *H pylori* infection, eosinophilic GI disease, celiac disease (CD), and CrD. Endoscopic diagnosis of active *H pylori* infection may be achieved by histologic examination of gastric biopsies or measurement of urease activity on gastric tissue specimens. Additional noninvasive methods of diagnosis of active *H pylori* infection include evaluation of breath for radiolabeled carbon dioxide after administration of radiolabeled urea by mouth and detection of *H pylori* antigen in the stool. False-negative results for the latter two tests have been described when the patient is taking a PPI. Serum antibodies against *H pylori* have poor sensitivity and specificity, and do not prove that there is active infection. For severe or recurrent ulcerations not caused by *H pylori*, stress, or medications, a serum gastrin level may be considered to evaluate for a gastrin-secreting tumor (Zollinger-Ellison syndrome), though mild to moderate elevation in gastrin levels can be seen with the use of PPI drugs. Upper GI barium radiographs may show an ulcer crater. Radiologic signs suggestive of peptic disease in adults (duodenal spasticity and thick irregular folds) are not reliable indicators in children.

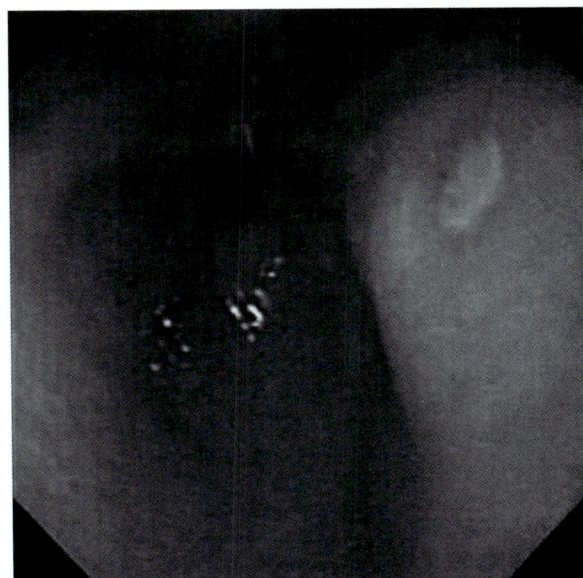

▲ **Figure 21–4.** Gastric ulcer. White exudate coats the ulcer bed of antral ulcer that is surrounded by an erythematous margin.

▶ Treatment

Treatment of symptomatic *H pylori* infection requires eradication of the organism. Standard first-line triple therapy for eradication of *H pylori* has traditionally been a 7- to 10-day treatment course involving simultaneous administration of two oral antibiotics (most commonly, amoxicillin and clarithromycin) and PPI. However, rising rates of resistance to clarithromycin have rendered this combination ineffective in certain parts of the world. As a result, alternative combinations of antimicrobials (metronidazole and tetracycline) have been evaluated. The addition of bismuth to two antibiotics and PPI (bismuth quadruple therapy) may increase efficacy. Because resistance to antibiotics varies greatly by country, regional antibiotic resistance patterns for *H pylori* should be a guide in selecting initial therapy (though often unavailable). Antimicrobial susceptibility testing can be performed on gastric biopsy specimens using a variety of techniques. Test of cure can be achieved by either the urease breath test or fecal *H pylori* antigen test.

Eosinophilic gastrointestinal disease (EGID) is now recognized as a common source of mucosal disease in the stomach and duodenum. Emerging data suggest that this may be the second most common source of gastric and duodenal ulceration in pediatrics after *H pylori*. Gross endoscopic findings are variable, with limited sensitivity, and thus biopsy is indicated in symptomatic patients, even with normal appearing mucosa. PPIs alone or in combination with diet and corticosteroids have been used with variable success. Emerging data suggest potential efficacy of dietary elimination, and there are numerous clinical trials evaluating the role of biologic therapies in the treatment of EGID.

Aguilera MI et al: *Helicobacter pylori* infection in children. BMJ Paediatr Open 2020 Aug 3;4(1):e000679. doi: 10.1136/bmjpo-2020-000679 [PMID: 32818155].

Mousavi T et al: The pharmacotherapeutic management of duodenal and gastric ulcers. Expert Opin Pharmacother 2022 Jan;23(1):63–89. doi: 10.1080/14656566.2021.1959914. Epub 2021 Aug 26 [PMID: 34435515].

Egan M, Furuta GT: Eosinophilic gastrointestinal diseases beyond eosinophilic esophagitis. Ann Allergy Asthma Immunol 2018 Aug;121(2):162–167. doi: 10.1016/j.anai.2018.06.013. Epub 2018 Jun 22 [PMID: 29940308].

Joo JY, Cho JM, Yoo IH, Yang HR: Eosinophilic gastroenteritis as a cause of non-*Helicobacter pylori*, non-gastrotoxic drug ulcers in children. BMC Gastroenterol 2020 Aug 20;20(1):280. doi: 10.1186/s12876-020-01416-7 [PMID: 32819298].

Korotkaya Y et al: *Helicobacter pylori* in pediatric patients. Pediatr Rev 2020 Nov;41(11):585–592. doi: 10.1542/pir.2019-0048 [PMID: 33139411].

Pesek RD et al; Consortium of Eosinophilic Gastrointestinal Disease Researchers (CEGIR): Association between endoscopic and histologic findings in a multicenter retrospective cohort of patients with non-esophageal eosinophilic gastrointestinal disorders. Dig Dis Sci 2020 Jul;65(7):2024–2035. doi: 10.1007/s10620-019-05961-4. Epub 2019 Nov 26 [PMID: 31773359].

Peterson K et al: Emerging therapies for eosinophilic gastrointestinal diseases. J Allergy Clin Immunol Pract 2021 Sep;9(9):3276–3281. doi: org/10.1016/j.jaip.2021.07.031 [PMID: 34343695].

CONGENITAL DIAPHRAGMATIC HERNIA

ESSENTIALS OF DIAGNOSIS & TYPICAL FEATURES

▶ Congenital diaphragmatic hernia (CDH) is often diagnosed prenatally by screening ultrasound.

▶ Postnatal challenges include pulmonary hypoplasia and cardiovascular dysfunction.

▶ After surgical repair, chronic pulmonary disease and GERD can be lifelong morbidities.

Herniation of abdominal contents through the diaphragm complicates 2.3–2.8 per 10,000 live births, usually through a posterolateral defect involving the left side of the diaphragm (foramen of Bochdalek). In about 27% of cases, the diaphragmatic defect is retrosternal (foramen of Morgagni). Bilateral defects occur only rarely, in 3% of cases, and are more likely to result in stillbirth. The herniation of abdominal contents into the thoracic cavity can lead to pulmonary hypoplasia and significant cardiovascular dysfunction including severe persistent pulmonary hypertension after birth.

The eventration of the diaphragm, a subtype of CDH, produces a milder phenotype or may be asymptomatic. In this disorder, a leaf of the diaphragm with hypoplastic muscular elements balloons into the chest.

Diagnosis of CDH is typically made prenatally by ultrasound, although over one-third are not identified on routine prenatal ultrasound. While 60% have isolated CDH, approximately 17% have associated congenital malformations, most commonly cardiovascular structural defects. With improved care of the immediate complications of cardiopulmonary disease in the newborn period using inhaled nitric oxide, high-frequency oscillatory ventilation, and extracorporeal membrane oxygenation (ECMO), survival has improved for infants with CDH up to 70%–90% in some centers. Antenatal intervention with fetoscopic endoluminal tracheal occlusion (FETO) may improve survival in CDH with the "plug-unplug sequence" where the fetal trachea is occluded with a balloon around 27–32 weeks' gestation to induce lung growth, then the balloon is removed around 34 weeks gestation to promote lung maturation and surfactant production. Operative repair of the diaphragmatic defect is usually performed in the newborn period once cardiopulmonary stabilization is achieved, increasingly via laparoscopic and thoracoscopic minimally invasive approaches. Long-term health issues in CDH survivors include chronic pulmonary disease, pulmonary hypertension, neurodevelopmental delays, hearing loss, and GERD.

CONGENITAL DUODENAL OBSTRUCTION

▶ General Considerations

Obstruction is generally classified by intrinsic and extrinsic causes, although rare cases of simultaneous intrinsic and extrinsic anomalies have been reported.

Etiologies of extrinsic duodenal obstruction include congenital peritoneal bands associated with intestinal malrotation, annular pancreas, or duodenal duplication. Intrinsic duodenal obstruction is more common and is typically associated with congenital atresia, stenosis, or mucosal webs (so-called "wind-sock deformity"). In about two-thirds of patients with congenital duodenal obstruction, there are other associated anomalies.

▶ Imaging Studies

Diagnosis of congenital duodenal obstructions is often made prenatally by ultrasound. Prenatal diagnosis predicts complete obstruction in 77% of cases and is associated with polyhydramnios, prematurity, and higher risk of maternal-fetal complications. A "double bubble" (ie, gaseous distention of the stomach and proximal duodenum) may be seen on ultrasound and/or postnatal abdominal plain radiographs. With protracted vomiting, there is less air in the stomach and less abdominal distention. Absence of distal intestinal gas suggests atresia or severe extrinsic obstruction, whereas a pattern of intestinal air scattered over the lower abdomen may indicate partial duodenal obstruction. Barium enema may be helpful in determining the presence of malrotation or atresia in the lower GI tract, as well as evaluating for radiographic evidence of Hirschsprung disease, which may also present with abdominal distension and vomiting.

▶ Clinical Findings

A. Duodenal Atresia

Maternal polyhydramnios is common with fetal duodenal atresia and often leads to prenatal diagnosis by ultrasonography. Vomiting (usually bile-stained) and epigastric distention begin within a few hours of birth. Meconium may be passed normally. Duodenal atresia is often associated with other congenital anomalies (30%), including esophageal atresia, intestinal atresias, and cardiac and renal anomalies. Preterm birth (25%–50%) and Down syndrome (20%–30%) are also associated with duodenal atresia.

B. Duodenal Stenosis and web

Duodenal luminal narrowing (stenosis) or intraluminal mucosal membrane (web) may lead to either complete or incomplete obstruction. Onset of obvious obstructive symptoms may be delayed for weeks or years. Although the stenotic area is usually distal to the ampulla of Vater, the vomitus does not always contain bile.

C. Annular Pancreas

Annular pancreas is a rotational defect in which normal fusion of the dorsal and ventral pancreatic anlagen does not occur, and a ring of pancreatic tissue encircles the duodenum. The presenting symptom is duodenal obstruction. Down syndrome and congenital anomalies of the GI tract are commonly associated. Polyhydramnios is common. Symptoms may develop late in childhood or even in adulthood if the obstruction is not complete. Treatment consists of duodenoduodenostomy or duodenojejunostomy without operative dissection or division of the pancreatic annulus. Pancreatic function is normal.

▶ Treatment & Prognosis

In almost all settings, surgical intervention (either laparoscopic or open) is required for congenital duodenal obstructive lesions. Typically, duodenoduodenostomy is performed to bypass the area of stenosis or atresia. For duodenal stenoses, however, there have been isolated reports of successful endoscopic treatment with balloon dilation. Thorough surgical exploration is typically done to ensure that no lower GI tract anomalies are present. More recent reports document the safety and utility of a laparoscopic approach. The mortality rate is increased in infants with preterm birth, Down syndrome, and associated congenital anomalies. Duodenal dilation and hypomotility from antenatal obstruction may cause duodenal dysmotility with obstructive symptoms even after surgical treatment. Placement of transanastomotic feeding tubes at the time of the initial repair has been found to result in more rapid progression to full enteral feeds and decreased need for parenteral nutrition (PN). The overall prognosis for these patients is good, though the mortality risk is higher in patients with additional anomalies.

Adams SD, Stanton MP: Malrotation and intestinal atresias. Early Hum Dev 2014 Dec;90(12):921–925 [PMID: 25448782].

Brinkley MF, Tracy ET, Maxfield CM: Congenital duodenal obstruction: causes and imaging approach. Pediatr Radiol 2016 Jul;46(8):1084–1895. doi: 10.1007/s00247-016-3603-1. Review [PMID: 27324508].

Morris G, Kennedy A Jr: Small bowel congenital anomalies: a review and update. Surg Clin North Am 2022 Oct;102(5):821–835. doi: 10.1016/j.suc.2022.07.012. Epub 2022 Sep 13 [PMID: 36209748].

DISORDERS OF THE SMALL INTESTINE

INTESTINAL ATRESIA & STENOSIS

Excluding anal anomalies, intestinal atresia or stenosis accounts for one-third of all cases of neonatal intestinal obstruction (see Chapter 2). Antenatal ultrasound can identify intestinal atresia in utero; polyhydramnios occurs in most affected pregnancies. Sensitivity of antenatal ultrasound is greater in more proximal atresias. Other congenital anomalies may be present in up to 54% of cases. Approximately half of affected infants are delivered preterm. Occult congenital cardiac anomalies have been reported in as many as 30% of apparently isolated atresia cases. In one large population-based study, the prevalence was 2.9 per 10,000 births, although there is some evidence that the prevalence may be increasing. The localization and relative incidence of atresias and stenoses are listed in Table 21–1. Although jejunal and ileal atresias are often grouped together, there are data to suggest that jejunal atresias are associated with increased morbidity and mortality compared to ileal atresia. These differences may be related to increased compliance of the jejunal wall, resulting in more proximal dilation and subsequent loss in peristaltic activity.

Bile-stained vomitus and abdominal distention begin in the first 48 hours of life. Multiple sites in the intestine may be affected. In addition to stenoses, the overall length of the small intestine may be significantly shortened. Radiographic features include dilated loops of small bowel and absence of colonic gas. Barium enema reveals narrow-caliber microcolon because of lack of intestinal flow distal to the atresia. In over 10% of patients with intestinal atresia, the mesentery is absent, and the superior mesenteric artery (SMA) cannot be identified beyond the origin of the right colic and ileocolic arteries. The ileum coils around one of these two arteries, giving rise to the so-called Christmas tree deformity on contrast radiographs. The tenuous blood supply often compromises surgical anastomoses.

The differential diagnosis of intestinal atresia includes Hirschsprung disease, paralytic ileus secondary to sepsis, midgut volvulus, and meconium ileus. Surgery is mandatory. Postoperative complications include short bowel syndrome (SBS) in 15% and small bowel hypomotility secondary to antenatal obstruction. Overall mortality has been reported at 8%, with increased risk in low-birthweight and premature infants.

Adams SD, Stanton MP: Malrotation and intestinal atresias. Early Hum Dev 2014 Dec;90(12):921–925 [PMID: 25448782].
Morris G, Kennedy A Jr: Small bowel congenital anomalies: a review and update. Surg Cin North Am 2022 Oct;102(5): 821–835. doi: 10.1016/j.Suc.2022.07.012. Epub 2022 Sep 13 [PMID: 36209748].

INTESTINAL MALROTATION

▶ General Considerations

The midgut extends from the duodenojejunal junction to the mid-transverse colon. It is supplied by the SMA, which runs in the root of the mesentery. During gestation, the midgut elongates into the umbilical sac, returning to an intra-abdominal position during the 10th week of gestation. The root of the mesentery rotates in a counterclockwise direction during retraction causing the colon to cross the abdominal cavity ventrally. The cecum moves from the left to the right lower quadrant, and the duodenum crosses dorsally becoming partly retroperitoneal. When rotation is incomplete, the dorsal fixation of the mesentery is defective and shortened, so that the bowel from the ligament of Treitz to the mid-transverse colon may rotate around its narrow mesenteric root and occlude the SMA (volvulus). Up to 1% of the general population may have intestinal malrotation, which is diagnosed in the first year of life in 70%–90% of patients. The remainder are diagnosed later in life or on autopsy.

▶ Clinical Findings

A. Symptoms and Signs

Malrotation with volvulus accounts for 10% of neonatal intestinal obstructions. Most infants present in the first 3 weeks of life with bile-stained vomitus or with overt small bowel obstruction. Intrauterine volvulus may cause intestinal obstruction or perforation at birth. The neonate may present

Table 21–1. Localization and relative frequency of congenital gastrointestinal atresias and stenoses.

	Area Involved	Type of Lesion	Relative Frequency (%)
Pylorus		Atresia; web or diaphragm	1
Duodenum	80% are distal to the ampulla of Vater	Atresia, stenosis; web or diaphragm	45
Jejunoileal	Proximal jejunum and distal ileum	Atresia (multiple in 6%–29%); stenosis	50
Colon	Left colon and rectum	Atresia (usually associated with atresias of the small bowel)	5–9

with ascites or meconium peritonitis. Later presenting signs include intermittent intestinal obstruction, malabsorption, protein-losing enteropathy, or diarrhea. Associated congenital anomalies, especially cardiac, occur in over 25% of symptomatic patients. Many of these may be found in a subgroup of malrotation patients with heterotaxy syndromes, with associated asplenia or polysplenia. Older children and adults with undiagnosed malrotation typically present with chronic GI symptoms of nausea, vomiting, diarrhea, abdominal pain, dyspepsia, bloating, and early satiety.

B. Imaging

An upper GI series is considered the gold standard for diagnosis, with a reported sensitivity of 96%, and classically shows the duodenojejunal junction and the jejunum on the right side of the spine. The diagnosis of malrotation can be further confirmed by barium enema, which may demonstrate a mobile cecum located in the midline, right upper quadrant, or left abdomen. Plain films of the abdomen in the newborn period may show a "double-bubble" sign, resulting in a misdiagnosis of duodenal atresia. CT scan and ultrasound of the abdomen may be used to make the diagnosis as well and are characterized by the "whirlpool sign" denoting midgut volvulus. Reversal of the normal position of the SMA and superior mesenteric vein (SMV) may be seen in malrotation, though normal position may be found in up to 29% of patients. Identification of the third portion of the duodenum within the retroperitoneum makes malrotation very unlikely.

Treatment & Prognosis

Surgical treatment of malrotation is the Ladd procedure. In young infants the Ladd procedure should be performed even if volvulus has not occurred. The duodenum is mobilized, the short mesenteric root is extended, and the bowel is then fixed in a more normal distribution. Because volvulus can occur at any age, surgical repair is usually recommended, even in asymptomatic children. Laparoscopic repair of malrotation is possible but is technically difficult and is never performed in the presence of volvulus.

Midgut volvulus is a surgical emergency as occlusion of the SMA leads to bowel necrosis. When necrosis is extensive, a two-stage surgical intervention is recommended. The first operation includes only reduction of the volvulus with lysis of mesenteric bands. A second operation, 24–48 hours later, is done to resect necrotic bowel. The delay between surgeries is typically undertaken in the hope that more bowel can be salvaged. The prognosis is guarded if perforation, peritonitis, or extensive intestinal necrosis is present. Mid-gut volvulus is one of the most common indications for small bowel transplant in children, responsible for 10% of cases in a recent series.

Adams SD, Stanton MP: Malrotation and intestinal atresias. Early Hum Dev 2014 Dec;90(12):921–925 [PMID: 25448782].

Langer JC: Intestinal rotation abnormalities and midgut volvulus. Surg Clin North Am 2017 Feb;97(1):147–159. doi: 10.1016/j.suc.2016.08.011. Review [PMID: 27894424].
Morris G, Kennedy A Jr: Small bowel congenital anomalies: a review and update. Surg Clin North Am 2022 Oct;102(5): 821–835. doi: 10.1016/j.suc.2022.07.012. Epub 2022 Sep 13 [PMID: 36209748].

SHORT BOWEL SYNDROME

General Considerations

Short bowel syndrome (SBS) is defined as a condition resulting from reduced intestinal absorptive surface that leads to alteration in intestinal function that compromises normal growth, fluid/electrolyte balance, or hydration status. Most pediatric patients with SBS have undergone neonatal surgical resection of intestine. The most common etiologies in children are necrotizing enterocolitis (45%); intestinal atresias (23%); gastroschisis (15%); volvulus (15%); and, less commonly, congenital short bowel, long-segment Hirschsprung disease, and ischemic bowel. In many instances, infants with SBS require PN in order to provide adequate caloric, fluid, and electrolyte delivery in the setting of insufficient intestinal absorptive function. The requirement of supplemental PN for more than 2–3 months in the setting of SBS or any other underlying disorder qualifies the diagnosis of intestinal failure (IF).

Many factors, including patient's gestational age, postsurgical anatomy (including residual small bowel length and presence of ileocecal valve and/or colon), presence of small bowel bacterial overgrowth, and underlying etiology leading to intestinal resection influence the process and likelihood of bowel adaptation and enteral autonomy. No specific anatomic bowel length measurements offer 100% certainty in predicting clinical outcomes in SBS.

Symptoms & Signs

Typical signs for the patient with SBS are related to their underlying malabsorptive state, including diarrhea, dehydration, electrolyte or micronutrient deficiency states, and growth failure. Patients with SBS are also at risk for small bowel obstruction, bowel dilation and dysmotility (with secondary small bowel bacterial overgrowth), hepatobiliary disorders including cholelithiasis, nephrolithiasis due to calcium oxalate stones, oral feeding challenges, and GI mucosal inflammatory problems including noninfectious colitis and anastomotic ulcerations. For patients with IF, complications related to underlying PN therapy are common and can be life threatening (see Chapter 11).

Treatment & Prognosis

Treatment of SBS should promote growth and adaptation while minimizing and/or treating complications of the underlying intestinal disorder or PN therapy. Outcomes are improved when intestinal rehabilitation is undertaken by a multidisciplinary team approach, involving gastroenterology, nutrition, and surgery. Enteral nutrition should be adjusted to favor absorption, commonly requiring continuous delivery of an elemental formula through a gastrostomy tube. Commonly prescribed pharmacologic adjuncts include acid suppressive therapy, antimotility and antidiarrheal agents, and antibiotics for the treatment of small bowel bacterial overgrowth. Recently, a glucagon-like peptide-2 analogue (teduglutide) has been approved for use in pediatric patients. This therapy reduced the volume of PN prescribed in patients with IF/SBS and offers the potential to accelerate intestinal adaptation and PN weaning.

Management for the patient with SBS and IF should include strategies to manage or prevent complications related to PN therapy, including infection and liver disease. Antimicrobial lock solutions distilled into central venous catheters using either ethanol or antibiotics may have a role in reducing infection rates. Compelling evidence over the past several years suggests that modification of parenteral lipid solution, either through reduction in dose of soy-based intralipid or replacement with a third-generation lipid solution (Omegaven or SMOF lipid), improves outcomes associated with PN-associated liver disease (PNALD) in pediatric patients.

Autologous bowel reconstructive surgery (bowel lengthening) should be considered in a patient who is failing to advance enterally and has anatomy amenable to surgical intervention. Both the serial transverse enteroplasty (STEP) procedure and longitudinal intestinal lengthening and tailoring (Bianchi) procedure have been successful in allowing weaning from TPN in up to 50% of patients in reported series. In recent years, the STEP procedure has gained favor as being potentially less technically demanding and repeatable, if the bowel dilates sufficiently after the initial procedure.

When medical, nutritional, and surgical management fails, intestinal transplantation may be considered for a child with refractory and life-threatening complications of IF. Current outcome data after pediatric intestinal transplantation suggest 1- and 3-year survival rates of 83% and 60%, respectively.

Duggan CP, Jaksic T: Pediatric intestinal failure. N Engl J Med 2017 Aug 17;377(7):666–675 [PMID: 28813225].

Jaksic T: Current short bowel syndrome management: an era of improved outcomes and continued challenges. J Pediatr Surg 2023 May;58(5):789–798. doi: 10.1016/j.jpedsurg.2023.01.011. Epub 2023 Jan 20 [PMID: 36870826].

Lee EJ, Mazariegos GV, Bond GJ: Pediatric intestinal transplantation. Semin Pediatr Surg 2022 Jun;31(3):151181. doi: 10.1016/j.sempedsurg.2022.151181. Epub 2022 May 20 [PMID: 35725057].

Oliveira SB, Cole CR: Insights into medical management of pediatric intestinal failure. Semin Pediatr Surg 2018 Aug;27(4): 256–260. doi: 10.1053/j.sempedsurg.2018.07.006. Epub 2018 Jul 29 [PMID: 30342600].

Wendel D, Cole CR, Cohran VC: Approach to intestinal failure in children. Curr Gastroenterol Rep 2021 Apr 15;23(6):8. doi: 10.1007/s11894-021-00807-4 [PMID: 33860385].

INTUSSUSCEPTION

ESSENTIALS OF DIAGNOSIS & TYPICAL FEATURES

► Intussusception is the most common cause of bowel obstruction in the first 2 years of life.

► The most common location for intussusception is ileocolic, and 85% of cases are idiopathic.

► Ultrasound is the most sensitive and specific diagnostic modality for intussusception.

► Air enema is the best therapeutic approach in a stable patient, successfully reducing 75% of cases.

Intussusception occurs when one segment of the intestine telescopes into another. Intussusception can occur anywhere along the small and large bowel, often starting just proximal to the ileocecal valve and extending for varying distances into the colon. It is the most frequent cause of intestinal obstruction in the first 2 years of life and is three times more common in males. Obstruction and ischemia occur from swelling, hemorrhage, vascular compromise, and necrosis of the intussuscepted ileum. The likelihood of identifying a cause of intussusception increases with a patient's age, but 85% are idiopathic in children. Implicated primary causes of intussusception include small bowel polyp, Meckel diverticulum, omphalomesenteric remnant, duplication cyst, lymphoma, lipoma, parasites, foreign bodies, and, most commonly, viral enteritis with hypertrophy of Peyer patches. Intussusception of the small bowel can also be seen in CD, cystic fibrosis, and Henoch-Schönlein purpura. In children older than 6 years, lymphoma is the most common cause of intussusception.

► Clinical Findings

Classically, a previously healthy infant 3–12 months old develops recurring paroxysms of abdominal pain with screaming and drawing up the knees. Vomiting and diarrhea occur next in 90% of cases, and bloody bowel movements with mucus (described as "currant jelly stools") appear in half within the next 12 hours. The child is characteristically lethargic between paroxysms and may be febrile. The abdomen is tender and often distended. A sausage-shaped mass may be palpated, usually in the upper mid abdomen.

In older children, sudden attacks of abdominal pain may be related to chronic recurrent intussusception with spontaneous reduction between.

Diagnosis & Treatment

The constellation of abdominal pain, lethargy, vomiting, and a suspicious abdominal radiograph was found to have a sensitivity of 95% in identifying intussusceptions in children. Abdominal radiographs alone, however, have poor sensitivity for diagnosing intussusception, whereas abdominal ultrasound has 98%–100% sensitivity. Barium enema and air enema are both diagnostic and therapeutic, but reduction of the intussusception by barium enema should not be attempted if signs of strangulated bowel, perforation, or toxicity are present. Air insufflation of the colon under fluoroscopic guidance is a safe alternative to barium enema with excellent diagnostic sensitivity and specificity without the risk of contaminating the abdominal cavity with barium. Rates of successful reduction by air enema approach 75%, and when initial enema reduction is successful, recurrence of intussusception within 24–48 hours occurs in less than 5% of patients. The rate of perforation with either liquid or air enema is approximately 1%, but if ischemic damage to the intestine is suspected based on symptom severity (shock or sepsis), the risk of perforation increases, and surgical reduction is preferred. Surgery is thus required for extremely ill patients including those with evidence of bowel perforation, or after unsuccessful hydrostatic or pneumatic reduction. Surgeons can intraoperatively identify a lead point such as Meckel diverticulum, lymphoma, or small bowel polyp. Surgical reduction of intussusception is associated with an even lower recurrence rate than pneumatic reduction.

Prognosis

Successful reduction by enema is less likely when symptoms have been present over 24 hours. Having symptoms greater than 24 hours increases the risk of subsequent bowel resection from 17% to 39% in patients needing surgery. Overall mortality rate with treatment is 1%–2%.

Gray MP et al: Recurrence rates after intussusception enema reduction: a meta-analysis. 2014 Jul;134(1):110–119. doi: 10.1542/peds.2013-3102 [PMID: 24935997].

INGUINAL HERNIA

Inguinal hernias may present at any age, are most often indirect, and occur 9x more frequently in boys. The incidence in preterm male infants is 5% overall, with higher incidence (30%) in male infants weighing 1000 g or less.

Clinical Findings

In most cases, a hernia is a painless inguinal swelling. Parents may be the only one to see the mass, as it may retract when the infant is active, cold, frightened, or agitated. Clinical clues include inguinal fullness after coughing or long periods of standing, or presence of a firm, globular, and tender swelling, sometimes associated with vomiting and abdominal distention. Sometimes a herniated loop of intestine may become partially obstructed causing severe pain. Rarely, bowel becomes trapped in the hernia sac, and complete intestinal obstruction occurs, with gangrene of the hernia contents or testis. A suggestive history often is the only criterion for diagnosis, along with the "silk glove" feel of the rubbing together of the two walls of the empty hernia sac.

Differential Diagnosis

Inguinal lymph nodes may be mistaken for a hernia but are usually multiple with more discrete borders. A hydrocele of the spermatic cord should transilluminate. An undescended testis is usually mobile in the canal with absence of the gonad in the scrotum.

Treatment

Incarceration of an inguinal hernia is more likely to occur in boys or when younger than 10 months. Manual reduction of incarcerated inguinal hernias can be attempted after the sedated infant is placed in the Trendelenburg position with an ice bag on the affected side. Manual reduction is contraindicated if incarcerated for more than 12 hours or if bloody stools are noted. Surgery is indicated if a hernia has ever incarcerated and is often undertaken preventatively in higher risk children.

Esposito C et al: Laparoscopic versus open inguinal hernia repair in pediatric patients: a systematic review. J Laparoendosc Adv Surg Tech A 2014 Nov;24(11):811–818 [PMID: 25299121].
Gause CD et al: Laparoscopic versus open inguinal hernia repair in children ≤3: a randomized controlled trial. Pediatr Surg Int 2017 Mar;33(3):367–376. doi: 10.1007/s00383-016-4029-4 [PMID: 28025693].

UMBILICAL HERNIA

Umbilical hernias are most common in full-term Black infants. Small bowel may very rarely incarcerate in small-diameter umbilical hernias, but most umbilical hernias regress spontaneously if the fascial defect has a diameter of less than 1 cm. Generally, asymptomatic umbilical hernias are managed expectantly with no intervention until age 4–5 years, then are treated surgically if persistent.

PATENT OMPHALOMESENTERIC DUCT

ESSENTIALS OF DIAGNOSIS & TYPICAL FEATURES

▶ Persistent umbilical discharge in an infant may represent a patent omphalomesenteric duct.

▶ Ultrasound is the preferred diagnostic method for patent omphalomesenteric duct.

▶ Surgical excision of the omphalomesenteric remnant is required.

The omphalomesenteric duct connects the fetal yolk sac to the developing gut and is usually obliterated early in embryologic development. When this fails, a structure from the embryonic duct remnant connects the ileum to the undersurface of the umbilicus. If the remnant is patent, it can lead to herniation of intestinal contents into the umbilical cord or lead to fecal discharge from the umbilicus. A fibrous cord may become the focal point for volvulus and small bowel obstruction, or a cause of chronic abdominal pain. Mucoid umbilical discharge may indicate a mucocele in the omphalomesenteric remnant, opening at the umbilicus. A closed mucocele may protrude through the umbilicus and appear as a firm, bright red, polypoid mass that may be mistaken for an umbilical granuloma. Ultrasound or abdominal CT can help confirm the diagnosis of an omphalomesenteric duct remnant, and surgical excision of omphalomesenteric remnants is indicated.

Kadian YS, Verma A, Rattan KN, Kajal P: Vitellointestinal duct anomalies in infancy. J Neonatal Surg 2016 Jul 3;5(3):30. doi: 10.21699/jns.v5i3.351 [PMID: 27433448].

Kelly KB et al: Pediatric abdominal wall defects. Surg Clin North Am 2013 Oct;93(5):1255–1267 [PMID: 24035087].

Zens T, Nichol PF, Cartmill R, Kohler JE: Management of asymptomatic pediatric umbilical hernias: a systematic review. J Pediatr Surg 2017 Nov;52(11):1723–1731. doi: 10.1016/J. Jpedsurg.2017.07.016. Epub 2017 Jul 24 [PMID: 28778691].

MECKEL DIVERTICULUM

Meckel diverticulum is the most common form of omphalomesenteric duct remnant. It occurs in 1.5% of the population and is asymptomatic for most. If complications occur, they are three times more common in males than in females. More than 50% of complications occur in the first 2 years of life.

▶ Clinical Findings

A. Symptoms and Signs

Forty to 60% of symptomatic patients have painless episodes of maroon or melanotic rectal bleeding. Bleeding is due to ileal ulcers adjacent to the diverticulum caused by acid secreted from heterotopic gastric tissue. It may be large enough in volume to cause shock and anemia. Occult bleeding is less common. Intestinal obstruction occurs in 25% of symptomatic patients due to ileocolonic intussusception. Intestinal volvulus may occur around a fibrous remnant of the vitelline duct extending from the tip of the diverticulum to the abdominal wall. Meckel diverticula may be trapped in an inguinal hernia.

B. Imaging

Diagnosis of Meckel diverticulum is made with a Meckel scan. Technetium-99m (^{99m}Tc) is taken up by the heterotopic gastric mucosa in the diverticulum and outlines the diverticulum on a nuclear scan. Giving pentagastrin or famotidine before administering the radionuclide increases ^{99m}Tc uptake and retention by the heterotopic gastric mucosa that increases the sensitivity of the test.

▶ Treatment & Prognosis

Treatment is surgical and the prognosis for Meckel diverticulum is good.

ACUTE APPENDICITIS

▶ General Considerations

Acute appendicitis is the most common indication for emergency abdominal surgery in childhood. The frequency increases with age and peaks between 15 and 30 years. Obstruction of the appendix by fecalith (25%) is a common predisposing factor. Parasites may rarely cause obstruction (especially ascarids). Most of the remaining cases are idiopathic. The incidence of perforation is high in childhood (40%), especially in children younger than 2 years, in whom pain is often poorly localized and symptoms nonspecific. To avoid delay in diagnosis, it is important to maintain close communication with parents and perform a thorough initial physical examination with sequential examinations at frequent intervals over several hours to correctly interpret the evolving symptoms and signs.

▶ Clinical Findings

A. Symptoms and Signs

Patients typically present early with periumbilical abdominal pain, which then migrates to the lower right quadrant. Anorexia, vomiting, pain with movement, fever can also occur. Contrary to the vomiting of acute gastroenteritis, which usually precedes abdominal pain, vomiting in appendicitis usually follows the onset of pain. The clinical picture is frequently atypical, especially in young children and infants. Serial examinations are critical in differentiating appendicitis from the many other conditions that transiently mimic its symptoms.

B. Laboratory Findings

The white blood cell count is seldom higher than 15,000/μL. The combination of elevated C-reactive protein (CRP) and leukocytosis has been reported to have positive predictive value of 92% for acute appendicitis, although having normal values for both measures does not exclude the diagnosis.

C. Imaging

In experienced hands, ultrasonography of the appendix shows a noncompressible, thickened appendix in 93% of cases. Abdominal CT after rectal instillation of contrast may be diagnostic. An otherwise normal abdominal CT scan with a nonvisualized appendix has still been reported to have a negative predictive value of 99%. Analysis of diagnostic strategies for pediatric patients with suspected appendicitis has shown abdominal ultrasound, followed by CT scan for negative studies, to be the most cost-effective diagnostic approach.

▶ Differential Diagnosis

Acute gastroenteritis, pneumonia, urinary tract infection, nephrolithiasis, and pelvic inflammatory disease may mimic appendicitis. Acute gastroenteritis with *Yersinia enterocolitica* may present as pseudoappendicitis in 17% of cases. Other medical and surgical conditions causing acute abdomen should also be considered (see Table 21–7).

▶ Treatment & Prognosis

Exploratory laparotomy or laparoscopy is indicated when the diagnosis of acute appendicitis cannot be ruled out after a period of close observation. Treatment for appendicitis is appendectomy, however non operative management with antibiotics is an alternative for patients with low risk of perforation. The mortality rate is less than 1% during childhood, despite the high incidence of perforation.

Lipsett SC, Monuteaux MC, Shanahan KH, Bachur RG: Nonoperative management of uncomplicated appendicitis. Pediatrics. 2022 May 1;149(5):e2021054693. doi: 10.1542/peds.2021-054693 [PMID: 35434736].

Minneci PC et al; Midwest Pediatric Surgery Consortium: Association of nonoperative management using antibiotic therapy vs laparoscopic appendectomy with treatment success and disability days in children with uncomplicated appendicitis. JAMA 2020 Aug 11;324(6):581–593. doi: 10.1001/jama.2020.10888 [PMID: 32730561].

DUPLICATIONS OF THE GASTROINTESTINAL TRACT

Enteric duplications are congenital spherical or tubular structures found mostly in the ileum but also occurring in the duodenum, rectum, and esophagus. Most duplications do not communicate with the intestinal lumen. Symptoms of vomiting, abdominal distention, colicky abdominal pain, rectal bleeding, partial or total intestinal obstruction, or an abdominal mass may start in infancy. Diarrhea and malabsorption may result from bacterial overgrowth in communicating duplications. Physical examination may reveal a rounded, smooth, movable mass, and barium radiograph or CT of the abdomen may show a noncalcified cystic mass displacing other organs. Technetium-99m scan may help identify duplications containing gastric mucosa. Duplications of the ileum can give rise to an intussusception. Prompt surgical treatment is indicated.

Erginel B et al: Enteric duplication cysts in children: a single-institution series with forty patients in twenty-six years. World J Surg 2017 Feb;41(2):620–624. doi: 10.1007/s00268-016-3742-4 [PMID: 27734079].

▼ DISORDERS OF THE COLON

CONGENITAL AGANGLIONIC MEGACOLON (HIRSCHSPRUNG DISEASE)

▶ General Considerations

Hirschsprung disease results from an absence of ganglion cells in the mucosal and muscular layers of the colon. Neural crest cells fail to migrate into the gut mesodermal layers during gestation. The absence of ganglion cells results in failure of the colonic muscles to relax. In 80% of individuals, aganglionosis is restricted to the rectosigmoid colon (short-segment disease); in 15%–20%, aganglionosis extends proximal to the sigmoid colon (long-segment disease); in about 5%, aganglionosis affects the entire colon (total colonic aganglionosis). Segmental aganglionosis is possible but rare.

Aganglionic segments have normal or slightly narrowed caliber with dilation of the normal colon proximal to the aganglionic segment. The mucosa of the dilated colonic segment may become thin and inflamed, causing diarrhea, bleeding, and protein loss (enterocolitis).

A familial pattern has been described, particularly in total colonic aganglionosis. The incidence of Hirschsprung disease is 1 in 5000 live births and is four times more common in boys than girls. A chromosomal abnormality is present in approximately 12% of individuals with Hirschsprung disease. Mutations in the RET proto-oncogene have been identified in about 15% of nonsyndromic cases. The most common chromosomal abnormality associated with Hirschsprung disease is Down syndrome; 2%–10% of individuals with Down syndrome may be affected.

▶ Clinical Findings

A. Symptoms and Signs

Failure of the newborn to pass meconium, followed by vomiting, abdominal distention, and reluctance to feed suggest the diagnosis of Hirschsprung disease. Enterocolitis manifested by fever, dehydration and explosive diarrhea is reported in approximately 50% of affected newborns. Enterocolitis may lead to inflammatory and ischemic changes in the colon, with perforation and sepsis. In some patients, especially those with short segments involved, symptoms are not obvious at birth. In later infancy, alternating obstipation, difficulty passing feces, and diarrhea predominate. The older child is more likely to have constipation alone. Symptoms can include foul-smelling or ribbon-like stools, a distended abdomen, intermittent bouts of intestinal obstruction, hypoproteinemia, and failure to thrive. Encopresis is rare. On digital rectal examination, the anal canal and rectum are devoid of fecal material despite obvious retained stool on abdominal examination or radiographs. If the aganglionic segment is short, there may be a gush of flatus and stool as the finger is withdrawn on rectal examination.

B. Laboratory Findings

On rectal suction biopsy samples, ganglion cells are absent in both the submucosal and muscular layers of the affected bowel. Special stains may show nerve trunk hypertrophy and increased acetylcholinesterase activity.

C. Imaging

Plain abdominal radiographs may reveal dilated proximal colon and absence of gas in the pelvic colon. Barium enema using a catheter without a balloon and with the tip inserted barely beyond the anal sphincter usually demonstrates a narrow distal segment with a sharp transition to the proximal dilated (normal) colon. Transition zones may not be seen in neonates since the normal proximal bowel has not had time to become dilated.

D. Special Examinations

Rectal manometric testing reveals failure of rectoanal inhibitory reflex (*RAIR*), relaxation of the internal anal sphincter after distention of the rectum in patients with Hirschsprung disease, regardless of the length of the aganglionic segment.

▶ Differential Diagnosis

Hirschsprung disease accounts for 15%–20% of cases of neonatal intestinal obstruction. In childhood, Hirschsprung disease must be differentiated from retentive constipation, hypothyroidism, intestinal pseudo-obstruction, and other motility disorders.

▶ Treatment & Prognosis

Treatment is surgical to resect the affected aganglionic segment. Depending on the child's size and state of health, this may be performed in stages such as an initial diverting colostomy (or ileostomy), to allow the dilated bowel to decompress or may be done in a single surgery. At the time of definitive surgery, the transition zone between ganglionated and nonganglionated bowel is identified. Aganglionic bowel is resected, and a pull-through of ganglionated bowel to the preanal rectal remnant is made.

Complications after surgery include fecal retention, fecal incontinence, anastomotic breakdown, or anastomotic stricture. Postoperative obstruction may result from inadvertent retention of a distal aganglionic colon segment or postoperative destruction of ganglion cells secondary to vascular impairment. Neuronal dysplasia of the remaining bowel may produce a pseudo-obstruction syndrome. Enterocolitis occurs postoperatively in 15% of patients. Recent studies have shown that patients have an altered microbiome even after surgical correction. The role this may play in enterocolitis or other long-term issues for children is still under investigation.

Davidson JR et al: Long-term surgical and patient-reported outcomes of Hirschsprung disease. J Pediatr Surg 2021 Sep;56(9):1502–1511. doi: 10.1016/j.jpedsurg.2021.01.043. Epub 2021 Feb 13 [PMID: 33706942].

Tilghman JM et al: Molecular genetic anatomy and risk profile of Hirschsprung's disease. N Engl J Med 2019 Apr 11; 380(15):1421–1432. doi: 10.1056/nejmoa1706594 [PMID: 30970187].

CONSTIPATION

Chronic constipation in childhood is defined as two or more of the following characteristics for 2 months: (1) fewer than three bowel movements per week; (2) more than one episode of encopresis per week; (3) impaction of the rectum with stool; (4) passage of stool so large it obstructs the toilet; (5) retentive posturing and fecal withholding; and (6) pain with defecation. Retention of feces in the rectum can result in overflow incontinence (encopresis) in 60% of children with constipation. Most constipation in childhood is a result of voluntary or involuntary retentive behavior (chronic retentive constipation). About 2% of healthy primary school children have chronic retentive constipation. The ratio of males to females may be as high as 4:1.

▶ Clinical Findings

Infants younger than 3 months often grunt, strain, and turn red in the face while passing normal stools, which is referred to as infant dyschezia. Failure to appreciate this normal developmental pattern may lead to the unnecessary use of laxatives or rectal stimulation. Infants and children may, however, develop the ability to ignore the sensation of rectal fullness and retain stool. Many factors reinforce this behavior, which results in impaction of the rectum and overflow incontinence. Among these are painful defecation; skeletal muscle weakness; psychological issues, especially those relating to control and authority; modesty and distaste for school bathrooms; medications; and other factors listed in

Table 21–2. Causes of constipation.

Functional or retentive causes	Abnormalities of myenteric
Dietary causes	**ganglion cells**
Undernutrition, dehydration	Hirschsprung disease
Excessive milk intake	Waardenburg syndrome
Lack of bulk	Multiple endocrine
Cathartic abuse	neoplasia 2a
Drugs	**Hypo- and hyperganglionosis**
Narcotics	von Recklinghausen disease
Antihistamines	Multiple endocrine
Some antidepressants	neoplasia 2b
Vincristine	Intestinal neuronal dysplasia
Structural defects of	Chronic intestinal
gastrointestinal tract	pseudo-obstruction
Anus and rectum	**Spinal cord defects**
Fissure, hemorrhoids,	**Metabolic and endocrine**
abscess	**disorders**
Anterior ectopic anus	Hypothyroidism
Anal and rectal stenosis	Hyperparathyroidism
Presacral teratoma	Renal tubular acidosis
Small bowel and colon	Diabetes insipidus
Tumor, stricture	(dehydration)
Chronic volvulus	Vitamin D intoxication
Intussusception	(hypercalcemia)
Smooth muscle diseases	Idiopathic hypercalcemia
Scleroderma and	**Skeletal muscle weakness or**
dermatomyositis	**incoordination**
Systemic lupus erythematosus	Cerebral palsy
Chronic intestinal	Muscular dystrophy/
pseudo-obstruction	myotonia

Reproduced with permission from Silverman A, Roy CC: *Pediatric Clinical Gastroenterology*, 3rd ed. Philadelphia, PA: Mosby; 1983.

Table 21–2. The dilated rectum gradually becomes less sensitive to fullness, thus perpetuating the problem.

▶ Differential Diagnosis

One must distinguish between chronic retentive constipation from Hirschsprung disease as summarized in Table 21–3.

▶ Treatment

In children with poor diets increased intake of high-residue foods such as bran, whole wheat, fruits and vegetables, and water may be sufficient therapy in mild constipation. If diet change alone is ineffective, medications may be required. Polyethylene glycol solution (MiraLax), 0.8–1 g/kg/day, lactulose 1–2 g/kg/day, and milk of magnesia (400–1200 mg/day for 2- to 5-years-old; 1200–2400 mg/day for 6–11 years old) are safe stool softeners in infants and children. Stimulant laxatives such as Senna or Bisacodyl can be considered as an additional or second-line treatment. If encopresis is present, treatment should start with relieving fecal impaction. Disimpaction can be achieved in several ways, including medications such as saline enemas, and nonabsorbable osmotic

Table 21–3. Differentiation of retentive constipation and Hirschsprung disease.

	Retentive Constipation	Hirschsprung Disease
Onset	2–3 y	At birth
Abdominal distention	Rare	Present
Nutrition and growth	Normal	Poor
Soiling and retentive behavior	Intermittent or constant	Rare
Rectal examination	Ampulla full	Ampulla may be empty
Rectal biopsy	Ganglion cells present	Ganglion cells absent
Rectal manometry	Normal rectoanal reflex	Nonrelaxation of internal anal sphincter after rectal distention
Barium enema	Distended rectum	Narrow distal segment with proximal megacolon

agents such as polyethylene glycol and milk of magnesia. Effective stool softeners should thereafter be given regularly in doses sufficient to induce very soft daily bowel movements. After several weeks to months of regular soft stools, stool softeners can be tapered and stopped. Recurrence of encopresis is common and should be treated promptly with a short course of stimulant laxatives or an enema. Psychology consultation may be indicated for patients with resistant symptoms or severe emotional disturbances.

Pärtty A, Rautava S, Kalliomäki M: Probiotics on pediatric functional gastrointestinal disorders. Nutrients 2018 Nov 29;10(12): 1836 [PMID: 30501103].

Shin A, Preidis GA, Shulman R, Kashyap PC: The gut microbiome in adult and pediatric functional gastrointestinal disorders. Clin Gastroenterol Hepatol 2019 Jan;17(2):256–274 [PMID: 30153517].

Tabbers MM et al: Evaluation and treatment of functional constipation in infants and children: evidence-based recommendations from ESPGHAN and NASPGHAN. J Pediatr Gastroenterol Nutr 2014 Feb;58(2):258–274 [PMID: 24345831].

ANAL FISSURE

Anal fissure is a slit-like tear in the squamous epithelium of the anus, which usually occurs secondary to the passage of large, hard fecal masses, typically at the superior and inferior aspects of the anus. Anal stenosis, anal crypt abscess, and trauma can be contributory factors. Sexual abuse must be considered in children with large, irregular, or multiple anal fissures.

Anal fissures may be the presenting sign of inflammatory bowel disease (IBD) in older children.

The infant or child with anal fissure typically cries with defecation and will try to hold back stools. Sparse, bright red bleeding is seen on the outside of the stool or on the toilet tissue following defecation. Fissures can often be seen if patients are examined in a knee-chest position with the buttocks spread apart. When a fissure cannot be identified, it is essential to rule out other causes of rectal bleeding such as juvenile polyp, hemorrhoids, perianal inflammation due to group A β-hemolytic streptococcus, or IBD. Anal fissures should be treated promptly to break the constipation, fissure, pain, retention, and constipation cycle.

CONGENITAL ANORECTAL ANOMALIES

1. Anterior Displacement of the Anus

Anterior displacement of the anus is a common anomaly of infant girls. Its usual presentation in infants is constipation and straining with stool with the introduction of solids. On physical examination, the anus looks normal but is ventrally displaced, located close to the vaginal fourchette (in females) or to the base of the scrotum (in males). The diagnosis is made in girls if the distance from the vaginal fourchette to the center of the anal opening is less than 34% of the total distance from fourchette to coccyx. In boys, the diagnosis is made if the distance from the base of the scrotum to the anal aperture is less than 46% of the total distance from scrotum to coccyx. On internal digital examination a posterior "rectal shelf" will often be appreciated. In severe anterior displacement, when the anal opening is located less than 10% of the distance from the vaginal fourchette to the coccyx, the anal sphincter muscle may not completely encircle the anal opening and severe obstipation like that seen in imperforate anus may occur. Surgery is not needed in most cases. Stool softeners or occasional glycerin suppositories usually relieve straining with defecation. This problem improves significantly by age 3–4 years as normal toddler lordosis disappears.

2. Anal Stenosis

Anal stenosis usually presents in the newborn period. The anal aperture may be very small and filled with a dot of meconium. Defecation is difficult, with ribbon-like stools, blood and mucus per rectum, fecal impaction, and abdominal distention. Anal stenosis occurs in about 3 of 10,000 live births, with slightly more males affected. Anal stenosis may not be apparent at birth because the anus looks normal. Rectal bleeding in a straining infant often leads to a rectal examination, which reveals a tight ring in the anal canal. Dilation of the anal ring is usually curative but may have to be repeated daily for several weeks.

3. Imperforate Anus

Imperforate anus typically develops during the fifth to seventh week of pregnancy and occurs in 1 of 5000 live births,

slightly more common males. Almost 50% of babies with imperforate anus have additional defects, often in association with a particular syndrome.

Defects are generally classified as low (rectoperineal malformation) where the rectum may not connect to the anus, a membrane may be present over the anal opening, or the anal opening may be narrow or misplaced. A high lesion is classified where the rectum may connect to part of the urinary tract or the reproductive system through a fistula. Infants with low imperforate anus fail to pass meconium. There may be a greenish bulging membrane obstructing the anal aperture. Perforation of the anal membrane is a relatively simple surgical procedure. A skin tag shaped like a "bucket handle" is seen on the perineum of some males below which a stenotic aperture can be seen. Eighty to 90% of patients with low imperforate anus are continent after surgery.

In high imperforate anus, physical examination usually shows no anal musculature. There may be a rectoperineal, rectovesicular, rectourethral, or rectovaginal fistula; hypoplastic buttocks; cloacal anomalies; and sometimes evidence of distal neurologic deficit. It is critical in these cases to fully evaluate the complex anatomy and neurologic function before attempting corrective surgery. A diverting colostomy is usually performed to protect the urinary tract and relieve obstruction. After reparative surgery, only 30% of patients with high imperforate anus achieve fecal continence.

Levitt MA, Pena A: Outcomes from the correction of anorectal malformations. Curr Opin Pediatr 2005;17:394 [PMID: 15891433].
Reisner SH, Sivan Y, Nitzan M, Merlob P: Determination of anterior displacement of the anus in newborn infants and children. Pediatrics 1984;73:216–217 [PMID: 6694879].

CLOSTRIDIUM DIFFICILE INFECTION IN CHILDREN

 ESSENTIALS OF DIAGNOSIS & TYPICAL FEATURES

► *C difficile* in children leads to a spectrum of clinical disease, from asymptomatic colonization to severe pseudomembranous colitis with fever, severe abdominal pain, and bloody diarrhea.

► Risk factors for *C difficile* disease include previous antibiotic use and a variety of chronic diseases, including immunodeficiency, cystic fibrosis, Hirschsprung disease, IBD, oncologic process, and solid-organ transplant.

► Incidence of community-acquired *C difficile* disease in healthy hosts is increasing

Pathogenesis

C difficile is a spore-forming gram-positive bacillus that causes human disease via the secretion of enterotoxins that cause necrotizing inflammation of the colon. Interestingly, asymptomatic *C difficile* colonization of the human GI tract occurs commonly in infants and can occur in older children and adults as well. To some extent, *C difficile* may reside in balance with the constituent intestinal microbiome in a healthy host. Disruption of normal commensal intestinal bacteria or interruption of host immune defense, via intestinal injury or host immune suppression, then appears to give *C difficile* a potential foothold in the human gut where it can lead to disease. Hospitalization is a critical risk factor for *C difficile* disease. Additional risk factors in children include previous antibiotic use and a variety of chronic diseases including IBD, cystic fibrosis, Hirschsprung disease, history of solid-organ transplant, oncologic process, and immunodeficiency.

In recent years there has been an alarming increase in the incidence, morbidity, and mortality of *C difficile* reported in Europe, Canada, and the United States. At least a portion of this increase seems to be due to the expansion of a new strain of *C difficile*, identified as the North American Pulsed Field type 1 (NAP1) *C difficile*, which has been found to have increased toxin production, sporulation, and antibiotic resistance. Surveillance from children's hospitals seems to mirror the increase in incidence of *C difficile* in adults but not necessarily the increase in morbidity and mortality.

Clinical Findings

C difficile disease in children represents a spectrum of clinical symptoms, ranging from asymptomatic colonization to persistent, watery diarrhea to pseudomembranous colitis. Recognizing that antibiotic exposure remains a critical risk factor, the onset of colitis ranges from 1 to 14 days after initiation of antibiotic therapy to as many as 30 days after antibiotics have been discontinued. Clindamycin was one of the first antibiotics associated with pseudomembranous colitis, but all antibiotics are now recognized to be potential causes. In pediatric patients, amoxicillin and cephalosporins are commonly associated with *C difficile*–associated pseudomembranous enterocolitis, probably because of their widespread use.

The patient with pseudomembranous colitis characteristically has fever, abdominal distention, tenesmus, diarrhea, and generalized abdominal tenderness. Chronic presentations with low-grade fever, diarrhea, and abdominal pain have been described. Diarrheal stools contain sheets of neutrophils and sometimes gross blood. Plain abdominal radiographs show a thickened colon wall and ileus. Endoscopically, the colon appears to be covered with small, raised white plaques (pseudomembranes) with areas of apparently normal bowel in between (Figure 21–5). Biopsy specimens show "exploding crypts or volcano lesion"—an eruption of white cells that appears to be shooting out of affected crypts.

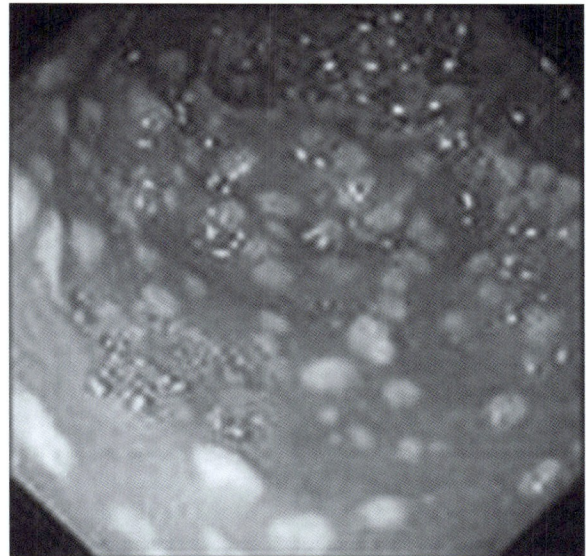

▲ **Figure 21–5.** *Clostridium difficile*–associated pseudomembranes. Colonic mucosa is covered with plaques coated with white exudates.

Stool cultures often show overgrowth of *Staphylococcus aureus*, which is probably an opportunistic organism growing in the necrotic tissue. *C difficile* can be cultured in specialized laboratories. Identification of stool toxins is the usual method of diagnosis. Use of real-time polymerase chain reaction (PCR) for toxin identification has been replacing more traditional enzyme immunoassay (EIA) methods of stool toxin detection, because of improved sensitivity. Interpretation of *C difficile* diagnostic testing in infants remains controversial because asymptomatic colonization is well recognized in the first year of life.

Treatment

Standard treatment of pseudomembranous colitis consists of stopping antibiotics and instituting therapy with oral metronidazole (30 mg/kg/day) or vancomycin (30–50 mg/kg/day). Recent evidence suggests the safety and efficacy of fidaxomicin in pediatric patients with refractory disease, and ongoing work is underway to determine optimal approach to second- and third-line treatment courses. Metronidazole can be given intravenously for patients with vomiting or ileus. Relapse occurs after treatment in 10%–50% of patients because of exsporulation of residual spores in the colon. Spores are very hardy and may remain viable on inanimate surfaces for up to 12 months. Retreatment with the same antibiotic regimen is usually effective, but multiple relapses are possible and may be a significant management problem. Adjunctive strategies, such as *Saccharomyces boulardii* probiotic therapy, cholestyramine as a toxin-binder, and pulsed courses of antibiotics, have been used for refractory disease. Fecal bacteriotherapy, known popularly as *fecal microbiota transplantation*, is now a widely accepted and effective treatment of recurrent *C difficile* infection in adults and pediatrics, with efficacy similar or improved compared to prolonged vancomycin taper. As clinical experience increases with this novel therapy, a more accurate understanding of appropriate indications, contraindications, and potential risks may be further realized.

Adams DJ, Barone JB, Nylund CM: Community-associated *Clostridioides difficile* infection in children: a review of recent literature. J Pediatric Infect Dis Soc 2021 Nov17;10(Suppl 3): S22–S26. doi: 10.1093/jpids/piab064 [PMID: 34791398].

Borali E, De Giacomo C: *Clostridium difficile* infection in children: a review. J Pediatr Gastroenterol Nutr 2016 Dec;63(6): e130–e140 [PMID: 27182626].

Davidovics ZH et al; FMT Special Interest Group of the North American Society of Pediatric Gastroenterology Hepatology, Nutrition, the European Society for Pediatric Gastroenterology Hepatology, Nutrition: Fecal microbiota transplantation for recurrent *Clostridium difficile* infection and other conditions in children: a joint position paper from the North American Society for Pediatric Gastroenterology, Hepatology, and Nutrition and the European Society for Pediatric Gastroenterology, Hepatology, and Nutrition. J Pediatr Gastroenterol Nutr 2019 Jan;68(1):130–143 [PMID: 30540704].

Oliver MB, Vaughn BP. Fidaxomicin use in the pediatric population with *Clostridioides difficile*. Clin Pharmacol 2022 Sep 23;14:91–98. doi: 10.2147/CPAA.S273318 [PMID: 36177387].

Wolf J et al: Safety and efficacy of fidaxomicin and vancomycin in children and adolescents with *Clostridioides (Clostridium) difficile* infection: a phase 3, multicenter, randomized, single-blind clinical trial (SUNSHINE). Clin Infect Dis 2020 Dec 17;71(10): 2581–2588 [PMID: 31773143].

DISORDERS OF THE PERITONEAL CAVITY

PERITONITIS

Primary bacterial peritonitis accounts for less than 2% of childhood peritonitis. The most common causative organisms are *Escherichia coli*, other enteric organisms, hemolytic streptococci, and pneumococci. Primary peritonitis occurs in patients with splenectomy, splenic dysfunction, or ascites (nephrotic syndrome, advanced liver disease, kwashiorkor). It can also occur in infants with pyelonephritis or pneumonia.

Secondary peritonitis is much more common. It is associated with peritoneal dialysis, abdominal trauma, or ruptured viscus. The organisms associated with secondary peritonitis vary with the cause. Organisms such as *Staphylococcus epidermidis* and *Candida* may cause secondary peritonitis in patients receiving peritoneal dialysis. Multiple enteric organisms may be isolated after abdominal injury, bowel perforation, or ruptured appendicitis.

Symptoms of peritonitis include abdominal pain, fever, nausea, vomiting, acidosis, and shock. The abdomen is tender, rigid, and distended, with involuntary guarding. Bowel sounds may be absent. Most peritonitis is a medical emergency. In patients receiving peritoneal dialysis, peritonitis can be a chronic infection causing milder symptoms.

Leukocyte count is high initially ($> 20,000/\mu L$) and later it may fall to neutropenic levels, especially in primary peritonitis. Abdominal imaging can confirm the presence of ascites. Bacterial peritonitis should be suspected if paracentesis fluid contains more than 500 leukocytes/μL or lactate greater than 32 mg/dL; if it has a pH less than 7.34; or if the pH is over 0.1 pH unit less than arterial blood pH. Diagnosis is made by Gram stain and culture, preferably of 5–10 mL of fluid for optimal yield.

Antibiotic treatment and supportive therapy for dehydration, shock, and acidosis are indicated. Surgical treatment of the underlying cause of secondary peritonitis is critical. Removal of infected peritoneal dialysis catheters in patients with secondary peritonitis is sometimes necessary and almost always required if *Candida* infection is present.

European Association for the Study of the Liver: EASL clinical practice guidelines on the management of ascites, spontaneous bacterial peritonitis and hepatorenal syndrome in cirrhosis. J Hepatol 2010 Sep;53(3):397–417 [PMID: 20633946].

CHYLOUS ASCITES

Both congenital and acquired lymphatic obstructions cause chylous ascites, diarrhea, and, in some circumstances, failure to thrive. The abdomen is distended, with a fluid wave and shifting dullness. Unilateral or generalized peripheral edema may be present.

Neonatal chylous ascites may be due to congenital infection or developmental abnormality of the lymphatic system (intestinal lymphangiectasia). If the thoracic duct is involved, chylothorax may be present. Later in life, chylous ascites may result from congenital lymphangiectasia, retroperitoneal or lymphatic tumors, peritoneal bands, abdominal trauma, intestinal malrotation or infection, or it may occur after cardiac or abdominal surgery.

Laboratory findings include hypoalbuminemia, hypogammaglobulinemia and lymphopenia. Ascitic fluid contains lymphocytes and has the biochemical composition of chyle if the patient has just been fed; otherwise, it is indistinguishable from ascites secondary to cirrhosis. Chylous ascites must be differentiated from ascites due to liver disease and in the older child, from constrictive pericarditis, chronically elevated right heart pressure, malignancy, infection, or inflammatory diseases causing lymphatic obstruction. In the newborn, urinary ascites from anatomic abnormalities of the kidney or collecting system must be considered.

Chylous ascites is associated with fat malabsorption and protein loss with resultant edema. Little can be done to correct congenital abnormalities due to hypoplasia, aplasia, or ectasia of the lymphatics unless they are surgically resectable. More recently, somatostatin and fibrin glue have been tried with varying success. Treatment is supportive, consisting mainly of a high-protein diet and careful attention to infections. Shunting peritoneal fluid into the venous system is sometimes effective. A fat-free diet supplemented with medium-chain triglycerides decreases the formation of chylous ascites. Infusions of albumin generally provide only temporary relief and are rarely used for chronic management. In the neonate, congenital chylous ascites may spontaneously disappear following one or more paracenteses and a medium-chain triglyceride diet.

Kassem R et al: Chylous ascites in an infant treated surgically with fibrin glue after failed medical treatment—a case report. J Pediatr Surg Case Rep 2017;19:25–27. 10.1016/j.epsc.2017.02.00

Moreira D de A et al: Congenital chylous ascites: a report of a case treated with hemostatic cellulose and fibrin glue. J Pediatr Surg 2013 Feb;48(2):e17–e19 [PMID: 23414895].

Olivieri C, Nanni L, Masini L, Pintus C: Successful management of congenital chylous ascites with early octreotide and total parenteral nutrition in a newborn. BMJ Case Rep 2012 Sep 25;2012:bcr2012006196 [PMID: 23010459].

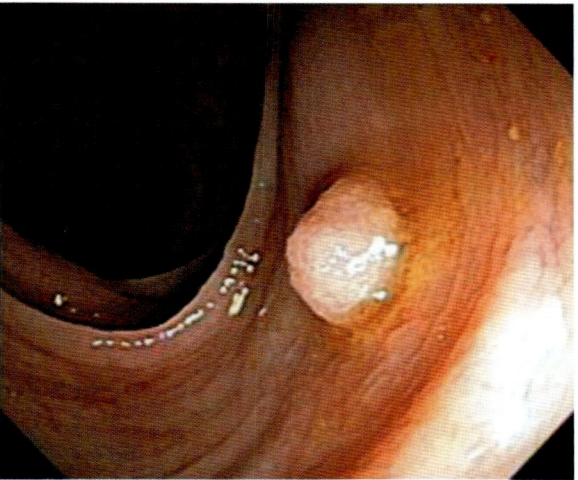

▲ **Figure 21–6.** Juvenile polyp. Solitary, smooth polyp, with erythematous pattern that lies on the surface of a normal colonic mucosa.

GASTROINTESTINAL TUMORS & MALIGNANCIES

JUVENILE POLYPS

Juvenile polyps belong to the hamartomatous category of polyps and are usually pedunculated and solitary in children who have the common type of sporadic juvenile polyps (Figure 21–6). The head of the polyp is composed of hyperplastic, glandular and vascular elements, often with cystic transformation. Juvenile polyps are benign; and 80% occur in the rectosigmoid. Juvenile polyps are the most common type of intestinal polyps in children and occur most commonly between ages 3 and 5 years of age and rarely before 1 year. The painless passage of small amounts of bright red blood with mucus on a normal or constipated stool is the most frequent manifestation. Abdominal pain is rare, but low-lying polyps may prolapse during defecation. Colonoscopy is diagnostic and therapeutic when polyps are suspected. After removal of a single juvenile polyp by electrocautery, nothing further should be done if histologic findings confirm the diagnosis. Recurrence of juvenile polyps is low. Other polyposis syndromes are summarized in Table 21–4.

Rarely, many juvenile polyps may be present in the colon, causing anemia, diarrhea with mucus, and protein loss. An individual may be diagnosed with juvenile polyposis syndrome (JPS) if there are five or more juvenile polyps in the colon, multiple juvenile polyps elsewhere in the GI tract, or any number of juvenile polyps with a family history of JPS. JPS does confer an increased risk of colorectal cancer and surveillance with endoscopy is required. Other hamartomatous polyp syndromes include Peutz-Jeghers syndrome and the PTEN hamartoma tumor syndrome. Peutz-Jeghers syndrome is associated with polyps commonly in the small intestine and colon but can also been seen in the stomach and in other organs. A distinctive mucocutaneous pigmentation (freckling) may appear along the vermillion border of the lips, buccal mucosa, and hands and feet but can disappear by age 5. Due to the higher risk of both GI and non-GI malignancies, routine cancer surveillance is necessary. In addition, 50% will develop intussusception at some point in their lifetime. Prompt investigation for intussusception is needed in the case of symptoms suggesting intestinal obstruction. Phosphatase and tensin homolog (PTEN) hamartoma syndrome involves a spectrum of hamartomatous conditions that are associated with mutations in the *PTEN* gene such as Cowden syndrome, Bannayan-Riley-Ruvalcaba syndrome, and Proteus syndrome.

Barnard J: Screening and surveillance recommendations for pediatric gastrointestinal polyposis syndrome. J Pediatr Gastroenterol Nutr 2009 Apr;48(Suppl 2):575–578 [PMID: 19300132].

Gorji L, Albrecht P: Hamartomatous polyps: diagnosis, surveillance, and management. World J Gastroenterol 2023 Feb 28; 29(8):1304–1314 [PMID: 36925460].

Thakkar K, Fishman DS, Gilger MA: Colorectal polyps in childhood. Curr Opin Pediatr 2012 Oct;24(5):632–637. doi: 10.1097/MOP.0b013e328357419f [PMID: 22890064].

Table 21–4. Gastrointestinal polyposis syndromes

	Location	Number	Histology	Extraintestinal Findings	Malignant Potential	Recommended Therapy
Juvenile polyps	Colon	Single (70%) Several (30%)	Hyperplastic, hamartomatous	None	None	Remove polyp if continuous bleed-ing or prolapse.
Juvenile polypo-sis syndrome[a]	Colon, stomach, small bowel	≥ 5	Hyperplastic, hamartoma-tous, can have focal adenoma-tous change	Telangiectasia with JPS-HHT	Up to 50%	Remove all polyps. Consider colectomy if very numerous or adenomatous.
PTEN hamar-toma tumor syndrome[a]	Colon, stomach, small bowel	Multiple	Hyperplastic, hamartomatous	Skin, eyes, GU, CNS. Cancers especially for breast, thyroid, and endometrium	10% colorec-tal cancer risk	Surveillance colonoscopies starting in adulthood.
Peutz-Jeghers syndrome[a]	Small bowel, stomach, colon	Multiple	Hamartomatous	Pigmented cutaneous and oral macules; ovarian cysts and tumors; bony exostoses	2%–3%	Remove accessible polyps or those causing obstruction or bleeding.
Cronkhite-Canada syndrome	Stomach, colon; less commonly, esophagus and small bowel	Multiple	Hamartomatous	Alopecia; ony-chodystrophy; hyperpigmentation	Rare	None.
Familial adenomatous polyposis[a]	Colon; less commonly, stomach and small bowel	Multiple	Adenomatous	Osteomas, hepato-blastoma ,desmoid tumors, dental anomalies, con-genital hypertrophy retinal pigment epi-thelium (CHRPE)	95%–100%	Colectomy when unable to control endoscopically or when concerning pathology, often by age 18 y.

[a]Autosomal dominant.

CANCERS OF THE ESOPHAGUS, SMALL BOWEL, & COLON

Esophageal cancer is rare in childhood. Cysts, leiomyomas, and hamartomas predominate. Caustic injury of the esopha-gus increases the very long-term risk of squamous cell carci-noma. Chronic peptic esophagitis is associated with Barrett esophagus, a precancerous lesion. Simple GE reflux in infancy without esophagitis is not a risk for esophageal cancer.

The most common gastric or small bowel cancer in chil-dren is lymphoma or lymphosarcoma. Intermittent abdomi-nal pain, abdominal mass, intussusception, or a celiac-like presentation may be present. Carcinoid tumors are usually benign and most often an incidental finding in the appendix. The carcinoid syndrome (flushing, sweating, hypertension, diarrhea, and vomiting), associated with serotonin secretion, only occurs with rare metastatic carcinoid tumors. Colonic adenocarcinoma is rare in childhood. Children with a fam-ily history of colon cancer, chronic ulcerative colitis (UC), or familial polyposis syndromes including familial adeno-matous polyposis (FAP) or JPS are at greater risk. Accu-rate and complete family history is important to determine which children may be at higher risk and thus require further genetic evaluation or endoscopic surveillance.

MESENTERIC CYSTS

Mesenteric and omental cysts are rare intra-abdominal masses in children. These cysts are thin-walled and contain serous, chylous, or hemorrhagic fluid. They are commonly located in the small bowel mesentery but are also found in the mesocolon. Most mesenteric cysts cause no symptoms and are found incidentally, although traction on the mesen-tery may lead to colicky abdominal pain. Volvulus may occur around a cyst, and hemorrhage into a cyst may be mild or hemodynamically significant. A rounded mass can occasion-ally be palpated or seen on radiograph displacing adjacent intestine. Abdominal ultrasonography is usually diagnostic.

Surgical removal is indicated when a cyst is identified. Malignant transformation of mesenteric cysts has been reported in adults, and therefore surgical removal is indicated even in asymptomatic cases.

Tan JJ, Tan KK, Chew SP: Mesenteric cysts: an institution experience over 14 years and review of the literature. World J Surg 2009 Sep;33(9):1961–1965 [PMID: 19609826].

INTESTINAL HEMANGIOMAS & VASCULAR MALFORMATIONS

GI hemangiomas and vascular malformations are uncommon causes of bleeding. Like their skin counterparts, intestinal hemangiomas are typically not present at birth. They tend to appear in the first two months of life, can cause bleeding in the first year as they undergo a rapidly proliferating growth phase, and then can involute. Vascular malformations include capillary, arterial, venous, and mixed lesions, and are present from birth with risk of bleeding throughout life. The physically largest subtype of vascular lesion is the cavernous malformation, which may protrude into the lumen as a polypoid lesion or may invade the intestine from mucosa to serosa.

▶ Clinical Presentation

Intestinal vascular lesions are most often found in the small bowel. These lesions may cause acute or occult blood loss or may present as intussusception, intestinal narrowing, or intramural hematoma. Thrombocytopenia and consumptive coagulopathy are complications of rapidly growing hemangiomas. Intestinal vascular lesions are usually found in isolation, but associated syndromes include the blue rubber bleb nevus syndrome (BRBNS), the Osler-Rendu-Weber syndrome, and the Klippel-Trenaunay-Weber syndrome. The diagnosis of GI bleeding can be challenging, particularly when bleeding is occult or intermittent. Physical examination is typically not helpful unless there are other skin hemangiomas present in the young child that may point to an intestinal hemangioma. Vascular protocols with CT or magnetic resonance imaging (MRI) may identify larger vascular lesions. Endoscopic techniques remain crucial to the diagnosis of intestinal vascular lesions. Video capsule endoscopy (CE) and small bowel enteroscopy techniques have allowed for diagnosis and potential therapy of small bowel vascular lesions that were previously inaccessible using conventional endoscopy.

▶ Treatment

Vascular malformations of the skin and liver have been treated medically with corticosteroids, propranolol, sirolimus, angiotensin-converting enzyme inhibitors, interferon, and vincristine. There is relatively little experience with using these medical techniques for intestinal hemangiomas. Endoscopic techniques for treatment of vascular lesions include banding, submucosal injections of sclerosants, and electrocautery methods. Vascular embolization is a consideration for rapid blood loss in the setting of GI vascular malformations. Finally, surgical resection of the vascular lesion and surrounding bowel may be required for lesions in the mid-small bowel that are not accessible by endoscopy or for large lesions that are not amenable to endoscopic therapies.

Yoo S: GI-associated hemangiomas and vascular malformations. Clin Colon Rectal Surg 2011 Sep;24(3):193–200 [PMID: 22942801].

MAJOR GASTROINTESTINAL SYMPTOMS & SIGNS

ACUTE ABDOMEN

An acute abdomen is a constellation of findings indicating an intra-abdominal process that may require surgery. When this develops, a high degree of urgency exists to identify an underlying cause. The localized or generalized pain of an acute abdomen intensifies over time and is rarely relieved without definitive treatment. The abdomen may be distended and tense, and bowel sounds are often reduced or absent. Patients appear ill and are reluctant to be examined or moved. The acute abdomen is usually a result of infection of intra-abdominal or pelvic organs, but can also occur with intestinal obstruction, appendicitis, intestinal perforation, inflammatory conditions, trauma, and some metabolic disorders. Some of the conditions causing acute abdomen are listed in Table 21–7. Reaching a timely and accurate diagnosis is critical and requires skill in physical diagnosis, recognition of the symptoms of a large number of conditions, and a judicious selection of laboratory and radiologic tests.

ACUTE DIARRHEA

Viruses are the most common cause of acute gastroenteritis in developing and developed countries. Bacterial and parasitic enteric infections are discussed in Chapters 42 and 43. Of the viral agents causing enteric infection, rotavirus and caliciviridae (*Norovirus* and *Sapovirus*) are the most common, followed by enteric adenovirus, and astrovirus. As with most viral pathogens, rotavirus affects the small intestine, causing voluminous watery diarrhea without leukocytes or blood. In the United States, rotavirus primarily affects infants between 3 and 15 months of age. The peak incidence in the United States is in the winter with sporadic cases occurring at other times. The virus is transmitted via the fecal-oral route and survives for hours on hands and for days on environmental surfaces. Rotavirus had been the most common viral source accounting for between one-third and two-thirds of gastroenteritis related hospitalizations prior to vaccine introduction. In the post vaccine era, the United States and many other industrialized countries have seen a sharp decline in the number and severity of gastroenteritis cases caused by rotavirus.

1. Rotavirus Infection

The incubation period for rotavirus is 1–3 days. Symptoms caused by rotavirus are like other viral pathogens. Vomiting is the first symptom in 80%–90% of patients, followed within 24 hours by low-grade fever and watery diarrhea. Diarrhea usually lasts 4–8 days but may last longer in young infants or immunocompromised patients. Fever is present in up to a third of patients. Rotavirus and adenoviruses can be detected in feces using EIA or latex agglutination. The specific identification of rotavirus is not required in every case, however, as treatment is nonspecific. Additional laboratory testing is also generally unnecessary but, when obtained, will usually show a normal white blood cell count. Metabolic acidosis can occur from bicarbonate loss in the stool, ketosis from poor intake, and in severe cases lactic acidemia occurs from hypotension and hypoperfusion. Stools do not contain blood or white blood cells.

As with most other viral causes of acute diarrhea, treatment is nonspecific and supportive. Replacement of fluid and electrolyte deficits, along with ongoing losses, especially in small infants is necessary (oral and intravenous therapies are discussed in Chapter 23.) The use of oral rehydration solutions is appropriate in most cases. The use of clear liquids or hypocaloric (dilute formula) diets for more than 48 hours is not advisable. Early initiation of refeeding is recommended. Intestinal lactase levels may be reduced during rotavirus infection. Therefore, the brief use of a lactose-free diet may be associated with a shorter period of diarrhea but is not critical to successful recovery in healthy infants. Reduced fat intake during recovery may decrease nausea and vomiting.

Antidiarrheal medications are ineffective (kaolin-pectin combinations) and in some circumstances can be dangerous (loperamide, tincture of opium, diphenoxylate with atropine). Bismuth subsalicylate preparations may reduce stool volume but are not critical to recovery and are generally not recommended especially in young children due to the salicylate component and potential risk of Reye syndrome. Oral immunoglobulin or specific antiviral agents have occasionally been reported to limit duration of disease in immunocompromised patients.

Most children are infected with rotavirus more than once, with the first infection being the most severe. Some protective immunity is imparted by the first infection. As treatment for rotavirus is nonspecific, prevention of illness is critical. Prevention of infection occurs primarily by good hygiene and prevention of fecal-oral contamination. Two rotavirus vaccines are commercially available, which are administered in multiple doses typically from 2 to 6 months of age.

2. Other Viral Infections Causing Acute Diarrhea

Other viral pathogens causing diarrhea in children can be identified in stool by electron microscopy, viral culture, or enzyme-linked immunoassay. Depending on the geographic area, after rotavirus the next most common viral pathogens in infants are norovirus, or enteric adenovirus.. The symptoms of enteric adenovirus infection are like those of rotavirus, but infection is not seasonal and the incubation period more prolonged (8–10 days) with more prolonged duration of illness of typically 8–10 days.

Norovirus is now thought to be the leading source of community acquired diarrhea and is highly contagious. Norovirus is a small RNA virus that mainly causes vomiting but can also cause diarrhea in older children and adults, usually in common source outbreaks. The duration of symptoms is short, usually 24–48 hours. Other potentially pathogenic viruses include astroviruses, corona-like viruses, and other small round viruses. Several norovirus vaccines are currently undergoing clinical trials with promising results.

Cytomegalovirus (CMV) rarely causes diarrhea in immunocompetent children but may cause erosive enteritis or colitis in immunocompromised hosts. CMV enteritis is particularly common after solid-organ and bone marrow transplant and in the late stages of human immunodeficiency virus (HIV) infection but can be seen in patients taking immunosuppressive medication. Ten percent of children presenting with COVID-19 illness present with GI manifestations including diarrhea.

A diversity of opinions exists regarding the use of probiotics in treating gastroenteritis. The Centers for Disease Control and Prevention states that probiotics are "not recommended," while The European Society for Pediatric Gastroenterology, Hepatology, and Nutrition previously "strongly" recommended use, now allows use with weak evidence and confidence for specific strains. The most recent Cochrane review stated: "Probiotics probably make little or no difference to the number of people who have diarrhoea lasting 48 hours or longer, and we are uncertain whether probiotics reduce the duration of diarrhoea." Probiotics should be used with caution in immunocompromised or seriously ill children, in particular those with a central venous catheter.

Bernstein DT: Rotavirus overview. Pediatric Infect Dis J 2009 Mar;28(Suppl 3):S50–S53 [PMID: 19252423].

Collinson S et al: Probiotics for treating acute infectious diarrhoea. Cochrane Database Syst Rev 2020 Dec 8;12:CD003048. doi: 10.1002/14651858.CD003048.pub4 [PMID: 33295643].

Freedman SB et al; PERC PROGUT Trial Group: Multicenter trial of a combination probiotic for children with gastroenteritis. N Engl J Med 2018 Nov 22;379(21):2015–2026. doi: 10.1056/NEJMoa1802597 [PMID: 30462939].

Patel NA: Pediatric COVID-19: systematic review of the literature. Am J Otolaryngol 2020 Sep–Oct;41(5):102573. doi: 10.1016/j.amjoto.2020.102573. Epub 2020 Jun 6 [PMID: 32531620].

Shane AL et al: 2017 Infectious Diseases Society of America clinical practice guidelines for the diagnosis and management of infectious diarrhea. Clin Infect Dis 2017 Nov 29;65(12):e45–e80 [PMID: 29194529].

Suez J et al: The pros, cons, and many unknowns of probiotics. Nat Med 2019;25(5):716–729 [PMID: 31061539].

Szajewska et al; ESPGHAN Special Interest Group on Gut Microbiota and Modifications: Probiotics for the management of pediatric gastrointestinal disorders: position paper of the ESPGHAN Special Interest Group on Gut Microbiota and Modifications. J Pediatr Gastroenterol Nutr 2023 Feb;76(2):232–247. doi: 10.1097/MPG.0000000000003633 [PMID: 36219218].

CHRONIC DIARRHEA

Bowel habits are variable, making the diagnosis of chronic diarrhea difficult. Some healthy infants may have five to eight stools daily. A gradual or sudden increase in the number and volume of stools to more than 15 g/kg/day combined with an increase in fluidity should raise a suspicion for organic cause of chronic diarrhea. Diarrhea may result from (1) interruption of normal cell transport processes for water, electrolytes, or nutrients; (2) decreased surface area available for absorption due to shortened bowel length or mucosal disease; (3) increased intestinal motility; (4) increase in unabsorbable, osmotically active molecules in the intestinal lumen; (5) increased intestinal permeability, causing more water and electrolyte loss; and (6) stimulation of enterocyte secretion by toxins or cytokines. The most common entities causing chronic diarrhea are listed below. Malabsorption syndromes, which also cause chronic or recurrent diarrhea, are considered separately.

1. Causes of Chronic Diarrhea

A. Antibiotic Therapy

Acute and chronic diarrhea is reported in up to 60% of children receiving antibiotics, usually from eradication of normal gut flora and overgrowth of other organisms. Only a small fraction of these patients have *C difficile*–related pseudomembranous enterocolitis. Most antibiotic-associated diarrhea is watery, not associated with systemic symptoms, and decreases after antibiotic therapy stops. Some data suggest that probiotic use may decrease the incidence and severity of this diarrhea by helping restore intestinal microbial balance.

B. Extraintestinal Infections

Infections of the urinary tract and upper respiratory tract (especially otitis media) are sometimes associated with diarrhea through poorly understood mechanisms. Antibiotic treatment of the primary infection, toxins released by infecting organisms, and local irritation of the rectum (in patients with bladder infection) may play a role.

C. Malnutrition

Decreased bile acid synthesis, decreased pancreatic enzyme output, decreased disaccharidase activity, altered motility, and changes in the intestinal flora all may contribute to diarrhea in malnourished patients. Protein-calorie malnutrition can result in villous atrophy and malabsorption. In addition, severely malnourished children are at higher risk of enteric infections because of depressed cellular and humoral immune functions.

D. Diet and Medications

Relative deficiency of pancreatic amylase in young infants causes osmotic diarrhea after starchy foods. Fruit juices, especially those high in fructose or sorbitol, produce diarrhea because these osmotically active sugars are poorly absorbed. Intestinal irritants (spices and foods high in fiber) and foods that contain or release histamine (eg, citrus fruits, tomatoes, fermented cheeses, red wines, and scombroid fish such as tuna or mahi mahi) may also cause diarrhea.

FODMAPs (Fermentable, Oligo-, Di-, Mono-saccharides And Polyols) are a group of poorly absorbed short-chain carbohydrates. Lactose and fructose are classic examples of FODMAPs. Malabsorption of higher FODMAP foods can cause symptoms of chronic intermittent diarrhea as well as bloating, gassiness, and abdominal pain in people with irritable bowel syndrome, and removal of certain FODMAPs from the diet may improve symptoms.

Laxative abuse from eating disorders or Factitious Disorder Imposed on Another (previously known as Munchausen syndrome by proxy) can cause unpredictable diarrhea. A high concentration of magnesium in the stool may indicate the overuse of milk of magnesia or other magnesium-containing laxatives, but detection of other laxative preparations is not routinely available, so a high index of suspicion is required.

E. Allergic Diarrhea

Diarrhea resulting from allergy or intolerance to dietary proteins, especially cow's milk and soy proteins, is a frequently entertained but rarely proven diagnosis, especially in infants younger than 12 months.

In contrast to the self-limited cow's milk protein hypersensitivity of infancy, infants and older children may develop more severe diarrhea caused by a systemic allergic reaction. For instance, food protein–induced enterocolitis syndrome (FPIES) is a life-threatening condition occurring during infancy manifested by large-volume diarrhea, acidosis, and hypotensive shock after eating common food proteins such as milk or soy. Patients often require hospitalization for initial volume resuscitation, followed by strict avoidance of allergens with reintroduction only performed in a controlled setting by an experienced allergist.

Infants and children may develop an enteropathy secondary to dietary proteins, resulting in flattening of small bowel villi, steatorrhea, hypoproteinemia, occult GI blood loss, and chronic diarrhea. Milk protein is the most common cause of enteropathy. Skin testing is not reliable since it detects circulating antibodies, not the T-cell–mediated responses that are likely responsible for these food sensitivity reactions. Double-blind oral challenge with the suspected food under careful observation is often necessary to confirm this intestinal protein allergy, as small bowel biopsy findings are nonspecific. Consultation with an allergist is recommended for long-term management of patients with this disease.

Anaphylactic, immunoglobulin E (IgE)–mediated reactions to food scan occur in both young and older children. Soon after ingestion, the patient develops vomiting, then diarrhea, pallor, and hypotension. In these cases, radioallergosorbent test (RAST) and skin testing are positive. Food challenges should be undertaken in a setting in which resuscitation can be performed as there is often a progressively more severe reaction with subsequent ingestions. The close association between ingestion of a specific food and symptoms usually leaves little doubt about the diagnosis.

F. Chronic Nonspecific Diarrhea

Chronic nonspecific diarrhea, also called toddler's diarrhea, is the most common cause of loose stools in otherwise thriving children. The typical patient is a healthy, thriving child aged 6–20 months old who has three to six loose, nonbloody stools per day while awake. They grow normally and may have a family history of functional bowel disease. No organic etiology is found for their diarrhea, with negative stool tests for blood, white blood cells, fat, parasites, and bacterial pathogens. Diarrhea may worsen with a low-residue, low-fat, or high-carbohydrate diet and during periods of stress or infection. Excessive fruit or juice ingestion seems to worsen symptoms. This syndrome resolves spontaneously usually by age 3½ years or after potty training. Possible causes of this diarrhea include abnormalities of bile acid absorption in the terminal ileum, excess intake of osmotically active carbohydrates, and abnormal motor function. A change in dietary fiber (either increasing fiber if deficient or decreasing fiber if excessive), a slight increase in dietary fat, and restriction of osmotically active carbohydrates like fruit juices will often help control symptoms. If these measures fail, loperamide or cholestyramine can be used for symptomatic relief.

G. Immunologic Causes of Chronic Diarrhea

Chronic diarrhea is common in immune deficiency states, especially immunoglobulin A (IgA) deficiency and T-cell abnormalities, either due to an associated autoimmune enteropathy or due to chronic infection. Common bacterial, viral, fungal, or parasitic organisms usually considered nonpathogenic (rotavirus, *Blastocystis hominis*, *Candida*) or unusual organisms (CMV, *Cryptosporidium*, *Isospora belli*, *Mycobacterium* spp., microsporidia) can cause diarrhea in immunodeficient patients. Specific treatments are available for many of the unusual pathogens causing diarrhea in the immunocompromised host so a vigorous diagnostic search for specific pathogens is warranted in these individuals.

Over half of patients with common variable immune deficiency have enteropathy characterized by intestinal villous atrophy, often with prominent lymphonodular hyperplasia of the small intestine. Patients with congenital or Bruton-type agammaglobulinemia usually have diarrhea and abnormal intestinal morphology. Patients with isolated IgA deficiency are more likely to have CD, lymphonodular hyperplasia, or giardiasis. Patients with isolated defects of cellular immunity, combined cellular and humoral immune incompetence, and HIV infection may have severe chronic diarrhea leading to malnutrition, often without identifiable cause. Chronic granulomatous disease may be associated with symptoms characteristic of IBD.

H. Other Causes of Chronic Diarrhea

Most infections of the GI tract are acute and resolve spontaneously or with specific antibiotic therapy. Organisms most prone to cause chronic or recurrent diarrhea in immunocompetent children are *Giardia lamblia*, *Entamoeba histolytica*, *Salmonella* species, and *Yersinia*. Some patients may develop postinfectious diarrhea, with persistent diarrhea despite the eradication of the offending organism. Bacterial overgrowth of the small bowel can cause diarrhea in patients with SBS, undergoing chemotherapy, or with anatomic abnormalities.

Pancreatic insufficiency due to cystic fibrosis or Shwachman-Diamond syndrome may result in chronic diarrhea, typically in conjunction with failure to thrive. Certain tumors (neuroblastoma, ganglioneuroma, metastatic carcinoid, pancreatic VIPoma, or gastrinoma) may secrete substances such as gastrin and vasoactive intestinal polypeptide (VIP) that promote small intestinal secretion of water and electrolytes, causing diarrhea. Increased or disordered intestinal motility from hyperthyroidism or irritable bowel syndrome may also present with diarrhea.

Dennehy PH: Acute diarrheal disease in children: epidemiology, prevention, and treatment. Infect Dis Clin North Am 2005 Sep;19(3):585–602 [PMID: 16102650].

Grimwood K et al: Acute and persistent diarrhea. Pediatr Clin North Am 2009 Dec;56(6):1343–1361 [PMID: 19962025].

GASTROINTESTINAL BLEEDING

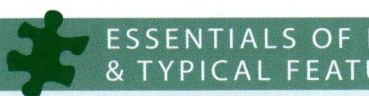

ESSENTIALS OF DIAGNOSIS & TYPICAL FEATURES

▶ Stabilization should be the priority in management of acute pediatric gastrointestinal bleeding (GIB), with large-bore IV access, available blood products, and potential intubation.

▶ Careful history, physical examination, and targeted laboratory evaluation should differentiate upper versus lower GIB.

▶ Endoscopic evaluation in an appropriately stabilized patient with evidence of ongoing bleeding can be of both diagnostic and therapeutic benefit.

Initial evaluation of a child with GI bleeding requires careful history, physical examination, and targeted laboratory investigation to identify the bleeding source. However, in large-volume, acute GI bleeding the primary focus should be stabilizing the patient by providing adequate hemodynamic support.

▶ History

Several substances mimic hematochezia or melena. The presence of blood should be confirmed chemically with guaiac testing. Coughing, tonsillitis, lost teeth, menarche, or epistaxis may cause what appears to be occult or overt GI bleeding. In infants, breast milk swallowed with blood from cracked nipples can present with hematemesis. A careful history of the specifics surrounding the bleeding is critical, including the site, volume and color of blood, history of NSAID use, and use of other medications. Inquiry about associated dysphagia, epigastric pain, or retrosternal pain should be made and, if present, suggest GER or a peptic cause of bleeding (Table 21–5).

Other important aspects of the history include foreign-body/caustic ingestion, history of chronic illnesses (especially liver/biliary disease), personal or family history of food allergy/atopy, associated symptoms (pain, vomiting, diarrhea, fever, weight loss), and family history of GI disorders (IBD, CD, liver disease, bleeding/coagulation disorder). In the presence of massive upper GI bleeding in the toddler, a high index of suspicion for button battery injury must be maintained despite the lack of any known history of ingestion. Other, more obscure causes of GI bleeding in children include Dieulafoy syndrome and heterotopic pancreas. Table 21–6 lists more common causes of GI bleeding by age and presentation.

Table 21–5. Identification of sites of gastrointestinal bleeding.

Symptom or Sign	Location of Bleeding Lesion
Effortless bright red blood from the mouth	Nasopharyngeal or oral lesions; tonsillitis; esophageal varices; lacerations of esophageal or gastric mucosa (Mallory-Weiss syndrome)
Vomiting of bright red blood or of "coffee grounds"	Lesion proximal to ligament of Treitz
Melanotic stool	Lesion proximal to ligament of Treitz, upper small bowel. Blood loss in excess of 50–100 mL/24 h
Bright red or dark red blood in stools	Lesion in the ileum or colon (massive upper gastrointestinal bleeding may also be associated with bright red blood in stool)
Streak of blood on outside of a stool	Lesion in the rectal ampulla or anal canal

▶ Physical Examination

The first objective of the examination is to determine if the child is acutely or chronically ill and initiate supportive measures as needed. Physical signs of portal hypertension, intestinal obstruction, or coagulopathy are particularly important. The nasal passages should be inspected for signs of recent epistaxis, the vagina for menstrual blood, and the anus for fissures and hemorrhoids. Skin examination should assess for hemangiomas, eczema, petechiae, or purpura. Clinical assessment of vital signs and perfusion should be assessed to establish the need for transfusion.

▶ Laboratory Findings

Initial laboratory tests should include a complete blood cell count (CBC), prothrombin time (PT), and partial thromboplastin time (PTT), at minimum. In specific cases, it may be prudent to add a liver profile (with suspected variceal bleeding), erythrocyte sedimentation rate (ESR)/CRP (with possible IBD), and blood urea nitrogen (BUN)/creatinine (for possible hemolytic uremic syndrome). A BUN to creatinine ratio of more than 30 has been shown to indicate a 10-fold increase in the risk of upper versus lower GI bleeding. Low MCV in association with anemia suggests chronic GI losses and may warrant addition of iron studies. Serial determination of hematocrit is essential to assess ongoing bleeding. Detection of blood in the gastric aspirate confirms a bleeding site proximal to the ligament of Treitz. However, its absence does not rule out the duodenum as the source. Testing the

Table 21–6. Differential diagnosis of gastrointestinal bleeding in children by symptoms and age at presentation.

	Infant	Child (2–12 y)	Adolescent (> 12 y)
Hematemesis	Swallowed maternal blood Peptic esophagitis Mallory-Weiss tear Gastritis Gastric ulcer Duodenal ulcer	Epistaxis Peptic esophagitis Caustic ingestion Mallory-Weiss tear Esophageal varices Gastritis Gastric ulcer Duodenal ulcer Hereditary hemorrhagic telangiectasia Hemobilia Henoch-Schönlein purpura	Esophageal ulcer Peptic esophagitis Mallory-Weiss tear Esophageal varices Gastric ulcer Gastritis Duodenal ulcer Hereditary hemorrhagic telangiectasia Hemobilia Henoch-Schönlein purpura
Painless melena	Duodenal ulcer Duodenal duplication Ileal duplication Meckel diverticulum Gastric heterotopia[a]	Duodenal ulcer Duodenal duplication Ileal duplication Meckel diverticulum Gastric heterotopia[a]	Duodenal ulcer Leiomyoma (sarcoma)
Melena with pain, obstruction, peritonitis, perforation	Necrotizing enterocolitis Intussusception[b] Volvulus	Duodenal ulcer Hemobilia[c] Intussusception[b] Volvulus Ileal ulcer (isolated)	Duodenal ulcer Hemobilia[c] Crohn disease (ileal ulcer)
Hematochezia with diarrhea, crampy abdominal pain	Infectious colitis Pseudomembranous colitis Eosinophilic colitis Hirschsprung enterocolitis	Infectious colitis Pseudomembranous colitis Granulomatous (Crohn) colitis Hemolytic-uremic syndrome Henoch-Schönlein purpura Lymphonodular hyperplasia	Infectious colitis Pseudomembranous colitis Granulomatous (Crohn) colitis Hemolytic-uremic syndrome Henoch-Schönlein purpura
Hematochezia without diarrhea or abdominal pain	Anal fissure Eosinophilic colitis Rectal gastric mucosa heterotopia Colonic hemangiomas	Anal fissure Solitary rectal ulcer Juvenile polyp Lymphonodular hyperplasia	Anal fissure Hemorrhoid Solitary rectal ulcer Colonic arteriovenous malformation

[a]Ectopic gastric tissue in jejunum or ileum without Meckel diverticulum.
[b]Classically, "currant jelly" stool.
[c]Often accompanied by vomiting and right upper quadrant pain.
Reproduced with permission from Treem WR: Gastrointestinal bleeding in children. Gastrointest Endosc Clin N Am 1994;4(1):75–97.

stool for occult blood will help monitor ongoing losses. In a large study of over 600 cases of pediatric upper GI bleeding, only 4% who were found to have a significant drop in hemoglobin levels that required transfusion, emergent endoscopic or surgical intervention. In this series, having one or more risk factors, including melena, hematochezia, unwell appearance, and/or large amount of fresh blood in the emesis, had a sensitivity of 100% in identifying the significant bleeds. Elevation of fecal calprotectin levels are associated with bleeding from both IBD and juvenile polyposis.

▶ Imaging Studies

In infants with acute onset of bloody stools, multiple-view plain x-rays of the abdomen are helpful in assessing for pneumatosis intestinalis or signs of obstruction. Children younger than 2 years with a history and examination suggestive of intussusception should undergo air or water-soluble contrast enema. Painless, large-volume bleeding may prompt performance of a Technetium-99 nuclear scan to assess for a Meckel diverticulum. Pretreatment with an H_2-receptor antagonist may be helpful in increasing the sensitivity of this study; however, a negative scan does not preclude the diagnosis. CT scan of the abdomen with oral and IV contrast may be indicated to look for structural and inflammatory causes of bleeding. More recently, CT enterography has been proposed as a useful tool in cases of lower GI bleeding in children. Persistent bleeding without a clear source may prompt consideration of a radioisotope-tagged red blood cell (RBC) scan with ^{99m}Tc-sulfur colloid, though the bleeding must be active at the time of the study, with a rate of at least 0.1 mL/min. Angiography is generally less sensitive, requiring bleeding rate of 1–2 mL/min.

▶ Treatment

In severe bleeding, the ABCs of resuscitation should be performed. Adequate IV access is critical in these cases. If a hemorrhagic diathesis is detected, vitamin K and additional blood products should be administered to correct any underlying coagulopathy. In severe bleeding, the need for volume replacement is monitored by measurement of central venous pressure. In less severe cases, vital signs, serial hematocrits, and gastric aspirates are sufficient.

In suspected upper GI bleeding, gastric lavage with saline should be performed, but there is no value of lavage in controlling bleeding. After stabilization, EGD may be considered to identify the bleeding site, and performance of endoscopy has been associated with lower readmission rates after an initial GI bleeding event. A large retrospective study of endoscopy performed for upper GI bleeding in children found that a definitive source for bleeding was identified in 57%, with a suspected source in another 30%. Risk factors for a nondiagnostic endoscopy in this series were a history of bleeding of less than 1 month and a delay of greater than 48 hours between presentation and endoscopy. Acid suppression with intravenous H_2-antagonists or preferably PPIs may be helpful in suspected peptic causes of bleeding. Colonoscopy may identify the source of bright red rectal bleeding, but it should be performed emergently only if the bleeding is severe and if abdominal radiographs show no signs of obstruction. Colonoscopy on an unprepped colon is often inadequate for making a diagnosis. CE may help identify the site of bleeding if colonoscopy and upper endoscopy findings are negative and is one of the most common indications for CE. Push or balloon enteroscopy may be helpful to perform therapeutic interventions, obtain biopsies, or mark small bowel lesions (prior to laparotomy/laparoscopy) identified on CE. Use of balloon enteroscopy in conjunction with CE in children with occult GI bleeding has been found to have a diagnostic yield of 95%.

Persistent vascular bleeding (varices [Figure 21–7], vascular anomalies) may be relieved temporarily using intravenous octreotide (1–4 mcg/kg/h) for up to 48 hours with careful monitoring of glucose homeostasis. Severe bleeding from esophageal varices may be stopped by compression with a Sengstaken-Blakemore tube. Endoscopic sclerosis or banding of bleeding varices are both effective, with equivalent success rates (87%–89%) and complication rates (10%–19%) between methods. Use of cyanoacrylate for gastric varices in children has been shown to be safe and effective in small, single-center studies.

If conservative measures are ineffective in stopping ulcer bleeding, endoscopic therapy with argon plasma coagulation, local injection of epinephrine, electrocautery, or application of hemostatic clips may be used. Newer, over-the-scope clips

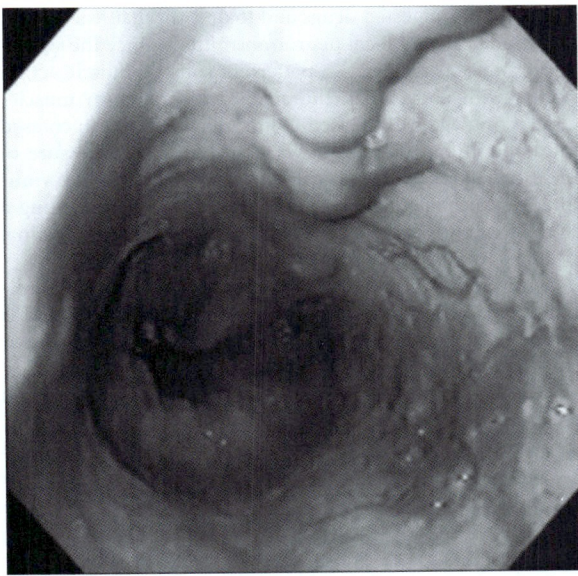

▲ **Figure 21–7.** Esophageal varices. Serpiginous esophageal varix extending to the esophageal lower esophageal sphincter.

have recently been shown to be safe and effective in pediatric patients as young as 4 years of age and as small as 17.4 kg. Though there are limited studies published in children, the use of hemostatic powder shows promise as effective and less technically challenging than other forms of endoscopic hemostasis. As in adults, the use of only one modality in nonvariceal bleeding has been shown to increase the risk of rebleeding. If bleeding remains refractory to therapy, emergency surgery may be necessary. Alternatively, endovascular therapy with selective coiling of involved vessels has been shown to be effective in children with refractory bleeding.

Thomson M, Urs A, Narula P, Prithviraj R, Belsha D: The use and safety of a novel haemostatic spray in the endoscopic management of acute nonvariceal upper gastrointestinal bleeding in children. J Pediatr Gastroenterol Nutr 2018 Sep;67(3):e47–e50. doi: 10.1097/MPG.0000000000001967 [PMID: 29570557].

Tran P, Carroll J, Barth BA, Channabasappa N, Troendle DM: Over the scope clips for treatment of acute nonvariceal gastrointestinal bleeding in children are safe and effective. J Pediatr Gastroenterol Nutr 2018;67(4):458–463 [PMID: 29927862].

VOMITING

Vomiting is an extremely complex activity that is triggered by stimulation of chemoreceptors and mechanoreceptors in the wall of the GI tract, activated by contraction and distension. The nucleus of the solitary tract is the key CNS site for emetic response. Vagal afferents from the gut to brain are stimulated by ingested drugs and toxins, mechanical stretch, inflammation, and local neurotransmitters. Once the vomiting response is triggered, a pattern of somatic muscle action occurs with abdominal, thoracic, and diaphragm muscles contracting against a closed glottis. The resulting increased intra-abdominal pressure reverses the negative pressure of the esophagus and forces gastric contents upward. The vomiting response also alters intestinal motility by generating a retroperistaltic contractile complex that moves intestinal contents toward the esophagus.

Vomiting is the presenting sign of many pediatric conditions. The most common cause of vomiting in childhood is acute viral gastroenteritis. However, obstruction and acute or chronic inflammation of the GI tract are also major causes. CNS inflammation, increased intracranial pressure, or mass effect may cause vomiting. The area postrema in the brainstem can also trigger vomiting without input from the vagal afferents. Metabolic derangements associated with inborn errors of metabolism, sepsis, and drug intoxication can stimulate either the area postrema or the brain directly to promote vomiting.

Control of vomiting with medication is rarely necessary in acute gastroenteritis, but it may relieve nausea and vomiting and decrease the need for intravenous fluids and/or hospitalization. Antihistamines and anticholinergics are appropriate for motion sickness because of their labyrinthine effects. 5-HT_3–receptor antagonists (ondansetron, granisetron) are useful for vomiting associated with surgery and chemotherapy. Ondansetron has been found to be the best intervention for cessation of vomiting and prevention of hospitalization. Benzodiazepines, corticosteroids, and substituted benzamides are also used in chemotherapy-induced vomiting. Butyrophenones (droperidol, haloperidol) are powerful drugs that block the D_2 receptor in the area postrema and are used for intractable vomiting in acute gastritis, chemotherapy, and after surgery.

Levine DA: Anti-emetics for acute gastroenteritis in children. Curr Opin Pediatr 2009 Jun;21(3):294–298 [PMID: 19381093].

Niño-Serna L, Acosta-Reyes J, Veroniki AA, Florez ID: Antiemetics in children with acute gastroenteritis: a meta-analysis. Pediatrics 2020 Apr;145(4):e20193260 [PMID: 32132152].

Zhong W et al: Mechanisms of nausea and vomiting: current knowledge and recent advances in intracellular emetic signaling systems. Int J Mol Sci 2021 May 28;22(11):5797. doi: 10.3390/ijms22115797 [PMID: 34071460].

Cyclic Vomiting Syndrome

▶ Clinical Findings

Cyclic vomiting syndrome (CVS) is defined as three or more recurrent episodes of stereotypical vomiting in children usually older than 1 year. The emesis is forceful and frequent, occurring up to six times per hour for up to 72 hours or more.

Episode frequency ranges from two to three per month to less than one per year. Nausea, retching, and small-volume bilious emesis continue even after the stomach is emptied. Hematemesis secondary to forceful vomiting and a Mallory-Weiss tear (tear or laceration of the mucous membrane at the GE junction) may occur. Patients experience abdominal pain, anorexia, and, occasionally, diarrhea. Autonomic symptoms, such as pallor, sweating, temperature instability, and lethargy, are common and give the patient a very ill appearance. The episodes end suddenly, often after a period of sleep. In some children, dehydration, electrolyte imbalance, and shock may occur. Between episodes, the child is completely healthy.

The cause of CVS is unknown; however, a relationship to migraine headaches has long been recognized. Family history is positive for migraine in 50%–70% of cases, and many patients develop migraine headaches as adults. Research suggests that abnormalities of neurotransmitters and hormones provoke CVS. About one-quarter of patients have typical migraine symptoms during episodes: premonitory sensation, headache, photophobia, and phonophobia. Identifiable triggers are similar to migraines and include infection, positive or negative emotional stress, diet (chocolate, cheese, monosodium glutamate), menses, sleep deprivation, or motion sickness.

▶ Differential Diagnosis

Conditions that mimic CVS include drug toxicity, increased intracranial pressure, seizures, brain tumor, Chiari malformation, recurrent sinusitis, choledochal cyst, gallstones, recurrent small-bowel obstruction, IBD, familial pancreatitis, obstructive uropathy, recurrent urinary infection, diabetes, mitochondrial diseases, disorders of fatty and organic acid metabolism, adrenal insufficiency, and Factitious Disorder Imposed on Another (FDIA). Chronic marijuana use has been associated with chronic vomiting (cannabinoid hyperemesis syndrome) and can mimic CVS.

▶ Treatment

Avoidance of triggers prevents episodes in some patients. Sleep can also end an episode although some children awaken and resume vomiting. Diphenhydramine or lorazepam is used at the onset of spells in some children to reduce nausea and induce sleep. Early use of antimigraine medications (sumatriptan), antiemetics (ondansetron), or antihistamines can abort spells in some patients. Intravenous fluids may be required to end it. Several approaches may be tried before an effective therapy is found. Preventing spells with prophylactic propranolol, amitriptyline, antihistamines, or anticonvulsants are effective in some patients with frequent or disabling spells. Some patients require the additions of the mitochondrial-targeted cofactors coenzyme Q10 and L-carnitine to help manage their vomiting episodes. Other agents such as aprepitant may be considered when vomiting is refractory to initial treatments.

Blohm E, Sell P, Neavyn M: Cannabinoid toxicity in pediatrics. Curr Opin Pediatr 2019 Apr;31(2):256–261 [PMID: 30694824].

Kovacic K, Sood M, Venkatesan T: Cyclic vomiting syndrome in children and adults: what is new in 2018? Curr Gastroenterol Rep 2018 Aug 29;20(10):46 [PMID: 30159612].

Tillman EM, Harvath EM: Cyclic vomiting syndrome in pediatric patients: a review of therapeutics. J Pediatr Pharmacol Ther 2022;27(1):12–18. doi: 10.5863/1551-6776-27.1.12. Epub 2021 Dec 22 [PMID: 35002554].

ABDOMINAL PAIN

Approximately 2%–4% of all pediatric office visits occur because of unexplained recurrent abdominal pain. Functional GI disorders (FGID) have been reported in roughly 10%–30% of children/adolescents and 30%–40% of infants and toddlers. A recent study found that roughly 50% of new patients younger than 4 years and 75% of patients older than 4 years seen in an ambulatory GI clinic met criteria for at least one FGID. Criteria were published in 2016 in order to incorporate new findings in the literature including new information on gut-brain interactions and microenvironments. The descriptive term "recurrent abdominal pain" has been discarded for the more meaningful terms. For patients with significant pain, the term *functional abdominal pain disorder* (FAPD) is used. This term encompasses several entities: functional dyspepsia (with subtypes of epigastric pain vs postprandial distress), irritable bowel syndrome (characterized by altered form and frequency of stools and improvement with defecation), abdominal migraines, and functional abdominal pain.

▶ Clinical Findings

A. Symptoms and Signs

Children with functional abdominal pain experience recurrent attacks of abdominal pain or discomfort at least once per week for at least 2 months. Classifications of abdominal pain depend on the characteristics of the pain such as location of pain, association with bowel habits, and associated symptoms. The pain is usually localized to the periumbilical area but may also be more generalized. The pain occurs primarily during the day but may prevent children from falling asleep at night. It may be associated with pallor, nausea, or vomiting, and also with dramatic reactions such as frantic crying, clutching the abdomen, and doubling over. Parents may become alarmed and take their children into the emergency departments, where the evaluation is negative for an acute abdomen. School attendance may suffer, and enjoyable family events may be disrupted.

Alarm symptoms that suggest an organic etiology include dysphagia, persistent vomiting, GI blood loss, associated rashes, or joint complaints, nocturnal stooling, weight loss, stunting of growth, and fevers.

Functional abdominal pain usually bears little relationship to bowel habits and physical activity. However, some patients have a constellation of symptoms suggestive of irritable bowel syndrome, including bloating, postprandial pain, lower abdominal discomfort, and erratic stool habits with a sensation of obstipation or incomplete evacuation of stool. A precipitating or stressful situation in the child's life at the time the pains began can sometimes be elicited. School phobia may be a precipitant.

A careful and thorough physical examination that includes a rectal examination is essential and usually normal. Complaints of abdominal tenderness elicited during palpation may be inconsistent, out of proportion to visible signs of distress, and distractible.

B. Laboratory Findings

CBC, sedimentation rate, and stool test for occult blood are usually a sufficient evaluation. Extraintestinal sources such as kidney, spleen, and genitourinary tract may require assessment. In the adolescent female patient, ultrasound of the abdomen and pelvis may be helpful to detect gallbladder or ovarian pathology. If the pain is atypical, further testing suggested by symptoms and family history should be done. This may include additional imaging studies or endoscopic analysis. Any concern for lower tract inflammation and IBD may prompt consideration for the use fecal inflammatory markers such as lactoferrin and calprotectin.

▶ Differential Diagnosis

Lactose intolerance usually causes abdominal distention, gas, and diarrhea with milk ingestion. At times, however, abdominal discomfort may be the only symptom. The incidence of peptic gastritis or EoE, duodenitis, and ulcer disease is probably underappreciated. Though esophageal eosinophilia typically presents with dysphagia and primarily esophageal symptoms in adolescents and adults, it can present with abdominal pain in younger children. Abdominal migraine and cyclic vomiting are conditions with an episodic character often associated with headaches or vomiting. For a list of disorders causing an acute abdomen, see Table 21–7.

▶ Treatment & Prognosis

Treatment of FAPD consists of reassurance based on a thorough history and physical examination and a sympathetic, age-appropriate explanation of the nature of functional pain. It is important to acknowledge that the child is experiencing pain. The concept of "visceral hyperalgesia" or increased pain signaling from physiologic stimuli such as gas, acid secretion, or stool is one that parents can understand and helps them respond appropriately to the child's complaints. A child's abdominal pain may be compared to usual headaches that another person may experience, in that the workup can be

Table 21–7. Differential diagnosis of acute abdomen.

Gastrointestinal causes	Hepatobiliary causes
Appendicitis	Cholecystitis
Bowel obstruction	Cholangitis
Perforated ulcer	Hepatic abscess
Ischemic colitis	Splenic rupture
Volvulus	Splenic infarction
Intussusception	**Urologic/gynecologic causes**
Pancreatitis	Acute cystitis
Incarcerated hernia	Nephrolithiasis
Toxic megacolon	Ruptured ectopic pregnancy
Abdominal vasculitis	Ovarian torsion
Intra-abdominal abscess	Testicular torsion
Other causes	Acute salpingitis
Diabetic ketoacidosis	Pelvic inflammatory disease
Lead poisoning	
Porphyria	
Abdominal sickle cell crisis	

normal even though there is pain. Reassurance without education is rarely helpful. Regular activity should be resumed, especially school attendance. Therapy for psychosocial stressors, including biofeedback therapy, may be necessary. In specific patients, targeted therapy based on symptoms may be helpful. For abdominal migraines, treatments for migraine headaches may also be of benefit.

Numerous dietary modifications have been proposed as treatment for functional disorders, but data are lacking as to their effectiveness. For instance, restriction of lactose and fructose and low FODMAP diets may benefit some patients, whereas a positive impact of fiber, prebiotics, and probiotics on symptoms has not been shown.

Likewise, pharmacologic studies of pediatric patients with FAPD have been underpowered and yielded inconsistent results. For instance, peppermint oil has shown benefit in reducing frequency and severity of pain, a finding that may be attributed to inhibition of calcium channels and reduction in colonic spasm. In contrast, although studies examining the impact of antispasmotic medications in adults have shown promise, these have yet to be replicated in children. The use of cyproheptadine may benefit some patients.

The most recent Cochrane review found no convincing data on the use of drugs to treat FAPD in children. Interestingly, pooled data from a recent systematic review examining the placebo effect show improvement in pain scales in 41% and resolution of pain in 17%.

In contrast, biopsychosocial therapy, cognitive behavioral therapy, and hypnosis may offer benefit. In a recent meta-analysis including more than 2000 patients, psychological therapies were more effective than control treatments (placebo, supportive therapy, physician's "usual management") for alleviating chronic abdominal pain in adults and children.

Beinvogl B et al: Multidisciplinary treatment reduces pain and increases function in children with functional gastrointestinal disorders. Clin Gastroenterol Hepatol 2019 Apr;17(5):994–996 [PMID: 30055266].

Black CJ et al: Efficacy of psychological therapies for irritable bowel syndrome: systematic review and network meta-analysis. Gut 2020;69:1441–1451. doi: 10.1136/gutjnl-2020-321191 [PMID: 32276950].

Rouster AS et al: Functional gastrointestinal disorders dominate pediatric gastroenterology outpatient practice. J Pediatr Gastroenterol Nutr 2016 Jun;62(6):847–851. doi: 10.1097/MPG.0000000000001023 [PMID: 26513617].

Thapar N et al: Paediatric functional abdominal pain disorders. Nat Rev Dis Primers 2020 Nov 5;6(1):89. doi: 10.1038/s41572-020-00222-5 [PMID: 33154368].

MALABSORPTION SYNDROMES

Malabsorption of ingested food has many causes (Table 21–8). Shortened small intestinal length (usually via surgical resection) and mucosal damage (CD) both reduce surface area. Impaired gut motility interferes with normal propulsive movements leading to ineffective mixing of food with pancreatic and biliary secretions. This, in turn, permits anaerobic bacterial overgrowth. Bacterial overgrowth may lead to increased carbohydrate fermentation, acidic diarrhea., and increased bacterial bile acid deconjugation leading to fat malabsorption. Impaired intestinal lymphatic (congenital lymphangiectasia) or venous drainage also causes malabsorption.

Table 21–8. Malabsorption syndromes.

Intraluminal abnormalities	Graft-vs-host disease
Acid hypersecretion (eg, Zollinger-Ellison syndrome)	Mucosal injury
	Celiac disease
Exocrine pancreatic insufficiency	Allergic enteropathy
Cystic fibrosis	IBD
Shwachman syndrome	Radiation enteritis
Malnutrition	Enzyme deficiency
Enzyme deficiency	Lactase deficiency
Enterokinase deficiency	Sucrase-isomaltase deficiency
Trypsinogen deficiency	Short bowel syndrome
Co-lipase deficiency	**Vascular abnormalities**
Decreased intraluminal bile acids	Ischemic bowel
Chronic parenchymal liver disease	Vasculitis: lupus, mixed connective tissue disorder
Biliary obstruction	Congestive heart failure
Bile acid loss (short gut, ileal disease)	Intestinal lymphangiectasia
Bile acid deconjugation by bacterial overgrowth	**Metabolic genetic disease**
	Abetalipoproteinemia
	Congenital secretory diarrheas
Mucosal abnormalities	Lysinuric protein intolerance
Infection (eg, *Giardia*, *Cryptosporidium*)	Cystinosis

Remember Conv

Diseases reducing pancreatic exocrine function (cystic fibrosis, Shwachman syndrome) or the production and flow of biliary secretions (biliary atresia) cause nutrient malabsorption. Malabsorption of specific nutrients may also be genetically determined (acrodermatitis enteropathica, disaccharidase deficiency, abetalipoproteinemia).

Clinical Findings

Diarrhea, vomiting, anorexia, abdominal pain, failure to thrive, and abdominal distention are common. With fat malabsorption, stools are typically bulky, foul, greasy, and pale. Identification of fecal microscopic fat globules may be useful. For example, neutral fat is seen in pancreatic insufficiency such as cystic fibrosis and "split fat" fatty acids are seen in mucosal injury such as CD. In contrast, osmotic diarrhea stools are loose, watery, and acidic.

Long-standing fat malabsorption leads to deficiencies of the fat-soluble vitamins (A, D, E, K). Deficiency of vitamin K causes prolonged PT. Loss of serum proteins is suggested by elevated fecal α1-antitrypsin levels. Disaccharide or monosaccharide malabsorption manifests by acidic stool with pH less than 5.5 due to lactic acid and reducing substances. Specific enzyme deficiencies may be evaluated by breath hydrogen test (lactose intolerance), or specific disaccharidase activity measurement from small intestinal biopsy. Other helpful tests include fecal elastase and cystic fibrosis gene testing for exocrine pancreatic insufficiency, and intestinal mucosal biopsy for CD, lymphangiectasia, and IBD. Common disorders associated with malabsorption in pediatric patients are detailed below.

1. Protein-Losing Enteropathy

Loss of plasma proteins into the GI tract leads to protein-losing enteropathy and occurs in association with a myriad of conditions (Table 21–9).

Clinical Findings

Signs and symptoms are mainly caused by hypoproteinemia or fat malabsorption: edema, ascites, poor weight gain, anemia, lymphopenia, and deficiencies of fat-soluble vitamins and minerals. Serum albumin and globulins may decrease. Fecal α_1-antitrypsin is elevated (> 3 mg/g dry weight stool; slightly higher in breast-fed infants).

Differential Diagnosis

Hypoalbuminemia may be due to increased catabolism, poor protein intake, impaired hepatic protein synthesis, or congenital malformations of lymphatics.

Treatment

Albumin infusion, diuretics, and a high-protein, low-fat diet may control symptoms. Nutritional deficiencies should be corrected, and the underlying cause treated.

Table 21–9. Disorders associated with protein-losing enteropathy.

Cardiac disease
Congestive heart failure
Constrictive pericarditis
Cardiomyopathy
Post-Fontan procedure with elevated right atrial pressure
Lymphatic disease
Primary congenital lymphangiectasia
Secondary lymphangiectasia
Malrotation
Malignancy: lymphoma, retroperitoneal tumor
Other: sarcoid, arsenic poisoning
Inflammation
Giant hypertrophic gastritis (Ménétrier disease), often secondary to cytomegalovirus infection or *Helicobacter pylori*
Infection: TB, *Clostridium difficile*, parasite (eg, *Giardia*), bacteria (eg, *Salmonella*)
Allergic enteropathy
Celiac disease
Radiation enteritis
Graft-vs-host disease
Inflammatory bowel disease
Hirschsprung disease
Necrotizing enterocolitis
Vascular disorders
Systemic lupus erythematosus and mixed connective tissue disorder

2. Celiac Disease (Gluten Enteropathy)

Celiac disease (CD) is an immune-mediated enteropathy triggered by gluten, a protein in wheat, rye, and barley. CD presents any time after gluten is introduced in the diet. Disease frequency approaches 1 in 100. Risk factors include type 1 diabetes (4%–10%), Down syndrome (5%–12%), Turner syndrome (4%–8%), IgA deficiency (2%–8%), autoimmune thyroiditis (8%), and family history of CD (5%–10%). Almost all CD patients express HLA-DQ2 or DQ8 tissue antigens.

Clinical Findings

A. Symptoms and Signs

Gastrointestinal manifestations—In the classic form of CD, symptoms begin soon after gluten is introduced in the diet, typically between 6 and 24 months of age. Chronic diarrhea, abdominal distention, irritability, anorexia, vomiting, and poor weight gain are typical. Celiac crisis manifested by dehydration, hypotension, hypokalemia, and explosive diarrhea, is rare. Older children may have oral ulcers, abdominal pain, vomiting, diarrhea, and bloating.

Nongastrointestinal manifestations—Adolescents with CD may present with delayed puberty or short stature. Female patients may have delayed menarche. CD should

be considered in children with unexplained iron-deficiency anemia, decreased bone mineral density, elevated liver function enzymes, arthritis, epilepsy with cerebral calcifications, or intensely pruritic rash called dermatitis herpetiformis.

B. Laboratory Findings

Serologic and genetic testing—Patients suspected of CD should be screened with serum IgA and tissue transglutaminase (TTG) IgA, which is highly sensitive and specific. For patients with IgA deficiency, the deamidated gliadin peptide IgG or the IgG-based versions of the TTG or antiendomysial antibodies should also be sent. Testing for HLA-DQ2 and DQ8 has a high negative predictive value, and family members who test negative are unlikely to ever develop CD.

Stools—May have fatty acid globules or be acidic.

Hypoalbuminemia—Can be severe enough to lead to edema.

Anemia—Low MCV and evidence of iron deficiency is common.

C. Biopsy Findings

Characteristic histologic findings on light microscopy are villous atrophy with increased numbers of intraepithelial lymphocytes.

▶ Differential Diagnosis

The differential diagnosis includes food allergy, non-celiac gluten sensitivity, CrD, postinfectious diarrhea, primary lactose intolerance, functional abdominal pain, irritable bowel syndrome, immunodeficiencies, and graft-versus-host disease.

▶ Treatment

Treatment is strict dietary gluten restriction for life. All sources of wheat, rye, and barley are eliminated. Most, but not all, patients tolerate oats.

▶ Prognosis

A gluten-free diet leads to mucosal healing, absence (or low titers) of celiac related antibodies and normal growth. Individuals with poor adherence to gluten-free diet may be at increased risk for fractures, iron deficiency anemia, infertility, and enteropathy-associated T-cell lymphoma.

Celiac Disease Foundation: www.celiac.org. Beyond Celiac: www.beyondceliac.org.

Rubio-Tapia A et al: American College of Gastroenterology guidelines update: diagnosis and management of celiac disease. Am J Gastroenterol 2023;11859–11876 [PMID 36602836].

3. Carbohydrate Malabsorption

Carbohydrate malabsorption is typically a nonimmune-mediated intolerance to dietary carbohydrates due to a deficiency in an enzyme or transporter, or due to excess consumption overloading a functional transporter. These systems are located on the small bowel epithelial brush border. The non-absorbed molecules cause osmotic diarrhea and are fermented in the gut producing gas. As a result, clinical symptoms include abdominal distention, bloating, flatulence, abdominal discomfort, nausea, and watery diarrhea. Stools are liquid, and acidic, and will test positive for reducing substances. Diagnostic tests are breath tests looking for malabsorption of specific carbohydrates (including lactose, sucrose, or fructose), genetic tests (lactase deficiency, sucrase-isomaltase deficiency), and disaccharide activity assays on mucosal biopsy specimens. Symptoms resolve with dietary avoidance or with enzyme supplementation (eg, lactase or sacrosidase).

A. Disaccharidase Deficiency

Oligosaccharides (from breakdown of starches) and disaccharides, (sucrose and lactose), are the most important dietary carbohydrates and require hydrolysis by intestinal brush border disaccharidases for absorption. Disaccharidase levels are highest in the jejunum and proximal ileum. Characteristics of primary disaccharidase deficiency include permanent disaccharide intolerance, absence of intestinal injury, and positive family history.

B. Lactase Deficiency

All human ethnic groups are lactase-sufficient at birth making congenital lactase deficiency extremely rare. Genetic or familial lactase deficiency appears after 5 years of age and develops in virtually all Asians, Alaskan natives, Native Americans, 80% of Africans, 70% of African Americans, and 30%–60% of Caucasian Americans. Transient or secondary lactase deficiency caused by mucosal injury such as acute viral gastroenteritis is common and resolves within a few weeks.

C. Sucrase-Isomaltase Deficiency

This condition is inherited in a rare autosomal recessive fashion and found most in Greenland, Iceland, and among Alaskan natives. Infants may present with abdominal distention, failure to thrive, and watery, acidic diarrhea.

D. Monosaccharide Malabsorption

The most important monosaccharides are fructose, glucose, and galactose.

Glucose-galactose malabsorption is a rare disorder in which the sodium-glucose transport protein is defective.

Transport of glucose in the intestinal epithelium and renal tubule is impaired. Diarrhea begins with the first feedings, accompanied by reducing sugar in the stool and acidosis. Glycosuria and aminoaciduria may develop, and the glucose tolerance test is abnormal. Small bowel histology appears normal. Diarrhea subsides promptly on withdrawal of glucose and galactose from the diet. The acquired, transient form of glucose-galactose malabsorption occurs mainly in infants younger than 6 months, usually following acute viral or bacterial enteritis, and may require short-term PN. A carbohydrate-free base formula is used with added fructose. The prognosis is good if diagnosed early. Tolerance for glucose and galactose improves with age.

Fructose malabsorption occurs when fructose is in excess of glucose, often with consumption of high-fructose corn syrup.

4. Intestinal Lymphangiectasia

This form of protein-losing enteropathy results from obstruction of intestinal lymphatics and leakage of lymph into the bowel lumen. Congenital lymphangiectasia is associated with abnormalities of the lymphatics in the extremities. Malrotation with volvulus can also cause intestinal lymphangiectasia.

Clinical Findings

Peripheral edema, diarrhea, abdominal distention, chylous effusions, and repeated infections are common. Laboratory findings include low calcium, magnesium, albumin, immunoglobulin levels, lymphocytopenia, and elevated fecal α_1-antitrypsin. Imaging may show bowel wall edema, and biopsy may reveal dilated lacteals in the villi and lamina propria. If only the lymphatics of the deeper layers of bowel or intestinal mesenteries are involved, laparotomy may be necessary to establish the diagnosis. CE shows diagnostic brightness secondary to the fat-filled lacteals.

Differential Diagnosis

Causes of protein losing enteropathy should be considered.

Treatment & Prognosis

A high-protein diet (up to 6–7 g/kg/day) enriched with medium-chain triglycerides usually allows for adequate nutrition and growth. Vitamin and calcium supplements are often needed. PN supplementation may be needed temporarily. Surgery may be curative if the lesion is localized to a small area of the bowel or in cases of constrictive pericarditis or obstructing tumors. IV albumin and immune globulin may be needed but usually not chronically. The serum albumin may not normalize. The prognosis is not favorable, although remission may occur with age. Malignant degeneration of the abnormal lymphatics may occur, and intestinal B-cell lymphoma may develop.

5. Cow's Milk Protein Intolerance

Milk protein intolerance refers to nonallergic food sensitivity and is more common in males than females and in young infants with a family history of atopy. The estimated prevalence is 0.5%–1.0%. Symptoms may occur while an infant is still exclusively breast-fed. Typically, a healthy, well appearing infant develops flecks of blood in the stool or loose mucoid, blood-streaked stools when fed formula or breast milk with cow's milk protein. Skin testing is not reliable or indicated as this is not thought to be an IgE-mediated disease. Treatment is a diet without cow's milk protein. Maternal avoidance of milk protein will often suffice if breast-fed. If formula-fed, substituting an alternative protein formula (soy or a protein hydrolysate formula) for the cow's milk–based formula is indicated. Cow's milk protein intolerance is self-limited, usually disappearing by 8–12 months of age. Histology, not required for diagnosis, shows mild lymphonodular hyperplasia, mucosal edema, and eosinophilia on rectal biopsy.

In older children, milk protein sensitivity may induce eosinophilic gastroenteritis with protein-losing enteropathy, iron deficiency, hypoalbuminemia, and hypogammaglobulinemia. A celiac-like syndrome with villous atrophy, malabsorption, hypoalbuminemia, occult blood in the stool, and anemia can occur.

6. Pancreatic Insufficiency

The most common cause of pancreatic exocrine insufficiency in childhood is cystic fibrosis. Decreased secretion of pancreatic digestive enzymes is caused by obstruction of the exocrine ducts by thick secretions, which destroys pancreatic acinar cells. Other conditions associated with exocrine pancreatic insufficiency are discussed in Chapter 22.

7. Other Genetic Disorders Causing Malabsorption

A. Abetalipoproteinemia

Abetalipoproteinemia is a rare autosomal recessive condition in which the secretion of triglyceride-rich lipoproteins from the small intestine (chylomicrons) and liver (very low-density lipoproteins) is limited or absent. Profound steatosis of intestinal enterocytes (and hepatocytes) and severe fat malabsorption occur. Deficiencies of fat-soluble vitamins develop with neurologic complications of vitamin E deficiency and atypical retinitis pigmentosa. Serum cholesterol level is very low, and red cell membrane lipids are abnormal, causing acanthosis of red blood cells, two findings that may be the key to diagnosis.

B. Acrodermatitis Enteropathica

Acrodermatitis enteropathica is an autosomal recessive condition in which the intestine has a selective inability to absorb zinc. The condition usually becomes obvious at the time of weaning from breast-feeding and is characterized by rash on the extremities, rashes around the body orifices, eczema, profound failure to thrive, steatorrhea, diarrhea, and immune deficiency. Zinc supplementation by mouth results in rapid improvement.

INFLAMMATORY BOWEL DISEASE

▶ General Considerations

IBD, a chronic relapsing inflammatory disease, is most commonly differentiated into CrD and UC. The etiology of IBD is multifactorial, involving a complex interaction of environmental and genetic factors leading to maladaptive immune responses to flora in the GI tract. Between 5% and 30% of patients identify a family member with IBD. Very early onset IBD, before age 2–5 years, is more likely to be monogenic and severe.

▶ Clinical Findings

A. Symptoms and Signs

Inflammation causes abdominal pain, diarrhea, bloody stools, fever, anorexia, fatigue, and weight loss. CrD may present when strictures cause abdominal pain and intestinal obstruction, or as a penetrating/fistulizing form with abscess, perianal disease, or symptoms similar to acute appendicitis. CrD can affect any part of the GI tract from lips to anus. Childhood CrD most often affects the terminal ileum and colon and may be patchy in distribution. UC usually presents with diarrhea that becomes bloody and is limited to the colon. In children, UC typically involves the entire colon (pancolitis). The younger the age at onset, the more severe the course is likely to be.

Extraintestinal manifestations are common in both forms of IBD and may precede the intestinal complaints. These include uveitis, recurrent oral aphthous ulcers, arthritis, growth and pubertal delay, liver involvement (typically primary sclerosing cholangitis), rash (erythema nodosa and pyoderma gangrenosum), and iron deficiency anemia.

B. Diagnostic Testing

Diagnosis is based on symptoms, relapsing course, radiographic, endoscopic, and histologic findings, and exclusion of other disorders. No single test is diagnostic. Patients often have low hemoglobin, iron, and serum albumin levels, and elevated ESR, CRP and fecal calprotectin. Abdominal imaging with CT, magnetic resonance enterography, ultrasound and video capsule may reveal small bowel disease and exclude other etiologies. Findings include thickening of the bowel wall, strictures mucosal ulceration, enteric fistulas, and mucosal and mural edema.

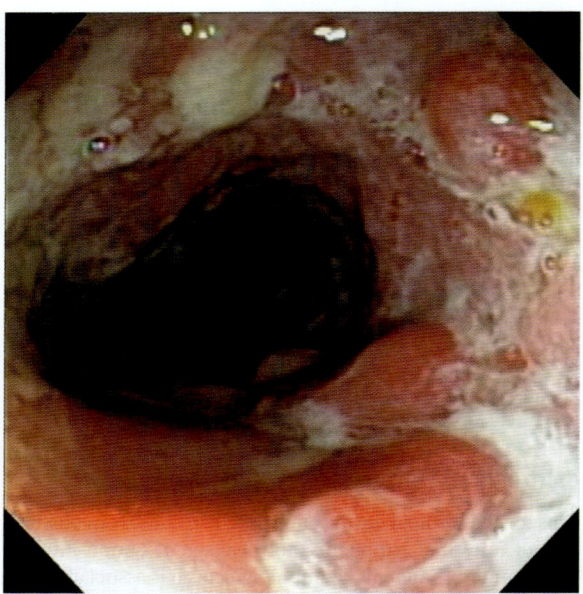

▲ **Figure 21–8.** Crohn colitis. White exudate overlies deep long serpiginous ulceration.

Upper endoscopy and ileocolonoscopy are the most useful diagnostic modalities, revealing severity and extent of upper intestinal, ileal, and colonic involvement. Granulomas are found in 25%–50% of CrD cases. Deep linear ulcers, white exudate, aphthous lesions (Figure 21–8), patchy involvement, and perianal disease suggest CrD. Superficial and continuous involvement of the colon sparing the upper GI tract is typical of UC (Figure 21–9).

▶ Differential Diagnosis

When extraintestinal symptoms predominate, CrD can be mistaken for rheumatoid arthritis, systemic lupus erythematosus or other vasculitides, CD, or hypopituitarism. The acute onset of ileocolitis may be mistaken for intestinal obstruction, appendicitis, lymphoma, infection. Malabsorption symptoms suggest CD, peptic ulcer, *Giardia*, food protein allergy, anorexia nervosa, or growth failure from endocrine causes. Perianal disease suggests child abuse. Crampy diarrhea and blood in the stool can also occur with enteric infections. Mild IBD mimics irritable bowel syndrome, or lactose intolerance. Consider Behçet disease if there are deep intestinal ulcers, oral aphthous ulcerations along with at least two of the following: genital ulcers, synovitis, posterior uveitis, meningoencephalitis, and pustular vasculitis. Chronic granulomatous disease, tuberculosis and sarcoidosis also cause granulomas.

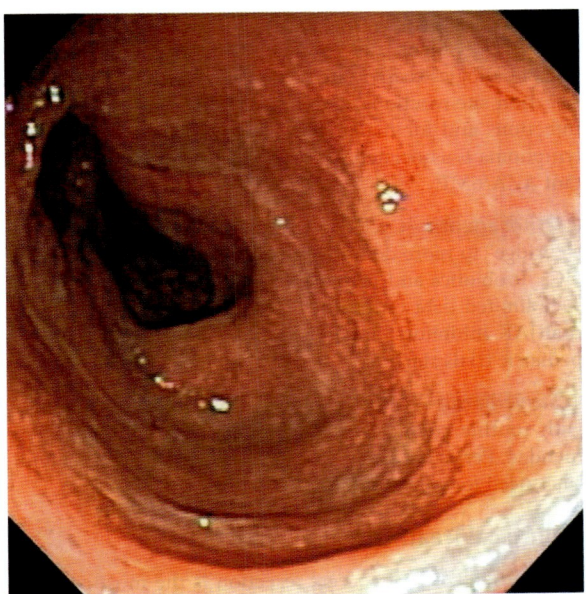

▲ **Figure 21–9.** Ulcerative colitis. Colonic mucosa is uniformly involved with loss of surface vasculature and presence of multiple aphthous ulcers.

▶ Complications

A. Crohn Disease

Nutritional complications include growth and pubertal delay, decreased bone mineralization, and specific nutrient deficiencies, including iron, calcium, zinc, vitamin B_{12}, and vitamin D. Prolonged corticosteroid therapy may impact growth and bone mineral density. Intestinal obstruction, fistulae, abdominal abscess, perianal disease, pyoderma gangrenosum, arthritis, and amyloidosis can occur. Crohn colitis increases risk for colon adenocarcinoma.

B. Ulcerative Colitis

Diagnosis can be difficult, as even with the typical presentation of UC, up to 35% will eventually be diagnosed instead with CrD. Arthritis, uveitis, pyoderma gangrenosum, and malnutrition can occur. Growth failure and delayed puberty are less common than in CrD, while liver disease (chronic active hepatitis, sclerosing cholangitis) is more common. Adenocarcinoma of the colon occurs with an incidence of 1%–2% per year after the first 7–8 years of disease in patients with pancolitis and is significantly higher in patients with UC and sclerosing cholangitis.

▶ Treatment

A. Medical Treatment

Therapy for pediatric IBD involves induction and maintenance of remission and addressing nutritional deficiencies to promote normal growth and development. Treatment includes diet, anti-inflammatory, immunomodulatory, antidiarrheal, antibiotic, and biological medications. No medical therapy is uniformly effective in all patients. In severe CrD, growth hormone may be needed to attain full height potential.

1. Nutrition and Diet—Ensuring adequate nutrition for replenishing deficits and promoting normal growth (including pubertal growth) can be challenging. In addition to total calories, micronutrients, iron, calcium, and vitamin deficiencies should be replenished. Restrictive or bland diets are avoided because they usually result in poor intake. A high-protein, high-carbohydrate diet with normal amounts of fat is recommended. Low-fiber diets may reduce symptoms during active colitis. In severe CrD, supplemental calories from formulas taken orally or by NG tube promote catch-up growth.

Specific diets can be effective for induction and maintenance but may be difficult to adhere to over time. For CrD, enteral nutrition with liquid formula providing more than 85% of caloric needs is an effective induction therapy and promotes linear growth. Other diets, such as the Crohn disease elimination, specific carbohydrate and paleo are popular in mild disease. Diet therapies are less effective in UC.

2. Aminosalicylates (ASA)—Multiple preparations of 5-ASA derivatives can induce and maintain remission in mild CrD and UC. Common preparations including 5-ASA products such as sulfasalazine (50 mg/kg/day), or balsalazide (0.75–2.5 g PO tid) or mesalamine products (adult dose range 2.4–4.8 g/day), are available in tablets, granules, and delayed release formulations targeting specific locations in the GI tract. Side effects include skin rash; nausea; headache and abdominal pain; hair loss; diarrhea; and rarely nephritis, pericarditis, serum sickness, hemolytic anemia, aplastic anemia, and pancreatitis. Sulfasalazine, in which sulfa delivers the 5-ASA, may cause sulfa-related side effects including photosensitivity and rash.

3. Corticosteroids—Patients with moderate to severe CrD and UC generally respond quickly to corticosteroids. Methylprednisolone (1 mg/kg/day) may be given intravenously when disease is severe. For moderate disease, prednisone (1 mg/kg/day, orally in one to two divided doses), or budesonide in preparations targeting the ileocecal area or colon may quickly improve symptoms but should be tapered over 4–8 weeks. Budesonide, due to "single pass" liver clearance, may have less side effects than prednisone. Steroid dependence is an indication for escalating therapy. Corticosteroid enemas and foams are useful topical agents for distal proctitis or left-sided colitis. While on systemic corticosteroids, consideration should be given to calcium and vitamin D supplementation as well as acid suppression to prevent gastritis. Due to side effects and incomplete healing, corticosteroids should be used sparingly.

4. Immunomodulators: azathioprine (AZA), 6-mercaptopurine (6MP), and methotrexate (MTX)—Immunomodulators are used in moderate to severe disease, when steroid-dependent, and in conjunction with biologics. AZA (2–3 mg/kg/day PO) or 6MP (1–2 mg/kg/day PO) dosing can be optimized based on the activity of the enzyme thiopurine methylene transferase (TPMT), which should be measured before starting therapy (genotype or enzyme activity). Korean and Chinese patients may have an enzyme deficiency (NUDT) in which AZA and 6MP are avoided. When adherence may be an issue, or when dose adjustments may be necessary, AZA or 6MP metabolites may be measured. Maximum therapeutic efficacy may not be seen for 2–3 months after beginning treatment. Side effects include pancreatitis, hepatotoxicity, and bone marrow suppression.

MTX is effective in CrD but not UC, and with onset of action within 2–3 weeks. Weekly oral or intramuscular dosage ranges from 15 mg/m^2 up to 25 mg. The most common side effect is nausea, managed with folate 1 mg a day; serious adverse events include bone marrow, liver, lung, kidney toxicities and teratogenicity.

5. Antibiotics—Metronidazole (15–30 mg/kg/day in three divided doses) and ciprofloxacin treat perianal CrD and bacterial overgrowth. Peripheral neuropathy may occur with the prolonged use of metronidazole.

6. Biologicals—Biologicals are used with increasing frequency and early use is associated with better response. Antibody against tumor necrosis factor-α (TNFα) is used for moderate to severe CrD and UC, and for fistulizing or penetrating disease. Formulations are available for IV (infliximab) or intramuscular (adalimumab, golimumab, certolizumab) administration. Disease recurrence is usually within 12 months of stopping therapy. New biologicals include vedolizumab, an alpha4/beta7 anti-integrin, ustekinumab, an anti IL12/23 agent, and risankizumab, an IL-23 antagonist. Use of biologics is associated with risk for infusion reactions, injection site reactions, and increased risk for opportunistic infections and for malignancy. Rarely, hepatosplenic T-cell lymphoma is associated with anti-TNF agents and concomitant AZA/6MP.

7. Other agents—Cyclosporine or tacrolimus may be used as a "bridge" to more definitive therapy (such as colectomy for UC). Probiotics and prebiotics are frequently used but with very limited data on efficacy. Tofacitinib and upadacitinib, oral JAK inhibitors, are approved for adults with UC, with pediatric trials starting.

8. Surveillance—After 7–8 years of colitis, cancer screening with routine colonoscopy and multiple biopsies is recommended. Persistent metaplasia, aneuploidy, or dysplasia indicates need for colectomy.

B. Surgical Treatment

1. Crohn disease—Ileocecal resection is the most common surgery, but recurrence is expected. Indications for surgery in CrD include stricture, obstruction, uncontrollable bleeding, perforation, abscess, fistula, and failure of medical management.

2. Ulcerative colitis—Total colectomy is curative and is recommended for patients with steroid dependence or steroid resistance, uncontrolled hemorrhage, toxic megacolon, high-grade dysplasia, or malignant tumors; elective colectomy may be chosen for prevention of colorectal cancer after 7–8 years of disease. Liver disease associated with IBD is not improved by colectomy.

Web Resources

http://www.crohnscolitisfoundation.org/.

Liver & Pancreas

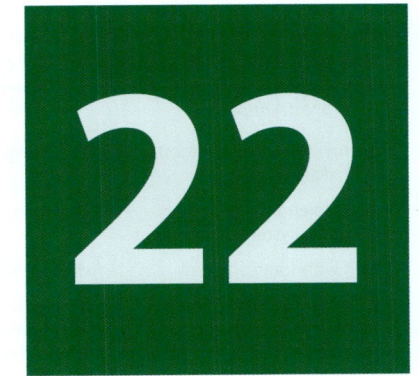

Ronald J. Sokol, MD

Julia M. Boster, MD, MSCS

Amy G. Feldman, MD, PhD

Jacob A. Mark, MD

Cara L. Mack, MD

Shikha S. Sundaram, MD, MSCI

LIVER DISORDERS

NEONATAL CHOLESTATIC JAUNDICE

Key clinical features of disorders causing prolonged neonatal cholestasis are (1) jaundice with elevated serum conjugated (or direct) bilirubin fraction (> 1.0 mg/dL and > 20% of total bilirubin), (2) variably acholic stools, (3) dark urine, and (4) hepatomegaly.

Neonatal cholestasis, with decreased bile flow, is caused by both intrahepatic and extrahepatic diseases. Specific clinical clues (Table 22–1) distinguish these two major categories of jaundice in 85% of cases. Patients with intrahepatic cholestasis frequently appear ill and fail to thrive, whereas infants with extrahepatic cholestasis (eg, biliary atresia [BA]) typically do not appear ill, have stools that are usually completely acholic, and have an enlarged, firm liver. Histologic examination of percutaneous liver biopsy specimens increases the accuracy of differentiation to 85%–90% (Table 22–2).

INTRAHEPATIC CHOLESTASIS

ESSENTIALS OF DIAGNOSIS & TYPICAL FEATURES

► Elevated total and conjugated/direct bilirubin.

► Hepatomegaly and dark urine.

► Patency of extrahepatic biliary tree.

▶ General Considerations

Intrahepatic cholestasis is characterized by impaired hepatocyte secretion of bile and patency of the extrahepatic biliary system. A specific cause can be identified in about 60%–80% of cases, the remainder being labeled as idiopathic neonatal hepatitis or transient neonatal cholestasis. Patency of the extrahepatic biliary tract is suggested by pigmented stools and lack of bile duct proliferation and portal tract bile plugs on liver biopsy. Patency can also be determined, when clinically indicated, by cholangiography carried out either intraoperatively, percutaneously by transhepatic cholecystography, or by endoscopic retrograde cholangiopancreatography (ERCP) using a pediatric-size side-viewing endoscope. Magnetic resonance cholangiopancreatography (MRCP) in infants is of limited use and highly dependent on the operator and equipment.

1. Perinatal or Neonatal Hepatitis Resulting from Infection

This diagnosis is considered in infants with jaundice, hepatomegaly, vomiting, lethargy, fever, and petechiae. It is important to identify perinatally acquired viral, bacterial, or protozoal infections (Table 22–3) as they may be treatable. Infection may occur transplacentally, by ascent through the cervix into amniotic fluid, from swallowed contaminated fluids (maternal blood, urine, vaginal secretions) during delivery, from blood transfusions administered in the early neonatal period, or from breast milk or post-natal environmental exposure. Infectious agents include herpes simplex virus (HSV), varicella virus, picornaviruses (enteroviruses and human echoviruses), cytomegalovirus (CMV), rubella virus, adenovirus, parvovirus, human herpesvirus type 6 (HHV-6), hepatitis B virus (HBV), human immunodeficiency virus (HIV), *Treponema pallidum*, and *Toxoplasma gondii*. Although hepatitis C may be transmitted vertically, it rarely causes neonatal cholestasis. The degree of liver cell injury caused by these agents is variable, ranging from massive hepatic necrosis (herpes simplex, picornavirus) to focal necrosis and mild inflammation (CMV, HBV). Serum bilirubin, alanine aminotransferase (ALT), aspartate aminotransferase (AST), alkaline phosphatase, and bile acids are typically elevated. The infant is jaundiced, may have petechiae or rash, and generally appears ill.

Table 22–1. Characteristic clinical features of intrahepatic and extrahepatic neonatal cholestasis.

Intrahepatic	Extrahepatic
Preterm infant, small for gestational age, appears ill	Full-term infant, seems well
Hepatosplenomegaly, other organ or system involvement	Hepatomegaly (firm to hard)
Stools with some pigment	Acholic stools
Associated cause identified (infections, metabolic, familial, etc)	Polysplenia or asplenia syndromes, midline liver (10% of biliary atresia)

► Clinical Findings

A. Symptoms and Signs

Clinical symptoms typically present in the first 2 weeks of life but may appear as late as age 2–3 months. Poor oral intake, poor sucking reflex, lethargy, hypotonia, and vomiting are frequent. Stools may be normal to pale in color but are seldom acholic. Dark urine stains the diaper. Firm hepatomegaly may be present, and splenomegaly is variably present. Macular, papular, vesicular, or petechial rashes may occur. Unusual presentations include neonatal liver failure, hypoproteinemia, anasarca (nonhemolytic hydrops), and hemorrhagic disease of the newborn.

B. Diagnostic Studies

Neutropenia, thrombocytopenia, and mild hemolysis are common. Mixed hyperbilirubinemia, elevated aminotransferases with near-normal alkaline phosphatase and γ-glutamyl transpeptidase (GGT), prolongation of clotting studies, mild acidosis, and elevated cord serum immunoglobulin M (IgM) suggest congenital infection. Nasopharyngeal washings,

Table 22–2. Characteristic histologic features of intrahepatic and extrahepatic neonatal cholestasis.

	Intrahepatic	Extrahepatic
Giant cells	+++	+
Lobules	Disarray	Normal
Portal reaction	Inflammation, minimal fibrosis	Fibrosis, lymphocytic infiltrate
Neoductular proliferation	Rare	Marked
Other	Steatosis, extramedullary hematopoiesis, iron deposition	Portal bile duct plugging, bile lakes

urine, stool, serum, and cerebrospinal fluid (CSF) may be cultured for virus and/or tested for pathogen-specific nucleic acids. Specific IgM antibody may be useful, as are long-bone radiographs to determine the presence of "celery stalking" in the metaphyseal regions of the humeri, femurs, and tibias. When indicated, computed tomography (CT) scans can identify intracranial calcifications (especially with CMV and toxoplasmosis). Hepatobiliary scintigraphy shows decreased hepatic clearance of the circulating isotope with intact excretion into the gut. Gallbladder is present on ultrasonography. Careful ophthalmologic examination may be useful for diagnosis of HSV, CMV, toxoplasmosis, and rubella.

A percutaneous liver biopsy may be useful in distinguishing infectious cholestasis but may not identify a specific infectious agent (see Table 22–2). Exceptions are the typical inclusions of CMV in hepatocytes or bile duct epithelial cells, the presence of multinucleated giant cells and intranuclear acidophilic inclusions of herpes simplex or varicella-zoster virus, the presence of adenovirus basophilic intranuclear inclusions, or positive immunohistochemical stains for several viruses. Variable degrees of lobular disarray characterized by focal necrosis, multinucleated giant-cell transformation, and ballooned pale hepatocytes with loss of cord-like arrangement of liver cells are usual. Intrahepatocytic and canalicular cholestasis may be prominent. Portal changes are not striking, but modest neoductular proliferation and mild fibrosis may occur. Viral cultures, immunohistochemical stains, or polymerase chain reaction (PCR) testing of biopsy material may be helpful.

► Differential Diagnosis

Great care must be taken to distinguish infectious causes of intrahepatic cholestasis from genetic or metabolic disorders because the clinical presentations are similar and may overlap. Galactosemia, hereditary fructose intolerance, and tyrosinemia must be investigated promptly because specific therapy is available. These infants may also have concomitant gram-negative bacteremia. Cystic fibrosis, α_1-antitrypsin deficiency, bile acid synthesis defects, progressive familial intrahepatic cholestasis (PFIC), mitochondrial respiratory chain disorders, and gestational alloimmune liver disease (GALD) must also be considered. Specific physical features may suggest Alagille syndrome, arthrogryposis/renal dysfunction/cholestasis (ARC) syndrome, or Zellweger syndrome. Idiopathic neonatal hepatitis (transient neonatal cholestasis) can be indistinguishable from infectious causes.

► Treatment

Infections with HSV, varicella, CMV, parvovirus, and toxoplasmosis have specific treatments (see Table 22–3). Penicillin for suspected syphilis, specific antiviral therapy, or antibiotics for bacterial hepatitis or urinary tract infections need to be administered promptly. Intravenous dextrose

Table 22–3. Infectious causes of neonatal hepatitis.

Infectious Agent	Diagnostic Tests	Specimens	Treatment
Cytomegalovirus	Culture and PCR, liver histology, IgM/[a]IgG	Urine, blood, liver, saliva	Ganciclovir (Foscarnet)[b]
Herpes simplex	PCR and culture, liver histology, Ag (skin)	Liver, blood, eye, throat, rectal, CSF, skin	Acyclovir
Rubella	Culture, IgM/[a]IgG	Liver, blood, urine	Supportive
Varicella	Culture, PCR, Ag (skin)	Skin, blood, CSF, liver	Acyclovir (Foscarnet)[b]
Parvovirus	Serum IgM/[a]IgG, PCR	Blood	Supportive, IVIG
Enteroviruses	Culture and PCR	Blood, urine, CSF, throat, rectal, liver	IVIG may have value; investigational drugs being tested
Adenovirus	Culture and Whole Blood PCR	Nasal/throat, rectal, blood, liver, urine	No established therapy, Cidofovir or IVIG may have value
Hepatitis B virus (HBV)	HBsAg, HBcAg IgM, HBV DNA	Serum	Supportive for acute infection
Hepatitis C virus (HCV)	HCV PCR, HCV IgG	Serum	Supportive for acute infection
Treponema pallidum	Serology	Serum, CSF	Penicillin
Toxoplasma gondii	IgM/[a]IgG, PCR, culture	Serum, CSF, liver	See Chapter 43, Parasites
Mycobacterium tuberculosis	Chest radiograph, liver tissue histologic stains, culture or PCR, gastric aspirate stain, culture or PCR	Serum, liver, gastric aspirate	INH, pyrazinamide, rifampin, ethambutol (if multiple drug-resistant TB is present, consult a specialist)
Bacterial infection	Cultures or PCR and other rapid methods	Blood, urine, other tissues or surfaces	Appropriate antibiotics

Ag, viral antigen testing; CSF, cerebrospinal fluid; HBcAg, hepatitis B core antigen; HBsAg, hepatitis B surface antigen; IgG, immunoglobin G; IgM, immunoglobin M; INH, isoniazid; IVIG, intravenous immune globulin; PCR, polymerase chain reaction test for viral DNA or RNA; PPD, purified protein derivative; TB, tuberculosis.

[a]IgG = positive indicates maternal infection and transfer of antibody trans-placentally; negative indicates unlikelihood of infection in mother and infant.

[b]Use foscarnet for resistant viruses, which should be rare in the neonate. Treat only if symptomatic.

is needed if feedings are not well tolerated. The consequences of cholestasis are treated as indicated (Table 22–4). Vitamin K orally or by injection and vitamins A, D, and E orally should be provided. Choleretics (ursodeoxycholic acid [UDCA]) are used if cholestasis persists. Corticosteroids are contraindicated.

▶ Prognosis

Multiple organ involvement portends a poor outcome. Hepatic or cardiac failure, intractable acidosis, or intracranial hemorrhage is associated with fatal outcome in herpesvirus, adenovirus, or enterovirus infections, and occurs occasionally in CMV or rubella infection. HBV rarely causes fulminant neonatal hepatitis; most infected infants are immunotolerant to hepatitis B. The neonatal liver usually recovers without fibrosis after acute infections. Chronic cholestasis, although rare following infections, may lead to dental enamel hypoplasia, failure to thrive, biliary rickets, severe pruritus, and xanthoma.

Bilavsky E, Schwarz M, Bar-Sever Z, Pardo J, Amir J: Hepatic involvement in congenital cytomegalovirus infection—infrequent yet significant. J Viral Hepat 2014 Dec 12. doi: 10.1111/jvh.12374 [PMID: 25496231].

Feldman AG, Sokol RJ: Neonatal cholestasis: emerging molecular diagnostics and potential novel therapeutics. Nat Rev Gastroenterol Hepatol 2019 Jun;16(6):346–360 [PMID: 30903105].

Goel A et al: Detection of cytomegalovirus in liver tissue by polymerase chain reaction in infants with neonatal cholestasis. Pediatr Infect Dis J 2018 Jul;37(7):632–636 [PMID: 29389827].

2. Specific Infectious Agents

A. Neonatal Hepatitis B Virus Disease

Vertical transmission of HBV may occur at any time during perinatal life. Most cases are acquired from mothers who are asymptomatic carriers of HBV. Although HBV has been found in most body fluids, including breast milk, neonatal transmission occurs primarily from exposure to maternal blood at delivery and only occasionally transplacentally

Table 22–4. Treatment of complications of chronic cholestatic liver disease.

Indication	Treatment	Dose	Toxicity
Intrahepatic cholestasis	Phenobarbital	3–10 mg/kg/day	Drowsiness, irritability, interference with vitamin D metabolism
	Cholestyramine or colestipol hydrochloride	250–500 mg/kg/day	Constipation, acidosis, binding of drugs, increased steatorrhea
	Ursodeoxycholic acid	15–20 mg/kg/day	Transient increase in pruritus
Pruritus	Phenobarbital	3–10 mg/kg/day	Drowsiness, irritability, interference with vitamin D metabolism
	Cholestyramine or colestipol	250–500 mg/kg/day	Constipation, acidosis, binding of drugs, increased steatorrhea
	Diphenhydramine hydrochloride	5–10 mg/kg/day	Drowsiness
	Hydroxyzine	2–5 mg/kg/day	Drowsiness
	Ultraviolet light B	Exposure as needed	Skin burn
	Rifampicin	10 mg/kg/day	Hepatotoxicity, bone marrow suppression
	Ursodeoxycholic acid	15–20 mg/kg/day	Transient increase in pruritus
	Naltrexone	1 mg/kg/day	Irritability, vomiting
	Plasmapheresis	Each 2–4 wk	Central venous access, expensive
Steatorrhea	Formula containing medium-chain triglycerides (eg, Pregestimil or Alimentum)	120–150 kcal/kg/day for infants	Expensive
	Oil supplement containing medium-chain triglycerides	1–2 mL/kg/day	Diarrhea, aspiration
Malabsorption of fat-soluble vitamins	Vitamin A	10,000–25,000 U/day	Hepatitis, pseudotumor cerebri, bone lesions
	Vitamin D_2 or D_3	800–8000 U/day (up to 1000 U/kg/day for infants)	Hypercalcemia, hypercalciuria
	25-hydroxy-cholecalciferol	3–5 mcg/kg/day	Hypercalcemia, hypercalciuria
	1,25-dihydroxy-cholecalciferol	0.05–0.2 mcg/kg/day	Hypercalcemia, hypercalciuria
	Vitamin E (oral)	25–200 IU/kg/day	
	Vitamin E (oral, TPGS[a])	15–25 IU/kg/day	Potentiation of vitamin K deficiency
	Vitamin E (intramuscular)	1–2 mg/kg/day	Potentiation of vitamin K deficiency
	Vitamin K (oral)	2.5 mg twice per wk up to 5 mg/day	
	Vitamin K (intramuscular)	2–5 mg each 4 wk	Muscle calcifications
Malabsorption of other nutrients	Multiple vitamin	One to two times the standard dose	
	Calcium	25–100 mg/kg/day	Hypercalcemia, hypercalciuria
	Phosphorus	25–50 mg/kg/day	Gastrointestinal intolerance
	Zinc	1 mg/kg/day	Interference with copper and iron absorption
			Gastrointestinal intolerance

[a]D-α-Tocopheryl polyethylene glycol-1000 succinate.

(< 5%–10% of cases). In chronic HB surface antigen (HBsAg)–carrier mothers, neonatal acquisition risk is greatest if the mother: (1) is also HB "e" antigen (HBeAg)–positive and HB "e" antibody (HBeAb)–negative, (2) has high serum levels of hepatitis B core antibody (HBcAb), or (3) has high blood levels of HBV DNA (> 10^7 copies/mL). The infant has a 70%–90% chance of acquiring HBV at birth from an HBsAg/HBeAg-positive mother if the infant does not receive prophylaxis. Most infected infants develop a prolonged asymptomatic immune-tolerant phase of HBV infection. Fulminant hepatic necrosis and liver failure rarely occur in infants. Other patients develop immune active chronic hepatitis with focal hepatocyte necrosis and a mild portal inflammatory response. Chronic hepatitis may persist for years, with serologic evidence of persisting HBeAg and mildly elevated or normal serum aminotransferases. Most infected infants have only mild biochemical evidence, if any, of liver injury and do not appear ill. Most infants remain asymptomatic in an immune-tolerant state of HBV infection; 3%–5% per year develop acute or chronic hepatitis (see section Hepatitis B).

To prevent perinatal transmission, all infants of mothers who are HBsAg-positive (regardless of HBeAg status) should receive hepatitis B immunoglobulin (HBIG) and hepatitis B vaccine within the first 24 hours after birth and vaccine again at ages 1 and 6 months (see Chapter 10). This prevents HBV infection in 85%–95% of infants. If not given at birth, HBIG can be administered as late as 7 days postpartum, as long as the infant has received the vaccine. Universal HBV immunization during infancy is recommended for all infants at birth regardless of maternal HBV status. Universal screening of pregnant women for HBsAg is conducted to determine which infants will also need HBIG. Pregnant women with greater than 200,000 IU/mL of HBV DNA should be considered for third trimester anti-viral therapy to lower HBV levels and reduce risk for vertical transmission.

B. Neonatal Bacterial Hepatitis

Most bacterial liver infections in newborns are acquired by transplacental invasion from amnionitis with ascending spread from maternal vaginal or cervical infection. Onset is abrupt, usually within 48–72 hours after delivery, with signs of sepsis and often shock. Jaundice appears early with direct hyperbilirubinemia. The most common organisms involved are *Escherichia coli*, *Listeria monocytogenes*, and group B streptococci. Neonatal liver abscesses caused by *E coli* or *Staphylococcus aureus* may result from omphalitis or umbilical vein catheterization. These infections require specific antibiotics in optimal doses and combinations and, rarely, surgical or interventional radiologic drainage. Deaths are common, but survivors show no long-term consequences of liver disease.

C. Neonatal Jaundice With Urinary Tract Infection

Urinary tract infections typically present with cholestasis between the second and fourth weeks of life. Lethargy, fever, poor appetite, jaundice, and hepatomegaly may be present. Except for mixed hyperbilirubinemia, other liver function tests (LFTs) are only mildly abnormal. Leukocytosis is frequently present, and infection is confirmed by urine culture. The liver impairment is caused by the action of endotoxin and cytokines on bile secretion.

Treatment of the infection leads to resolution of the cholestasis without hepatic sequelae. Metabolic liver diseases, such as galactosemia and tyrosinemia, may present with gram-negative bacterial urinary tract infection and must be excluded.

Cheung KW, Seto MTY, Lao TT: Prevention of perinatal hepatitis B virus transmission. Arch Gynecol Obstet 2019 Aug;300(2):251–259 [PMID: 31098821].

Harris JB, Holmes AP: Neonatal herpes simplex viral infections and acyclovir: an update. J Pediatr Pharmacol Ther 2017 Mar–Apr;22(2):88–93 [PMID: 24869532].

Terrault NA et al: Update on prevention, diagnosis, and treatment of chronic hepatitis B: AASLD 2018 hepatitis B guidance. Hepatology 2018 Apr;67(4):1560–1599 [PMID: 29405329].

Zeng QL et al: Tenofovir alafenamide to prevent perinatal hepatitis B transmission: a multicenter, prospective, observational study. Clin Infect Dis 2021 Nov 2;73(9):e3324–e3332 [PMID: 33395488].

3. Intrahepatic Cholestasis Resulting From Inborn Errors of Metabolism, Familial, & "Toxic" Causes

Cholestasis caused by specific enzyme and transporter deficiencies, other genetic disorders, or certain toxins share findings of intrahepatic cholestasis (jaundice, hepatomegaly, and normal to completely acholic stools). Specific genetic conditions have characteristic clinical signs, and many can be identified by genotyping.

A. Inborn Errors of Metabolism

Establishing the specific diagnosis as early as possible is important because dietary or pharmacologic treatment may be available (Table 22–5), and parents of the affected infant should be offered genetic counseling. For some disorders, prenatal genetic diagnosis is available.

Cholestasis caused by inborn errors of metabolism (eg, galactosemia, hereditary fructose intolerance, and tyrosinemia) is frequently accompanied by vomiting, lethargy, poor feeding, hypoglycemia, or irritability. The infants often appear septic; gram-negative bacteria can be cultured from blood in up to 25%–50% of symptomatic cases, especially in galactosemia with cholestasis. Neonatal screening programs for galactosemia and tyrosinemia usually detect the disorder before cholestasis develops. Other metabolic and genetic causes of neonatal intrahepatic cholestasis are outlined in Table 22–5. Treatment of these disorders is discussed in Chapter 36.

B. "Toxic" Causes of Neonatal Cholestasis

1. Neonatal ischemic-hypoxic conditions—Perinatal events that result in hypoperfusion or hypoxia of the gastrointestinal system are sometimes followed within 1–2 weeks by cholestasis. This occurs in infants with birth asphyxia, acute cardiac dysfunction, severe hypoxia, hypoglycemia, shock, and acidosis. When these perinatal conditions develop in association with gastrointestinal lesions, such as ruptured omphalocele, gastroschisis, or necrotizing enterocolitis, a subsequent cholestatic picture is common (25%–50% of cases). Mixed hyperbilirubinemia, elevated alkaline phosphatase and GGT values, and variable elevation of the aminotransferases are common. Stools are seldom persistently acholic.

The mainstays of treatment are choleretics (UDCA), introduction of enteral feedings using special formulas as soon as possible, and nutrient supplementation until the cholestasis resolves (see Table 22–4). As long as no severe intestinal problem or ongoing sepsis is present (eg, short gut syndrome or intestinal failure) and the infant is weaned off parenteral nutrition within 1–2 months, resolution of the hepatic abnormalities without subsequent hepatic fibrosis is the rule, although this may take many weeks.

2. Parenteral nutrition-associated cholestasis (PNAC)—Cholestasis may develop after 1–2 weeks in premature

Table 22–5. Metabolic and genetic causes of neonatal cholestasis.

Disease	Inborn Error	Hepatic Pathology	Diagnostic Studies
Galactosemia	Galactose-1-phosphate uridyltransferase	Cholestasis, steatosis, necrosis, pseudoacini, fibrosis	Galactose-1-phosphate uridyltransferase assay of red blood cells or genotyping[a]
Fructose intolerance	Fructose-1-phosphate aldolase	Steatosis, necrosis, pseudoacini, fibrosis	Liver fructose-1-phosphate aldolase assay or genotyping[a]
Tyrosinemia	Fumarylacetoacetase	Necrosis, steatosis, pseudoacini, portal fibrosis	Urinary succinylacetone, fumarylacetoacetase assay of red blood cells
Cystic fibrosis	Cystic fibrosis transmembrane conductance regulator gene	Cholestasis, neoductular proliferation, excess bile duct mucus, portal fibrosis	Sweat chloride test and genotyping[a]
Hypopituitarism	Deficient production of pituitary hormones	Cholestasis, giant cells	Thyroxin, TSH, cortisol levels
α_1-Antitrypsin deficiency	Abnormal α_1-antitrypsin molecule (PiZZ or PiSZ phenotype)	Giant cells, cholestasis, steatosis, neoductular proliferation, fibrosis, PAS-positive diastase–resistant cytoplasmic globules	Serum α_1-antitrypsin phenotype or genotype
Gaucher disease	β-Glucosidase	Cholestasis, cytoplasmic inclusions in Kupffer cells (foam cells)	β-Glucosidase assay in leukocytes or genotyping[a]
Niemann-Pick type C disease	Lysosomal sphingomyelinase	Cholestasis, cytoplasmic inclusions in Kupffer cells	Sphingomyelinase assay of leukocytes or liver or fibroblasts (type C); genotyping[a]
Glycogen storage disease type IV	Branching enzyme	Fibrosis, cirrhosis, PAS-diastase–resistant cytoplasmic inclusions	Branching enzyme analysis of leukocytes or liver, genotyping[a]
Gestational alloimmune liver disease (GALD)	Transplacental alloimmunization	Giant cells, portal fibrosis, hemosiderosis, cirrhosis	Histology, iron stains on lip biopsy, chest and abdominal MRI
Peroxisomal disorders (eg, Zellweger syndrome)	Deficient peroxisomal enzymes or assembly	Cholestasis, necrosis, fibrosis, cirrhosis, hemosiderosis	Plasma very-long-chain fatty acids, qualitative bile acids, plasmalogen, pipecolic acid, liver electron microscopy, genotyping[a]
Bile acid synthesis and metabolism disorders	Nine enzyme deficiencies defined	Cholestasis, necrosis, giant cells	Urine, serum, duodenal fluid analyzed for bile acids by fast atom bombardment–mass spectroscopy, genotyping[a]
Byler disease (PFIC type I)	FIC-1 (ATP8B1) gene	Cholestasis, necrosis, giant cells, fibrosis	Histology, family history, normal cholesterol, low or normal γ-glutamyl transpeptidase, genotyping[a]
PFIC type II PFIC type III	BSEP (ABCB11) gene MDR3 (ABCB4) gene	Cholestasis, necrosis, giant cells, fibrosis Cholestasis, bile duct proliferation, portal fibrosis	Histology, family history, normal cholesterol, low or normal γ-glutamyl transpeptidase, genotyping[a] Elevated GGTP, genotyping[a]
TJP2 deficiency (PFIC type IV)	TJP2 gene	Cholestasis, necrosis, giant cells, fibrosis	Genotyping[a]
FXR deficiency (PFIC type V)	NRIH4 gene	Cholestasis, necrosis, giant cells, fibrosis	Genotyping[a]
MYO5B deficiency (PFIC type VI)	MYO5B gene	Cholestasis, necrosis, giant cells, fibrosis	Genotyping[a]

(Continued)

Table 22–5. Metabolic and genetic causes of neonatal cholestasis. (*Continued*)

Disease	Inborn Error	Hepatic Pathology	Diagnostic Studies
Arthrogryposis/renal dysfunction/cholestasis syndrome	*VPS33B* and *VIPAR* genes	Cholestasis, fibrosis	Genotyping[a]
Alagille syndrome (syndromic paucity of interlobular bile ducts)	*JAGGED1* and *NOTCH2* mutations	Cholestasis, paucity of interlobular bile ducts, increased copper levels	Three or more clinical features, liver histology, genotyping[a]
Mitochondrial hepatopathies (respiratory chain diseases and mtDNA depletion syndrome)	*POLG, BCS1I, SCO1, DGUOK,* Twinkle and *MPV17, TRMU,* and other gene mutations	Cholestasis, steatosis, portal fibrosis, abnormal mitochondria on electron microscopy	mtDNA depletion studies, respiratory chain studies on liver or muscle, genotyping[a]

IV, intravenous; MDR3, multiple-drug resistance protein type 3; MRI, magnetic resonance imaging; mtDNA, mitochondrial DNA; PAS, periodic acid–Schiff; PFIC, progressive familial intrahepatic cholestasis; TSH, thyroid-stimulating hormone.
[a]Performed on leukocyte DNA.

newborns receiving parenteral nutrition, especially those with necrotizing enterocolitis. Even full-term infants with significant intestinal atresia, resections, gastroschisis, congenital absorptive deficiencies, or dysmotility (all potential causes of intestinal failure) may develop PNAC, also called intestinal failure-associated cholestasis. Contributing factors include toxicity of intravenous soy lipid emulsions (eg, plant sterols), diminished stimulation of bile flow from prolonged absence of feedings, frequent episodes of bacterial or fungal infection, small intestinal bacterial overgrowth with impaired barrier function and translocation of intestinal bacteria and their cell wall products, missing nutrients or antioxidants, photooxidation of amino acids, and the "physiologic cholestatic" propensity of the infant. Activation of innate immune pathways in the liver by endotoxin and plant sterols, as well as reduced ileal secretion of FGF19 due to resections or dysfunction, appears to be involved. Histology of the liver may be identical to that of BA. Early introduction of feedings, surgical/medical therapies to induce intestinal adaptation (eg, GLP-2 analogue therapy), prevention of central line–associated bloodstream infections (CLABSIs), and modifications of intravenous lipid emulsions (substituting for soy-oil lipid emulsions with fish oil lipid emulsions or mixed lipid emulsions) have reduced the frequency/severity of this disorder. The prognosis is generally good; however, infants with intestinal failure may progress to cirrhosis, liver failure, or rarely hepatocellular carcinoma, requiring liver and intestinal, or multivisceral transplantation. Oral erythromycin as a promotility agent may reduce the incidence of cholestasis in very-low-birth-weight infants. Substituting intravenous fish oil–based lipid emulsions or multiple constituent lipid emulsions, or reducing the amount of soy oil–based lipid emulsions, may reverse PNAC and prevent the need for liver transplantation and delay the need for intestinal transplantation.

3. Inspissated bile syndrome—This syndrome is the result of accumulation of bile in canaliculi and in the small- and medium-sized bile ducts in hemolytic disease of the newborn (Rh, ABO) and in some infants receiving parenteral nutrition. The same mechanisms may cause intrinsic obstruction of the common bile duct. An ischemia-reperfusion injury may also contribute to cholestasis in Rh incompatibility. Stools may become acholic and levels of bilirubin, primarily conjugated, may reach 40 mg/dL. If inspissation of bile occurs within the extrahepatic biliary tree, differentiation from BA may be difficult. Although most cases improve slowly over 2–6 months, persistence of complete cholestasis (acholic stools) for more than 1–2 weeks requires further studies (ultrasonography, liver biopsy) with possible cholangiography. Irrigation of the common bile duct is sometimes necessary to dislodge the obstructing inspissated biliary material.

El Kasmi KC et al: Phytosterols promote liver injury and Kupffer cell activation in parenteral nutrition-associated liver disease. Sci Transl Med 2013 Oct 9;5(206):206ra137 [PMID: 24107776].
Khalaf RT, Sokol RJ: New insights into intestinal failure associated liver disease in children. Hepatology 2020 Apr;71(4):1486–1498 [PMID: 32003009].
Secor JD, Yu L, Tsikis S, Fligor S, Puder M, Gura KM: Current strategies for managing intestinal failure-associated liver disease. Expert Opin Drug Saf 2021 Mar;20(3):307–320 [PMID: 33356650].

4. Idiopathic Neonatal Hepatitis (INH; Transient Neonatal Cholestasis)

This idiopathic type of cholestatic jaundice, which has a typical liver biopsy appearance of giant cell hepatitis, historically accounted for up to 20%–40% of cases of neonatal intrahepatic cholestasis but is decreasing in frequency as new genetic causes of cholestasis are discovered. The degree of cholestasis is variable, and the disorder may be indistinguishable from extrahepatic causes in 10% of cases. Viral infections, α_1-antitrypsin deficiency, Alagille syndrome, Niemann-Pick type C disease (NPC), PFIC and other genetic disorders, citrin deficiency, GALD, mitochondrial disorders, and bile acid synthesis defects may present with similar clinical and histologic features and should be excluded. In idiopathic neo-natal hepatitis, PFIC types I and II, ARC syndrome, and bile acid synthesis defects, GGT levels are normal or low. Electron microscopy of the liver biopsy and genotyping will help dis-tinguish NPC and PFIC. It is likely that a heterozygous state or mild missense mutations for known or yet to be discov-ered causative genes are responsible for the vast majority of idiopathic cases.

Intrauterine growth retardation, prematurity, poor feed-ing, emesis, poor growth, and partially or intermittently acholic stools are characteristic of INH. Serious hemorrhage from vitamin K deficiency may also be present. Patients with neonatal lupus erythematosus may present with giant-cell hepatitis; however, thrombocytopenia, rash, or congenital heart block is usually also present.

In cases of suspected INH (diagnosed in the absence of infectious, known genetic, metabolic, and toxic causes and characteristic liver biopsy findings) that persist, genetic test-ing (targeted gene panels or whole exome sequencing) should be obtained, and patency of the biliary tree may need to be verified to exclude extrahepatic disorders. HIDA scanning and ultrasonography may be helpful in this regard if stools are acholic. Liver biopsy findings are usually diagnostic after age 6–8 weeks (see Table 22–2) but may be misleading before age 6 weeks as there is overlap with BA histology. Failure to detect patency of the biliary tree, nondiagnostic liver biopsy findings, or persisting complete cholestasis (acholic stools) are indications for intraoperative cholangiography performed by an experienced surgeon, ERCP, or percutaneous transhepatic cholecystography. Occasionally, a small but patent (hypoplas-tic) extrahepatic biliary tree is demonstrated (as in Alagille syndrome). It is probably the result, rather than the cause, of diminished bile flow, so surgical reconstruction of hypoplastic biliary trees in Alagille syndrome should not be attempted.

Therapy should include choleretics, a special formula with medium-chain triglycerides (eg, Pregestimil, Alimen-tum) or breast milk (if growth is adequate), and supplemental fat-soluble vitamins in water-soluble form (see Table 22–4). This therapy is continued as long as significant cholestasis remains (conjugated bilirubin > 1 mg/dL). Fat-soluble vita-min serum levels and INR should be monitored at regular intervals while supplements are given and repeated at least once after their discontinuation.

Around 80% of patients recover without significant hepatic fibrosis. However, failure to resolve the cholestatic picture by age 6–12 months is associated with progressive liver dis-ease and evolving cirrhosis, most likely caused by known or yet to be defined underlying genetic/metabolic disorders.

Liver transplantation has been successful when signs of hepatic decompensation are noted (rising bilirubin, coagu-lopathy, intractable ascites).

Hertel PM et al: Presentation and outcomes of infants with idiopathic cholestasis: a multicenter prospective study. J Pediatr Gastroenterol Nutr 2021 Oct 1;73(4):478–484 [PMID: 34310436].
Liu LY et al: Association of variants of ABCB11 with transient neonatal cholestasis. Pediatr Int 2013;55:138–344 [PMID: 23279303].
Yan YY et al: Abnormal bilirubin metabolism in patients with sodium taurocholate cotransporting polypeptide deficiency. J Pediatr Gastroenterol Nutr 2020 Nov;71(5):e138–e141 [PMID: 33093374].

5. Paucity of Interlobular Bile Ducts

Forms of intrahepatic cholestasis caused by decreased num-bers of interlobular bile ducts (< 0.5 bile ducts per portal tract) are classified according to whether they are associated with other malformations. Alagille syndrome (syndromic paucity or arteriohepatic dysplasia) is caused by mutations in the gene *JAGGED1*, located on chromosome 20p, which codes for a ligand of the notch receptor, or more rarely in the gene *NOTCH2*. Alagille syndrome is recognized by the characteristic facies, which become more obvious with age. The forehead is prominent with deep-set eyes and sometimes hypertelorism. The chin is small and slightly pointed and ears are prominent. The stool color varies with the severity of cholestasis. Pruritus begins by age 6 months. Firm, smooth hepatomegaly may be present, or the liver may be of normal size. Cardiac murmurs are present in 90% of patients, and butterfly vertebrae (incomplete fusion of the vertebral body or anterior arch) are present in 50%. Xanthomas may develop in those with severe hypercholesterolemia.

Conjugated hyperbilirubinemia may be mild to severe (2–15 mg/dL). Serum alkaline phosphatase, GGT, and cho-lesterol may be markedly elevated, especially early in life. Serum bile acids are always elevated, aminotransferases are mildly to moderately increased, but clotting factors and other liver proteins are usually normal.

Cardiac involvement includes peripheral pulmonary artery, branch pulmonary artery, or pulmonary valvular ste-noses, atrial septal defect, coarctation of the aorta, and tetral-ogy of Fallot. Up to 10%–15% of patients have intracranial vascular or cystic abnormalities or may develop intracranial hemorrhage or stroke in childhood.

Eye findings (posterior embryotoxon or a prominent Schwalbe line in 50%–90%) are common and renal abnor-malities (dysplastic kidneys, renal tubular ectasia, single kid-ney, renal tubular acidosis, hematuria) may occur in 40% of patients. Growth retardation with normal to increased levels of growth hormone (growth hormone resistance) is common. Although variable, the intelligence quotient is frequently low. Hypogonadism with micropenis may be present. A weak, high-pitched voice may develop. Neurologic disorders resulting from vitamin E deficiency (areflexia, ataxia, ophthalmoplegia), which may eventually develop in unsupplemented children, may be profound.

In the nonsyndromic form, paucity of interlobular bile ducts occurs associated with α_1-antitrypsin deficiency, Zellweger syndrome, in association with lymphedema (Aagenaes syndrome), PFIC, cystic fibrosis, CMV or rubella infection, and inborn errors of bile acid metabolism.

High doses (250 mg/kg/day) of cholestyramine may control pruritus, lower cholesterol, and clear xanthomas. UDCA (15–20 mg/kg/day) appears to be more effective and causes fewer side effects than cholestyramine. Rifampicin (10 mg/kg/day) may also reduce pruritus. Naltrexone (1 mg/kg/day) is occasionally required. Partial external or internal biliary diversion or ileal exclusion surgery may reduce pruritus and xanthomas in about half of severe cases, as long as significant hepatic fibrosis is absent. Unremitting pruritus may indicate the need for liver transplantation. The addition of newer ileal bile acid transporter (IBAT) inhibitors effectively reduces pruritus in 70%–90% of patients and may delay or avoid biliary diversion surgery or liver transplantation in childhood. Nutritional therapy to prevent wasting and deficiencies of fat-soluble vitamins is of particular importance because of the severity of cholestasis (see Table 22–4).

Prognosis is more favorable in the syndromic than in the nonsyndromic varieties. In the former, only 40%–50% of patients have significant complications, whereas over 70% of patients with nonsyndromic varieties progress to cirrhosis. Many of this latter group likely have genetic forms of PFIC that have yet to be identified. In Alagille syndrome, cholestasis may improve by age 2–4 years, with minimal residual hepatic fibrosis. Survival into adulthood despite raised serum bile acids, aminotransferases, and alkaline phosphatase occurs in about 50% of cases, however progressive portal hypertension may ensue. Several patients have developed hepatocellular carcinoma. Hypogonadism has been noted, however, fertility is not often affected. Cardiovascular anomalies and intracranial vascular lesions may shorten life expectancy. Some patients have persistent, severe cholestasis, rendering their quality of life poor. Recurrent bone fractures may result from metabolic bone disease. Liver transplantation has been successful under these circumstances. Intracranial hemorrhage, moyamoya disease, or stroke may occur in up to 10%–12% of affected children. IBAT inhibitors are now approved in many countries as agents to reduce pruritus and serum bile acid levels and possibly to improve long-term outcomes.

Kamath BM et al: Fat-soluble vitamin assessment and supplementation in cholestasis. Clin Liver Dis 2022 Aug;26(3):537–553 [PMID: 35868689].

Kamath BM et al: Outcomes of childhood cholestasis in Alagille syndrome: results of a multicenter observational study. Hepatol Commun 2020 Jan 22;4(3):387–398 [PMID: 33313463].

Kohut TJ et al: Alagille syndrome: a focused review on clinical features, genetics, and treatment. Semin Liver Dis 2021 Jul 2. doi: 10.1055/s-0041-1730951. Online ahead of print [PMID: 34215014].

Shneider BL et al: Impact of long-term administration of maralixibat on children with cholestasis secondary to Alagille syndrome. Hepatol Commun 2022 Aug;6(8):1922–1933 [PMID: 35672955].

6. Progressive Familial Intrahepatic Cholestasis (Byler Disease, Byler Syndrome, & Others)

Progressive familial intrahepatic cholestasis (PFIC) is an expanding group of genetic disorders presenting as pruritus, diarrhea, jaundice, fat-soluble vitamin deficiencies, and failure to thrive in the first 6–12 months of life. PFIC type I (Byler disease), caused by biallelic mutations in *ATP8B1* coding FIC1, an aminophospholipid transporting ATPase, is associated with low to normal serum levels of GGT and cholesterol and elevated levels of bilirubin, aminotransferases, and bile acids. Pancreatitis and hearing loss may develop. Liver biopsy demonstrates cellular cholestasis, sometimes with a paucity of interlobular bile ducts and centrilobular fibrosis that progresses to cirrhosis. Giant cells are absent. Electron microscopy may show characteristic granular "Byler bile" in canaliculi. Diagnosis is established by genotyping by targeted gene panels, whole exome or whole genome sequencing. Treatment includes administration of UDCA, antipruritics, partial biliary diversion or ileal exclusion if the condition is unresponsive to medical therapy and advanced fibrosis is absent, and liver transplantation if progressive and unresponsive to these therapies. With partial biliary diversion or ileal exclusion surgery, many patients show improved growth and liver histology, reduction in symptoms, and, thus, avoid or delay liver transplantation. Following liver transplantation, chronic diarrhea and fatty liver may complicate recovery. IBAT inhibitors are effective in reducing pruritus and improving growth in up to 40%–50% of patients and may replace biliary diversion surgery in the treatment algorithm. IBAT inhibitors (maralixibat and odevixibat) have been approved in many countries.

PFIC type II is caused by biallelic mutations in *ABCB11* coding the bile salt export pump (BSEP), the adenosine triphosphate–dependent canalicular bile salt transport protein. These patients are clinically and biochemically similar to PFIC type I patients (eg, low GGT cholestasis), but liver histology includes numerous multinucleated "giant cells", AST and ALT are more elevated, and they lack the extrahepatic features. There is an increased incidence of hepatocellular carcinoma in patients with severe (protein truncating) *ABCB11* mutations. Treatment is similar to PFIC type I although close monitoring for hepatocellular carcinoma is essential. IBAT inhibitors are effective in 50% of patients and may avoid partial biliary diversion. Following liver transplantation, recurrent disease has been described in patients who developed autoantibody-mediated BSEP dysfunction.

PFIC type III is caused by mutations in *ABCB4* coding the multiple drug resistance protein type 3 (MDR3), a canalicular protein that pumps phospholipid into bile. Serum GGT and bile acid levels are both elevated, bile duct proliferation and portal tract fibrosis are seen in liver biopsies (resembling BA), and bile phospholipid levels are low. Treatment requires UDCA and is otherwise similar to that of other forms of PFIC except that partial biliary diversion is not recommended and liver transplantation is inevitable for most patients. *ABCB4* variants are also associated with intrahepatic cholestasis of pregnancy, drug hepatotoxicity and cholelithiasis in adults.

PFIC type IV is a low GGT form of neonatal cholestasis caused by mutations in tight junction protein 2 (*TJP2*) with rapid progression to cirrhosis and need for liver transplantation in early childhood. PFIC type V (FXR deficiency) and type VI (*MYO5B* deficiency) resemble clinically the other low GGT PFICs; however, FXR deficiency is more severe and presents early and *MYO5B* deficiency may be associated with chronic diarrhea (microvillus inclusion disease). Other genes have been identified in small numbers of PFIC-like cases (eg, *OSTα/β*, *UNC45*, *USP53*, *ABCC12*). Up to one-third of PFIC patients have negative genotyping for the above genes and likely have yet-to-be discovered genetic etiologies.

Bile acid synthesis defects are clinically similar to PFIC types I and II, with low serum levels of GGT and cholesterol; however, the serum levels of total and primary bile acids are inappropriately normal or low, pruritus is generally absent, and urine bile acid analysis or genotyping may identify a synthesis defect. Milder defects cause fat-soluble vitamin deficiency without severe liver disease. Treatment of most bile acid synthesis defects is with oral cholic acid and for conjugation defects with oral glycocholic acid.

Feldman AG, Sokol RJ: Neonatal cholestasis: emerging molecular diagnostics and potential novel therapeutics. Nat Rev Gastroenterol Hepatol 2019 Jun;16(6):346–360 [PMID: 30903105].

Sambrotta M et al: Mutations in TJP2 cause progressive cholestatic liver disease. Nat Genet 2014 Apr;46(4):326–328 [PMID: 24614073].

Thompson RJ et al: Odevixibat treatment in progressive familial intrahepatic cholestasis: a randomised, placebo-controlled, phase 3 trial. Lancet Gastroenterol Hepatol 2022 Sep;7(9):830–842 [PMID: 35780807].

Wang K et al: Analysis of surgical interruption of the enterohepatic circulation as a treatment for pediatric cholestasis. Hepatology 2017;65:1645–1654 [PMID: 28027587].

EXTRAHEPATIC NEONATAL CHOLESTASIS

Extrahepatic neonatal cholestasis is characterized by complete and persistent cholestasis (acholic stools) in the first 1–3 months of life; lack of patency of the extrahepatic biliary tree demonstrated by intraoperative, percutaneous transhepatic, or endoscopic cholangiography; firm to hard hepatomegaly; and typical features on histologic examination of liver biopsy tissue (see Table 22–2). Causes include BA, choledochal cyst (CDC), spontaneous perforation of the extrahepatic ducts, neonatal sclerosing cholangitis, stones, and intrinsic or extrinsic obstruction of the common duct.

1. Biliary Atresia

► General Considerations

BA is a progressive fibroinflammatory obliteration of the lumen of all, or part of, the extrahepatic biliary tree presenting within the first 3 months of life. BA occurs in 1:6600 (Taiwan)–1:18,000 (Europe) births, and in the United States the incidence is approximately 1:12,000. The incidence is highest in Asians, African Americans, and preterm infants, and there is a slight female predominance. There are four types of BA: isolated BA (84% of cases), BA with at least one malformation but without laterality defects (6%; CV, GI, or GU defects), BA splenic malformation (BASM) syndrome associated with laterality defects and polysplenia or asplenia (4%–10%), and cystic BA, which includes a hilar CDC. The etiology of BA is likely multifactorial, encompassing an initial viral, toxin, or environmental injury to the bile duct epithelium that likely occurs prenatally, leading to inflammatory and autoimmune responses targeting the bile ducts, and culminating in aggressive fibrosis and obstruction of the biliary system. There are also rare genetic forms of BA, such as that caused by pathologic variants in *PKD1L1*.

► Clinical Findings

A. Symptoms and Signs

All infants with BA have jaundice that may be noted in the newborn period or by age 2–3 weeks. Therefore, all jaundiced infants 2 weeks of age or older should have conjugated bilirubin measured to identify cholestasis. Stools are pale yellow, gray, or acholic. Firm hepatomegaly is common at diagnosis and infants are at risk for failure to thrive due to fat malabsorption. Symptoms of portal hypertension (splenomegaly, ascites, variceal bleeding) and malnutrition may develop in the first year of life. Pruritus, digital clubbing, bone fractures, and variceal bleeding complications may occur in infancy or later in childhood.

B. Laboratory Findings and Imaging

No single laboratory test will consistently differentiate BA from other causes of obstructive jaundice. Although BA is suggested by persistent elevation of serum GGT in addition to conjugated/direct bilirubin, elevated GGT can be seen with other causes of cholestasis and occasional children with BA will have normal GGT. Serum levels of matrix metalloproteinase 7 (MMP7), combined with elevated GGT, may be a more predictive biomarker for BA than GGT alone. Generally, aminotransferases are only moderately elevated in BA and serum albumin and blood clotting factors are normal early in the disease. Ultrasonography of the biliary system should be performed to exclude the presence of CDC and identify intra-abdominal anomalies associated with BA. In the majority of cases of BA, the gallbladder is not visualized or is small; however, the presence of a normal appearing gallbladder on ultrasound does not exclude BA. Cholangiography consistently demonstrates complete obstruction of the extrahepatic biliary tree at some level.

Differential Diagnosis

The major diagnostic dilemma is distinguishing between BA and infections, bile duct paucity, genetic and metabolic liver diseases (particularly α_1-antitrypsin deficiency and PFIC), CDC, neonatal sclerosing cholangitis, or intrinsic bile duct obstruction (inspissated bile syndrome). Although spontaneous perforation of extrahepatic bile ducts leads to jaundice and acholic stools, these infants are usually quite ill with chemical peritonitis from biliary ascites.

The diagnosis of BA is suggested in the infant with acholic stools based on liver histology showing obstruction (bile duct plugs, bile duct proliferation, and portal fibrosis) or elevated serum MMP7. Once the diagnosis of α_1-antitrypsin deficiency and Alagille syndrome are excluded, a cholangiogram (intraoperative [IOC], endoscopic or transhepatic cholecystographic) to exclude the diagnosis of BA should be performed as soon as possible since outcomes are improved if surgical intervention is taken before 30–60 days of life. Radiographic visualization of cholangiographic contrast in the duodenum excludes obstruction to the distal extrahepatic ducts. In the majority of cases of BA, the entire extrahepatic biliary system including the gallbladder is obstructed and no cholangiographic contrast will be visible within the biliary tree.

Treatment

In the absence of surgical correction or transplantation, biliary cirrhosis, hepatic failure, and death occur uniformly by age 18–24 months. The standard procedure, hepatoportoenterostomy (Kasai procedure), to achieve drainage of bile from liver to intestine is performed at the time of IOC and is best done in specialized centers where experienced surgical, pediatric, and nursing personnel are available. For best results, surgery should be performed as early as possible (ideally before 30–45 days of life); the Kasai procedure should generally not be undertaken in infants older than 4 months or with advanced cirrhosis because the likelihood of achieving bile drainage at this age is very low. Orthotopic liver transplantation is indicated for patients who do not undergo the Kasai procedure, who fail to drain bile after the Kasai procedure, or who progress to end-stage biliary cirrhosis despite surgical treatment.

Supportive medical treatment consists of vitamin and caloric support (vitamins A, D, E, and K supplements and formulas containing high amounts of medium-chain triglycerides [eg, Pregestimil or Alimentum]) (see Table 22–4). Nasogastric tube feedings or parenteral nutrition may be required in patients failing oral caloric supplementation. Monitoring of serum fat-soluble vitamin levels is essential to ensure adequate supplementation. UDCA as a choleretic agent is routinely given post-Kasai and continued up to 3 years of age. UDCA should not be used in the setting of a "failed Kasai" whereby bile flow is not established, as UDCA in this setting is potentially hepatotoxic. Suspected ascending cholangitis (based on fever, jaundice, acholic stools, abdominal pain, leukocytosis, elevated bilirubin, and liver enzymes) should be treated promptly with antibiotics effective against gram-negative bacterial infections. Antibiotic prophylaxis (eg, trimethoprim-sulfamethoxazole) may reduce the recurrence rate of cholangitis. Ascites can be managed initially with spironolactone; furosemide is added in severe or unresponsive cases. There is currently no therapy that has been proven to prevent the progression of biliary disease and portal fibrosis that occurs in the majority of patients post-Kasai, although the use of corticosteroids is popular at some centers.

Prognosis

Outcomes post-Kasai include failure to reestablish bile flow in one-third and improvement in bile flow in up to two-thirds of patients. Approximately 50% of BA patients will require liver transplantation in the first 2 years of life, some despite achieving good bile drainage. The best predictor of the need for liver transplant in the first 2 years is the total serum bilirubin value at 3 months post-Kasai: if the total bilirubin is less than 2 mg/dL, it is unlikely that child will need transplant in the first 2 years; if the bilirubin is greater than 6 mg/dL, a liver transplant will likely be necessary in the first 2 years. Even in the setting of reestablished bile flow following Kasai surgery, approximately 80% of all BA patients will progress to biliary cirrhosis and need a liver transplantation at some point in childhood. Serum bile acid levels measured 6 months after Kasai surgery may predict subsequent outcome. Death is usually caused by liver failure, sepsis, intractable variceal bleeding, or respiratory failure secondary to intractable ascites. Esophageal variceal hemorrhage develops in 20%–40% of patients, yet terminal hemorrhage is unusual. Occasional long-term survivors develop hepatopulmonary syndrome (intrapulmonary right to left shunting of blood resulting in hypoxia) or portopulmonary hypertension (pulmonary arterial hypertension in patients with portal hypertension). Liver transplantation is indicated for all of the above-noted complications and long-term survival posttransplant is over 90%.

Kamath BM et al: Fat-soluble vitamin assessment and supplementation in cholestasis. Clin Liver Dis;2022 Aug;26(3):537–553 [PMID: 35868689].

Feldman AG, Sokol RJ: Neonatal cholestasis: emerging molecular diagnostics and potential novel therapeutics. Nat Rev Gastroenterol Hepatol 2019 Jun;16(6):346–360 [PMID: 30903105].

Sundaram SS et al: Biliary atresia: indications and timing of liver transplantation and optimization of pretransplant care. Liver Transpl 2017;23(1):96–109 [PMID: 27650268].

Thomas H: Biliary tract: MMP7—a diagnostic biomarker for biliary atresia. Nat Rev Gastroenterol Hepatol 2018;15:68 [PMID: 29235550].

2. Choledochal Cyst

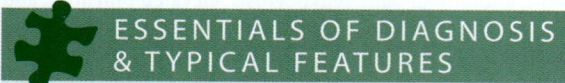

> ### ESSENTIALS OF DIAGNOSIS & TYPICAL FEATURES

> ▶ Abnormal abdominal ultrasound or other imaging with cyst of the biliary tree.

▶ Clinical Features

A. Symptoms and Signs

Choledochal cysts (CDCs) are cystic lesions of all or part of the extrahepatic biliary system, which in rare cases can include the intrahepatic bile duct branches. Abdominal ultrasound imaging will detect cases of CDC. In most cases presenting in infancy, the clinical manifestations and basic laboratory findings are indistinguishable from those associated with BA. Furthermore, a rare form of BA, termed "cystic biliary atresia" can mimic a CDC in the neonatal period. Clues to the diagnosis of CDC (vs cystic BA) include the presence of intrahepatic biliary dilation and a normal or distended gallbladder. In older children, CDC presents as recurrent episodes of right upper quadrant abdominal pain, fevers, vomiting, obstructive jaundice, pancreatitis, or as a right abdominal mass. Infants and children with CDC are at increased risk for developing bacterial cholangitis. CDCs represent only 2%–5% of cases of extrahepatic neonatal cholestasis; the incidence is higher in girls and patients of Asian descent.

B. Diagnosis and Treatment

▶ Diagnosis

Ultrasonography is used to screen for CDC, and an MRCP will confirm the diagnosis and the extent of the cystic lesion (Figure 22–1).

▶ Treatment

Timely surgery is indicated once abnormalities in clotting factors have been corrected and bacterial cholangitis, if present, has been treated with intravenous antibiotics. Excision of the cyst and its mucosa and choledocho–Roux-en-Y jejunal anastomosis are recommended. Anastomosis of cyst to jejunum

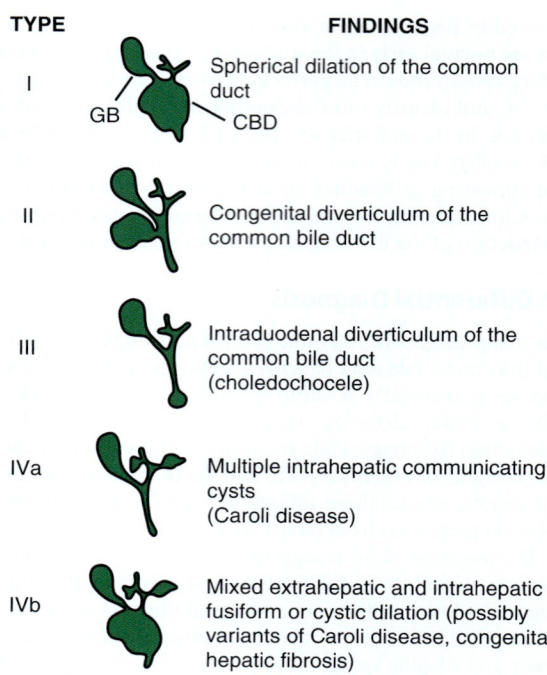

TYPE		FINDINGS
I		Spherical dilation of the common duct
II		Congenital diverticulum of the common bile duct
III		Intraduodenal diverticulum of the common bile duct (choledochocele)
IVa		Multiple intrahepatic communicating cysts (Caroli disease)
IVb		Mixed extrahepatic and intrahepatic fusiform or cystic dilation (possibly variants of Caroli disease, congenital hepatic fibrosis)

▲ **Figure 22–1.** Classification of cystic dilation of the bile ducts. Types I, II, and III are extrahepatic CDCs. Type IVa is solely intrahepatic, and type IVb is both intrahepatic and extrahepatic.

or duodenum is not recommended due to the continued risks of cholangitis and bile duct carcinoma (cholangiocarcinoma).

▶ Prognosis

If an isolated extrahepatic cyst is encountered, the outcome is generally excellent, with resolution of the jaundice and return to normal liver architecture after cyst excision. However, bouts of ascending cholangitis may occur, particularly if intrahepatic cysts are present or stricture of the anastomotic site develops. The risk of cholangiocarcinoma developing within the cyst is about 5%–15% in adulthood.

Aspelund G et al; American Academy of Pediatrics Section on Surgery's Delivery of Surgical Care Committee: Transitional care for patients with surgical pediatric hepatobiliary disease: choledochal cysts and biliary atresia. J Gastroenterol Hepatol 2019 Jun;34(6):966–974 [PMID: 30552863].

Soares KC et al: Pediatric choledochal cysts: diagnosis and current management. Ped Surg Int 2017;33(6):637–650 [PMID: 28364277].

3. Spontaneous Perforation of the Extrahepatic Bile Ducts

The sudden appearance of obstructive jaundice, acholic stools, and abdominal enlargement with ascites in a sick newborn is suggestive of this condition. The liver is usually normal in size, and a yellow-green discoloration can often be discerned under the umbilicus or in the scrotum. In 24% of cases, stones or sludge obstructs the common bile duct. HIDA scan or ERCP shows leakage from the biliary tree, and ultrasonography confirms ascites or fluid around the bile duct.

Treatment is surgical. Simple drainage, without attempts at oversewing the perforation, is sufficient in primary perforations. A diversion anastomosis is constructed in cases associated with CDC or stenosis. The prognosis is generally good.

Jeanty C et al: Spontaneous biliary perforation in infancy: management strategies and outcomes. J Pediatr Surg 2015;50(7): 1137–1141 [PMID: 25783338].

OTHER NEONATAL HYPERBILIRUBINEMIC CONDITIONS (NONCHOLESTATIC NONHEMOLYTIC)

Two other groups of disorders are associated with hyperbilirubinemia: (1) unconjugated hyperbilirubinemia is characteristic of breast-feeding and breast milk jaundice, congenital hypothyroidism, red blood cell hemolysis, upper intestinal obstruction, Gilbert disease, Crigler-Najjar syndrome, and drug-induced hyperbilirubinemia; and (2) conjugated noncholestatic hyperbilirubinemia is characteristic of Dubin-Johnson syndrome and Rotor syndrome.

1. Unconjugated Hyperbilirubinemia

A. Breast Milk Jaundice

Jaundice at 2 weeks of age is relatively common affecting up to 15% of newborns. Enhanced β-glucuronidase activity in breast milk is one factor that increases absorption of unconjugated bilirubin. Substances (eg, L-aspartic acid) in casein hydrolysate formulas inhibit this enzyme. The increased enterohepatic shunting of unconjugated bilirubin exceeds the normal conjugating capacity in the liver of these infants. The mutation for Gilbert syndrome (UDP-glucuronyltransferase 1A1 [UGT1A1]) predisposes to breast milk jaundice and to more prolonged jaundice. Neonates who carry the 211 and 388 variants in the UGT1A1 and OATP 2 genes, respectively, or the UGT1A1*6 allele and feed with breast milk, are at high risk to develop severe hyperbilirubinemia. Low volumes of ingested breast milk may also contribute to jaundice in the first week of life. Finally, breast milk may suppress UGT1A1 expression in the infant's intestines, which may also lead to unconjugated hyperbilirubinemia.

Hyperbilirubinemia does not usually exceed 20 mg/dL, with most cases in the range of 10–15 mg/dL. Jaundice is noticeable by the fifth to seventh day of breast-feeding. It may accentuate the underlying physiologic jaundice, especially early, when total fluid intake may be less than optimal.

Except for jaundice, the physical examination is normal; urine does not stain the diaper, and the stools are golden yellow.

The jaundice peaks before the third week of life and clears before age 3 months in almost all infants, even when breast-feeding is continued. All infants who remain jaundiced past age 2–3 weeks should have measurement of conjugated bilirubin to exclude cholestasis and hepatobiliary disease.

Kernicterus has rarely been reported in association with this condition. In special situations, breast-feeding may be discontinued temporarily and replaced by formula feedings for 2–3 days until serum bilirubin decreases by 2–8 mg/dL. Cow's milk formulas inhibit the intestinal reabsorption of unconjugated bilirubin. When breast-feeding is reinstituted, the serum bilirubin may increase slightly, but not to the previous level. Phototherapy is not indicated in the healthy full-term infant with this condition unless bilirubin levels meet high-risk levels as defined by the American Academy of Pediatrics.

Bratton S, Stern M: Breast milk jaundice. StatPearls [Internet]. Treasure Island, FL: StatPearls Publishing; 2019 Jan–2019 Nov [PMID: 30726019].
Maruo Y et al: Bilirubin uridine diphosphate-glucuronosyltransferase variation is a genetic basis of breast milk jaundice. J Pediatr 2014 Jul;165(1):36–41 [PMID: 24650397].
Preer GL, Philipp BL: Understanding and managing breast milk jaundice. Arch Dis Child Fetal Neonatal Ed 2011;96:F461 [PMID: 20688866].

B. Congenital Hypothyroidism

Although the differential diagnosis of indirect hyperbilirubinemia should always include congenital hypothyroidism, the diagnosis is usually identified by the newborn screening results or by clinical and physical clues. Jaundice clears quickly with replacement thyroid hormone therapy, although the mechanism is unclear. Hypopituitarism can also present with neonatal cholestasis and can be associated with septo-optic dysplasia, a congenital malformation syndrome featuring underdevelopment of the optic nerve, pituitary gland dysfunction, and absence of the septum pellucidum.

Tiker F: Congenital hypothyroidism and early severe hyperbilirubinemia. Clin Pediatr (Phila) 2003;42:365 [PMID: 12800733].

C. Upper Intestinal Obstruction

The association of indirect hyperbilirubinemia with high intestinal obstruction (eg, duodenal atresia, annular pancreas, pyloric stenosis) in the newborn has been observed; the mechanism is unknown. Diminished levels of hepatic glucuronyltransferase are found on liver biopsy in pyloric stenosis, and genetic studies suggest that this indirect hyperbilirubinemia may be an early sign of Gilbert syndrome. Treatment is that of the underlying obstructive condition (usually surgical). Jaundice disappears once adequate nutrition is achieved.

Hua L et al: The role of UGT1A1'28 mutation in jaundiced infants with hypertrophic pyloric stenosis. Pediatr Res 2005;58:881 [PMID: 16257926].

D. Gilbert Syndrome

Gilbert syndrome is a common form of familial hyperbilirubinemia present in 3%–7% of the population. It is associated with a partial reduction of hepatic bilirubin uridine diphosphate-glucuronyltransferase activity. Affected infants may have more rapid increase in jaundice in the newborn period, accentuated breast milk jaundice, and jaundice with intestinal obstruction. During puberty and beyond, mild fluctuating jaundice, especially with illness and vague constitutional symptoms, is common. Shortened red blood cell survival in some patients is thought to be caused by reduced activity of enzymes involved in heme biosynthesis (protoporphyrinogen oxidase). Reduction of hyperbilirubinemia has been achieved in patients by administration of phenobarbital (5–8 mg/kg/day), although this therapy is not needed.

The disease is inherited as an abnormality of the promoter region of uridine diphosphate-glucuronyltransferase-1 (UDGT1) coded by UGT1A1; however, another factor appears to be necessary for disease expression. The homozygous (16%) and heterozygous states (40%) are common. Males are affected more often than females (4:1) for reasons that are not clear. Serum unconjugated bilirubin is generally less than 3–6 mg/dL, although unusual cases may exceed 8 mg/dL. The findings on liver biopsy and most LFTs are normal. An increase of 1.4 mg/dL or more in the level of unconjugated bilirubin after a 2-day fast (300 kcal/day) is consistent with the diagnosis of Gilbert syndrome. Gilbert syndrome, conferred by the donor liver, can occur following liver transplantation. Genetic testing is available but rarely needed. No treatment is necessary.

Erlinger S et al: Inherited disorders of bilirubin transport and conjugation: new insights into molecular mechanisms and consequences. Gastroenterology 2014 Jun;146(7):1625–1638 [PMID: 24704527].

Kathemann S et al: Gilbert syndrome—a frequent cause of unconjugated hyperbilirubinemia in children after orthotopic liver transplantation. Pediatr Transplant 2012;16:20 [PMID: 22360405].

Travan L et al: Severe neonatal hyperbilirubinemia and UGT1A1 promoter polymorphism. J Pediatr 2014 Jul;165(1):42–45 [PMID: 24726540].

E. Crigler-Najjar Syndrome

Infants with type 1 Crigler-Najjar syndrome usually develop rapid severe unconjugated hyperbilirubinemia (> 30–40 mg/dL) with neurologic consequences (kernicterus). The deficiency in UGT1A1 is inherited in an autosomal recessive pattern. Genetic testing of UGT1A1 is definitive. Prompt recognition of this entity and treatment with exchange transfusions are required, followed by phototherapy. Phenobarbital administration does not significantly alter these findings, nor does it lower serum bilirubin levels. A combination of aggressive phototherapy and cholestyramine may keep bilirubin levels below 25 mg/dL. Liver transplantation is curative and may prevent kernicterus if performed early. Hepatocyte transplantation through the portal vein has been tried but is hampered by the requirement of multiple infusions of cells over time.

A milder form (type 2) with both autosomal dominant and recessive inheritance is rarely associated with neurologic complications. Hyperbilirubinemia is less severe, and the bile is pigmented and contains small amounts of bilirubin monoglucuronide and diglucuronide. Patients with this form respond to phenobarbital (4 mg/kg/day in infants) with lowering of serum bilirubin levels. An increased proportion of monoconjugated and diconjugated bilirubin in the bile follows phenobarbital treatment. Liver biopsy findings and aminostransferases are consistently normal in both types.

Aronson SJ et al. Disease burden and management of Crigler-Najjar syndrome: report of a World Registry. Liver Int 2022 Jul;42(7):1593–1604 [PMID: 35274801].

Strauss KA et al: Crigler-Najjar syndrome type 1: pathophysiology, natural history and therapeutic frontier. Hepatology 2020 Jun;71(6):1923–1939 [PMID: 31553814].

F. Drug-Induced Hyperbilirubinemia

Vitamin K_3 (menadiol) may elevate indirect bilirubin levels by causing hemolysis. Vitamin K_1 (phytonadione) can be used safely in neonates. Carbamazepine can cause conjugated hyperbilirubinemia in infancy. Rifampin and antiretroviral protease inhibitors (PIs; atazanavir) may cause unconjugated hyperbilirubinemia. Pancuronium bromide and chloral hydrate have been implicated in causing neonatal jaundice. Other drugs (eg, ceftriaxone, sulfonamides) may displace bilirubin from albumin, potentially increasing the risk of kernicterus—especially in the sick premature infant.

2. Conjugated Noncholestatic Hyperbilirubinemia (Dubin-Johnson Syndrome & Rotor Syndrome)

These diagnoses are suspected when persistent or recurrent conjugated hyperbilirubinemia and jaundice occur and aminotransferases are normal. The basic defect in Dubin-Johnson syndrome is in the multiple organic anion transport protein 2 (MRP2) of the bile canaliculus, causing impaired hepatocyte excretion of conjugated bilirubin into bile. A variable degree of impairment in uptake and conjugation complicates the clinical picture. Transmission is autosomal recessive, so a positive family history is occasionally obtained. In Rotor syndrome, the defect lies in hepatic uptake and storage of bilirubin. OATP1B1 (coded by SLCO1B1) and OATP1B3

(*SLCO1B3*) are the two transporters that are deficient. Bile acids are metabolized normally, so that cholestasis does not occur. Bilirubin values range from 2 to 5 mg/dL, and other aminotransferases are normal.

In Rotor syndrome, the liver is normal; in Dubin-Johnson syndrome, it is darkly pigmented on gross inspection and may be enlarged. Microscopic examination reveals numerous dark-brown pigment granules consisting of polymers of epinephrine metabolites, especially in the centrilobular regions. However, the amount of pigment varies within families, and some jaundiced family members may have no demonstrable pigmentation in the liver. Otherwise, the liver is histologically normal. Oral cholecystography fails to visualize the gallbladder in Dubin-Johnson syndrome but is normal in Rotor syndrome. Differences in the excretion patterns of bromosulfophthalein, in results of HIDA cholescintigraphy, in urinary coproporphyrin I and III levels, and in the serum pattern of monoglucuronide and diglucuronide conjugates of bilirubin can help distinguish between these two conditions. Clinical genotyping of *MRP2*, *SLCO1B1*, and *SLCO1B3* is available. No treatment is needed for either condition. Choleretic agents (eg, UDCA) may reduce the cholestasis in infants with Dubin-Johnson syndrome.

Jirsa M et al: Rotor syndrome. In: Pagon RA et al. (eds): *GeneReviews* [Internet]. 2012 Dec 13 [PMID: 23236639].
Keppler D: The roles of MRP2, MRP3, OATP1B1, and OATP1B3 in conjugated hyperbilirubinemia. Drug Metab Dispos 2014 Apr;42(4):561–565 [PMID: 24459177].

HEPATITIS VIRUS ABBREVIATIONS

HAV	Hepatitis A virus
HBV	Hepatitis B virus
HBcAg	HBV core antigen
Anti-HBs	Antibody to HBsAg
Anti-HBc IgM	IgM antibody to HBcAg
HCV	Hepatitis C virus
HDV	Hepatitis D (delta) virus
HEV	Hepatitis E virus
Anti-HAV IgM	IgM antibody to HAV
HBsAg	HBV surface antigen
HBeAg	HBV e antigen
Anti-HBc	Antibody to HBcAg
Anti-HBe	Antibody to HBeAg
Anti-HCV	Antibody to HCV
Anti-HDV	Antibody to HDV
Anti-HEV	Antibody to HEV

HEPATITIS A

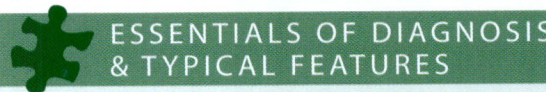

ESSENTIALS OF DIAGNOSIS & TYPICAL FEATURES

► Gastrointestinal upset (anorexia, vomiting, diarrhea).
► Jaundice.
► Liver tenderness and enlargement.
► Abnormal aminotransferases.
► Local epidemic of hepatitis A infection.
► Positive anti–hepatitis A virus (HAV) IgM antibody.

Pathogenesis

Hepatitis A virus (HAV) infection occurs in both epidemic and sporadic fashion and is transmitted by the fecal-oral route (Table 22–6). HAV particles are found in stool during the acute phase of hepatitis A infection. Epidemic outbreaks are caused by contaminated food or water supplies, including by food handlers, while sporadic cases usually result from contact with an infected individual. Transmission through blood products obtained during the viremic phase is a rare event, although it has occurred in a newborn nursery.

Prevention

Isolation of an infected patient during initial phases of illness is indicated, although most patients with hepatitis A are noninfectious by the time the disease becomes overt. Stool, diapers, and other fecally stained clothing should be handled with care for 1 week after the appearance of jaundice.

Hepatitis A vaccines are licensed for age 12 months and above and given on a two-dose schedule. Vaccination is routinely recommended in children 12–23 months of age (or in those 2–18 years who have not yet received the vaccine) regardless of risk factors and should be emphasized in those at higher risk for severe infection (people with chronic liver disease, people experiencing homelessness, or those traveling to an endemic area). The HAV vaccine is highly immunogenic, with at least 95% of healthy people demonstrating protective antibodies after one dose and 99% after a second dose. When an emigrant child from an endemic area is adopted, the immediate family members should be immunized.

Exposed susceptible persons younger than 12 months or older than 40 years, and anyone who is immunocompromised or has chronic liver disease is recommended to receive immune globulin, 0.02 mL/kg intramuscularly. Illness is prevented in more than 85% of individuals if immune globulin is given within 2 weeks of exposure. For immunocompetent individuals 12 months to 40 years old, HAV vaccine is recommended following exposure. Infants younger than 12 months

Table 22–6. Hepatitis viruses.

	HAV	HBV	HCV	HDV	HEV
Type of virus	Enterovirus (RNA)	Hepadnavirus (DNA)	Flavivirus (RNA)	Delta virus (RNA)	Hepevirus (RNA)
Transmission routes	Fecal-oral	Parenteral, sexual, vertical	Parenteral, sexual, vertical	Parenteral, sexual	Fecal-oral
Incubation period (days)	15–40	45–160	30–150	20–90	14–65
Diagnostic test	Anti-HAV IgM	HBsAg, anti-HBc IgM, DNA PCR	Anti-HCV, RNA PCR	Anti-HDV	Anti-HEV IgM, HEV PCR
Mortality rate (acute)	0.1%–0.2%	0.5%–2%	1%–2%	2%–20%	1%–2% (10%–20% in pregnant women)
Carrier state	No	Yes	Yes	Yes	Rare (in immuno-compromised)
Vaccine available	Yes	Yes	No	Yes (HBV)	Yes (not widely available)
Treatment	None	Preferred: Entecavir or Tenofovir	Combination of Sofosbuvir/ Ledipasvir; Sofosbuvir/ Velpatasvir; or Glecaprevir/Pibrentasvir	Treatment for HBV	None

HAV, hepatitis A virus; HBc, hepatitis B core; HBsAg, hepatitis B surface antigen; HBV, hepatitis B virus; HDV, hepatitis D (delta) virus; HEV, hepatitis E virus; PCR, polymerase chain reaction.

traveling to endemic disease areas should receive HAV vaccine, which does not count towards the routine two-dose series, or immunoglobulin (for trips > 3 months in duration) as prophylaxis. Older individuals should receive the HAV vaccine and immunoglobulin.

▶ Clinical Findings

A. History

Historical risk factors may include direct exposure to a previously jaundiced individual or recently arrived individual from a high-prevalence country, consumption of seafood, contaminated water or imported fruits or vegetables, attendance in a day care center, or recent travel to an endemic area. Following an incubation period of 15–40 days, nonspecific symptoms of nausea, fever, malaise, or anorexia usually precede the development of jaundice by 5–10 days. In developing countries, hepatitis A is common, and most children are exposed by age 10 years, while only 20% are exposed by age 20 years in developed countries.

B. Symptoms and Signs

The overt form of the disease is easily recognized by the clinical manifestations. However, two-thirds of children are asymptomatic, and two-thirds of symptomatic children are anicteric. Therefore, the presenting symptoms in children with HAV often resemble gastroenteritis.

Fever, anorexia, vomiting, headache, and abdominal pain are typical and dark urine precedes jaundice, which peaks in 1–2 weeks and then begins to subside. The stools may become light- or clay-colored. Clinical improvement can occur as jaundice develops. Tender hepatomegaly and jaundice are typically present in symptomatic children; splenomegaly is variable.

C. Laboratory Findings

Serum aminotransferases and conjugated and unconjugated bilirubin levels are elevated. Although unusual, hypoalbuminemia, hypoglycemia, and marked prolongation of PT (international normalized ratio [INR] > 2.0) are poor prognostic findings. Diagnosis is made by a positive anti-HAV IgM, whereas anti-HAV IgG persists after recovery and indicates prior infection or vaccination.

Percutaneous liver biopsy is rarely indicated as the diagnosis can be made on serology, as above. "Balloon cells" and acidophilic bodies are characteristic histologic findings but are nonspecific to HAV infection. Liver cell necrosis may be diffuse or focal, with accompanying infiltration of inflammatory cells containing polymorphonuclear leukocytes, lymphocytes, macrophages, and plasma cells, particularly in portal areas. Some bile duct proliferation may be seen in the perilobular portal areas alongside areas of bile stasis. Regenerative liver cells and proliferation of reticuloendothelial cells are present.

Differential Diagnosis

Before jaundice appears, the symptoms are those of non-specific viral enteritis. Other diseases with somewhat similar onset include infectious mononucleosis (EBV), leptospirosis, drug-induced hepatitis, Wilson disease, autoimmune hepatitis (AIH), and infection with other hepatitis viruses. Acquired CMV disease may also mimic HAV, although lymphadenopathy is usually present in the former.

Treatment

No specific treatment measures are required beyond supportive care. New drugs and elective surgery should be avoided during acute infection. Hospitalization is recommended for children with coagulopathy, encephalopathy, or severe vomiting and evaluation for liver transplantation considered if a patient is not demonstrating improvement in liver function. Hospitalization rates for hepatitis A have decreased over the decades, with those who require hospitalization being older adults or those with underlying liver disease and/or comorbid conditions.

Prognosis

Around 99% of children recover without sequelae. Although the great majority of children with HAV hepatitis are asymptomatic or have mild disease and recover completely, some will develop acute liver failure (ALF) leading to death or requiring liver transplantation. Persons with underlying chronic liver disease have an increased risk of death. The prognosis is poor if hepatic coma or ascites develop; liver transplantation is indicated under these circumstances and is lifesaving. Incomplete resolution can cause a prolonged hepatitis, but resolution invariably occurs without long-term hepatic sequelae. Rare cases of aplastic anemia following acute infectious hepatitis have been reported. A benign relapse of symptoms may occur in 10%–15% of cases after 6–10 weeks of apparent resolution. Chronic infection does not occur.

Hepatitis A in Red Book: *2021–2024 Report of the Committee on Infectious Diseases.* 32nd ed. Elk Grove Village, IL. American Academy of Pediatrics; 2021.

Herzog C et al: Hepatitis A vaccination and its immunologic and epidemiologic long-term effects—a review of the evidence. Hum Vaccin Immunother 2021;17(5):1496–1519 [PMID: 33325760].

Lee HW et al: Clinical factors and viral load influencing severity of acute hepatitis A. PLoS One 2015 Jun 19;10(6) [PMID: 26090677].

Murphy TV et al: Progress toward eliminating hepatitis A disease in the United States. MMWR Supple 2016 Feb 12;65(1):29–41 [PMID: 26916458].

HEPATITIS B

ESSENTIALS OF DIAGNOSIS & TYPICAL FEATURES

► The vast majority of patients with vertically acquired HBV infection will be asymptomatic and have a normal physical examination.

► Acute HBV infection may be associated with anorexia, vomiting, diarrhea, jaundice, tender hepatomegaly, and abnormal aminotransferases.

► Serologic evidence of hepatitis B disease: positive HBsAg, HBeAg, anti-HBc IgM.

► History of parenteral, sexual, or household exposure or maternal HBsAg positivity.

General Considerations

HBV is a DNA virus with an incubation period of 45–160 days (see Table 22–6). HBV is either acquired perinatally from a mother with hepatitis B infection, or later in life from exposure to contaminated blood through shared needles, needle sticks, skin piercing, tattoos, or sexual transmission.

Pathophysiology

The HBV particle is composed of a core and a double outer shell where the surface antigen (HBsAg) is located. The nomenclature for the viral antigens and antibodies is found in the table of Hepatitis Virus Abbreviations provided above. Hepatitis B e antigen (HBeAg), a truncated soluble form of the core antigen (HBcAg), correlates with active virus replication. Persistence of HBeAg is a marker of infectivity, whereas the appearance of anti-HBe generally implies a lower level of viral replication. However, HBV mutant viruses (precore mutant) may replicate with negative HBeAg tests and positive tests for anti-HBe antibody (known as HBeAg-negative chronic hepatitis). Such cases are associated with a more virulent form of hepatitis. Circulating HBV DNA (measured by PCR) also indicates viral replication.

Prevention

HBV vaccination is the preferred method for prevention. Universal immunization of all infants is recommended. Other control methods include screening of blood donors and pregnant women, use of properly sterilized needles and surgical equipment, avoidance of sexual contact with carriers, general adoption of safe sex practices, and vaccination of household contacts, sexual partners, medical personnel, and those at high risk. For postexposure prophylaxis, HBV vaccine is given alone (see Chapter 10) or together with administration of hepatitis B immune globulin (HBIG) (0.06 mL/kg intramuscularly as soon as possible after exposure, up to 7 days). The risk of vertical transmission is dramatically reduced with the combination of newborn vaccination and HBIG administration. Hepatitis B vaccine should be given to all infants born to HBsAg-negative mothers in the first 24 hours of birth and HBIG should be given in the first 12 hours of birth (in addition to the vaccine) in all infants of HBsAg-positive mothers. For infected pregnant women with high viral loads, use of oral antivirals in the last half of pregnancy combined with postdelivery prophylaxis in the newborn can further reduce perinatal prophylaxis failures from 5% to 1.5%.

Clinical Findings

A. Symptoms and Signs

Most infants and young children are asymptomatic, especially if the infection is acquired vertically. Symptoms of acute HBV infection may include fever, malaise, and mild gastrointestinal upset. Visible jaundice is usually the first significant finding and hepatomegaly is frequently present. Rare presentations include immune complex-mediated rash, arthritis, glomerulonephritis, or nephrotic syndrome.

B. Laboratory Findings

The diagnosis of acute HBV infection is confirmed by the presence of HBsAg and anti-HBc IgM. Recovery from acute infection is accompanied by HBsAg clearance and appearance of anti-HBs and anti-HBc IgG. Individuals who are immune by vaccination are positive for anti-HBs but are negative for anti-HBc IgG. Chronic infection is defined as the presence of HBsAg for at least 6 months. Vertical transmission to newborns is documented by positive HBsAg (serologies should not be used in infancy as these will reflect maternal antibody). The various phases of chronic HBV infection are shown in Table 22–7.

Differential Diagnosis

The differentiation between HAV and HBV disease is aided by a history of parenteral exposure, a HBsAg-positive parent, or a long incubation period. HBV, hepatitis C virus (HCV) infection, and Epstein-Barr virus (EBV) infection are differentiated serologically. Other diseases to consider in the differential diagnosis include AIH, Wilson disease, hemochromatosis, nonalcoholic fatty liver disease (NAFLD), or α_1-antitrypsin deficiency.

Treatment

No treatment is recommended in the setting of uncomplicated acute HBV infection. In the rare instance of severe infection with ALF, treatment with a nucleos(t)ide analogue should be considered. There is no therapy that is highly curative for chronic hepatitis B, but the goal of treatment is to prevent progression to cirrhosis, liver failure, and development of hepatocellular carcinoma. For children with vertically acquired HBV infection and normal aminotransferases and physical examination (immunotolerant phase), treatment does not decrease viral load and is not recommended. For chronic infection with elevated LFTs for more than 6 months (immunoactive phase), nucleos(t)ide therapy may be helpful. Preferred antiviral therapy in pediatrics includes entecavir or tenofovir. A significant decrease in viral load with these nucleos(t)ide therapies can be seen in up to 75% of treated children, with minimal side effects, but may require long-term treatment. Updated practice guidelines and information on Food and Drug Administration (FDA) medication approval are available at the American Association for the Study of Liver Disease website (https://www.aasld.org/practice-guidelines/chronic-hepatitis-b). Liver transplantation is successful in ALF due to hepatitis B; however, reinfection is common following liver transplantation for chronic hepatitis B unless long-term HBIG or antivirals are used.

Prognosis

In older children or adults who acquire acute hepatitis B infection, 90%–95% will clear the virus and not progress to chronic infection. Individuals who have cleared HBV (HBsAg negative, anti-HBcIgG positive) are at risk for reactivation of HBV infection with significant immunosuppression (eg, chemotherapy). Infants who acquire HBV via vertical transmission

Table 22–7. Phases of chronic hepatitis B infection.

Phase	HBeAg/Anti-HBeAb	HBsAg/Anti-HBsAb	ALT	HBV DNA
Immune tolerant	Positive/negative	Positive/negative	Normal	> 20,000 IU/mL
Immune active	Positive/negative	Positive/negative	Elevated	High
Chronic HBsAg carrier	Negative/positive	Positive/negative	Normal	< 2000 IU/mL
HBeAg negative hepatitis/ reactivation	Negative/positive	Positive/negative	Elevated	> 2000 IU/mL
HBsAg clearance	Negative/positive	Negative/positive	Normal	Undetectable

are much more likely to develop chronic infection, with persistence of perinatally acquired HBsAg positivity in 70%–90% of infants without immunoprophylaxis or vaccination. The presence of HBeAg in a HBsAg carrier indicates ongoing viral replication. However, 1%–2% of children infected at birth will show spontaneous seroconversion of HBeAg each year. Chronic HBV disease predisposes the patient to development of hepatocellular carcinoma. Once chronic HBV infection is established, surveillance for development of hepatocellular carcinoma with serum α-fetoprotein (AFP) is performed biannually and ultrasonography every 1–3 years. Routine HBV vaccination of newborns in endemic countries has greatly reduced the incidence of ALF, chronic hepatitis, and hepatocellular carcinoma.

Defresne F, Sokol E: Chronic hepatitis B in children: therapeutic challenges and perspectives. J Gastroenterol Hepatol 2017: 368–371 [PMID: 27262164].
Hepatitis A in Red Book: *2021–2024 Report of the Committee on Infectious Diseases*. 32nd ed. Elk Grove Village, IL. American Academy of Pediatrics; 2021.
Jonas M et al: Antiviral therapy in management of chronic hepatitis B viral infection in children: a systematic review and meta-analysis. Hepatology 2016;63:307 [PMID: 26566163].
Terrault NA et al: Update on prevention, diagnosis, and treatment of chronic hepatitis B: AASLD 2018 hepatitis B guidance. Hepatology 2018;67:1560–1599 [PMID: 29405329].

HEPATITIS C

General Considerations

HCV is the most common cause of non–HBV-related chronic hepatitis. HCV is a single-stranded RNA flavivirus with at least seven genotypes (see Table 22–6). Risk factors in adults and adolescents include the illicit use of intravenous drugs and occupational or sexual exposure. The risk of acquiring HCV from a blood transfusion in the United States is currently less than 1 per 2 million units of blood transfused. Most cases in children are associated with vertical transmission from an infected mother with transmission from household contacts being quite rare. Vertical transmission from HCV-infected mothers occurs more commonly in those mothers who are also HIV-positive (15%–20%) compared with those who are HIV-negative (5%–6% risk of perinatal transmission). Approximately 1% of the United States population has chronic HCV infection.

Prevention

At present, the only effective means of prevention is avoidance of exposure through elimination of risk-taking behaviors such as the illicit use of intravenous drugs. There is no effective prevention for vertical transmission, but avoidance of fetal scalp monitoring in infants of mothers with HCV has been suggested. Elective Caesarean section is not recommended for HCV-monoinfected women, as it confers no reduction in mother-to-infant HCV transmission. Breastfeeding does not promote HCV transmission from mother to infant. However, it is advised to avoid breast-feeding if the nipples are bleeding, if mastitis is present or if the mother is experiencing a flare of hepatitis with jaundice postpartum. There is no vaccine and no benefit from using immune globulin in infants born to infected mothers. In mothers with HIV coinfection, control of HIV viremia with antiretroviral therapy may reduce rates of HCV transmission to the infant.

Clinical Findings

A. Symptoms and Signs

The majority of childhood cases, especially those acquired vertically, are asymptomatic despite development of chronic hepatitis. The incubation period is 1–5 months, with insidious onset of symptoms. Flu-like prodromal symptoms and jaundice occur in less than 25% of cases. Hepatosplenomegaly is variable. Ascites, clubbing, palmar erythema, and spider angiomas are rare and indicate progression to cirrhosis. In adults, chronic HCV infection has been associated with mixed cryoglobulinemia, polyarteritis nodosa, a sicca-like syndrome, and membranoproliferative glomerulonephritis, as well as hepatocellular carcinoma.

B. Laboratory Findings

Since anti-HCV IgG crosses the placenta, testing anti-HCV IgG is not informative until the infant is 18 months old, at which time antibody testing should be performed. Patients older than 18 months with positive anti-HCV IgG should have subsequent testing for serum HCV RNA to determine if active infection is present. Serum HCV RNA can be tested prior to 18 months of age but should not be tested before 2 months old. If serum HCV RNA is positive in infancy, it should be rechecked at 12 months of age to determine presence of chronic infection. Fluctuating mild to moderate elevations of aminotransferases over long periods are characteristic of chronic HCV infection; however, normal aminotransferases are common in children. Cirrhosis in adults generally requires 20–30 years of chronic HCV infection, but it has occasionally developed sooner in children.

Differential Diagnosis

HCV disease should be distinguished from HAV and HBV disease by serologic testing. Other causes of chronic hepatitis in children should be considered, including Wilson disease, α1-antitrypsin deficiency, AIH, primary sclerosing cholangitis (PSC), drug-induced hepatitis, or steatohepatitis.

Treatment

The treatment for chronic HCV has rapidly changed because of direct-acting antiviral (DAA) therapies, which when used for 8–24 weeks result in HCV eradication rates of more than 90%. A website from the American Association for the Study of Liver Diseases and the Infectious Diseases Society of America provides up-to-date guidance for suggested therapies in this era of rapidly evolving approval of new drugs for HCV (http://www.hcvguidelines.org). The use of subcutaneous injections of pegylated interferon-α and oral ribavirin is no longer recommended. The combination of sofosbuvir plus ledipasvir (Harvoni) once daily for 12 weeks for the treatment of genotype 1, 4, 5, or 6, with weight-based dosing, is available for children at least 3 years of age. Children aged 3 years or older with any genotype can be treated with a weight-based regimen of 8 weeks of a Glecaprevir/Pibrentasvir combination or 12 weeks of Sofosbuvir/Velpatasvir. End-stage liver disease secondary to HCV responds well to liver transplantation, although reinfection of the transplanted liver is very common. The new DAA therapies appear to be effective at eradicating HCV post-liver transplant as well.

▶ Prognosis

Following an acute infection with HCV, 70%–80% of adults and older children develop a chronic infection. Around 20% of adults with chronic HCV develop cirrhosis by 30 years. Infants infected by vertical transmission have a high rate of spontaneous clearance, approaching 25%–40%. Most have spontaneous resolution by 24 months of age, but some may have spontaneous resolution as late as 7 years after vertical infection. The majority of children with chronic HCV have mild inflammation and fibrosis on liver biopsy, although cirrhosis may develop rapidly in rare cases. Limited 30-year follow-up of infants exposed to HCV by transfusion suggests a lower rate of progression to cirrhosis compared to adults. The prognosis for infants infected at birth with concomitant HIV infection is unknown, but the course appears benign for the first 10 years of life.

AASLD/IDSA: Recommendations for testing, managing and treating hepatitis C. http://www.hcvguidelines.org. Accessed March 2, 2023.

Leung DH et al: Hepatitis C in 2020: a North American Society for Pediatric Gastroenterology, Hepatology and Nutrition Position Paper. J Pediatr Gastroenterol Nutr 2020 Sep;71(3):407–417 [PMID: 32826718].

Squires JE et al: Hepatitis C virus infection in children and adolescents. Hepatol Commun 2017 Mar;23(1):87-98. [PMID: 29404447].

HEPATITIS D (DELTA AGENT)

Hepatitis D virus (HDV) requires the presence of HBsAg to be infectious (see Table 22–6) and thus HDV infection can occur only in the presence of HBV infection. Transmission is by parenteral exposure or intimate contact. HDV is rare in North America, but its prevalence is higher in Africa, South America, Central Asia, and parts of Eastern Europe and the Middle East. HDV can infect simultaneously with HBV, causing acute hepatitis, or can superinfect a patient with chronic HBV infection, predisposing the individual to chronic hepatitis or fulminant hepatitis. In children, the association between chronic HDV coinfection with HBV and chronic hepatitis and cirrhosis is strong. Vertical HDV transmission is rare. HDV is detected by anti-HDV IgG, which indicates active or previous infection; active infection is confirmed by detecting HDV RNA by PCR or by detecting HDV IgM antibody. Testing should be considered in patients with known HBV infection who either have an unusually severe or protracted course of hepatitis or those with specific risk factors (injection drug use, men who have sex with men, coinfection with HCV or HIV, high-risk sexual practices, or emigration from an endemic area). Treatment has historically been limited to interferon therapy, although new drugs are emerging.

Urban S et al. Hepatitis D virus in 2021: virology, immunology and new treatment approaches for a difficult-to-treat disease. Gut 2021;70:1782–1794 [PMID: 34103404].

Wranke A, Wedemeyer H: Antiviral therapy of hepatitis delta virus infection—progress and challenges towards cure. Curr Opin Virol 2016;20:112 [PMID: 27792905].

HEPATITIS E

Hepatitis E virus (HEV) infection causes acute hepatitis (see Table 22–6). The World Health Organization estimates that one-third of the world's population has been exposed to HEV. The routes of HEV transmission include fecal-oral (consumption of contaminated water and food), vertical, person-to-person, and, rarely, parenteral transmission. Epidemics occur mainly in resource poor regions secondary to contamination of drinking water; however, HEV has increasingly been recognized as endemic in some developed regions where infections occur through zoonotic transmission or contaminated blood products. The majority of cases are asymptomatic; if symptomatic, the clinical manifestations resemble those of HAV infection. HEV infection in pregnancy is associated with a high mortality (10%–20%), particularly when acquired in the third trimester. HEV infection in individuals with chronic liver disease can cause acute deterioration. Immunocompromised individuals infected with HEV are at increased risk for the development of chronic infection, with higher rates of ALF and rapid onset of cirrhosis. Diagnosis is by detecting anti-HEV IgM antibody or HEV PCR. HEV is usually self-limited. Treatment is supportive care for healthy individuals and lowering of immunosuppressive medications and ribavirin in immunosuppressed individuals. An efficacious vaccine for HEV infection exists but has not been widely implemented.

Kamar N et al: Hepatitis E virus infection. Nat Rev Dis Primers 2017 Nov l6;3:17086 [PMID: 29154369].

Lynch JA et al: Hepatitis E vaccine—Illuminating the barriers to use. PLoS 2023;17:e0010969 [PMID: 36602994].

OTHER HEPATITIS VIRUSES

Other viruses, including enterovirus, adenovirus, coronavirus, parvovirus, varicella, influenza, CMV, HSV, HHV-6, and HIV may cause severe acute hepatitis or ALF in children. Non-viral infections that may also cause acute hepatitis include brucella, Q-fever, and leptospirosis, as well as sepsis of any etiology. Infectious mononucleosis (EBV) is commonly associated with self-resolving acute hepatitis, although rare cases of EBV-associated ALF have been reported. Primary EBV infection in an immunocompromised solid organ transplant recipient may result in a lymphoproliferative disorder. Although some of the above viruses can be treated with specific antiviral therapies, the cornerstone of management for viral hepatitis is supportive care. Liver transplantation is considered in cases of ALF.

Jha HC et al: Epstein-Barr virus: diseases linked to infection and transformation. Front Microbiol 2016;7:1602 [PMID: 27826287].

Shwarz KB et al: Analysis of viral testing in nonacetaminophen pediatric acute liver failure. J Pediatr Gastroenterol Nutr 2014;59:616–623 [PMID: 25340974].

ACUTE LIVER FAILURE

ESSENTIALS OF DIAGNOSIS & TYPICAL FEATURES

▶ Acute hepatitis with deepening jaundice.
▶ Extreme elevation of AST and ALT.
▶ Prolonged PT and INR.
▶ Encephalopathy and cerebral edema.
▶ Asterixis.

▶ General Considerations

Acute liver failure (ALF) is defined as acute liver dysfunction associated with significant hepatic synthetic dysfunction evidenced by vitamin K–resistant coagulopathy (INR > 2.0) within 8 weeks of onset of liver injury. This is often associated with encephalopathy, but in young children, encephalopathy may be difficult to detect. Without liver transplantation, mortality approaches 40% in children. In many cases, an identifiable cause is not found but

Table 22–8. Common identifiable causes of acute liver failure by age.[a]

Neonates	Infections: herpesviruses and enteroviruses. Metabolic: neonatal iron storage disease/GALD, galactosemia, fructosemia, tyrosinemia, FAO, mitochondrial disorders. Ischemia: congenital heart disease.
Infants 1–24 mo	Infections: HAV, HBV. Metabolic: FAO, mitochondrial disorders, tyrosinemia, fructosemia, bile acid synthesis defects. Drug: acetaminophen, valproate. Immune: AIH, HLH.
Children	Infections: EBV, HAV. Metabolic: FAO, Wilson disease. Drug: acetaminophen, valproate, others. Immune: AIH.
Adolescents	Infections: EBV, HAV. Metabolic: FAO, Wilson disease, acute fatty liver of pregnancy. Drug: acetaminophen, valproate, herbs, "ecstasy," others. Immune: AIH.

AIH, autoimmune hepatitis; EBV, Epstein-Barr virus; GALD, gestational alloimmune liver disease; FAO, fatty acid oxidation defects; HAV, hepatitis A; HBV, hepatitis B; HLH, hemophagocytic lymphohistiocytosis.
[a]Unknown/Indeterminate cause of ALF remains the most common etiology.

is postulated to be an unusually virulent infectious agent or aggressive host immune response. Common identifiable causes of ALF are shown in Table 22–8.

▶ Clinical Findings

A. History

In some patients, ALF presents with the rapid development of deepening jaundice, bleeding, confusion, and progressive encephalopathy, while others are asymptomatic at the onset and then suddenly become severely ill during the second week of the disease. Jaundice, fever, anorexia, vomiting, and abdominal pain are the most common symptoms. A careful history of drug and toxin exposure may identify a drug-induced cause.

B. Symptoms and Signs

Children may present with flu-like symptoms, including malaise, myalgias, jaundice, nausea, and vomiting. Tender hepatomegaly is common, which may be followed by progressive shrinking of the liver, often with worsening hepatic function. Other physical findings (splenomegaly, spider hemangiomata) should suggest an underlying chronic liver disease. A disturbed sleep wake cycle, hyperreflexia, and positive extensor plantar responses are seen in the early stages of hepatic encephalopathy.

C. Laboratory Findings

Characteristic findings include elevated serum bilirubin levels (usually > 10 mg/dL), sustained elevations of AST and ALT (often > 3000 U/L), low serum albumin, hypoglycemia, and prolonged PT and INR. Blood ammonia levels may become elevated. Prolonged PT from disseminated intravascular coagulation (DIC) can be differentiated by determination of factor V (low in ALF and DIC) and VIII (normal to high in ALF and low in DIC). Rapid decreases in AST and ALT, together with shrinking hepatomegaly, due to massive necrosis and collapse, combined with worsening coagulopathy portend a poor prognosis.

▶ Differential Diagnosis

Severe hepatitis, with or without coagulopathy, due to infections, metabolic disease, AIH or drug toxicity can initially mimic ALF. Acute leukemia, cardiomyopathy, and Budd-Chiari syndrome can mimic severe hepatitis. Patients with Reye syndrome or urea cycle defects are typically anicteric.

▶ Complications

The development of renal failure and depth of hepatic coma are major prognostic factors. Patients in stage 4 coma (unresponsiveness to verbal stimuli, decorticate or decerebrate posturing) rarely survive without liver transplantation and may have residual central nervous system deficits even after transplant. Cerebral edema, which usually accompanies coma, is frequently the cause of death. Extreme prolongation of PT or INR greater than 3.5 predicts poor recovery, except with acetaminophen overdose. Sepsis, hemorrhage, renal failure, and cardiorespiratory arrest are common terminal events.

▶ Treatment

Excellent critical care is paramount, including careful management of hypoglycemia, bleeding and coagulopathy, hyperammonemia, cerebral edema, and fluid balance, while systematically investigating for potentially treatable causes. Several therapies have failed to affect outcome, including exchange transfusion, plasmapheresis with plasma exchange, total body washout, charcoal hemoperfusion, and hemodialysis using a special high-permeability membrane. While spontaneous survival may occur in up to 50% of patients, liver transplant may be lifesaving in patients without signs of spontaneous recovery. Therefore, early transfer of patients in ALF to centers where liver transplantation can be performed is recommended. Criteria for deciding when to perform transplantation are not firmly established; however, serum bilirubin over 20 mg/dL, INR greater than 4, and factor V levels less than 20% indicate a poor prognosis. Prognosis is better for acetaminophen ingestion, particularly when

N-acetylcysteine treatment is given. *N*-acetylcysteine is not recommended in non–acetaminophen-induced liver failure, as it does not improve survival and may, in fact, negatively impact survival in those younger than 2 years. The role of immunosuppressants, including corticosteroids are currently being studied in a multicenter randomized control trial. Acyclovir is essential in herpes simplex or varicella-zoster virus infection. For hyperammonemia, oral antibiotics such as neomycin or rifaximin, and lactulose (1–2 mL/kg three or four times daily) are used to reduce blood ammonia levels and trap ammonia in the colon.

Close monitoring of fluid and electrolytes is mandatory and requires a central venous line. Adequate dextrose should be infused (6–8 mg/kg/min) to maintain normal blood glucose and cellular metabolism. Diuretics, sedatives, and tranquilizers should be used sparingly. Comatose patients should be intubated, given mechanical ventilatory support, and monitored for signs of infection. Coagulopathy accompanied by bleeding is treated with fresh-frozen plasma, recombinant factor VIIa, other clotting factor concentrates, and platelet infusions. Hemodialysis may help stabilize a patient while awaiting liver transplantation. Monitoring for increased intracranial pressure (hepatic coma stages 3 and 4) in patients awaiting liver transplantation is advocated by some. Continuous venous-venous dialysis may be helpful to maintain fluid balance.

▶ Prognosis

Prognosis is primarily dependent on the etiology of ALF and depth of coma. Only 20%–30% of children with stage 3 or 4 hepatic encephalopathy will have a spontaneous recovery. Children with acute acetaminophen toxicity have a high rate of spontaneous survival, while only 40% of children with indeterminate ALF (of unknown etiology) will have a spontaneous recovery. One large study suggests that the spontaneous recovery rate is about 40%–50% when all causes of ALF are combined; 30% of patients will receive a liver transplant; and 20% will die without a transplant. Exchange transfusions or other modes of heroic therapy do not improve survival. Indeterminate ALF, non-acetaminophen drug-induced ALF, and ALF in infants are associated with a poorer prognosis. Acetaminophen and AIH etiologies of ALF and rising levels of factors V and VII, coupled with rising levels of serum AFP, may signify a more favorable prognosis. The 1-year survival rate in patients who undergo liver transplantation for ALF is 60%–85%.

Sabapathy DG et al: Acute liver failure in children. Pediatr Clin North Am 2022 Jun;69(3):465–495 [PMID: 35667757].
Squires JE et al: NASPGHAN position paper on the diagnosis and management of pediatric acute liver failure. JPGN 2022 Jan 1; 74(1):138–158 [PMID: 34247674].

AUTOIMMUNE HEPATITIS

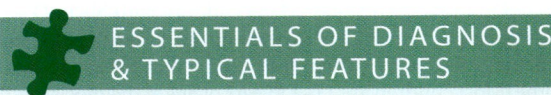

ESSENTIALS OF DIAGNOSIS & TYPICAL FEATURES

- ▶ Acute or chronic hepatitis.
- ▶ Hypergammaglobulinemia.
- ▶ Positive antinuclear antibody (ANA), anti–smooth muscle (or actin) antibody (ASMA), or anti–liver-kidney microsomal (LKM) antibody.

▶ Clinical Findings

A. History

Autoimmune hepatitis (AIH) is a progressive inflammatory disorder. It is characterized histologically by portal tract inflammation (often with plasma cells) that extends into the parenchyma (known as "interface hepatitis"); serologically by the presence of non–organ-specific autoantibodies; biochemically by elevated aminotransferases and serum IgG; and clinically by response to immunosuppressive treatment in the absence of other known causes of liver disease. A family history of autoimmune diseases is present in approximately 40% of cases.

B. Symptoms and Signs

Pediatric patients are often asymptomatic early in the disease process and come to medical attention based on an incidental finding of elevated liver tests. In those with symptoms, lethargy as well as malaise are common symptoms, and patients may also complain of jaundice, recurrent fevers, abdominal pain, or distension. Other complaints at the time of presentation may include a recurrent rash, arthritis, chronic diarrhea, or amenorrhea. Hepatomegaly and/or splenomegaly may be found on examination. In more advanced cases, jaundice and ascites may develop. Cutaneous signs of chronic liver disease may be noted (eg, spider angiomas, palmar erythema, and digital clubbing). In approximately10% of cases, AIH patients present with an acute presentation resembling ALF.

C. Laboratory Findings

Liver tests reveal moderate elevations of serum AST, ALT, and variable elevations of alkaline phosphatase, bilirubin, and total IgG. Two subtypes of disease have been described based on the autoantibodies present: type 1 AIH: ANA and/or ASMA (anti-actin); type 2 AIH: anti-LKM (anti–liver-kidney microsomal). Type 1 AIH is the most common form of AIH in the United States. Type 2 AIH is more common in Europe, presents at a younger age, and is more likely to present with ALF compared to type 1. A genetic susceptibility to AIH is

suggested by the increased incidence of the histocompatibility alleles HLA DR*0301 (type 1 AIH) or HLA DR*0701 (type 2 AIH). Liver biopsy remains the gold standard in diagnosis, revealing the typical histologic picture of interface hepatitis: a dense infiltration of the portal tracts consisting mainly of lymphocytes and plasma cells that extends into the liver lobules with destruction of the hepatocytes at the periphery of the lobule and erosion of the limiting plate. There may be bridging fibrosis or cirrhosis evident as well.

▶ Differential Diagnosis

Laboratory and histologic findings differentiate other types of chronic hepatitis (eg, HBV, HCV; steatohepatitis; Wilson disease; α_1-antitrypsin deficiency; PSC). PSC occasionally presents in a manner similar to AIH, including the presence of autoantibodies. Up to 30% of pediatric patients have an "overlap syndrome" of AIH and PSC. Drug-induced chronic hepatitis (minocycline, isoniazid, methyldopa, pemoline) should be ruled out. In addition, minocycline has been reported as a potential "trigger" of type 1 AIH.

▶ Complications

Untreated disease that continues for months to years eventually results in cirrhosis, with complications of portal hypertension such as esophageal varices and ascites, and liver synthetic dysfunction. Untreated AIH can also lead to liver failure.

▶ Treatment

Corticosteroids (prednisone, 2 mg/kg/day or budesonide, 9 mg daily) as induction therapy decreases the mortality rate during the early active phase of the disease. Recent data suggest that oral budesonide may be as efficacious as prednisone at inducing remission with less steroid side effects. Budesonide should not be used in the setting of acute severe AIH or AIH with cirrhosis (due to limited efficacy with these modes of presentation). Maintenance therapy with azathioprine or 6-mercaptopurine (6-MP), 1–2 mg/kg/day, is recommended to facilitate weaning off of steroids. Thiopurine methyltransferase activity in red blood cells or genotype should be assessed prior to starting azathioprine or 6-MP to prevent extremely high blood levels and severe bone marrow toxicity. Steroids are reduced over a 3- to 6-month period and azathioprine is continued for at least 2 years. At that point, if AST and ALT have been consistently normal, one can consider a future wean off therapy. A liver biopsy must be performed before stopping azathioprine or 6-MP therapy to ensure histologic remission; if any inflammation persists, azathioprine or 6-MP is continued. The majority of pediatric patients will require chronic azathioprine or 6-MP therapy, but up to 30% can stop therapy eventually. Mycophenolate mofetil can be substituted for azathioprine or 6-MP if there is a contraindication or side effect from these medications.

The calcineurin inhibitors tacrolimus is often highly effective in cases refractory to standard therapies. Liver transplantation is indicated when disease progresses to decompensated cirrhosis or in cases presenting in ALF that do not respond to steroid therapy.

► Prognosis

The prognosis for AIH has improved significantly with early initiation of therapy; approximately 90% of patients with type 1 AIH will enter remission. Some studies report permanent remission (normal histologic findings) in up to 30% of patients. Relapses (seen clinically and histologically) occur in 40%–50% of patients after cessation of therapy; remissions follow repeat treatment. Complications of portal hypertension (bleeding varices, ascites, spontaneous bacterial peritonitis, and hepatopulmonary syndrome) require specific therapy or liver transplant. Disease recurs after transplantation in approximately 20% of cases and is treated by adding azathioprine or mycophenolate mofetil to the post-transplant immunosuppressant regimen.

Mack CL et al: Diagnosis and management of autoimmune hepatitis in adults and children: 2019 practice guidance and guidelines from the American Association for the Study of Liver Diseases. Hepatology 2020;72(2):671–722 [PMID: 31863477].

Mieli-Vergani G et al: Autoimmune hepatitis. Nat Rev Dis Primers 2018;12(4):18017 [PMID: 29644994].

Vierling JM et al: Immunosuppressive treatment regimens in autoimmune hepatitis: systematic reviews and meta-analyses supporting American Association for the Study of Liver Diseases guidelines. Hepatology 2020 Aug;72(2):753–769 [PMID: 32500593].

NONALCOHOLIC FATTY LIVER DISEASE

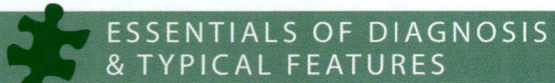

ESSENTIALS OF DIAGNOSIS & TYPICAL FEATURES

► Hepatomegaly in patient with BMI more than 95th percentile.

► Elevated ALT > AST.

► Histologic evidence of fat in the liver, which may be accompanied by inflammation, hepatocyte ballooning degermation, and fibrosis.

Nonalcoholic fatty liver disease (NAFLD), a clinicopathologic condition of abnormal hepatic fat deposition in the absence of alcohol consumption, is the most common cause of abnormal aminotransferases in the United States. NAFLD ranges from bland steatosis to fat and inflammation, with or without scarring (also referred to as nonalcoholic steatohepatitis, NASH) to cirrhosis. Trends in NAFLD parallel trends in obesity, with up to 10% of all children, and 38% of obese children affected in the United States. Many children with NAFLD are also affected by type 2 diabetes mellitus, hypertension, hyperlipidemia, obstructive sleep apnea, and the metabolic syndrome. Most children are 11–13 years of age at diagnosis, with males (ratio of 2:1) and Hispanics at highest risk.

► Prevention

The most effective therapy is prevention of the overweight or obese state.

► Clinical Findings

A. History

Most patients with NAFLD are asymptomatic and discovered upon routine screening. Some may complain of fatigue or right-upper quadrant pain. Obesity and insulin resistance are known risk factors. Moderate sleep apnea is also common in children with NAFLD. NAFLD screening (using ALT) should be considered in children beginning at age 9–11 years if they are obese or overweight with additional risk factors.

B. Symptoms and Signs

Patients with NAFLD may present with asymptomatic soft hepatomegaly, though abdominal adiposity may make this difficult to assess. Physical findings of insulin resistance (acanthosis nigricans and a buffalo hump) are frequently present.

C. Laboratory Findings

Serum aminotransferases will not identify bland steatosis, so NAFLD patients may have completely normal AST and ALT. If elevated, the AST and ALT are typically elevated less than two times the upper limit of normal, with an ALT:AST ratio of greater than 1. Alkaline phosphatase and GGT may be mildly elevated, but bilirubin is normal. Hyperglycemia and hyperlipidemia are also common. If performed, the liver biopsy may show micro- or macrovesicular steatosis, hepatocyte ballooning, Mallory bodies, and lobular or portal inflammation. In addition, varying degrees of fibrosis from portal focused to cirrhosis may be present. Obstructive sleep apnea and hypoxia appear to contribute to NAFLD disease severity. There are no established reliable biochemical predictors of the degree of hepatic fibrosis. Currently, surrogate markers and scores developed to predict NAFLD are not accurate enough, nor sufficiently validated, to be used in the clinical setting.

D. Imaging

Ultrasonography, CT scan, or MRI can be used to confirm fatty infiltration of the liver. Ultrasound, however, is of lower cost and lacks radiation exposure, although it may be insensitive with severe central adiposity or when less than 30% steatosis is present. Currently, radiologic imaging cannot distinguish bland steatosis from the more severe NASH, nor reliably identify fibrosis. Transient elastography and MR elastography are increasingly available as clinical tools that show promise in accurately estimating both hepatic fat and fibrosis.

▶ Differential Diagnosis

Steatohepatitis is also associated with Wilson disease, hereditary fructose intolerance, tyrosinemia, HCV hepatitis, cystic fibrosis, fatty acid oxidation defects, Reye syndrome, respiratory chain defects, total parenteral nutrition associated liver disease, and toxic hepatopathy (ethanol and others). Other causes of chronic hepatitis to be considered include α_1-antritrypsin deficiency, AIH, and lysosomal acid lipase deficiency.

▶ Complications

Untreated, NAFLD with hepatic inflammation can progress to cirrhosis with complications that include portal hypertension. Dyslipidemia, hypertension, insulin resistance, and obstructive sleep apnea are more common in children and adolescents with NAFLD.

▶ Treatment

Multiple potential therapies, including metformin, UDCA, and lipid-lowering agents, have been tested without therapeutic success. Therefore, treatment is focused on lifestyle modifications, through both dietary changes and exercise, to induce slow weight loss. A 7%–10% decrease in body weight can significantly improve NAFLD. Vitamin E, an antioxidant, has shown promise in clinical trials in improving histologically confirmed NASH.

▶ Prognosis

Although untreated NAFLD can progress to cirrhosis and liver failure; there is a very high response rate to weight reduction. However, success in achieving long-term weight reduction is low in children and adults.

Rinella ME et al: AASLD practice guidance on the clinical assessment and management of nonalcoholic fatty liver disease. Hepatology 2023;77(5):1797–1835 [PMID: 36727674].

Sundaram SS: Obstructive sleep apnea and hypoxemia are associated with advanced liver histology in pediatric nonalcoholic fatty liver disease. J Pediatr 2014;164:699 [PMID: 24321532].

Vos MB et al: NASPGHAN clinical practice guideline for the diagnosis and treatment of nonalcoholic fatty liver disease in children: recommendations from the expert committee on NAFLD (ECON) and the North American Society of Pediatric Gastroenterology, Hepatology and Nutrition (NASPGHAN). J Pediatr Gastroenterol Nutr 2017 Feb;64(2)319–334. [PMID: 28107283].

Xanthakos SA: Nonalcoholic steatohepatitis in children. Clin Liver Dis 2022 Aug; 26(3):439–460 [PMID: 35868684].

α_1-ANTITRYPSIN DEFICIENCY LIVER DISEASE

ESSENTIALS OF DIAGNOSIS & TYPICAL FEATURES

▶ Serum α_1-antitrypsin level < 50–80 mg/dL.

▶ Identification of a specific protease inhibitor (PI) phenotype (PIZZ, PISZ) or genotype.

▶ Detection of PAS positive, diastase-resistant glycoprotein deposits in periportal hepatocytes.

▶ Family history of early-onset pulmonary disease or liver disease.

▶ General Considerations

The disease is caused by a deficiency in α_1-antitrypsin, a PI made in the liver, predisposing patients to chronic liver disease, and an early onset of pulmonary emphysema. Liver disease is associated only with the Pi phenotypes ZZ and SZ. The accumulation of misfolded aggregates of α_1-antitrypsin protein in the liver causes liver injury by unclear mechanisms. α_1-antitrypsin is a common genetic disorder affecting up to 1 in 1600 to 1 in 2000 live births, especially among those of Northern European heritage.

▶ Clinical Findings

A. Symptoms and Signs

α_1-antitrypsin deficiency should be considered in all infants with neonatal cholestasis. About 10%–20% of affected individuals present with neonatal cholestasis. Serum GGT is usually elevated. Jaundice, acholic stools, and malabsorption may also be present. Infants are often small for gestational age, and may have pruritus, hepatosplenomegaly, ascites, and/or easy bleeding and bruising. The family history may be positive for emphysema or cirrhosis.

Toddlers and older children may present with signs of chronic liver disease, including failure to thrive, hepatosplenomegaly, gastrointestinal bleeding, or ascites. Very few children have significant pulmonary involvement. Most affected children are completely asymptomatic, with no laboratory or clinical evidence of liver or lung disease.

B. Laboratory Findings

Serum α_1-antitrypsin level is low (< 50–80 mg/dL) in homozygotes (PiZZ). Specific Pi phenotyping or genotyping should be done to confirm the diagnosis. Liver tests often reflect underlying hepatic pathologic changes. Hyperbilirubinemia (mixed) and elevated aminotransferases, alkaline phosphatase, and GGT are present early. Hyperbilirubinemia generally resolves, while aminotransferase and GGT elevation may persist. Signs of cirrhosis and hypersplenism may develop even when liver tests are normal.

Liver biopsy findings after age 6 months show diastase resistant, periodic acid–Schiff staining intracellular globules, particularly in periportal zones. These may be absent prior to age 6 months, but when present, are characteristic of α$_1$-antitrypsin deficiency.

Differential Diagnosis

In newborns, other specific causes of neonatal cholestasis need to be considered, including BA. In older children, other causes of insidious cirrhosis (eg, HBV or HCV infection, AIH, Wilson disease, cystic fibrosis, and glycogen storage disease) should be considered.

Complications

Of all infants with PiZZ α$_1$-antitrypsin deficiency, only 15%–20% develop liver disease in childhood, and many have clinical recovery. A history of neonatal cholestasis is predictive of future portal hypertension. Thus, other genetic or environmental modifiers must be involved. An associated abnormality in the microsomal disposal of accumulated aggregates may contribute to the liver disease phenotype. The complications of portal hypertension, cirrhosis, and chronic cholestasis predominate in affected children. An increased susceptibility to hepatocellular carcinoma has been noted in cirrhosis associated with α$_1$-antitrypsin deficiency. α$_1$-antitrypsin deficiency is the most common genetic cause of pediatric liver disease and the most frequent inherited indication for liver transplantation in the pediatric population.

Early-onset pulmonary emphysema occurs in young adults (age 30–40 years), particularly in smokers.

Treatment

There is no specific treatment for the liver disease of this disorder. The neonatal cholestatic condition is treated with choleretics, medium-chain triglyceride–containing formula, and water-soluble preparations of fat-soluble vitamins (see Table 22–4). UDCA may reduce AST, ALT, and GGT, but its effect on outcome is unknown. Portal hypertension, esophageal bleeding, ascites, and other complications are treated as described elsewhere. Hepatitis A and B vaccines should be given to children with α$_1$-antitrypsin deficiency. Genetic counseling is indicated when the diagnosis is made. Diagnosis by prenatal screening is possible. Liver transplantation, performed for end-stage liver disease cures the deficiency with excellent long-term survival and prevents the development of pulmonary disease. Pediatric patients should be referred to a pulmonologist by 18 years of age for education and to establish baseline pulmonary

function tests (PFTs). Passive and active cigarette smoke exposure should be eliminated to help prevent pulmonary manifestations, and obesity should be avoided. Replacement of the protein by infusion therapy is used to prevent or treat pulmonary disease in affected adults. In the future, novel treatments including chemical chaperones, autophagy inducers, hepatocyte transplantation, and gene transfer therapy may be available.

Prognosis

Of those patients presenting with neonatal cholestasis, approximately 10%–25% will need liver transplantation in the first 5 years of life, 15%–25% during childhood or adolescence, and 50%–75% will survive into adulthood with variable degrees of liver fibrosis. Neonatal cholestasis is not predictive of severe disease (including portal hypertension and need for liver transplantation) later in life. Liver failure can be expected 5–15 years after development of cirrhosis. Recurrence or persistence of hyperbilirubinemia along with worsening coagulation studies indicates the need for evaluation for liver transplantation. Decompensated cirrhosis caused by this disease is an indication for liver transplantation. Pulmonary involvement is prevented by liver transplantation. Heterozygotes may have a slightly higher incidence of liver disease. The exact relationship between low levels of serum α$_1$-antitrypsin and the development of liver disease is unclear. Emphysema develops because of a lack of inhibition of neutrophil elastase, which destroys pulmonary connective tissue.

Feldman AG, Sokol RJ: Alpha-1-antitrypsin deficiency: an important cause of pediatric liver disease. Lung Health Prof Mag 2013;4(2):8–11 [PMID: 27019872].

Teckman J et al: Longitudinal outcomes in young patients with alpha-1-antitrypsin deficiency with native liver reveal that neonatal cholestasis is a poor predictor of future portal hypertension. J Peds 2020;227:81–86 [PMID: 32663593].

WILSON DISEASE (HEPATOLENTICULAR DEGENERATION)

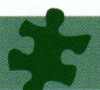

ESSENTIALS OF DIAGNOSIS & TYPICAL FEATURES

- ► Acute or chronic liver disease.
- ► Deteriorating neurologic status.
- ► Kayser-Fleischer rings.
- ► Elevated liver copper.
- ► Abnormalities in levels of ceruloplasmin and serum and urine copper.

General Considerations

Wilson disease is caused by mutations in the gene *ATP7B* on chromosome 13 coding for a specific P-type adenosine triphosphatase involved in copper transport. This results in impaired biliary excretion of copper and incorporation of copper into ceruloplasmin by the liver. The accumulated hepatic copper causes oxidative (free-radical) damage to the liver. Subsequently, copper accumulates in the basal ganglia and other tissues. The disease should be considered in all children older than 1–2 years with evidence of liver disease (especially with hemolysis) or with suggestive neurologic signs. A family history is often present, and 25% of patients are identified by screening asymptomatic homozygous family members. The disease is autosomal recessive and occurs in 1:30,000 live births in all populations.

Clinical Findings

A. Symptoms and Signs

Hepatic involvement may present as ALF, acute hepatitis, chronic liver disease, cholelithiasis, fatty liver disease, or cirrhosis with portal hypertension. Findings may include jaundice, hepatomegaly early in childhood, splenomegaly, and Kayser-Fleischer rings. The disease is generally considered after 3 years of age. However, liver involvement occurs early in life and may be present by age 1–2 years. The later onset of neurologic or psychiatric manifestations after age 10 years may include tremor, dysarthria, and drooling. Deterioration in school performance can be the earliest neurologic expression of disease. The Kayser-Fleischer ring, usually present if there is neurologic involvement, is a brown band at the junction of the iris and cornea, generally requiring slit-lamp examination for detection. Absence of Kayser-Fleischer rings does not exclude this diagnosis.

B. Laboratory Findings

The laboratory diagnosis can be challenging. Plasma ceruloplasmin levels are usually less than 15–20 mg/dL. (Normal values are 23–43 mg/dL.) Low values, however, occur normally in infants younger than 3 months, and in at least 10%–20% of homozygotes the levels may be within the lower end of the normal range (20–30 mg/dL), particularly since immunoassays are commonly used to measure ceruloplasmin. Rare patients with higher ceruloplasmin levels have been reported. Serum copper levels are low, but the overlap with normal is too great for satisfactory discrimination. In acute fulminant Wilson disease, serum copper levels are elevated markedly, owing to hepatic necrosis and release of copper. The presence of anemia, hemolysis, very high serum bilirubin levels (> 20–30 mg/dL), low alkaline phosphatase, and low acid are characteristic of acute Wilson disease. Urine copper excretion in children older than 3 years is normally less than 30 mcg/day; in Wilson disease, it is generally greater than 100 mcg/day,

although it can be as low as less than 40 mcg/day. Finally, the tissue content of copper from a liver biopsy, normally less than 40–50 mcg/g dry tissue, is greater than 250 mcg/g in the majority of Wilson disease patients but may be as low as greater than 75 mcg/day. Glycosuria and aminoaciduria have been reported. Hemolysis and gallstones may be present; bone lesions simulating those of osteochondritis dissecans have also been found.

The coarse nodular cirrhosis, macrovesicular steatosis, and glycogenated nuclei in hepatocytes seen on liver biopsy may distinguish Wilson disease from other types of cirrhosis. Early in the disease, vacuolation of liver cells, steatosis, and lipofuscin granules can be seen, as well as Mallory bodies. The presence of Mallory bodies in a child is strongly suggestive of Wilson disease. Stains for copper may sometimes be negative despite high copper content in the liver. Therefore, quantitative liver copper levels must be determined biochemically on biopsy specimens. Electron microscopy findings of abnormal mitochondria may be helpful.

Differential Diagnosis

During the icteric phase, acute or chronic viral hepatitis, α_1-antitrypsin deficiency, AIH, and drug-induced hepatitis are other diagnostic possibilities. Nonalcoholic steatohepatitis may have similar histology and be confused with Wilson disease in overweight patients. Laboratory testing for plasma ceruloplasmin, 24-hour urine copper excretion, liver quantitative copper concentration, and a slit-lamp examination of the cornea will help differentiate Wilson disease from the other causes in most patients. Urinary copper excretion during penicillamine challenge (500 mg twice a day in the older child or adult) may also be helpful. Genetic testing of *ATP7B* is available and is helpful if two disease-causing mutations are present. Other copper storage diseases that occur in early childhood include Indian childhood cirrhosis, Tyrolean childhood cirrhosis, and idiopathic copper toxicosis. However, ceruloplasmin concentrations are normal to elevated in these conditions.

Complications

Cirrhosis, hepatic coma, progressive neurologic degeneration, and eventual death are the rule in the untreated patient. The complications of portal hypertension (variceal hemorrhage, ascites) may be present at diagnosis. Progressive central nervous system disease and terminal aspiration pneumonia were common in untreated older people. Acute hemolytic disease may result in acute renal failure. Profound jaundice and coma, hemolysis, and oliguric acute kidney injury may be a part of the presentation of acute fulminant Wilson disease.

Treatment

Copper chelation with D-penicillamine or trientine hydrochloride, 750–1500 mg/day orally, is the treatment of choice, whether or not the patient is symptomatic. The target dose for children is 20 mg/kg/day; begin with 250 mg/day and increase the dose weekly by 250 mg increments. Strict dietary restriction of copper intake is not practical; however, selected high copper foods should be minimized. Supplementation with zinc acetate (25–50 mg orally, three times daily) may reduce copper absorption but should not be given at same time as copper chelators. Copper chelation or zinc therapy is continued for life, although doses of chelators may be reduced transiently at the time of surgery or early in pregnancy. Vitamin B$_6$ (25 mg) is given daily during therapy with penicillamine to prevent optic neuritis. In some countries, after a clinical response to penicillamine or trientine, zinc therapy is substituted and continued for life. Derivatives of tetrathiomolybdate are being tested as an alternative therapy. Nonadherence with any of the drug regimens (including zinc therapy) can lead to sudden fulminant liver failure and death within months.

Liver transplantation is indicated for all cases of acute fulminant disease (with hemolysis and renal failure), for progressive hepatic decompensation despite several months of therapy, and severe progressive hepatic insufficiency in patients who inadvisedly discontinue penicillamine, triene, or zinc therapy. Gene replacement therapies are investigational and undergoing early phase clinical trials.

▶ **Prognosis**

The prognosis of untreated Wilson disease is poor. The fulminant presentation is fatal without liver transplantation in almost all cases. Copper chelation reduces hepatic copper content, reverses many of the liver lesions, and can stabilize the clinical course of established cirrhosis. Neurologic symptoms generally respond to therapy, although occasional patients have progression during chelation, but improve following liver transplantation. All siblings should be immediately screened and homozygotes treated with copper chelation or zinc acetate therapy, even if asymptomatic. Recent data suggest that zinc monotherapy may not be as effective for hepatic Wilson disease as copper chelation. Genetic testing (ATP7B genotyping) is available if there is any doubt about the diagnosis and is particularly useful for screening all family members.

Saroli Palumbo C, Schilsky ML: Clinical practice guidelines in Wilson disease. Ann Transl Med 2019 Apr;7(Suppl 2):S65 [PMID: 31179302].

Schilsky ML et al: A multidisciplinary approach to the diagnosis and management of Wilson disease: 2022 practice guidance on Wilson disease from the American Association for the Study of Liver Diseases. Hepatology 2022 Dec 7. doi: 10.1002/hep.32801. Online ahead of print [PMID: 36151586].

Socha P et al: Wilson's disease in children: a position paper by the Hepatology Committee of the European Society for Paediatric Gastroenterology, Hepatology and Nutrition. J Pediatr Gastroenterol Nutr 2018 Feb;66(2):334–344 [PMID: 29341979].

DRUG-INDUCED LIVER DISEASES

▶ **General Considerations**

Drug-induced liver injury (DILI) may be predictable or unpredictable. Predictable hepatotoxins cause liver injury in a dose-dependent manner. Unpredictable hepatotoxins cause liver injury in an idiosyncratic manner, which may be influenced by the genetic and environmental characteristics of particular individuals. DILI has been described with a wide variety of medications, including antihypertensives, acetaminophen, anabolic steroids, antibiotics, anticonvulsants, antidepressants, antituberculosis medications, antipsychotics, antivirals, herbals, dietary supplements, check point inhibitors, and weight loss agents.

▶ **Symptoms**

Many people with DILI are asymptomatic and only detected because aminotransferases are performed for other reasons. If symptomatic, indicating more severe DILI, patients may have malaise, anorexia, pruritus, nausea and vomiting, right-upper quadrant pain, jaundice, acholic stools, and dark urine. If the DILI is a hypersensitivity reaction, fever and rash may also occur.

When submassive hepatic necrosis and fulminant failure occur, mortality can exceed 50%.

▶ **Diagnosis**

No specific testing for DILI is available, with diagnosis requiring a causality assessment. This assessment should determine if the patient was exposed to the drug during a logical time period, if the drug has previously been reported to cause DILI, and if the symptom complex is consistent with DILI. In addition, other explanations for liver injury should be sought, including viral hepatitis, AIH, and alcohol use. Finally, removal of the offending agent typically results in clinical and laboratory improvement, further proving causality.

▶ **Treatment**

Primary therapy is supportive care, discontinuation of the offending drug, and avoiding reexposure. This typically results in rapid and complete resolution of symptoms. However, DILI severe enough to cause ALF has a poor prognosis without urgent liver transplant. Specific therapies for some DILI etiologies include N-acetylcysteine for acetaminophen poisoning and L-carnitine for valproic acid hepatotoxicity. The use of UDCA may speed resolution of jaundice. The use of corticosteroids for DILI remains controversial but may have a role in immune-mediated disease. An NIH-sponsored website provides up-to-date information about each drug and herbal substance associated with DILI (LiverTox).

Garcia-Cortes et al: Drug-induced liver injury: an update. Arch Toxicology 2020 Oct;94(10):3381–3407 [PMID: 32852569].
LiverTox: Clinical and research information on drug-induced liver injury. http://www.livertox.nih.gov/. Accessed August 1, 2017.

CIRRHOSIS

ESSENTIALS OF DIAGNOSIS & TYPICAL FEATURES

- ▶ Underlying liver disease.
- ▶ Nodular, hard liver and splenomegaly.
- ▶ Nodular liver on abdominal imaging.
- ▶ Liver biopsy demonstrating cirrhosis.

▶ General Considerations

Cirrhosis is defined by the World Health Organization as a diffuse process whereby the architecture of the liver has been replaced by structurally abnormal nodules due to fibrosis. It may be micronodular or macronodular in appearance. The resulting vasculature distortion leads to increased resistance to blood flow, producing portal hypertension, and its consequences.

Many liver diseases may progress to cirrhosis in children, including metabolic and genetic disorders, infectious diseases, autoimmune and inflammatory diseases, cholestatic diseases and biliary malformations, vascular lesions, and drugs/toxins. In the first year of life, BA and genetic-metabolic diseases are the most common cause of cirrhosis. In older children, cirrhosis is most commonly caused by chronic viral hepatitis, Wilson disease, PSC, AIH, and α1-antitrypsin deficiency. Regardless of etiology, cirrhosis can lead to liver failure and death.

▶ Clinical Findings

A. History

Many children with cirrhosis may be asymptomatic early in the course. Malaise, loss of appetite, failure to thrive, and nausea are frequent complaints, especially in anicteric varieties. Easy bruising may be reported. Jaundice may or may not be present.

B. Symptoms and Signs

The first indication of underlying liver disease may be splenomegaly, ascites, gastrointestinal hemorrhage, or hepatic encephalopathy. Variable hepatomegaly, spider angiomas, warm skin, palmar erythema, or digital clubbing may be present. A small, shrunken liver may be present. Most often, the liver is enlarged slightly, especially in the subxiphoid region, where it has a firm to hard quality and an irregular edge. Splenomegaly generally precedes other complications of portal hypertension. Ascites, gynecomastia in males, digital clubbing, pretibial edema, and irregularities of menstruation in females may be present. In biliary cirrhosis, patients often also have jaundice, dark urine, pruritus, hepatomegaly, and sometimes xanthomas. Malnutrition and failure to thrive due to steatorrhea may be more apparent in biliary cirrhosis.

C. Laboratory Findings

Mild abnormalities of AST and ALT are often present, with a decreased level of albumin. PT is prolonged and may be unresponsive to vitamin K administration. Burr and target red cells may be noted on the peripheral blood smear. Anemia, thrombocytopenia, and leukopenia are present if hypersplenism exists. However, blood tests may be normal in patients with cirrhosis. In biliary cirrhosis, increased levels of conjugated bilirubin, bile acids, GGT, alkaline phosphatase, and cholesterol are common.

D. Imaging

Hepatic ultrasound, CT, or MRI may demonstrate abnormal hepatic texture and nodules. In biliary cirrhosis, abnormalities of the biliary tree may be apparent. Transient or magnetic resonance elastography will demonstrate increased liver stiffness.

E. Pathologic Findings

Liver biopsy findings of regenerating nodules and surrounding fibrosis are hallmarks of cirrhosis. Pathologic features of biliary cirrhosis also include canalicular and hepatocyte cholestasis, as well as plugging of bile ducts. The interlobular bile ducts may be increased or decreased, depending on the cause and the stage of the disease process.

▶ Differential Diagnosis

In children, multiple diseases can result in cirrhosis, including biliary obstruction (BA, CDC, bile duct stenosis), inborn errors of metabolism and genetic conditions (PFIC, α1-antitrypsin deficiency, galactosemia, fructosemia, GSD types III and IV, cystic fibrosis, mitochondrial hepatopathies, Wilson disease), viral (HBV, HCV) and parasitic infections (*Opisthorchis sinensis*, *Fasciola*, Schistosoma, and *Ascaris*), chronic drug and toxin exposure, AIH, PSC, vascular alterations, and NAFLD. Most cases of biliary cirrhosis result from congenital abnormalities of the bile ducts (BA, CDC), tumors of the bile duct, Caroli disease, progressive familial intrahepatic cholangitis, PSC, paucity of the intrahepatic bile ducts, and cystic fibrosis. The evolution to cirrhosis may be insidious, with no recognized icteric phase. At the time of diagnosis of cirrhosis, the underlying liver disease may be active, with abnormal aminotransferases; or it may be quiescent, with normal aminotransferases.

Complications

Major complications of cirrhosis in childhood include progressive nutritional disturbances, hormonal disturbances, infections, and the evolution of portal hypertension and its complications (GI bleeding, ascites, and encephalopathy). Hepatocellular carcinoma occurs with increased frequency in the cirrhotic liver, especially in patients with the chronic form of hereditary tyrosinemia or after long-standing HBV or HCV disease. Some children with cirrhosis may develop hepatopulmonary syndrome characterized by intrapulmonary vasodilation and hypoxia, portal-pulmonary hypertension, or hepatorenal syndrome characterized by progressive deterioration of renal function.

Treatment

At present, there is no proven medical treatment for cirrhosis, but whenever a treatable disease is identified (eg, Wilson disease, galactosemia, AIH) or an offending agent eliminated (HBV, HCV, drugs, toxins), disease progression can be altered; occasionally regression of fibrosis has been noted. Cirrhosis from HCV and HBV may be reversed by successful antiviral therapy. Children with cirrhosis should receive the hepatitis A and B vaccines and be monitored for the development of hepatocellular carcinoma with serial serum AFP determinations and abdominal ultrasound for hepatic nodules annually. Liver transplantation may be appropriate in patients with cirrhosis caused by a progressive disease; evidence of worsening hepatic synthetic function; or complications of cirrhosis that are no longer manageable.

Prognosis

Cirrhosis has an unpredictable course. Without transplantation, affected patients may die from liver failure within 10–15 years. Patients with a rising bilirubin, a vitamin K–resistant coagulopathy, or diuretic refractory ascites usually survive less than 1–2 years. The terminal event in some patients may be generalized hemorrhage, sepsis, or cardiorespiratory arrest. For patients with biliary cirrhosis, the prognosis is similar, except for those with surgically corrected lesions that result in regression or stabilization of the underlying liver condition. With liver transplantation, the long-term survival rate is 70%–90%.

Hsu EK, Murray KF: Cirrhosis and chronic liver failure. In: Suchy FJ, Sokol RJ, Balistreri WF (eds): *Liver Disease in Children*. 4th ed. Cambridge University Press; 2014:51–67.

Pinto RB, Schneider AC, da Silveira TR: Cirrhosis in children and adolescents: an overview. World J Hepatol 2015 Mar 27; 7(3):392–405. doi: 10.4254/wjh.v7.i3.392 [PMID: 25848466].

PORTAL HYPERTENSION

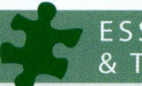

ESSENTIALS OF DIAGNOSIS & TYPICAL FEATURES

► Splenomegaly.
► Recurrent ascites.
► Variceal hemorrhage.
► Hypersplenism.

General Considerations

Portal hypertension is defined as an increase in the portal venous pressure to greater than 5 mm Hg above that of the inferior vena caval pressure. Portal hypertension is most commonly a result of cirrhosis. Portal hypertension may be divided into prehepatic, suprahepatic, and intrahepatic causes (Table 22–9). Although the specific lesions vary somewhat in their clinical signs and symptoms, the consequences of portal hypertension are common to all.

Table 22–9. Causes of portal hypertension.

Prehepatic	Intrahepatic	Posthepatic

Portal vein thrombosis, stenosis or obstruction (can be congenital or acquired)
Splenic vein thrombosis
	Pre-sinusoidal:
	  Congenital hepatic fibrosis
	  Nodular regenerative hyperplasia
	  Schistosomiasis
	Sinusoidal:
	  Cirrhosis
	  Infiltrative liver disease
	Post-sinusoidal:
	  Sinusoidal obstructive syndrome
		Hepatic vein thrombosis/obstruction (Budd-Chiari syndrome)
		Inferior vena cava web/band/stricture/ thrombosis
		Constrictive pericarditis
		Congestive heart failure

A. Prehepatic Portal Hypertension

Prehepatic portal hypertension from acquired abnormalities of the portal and splenic veins accounts for 30%–50% of cases of variceal hemorrhage in children. A history of neonatal omphalitis, sepsis, dehydration, or umbilical vein catheterization may be present. Causes in older children include local trauma, peritonitis (pylephlebitis), hypercoagulable states, and pancreatitis. Symptoms may occur before age 1 year, but in most cases the diagnosis is not made until age 3–5 years. Patients with a positive neonatal history tend to be symptomatic earlier.

A variety of portal or splenic vein malformations, some of which may be congenital, have been described to cause pre-hepatic portal hypertension, including defects in valves and atretic segments. Cavernous transformation of the portal vein is the result of attempted collateralization around the thrombosed portal vein rather than a congenital malformation. The site of the venous obstruction may be anywhere from the hilum of the liver to the hilum of the spleen.

B. Suprahepatic Vein Occlusion or Thrombosis (Budd-Chiari Syndrome)

No cause can be demonstrated in most instances of suprahepatic vein occlusion or thrombosis in children, while tumor, medications, and hypercoagulable states are common causes in adults. The occasional association of hepatic vein thrombosis in inflammatory bowel disease favors the presence of endogenous toxins traversing the liver. Vasculitis leading to endophlebitis of the hepatic veins has also been described.

In addition, hepatic vein obstruction may be secondary to tumor, abdominal trauma, hyperthermia, or sepsis, or it may occur following the repair of an omphalocele or gastroschisis. Congenital vena caval bands, webs, a membrane, or stricture above the hepatic veins are sometimes causative. Hepatic vein thrombosis may be a complication of oral contraceptive medications. Underlying thrombotic conditions (deficiency of antithrombin III, protein C or S, or factor V Leiden; antiphospholipid antibodies; or mutations of the prothrombin gene) are common in adults.

C. Intrahepatic Portal Hypertension

1. Cirrhosis—See previous section.

2. Sinusoidal obstruction syndrome (acute stage)—This entity occurs most frequently in bone marrow or stem cell transplant recipients. Additional causes include high dose thiopurines, ingestion of pyrrolizidine alkaloids ("bush tea") or other herbal teas, and a familial form of the disease occurring in congenital immunodeficiency states. The acute form of the disease generally occurs in the first month after bone marrow transplantation and is heralded by the triad of weight gain (ascites), tender hepatomegaly, and jaundice.

3. Congenital hepatic fibrosis—This is a rare autosomal recessive cause of intrahepatic presinusoidal portal hypertension (Table 22–10). Liver biopsy is generally diagnostic, demonstrating Von Meyenburg complexes (abnormal clusters of ectatic bile ducts). On angiography, the intrahepatic branches of the portal vein may be duplicated. Autosomal

Table 22–10. Treatment of complications of portal hypertension.

Complication	Diagnosis	Treatment
Bleeding esophageal varices	Endoscopic verification of variceal bleeding.	Endosclerosis or variceal band ligation. Octreotide, 1 mcg/kg bolus followed by 1-3 mcg/kg/h infusion. Pediatric Sengstaken-Blakemore tube. Surgical portosystemic shunt, TIPS, OLT. Propranolol (nonselective β-blockers) may be useful to prevent recurrent bleeding in select patients but caution that limited ability to compensate with increased cardiac output if they bleed.
Ascites	Clinical examination (fluid wave, shifting dullness), abdominal ultrasonography.	Sodium restriction (1–2 mEq/kg/day), spironolactone (3–5 mg/kg/day), furosemide (1–4 mg/kg/day), intravenous albumin (0.5–1 g/kg per dose), paracentesis, TIPS, surgical portosystemic shunt, OLT.[a]
Hepatic encephalopathy	Abnormal neurologic examination, elevated plasma ammonia.	Protein restriction (0.5–1 g/kg/day), intravenous glucose (6–8 mg/kg/min), neomycin (2–4 g/m² BSA PO in four doses), rifaximin (200 mg three times a day in children > 12 y), lactulose (1 mL/kg per dose [up to 30 mL] every 4–6 h PO), plasmapheresis, hemodialysis, OLT.[a]
Hypersplenism	Low WBC count, platelets, and/or hemoglobin. Splenomegaly.	No intervention, partial splenic embolization, surgical portosystemic shunt, TIPS, OLT. Splenectomy may worsen variceal bleeding.

BSA, body surface area; OLT, orthotopic liver transplantation; PO, by mouth; TIPS, transjugular intrahepatic portosystemic shunt; WBC, white blood cell.
[a]In order of sequential management.

recessive polycystic kidney disease is frequently associated with this disorder.

4. Other rare causes—Hepatoportal sclerosis (idiopathic portal hypertension, noncirrhotic portal fibrosis), focal nodular regeneration of the liver, and schistosomal hepatic fibrosis are also rare causes of intrahepatic presinusoidal portal hypertension.

▶ Clinical Findings

A. Symptoms and Signs

For prehepatic portal hypertension, splenomegaly in an otherwise well child is the most common physical sign. Ascites may be noted. The usual presenting symptoms are hematemesis and melena.

The presence of prehepatic portal hypertension may be suggested by (1) a history of severe infection in the newborn period or early infancy—especially omphalitis, sepsis, gastroenteritis, severe dehydration, or prolonged or difficult umbilical vein catheterizations; (2) no previous evidence of liver disease; (3) a history of well-being prior to onset or recognition of symptoms; and (4) normal liver size and liver tests with splenomegaly.

Most patients with suprahepatic portal hypertension present with abdominal pain, tender hepatomegaly of acute onset, and ascites. Jaundice is present in only 25% of patients. Vomiting, hematemesis, and diarrhea are less common. Cutaneous signs of chronic liver disease are often absent, as the obstruction is usually acute. Distended superficial veins on the back and the anterior abdomen, along with dependent edema, are seen when inferior vena cava obstruction affects hepatic vein outflow. Absence of hepatojugular reflux (jugular distention when pressure is applied to the liver) is a helpful clinical sign. The symptoms and signs of intrahepatic portal hypertension are generally those of cirrhosis (see section Cirrhosis).

B. Laboratory Findings and Imaging

Most other common causes of splenomegaly or hepatosplenomegaly may be excluded by appropriate laboratory tests, such as EBV and hepatitis serologies, blood smear examination, bone marrow studies, and LFTs. In prehepatic portal hypertension, liver tests are generally normal. In Budd-Chiari syndrome and veno-occlusive disease, mild to moderate hyperbilirubinemia with modest elevations of AST, ALT, and PT/INR are often present. Significant early increases in fibrinolytic parameters (especially plasminogen activator inhibitor 1) have been reported in veno-occlusive disease. Hypersplenism with mild leukopenia and thrombocytopenia is often present. Upper endoscopy may reveal varices in symptomatic patients.

Doppler-assisted ultrasound scanning of the liver, portal vein, splenic vein, inferior vena cava, and hepatic veins may assist in defining the vascular anatomy. In prehepatic portal hypertension, abnormalities of the portal or splenic vein may be apparent, whereas the hepatic veins are normal. However, cavernous transformation can sometimes erroneously appear as normal portal inflow on ultrasonography. Therefore, if there is high suspicion for pre-hepatic portal hypertension, CT angiography/venography scan should be obtained. When noncirrhotic portal hypertension is suspected, angiography/venography is often diagnostic. Selective arteriography or MRI of the superior mesenteric artery is recommended prior to surgical shunting to determine the patency of the superior mesenteric vein.

For suprahepatic portal hypertension, an inferior vena cavogram using catheters from above or below the suspected obstruction may reveal an intrinsic filling defect, an infiltrating tumor, or extrinsic compression of the inferior vena cava by an adjacent lesion. A large caudate lobe of the liver suggests Budd-Chiari syndrome. Care must be taken in interpreting extrinsic pressure defects of the subdiaphragmatic inferior vena cava if ascites is significant.

Simultaneous wedged hepatic vein pressure and hepatic venography are useful to demonstrate obstruction to major hepatic vein ostia and smaller vessels. In the absence of obstruction, reflux across the sinusoids into the portal vein branches can be accomplished. Pressures should also be taken from the right heart and supradiaphragmatic portion of the inferior vena cava to eliminate constrictive pericarditis and pulmonary hypertension from the differential diagnosis.

▶ Differential Diagnosis

All causes of splenomegaly must be included in the differential diagnosis. The most common ones are infections, immune thrombocytopenic purpura, blood dyscrasias, lipidosis, reticuloendotheliosis, cirrhosis of the liver, and cysts or hemangiomas of the spleen. When hematemesis or melena occurs, other causes of gastrointestinal bleeding are possible, such as gastric or duodenal ulcers, tumors, duplications, and inflammatory bowel disease. Because ascites is almost always present in suprahepatic portal hypertension, cirrhosis resulting from any cause must be excluded. Other suprahepatic (cardiac, pulmonary) causes of portal hypertension must also be ruled out. Although ascites may occur in prehepatic portal hypertension, it is uncommon.

▶ Complications

The major manifestation and complication of portal hypertension is bleeding from esophageal varices. Fatal exsanguination is uncommon, but hypovolemic shock or resulting anemia requires prompt treatment. Hypersplenism with leukopenia and thrombocytopenia occurs, but seldom causes major symptoms. Without treatment, complete and persistent hepatic vein obstruction in suprahepatic portal hypertension leads to liver failure, coma, and death. A nonportal type of cirrhosis may develop in the chronic form of hepatic veno-occlusive disease in which small- and medium-sized hepatic veins are affected. Death from renal failure may occur in rare cases of congenital hepatic fibrosis.

▶ Treatment

Definitive treatment of noncirrhotic portal hypertension is lacking. Aggressive medical treatment of the complications of prehepatic portal hypertension is generally quite effective. Excellent results are also seen with either a portosystemic shunt or the meso-rex (mesenterico–left portal bypass) shunt. When possible (there must be an open left portal vein and no underlying liver disease on biopsy), the Meso-Rex shunt is the preferred technique. The risk of veno-occlusive disease may be decreased by the prophylactic use of UDCA or defibrotide prior to conditioning for bone marrow transplantation. Treatment with defibrotide and withdrawal of the suspected offending agent, if possible, may increase the chance of recovery. Transjugular intrahepatic portosystemic shunts have been successful in bridging to recovery in veno-occlusive disease. For suprahepatic portal hypertension, efforts should be directed at correcting the underlying cause, if possible. Either surgical or angiographic relief of obstruction should be attempted if a defined obstruction of the vessels is apparent. Liver transplantation, if not contraindicated, should be considered early if direct correction is not possible. In most cases, management of portal hypertension is directed at management of the complications (see Table 22–10).

▶ Prognosis

For prehepatic portal hypertension, the prognosis depends on the site of the block, the effectiveness of variceal eradication, the availability of suitable vessels for shunting procedures, and the experience of the surgeon. In patients treated medically, bleeding episodes may diminish with adolescence. Portacaval encephalopathy is unusual after shunting except when protein intake is excessive, but neurologic outcome may be better in patients who receive a Meso-Rex shunt when compared with medical management alone. The mortality rate of hepatic vein obstruction is very high (95%). In veno-occlusive disease, the prognosis is better, with complete recovery possible in 50% of acute forms and 5%–10% of subacute forms.

Bass LM et al: Risk of variceal hemorrhage and pretransplant mortality in children with biliary atresia. Hepatology 2022 Sep;76(3):712–726 [PMID: 35271743].

Chapin C, Bass LM: Cirrhosis and portal hypertension in the pediatric population. Clin Liver Dis 2018;22(4):735–752 [PMID: 30266160].

Lautz TB et al. Advantages of the meso-Rex bypass compared with portosystemic shunts in the management of extrahepatic portal vein obstruction in children. J Am Coll Surg 2013 Jan;216(1):83–89 [PMID: 23177370].

BILIARY TRACT DISEASE

ESSENTIALS OF DIAGNOSIS & TYPICAL FEATURES

▶ Episodic right-upper quadrant abdominal pain.

▶ Elevated bilirubin, alkaline phosphatase, and GGT.

▶ Stones or sludge seen on abdominal imaging.

1. Cholelithiasis

▶ General Considerations

Gallstones may develop at all ages in the pediatric population and in utero. Gallstones may be divided into cholesterol stones (> 50% cholesterol) and pigment (black [sterile bile] and brown [infected bile]) stones. Pigment stones are the predominate type in the first decade of life, while cholesterol stones account for up to 90% of gallstones in adolescence. The process is reversible in some patients.

▶ Clinical Findings

A. History

Most symptomatic gallstones are associated with acute or recurrent episodes of moderate to severe, sharp right upper quadrant, or epigastric pain. The pain may radiate substernally or to the right shoulder. Nausea and vomiting may occur during attacks. Pain episodes often occur postprandially, especially after ingestion of fatty foods. If gallstones become impacted in the bile duct they may cause jaundice, elevation in AST, ALT and GGT, cholangitis, and can sometimes obstruct the pancreatic duct causing pancreatitis. Risk factors for gallstones include patients with hemolytic disease; females; teenagers; pregnancy; obesity; rapid weight loss; portal vein thrombosis; certain racial or ethnic groups, particularly Native Americans (Pima Indians) and Hispanics; Crohn disease or prior ileal resection; cystic fibrosis; Wilson disease; prolonged parenteral nutrition; and bile acid transporter defects. Other less certain risk factors include a positive family history, use of birth control pills, and diabetes mellitus.

B. Symptoms and Signs

During acute episodes of pain, tenderness is present in the right-upper quadrant or epigastrium, with a positive inspiratory arrest (Murphy sign), usually without peritoneal signs. Evidence of underlying hemolytic disease in addition to scleral icterus may include pallor (anemia), splenomegaly, tachycardia, and high-output cardiac murmur. Fever is unusual in uncomplicated cases and should raise concern for cholangitis or cholecystitis.

C. Laboratory Findings

Laboratory tests are usually normal unless calculi have lodged in the extrahepatic biliary system (choledocholithiasis), in which case the serum bilirubin and GGT (or alkaline phosphatase) may be elevated. Lipase and/or amylase levels may be increased if stone obstruction occurs at the major papilla and causes gallstone pancreatitis.

D. Imaging

Ultrasound evaluation is the best initial imaging technique to identify abnormal intraluminal contents (stones, sludge) in the gallbladder. For patients with cholelithiasis and signs of potential stones in the common bile duct (dilation of common bile duct, elevation in AST, ALT, total and/or direct bilirubin), ultrasound is not sufficiently sensitive to rule out choledocholithiasis. In indeterminate cases, MRCP or endoscopic ultrasound should be considered and ERCP for therapy of choledocholithiasis.

▶ Differential Diagnosis

Other abnormal conditions of the biliary system with similar presentation are summarized in Table 22–11. Liver disease (hepatitis, abscess, or tumor) can cause similar symptoms or signs. Functional dyspepsia or other functional GI disorders, peptic disease, reflux or eosinophilic esophagitis, paraesophageal hiatal hernia, cardiac disease, and pneumomediastinum must be considered when the pain is epigastric or substernal in location. Renal or pancreatic disease is a possible explanation if the pain is localized to the right flank or mid back. Subcapsular or supracapsular lesions of the liver (abscess, tumor, or hematoma) or right-lower lobe infiltrate may also be a cause of nontraumatic right shoulder pain.

▶ Complications

Major problems are related to stone impaction in either the cystic or common bile duct, which may lead to stricture formation or perforation and subsequent bile leak. Stones impacted at the level of the major ampulla can cause gallstone pancreatitis.

▶ Treatment

Symptomatic cholelithiasis is treated by cholecystectomy. Intraoperative cholangiography via the cystic duct or preoperative endoscopic ultrasound can be considered in select patients so that the physician can be certain the biliary system is free of retained stones. Calculi in the extrahepatic bile ducts may be removed via ERCP.

Gallstones developing in infants and children on parenteral nutrition can be followed by ultrasound examination. Most infants are asymptomatic, and their stones will resolve in 3–36 months. Gallstone dissolution using cholelitholytics (UDCA) may be useful in this setting. Asymptomatic gallstones in otherwise healthy patients do not usually require treatment, as less than 20% will eventually cause problems.

▶ Prognosis

The prognosis is excellent in uncomplicated cases that come to standard or laparoscopic cholecystectomy.

Fradin K et al: Obesity and symptomatic cholelithiasis in childhood: epidemiologic and case-control evidence for a strong relation. J Pediatr Gastroenterol Nutr 2014;58:102–106 [PMID: 23969538].

Langballe KO, Bardram L: Cholecystectomy in Danish children—a nationwide study. J Pediatr Surg 2014;49:626–630 [PMID: 24726126].

Svensson J et al: Gallstone disease in children. Semin Pediatr Surg 2012;21:255 [PMID: 22800978].

2. Primary Sclerosing Cholangitis

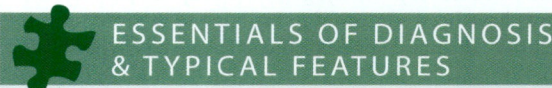

ESSENTIALS OF DIAGNOSIS & TYPICAL FEATURES

- ▶ Pruritus and jaundice.
- ▶ Elevated GGT.
- ▶ Associated with inflammatory bowel disease.
- ▶ Abnormal ERCP or MRCP.

▶ General Considerations

Primary sclerosing cholangitis (PSC) is a progressive liver disease characterized by chronic inflammation and fibrosis of the intrahepatic and/or extrahepatic bile ducts, leading to fibrotic strictures and saccular dilations of all or parts of the biliary tree. The etiology of PSC is likely multifactorial, including genetic predispositions, with alterations in innate and autoimmunity. PSC is more common in males, and has a strong relationship to inflammatory bowel disease, particularly ulcerative colitis. A PSC-like condition can also be seen with histiocytosis X, AIH, IgG4 cholangiopathy/autoimmune pancreatitis, sicca syndromes, congenital and acquired immunodeficiency syndromes, and cystic fibrosis. Secondary sclerosing cholangitis due to Cryptosporidia may occur in immunodeficiency syndromes.

▶ Clinical Findings

A. Symptoms and Signs

PSC often has an insidious onset and may be asymptomatic. Clinical symptoms may include abdominal pain, fatigue, pruritus, jaundice, and weight loss. Acholic stools, steatorrhea, hepatomegaly, and splenomegaly can occur.

Table 22–11. Biliary tract diseases of childhood.

	Acute Hydrops/Transient Dilation of Gallbladder[a,b]	Choledochal Cyst[c] (see Figure 22–1)	Acalculous Cholecystitis[d]	Caroli Disease[e] (Idiopathic Intrahepatic Bile Duct Dilation)	Congenital Hepatic Fibrosis[f]	Biliary Dyskinesia[g] and Functional Dyspepsia
Predisposing or associated conditions	Premature infants with prolonged fasting or systemic illness. Hepatitis. Abnormalities of cystic duct. Kawasaki disease. Bacterial sepsis, EBV.	Congenital lesion. Female sex. Asians. Rarely with Caroli disease or congenital hepatic fibrosis.	Systemic illness, sepsis (*Streptococcus, Salmonella, Klebsiella*, etc), EBV or HIV infection. Gallbladder stasis, obstruction of cystic duct (stones, nodes, tumor).	Congenital lesion. Also found in congenital hepatic fibrosis or with choledochal cyst. Female sex. Autosomal recessive polycystic kidney disease.	Familial (autosomal recessive), 25% with autosomal recessive polycystic kidney disease (PKHD1 mutation). Choledochal cyst. Caroli disease. Meckel-Gruber, Ivemark, or Jeune syndrome.	School ages and adolescents.
Symptoms	Absent in premature infants. Vomiting, abdominal pain in older children.	Abdominal pain, vomiting, jaundice.	Acute severe abdominal pain, vomiting, fever.	Recurrent abdominal pain, vomiting. Fever, jaundice when cholangitis occurs.	Hematemesis, melena from bleeding esophageal varices.	Intermittent epigastric or RUQ pain.
Signs	RUQ abdominal mass. Tenderness in some.	Icterus, acholic stools, dark urine in neonatal period. RUQ abdominal mass or tenderness in older children.	Tenderness in mid and right upper abdomen. Occasional palpable mass in RUQ.	Icterus, hepatomegaly.	Hepatosplenomegaly.	Usually normal examination.
Laboratory abnormalities	Most are normal. Increased WBC count during sepsis (may be decreased in premature infants). Abnormal LFTs in hepatitis.	Conjugated hyperbilirubinemia, elevated GGT, slightly increased AST. Elevated pancreatic serum amylase common.	Elevated WBC count, normal or slight abnormality of LFTs.	Abnormal LFTs. Increased WBC count with cholangitis. Urine abnormalities if associated with congenital hepatic fibrosis.	Low platelet and WBC count (hypersplenism), slight elevation of AST, GGT. Inability to concentrate urine.	Usually normal.
Diagnostic studies most useful	Gallbladder US.	Gallbladder US, MRCP, endoscopic US.	Scintigraphy to confirm nonfunction of gallbladder. US or abdominal CT scan to rule out other neighboring disease.	Transhepatic cholangiography, MRCP, ERCP, scintigraphy, US	Liver biopsy. US of liver and kidneys. Upper endoscopy.	Normal US, HIDA scans have not predicted improvement after cholecystectomy in pediatrics.

(Continued)

Table 22–11. Biliary tract diseases of childhood. (*Continued*)

	Acute Hydrops/Transient Dilation of Gallbladder[a,b]	Choledochal Cyst[c] (see Figure 22–1)	Acalculous Cholecystitis[d]	Caroli Disease[e] (Idiopathic Intrahepatic Bile Duct Dilation)	Congenital Hepatic Fibrosis[f]	Biliary Dyskinesia[g] and Functional Dyspepsia
Treatment	Treatment of associated condition. Needle or tube cystostomy rarely required. Cholecystectomy seldom indicated.	ERCP if acute obstruction. Definitive treatment is surgical resection and Cholecystectomy.	Broad-spectrum antibiotic coverage, then cholecystectomy.	Antibiotics and surgical or endoscopic drainage for cholangitis. Liver transplantation for some. Lobectomy for localized disease.	Treatment of portal hypertension. Liver and kidney transplantation for some.	Symptomatic therapy. Cholecystectomy may be considered in well-selected cases.
Complications	Perforation with bile peritonitis rare.	Progressive biliary cirrhosis. Increased incidence of cholangiocarcinoma. Cholangitis in some.	Perforation and bile peritonitis, sepsis, abscess or fistula formation. Pancreatitis.	Sepsis with episodes of cholangitis, biliary cirrhosis, portal hypertension. Intraductal stones. Cholangiocarcinoma.	Bleeding from varices. Splenic rupture, severe thrombocytopenia. Progressive renal failure.	Continued pain after surgery. Complications from surgery.
Prognosis	Excellent with resolution of underlying condition. Consider cystic duct obstruction if disorder fails to resolve.	Depends on anatomic type of cyst, associated condition, and success of surgery. Liver transplantation required in some.	Good with early diagnosis and treatment.	Poor, with gradual deterioration of liver function. Multiple surgical drainage procedures expected. Liver transplantation should improve long-term prognosis.	Good in absence of serious renal involvement and with control of portal hypertension. Slightly increased risk of cholangiocarcinoma.	Similar to other functional gastrointestinal disorders. Unclear if surgery is beneficial for biliary dyskinesia.

AST, aspartate aminotransferase; CCK, cholecystokinin; CT, computed tomography; EBV, Epstein-Barr virus; ERCP, endoscopic retrograde cholangiopancreatography; GGTx, γ-glutamyl transpeptidase; HIDA, hepatobiliary iminodiacetic acid; HIV, human immunodeficiency virus; LFT, liver function test; MRCP, magnetic resonance cholangiopancreatography; RUQ, right upper quadrant; US, ultrasound; WBC, white blood cell.

[a]Crankson S et al: Acute hydrops of the gallbladder in childhood. Eur J Pediatr 1992;151:318 [PMID: 9788647].

[b]Mathai SS et al: Gall bladder hydrops—a rare initial presentation of Kawasaki disease. Indian J Pediatr 2013;80:616–617 [PMID: 23180399].

[c]Ronnekeiv-Kelly SM, Soares KC, Ejaz A, Pawlik TM: Management of choledochal cysts. Curr Opin Gastroenterol 2016 May;32(3):225–231 [PMID: 26885950].

[d]Imamoglu M et al: Acute acalculous cholecystitis in children: diagnosis and treatment. J Pediatr Surg 2002;37:36 [PMID: 11781983].

[e]Liang JJ, Kamath PS: Caroli syndrome. Mayo Clin Proc 2013;88(6):e59 [PMID: 23726409].

[f]Hoyer PF: Clinical manifestations of autosomal recessive polycystic kidney disease. Curr Opin Pediatr 2015 Apr;27(2):186–192 [PMID: 25689455].

[g]Santucci NR, Hyman PE, Harmon CM, Schiavo JH, Hussain SZ: Biliary dyskinesia in children: a systematic review. J Pediatr Gastroenterol Nutr 2017 Feb;64(2):186–193 [PMID: 27472474].

B. Laboratory Findings

The earliest finding may be asymptomatic elevation of the GGT. Subsequent laboratory abnormalities include elevated levels of alkaline phosphatase and bile acids. Later, cholestatic jaundice and elevated AST and ALT may occur. Markers of autoimmune liver disease (ANA and ASMA) are often found but are not specific for PSC and may actually be due to concurrent overlap with AIH (overlap syndrome or autoimmune cholangitis).

C. Diagnosis

Ultrasound is often normal in PSC but may detect dilated bile ducts related to dominant biliary strictures. MRCP is the diagnostic study of choice for medium/large duct PSC, demonstrating irregularities of the biliary tree, including saccular dilation of normal intrahepatic bile ducts with segmental strictures ("beads on a string"), dominant strictures of large ducts, or "pruning" of the smaller bile duct branches. ERCP may be more sensitive for the diagnosis of irregularities of the intrahepatic biliary tree and allow for therapeutic interventions. In approximately 15% of cases, the MRCP will be normal and the disease manifests only in the small bile ducts ("small duct PSC"). Small duct PSC is diagnosed based on the liver histology finding of concentric fibrosis surrounding the bile ducts ("onion skinning").

▶ Differential Diagnosis

The differential diagnosis includes infectious hepatitis, secondary sclerosing cholangitis, AIH, PFIC type III, cystic fibrosis, CDC, or other anomalies of the biliary tree, including Caroli disease (see Table 22–10).

▶ Complications

Complications include refractory pruritus, bacterial cholangitis, biliary fibrosis, cirrhosis, and complications of portal hypertension. Slow progression to end-stage liver disease is likely, and patients are at increased risk of cholangiocarcinoma. The Sclerosing Cholangitis Outcomes in Pediatrics (SCOPE) Index has been developed as a pediatric specific prognostic tool for PSC, using routinely obtained clinical data (total bilirubin, albumin, platelet count, GGT, and cholangiography) to predict the risk of portal hypertension, hepatobiliary complication, liver transplant and death over a 5-year time period.

▶ Treatment

Treatment of PSC focuses on supportive care. UDCA (15–20 mg/kg/day) is often used in pediatrics, though high doses may worsen disease in adults. Long-term outcomes in children with PSC may not be improved, however, by UDCA or oral vancomycin. Pruritus may improve with UDCA, rifampin, or naltrexone. Patients with autoimmune sclerosing cholangitis or IgG4 cholangitis should benefit from treatment with corticosteroids. Antibiotic treatment of cholangitis and dilation and stenting of dominant bile duct strictures can reduce symptoms. Liver transplantation is effective for patients with end-stage complications, but the disease may recur in up to 20% after transplant.

▶ Prognosis

The majority of patients will eventually require liver transplantation in adulthood; however, the rate of progression is variable. PSC is the fifth leading indication for liver transplantation in adults in the United States.

Deneau MR et al: The Sclerosing Cholangitis Outcomes in Pediatrics (SCOPE) Index: a prognostic tool for Children. Hepatology 2021 Mar; 73(3):1074–1087 [PMID: 32464706].
Mieli-Vergani G, Vergani D: Sclerosing cholangitis in children and adolescents. Clin Liver Dis 2016;20(1):99–111 [PMID: 26593293].

3. Other Biliary Tract Disorders

For a schematic representation of the various types of CDCs, see Figure 22–1. For summary information on acute hydrops, CDC, acalculous cholecystitis, Caroli disease, biliary dyskinesia, and congenital hepatic fibrosis, see Table 22–11.

PYOGENIC & AMEBIC LIVER ABSCESS

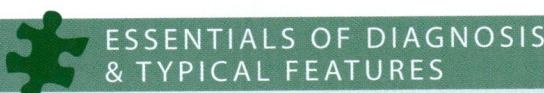

ESSENTIALS OF DIAGNOSIS
& TYPICAL FEATURES

► Fever and painful hepatomegaly.
► Ultrasound of liver demonstrating an abscess.
► Positive serum ameba antibody or positive bacterial culture of abscess fluid.

▶ General Considerations

Pyogenic liver abscesses are much more common than amebic liver abscesses and constitute the majority of hepatic abscesses in children. Pediatric liver abscesses in general are uncommon in developed countries but remain a significant issue in developing countries. Common pathogens for pyogenic abscesses include S aureus, Klebsiella pneumoniae, Streptococcus species, polymicrobial infection, and rarely candida. The resulting lesion tends to be solitary and located in the right hepatic lobe. Unusual causes include omphalitis, subacute infectious endocarditis, pyelonephritis, Crohn disease, and perinephric abscess. In immunocompromised patients, S aureus, gram-negative organisms, and fungi may seed the liver from the arterial system. Multiple pyogenic liver abscesses are associated with severe sepsis. Children receiving anti-inflammatory and immunosuppressive agents and children with defects in white blood cell function (chronic granulomatous disease) are prone to pyogenic hepatic abscesses, especially those caused by *S aureus*.

Amebic liver abscess can occur when *Entamoeba histolytica* invasion occurs via the large bowel, although a history of diarrhea (colitis-like picture) is not always obtained.

► Clinical Findings

A. History

With any liver abscess, nonspecific complaints of fever, chills, malaise, and abdominal pain are frequent. Although amebic liver abscess is rare in children, there is an increased risk associated with travel in areas of endemic infection within 5 months of presentation.

B. Symptoms and Signs

The dominant complaint is a constant dull pain over an enlarged liver that is tender to palpation. Some patients experience jaundice in addition to fever and chills. Weight loss may be present when the diagnosis is delayed. An elevated hemidiaphragm with reduced or absent respiratory excursion may be demonstrated on physical examination and confirmed by imaging.

Fever and abdominal pain are the two most common symptoms of amebic liver abscess. Abdominal tenderness and hepatomegaly are present in over 50%. An occasional prodrome may include cough, dyspnea, and shoulder pain when rupture of the abscess into the right chest occurs.

C. Laboratory Findings

Laboratory studies show leukocytosis and elevated inflammatory markers. LFTs may be normal or reveal mild elevation of transaminases, bilirubin, and alkaline phosphatase. Blood cultures may be positive and helpful in identifying an organism and guiding treatment; however, the majority of patients will have negative blood cultures. The distinction between pyogenic and amebic abscesses in developed countries is best made by enzyme immunoassay (EIA) testing (which is positive in > 95% of patients with amebic liver disease) and the prompt clinical response of the latter to anti-amebic therapy (metronidazole followed by an amebicide). Examination of material obtained by needle aspiration of the abscess using ultrasound guidance is often diagnostic and guides antimicrobial therapy in the setting of a pyogenic abscess. With amebic abscesses, on the other hand, abscess aspirates are frequently nondiagnostic and the diagnosis is better made serologically.

D. Imaging

Ultrasound is the most useful initial diagnostic aid in evaluating pyogenic and amebic abscesses, detecting lesions as small as 1–2 cm. MRI or CT may be useful in differentiating tumors or hydatid cysts. Consolidation of the right lower lobe of the lung is common (10%–30% of patients) in amebic abscess.

► Differential Diagnosis

Hepatitis, hepatoma, hydatid cyst, gallbladder disease, or biliary tract infections can mimic liver abscess. Hydatid cysts, caused by infection with *Echinococcus*, can be distinguished from pyogenic or amebic abscess by serologic testing, but hydatid infection is rare in North America. Subphrenic abscesses, empyema, and pneumonia may give a similar picture. Inflammatory disease of the intestines or the biliary system may be complicated by liver abscess.

► Complications

Spontaneous rupture of the abscess may occur with extension of infection into the subphrenic space, thorax, peritoneal cavity, and, occasionally, the pericardium. Bronchopleural fistula with large sputum production and hemoptysis can develop in severe cases. An amebic liver abscess may be secondarily infected with bacteria (in 10%–20% of patients). Metastatic hematogenous spread to the lungs and the brain has been reported.

► Treatment

Small bacterial liver abscesses (< 5 cm) or those with a solid appearance can be treated medically. Ultrasound- or CT-guided percutaneous needle aspiration for aerobic and anaerobic culture with simultaneous placement of a catheter for drainage, combined with appropriate antibiotic therapy, is the treatment of choice for solitary larger or liquid pyogenic liver abscesses. Multiple liver abscesses may also be treated successfully by this method. Surgical intervention may be indicated if rupture occurs outside the capsule of the liver or if enterohepatic fistulae are suspected.

Amebic abscesses in uncomplicated cases should be treated with oral metronidazole, 35–50 mg/kg/day, in three divided doses for 10 days. This should be followed by a course of an enteral amebicide (eg, iodoquinol, diloxanide furoate, or paromomycin) to eradicate potential intestinal amebic infection. Needle aspiration or surgical drainage is indicated for failure of medical management or cysts greater than 10 cm. Although symptomatic improvement typically occurs within days, resolution of the abscess cavity occurs over 3–6 months.

► Prognosis

With drainage and antibiotics, the cure rate is about 90%. Mortality have improved, but remain at 4% for pyogenic liver abscess, especially with extrahepatic complications, and less than 1% for amebic abscess.

Jain M, Jain J, Gupta S: Amebic liver abscess in children-experience from Central India. Indian J Gastroenterol 2016 May;35(3): 248–249 [PMID: 27260285].

Pai-Jui Y et al: Pediatric Liver Abscess: Trends in Incidence, Etiology, and Outcomes Based on 20-Years of Experience at a Tertiary Center. Front Pediatr 2020;8:111 [PMID: 32266189].

Roy Choudhury S, Khan NA, Saxena R, Yadav PS, Patel JN, Chadha R: Protocol-based management of 154 cases of pediatric liver abscess. Pediatr Surg Int 2017 Feb;33(2):165–172 [PMID: 27826650].

LIVER TUMORS

ESSENTIALS OF DIAGNOSIS & TYPICAL FEATURES

▶ Abdominal enlargement and pain, weight loss, anemia, although many tumors present asymptomatically or with palpable mass only.

▶ Hepatomegaly with or without a definable mass.

▶ Mass lesion on imaging studies.

▶ Laparotomy and tissue biopsy.

▶ General Considerations

Primary neoplasms of the liver represent 0.3%–5% of all solid tumors in children. Of these, two-thirds are malignant, with hepatoblastoma being most common (79% of all pediatric liver cancers). Hepatoblastoma typically occurs in children ages 6 months to 3 years, with a male predominance. Most children present with an asymptomatic abdominal mass, though with more advanced disease, weight loss, anorexia, abdominal pain, and emesis may occur. Children with Beckwith-Wiedemann syndrome and familial adenomatosis polyposis coli are at increased risk of hepatoblastoma and should undergo routine screening with AFP determinations and abdominal ultrasound until the age of 5 years. In addition, low-birth-weight infants (< 1000 g) have a 15 times increased risk of hepatoblastoma, as compared to infants weighing more than 2500 g.

Hepatocellular carcinoma most commonly occurs between the ages of 10 and 12 years and is more common in males. Children are more likely than adults to have advanced disease at presentation, and therefore be symptomatic, with abdominal distension, pain, anorexia, and weight loss. Patients with chronic HBV or HCV infection, cirrhosis, glycogen storage disease type I, tyrosinemia, PFIC, and α_1-antitrypsin deficiency are at increased risk for developing hepatocellular carcinoma. As compared to adult HCC, which occurs in the setting of cirrhosis in the vast majority of cases, pediatric HCC is more likely to occur in a patient with no predisposing liver disease and may be of a somewhat different biology.

Other rare primary hepatic malignancies in childhood include rhabdoid sarcoma, embryonal sarcoma, cholangiocarcinoma, and angiosarcoma. Additionally, Wilms tumor, neuroblastoma, and lymphoma may present with metastases in the liver.

▶ Clinical Findings

A. History

Noticeable abdominal distension, with or without pain, is the most constant feature. A parent may note a bulge in the upper abdomen or report feeling a hard mass. Constitutional symptoms (eg, anorexia, weight loss, fatigue, fever, and chills) may be present. Jaundice or pruritus may occur with obstruction of the biliary tree. Virilization has been reported as a consequence of gonadotropic activity of tumors. Feminization with bilateral gynecomastia may occur in association with high estradiol levels in the blood, the latter a consequence of increased aromatization of circulating androgens by the liver.

B. Symptoms and Signs

Weight loss, pallor, and abdominal pain in association with a large abdomen are common. Physical examination reveals hepatomegaly with or without a definite tumor mass, usually to the right of the midline. In the absence of cirrhosis, signs of chronic liver disease are usually absent.

C. Laboratory Findings

Normal or near-normal liver tests are the rule. Anemia frequently occurs, especially in cases of hepatoblastoma. AFP levels are typically quite elevated, especially in hepatoblastoma. One notable exception is with the fibrolamellar subtype of HCC that is typically associated with normal AFP levels.

D. Imaging

Ultrasonography, CT, and MRI are useful for diagnosis, staging, and following tumor response to therapy. A chest CT is generally a part of the preoperative workup to evaluate metastatic disease.

▶ Differential Diagnosis

In the absence of a palpable mass, the differential diagnosis is that of hepatomegaly with or without anemia or jaundice. When a mass is identified, AFP can help differentiate benign and malignant tumors, as can characteristic features on MRI. Histopathologic assessment of the tumor is the cornerstone of diagnosis when there is a concern for a primary hepatic malignancy. While a laparoscopic approach for surgical biopsy is an option, a percutaneous approach typically yields adequate tissue with fewer associated complications. The histologic differentiation between hepatoblastoma (HB) and HCC is not always clear, as significant morphologic overlap between the two types of malignancy can exist in one tumor.

▶ Complications

With progressive enlargement of the tumor, abdominal discomfort, ascites, respiratory difficulty, and widespread metastases (especially to the lungs and the abdominal lymph nodes) may occur. Rupture of the neoplastic liver and intraperitoneal hemorrhage have been reported.

▶ Treatment

Complete surgical resection is essential in the treatment of HB, however about 60% of HB tumors are unresectable at the time of diagnosis. Fortunately, HB is a relatively chemoresponsive malignancy and adjuvant chemotherapy reduces tumor size in a majority of patients to allow for resection (see Chapter 31 for additional discussion). In those tumors that remain unamenable to conventional resection after chemotherapy, liver transplantation is a consideration. Lung metastases may also resolve with chemotherapy alone, but occasionally require surgical resection. Survival outcomes following liver transplantation for HB have improved over the decades with advances in surgical and chemotherapeutic approaches. Treatment for most children with HB is determined by the current Pediatric Hepatic International Tumor Trial (PHITT).

Radiotherapy and chemotherapy have been disappointing in the treatment of hepatocellular carcinoma, although newer immunotherapies continue to emerge. The Milan and UCSF criteria developed in adult HCC to predict survival after, and thus utility of, liver transplantation for HCC have not been studied in children.

▶ Prognosis

If the tumor is completely removed, the survival rate for hepatoblastoma is 90%. The prognosis depends on a number of factors including tumor histology and tumor extent (with larger, more extensive tumors associated with a higher risk of recurrence and death). In well-selected candidates with unresectable HB, liver transplant outcomes are quite favorable. Survival after liver transplant for HB exceeds 80%, which is only mildly inferior to pediatric liver transplant for non-malignant indications.

The prognosis for pediatric HCC is not as favorable, likely attributable to inadequate response to chemo- and radiotherapies as well as the extensive tumor burden that is typical in children. The survival rate may be better for patients in whom the tumor is incidental to another disorder (tyrosinemia, BA, cirrhosis) or is less than 7 cm diameter without

vascular invasion. Survival following liver transplantation for pediatric HCC has also improved over the decades, with recent reports of 3-year survival exceeding 60%. In HBV-endemic areas, childhood HBV vaccination has reduced the incidence of hepatocellular carcinoma.

Boster JM et al. Predictors of survival following liver transplantation for pediatric hepatoblastoma and hepatocellular carcinoma: experience from the Society of Pediatric Liver Transplantation (SPLIT). Am J Transplant 2022 May;22(5):1396–1408 [PMID: 34990053].

Khanna R et al: Pediatric hepatocellular carcinoma. World J Gastroenterol 2018 Sep;24(35): 3980–3999 [PMID: 30254403].

Meyers RL et al: Hepatoblastoma state of the art: pre-treatment extent of disease, surgical resection guidelines and the role of liver transplantation. Curr Opin Pediatr 2014 Feb;26:29 [PMID: 24362406].

Ranganathan S et al: Hepatoblastoma and pediatric hepatocellular carcinoma: an update. Pediatr Dev Pathol 2020;23:79–95 [PMID: 31554479].

LIVER TRANSPLANTATION

Orthotopic liver transplantation is indicated in children with end-stage liver disease, acute fulminant hepatic failure, non-resectable liver tumors, or complications from metabolic liver disorders. Approximately 600 pediatric liver transplants are performed annually, with excellent 1-year (83%–91%) and 5-year (82%–84%) survival rates. The multitude of immunosuppression options, ability to individualize immunosuppression, improved candidate selection, refinements in surgical techniques, anticipatory monitoring for complications (eg, CMV and EBV infections, hypertension, renal dysfunction, and dyslipidemias), and experience in postoperative management have contributed to improved outcomes over time. The major indications for childhood transplantation are shown in Table 22–12.

Table 22–12. Indications for pediatric liver transplantation.

Biliary atresia (failed Kasai, repeated episodes of cholangitis, decompensated cirrhosis)
Metabolic diseases (eg, decompensated α_1-antitrypsin deficiency, Wilson disease, urea cycle defects)
Non-biliary atresia cholestatic disorders with intractable pruritus, growth failure or decompensated cirrhosis (eg, Alagille syndrome, PFIC)
Acute liver failure
Decompensated cirrhosis (autoimmune hepatitis, hepatitis B and C, primary sclerosing cholangitis)
Hepatic malignancies (unresectable hepatoblastoma, HCC, others)
Others

Children who are potential candidates for liver transplantation should be referred to a pediatric transplant center early for evaluation. In addition to full-sized cadaveric organs, children may also receive reduced segment or split cadaveric livers and live donor transplants (from directed or non-directed donors), all of which have expanded the potential donor pool. Lifetime immunosuppression therapy, using combinations of tacrolimus, prednisone, azathioprine, mycophenolate mofetil, or sirolimus, with its incumbent risks, is generally necessary to prevent rejection. A select group of patients may be eligible for complete immunosuppression withdrawal. The minimal amount of immunosuppression that will prevent allograft rejection should be chosen. The overall quality of life for children with a transplanted liver appears to be excellent. There is an increased risk (up to 25%) of renal dysfunction and low intelligence scores. The lifelong risk of EBV-induced lymphoproliferative disease, which is approximately 5%, is related to age and EBV exposure status at time of transplantation, and intensity of immunosuppression.

Kohli R et al: Liver transplantation in children: state of the art and future perspectives. Arch Dis Child 2018 Feb;103(2):192–198 [PMID: 28918383].

Kwong AJ et al: OPTN/SRTR 2020 annual data report: liver. Am J Transplant 2022 Mar;22 (Suppl 2):204–309 [PMID: 35266621].

PANCREATIC DISORDERS

ACUTE PANCREATITIS

ESSENTIALS OF DIAGNOSIS & TYPICAL FEATURES

Two out of three of the following:

▶ Abdominal pain, nausea, vomiting, or upper back pain.

▶ Elevated serum lipase and/or amylase ≥ 3 times the upper limit of normal.

▶ Evidence of pancreatic inflammation by imaging (CT, ultrasound, or MRI).

▶ General Considerations

The incidence of acute pancreatitis in children is about 1 per 10,000. Acute pancreatitis is defined as at least two of the following three: abdominal pain consistent with acute pancreatitis; amylase and/or lipase greater than three times the upper limit of normal; and US, CT, or MRI imaging consistent with acute pancreatitis. Most identified causes of acute pancreatitis are due to obstruction of pancreatic flow, the result of drugs, viral infections, systemic diseases, or abdominal trauma. More than 20% are idiopathic. Causes of pancreatic obstruction include stones, CDCs, tumors of the duodenum, pancreas divisum, and ascariasis. Acute pancreatitis has been seen following treatment with many different medications. Some, such as asparaginase and valproic acid, are definitively causal for some patients. Causality is more difficult to determine with other medications that are commonly used, such as NSAIDs, systemic steroids, and acetaminophen. Acute pancreatitis may also occur as a result of systemic illnesses such as hemolytic uremic syndrome, systemic lupus erythematosus, diabetes mellitus (especially during an episode of diabetic ketoacidosis (DKA)), Crohn disease, glycogen storage disease type I, hypertriglyceridemia, hyperparathyroidism, Henoch-Schönlein purpura, Reye syndrome, organic acidopathies, Kawasaki disease, chronic renal failure; during rapid refeeding in cases of malnutrition; following spinal fusion surgery; and certain genetic mutations. Alcohol-induced pancreatitis should be considered in adolescents.

▶ Clinical Findings

A. History

The common presenting picture is acute onset of persistent (hours to days), moderate to severe upper abdominal and midabdominal pain occasionally referred to the back, frequently associated with vomiting or nausea.

B. Symptoms and Signs

The abdomen is tender, but not rigid. Abdominal distention is common in infants and younger children, and classic symptoms of abdominal pain, tenderness, and nausea are less common in this age group. Jaundice is unusual. Ascites may be noted, and a left-sided pleural effusion is present in some patients. Periumbilical and flank bruising are rare and indicate hemorrhagic pancreatitis.

C. Laboratory Findings

An elevated serum amylase or lipase (more than three times normal) is the key laboratory finding. The elevated serum lipase persists longer than serum amylase. Infants younger than 6 months may not have an elevated amylase or lipase. In this setting, an elevated immunoreactive trypsinogen may be more sensitive. Measuring pancreatic lipase can help differentiate nonpancreatic causes (eg, salivary, intestinal, or tubo-ovarian) of serum lipase elevation. Leukocytosis, hyperglycemia (serum glucose > 300 mg/dL), hypocalcemia, falling hematocrit, rising blood urea nitrogen, and acidosis may occur in severe cases.

D. Imaging

Ultrasonography is the initial imaging of choice, primarily to assess for biliary tract disease leading to pancreatitis. The pancreas (especially the body and tail) is often difficult to image with ultrasound due to overlying gas. CT scan images the pancreas more consistently and is better for detecting pancreatic phlegmon, pseudocyst, or necrosis. ERCP or MRCP may be useful in confirming patency of the main pancreatic duct in cases of abdominal trauma; in recurrent acute pancreatitis; or in revealing stones, ductal strictures, and pancreas divisum.

▶ Differential Diagnosis

The many other causes of acute upper abdominal pain include gastritis, peptic ulcer disease, duodenal ulcer, hepatitis, liver abscess, cholelithiasis, cholecystitis, choledocholithiasis, acute gastroenteritis, functional gastrointestinal disorders such as functional dyspepsia, atypical appendicitis, pneumonia, volvulus, intussusception, and nonaccidental trauma.

▶ Complications

Early complications include shock, fluid and electrolyte disturbances, ileus, acute respiratory distress syndrome, and acute kidney injury. Hypervolemia due to fluid resuscitation and renal insufficiency related to renal tubular necrosis may occur. Early predictors of a more aggressive course include renal dysfunction, significant fluid requirements, and multisystem organ dysfunction. Patients can develop pancreatic fluid collections (pseudocysts are completely fluid filled and walled off while necrotic cavities contain fluid and solid necrotic debris) that may be asymptomatic or present with recurrence of abdominal pain, vomiting, or nausea. Up to 60%–70% of pseudocysts resolve spontaneously, and intervention is dependent on symptoms, not size. Infection, hemorrhage, rupture, or fistulization may occur. Mature symptomatic fluid collections may be treated with endoscopic ultrasound-guided cystogastrostomy. Chronic pancreatitis and exocrine or endocrine pancreatic insufficiency are rare sequelae of acute pancreatitis.

▶ Treatment

Medical management includes careful attention to pain control, fluid, electrolytes, and respiratory status. There is increasing evidence that lactated ringers may be preferred for initial volume expansion in acute pancreatitis. Pain should be aggressively treated with opioid and non-opioid medications. Historically patients were kept NPO, but more recent studies have shown that early enteral nutrition by mouth decreases hospital length of stay in mild-moderate pediatric pancreatitis. Early supplemental enteral nutrition via nasogastric or nasojejunal tube has improved outcomes compared to parenteral nutrition in severe pancreatitis. Broad-spectrum antibiotic coverage is not routinely recommended. Drugs known to produce acute pancreatitis should be discontinued. Surgical treatment is reserved for traumatic disruption of the gland, anatomic obstructive lesions, and unresolved or infected pseudocysts or abscesses not amenable to endoscopic or radiographically-guided drainage. Endoscopic decompression of the biliary system reduces the morbidity associated with pancreatitis caused by obstruction of the common bile duct.

▶ Prognosis

In the pediatric age group, prognosis is good with conservative management with mortality less than 0.4%. Up to 42% of children hospitalized with their initial episode of acute pancreatitis will have one or more subsequent admissions for pancreatitis.

Abu-El-Haija et al: Management of acute pancreatitis in the pediatric population: a clinical report from the North American Society for Pediatric Gastroenterology, Hepatology and Nutrition Pancreas Committee. J Pediatr Gastroenterol Nutr 2018 Jan;66(1):159–176. doi: 10.1097/MPG.0000000000001715 [PMID: 29280782].

Farrell PR, Farrell LM, Hornung L, Abu-El-Haija M: Use of lactated Ringer's solution compared with normal saline is associated with shorter length of stay in pediatric acute pancreatitis. Pancreas 2020 Mar;49(3):375–380. doi: 10.1097/MPA.0000000000001498 [PMID: 32132512].

Pant C, Sferra TJ, Lee BR, Cocjin JT, Olyaee M: Acute recurrent pancreatitis in children: a study from the pediatric health information system. J Pediatr Gastroenterol Nutr 2016 Mar;62(3):450–452. doi: 10.1097/MPG.0000000000001058 [PMID: 26704865].

CHRONIC PANCREATITIS

Chronic pancreatitis does not imply long-standing pancreatitis but denotes that the pancreas has permanent parenchymal or ductal changes from inflammation. The causes are similar to acute pancreatitis, but children with chronic pancreatitis are more likely to have underlying genetic or anatomic risk factors for pancreatitis.

▶ Clinical Findings

A. History

The diagnosis often is delayed by the nonspecificity of symptoms and the lack of persistent laboratory abnormalities. There is usually a prolonged history of recurrent upper abdominal pain and/or nausea of variable severity. Radiation of the pain into the back is a frequent complaint.

B. Symptoms and Signs

Fever and vomiting are rare. Diarrhea, due to steatorrhea, and symptoms of diabetes may develop later in the course.

Malnutrition due to acquired exocrine pancreatic insufficiency may also occur.

C. Laboratory Findings

Serum amylase and lipase levels are usually elevated during early acute attacks but are often normal in the chronic phase. Pancreatic insufficiency may be difficult to diagnose, but initial screening can be performed by measuring fecal pancreatic elastase 1. Increasingly, multiplex genetic testing panels are used to screen for the expanding number of identified genetic causes for chronic pancreatitis. Some identified genes include those for cationic trypsinogen (PRSS1), the pancreatic secretory trypsin inhibitor, the cystic fibrosis transmembrane conductance regulator (CFTR), carboxypeptidase A1, and chymotrypsin C. Screening for pancreatogenic (type 3c) diabetes should be considered. Sweat chloride should be checked for cystic fibrosis.

D. Imaging

Strict diagnostic criteria for chronic pancreatitis are primarily based on imaging and include pancreatic duct stricture(s), dilation, and pancreatic stones. CT may detect calcified stones that are easily missed on MRCP. MRCP or ERCP can show ductal dilation, stones, strictures, or stenotic segments. Endoscopic ultrasound may show early changes of chronic pancreatitis.

▶ Differential Diagnosis

Other causes of recurrent abdominal pain must be considered. Specific causes of pancreatitis such as autoimmune pancreatitis, hyperparathyroidism, systemic lupus erythematosus, systemic infectious diseases, traumatic pancreatitis, and ductal obstruction by tumors, stones, or helminths must be excluded by appropriate tests.

▶ Complications

Disabling abdominal pain, exocrine pancreatic insufficiency, malnutrition, pancreatic pseudocysts, and diabetes are the most frequent long-term complications. Pancreatic carcinoma occurs more frequently in adults with chronic pancreatitis, and the risk is higher in patients with PRSS1 mutations and those who smoke cigarettes.

▶ Treatment

Medical management of acute attacks is indicated (see section Acute Pancreatitis). If ductal obstruction is strongly suspected, endoscopic therapy (balloon dilation, stenting, stone removal, or sphincterotomy) should be pursued. Relapses occur in most patients. There are no proven therapies that modify the course of chronic pancreatitis. Pancreatic enzyme therapy should be used in patients with exocrine insufficiency. Mature fluid collections may be drained with endoscopic ultrasound-guided cystogastrostomy. If this is unavailable, interventional radiology or surgical approaches can be used to drain symptomatic collections.

Surgical treatment includes pancreatic ductal decompression procedures as well as total pancreatectomy and islet cell autotransplantation (TPIAT). TPIAT is performed in specialized centers. It is curative for the pancreatic inflammation, resolves the risk of pancreatic cancer, and may significantly improve or resolve pain. However, it carries risks of surgical morbidity, causes lifelong exocrine insufficiency, and many patients require lifelong insulin. Previous pancreatic surgery decreases the amount of islet cells that can be isolated from the pancreas and increases the risk of diabetes after TPIAT.

▶ Prognosis

In the absence of a correctable lesion, the prognosis is poor. Disabling episodes of pain, pancreatic insufficiency, diabetes, and pancreatic cancer may ensue. Disabling disease increases the risk of narcotic addiction and suicide in teenagers. TPIAT may significantly improve quality of life in pediatric patients with severe chronic pancreatitis pain. Given the complexity of chronic pancreatitis, a multidisciplinary approach is recommended, and referral to centers with expertise with management of pancreatic disorders should be strongly considered.

Awano H et al: Childhood-onset hereditary pancreatitis with mutations in the CT gene and SPINK1 gene. Pediatr Int 2013;55:646–649 [PMID: 24134754].

Ceppa EP et al: Hereditary pancreatitis: endoscopic and surgical management. J Gastrointest Surg 2013;17:847–856 [PMID: 23435738].

Uc A et al: Analysis of INSPPIRE-2 Cohort: risk factors and disease burden in children with acute recurrent or chronic pancreatitis. J Pediatr Gastroenterol Nutr 2022;75(5):643–649 [PMID: 35976273].

GASTROINTESTINAL & HEPATOBILIARY MANIFESTATIONS OF CYSTIC FIBROSIS

Pulmonary and pancreatic involvement dominate the clinical picture for most patients with cystic fibrosis (see Chapter 19), however, various other organs can be involved. Table 22–13 lists the important gastrointestinal, pancreatic, and hepatobiliary conditions that may affect patients with cystic fibrosis along with their clinical findings, incidence, most useful diagnostic studies, and preferred treatment. The development of highly effective CFTR modulator therapies is rapidly changing the course of CF for eligible patients. GI manifestations may be improved with modulator therapy, but monitoring for liver toxicity is required as there have been some cases of severe DILI from modulator therapies. In addition to the listed conditions, children with cystic fibrosis can develop functional gastrointestinal disorders like any other children.

Table 22–13. Gastrointestinal and hepatobiliary manifestations of cystic fibrosis.

Organ	Condition	Symptoms	Age at Presentation	Prevalence (%)	Diagnostic Evaluation	Management
Esophagus	Gastroesophageal reflux, esophagitis	Heartburn, dysphagia, epigastric pain, hematemesis.	All ages.	10–20	Endoscopy and biopsy, overnight pH study.	H_2 blockers, PPIs, surgical anti-reflux procedure.
	Varices in those with cirrhosis	Hematemesis, melena.	Childhood and adolescents.	3–5	Endoscopy.	Endosclerosis, band ligation, drugs (see text), TIPS, surgical shunt, liver transplantation (see Table 22–9).
Stomach	Gastritis	Upper abdominal pain, vomiting, hematemesis.	School age and older.	10–25	Endoscopy and biopsy.	H_2 blockers, PPIs.
	Hiatal hernia	Reflux symptoms (see above), epigastric pain.	School age and older.	3–5	UGI; endoscopy.	As above. Surgery in some.
Intestine	Meconium ileus	Abdominal distention, bilious emesis.	Neonate.	10–15	Radiologic studies, plain abdominal films; contrast enema shows microcolon.	Dislodgement of obstruction with Gastrografin enema. Surgery if unsuccessful or if case complicated by atresia, perforation, or volvulus.
	Distal intestinal obstruction syndrome	Abdominal pain, acute and recurrent; distention; occasional vomiting.	Any age, usually school age through adolescence.	5–10	Palpable mass in right lower quadrant; radiologic studies.	Gastrografin enema, intestinal lavage solution, diet, bulk laxatives, adjustment of pancreatic enzyme intake.
	Intussusception	Acute, intermittent abdominal pain; distention; emesis.	Infants through adolescence.	1–3	Radiographic studies, barium enema.	Reduction by barium or air enema or surgery if needed. Diet. Bulk laxatives. Adjustment of pancreatic enzyme intake.
	Rectal prolapse	Anal discomfort, rectal bleeding.	Infants and children to age 4–5 y.	15–25	Visual mass protruding from anus.	Manual reduction, adjustment of pancreatic enzyme dosage, reassurance as problem usually resolves by age 3–5 y.
	Carbohydrate intolerance	Abdominal pain, flatulence, continued diarrhea with adequate enzyme replacement therapy.	Any age.	10–25	Intestinal mucosal biopsy and disaccharidase analysis. Lactose breathe hydrogen test.	Reduce lactose intake; lactase; reduction of gastric hyperacidity if mucosa shows partial villous atrophy. Beware concurrent celiac disease or *Giardia* infection.
	Small bowel bacterial overgrowth	Abdominal pain, flatulence, continued diarrhea with adequate enzyme replacement therapy.	Any age: Higher risk with previous intestinal surgery.	Unknown	Culture of duodenal fluid, glucose breath hydrogen test.	Probiotic therapy, oral antibiotics (metronidazole, trimethoprim-sulfamethoxazole, Rifaximin).
Pancreas	Total exocrine insufficiency	Diarrhea, steatorrhea, malnutrition, failure to thrive. Fat-soluble vitamin deficiency.	Neonate through infancy.	85–90	72-h fecal fat evaluation, fecal pancreatic elastase, direct pancreatic function tests.	Pancreatic enzyme replacement; may need elemental formula, fat-soluble vitamin supplements.

	Clinical features	Age	%	Diagnosis	Treatment
Pancreatic sufficiency (partial exocrine insufficiency)	Occasional diarrhea, mild growth delay.	Any age.	10–15	72-h fecal fat evaluation, direct pancreatic function tests, fecal pancreatic elastase.	Pancreatic enzyme replacement in selected patients. Fat-soluble vitamin supplements as indicated by biochemical evaluation.
Pancreatitis	Recurrent abdominal pain, vomiting.	Older children through adolescence. Primarily in patients with partial pancreatic sufficiency.	0.1	Increased serum lipase and amylase, CT, MRCP, ERCP.	Endoscopic removal of sludge or stones if present, endoscopic papillotomy.
Diabetes	Weight loss, polyuria, polydipsia.	Older children through adolescence.	Increases with age up to 35%	Glucose tolerance test and insulin levels.	Diet, insulin.
Pancreatic cystosis	Usually asymptomatic, can present with abdominal pain or mass effect	Older children through adolescence	8	MRI.	Usually not indicated. Surgical or endoscopic treatment if mass effect or hemorrhage
Liver — Steatosis	Hepatomegaly, often in setting of malnutrition, elevated ALT.	Neonates and infants, but can be seen at all ages.	20–60	US showing homogeneous increased echogenicity. Liver biopsy.	Improved nutrition, replacement of pancreatic enzymes, vitamins, and essential fatty acids.
Hepatic fibrosis	Hepatomegaly, firm liver. May have abnormal AST, ALT.	Infants and older patients.	10–70	US showing heterogeneous echogenicity. Liver biopsy.	As above. UDCA
Cirrhosis	Hepatosplenomegaly, hematemesis from esophageal varices; hypersplenism, jaundice, ascites late in course.	Infants through adolescence.	5–10	US showing nodular liver, signs of portal hypertension. Liver biopsy, endoscopy.	Improved nutrition, UDCA endosclerosis or band ligation of varices, or partial splenic embolization, liver transplantation.
Neonatal jaundice	Cholestatic jaundice hepatomegaly; often seen with meconium ileus.	Neonates.	0.1–1	Sweat chloride test, liver biopsy.	Nutritional support, special formula with medium-chain triglyceride–containing oil, pancreatic enzyme replacement, vitamin supplements.
Gallbladder — Microgallbladder	None.	Congenital, presents at any age.	30	US or hepatobiliary scintigraphy.	None needed.
Cholelithiasis	Recurrent right upper quadrant abdominal pain, rarely jaundice.	School age through adolescence.	1–10	US.	Surgery if symptomatic and low-risk, trial of cholelitholytics in others.
Extrahepatic bile ducts — Intraluminal obstruction (sludge, stones, tumor)	Jaundice, hepatomegaly, abdominal pain.	Neonates, then older children through adolescence.	Rare in neonates (< 0.1)	US and hepatobiliary scintigraphy, MRCP.	Surgery in neonates; ERCP in older patients or surgery.
Extraluminal obstruction (intrapancreatic compression, tumor)	As above.	Older children to adults.	Rare (< 1)	As above.	Surgical biliary drainage procedure or ERCP.

ALT, alanine aminotransferase; AST, aspartate aminotransferase; CT, computed tomography; ERCP, endoscopic retrograde cholangiopancreatography; MRCP, magnetic resonance cholangiopancreatography; PPI, proton pump inhibitor; TIPS, transjugular intrahepatic portosystemic shunt; UDCA, ursodeoxycholic acid; UGI, upper gastrointestinal; US, abdominal ultrasound.

Flass T, Narkewicz MR: Cirrhosis and other liver disease in cystic fibrosis. J Cyst Fibros 2013;12:116 [PMID: 23266093].

Nichols DA et al: PROMISE: working with the CF community to understand emerging clinical and research needs for those treated with highly effective CFTR modulator therapy. J Cyst Fibros 2021;20:2, 205–212 [PMID: 33619012].

Somaraju UR, Solis-Moya A: Pancreatic enzyme replacement therapy for people with cystic fibrosis. Cochrane Database Syst Rev 2014;10:CD008227 [PMID: 25310479].

SYNDROMES WITH PANCREATIC EXOCRINE INSUFFICIENCY

Several syndromes are associated with exocrine pancreatic insufficiency. Patients present with failure to thrive, diarrhea, fatty stools, and an absence of respiratory symptoms. Laboratory findings include low fecal pancreatic elastase 1; high fecal fat content with 72-hour fecal fat analysis using a standardized high-fat diet; and low to absent pancreatic lipase, amylase, and trypsin levels on endoscopic duodenal fluid aspiration. Each disorder has several associated clinical features that aid in the differential diagnosis. In Shwachman-Diamond syndrome, pancreatic exocrine hypoplasia with widespread fatty replacement of the glandular acinar tissue is associated with neutropenia because of maturational arrest of the granulocyte series. Metaphyseal dysostosis and an elevated fetal hemoglobin level are common; immunoglobulin deficiency and hepatic dysfunction are also reported. CT of the pancreas demonstrates widespread fatty replacement. In Shwachman-Diamond syndrome, pancreatic exocrine insufficiency usually improves with age. Increased infections may result from chronic neutropenia and reduced neutrophil mobility. An increased incidence of leukemia has been noted in these patients. Thus, patients with myelodysplasia syndrome should be considered for hematopoietic stem cell transplantation.

Genotyping of the *SBDS* gene is available. Serum immunoreactive trypsinogen levels are extremely low.

Other associations of exocrine pancreatic insufficiency include (1) aplastic alae, aplasia cutis, deafness (Johanson-Blizzard syndrome); (2) sideroblastic anemia, developmental delay, seizures, and liver dysfunction (Pearson marrow pancreas syndrome); (3) duodenal atresia or stenosis; and (5) pancreatic hypoplasia or agenesis.

The complications and sequelae of exocrine pancreatic insufficiency are malnutrition, diarrhea, and growth failure. The degree of steatorrhea may vary by age and degree of pancreatic function. Intragastric lipolysis by lingual lipase may compensate in patients with low or absent pancreatic function.

Pancreatic enzyme and fat-soluble vitamin replacement are required therapy in most patients.

Almashraki N, Abdulnabee MZ, Sukalo M, Alrajoudi A, Sharafadeen I, Zenker M: Johanson-Blizzard syndrome. World J Gastroenterol 2011;17:42–47 [PMID: 22072859].

Dror Y et al: Draft consensus guidelines for diagnosis and treatment of Shwachman-Diamond syndrome. Ann N Y Acad Sci 2011;1242:40 [PMID: 22191555].

ISOLATED EXOCRINE PANCREATIC ENZYME DEFECT

Premature infants and most newborns produce little, if any, pancreatic amylase following meals or exogenous hormonal stimulation. This temporary physiologic insufficiency may persist for the first 3–6 months of life and cause diarrhea when complex carbohydrates (cereals) are introduced early in the diet.

Congenital pancreatic lipase deficiency and congenital colipase deficiency are extremely rare disorders, causing diarrhea and variable malnutrition with malabsorption of dietary fat and fat-soluble vitamins. In these cases, the sweat chloride level is normal, and neutropenia is absent. Treatment is oral replacement of pancreatic enzymes and a low-fat diet or formula containing medium-chain triglycerides.

Exocrine pancreatic insufficiency of proteolytic enzymes (eg, trypsinogen, trypsin, chymotrypsin) is caused by enterokinase deficiency, a duodenal mucosal enzyme required for activation of the pancreatic proenzymes. Affected patients present with malnutrition associated with hypoproteinemia and edema. Similar to lipase and colipase deficiencies, the sweat test and neutrophil counts are normal. Patients with enterokinase deficiency respond to pancreatic enzyme replacement therapy and feeding formulas that contain a casein hydrolysate (eg, Nutramigen, Pregestimil). Some patients may have transient exocrine pancreatic insufficiency that resolves with time.

Scheers I, Berardis S: Congenital etiologies of exocrine pancreatic insufficiency. Front in Pediatr 2022:10:909925 [PMID: 35935370].

PANCREATIC TUMORS

Pancreatic tumors, whether benign or malignant, are rare. The majority of patients with malignant tumors present with abdominal pain or are found incidentally. The most common pediatric pancreatic tumors are solid pseudopapillary tumors (found predominantly in adolescent females), and neuroendocrine tumors (PNET) (insulinoma, gastrinoma, glucagonoma, VIPoma, and nonfunctioning PNET). PNETs present in the pancreas in pediatric patients should prompt evaluation for MEN1 syndrome. NET can produce diverse symptoms if they are producing biologically active polypeptides or can be asymptomatic. The clinical features of these tumors are summarized in Table 22–14. The differential diagnosis of pancreatic tumors includes Wilms tumor, neuroblastoma, pancreatic blastoma, and lymphoma. Endoscopic

Table 22–14. Pancreatic tumors.

	Age	Major Findings	Diagnosis	Treatment	Associated Conditions
Solid pseudo-papillary tumor	Adolescents, usually female	Single solid mass in pancreas found incidentally or in evaluation of abdominal pain	CT scan, MRI, EUS	Surgery	
Adenocarcinoma	Older adolescents	Epigastric pain, mass, weight loss, anemia, biliary obstruction	CT scan, MRI, EUS	Chemotherapy, surgery	Chronic pancreatitis
Lymphoma	Any age	Solid round tumors, enlarged lymph nodes	CT scan, MRI, EUS	Chemotherapy	
Pancreatic blastoma	2–20, mean 7 y	Heterogeneous, may appear pancreatic or liver origin on imaging, metastases	CT scan, MRI, EUS	Chemotherapy, surgery	
Pancreatic Neuroendocrine Tumors					
Nonfunctioning	Any age	Incidental finding, abdominal pain	CT scan, EUS, MRI	Observation or surgery depending size	MEN1
Insulinoma	Any age	Hypoglycemia, seizures; high serum insulin; weight gain; abdominal pain and mass infrequent	CT scan, MRI, PET, EUS, SRS	Surgery, diazoxide, SSTA	MEN1
Gastrinoma	> 5–8 y	Male sex, gastric hypersecretion, peptic symptoms, multiple ulcers, gastrointestinal bleeding, anemia, diarrhea	Elevated fasting gastrin and post secretin suppression test (> 300 pg/mL), CT scan, MRI, EUS, SRS, laparotomy	PPI, surgical resection, total gastrectomy, SSTA	Zollinger-Ellison syndrome, MEN1, neurofibromatosis
VIPoma	Any age (more common 2–4 y old)	Secretory diarrhea, hypokalemia, hypochlorhydria, weight loss, flushing	Elevated VIP levels (> 75 pg/mL); sometimes, elevated serum gastrin and pancreatic polypeptide; CT, EUS, SRS	Surgery, SSTA, IV fluids	
Glucagonoma	Older patients	Diabetes, necrolytic migratory erythema, diarrhea, anemia, thrombotic events, depression	Elevated glucagon, hyperglycemia, gastrin, VIP, CT, MRI, EUS, SRS	Surgery, SSTA	

CT, computed tomography; EUS, endoscopic ultrasound; IV, intravenous; MEN1, multiple endocrine neoplasia syndrome type I; MRI, magnetic resonance imaging; NET, neuroendocrine tumor; PET, positron emission tomography; PPI, proton pump inhibitor; SRS, somatostatin-receptor scintigraphy; SSTA, somatostatin analogue; VIP, vasoactive intestinal polypeptide.

ultrasonography with fine needle biopsy can aid in making definitive diagnoses and guiding surgical planning.

Klimstra DS, Adsay V: Acinar neoplasms of the pancreas—a summary of 25 years of research. Semin Diagn Pathol 2016;33(5):307–318 [PMID: 27320062].

Rojas Y et al: Primary malignant pancreatic neoplasms in children and adolescents: a 20 year experience. J Pediatr Surg 2012;47:2199 [PMID: 23217876].

REFERENCES

Kleinman R et al (eds): *Walker's Pediatric Gastrointestinal Disease: Physiology, Diagnosis, Management.* 6th ed. BC Decker; 2018.

SuchyFJ, SokolRJ, BalistreriWF (eds): *Liver Disease in Children.* 5th ed. Cambridge University Press; 2021.

Wyllie R, Hyams JS (eds): *Pediatric Gastrointestinal and Liver Disease.* 6th ed. Elsevier; 2020.

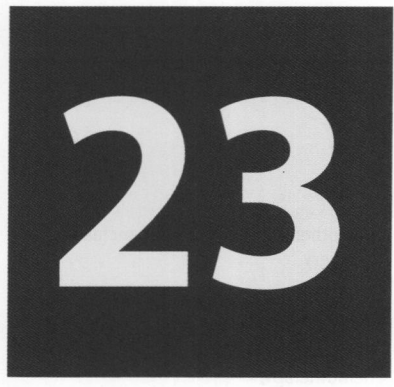

23

Fluid, Electrolyte, & Acid–Base Disorders & Therapy

Melisha G. Hanna, MD, MS

Margret E. Bock, MD, MS

REGULATION OF BODY FLUIDS, ELECTROLYTES, & TONICITY

Total body water (TBW) constitutes 50%–75% of the total body mass, depending on age, sex, and fat content. After an initial brisk postnatal diuresis, the TBW slowly decreases to the adult range near puberty. Values vary with differing amounts of body fat; muscle has higher water content than fat. TBW, for example, decreases with increasing obesity. TBW is divided into the intracellular and extracellular spaces, separated by cell membranes (Figure 23–1). Intracellular fluid (ICF) accounts for two-thirds of the TBW and extracellular fluid (ECF) for one-third. The ECF is further compartmentalized into plasma (intravascular) volume and interstitial fluid (ISF). Size of ECF components vary by age—being larger in infants and young children.

The principal constituents of plasma are sodium, chloride, bicarbonate, and protein (primarily albumin). The ISF is like plasma but lacks significant amounts of protein. Conversely, the ICF is rich in potassium, magnesium, phosphates, sulfates, and protein.

An understanding of osmotic shifts between the ECF and ICF is fundamental to understanding disorders of fluid balance. Iso-osmolality is generally maintained between fluid compartments. Because the cell membrane is water-permeable, abnormal fluid shifts occur if the concentration of solutes that cannot permeate the cell membrane in the ECF does not equal the concentration of such solutes in the ICF. Thus, NaCl, mannitol, and glucose (only in the setting of hyperglycemia) remain restricted to the ECF space and contribute effective osmoles by obligating water to remain in or be drawn into the ECF compartment. In contrast, a freely permeable solute such as urea does not contribute effective osmoles because it is not restricted to the ECF and readily crosses cell membranes. Tonicity, or effective osmolality, differs from measured osmolality as it accounts only for osmotically active impermeable solutes (effective osmoles) rather than all osmotically active solutes (ineffective osmoles), including those that are permeable to cell membranes. Serum osmolality may be estimated by the following formula:

$$mOsm/kg = 2[Na^+(mEq/L)] + \frac{Glucose\,(mg/dL)}{18} + \frac{BUN\,(mg/dL)}{2.8}$$

Although osmolality and osmolarity differ, the former being an expression of osmotic activity per weight (kg) and the latter per volume (L) of solution, for clinical purposes they are similar and occasionally used interchangeably. Oncotic pressure, or colloid osmotic pressure, represents the osmotic activity of macromolecular constituents such as albumin in the plasma and body fluids, resulting in fluid being drawn back into the vascular space. The importance of albumin in maintaining intravascular volume status is reflected in the setting of the nephrotic syndrome, protein losing enteropathy, hepatic failure, and other low serum albumin (and low oncotic pressure) states wherein fluids accumulate in the interstitial compartment leading to edema.

ECF volume and tonicity are directly affected by changes in body sodium content. These changes may be sensed by central osmoreceptors, peripheral volume-sensitive receptors, components of the renin-angiotensin-aldosterone

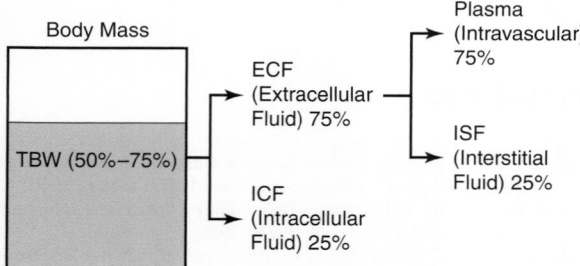

▲ **Figure 23–1.** Distribution of total body water.

system (RAAS), and the sympathetic nervous system. Thirst, vasopressin or antidiuretic hormone (ADH), the RAAS, and atrial and brain natriuretic peptide (ANP and BNP) exert their influence by affecting either water/salt intake or renal water and sodium handling.

Thirst

Water intake is commonly determined by cultural and behavioral factors. Thirst is physiologically stimulated by two main triggers: (1) when plasma osmolality reaches 280–290 mOsm/kg, a level at which ADH release induces maximal antidiuresis and (2) when significant volume is lost (ie, as a result of bleeding, diarrhea, emesis, or polyuria). The osmotic threshold for thirst is slightly higher than for ADH release. Thirst provides control over a wide range of fluid states and allows maintenance of appropriate intravascular volume, together with vasoconstriction, even in settings of extreme volume loss. An adequate thirst mechanism is central to maintaining adequate fluid balance. The most potent hormonal stimulus for thirst is angiotensin II (released via the RAAS in response to hypovolemia and hypotension)– which in turn acts directly on the subfornical organ in the hypothalamus of the brain.

Antidiuretic Hormone

In the kidney, ADH increases water reabsorption in the cortical and medullary collecting ducts, leading to formation of concentrated urine. In the absence of ADH, dilute urine is produced. Typically, ADH secretion is regulated by the tonicity of body fluids rather than intravascular fluid volume; it becomes detectable at a plasma osmolality of 280 mOsm/kg or greater. Tonicity may, however, be sacrificed to preserve ECF volume (ie, with hyponatremic dehydration), wherein ADH secretion and renal water retention are maximal, despite comparatively lower plasma osmolality.

Renin-Angiotensin-Aldosterone

Aldosterone is released from the adrenal cortex in response to (1) decreased effective circulating volume and resultant stimulation of the renin-angiotensin-aldosterone axis, (2) increasing plasma K^+ (3) acidosis, and (4) stimulation of atrial stretch receptors. Aldosterone enhances renal tubular reabsorption of Na^+ in exchange for K^+, and to a lesser degree H^+. At a constant osmolality, retention of Na^+ leads to expansion of ECF volume and suppression of aldosterone release.

Atrial Natriuretic Peptide & Brain Natriuretic Peptide

ANP, a polypeptide hormone secreted principally by the cardiac atria in response to atrial dilation, contributes to regulation of blood volume and blood pressure. ANP inhibits renin secretion and aldosterone synthesis and causes an increase in glomerular filtration rate and renal sodium excretion. ANP also guards against excessive plasma volume expansion in the face of increased ECF volume by shifting fluid from the vascular to the interstitial compartment. ANP inhibits angiotensin II and norepinephrine-induced vasoconstriction and acts in the brain to decrease the desire for salt and inhibit the release of ADH. Thus, the net effect of ANP is a decrease in blood volume and blood pressure associated with natriuresis and diuresis.

BNP (also known as B-type natriuretic peptide) similarly is a polypeptide hormone secreted by cardiac myocytes in cardiac ventricles in response to ventricular dilatation. BNP also binds to the ANP factor receptor; its physiologic actions are like those of ANP—decreasing central venous pressure and systemic vascular resistance and increasing natriuresis and subsequent diuresis.

Danziger J, Zeidel ML: Osmotic homeostasis. Clin J Am Soc Nephrol 2015 May 7;10(5):852–862 [PMID: 25078421].

Finberg L et al: *Water and Electrolytes in Pediatrics: Physiology, Pathophysiology and Treatment.* 2nd ed. WB Saunders; 1993.

Friedman A: Fluid and electrolyte therapy: a primer. Pediatr Nephrol 2010;25:842–846 [PMID: 19444484].

Friis-Hensen B: Body water compartments in children changes during growth and related changes in body composition. Pediatrics 1961;28:169–181.

ACID–BASE BALANCE

The pH of arterial blood is maintained between 7.38 and 7.42 to ensure that pH-sensitive enzyme systems function normally. Acid–base balance is maintained by interaction of the lungs, kidneys, and systemic buffering systems. Over 50% of the blood's buffering capacity is provided by the carbonic acid–bicarbonate system, roughly 30% by hemoglobin, and the remainder by phosphates and ammonium. The carbonic acid–bicarbonate system, depicted chemically as

$$CO_2 + H_2O \leftrightarrow H_2CO_3 \leftrightarrow H^+ + HCO_3^-$$

interacts via the lungs and kidneys, and in conjunction with the nonbicarbonate systems, to stabilize systemic pH. The concentration of dissolved CO_2 in blood is established by the respiratory system and that of HCO_3^- by the kidneys. Disturbances in acid–base balance are initially stabilized by chemical buffering, compensated for by pulmonary or renal regulation of CO_2, and ultimately corrected when the primary cause of the acid–base disturbance is eliminated.

Renal regulation of acid–base balance is accomplished by (1) the reabsorption of filtered HCO_3^-, primarily in the proximal tubule (predominantly as a result of sodium-hydrogen exchange by the proximal tubules) and (2) the excretion of H^+ or HCO_3^- in the distal nephron to match the net input of acid or base. When urine is alkalinized (such as in response

Table 23–1. Caloric and water needs per unit of body weight.

Body Weight (kg)	kcal/kg	mL of Water/kg	IVF Rate/h
3–10	100	100	4mL/kg/h
11–20	1000 kcal + 50 kcal/kg for each kg > 10 kg	1000 mL + 50 mL/kg for each kg > 10 kg	4 mL/kg/h (first 10kg) + 2 mL/kg/h
> 20	1500 kcal + 20 kcal/kg for each kg > 20 kg	1500 mL + 20 mL/kg for each kg > 20 kg	4 mL/kg/h (first 10kg) + 2 mL/kg/h (second 10kg) + 1 mL/kg/h

Data from Holliday MA, Segar WE: The maintenance need for water in parenteral fluid therapy. Pediatrics 1957 May;19(5):823–832.

to respiratory or metabolic alkalosis, ingestions or following meals) filtered HCO_3^- is ultimately lost in the urine. However, urinary alkalinization will not occur if there is a deficiency of urine Na^+ or K^+, as electroneutrality must be maintained. In contrast, the urine may be acidified if an absolute or relative decrease occurs in systemic HCO_3^-. In this setting, proximal tubular HCO_3^- reabsorption and distal tubular H^+ excretion are maximal. A "paradoxical aciduria" with low urinary pH may be seen in the setting of hypokalemic metabolic alkalosis and systemic K^+ depletion wherein H^+ is exchanged and excreted in preference to K^+ in response to mineralocorticoid.

Hamm LL, Nakhoul N, Hering-Smith KS: Acid-base homeo-stasis. Clin J Am Soc Nephrol 2015;10(12):2232–2242 [PMID: 26597034].

Online resource for the physiology of acid-base and electrolyte disorders: http://www.rosebook.club.

Seifter JL: Integration of acid-base and electrolyte disorders. N Engl J Med 2014;371:1821–1831 [PMID: 25372090].

Shaw I, Gregory K: Acid-base balance: a review of normal physiology. BJA Educ 2022;22(10):396–401.

FLUID & ELECTROLYTE MANAGEMENT

Therapy of fluid and electrolyte disorders should be phased to (1) expand the ECF volume and restore tissue perfusion in settings of hypovolemia, (2) replenish fluid and electrolyte deficits while correcting attendant acid–base abnormalities, and (3) meet the patient's nutritional needs, and (4) replace ongoing losses.

The cornerstone of fluid and electrolyte management involves a detailed understanding of "maintenance" fluid and electrolyte requirements. "Maintenance" requirements call for provision of enough water, glucose, and electrolytes to prevent deterioration of body stores for an euvolemic patient under normal conditions. During short-term paren-teral therapy, sufficient glucose is provided to prevent ketosis and limit protein catabolism, although this usually provides little more than 20% of the patient's true caloric needs. Prior to the administration of "maintenance" fluids, it is impor-tant to carefully consider the patient's volume status and to

determine whether intravenous (IV) fluids are truly needed, and if so, what volume resuscitation goals are.

Various models have been devised to facilitate calcula-tion of "maintenance" requirements based on body surface area, weight, and caloric expenditure. A system based on caloric expenditure is most helpful because 1 mL of water is needed for each kilocalorie expended. The system presented in Table 23–1 is based on caloric needs and is applicable to children weighing more than 3 kg.

As depicted in Table 23–1, a child weighing 30 kg would need 1700 kcal or 1700 mL of water daily. If the child received parenteral fluids for 2 days, the fluid would usually contain 5% glucose, which would provide 340 kcal/day or 20% of the maintenance caloric needs. Maintenance fluid requirements take into account normal insensible water losses (Table 23–2) and water lost in sweat, urine, and stool, and assume the patient to be afebrile, at their true dry weight, and relatively inactive. Thus, if excessive losses occur, standard "main-tenance fluids" will be inadequate. In contrast, if losses are reduced for any reason, standard "maintenance fluid" admin-istration would be excessive. Maintenance requirements are greater for low-birthweight and preterm infants. Table 23–3 lists other factors that commonly alter fluid and caloric needs.

Physiologic electrolyte losses occur primarily through the urinary tract and to a lesser degree via the skin and stool. Maintenance sodium and potassium electrolyte needs have historically been approximated to be in the 3 mEq Na/100 kcal and 2 mEq K/100 kcal range, leading to the common use of hypotonic IV fluids with 77 mEq/L of sodium (½ normal saline) and 20 mEq/L of potassium. Over the past 10 years, many authors have drawn attention to the serious problem of hospital-acquired hyponatremia in children with the use of hypotonic IV solutions; notably, hyponatremia is the most common electrolyte abnormality in children and affects

Table 23–2. Insensible losses.

Infant	20–30 mL/kg/day
Children, adults, and adolescents	400 mL/m²/day

Table 23–3. Alterations of fluid requirements.

Increased Requirements	
Factor	**Altered Requirement**
Fever	12% per degree > 38°C
Hyperventilation	10–60 mL/100 kcal
Sweating	10–25 mL/100 kcal
Hyperthyroidism	Variable: 25%–50%
Hyperosmolar states (eg, diabetic ketoacidosis)	Variable, assess volume status (see Chapter 35)
Gastrointestinal loss (vomiting, diarrhea, NG output)	Monitor and analyze output. Adjust therapy accordingly.
Decreased Requirements	
Factor	**Altered Requirement**
Hypothermia	Variable
Increased environmental humidity	Variable
Hypometabolic states	Variable
Anuric/oliguric renal failure	Restrict to insensible losses plus urine output

approximately 25% of hospitalized pediatric patients. Furthermore, the astute clinician will bear in mind the dynamic nature of clinical context in treating patients and that the choice of IV solution (Table 23–4) and rate of infusion must be made on an individual basis and must be reassessed often. A child with profound water loss from stool and hypernatremia who is placed on hypotonic IV fluids and whose diarrhea ceases but is continued on hypotonic solution without close monitoring of serum electrolytes is at risk for the devastating clinical consequences related to sequelae of rapid changes in sodium balance. Similarly, a child with hypertension and chronic kidney disease, if placed on isotonic maintenance fluids, is at risk for development of significant salt and water retention and resultant worsening blood pressure control. In recent years, there also has been a trend for total parenteral nutrition solution sodium and other electrolytes to be calculated and ordered on a milliequivalents-per-kilogram basis rather than the more classic milliequivalents-per-liter basis (eg, 2 mEqNa/kg/TPN volume vs 0.2 or 0.45 "normal saline"). If the administered fluid volume is decreased in this setting, as the child is weaned from supplemental IV fluids to enteral intake, the sodium and other electrolytes will need to be reduced accordingly to avoid changes in IV fluid tonicity that can result in hypernatremia or other electrolyte derangements.

Patient weight, total output (including urinary output, emesis, stool output, blood draws, surgical drain outputs, etc), and total fluid input should be monitored daily during hospitalization. Electronic medical records may calculate the net total volume in a 24-hour period, but this should be interpreted cautiously as it does not account for the patient's insensible losses; obtaining daily weights is a cornerstone of appropriate monitoring of fluid and electrolyte balance. If fluid or electrolyte balance is abnormal, serial determination of serum electrolyte concentrations, blood urea nitrogen, and creatinine are necessary, for example in patients with significant burns, anuria, oliguria, or persistent abnormal stool, urine, or body fluid losses. Serial labs should also be monitored in patients receiving IV fluids or parental nutrition.

Table 23–4. Composition of common intravenous fluid solutions

Fluid	Osmolarity (mOsm/L)	Dextrose (g/L)	Na+ (mEq/L)	Cl− (mEq/L)	K+ (mEq/L)	Ca++ (mEq/L)	Mag++ (mEq/L)	Acetate (mEq/L)	Gluconate (mEq/L)	Lactate (mEq/L)
Plasma-Lyte 148	547	50	140	98	5	0	3	27	23	0
Plasma-Lyte A	294	0	140	98	5	0	3	27	23	0
D5 Lactated Ringer (LR)	560	50	130	109	4	3	0	0	0	28
Lactated Ringer (LR)	273	0	130	109	4	3	0	0	0	28
D5W	253	50	0	0	0	0	0	0	0	0
D5 0.2 NS	330	50	38	38	0	0	0	0	0	0
D5 0.45 NS	406	50	77	77	0	0	0	0	0	0
D5 0.9 NS	560	50	154	154	0	0	0	0	0	0
Normal saline (NS)	308	0	154	154	0	0	0	0	0	0
Hypertonic saline (3% NaCl)	1026	0	513	513	0	0	0	0	0	0

DEHYDRATION

Depletion of body fluids is one of the most encountered problems in clinical pediatrics. The clinical evaluation of a child with dehydration, or volume contraction, should focus on the composition and volume of fluid intake and losses (vomiting, diarrhea, urine, "insensible losses"). A timely assessment of acute weight loss is central to calculating the magnitude of volume depletion. Important clinical features in estimating the degree of dehydration include the capillary refill time, postural blood pressure, and heart rate changes; dryness of the lips and mucous membranes; lack of tears; lack of external jugular venous filling when supine; a sunken fontanelle in an infant; oliguria; and altered mental status (Table 23–5). Children generally respond to a decrease in circulating volume with a compensatory increase in pulse rate and may maintain their blood pressure in the face of severe dehydration. A low or falling blood pressure is, therefore, a late sign of shock in children, and when present should prompt emergent treatment. Salient laboratory parameters include a high urine-specific gravity (in the absence of an underlying renal concentrating defect as seen in diabetes insipidus or chronic obstructive or reflux nephropathy), a low urinary [Na^+] excretion (< 20 mEq/L) or fractional excretion of sodium less than 0.1%, and an elevated hematocrit or serum albumin level secondary to hemoconcentration.

Emergent intravenous therapy is indicated when there is evidence of compromised perfusion (inadequate capillary refill, tachycardia, poor color, oliguria, or hypotension). The initial goal is to rapidly expand the plasma volume and to prevent circulatory collapse. A 20-mL/kg bolus of isotonic fluid should be given intravenously as rapidly as possible. Either colloid (5% albumin) or crystalloid (normal saline, Ringer lactate, or Plasma-Lyte) may be used. Colloid is particularly useful in hypernatremic patients in shock, in malnourished infants, or in children with active nephrotic syndrome presenting with severe TBW and intravascular volume contraction. If no intravenous site is available, fluid may be administered via interosseous access into the marrow space. If there is no response to the first fluid bolus, a second bolus may be given. When adequate tissue perfusion is demonstrated by improved capillary refill, decreased pulse rate and improved mental status, deficit replacement may be instituted. If adequate perfusion is not restored after 40 mL/kg of isotonic fluids, other pathologic processes must be considered such as sepsis, occult hemorrhage, or cardiogenic shock. Isotonic dehydration may be treated by providing half of the remaining fluid deficit over 8 hours and the second half over the ensuing 16 hours in the form of 5% dextrose with isotonic fluid containing 20 mEq/L of KCl. In the presence of metabolic acidosis, the addition of sodium or potassium acetate or bicarbonate may be considered. Serum potassium and calcium concentrations should be closely monitored, as these can decrease significantly with resolution of acidosis. Maintenance fluids and replacement of ongoing losses should also be provided. Given data demonstrating morbidity and mortality found with administration of hypotonic fluids, in 2018 the American Academy of Pediatrics put out a key action statement as follows: "Children between 28 days to 18 years of age requiring maintenance IVF should receive

Table 23–5. Clinical manifestations of dehydration.

Clinical Signs	Degree of Dehydration		
	Mild	Moderate	Severe
Decrease in body weight	3%–5%	6%–10%	11%–15%
Skin			
Turgor	Normal ±	Decreased	Markedly decreased
Color	Normal	Pale	Markedly decreased
Mucous membranes	Dry	⟶	Mottled or gray; parched
Hemodynamic signs			
Pulse	Normal	Slight increase	Tachycardia
Capillary refill	2–3 s	3–4 s	> 4 s
Blood pressure	Normal	⟶	Low
Perfusion	Normal	⟶	Circulatory collapse
Fluid loss			
Urinary output	Mild oliguria	Oliguria	Anuria
Tears	Decreased		Absent
Urinary indices			
Specific gravity	> 1.020	⟶	Anuria
Urine [Na^+]	< 20 mEq/L	⟶	Anuria

Table 23–6. Typical electrolyte compositions of various body fluids.

	Na⁺ (mEq/L)	K⁺ (mEq/L)	HCO₃⁻ (mEq/L)
Diarrhea	10–90	10–80	40
Gastric	20–80	5–20	0
Small intestine	100–140	5–15	40
Ileostomy	45–135	3–15	40

Data from Winters RW: *Principles of Pediatric Fluid Therapy.* 2nd ed. Philadelphia, PA: Lippincott Williams & Wilkins; 1973.

isotonic solutions with appropriate potassium chloride and dextrose." Typical electrolyte compositions of various body fluids are depicted in Table 23–6, although it may be necessary to measure the specific constituents of a patient's fluid losses to guide therapy. If the patient is unable to eat for a prolonged period, nutritional needs must be met through hyperalimentation or enteral tube feedings.

Oral rehydration may be provided to children with mild to moderate dehydration. Commercially available solutions provide 45–75 mEq/L of Na⁺, 20–25 mEq/L of K⁺, 30–34 mEq/L of citrate or bicarbonate, and 2%–2.5% of glucose (Table 23–7). Clear liquid beverages found in the home, such as broth, soda, juice, and tea are inappropriate for the treatment of dehydration. Frequent small aliquots (5–15 mL) of appropriate rehydration solutions should be given to provide approximately 50 mL/kg over 4 hours for mild dehydration and up to 100 mL/kg over 6 hours for moderate dehydration. Oral rehydration is contraindicated in children with altered levels of consciousness or respiratory distress who cannot drink freely; in children suspected of having an acute surgical abdomen; in infants with greater than 10% volume depletion; in children with hemodynamic instability; and in the setting of severe hyponatremia ([Na⁺] < 120 mEq/L) or hypernatremia ([Na⁺] > 160 mEq/L), or other significant electrolyte derangements. Failure of oral rehydration due to persistent vomiting or inability to keep up with losses mandates intravenous therapy. Successful oral rehydration requires explicit instructions to caregivers and close clinical follow-up of the child.

Table 23–7. Composition of oral rehydration solutions.

Fluid	Carbohydrate (g/L)	Na⁺ (mEq/L)	HCO₃⁻ (mEq/L)	K⁺ (mEq/L)
Pedialyte	25	45	30	20
Enfalyte	30	50	30	25
WHO (2002)	13.5	75	30	20

The type of dehydration is often characterized by the serum [Na⁺]. If relatively more solute is lost than water, the [Na⁺] falls, and hyponatremic dehydration ([Na⁺] < 130 mEq/L) ensues. This is important clinically because hypotonicity of the plasma contributes to further volume loss from the ECF into the intracellular space. Thus, tissue perfusion is more significantly impaired for a given degree of hyponatremic dehydration than for a comparable degree of isotonic or hypertonic dehydration. It is important to note, however, that significant solute losses also occur in hypernatremic dehydration. Furthermore, because plasma volume is somewhat protected in hypernatremic dehydration, the clinician may underestimate the severity of dehydration. Electrolyte and water deficits in moderate to severe dehydration are common. The three broad groups of dehydration include isotonic, hypotonic and hypertonic. In children, isotonic dehydration is characterized by 100–150 mL/kg water losses, 8–10 meq/kg sodium losses, 8–10 meq/kg potassium losses and 16–20 meg/kg of chloride losses. Hypotonic dehydration is characterized by 50–100/kg water losses, 10–14 meq/kg sodium losses, 10–14 meq/kg potassium losses and 20–28 meg/kg of chloride losses. Finally, hypertonic dehydration is characterized by 120–180 mL/kg water losses, 2–5 meq/kg sodium losses, 3–5 meq/kg potassium losses and 4–10 meg/kg of chloride losses.

HYPONATREMIA

Hyponatremia may be factitious in the presence of high plasma lipids or proteins, which decrease the percentage of plasma volume that is water. Hyponatremia in the absence of hypotonicity also occurs when an osmotically active solute, such as glucose or mannitol, is added to the ECF. Water drawn from the ICF dilutes the serum [Na⁺] despite isotonicity or hypertonicity.

Patients with hyponatremic dehydration generally demonstrate typical signs and symptoms of dehydration (see Table 23–5), as the vascular space is compromised as water leaves the ECF to maintain osmotic neutrality. The treatment of hyponatremic dehydration must address both sodium and fluid deficits. The magnitude of the sodium deficit may be calculated by the following formula:

$$\text{Na}^+ \text{ deficit} = (\text{Na}^+ \text{ desired} - \text{Na}^+ \text{ observed}) \times \text{Bodyweight (kg)} \times 0.6$$

Half of the deficit is replenished in the first 8 hours of therapy, and the remainder is given over the following 16 hours. Maintenance and replacement fluids should also be provided. The deficit plus maintenance calculations often approximate 5% dextrose with 0.45% or higher saline. The rise in serum [Na⁺] should target a goal of 4–6 mEq/L over 24 hours and should not exceed 0.5 mEq/L/h unless the patient demonstrates central nervous system (CNS) symptoms that warrant more rapid initial correction. Correction of the serum [Na$^+$] should not exceed to 8 mEq/L over 24 hours to avoid potential complications. The dangers of rapid correction of hyponatremia include cerebral dehydration and injury due to fluid shifts from the ICF compartment, a condition known as osmotic demyelination syndrome (ODS). In patients with hyponatremia who experience a rapid correction of the serum [Na$^+$], therapeutic relowering of the serum [Na$^+$] with free water or desmopressin may be considered when risk factors for developing ODS are present or the patient is exhibiting signs of ODS.

In cases of severe hyponatremia (serum [Na$^+$] < 120 mEq/L) with CNS symptoms, IV hypertonic saline (3% NaCl) may be given to raise the [Na$^+$] by 5 mEq/L to alleviate CNS manifestations and sequelae. In general, 1 mL/kg of 3% NaCl will raise the serum [Na$^+$] by about 1 mEq/L. If hypertonic saline is administered, estimated Na$^+$ and fluid deficits should be adjusted accordingly. Further correction should proceed slowly, as outlined earlier.

Hypovolemic hyponatremia also occurs in cystic fibrosis, renal dysplasia, adrenal insufficiency, and cerebral salt-wasting (CSW). CSW is associated with CNS insults, most commonly subarachnoid hemorrhage, and is characterized by an inappropriate natriuresis (urinary [Na$^+$] > 40 mEq/L) in a patient with high urine output and a contracted effective circulatory blood volume in the absence of other causes for Na$^+$ excretion. This must be distinguished from the syndrome of inappropriate secretion of ADH (SIADH), which may also manifest in CNS conditions and pulmonary disorders (Table 23–8). In contrast to CSW, SIADH is characterized by euvolemia or mild volume expansion and relatively low urine output due to ADH-induced water retention. Urinary [Na$^+$] is high in both conditions, though generally higher in CSW. The treatment of CSW involves replacement of urinary salt and water losses, whereas the treatment of SIADH involves water restriction. It is also important to remember that patients with SIADH are not necessarily oliguric and that their urine does not need to be maximally concentrated but merely inappropriately concentrated for their degree of serum tonicity.

Hypervolemic hyponatremia may occur in edematous disorders such as nephrotic syndrome, congestive heart failure, and cirrhosis, wherein water is retained in excess of salt. Treatment involves restriction of Na$^+$ and water and correction of the underlying disorder. Hypervolemic hyponatremia due to water intoxication is characterized by a maximally dilute urine and is also treated with water restriction.

HYPERNATREMIA

Although diarrhea is commonly associated with hyponatremic or isonatremic dehydration, hypernatremia may develop in the presence of persistent fever, decreased fluid intake, or improperly mixed rehydration solutions. Extreme care is required to treat hypernatremic dehydration appropriately to avoid CNS complications. If the serum [Na$^+$] falls precipitously, the osmolality of the ECF drops more rapidly than that of the CNS and water shifts from the ECF compartment into the CNS to maintain osmotic neutrality. If hypertonicity is corrected too rapidly, cerebral edema, seizures, and CNS injury may occur. Thus, following the initial restoration of adequate tissue perfusion using isotonic fluids, a gradual decrease in serum [Na$^+$] is desired for patients with chronic hypernatremia (> 48 hours or unknown duration) or acute severe hypernatremia (serum [Na$^+$] >160 mEq/L). Correction should not exceed a reduction of 8-10 mEq/L over 24 hours or a drop of greater than 0.5 mEq/L/h. This is commonly achieved using 5% dextrose with 0.2% saline to replace the calculated fluid deficit over 48 hours or longer depending on the severity and chronicity of the fluid losses. Maintenance and replacement fluids should also be provided. If the serum [Na$^+$] is not correcting appropriately, the free water deficit may be estimated as 4 mL/kg of free water for each milliequivalent of serum [Na$^+$] above 145 mEq/L and provided as 5% dextrose. If metabolic acidosis is also present, it must be corrected slowly to avoid CNS irritability. Potassium is provided as indicated. Electrolyte concentrations should be assessed every 2 hours to control the decline in serum [Na$^+$]. Elevations of blood glucose and blood urea nitrogen may worsen the hyperosmolar state in hypernatremic dehydration

Table 23–8. SIADH and cerebral salt wasting.

	Serum Na$^+$	Serum Osmolality	Urine Na$^+$	Urine Output	Urine Osmolality	Volume Status	Treatment
SIADH	< 135 mEq/L	< 280 mOsm/kg	> 40 mEq/L	Low	> 100 mOsm/kg[a]	Euvolemia or mild volume expansion	Water restriction
Cerebral salt-wasting	< 135 mEq/L	< 280 mOsm/kg	> 40 mEq/L	High	Variable[b]	Hypovolemia	Sodium and water replacement

[a]Urine is inappropriately concentrated when it should be maximally dilute with a urine osmolality of <100 mOsm/kg.
[b]May be normal or maximally dilute with a urine osmolality of <100 mOsm/kg.

and should also be monitored closely. Hyperglycemia is often associated with hypernatremic dehydration and may necessitate lower intravenous glucose concentrations (eg, 2.5%).

Patients with diabetes insipidus, whether nephrogenic or central in origin, are prone to develop profound hypernatremic dehydration as a result of unremitting urinary-free water losses (urine-specific gravity < 1.010), particularly during superimposed gastrointestinal illnesses associated with vomiting or diarrhea. Treatment involves restoration of fluid and electrolyte deficits as described earlier as well as replacement of excessive water losses. Formal water deprivation testing to distinguish responsiveness to ADH should only be done during wake periods in an inpatient hospitalization after restoration of normal fluid volume status. The evaluation and treatment of nephrogenic and central diabetes insipidus are discussed in detail in Chapters 24 and 34, respectively.

Hypervolemic hypernatremia (salt poisoning), associated with excess total body salt and water, may occur because of improperly mixed formula, excessive NaCl or NaHCO$_3$ administration, or as a feature of primary hyperaldosteronism. Treatment includes the use of diuretics, and potentially, concomitant water replacement or dialysis.

POTASSIUM DISORDERS

The predominantly intracellular distribution of potassium is maintained by the actions of Na$^+$-K$^+$-ATPase in the cell membranes. Potassium is shifted into the ECF and plasma by acidemia and into the ICF in the setting of alkalosis, hypochloremia, or in conjunction with insulin-induced cellular glucose uptake. The ratio of intracellular to extracellular K$^+$ is the major determinant of the cellular resting membrane potential and contributes to the action potential in neural and muscular tissue. Abnormalities of K$^+$ balance are potentially life threatening. In the kidney, K$^+$ is filtered at the glomerulus, reabsorbed in the proximal tubule, and excreted in the distal tubule. Distal tubular K$^+$ excretion is regulated primarily by the mineralocorticoid aldosterone. Renal K$^+$ excretion is primarily dependent on the urinary flow rate and continues for significant periods even after the intake of K$^+$ is decreased. Thus, by the time urinary [K$^+$] decreases, the systemic K$^+$ pool has been depleted significantly. In general, the greater the urine flow the greater the urinary K$^+$ excretion.

The causes of hypokalemia are primarily renal in origin. Gastrointestinal losses through nasogastric suction or vomiting reduce total body K$^+$ to some degree. However, the resultant volume depletion results in an increase in plasma aldosterone, promoting renal excretion of K$^+$ in exchange for Na$^+$ reclamation to preserve circulatory volume. Diuretics (especially thiazides and loop diuretics), mineralocorticoids, and intrinsic renal tubular diseases (eg, Bartter syndrome) enhance the renal excretion of K$^+$. Systemic K$^+$ depletion

in hypokalemic metabolic acidosis may lead to "paradoxical aciduria" and low urine pH wherein H$^+$ is preferentially exchanged for Na$^+$ in response to aldosterone. Clinically, hypokalemia is associated with neuromuscular excitability, decreased peristalsis or ileus, hyporeflexia, paralysis, rhabdomyolysis, and arrhythmias. Electrocardiographic changes include flattened T waves, a shortened PR interval, and the appearance of U waves. Arrhythmias associated with hypokalemia include premature ventricular contractions; atrial, nodal, or ventricular tachycardia; and ventricular fibrillation.

The priority in the treatment of hypokalemia is the restoration of an adequate serum [K$^+$]. Providing maintenance amounts of K$^+$ is usually sufficient; however, when the serum [K$^+$] is dangerously low and in the presence of arrhythmias, extreme muscle weakness, or respiratory compromise, intravenous K$^+$ should be given. If the patient is hypophosphatemic ([Po$_4$$^{3-}$] < 2 mg/dL), a phosphate salt may be used. If K$^+$ must be administered intravenously, it should not be given faster than a rate of 0.3 mEq/kg/h; it is imperative that the patient have a cardiac monitor. Oral K$^+$ supplements may be needed for weeks to replenish depleted body stores.

Hyperkalemia is caused by decreased renal K$^+$ excretion, mineralocorticoid deficiency or unresponsiveness, or K$^+$ release from the ICF compartment. Clinically, hyperkalemia is characterized by muscle weakness, paresthesias, and tetany; ascending paralysis; and arrhythmias. Electrocardiographic changes include peaked T waves, widening of the QRS complex, and arrhythmias such as sinus bradycardia or sinus arrest, atrioventricular block, nodal or idioventricular rhythms, and ventricular tachycardia or fibrillation. An EKG should be obtained when significant hyperkalemia is suspected. If the serum [K$^+$] is less than 6 mEq/L, discontinuing K$^+$ supplementation may be sufficient if there is no ongoing K$^+$ source, such as cell lysis, and if urine output continues. If the serum [K$^+$] is greater than 6 mEq/L or if potentiating factors such as renal failure are present, more aggressive therapy is needed (Table 23–9). If electrocardiographic changes or arrhythmias are present, treatment must be initiated promptly. Initial treatment consists of cardiac membrane stabilization and rapid intracellular shifting of K$^+$. Intravenous calcium gluconate will rapidly ameliorate depolarization and may be repeated after 5 minutes if electrocardiographic changes persist. Calcium should be given only with a cardiac monitor in place and should be discontinued if bradycardia develops. Administering Na$^+$ and increasing systemic pH with bicarbonate therapy will shift K$^+$ from the ECF to the ICF compartment, as will therapy with a β-agonist such as albuterol. Administration of IV glucose and insulin may be needed as a simultaneous drip given over 2 hours with monitoring of the serum glucose level every 15 minutes.

The therapies outlined above provide transient benefits, and K$^+$ will remain elevated unless other interventions are used to decrease total body potassium. Therapy must be given to reduce K$^+$ to normal levels by renal potassium

Table 23–9. Drugs for the treatment of hyperkalemia in children.

Drug	Actions	Notes
Calcium gluconate (10% solution)	Cardiac membrane stabilization. Does not alter the serum K⁺ level.	Cardiac monitoring needed. May repeat dose if ECG changes persist. Discontinue if bradycardia develops.
Albuterol (nebulized)	Transient shift of K⁺ from the ECF to the ICF compartment.	May repeat for 1 additional dose. Tachycardia may limit dosing.
Sodium bicarbonate	Transient shift of K⁺ from the ECF to the ICF compartment.	Avoid use if alkalosis or hypocalcemia is present. May cause hypernatremia, hypocalcemia.
Insulin (regular)	Transient shift of K⁺ from the ECF to the ICF compartment.	Must be given with a glucose infusion to prevent severe hypoglycemia. Diabetic patients may not require glucose infusion. Requires close monitoring of serum glucose.
Sodium polystyrene sulfonate	Ion exchange resin that exchanges K⁺ for Na⁺. Will decrease total body K⁺.	Do not use in neonates and patients with bowel hypomotility or bowel obstruction due to risk of intestinal necrosis. May cause hypernatremia, hypocalcemia, and hypomagnesemia.
Furosemide	Diuretic that increases renal K⁺ excretion. Will decrease total body K⁺.	May need higher doses in patients with acute kidney injury and chronic kidney disease to achieve desired effect.

excretion using diuretics, fecal potassium excretion using ion exchange resins such as sodium polystyrene sulfonate, or potassium removal by dialysis.

Feld LG et al: Clinical practice guideline: maintenance intravenous fluids in children. Pediatrics 2018;142(6):e20183083 [PMID: 30478247].

Montford JR, Linas S: How dangerous is hyperkalemia? J Am Soc Nephrol 2017;28(11):3155–3165 [PMID: 28778861].

Online resource for electrolyte cases: http://www.skeletonkey.group.

Palmer BF: Regulation of potassium homeostasis. Clin J Am Soc Nephrol 2015;10(6):1050–1060 [PMID: 24721891].

Rondon-Berrios H: Therapeutic relowering of plasma sodium after overly rapid correction of hyponatremia. Clin J Am Soc Nephrol 2020;15(2):282–228 [PMID: 31601554].

Sterns RH: Disorders of plasma sodium—causes, consequences, and correction. N Engl J Med 2015;372:55–65 [PMID: 25551526].

Sterns RH: Treatment of severe hyponatremia. Clin J Am Soc Nephrol 2018;13(4):641–649 [PMID: 29295830].

ACID–BASE DISTURBANCES

When evaluating a disturbance in acid–base balance, the systemic pH, partial carbon dioxide pressure (P_{CO_2}), serum HCO_3^-, and anion gap must be considered. The anion gap, $[Na^+ - (Cl^- + HCO_3^-)]$, is an expression of the unmeasured anions in the plasma and is normally 12 ± 4 mEq/L. An increase above normal suggests the presence of an unmeasured anion, such as occurs in diabetic ketoacidosis, lactic acidosis, and salicylate intoxication. Although the base excess (or deficit) is also used clinically, it is important to recall that this expression of acid–base balance is influenced by the renal response to respiratory disorders and cannot be interpreted independently (as in a compensated respiratory acidosis, wherein the base excess may be quite large).

METABOLIC ACIDOSIS

Metabolic acidosis is characterized by a primary decrease in serum $[HCO_3^-]$ and systemic pH due to the loss of HCO_3^- from the kidneys or gastrointestinal tract, the addition of an acid from external sources or via altered metabolic processes, or the rapid dilution of the ECF with non-bicarbonate–containing solution (usually normal saline). When HCO_3^- is lost through the kidneys or gastrointestinal tract, Cl^- must be reabsorbed with Na^+ disproportionately, resulting in a hyperchloremic acidosis with a normal anion gap. Thus, a normal anion gap acidosis in the absence of diarrhea or other bicarbonate-rich gastrointestinal losses suggests the possibility of renal tubular acidosis (see Chapter 24). In contrast, acidosis that results from the addition of an unmeasured acid is associated with a high anion gap. Examples are diabetic ketoacidosis, lactic acidosis, starvation, uremia, toxin ingestion (salicylates, ethylene glycol, or methanol), and certain inborn errors of organic or amino acid metabolism. Dehydration may also result in a high anion gap acidosis as a result of inadequate tissue perfusion, decreased O_2 delivery, and subsequent lactic and keto acid production. Respiratory compensation is accomplished through an increase in minute ventilation and a decrease in P_{CO_2}.

The ingestion of unknown toxins or the possibility of an inborn error of metabolism (see Chapter 36) must be considered in children without an obvious cause for a high anion gap acidosis. Unfortunately, some hospital laboratories fail to include ethylene glycol or methanol in their standard toxicology screens, so assay of these toxins must be requested specifically. This is of critical importance when therapy with fomepizole (4-methylpyrazole) must be considered for either ingestion and instituted promptly to avoid profound toxicity. Salicylate intoxication has a stimulatory effect on the respiratory center of the CNS; thus, patients may initially present with respiratory alkalosis or mixed respiratory alkalosis and widened anion gap acidosis.

Most types of metabolic acidosis will resolve with correction of the underlying disorder, improved renal perfusion, and acid excretion. Intravenous $NaHCO_3$ administration may be considered in the setting of metabolic acidosis when the pH is less than 7.2, but only if adequate ventilation is ensured. The dose (in milliequivalents) of $NaHCO_3$ may be calculated as

$$\text{Weight (kg)} \times \text{Base deficit} \times 0.3$$

and given as a continuous infusion over 1 hour. The effect of NaHCO3 in lowering serum potassium and ionized calcium concentrations must also be considered and monitored.

METABOLIC ALKALOSIS

Metabolic alkalosis is characterized by a primary increase in $[HCO_3^-]$ and pH resulting from a loss of strong acid or gain of buffer base. The most common cause for a metabolic alkalosis is the loss of gastric juice via nasogastric suction or vomiting. This results in a Cl^- responsive alkalosis, characterized by a low urinary $[Cl^-]$ (< 20 mEq/L) indicative of a volume-contracted state that will be responsive to the provision of adequate Cl^- salt, usually in the form of normal saline. Cystic fibrosis may also be associated with a Cl^- responsive alkalosis due to the high losses of NaCl through the sweat. Congenital Cl^- losing diarrhea is a rare cause of Cl^- responsive metabolic alkalosis. Cl^- resistant alkalosis is characterized by a urinary $[Cl^-]$ greater than 20 mEq/Land is associated with Bartter syndrome, Cushing syndrome, and primary hyperaldosteronism, conditions associated with primary increases in urinary $[Cl^-]$, or volume-expanded states lacking stimuli for renal Cl^- reabsorption. Thus, the urinary $[Cl^-]$ is helpful in distinguishing the nature of a metabolic alkalosis but must be specifically requested in many laboratories because it is not routinely included in urine electrolyte panels. The serum $[K^+]$ is also low in these settings (hypokalemic metabolic alkalosis) owing to a combination of increased mineralocorticoid activity associated with volume contraction, the shift of K^+ to the ICF compartment, and preferential reabsorption of Na^+ rather than K^+ to preserve intravascular volume. A hypokalemic alkalosis seen in the setting of primary mineralocorticoid excess would be expected to be associated with systemic hypertension clinically, as observed in an adrenal adenoma and some forms of monogenic hypertension, including Liddle syndrome and apparent mineralocorticoid excess (AME).

RESPIRATORY ACIDOSIS

Respiratory acidosis develops when alveolar ventilation is decreased, increasing PCO_2 and lowering systemic pH. The kidneys compensate for respiratory acidosis by increasing HCO_3^- reabsorption, a process that takes several days to fully manifest. Patients with acute respiratory acidosis frequently demonstrate air hunger with retractions and the use of accessory respiratory muscles. Respiratory acidosis occurs in upper or lower airway obstruction, ventilation-perfusion disturbances, CNS depression, and neuromuscular defects. The goal of therapy is to correct or compensate for the underlying pathologic process to improve alveolar ventilation. Bicarbonate therapy is not indicated in a pure respiratory acidosis because it will worsen the acidosis by shifting the equilibrium of the carbonic acid–bicarbonate buffer system to increase PCO_2.

RESPIRATORY ALKALOSIS

Respiratory alkalosis occurs when hyperventilation results in a decrease in PCO_2 and an increase in systemic pH. Depending on the acuity of the respiratory alkalosis, there may be an associated compensatory loss of bicarbonate by the kidneys manifested as a low serum bicarbonate level and a normal anion gap that may be misinterpreted as a normal anion gap acidosis if all acid–base parameters are not considered. Patients may experience tingling, paresthesias, dizziness, palpitations, syncope, or even tetany and seizures due to the associated decrease in ionized calcium. Causes of respiratory alkalosis include psychobehavioral disturbances, CNS irritation from meningitis or encephalitis, salicylate intoxication, and iatrogenic overventilation in patients who are mechanically ventilated. Therapy is directed toward addressing the causal process.

Al-Jaghbeer M, Kellum JA: Acid-base disturbances in intensive care patients: etiology, pathophysiology and treatment. Nephrol Dial Transplant 2015 Jul;30(7):1104–1011 [PMID: 25213433].

Berend K, de Vries AP, Gans RO: Physiological approach to acid-base disturbances. N Engl J Med 2014;371:1434–1445 [PMID: 25295502].

Carmody JB, Norwood VF: A clinical approach to paediatric acid-base disorders. Postgrad Med J 2012;88:143–151 [PMID: 22267531].

White ML, Liebelt EL: Update on antidotes for pediatric poisoning. Pediatr Emerg Care 2006;22:740 [PMID: 17110870].

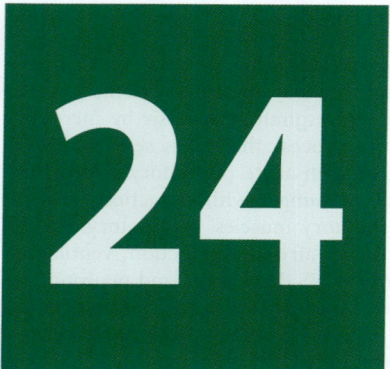

Kidney & Urinary Tract

Margret E. Bock, MD, MS

Eliza D. Blanchette, MD, MS

Melisha G. Hanna, MD, MS

EVALUATION OF THE KIDNEY & URINARY TRACT

HISTORY

When renal disease is suspected, the history should include the following:

1. Preceding acute or chronic illnesses (eg, urinary tract infection [UTI], pharyngitis, systemic lupus erythematosus [SLE])
2. Rashes or joint pain/swelling
3. Growth delay or failure to thrive
4. Polyuria, polydipsia, enuresis, urinary frequency, or dysuria
5. Hematuria, proteinuria, or discolored urine
6. Pain (abdominal, costovertebral angle, or flank)
7. Sudden weight gain or loss or edema
8. Drug or toxin exposure
9. Perinatal history including prematurity, prenatal ultrasonographic studies, oligo- or polyhydramnios, birth asphyxia, dysmorphic features and other congenital anomalies, voiding patterns, and umbilical artery catheterization
10. Family history of kidney disease, hypertension, deafness, dialysis, or kidney transplantation

PHYSICAL EXAMINATION

Important aspects of the physical examination include the height, weight, and growth percentiles. Blood pressure (BP) should be measured in a quiet setting with a manual cuff of the appropriate size in the right upper extremity, ideally with the child seated with feet flat on the ground and after 3–5 minutes of rest. The cuff should have a bladder length that is 80%–100% and a width that is 40% of the circumference of the upper arm. Peripheral pulses should be assessed, and presence of skin lesions (café au lait, ash leaf spots, purpura, or rash), pallor, edema, or skeletal deformities should be evaluated. Anomalies of the ears, eyes, or external genitalia may be associated with renal anomalies or disease. The abdomen should be palpated and auscultated, with attention to nephromegaly, abdominal masses, musculature, ascites, or bruits.

LABORATORY EVALUATION OF RENAL FUNCTION

Serum Analysis

The standard indicators of renal function are serum levels of blood urea nitrogen (BUN) and creatinine; their ratio is normally about 10:1. The BUN to creatinine ratio may increase when renal perfusion or urine flow is decreased, as in urinary tract obstruction or dehydration. Because serum BUN levels are more affected by these and other factors such as nitrogen intake, catabolism, and the use of corticosteroids, the serum creatinine is the more reliable single indicator of glomerular function. Normative values for serum creatinine relate to muscle mass, and the generation of creatinine may be affected by age, sex, malnutrition, chronic illness, and amputation. At birth, serum creatinine reflects the mother's creatinine level and declines over the first 1–2 weeks to reach a normal level for age. Serum cystatin C, a cysteine protease inhibitor that is produced by all nucleated cells and released in the blood, is an additional indicator of glomerular function, and levels are not affected by sex, height, or muscle mass. Cystatin C assays are less reliable in certain clinical settings, such as with corticosteroid administration or thyroid disease. Less precise but nonetheless important indicators of possible renal disease are abnormalities of serum electrolytes, bicarbonate, pH, calcium, phosphorus, magnesium, albumin, or complement.

Glomerular Filtration Rate

The endogenous creatinine clearance (C_{Cr}) in milliliters per minute estimates the glomerular filtration rate (GFR).

A 24-hour urine collection is the "classic" approach for determining C_{Cr}; however, it is often difficult to accurately obtain in the pediatric population, particularly in children who are not continent. Total daily creatinine excretion should be 15–25 mg/kg, with normal values higher in males than in females, reflective of differences in muscle mass. Values on either side of this range suggest collections that were either inadequate or excessive. The following formula requires measurements of plasma or serum creatinine (P_{Cr}) in mg/dL, urine creatinine (U_{Cr}) in mg/dL, and urine volume (V) expressed as mL/min:

$$C_{Cr} = \frac{U_{Cr}V}{P_{Cr}}$$

Because accepted ranges of normal C_{Cr} are based on adult parameters, correction to a standard body surface area of 1.73 m² is needed in children:

$$\text{"Corrected" } C_{Cr} = \frac{\text{Patient's } C_{Cr} \times 1.73\, m^2}{\text{Patient's body surface area}}$$

Normative values for GFR change with age, and children do not reach adult levels of GFR (90–120 mL/min/1.73 m²) until approximately 2 years of age. Levels below 90 mL/min/1.73 m² in children older than 2 years may indicate underlying kidney disease.

A quick approximation of estimated GFR (eGFR) in children can be accomplished using validated equations. These are useful only when the creatinine is stable and should not be used in patients with acute kidney injury (AKI). The "Bedside Schwartz" equation provides an eGFR based on plasma or serum creatinine level and length in centimeters:

$$\text{eGFR (mL/min/1.73 m}^2) = 0.413 \times \text{height (cm)}/P_{Cr} \text{ (mg/dL)}$$

This formula was developed in children with chronic kidney disease (CKD) and has also been validated in children with normal renal function. When cystatin C (cysC) has been assessed, the creatinine-cystatin C–based CKiD equation may be utilized to include this variable and BUN:

$$\text{eGFR (mL/min/1.73 m}^2) = 39.8 \times [\text{height (m)}/P_{Cr}(\text{mg/dL})]^{0.456}$$
$$\times [1.8/\text{cysC (mg/L)}]^{0.418} \times [30/\text{BUN}]^{0.079}$$
$$\times [1.076^{\text{ male}}] [1.00^{\text{ female}}] \times [\text{ht (m)}/1.4]^{0.179}$$

This calculation may be useful as a confirmatory test in circumstances when eGFR based on serum creatinine is less accurate (eg, low muscle mass) or when the clinical scenario warrants a secondary test. The CKiD under 25 eGFR equations for use in children and young adults with CKD have been developed with additional data from the Chronic Kidney Disease in Children Study (CKiD). These equations use age- and sex-dependent variables, and there is an online tool available to facilitate calculation: https://ckid-gfrcalculator.shinyapps.io/eGFR/.

Urine Concentrating Ability

Inability to concentrate urine causes polyuria, polydipsia, or enuresis. The first morning void should be concentrated (specific gravity ≥ 1.020), presuming cessation of fluid intake overnight. Thus, determination of the specific gravity of a first morning void is an easy and helpful test of the kidney's concentrating ability.

Urinalysis

Commercially available dipsticks can be used to screen urine for blood, leukocytes, nitrites, protein, and specific gravity and to approximate the urine pH. Positive results for blood should always be confirmed by microscopy, which is also the only way to determine if there is significant crystalluria or casts. Hematuria is present when there are more than 5 red blood cells/high-powered field (RBCs/hpf). Significant proteinuria (≥30 mg/dL) detected by dipstick should be confirmed by quantitation. In pediatrics, this is customarily accomplished by measuring the ratio of protein (mg/dL)/creatinine (mg/dL) in a random urine sample, rather than a 24-hour urine collection. A urine protein/creatinine ratio (UPC) above 0.2 is abnormal and a ratio more than 2 is considered nephrotic range proteinuria.

In children with asymptomatic hematuria, an evaluation for a renal origin will yield the most results, although urologic etiologies should also be considered. The presence of urinary RBC casts suggests glomerulonephritis (GN), but the absence of casts does not exclude this diagnosis. Urine RBC morphology may be helpful, with dysmorphic RBC arising from the kidneys. Anatomic abnormalities such as cystic disease with cyst rupture may also cause hematuria. Benign hematuria, including benign familial hematuria/thin glomerular basement membrane disease, is diagnosed by exclusion. Hematuria can also be observed in the setting of hypercalciuria or urolithiasis. Figure 24–1 suggests an approach to the renal workup of hematuria.

An initial approach to the evaluation of proteinuria and differential diagnosis is shown in Figure 24–2. In the evaluation of asymptomatic proteinuria, orthostatic or postural proteinuria should be excluded. This can be accomplished simply by comparing the UPC of urine formed in the supine position (the first morning void accumulated in the bladder while sleeping) to a sample obtained during daily ambulation. If the first morning urine sample is normal and proteinuria is occurring only during upright posture, this demonstrates postural/orthostatic proteinuria. Such patients typically show resolution of orthostatic proteinuria over time, but rarely an orthostatic pattern can be seen initially in GN, thus warranting ongoing follow-up. If both samples are abnormal, proteinuria would be considered "persistent" and additional workup and referral to nephrology are warranted. Combined proteinuria and hematuria are characteristic of more significant glomerular disease (see Figure 24–1).

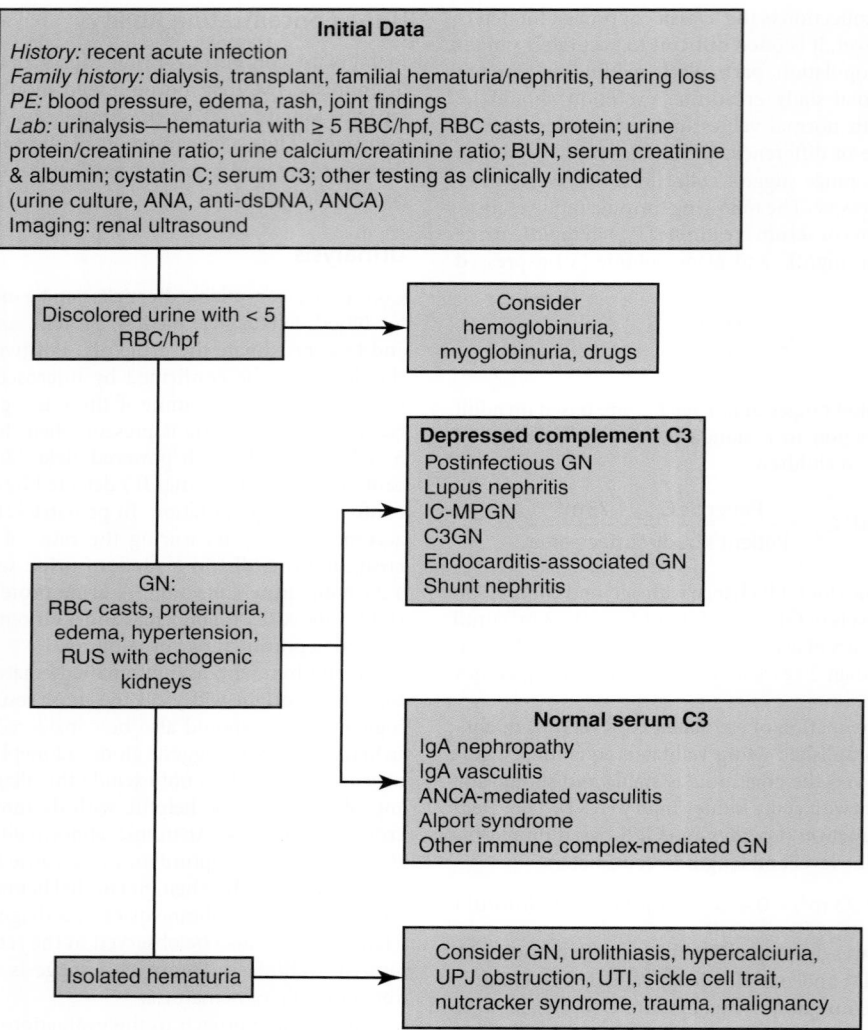

Initial Data
History: recent acute infection
Family history: dialysis, transplant, familial hematuria/nephritis, hearing loss
PE: blood pressure, edema, rash, joint findings
Lab: urinalysis—hematuria with ≥ 5 RBC/hpf, RBC casts, protein; urine protein/creatinine ratio; urine calcium/creatinine ratio; BUN, serum creatinine & albumin; cystatin C; serum C3; other testing as clinically indicated (urine culture, ANA, anti-dsDNA, ANCA)
Imaging: renal ultrasound

Discolored urine with < 5 RBC/hpf

Consider hemoglobinuria, myoglobinuria, drugs

GN: RBC casts, proteinuria, edema, hypertension, RUS with echogenic kidneys

Depressed complement C3
Postinfectious GN
Lupus nephritis
IC-MPGN
C3GN
Endocarditis-associated GN
Shunt nephritis

Normal serum C3
IgA nephropathy
IgA vasculitis
ANCA-mediated vasculitis
Alport syndrome
Other immune complex-mediated GN

Isolated hematuria

Consider GN, urolithiasis, hypercalciuria, UPJ obstruction, UTI, sickle cell trait, nutcracker syndrome, trauma, malignancy

▲ **Figure 24–1.** Approach to the evaluation of hematuria. ANA, antinuclear antibody; ANCA, antineutrophil cytoplasmic antibody; BUN, blood urea nitrogen; C3, complement; C3GN, C3 glomerulopathy; dsDNA, double-stranded DNA; GN, glomerulonephritis; hpf, high-power field; HSP, Henoch-Schönlein purpura; IC-MPGN, immune-complex membranoproliferative glomerulonephritis; IgA, immunoglobulin A; RBC, red blood cell; RUS, renal ultrasound; UPJ, ureteropelvic junction; UTI, urinary tract infection.

Special Tests of Renal Function

Measurements of urinary sodium, creatinine, and osmolality are useful in differentiating prerenal from renal causes of AKI. The physiologic response to decreased renal perfusion is decreased urinary output, increased urine osmolality, increased urinary solute concentration (eg, creatinine), and decreased urinary sodium (usually < 20 mEq/L).

The presence of certain substances in urine may suggest tubular dysfunction. For example, urine glucose should be less than 5 mg/dL in the setting of normal serum glucose concentration. Hyperphosphaturia occurs with significant proximal tubular abnormalities (eg, Fanconi syndrome). Measurement of the phosphate concentration of a 24-hour urine specimen and evaluation of tubular reabsorption of phosphorus (TRP) will help document renal tubular diseases

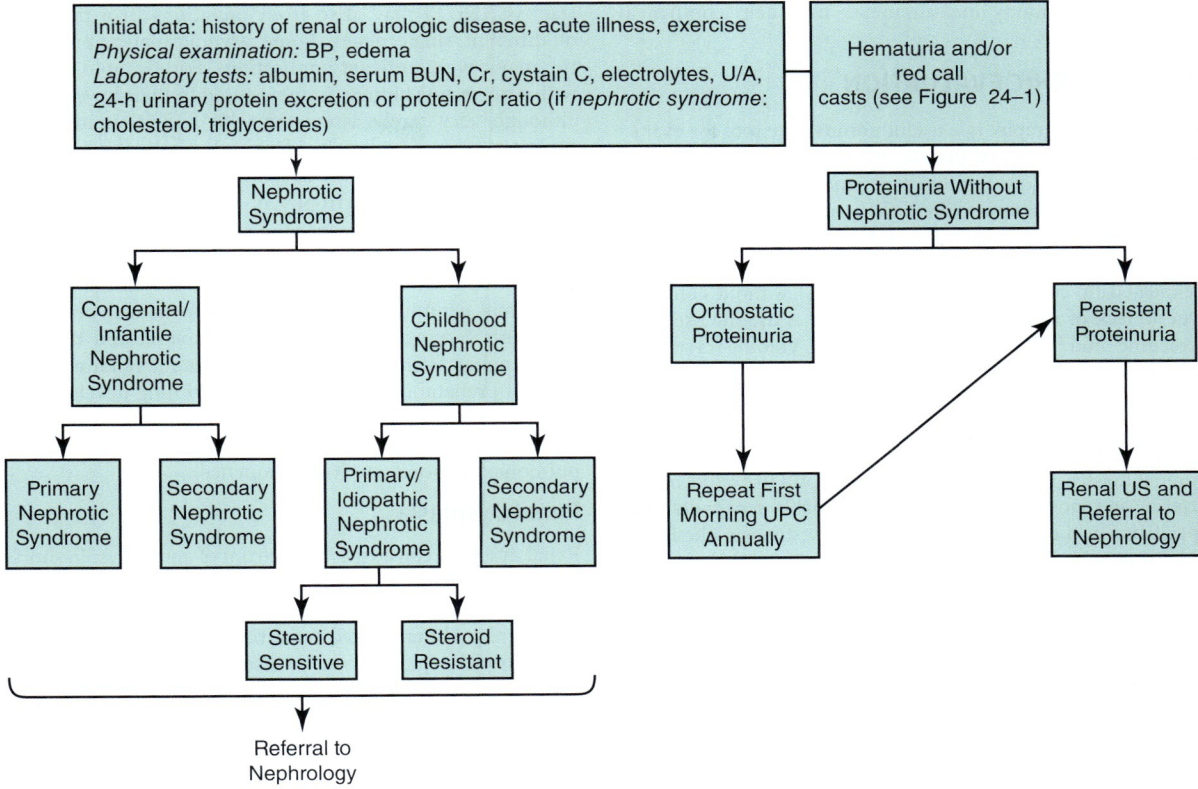

▲ Figure 24–2. Initial approach to the evaluation of proteinuria and an algorithm for developing a differential diagnosis. BP, blood pressure; Cr, creatinine; hpf, high-power field; RBC, red blood cell; U/A, urinalysis; UPC, urine protein/creatinine ratio; US, ultrasound.

as well as hyperparathyroid states. TRP (expressed as percentage of reabsorption) is calculated as follows:

$$TRP = 100\left[1 - \frac{S_{Cr} \times Upo_4}{Spo_4 \times U_{Cr}}\right]$$

where S_{Cr} = serum creatinine, U_{Cr} = urine creatinine, Spo_4 = serum phosphate, and Upo_4 = urine phosphate, with values for creatinine and phosphate expressed in mg/dL. A TRP value of 85% or greater is considered normal in children.

A quantitative increase in urinary excretion of amino acids is seen in generalized proximal tubular disease. Defective proximal tubular reabsorption of bicarbonate can be seen in isolated renal tubular acidosis (RTA), Fanconi syndrome, and chronic renal failure.

Urinary Biomarkers

Urinary markers of AKI, most often of tubular damage, have become more clinically available. They include urinary neutrophil gelatinase-associated lipocalin (NGAL),

an iron-transporting protein that is almost completely reabsorbed by normal renal tubules. NGAL levels increase after acute ischemic/nephrotoxic insults and have been found to be sensitive markers of AKI.

LABORATORY EVALUATION OF IMMUNOLOGIC FUNCTION

Many parenchymal renal diseases are thought to be caused by immunologic mechanisms, such as deposition of circulating antigen-antibody complexes that are directly injurious or incite injurious responses and formation of antibody directed against the glomerular basement membrane (rare in children). Serum C3 and C4 complement concentrations should be measured when immune-mediated renal injury or GN is suspected. Where clinically indicated, antinuclear antibodies (ANAs), antineutrophil cytoplasmic antibodies (ANCAs), hepatitis B surface antigen, and hepatitis C antibody should be obtained. In rare cases, cryoglobulins (very rare in childhood), C3 nephritic factor and other assessment of complement function, or anti-glomerular basement membrane (anti-GBM) antibody measurements may help confirm a specific diagnosis.

RADIOGRAPHIC EVALUATION

Renal ultrasonography is a useful noninvasive tool for evaluating renal parenchymal disease, urinary tract abnormalities, and renal blood flow. Radioisotope studies provide information about renal anatomy, blood flow, and integrity and function of the glomerular, tubular, and collecting systems. Renal stones are often visualized by ultrasonography but are best delineated by computed tomography (CT) without contrast. Due to lack of radiation, ultrasonography is usually used for screening and follow-up of urolithiasis. Voiding cystourethrography (VCUG) is indicated when vesicoureteral reflux (VUR) or bladder outlet obstruction (eg, to visualize the posterior urethra) is suspected. Magnetic resonance imaging (MRI) or CT are useful for identification and delineation of renal or adrenal masses. Doppler ultrasound is helpful to exclude renal arterial or venous thrombosis but of variable sensitivity and specificity in the diagnosis of renal artery stenosis; the latter condition is better assessed by MR or CT angiography. Intrarenal arterial stenosis may require direct renal arteriography.

RENAL BIOPSY

Histologic information that includes light, immunofluorescence, and electron microscopy is valuable in select cases to diagnose, guide treatment, and inform prognosis. The need for a renal biopsy should be determined by a pediatric nephrologist.

Bignall ONR, Dixon BP: Management of hematuria in children. Curr Treat Options Pediatr 2018 Sep;4(3):333–349 [PMID: 30128264].

Brown DD, Reidy KJ: Approach to the child with hematuria. Pediatr Clin North Am 2019 Feb;66(1):15–30 [PMID: 30454740].

Malhotra R, Siew ED: Biomarkers for the acute detection and acute prognosis of acute kidney injury. Clin J Am Soc Nephrol 2017;12(1):149–173 [PMID: 27827308].

Mian AN, Schwartz GJ: Measurement and estimation of glomerular filtration rate in children. Adv Chronic Kidney Dis 2017 Nov;24(6):348–356 [PMID: 29229165].

Pierce CB, Muñoz A, Ng DK, Warady BA, Furth SL, Schwartz GJ: Age and sex dependent clinical equations to estimate glomerular filtration rates in children and young adults with chronic kidney disease. Kidney Int 2021;99(4):948–956 [PMID: 33301749].

Viteri B, Calle-Toro JS, Furth S, Darge K, Hartung EA, Otero H: State-of-the-art renal imaging in children. Pediatrics 2020; 145(2):e20190829 [PMID: 31915193].

CONGENITAL ANOMALIES OF THE URINARY TRACT

RENAL PARENCHYMAL ANOMALIES

About 10% of children have congenital anomalies of the genitourinary tract, which range in severity from asymptomatic to lethal. Congenital anomalies of the kidney and urinary tract (CAKUT) may arise from mutations in a multitude of different single genes. Some asymptomatic abnormalities may have significant implications. For example, patients with a horseshoe kidney (kidneys fused in their lower poles), although very rarely associated with reduction in kidney function, have a higher incidence of renal calculi. Unilateral agenesis or multicystic dysplasia is usually accompanied by compensatory hypertrophy of the contralateral kidney, and thus is typically associated with normal renal function. Supernumerary kidneys are often of no significance while ectopic kidneys have an increased incidence of VUR. Abnormal genitourinary tract development can be associated with varying degrees of renal dysplasia and dysfunction ranging from mild to severe. Bilateral renal agenesis, without prenatal intervention to support lung development, is associated with anhydramnios, abnormal facies and limb anomalies from fetal compression, and perinatal death from pulmonary hypoplasia (Potter sequence).

Renal Dysplasia

Renal dysplasia constitutes a spectrum of anomalies. In simple hypoplasia, which may be unilateral or bilateral, the affected kidneys are smaller than normal. In some forms of dysplasia, immature undifferentiated renal tissue persists. The number of functional nephrons may be insufficient to sustain normal renal function once the child reaches a critical body size. The lack of adequate renal tissue is not always readily discernible in the newborn period in the presence of normal or often increased urine production. Other forms of renal dysplasia include oligomeganephronia (presence of only a few large glomeruli) and cystic dysplasia (characterized by renal cysts).

Polycystic Kidney Disease

Simple renal cysts are rare in children, and the presence of multiple simple cysts should raise concern for underlying polycystic kidney disease. Both forms of polycystic kidney disease, autosomal recessive (ARPKD) and dominant (ADPKD), are increasingly diagnosed by prenatal ultrasound.

In its most severe form, ARPKD kidneys are dysfunctional in utero, and newborns may demonstrate Potter sequence. In less severe cases, kidney enlargement by cysts may initially be recognized when nephromegaly is noted on physical examination. Hypertension is an early problem in ARPKD. The rate of progression of CKD varies in ARPKD, but many children with a neonatal renal presentation reach end-stage renal disease (ESRD) by school age. Studies suggest wide variation in phenotype, even within families. Some patients present in early adulthood with liver dysfunction from congenital hepatic fibrosis with moderate nephromegaly and mild to moderate CKD.

With advances in radiographic imaging, ADPKD is being diagnosed earlier in life, including prenatally. Children with ADPKD can manifest many of the same findings as adults with ADPKD, such as enlarged kidneys, pain, hematuria, proteinuria, hypertension, kidney stones, and extrarenal cysts (pancreas, spleen, liver), although advanced CKD and intracranial aneurysms are rare in childhood. Routine monitoring for hypertension is indicated in children with or known to be at risk for ADPKD. Because cysts grow over time, a normal renal ultrasound does not exclude ADPKD in an at-risk child (ie, parent known to have ADPKD). Approximately one-half of patients with ADPKD reach ESRD by 60 years of age. Rarely ADPKD can present with Potter sequence or severe neonatal manifestations.

Medullary Cystic Disease/Nephronophthisis

Medullary cystic disease and nephronophthisis are inherited conditions with similar renal morphology characterized by bilateral small corticomedullary cysts in normal to small kidneys with tubulointerstitial scarring leading to ESRD. Numerous causative genes have been identified in nephronophthisis, all of which encode for proteins expressed in the primary cilia of renal epithelial cells, leading to classification as ciliopathies. Children with nephronophthisis manifest impaired urinary concentration leading to polyuria and polydipsia with progressive CKD in childhood or adolescence. Extrarenal involvement including retinitis pigmentosa, hepatic fibrosis, skeletal defects, cerebellar vermis aplasia, or other abnormalities can help target specific gene analysis. Several forms of autosomal dominant medullary cystic disease exist, usually presenting with adult-onset renal failure and no extrarenal involvement. However, uromodulin-associated kidney disease with hyperuricemia and renal failure can be seen in adolescents and should be considered in patients presenting with gout and CKD.

Bergmann C, Guay-Woodford LM, Harris PC, Horie S, Peters DJM, Torres VE: Polycystic kidney disease. Nat Rev Dis Primers 2018;4(1):50 [PMID: 30523303].

McConnachie DJ, Stow JL, Mallett AJ: Ciliopathies and the kidney: a review. Am J Kidney Dis 2021;77(3):410–419 [PMID:33039432].

Murugapoopathy V, Gupta IR: A primer on congenital anomalies of the kidneys and urinary tracts (CAKUT). Clin J Am Soc Nephrol 2020;15(5):723–731 [PMID: 32188635].

Stonebrook E, Hoff M, Spencer JD: Congenital anomalies of the kidney and urinary tract: a clinical review. Curr Treat Options Pediatr 2019;5(3):223–235 [PMID: 32864297].

DISTAL URINARY TRACT ANOMALIES

Obstructive Uropathy

Obstruction at the ureteropelvic junction may be the result of intrinsic muscle abnormalities, aberrant vessels, or fibrous bands. The lesion can cause hydronephrosis and usually presents as prenatal hydronephrosis, an abdominal mass in the newborn, or recurrent abdominal pain with vomiting in an older child (Dietl's crisis). Obstruction can occur in other parts of the ureter, especially at the ureterovesical junction, causing proximal hydroureter and hydronephrosis. Renal radionuclide scan with furosemide "wash-out" will reveal or rule out ureteral obstruction as the cause of the hydronephrosis. Whether intrinsic or extrinsic, urinary tract obstruction should be relieved as soon as possible to minimize damage to the kidneys.

Severe bladder malformations such as exstrophy are clinically obvious and a surgical challenge. More subtle—but urgent in terms of diagnosis—is obstruction of urine flow from vestigial posterior urethral valves (PUVs). This anomaly, which occurs exclusively in males, may be detected prenatally with an enlarged muscular bladder and hydroureteronephrosis. Neonates may demonstrate a poor voiding stream or eventual UTI. The kidneys and bladder may be easily palpable. Although rare, ureteric perforation proximal to the obstruction may produce urinary ascites. Decompression of the bladder, most often accomplished via urethral catheterization, is critical in children with PUV to prevent irreversible kidney damage.

Eagle-Barrett (prune belly) syndrome is an association of urinary tract anomalies with cryptorchidism and absent abdominal musculature. Renal dysplasia and/or functional urinary tract obstruction may lead to ESRD. Timely urinary diversion is essential to sustain renal function.

The goals of care for children with urologic abnormalities resulting in severe compromise and destruction of renal tissue is to preserve remaining renal function, prevent UTI and potential related renal scarring, and treat complications of progressive CKD. Collaboration between the pediatric urologist and nephrologist, ideally in a multidisciplinary clinic, with early co-management and ongoing follow-up is essential.

Reflux Nephropathy

The retrograde flow of urine from the bladder into the ureter (VUR), when high grade, may cause renal scarring and subsequent CKD and hypertension, especially in the setting of UTIs. Hydronephrosis on renal ultrasound suggests the possibility of VUR or obstruction. Absence of hydronephrosis on ultrasonography does not, however, rule out the possibility of VUR. VUR is most often diagnosed with a VCUG. Low-grade VUR typically resolves spontaneously over time. Prophylactic antibiotics may be administered depending on the child's age, degree of VUR, and frequency of UTI but are typically not warranted in low-grade VUR. Surgery may be required for chronic severe reflux. Appropriate management of reflux nephropathy includes prevention and prompt treatment of UTI, monitoring and management of hypertension and complications of CKD, and consideration of angiotensin-converting enzyme (ACE) inhibition to prevent glomerular hyperfiltration.

American Urological Association Guidelines: https://www.auanet.org/.

HEMATURIA & GLOMERULAR DISEASE

HEMATURIA

Children with painful hematuria should be investigated for UTI or direct injury to the urinary tract. Dysuria is common in cystitis or urethritis; associated back pain and/or fever suggests the possibility of pyelonephritis, and colicky flank pain may indicate the passage of a stone. Bright red blood or clots in the urine can also be associated with bleeding disorders, trauma, arteriovenous malformations, and viral cystitis caused by adenovirus. Abdominal masses suggest the presence of urinary tract obstruction, cystic disease, or tumors of the renal or perirenal structures.

Asymptomatic hematuria requires clinical and diagnostic data to determine whether nephrology evaluation is needed. The diagnosis of hematuria should not rely solely on a urine dipstick evaluation for blood and must be verified by a microscopic RBC count (normal < 5 RBC/hpf). Evaluation for hypercalciuria as a cause of hematuria with a random urine calcium/creatinine ratio (both values in mg/dL) is one of the initial steps in the evaluation of hematuria. A value greater than 0.2 mg/mg requires verification with a 24-hour urine collection when possible (hypercalciuria is present with calcium excretion > 4 mg/kg/day) and should prompt referral to pediatric nephrology. Figure 24–1 delineates the outpatient approach to hematuria. The primary concern in the differential diagnosis of hematuria is the possible presence of glomerular disease.

GLOMERULONEPHRITIS

ESSENTIALS OF DIAGNOSIS & TYPICAL FEATURES

Classic features of GN:

▶ Hematuria

▶ Edema

▶ Hypertension

▶ RBC casts in the urine

The various types of glomerulonephritis (GN) have similar clinical manifestations. The defining features of GN include hematuria, urinary RBC casts, hypertension, and edema. Hematuria may be microscopic or gross (often coffee- or tea-colored). While RBC casts are often present, their absence does not exclude the diagnosis of GN. Urine protein excretion may range from normal (Pr/Cr ratio < 0.2 mg/mg) to nephrotic range (Pr/Cr ratio > 2 mg/mg). Edema (periorbital, facial, extremities, ascites) occurs due to salt and water

retention with impaired glomerular function and contributes to systemic hypertension, which is further exacerbated by the glomerular inflammation and associated renin production. Affected children require evaluation of BP, renal function, serum albumin, and urine protein excretion. Serum C3 concentration is helpful to distinguish certain types of GN (depressed in postinfectious and membranoproliferative (MPGN)/C3 glomerulopathy (C3GN), GN due to SLE, and GN related to ventriculoatrial shunt infection or endocarditis). Renal biopsy may be indicated for diagnostic purposes and to guide therapy.

Severe glomerular histopathologic and clinical entities such as anti-GBM antibody disease (Goodpasture syndrome), granulomatosis with polyangiitis (GPA), microscopic polyangiitis (MPA), and crescentic IgA nephropathy may be considered in the differential diagnosis of acute GN but are unusual in children. Many of these diagnoses may be rapidly progressive, and affected children often present with AKI.

Acute Postinfectious Glomerulonephritis

The diagnosis of postinfectious GN (PIGN) is supported by a recent history of infection, typically within the preceding 7–14 days and most commonly group A β-hemolytic streptococcal pharyngitis or impetigo. If a positive culture is not available, recent infection may be supported by elevated antistreptococcal antibodies. However, documentation of elevated antistreptococcal antibodies alone does not confirm that GN is poststreptococcal in nature. Postinfectious GN is associated with depressed serum C3 complement and normal serum C4. The manifestations range from asymptomatic microhematuria to gross hematuria with nephrotic range proteinuria and AKI.

Typical postinfectious GN requires no specific treatment. Antibiotic therapy is indicated if an active infection is documented. Disturbances in renal function and resulting hypertension require close monitoring. Reduction in salt intake, diuretics, and other antihypertensive drugs, such as calcium channel blockers (CCBs), are used to address edema and hypertension. In cases of severe renal failure, dialysis may be necessary. Corticosteroids may also be considered for severe GN. In most cases, full recovery occurs and complement levels return to normal in 6–8 weeks, but microscopic hematuria may persist for as long as a year.

IgA Nephropathy

IgA nephropathy is the most common cause of GN and typically presents with asymptomatic gross hematuria, with or without proteinuria, concurrently with a minor acute illness or other stressful occurrence. IgA nephropathy may be accompanied by flank pain or dysuria; serum complement is normal. Gross hematuria typically resolves within days, and there are no serious sequelae in 85% of children. Treatment is not generally indicated, and the prognosis is generally good. Prognosis is guarded, however, if proteinuria, hypertension, or AKI occurs. In such instances, although no treatment is universally accepted, corticosteroids and other immunosuppressive drugs are used after confirmatory kidney biopsy. Omega-3 fatty acids from fish oils are also thought to be helpful by inhibiting macrophage infiltration of the glomerular mesangium.

IgA Vasculitis

IgA vasculitis, formerly known as Henoch-Schönlein purpura (HSP), is typically a clinical diagnosis based on the presence of a purpuric rash found primarily, but not exclusively, on the dependent surfaces of the lower extremities and buttocks, in addition to one or more of the following clinical manifestations: arthritis or arthralgias, abdominal pain, and renal involvement (hematuria, proteinuria). Hypertension may also be present. Renal involvement ranges from none to mild GN with microhematuria to severe GN with associated nephrosis and AKI. Ninety percent of children who will develop nephritis present by 8 weeks and 97% within the first 6 months after diagnosis; screening for renal involvement, therefore, should occur at regular intervals during this time. Kidney biopsy is rarely required but should be performed when there is severe renal involvement. Lupus- and ANCA-associated vasculitis should be considered in the appropriate setting, particularly in adolescents. The renal histologic lesion of IgA vasculitis is identical to that of IgA nephropathy. IgA vasculitis is usually self-limited. Joint and abdominal pains respond to treatment with short courses of corticosteroids. More severe renal involvement is associated with worse long-term prognosis, including potential for progression to ESRD. There is no universally accepted treatment for renal involvement, but corticosteroids and other immunosuppressive agents are often administered (see also Chapter 30).

Immune Complex Membranoproliferative Glomerulonephritis and C3 Glomerulopathy

Membranoproliferative glomerulonephritis (MPGN), a hypocomplementemic form of GN, is classified into immune complex MPGN (IC-MPGN) and C3 glomerulopathy (C3GN). In contrast to adults in whom IC-MPGN is most often associated with chronic infections and autoimmune disease, the disease in children is most often idiopathic. C3GN is caused by underlying dysregulation of the alternative complement pathway and, in children, is usually related to the presence of autoantibodies to complement (eg, C3 nephritic factor) or genetic mutations in complement-related genes. There is a wide phenotypic spectrum of these conditions. They typically are associated with depressed serum C3, and diagnosis is established by kidney biopsy. Treatment consists of corticosteroids and other immunosuppressive agents that may include targeted blockade of components of the complement system.

Lupus Nephritis

The diagnosis of SLE is based on its numerous clinical features and abnormal laboratory findings that include a positive ANA test, depressed serum complements C3 and C4, and increased serum antibodies to double-stranded DNA. Renal involvement occurs in more than 50% of children with SLE; more severe cases are accompanied by AKI and hypertension. Renal disease should be assessed by renal biopsy to establish the class of lupus nephritis and direct therapy. Lupus nephritis requires treatment with various combinations of immunosuppressive drugs, including prednisone, azathioprine, cyclophosphamide, mycophenolate, tacrolimus or volcosporin, rituximab, and belimumab. ESRD develops in 10%–15% of patients with childhood SLE.

Hereditary Glomerulonephritis

The most common hereditary GN is Alport syndrome, due to mutations in type IV collagen found in basement membranes of the glomeruli, cochlea, and lens, and characterized by progressive GN, high-frequency sensorineural hearing loss, and lens abnormalities. Although the condition can be inherited in autosomal dominant or recessive manners, the vast majority of cases are X-linked and males are typically more severely affected. Males with X-linked disease and children with autosomal recessive disease typically present early with persistent microhematuria and recurrent gross hematuria associated with intercurrent illness, followed by chronic proteinuria and then deterioration in renal function with ESRD usually occurring in the second to third decade of life. Females with X-linked Alport syndrome have a wide spectrum of manifestations, from asymptomatic hematuria to ESRD. A family history may be present, but there is a spontaneous mutation rate of about 20%. Although there is no cure for this disorder, early initiation of ACE inhibitors (ACEIs) has been shown to improve renal outcomes.

Eison TM, Ault BH, Jones DP, Chesney RW, Wyatt RJ: Post-streptococcal acute glomerulonephritis in children: clinical features and pathogenesis. Pediatr Nephrol 2011;26(2):165–180 [PMID: 20652330].

Hastings MC et al: IgA vasculitis with nephritis: update of the pathogenesis with clinical implications. Pediatr Nephrol 2022;37(4):719–733 [PMID: 33818625].

Kashtan CE, Gross O: Clinical practice recommendations for the diagnosis and management of Alport syndrome in children, adolescents, and young adults—an update for 2020. Pediatr Nephrol 2021;36(3):711–719 [PMID: 33159213].

Kidney Disease Improving Global Outcomes (KDIGO) Glomerulonephritis guidelines: https://kdigo.org.

Oni L, Wright RD, Beresford MW, Tullus K: Kidney outcomes for children with lupus nephritis. Pediatr Nephrol 2021;36(6):1377–1385 [PMID: 32725543].

Smith RJH et al: C3 glomerulopathy—understanding a rare complement-driven renal disease. Nat Rev Nephrol 2019;15:129–143 [PMID: 30692664].

TUBULOINTERSTITIAL DISEASE

ACUTE INTERSTITIAL NEPHRITIS

Acute interstitial nephritis is characterized by diffuse or focal inflammation and edema of the renal interstitium and secondary involvement of the tubules. The condition is most commonly drug-related (eg, β-lactam–containing antibiotics or nonsteroidal anti-inflammatory drugs [NSAIDs]), but infectious etiologies, including Epstein-Barr virus, also occur. Fever, rash, and eosinophilia may occur in drug-associated cases. Urinalysis usually reveals leukocyturia and, potentially, mild hematuria and proteinuria, or it can be entirely bland. Hansel staining of the urinary sediment may demonstrate eosinophils, although this is not specific to acute interstitial nephritis and is infrequently performed clinically. The inflammation can cause significant deterioration of renal function and systemic hypertension. The association between tubulointerstitial nephritis and uveitis (TINU) is occasionally seen in childhood. If the diagnosis is unclear, a kidney biopsy may be performed to demonstrate characteristic tubular and interstitial inflammation. Immediate identification and removal of the causative agent, whenever possible, is imperative and may be all that is necessary. Treatment with corticosteroids or other immunomodulatory agents may be needed in patients with severe AKI or associated nephrotic syndrome. Dialysis support is occasionally required.

Perazella MA: Clinical approach to diagnosing acute and chronic tubulointerstitial disease. Adv Chronic Kidney Dis 2017 Mar;24(2):57–63 [PMID: 28284380].

PROTEINURIA & RENAL DISEASE

Urine is rarely completely protein free, but the average excretion is well below 150 mg/24 h. Small increases in urinary protein, transient proteinuria, can accompany febrile illnesses or exertion and in some cases occur while in the upright posture (orthostatic proteinuria). An algorithm for investigation of isolated proteinuria is presented in Figure 24–2.

CONGENITAL & INFANTILE NEPHROSIS

Congenital and infantile nephrosis, also known as congenital and infantile nephrotic syndrome, is a rare set of diseases that present within the first year of life. Congenital typically refers to onset within the first 3 months of life and infantile typically within 3–12 months of life. Most cases are caused by monogenic mutations, but some are caused by congenital infections or mercury poisoning. Five main genetic mutations account for the majority of congenital and infantile nephrotic syndrome. Congenital nephrotic syndrome of the Finnish type is a rare autosomal recessive disorder caused by genetic mutations in NPHS1. Mutations in NPHS2 typically cause autosomal recessive familial focal segmental glomerulosclerosis

(FSGS) but can also present similarly to Finnish type congenital nephrotic syndrome. Mutations in WT1 (Wilms tumor-1) typically lead to characteristic diffuse mesangial sclerosis on kidney biopsy and are associated with Denys-Drash syndrome (male pseudo-hermaphroditism, rapidly progressive glomerulopathy and risk of Wilms tumor) and Frasier syndrome (male pseudo-hermaphroditism and gonadoblastoma without Wilms tumor). Mutations in PLCE1 may manifest as congenital nephrotic syndrome, and mutations in LAMB2 are associated with Pierson syndrome (congenital nephrotic syndrome with ocular anomalies).

Infants with congenital nephrosis, especially the Finnish type, may have markedly elevated maternal serum α-fetoprotein concentration, a large placenta, wide cranial sutures, and delayed ossification. Progressive edema may be seen after the first few weeks of life. Massive urine protein losses may lead to recurrent infection due to hypogammaglobulinemia (urinary loss of immunoglobulin G), thrombosis (urinary loss of antithrombin III, protein C and S), clinical hypothyroidism (urinary loss of thyroid-binding globulin), and severe hyperlipidemia. Children with large protein losses usually require nightly albumin infusions. They may also be managed with intravenous immunoglobulin (IVIG) infusions, although their utility is unclear, as the majority of the IVIG is lost in the urine within hours. These infants also require intensive nutritional care and high protein diets. Nephrectomies may be required to prevent complications of high-grade protein loss. Progressive renal failure requiring dialysis and transplantation is anticipated. The exception is Co-Q2 nephropathy, a group of mitochondrial diseases that cause congenital nephrotic syndrome that can be effectively treated with high dose Co-Q10 supplementation.

Boyer O et al: Management of congenital nephrotic syndrome: consensus recommendations of the ERKNet-ESPN Working Group. Nat Rev Nephrol 2021 Apr;17(4):277–289 [PMID: 33514942].
Starr MC et al: COQ2 nephropathy: a treatable cause of nephrotic syndrome in children. Pediatr Nephrol 2018 Jul;33(7):1257–1261. doi: 10.1007/s00467-018-3937-z. Epub 2018 Apr 10 [PMID: 29637272].

IDIOPATHIC NEPHROTIC SYNDROME OF CHILDHOOD

ESSENTIALS OF DIAGNOSIS & TYPICAL FEATURES

Classic features of nephrotic syndrome:

▶ Proteinuria

▶ Hypoalbuminemia

▶ Edema

▶ Hyperlipidemia

Clinical Findings

Affected patients are generally < 10 years at onset. Typically, periorbital swelling is noted, often following intercurrent illness. Within a few days, increasing edema—even anasarca—becomes evident. Most children have few complaints other than vague malaise or abdominal pain. With significant hypoalbuminemia, some children experience symptoms of intestinal malabsorption, and, with marked edema, dyspnea due to pleural effusions or massive ascites may occur.

Despite heavy proteinuria, the urine sediment is usually normal, although microscopic hematuria may be present. Gross hematuria is occasionally seen, more often with FSGS than with minimal change disease (MCD), the most common cause of idiopathic nephrotic syndrome in children. Plasma albumin concentration is low and lipid levels are increased. Kidney function is generally normal in children with MCD. When azotemia occurs, it is usually secondary to intravascular volume depletion.

Complications

Infections (eg, peritonitis, sepsis), frequently caused by encapsulated bacteria such as *Streptococcus pneumoniae*, sometimes occur. Hypercoagulability may lead to thromboembolic phenomena such as deep venous thrombosis, renal vein thrombosis, or sagittal sinus thrombosis. Hypertension may be present, and AKI can result from decreased renal perfusion. Hyperlipidemia resolves when affected children enter remission but is of concern in treatment-resistant nephrotic syndrome.

Treatment & Prognosis

When the diagnosis of idiopathic nephrotic syndrome is made, corticosteroid treatment should be started, as this will induce remission in the vast majority of children. Prednisone, 60 mg/m^2 or 2 mg/kg/day (maximum, 60 mg/day), is given for 6 weeks as a single daily dose. A dose of 40 mg/m^2 or 1.5 mg/kg/day is then administered on an alternate-day schedule for 6 weeks. Thereafter, corticosteroids are discontinued, or the dose is tapered gradually and discontinued over the ensuing few months. The goal of this regimen is disappearance of proteinuria. If remission is not achieved during the initial 6 weeks of corticosteroid treatment, steroid-sparing therapy and kidney biopsy should be considered. If remission is achieved but followed by relapse, the treatment course may be repeated. A renal biopsy is often considered when there is little or no response to treatment or in children older than 12 years due to decreased likelihood of MCD.

Careful clinical assessment of intravascular volume status is indicated to guide diuretic therapy in children with idiopathic nephrotic syndrome. While those with obvious evidence of volume overload will benefit from diuretics, some children will show evidence of intravascular volume depletion due to third space fluid leak. The latter group will experience hypotension and prerenal azotemia with aggressive diuresis; thus, careful restoration of compromised circulating volume with intravenous 25% albumin infusion with consideration of a diuretic such as furosemide is most helpful in mobilizing edema. Infections such as peritonitis should be treated promptly to reduce morbidity. Immunization with pneumococcal conjugate and polysaccharide vaccines is advised due to the increased risk of invasive pneumococcal disease.

Resolution of proteinuria with corticosteroid treatment suggests a good prognosis. Early relapse usually heralds a prolonged series of relapses; frequent relapses increase corticosteroid exposure and should lead to consideration of alternate immunosuppressive therapy to maintain remission. Calcineurin inhibitors (most commonly tacrolimus), mycophenolate mofetil, and rituximab are currently used as steroid-sparing agents. Children who fail to respond to corticosteroids have a more guarded long-term prognosis for renal function yet may still attain remission with alternative immunosuppressive agents.

FOCAL SEGMENTAL GLOMERULOSCLEROSIS

Focal segmental glomerulosclerosis (FSGS) is a cause of idiopathic nephrotic syndrome in children but can also cause chronic asymptomatic proteinuria. Active nephrotic syndrome is treated as above (see Idiopathic Nephrotic Syndrome of Childhood section); the benefits of chronic immunosuppressive therapy are less clear in the asymptomatic child. The response of FSGS to corticosteroid treatment is variable, and up to 15%–20% of FSGS progresses to end-stage renal failure. Recurrence of FSGS is common following renal transplantation. Fortunately, most children respond well to treatment with plasmapheresis and/or rituximab after kidney transplantation.

MEMBRANOUS NEPHROPATHY

Although most often idiopathic, membranous nephropathy (MN) can be found in association with infections, including hepatitis B, hepatitis C, and congenital syphilis; with immunologic disorders such as autoimmune thyroiditis and SLE (in contrast to other forms of lupus nephritis, serum C3 is often normal with membranous lupus); and with administration of drugs such as penicillamine. Patients with idiopathic MN have autoantibodies to podocyte antigens, including phospholipase A2 receptor (PLA2R), thrombospondin type-1 domain-containing 7A (THSD7A), neural epidermal growth factor-like 1 (NELL1), and others.

MN occurs more often in older children and adults. The onset may be insidious or may resemble that of idiopathic nephrotic syndrome of childhood. Proteinuria in MN may respond poorly to corticosteroid therapy and secondary immunomodulatory agents are often prescribed. Historically, alkylating agents such as cyclophosphamide were used with corticosteroid therapy, while more recently calcineurin inhibitors, mycophenolate mofetil and rituximab have been explored with some success. The diagnosis is made by renal biopsy, although patients with positive serum anti-PLA2R antibodies may not need a biopsy.

Ronco P et al: Membranous nephropathy. Nat Rev Dis Primers 2021;7:69 [PMID: 34593809].

Trautmann A et al: IPNA clinical practice recommendations for the diagnosis and management of children with steroid-resistant nephrotic syndrome. Pediatr Nephrol 2020;35:529–1561 [PMID: 32382828].

Trautmann A et al: IPNA clinical practice recommendations for the diagnosis and management of children with steroid-sensitive nephrotic syndrome. Pediatr Nephrol 2023;38:877–919 [PMID: 36269406].

DISEASES OF THE RENAL VESSELS

RENAL VEIN THROMBOSIS

In newborns, renal vein thrombosis may complicate sepsis or dehydration. It may be observed in infants of diabetic mothers, may be associated with umbilical vein catheterization, or may result from any condition that produces a hypercoagulable state (eg, clotting factor deficiency or thrombocytosis). Renal vein thrombosis is less common in older children and adolescents, but may develop following trauma, with a procoagulant state (such as antiphospholipid antibody positivity in SLE or treatment-resistant nephrotic syndrome), or without any apparent predisposing factors. Spontaneous renal vein thrombosis has been associated with MN.

▶ Clinical Findings

Renal vein thrombosis in newborns is generally characterized by the sudden development of an abdominal mass. If the thrombosis is bilateral, oliguria may be present. In older children, flank pain, sometimes with a palpable mass, is a common presentation. No single laboratory test is diagnostic of renal vein thrombosis. Hematuria usually is present and may occasionally be gross in nature; proteinuria is less constant. In the newborn, thrombocytopenia may be found, but it is rare in older children. The diagnosis is made by ultrasonography and Doppler flow studies.

▶ Treatment

Anticoagulation with heparin is the treatment of choice in newborns and older children. In the newborn, a course of heparin combined with treatment of the underlying problem is usually all that is required; risks of systemic anticoagulation in the newborn, particularly if preterm, must be considered. Evaluation for thrombophilia may be indicated. In children

with an identified condition that predisposes to recurrence, longer-term anticoagulation may be required.

▶ Course & Prognosis

The mortality rate in newborns from renal vein thrombosis depends on the underlying cause. Extension into the vena cava with pulmonary emboli is possible. With unilateral renal venous thrombosis at any age, the prognosis for adequate renal function is good. Bilateral disease is more concerning, and long-term renal follow-up focusing on renal function and growth is warranted in such children. Renal vein thrombosis may rarely recur in the same kidney or in the other kidney years after the original episode.

RENAL ARTERIAL DISEASE

Arterial disease (eg, fibromuscular dysplasia, congenital renal artery or mid-aortic stenosis, Takayasu arteritis) is a rare cause of hypertension in children. Although few clinical clues are specific to underlying arterial lesions, they should be suspected in children with severe hypertension, onset at or before age 10 years, or hypertension that is increasingly difficult to control. The diagnosis is established by MR or CT angiography and confirmed by renal arteriography or direct intraoperative visualization. When vasculitis is present, immunosuppressive treatment is the first approach. Other lesions may be approached by transluminal angioplasty or surgery (see Hypertension section), but repair may be technically impossible in small children, for whom medical management is indicated pending somatic growth. Although thrombosis of renal arteries is rare, it should be considered in a patient with acute onset of hypertension and hematuria in an appropriate setting (eg, in association with hyperviscosity or umbilical artery catheterization). Early diagnosis and treatment provide the best chance of reestablishing renal blood flow.

HEMOLYTIC-UREMIC SYNDROME

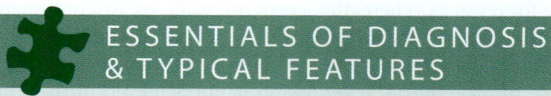

ESSENTIALS OF DIAGNOSIS & TYPICAL FEATURES

Classic features of hemolytic-uremic syndrome (HUS):
► Microangiopathic hemolytic anemia
► Thrombocytopenia
► Acute kidney injury

HUS is the most common cause of AKI in childhood. The diarrhea-associated form is usually the result of infection with Shiga toxin–producing strains of *Escherichia coli* (STEC) or, less commonly, shigella. Undercooked ground beef or unpasteurized foods are common sources. Many serotypes of Shiga toxin-producing bacteria cause HUS, but the most common pathogen in the United States is *E. coli* O157:H7. Bloody diarrhea is the usual presenting complaint, followed by hemolysis, thrombocytopenia, and AKI. Circulating toxin causes endothelial damage, which leads to platelet deposition/consumption and microvascular occlusion with subsequent hemolysis. Similar microvascular endothelial activation may also be triggered by drugs (eg, calcineurin inhibitors or mammalian target of rapamycin inhibitors); viruses (human immunodeficiency virus [HIV]); and pneumococcal infections, in which bacterial neuraminidase exposes the Thomsen-Friedenreich antigen on RBCs, platelets, and endothelial cells, with associated cell lysis. Rare cases, referred to as atypical HUS, are caused by genetically mediated complement dysregulation (eg, factor H deficiency).

Clinical Findings

HUS due to *E. coli* or shigella begins with a prodrome of abdominal pain, diarrhea (frequently bloody), and vomiting. Children with pneumococcus-associated HUS typically have documented pneumococcal pneumonia, sepsis, or meningitis. Children with atypical HUS associated with complement dysregulation often develop an episode of HUS following intercurrent illness and present with malaise and pallor. Hypertension and seizures develop in some children—especially those who develop severe renal failure and fluid overload. There may also be significant endothelial involvement affecting the central nervous system (CNS), heart, and pancreas. Anemia may be profound, and RBC fragments (schistocytes) are seen on blood smears. A high reticulocyte count, increased lactate dehydrogenase, and low haptoglobin are all consistent with hemolysis, but an elevated reticulocyte count may not be noted in the presence of renal failure. Thrombocytopenia is often severe, while other coagulation abnormalities are less consistent. Serum fibrin split products are often present, but fulminant disseminated intravascular coagulation is rare. Hematuria and proteinuria are often present, and hemoglobinuria is occasionally observed due to marked RBC hemolysis.

Complications

Complications of AKI occur. Neurologic problems, particularly seizures, and posterior reversible encephalopathy syndrome (PRES), may result from hyponatremia, hypertension, or CNS vascular disease. Despite thrombocytopenia, many children are prone to thrombosis due to the underlying endothelial damage.

Treatment

Meticulous attention to fluid and electrolyte status is crucial. The use of antimotility agents and antibiotics for HUS caused by gastrointestinal infection is believed to worsen the disease. RBC transfusions are often necessary and have also been associated with improved prognosis. Platelet transfusions should be avoided unless there is active bleeding. Atypical HUS due to complement dysregulation is treated with the anti-C5a monoclonal antibody, eculizumab, or with the longer acting C5 inhibitor, ravulizumab. Whether eculizumab may be of benefit in other forms of HUS remains to be determined. Plasma infusions should be avoided in pneumococcal HUS as it provides the patient with anti–Thomsen-Friedenreich antibody, further driving the HUS process. Although no therapy is universally accepted, strict control of hypertension and fluid balance, adequate nutrition support, and the timely use of dialysis reduce morbidity and mortality. If renal failure is non-oliguric and if urine output is sufficient to ensure against fluid overload and electrolyte abnormalities, management of renal failure without dialysis is possible.

Course & Prognosis

Most commonly, children with STEC HUS recover from the acute episode within 2–3 weeks. Residual renal disease (including hypertension, proteinuria, or CKD) occurs in about 30%, and end-stage renal failure occurs in about 15%. The risk of ESRD is higher in children with atypical or pneumococcal-induced HUS. Follow-up of children recovering from HUS should include serial determinations of renal function, with frequency dictated by the etiology, course, and subsequent findings, and routine monitoring of BP. Overall mortality (about 3%–5%) is most likely in the early phase, primarily from CNS or cardiac complications. As with most renal conditions, chronic proteinuria, hypertension, or abnormal renal function are associated with worse long-term renal prognosis.

Boyer O, Niaudet P: Hemolytic-uremic syndrome in children. Pediatr Clin North Am 2022 Dec;69(6):1181–1197. doi: 10.1016/j.pcl.2022.07.006. Epub 2022 Oct 29 [PMID: 36880929].
Harkins VJ, McAllister DA, Reynolds BC: Shiga-toxin *E. coli* hemolytic uremic syndrome: review of management and long-term outcome. Curr Pediatr Rep 2020;8:16–25 [PMID: 36595068].

RENAL FAILURE

ACUTE KIDNEY INJURY

The term "acute kidney injury" (AKI) denotes the sudden inability to excrete urine of sufficient quantity (decrease in urine output) or composition (increase in serum creatinine), or both. Explanations are typically divided into prerenal (decrease in blood flow to kidneys), renal (intrinsic kidney problems), and postrenal (blockage of urine outflow) causes (Table 24–1). Criteria for diagnosing AKI (KDIGO guidelines) include (a) increase in serum creatinine greater than 0.3 mg/dL in 48 hours, (b) increase in serum creatinine

Table 24–1. Classification of AKI.

Prerenal
  Intravascular volume depletion (gastrointestinal, skin, or renal losses; significantly diminished intake; hemorrhage)
  Diminished effective circulating volume (low-output cardiac failure, nephrotic syndrome, capillary leak, cirrhosis)
  Aortic or renal vessel injury
  Renal arterial thrombosis

Renal
  Hemolytic-uremic syndrome
  Renal vascular thrombosis
  Glomerulonephritis
  Nephrotoxins
  Acute tubular necrosis
  Renal (cortical) necrosis
  Tubular crystalluria (sulfonamide uric acid, tumor lysis)
  Pigment nephropathy (ATN)
  Contrast nephropathy
  Interstitial nephritis
  Trauma

Postrenal
  Obstruction due to tumor, hematoma, posterior urethral valves, ureteropelvic junction stricture, ureterovesical junction stricture, ureterocele, other bladder outlet, narcotic-induced urinary retention, stones, obstructed bladder catheter

Note: Any of the prerenal etiologies of renal failure can evolve into acute tubular nephropathy when prolonged.

more than 1.5 times baseline as compared to a measurement 7 days prior, or (c) decrease in urine volume to less than 0.5 mL/kg/h × 6 hours.

► Clinical Findings

The hallmark of early AKI is oliguria with subsequent variable rise in serum creatinine and BUN; these observations are more likely to be recognized in a hospitalized patient. Although an exact etiologic diagnosis may be unclear at the onset, classifying AKI as outlined in Table 24–1 is helpful in determining if an immediately reversible cause is present. Staging of the severity of AKI is most commonly done with the KDIGO criteria (Table 24–2).

A. Prerenal Causes

The most common cause of acute decreased renal function in children is compromised renal perfusion. It is usually secondary to true intravascular volume depletion, critical hypotension or a decrease in effective circulating volume, as may be seen in cardiac failure, cirrhosis, or nephrotic syndrome. Alternatively, compromised renal perfusion may be caused by local changes to blood supply of the kidneys, resulting from either artery stenosis or renal vein thrombosis. A detailed history (assessing for vomiting, diarrhea, acute

Table 24–2. KDIGO criteria of AKI.

Stage	Serum Creatinine	Urine Output
1	1.5–1.9 times baseline OR ≥ 0.3 mg/dL increase	< 0.5 mL/kg/h for 6–12 h
2	2.0–2.9 times baseline	< 0.5 mL/kg/h for ≥ 12 h
3	3.0 times baseline OR Increase in serum creatinine to ≥ 4.0 mg/dL OR Initiation of renal replacement therapy OR In patient aged < 18 y, decrease in eGFR to < 35 mL/min per 1.73 m^2	< 0.3 mL/kg/h for ≥ 24 h OR Anuria for ≥ 12 h

AKI, acute kidney injury; eGFR, estimated glomerular filtration rate; KDIGO, Kidney Disease Improving Global Outcomes.

febrile illnesses) and physical examination (change in weight, presence of edema or ascites) will aid in diagnosis. Table 24–3 lists the urinary indices helpful in distinguishing these "prerenal" conditions from true renal parenchymal insult, such as acute tubular necrosis.

B. Renal Causes

Causes of AKI intrinsic to the kidneys include acute glomerulonephritides, HUS, acute interstitial nephritis, and nephrotoxic injury each affecting one or more anatomic parts of the kidneys: the glomerulus, tubules or interstitium. The diagnosis of acute tubular necrosis, which is reserved for those cases

Table 24–3. Urine studies for differentiating prerenal failure from renal parenchymal insults such as acute tubular necrosis.

	Prerenal Failure	Acute Tubular Necrosis
Urine osmolality	> 500	< 350
Urine-specific gravity	> 1.020	~ 1.010
Urine sodium	< 20 mEq/L	> 40 mEq/L
Fractional excretion of sodium	< 1%	> 3%
Ratio of urine creatinine to plasma creatinine	> 40:1	< 20:1
Ratio of blood urea nitrogen (BUN) to plasma creatinine	> 20:1	< 10–15

Note: Urine osmolality and sodium concentration should be interpreted in light of the child's age-related capacity for these parameters (eg, newborns have limited urinary concentrating capacity and excrete more sodium than older children).

in which renal ischemic insult is believed to be the likely cause, should be considered when correction of prerenal or postrenal problems does not improve renal function and there is no evidence of de novo renal disease. Muddy brown casts seen with urine microscopy is a characteristic finding. Rhabdomyolysis and tumor lysis syndrome are examples of nephrotoxic kidney injury, as are exposures to medications such as calcineurin inhibitors – all causing direct damage to the tubules.

C. Postrenal Causes

Postrenal failure in pediatric patients is usually due to congenital urologic anatomic abnormalities and is accompanied by varying degrees of renal insufficiency. One should always keep in mind the possibility of acute urinary tract obstruction in AKI, especially in the setting of anuria of acute onset. This is best evaluated by non-invasive imaging – specifically renal and bladder ultrasonography. Whatever the cause, ensuring urine drainage is the first step toward reversibility of oliguria. This is most effectively achieved with placement of a foley catheter via the urethra, a suprapubic tube, or percutaneous nephrostomy tubes if the lower urinary tract needs to be circumvented.

▶ Complications

The severity of the complications of AKI depends on the degree of renal functional impairment and oliguria. Common complications include (1) fluid overload (hypertension, congestive heart failure, and pulmonary edema), (2) electrolyte disturbances (hyperkalemia, hyperphosphatemia), (3) metabolic acidosis, (4) uremia, and (5) death. Patients who experience AKI are at increased risk for developing chronic kidney disease.

▶ Treatment

Prerenal and/or postrenal factors should be excluded and rectified. Normal circulating volume should be maintained, and normal BP and cardiac performance established with appropriate fluid or pressor support. Input and output should be strictly measured, with input adjusted as reduction in output dictates. Placement of a Foley bladder catheter can aid in timely measurement of output. However, in cases where oligo/anuric renal failure is well established (ie, insignificant urine volume), the foreign body should be removed to minimize bladder infection risk. Measurement of central venous pressure may be indicated. Routine assessment of weight is helpful to assess fluid balance in children in whom this is possible. Increasing urine output with diuretics, such as furosemide (1–2 mg/kg per dose, intravenously, maximum of 200 mg every 6 hours or 4 mg/kg/day), can be attempted. The effective dose will depend on the amount of functional compromise. If a response does not occur within 1 hour and the urine output remains low (< 0.5 mL/kg/h), the furosemide dose should

be maximized and a continuous infusion may be considered. In some cases, the addition of a long-acting thiazide diuretic, such as metolazone, may improve the response. If no diuresis occurs with maximum dosing, further administration of diuretics should cease and fluid intake should be restricted accordingly. The child should be monitored closely for indications for acute dialysis. All medication dosages should be adjusted as appropriate for the degree of renal clearance.

A. Acute Dialysis: Indications

Immediate indications for dialysis are (1) hyperkalemia refractory to medical management; (2) metabolic acidosis recalcitrant to medical management; (3) fluid overload (which may be manifest as significant hypertension, congestive heart failure, pulmonary edema, or simply inability to provide appropriate medication and nutritional support due to fluid restriction); (4) symptoms of uremia, usually manifested in children by CNS depression (rare); (5) ingestions of drugs/substances removed by hemodialysis (eg, lithium); and (6) hyperammonemia.

B. Methods of Dialysis

Dialysis can be achieved either through the use of the peritoneum—a vascular partially permeable membrane—(peritoneal dialysis) or through filtration of blood via an extracorporeal filter (hemodialysis). Peritoneal dialysis is often preferred in children because of ease of performance and patient tolerance. Although peritoneal dialysis is technically less efficient than hemodialysis (per hour of treatment), hemodynamic stability and metabolic control can be better sustained because this technique can be applied on a relatively continuous basis. Hemodialysis should be considered (1) if rapid removal of toxins is desired, (2) if the hemodynamic status will tolerate the intermittent solute and fluid removal, or (3) if impediments to efficient peritoneal dialysis are present (eg, postoperative abdomen, adhesions). If vascular access and potential usage of anticoagulation are not impediments, a slow, continuous form of dialysis, continuous renal replacement therapy (CRRT) may be applied in hemodynamically unstable, critically ill patients, including those on extracorporeal membrane oxygenation. Typically, either systemic or regional anticoagulation is provided to maintain the extracorporeal circuit. Nutritional support and medication doses should be reviewed and adjusted accordingly for patients receiving dialytic therapies.

C. Dialysis Management and Complications

Intravascular volume depletion can be observed in any dialytic therapy; thus, close attention to the patient's hemodynamic status (assessment of weight, BP) with adjustment in dialytic fluid removal is indicated. Significant intravascular volume depletion can contribute to acute tubular nephropathy and limit the timely recovery of intrinsic renal function.

Complications specific to peritoneal dialysis include peritonitis and technical complications such as dialysate leakage or respiratory compromise from intra-abdominal dialysate fluid. Peritonitis risk can be diminished by strict aseptic technique. Peritoneal fluid cultures and cell counts should be obtained as clinically indicated. Leakage is reduced by good catheter placement technique and appropriate intra-abdominal dialysate volumes. Adjustment of the electrolyte concentration of dialysate is important to maintain electrolyte balance. Potassium and phosphate, absent from standard dialysate solutions, can be added to the dialysate as clinically required. Several antibiotics can be added to the dialysate for intraperitoneal administration with associated systemic absorption for treatment of peritonitis or when systemic antibiotic treatment is indicated but vascular access is limited. Correction of fluid overload is accomplished with high osmolar dialysis fluids, resulting in an increase in ultrafiltration. Higher dextrose concentrations (maximum 4.25%) can correct fluid overload rapidly at the risk of causing hyperglycemia. Fluid removal may also be increased with more frequent exchanges of the dialysate, but rapid osmotic transfer of water may result in hypernatremia. Because fluid removal is dependent on many factors (osmolar load of dialysate, individual peritoneal membrane transport characteristics, peritoneal membrane perfusion), it is not possible to exactly control the hourly rate of fluid removal during peritoneal dialysis as can be done with CRRT.

Even in small infants, hemodialysis can rapidly correct major metabolic and electrolyte disturbances as well as volume overload. The process is highly efficient. Careful monitoring of appropriate biochemical parameters is important. Note that during or immediately following the procedure, blood sampling will produce misleading results because equilibration between extravascular compartments and the blood will not yet have been achieved. Appropriate vascular access must be maintained (eg, via a hemodialysis catheter or arteriovenous fistula/graft). Systemic anticoagulation, usually with heparin, is typically required. Hemodialysis is generally intermittent, daily to three times per week. If need be, CRRT may be used to maintain more minute-to-minute, continuous metabolic and fluid control, especially in the hemodynamically unstable or septic patient.

▶ Course & Prognosis

The course and prognosis of AKI vary with the etiology. When acute tubular necrosis is the cause of AKI, the concomitant oliguria usually lasts about 10 days. Should anuria or oliguria last longer than 6 weeks this is concerning for progression to cortical necrosis and limited renal recovery. The diuretic phase of recovery from AKI due to acute tubular necrosis begins with an increase in urinary output to large volumes of isosthenuric urine containing sodium levels of 80–150 mEq/L. The associated polyuria may persist for several days or weeks; appropriate hydration to prevent prerenal azotemia or acute tubular

necrosis should be ensured. Urinary abnormalities usually disappear completely within a few months.

Regardless of etiology of AKI, if renal recovery does not ensue within about 6 weeks of oligoanuria, arrangements should be made for chronic dialysis. Some children requiring prolonged (> 1 month) dialysis support will demonstrate recovery to varying degrees of CKD but are at high risk for eventual progression to ESRD. All children with history of KDIGO stage II or higher AKI are at increased risk for further AKI, hypertension, and CKD. Their risk of CKD is increased with increased severity of AKI and with repeated episodes of AKI. Children who have experienced significant AKI require long-term follow-up with a nephrologist.

John JC, Taha S, Bunchman TE: Basics of continuous renal replacement therapy in pediatrics. Kidney Res Clin Pract 2019 Dec 31; 38(4):455–461 [PMID: 31661769].

Ricci Z, Goldstein SL: Pediatric continuous renal replacement therapy. Contrib Nephrol 2016;187:121–130 [PMID: 26881430].

Ronco C, Bellomo R, Kellum JA: Acute kidney injury. Lancet 2019;394(10212):1949–1964 [PMID: 31777389].

Sigurjonsdottir VK, Chaturvedi S, Mammen C, Sutherland SM: Pediatric acute kidney injury and the subsequent risk for chronic kidney disease: is there cause for alarm? Pediatr Nephrol 2018 Nov;33(11):2047–2055 [PMID: 29374316].

Sutherland SM, Kwiatkowski DM: Acute kidney injury in children. Adv Chronic Kid Dis 2017 Nov;24(6):380–387 [PMID: 29229169].

CHRONIC KIDNEY DISEASE

Chronic kidney disease (CKD) in children most commonly results from congenital abnormalities of the kidneys or urinary tract (CAKUT). Renal hypoplasia/dysplasia, obstructive uropathy (including PUVs and ureteropelvic junction obstruction), or severe VUR without (or despite) surgical intervention is often associated with progressive renal insufficiency. In older children, the chronic glomerulonephritides and nephroses, irreversible nephrotoxic injury, or HUS may also cause CKD.

▶ Complications

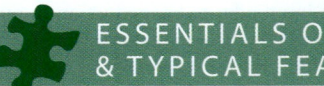

ESSENTIALS OF DIAGNOSIS & TYPICAL FEATURES

Complications of CKD:

► Anemia

► Hyperphosphatemia/secondary hyperparathyroidism

► Metabolic acidosis

► Growth failure

► Hypertension

► Uremia

Any remaining unaffected renal tissue can compensate for gradual loss of functioning nephrons in progressive CKD, but complications of renal insufficiency appear when this compensatory ability is overwhelmed. In children who have structural kidney lesions (such as renal hypoplasia or dysplasia) associated with impaired urinary concentration, polyuria, and dehydration are more likely to be problems than fluid overload until very late in the course of renal insufficiency. Some of these children can continue to produce generous volumes of poor-quality urine even though they require dialysis. A salt-wasting state can also occur. In contrast, children who develop chronic renal failure due to glomerular disease or renal injury will characteristically retain sodium and water with associated hypertension and eventual loss of urine output.

Metabolic acidosis and growth retardation occur early in chronic renal failure. Disturbances in calcium, phosphorus, and vitamin D metabolism leading to renal osteodystrophy and rickets require prompt attention. Increases in parathyroid hormone (PTH) occur in response to decreased serum calcium from lack of renally activated vitamin D. Rising serum phosphorus also potently induces an increase in the PTH level and in fibroblast growth factor 23 (FGF23) production by osteoblasts that improve renal tubular excretion of phosphorous and can maintain normal serum calcium and phosphate levels early in the course, but at the expense of the skeleton. Anemia due to decreased erythropoietin production and iron deficiency can occur relatively early on as well.

Symptoms such as anorexia, nausea, and malaise occur late in chronic renal failure (generally <30% renal function). These symptoms can be minimized if chronic renal failure has been detected early and associated complications treated, but refractory symptoms are indications for renal replacement therapy. CNS abnormalities such as confusion and lethargy are very late symptoms, followed even later by stupor and coma. Such findings are unusual as children usually seek medical attention before deteriorating to this point, and the rise in BUN is typically gradual. Other late complications of untreated chronic renal failure are platelet dysfunction and bleeding tendencies, pericarditis, and chronic fluid overload leading to congestive heart failure, pulmonary edema, and worsening hypertension.

▶ Treatment

A. Management of Complications

Treatment of CKD is primarily aimed at controlling associated complications. Acidosis may be treated with sodium citrate or bicarbonate, as long as the added sodium does not aggravate hypertension. Sodium restriction is advisable when hypertension is present. Hyperphosphatemia is controlled by dietary restriction and dietary phosphate binders (eg, calcium carbonate, sevelamer). Supplementation with vitamin D (cholecalciferol or ergocalciferol) is typically required and supplementation with calcitriol is indicated with severe elevations of PTH. These measures target the prevention of renal osteodystrophy or rickets. Dietary potassium restriction will be necessary as the GFR falls. Caloric intake must be optimized to provide the child's daily requirements for growth. Routine input from a renal dietitian is integral with more advanced stages of CKD. Protein restriction in children is not recommended; rather, appropriate quantities of protein required for age and growth are targeted as part of dietary plans.

Renal function must be monitored regularly with markers including creatinine, BUN and cystatin C. Serum electrolytes, calcium, phosphorus, intact PTH, 25-OH-vitamin D, iron and ferritin, and hemoglobin and hematocrit levels can be monitored to guide changes in fluid and dietary management as well as dosages of phosphate binder, citrate buffer, vitamin D supplements, BP medications, iron supplements, and epoetin alfa. Linear growth failure, seen in advanced stages of CKD due to relative resistance to growth hormone and functional deficiency of insulin-like growth factors, may be overcome with ensuring adequate caloric intake and daily subcutaneous human recombinant growth hormone to target an adult height in the low-normal range. Care must be taken to avoid medications that aggravate hypertension; increase the body burden of sodium, potassium, or phosphate; or increase production of BUN. Successful management relies greatly on education of the patient and family. Attention must also be directed towards psychosocial needs of the patient and family as they adjust to chronic illness and eventual need for dialysis and/or kidney transplantation. The multidisciplinary nephrology team works with each child/family to determine appropriate timing for chronic dialysis and/or kidney transplantation.

B. Dialysis and Transplantation

Chronic peritoneal dialysis (home-based) and hemodialysis provide lifesaving treatment for children until kidney transplantation. The best measure of success of chronic dialysis is the level of physical and psychosocial rehabilitation achieved, including continued participation in day-to-day activities and school attendance. The goal for all children with chronic or end-stage kidney disease is to achieve kidney transplantation, using dialysis as a lifesaving bridge when necessary. Preemptive kidney transplantation in a child with known progressing CKD should be considered, if possible, given improved long-term graft and patient survival compared to peers transplanted after receiving dialysis.

At present, the graft survival rate for living donor kidney transplants is 97.2% at 1 year and 87.1% at 5 years. With deceased donor transplantation, graft survivals are 92.5%, and 75.6%, respectively. Patient survival remains well above 95% at 5 years after transplant. Adequate growth and well-being are directly related to immunologic acceptance of the graft, graft function, and medication side effects.

Chua A et al; NAPRTCS investigators: Kidney transplant practice patterns and outcome benchmarks over 30 years: the 2018 report of the NAPRTCS. Pediatr Transplant 2019 Dec;23(8):e13597 [PMID: 31657095].

De Galasso L, Picca S, Guzzo I: Dialysis modalities for the management of pediatric acute kidney injury. Pediatr Nephrol 2020 May;35(5):753–765 [PMID: 30887109].

Etesami K, Lestz R, Hogen R: Pediatric kidney transplantation in the United States. Curr Opin Organ Transplant 2020 Aug;25(4): 343–347 [PMID: 32692040].

2022 Annual Data Report: NIDDK, USRDS. www.usrds-adr.niddk.nih.gov/2022.

HYPERTENSION

Hypertension in children is often of renal origin, although the prevalence of obesity-related hypertension is rapidly rising. Systemic hypertension is anticipated as a complication of known renal parenchymal disease, but it may be first identified on routine physical examination in an otherwise healthy-appearing child. Increased understanding of the roles of water and salt retention and overactivity of the renin-angiotensin system has done much to guide therapy; nevertheless, not all forms of hypertension can be explained by these two mechanisms.

The causes of renal hypertension in the newborn period include: (1) congenital anomalies of the kidneys, urinary tract or renal vasculature, (2) obstruction of the urinary tract, (3) thrombosis of renal vasculature, (4) volume overload, and (5) sequelae of AKI. Paradoxical elevations of BP have been reported in clinical situations in which chronic diuretic therapy is used, such as bronchopulmonary dysplasia. Chronic hypoxia may play a role in vascular alterations, similar to what is seen with hypertension in older children with obstructive sleep apnea. Umbilical artery catheterization and associated thrombosis of the renal vasculature continue to be a contributor to hypertension in infants and young children.

All infants and children with hypertension require careful evaluation to exclude a secondary cause of hypertension. These can include renal parenchymal or renovascular (renal arterial or venous thrombosis, congenital vascular stenosis) disease, other vascular diseases (vasculitis, aortic coarctation), endocrine disorders (thyroid disease, cortisol excess, pheochromocytoma, congenital adrenal hyperplasia), monogenic hypertension (glucocorticoid remediable aldosteronism, Liddle syndrome, etc.), primary hyperaldosteronism, or history of prematurity. The most recognized risk factors for hypertension in children and adolescents with history of prematurity are reduced nephron mass, umbilical artery catheterization, and history of AKI in the neonatal period. The family history of hypertension and cardiovascular disease should be reviewed with particular attention to early-onset hypertension. Primary or essential hypertension is becoming increasingly common with an increasing prevalence of obesity, high salt/sugar diet and limited routine exercise.

▶ Clinical Findings

The current definition of hypertension in children is based on the normative distribution of BP in healthy children. A child younger than 13 years is normotensive if the average recorded systolic and diastolic BPs are lower than the 90th percentile for age, sex, and height. The 90th percentile in the newborn period is approximately 85–90/55–65 mm Hg for both sexes. In the first year of life, the acceptable levels (90th percentile) are 90–100/60–67 mm Hg. Incremental increases with growth occur, gradually approaching young adult 90th percentile ranges of 100–120/65–80 mm Hg in the late teens. In children >1 and <13 years, a BP of = 90th percentile to < 95th percentile or 120/80 mm Hg to < 95th percentile (whichever is lower) is consistent with elevated BP while a BP 95th percentile to < 95th percentile + 12 mm Hg, or 130/80–139/89 mm Hg (whichever is lower) is consistent with stage 1 hypertension. A BP between the 90-95th percentile or exceeding 120/80 in adolescents (=13 years) is consistent with elevated BP while a BP >130/80 is consistent with stage 1 hypertension. For measurement of BP, the cuff should be wide enough to cover two-thirds of the upper arm and should encircle the arm completely without an overlap in the inflatable bladder, and, ideally, the child should be sitting quietly for 5 minutes with feet flat on the floor before BP is measured in the right arm (upon which norms are based). Although an anxious child may have an elevation in BP, abnormal readings must not be too hastily attributed to this cause. Repeat measurement is helpful, especially after the child has been consoled. Manual auscultated BP measurement in all four extremities should be pursued when automated readings are elevated. In cases where more detailed assessment is needed, 24-hour ambulatory BP monitoring can be valuable for diagnosing white coat hypertension or loss of normal 24-hour variation in BPs and remains the gold standard for diagnosis of hypertension.

Routine laboratory studies for evaluation of hypertension include serum BUN, creatinine, and electrolytes and urinalysis. Abnormal BUN and creatinine would support underlying renal disease as the cause, and serum electrolytes demonstrating hypokalemic alkalosis suggest excess mineralocorticoid effect. Routine assessment of serum lipids, glucose, A_{1C} hemoglobin, thyroid function tests, renin, and aldosterone is indicated. Screening of plasma/urine catecholamines and metanephrines and/or serum cortisol should be obtained as clinically indicated. Pheochromocytoma is unusual but should be suspected with episodic severe hypertension associated with tachycardia and flushing. Echocardiogram has been recommended for routine assessment of hypertension in children and may be of value for excluding secondary left ventricular hypertrophy. Careful assessment of distal pulses and four extremity BPs is necessary to exclude aortic coarctation clinically; this can be further evaluated by confirmatory echocardiogram. Renal ultrasonography with Doppler flow is

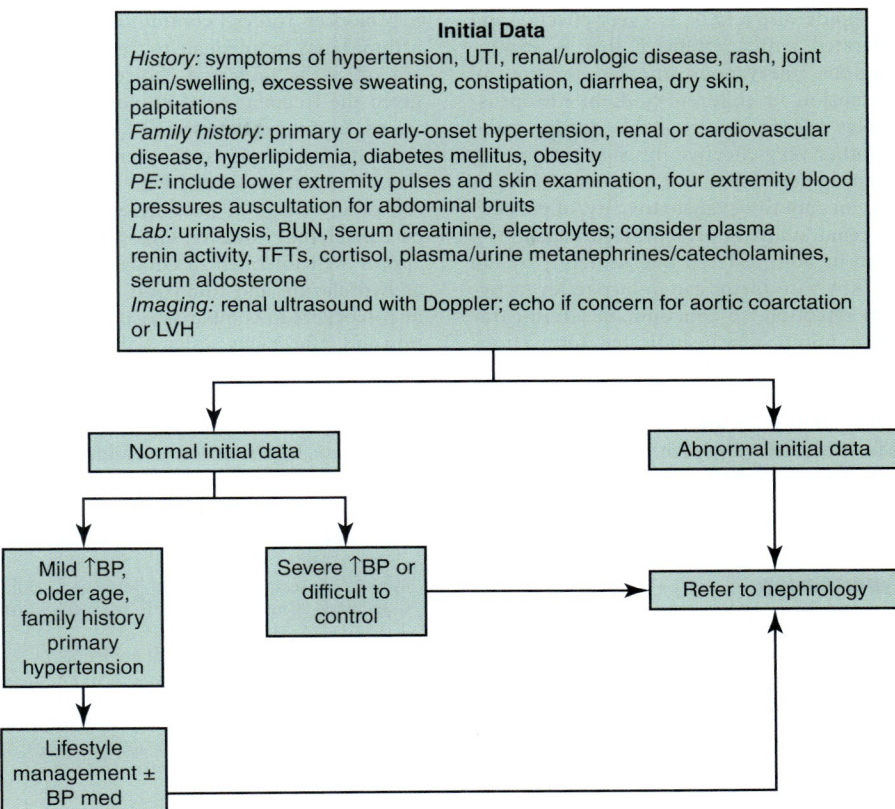

Initial Data

History: symptoms of hypertension, UTI, renal/urologic disease, rash, joint pain/swelling, excessive sweating, constipation, diarrhea, dry skin, palpitations

Family history: primary or early-onset hypertension, renal or cardiovascular disease, hyperlipidemia, diabetes mellitus, obesity

PE: include lower extremity pulses and skin examination, four extremity blood pressures auscultation for abdominal bruits

Lab: urinalysis, BUN, serum creatinine, electrolytes; consider plasma renin activity, TFTs, cortisol, plasma/urine metanephrines/catecholamines, serum aldosterone

Imaging: renal ultrasound with Doppler; echo if concern for aortic coarctation or LVH

- Normal initial data
  - Mild ↑BP, older age, family history primary hypertension
    - Lifestyle management ± BP med
  - Severe ↑BP or difficult to control
- Abnormal initial data
  - Refer to nephrology

▲ **Figure 24–3.** Approach to the outpatient workup of hypertension. BP, blood pressure; BUN, blood urea nitrogen; LVH, left ventricular hypertrophy; TFT, thyroid function test; UTI, urinary tract infection.

helpful in assessing for renal scarring, urinary tract obstruction, or renovascular flow disturbances. However, the sensitivity and specificity of Doppler ultrasound for renal artery stenosis vary widely between institutions, and renal MR or CT angiography is indicated when there is high suspicion for renal artery stenosis. A renal biopsy (which rarely reveals the cause of hypertension unless clinical evidence of renal disease is present) should be undertaken with special care in the hypertensive patient and preferably after pressures have been controlled by therapy. Figure 24–3 presents a suggested approach to the outpatient workup of hypertension.

▶ **Treatment**

A. Acute Hypertensive Emergencies

A hypertensive emergency exists when CNS signs of hypertension appear, such as papilledema, encephalopathy, or seizures. Associated symptoms may include headache, emesis, or changes in vision. Retinal hemorrhages or exudates also

indicate a need for prompt BP control. Children with acute hypertensive emergencies require management in the intensive care setting with consideration of continuous arterial BP monitoring and intravenous antihypertensive therapy. It is recommended that the BP in acute hypertensive emergency be reduced by no more than 25% in the first 6–8 hours, with complete normalization over the subsequent 12–24 hours. In addition to controlling emergent hypertension, medications for sustained control should also be initiated so that normal BP will be maintained when the emergent measures are discontinued. The primary classes of useful antihypertensive drugs are (1) ACEIs and angiotensin receptor blockers, (2) CCBs, (3) α- and β-adrenergic blockers, (4) diuretics, and (5) vasodilators.

Sublingual nifedipine is a rapid-acting CCB that can be administered to acutely decrease severe hypertension. However, its use has fallen out of favor for acute management of hypertension due to risk of severe hypotension and has been replaced by isradipine, another short-acting CCB.

Alternatively, nicardipine, also a CCB, is a very effective and generally well-tolerated antihypertensive that is administered via continuous intravenous infusion for control of systemic hypertension in children. Sodium nitroprusside, which promotes release of nitric oxide causing rapid vasodilation, is another very effective infusion for gaining control of malignant hypertension, but long-term usage is limited by concern for rare thiocyanate toxicity, of particular concern when renal failure is present. Hydralazine is a vasodilator that can be administered intermittently by the intravenous route. Any vasodilator can induce reflex tachycardia and sodium retention, so concomitant administration of a β-blocker or diuretic may be indicated. Intravenous forms of β-blockers such as esmolol or labetalol (both available as continuous infusions) are useful when there are no cardiac or respiratory contraindications to their use. Finally, diuretics such as furosemide or hydrochlorothiazide can be useful in the acute setting when there is evidence of intravascular volume overload as they induce diuresis and/or natriuresis.

B. Sustained Hypertension

For children with sustained hypertension, reductions in BP toward goal measurements based on age, gender, and height should be undertaken by no more than 25% for each 24–48-hour period to prevent loss of adequate cerebral and renal perfusion pressure. Several choices are available for treatment (Table 24–4). A single drug such as an ACEI or a β-blocker (unless contraindicated, eg, with underlying asthma) may be adequate to treat mild hypertension. ACEIs are often the preferred choice of pediatric nephrologists given the frequent renal etiology of hypertension. Diuretics are useful in the setting of renal insufficiency or in the context of systemic corticosteroid therapy, both situations that are often associated with sodium and fluid retention; the disadvantage of possible electrolyte imbalance should be considered, however. CCBs are increasingly useful and appear well tolerated in children. Direct vasodilators such as hydralazine and minoxidil often require diuretics and/or β-blockers to combat associated sodium and fluid retention and reflex tachycardia. Although minoxidil is extremely effective in control of hypertension of a variety of etiologies, hirsutism is a significant side effect. The advice of a pediatric nephrologist should be sought in the management of acute and chronic hypertension in children.

Ferguson MA, Flynn JT: Rational use of antihypertensive medications in children. Pediatr Nephrol 2014;29(6):979–988 [PMID: 23715784].

Flynn JT: Assessment of blood pressure in children: it's all in the details. J Clin Hypertens (Greenwich) 2013;15(11):772–773 [PMID: 24283595].

Flynn JT et al: Clinical practice guideline for screening and management of high blood pressure in children and adolescents. Pediatrics 2017;140(3) [PMID: 28827377].

Raina R et al: Hypertensive crisis in pediatric patients: an overview. Front Pediatr 2020 Oct 20;8:588911 [PMID: 33194923].

Table 24–4. Antihypertensive drugs for ambulatory treatment in children ages 1–17 years.

Class	Drug	Oral Dose	Major Side Effects[a]
Angiotensin-converting enzyme inhibitor	Captopril	1–6 mg/kg/day ÷ tid	Rash, hyperkalemia, cough, decreased GFR
	Lisinopril	0.1–0.6 mg/kg/day ÷ qd–bid	
Calcium channel blocker	Amlodipine	0.1–0.6 mg/kg/day ÷ qd–bid	Higher doses relative to body weight may be required in younger children; headache, facial flushing, pretibial edema
	Nifedipine, extended-release	0.5–3 mg/kg/day ÷ tid	Flushing, tachycardia
Diuretic	Furosemide	0.5–20 mg/kg/day ÷ qd–qid (maximum 5 mg/kg/dose up to 200 mg)	Potassium and volume depletion
	Hydrochlorothiazide	1–3 mg/kg/day ÷ qd–bid	Potassium and volume depletion, hyperuricemia
Sympathetic nervous system blockade	Propranolol	0.6–4 mg/kg/day ÷ bid–tid (maximum 640 mg/day)	Syncope, bradycardia; use with caution in asthma or overt heart failure
	Metoprolol	1–6 mg/kg/day ÷ qd–bid (maximum 200 mg/day)	Syncope, bradycardia; use with caution in asthma or overt heart failure
Vasodilator	Hydralazine	0.75–7.5 mg/kg/day ÷ tid–qid (maximum 200 mg/day)	Lupus-like syndrome in slow acetylators; tachycardia, fluid retention, headache
	Minoxidil	0.3–1 mg/kg/day ÷ qd–bid	Tachycardia, fluid retention, hirsutism

bid, twice a day; GFR, glomerular filtration rate; qd, daily; qid, four times a day; tid, three times a day.
[a]Not all side effects are listed.

INHERITED OR DEVELOPMENTAL DEFECTS OF THE KIDNEYS

There are many developmental, hereditary, or metabolic defects of the kidneys and collecting system (Table 24–5). Their clinical consequences include metabolic abnormalities, failure to thrive, nephrolithiasis, renal glomerular or tubular dysfunction, and chronic renal failure.

DISORDERS OF THE RENAL TUBULES

RTAs are a set of tubular defects that are classified based on clinical presentation and pathophysiologic mechanisms: (1) the classic form (type I or distal RTA), (2) the bicarbonate-wasting form (type II or proximal RTA), and (3) type IV or hyperkalemic RTA, which is associated with hyporeninemic hypoaldosteronism or inherited in an autosomal manner. Types I and II and their variants are encountered most frequently in children. Type III is described historically as a combination of types I and II. Other primary tubular disorders in childhood, such as glycinuria, hyperuricosuria, or renal glycosuria, may result from a defect in a single tubular transport pathway (see Table 24–5).

Distal Renal Tubular Acidosis (Type I)

The most common form of distal RTA in childhood is the hereditary form. The clinical presentation includes failure to thrive, anorexia, vomiting, and dehydration. Hyperchloremic metabolic acidosis, hypokalemia, and inability to reduce urinary pH to less than 5.3 are found. Concomitant hypercalciuria may lead to nephrocalcinosis, nephrolithiasis, and renal failure. Some of the other entities listed in Table 24–5 may also be responsible for distal RTA. Acquired distal RTA is less common in childhood and is most commonly due to autoimmune diseases (Sjogren syndrome, SLE, rheumatoid arthritis), sickle cell disease, renal transplantation, or exposure to medications (eg, amphotericin B, ifosfamide).

Distal RTA results from a defect in the distal nephron in the tubular transport of hydrogen ion or in the maintenance of a steep enough gradient for proper excretion of hydrogen ion. Historically, the diagnosis could be established with an

Table 24–5. Inherited or developmental defects of the urinary tract.

Cystic diseases of genetic origin	Hereditary amyloidosis (familial Mediterranean fever, heredo-familial urticaria with deafness and neuropathy, primary familial amyloidosis with polyneuropathy)
Polycystic disease	
Autosomal recessive	**Hereditary renal diseases associated with tubular transport defects**
Autosomal dominant	Hartnup disease
Other syndromes that include either form	Oculocerebrorenal syndrome of Lowe
Nephronophthisis	Cystinosis (infantile, adolescent, adult types)
Medullary cystic kidney disease	Wilson disease
Glomerulocystic kidney disease	Galactosemia
Renal cysts and diabetes (HNF1-β)	Hereditary fructose intolerance
Dysplastic renal diseases	Renal tubular acidosis
Renal agenesis	Hereditary tyrosinemia
Renal hypoplasia	Renal glycosuria
Renal dysplasia	Vitamin D–resistant rickets
Cystic renal dysplasia	Pseudohypoparathyroidism
Multicystic dysplastic kidney	Nephrogenic diabetes insipidus
Oligomeganephronia	Bartter syndrome
Hereditary diseases associated with nephritis	Gitelman syndrome
Hereditary nephritis with deafness and ocular defects (Alport syndrome)	Liddle syndrome
Nail-patella syndrome	Hypouricemia
Familial hyperprolinemia	**Hereditary diseases associated with lithiasis**
Hereditary osteolysis with nephropathy	Hyperoxaluria
Hereditary diseases associated with intrarenal deposition of metabolites	L-Glyceric aciduria
Fabry disease	Xanthinuria
Zellweger syndrome	Lesch-Nyhan syndrome and variants, gout
Various storage diseases (eg, G_{M1} Hurler syndrome, Niemann-Pick disease, familial metachromatic leukodystrophy, glycogenosis type I [von Gierke disease], glycogenosis type II [Pompe disease])	Nephropathy due to familial hyperparathyroidism
	Cystinuria (types I, II, III)
	Glycinuria
	Dent disease

acid loading test, but this is rarely pursued currently. Instead, the findings of RTA with persistent elevation in urine pH despite acidosis, hypercalciuria or nephrocalcinosis, and relatively low requirement of alkali to normalize serum pH and bicarbonate concentration (1–3 mEq/kg/day), support a distal defect. Moreover, urinary citrate levels are uniquely low in distal RTA due to increased reabsorption of citrate by the proximal tubule in response to acidosis. Some forms of genetic distal RTA are associated with hearing loss. Correction of acidosis with citrate or, less commonly, bicarbonate reduces complications and improves growth. Distal RTA is often permanent. If renal damage from calcinosis is prevented, the prognosis with treatment is good.

Proximal Renal Tubular Acidosis (Type II)

Proximal RTA, the most common form of RTA in childhood, is characterized by failure to reabsorb bicarbonate appropriately in the proximal tubule with associated reduced serum bicarbonate concentration and normal anion gap hyperchloremic metabolic acidosis. Once a steady state is reached, the intact distal nephron appropriately excretes hydrogen ion, leading to a low urine pH. There are both hereditary and acquired types of proximal RTA; hereditary forms occur with autosomal recessive, autosomal dominant, or sporadic inheritance. Patients with autosomal recessive proximal RTA may present with CNS calcification, short stature, and cataracts.

In the newborn, proximal RTA can be considered an aspect of renal immaturity that improves with increasing gestational age. Proximal RTA in infants may be an isolated defect and accompanied by failure to thrive and, sometimes, hypokalemia. Secondary forms may result from reflux or drug exposures that result in tubular injury (eg, lead, tenofovir). Due to bicarbonate wasting, children with proximal RTA typically require large doses of alkali (5–20 mEq/kg/day citrate/bicarbonate) to achieve normal serum pH and bicarbonate concentration.

▶ Evaluation & Treatment

The diagnosis of RTA is made with the finding of a normal anion gap, hyperchloremic metabolic acidosis in the absence of diarrhea or intravascular volume depletion. A concomitant urine pH is helpful in many cases, as it is elevated in distal RTA despite the metabolic acidosis. The finding of hypophosphatemia or glycosuria should lead to further investigation of proximal tubular function (eg, Fanconi syndrome). A renal ultrasound should be obtained to exclude urinary tract obstruction (which can be seen with proximal or distal RTA) and nephrocalcinosis (seen in distal RTA). A urine calcium/creatinine ratio may be helpful in the latter condition. In either proximal or distal RTA, citrate or bicarbonate supplementation is provided; citrate solutions are more effective and often better tolerated. Sodium citrate (1 mEq/mL of Na^+ and citrate) or potassium citrate (2 mEq/mL

of citrate and 1 mEq/mL each of Na^+ and K^+) is administered two to three times per day to target a trough serum bicarbonate level of 20–24 mEq/L. Potassium supplementation may be required (and can often be accomplished simply with a change from sodium citrate to potassium citrate) because the added sodium load presented to the distal tubule may exaggerate potassium losses.

The prognosis is excellent in cases of isolated proximal RTA, especially when related to renal immaturity. Alkali therapy can usually be discontinued after several months to a few years. Growth should be normal, and the gradual increase in the serum bicarbonate level to greater than 24 mEq/L heralds the normalization of the threshold for proximal tubular bicarbonate reabsorption. If the defect is part of Fanconi syndrome or distal RTA, the prognosis depends on the underlying disorder or syndrome.

Soleimani M, Tastegar A: Pathophysiology of renal tubular acidosis: core curriculum 2016. AJKD 2016;68(3):488–498 [PMID: 27188519].

GENETIC TUBULAR DISORDERS

Familial Fanconi Syndromes

Fanconi syndrome refers to a group of conditions characterized by inappropriate reabsorption of small molecules (including phosphorus, glucose, potassium, bicarbonate, glucose, uric acid, amino acids) by the proximal tubules of the kidney. The most common forms of familial Fanconi syndromes are cystinosis and Wilson disease but also include Lowe (oculorenal) syndrome, Fanconi Bickel syndrome, and Dent disease. Different forms of Fanconi syndrome can affect different parts of the proximal tubule, resulting in varying phenotypes.

Cystinosis, most often transmitted via autosomal recessive inheritance, is the most common cause of Fanconi syndrome in children and results from mutations in the *CTNS* gene, which encodes the cystine transporter. There are three types of cystinosis: adult, adolescent, and infantile. The adult form is characterized by ocular cystinosis without renal involvement. In the adolescent and infantile types, cystine accumulation in lysosomes causes cell death in numerous organs, including the kidneys. The infantile type is most common and the most severe. Characteristically, children present in the first or early second year of life with Fanconi syndrome, polyuria and polydipsia, and failure to thrive. If left untreated, ESRD is reached by 7–10 years of age in the infantile form. Whenever the diagnosis of cystinosis is suspected, slit-lamp examination of the corneas should be performed. Cystine crystal deposition causes an almost pathognomonic ground-glass "dazzle" appearance. Increased white blood cell cystine levels are diagnostic. Treatment with oral cysteamine aids in the metabolic conversion of cystine (unable to exit cells) to cysteine (able to exit cells) and delays intracellular accumulation and associated complications, which include Fanconi syndrome with salt-wasting and functional nephrogenic diabetes insipidus (NDI), proximal RTA, hypophosphatemic rickets, eventual progression to ESRD, hypothyroidism, ocular cystinosis with eventual blindness, and neurologic deterioration. The condition does not recur in transplanted kidneys, but ongoing cysteamine therapy is required to prevent complications in other organs.

Emma F et al: Nephropathic cystinosis: an international consensus document. Nephrol Dial Transplant 2014;29(Suppl 4):iv87–iv94 [PMID: 25165189].
Foreman JW: Fanconi syndrome. Pediatr Clin North Am 2019 Feb;66(1):159–167 [PMID: 30454741].

Oculocerebrorenal Syndrome (Lowe Syndrome)

Lowe syndrome results from various mutations in the *OCRL1* gene, which codes for a Golgi apparatus phosphatase. Affected males have anomalies involving the eyes, brain, and kidneys. The physical stigmata and degree of intellectual disability vary with the location of the mutation. In addition to congenital cataracts and buphthalmos, the typical facies include prominent epicanthal folds, frontal prominence, and a tendency to scaphocephaly. Muscle hypotonia is prominent. Renal abnormalities are tubular and include hypophosphatemic rickets with low serum phosphorus levels, low to normal serum calcium levels, elevated serum alkaline phosphatase levels, proximal RTA, and aminoaciduria. Treatment includes alkali therapy, phosphate replacement, and vitamin D support. Glomerulosclerosis likely results from progressive renal tubular injury and may lead to chronic renal failure and ESRD between the second and fourth decades of life.

Hypokalemic Alkalosis (Bartter Syndrome, Gitelman Syndrome, & Liddle Syndrome)

A number of genetic tubular disorders result in hypokalemic metabolic alkalosis. Bartter syndrome is characterized by severe hypokalemic, hypochloremic metabolic alkalosis, extremely high levels of circulating renin and aldosterone, and a paradoxical absence of hypertension. On renal biopsy (rarely pursued in the current era), a striking juxtaglomerular hyperplasia is seen. A neonatal form of Bartter syndrome is thought to result from mutations in two genes (*NKCC2*, *ROMK*) affecting nephron Na^+-K^+ or K^+ transport. These patients typically have a history of polyhydramnios and following birth have recurrent life-threatening episodes of fever and dehydration with the aforementioned electrolyte and acid–base disturbances, hypercalciuria, and early-onset nephrocalcinosis. Classic Bartter syndrome presenting in infancy with polyuria and growth retardation (but not nephrocalcinosis) is thought to result from mutations in a chloride channel gene. A novel transient antenatal form (associated with MAGED2 mutations) has also recently been identified. Gitelman syndrome occurs in older children and features episodes of muscle weakness and tetany associated with severe hypokalemia and hypomagnesemia. These children have hypocalciuria. Treatment with prostaglandin inhibitors and potassium-conserving diuretics (eg, amiloride) and potassium and magnesium supplements, where indicated, is beneficial in Bartter and Gitelman syndrome. These are lifelong conditions that require ongoing electrolyte supplementation and may progress to ESRD (more commonly in Bartter syndrome).

Liddle syndrome is associated with constitutive activation of the epithelial sodium channel with associated salt and water retention. Thus, the initial presenting abnormality is often hypertension associated with hypokalemia and metabolic alkalosis. Serum renin and aldosterone are suppressed due to the sodium and fluid retention. Treatment in Liddle syndrome is with a low-sodium diet and blockade of the epithelial sodium channel with amiloride or triamterene. Spironolactone is ineffective in this condition as aldosterone is typically suppressed.

NEPHROGENIC DIABETES INSIPIDUS

Hereditary nephrogenic (vasopressin-resistant) diabetes insipidus (NDI) is most often caused by X-linked mutations in the *AVPR2* gene that encodes the vasopressin V_2 receptor. Autosomal (recessive and dominant) forms of NDI occur less commonly due to mutations of the *AQP2* gene that codes for the collecting tubule water channel protein aquaporin-2. Affected children often have a profound impairment in maximal urinary concentrating capacity, which rarely exceeds 100 mOsm/kg H_2O. Genetic counseling and mutation testing are available. Acquired NDI is observed in numerous conditions including sickle cell anemia, chronic pyelonephritis, hypokalemia, hypercalcemia, Fanconi syndrome, obstructive uropathy, chronic renal insufficiency, and lithium treatment.

The symptoms of NDI include polyuria and polydipsia. In severe cases, water intake is preferred to formula, leading to failure to thrive. In some children, particularly if the solute intake is unrestricted, adjustment to an elevated serum osmolality may develop. Children with genetic NDI are particularly susceptible to episodes of dehydration, fever, vomiting, and hypernatremia when access to free water is limited.

NDI can be suspected on the basis of a history of polydipsia and polyuria, for which the differential diagnosis includes hyperglycemia and primary polydipsia, which occurs in children as young as infancy. The family history may be informative in hereditary cases while the patient's medical history, medications, and serum chemistries can help identify a source of acquired NDI. The diagnosis is confirmed by a water deprivation test, during which serum and urine osmolality are assessed and either arginine vasopressin or desmopressin administered to evaluate tubular response.

When hereditary NDI is suspected, a water deprivation test should be performed in a controlled hospital setting, as the restriction of water intake in such children can lead to severe intravascular volume depletion and hyperosmolality.

In infants with NDI, it is usually best to allow water on demand and to restrict salt intake. Caregivers must be aware of the risks of dehydration and hypernatremia if fluid intake is restricted either due to lack of availability or inability to keep fluids down (eg, vomiting). A low-salt diet limits the amount of urine that must be produced for daily solute excretion. Due to the need for high-volume free-water intake, caloric intake may be limited and affected children often benefit from routine follow-up with a renal dietitian. Treatment with hydrochlorothiazide decreases urine volume by limiting the amount of free water delivered to the distal nephron for excretion. Prostaglandin inhibitors such as indomethacin are also efficacious, by decreasing renal blood flow and GFR and preventing reclamation of the AQP2 water channel from the collecting duct cell apical membrane.

Bockenhauer D, Bichet DG: Urinary concentration: different ways to open and close the tap. Pediatr Nephrol 2014;29(8):1297–1303 [PMID: 23736674].

Cunha T, Heilberg P: Bartter syndrome: causes, diagnosis and treatment. Inter J Neph Renovasc Dis 2018;11:2910301 [PMID: 30519073].

Laghmani K et al: Polyhydramnios, transient antenatal Bartter's syndrome and MAGED2 mutations. New Engl J Med 2016;374:1853–1863 [PMID: 27120771].

Wong LM, Man SS: Water deprivation test in children with polyuria. J Pediatr Endocrinol Metab 2012;25(9–10):869–874 [PMID: 23426815].

NEPHROLITHIASIS

Although more common in adults, the incidence of nephrolithiasis in children increased by 6%–10% annually in the last 20 years—currently the incidence is 36–57/100,000 children in the United States. The increased incidence may be related to increases in obesity and high salt/sugar diets. Stones in children are most often calcium oxalate and calcium phosphate in composition, resulting most commonly from hypercalciuria or hypocitraturia. Renal calculi in children may also result from products of hereditary errors of metabolism, such as cystine in cystinuria, glycine in hyperglycinuria, urates in Lesch-Nyhan syndrome, and oxalates in primary hyperoxaluria. These diagnoses are best established via 24-hour urine collection to assess for common biochemical risk factors for stone formation. Large stones are often seen in children with spina bifida who have paralyzed lower limbs or in any situation in which immobilization promotes calcium mobilization from the bones or there is recurrent UTI with urease-producing organisms (struvite calculi). Most cases are initially addressed with attention toward maintaining optimal hydration and targeting the inciting cause of stone formation with appropriate medical therapy. Surgical removal of stones or lithotripsy should be considered for obstruction, intractable severe pain, and chronic infection.

Gellin C: Urinary tract stones. Pediatr Rev (AAP) 2019;40(3):154–156 [PMID: 30824503].

Schott C, Pourtousi A, Connaughton DM: Monogenic causes of pediatric nephrolithiasis. Front Urol 2:1075711.

Cystinuria

Cystinuria is primarily an abnormality of amino acid transport across both the enteric and proximal renal tubular epithelium. There are at least three biochemical types. In the first type, the bowel transport of basic amino acids and cystine is impaired, but transport of cysteine is not impaired. In the renal tubule, basic amino acids are again rejected by the tubule, but cystine absorption appears to be normal. The reason for cystinuria remains obscure. Heterozygous individuals have no aminoaciduria. The second type is similar to the first except that heterozygous individuals excrete excess cystine and lysine in the urine, and cystine transport in the bowel is normal. In the third type, only the nephron is involved, and the only clinical manifestations are related to stone formation: ureteral colic, dysuria, hematuria, proteinuria, and secondary UTI. Urinary excretion of cystine, lysine, arginine, and ornithine is increased.

The most reliable way to prevent stone formation is to maintain a constantly high free-water clearance via generous fluid intake. Alkalinization of the urine is also helpful. If these measures do not prevent significant renal lithiasis, the use of tiopronin is recommended.

Servais A et al: Cystinuria: clinical practice recommendation. Kidney Int 2021 Jan;99(1):48–58 [PMID: 32918941].

Primary Hyperoxaluria

Oxalate in humans is derived from oxidative deamination of glycine to glyoxylate, the serine-glycolate pathway, and from ascorbic acid. Type I primary hyperoxaluria is a deficiency of liver-specific peroxisomal alanine–glyoxylate aminotransferase. Type II primary hyperoxaluria is glyoxylate reductase deficiency. Type III primary hyperoxaluria is associated with increased mitochondrial 4-hydroxy-2-oxoglutarate aldolase activity; this type appears to be milder than types I or II. Secondary hyperoxaluria with associated urolithiasis can also occur due to excessive absorption of dietary oxalate as a consequence of severe ileal disease or ileal resection.

Excess oxalate combines with calcium to form insoluble deposits in the kidneys, lungs, eyes and other tissues beginning in childhood. The joints are occasionally involved, but the main effect is on the kidneys, where progressive oxalate deposition leads to fibrosis and eventual renal failure.

A low-oxalate diet with normal calcium intake and high fluid intake is recommended. High-dose pyridoxine can be administered in type I primary hyperoxaluria as it is a cofactor for the defective pathway. While the prognosis of type I primary hyperoxaluria was previously poor, with half of patients developing ESRD by 15 years of age, recent approval of Lumasiran, an RNA interference therapeutic that decreases oxalate production, has yielded encouraging results including decreasing serum oxalate levels to near normal after 6 months of treatment. Renal transplantation is not very successful because of destruction of the transplant kidney by continued oxalate overproduction. However, encouraging results have been obtained with concomitant liver transplantation that corrects the metabolic defect. Types II and III primary hyperoxaluria appear to have better long-term renal outcomes.

Garrelfs SF et al: Lumasiran, an RNAi therapeutic for primary hyperoxaluria type 1. New Engl J Med 2021;384:1216–1226 [PMID: 33789010].

URINARY TRACT INFECTIONS

It is estimated that 8% of girls and 2% of boys will acquire UTIs in childhood. Girls older than 6 months have UTIs far more commonly than boys, whereas uncircumcised boys younger than 3 months have more UTIs than girls. Circumcision reduces the risk of UTI, especially due to VUR, in boys.

Pathogenesis

Most UTIs are ascending infections. The density of distal urethral and periurethral bacterial colonization with uropathogenic bacteria correlates with the risk of UTI in children. Specific adhesins present on the fimbria of uropathogenic bacteria allow colonization of the uroepithelium in the urethra and bladder and increase the likelihood of UTI. The organisms most commonly responsible are fecal flora, most frequently E. coli (> 85%), klebsiella species, proteus species, other gram-negative bacteria, and, less frequently, enterococcus or coagulase-negative staphylococci. Dysfunctional voiding, uncoordinated relaxation of the urethral sphincter during voiding, leads to incomplete emptying of the bladder, which increases the risk of UTI. Similarly, other conditions that interfere with complete emptying of the bladder, such as constipation, VUR, urinary tract obstruction, or neurogenic bladder, increase the risk of UTI. Poor perineal hygiene, structural abnormalities of the urinary tract, catheterization or other instrumentation of the urinary tract, and sexual activity increase the risk as well. When infection reaches the kidneys (pyelonephritis), the inflammatory response may produce renal parenchymal scars that can contribute to hypertension, renal disease, and renal failure later in life.

Clinical Findings

A. Symptoms and Signs

Newborns and infants with UTI have nonspecific symptoms and signs, including fever, hypothermia, jaundice, poor feeding, irritability, vomiting, and failure to thrive, and they may present with sepsis. Strong, foul-smelling, or cloudy urine may be noted. Preschool children may have abdominal or flank pain, vomiting, fever, urinary frequency, dysuria, urgency, or enuresis. School-aged children commonly have classic signs of cystitis (frequency, dysuria, and urgency) or pyelonephritis (fever, vomiting, and flank pain). Costovertebral tenderness is unusual in young children but may be demonstrated by school-aged children. Physical examination should include BP determination and abdominal and genitourinary examination. Urethritis, poor perineal hygiene, herpes simplex virus infection, or other genitourinary infections may be apparent.

B. Laboratory Findings

Screening urinalysis indicates pyuria (> 5 WBCs/hpf) in most children with UTI, but sterile pyuria can also be seen without UTI due to white cells from the urethra or vagina or from a renal inflammatory process. The leukocyte esterase test correlates well with pyuria but has a similar false-positive rate for UTI. The detection of urinary nitrite by dipstick is highly correlated with enteric organisms being cultured from urine. Most young children (70%) with UTI have negative nitrite tests, however, because they empty their bladders frequently and it requires several hours for bacteria to convert ingested nitrates to nitrite in the bladder. Additionally, some organisms that cause UTIs such as enterococci and staphylococci do not convert nitrate to nitrite.

The gold standard for diagnosis remains the culture of a properly collected urine specimen. Collection of urine for urinalysis and culture is difficult in children due to frequent contamination of the sample. In toilet-trained, cooperative, older children, a midstream, clean-catch method is usually satisfactory. Although cleaning of the perineum does not improve specimen quality, straddling of the toilet to separate the labia in girls, retraction of the foreskin in boys, and collecting midstream urine significantly reduce contamination. In infants and younger children, bladder catheterization or suprapubic collection is necessary in most cases to avoid contaminated samples. Bagged urine specimens are helpful only if negative. Specimens that are not immediately cultured should be refrigerated during transport. Any growth is considered significant from a suprapubic culture. Quantitative recovery of 10^5 cfu/mL or greater is considered significant from clean-catch specimens, and 10^4–10^5 cfu/mL is considered significant from catheterized specimens. Usually, the recovery of multiple organisms indicates contamination.

Asymptomatic bacteriuria is detected in 0.5%–1.0% of children who are screened with urine culture. Asymptomatic bacteriuria, as seen commonly in children requiring chronic bladder catheterization, is believed to represent colonization of the urinary tract with non-uropathogenic bacteria. Treatment in such cases may increase the risk of symptomatic UTI by eliminating nonpathogenic colonization. Screening urine cultures in asymptomatic children are, therefore, generally discouraged.

C. Imaging

The type and timing of imaging studies in infants and children after first UTI remain controversial. Updated American Academy of Pediatrics guidelines no longer recommend routine VCUG or Lasix renogram in infants between 2 and 24 months after a first UTI. However, renal ultrasound, a non-invasive study, should be completed in all infants after a first febrile UTI to screen for congenital urologic anomalies. The finding of significant hydronephrosis or other concerning urinary tract abnormalities on screening ultrasound warrants further imaging. The sensitivity of renal ultrasound for detection of significant VUR varies widely in medical literature. VUR, a congenital abnormality present in about 1% of the population beyond infancy, is graded using the international scale (I—reflux into ureter; II—reflux to the kidneys; III—reflux to kidneys with dilation of ureter only; IV—reflux with dilation of ureter and mild blunting of renal calyces; V—reflux with dilation of ureter and blunting of renal calyces). Reflux is detected in 30%–50% of children presenting with a UTI at 1 year of age and younger. The natural history of reflux is to improve, and 80% of reflux of grades I, II, or III will resolve or significantly improve within 3 years following detection. Thus, significant debate exists regarding appropriate radiographic imaging for UTI and best management of VUR, including indications for and value of surgical intervention and/or prophylactic antibiotics.

▶ Treatment

A. Antibiotic Therapy

Very young children (age < 3 months) and children with dehydration, toxicity, or sepsis are generally admitted to the hospital and initially treated with parenteral antimicrobials. Older infants and children who are not seriously ill can be treated as outpatients. Initial antimicrobial therapy is based on prior history of infection and antimicrobial use, as well as presumed location of the infection within the urinary tract.

Most uncomplicated cystitis can be treated with amoxicillin, trimethoprim-sulfamethoxazole, or a first-generation cephalosporin. These antimicrobials are concentrated in the lower urinary tract and are associated with high cure rates. Knowledge of rates of antimicrobial resistance in the local community is helpful in choosing an antibiotic. More seriously ill children are initially treated parenterally with a third-generation cephalosporin or, less commonly, an aminoglycoside. The initial antimicrobial choice is adjusted after culture and susceptibility results are known. The recommended duration of antimicrobial therapy for uncomplicated cystitis is 7–10 days. For sexually mature teenagers with cystitis, fluoroquinolones such as ciprofloxacin and levofloxacin for 3 days are effective and cost-effective. Short-course therapy of cystitis is not recommended in children, because differentiating upper and lower tract disease may be difficult and higher failure rates are reported in most studies of short-course therapy.

Acute pyelonephritis is usually treated for 10 days. In nontoxic children older than 3 months of age who are not vomiting, oral treatment with an appropriate agent can be used. In sicker children, parenteral therapy may be required initially. Most of these children can complete therapy orally once symptomatic improvement has occurred. A repeat urine culture 24–48 hours after beginning therapy or after completion of antibiotic therapy is not needed if the child is improving and doing well.

B. Prophylactic Antimicrobials

Selected children with frequently recurring UTI may benefit from prophylactic antimicrobials. In children with high-grade VUR, prophylactic antimicrobials may be beneficial in reducing UTI, as an alternative to surgical correction, or in the interval prior to surgical therapy, which some experts recommend for higher-grade reflux (particularly grade V). Children with dysfunctional voiding may also benefit from prophylactic antimicrobials; however, addressing the underlying dysfunctional voiding is most important. Trimethoprim—sulfamethoxazole and nitrofurantoin are approved for prophylaxis. The use of broader-spectrum antimicrobials leads to colonization and infection with resistant strains.

Subcommittee on Urinary Tract Infection, Steering Committee on Quality Improvement and Management; Roberts KB: Urinary tract infection: clinical practice guidelines for the diagnosis and management of the initial UTI in febrile infants and children 2 to 24 months. Pediatrics 2011;128(3):595–610 [PMID: 21873693].

't Hoen LA et al: Update of the EAU/ESPU guidelines on urinary tract infections in children. J Pediatr Urol 2021 Apr;17(2): 200–207. Erratum in: J Pediatr Urol. 2021 Aug;17(4):598 [PMID: 33589366].

Neurologic & Muscular Disorders

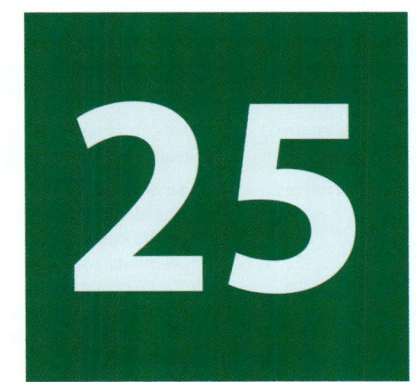

Ricka Messer, MD, PhD

Elizabeth Troy, MD

Diana Walleigh, MD

Melissa Wright, MD, PhD

NEUROLOGIC ASSESSMENT & NEURODIAGNOSTICS

HISTORY & EXAMINATION

History

Even in this era of increasingly sophisticated neurodiagnostic testing, the assessment and diagnosis of a child with a possible neurologic disorder still hinges on a detailed history and examination. In particular, the progression of the neurologic signs and symptoms (acute vs chronic, progressive vs static, episodic vs continuous) can direct the evaluation. Episodic events, such as headaches or seizures, warrant emphasis on the symptoms preceding, during, and succeeding the event. Neurologic symptoms may be associated with other organ system involvement, such as joint pain, changes in appetite or bowel/bladder habits, or a preceding viral illness. Birth history should include assessment of fetal movement and whether the infant was breech or vertex. A thorough past medical history and family history can illuminate risk factors for certain neurologic disorders. Social history should include school performance, preferred activities, and travel history.

Neurologic Examination

The hallmark of neurologic diagnosis is *localization*, determining where within the nervous system the "lesion" is located. While not all childhood neurologic disorders are easily localized, even narrowing down to, for example, a central versus peripheral origin, can guide further evaluation and treatment. Localization begins with the general physical examination (see Chapter 9). Growth parameters should be noted, particularly head circumference, since macro- or microcephaly are often associated with neurologic disorders (see Chapter 3). Developmental assessments, using a small toy or an appropriate screening tool, are fundamental for infants and young children (see Chapter 3). Expected infant reflexes and other age-related examination findings are included in Chapter 2.

Table 25–1 outlines key components of the neurologic examination—mental status, cranial nerves, motor (including tone, muscle bulk, and strength), reflexes, sensation, coordination, and gait. Much of the examination of the frightened or active child is, by necessity, observational, and the examiner must capitalize on moments of opportunity while maintaining a systematic approach to avoid overlooking a key component. Playing games engages a toddler or preschooler; activities such as throwing a ball, stacking blocks, jumping, and drawing can reduce anxiety and allow assessment of motor coordination, balance, and handedness. In the older child, "casual" conversation can reveal both language and cognitive abilities.

DIAGNOSTIC EVALUATIONS

Electroencephalography

Electroencephalography (EEG) is a noninvasive method for recording neuronal electrical activity. EEG background patterns vary by both age (infant, toddler, or adolescent) and clinical state (awake, drowsy, or asleep). EEG may be difficult to obtain if the child is unable to cooperate, but sedating medications, such as benzodiazepines, can alter the EEG and decrease the likelihood of recording abnormalities. Normal patterns, such as spindles or other sleep architecture while asleep or a posterior dominant rhythm (PDR) during wakefulness, can be positive prognostic indicators. In contrast, abnormally slow or disorganized backgrounds may suggest neurodevelopmental issues or acute brain dysfunction. Interictal (between seizures) "epileptiform activity" can indicate an increased risk for seizures or, in some cases, can be diagnostic for a particular type of epilepsy, although children without epilepsy can also have abnormal backgrounds and/or epileptiform discharges.

Table 25–1. Neurologic examination: toddler age and up.

Category	Operation	Assesses
Mental status	Level of consciousness; level of awareness; orientation, language, development/cognition; affect	Cortical and subcortical pathways, executive functioning
Cranial nerves	CN I: Smell (usually omitted) CN II: Pupillary light reflex (sensory), visual acuity, visual fields, fundi CN III, IV, VI: Pupillary light reflex (motor), eye opening, extraocular movements, convergence CN V: Facial sensation (upper, middle, lower; V_1, V_2, V_3); muscles of mastication (jaw clench) CN VII: Upper—eye closure, brow raise; Lower—smile, grimace, show teeth CN VIII: Finger rub at each ear CN IX, X: Palate elevation (gag—often omitted); strength of vocalizations CN XI: Head turn (sternocleidomastoid) and shoulder shrug (trapezius) CN XII: Tongue protrusion and bulk	Cortical pathways, brainstem (midbrain, pons, medulla), and peripheral cranial nerves
Motor	Tone: head control, body posture, passive range of motion of the limbs Muscle bulk: palpate for atrophy, pseudohypertrophy, or fibrosis Strength: proximal (shoulders/hips) to distal (fingers/wrists, toes/ankles). Grading: 0 = no movement, 1 = trace movement, 2 = movement in lateral plane but not against gravity, 3 = against gravity, 4 (4–/4/4+) = some resistance to examiner with mild weakness, 5 = normal strength	*Upper motor neurons*: motor cortex, corticospinal tracts → Lesions cause hypertonia *Lower motor neurons*: anterior horn cells in the spinal cord, spinal nerve roots, peripheral nerves → Lesions cause hypotonia
Reflexes	Tendon stretch reflexes: biceps, triceps, brachioradialis, patella, Achilles. Grading: 0 = reflex absent; 1 = reflex present only with augmentation maneuver; 2 = reflex present without spread to adjacent muscle groups (if movement is large amplitude, can describe as "brisk"); 3 = reflex spreads to adjacent muscle groups; 4 = clonus Primitive and superficial reflexes	Corticospinal tracts → Lesions cause hyperreflexia Spinal cord and peripheral nerves → Lesions cause hyporeflexia
Gait	Assess casual stance for excessively wide base. Walking, running, walking on heels/toes, tandem gait	Cerebellum (vermis), spinocerebellar tracts, sensory pathways, motor system, others
Coordination (truncal, limb)	Smooth pursuit (eye movements); reaching for objects; finger-to-nose and heel-to-shin movements; rapid alternating movements. Note other abnormal movements (such as tics).	Cerebellum (hemisphere or vermis), sensory pathways, others
Sensory	Light touch, vibration (with tuning fork), proprioception, pinprick (often skipped in pediatrics) temperature (cold tuning fork) Romberg test: truncal balance and recovery (proprioception)	Peripheral nerves Posterior columns (light touch, vibration, proprioception) Spinothalamic tracts (pain/temp) Thalamus; parietal lobe

Routine EEGs obtained in the outpatient setting are typically brief (20–40 minutes). Therefore, events of interest are usually not recorded. Prolonged ambulatory EEG (obtained over 24–72 hours) can be useful in capturing events to determine if they are epileptic seizures but does not include video. Adding a full montage EEG to a nocturnal polysomnogram (sleep study) can help differentiate nonepileptic sleep-related events from nocturnal epileptic seizures. Continuous video-EEG recording, obtained during an inpatient admission to an epilepsy monitoring unit (EMU), also allows spell characterization, as well as assessment of patients with medically intractable epilepsy. Localization of the seizure focus by EEG recording during seizures (the "ictal period") can determine candidacy for surgical resection. In addition, prolonged or continuous inpatient video-EEG recordings have numerous applications during acute neurologic conditions, such as altered mental status, status epilepticus, hypoxic-ischemic encephalopathy (HIE), or traumatic brain injury.

Evoked Potentials

Visual, auditory, or somatosensory evoked potentials (SSEP) are obtained by repetitive stimulation of the retina by light flashes, the cochlea by sounds, or a nerve by galvanic stimuli.

These stimuli result in cortical-evoked potentials that can be recorded with scalp electrodes for specific situations. Visual evoked potentials may be helpful in evaluating patients with optic neuritis, multiple sclerosis (MS), or other demyelinating diseases. Brainstem auditory evoked responses (BAER) are routinely used to screen for hearing impairment in neonates. SSEP monitoring is critical for identifying potentially reversible spinal cord injury during spinal surgery.

Lumbar Puncture

Cerebrospinal fluid (CSF) can be obtained by inserting a small-gauge needle through the L3–L4 intervertebral space into the thecal sac, while the patient is lying in a lateral recumbent position. Radiographic guidance and sedation may be necessary in some patients. After an opening pressure is measured, fluid is removed to examine for evidence of infection, inflammation, or metabolic disorders (Table 25–2). Special staining techniques can be used for mycobacterial and fungal infections, and further testing can be performed for specific viral agents, antibody titer determinations, cytopathologic studies, lactate and pyruvate concentrations, amino acid levels, and neurotransmitter analysis.

Genetic/Metabolic Testing

Genetic testing and, to a lesser degree, metabolic testing can play an important role in the diagnosis of a variety of neurologic disorders. Published testing algorithms typically recommend beginning with targeted gene testing (either single gene or gene panels) before moving to chromosomal microarray, which could then be followed by clinical (whole) exome sequencing (WES). However, in practice, utilization of WES is rapidly expanding (see Chapter 37) and, in some cases, is an affordable alternative to extensive biochemical, single gene, and gene panel testing. Recent studies suggest that WES has a diagnostic yield of 20%–40% for neurologic conditions including developmental delay/intellectual disability, neuromuscular disorders, movement disorders, and epilepsy. Given the complexity and fast-paced progress of genetic evaluations, consider consulting a genetics expert prior to initiating testing.

Nerve Conduction Studies & Electromyography Testing

Nerve conduction studies (NCS) and electromyography (EMG) testing can assess for disorders of the lower motor neurons, peripheral nerves, neuromuscular junction, and muscle. NCS is performed by applying small currents (shocks) to peripheral nerves and calculating the response amplitude and conduction velocity. EMG requires placement of recording electrodes (needles) into selected muscles to record spontaneous and volitional electrical activity. For more details, refer to the section Disorders of Childhood Affecting Muscles.

PEDIATRIC NEURORADIOLOGIC PROCEDURES

Computed Tomography

Computed tomography (CT) allows rapid visualization of intracranial contents by obtaining a series of cross-sectional X-ray images, often without sedation. CT scans have high sensitivity (88%–96% of lesions $> 1–2$ cm can be seen) but low specificity (tumor, infection, or infarct may look similar). CT is particularly helpful in identifying "blood" (hemorrhage), "bones" (skull fractures or calcifications), and "bullets" (and other foreign bodies)—all of which appear "hyperdense" (bright), as well as for measuring ventricular size. "Hypodense" (dark) lesions are nonspecific and can indicate ischemic stroke, contusion, demyelinating disorders, infection, or edema. Intravenous injection of iodized contrast allows visualization of the arteries (CTA) or veins (CTV). A single head CT scan is approximately 2 milli sieverts (mSv; typical chest X-ray PA view = 0.02 mSv), which equates to approximately 8 months of exposure to naturally occurring environmental radiation. The risk of malignancy is thought to be 1 brain tumor per 10,000 patients in the 10 years following CT exposure, and the lifetime risk of brain tumor after head CT is likely higher, particularly in younger children.

Magnetic Resonance Imaging

Magnetic resonance imaging (MRI) utilizes powerful electromagnetic fields and radiofrequency currents to create high-resolution images of soft tissues without ionizing radiation. MRI signals vary with the ratio of water to protein and lipid in tissue, as well as with the particular MRI sequence (T1, T2, etc), allowing detection of various neurologic disorders, including tumors, ischemic and hemorrhagic lesions, vascular disorders, inflammation, demyelination, infection, metabolic disorders, and degenerative processes.

MRI T1 sequences yield excellent anatomical characterization. Although myelination progresses from infancy into young adulthood, by 2–3 years of age, the gray matter should appear "hypointense" (dark) compared to the "hyperintense" (bright) myelinated white matter on T1. T2 and FLAIR (fluid-attenuation inversion recovery) sequences allow better visualization of pathology, such as demyelinating lesions. Perfusion-weighted imaging, apparent diffusion coefficient (ADC), and diffusion-weighted imaging (DWI), which measure the motion of water molecules, identify ischemic and cytotoxic edema in acute stroke and toxic/metabolic disorders. Contrast is typically used only if inflammation (including demyelination) or infection are suspected. Magnetic resonance angiography (MRA) or magnetic resonance venography (MRV) visualize large extra- and intracranial blood vessels, though they are not as sensitive as CT or conventional angiography. Magnetic resonance spectroscopy (MRS) assesses biochemical changes, increased cellular activity, and

Table 25–2. Characteristics of cerebrospinal fluid in the normal child and in central nervous system infections and inflammatory conditions.

Condition	Initial Pressure (cm H₂O)	Appearance	Cells/µL	Protein (mg/dL)	Glucose (mg/dL)	Other Tests	Comments
Normal	< 16	Clear	Newborns: up to 30 WBCs Others: 0–5 WBC; RBCs should be rare	Newborns: up to 150 (lumbar); Infants: up to 65 (lumbar); Others: 15–35 (lumbar), 5–15 (ventricular)	50–80 (two-thirds of blood glucose); may be increased after seizure	CSF-IgG index[a] less than 0.7[a]; LDH 2–27 U/L	Infants: CSF protein may be up to 170 mg/dL; seizures do not cause an increase in CSF WBCs
Bloody tap	Normal or low	Bloody (sometimes with clot)	One additional WBC per 700 RBCs[b]; RBCs not crenated	One additional milligram per 800 RBCs[b]	Normal	RBC number should decrease between 1st and 3rd tubes	Spin down fluid, supernatant will be clear and colorless[c]
Bacterial meningitis, acute	20–75+	Opalescent to purulent	Up to thousands of WBCs, mostly PMNs (Very early, there may be few WBCs)	Up to hundreds	Decreased; may be none (Very early, it may be normal)	Gram stain, smear and culture mandatory; PCR; LDH greater than 24 U/L	PCR often positive for meningococci and pneumococci in plasma and/or CSF
Bacterial meningitis, partially treated	Usually increased	Clear or opalescent	WBCs usually increased, PMNs usually predominate	Elevated	Normal or decreased	LDH usually greater than 24 U/L; PCR may still be positive	Smear and culture may be negative if antibiotics have been in use
Tuberculous meningitis	15–75+	Opalescent; fibrin web or pellicle	250–500 WBCs, mostly lymphocytes (Early, more PMNs)	45–500; parallels cell count; increases over time	Decreased; may be none	Smear for acid-fast organism: CSF culture; PCR	Consider AIDS, a common comorbidity of tuberculosis
Fungal meningitis	Increased	Variable; often clear	10–500 WBCs, mostly lymphocytes (Early, more PMNs)	Elevated and increasing	Decreased	India ink preparations, cryptococcal antigen, PCR, culture, immunofluorescence tests	Often superimposed in patients who are debilitated or on immunosuppressive therapy
Aseptic meningo-encephalitis (viral meningitis or encephalitis)	Normal or slightly increased	Clear unless cell count > 300/µL	None to a few hundred WBCs, mostly lymphocytes (Early, more PMNs)	20–125	Normal; may be low in mumps, herpes, or other viral infections	CSF, stool, blood, throat washings for viral cultures; LDH less than 28 U/L; PCR for HSV, CMV, EBV, enterovirus, etc	Acute and convalescent antibody titers; in mumps or enterovirus infection, can see up to 1000 lymphocytes;

Condition	Pressure	Appearance	Cell count	Protein (mg/dL)	Glucose	Special tests	Comments
Parainfectious encephalomyelitis (ADEM) and other demyelinating disorders (such as MS)	8–45, usually increased	Usually clear	0–50+ WBCs, mostly lymphocytes; often normal in MS	15–75	Normal	CSF-IgG index, oligoclonal bands variable (often positive in MS)	No organisms; fulminant cases can resemble bacterial meningitis
Polyneuritis (including Guillain-Barre syndrome)	Normal and occasionally increased	Early: normal; late: xanthochromic if protein high	Normal to slightly increased WBCs	Early: normal; late: 45–1500	Normal	CSF-IgG index may be increased; oligoclonal bands variable	Try to find cause (viral infections, toxins, lupus, diabetes, etc)
Meningeal carcinomatosis	Often elevated	Clear to opalescent	Cytologic identification of tumor cells	Often mildly to moderately elevated	Often depressed	Cytopathology and/or flow cytometry	Seen with leukemia, medulloblastoma, meningeal melanosis, histiocytosis X
Brain abscess	Normal or increased	Usually clear	5–500 WBCs in 80%, mostly PMNs	Usually slightly increased	Normal; occasionally decreased	Imaging study of brain (MRI)	Cell count related to proximity to meninges; findings as in purulent meningitis if abscess ruptures

ADEM, acute disseminated encephalomyelitis; AIDS, acquired immunodeficiency syndrome; CMV, cytomegalovirus; CSF, cerebrospinal fluid; EBV, Epstein-Barr virus; HSV, herpes simplex virus; IL-8, interleukin 8; LDH, lactate dehydrogenase; MRI, magnetic resonance imaging; MS, multiple sclerosis; PCR, polymerase chain reaction; PMN, polymorphonuclear neutrophil; RBC, red blood cell; TNF, tumor necrosis factor; WBC, white blood cell.

[a]CSF-IgG index = (CSF IgG/serum IgG)/(CSF albumin/serum albumin).

[b]Many studies document pitfalls in using these ratios due to WBC lysis. Clinical judgment and repeat lumbar punctures may be necessary.

oxidative metabolism, for example, in brain tumors or after neonatal HIE. To avoid movement artifact, sedation is necessary for children who are unable to lie still for 45 minutes. However, "ultrafast" MRI protocols are increasingly used to rule out neurologic emergencies, including hemorrhage and hydrocephalus, avoiding unnecessary radiation from CT.

Specialized Neuroimaging

Additional neuroimaging techniques can provide detailed anatomical and functional characterization of lesions, such as brain tumors or seizure foci (epileptogenic brain regions that generate seizures). In general, these are performed only by a multidisciplinary clinical and/or research team. **Functional MRI (fMRI)** assesses blood oxygenation changes throughout the brain, while the patient performs language or motor tasks to localize specific brain functions. **Diffusion tensor imaging (DTI)** identifies the axonal tracts of neurologic pathways, such as the optic radiations or motor system. **Positron emission tomography (PET)** uses radiolabeled substrates, such as intravenously administered fluorodeoxyglucose, to measure the metabolic rate throughout the brain. When performed during a seizure (the ictal state), seizure foci can be three-dimensionally reconstructed for surgical planning. **Single-photon emission computed tomography (SPECT)** allows three-dimensional visualization of cerebral blood flow using a radioactive tracer (typically technetium-99m). Metabolically active areas, such as seizure foci or tumors, may demonstrate increased blood flow, while vascular regions at risk may show decreased cerebral blood flow. **Conventional cerebral angiography** utilizes traditional X-rays and catheterization, typically via the femoral vessels under sedation, to visualize the cerebral blood vessels. This detailed anatomical characterization may be useful in the diagnosis of cerebral aneurysms and other vascular malformations, as well as surgical planning for brain tumors.

Ultrasonography

In infants with an open fontanelle, head ultrasonography (US) is an excellent tool for rapidly assessing brain structures with portable equipment, without ionizing radiation or need for sedation. Intracranial hemorrhage, ventriculomegaly, ischemia, malformations, and calcifications can be well visualized with US, though full characterization may require other imaging modalities.

Cakir B et al: Inborn errors of metabolisms presenting in childhood. J Neuroimaging 2011;21(2):e117−e133 [PMID: 21435076].

Fogel BL: Genetic and genomic testing for neurological disease in clinical practice. Handb Clin Neurol 2018:147:11−22 [PMID: 29325607].

Haslam RHA: Clinical neurological examination of infants and children. Handb Clin Neurol 2013:111:17−25 [PMID: 23622147].

Michelson DJ et al: Evidence report: genetic and metabolic testing on children with global developmental delay: report of the Quality Standards Subcommittee of the American Academy of Neurology and the Practice Committee of the Child Neurology Society. Neurology 2011 Oct 25;77(17):1629−1635 [PMID: 21956720].

Orman G, Rossi A, Meoded A, Huisman TAGM: Children with acute neurological emergency. In: *Diseases of the Brain, Head and Neck, Spine 2020−2021: Diagnostic Imaging*. Cham (CH): Springer; 2020. Chapter 14. [PMID: 32119241].

DISORDERS AFFECTING THE NERVOUS SYSTEM IN INFANTS & CHILDREN

ALTERED STATES OF CONSCIOUSNESS (COMA)

ESSENTIALS OF DIAGNOSIS & TYPICAL FEATURES

► Acute onset of reduced or altered arousal, attentiveness, or cognitive functions can be caused by numerous etiologies, many of which are treatable.

Consciousness encompasses both the patient's level of wakefulness and ability to interact with the environment. The neurologic substrate for consciousness is the ascending reticular activating system (RAS), comprising the reticular formation in the brainstem, thalamic intralaminar nuclei, and portions of the hypothalamus. Dysfunction of the cerebral cortex, especially bilateral lesions, can also cause coma.

► Clinical Findings

Many terms, including obtundation, lethargy, somnolence, stupor, and coma, are used to describe the continuum from fully alert and aware to complete unresponsiveness. While providers can use a scale, such as the Glasgow coma scale (see Chapter 12), qualitative descriptions such as, "opens eyes with painful stimulus, but does not respond to voice" may better help subsequent observers evaluate the severity of the disorder of consciousness (DoC; Table 25–3).

- *Minimally conscious state* (MCS) denotes patients who demonstrate sleep-wake cycles and some residual degree of interaction with the environment, such as purposeful movements. Thus, MCS involves "partial preservation of consciousness."

- *Vegetative state/Unresponsive wakefulness syndrome (VS/UWS)* denotes a condition in which the patient has sleep-wake cycles but no awareness of self or the environment, often described as "wakefulness without awareness." When this condition lasts greater than 3 months for

Table 25–3. The spectrum of consciousness/unconsciousness.

	Conscious	MCS	VS/UWS	Coma	Brain Death
Awake?	Yes	Yes	Yes	No	No
Aware?	Yes	Partially	No	No	No
Motor responses?	Present	Present	Present	Absent	Absent
Brainstem reflexes?	Present	Present	Present	Present	Absent

MCS, minimally conscious state; VS/UWS, vegetative state/unresponsive wakefulness state.

non-traumatic etiologies or greater than 12 months for traumatic causes, the term "chronic VS/UWS", followed by the duration, is preferred over the previous term of "permanent vegetative state." This is in recognition that recovery has been reported up to 24 months after the initial injury, with some patients even regaining functional independence.

- *Coma* is defined by the complete absence of wakefulness and interaction with the environment for at least 1 hour. When coma persists, evaluation for the presence of sleep-wake cycles or absence of all brain function can further delineate the severity.
- *Brain death* (death by neurologic criteria) refers to patients in a coma who have cessation of all brain function, including cortical activity, brainstem reflexes, and spontaneous respirations. See Chapter 14 for details of the brain death evaluation.

Diagnostic Evaluation

Medical causes, including anoxia/ischemia/stroke, infection, toxidromes, seizures, metabolic disturbances, and hypothermia/hyperthermia, account for 90% of cases of coma in children. Structural causes, such as trauma, neoplasm, and increased intracranial pressure (ICP), comprise the remaining 10%. Infection is the most common cause (30%), and blood cultures and lumbar puncture (LP) are often necessary. A detailed history and examination will often reveal the cause of an altered state of consciousness. When this is not the case complete blood count, serum urea nitrogen and creatinine (to evaluate kidney function), liver enzymes, and ammonia should be obtained. Urine, blood, and even gastric contents can be evaluated by toxin screens, with considerations for pesticides, lead, salicylates, and other medications within the home, as well as illicit substances. Hypoglycemia, diabetic ketoacidosis, and hyperglycemic nonketotic coma should be investigated. Additional testing might include oxygen and carbon dioxide partial pressures to evaluate for carbon monoxide poisoning, or extensive metabolic evaluations such as plasma porphyrins and amino acid concentrations, and urine organic acids. If head trauma, intracranial hemorrhage, or increased ICP is suspected, an emergency CT scan or MRI is

necessary. EEG should be obtained if seizures are suspected and, in some cases, may add prognostic information.

Differential Diagnosis

Diagnostic errors occur in up to 40% of patients with DoC, due to both overestimation of the severity of DoC, as well as lack of recognition of the following conditions:

- *Locked-in syndrome* describes patients who are conscious (awake and aware) but cannot demonstrate interactiveness with their environment due to a massive loss of motor function, typically from a lesion in the pons. Vertical eye movements may be preserved.
- *Akinetic-mutism* denotes a patient who is awake and aware, but does not speak, initiate movements, or follow commands, typically due to lesions of the frontal lobes.
- *Catatonia* refers to patients with abnormal alertness and awareness (though typically not completely absent) secondary to psychiatric illness. Patients often retain the ability to maintain trunk and limb postures.

Treatment

As with any emergency, the clinician must first stabilize the comatose child using the ABCs of resuscitation. A thorough trauma evaluation is key; treatment of trauma is discussed in detail in Chapter 12. Bradycardia, high blood pressure, and irregular breathing (Cushing triad) or midbrain dysfunction, such as third nerve palsy (with the eye deviated down and out) or a "blown" pupil (large, fixed/unreactive pupil), indicate increased ICP and impending brain herniation and, thus, require prompt neurosurgical consultation. Initial treatment of impending herniation includes elevating the head of the bed to 15–30 degrees and providing moderate hyperventilation. The use of mannitol, hypertonic saline, pharmacologic coma, hypothermia, and drainage of CSF are covered in detail in Chapter 14.

Subacute-chronic treatment and prognosis data are lacking for children with DoC; therefore, guidelines for adult patients are often extrapolated to the pediatric population. In general, clinicians should avoid implying that patients with DoC have a universally poor prognosis, particularly during the first 28 days postinjury. Ongoing management should include serial assessments, avoidance of common medical complications, considerations for specialized facilities, and, in some cases, a trial of amantadine, a neurostimulant medication. Hyperbaric oxygen and stem cell therapy are not currently recommended, though studies are underway. Ongoing discussions of long-term prognosis may benefit from involvement of specialists familiar with the nuances of recovery from DoC.

Giacino JT et al: Comprehensive systematic review update summary: disorders of consciousness. Neurology 2018;91:461–470 [PMID: 30089617].

Giacino JT et al: Practice guideline update recommendations summary: disorders of consciousness. Neurology 2018;91:450–460 [PMID: 30089618].

Rabinstein A: Coma and brain death. Continuum 2018;24(6):1708–1731 [PMID: 30516602].

SEIZURES & EPILEPSY

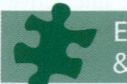

ESSENTIALS OF DIAGNOSIS & TYPICAL FEATURES

▶ Seizures occur due to abnormal synchronized electrical activity within the brain, associated with transient motor, sensory, or cognitive abnormalities.

▶ Epilepsy is defined as two unprovoked seizures or a single seizure with an EEG and/or risk factors suggesting high risk for recurrent events.

▶ Febrile seizures are provoked by a minor febrile illness in children aged 6 months to 6 years.

A seizure is a sudden, transient disturbance of brain activity, manifested by involuntary motor, sensory, autonomic, or cognitive phenomena, alone or in any combination, often accompanied by alteration of consciousness. Seizures can be provoked by any factor that disturbs brain function, including acute metabolic, traumatic, anoxic, or infectious insults to the brain (classified as symptomatic or provoked seizures). Seizures can also occur spontaneously without an acute central nervous system (CNS) insult (unprovoked seizures), often related to structural abnormalities or genetic disorders.

Epilepsy is defined as two seizures separated by at least 24 hours, or a single seizure associated with a greater than 60% risk of recurrence or the diagnosis of an epilepsy syndrome. The chance of having a second seizure after an initial unprovoked episode in a child is about 50%. The risk of recurrence after a second unprovoked seizure is 85%. During childhood, the incidence of epilepsy is highest in the newborn period. Prevalence flattens out after age 10–15 years. Up to 70% of children with epilepsy will achieve seizure remission with their first appropriate medication.

▶ Classification

The International League Against Epilepsy (ILAE; www.ilae.org) has established classifications of seizures and epilepsy syndromes. Seizures are classified as *focal*, previously called partial (with suspected seizure onset that can be localized to one part of the brain), *generalized* (involving the whole brain or a network of the brain), or *unknown* if it is not clear if they are focal or generalized.

Several types of generalized seizures are recognized with *ILAE seizure classification*: tonic-clonic (stiffening-shaking), absence (typical, atypical, and with special features), myoclonic (twitching/jerking), atonic (sudden loss of tone), myoclonic atonic (jerk followed by sudden loss of tone), tonic, and clonic seizures. ILAE nomenclature for focal seizures is based on the presentation of the seizure, such as "with or without alteration of awareness" and "motor" vs "nonmotor (autonomic, emotional, or sensory)" seizure.

Epilepsy syndromes are defined by the nature of the seizures, age of onset, EEG findings, and other clinical factors. The 2017 *ILAE terminology for epilepsy syndromes* reflects our growing understanding of underlying etiology and allows for a hierarchical classification approach, identical to the seizure guidelines. In parallel, patients may have an etiologic diagnosis (structural, genetic, infectious, etc) and may have comorbid diagnoses (ADHD, depression, anxiety, etc). Characterizing the seizure and/or subsequent epilepsy syndrome (Table 25–4) is necessary for accurate diagnosis, determines further evaluation and treatment, assists with prognostication, and facilitates research of specific syndromes.

1. Seizures & Epilepsy in Childhood

▶ Clinical Findings

Seizures are stereotyped, paroxysmal clinical events; the key to diagnosis is usually in the history. Not all paroxysmal/sudden events are epileptic. Careful questioning regarding prior events may identify previously unrecognized seizures or provide clues that the events are nonepileptic, such as with syncopal events or stereotypies. Events prior to, during, and after the seizure need to be ascertained. Videos of events are extremely useful. Although observers often primarily recall only the generalized convulsive activity, careful questions can unveil additional details, such as a focal onset. An aura may precede the clinically apparent seizure. The family may note alterations in behavior, or the patient may describe a feeling of extreme fear, happiness, or anxiety, an odd or unusual taste or smell, or a rising feeling in the abdomen. The specific symptoms may help define the location of seizure onset (eg, déjà vu suggests temporal lobe onset).

Table 25–4. Characteristics of childhood seizures and epilepsy syndromes.

Seizure-Type Epilepsy Syndrome	Age at Onset	Clinical Manifestations	Causative Factors	EEG Pattern	Other Diagnostic Studies	Treatment and Comments
Absence seizures (previously called petit mal)		Lapses of consciousness or vacant stares, lasting 3–10 s, often in clusters. Can have automatisms of face and hands.	Depends on epilepsy syndrome.	3-Hz spike and slow wave; hyperventilation may provoke discharges or seizures.	Typically not necessary	Ethosuximide is often effective; other agents may be used.
Focal seizures (previously called simple or complex partial seizures)	Any age	Seizure may involve any part of body; may spread in fixed pattern. Can include staring.	Often unknown; brain tumor, trauma, vascular pathology, possibly genetic, meningitis, cortical malformations (dysplasia), etc.	EEG may be normal; focal spikes or slow waves in appropriate cortical region.	MRI, repeat if seizures poorly controlled or progressive.	Oxcarbazepine, lamotrigine, and levetiracetam as first line; topiramate, zonisamide, and lacosamide as second line. Surgery may be an option.
Generalized tonic-clonic seizures (GTCs; previously called grand mal)	Any age	Loss of consciousness; tonic-clonic movements. Incontinence in 15%. Postictal confusion and somnolence.	May be seen with metabolic disturbances, trauma, infection, intoxication, degenerative disorders, brain tumors. Can be genetic.	Bilateral synchronous, symmetric multiple high-voltage spikes, spike waves.	Metabolic, imaging and infectious evaluation may be appropriate.	Levetiracetam, lamotrigine, zonisamide, or valproic acid
Neonatal seizures	Birth–2 wk	Can be any seizure type, can be very subtle.	Neurologic insults (hypoxia/ischemia; intracranial hemorrhage); hypoglycemia, hypocalcemia, hyperand hyponatremia. Drug withdrawal. Pyridoxine deficiency. Other metabolic disorders. CNS infections. Structural abnormalities. Genetic causes are increasingly recognized.	Focal spikes or slow rhythms; multifocal discharges. Electroclinical dissociation (electrical seizure without clinical manifestations) may occur.	Lumbar puncture; CSF PCR for herpes, enterovirus; serum and CSF glucose, serum Ca^{2+}, PO_4^{3-}, Mg^{2+}, BUN, ammonia, amino acids, organic acids, TORCHS, other metabolic testing if suspected. Ultrasound or CT/MRI.	Benzodiazepines, phenobarbital, phenytoin IV. Recent experience with levetiracetam and topiramate. B6 (pyridoxine) trial. Treat underlying disorder.

(Continued)

Table 25-4. Characteristics of childhood seizures and epilepsy syndromes. (*Continued*)

Seizure-Type Epilepsy Syndrome	Age at Onset	Clinical Manifestations	Causative Factors	EEG Pattern	Other Diagnostic Studies	Treatment and Comments
Epileptic spasms (aka infantile spasms or West syndrome)	3–18 mo, usually about 6 mo	Abrupt, usually (but not always) symmetric; adduction or flexion of head and trunk, or extensor movements (similar to Moro reflex). Occur in clusters typically upon awakening. Associated with developmental regression or plateau.	Etiology identified in approximately two-thirds, structural, metabolic, or genetic. Tuberous sclerosis in 5%–10%. Trisomy 21 in 2.5%–3.1%, TORCHS, and other genetic mutations.	Hypsarrhythmia (chaotic high-voltage slow waves or random spikes) [90%]; other abnormalities in 10%. Rarely normal at onset. EEG improvement is required for treatment efficacy.	Funduscopic and skin examination, MRI. Other testing if clinical suspicion (amino and organic acid screen, TORCHS screen, microarray). Consider epilepsy gene panels.	ACTH, prednisolone, or vigabatrin (especially if tuberous sclerosis). Early treatment improves outcomes.
Lennox-Gastaut syndrome (LGS)	Any time in childhood (usually 2–7 y)	Multiple seizure types including tonic, myoclonic (shock-like jerks or contractions of muscle groups); atonic ("drop attacks") and atypical absence.	Multiple causes, usually resulting in diffuse neuronal damage. History of infantile spasms; prenatal or perinatal brain injury; meningitis; CNS degenerative disorders; structural abnormalities.	Atypical slow (1–2.5 Hz) spike-wave complexes and bursts of high-voltage generalized spikes, often with diffusely slow background frequencies. Electrodecrement and fast spikes during sleep.	Dictated by index of suspicion: MRI; genetic testing; inherited metabolic disorders, neuronal ceroid lipofuscinosis, lysosomal enzymes. Skin or conjunctival biopsy for electron microscopy.	Difficult to treat, typically requires multiple medications. Avoid carbamazepine and oxcarbazepine.
Dravet syndrome	First to second year of life	Initially prolonged febrile seizure that may be hemiconvulsions; after 1 y of age with multiple seizure types; typically sensitive to change in temperature. May also have abnormal gait.	85% with SCN1A mutation others with SCN1B or GABA receptor mutations.	Multifocal epileptiform discharges, generalized epileptiform discharges, and slowing.	Genetic testing.	Can be difficult to treat, consider Dravet-specific medications (stiripentol and fenfluramine). Avoid maintenance Na channel blockers such as phenytoin, carbamazepine, oxcarbazepine.
Epilepsy with myoclonic atonic seizures (Doose syndrome)	Any time in childhood (usually 2–7 y)	Multiple seizure types including atonic, myoclonic atonic, atypical absence, tonic and generalized tonic-clonic	Rarely is etiology found, likely genetic, < 5% with SCN1A mutation; large percentage with family history of febrile seizures.	Generalized spike wave discharges, central theta slowing.	Genetic testing.	Can be difficult to treat, consider ketogenic diet. Avoid phenytoin, carbamazepine, oxcarbazepine, and gabapentin.

Syndrome	Age	Clinical features	Etiology	EEG	Imaging	Treatment
Childhood absence epilepsy (previously called petit mal)	3–12 y	Absence seizures (often several/day); clonic activity in 30%–45%. Often mimics focal seizures but no aura or postictal confusion.	Presumed genetic. Abnormal thalamocortical circuitry.	EEG always abnormal. 3-Hz spike and slow wave discharges, provoked by hyperventilation. EEG normalization correlates with seizure control.	Hyperventilation often provokes attacks. Imaging studies rarely of value.	Ethosuximide most effective and best tolerated; valproic acid, lamotrigine, levetiracetam.
Juvenile absence epilepsy	10–15 y	Absence seizures, less frequent than in childhood absence epilepsy. Greater risk of convulsive seizures.	Presumed genetic.	3–6-Hz generalized spike wave discharges.	Not always triggered by hyperventilation.	Same as childhood absence epilepsy but may be more difficult to treat.
Self-limited Epilepsy with Centrotemporal Spikes SeLECTS (previously called benign rolandic epilepsy or benign epilepsy with centrotemporal spikes, BECTS)	5–16 y	Focal seizures affect the face, tongue, hand +/– secondary generalization. Usually nocturnal or early AM. Similar seizure patterns may be observed in patients with focal cortical lesions. Almost always remits by puberty.	Presumed genetic. Seizure history or abnormal EEG findings in relatives of 40% of affected probands, suggesting a single autosomal dominant gene, possibly with age-dependent penetrance.	Centrotemporal spikes or sharp waves ("rolandic discharges") appearing against a normal EEG background.	Seldom need CT or MRI.	Often no medication is necessary, especially if seizures are exclusively nocturnal and infrequent. Oxcarbazepine, lamotrigine or levetiracetam. (See focal seizures.)
Juvenile myoclonic epilepsy (JME)	Usually between 12 and 18 y	Early morning myoclonic seizures (small jerks of neck and shoulder muscles), GTCs, sometimes absence seizures. Typically developing. Rarely resolves (20%–25%) but usually remits on medications.	Presumed genetic. 40% of relatives have myoclonias, especially in females; 15% have an abnormal EEG pattern.	Interictal EEG shows generalized spike-and-wave sequences or 4-6-Hz polyspike-and-wave discharges.	Imaging not necessary. If course is unfavorable, consider progressive myoclonic epilepsy syndromes (neurodegenerative disorders).	Valproic acid, lamotrigine or levetiracetam.
Febrile seizures	6 mo–6 y (peak 6–18 mo); most common childhood seizure (incidence 2%–5%)	Usually generalized seizures, rarely focal in onset. May lead to status epilepticus. Recurrence risk of second febrile seizure 30% (50% if < 1 y of age); Higher risk of subsequent epilepsy if febrile status epilepticus.	Nonneurologic febrile illness. Risk factors: positive family history, day care, developmental delay, prolonged neonatal hospitalization. Some minor illnesses can provoke seizures even without fever (eg, GI-illness provoked seizures).	Normal interictal EEG, especially when obtained at least 1 wk after seizure. Therefore, not useful unless complicating features.	Lumbar puncture in infants or whenever suspicion of meningitis exists.	Treat underlying illness, fever. Diazepam rectally for prolonged (more than 5 min) seizure. Prophylaxis rarely needed.

ACTH, adrenocorticotropic hormone; BUN, blood urea nitrogen; CNS, central nervous system; CSF, cerebrospinal fluid; CT, computed tomography; EEG, electroencephalogram; MRI, magnetic resonance imaging; PCR, polymerase chain reaction; TORCHS, toxoplasmosis, other infections, rubella, cytomegalovirus, herpes simplex, and syphilis; VNS, vagus nerve stimulation.

The behavior and movements of the child during the actual seizure activity are key to classifying the seizure type. The parent may report lateralized motor activity (eg, the child's eyes may deviate to one side, or the child may experience posturing of a limb) without impaired awareness, suggestive of focal motor seizures (previously termed simple partial seizures). Automatisms, such as blinking, chewing, or hand movements, associated with staring or "zoning out" (partially impaired awareness) also support a diagnosis of focal motor seizures (previously termed complex partial seizures).

In contrast, generalized convulsive seizures usually manifest with acute, complete loss of consciousness and whole body (generalized) motor activity. Tonic posturing, tonic-clonic activity, or myoclonus may occur. In children with absence seizures, which are a generalized type of seizure, behavioral arrest may be associated with staring and automatisms, making it difficult to differentiate between absence seizures and focal seizures. Postictal states (after the seizure) can also be helpful in diagnosis. After many focal seizures and most generalized convulsive seizures, postictal sleepiness typically occurs, while absence, myoclonic, or atonic seizures do not typically cause postictal changes.

▶ Diagnostic Evaluation

Many factors determine the extent and urgency of the diagnostic evaluation, such as the child's age, the severity and type of seizure, whether the child is ill or injured, and the clinician's suspicion about the underlying cause. Seizures in early infancy often have an underlying cause that is structural, genetic, or metabolic and will guide prognosis and management. Therefore, the younger the child, the more extensive the diagnostic assessment should be. Any child younger than 3 years with new onset of *unprovoked* seizures should be evaluated with an EEG and MRI, although the need is not emergent.

Metabolic abnormalities are seldom found in the well child with seizures. Unless there is a high clinical suspicion of serious medical conditions (eg, significant diarrhea/dehydration, uremia, hyponatremia, hypocalcemia, or hypoglycemia), routine laboratory tests are typically not necessary. Special studies may be necessary in circumstances that suggest an acute systemic etiology for a seizure, for example, in the presence of apparent renal failure, sepsis, or substance abuse. Emergent brain imaging is usually not needed without evidence of trauma or acute physical abnormalities on examination.

Routine EEG is useful primarily for defining interictal activity (between seizures), except for the fortuitous recording of a clinical seizure or in situations when seizures are easily provoked, such as childhood absence epilepsy. Ultimately, a seizure is a clinical phenomenon. An EEG showing epileptiform activity may confirm and clarify the clinical diagnosis (for instance, defining an epilepsy syndrome), but it is not always diagnostic (see section Electroencephalography under Diagnostic Evaluation).

▶ Differential Diagnosis

The diagnosis of epilepsy will carry profound implications for the patient; thus, sufficient proof and accuracy are imperative. Various nonepileptic paroxysmal events are outlined in Table 25–5, and many of these are described in more detail in Chapter 3. Nonepileptic spells are less common in children than in adults but must be considered, even in the young or cognitively impaired child. More common seizure mimics include inattention in school-aged children, while infants and toddlers tend to have stereotypies, sleep-related movements, self-gratification syndrome (sometimes called infantile masturbation), and gastroesophageal reflux. Identifying life-threatening disorders, such as prolonged QT syndrome, as the cause of a patient's spells is of utmost importance.

▶ Complications & Sequelae

A. Psychosocial Impact

Mood disturbances, especially depression but also anxiety, anger, and feelings of guilt and inadequacy, often occur in the patient, as well as the parents of a child with epilepsy. Actual or perceived stigmas as well as issues regarding disclosure are common. School-aged children and adults with epilepsy have an increased risk of suicide. The discussion of comorbid mental health concerns should start at the time of diagnosis.

B. Cognitive Impairment

Epileptic encephalopathy, in which seizures are associated with intellectual decline, does occur, particularly in young children with epilepsies such as infantile spasms (West syndrome), Dravet syndrome, and Lennox-Gastaut syndrome. However, any child living with epilepsy, particularly with untreated or poorly controlled seizures, can develop reduced cognition and memory. The impact of persistent focal seizures depends on the location of the seizure onset. For example, persistent temporal lobe seizures in adults are associated with memory dysfunction. In general, interictal epileptiform activity is not felt to contribute to cognitive impairment; however, increased epileptiform burden has been associated with mild cognitive problems in some disorders previously thought to be benign, such as self-limited epilepsy with centrotemporal spikes, formally BECTS. Continuous epileptiform activity in sleep is associated with Landau-Kleffner syndrome (acquired epileptic aphasia) and electrical status epilepticus in sleep (ESES), both of which are associated with cognitive decline and developmental/behavioral regression. Some antiseizure medications (ASMs), such as phenobarbital, topiramate, and zonisamide, may produce reversible cognitive impairment.

C. Injury and Death

Children with epilepsy are at far greater risk of injuries than the general pediatric population. Direct physical injuries are

Table 25–5. Nonepileptic paroxysmal events.

Breath-holding attacks (cyanotic and pallid) Cyanotic: Age 6 mo–3 y. Always precipitated by trauma or emotion. Cyanosis; sometimes tonic or clonic movements convulsion (anoxic seizure). Patient may sleep following attack. Family history positive in 30%. Electroencephalogram (EEG) is not useful. Anti- medication treatment is not necessary, but if the patient is iron-deficient, supplementation may reduce events. Pallid: Usually, no apparent precipitant, although fright may precipitate. Pallor; may be followed by anoxic seizure. Vagally mediated (heartbeat slows), like adult syncope. EEG is not useful.	**Benign sleep myoclonus** Common in infants and may last into adulthood. Focal or generalized jerks (the latter also called hypnic or sleep jerks) may look like myoclonic seizures but can persist from onset of sleep all night. A video record for review can aid in diagnosis. EEG taken during jerks is normal, proving that these jerks are not myoclonic seizures. Treatment is reassurance.
Tics (Tourette syndrome) Simple or complex stereotyped jerks or movements, coughs, grunts, sniffs. Worse at rest or with stress. May be suppressed. Patients may experience a premonitory urge. Diagnosis is clinical. Magnetic resonance imaging (MRI) and EEG are not necessary.	**Shuddering spells** Shuddering or shivering attacks can occur in infancy and early childhood. Shivering/shuddering may be very frequent. EEG is normal. There is no change in consciousness. **Gastroesophageal reflux (Sandifer syndrome)** Reflux of acid gastric contents may cause pain that cannot be described by the infant. Unusual posturing (dystonic or other) of head and neck or trunk may occur, an apparent attempt to stretch the esophagus or close the opening. There is no loss of consciousness, but eye rolling, apnea, and occasional vomiting may simulate a seizure. EEG during an episode may be necessary to distinguish from seizures.
Parasomnias (night terrors, sleep talking, sleep walking) Ages 3–10 y. Usually occurs in first sleep cycle (30–90 min after going to sleep), with crying, screaming, and autonomic symptoms (pupils dilated, perspiration). May last a few minutes or be more prolonged. Child goes back to sleep and has no recall of event. Sleep talking and walking are fragmentary arousals; EEG during spells shows arousal from deep sleep, though behavior seems wakeful. Child needs to be protected from injury and gradually settled down and taken back to bed.	**Infantile masturbation/self-gratification movements** Usually in toddlers, repetitive rocking, leg stiffening, or rubbing motions, accompanied by zoning out and autonomic symptoms, may simulate seizures. Observation by a skilled individual, sometimes even in a hospital setting, may be necessary to distinguish from seizures. EEG is normal, including during attacks. Interpretation and reassurance are the only necessary treatments.
Nightmares Nightmares or vivid dreams occur in subsequent cycles of sleep, often in the early morning hours, and are partially recalled the next day. The bizarre and frightening behavior may sometimes be confused with focal onset seizures but occurs during REM (rapid eye movement) sleep; whereas epileptic seizures usually do not.	**Nonepileptic seizures/spells (NES)** Episodes may involve writhing, pelvic thrusting, bizarre jerking, thrashing, or sudden unresponsiveness. Spells may need to be seen, video-recorded, or captured on EEG to distinguish from epileptic seizures, but sometimes the history is convincing. NES can occur in children with or without developmental delays and is common in children with epilepsy. **Temper tantrums and rage attacks** Child often reports amnesia for events during spell. Attacks are usually precipitated by frustration or anger, often directed either verbally or physically, and subside with behavior modification and isolation. Following a focal seizure, severe agitation can occur.
Migraine On occasion, migraine can be associated with an acute confusional state. Usual migraine prodrome of nausea/vomiting, dizziness, or visual symptoms is present, followed by headache, then confusion. Prior history of typical migraines may aid in diagnosis. A severe headache with vomiting as the child comes out of spell may aid in distinguishing the attack from seizure. However, some patients may experience post-ictal headaches after seizures.	**Staring spells** Teachers often make referrals for absence seizures in children who stare or seem preoccupied at school. A lack of spells at home is helpful. If the events are interruptible by a firm command or touch, they are unlikely to be seizures. EEG is sometimes necessary to rule out absence of focal seizures.

particularly frequent in atonic seizures ("drop attacks"), at times necessitating protective headgear, but are less common with other seizure types. Drowning, injuries related to working in kitchens, injuries while driving, and falls from heights remain potential risks for all children with epilepsy - highlighting the need for seizure precautions, especially water safety at all times and driving restrictions until seizure-freedom is achieved. Showers are recommended over bathing.

The greatest fear of a parent of a child with new-onset epilepsy is the possibility of death or brain injury. Children with epilepsy do have an increased risk of premature death, but most deaths are related to the underlying neurologic disorder rather than the seizures. Sudden unexpected death with epilepsy (SUDEP) is a rare event in children, occurring in only 1–2:10,000 patient-years. The greatest risk factor for SUDEP is medically uncontrolled epilepsy. The etiology of SUDEP is not yet known, and the only proven strategy to prevent SUDEP is seizure control.

► **Treatment**

A. First Aid

Caregivers should be instructed to protect the patient against injury. Turning the child to the side is useful for

Table 25–6. Home/school seizure rescue medication options and their indications.

Medication	Route	Prolonged Seizure	Seizure Clusters	Dosing Guidance (Round to Convenient Dose)
Diazepam (Diastat)	Rectal	Y	Y	6 mo–adults; dosing is both age- and weight-based
Diazepam (Valtoco)	Intranasal	Y	Y	6 y–adults; dosing is both age- and weight-based
Midazolam (Versed; Nayzilam)	Intranasal	Y	Y	Patients > 10 kg; 0.2–0.3 mg/kg/dose
Clonazepam (Klonopin)	Oral disintegrating tablet	N	Y	Infants–adults; 0.01–0.03 mg/kg/dose

preventing aspiration. Placing any objects in the mouth of a convulsing patient or trying to restrain tonic-clonic movements may cause worse injuries. Parents are often concerned that cyanosis occurs during generalized convulsive seizures, but clinically significant hypoxia, even with cyanosis is rare. Mouth-to-mouth resuscitation is rarely necessary and is unlikely to be helpful.

For prolonged seizures (those lasting over 5 minutes) or seizure clusters of more than six seizures in 1 hour, acute home treatment with benzodiazepines, such as rectal diazepam gel (Diastat), intranasal diazepam (Valtoco), or intranasal midazolam (Versed, Nayzilam), may be administered to prevent the development of status epilepticus and have proven to be safe even when administered by nonmedical professionals (Table 25–6).

B. Antiseizure Medications (ASMs)

1. Treatment strategy—The ideal treatment of acute symptomatic (provoked) seizures is the correction of specific causes. However, even when a biochemical disorder, tumor, meningitis, or another specific cause is being treated, short-term ASMs may be necessary. The child with a single unprovoked seizure has a 50% chance of seizure recurrence. Thus, daily antiseizure medications (ASMs) are not necessary until the diagnosis of epilepsy is established.

2. Drug selection—Several issues should be considered when choosing ASMs, which are no longer called antiepileptic drugs (AEDs) because no ASM actually prevents or cures epilepsy. Some ASMs are effective for focal seizures but can make generalized seizures worse (eg, oxcarbazepine and carbamazepine), while other medications are broad-spectrum, effective for most seizure types. The seizure type and epilepsy syndrome, as well as potential side effects, will determine which drug to initiate, taking into account the Epilepsy Foundation's motto of "no seizures and no side effects" whenever possible. If monotherapy fails, a second, and when necessary, a third medication may be required to help reduce seizure frequency. Care must be taken when using multiple ASMs, which increases the chance of side effects. ASMs with different mechanisms of action may have improved combined tolerability and effectiveness.

3. Long-term management and discontinuation of treatment—Therapy should be continued until the patient is free of seizures for at least 1–2 years. In about 75% of patients, seizures will not recur following discontinuation of medication after 2 years of remission. Variables such as younger age at onset, normal EEG, undetermined etiology, and ease of controlling seizures carry a favorable prognosis; whereas, identified etiology, later onset, continued epileptiform discharges on EEG, difficulty in establishing seizure control, polytherapy, generalized tonic-clonic or myoclonic seizures, and an abnormal neurologic examination are associated with a higher risk of future recurrence. Most ASMs (except barbiturates and benzodiazepines) can be withdrawn over 6–8 weeks.

Recurrent seizures affect up to 25% of children who attempt withdrawal from medications, typically within 6–12 months of discontinuing medications. Therefore, seizure safety and precautions, including driving restrictions, need to be reinstituted during medication withdrawal. If seizures recur during or after withdrawal, ASM therapy should be reinstituted and maintained for at least another 1–2 years. Most children will again achieve remission of their seizures.

C. Specific and Alternative Treatments

1. Ketogenic diet—Fasting has been described to stop seizures for centuries, and a diet high in fat and low in protein and carbohydrates will result in ketosis and simulate a fasting state. Such a diet has been observed to decrease and even control seizures in some children, though the mechanism of action is unknown. In certain types of genetic epilepsies, the ketogenic diet is the treatment of choice. Potential adverse effects include acidosis and hypoglycemia, particularly upon initiation of the diet, which is typically done via admission to an experienced ketogenic diet center. Close follow-up and monitoring can help prevent other potential complications, such as renal stones, pancreatitis, and acidosis. In addition, vitamin and minerals need to be followed carefully, and potentially supplemented, to avoid deficiencies, especially carnitine, iron, and vitamin D.

The ketogenic diet requires careful adherence and the full cooperation of all family members. The increased use of the ketogenic diet and family support groups have increased the number of palatable recipes for patients and families on the ketogenic diet. A modified Atkins diet or a low-glycemic index diet can also be effective in older and higher functioning children who will not tolerate the ketogenic diet or for specific genetic diseases, such as Angelman syndrome. Families must be cautioned that abrupt withdrawal (accidental or purposeful) of the diet can precipitate seizures and even status epilepticus.

2. Adrenocorticotropic hormone (ACTH) and corticosteroids—

Treatment with ACTH or oral corticosteroids is the standard of care for infantile spasms. Duration of therapy is guided by cessation of clinical seizures and normalization of the EEG. Vigabatrin is an alternative treatment that is also considered standard of care for infantile spasms and has been shown to be superior for infantile spasms resulting from tuberous sclerosis. All other treatments for infantile spasms have a lower likelihood of being effective.

Precautions: Side effects can occur in up to 90% of patients. It is important to guard against infections, provide gastrointestinal (GI) prophylaxis, follow for possible hypertension, and discuss the likelihood of significant weight gain. ACTH and oral corticosteroids should not be withdrawn suddenly to avoid adrenal crisis. In some areas, prophylaxis against *Pneumocystis* infection may be required. Partnering with a medical home can be very helpful in surveillance, such as monitoring blood pressure, weight, and potential adverse effects.

3. Implantable devices

- **Vagus nerve stimulator (VNS)** is a pacemaker-like device that is implanted below the clavicle and attached to the left vagus nerve. A cycle of electrical stimulation of the nerve is established, which has an antiseizure effect, reducing seizures by at least 50% in over half the children treated. In addition, an emergency mode that is automatically triggered by abrupt tachycardia or manually activated by swiping a magnet over the device may interrupt a seizure.

- **Responsive neurostimulation (RNS)** is a cranially implantable programmable device for patients with refractory epilepsy with no more than two epileptic foci. RNS detects previously identified brain wave patterns and interrupts them, preventing the patient from having a clinical seizure.

- **Deep brain stimulation (DBS)** is another programmable implantable cranial device that can be used for refractory epilepsy. It works by electrical stimulation of the thalamic nuclei. The proposed mechanism of action is focal modulation of specific functional circuits that may exert control on seizure generators.

D. Epilepsy Surgery

Epilepsy surgery is an appropriate treatment option for adults and children with medication resistant ("refractory") epilepsy, defined as failure of two drugs alone or as combination therapy to control seizures. Evaluation for possible surgical treatment should begin as soon as a child with epilepsy is not responding to standard therapy. Advances in technology allow for identification and removal of the region of seizure onset (epileptogenic focus), even in young infants. The evaluation and surgery should be performed at a center with a dedicated neurosurgeon, epileptologists, neuropsychologists, and neuroradiologists with experience in epilepsy surgery. With surgical resection of a seizure focus, the chance of seizure freedom can be up to 95%. Some children with generalized seizures may qualify for palliative surgeries, such as corpus callosotomy, that aim to reduce seizure burden but are not expected to make the patient seizure free.

E. General Management of the Child With Epilepsy

1. Education—The initial diagnosis of epilepsy is often devastating for families. The clinical team must be prepared to help the patient and guardians understand the nature of epilepsy and its management, including prognosis, safety issues, and treatment options. Excellent patient educational materials are available, both in print and online (www.epilepsy.com). The Epilepsy Foundation's local chapter and other community organizations can provide guidance and other services. Support groups and epilepsy summer camps are also available in many regions.

2. Privileges and precautions in daily life—Patients with epilepsy should be encouraged to live as normal a life as possible. Children should engage in physical activities appropriate to their age. Patients should be supervised closely when swimming, and protective gear should be worn (eg, a harness while rock-climbing, a helmet while biking). There are no absolute contraindications to any sports, although some physicians recommend against contact sports. Exercise may decrease overall seizure burden and help maintain good bone health, which can be negatively impacted by ASMs. Sleep deprivation and alcohol should be avoided as they are triggers for seizures for patients with epilepsy. Prompt attention should be given to intercurrent illnesses that can also trigger seizures.

Although every effort should be made to control seizures, treatment must not interfere with a child's ability to function normally. A child may do better having an occasional mild seizure than being so heavily sedated that function at home, in school, or at play is impaired. Therapy and medication adjustment often require much art and fortitude on the part of the provider, patient, and family.

3. Driving—Driving restrictions for persons with epilepsy and other disturbances of consciousness vary from state to state. In most states, a learner's permit or driver's license will be issued to an individual with epilepsy if he or she has been seizure-free for at least 6–12 months, provided that the treatment or underlying neurologic problems do not interfere with the ability to drive. A guide to this and other legal matters pertaining to persons with epilepsy is published by the Epilepsy Foundation.

4. Pregnancy—Contraception (especially interaction of oral contraceptive with some ASMs), the potential teratogenicity of ASMs, and the management of pregnancy should be discussed as soon as appropriate with adolescents with epilepsy who may become pregnant. Daily vitamins, including high-dose folic acid, can be protective against neural tube defects. All ASMs appear to have some risk for teratogenicity, although valproate carries a particularly high risk for spinal dysraphism, as well as being associated with cognitive issues in children exposed to valproate in utero. Management by an obstetrician conversant with the use of ASMs in pregnancy is appropriate for pregnant teenagers with epilepsy. Patients should be cautioned against discontinuing their ASMs during pregnancy.

5. School intervention and seizure response plans—Schools are required by federal law to work with guardians to establish a seizure action plan for their child with epilepsy, but some may be hesitant to administer seizure rescue medication. Seizure action plan templates are available at https://www.epilepsy.com/living-epilepsy/toolbox/seizure-forms and usually require the approval of the child's provider, which may relieve the school's concerns. School authorities should be encouraged to avoid needless restrictions and to address the emotional and educational needs of all children with disabilities, including epilepsy.

2. Status Epilepticus

Historically, status epilepticus has been defined as a clinical or electrical seizure or a series of seizures without complete recovery lasting at least 30 minutes. After 30 minutes of seizure activity, hypoxia and acidosis occur, with depletion of energy stores, cerebral edema, and possible structural damage. Eventually, high fever, hypotension, respiratory depression, and even death may occur. Status epilepticus is a medical emergency. The ILAE recommends utilizing a threshold of 5 minutes to define a prolonged seizure that may benefit from intervention, such as benzodiazepines, to prevent status epilepticus.

Status epilepticus is classified as (1) convulsive (the common generalized tonic-clonic type) or (2) nonconvulsive (characterized by altered mental status or behavior with subtle or absent motor components). Absence status, or spike-wave stupor, and focal status epilepticus are examples of the nonconvulsive type, which typically requires an EEG to diagnose. Status epilepticus that has not responded to two medications is considered refractory status epilepticus and often requires care in an intensive care unit. For treatment options, see Table 25–7.

Table 25–7. Status epilepticus treatment.

1. ABCs (if conscious) or CAB (if unconscious)
   a. Airway: maintain oral airway; intubation may be necessary.
   b. Breathing: oxygenation and ventilation.
   c. Circulation: assess pulse, blood pressure; support with IV fluids, drugs. Monitor vital signs.
2. Start glucose-containing IV (unless patient is on ketogenic diet); evaluate serum glucose, electrolytes, HCO_3^-, CBC, BUN, anticonvulsant levels.
3. Consider arterial blood gases, pH.
4. Give 50% glucose if serum glucose low (1–2 mL/kg).
5. Begin IV antiseizure medications; goal is to control status epilepticus within 5–60 min.
   a. First-line therapies (IV benzodiazepines): Diazepam 0.2 mg/kg (max 10 mg); may repeat in 5 min; lorazepam 0.1 mg/kg (max 4 mg; longer-acting than diazepam), may repeat in 5 min; OR midazolam 0.1–0.2 mg/kg. For non-IV options, consider intramuscular agents or see Table 25–6 for nasal/enteral/rectal agents.
   b. Second-line therapies: Fosphenytoin 20 mg PE/kg IV (max 1500 mg), may give additional 10 mg PE/kg if seizures continue after 10 min; levetiracetam 60 mg/kg (max 4500 mg) over 15 min; valproate sodium 40 mg/kg (max 3000 mg) over 15 min, but avoid in children < 2 years old; OR phenobarbital 20 mg/kg (max 1000), may give additional 10 mg/kg if seizures continue after 10 min. If seizures persist 10–20 min after second-line agent finishes infusing, strongly consider advancing to a continuous infusion agent rather than trying additional second-line agents.
   c. Third-line therapies (continuous infusions): midazolam, pentobarbital, ketamine, or propofol. Frequent boluses may be needed to establish seizure control and are preferred over frequent rate increases. EEG and ICU admission are typically necessary at this point.
6. Correct metabolic perturbations (eg, low sodium, acidosis). Administer fluids if needed.
7. Consider underlying causes:
   a. Structural disorders or trauma: MRI or CT scan.
   b. Infection: lumbar puncture, blood culture, antibiotics.
   c. Metabolic disorders: consider lactic acidosis, toxins, and uremia if child is being treated with chronic ASMs, obtain medication levels. Toxin screen.

ASM, antiseizure drug; BUN, blood urea nitrogen; CBC, complete blood count; CT, computed tomography; EEG, electroencephalography; ICU, intensive care unit; IM, intramuscularly; IV, intravenously; MRI, magnetic resonance imaging.

3. Febrile Seizures

▶ Clinical Findings

Febrile seizures occur in 2%–5% of children. Criteria include (1) age 6 months to 6 years (most occur between 6 and 18 months), (2) fever of greater than 38.8°C, and (3) non-CNS infection. More than 90% of febrile seizures are generalized, last less than 5 minutes, and occur early in the illness. Often the fever is not noted until after the seizure occurs. Acute respiratory illnesses are most associated with febrile seizures. Gastroenteritis, especially when caused by *Shigella*, *Campylobacter*, or GI viruses can also provoke seizures, even in the absence of fever, and seizures may occur up to 3 days after GI symptoms begin; these GI-illness-provoked seizures have a similar outcome to febrile seizures. Febrile seizures are termed complex if the patient had multiple seizures in 24 hours, if a single seizure lasted more than 15 minutes, or if a single seizure was focal. Febrile status epilepticus describes a febrile seizure that lasts 30 minutes or longer. Human herpesvirus type 6 (HHV-6) and type 7 (HHV-7) are common causes for febrile status epilepticus, accounting for one-third of cases, though these are not typically tested for clinically since they do not change management.

▶ Diagnostic Evaluation

The child with a febrile seizure must be evaluated for the source of the fever.. In particular, CNS infection must be considered, even if the child has had a prior febrile seizure. History and the examination should guide the workup, and any treatment-amenable infection should be addressed. Signs of meningitis (eg, bulging fontanelle, stiff neck, stupor, and irritability) may be absent, especially in a child younger than 18 months. Routine studies such as serum electrolytes, glucose, calcium, skull radiographs, or brain imaging are seldom helpful unless warranted based on clinical history or suspicion of abuse. LP should be considered if the child is younger than 18 months, has been pretreated with antibiotics, or is under immunized. Seizure is not an acceptable explanation for CSF pleocytosis; a recent study demonstrated that 96% of children with febrile status epilepticus who received an LP had 0–2 CSF WBCs. Occasionally, observation in the emergency department for several hours obviates the need for LP, but in general, one should have a low threshold for performing this potentially life-saving test.

EEG may be considered if the febrile seizure is complicated, focal, or otherwise unusual, but has little predictive value for later epilepsy. In simple febrile seizures, the EEG is usually normal. Unless acutely indicated, the EEG should be done at least a week after the illness to avoid transient changes due to fever or the seizure itself.

▶ Treatment

Prophylactic ASMs are not recommended after a febrile seizure. Though some agents have demonstrated efficacy in preventing febrile seizures, the side effects were not felt to outweigh the possible benefit. Measures to control fever such as sponging, tepid baths, or antipyretics including ibuprofen and acetaminophen are ineffective at preventing recurrent febrile seizures and, thus, should not be recommended solely for this purpose.

▶ Prognosis

Recurrent febrile seizures occur in 30%–50% of cases; therefore, families should be prepared to expect more seizures. The likelihood of later epilepsy is influenced by the overall presentation—simple febrile seizures carry a 1%–3% risk, complex seizures confer a 5%–7% risk, and febrile status epilepticus is associated with later epilepsy in up to 25% of cases. Additional factors that may raise the risk of epilepsy include abnormal neurologic status preceding the seizures (eg, cerebral palsy [CP] or intellectual disability), early onset of febrile seizure (before age 1 year), and a family history of epilepsy. Cognitive function is not significantly different from that of siblings without febrile seizures.

Duffner P et al: Clinical Practice Guideline—febrile seizures: guideline for the neurodiagnostic evaluation of the child with a simple febrile seizure. Pediatrics 2015;127(2):389–394 [PMID: 21285335].

Glauser T et al: Evidence-based guideline: treatment of convulsive status epilepticus in children and adults: report of the Guideline Committee of the American Epilepsy Society. Epilepsy Curr 2016;16(1):48–61 [PMID: 26900382].

Kossoff E et al: Optimal clinical management of children receiving dietary therapies for epilepsy: updated recommendations of the international ketogenic diet study group. Epilepsia Open 2018;3(2):175–192 [PMID: 29881797].

Messer R, Knupp KG: Infantile spasms: opportunities to improve care. Semin Neurol 2020;40(2):236–240 [PMID: 32143232].

Nasser Z et al: Deep brain stimulation and drug-resistant epilepsy: a review of the literature. Font Neurol 2019; 10:601 [PMID: 31244761].

Perucca E et al: 30 years of second-generation antiseizure medications: impact and future perspectives. Lancet Neurol 2020; 19(6):544–556 [PMID: 32109411].

Rugg-Gunn F, Miserocchi A, McEvoy A: Epilepsy surgery. Pract Neurol 2020;20(1):4–14 [PMID: 31420415].

Scheffer IE et al: ILAE classification of the epilepsies: position paper of the ILAE Commission for Classification and Terminology. Epilepsia 2017;58(4):512–521 [PMID: 28276062].

Sillanpää M, Shinnar S: SUDEP and other causes of mortality in childhood-onset epilepsy. Epilepsy Behav 2013;28(2):249–255 [PMID: 23746924].

Skarpass T et al: Brain-responsive neurostimulation for epilepsy (RNS® System). Epilepsy Res 2019 Jul;153:68–70 [PMID: 30850259].

SLEEP DISORDERS

ESSENTIALS OF DIAGNOSIS & TYPICAL FEATURES

- ▶ Narcolepsy is characterized by inappropriate daytime sleep with or without cataplexy, defined as sudden loss of tone with preservation of consciousness.

- ▶ Benign sleep myoclonus is common in infants and can be identified by muscle jerks in sleep that stop upon awakening.

Sleep and its development are reviewed in Chapter 3. Sleep disorders can originate from abnormalities within the respiratory system, the neurologic system, and the coordination (or lack thereof) between these two systems. Chapter 3 also discusses behavioral considerations in the treatment of sleep disorders. Respiratory abnormalities that are associated with sleep, such as obstructive sleep apnea, are described in Chapter 19. This discussion focuses on neurologic features of several pediatric sleep disorders.

1. Narcolepsy

Narcolepsy, a primary disorder of sleep, is characterized by chronic, inappropriate daytime sleep that occurs regardless of activity or surroundings and is not relieved by increased sleep at night. Half of individuals affected by narcolepsy experience their initial symptoms in childhood, typically around/after puberty. The *International Classification of Sleep Disorders*, 3rd Edition (ICSD-3) describes two forms of narcolepsy:

- Type 1 (narcolepsy with cataplexy): In addition to narcolepsy, patients develop cataplexy, a transient partial or total loss of muscle tone, often triggered by laughter, or other heightened emotional states. Consciousness is preserved during these spells, which can last several minutes in duration. The pathophysiology of type 1 is deficiency of hypocretin-1 (orexin), a peptide essential for maintaining alertness.

- Type 2 (narcolepsy without cataplexy): In addition to narcolepsy, patients may experience hypnagogic or hypnopompic hallucinations and sleep paralysis, but they do not have cataplexy. Hypnagogic hallucinations are intense visual or auditory hallucinations noted while falling asleep, whereas hypnopompic hallucinations occur while waking from sleep. Sleep paralysis is a brief loss of voluntary muscle control, typically occurring at sleep-wake transitions and lasting for minutes. Hypocretin-1 levels are normal.

Nocturnal polysomnography and multiple sleep latency testing (MSLT) can demonstrate the abnormally short latency between sleep onset and transition into rapid eye movement (REM) sleep that is diagnostic for narcolepsy. Human leukocyte antigen (HLA) subtypes DQB1*0602 and DRB1*1501 are associated with narcolepsy, as well as absence of a hypothalamic neuropeptide, hypocretin, which can be measured in CSF. Sleep hygiene and behavior modification are used to treat patients with narcolepsy. Medications used for narcolepsy and cataplexy are off-label in children but include some CNS stimulants and antidepressants.

2. Benign Sleep Myoclonus

Benign sleep myoclonus is characterized by clusters of myoclonic jerks, usually bilateral and synchronous, which may last seconds to 20 minutes, occur only during sleep, and stop abruptly when the child is aroused. It is a benign condition that is frequently confused with epileptic seizures. Onset is typically in the first 2 weeks of life and improves spontaneously in the first months of life, although older children and adults may have infrequent isolated myoclonic jerks in sleep, rather than frequent clusters.

3. Parasomnias

Parasomnias are complex movements and behaviors that occur in association with various sleep stages or the transition between sleeping and waking. These are discussed in more detail in Chapter 3. The non-REM parasomnias consist of partial arousals, disorientation, and motor disturbances and include sleepwalking (somnambulism), sleep talking, confusional arousals, and night terrors, among others. The REM sleep parasomnias include nightmares, hypnagogic, and hypnopompic hallucinations (as can occur in narcolepsy), and REM sleep behavior disorder, which is characterized by physical and sometimes violent movements during the dream state and is primarily seen in adulthood.

4. Restless Legs Syndrome

Restless legs syndrome refers to a feeling of needing to move the legs (dysesthesia) that often starts when resting at night. Movement of the legs temporarily relieves the symptoms, though this can interfere with the ability to fall asleep. This disorder can be familial; therefore, a detailed family history may be helpful. Occasionally, iron deficiency has been noted in adults and children with the disorder; in these cases, improvement has occurred with ferrous sulfate treatment. These are discussed in more detail in Chapter 3.

American Academy of Sleep Medicine: *International Classification of Sleep Disorders*. 3rd ed. Darien, IL: American Academy of Sleep Medicine; 2014.

Aurora RN et al: Practice parameters for the non-respiratory indications for polysomnography and multiple sleep latency testing for children. Sleep 2012;35(11):1467–1473 [PMID: 23115395].

Caraballo RH et al: The spectrum of benign myoclonus of early infancy: clinical and neurophysiologic features in 102 patients. Epilepsia 2009;50(5):1176–1183 [PMID: 19175386].

Hoban T: Sleep disorders in children. Ann N Y Acad Sci 2010; 1184(1);1–14 [PMID: 20146688].

PRIMARY HEADACHE DISORDERS

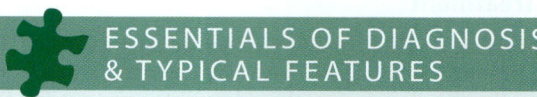

ESSENTIALS OF DIAGNOSIS & TYPICAL FEATURES

► Migraines are unilateral/bilateral, moderate-severe, pulsating headaches that are associated with nausea/vomiting, photo/phonophobia, and are worsened by physical activity.

▶ Tension-type headaches are bilateral, mild-moderate, pressure or tightening headaches that are not worsened by physical activity.

▶ Red flags include new or different headache pattern, overnight or early morning headache, positional headache, papilledema, neurologic deficits, or fever.

Headache is the most common neurologic symptom leading children and adolescents to seek medical care. The prevalence of migraine is higher in females, increasing throughout childhood with 25% of adolescents experiencing migraine. The prevalence of tension-type headache is likely more frequent, but as children typically do not present to care for tension-type headaches, the true prevalence is unclear.

▶ Clinical Findings

The International Classification of Headache Disorders provides a framework for primary headaches, including migraine, tension-type headache, and trigeminal autonomic cephalalgia. Clinical features of migraine without aura and tension-type headache are compared in Table 25–8. The most common aura is visual followed by sensory and is described as a fully reversible unilateral positive symptom that spreads over 5 minutes and resolves within 60 minutes. Other pediatric migraine phenotypes include benign paroxysmal torticollis, benign paroxysmal vertigo, and cyclic vomiting. Prior history of these periodic syndromes may be discovered in patients with migraine. Triggers of headache include physical or emotional stress, inadequate sleep or fluid

Table 25–8. Classification of migraine without aura and tension-type headache.

	Migraine Without Aura	Tension-Type Headache
Duration	2–72 h[a]	30 min to 7 days
	At least two of:	At least two of:
Location	Unilateral/bilateral[a]	Bilateral
Quality	Pulsating	Pressure or tightening
Intensity	Moderate to severe	Mild to moderate
Physical activity	Worsens headache	No effect
Associated factors	At least one of:	Both of:
	Nausea and/or vomiting	No nausea or vomiting
	Photophobia and phonophobia	No more than one of photophobia or phonophobia

[a]Modified for children based on the ICHD-III classification criteria.

Table 25–9. Red flags for children with headaches.

Age < 5 y
Explosive onset or progressive headache
Awakening at night or early morning with or without vomiting
Worsens with Valsalva maneuver
Positional headache (worse with lying or standing)
Papilledema
Focal neurologic deficit (including diplopia)
Unexplained fever or other systemic signs
Neurocutaneous stigmata (such as café-au-lait spots)

intake, menstrual cycle, and barometric shifts. Trigeminal autonomic cephalalgias, including paroxysmal hemicrania and cluster headache, are exceedingly rare in children. They present as recurrent, severe, unilateral headaches that are associated with autonomic dysfunction, such as lacrimation, rhinorrhea, facial sweating, miosis, or ptosis.

▶ Diagnostic Evaluation

A complete history and physical examination are crucial to distinguish between a primary and secondary headache. Migrainous symptoms are known to occur in secondary headaches; thus, the presence of such symptoms does not ensure the diagnosis of a primary headache. Red flag symptoms of headache are outlined in Table 25–9. Of these, abnormalities on the neurologic or funduscopic examination are the most common features associated with abnormalities on neuroimaging, but others may also guide the need for further workup. For primary headache disorders, routine laboratory testing and neuroimaging are not indicated.

▶ Differential Diagnosis

Table 25–10 outlines various etiologies of secondary headaches. In general, the most common cause of a secondary

Table 25–10. Differential diagnosis of secondary headaches.

Intracranial Causes	Systemic or Other Causes
Arterial dissection	Anemia
Cerebral venous sinus thrombosis	Asthenopia (eye strain)
Chiari malformation	Hypercapnia
CNS vasculitis	Hypertension
Head trauma	Hypoxia
Hemorrhagic stroke	Medication overuse headache
Hydrocephalus	Mitochondrial disorders
Intracranial hypotension	Sinusitis
Intracranial infection	Sleep apnea
Ischemic stroke	Substance use or withdrawal
Primary intracranial hypertension	Systemic infection
Tumor	Temporomandibular joint (TMJ) dysfunction
	Thyroid dysfunction

headache is a viral illness. Features that raise the suspicion for increased ICP are overnight or early morning headache with emesis, pulsatile tinnitus, worsening pain when supine, transient visual obscurations, and diplopia. If symptoms of increased ICP occur with fever and encephalopathy or meningismus, additional testing should be done to evaluate for CNS infection. Patients with sinusitis commonly have a frontal headache, and the history and physical examination may not be sufficient to rule out an intracranial complication. In this population, it is important to consider neuroimaging.

CNS vasculitis is a rare cause of headache in the pediatric population and is typically secondary to a systemic inflammatory process. Patients present with headache and usually have focal neurologic deficits with personality changes. Headache due to vascular malformation is most commonly caused by hemorrhage. If due to rupture of aneurysm, patients will have severe headache with meningismus. If due to rupture of arteriovenous malformation, patients will present with encephalopathy and focal neurologic deficits. Head CT should be obtained urgently in both conditions. Arachnoid cysts are common incidental findings seen on imaging and rarely contribute to headaches. Chiari malformation type I is commonly noted as an incidental finding in patients with headaches, and it is important to identify if the Chiari malformation type I is symptomatic (see section Chiari Malformations). Worrisome features include occipital or neck pain, onset with Valsalva, duration of less than 5 minutes, and associated with signs of brainstem, cerebellar, or cervical spine dysfunction.

Seizure is a unique diagnostic consideration, as headache is a common postictal phenomenon. Supportive features for seizures as a cause of headache include alteration of awareness, abrupt onset, and visual symptoms that are complex, multicolored, or last 30–90 seconds. Medication-overuse headache (previously termed rebound headache) can be seen if patients use abortive medications more than three times per week. For patients who are on other medications, consider whether headache could be a medication side effect. Toxins or drug use can also lead to headache. Posttraumatic headaches can be seen within 2 weeks following a closed head injury. Sleep apnea is in the differential for morning headaches that resolve over the course of the day. A proper eye and dental examination can rule out eye strain (asthenopia) and temporomandibular joint dysfunction.

▶ **Complications**

A minority of patients with episodic migraine or tension-type headache progress to a chronic headache, which is defined as greater than 15 headache days per month for more than 3 consecutive months. The most important risk factor to consider is medication overuse. When the offending medications are withdrawn, 50% of patients will revert to episodic headache. Common co-morbidities of headache include anxiety, depression, sleep disruption, and dizziness/vertigo. Comprehensive care of headache patients includes evaluation for these conditions to further limit headache disability, including poor school attendance, academic performance, and peer relationships.

▶ **Treatment**

Lifestyle modifications, including adequate sleep, regular nutritious meals, ample fluid intake, consistent exercise, and limiting stress, are important for all headache types. It can be helpful for families to identify a single issue to improve on by setting small, achievable goals. Heat or cold packs, massage, biofeedback, dry needling, acupuncture, and relaxation via yoga or meditation can be helpful for all headache types. Medications for headache are divided into two categories—rescue and preventative. In general, rescue medications should be used no more than 3 times per week to avoid medication overuse headache.

A. Migraine Headache Treatment

Rescue treatment for pediatric migraine is approached in a stepwise fashion and should be initiated at first sign of pain. First line is an oral analgesic, and ibuprofen is typically more effective than acetaminophen. Ondansetron is commonly used for nausea with migraine and often is administered prior to an analgesic. The only triptan approved for children by the Food and Drug Administration (FDA) is rizatriptan, but others are frequently prescribed off-label and have shown benefit. Common side effects are jaw or chest tightness, paresthesias, and drowsiness. Use is contraindicated in patients with cardiac, cerebrovascular, or peripheral vascular disease.

For migraine refractory to home management, patients should present to the emergency department or infusion center for intravenous medication. A combination of normal saline bolus, ketorolac, and a dopamine receptor antagonist, of which prochlorperazine is most effective, is typically the first line. Diphenhydramine can be given to prevent an acute dystonic reaction. If not effective, dihydroergotamine (DHE) is the next step. The most common side effect is nausea, and headache can worsen with the first few doses. Other options are intravenous valproic acid or ketamine and occipital nerve block.

Patients who experience migraine one or more days per week warrant a daily preventative medication. Nutraceuticals, such as magnesium, riboflavin, and feverfew, have limited data to support use. Cyproheptadine is the most common medication used in pre-pubertal children. Common side effects are drowsiness and weight gain. Topiramate and amitriptyline are the most common preventatives in pubertal children. Common side effects for topiramate are weight loss, paresthesias, and cognitive slowing, while rare side effects are glaucoma and kidney stones. Common side effects for amitriptyline are drowsiness, weight gain, and constipation while rare side effects are prolonged QTc. These medications are dosed at night to use the side effect of drowsiness to the patient's benefit. All have the potential to worsen mood symptoms, although typically as headache improves, mood follows. Calcitonin gene–related peptide (CGRP) antagonists, such as fremanezumab and galcanezumab, are monthly injectable preventative medications are that not FDA-approved in the pediatric population but are frequently prescribed to those who have failed oral medications. They are well tolerated with most common side effects being nausea or injection site reaction. Onabotulinum toxin A is a series of 31 injections performed every 12 weeks and is FDA-approved for chronic migraine.

B. Tension-Type Headache Treatment

Tension-type headaches respond well to over-the-counter analgesics, such as acetaminophen and ibuprofen. Prevention focuses on non-pharmacologic treatments, such as physical therapy, cognitive behavioral therapy, and relaxation through meditation, massage, and yoga. Daily preventative medications are rarely needed for tension-type headache.

► Prognosis

Most children with pediatric headache will continue to have migraine or tension-type headache into adulthood, but the frequency and intensity of headaches will wax and wane. In females, increased hormones, either in puberty or pregnancy, can have a significant positive or negative impact on headache frequency. The presence of chronic migraine is likely associated with increased risk for continued headache into adulthood, but more studies are needed to investigate other risk factors.

Headache Classification Committee of the International Headache Society: The International Classification of Headache Disorders, 3rd ed. Cephalalgia 2018;38(1):1–211 [PMID: 29368949].

Oskoui M et al: Practice guideline update summary: pharmacologic treatment for pediatric migraine prevention: report of the Guideline Development, Dissemination, and Implementation Subcommittee of the American Academy of Neurology and the American Headache Society. Neurology 2019 Sep 10; 93(11):500–509 [PMID: 31413170].

Oskoui M et al: Practice guideline update summary: acute treatment of migraine in children and adolescents: report of the Guideline Development, Dissemination, and Implementation Subcommittee of the American Academy of Neurology and the American Headache Society. Neurology 2019 Sep 10;93(11):487–499 [PMID: 31413171].

Yonker M: Secondary headaches in children and adolescents: what not to miss. Curr Neurol Neurosci Rep 2018 Jul 30;18(9):61 [PMID: 30058035].

INTRACRANIAL HYPERTENSION

ESSENTIALS OF DIAGNOSIS & TYPICAL FEATURES

► Signs and symptoms of increased ICP include progressive positional headache, pulsatile tinnitus, vision changes, and papilledema.

► Brain MRI may demonstrate secondary findings of increased ICP.

► LP demonstrates elevated opening pressure with normal CSF studies.

► Pathogenesis

Intracranial hypertension is the buildup of pressure around the brain and is frequently associated with headache and vision changes. It can be either primary or secondary in etiology. Primary intracranial hypertension, also known as pseudotumor cerebri or idiopathic intracranial hypertension (IIH), is characterized by increased ICP in the absence of hydrocephalus, mass, traumatic brain injury, or other identifiable cause. The pathogenesis of primary intracranial hypertension is poorly understood, but risk factors include female sex, obesity, and puberty. Secondary intracranial hypertension can be medication induced, due to impaired venous drainage, or associated with other chronic medical conditions.

► Clinical Findings

Presenting features include headache worsened by supine position or Valsalva maneuvers, pulsatile tinnitus, and vision changes, such as enlarging blind spot, constriction of visual fields, or reduction in visual acuity. Transient visual obscurations, or loss of vision lasting seconds, also can occur. Papilledema is seen on examination in almost all patients, and patients can have diplopia with an abducens or lateral gaze palsy.

► Diagnostic Evaluation

All patients with suspicion for increased ICP should receive imaging, and an MRI of the brain is the preferred modality. Patients with risk factors for CSVT should also have an MR venogram. In IIH, MRI of the brain parenchyma is normal, while secondary findings of increased ICP can be seen (Figure 25–1). An LP should be performed in the lateral decubitus position to confirm the presence of increased pressure, defined as greater than 28 cm H_2O in children, and basic CSF studies should be performed to rule out infection and inflammation.

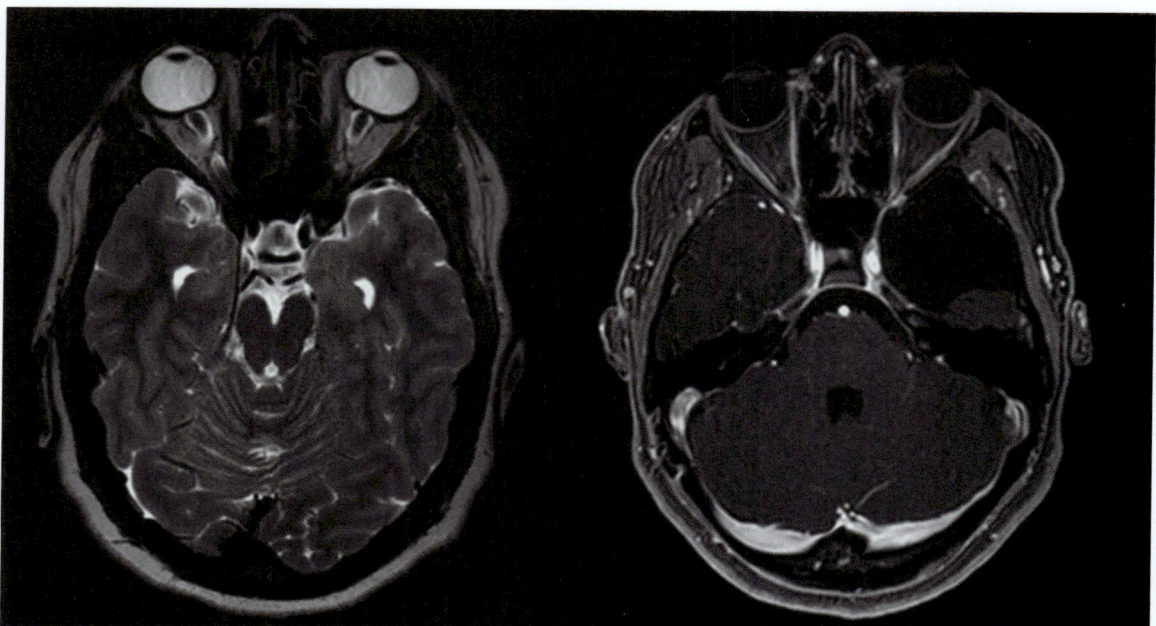

▲ **Figure 25–1.** Secondary findings of increased intracranial pressure seen on axial brain MRI—distension of optic nerve sheaths with flattening of posterior sclera (left) and narrowing of bilateral transverse venous sinuses (right).

▶ Differential Diagnosis

Hydrocephalus, tumor, and other mass lesion must be ruled out with imaging. Etiologies of secondary intracranial hypertension (Table 25–11) should be investigated.

Table 25–11. Conditions associated with secondary intracranial hypertension.

Medications	Cerebrovenous Conditions
Hormonal therapy, including chronic steroids and growth hormone	Cerebral venous sinus thrombosis
Steroid withdrawal	Otitis or mastoid infection
Use of tetracyclines, including minocycline	**Other Medical Conditions**
Hypervitaminosis A and use of retinoids	Chronic hypercapnia
Endocrine	Anemia
Hypocalcemia	Iron deficiency
Hyperthyroidism	Renal failure
Adrenal insufficiency	Systemic lupus erythematosus
	Down syndrome
	Turner syndrome

▶ Treatment

Treatment of intracranial hypertension is aimed at correcting the underlying condition or modifiable risk factors, including weight loss for obese patients or discontinuation of provoking medication. Sequential ophthalmologic evaluation is important to ensure papilledema resolves and visual field deficits improve. Most patients benefit from a 6-month course of acetazolamide or topiramate to decrease CSF production and prevent recurrence. In a minority of patients who do not respond to medical management, neurosurgical intervention such as shunt placement or optic nerve fenestration is considered.

▶ Prognosis

Headache will fully resolve in most patients with appropriate reduction in ICP, but recurrence is seen in up to 20%. Permanent visual disability occurs in a quarter of patients and is associated with moderate to severe papilledema at presentation. This highlights the urgency to promptly identify and treat intracranial hypertension.

Avery RA et al: Reference range for cerebrospinal fluid opening pressure in children. N Engl J Med 2010 Aug 26;363(9):891–893 [PMID: 20818852].

Friedman DI, Liu GT, Digre KB: Revised diagnostic criteria for the pseudotumor cerebri syndrome in adults and children. Neurology 2013 Sep 24;81(13):1159–1165 [PMID: 23966248].

Gospe SM 3rd, Bhatti MT, El-Dairi MA: Anatomic and visual function outcomes in paediatric idiopathic intracranial hypertension. Br J Ophthalmol 2016 Apr;100(4):505–509 [PMID: 26269534].

Kohli AA et al: Magnetic resonance imaging findings in pediatric pseudotumor cerebri syndrome. Pediatr Neurol 2019 Oct;99:31–39 [PMID: 31303369].

ARTERIAL ISCHEMIC STROKE

ESSENTIALS OF DIAGNOSIS & TYPICAL FEATURES

▶ Perinatal arterial ischemic stroke (AIS) occurs in neonates younger than 28 days; patients may present with seizures in the neonatal period or chronic focal deficits later in infancy/toddlerhood.

▶ Childhood AIS occurs in children between 28 days and 18 years old; patients may present with acute onset focal seizures or neurologic deficits.

▶ Acute ischemic strokes are often not apparent on CT but will demonstrate restricted diffusion on brain MRI.

▶ Urgent vascular imaging can identify large vessel occlusions (LVOs) that may benefit from intra-arterial therapy (thrombectomy).

Pediatric AIS is subdivided into two categories: perinatal AIS (28 weeks' gestation to 28 days of life) and childhood AIS (28 days to 18 years of age).

1. Perinatal Arterial Ischemic Stroke

Perinatal arterial ischemic stroke (AIS) is more common than childhood ischemic stroke, affecting up to 1:3000 live births, with two distinct presentations: acute and delayed. Most patients with an acute presentation develop neonatal seizures during the first week of life, particularly focal motor seizures of the contralateral arm and/or leg, due to the predilection of perinatal ischemic stroke to occur in the middle cerebral artery. Diffusion-weighted abnormalities on MRI confirm an acute perinatal ischemic stroke during the first week of life. Patients with "presumed perinatal AIS" present with delayed symptoms, typically hemiparesis, which became notable at 4–8 months. Imaging demonstrates evidence of a remote injury, such as encephalomalacia.

Acute treatment of a perinatal AIS is usually limited to supportive care, including normalizing glucose levels, monitoring blood pressure, optimizing oxygenation, and managing seizures. Treatable causes such as infection, cardiac embolus, metabolic derangement, and inherited thrombophilia must be ruled out. Unless an embolic source is identified, aspirin and anticoagulation are rarely prescribed.

Long-term management of perinatal AIS includes identifying risk factors, such as testing for prothrombotic abnormalities, particularly once the patient has reached at least 6 months of age. Maternal risk factors such as infertility, preeclampsia, smoking, and autoimmune disease may be associated with perinatal AIS.

Historically, the prognosis for children with perinatal ischemic strokes has been considered better than for children or adults with ischemic strokes, presumably because of the plasticity of the neonatal brain. Although 20%–40% of patients have no neurologic deficits, 40%–60% will have long-term motor impairment, particularly hemiplegic CP. Cognitive deficits are seen in up to 25% of children with perinatal AIS, and 10%–40% develop epilepsy. Ischemic stroke recurs in 3% of neonates and is usually associated with a prothrombotic abnormality or an underlying illness, such as cardiac malformation or infection. Long-term management is largely rehabilitative, including constraint therapy, in which the stronger limb is temporarily physically constrained to promote use of the weaker limb.

2. Childhood Arterial Ischemic Stroke

Childhood AIS affects 1.6 per 100,000 children per year and is associated with poor outcomes, including death (10%), neurologic deficits or seizures (70%–75%), and recurrent ischemic stroke (20%). Childhood AIS is a neurologic emergency, following the adage "time is brain." Recanalization with thrombolytic agents (such as intravenous tissue plasminogen activator [tPA] or tenecteplase/TNKase) and intra-arterial therapy (such as mechanical thrombectomy) have consistently shown benefit in adults who present within 24 hours and have evidence of "large vessel occlusion" (LVO, occlusion of the internal carotid artery/ICA or proximal middle cerebral artery/MCA) or basilar artery occlusion on imaging. As these interventions are increasingly utilized in children, urgent consultation with a pediatric neurologist and neuroimaging should be obtained for any patient with concern for acute ischemic stroke.

▶ Clinical Findings

Manifestations of AIS in childhood vary according to the involved vascular territory. Children may present with hemiplegia, aphasia, or vertigo, similar to ischemic stroke in adults. Symptoms may develop over a period of minutes, but at times, symptoms may evolve over several hours. Unlike in adults, new-onset focal seizure accompanied by focal neurologic deficits is a common presentation of childhood AIS.

Clinicians should carefully determine the last time that someone observed that the patient was symptom-free—the "last known well" (LKW), which is often different than the time that the symptoms were first noticed. All clinical trials have utilized LKW to determine appropriate treatment windows. Physical examination of the patient initially focuses on identifying the specific deficits related to impaired cerebral blood flow. The Pediatric National Institutes of Health Stroke Scale (NIHSS) is a rapid neurologic examination designed to identify acute arterial stroke in children. An NIHSS of at least 6 is particularly concerning for LVO. The evaluation should also include a thorough history of prior illnesses, preceding viral infection, minor head or neck trauma, and familial clotting tendencies, as well as any predisposing cardiac, vascular, or hematologic disorders (Table 25–12). Additional examination findings, such as retinal hemorrhages, splinter hemorrhages in the nail beds, cardiac murmurs, rash, fever, neurocutaneous stigmata, and signs of trauma may point to a specific etiology.

Table 25–12. Etiologic risk factors for ischemic and/or hemorrhagic ischemic stroke.

Cardiac Disorders	Hematologic Disorders
Structural heart disease	Iron deficiency anemia
Valvular disease, including endocarditis	Polycythemia
Cardiomyopathy	Thrombotic thrombocytopenia
Arrhythmias	Thrombocytopenic purpura
Vascular Disorders	Leukemia
Cervical/cerebral arterial dissection	Hemoglobinopathies, including Sickle cell disease
Moyamoya	Coagulation defects
Fibromuscular dysplasia	Hemophilia
Connective tissue diseases	Vitamin K deficiency
Arteriovenous malformation	Hypercoagulable states
Arterial aneurysm	Prothrombin gene mutation
Dural sinus and cerebral venous sinus thrombosis	Methylenetetrahydrofolate reductase mutation
Focal cerebral arteriopathy	Antithrombin III deficiency
Vasculitis	Protein C and S deficiencies
Polyarteritis nodosa	Factor VIII elevation
Systemic lupus erythematosus	Lipoprotein (a) derangements
Drug abuse (amphetamines)	Hypercholesterolemia, hypertriglyceridemia
Infection (varicella, herpes simplex, HIV)	Factor V Leiden deficiency
Homocystinuria/ homocystinemia	Antiphospholipid antibodies
Diabetes	Systemic lupus erythematosus
Nephrotic syndrome	Pregnancy
Systemic hypertension	Use of oral contraceptives

Diagnostic Evaluation

In the acute phase, complete blood count, complete metabolic panel, prothrombin time/partial thromboplastin time (PT/PTT), and a pregnancy test, as well as brain imaging, should be obtained emergently. Additional urgent testing to consider includes disseminated intravascular coagulation (DIC) panel, fibrin split products, erythrocyte sedimentation rate, C-reactive protein, anti–factor Xa activity, chest radiography, electrocardiogram (ECG), and urine toxicology.

Urgent brain imaging with CT/CTA and/or MRI/MRA is critical to evaluate for LVO or vascular abnormalities. Importantly, CT scans are often normal within the first 24 hours of an ischemic stroke and are primarily performed to exclude intracranial hemorrhage, which may influence eligibility for anticoagulation, thrombolytic agents, or mechanical thrombectomy. Especially in pediatric patients, for whom stroke "mimics" are common, MRI with DWI is ultimately necessary to determine whether an AIS has occurred. Up to 80% of pediatric patients with AIS will have vascular abnormalities on imaging, including transient cerebral arteriopathy, focal cerebral arteriopathy (FCA), arteriopathy associated with sickle cell disease, moyamoya disease, arterial dissection, aneurysm, fibromuscular dysplasia, and vasculitis. Many of these conditions are not amenable to thrombolytic therapies, further underscoring the importance of consultation with a pediatric neurologist.

Subsequent studies can be carried out systematically, with particular attention to disorders involving the heart, blood vessels, platelets, red cells, hemoglobin, and coagulation proteins. Twenty to 50% of pediatric ischemic stroke patients have a prothrombotic state. Congenital heart disease is the most common predisposing condition, followed by hematologic and neoplastic disorders, though most patients are not found to have a specific disorder. ECG and echocardiography with bubble study (to evaluate for patent foramen ovale) are useful in evaluating stroke etiology, particularly when hypotension or cardiac arrhythmias complicate the clinical course, and when the stroke is suspected to be embolic in nature.

Examination of CSF is indicated in patients with suspected infection, rheumatologic disease, or subarachnoid hemorrhage but is otherwise rarely helpful in the acute setting. Patients with seemingly idiopathic AIS may benefit from serum and CSF testing for HSV and VZV, both of which can cause stroke secondary to FCA, even years after the initial infection.

Differential Diagnosis

Common pediatric ischemic stroke "mimics" include hypoglycemia, prolonged focal seizures, a prolonged postictal paresis (Todd paralysis), acute disseminated encephalomyelitis (ADEM), meningitis, hemorrhagic stroke, encephalitis, hemiplegic migraine, ingestion, and brain abscess. In particular, migraine with focal neurologic deficits may be difficult to differentiate from ischemic stroke—urgent imaging is typically warranted. The possibility of drug abuse and other toxic exposures must be investigated in any patient with acute mental status changes.

Treatment

The initial management of pediatric ischemic stroke focuses on optimizing perfusion while quickly determining whether the patient is candidate for urgent intervention. Once hemorrhage, hydrocephalus, and intracranial mass have been ruled out, the patient should be positioned flat, and "permissive hypertension" is encouraged to promote cerebral blood flow. Neurology consultation should be obtained emergently, including discussion of the patient's LKW and NIHSS, so specific treatment can be tailored to the underlying pathogenesis and timeline.

In general, the Royal College of Physicians Pediatric Ischemic Stroke Working Group recommends aspirin 5 mg/kg daily as soon as the diagnosis is made. Long-term aspirin use in pediatric patients appears to be safe, though the American Heart Association (AHA) does recommend yearly flu shots and close monitoring for Reye syndrome. In cases of arterial dissection or cardioembolic events, anticoagulation with heparin should be considered, particularly if evidence of persistent thrombus is present (eg, on echo or CTA). Sickle cell patients require urgent exchange transfusion.

Recent guidelines for adults with acute ischemic stroke recommend intra-arterial treatment (such as mechanical thrombectomy) for patients with an LVO and less than 24 hours of symptoms, regardless of the size of the stroke. Although pediatric data are lacking, the use of thrombolytic agents (such as tPA) and intra-arterial interventions in pediatric patients will likely rapidly increase in the coming years.

Most patients with acute ischemic stroke should be admitted for 24–72 hours, and many require intensive care monitoring initially. When the ischemic stroke involves large portions of one hemisphere or portions of both hemispheres, serial neuroimaging is also warranted, due to the risk of fatal cerebral edema. Long-term management requires intensive rehabilitation aimed at improving the child's language, motor, educational, and psychological performance. Constraint therapy may be particularly helpful in cases of hemiparesis. Length of treatment with anticoagulation or antiplatelet agents is determined case by case.

Prognosis

The outcome of ischemic stroke in infants and children is variable, depending on the presence of underlying predisposing conditions and the vascular territory involved. Roughly one-third may have minimal or no deficits, one-third are moderately affected, and one-third are severely affected, although chronic cognitive and behavioral problems are common. Seizures may occur in 30%–50% of patients at some

point in their course. Stroke recurrence is 14%–20%, and is higher in some conditions, such as protein C deficiency, lipoprotein (a) abnormalities, and vascular abnormalities. Long-term follow-up with a pediatric neurologist and, if possible, a multidisciplinary ischemic stroke team, is indicated.

Barry M et al: What is the role of mechanical thrombectomy in childhood stroke? Pediatr Neurol 2019;95:19–25 [PMID: 30795888].

Powers WJ et al: 2019 American Heart Association/American Stroke Association Guidelines for the early management of patients with acute ischemic stroke: 2019 update to the 2018 Guidelines for the Early Management of Acute Ischemic Stroke. Stroke 2019;50(12):e344–e418 [PMID: 31662037].

Whitaker E, Cipolla M: Perinatal stroke. Handb Clin Neurol 2020;171:313–326 [PMID: 32736758].

ABNORMAL HEAD SIZE

The bones of the cranium rely on extrinsic forces from brain growth to stimulate skull growth. An accurate assessment of head growth is one of the most important aspects of the neurologic examination in a young child. An atypical head shape or a head circumference that is two standard deviations above or below the mean for age requires investigation.

1. Craniosynostosis

ESSENTIALS OF DIAGNOSIS & TYPICAL FEATURES

▶ Craniosynostosis is the premature fusion of one or multiple cranial sutures and can be isolated or associated with other systemic involvement.

▶ Craniosynostosis may require repair to preserve brain growth and optimize neurodevelopmental and visual outcomes.

Clinical Findings

Craniosynostosis is seen in 1 in 2000 live births. It is defined as the premature closure of one or more cranial sutures, and it leads to enhanced skull growth for sutures that are patent, resulting in an atypical but expected head shape. Eighty percent of cases occur in isolation as a single suture craniosynostosis, while the remainder are multisuture and are associated with increased risk of other skeletal, hearing, or airway abnormalities. Risk factors for craniosynostosis include intrauterine constraint, advanced parental age, tobacco use during pregnancy, and medical conditions such as hypothyroidism, hypophosphatasia, rickets, or mucopolysaccharidoses. Several well described genetic conditions are associated with multisuture involvement, including pathogenic variants in *FGFR1*, *FGFR2*, *FGFR3*, and *TWIST1*. Most cases

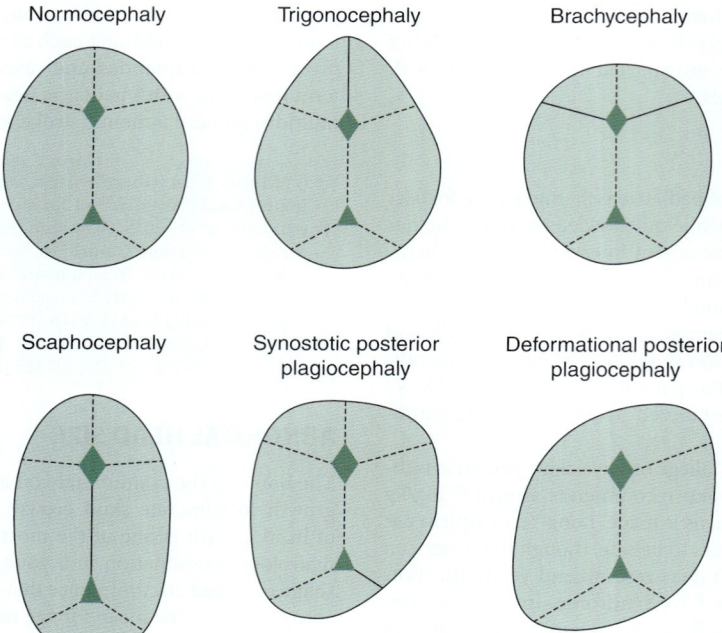

Normocephaly   Trigonocephaly   Brachycephaly

Scaphocephaly   Synostotic posterior   Deformational posterior
                 plagiocephaly   plagiocephaly

▲ **Figure 25–2.** Comparison of different types of craniosynostoses versus positional plagiocephaly. (Reproduced with permission from Mark W, Kline, et al. Craniosynostosis: Rudolph's pediatrics, 23rd ed. New York: McGraw Hill; 2018.)

are congenital and diagnosed clinically based on head shape, although the gold standard for diagnosis remains high-resolution CT with three-dimensional reconstruction. Sagittal suture craniosynostosis accounts for approximately 50% of cases, and it presents as scaphocephaly or the elongation of the skull in the anterior-posterior plane. Figure 25–2 depicts various types of craniosynostoses versus deformational positional plagiocephaly.

▶ Differential Diagnosis

Deformational positional plagiocephaly is the most common cause of an asymmetric head shape and results in a parallelogram shape, rather than the trapezoid shape seen with unilateral lambdoid craniosynostosis, which is quite rare. Supine sleep position remains important for preventing sudden infant death syndrome. Most positional plagiocephaly resolves by 2 years of age. Repositioning the head during naps, prone position when awake, and physical therapy for treatment of torticollis are effective treatments.

▶ Treatment

Surgical intervention is frequently required to optimize brain growth for patients with craniosynostosis. Timing of surgery is determined by the patient's age and severity of symptoms at presentation. An ongoing multidisciplinary approach is

commonly required to assess for developmental delay and oral, vision, and hearing abnormalities.

2. Microcephaly

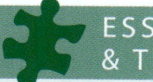
ESSENTIALS OF DIAGNOSIS & TYPICAL FEATURES

▶ Microcephaly is defined as head circumference more than two standard deviations below the mean for age and sex.
▶ Microcephaly is nearly always associated with neurodevelopmental disabilities.

Microcephaly is defined as occipitofrontal head circumference more than 2 standard deviations below the mean for age and sex (Figure 25–3). It is seen in 1–5 per 10,000 live births and is higher in low-income countries. Microcephaly is almost always associated with neurodevelopmental disabilities, and other system involvement frequently co-occurs. Primary microcephaly is present at birth while secondary microcephaly develops postnatally. Etiologies can be divided into acquired and genetic. Acquired etiologies are enumerated in Table 25–13. Nearly 2000 genetic etiologies have been described.

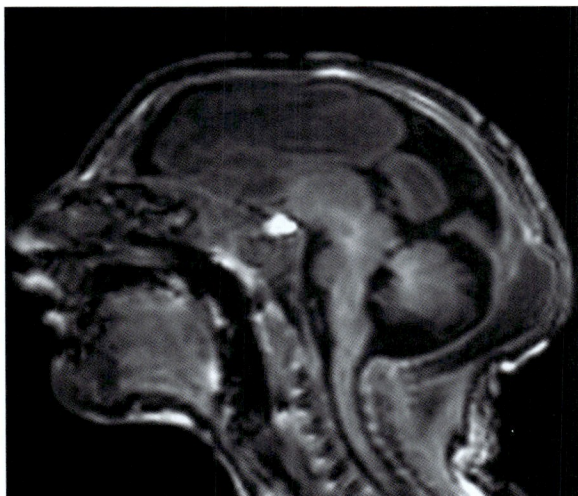

▲ **Figure 25–3.** Severe microcephaly with simplified gyral pattern and absent corpus callosum seen on sagittal brain MRI.

▶ Diagnostic Evaluation

If the history and physical examination do not yield a unifying cause a urine PCR for CMV and serologies for other infectious etiologies are done in the neonatal period. A brain MRI is pursued for characterization of brain parenchyma, specifically to assess for migrational abnormalities, white matter injury, and intracranial calcifications. In the absence of an acquired cause, genetic testing, specifically WES, is pursued.

Table 25–13. Acquired causes of microcephaly.

Causes	Examples
Intrauterine	
Infection	Cytomegalovirus, Zika, human immunodeficiency virus, rubella, herpes simplex, syphilis, toxoplasmosis
Radiation	Maternal pelvis in first and second trimesters
Maternal factors	Placental insufficiency, alcohol or cocaine use, maternal phenylketonuria, hypothyroidism, malnutrition
Perinatal	
Hypoxia	Hypoxic ischemic encephalopathy, abusive head trauma, stroke
Infections	Group B streptococci, enterovirus, herpes simplex
Other	Malnutrition, craniosynostosis, hypopituitarism, hypothyroidism, chronic illness

▶ Treatment

Treatment of microcephaly is based on symptomatic care. A referral to early intervention is placed as appropriate therapies is paramount to optimization of developmental outcomes. A multidisciplinary approach is often required as children can also have vision or hearing problems, feeding intolerance, or cardiac disease.

3. Macrocephaly

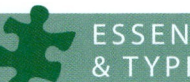

ESSENTIALS OF DIAGNOSIS & TYPICAL FEATURES

▶ Macrocephaly is defined as head circumference more than two standard deviations above the mean for age and sex.

▶ Macrocephaly may be associated with increased ICP.

Macrocephaly (Figure 25–3) is defined as an occipitofrontal head circumference more than 2 standard deviations above the mean for age and sex. This is more common than microcephaly with an estimated prevalence of 2%–5%. A complete history and physical examination are paramount as the differential diagnosis is broad. While CT head is pursued in urgent scenarios, an MRI brain is the preferred modality for characterization of the brain parenchyma.

▶ Differential Diagnosis

The substrates that account for head size are brain parenchyma, CSF, blood, and the skull, and the differential for macrocephaly can be approached by which component is in excess. The reassuring etiologies for macrocephaly are benign familial macrocephaly and benign enlargement of subarachnoid spaces (BESS). In the former, a prominent head circumference is identified at birth, and there is a significant family history of macrocephaly. Neurodevelopment is typical. In BESS, there is a rapid head growth at 6 months followed by stabilization at 18 months, and most children also have typical development.

Megalencephaly is due to either an abnormality in neuronal development or an accumulation of metabolic substances. When isolated to one hemisphere, it is termed *hemimegaloencephaly*. Over 500 genetic conditions have been associated with macrocephaly, and a portion are detailed in Table 25–14. Cortical development can be typical, but cortical malformations and posterior fossa abnormalities are often noted (see next section).

Hydrocephalus (Figure 25–4) is an urgent etiology for macrocephaly. Children present with signs and symptoms of increased ICP, and an external ventricular drain (EVD) or ventriculoperitoneal (VP) shunt is frequently required.

Table 25–14. Causes of megalencephaly.

Causes	Examples
Neurocutaneous conditions	Neurofibromatosis type 1, Tuberous Sclerosis, Noonan syndrome
Overgrowth conditions	*PIK3CA*-related including megalencephaly-capillary malformation (MCAP) and CLOVES, *mTOR*-related including megalencephaly-polymicrogyria-pigmentary mosaicism (MPPM), Sotos syndrome, PTEN hamartoma syndrome, Beckwith-Wiedemann syndrome
Other genetic disorders	Fragile X
Metabolic	
Organic acidurias	Glutaric aciduria type 1
Lysosomal	Mucopolysaccharidoses
Leukoencephalopathies	Canavan disease Alexander disease

A thickened skull can be seen in skeletal dysplasias, such as achondroplasia, vitamin D deficiency rickets, or β-thalassemia. Macrocephaly can also be associated with vascular malformations such as arteriovenous malformation (AVM).

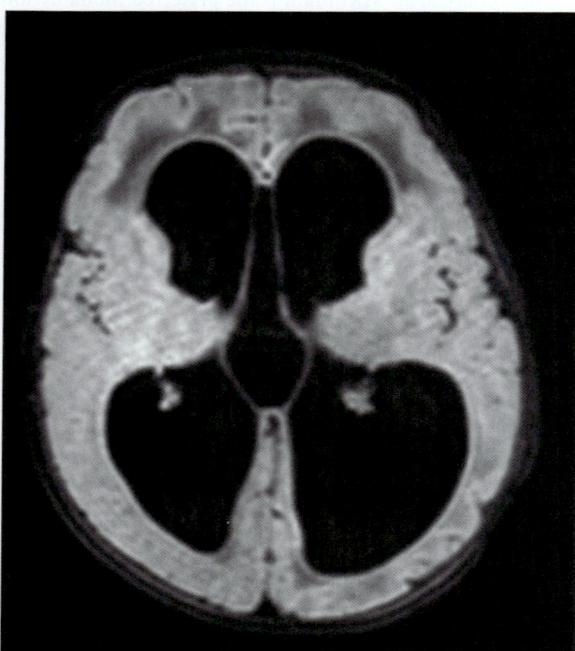

▲ **Figure 25–4.** Hydrocephalus with ventricular dilatation of lateral and third ventricles seen on axial brain MRI.

Accogli A et al: Diagnostic approach to macrocephaly in children. Front Pediatr 2022;9:794069 [PMID: 35096710].

Ashwal S et al: Practice parameter: evaluation of the child with microcephaly (an evidence-based review): report of the Quality Standards Subcommittee of the American Academy of Neurology and the Practice Committee of the Child Neurology Society. Neurology 2009;73(11):887–897 [PMID: 19752457].

Von der Hagen et al: Diagnostic approach to microcephaly in childhood: a two-center study and review of the literature. Dev Med Child Neurol 2014;56:732 [PMID: 24617602].

CONGENITAL MALFORMATIONS OF THE NERVOUS SYSTEM

Malformations of the nervous system occur in 3% of living neonates and represent 40% of infant mortality. Structural malformations of the CNS may result from infectious, toxic, genetic, metabolic, or vascular insults, and the degree of malformation is dictated by the gestational period when the injury occurs. During the first month of gestation, the neural plate appears, followed by formation and closure of the neural tube. Interruptions can result in a major absence of neural structures, such as anencephaly, or in a defect of neural tube closure, such as spina bifida, meningomyelocele, or encephalocele. Cellular proliferation and migration characterize neural development from 12 to 20 weeks of gestation. During this period, lissencephaly, pachygyria, agyria, and agenesis of the corpus callosum (ACC) may arise.

1. Abnormalities of Neural Tube Closure

Neural tube defects (NTDs) are one of the most common congenital malformations affecting the CNS. Folate supplementation decreased incidence by 50%–75% in developed countries, but NTDs continue to be a significant cause of infant morbidity and mortality in developing countries. The most common cranial NTDs are anencephaly and encephalocele. In anencephaly, all or a portion of the brain and skull do not form, whereas in encephalocele a portion of the brain and meninges herniates through a defect in the skull. Spina bifida, meningocele, and myelomeningocele are caudal NTDs with varying involvement of spinal cord and meninges.

The diagnosis of NTDs is apparent at the time of birth, and prenatal diagnostic accuracy is increasing as ultrasound technology improves. Risk factors for NTDs include folate deficiency, maternal obesity or diabetes, use of antiseizure medications during pregnancy, and chromosomal abnormalities, including trisomy 13 or 18.

Multidisciplinary care should include neurology, neurosurgery, orthopedic surgery, and rehabilitation. Anencephaly is universally fatal. Intrauterine or early life surgical closure is available for caudal NTDs. Morbidity of caudal NTDs is based on extent of spinal cord and peripheral nerve involvement. They merit long-term monitoring for lower extremity function, bowel and bladder difficulties, and orthopedic abnormalities. These children are also at risk for hydrocephalus.

2. Disorders of Cortical Development

Malformations of cortical development (MCD) are a heterogenous group of conditions due to disruption in neuronal proliferation and migration. Diagnosis is confirmed by pathology, but advances in neuroradiology and neurogenetics have led to a greater understanding of these entities. They are classified into diffuse or focal disruptions of the cortex. Sizeable MCDs are associated with epilepsy, CP, movement disorders, feeding difficulties, and significant neurodevelopmental disabilities.

A. Lissencephaly

Lissencephaly is an example of impaired neuronal migration. This severe malformation of the brain is characterized by a smooth cortical surface with abnormal sulci. On the most severe spectrum is agyria, which is the absence of sulci, whereas pachygyria is a thickened and simplified sulcal pattern. Patients with lissencephaly usually have microcephaly, intellectual disability, spastic quadriplegia, and medically refractory epilepsy, including infantile spasms. Autosomal dominant causes are *LIS1* and *RELN*. X-linked etiologies include *DCX* and *ARX*, which present in males with lissencephaly, but a milder variant discussed later called subcortical band heterotopia occurs in females. Cobblestone lissencephaly, which is due to over-migration of neurons, is associated with congenital muscular dystrophy as seen in Walker-Warburg syndrome, Fukuyama muscular dystrophy, and muscle-eye-brain disease.

B. Gray Matter Heterotopia

Gray matter heterotopia is the premature arrest of migration in typically formed neurons. The most common locations are periventricular and subcortical. A rare subtype is subcortical band heterotopia, which is a diffuse band of heterotopia that arrests in the white matter resembling a double cortex (Figure 25–5, left image). It is common for a single nodule to be incidentally identified on MRI of the brain. If robust or occurring with other CNS malformations, it is associated with epilepsy and a spectrum of neurodevelopmental outcomes.

C. Focal Cortical Dysplasia

Focal cortical dysplasia is an absence of appropriate neuronal organization in typical or atypical neurons. There are three subtypes, and type II is the most common. Tubers of tuberous sclerosis are a classic example. MRI findings are blurring of gray-white junction, alteration in cortical thickness, or transmantle sign, which is the persistence of fetal radial migration pattern. These lesions are highly associated with epilepsy and can be amenable to resection if medically intractable.

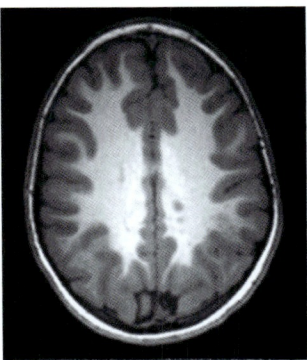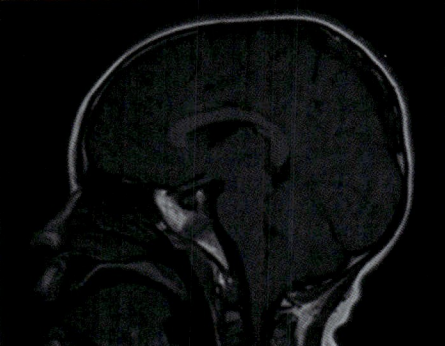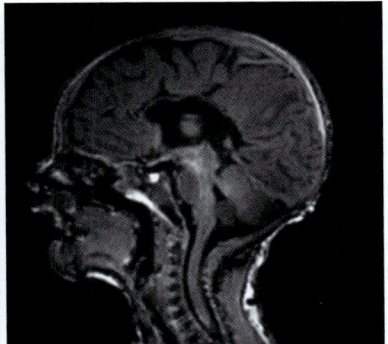

▲ **Figure 25–5.** Examples of congenital brain malformations (on brain MRI). Posterior predominant subcortical band heterotopia (left), Chiari 1 malformation with descent of cerebellar tonsils and crowding of craniocervical junction (center), and isolated agenesis of corpus callosum (right).

D. Polymicrogyria

Polymicrogyria is a postmigrational disorder characterized by numerous but very small gyri. It can be associated with schizencephaly, which is a cleft lined by grey matter extending from ventricle to cortical surface. Bilateral perisylvian polymicrogyria is the most common form and is associated with bulbar dysfunction, epilepsy, and cognitive deficits. Etiologies of polymicrogyria are subdivided into genetic, such as 22q11 deletion and numerous single gene pathogenic variants, and acquired, including early infectious or vascular injury.

3. Disorders of Cerebellum Development

A. Chiari Malformations

Chiari malformation type I consists of displacement of the caudal end of the cerebellar tonsils through the foramen magnum (Figure 25–5, center image). A newer entity is Chiari 1.5, which is the descent of cerebellar tonsils and lower brainstem through the foramen magnum. Due to disruption in CSF flow, these can be associated with a cervical or thoracic syrinx. These typically remain asymptomatic and do not require intervention. In rare circumstances, they can present with brief occipital headaches associated with lower cranial neuropathies and cerebellar signs which are provoked by straining, and this can require decompression of the posterior fossa for relief.

Chiari malformation II and III are likely distinct entities from Chiari 1 malformations, though there is considerable overlap in features. Chiari II malformation consists of displaced cerebellar vermis, fourth ventricle, and medulla through the foramen magnum plus an associated myelomeningocele. Chiari malformation III is characterized by herniation of the cerebellum through the foramen magnum with associated cervical spinal cord defect. Hydrocephalus is common in both Chiari II and III. These patients may also have hydromyelia, syringomyelia, and cortical dysplasia. The clinical manifestations are most commonly caused by associated hydrocephalus and meningomyelocele. In addition, dysfunction of the lower cranial nerves may be present. Up to 25% of patients have epilepsy.

B. Dandy-Walker Malformation

Dandy-Walker malformation is a rare condition that is characterized by aplasia of the cerebellar vermis, cystic enlargement of the fourth ventricle, and rostral displacement of the tentorium. Hydrocephalus commonly develops within the first few months of life. On physical examination, a rounded protuberance or exaggeration of the cranial occiput often exists. In the absence of hydrocephalus, few physical findings may be present to suggest neurologic dysfunction. Ataxia occurs in fewer than 20% of patients and is usually late in appearing. Patients are at risk for global developmental delay and other developmental disabilities. MRI of the brain confirms the diagnosis. Although presumed to be genetic in etiology, a specific cause is identified in a minority of patients.

4. Agenesis of the Corpus Callosum

Agenesis of the corpus callosum (ACC; Figure 25–5, right image) is the absence of central connecting fibers between the left and right hemispheres. It is seen in 1 in 5000 live births. When it occurs in isolation, up to 75% will have typical neurodevelopment. A genetic etiology is more likely to be identified if other brain malformations are seen or other systems are involved. These children are at increased risk for epilepsy, global developmental delay, and autism spectrum disorder.

Severino M et al: Definitions and classification of malformations of cortical development: practical guidelines. Brain 2020 Oct 1; 143(10):2874–2894 [PMID: 32779696].

NEUROCUTANEOUS DISORDERS

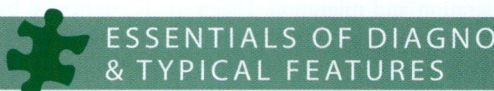

ESSENTIALS OF DIAGNOSIS & TYPICAL FEATURES

► Disruptions in fetal ectoderm formation can impact the epidermis, nervous tissue, and other organs; thus, skin abnormalities provide diagnostic clues for a variety of neurocutaneous disorders.

► Many neurocutaneous disorders carry significant risks for epilepsy, cognitive impairments, tumors, and other organ involvement.

Neurocutaneous disorders are diseases of the neuroectoderm that sometimes involve endoderm and mesoderm. Tissues that share a common embryologic origin may be impacted; thus, characteristic birthmarks can be a clue to brain or spinal cord involvement, eye disease, and other organ systems. Benign and even malignant tumors may also develop in these conditions. Table 25–15 summarizes the key features of various neurocutaneous disorders.

1. Neurofibromatosis Type 1

Neurofibromatosis type 1 (NF-1) is a multisystem disorder with a prevalence of 1:3000. Fifty percent of cases are due to new pathogenic variants in the *NF1* gene, which is located on chromosome 17q11.2 encoding neurofibromin. Two or more positive criteria are diagnostic (see Table 25–15), while others may appear over time. See Chapter 37 for additional information.

Table 25–15. Key features of neurocutaneous disorders.

Disease	Essentials of Diagnosis and Typical Features
Neurofibromatosis type 1	• Six or more café au lait spots > 5 mm in prepubertal individuals and > 15 mm in postpubertal individuals. • Peripheral nerve sheath tumors: 2 or more neurofibromas of any type or 1 plexiform neurofibroma • Freckling in the axillary or inguinal regions • Optic pathway glioma • Two or more Lisch nodules (iris hamartomas) • Distinctive bony lesions, such as sphenoid dysplasia or thinning of long bone, with or without pseudarthrosis • First-degree relative with neurofibromatosis type 1
Neurofibromatosis type 2	• Bilateral vestibular schwannomas • Other tumors of the brain and spinal cord • Posterior lens cataract
Tuberous sclerosis complex	• At least three hypomelanotic macules, each at least 5 mm in diameter • Angiofibromas, ungal fibromas, intraoral fibromas • Shagreen patch • CNS manifestations: subependymal nodules, cortical dysplasias, subependymal giant cell astrocytomas (SEGAS) • Cardiac rhabdomyomas and angiomyolipomas • Hamartomas
Sturge-Weber syndrome	• Port-wine birthmark • Capillary-venous malformation in the eye (choroidal angioma) and brain (leptomeningeal angioma)
Von Hippel-Lindau disease (VHL)	• Retinal, central nervous system, and renal hemangioblastomas • Visceral cysts • Less frequently, adrenal and extra-adrenal pheochromocytomas, pancreatic endocrine cancers, and endolymphatic sac tumors

▶ Clinical Findings

The most common presenting symptoms are cognitive or psychomotor problems. During the evaluation, provider may notice the classic skin findings. Café au lait spots are seen in most affected children by age 1 year. The typical skin lesion is 10–30 mm, ovoid, and smooth-bordered. Discrete well-demarcated neurofibromas or lipomas can occur at any age. Plexiform neurofibromas are congenital but are frequently detected during periods of rapid growth.

Clinicians should evaluate head circumference, blood pressure, vision, hearing, spine for scoliosis, and limbs for pseudoarthroses. The eye examination should include checking for strabismus, amblyopia, proptosis, iris (Lisch) nodules, optic atrophy, or papilledema. Short stature and precocious puberty are occasional findings. Parents should be examined in detail. Family history is important in identifying dominant gene manifestations.

▶ Diagnostic Evaluation

Genetic testing can be helpful in cases of clinical uncertainty. Selected patients require brain MRI with special attention to the optic nerves to rule out optic glioma. Hypertension necessitates evaluation of renal arteries for dysplasia and stenosis. Cognitive testing may be indicated. Scoliosis or limb abnormalities should be studied by appropriate imaging.

▶ Differential Diagnosis

Patients with McCune-Albright syndrome often have larger café au lait spots with precocious puberty, polyostotic fibrous dysplasia, and endocrinopathies. Legius syndrome has overlapping features of café au lait spots and inguinal/axillary freckling but is not associated with neurofibromas. A large solitary café au lait spot is usually innocent. Children with six or more café au lait spots and no other positive criteria should be followed; most will develop NF-1 by 8 years of age.

▶ Complications

Neurodevelopmental sequelae are common—40% have learning disabilities, and 8% have intellectual disability. Seizures, hearing impairment, short stature, early puberty, and hypertension occur in less than 25% of patients with NF-1. Optic gliomas occur in about 15%; these rarely cause functional problems and are usually nonprogressive. Patients have a 5% lifetime risk for developing various malignancies, which can be a cause of early death. Even benign tumors may cause significant morbidity and mortality. For example, plexiform neurofibromas can be disfiguring or impair spinal cord, renal, or pelvic/leg function. Strokes from NF-1 cerebral arteriopathy are rare; arteriopathy of renal arteries can cause reversible hypertension in childhood.

► Treatment

Genetic counseling is important as 50% of cases are familial. The disease may be progressive, but serious complications are only occasionally seen. Annual or semiannual visits are important in the early detection of school problems, as well as screening for bone, vision, hearing, puberty, cardiac (including hypertension), or neurologic abnormalities. Multidisciplinary clinics at medical centers around the United States can be excellent resources, and information is available from the National Neurofibromatosis Foundation (http://www.nf.org).

2. Neurofibromatosis Type 2

Neurofibromatosis type 2 (NF-2) is a dominantly inherited neoplasia syndrome manifested as bilateral vestibular schwannomas (VIII nerve tumors), which may present in childhood with loss of hearing. Other tumors of the brain and spinal cord are common: meningiomas, other cranial nerve schwannomas, and ependymomas. Posterior lens cataracts are also a risk. Café au lait spots are not part of NF-2. In 50% of patients, the pathogenic variant occurs de novo.

3. Tuberous Sclerosis

Tuberous sclerosis complex (TSC) is a dominantly inherited disease. Almost all individuals have deletions on chromosome 9 (*TSC1* gene) or 16 (*TSC2* gene). The gene products hamartin and tuberin have tumor-suppressing effects; therefore, patients with TSC are more susceptible to hamartomas in many organs and brain tubers and tumors.

► Clinical Findings

TSC has a wide phenotypic expression, from asymptomatic carriers to patients with refractory epilepsy and significant intellectual disability. Seizures in early infancy, such as infantile spasms, correlate with developmental delay. The triad of seizures, intellectual disability, and adenoma sebaceum occurs in only 33% of patients.

A. Dermatologic Features

Skin findings bring most patients to the physician's attention (see Table 25–15). Ninety-six percent of patients have one or more hypomelanotic macules, facial angiofibromas, ungual fibromas, or shagreen (leathery orange peel) patches. Adenoma sebaceum (facial skin hamartomas) may first appear in early childhood, often on the cheek, chin, and dry sites of the skin where acne is not usually seen. Ash-leaf spots are off-white hypomelanotic macules, are often oval or "ash leaf" in shape and follow dermatomes. A Wood lamp (ultraviolet light) shows the macules more clearly. The equivalent to an ash leaf spot in the scalp is poliosis

(whitened hair patch). Subungual and periungual fibromas are more common in the toes. Fibrous or raised plaques may resemble coalescent angiofibromas. Café au lait spots are occasionally seen.

B. Neurologic Features

Seizures are the most common neurologic sequela. Virtually any kind of symptomatic seizure (eg, atypical absence, partial complex, and generalized tonic-clonic seizures) may occur. Up to 20% of patients with infantile spasms have TSC. Thus, any patient presenting with infantile spasms should be evaluated for TSC. Intellectual disability occurs in up to 50% of patients referred to tertiary care centers; the incidence is probably much lower in randomly selected patients.

C. Other Organ Involvement

US of the kidneys should be done in any patient suspected of TSC, both to aid in diagnosis of renal cysts or angiomyolipomas and also to rule out renal obstructive disease. Rarely, cystic lung disease may occur. Cardiac rhabdomyomas may be detected on prenatal ultrasound examination or postnatal chest radiographs or echocardiograms. Rhabdomyomas typically regress with age; thus, symptomatic presentations due to outflow obstruction or conduction abnormalities can occur in the perinatal period. Retinal hamartomas are often near the optic disc and are usually asymptomatic. Cystic lesions can be found in the bones of the fingers or toes.

► Diagnostic valuation

Plain radiographs may detect areas of thickening within the skull, spine, and pelvis, and cystic lesions in the hands and feet. Chest radiographs may show lung honeycombing. Head CT scan may show the virtually pathognomonic calcified subependymal nodules; brain MRI may show hypomyelinating white matter lesions, brain tumors, widened gyri, or cortical tubers. EEG should be considered in any TSC patient with new-onset spells concerning for seizures.

► Treatment

Dysfunction of tuberin or hamartin has been proposed to disinhibit the "mammalian target of rapamycin" (mTOR), allowing abnormal cell proliferation. In April 2018, the FDA approved Everolimus, an mTOR inhibitor, for the adjunctive treatment of epilepsy in patients with TSC. Surgical removal of epileptiform tubers may be needed for refractory epilepsy. Ongoing studies are investigating whether mTOR inhibitors can shrink dysplasias/tubers, tumors, and adenoma sebacea. Skin lesions on the face may need dermabrasion or laser treatment. Genetic counseling is important since the offspring of affected individuals have a 50% chance of inheriting the disorder. The patient should be seen annually for counseling and reexamination in childhood.

4. Sturge-Weber Syndrome

Sturge-Weber syndrome (SWS) is a sporadic congenital neurovascular disease that consists of a facial port wine nevus involving the upper part of the face (in the first division of cranial nerve V), a venous angioma of the meninges in the occipitoparietal regions, and choroidal angioma. Rarely, the syndrome has been described without the facial nevus (type III, exclusive leptomeningeal angioma). Recently, SWS was determined to be caused by a mosaic somatic activating mutation in the *GNAQ* gene.

▶ Clinical Findings

In infancy, the eye may show congenital glaucoma or buphthalmos, with a cloudy, enlarged cornea. Initially, the facial nevus may be the only indication. Facial nevi can involve the lower face, mouth, lip, neck, and even torso. Over time, the patient may develop radiographic and clinical evidence of brain involvement. Seizures are common, particularly in infancy. Hemiparesis and/or hemiatrophy on the side contralateral to the cerebral lesion may occur. Cognitive impairment, headache and migraines, stroke, and stroke-like episodes are other neurologic manifestations.

▶ Diagnostic Evaluation

Radiologic studies may show calcification of the cortex; CT scan may show this much earlier than plain radiographic studies. MRI eventually shows underlying brain involvement—cortical atrophy, calcifications, and meningeal angiomatosis. EEG often shows voltage attenuation over the involved area in early stages; later, focal epileptiform abnormalities may be present. Careful ophthalmologic assessment to detect early glaucoma is indicated.

▶ Differential Diagnosis

The differential diagnosis includes PHACES syndrome: **P**osterior fossa malformation, segmental (facial) **H**emangioma, **A**rterial abnormalities, **C**ardiac defects, **E**ye abnormalities, and **S**ternal (or ventral) defects; often, only portions of that list are present.

▶ Treatment & Prognosis

Bilateral brain involvement is associated with poorer cognitive outcomes, whereas larger nevus size is strongly correlated with subsequent epilepsy, which can also impact neurodevelopment, indicating a need for prompt treatment. Rarely, surgical removal of the involved meninges and the involved portion of the brain, even hemispherectomy, may be indicated.

5. Von Hippel-Lindau Disease (VHL)

Von Hippel-Lindau disease is a rare, dominantly inherited neurocutaneous disorder. The diagnostic criteria include retinal or cerebellar hemangioblastoma with or without a positive family history, intra-abdominal cyst (kidneys, pancreas), or renal cancer. The patient may present with ataxia, slurred speech, and nystagmus due to hemangioblastoma of the cerebellum or with a medullary spinal cord. Retinal detachment may occur from hemorrhage or exudate in retinal vascular malformations. Rarely, a pancreatic cyst or renal tumor may be the presenting symptom.

Asthagiri AR et al: Neurofibromatosis type 2. Lancet 2009;373:1974. [Epub May 22] [PMID: 19476995].
Cotter JA: An update on the central nervous system manifestations of tuberous sclerosis complex. Acta Neuropathol 2019 Apr 11;139(4):613–624 [PMID: 30976976].
Day AM et al: Physical and family history variables associated with neurological and cognitive development in Sturge-Weber syndrome. Pediatr Neurol 2019;96:30–36 [PMID: 30853154].
Gutmann DH et al: Neurofibromatosis type 1. Nat Rev Dis Primers 2017;23:3 [PMID: 28230061].
Krueger DA, Northrup H; International Tuberous Sclerosis Complex Consensus Group: Tuberous sclerosis complex surveillance and management: recommendations of the 2012 International Tuberous Sclerosis Complex Consensus Conference. Pediatr Neurol 2013;49(4):255–265 [PMID: 24053983].
Maher ER, Neumann HP, Richard S: von Hippel-Lindau disease: a clinical and scientific review. Eur J Hum Genet 2011;19(6):617 [PMID: 21386872].

LEUKODYSTROPHIES OF INFANCY & CHILDHOOD

Leukodystrophies are a group of heterogenous conditions due to abnormalities of white matter in the CNS (Table 25–16). They present with developmental plateau then regression of cognitive, motor, and visual function. While each entity has a characteristic MRI pattern, age of onset, head size, and evidence of peripheral neuropathy, brainstem or cerebellar lesions, and other system involvement can refine the diagnosis. Rapid diagnosis by biochemical testing, specific gene testing, or WES in unclear cases is vital as disease-modifying therapies (DMT), including gene therapy, are available for a subset of leukodystrophies. As these conditions acquire DMTs, they are increasingly added to newborn screening.

Adang L: Leukodystrophies. Continuum 2022;28(4):1194–1216 [PMID: 35938662].

Table 25–16. Leukodystrophies of childhood.

Disease	Genetics	Clinical Presentation	Diagnostic Tests	Prognosis/Treatment
Aicardi-Goutières syndrome	AR or AD; Genes: *TREX1*, *RNASEH2A/B/C*, *SAMHD1*, *ADAR1*, *IFIH1*. *LSM11*, *RNU7-1*	Onset: birth or first few months of life Symptoms: acquired microcephaly, spasticity, dystonia, regression, irritability, seizures Other systems: sterile pyrexia, hepatomegaly, chilblains.	CSF ↑ interferon-α with leukocytosis CTH with calcifications MRI with frontotemporal white matter changes	Supportive treatment.
Alexander disease	AD; Gene: *GFAP*	Onset: neonates to adults Symptoms: regression, megalencephaly, seizures, ophthalmoplegia, ataxia, spasticity	MRI with frontal white matter, basal ganglia, and brainstem changes	Supportive treatment.
Canavan disease	AR; Gene: *ASPA*	Onset: neonates to teenagers Symptoms: macrocephaly, hypotonia, delay +/− regression, optic atrophy, irritability. Juvenile onset is mild. Ashkenazi Jews.	Urine ↑ N-acetylaspartic acid Path: spongiform degeneration. MRI with diffuse cortical white matter changes.	Supportive treatment. Promising trials underway for gene therapy.
Krabbe disease/ Globoid cell leukodystrophy	AR; Gene: *GALC* Enzyme: galacto-cerebrosidase	Onset: infants to young children Symptoms: regression, irritability, spasticity, peripheral neuropathy, gait changes, seizures.	Leukocytes ↓ enzyme CSF ↑ protein MRI with white matter changes and enhancement of cranial nerves and spinal roots	HSCT can halt progression. Promising trials underway for gene therapy.
Megalencephalic leukodystrophy with subcortical cysts	AR or AD; Genes: *MLC1*, *MLC2A*, *MLC2B*	Typical: Macrocephaly in the first year, predominantly motor delay and regression, ataxia, spasticity, epilepsy. Improving phenotype: Similar to above but improves.	MRI shows frontoparietal white matter abnormalities with anterior temporal cysts.	Supportive treatment.
Metachromatic leukodystrophy	AR; Gene: *ARSA* Enzyme: Arylsulfatase A	Late infantile: Motor symptoms > cognitive regression; juvenile to adult: behavioral/cognitive difficulties > motor regression. Other: peripheral neuropathy, spasticity, bulbar disease.	Urine ↑ sulfatide enzyme Leukocytes ↓ enzyme MRI with parieto-occipital predominance, spares U fibers.	Supportive treatment. Promising gene therapy trials are underway.
Pelizaeus-Merzbacher disease	XLR; Gene: *PLP1*	First few weeks of life, up until 5 years of age: Nystagmus, hypotonia > spasticity, poor vision, ataxia, seizures.	MRI with symmetric, confluent white matter signal abnormalities.	Supportive treatment.
Vanishing white matter/Childhood ataxia with CNS hypomyelination	AR; Gene: *EIF2B1*, *EIF2B2*, *EIF2B3*, *EIF2B4*, *EIF2B5*	Early onset: microcephaly, cataracts, encephalopathy, and multisystem involvement. Late onset: regression with infection/trauma, ataxia, spasticity, optic atrophy, ovarian failure.	MRI with diffuse white matter changes > cystic encephalomalacia	Supportive treatment.
X-linked adrenoleuko-dystrophy	XLR; Gene: *ABCD1*	3–12 years: ADHD and fine motor difficulties > progressive cognitive/motor regression, seizures. Adolescence to young adult: progressive spastic paraparesis. Systems: adrenal insufficiency	Serum ↑ very-long-chain fatty acids MRI with posterior predominant white matter changes	HSCT can halt progression. Gene therapy in trials. Steroids for adrenal insufficiency.

AD, autosomal dominant; AR autosomal recessive; CSF, cerebrospinal fluid; CNS, central nervous system; CTH, computed tomography head; FDA, US Food and Drug Administration; HSCT, hematopoietic stem cell transplantation; LBSL, leukoencephalopathy with brainstem and spinal cord involvement and elevated lactate; MRI, magnetic resonance imaging; XLR, X-linked recessive.

CEREBRAL PALSY

Cerebral palsy (CP) occurs in 0.2% of live births. It is a nonspecific clinical descriptor used to encapsulate a static impairment of motor development, affecting tone, strength, or coordination. Causes range from hypoxic ischemic injury and intracranial infection to brain malformations and genetic conditions. Although it is nonprogressive, the full degree of impairment may not be evident until the child is 3–4 years of age when motor expectations are more robust.

▶ Clinical Findings

There are four subtypes of CP. Spastic CP occurs in 80% of patients and is described based on the limb(s) affected, specifically monoplegia, hemiplegia, diplegia, and quadriplegia. The affected extremity may be smaller and shorter than the others. Ataxic CP accounts for 15% of cases. It is most common in an upper extremity. Athetoid or dyskinetic CP, manifesting as choreoathetosis or dystonia, account for 5% of cases, and persistent hypotonia without spasticity comprises less than 1% of cases. The most common comorbid neurologic conditions are epilepsy and intellectual disability, which are seen in 25% and 50%, respectively. Other common co-morbidities are vision impairment, language delay, autism spectrum disorder, and learning disabilities. The presence of other system involvement can be helpful in identifying the underlying cause for these patients.

▶ Diagnostic Evaluation

History and physical examination guide the workup. MRI brain is essential to understand the extent of cerebral involvement and may offer the etiology. Figure 25–6 shows sequela of periventricular white matter injury of prematurity. If the diagnosis is not apparent based on history, physical examination, and MRI, genetic testing is typically pursued.

▶ Treatment

A multidisciplinary approach is essential to the management of CP. Treatment is directed at maximizing the child's neurologic functioning with physical, occupational, and speech therapy. A task-specific approach to therapy can encourage neuroplasticity, and intensive constraint-induced movement therapy can benefit the affected extremity. Monitoring for orthopedic issues, neuropsychological testing to provide optimal school support, and treatment of spasticity and seizures are integral.

▶ Prognosis

The prognosis for patients with CP depends greatly on the child's cognitive abilities, severity of motor deficits, and etiology of CP. Severely affected children can have a shortened

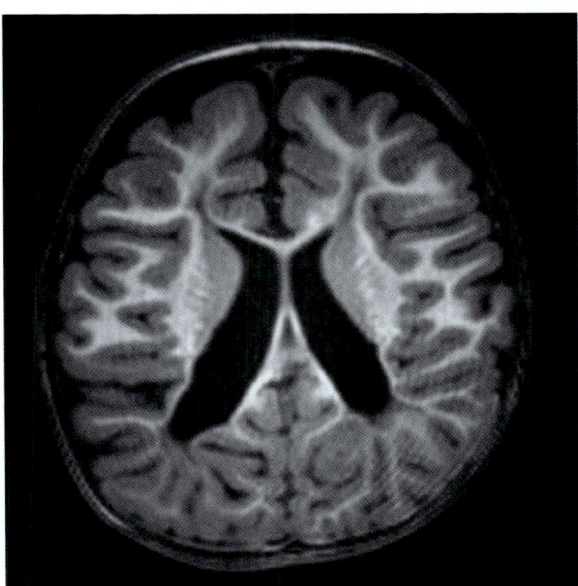

▲ **Figure 25–6.** Axial T1 MRI demonstrating posterior predominant periventricular white matter volume loss in a patient with spastic cerebral palsy due to white matter injury of prematurity.

lifespan, with infections, such as pneumonia or sepsis, as the most common cause of death. Patients with mild CP may improve with age, and a portion experience resolution of their motor deficits by 7 years of age.

Delgado MR et al: Practice parameter: pharmacologic treatment of spasticity in children and adolescents with cerebral palsy (an evidence-based review). Neurology 2010;74:336 [PMID: 20101040].

Novak I et al: State of the Evidence Traffic Lights 2019: systematic review of interventions for preventing and treating children with cerebral palsy. Curr Neurol Neurosci Rep 2020 Feb 21;20(2):3 [PMID: 32086598].

MOVEMENT DISORDERS

Movement disorders are conditions of excessive or slowed movements. The pathophysiology arises from dysfunction in the pathways amongst the motor cortex, basal ganglia, and cerebellum. The first step in evaluation is characterization of the movements, which guides the differential diagnosis and workup. Treatment is offered if the movements impact function. Children with movement disorders are also at risk for mood disorders, attention deficit/hyperactivity disorder (ADHD), obsessive compulsive disorder (OCD), and learning disabilities.

ATAXIAS OF CHILDHOOD

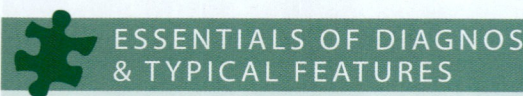

ESSENTIALS OF DIAGNOSIS & TYPICAL FEATURES

► Ataxia is defined as inability to coordinate a smooth trajectory for voluntary movements.

► It is most often due to cerebellar dysfunction but can be caused by abnormalities in almost any component of the nervous system.

► Acutely, serious causes such as ingestion, CNS infection, stroke, or intracranial mass must be excluded by history/examination or with LP and brain MRI.

► Chronically, brain MRI and genetic testing is highest yield in identifying the etiology.

► Clinical Findings

Ataxia is the inability to coordinate a smooth trajectory for voluntary movements. Ataxia localizes to the cerebellum, vestibular system, or sensory pathways. Lesions within the cerebellar vermis result in truncal and gait ataxia, while a lesion within a hemisphere will result in ipsilateral limb ataxia. Symptoms of cerebellar dysfunction also include nystagmus, dysarthria, irregularity in rapid movements, or over- or undershooting of visual targets. Swelling of the cerebellum can cause obstructive hydrocephalus or cranial neuropathies due to compression of the brainstem.

A detailed history and physical examination are important for differential diagnosis. Ataxia can be a false localizing sign for weakness, sensory abnormalities, or vestibular disturbances. Sensory ataxia is due to interruption of afferent pathways, ranging from myelopathy to radiculopathy to peripheral neuropathy. A distinction from cerebellar ataxia is worsening of symptoms when visual cues are removed. Vestibular ataxia is accompanied by nausea, vomiting, and nystagmus and typically has lateralizing symptoms. A helpful way to approach the evaluation of ataxia is based on the time course, specifically acute, subacute, recurrent, and chronic.

1. Acute & Subacute Ataxia

Acute cerebellar ataxia (ACA) and acute cerebellitis (Figure 25–7) fall along a spectrum of para-infectious etiologies of ataxia. ACA is the most common pediatric cause of acute ataxia (40% of cases) and affects children 2–4 years of age. Patients with either condition present with bilateral cerebellar signs, but the cardinal difference between ACA and acute cerebellitis is encephalopathy. If swelling is profound, acute cerebellitis can present with symptoms of increased

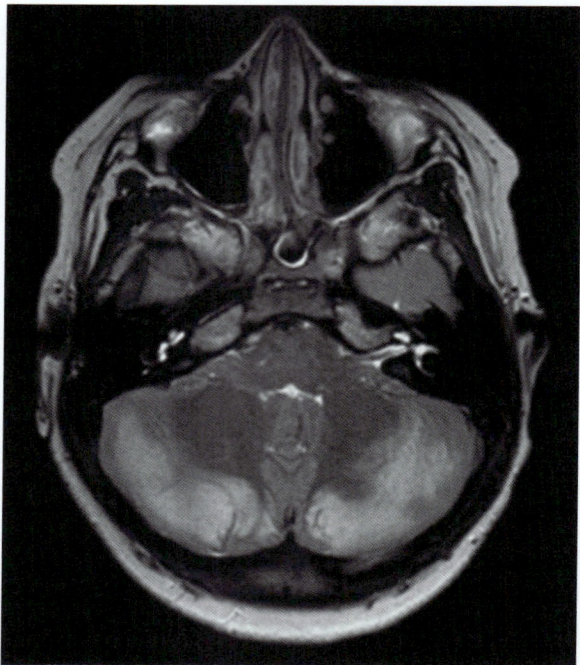

▲ **Figure 25–7.** Bilateral cerebellar edema (MRI T2 hyperintensities) causing compression of the fourth ventricle in a patient with acute cerebellitis.

ICP due to obstructive hydrocephalus. A preceding viral illness occurs in 80% of patients.

The second leading cause of acute ataxia in pediatrics is medication side effect or toxic ingestion (toxic cerebellar syndrome). Patients present with encephalopathy with bilateral cerebellar signs. ASMs are the most common prescribed medications that cause ataxia, whereas benzodiazepines, alcohol, marijuana, and dextromethorphan-containing cough syrups are common ingested medications. As many of these are not found on urine drug screens, a detailed history is required.

Sensory ataxia can present either acutely, subacutely, or even chronically. The classic example is spinal nerve root involvement due to acute inflammatory demyelinating polyneuropathy (AIDP), also called Guillain-Barre syndrome (GBS). Miller Fisher syndrome, which is a variant of GBS, is characterized by ataxia, areflexia, and ophthalmoplegia. Peripheral neuropathies, due to vitamin B_{12} or E deficiency or vitamin B_6 toxicity, can also lead to sensory ataxia. For all patients, it is important to watch for autonomic instability and bowel and bladder involvement.

Ataxia can be a presenting symptom of demyelinating disorders, though it is uncommon for ataxia to be the only symptom. Refer to later section Noninfectious Inflammatory Disorders of the Central Nervous System for more details.

Less common, but urgent, causes of acute or subacute ataxia include opsoclonus-myoclonus-ataxia syndrome (OMAS), posterior fossa tumor, and ischemic or hemorrhagic stroke. OMAS is a rare autoimmune condition that primarily affects young children. It is associated with neuroblastoma in up to 50% of patients, while others are triggered by a viral infection. Patients rarely exhibit all three symptoms. A high index of suspicion is required since treatment, which is a lengthy aggressive course of immunotherapy, is needed to prevent recurrence and cognitive decline. Posterior fossa tumors comprise up to 60% of childhood brain tumors. Most patients experience slowly progressive imbalance with signs of brainstem compression, such as ophthalmoplegia, but other children present acutely with obstructive hydrocephalus due to fourth ventricular compression. Though rare, stroke should be considered in the differential for acute ataxia. Risk factors include neck trauma, hyperextensibility, or family history of vasculopathy or coagulopathy. Patients typically have lateralizing signs, such as dysmetria, unidirectional nystagmus, significant vertigo, or sensation of being pulled to one side.

In vestibular disorders, patients can have unilateral ataxia and exquisite nausea, vertigo, and ocular motility abnormalities, such as skew deviation or nystagmus. In pediatrics, benign paroxysmal positional vertigo (BPPV) is uncommon, but labyrinthitis and vestibular neuritis are common. In functional ataxia, patients often lurch and stagger with ambulation but will have a narrow base and no other cerebellar signs.

2. Recurrent Ataxia

Migraine with brainstem aura, formerly termed complicated migraine or basilar migraine, can present with ataxia. Diagnostic criteria specify that patients must have at least one other brainstem or cerebellar sign, such as dysarthria, hypoacusis, or altered level of consciousness. In addition, hemiplegic migraine could present with false-localizing ataxia. For migraine, symptoms will progress over several minutes and will be followed by a headache with migrainous features. Benign paroxysmal vertigo of childhood is a migraine variant seen in younger children, which presents with discrete episodes of ataxia, pallor, and nausea.

Episodic ataxia (EA) is a heterogenous group of genetic conditions that present with recurrent episodes of ataxia with variable duration and frequency. Nystagmus, vertigo, tinnitus, and diplopia can also occur during ataxia episodes (ictally). Interictally, a portion of patients are free from neurologic manifestations, while others have developmental delay, learning disability, migraine, myokymia, or epilepsy. EAs are channelopathies, which are conditions caused by altered function of ion channels and membrane excitability, primarily in neurons. There are eight recognized EAs, and the most common pathogenic variants are *KCNA1* (EA1) and *CACNA1A* (EA2).

Inborn errors of metabolism should be strongly considered for both intermittent and chronic ataxia. The most common metabolic disorders known to cause ataxia include aminoacidopathies, urea cycle defects, and mitochondrial disease. Although ataxia can be a prominent symptom, it is uncommon to occur in isolation. For more details, refer to Chapter 36 on Inborn Errors of Metabolism.

3. Chronic Ataxia

Friedreich ataxia, described as the most common inherited ataxia, is an autosomal recessive condition due to a trinucleotide repeat expansion on the *FXN* gene. It typically presents in adolescents with ataxia, vibratory and proprioceptive loss, areflexia, positive Babinski, and progressive weakness that ultimately leads to loss of ambulation by young adulthood. It is a multisystem disorder with increased risk for optic atrophy, sensorineural hearing loss, hypertrophic cardiomyopathy, diabetes mellitus, and scoliosis.

Spinocerebellar ataxia is a heterogenous group of over 50 conditions with various inheritance patterns, of which autosomal dominant trinucleotide repeats are the most common. A portion are pure ataxia syndromes, whereas others are associated with optic atrophy, dystonia, myoclonus, parkinsonism, and cognitive decline.

Ataxia-telangiectasia is an autosomal recessive condition arising from a disruption in DNA repair, most commonly due to pathogenic variants in the *ATM* gene. Symptoms typically begin between 1 and 4 years of age and manifest with progressive ataxia, oculomotor apraxia, and conjunctival telangiectasias. Choreoathetosis and sensorimotor neuropathy are almost always present. Patients can have recurrent infections due to immunodeficiency and are at increased risk for malignancy with leukemia and lymphoma being the most common.

The list of genetic causes of progressive ataxia continues to expand. It is especially important to recognize other treatable causes of ataxia, such as ataxia with vitamin E deficiency, cerebrotendinous xanthomatosis, Refsum disease, glucose transporter type 1 deficiency, abetalipoproteinemia, and gluten ataxia.

▶ Diagnostic Evaluation

Red flags in the history or physical examination, including trauma, abrupt onset of symptoms, progressive or prolonged time course, positional headache, encephalopathy, seizures, or focal neurologic deficits, should prompt timely and targeted testing. In one study, for children older than 3 years who presented with more than 3 days of symptoms, brain imaging demonstrated urgent intracranial pathology in 10%–20%. Younger children and children with no more than 3 days of symptoms warrant close observation but may not need urgent brain imaging. LP should be performed if an inflammatory, demyelinating, or infectious etiology is being considered.

If a patient presents with chronic ataxia, treatable conditions must be investigated. If the patient has recurrent ataxia, workup is of highest yield while symptomatic. Basic labs to consider include complete blood count with peripheral smear, complete metabolic panel, and thyroid panel. Alpha-fetoprotein will screen for ataxia-telangiectasia. Testing for metabolic disease includes serum organic acids, urine organic acids, lactate, pyruvate, ammonia, very-long-chain fatty acids, acylcarnitine profile, lipid panel, phytanic acid, and biotinidase. Vitamin E, copper, and vitamin 12 are nutritional labs to consider. Genetic testing is typically done simultaneously with biochemical workup. LP for hypoglycorrhachia should be pursued if there is suspicion for glucose transporter type 1 deficiency. Brain MRI can investigate for cerebellar atrophy or signs of metabolic disease.

▶ Treatment

Treatment for ataxia is specific to the etiology. In acute ataxia, immunomodulatory therapy is frequently used. While treatment of ACA is typically supportive, high-dose methylprednisolone is commonly used in acute cerebellitis. Most patients fully recover from either condition. GBS is typically treated with IVIg, and patients typically make a full recovery within 6–12 months.

Treatment of EA is guided by the gene involved. Patients potentially respond to acetazolamide or a sodium channel blocker, such as carbamazepine. For patients with chronic progressive ataxia, the main treatment is supportive care, including school supports, therapies, and equipment, to facilitate cognitive development and independent function. Medications for epilepsy and tone are used when indicated.

Caffarelli M, Kimia AA, Torres AR: Acute ataxia in children: a review of the differential diagnosis and evaluation in the emergency department. Pediatr Neurol 2016 Dec;65:14–30 [PMID: 27789117].
Luetje M et al: Utility of neuroimaging in children presenting to a pediatric emergency department with ataxia. Pediatr Emerg Care 2019 May;35(5):335–340 [PMID: 30932991].

HYPERKINETIC MOVEMENT DISORDERS

1. Stereotypies

Stereotypies are repetitive movements that are fixed in morphology over time. Age of onset is 6 months to 3 years of age. Movements are provoked by excitement, frustration, concentration, or boredom. They can be interrupted by a caregiver, and awareness is maintained. Common stereotypies are head shaking and hand flapping, but the movements can be more complex and include vocalizations. Most patients are typically developing, but there is an increased prevalence in children with autism spectrum disorder and intellectual disability. Stereotypies are associated with an increased risk

for ADHD and anxiety. An EEG can be considered to rule out seizure, but since they are interruptible and provoked by emotion, additional workup is typically not required.

2. Tics

▶ Clinical Findings

Tics are nonrhythmic, involuntary movements that are stereotyped but evolve over time. They affect up to 20% of school-aged children, have a typical onset of 6–8 years, and are 4 times more common in male than female sex. The most common motor tic is eye blinking. Vocal tics range from throat clearing to sounds or words. Provisional tic disorder is motor or vocal tics lasting less than 1 year in duration, while persistent tic disorder is motor or vocal tics greater than 1 year in duration. Tourette syndrome is characterized by both motor and vocal tics lasting more than 1 year. For each of these diagnoses, onset must be prior to 18 years of age.

A premonitory urge or tension and brief suppressibility are classic features of tics but are not described by all children. Tics wax and wane in frequency and typically are exacerbated by stress. Up to 90% of patients have comorbidities. ADHD and OCD are the most common while anxiety, depression, and sleep and learning difficulties are also seen.

▶ Differential Diagnosis

The diagnosis of tics is clinical. Tics can easily be distinguished from seizures by presence of urge, suppressibility, and exacerbation in stressful situations. Pediatric autoimmune neuropsychiatric disorders associated with streptococcal infections (PANDAS) is a controversial diagnosis that can be considered in a prepubertal patient with recent streptococcal infection who has an abrupt, dramatic onset of tics, obsessions, or compulsions with other psychiatric symptoms, such as separation anxiety, emotional lability, or inattention. Stuttering is a common childhood speech disorder that is characterized by difficulty with the flow of speech rather than intrusive semi-voluntary sounds. Workup, including labs, imaging, and EEG, for tics is not typically required.

▶ Treatment & Prognosis

The cornerstone of treatment is education for the patient, family, and school about the nature of tic disorders. Although tics may be the presenting symptom, treatment of underlying anxiety, inattention, or sleep difficulties may have the most significant impact on tic frequency. Comprehensive Behavioral Intervention for Tics (CBIT) is a useful tool to help patients manage their tics. Most pediatric patients will have significant improvement or resolution of tics with time.

Pharmacologic treatment of tics is indicated if the tics are physically painful, disrupt relationships, or prevent the patient from focusing in school. First-line is clonidine or guanfacine, which can also be helpful in treatment of ADHD. Common side effects are drowsiness and lightheadedness. Topiramate is second-line but can be used first line in patients who have an elevated body mass index (BMI) or comorbid headaches or epilepsy. The only FDA-approved medications are haloperidol, pimozide, and aripiprazole, but given their side-effect profile, antipsychotics are reserved for patients with refractory tics.

3. Tremor

Tremor is an involuntary oscillatory movement across a joint axis. It is divided into rest and action. A rest tremor is present when all muscles are fully relaxed and is a classic feature of parkinsonism. An action tremor, which is the most common type of tremor, is present when a muscle is activated and can worsen when maintaining a posture or when approaching a target, as seen in intention tremor. The history and physical examination are integral in identifying red flags for tremor, including myoclonus, dystonia, seizures, cerebellar signs, or decline in cognitive function.

In pediatrics, the most common causes are enhanced physiologic tremor and essential tremor. Medications, such as bronchodilators, antidepressants, stimulants, antipsychotics, and ASMs, can exacerbate physiologic tremor. Essential tremor is a slowly progressive action tremor that is typically inherited in an autosomal dominant pattern. If red flags are not present in the history and neurologic examination is otherwise normal, laboratory studies and imaging are not required. If the history suggests, labs for hyperthyroidism or electrolyte derangements can be obtained.

Treatment for tremor can be either as needed or daily. Clonazepam is an excellent as needed medication. Propranolol and primidone are first-line for maintenance medications. Occupational therapy can also teach the patient strategies to reduce tremor.

4. Chorea, Athetosis, & Ballismus

▶ Clinical Findings

Chorea is a constant dance-like flow composed of fragments of semi-purposeful movements. Athetosis is a small, writhing movement, often involving distal extremities, whereas ballismus is a large amplitude jerk that typically occurs proximally. Athetosis and ballismus can co-occur with chorea. These involuntary movements interrupt purposeful movements. A cardinal examination finding of chorea is motor impersistence, the inability to sustain an isometric contraction, including milkmaid's sign (inability to sustain a grip on the examiner's fingers) or tongue darting (inability to maintain tongue protrusion). Chorea can persist during sleep and will worsen with purposeful movement.

▶ Differential Diagnosis

The age of onset, associated symptoms, and medical history are helpful in identifying the etiology. A brain MRI is obtained in any child who presents with chorea. The remainder of the workup, such as basic labs, autoimmune, or genetic, is guided by the clinical history.

Physiologic chorea is seen in typically developing infants as they are learning new motor milestones. Mild chorea as motor overflow can be seen in children with ADHD. Benign hereditary chorea is an autosomal dominant condition due to pathogenic variant in *NKX2.1* that is associated with gross motor delay, hypothyroidism, and pulmonary problems, such as idiopathic pulmonary fibrosis and asthma.

Acquired chorea can be seen in children with autoimmune disease or a prior injury. Sydenham chorea is the most common acquired form in children and is diagnostic for acute rheumatic fever. Other clinical features include emotional lability, hypotonia, and sleep disturbances. The symptoms develop several weeks following a streptococcal infection. Antistreptolysin O and anti-DNase titers can be helpful to identify a prior infection.

Chorea can also be a manifestation of antiphospholipid syndrome, systemic lupus erythematous, autoimmune encephalitis, or a prior brain injury. Subacute intermittent chorea can be a sign of moyamoya disease. Following hypoperfusion, chorea can wax and wane but should fully resolve with time. Postpump chorea can be seen in children following a cardiac procedure requiring time on bypass. Dyskinetic CP is described in the previous section.

Last, chorea can be a sign of a chronic condition. It is a presenting symptom in adult Huntington disease but is less common in juvenile Huntington disease, in which the initial features tend to be seizures and rigidity. Cognitive decline is seen in both at onset. Chorea can also be seen in Wilson disease, which can present in adolescents with psychiatric symptoms and new onset movement disorder.

▶ Treatment

Treatment of chorea relies on the underlying etiology. For Sydenham chorea, prophylactic antibiotics are required until age 40, and patients are followed by a cardiologist to monitor for valvular disease. Immunotherapy with either steroids or IVIg is rarely indicated. Chorea can be treated symptomatically with clonazepam, levetiracetam, or sodium valproate if symptoms are interfering with function. If due to Sydenham, postpump, or moyamoya, chorea typically resolves with time.

5. Myoclonus

▶ Clinical Findings

Myoclonus is a sudden jerk of one or more muscles caused by either a contraction or relaxation of the associated muscle. It is present at rest or with action but can also be reflex- or stimulus-induced. Myoclonus can be described based on location—axial, focal, multifocal, or generalized. Myoclonus localizes to the cortex, thalamus, brainstem, spinal cord, or peripheral nerve, with cortical and subcortical structures being more common. Myoclonus can occur in isolation or with other movement disorders, epilepsy, or learning difficulties.

▶ Differential Diagnosis

The differential for myoclonus is broad. Diagnostic considerations can be categorized based on phenotype—isolated myoclonus, myoclonus plus other neurologic signs, and myoclonus plus other systemic signs. Physiologic myoclonus is the most common and is seen with sleep, anxiety, or exercise. Essential myoclonus is on the spectrum of essential tremor, and these patients do not have a risk for epilepsy or cognitive involvement. Myoclonus-dystonia syndrome is a genetic condition with an autosomal dominant inheritance; 20% of patients have co-occurring dystonia. Genetic etiologies of myoclonus include *KCNC1*, *SAMD12*, and *SCARB2* in which patients have prominent myoclonus and are at risk for progressive cerebellar signs and learning difficulties.

Myoclonus can be difficult to clinically distinguish from myoclonic seizures and commonly co-occurs with epilepsy. EEG may be necessary. The classic presentation of juvenile myoclonic epilepsy, which is the most common myoclonic epilepsy, is a teenager who presents with early morning jerks of upper extremities. Doose and Dravet syndromes are epileptic encephalopathies that can have prominent myoclonic seizures. There are a variety of progressive myoclonic epilepsies, which are defined by prominent myoclonus, epilepsy, and cognitive impairment including regression.

Myoclonus can also be symptomatic of an acute neurologic or more global process. Autoimmune etiologies are associated with myoclonus, including acute inflammation seen in anti–*N*-methyl-D-aspartate receptor (NMDAR) encephalitis or a chronic symptom of demyelinating lesion in the brainstem. Myoclonus can be seen following a hypoxic injury to the cortex or subcortical structures. Medication side effect or toxidrome should also be considered.

▶ Treatment

As with any movement disorder, the treatment of myoclonus is based on whether the movements interfere with activity. The most common classes of medications are potentiators of GABA and ASMs. Clonazepam is best with spinal or peripheral etiologies, and levetiracetam and valproic acid are best for cortical or subcortical myoclonus. Botulinum toxin can also be considered if occurring in limited muscles.

6. Dystonia

▶ Clinical Findings

Dystonia is an involuntary sustained muscle contraction resulting in twisting or odd posture. Pain is a common symptom. Dystonia is described by the pattern of involvement, including focal, segmental, multifocal, hemi-dystonia, and generalized. An important examination clue is triggering or worsening of dystonia with attempted movement or the presence of a sensory trick, an amelioration of posture by placing a hand on the involved body part.

▶ Differential Diagnosis

Dystonia has both genetic and acquired causes. The list of genetic etiologies continues to expand although a cause is not identified in many cases. Dopa-responsive dystonia (DRD) is a genetic condition most commonly caused by pathogenic variant in *GCH1*. DRD typically presents in toddler or preschool years with diurnal worsening of dystonia in the distal lower extremities, and it is commonly misdiagnosed as CP. Paroxysmal kinesigenic or nonkinesigenic dyskinesias, of which dystonia is the most common phenotype, are stereotyped movements or postures that are provoked by exercise, stress, or caffeine. Frequency and duration can vary. Glucose transporter type 1 deficiency can manifest as exertion-induced dystonia.

CNS malformations or injury, especially of the basal ganglia or spinal cord, are a common cause of dystonia. Abnormalities of neurotransmitters, such as dopamine transporter deficiency, and metabolic conditions, such as glutaric acidemia, brain iron accumulation disorders, or mitochondrial conditions, should be considered in children with dystonia plus global developmental delay, hypotonia, and other movement disorders.

Brain MRI is a required part of the workup, but depending on pattern of dystonia, spine MRI should also be considered. The remainder of the workup, including serum or urine biochemical testing, LP for basic studies and neurotransmitters, and genetic testing, is guided by the history and physical examination.

▶ Treatment

If a treatable cause of dystonia is identified, it is important to initiate treatment early. Carbidopa-levodopa is first-line if DRD is suspected. In this condition, symptoms are exquisitely sensitive to low doses. Patients with other etiologies can have a partial response at higher doses. Other medications to consider are clonazepam, baclofen, levetiracetam, and trihexyphenidyl. Botox is helpful for focal dystonia. DBS and intrathecal baclofen are considered in refractory cases.

HYPOKINETIC MOVEMENT DISORDERS

Parkinsonism is defined as at least two of bradykinesia, rest tremor, and rigidity. In a typically developing child, the most common etiology is medication-induced, including first- or second-generation antipsychotics or dopamine receptor antagonists used for treatment of nausea. Juvenile Parkinson disease is a very rare condition that presents in school-aged children to young adults. Parkinsonism can be a symptom of other acquired or genetic etiologies and typically occurs in conjunction with other movements disorders such as myoclonus or dystonia. Treatment is removal of offending agent, if present. Otherwise, levodopa-carbidopa or amantadine are used.

Gewitz M: Revision of the Jones criteria for the diagnosis of acute rheumatic fever in the era of Doppler echocardiography: a scientific statement from the American Heart Association. Circulation 2015;131(20):1806–1818 [PMID: 25908771].

Pringsheim T et al: Practice guideline recommendations summary: treatment of tics in people with Tourette syndrome and chronic tic disorders. Neurology 2019 May 7;92(19):896–906 [PMID: 31061208].

Singer HS, Mink JW, Gilbert DL, Jankovic J. *Movement disorders in childhood*. 2nd ed. Elsevier Academic Press; 2016.

Zutt R et al: A novel diagnostic approach to patients with myoclonus. Nat Rev Neurol 2015 Dec;11(12):687–697 [PMID: 26553594].

INFECTIONS & INFLAMMATORY DISORDERS OF THE CENTRAL NERVOUS SYSTEM

Infections and inflammation of the CNS are among the most treatable neurologic conditions, but they also carry a high potential for catastrophic destruction of the nervous system. These conditions can involve the meninges (meningitis), brain parenchyma (encephalitis or cerebritis), spinal cord (myelitis), or nerve roots (radiculitis/radiculopathy). The cranial nerves or peripheral nerves can also be affected (neuritis/neuropathy), as well as the muscles (myositis).

CNS INFECTIONS

Clinical Findings

Chapters 40, 42, and 43 discuss specific viral, bacterial, and parasitic/mycotic pathogens in detail. Regardless of the causative microorganism, patients with CNS infections present with similar manifestations. These include systemic signs of infection, such as fever, malaise, chills, and organ dysfunction, and specific features suggesting CNS infection, including headache, stiff neck, fever or hypothermia, changes in mental status (ranging from hyperirritability to lethargy and coma), seizures, cranial nerve palsies, and focal sensory and motor deficits. Meningeal irritation is indicated by the presence of Kernig and Brudzinski signs. In very young infants, signs of meningeal irritation may be absent, and temperature instability and hypothermia are more common than fever. Infants may demonstrate a bulging fontanelle and an increased head circumference. Papilledema may eventually develop, particularly in older children and adolescents. Patients should be screened for factors that predispose them to CNS infection. Infections involving the sinuses or other structures in the head and neck region can result in direct extension of infection into the intracranial compartment. Open head injuries, neurosurgical procedures or hardware, immunodeficiency, or incomplete vaccination status may also increase the risk of intracranial infection.

Diagnostic Evaluation

Urgent LP is imperative when CNS infection is suspected. However, if the patient has focal neurologic deficits, papilledema, or signs of increased ICP, imaging should be obtained prior to LP. CSF should be examined for the presence of red and white blood cells, protein concentration, glucose concentration, bacteria, and other microorganisms; a sample should be cultured. Typical CSF findings in a variety of infectious and inflammatory disorders are shown in Table 25–2. In addition, serologic, immunologic, and nucleic acid detection (polymerase chain reaction [PCR]) tests may be performed on the spinal fluid. Many labs have multiplex PCR panels that allow for rapid testing of several pathogens, including HSV. In most instances, opening pressure should also be assessed, as many patients with CNS infection may have subclinical increased ICP. The patient's blood glucose should be checked at approximately the same time as the LP. Other serum studies, including a complete blood count, chemistry panel, and blood cultures, should be also obtained.

Neuroimaging with CT and MRI with and without contrast may be helpful in demonstrating the presence of brain abscess, meningeal inflammation, or secondary problems such as venous and arterial infarctions, hemorrhages, and subdural effusions. In addition, these procedures may identify sinus or other focal infections in the head or neck region that are related to the CNS infection.

Although often nonspecific, EEGs may be helpful for patients who had seizures at the time of presentation. In some instances, such as HSV, periodic lateralized epileptiform discharges (PLEDs) may be one of the earliest abnormalities to suggest the diagnosis. EEG may also show focal slowing over regions of infarcts or abscesses.

1. Bacterial Meningitis

Bacterial infections of the CNS may present acutely (symptoms evolving rapidly over 1–24 hours), subacutely (symptoms evolving over 1–7 days), or chronically (symptoms evolving over > 1 week). Although the term *meningitis* (inflammation of the meninges) is used to describe these infections, the brain parenchyma is often also inflamed (*encephalitis*), and blood vessel walls may be infiltrated by inflammatory cells (*vasculitis*), resulting in endothelial cell injury, vessel stenosis, and secondary ischemia and infarction.

Treatment

Broad-spectrum antibiotic coverage should be started immediately, even if LP will be delayed. Antimicrobial choice should match the likely pathogens encountered at a given age, as well as specific patient factors such as the presence of a VP shunt. See Chapter 39 for details of selecting antimicrobial coverage.

▶ Complications

Abnormalities of water and electrolyte balance result from either excessive or insufficient production of antidiuretic hormone and require careful monitoring and appropriate adjustments in fluid administration. Monitoring serum sodium closely during the first 1–2 days, and urine sodium if the inappropriate secretion of antidiuretic hormone is suspected, will usually reveal significant problems.

Seizures occur in 20%–30% of children with bacterial meningitis, typically early in the course. Persistent focal seizures or seizures associated with focal neurologic deficits strongly suggest a localized encephalitis, subdural effusion, abscess, or vascular lesion such as arterial infarct or cerebral venous sinus thrombosis.

Subdural effusions occur in up to one-third of young children with *Streptococcus pneumoniae* meningitis. These do not require treatment unless they are producing increased ICP or progressive mass effect. In most cases, the effusions are eventually sterilized with antibiotics; however, in some cases, aspiration of the fluid for documentation of sterilization or for relief of pressure should be considered.

Cerebral edema results in increased ICP, requiring treatment with dexamethasone, osmotic agents, diuretics, or hyperventilation; ICP monitoring may be needed.

Long-term sequelae of meningitis result from direct inflammatory destruction of brain cells, vascular injuries, or secondary gliosis. Focal motor and sensory deficits, visual impairment, hearing loss, seizures, hydrocephalus, and cranial nerve deficits can result. Sensorineural hearing loss can occur after viral or bacterial meningitis and may not be noted until months-years later. Early addition of dexamethasone to the antibiotic regimen may modestly decrease the risk of hearing loss in some children with *bacterial* meningitis. In addition, some patients with meningitis develop mild to severe cognitive impairment or behavioral issues.

2. Brain Abscess

Patients with brain abscess often appear to have systemic illness, similar to patients with bacterial meningitis, but they may also demonstrate focal neurologic deficits, papilledema, and other evidence of increased ICP or a mass lesion. Symptoms may be present for a week or more. Conditions predisposing to development of brain abscess include penetrating head trauma, chronic infection of the middle ear, mastoid, or sinuses (especially the frontal sinus), chronic dental or pulmonary infection, cardiovascular lesions allowing right-to-left shunting of blood (including AVMs), and endocarditis.

CT or MRI with contrast should be done prior to LP since significant midline shift or increased ICP from the abscess could result in herniation from the LP. Cultures from the CSF or the brain abscesses are often negative, but Gram stain may be informative. Antibiotics should be tailored to the patient's age and suspected source (see Chapter 39). With spread from

contiguous septic foci, streptococci, and anaerobic bacteria are most common. Staphylococci most often enter from trauma or spread from distant infections. Enteric organisms may form an abscess from chronic otitis. In their early stages, brain abscesses are areas of focal cerebritis and can be treated with antibiotic therapies alone. Encapsulated abscesses require surgical drainage.

Untreated cerebral abscesses lead to irreversible tissue destruction and may rupture into the ventricle, producing catastrophic deterioration in neurologic function. Because brain abscesses are often associated with systemic illness, the mortality rate is frequently high. Other poor prognostic indicators include rapid progression of disease and alteration of consciousness at the time of presentation. However, many patients can make a full recovery, even with multiple abscesses.

3. Viral Infections

Some viruses exhibit neurotropism, an affinity for specific CNS cell populations or regions. For example, **poliovirus and other enteroviruses (A71 and D68)** can selectively infect anterior horn cells and some intracranial lower motor neurons. **West Nile virus** is a mosquito-borne flavivirus that can afflict numerous nervous system regions, causing encephalopathy, paralysis, and even death from myelomeningoencephalitis and polyradiculitis.

Severe acute respiratory syndrome coronavirus 2 (SARS CoV-2), the cause of COVID-19, has been reported to cause various neurologic symptoms in pediatric patients. Common symptoms include anosmia, dysgeusia, and headache. Ischemic stroke, intracranial hemorrhage, acute symptomatic seizures, meningitis/encephalitis, inflammatory CNS lesions similar to acute demyelinating encephalomyelitis (ADEM), GBS, and cranial nerve palsies occur rarely. **Human immunodeficiency virus (HIV) infection** (see Chapters 33, 39, and 41) can cause a variety of neurologic syndromes, including subacute encephalitis, meningitis, myelopathy, polyneuropathy, and myositis. In addition, opportunistic CNS infections can occur in patients with HIV-induced immunosuppression. *Pneumocystis*, *Toxoplasma*, and CMV infections are particularly common. Patients with HIV can develop progressive multifocal leukoencephalopathy, caused by the John Cunningham (JC) virus, herpes simplex infections, and varicella-zoster infections. Neurologic abnormalities can also be the result of noninfectious neoplastic disorders, such as primary CNS lymphoma and metastatic lymphoma to the nervous system.

Although most viral infections of the nervous system have an acute or subacute course in childhood, chronic infections can occur. For example, **subacute sclerosing panencephalitis (SSEP)** is a chronic indolent infection caused by altered measles virus and is clinically characterized by progressive neurodegeneration and seizures that begin 7–10 years after infection. Risk is highest among patients infected with measles prior to the age of 2 years.

Treatment of most CNS viral infections is typically limited to symptomatic and supportive measures, except for HSV, and some cases of varicella-zoster virus infection, in which acyclovir is used (see section HSV of Chapter 40).

4. Other CNS Infections

A wide variety of other microorganisms, including *Toxoplasma*, mycobacteria, spirochetes, rickettsiae, amoebae, and mycoplasma, can cause CNS infections. CNS involvement in these infections is usually secondary to systemic infection or other predisposing factors. Appropriate cultures and serologic testing are required to diagnose these infections. Antimicrobial treatment for these infections is discussed in Chapter 39.

Boronat S: Neurologic care of COVID-19 in children. Front Neurol 2021;11:613831 [PMID: 33679571].

Zainel A, Mitchell H, Sadarangani M: Bacterial meningitis in children: neurological complications, associated risk factors, and prevention. Microorganisms 2021;9(3):535 [PMID: 33807653].

NONINFECTIOUS INFLAMMATORY DISORDERS OF THE CENTRAL NERVOUS SYSTEM

The full clinical and pathophysiologic spectrum of pediatric demyelinating disorders is ever-expanding. The salient features of ADEM, transverse myelitis, neuromyelitis optica (NMO), and MS are outlined in Table 25–17. Sarcoidosis, Behçet disease, and systemic lupus erythematosus are examples of atypical demyelinating disorders of the CNS. Autoimmune encephalopathy and, less commonly, paraneoplastic encephalopathy can cause severe neuropsychologic symptoms, seizures, and respiratory failure.

1. Acute Demyelinating Encephalomyelitis

Patients with acute demyelinating encephalomyelitis (ADEM) typically present with encephalopathy (confusion, irritability, lethargy) and multifocal neurologic deficits, such as weakness or ataxia, which have progressed over a few days. ADEM most commonly affects children 3–7 years of age. Fever can be present at the time of diagnosis, and many patients report an antecedent illness 1–3 weeks prior. MRI demonstrates diffuse, "fluffy" (indistinct margins) demyelinating lesions within the cerebral white matter, sometimes associated with deep grey matter lesions, which are T2 hyperintense. ADEM lesions can mimic those of MS but are typically larger and ill-defined and usually resolve within months of presentation. Serum studies should include anti-aquaporin 4 antibodies, to exclude NMO and anti-myelin oligodendrocyte (anti-MOG) antibodies, which are strongly associated with ADEM and indicate a higher risk of recurrence. CSF findings may be normal or mildly abnormal, with mild pleocytosis and elevated protein in 25%–50% of

Table 25–17. Prominent features of CNS inflammatory demyelination syndromes.

ADEM	Encephalopathy and fever; may also have headache, meningismus, or seizures. Half are serum MOG-IgG+. CSF typically negative for oligoclonal bands. Rarely, may recur within 3 mo (but consider other causes).
CIS	Solitary or multifocal MRI lesions without encephalopathy, not meeting criteria for multiple sclerosis. Examples include isolated optic neuritis or transverse myelitis.
MOGAD	Heterogenous presentations, including ADEM, optic neuritis, transverse myelitis, cranial neuropathies, and encephalitis. Can be monophasic or relapsing. Serum MOG-IgG+.
MS	Neurologic deficits without encephalopathy, can be difficult to localize. Requires clinical, laboratory, or radiographic evidence of dissemination in time and space. Consider excluding NMOSD and MOGAD, especially in children younger than 11 years. CSF often has positive oligoclonal bands. High risk of relapsing disease.
NMOSD	Longitudinally extensive transverse myelitis and/or optic neuritis, may also present with area postrema syndrome (intractable nausea), symptomatic narcolepsy, and other brainstem/cerebellar/cerebral symptoms. May be aquaporin-4-IgG+ in serum or be antibody negative. High risk of relapsing disease.

ADEM, acute disseminated encephalomyelitis; CIS, clinically isolated syndrome; MOG, myelin oligodendrocyte glycoprotein; MOGAD, MOG antibody-associated disease; MS, multiple sclerosis; NMOSD, neuromyelitis optica spectrum disorder.

cases. Oligoclonal bands can be seen in up to 20% of ADEM cases. High-dose intravenous methylprednisolone is the primary treatment for ADEM. IVIG or plasmapheresis may be necessary for refractory patients. Recurrence should raise suspicion for other causes. Most children make an excellent recovery, but some later develop MS.

2. Multiple Sclerosis (MS)

▶ Clinical Findings & Diagnostic Evaluation

Up to 10% of patients with MS are diagnosed before the age of 16 years. Risk factors may include exposure to Epstein-Barr virus, specific HLA subtypes, and obesity. Patients typically present with new-onset focal neurologic deficits, such as weakness, sensory changes, or loss of vision. Many patients have various, difficult to localize symptoms at presentation, which can be mistaken for a functional neurologic disorder. Fever, encephalopathy, involvement of the peripheral nervous system or other organ systems, elevated erythrocyte sedimentation rate, or marked CSF pleocytosis are atypical for pediatric MS. Brain MRI with and without contrast typically demonstrates multiple T2/FLAIR hyperintense lesions (areas of active demyelination), which may appear to fan out from the lateral ventricles on sagittal views (Dawson's fingers). Inactive lesions, if present, can appear T1 hypointense ("black holes").

The 2017 McDonald criteria for the diagnosis of MS require evidence of multiple, distinct episodes of demyelination, referred to as "dissemination in space and time," but these should be used cautiously for younger patients. For children at least 12 years old with an initial, non-ADEM clinical episode, MRI findings alone may meet dissemination in time and space. Dissemination in time may also be established by positive oligoclonal bands in the CSF. If these criteria are not met, the child is diagnosed with **clinically isolated syndrome (CIS)**, for example, optic neuritis or transverse myelitis. Approximately one-third of children with CIS will convert to MS.

▶ Treatment & Prognosis

Pediatric patients may experience more frequent relapses than adults. Treatment of acute relapses includes high-dose intravenous methylprednisolone and occasionally plasmapheresis. Pediatric patients tend to recover from relapses better than adults; however, due to the prolonged disease duration, the long-term risks of physical and cognitive disabilities are higher. Thus, early initiation of immunotherapy with disease-modifying treatments (DMTs) is critical. Fingolimod is the only FDA-approved DMT for children with MS; however, numerous injectable, oral, and infusion DMTs can be used off-label, and several pediatric clinical trials are underway.

3. Other CNS Demyelinating Disorders

NMO is most classically associated with longitudinally extensive transverse myelitis and optic neuritis, which may be bilateral. However, NMO can also cause intractable hiccups, nausea, and vomiting (area postrema syndrome), brainstem/cerebellar syndrome, seizures, and even narcolepsy. NMO is associated with aquaporin-4 antibodies in serum and/or CSF. Initial treatment includes initial high-dose steroids and plasmapheresis, followed by ongoing immunotherapy to prevent recurrences. **Myelin oligodendrocyte glycoprotein antibody-associated disease (MOGAD)** overlaps significantly with ADEM, NMO, optic neuritis, transverse myelitis, and encephalitis; thus, screening for serum anti-MOG antibodies in serum is important for any patient with demyelinating or unexplained inflammatory CNS disease. Atypical demyelinating diseases include systemic lupus erythematosus, Behcet syndrome, and Sjögren syndrome; these typically have characteristic systemic manifestations that facilitate diagnosis. Additional testing and screening for other organ involvement is important.

4. Autoimmune Encephalopathy/Encephalitis

Autoimmune encephalopathies are clinically heterogeneous, immune-mediated disorders with central and/or peripheral neurologic effects. These disorders are thought to result from misdirected immune response to shared epitopes between neuronal antigens and foreign or tumor antigens, with idiopathic, postinfectious (eg, post-HSV encephalitis), and neoplastic etiologies. NMDAR encephalitis is the most common cause of pediatric autoimmune encephalopathy. Ovarian or testicular teratomas must be excluded, though neoplasm is much rarer in pediatric patients than in adults. Behavioral changes, autonomic instability, insomnia, aphasia, seizures, and movement disorders are prominent. Various diagnostic criteria have been developed to assist in earlier diagnosis and treatment initiation. Immunotherapy, including high-dose steroids, IVIG, and/or plasmapheresis are beneficial. Second-line therapies include rituximab and/or cyclophosphamide.

Fadda G et al: Paediatric multiple sclerosis and antibody-associated demyelination: clinical, imaging, and biological considerations for diagnosis and care. Lancet Neurol 2021;20:136–49 [PMID: 33484648].

Pointon T et al: Evaluation of multiple consensus criteria for autoimmune encephalitis and temporal analysis of symptoms in a pediatric encephalitis cohort. Front Neurol 2022;13:952317 [PMID: 36237630].

Wang CX: Assessment and management of acute disseminated encephalomyelitis (ADEM) in the pediatric patient. Paediatr Drugs 2021;23(3):213–221 [PMID: 33830467].

▼ NEUROMUSCULAR SYNDROMES

SYNDROMES PRESENTING WITH ACUTE FLACCID PARALYSIS

▶ Pathogenesis

Flaccid paralysis can occur because of a lesion anywhere along the neuraxis. Neurotransmission is impaired in botulism and in tick paralysis. In neuropathies (nerve diseases) such as Guillan-Barre syndrome (GBS, also known as acute inflammatory demyelinating polyneuropathy [AIDP]), the axons undergo demyelination, inflammation, or even degeneration. Polio virus directly invades the lower motor neuron cell bodies in the spinal cord, while other viruses, such as enterovirus, cause spinal cord inflammation or dysfunction (myelitis/myelopathy). Autoimmune or postinfectious spinal cord demyelination causes transverse myelitis; spinal cord mass lesions or stroke can also cause sudden weakness. Acute myopathy (muscle disease—see next section) can be a rare cause of flaccid weakness. The most common causes of acute flaccid paralysis in children are described in Table 25–18.

Table 25–18. Acute flaccid paralysis in children.

	Acute Flaccid Myelitis	Guillain-Barré Syndrome (AIDP)	Botulism	Tick-Bite Paralysis	Transverse Myelitis
Etiology	Poliovirus types I, II, and III; vaccine strain poliovirus (rare); other enteroviruses, eg, EV-71; EV-68; West Nile virus.	Likely delayed hypersensitivity, with T-cell–mediated antiganglioside antibodies. Mycoplasma and viral infections (EBV, CMV), *Campylobacter jejuni*; hepatitis B; surgery, pregnancy can be precipitants.	*Clostridium botulinum* toxin causes block at neuromuscular junction. Under age 1, toxin from ingested spores or honey. At older ages toxin ingested in food. Rarely from wound infection.	Neurotoxin in tick saliva disrupts nerve function. Toxin typically produced 5-7 days after tick attachment.	Idiopathic transverse myelitis often postinfectious. May occur as part of multiple sclerosis, neuromyelitis optica spectrum disorder and anti-MOG antibody syndrome.
History	None, or inadequate polio immunization. May have preceding upper respiratory or GI symptoms. Often in summer and early fall epidemics.	Nonspecific respiratory or GI symptoms in preceding 1-3 weeks common. Any season, though slightly lower incidence in summer.	Infants: dusty environment (eg, construction area), honey. Older: food poisoning, with symptoms hours to days after ingesting contaminated food.	Exposure to ticks (dog tick in eastern United States; wood ticks). Irritability 12–24 h before onset of a rapidly progressive ascending paralysis.	May report nonspecific illness 1–2 wk prior to symptom onset.
Presenting complaints	May be febrile at time of paralysis. Meningeal signs, muscle tenderness, and spasms. Asymmetric weakness widespread or segmental (cervical, thoracic, lumbar). Bulbar symptoms may precede extremity weakness.	Symmetric weakness of legs, with rapid ascension to arms, trunk, and face. Paresthesias or pain may be significant. Fever uncommon. Can have facial weakness, diplopia, dysarthria, dysphagia.	Infancy: constipation, poor suck and weak cry due to bulbar weakness. Progressively "floppy." Respiratory weakness or failure. Older: blurred vision, diplopia, ptosis, choking, and weakness.	Rapid onset and progression of ascending flaccid paralysis; often accompanied by pain and paresthesias. Paralysis of upper extremities 2nd day after onset. Ataxia is common.	Back pain in about 30%–50%. Sensory loss below level of lesion accompanying rapidly developing paralysis. Sphincter difficulties common. Fever in 58%.
Findings	Flaccid weakness, usually asymmetric with decreased reflexes in affected limbs. Cranial nerve dysfunction; Encephalopathy possible, but not common;	Flaccid, usually symmetric weakness of the extremities, with variable respiratory and bulbar weakness. Reflexes lost early in course. Miller-Fisher variant: ophthalmoplegia, ataxia. Bulbar involvement may occur.	Both infants and older children usually appear alert, but with flaccid weakness, decreased/absent reflexes, ophthalmoparesis, ptosis, and weak/absent gag. Respiratory failure can occur early. Pupils typically dilated and nonreactive to light.	Flaccid, symmetric paralysis. Cranial nerve and bulbar (respiratory) paralysis, ataxia, sphincter dysfunction, and sensory deficits may occur. Occasional fever. Diagnosis rests on finding tick, which is especially likely to be on occipital scalp.	Paraplegia with areflexia below level of lesion early; later, may have hyperreflexia and spasticity. Sensory loss below and hyperesthesia or normal sensation above level of lesion. Paralysis of bladder and rectum.

(Continued)

Table 25–18. Acute flaccid paralysis in children. (*Continued*)

	Acute Flaccid Myelitis	Guillain-Barré Syndrome (AIDP)	Botulism	Tick-Bite Paralysis	Transverse Myelitis
CSF	Pleocytosis (20–500 + cells) with PMN predominance in 1st few days, later monocytic preponderance. Protein frequently elevated (50–150 mg/dL). Virus may be identified with encephalitis panel.	Cytoalbuminologic dissociation; 10 or fewer mononuclear cells with high protein after 1st week. Normal glucose. IgG may be elevated.	Normal.	Normal.	Usually normal opening pressure; CSF may show increased protein, pleocytosis with predominantly mononuclear cells, increased IgG.
EMG/NCS	EMG shows denervation after 10–21 days. No sensory NCS abnormalities.	NCSs may be normal early (within 1st week). Earliest changes: slowed to absent F or H reflexes. Demyelinating changes are typically seen 7–10 days after onset of symptoms.	EMG distinctive: BSAP (brief small abundant potentials). High-frequency stimulation may increase CMAP amplitude but is painful to perform in awake infant.	Nerve conduction velocity slowed; returns rapidly to normal after removal of tick.	Normal early. Can have evidence of denervation after 10–21 days.
Other studies	Polio virus in stool and throat. Enterovirus D68 or D71 in nasal secretions. West Nile: Serial serologic titers IgG, IgM; Hyponatremia in 30% MRI with T2 signal change in anterior gray matter or brainstem.	Search for specific cause such as infection, intoxication, autoimmune disease. Anti GM₁ antibodies seen in AMANᵃ. Anti-GQ1b antibodies seen in Miller-Fisher syndrome. Nerve root enhancement on MRI.	Infancy: stool culture, toxin. Rare serum toxin positive. Older: serum (or wound) toxin.	Leukocytosis, often with moderate eosinophilia.	MRI with T2 signal change in spinal cord, often with edema.
Course and prognosis	Paralysis usually maximal 3–5 days after onset. Transient bladder symptoms may occur. Outlook varies with extent and severity of involvement.	Course progressive over a few days to about 2 weeks then slowly improves. Morbidity greatest from respiratory failure (10%), autonomic crises (eg, widely variable blood pressure, arrhythmia), and superinfection. Full recovery is common except in severe or axonal cases.	Progressive descending weakness over days to 2 wk. Fatality 3%, usually due to complications from respiratory failure and intensive care. Full recovery likely if supported through first 4–8 wk.	Progressive weakness with mortality due to respiratory failure is common if tick is not removed.	May have complications from bowel or bladder dysfunction, respiratory failure with cervical lesion, or autonomic instability. Large degree of functional recovery possible.
Treatment	May trial IVIg but efficacy data are lacking. Mortality is greatest from respiratory failure and superinfection.	Plasmapheresis and IVIg can shorten the hospitalization. Relapses occasionally occur.	BIG intravenous shortens ICU stay. Respiratory and feeding support critical. Avoid aminoglycosides.	Removal of tick leads to rapid and complete recovery.	Corticosteroids, IVIg, and plasmapheresis may be used to shorten course.

AIDP, acute inflammatory demyelinating neuropathy; BIG, botulism immune globulin; CMAP, compound muscle action potentials; CMV, cytomegalovirus; CSF, cerebrospinal fluid; EBV, Epstein-Barr virus; EMG, electromyogram; EV-71, enterovirus 71; GI, gastrointestinal; ICU, intensive care unit; IVIg, intravenous immunoglobulin; MRI, magnetic resonance imaging; NCS, nerve conduction studies; PMN, polymorphonuclear neutrophil; SIDS, sudden infant death syndrome.
ᵃAMAN is acute motor axonal neuropathy (uncommon variant in the United States).

Clinical Findings

Acute flaccid paralysis presents with rapid onset (hours to days) of weakness with decreased muscle tone. Accompanying features that assist diagnosis are age, a history of preceding illness, rapidity of progression, cranial nerve findings, bowel and bladder changes, and the presence or absence of sensory findings (see Table 25–18). For example, fatigability when drinking from a bottle and constipation in an infant are suggestive of botulism. In GBS patients may initially present with ascending paresthesias, ill-defined pain, and loss of reflexes before they develop overt weakness. Patients with the Miller Fisher variant of GBS may present with ophthalmoplegia, ataxia, and loss of reflexes. Back pain, particularly wrapping around the chest or with a "hugging/squeezing" quality, is suggestive of a spinal cord lesion, such as in transverse myelitis or a spinal cord mass.

Diagnostic Evaluation

MRI is often necessary to evaluate for spinal cord inflammation and to rule out a mass lesion before CSF can be obtained. Evaluation of the spinal fluid for signs of inflammation or infection is often helpful. Viral cultures (CSF, throat, and stool) and titers aid in diagnosing poliomyelitis or acute flaccid myelitis. NCS and needle EMG can be helpful. In GBS, signs of a demyelinating neuropathy (decreased conduction velocities or response amplitudes) are seen on NCS in 50% of patients by 2 weeks and in 85% of patients by 3 weeks. Patients with botulism may have fibrillation potentials and increased compound muscle action potential amplitudes with high-frequency stimulation on EMG, though a clinical diagnosis of botulism can often be made. Elevation of muscle enzymes or even myoglobinuria may aid in diagnosis of acute myopathic weakness, and potassium abnormalities may be present in periodic paralysis.

Differential Diagnosis

In addition to the above common causes, other considerations include myopathy, spinal cord stroke, abscess, or epidural hemorrhage, which may present similarly to transverse myelitis. Myasthenic crisis, discussed under Disorders of Neuromuscular Transmission may present with acute weakness, but a careful history typically reveals the presence of chronic or subacute symptoms. Ingestion or systemic illness should be considered if weakness is accompanied by changes in mental status or markedly elevated creatine kinase (CK). Diagnostic considerations are further discussed in Table 25–18.

Complications

Complications from disorders causing acute flaccid paralysis are typically related to respiratory weakness, autonomic dysfunction, and bowel/bladder dysfunction. Attention to ventilation is essential, especially in patients with bulbar (oropharyngeal) weakness or early signs of respiratory failure. Patients with respiratory weakness may not show signs of increased work of breathing; increasing anxiety and a rise in blood pressure are early signs of hypoxia and hypercapnia. At the bedside, measurement of negative inspiratory force (NIF) is recommended at frequent intervals and may be more sensitive to early respiratory failure than blood gases. Intubation or noninvasive ventilation and careful suctioning of secretions should be considered early. Pneumonia is a frequent complication of respiratory or bulbar weakness and should be managed promptly. Autonomic crisis is a poorly understood but potentially fatal complication of GBS and acute spinal cord processes. Strict attention to vital signs to detect and treat hypotension or hypertension and cardiac arrhythmias in an intensive care setting is advisable early in the course and in severely ill patients.

Treatment

Supportive treatment is essential for any cause of acute flaccid weakness, including careful pulmonary care, fluids and nutrition, bladder and bowel care, prevention of decubitus ulcers, and in many cases, psychiatric support. Early involvement of physical, occupational, and speech therapy improves long-term recovery. Specific treatment is dependent on the cause of weakness.

Devia K et al: Acute idiopathic transverse myelitis in children: early predictors of relapse and disability. Neurology 2015 Jan 27; 84(4):341–349 [PMID: 25540303].

Murphy OC et al: Acute flaccid myelitis: cause, diagnosis, and management. Lancet 2021;397(10271):334–346 [PMID: 33357469].

Pifko E, Price A, Sterner S: Infant botulism and indications for administration of botulism immune globulin. Pediatr Emerg Care 2014;30(2):120 [PMID: 24488164].

DISORDERS OF CHILDHOOD AFFECTING MUSCLES

ESSENTIALS OF DIAGNOSIS & TYPICAL FEATURES

▶ Myopathies (diseases of muscle tissues) typically cause symmetric, proximal more than distal muscle weakness (positive Gowers sign, toe walking, waddling gait).

▶ Deep tendon reflexes are typically preserved early in the disease course and are typically lost in proportion to the degree of weakness later in the disease.

▶ Serum CK levels are normal to elevated.

▶ NCSs are generally normal; EMG demonstrates myopathic findings.

► Clinical Findings

Myopathies represent numerous diseases of muscle tissue, including congenital myopathies, muscular dystrophies, and acquired myopathies (Table 25–19). In general, proximal muscles are more affected. Reflexes may be preserved early in the course. Patients may have pseudohypertrophy (muscles that appear large due to fatty infiltrate and fibrosis), decreased muscle bulk, or even frank atrophy. Cramps, spasms, fatigue, and muscle stiffness can be seen. Some patients with Duchenne muscular dystrophy/Becker muscular dystrophy (DMD/BMD) may have a nonprogressive intellectual disability, with IQ scores one standard deviation below normal means. Some disorders are associated with systemic involvement, and cardiomyopathy is an important consideration.

► Diagnostic Evaluation

A. Serum Enzymes

Serum CK levels reflect muscle damage or "leaks" from muscle into plasma. Generally, CK levels are normal to mildly elevated in myopathies but may be markedly elevated (up to 50–100 times normal) in some muscular dystrophies, such as DMD, or in infectious or immune-mediated myositis. Medications and activity level may affect CK levels, for instance after an EMG, muscle biopsy, or exercise.

B. Genetic Testing

Genetic testing for myopathies and muscular dystrophies is rapidly improving and becoming widely available. Genetic testing should be guided by clinical findings and serum CK levels. Mutation analysis for DMD/BMD is considered the initial step if these disorders are suspected. Genetic characterization of suspected myopathies and muscular dystrophies is becoming increasingly important, as many therapies are being developed that target specific genetic changes. It is important to note, however, that a negative result does not exclude the possibility of a genetically mediated myopathy or muscular dystrophy.

C. Electrophysiologic Studies

NCSs are typically normal in muscle diseases; whereas, EMG shows short duration, polyphasic motor unit action potentials (MUAPs) that are increased in number for the strength of the contraction.

D. Muscle Biopsy

A muscle biopsy can be helpful in the diagnosis of a muscle disorder, if properly executed, though is becoming less common as genetic testing becomes more widely available. The timing of the biopsy and the specific muscle to biopsy should be carefully considered. Moderately affected muscles typically yield better results than strong or severely affected muscles and sites of prior needle EMG or injections should be avoided. Biopsies performed in the newborn period may be of limited utility as pathologic changes may not be evident in immature muscle.

► Complications

Though skeletal muscle weakness may be profound in muscle disorders, the greatest morbidity and mortality arises from cardiorespiratory complications. Advances in supportive care, especially noninvasive ventilation, cough assist, and secretion management, have had a tremendous impact in the care of these patients. Some myopathies and muscular dystrophies can affect cardiac function, and early involvement of a cardiac specialist is paramount. Other complications include delayed GI motility that can lead to debilitating constipation or pseudo-obstruction. Contractures are a particularly frustrating complication that can limit mobility, cause pain, and affect quality of life.

► Treatment & Prognosis

Treatment for patients with muscle disorders is predominantly supportive, and medications altering disease progression are limited but are an active area of investigation. A few examples of treatable myopathies/muscular dystrophies include DMD/BMD and Pompe disease.

Patients with DMD/BMD should be started on corticosteroids (prednisone, prednisolone, vamorolone, or deflazacort) between 4 and 8 years of age, when motor function begins to plateau or decline, to extend the period of independent ambulation by approximately 2.5 years and to preserve respiratory strength and cardiac function into the second decade. Novel steroids and other anti-inflammatory agents are under investigation. Additional treatments targeting specific mutations in DMD have been developed over the last decade, including commercial treatments with exon-skipping (eteplirsen, viltolarsen, casimersen, and golodirsen). Gene transfer therapies with microdystrophins have been approved for some patients.

In the past, the prognosis for infantile Pompe disease was uniformly grim, with death by age 1 year due to cardiomyopathy. However, enzyme replacement therapy (ERT) with recombinant acid alpha glucosidase changes the disease course and increases survival, though patients may still have residual or progressive weakness.

Gene-based treatments for myopathies and muscular dystrophies are an active area of research, and clinical trials for gene transfer therapies are underway for a number of these disorders. Thus, the treatment landscape for muscle diseases affecting children is rapidly changing. However, until curative treatments for muscle diseases are available, slowing the progressive deterioration in muscle strength and cardiorespiratory function and improving quality of life remain the emphasis of treatment.

Table 25–19. Muscular dystrophies, myopathies, myotonias, and anterior horn diseases of childhood.

Disease	Genetic Pattern	Age at Onset	Manifestation	Involved Muscles	Reflexes	Muscle Biopsy Findings	Other Diagnostic Tests	Treatment	Prognosis
Muscular dystrophies									
Dystrophinopathies (Duchenne muscular dystrophy and Becker muscular dystrophy)	X-linked recessive; Xp21; 30%–50% have no family history and are spontaneous mutations.	DMD: 2–6 y; BMD: childhood to adulthood.	Clumsiness, and delayed motor milestones are early signs. Difficulty climbing stairs. Walking on toes; waddling gait with excessive lumbar lordosis. Positive Gowers maneuver. Failure to thrive is common.	Proximal (pelvic > shoulder girdle) muscles; pseudohypertrophy typically of gastrocnemius. Progressive scoliosis, cardiomyopathy and respiratory weakness develop in the second decade.	Normal to decreased early, may be absent at late stages	Areas of degeneration and regeneration, variation in fiber size, inflammatory changes, proliferation of connective tissue. Immunostaining for dystrophin absent. Dystrophin may be reduced rather than absent in BMD.	Myopathic EMG. CK levels can be up to 50–100× normal, but decrease with increasing disease severity, as muscle replaced with fat/connective tissue. Genetic testing shows dystrophin gene deletion in 60%, duplication in 5%–15%, and point mutations, intronic deletions, or repeats in 20%–30%.	Management is largely supportive. Corticosteroids may prolong independent ambulation. Exon skipping treatments for some mutations. Close pulmonary and cardiac follow-up are needed due to risk of cardiorespiratory failure in 2nd–3rd decade of life. Treat osteoporosis with calcium and vitamin D.	DMD: use a wheelchair by 12 y; death from cardiorespiratory causes usually occurs by the 20s–30s. BMD: may remain ambulatory for 15–20 y after 1st symptoms; near normal life expectancy unless significant cardiac involvement.
Limb-girdle muscular dystrophy	Autosomal dominant, autosomal recessive, and X-linked forms.	Variable; early childhood to adulthood.	Weakness, with distribution according to type. Waddling gait, difficulty climbing stairs. Excessive lumbar lordosis.	Slowly progressive, symmetric proximal muscle involvement; characteristically involves shoulder and pelvic muscles.	Usually present	Necrosis and fiber splitting, increased endomysial connective tissue and inflammation, absent immunostaining for various proteins.	Myopathic EMG. CK often > 5000 IU/L. Leg MRI may show selective involvement (eg, peroneal muscles in Miyoshi myopathy). Genetic testing.	No curative treatments currently available but gene therapies being investigated for some subtypes. Physical therapy. Echocardiogram to screen for cardiomyopathy. PFTs to screen to respiratory weakness.	Variable by subtype.

(Continued)

Table 25–19. Muscular dystrophies, myopathies, myotonias, and anterior horn diseases of childhood. (*Continued*)

Disease	Genetic Pattern	Age at Onset	Manifestation	Involved Muscles	Reflexes	Muscle Biopsy Findings	Other Diagnostic Tests	Treatment	Prognosis
Facioscapulohumeral muscular dystrophy	Most are autosomal dominant inherited deletions of D4Z4 on 4q35	Usually late in 1st–5th decade depending on size of deletion.	Diminished facial movements, inability to close eyes, smile, or whistle. Difficulty raising arms over head. Weakness may be asymmetric.	Face, shoulder girdle muscles (biceps, triceps), asymmetric. Deltoid and forearm spared. 75% sensorineural hearing loss; 60% Coats disease	Present	Nonspecific myopathic changes: variation in fiber size, moderate increased endomysial connective tissue, mild inflammatory changes.	Myopathic EMG. CK mildly to moderately elevated (less than 1500 IU/L). Genetic testing confirms diagnosis.	No curative treatments available. Management of pain important. Identify and treat hearing loss, retinal telangiectasias, respiratory insufficiency (1% cases).	Variable and inversely related to age at symptom onset. Life-threatening bulbar, respiratory and cardiac problems rare, so life expectancy normal.
Congenital myopathies									
Centronuclear myopathy, central core disease, multiminicore disease, nemaline myopathy, and several others	Autosomal dominant, autosomal recessive, and X-linked recessive forms	Neonatal period to 12 mo.	Floppy infant; severe hypotonia, often with respiratory failure and feeding difficulties.	May have ptosis, ophthalmoplegia; moderate-severe symmetric distal and proximal weakness.	Mildly diminished or absent	Myopathic changes without inflammation. May have specific features such as cores or rods depending on subtype.	Myopathic EMG with fibrillations and complex repetitive discharges. Normal to mildly elevated CK. Genetic testing..	No curative treatments currently. Respiratory, nutritional support. Risk for malignant hyperthermia in some subtypes. Gene therapies under investigation.	Variable. Death in the neonatal period or early infancy with severe presentations; Mild-moderate presentations may improve in first several years then plateau.
CMDs									
Dystroglycanopathies (Fukuyama, Walker-Warburg, Muscle-eye-brain), Laminin α_2, collagen VI myopathies (Ullrich, Bethlem)	Autosomal recessive and autosomal dominant forms.	Birth to 12 mo.	Hypotonia, generalized weakness. Proximal contractures, distal hypermobility. May have severe intellectual disability and structural eye abnormalities.	Generalized and respiratory muscle weakness.	Mildly decreased to absent	Variable fiber size, internalized nuclei. May have reduced or absent staining of Laminin α_2, COLVI, or α-dystroglycan depending on subtype.	Myopathic EMG CK normal to 10x normal. May also have mild neuropathy. Brain MRI may show white matter changes, migrational abnormalities, lissencephaly, or cerebellar hypoplasia.	No curative treatments. Respiratory support often required early. Management of seizures, when present.	Variable. Most never walk or lose ability to walk early. Death by 1st–2nd decade secondary to respiratory failure in more severely affected patients.

Metabolic myopathies

| Pompe disease | Autosomal recessive; 17q23. | Classic infantile form: present by 6 mo of age. Juvenile: 2–18 y. | Infantile: Severe hypotonia, hepatomegaly, cardiomyopathy, hypoventilation. Juvenile: Proximal muscle weakness, head drop, | Proximal more than distal muscles, bulbar and respiratory muscles. Recurrent respiratory infections; nocturnal hypoventilation. Macroglossia. | Absent | Cytoplasmic lysosomal vacuoles stain positive with acid phosphatase. | Infantile: High CK (up to 10× normal). Juvenile: Mildly high CK. | Enzyme replacement therapy with alglucosidase alfa (Myozyme). Respiratory and nutritional support. Monitor cardiomyopathy. | Death by 2 y with untreated infantile form. Treatment significantly improves survival, cardiorespiratory status and motor skills. Some become non-ambulatory; most require ventilatory support. |

Ion channel disorders

| Hyperkalemic and hypokalemic periodic paralysis | Autosomal dominant. | Childhood, usually by 1st decade. | Episodic flaccid weakness, precipitated by rest after exercise, stress, fasting, carbohydrate rich meal, or cold depending on type. | Proximal and symmetric muscles, distal muscles may be involved if exercised. | Normal at baseline, may be absent with episodes | May see vacuoles and nonspecific myopathic changes, especially later in disease course. | NCS show increased CMAP amplitude after 5 min exercise. CK normal to 300 IU/L; attacks associated with high serum K⁺. | Many attacks are brief and do not need treatment; treat acute attack with carbohydrates for hyperkalemic form or with potassium for hypokalemic form. Chronic treatment varies by type. | Attacks may be more frequent with increasing age. Some patients develop slowly progressive weakness in adulthood. |

(Continued)

Table 25–19. Muscular dystrophies, myopathies, myotonias, and anterior horn diseases of childhood. (*Continued*)

Disease	Genetic Pattern	Age at Onset	Manifestation	Involved Muscles	Reflexes	Muscle Biopsy Findings	Other Diagnostic Tests	Treatment	Prognosis
Myotonic disorders									
DM1	Autosomal dominant, expanded CTG triplet repeat of DMPK gene on chromosome 19q13; anticipation can result in children being more affected than parents..	Often presents in the neonatal period (congenital) but can present through adulthood; some adults are diagnosed when their children are diagnosed.	Decreased fetal movement, neonates have respiratory insufficiency, difficulties sucking and swallowing. Older children and adults have difficulty releasing grip and "myotonic facies" due to atrophy and facial muscle weakness.	Generalized weakness; facial and pharyngeal involvement prominent; intellectual disability. Percussion myotonia on examination.	Decreased to absent	Mild myopathic changes, centralized nuclei, variation in fiber size, ring fibers.	Electrical myotonia on EMG but may not be present in neonatal period Normal or mildly elevated CK. Cataracts on slit-lamp examination. Reduced testosterone levels. Insulin resistance. ECG shows conduction defects, (eg, ventricular arrhythmias). Sleep study shows hypercapnia and hypoventilation.	No curative treatment. Avoid medications that predispose to arrhythmia (eg quinine, amitriptyline, digoxin). Arrhythmias may require pacemaker. Follow-up with pulmonology for risk of apnea, endocrinology for insulin resistance, and ophthalmology for cataracts. May have GI hypomotility, constipation, pseudo-obstruction.	Reduced survival to age 65; mean survival to 60 y. 50% utilize wheelchair before death, but most are ambulatory into adulthood.
Myotonia congenita (Thomsen disease)	Autosomal dominant or autosomal recessive on CLCN1 gene of chromosome 7q35.	Early infancy to adulthood.	Muscle hypertrophy. Difficulty relaxing muscles after contracting them, especially with cold or stress. Muscles may be stuck in contraction for seconds to minutes.	Mild fixed proximal muscle weakness or mild functional difficulties (like climbing stairs). Percussion myotonia on examination.	Normal	Usually normal though there may be absence of 2B fibers.	Myotonia and mild myopathic changes on EMG; CK may be slightly elevated 3–4x normal	Symptom treatment with quinine, mexiletine, Dilantin, carbamazepine, or acetazolamide. May improve with exercise. Worsened with β2 agonists, monocarboxylic amino acids, depolarizing muscle relaxants.	Normal life expectancy; muscle stiffness may interfere with activity but improves with exercise.

ASA, acetylsalicylic acid; CK, creatine kinase; CMD, congenital muscular dystrophy; CPT, carnitine palmityl transferase; CSF, cerebrospinal fluid; CT, computed tomography; DM1, myotonic dystrophy type 1; DMPK, dystrophia myotonica protein kinase; ECG, electrocardiogram; EMG, electromyogram; MRI, magnetic resonance imaging; PCR, polymerase chain reaction; SIDS, sudden infant death syndrome.

Benign acute childhood myositis (myalgia cruris epidemica) is characterized by transient severe muscle pain and weakness affecting mainly the calves and occurring 1–2 days following an upper respiratory tract infection. Symptoms are caused by direct invasion of skeletal muscle by virus and typically occur in children between the ages of 6 and 8 years. The course is usually self-limited, but management of rhabdomyolysis and myoglobinuria is occasionally warranted with IV fluids and pain management. Follow-up of serum CK levels is recommended to ensure that they return to normal. Patients with persistently elevated CKs or recurrent episodes of rhabdomyolysis require further workup for underlying disorders such as metabolic myopathies or muscular dystrophies.

Aartsma-Rus A et al: Evidence-based consensus and systematic review on reducing time to diagnosis of Duchenne muscular dystrophy. J Pediatr 2019;204:305–313 [PMID: 30579468].

Duan D et al: Duchenne muscular dystrophy. Nat Rev Dis Primers 2021;7(1):13 [PMID: 33602943].

Kishnani PS, Hwu WL: Introduction to the newborn screening, diagnosis, and treatment of Pompe disease guidance supplement. Pediatrics 2017;140(Suppl 1): S1–S3 [PMID: 29162672].

Kourakis S et al: Standard of care versus new-wave corticosteroids in the treatment of Duchenne muscular dystrophy: can we do better? Orphanet J Rare Dis 2021;16(1):117 [PMID: 33663533].

Nortiz G et al: Primary care and emergency department management of the patient with Duchenne. Pediatrics 2018;142(Suppl 2): 890–898 [PMID: 30275253].

Rosenberg T et al: Outcome of benign acute childhood myositis. Pediatr Emerg Care 2018;34(6):400–402 [PMID: 27548740].

Wang CH et al: Consensus statement on standard of care for congenital muscular dystrophies. J Child Neurol 2010; 25(12):1559–1581 [PMID: 21078917].

DISORDERS OF NEUROMUSCULAR TRANSMISSION

ESSENTIALS OF DIAGNOSIS & TYPICAL FEATURES

► Disorders of the neuromuscular junction typically cause fluctuating weakness, that comes on or increases with use (fatigue).

► Extraocular, bulbar, and respiratory muscles, in addition to appendicular muscles, are the most affected.

► Immune mediated diseases, such as myasthenia gravis, will demonstrate a positive response to neostigmine and edrophonium.

▶ General Considerations

Myasthenic syndromes are characterized by easy fatigability of muscles, particularly the extraocular, bulbar, and respiratory muscles. Three general categories of myasthenic syndromes are recognized: transient neonatal myasthenia, autoimmune myasthenia gravis, and congenital myasthenic syndromes.

▶ Clinical Findings

1. Neonatal (transient) myasthenia—This disorder occurs in 12%–19% of infants born to mothers with myasthenia gravis as a result of passive transfer of maternal acetylcholine receptor antibodies across the placenta. Neonates present before the third day of life with bulbar weakness, difficulty feeding, weak cry, and hypotonia.

2. Juvenile myasthenia gravis—This is the most common pediatric disorder of neuromuscular transmission. Like the adult form of myasthenia gravis, autoimmune juvenile myasthenia gravis is characterized by fatigable and sometimes asymmetric weakness. Unlike adult patients, who typically present with limb weakness, more than half of pediatric patients initially present with ocular symptoms (ptosis or ophthalmoplegia). Approximately 75% develop limb weakness or bulbar symptoms, such as difficulty chewing, dysphagia, or nasal voice, within 4 years. Symptoms of weakness tend to recur and remit and can be precipitated by illness or medications such as aminoglycoside antibiotics. Other autoimmune disorders, such as rheumatoid arthritis and thyroid disease, may co-occur.

3. Congenital myasthenic syndromes—These syndromes are a heterogenous group of hereditary/genetic, nonimmune disorders of presynaptic, synaptic, or postsynaptic neuromuscular transmission. Patients may present with mild motor delays, dramatic episodic apnea, constant and generalized weakness, or with more classic episodic/fatigable weakness. Onset of symptoms occurs before 2 years. The distinction between this group of disorders and acquired myasthenia gravis is important, as they are managed differently, but it may be clinically difficult to distinguish between the two. However, age of presentation under 2 years is highly suggestive of a congenital myasthenic syndrome.

▶ Diagnostic Evaluation

A. Cholinesterase inhibitor testing
(NEOSTIGMINE AND EDROPHONIUM TESTS)

Bedside testing with neostigmine, edrophonium, or pyridostigmine can confirm the presence of a neuromuscular disorder. This is done by administering the medication and watching for rapid improvement of easily observable clinical signs, such as dysarthria, ptosis, or ophthalmoplegia. Edrophonium is typically used in children, and the maximum effect occurs within 2 minutes. In newborns and very young infants, the neostigmine test may be preferable because the longer duration of its response permits better observation, especially of sucking and swallowing movements, but it may take 10 minutes for the effects to begin. The clinician should be prepared to suction secretions and administer atropine if necessary. Cholinesterase inhibitors must be used with caution in patients with suspected congenital myasthenic syndromes, as some forms may demonstrate a paradoxical worsening.

B. Laboratory Findings

1. Antibody testing—Serum acetylcholine receptor (AChR) binding, blocking, and modulating antibodies or serum muscle-specific kinase (MuSK) antibodies are often found in autoimmune juvenile myasthenia gravis and neonatal (transient) myasthenia. These antibodies are not found in congenital myasthenic syndromes, as these disorders are not immune-mediated. In juveniles, thyroid studies are appropriate, as concomitant thyroid disease is common.

2. Genetic testing—Commercial genetic testing is available for patients with congenital myasthenic syndromes, and genetic differentiation of the myasthenic syndrome is important to guide treatment.

C. Electrophysiologic Studies

Electrophysiologic studies may be helpful when myasthenic syndromes, and especially myasthenia gravis, are suspected. Repetitive stimulation of a motor nerve at slow rates of 2–3 Hz reveals a decrease in compound muscle action potentials in myasthenia gravis patients and in some, but not all, congenital myasthenic syndromes. Repetitive stimulation may be technically difficult to perform in infants and younger children, as it can be painful and requires cooperation. Single-fiber EMG in cooperative children is more sensitive, but it is technically challenging and time intensive.

D. Imaging

Chest radiograph and CT scan in older children with autoimmune myasthenia gravis may show thymic hyperplasia. Thymomas are rare in children.

▶ Treatment

A. General & Supportive Measures

In the newborn or child in myasthenic or cholinergic crisis (see the following section Complications), supportive care is essential, and the child should be monitored in a critical care setting. A careful search for signs of respiratory failure is crucial: simple bedside tests include evaluation of cough and counting to 20 in a single breath. Inability to do either or the presence of neck flexion weakness, nasal speech, and drooling are important indicators of impending respiratory problems.

B. Symptomatic Treatment: Anticholinesterase Inhibitors

Pyridostigmine is the first-line symptomatic treatment in patients with juvenile myasthenia gravis and mild weakness. Acetylcholinesterase inhibitors do not modify disease progression but transiently improve muscle strength. Pyridostigmine can worsen weakness in patients with some congenital myasthenic syndromes. Neostigmine is the drug of choice in newborns with neonatal (transient) myasthenia gravis, in whom prompt treatment may be lifesaving.

C. Immunomodulatory Treatment

Patients with autoimmune myasthenia gravis and severe weakness not responding to cholinesterase inhibitors alone require long-term treatment with immunomodulation. The mainstay of treatment is steroids, but some patients may require treatment with other immunosuppressants. IVIG and plasmapheresis are used for myasthenic crisis and occasionally for long-term management. Steroids, while helpful in long-term management, may transiently worsen symptoms if given at high doses during an acute exacerbation.

D. Surgical Treatment

There are few data for efficacy of thymectomy in the pediatric population. Some studies suggest that thymectomy within 2 years of diagnosis results in a higher rate of remission in Caucasian children.

▶ Complications

A. Myasthenic Crisis

Respiratory failure can develop swiftly due to critical weakness of respiratory muscles, bulbar muscles or both, during a myasthenic crisis. Patients may not appear to be in respiratory distress, due to inability to generate effortful movements. Crises are generally not fatal as long as patients receive timely respiratory support and appropriate immunotherapy. Certain medications may precipitate myasthenic crisis, including aminoglycoside antibiotics, muscle relaxants, and anesthetics.

B. Cholinergic Crisis

Cholinergic crisis may result from overmedication with anticholinesterase drugs. The resulting weakness may be similar to that of myasthenic crises, and the muscarinic side effects (diarrhea, sweating, lacrimation, miosis, bradycardia, and hypotension) may be difficult to appreciate. If suspected, cholinesterase inhibitors should be discontinued immediately, and improvement afterward suggests cholinergic crisis. As in myasthenic crisis, supportive respiratory care and appropriate immunotherapy should be given.

Prognosis

Prognosis for neonatal (transient) myasthenia in patients who receive good supportive care is generally excellent, with complete resolution of symptoms in 2–3 weeks as maternal antibodies decrease. The prognosis for congenital myasthenic syndromes is variable by subtype. Some subtypes show improvement in weakness with age. Others demonstrate life-threatening episodic apnea and life-long weakness. Patients with childhood and juvenile myasthenia gravis generally do well, with greater spontaneous remission rates than adult patients.

Hantai D et al: Congenital myasthenic syndromes. Curr Opin Neurol 2013;26(5):561–568 [PMID: 23995276].

Hennessey IA et al: Thymectomy for inducing remission in juvenile myasthenia gravis. Pediatr Surg Int 2011;27(6):591–594 [PMID: 21243366].

Liew WK et al: Comparison of plasmapheresis and intravenous immunoglobulin as maintenance therapies for juvenile myasthenia gravis. JAMA Neurol 2014;71(5):575–580 [PMID: 24590389].

Mehndiratta MM, Pandey S, Kuntzer T: Acetylcholinesterase inhibitor treatment for myasthenia gravis. Cochrane Database Syst Rev 2011;16(2):CD006986 [PMID: 21328290].

LESIONS OF THE CRANIAL & PERIPHERAL NERVES

1. Facial Weakness

ESSENTIALS OF DIAGNOSIS & TYPICAL FEATURES

► Central (upper motor neuron) versus peripheral (lower motor neuron) facial nerve lesions need to be distinguished to determine workup, treatment, and prognosis. Inability to raise the eyebrows indicates peripheral involvement of the facial nerve or lower motor neurons in the pons.

Pathogenesis

Idiopathic facial nerve palsy (Bell palsy) is the most common cranial mononeuropathy. Cranial nerve VII carries motor fibers to all muscles of facial expression, the stylohyoid, posterior belly of the digastric, and the stapedius, parasympathetic fibers supplying the soft palate, nasal mucosa, and the salivary and lacrimal glands, taste fibers to the anterior two-thirds of the tongue, and somatic sensory fibers supplying a small part of the external auditory meatus and the skin of the ear. Facial weakness can occur as the result of a lesion anywhere along the path of the nerve. Some cases are postinfectious, although increasing evidence suggests that Bell palsy is

a viral-induced cranial neuritis. It may be a presenting sign of HSV type 1 (HSV-1), Lyme disease, infectious mononucleosis, or GBS and is usually diagnosable by the history and physical examination.

Clinical Findings

Peripheral ("lower motor neuron") cranial nerve VII lesions or lesions of the facial nerve nuclei in the pons cause ipsilateral facial weakness that affects both the upper and lower facial muscles. Although the facial asymmetry is often striking, it can be surprisingly difficult to determine which side of the face is weak. The affected side will demonstrate inability to wrinkle the forehead, decreased eyebrow raise, and impaired eye closure. Inability to wrinkle the forehead may be demonstrated in infants and young children by getting them to follow a light moved vertically above the forehead. When smiling, the corner of the mouth will demonstrate decreased elevation on the weak side, whereas the unaffected corner may appear to "pull down" excessively. A key finding is that the nasolabial fold is flattened on the affected side. Some patients may have a widened palpebral fissure on the weak side, due to gravity pulling the lower lid down; the normal eye may falsely seem to have ptosis in comparison. The House-Brackmann scale is a useful tool for assessing the degree of upper and lower face weakness. Patients may also have decreased tearing and saliva production, hyperacusis, and absent taste sensation over the anterior two-thirds of the tongue on the affected side. Loss of taste may be demonstrated in cooperative children by age 4 or 5 years. In a younger child, the careful use of a tongue blade and something sour (eg, lemon juice) may enable the provider to note whether the child's face puckers up.

Differential Diagnosis

Varicella zoster infection can mimic idiopathic facial nerve palsy, and examination of the ear canal to rule out vesicular eruption is critical. Importantly, cranial nerve VII dysfunction can also be a sign of **brainstem tumor** or other **brainstem lesion**; thus, patients with additional neurologic deficits or atypical presentations should undergo brain MRI. A central "upper motor neuron" lesion, such as a **cortical stroke**, causes contralateral weakness of the lower face, sparing the forehead and orbicularis oculi muscles, which are bilaterally innervated.

Injuries to the facial nerve at birth occur in 0.25%–6.5% of consecutive live births. Forceps delivery is the cause in some cases; in others, the affected side of the face may have abutted against the sacral prominence in utero. Often, no cause can be established.

Asymmetric crying facies, in which one side of the lower lip depresses with crying (ie, the normal side) and the other does not, is suspected to be an autosomal dominantly inherited congenital malformation. Symptoms in the parent may be almost inapparent because the asymmetry often improves with age. EMG suggests congenital absence of the depressor angularis muscle of the lower lip but is rarely performed as it is technically challenging and uncomfortable for the infant. In 10% of cases, other major congenital defects, such as heart defects, accompany the palsy and should prompt evaluation for **22q11 deletion syndrome**.

Treatment & Prognosis

In the vast majority of cases, regardless of etiology, improvement begins within 1–3 weeks, and near or total recovery of function is observed within 3–4 months. Since eye closure or blinking are often impaired, eye drops or ointment should be used to protect the cornea during the day; at night, the lid should be taped shut with gauze and tape. Upward massage of the face for 5–10 minutes three or four times a day may help maintain muscle tone. Corticosteroids seem to improve outcomes in adults and are frequently used in children, though evidence in children is lacking. In the older child, acyclovir or valacyclovir (herpes antiviral agent) therapy or antibiotics (Lyme disease) may have a role. In the few children with permanent and cosmetically disfiguring facial weakness, plastic surgical intervention may be of benefit. New procedures, such as attachment of facial muscles to the temporal muscle and transplantation of cranial nerve XI, are being developed.

Gagyor I et al: Antiviral treatment for Bell's palsy (idiopathic facial paralysis). Cochrane Database Syst Rev 2019;9(9):CD001869 [PMID: 31486071].

George E, Richie MB, Glastonbury CM: Facial nerve palsy: clinical practice and cognitive errors. Am J Med 2020;133:1039–1044 [PMID: 32445717].

Madhok VB et al: Corticosteroids for Bell's palsy (idiopathic facial paralysis). Cochrane Database Syst Rev 2016;7(7):CD001942 [PMID: 27428352].

Rioja-Mazza et al: Asymmetric crying facies: a possible marker for congenital malformations. J Matern Fetal Neonatal Med 2005;18(4):275–277 [PMID: 16318980].

2. Peripheral Neuropathy

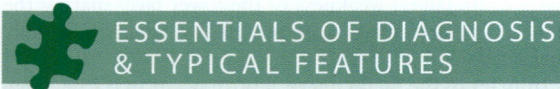

ESSENTIALS OF DIAGNOSIS & TYPICAL FEATURES

- ► Neuropathies (diseases of the nerves) typically cause weakness in the distal extremities.
- ► Reflexes are typically lost early in the disease course, out of proportion to the degree of weakness.
- ► Sensory changes usually accompany a neuropathy.

General Considerations

A careful history, including a pedigree, examination, and electrophysiologic testing of the patient and relatives are critical for determining whether a chronic polyneuropathy is genetic or acquired, which will determine management. **Hereditary neuropathies**, such as Charcot-Marie-Tooth disease, are the most common causes of chronic neuropathy in childhood. There may be a family history of gait or orthopedics abnormalities without a formal diagnosis of inherited neuropathy. Other genetic causes of polyneuropathies associated with systemic involvement include storage disorders or leukodystrophies. Acquired causes can include exposure to toxins known to cause neuropathies, such as lead, arsenic, or toluene, or use of medications such as vincristine. Neuropathies can be the late manifestations of systemic disorders like diabetes and autoimmune disorders. Treatment of these underlying disorders can improve or slow the progression of the neuropathy. AIDP, also known as GBS, has been discussed in another section, but a similar disorder, **chronic inflammatory demyelinating polyneuropathy** (CIDP) is an immune-mediated disorder with a slowly progressive course.

Clinical Findings

Peripheral nerve disorders typically progress in a distal to proximal fashion, with weakness and muscle atrophy occurring in the distal extremities first. Children can present with gait disturbances, such as tripping over their toes, and easy fatigability in walking or running, and less often, with weakness or clumsiness of the hands. Pain, tenderness, or paresthesia is mentioned less frequently and is more suggestive of an acquired neuropathy. On neurologic examination, the lower legs and hands are weaker than the thighs and upper arms. Reflexes are decreased in a distal to proximal fashion. Sensory deficits occur in a stocking-and-glove distribution. Trophic changes such as glassy or parchment skin and absent sweating may occur if the course has been chronic. Rarely, thickening of the ulnar and peroneal nerves may be felt. In sensory neuropathy, the patient may not feel minor trauma or burns, leading to traumatic injuries. Some hereditary neuropathies may have ataxia as a prominent finding, often overshadowing the neuropathy. Examples are Friedreich ataxia, adrenoleukodystrophy, and Krabbe disease.

Diagnostic Evaluation

Diagnosis of chronic polyneuropathies is made by electrophysiologic testing with EMG/NCS. CSF protein levels can be elevated, sometimes with an increased IgG index. Nerve biopsy, though rarely needed, may show varying patterns of abnormalities depending on the cause of the neuropathy. Muscle biopsy may show a denervation pattern. Some hereditary neuropathies are associated with identifiable and occasionally treatable metabolic errors (described in more detail in Chapter 36). Other laboratory studies directed toward specific causes mentioned above include screening for heavy metals and for metabolic, renal, or vascular disorders. Gene panels are commercially available for inherited neuropathies and may identify the few treatable inherited neuropathies.

Treatment & Prognosis

Therapy is directed at specific disorders whenever possible. In patients with CIDP, treatment includes corticosteroids, alone or in combination with other immunomodulatory treatments. Identification of secondary causes of CIDP is important, since other autoimmune disorders, thyroid disease, and infectious etiologies can be associated with CIDP. For chronic neuropathies, physical therapy and management of pain and discomfort are the mainstays of management.

The long-term prognosis varies with the cause and the ability to offer specific therapy. Children with CIDP typically have a more favorable outcome than adult patients. Genetic counseling of patients with inherited polyneuropathies is important for not only the patients, but their families as well. Generally, the course is one of slow progression of distal weakness, but the phenotypic and genotypic variability of the inherited polyneuropathies is broad.

Bordini BJ, Monrad P: Differentiating familial neuropathies from Guillain-Barre syndrome. Pediatr Clin North Am 2017;64(1): 231–252 [PMID: 27894447].

Harada Y et al: Pediatric CIDP: clinical features and response to treatment. J Clin Neuromuscul Dis 2017;19(2):57–65 [PMID: 29189550].

Shy M, Gutmann L: Update on Charcot-Marie-Tooth disease. Curr Opin Neurol 2015;28(5):462–467 [PMID: 26263471].

MOTOR NEURON DISORDERS

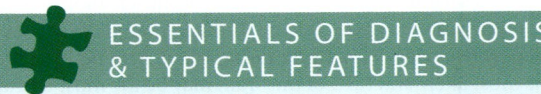

ESSENTIALS OF DIAGNOSIS & TYPICAL FEATURES

► Spinal muscular atrophy (SMA) is the most common cause of lower motor neuron disease.

► Weakness, hypotonia, absent reflexes, and fasciculations in an alert and bright-eyed child should suggest SMA.

► Commercially available treatments are available for SMA; therefore, early diagnosis is crucial to prevent permanent disability.

Pathogenesis

Spinal muscular atrophy (SMA) occurs in about 1 in 11,000 live births and is caused by autosomal recessive mutations in *SMN1*. The lack of survival motor neuron (SMN) protein results in progressive degeneration of the lower motor neurons in the spinal cord and brainstem. The phenotype is modified by the number of copies of *SMN2*, which encodes the same protein but contains an exonic splice enhancer that results in skipping of exon 7, leading to an unstable, truncated protein product that provides about 10%–20% of total SMN function.

Clinical Findings

SMA has a broad range of phenotypes, classified as type 0–4 by the patient's best functional ability. In general, the higher the copy number of *SMN2*, the milder the clinical phenotype. For instance, SMA type 1 patients typically have no more than 2 copies of *SMN2*, while types 3 and 4 patients have 4 or more copies. In SMA type 0, patients have prenatal onset of severe weakness and joint contractures. These patients often die in utero or shortly after birth. SMA type 1 is the most common type, and symptoms appear prior to 6 months of age. These patients appear normal at birth but develop progressive hypotonia and weakness in the first few weeks to months of life, and never achieve the ability to sit. They develop progressive difficulty with feeding and respiratory weakness. Without intervention, they die from respiratory failure by 2 years of age. Patients with SMA type 2 typically present between 6 and 18 months of age with delayed motor milestones. While they may achieve the ability to sit independently, they may later lose this ability. Patients with SMA type 3 achieve the ability to walk but typically lose that skill. Finally, patients with SMA type 4 present in adulthood with weakness. Patients with SMA have absent reflexes and tongue fasciculations, though fasciculations may be difficult to appreciate in milder forms of the disease. Many patients with SMA also demonstrate a tremor, which may be particularly noticeable in types 3 and 4. It is important to note that with early treatment of SMA becoming more common, classification of SMA (ie, type 0-4) is likely to change in the coming years.

Diagnostic Evaluation

Newborn screening is available for SMA in most states, but a negative screen does not exclude the diagnosis, since approximately 5% of patients carry mutations not detected by the screen. Commercially available genetic testing for *SMN1* deletions, duplications and sequence variants has allowed rapid diagnosis of SMA. Electrophysiologic testing and muscle biopsy are no longer used in the diagnosis of this disorder. Serum CK, if obtained, can be normal to mildly increased to the 500 IU/L range.

Differential Diagnosis

The diagnostic considerations for a hypotonic infant with absent reflexes include other primary neuromuscular disorders, such as **congenital myopathies**, **congenital muscular dystrophies**, and **congenital myasthenic syndromes**. Patients with CNS disorders are typically encephalopathic and have normal or increased reflexes, in contrast to patients with SMA, who appear bright-eyed and alert. Tongue fasciculations are rarely seen in children who do not have SMA.

Treatment & Prognosis

Historically, only supportive care was offered to patients with SMA. With rapid advancements in neuromuscular research, the treatment landscape has markedly changed. Nusinersen (Spinraza) is a commercially available antisense oligonucleotide that targets the *SMN2* gene product to include exon 7 and produce a full-length SMN protein. It is administered intrathecally, periodically for life. It has been shown to improve motor and respiratory function in patients. A similar medication, risdiplam (Evrysdi), can be given orally and was recently approved for children and infants of all ages. Gene therapy with onasemnogene abeparvovec-xioi (Zolgensma) replaces full-length *SMN1* as a single intravenous treatment and is approved for patients younger than 2 years. Early treatment results in dramatically better outcomes, underscoring the importance of early recognition and diagnosis. While targeted treatments are available, supportive care, monitoring and management of respiratory insufficiency, nutrition, and orthopedic issues remain crucial.

Finkel RS et al: Diagnosis and management of spinal muscular atrophy: part 1. Neuromuscul Disord 2018;28(3):197–207 [PMID: 29290580].

Finkel RS et al: Nusinersen versus sham control in infantile-onset spinal muscular atrophy. N Engl J Med 2017;377(18):1723–1732 [PMID: 29091570].

Mercuri E et al: Diagnosis and management of spinal muscular atrophy: part 2. Neuromuscul Disord 2018;28(2):103–115 [PMID: 29305137].

Nicolau S et al: Spinal muscular atrophy. Semin Pediatri Neurol 2021;37:100878 [PMID: 33892848].

THE FLOPPY INFANT

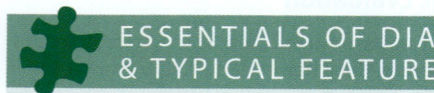

ESSENTIALS OF DIAGNOSIS & TYPICAL FEATURES

► Classic maneuvers to evaluate a floppy infant include checking vertical suspension, horizontal suspension, and traction response.

► Correct interpretation of neurologic findings in a hypotonic infant is dependent on a thorough knowledge of normal childhood development.

Pathogenesis

An infant may present with hypotonia due to dysfunction at any place along the neuroaxis, from the brain, spinal cord, nerve, neuromuscular junction, or muscle. Figure 25–8 provides a diagnostic algorithm for the "floppy infant" based on clinical features. Approximately 80% of hypotonic infants have a central rather than peripheral cause. Additionally, systemic disorders, metabolic disease, malnutrition and genetic disorders may cause an infant to appear "floppy." The evaluation of the hypotonic infant is therefore one of the most challenging diagnostic problems that a pediatrician is often faced with. The diagnostic workup requires a thorough knowledge of normal developmental milestones, careful assessment of the pre- and perinatal history, family history, developmental history, and evaluation of other systemic involvement.

Clinical Findings

In the young infant, horizontal suspension (ie, supporting the infant with a hand under the chest) normally results in the infant holding its head slightly up (45 degrees or less), the back straight or nearly so, the arms flexed at the elbows and slightly abducted, and the knees partly flexed. The "floppy" infant droops over the hand like an inverted U. The normal newborn attempts to keep the head in the same plane as the body when pulled up from supine to sitting by the hands (traction response). Marked head lag is characteristic of the floppy infant. Held under the armpits in vertical suspension, the hypotonic infant will slip through the examiner's hands. Hyperextensibility of the joints may or may not be present. Decreased antigravity movements of the extremities may help differentiate weakness (decreased strength) from hypotonia (decreased resting tone)—not all hypotonic infants are weak.

Diagnostic Evaluation

A general rule for diagnostic testing is to localize the etiology of the hypotonia. For instance, if a lower motor neuron or muscle etiology is suspected, genetic testing for SMA followed by a serum CK, EMG/NCS, and/or muscle biopsy may be appropriate as first-tier testing. If the hypotonia is accompanied by language or cognitive delay, a CNS or genetic disorder is most likely and MRI of the brain may be the most useful diagnostic test. See Table 25–7 for a diagnostic algorithm.

Differential Diagnosis

The most common etiology of hypotonia in the neonate is **HIE**. Dysmorphic features may suggest a genetic etiology such as **Down syndrome** or **Prader-Willi syndrome**, which results in dramatic hypotonia. Abnormalities of the hair or skin, which form from the neuroectoderm in development with the brain, may prompt an evaluation for brain malformations. Seizures, language difficulties, or cognitive delay may also accompany **brain malformations** and

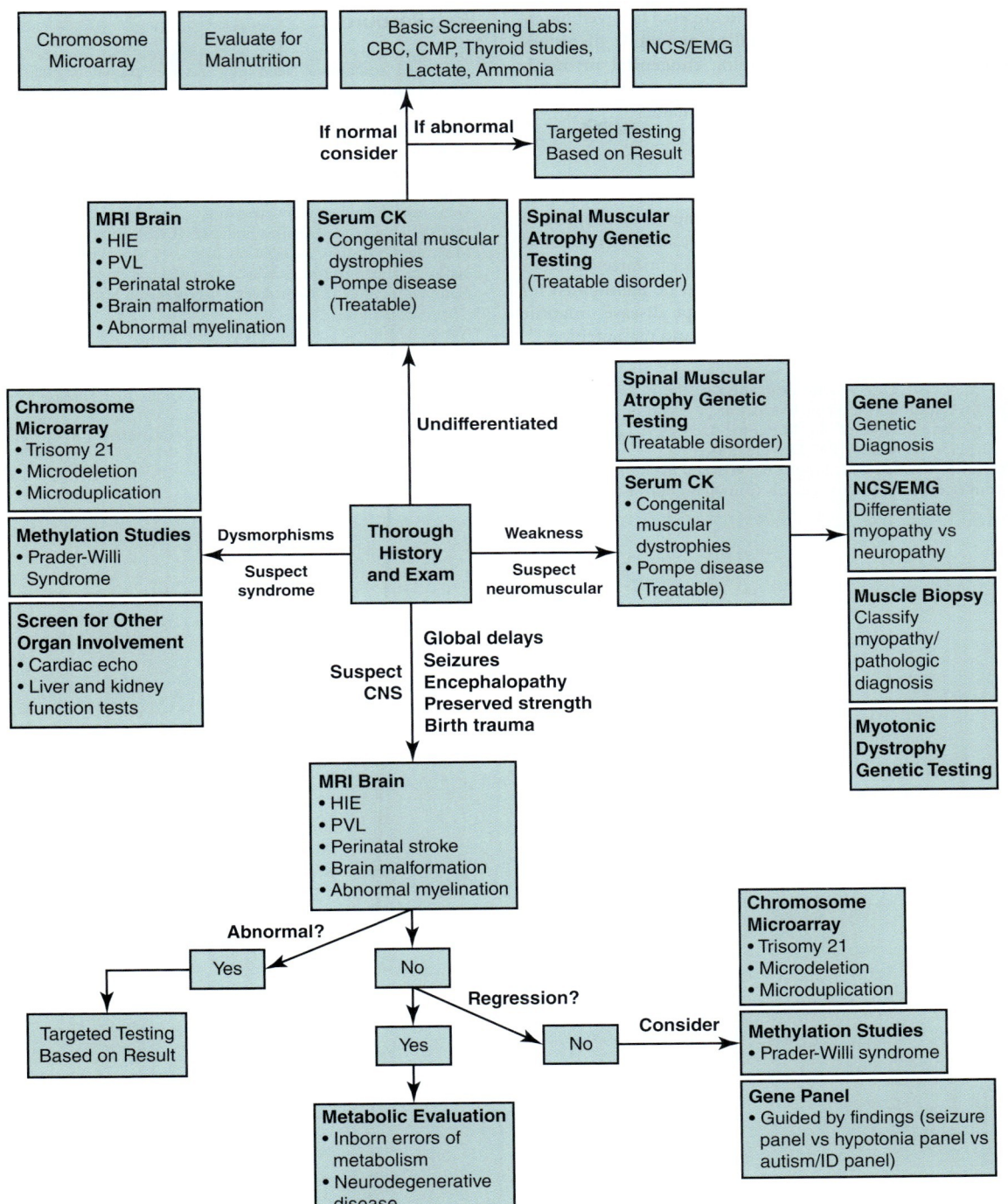

▲ **Figure 25–8.** Algorithm for evaluating the floppy infant. CBC, complete blood count; CMP, comprehensive metabolic panel; CNS, central nervous system; HIE, hypoxic-ischemic encephalopathy; NCS/EMG, nerve conduction studies/electromyography; PVL, periventricular leukomalacia.

other central causes of hypotonia. Regression in development is often a clue for **mitochondrial or metabolic disorders**. Neuromuscular disorders, including **congenital myotonic dystrophy** and **SMA**, can present as hypotonia with concomitant weakness and contractures in the infant.

Treatment

Treatment for many of these disorders is supportive. Physical and occupational therapy can facilitate some progress to a varying degree. Accompanying seizures and other systemic manifestations should be controlled to optimize development. A high index of suspicion should be maintained for treatable disorders such as SMA, Pompe disease, infantile botulism, inborn errors of metabolism, and malnutrition.

Lisi EC, Cohn RD: Genetic evaluation of the pediatric patient with hypotonia: perspective from a hypotonia specialty clinic and review of the literature. Dev Med Child Neurol 2011;53(7):586–599 [PMID: 2148198].

Mercuri E, Carmela PM, Brogna C: Neonatal hypotonia and neuromuscular conditions. Handb Clin Neurol 2019;162:435–448 [PMID: 31324324].

Web Resources

American Academy of Neurology Practice Parameters: http://www.aan.com.
American Epilepsy Society: http://www.aesnet.org.
Child Neurology Foundation: http://www.childneurologyfoundation.org.
Child Neurology Society: http://www.childneurologysociety.org.
Families of Spinal Muscular Atrophy: http://www.fsma.org/.
Gene tests: http://www.genetests.org.
International League Against Epilepsy (ILAE): https://www.ilae.org.
Muscular Dystrophy Association: http://www.mda.org.
National Ataxia Foundation http://www.ataxia.org.
National Institute of Neurologic Disorders and Stroke: http://www.ninds.nih.gov.
National Multiple Sclerosis Society http://nmss.org.
Neurofibromatosis Foundation: http://www.nf.org.
Tuberous Sclerosis Association: http://www.tsalliance.org.
Washington University, St. Louis, Neuromuscular Disease Center: http://neuromuscular.wustl.edu.
We Move: worldwide education and awareness for movement disorders: http://wemove.org.

Orthopedics

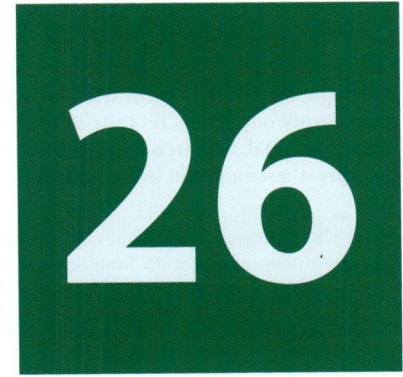

Jason T. Rhodes, MD, MS

Scott Miller, MS

Austin Skinner, BS

Alex Tagawa, BS

Sayan De, MD

26

INTRODUCTION

Orthopedics is the medical discipline that deals with disorders of the musculoskeletal system. Patients with orthopedic problems generally present with one or more of the following complaints: pain, swelling, loss of function, or deformity. Physical examination and radiographic imaging are vitally important features of orthopedic diagnosis.

DISTURBANCES OF PRENATAL ORIGIN

 ESSENTIALS OF DIAGNOSIS & TYPICAL FEATURES

- ▶ Conditions are present at birth (congenital).
- ▶ Multiple organ systems may be involved.
- ▶ Treatment is aimed at maximizing function.

CONGENITAL AMPUTATIONS & LIMB DEFICIENCIES

▶ Clinical Findings

A. Symptoms and Signs

The specific etiology of many congenital amputations is not clear, but a genetic association has been suggested. Some congenital amputations may be due to teratogens (eg, drugs or viruses), amniotic bands, or metabolic diseases (eg, maternal diabetes). Limb deficiencies are rare with an overall prevalence for all types of limb deficiencies of 0.79 per 1000. The most common cause of limb deficiencies is vascular disruption defects (prevalence of 0.22 per 1000). As a group, upper limb deficiencies occur more frequently than

lower limb deficiencies, but the single most frequent form of limb deficiency is congenital longitudinal deficiency of the fibula. Children with congenital limb deficiencies generally also have a high incidence of other congenital anomalies, including genitourinary, cardiac, and palatal defects. Deficiencies have a wide spectrum, ranging from mild limb length discrepancy to significant deformity. They usually consist of a partial absence of structures in the extremity along one side. For example, in radial club hand, the entire radius is absent, but the thumb may be either hypoplastic or completely absent. The effect on structures distal to the deficiency varies. Complex tissue defects are virtually always associated with longitudinal bone deficiency since associated nerves and muscles are not completely represented when a bone is absent.

▶ Treatment

The overall goal of treatment is to achieve a functional extremity. If the deficiency is in a weight-bearing limb, the treatment goal is to achieve mechanical function that is as equal as possible to the opposite side. For less severe deficiencies, methods to attain similar limb lengths include lengthening a limb using distraction osteogenesis (cutting bone and utilizing a distractor to slowly pull the two pieces of bone apart and allow healing to fill the gap created) or shortening a limb acutely or with guided growth (tethering or slowing the growth of one limb while allowing the other limb to continue to grow). More complex limb deformities may require reconstructive surgeries in coordination with lengthening procedures. During the duration of surgical and nonsurgical management, appropriate orthotic fitting is helpful to augment function. For certain severe limb differences, amputation is indicated as the child begins to stand and cruise to allow for early prosthetic fitting and a functional limb, facilitating timely ambulation in a developing child. In unilateral upper extremity amputation, the child may benefit from the use of a passive mitten-type prosthesis starting earlier than

6 months of age. Adaptive prostheses, which are designed specifically for a particular activity such as skiing, biking, or running sports, are used to participate in physical activity. Although myoelectric prostheses have technologic appeal, the majority of patients find the simplest construct to be the most functional. Children quickly learn how to function with their prostheses and can lead active lives.

Gold NB, Westgate MN, Holmes LB: Anatomic and etiological classification of congenital limb deficiencies. Am J Med Genet Part A 2011;155:1225–1235 [PMID: 21557466].

Hamdy RC, Makhdom AM, Saran N, Birch J: Congenital fibular deficiency. J Am Acad Orthop Surg 2014;22:246–255 [PMID: 24668354].

Koller A, Wetz HH. Hilfsmittel bei Fehlbildungen der oberen Extremitäten. Versorgungskonzepte im Wandel der Zeit [Management of upper limb deformities. Treatment concepts through the years]. Orthopade 2006 Nov;35(11):1137–1138, 1140–1142, 1144–1145. German. doi: 10.1007/s00132-006-1019-6 [PMID: 17061077].

DEFORMITIES OF THE EXTREMITIES

ESSENTIALS OF DIAGNOSIS & TYPICAL FEATURES

► Many represent normal physiologic growth patterns.

► Key to diagnosis is recognition of abnormal patterns that deviate from normal development.

► Treatment is varied depending on condition.

COMMON FOOT PROBLEMS

Metatarsus Adductus

► Clinical Findings

A. Symptoms and Signs

Metatarsus adductus, a common congenital foot deformity, is characterized by inward deviation of the forefoot. It is the most common foot abnormality, observed in newborns at a rate of 1–2 per 1000 live births. When the deformity is more rigid, it is characterized by a vertical crease in the medial aspect of the arch. Angulation occurs at the base of the fifth metatarsal causing prominence of this bone. Most flexible deformities are secondary to intrauterine positioning and usually resolve spontaneously. Several investigators have noticed that 10%–15% of children with metatarsus adductus have hip dysplasia; therefore, a careful hip examination is necessary. The etiology of rigid deformities is unknown.

► Treatment

Fully flexible deformity requires no treatment. If the deformity is rigid and cannot be manipulated past the midline, it is worthwhile to perform serial casting, with cast changes in 1- to 2-week intervals, to correct the deformity. Orthoses and corrective shoes do not improve symptoms; however, they can be used to maintain the correction obtained by casting.

Gonzales AS, Mendez MD: Intoeing (Pigeon Toes, Femoral Anteversion, Tibial Torsion, Metatarsus Adductus); National Center for Biotechnology Information, U.S. National Library of Medicine, 27 Oct 2018 [PMID: 29763169].

Williams CM, James AM, Tran T: Metatarsus adductus: development of a non-surgical treatment pathway. J Paediatr Child Health 2014;49(9):428–433 [PMID: 23647850].

Clubfoot (Talipes Equinovarus)

► Clinical Findings

A. Symptoms and Signs

Congenital talipes equinovarus (CTEV), or clubfoot, requires four clinical deformities for diagnosis: (1) high arch (cavus), (2) medial deviation of the forefoot (adductus), (3) inversion deformity of the heel (varus), and (4) plantar flexion of the ankle joint (equinus) (Figure 26–1). Clubfoot occurs in approximately 1–2 per 1000 live births. The three major categories of clubfoot are idiopathic, neurogenic, and those associated with syndromes such as arthrogryposis and Larsen syndrome. Infants with a clubfoot should be examined carefully for associated anomalies, especially of the spine. Idiopathic club feet can be transmitted between generations, suggesting a hereditary component.

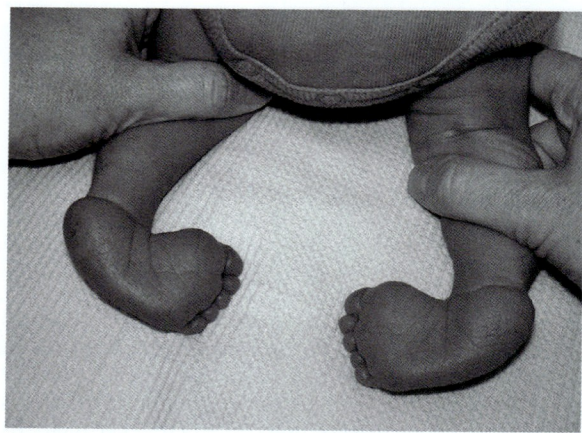

▲ **Figure 26–1.** Clubfoot in an infant.

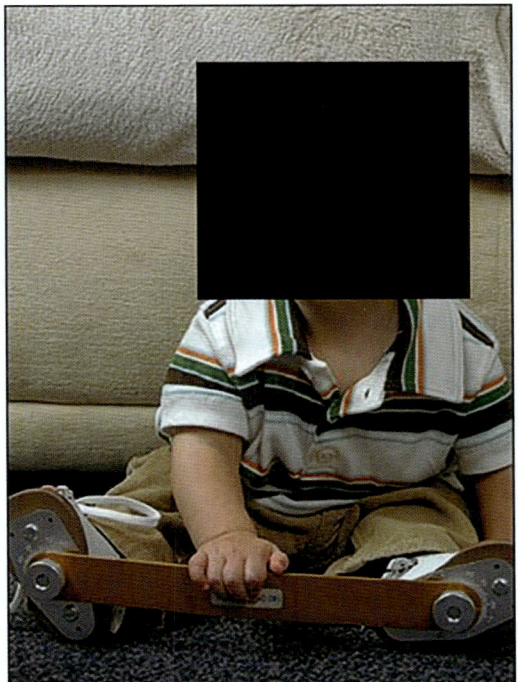

▲ **Figure 26–2.** Ponseti technique: utilizing a clubfoot brace to keep the fixed feet in the correct position.

▶ **Treatment**

Nonoperative management using the Ponseti technique or the French physiotherapy method yields good functional outcomes for children with clubfeet. The Ponseti technique is the more common method, utilizing serial manipulation with casting on a weekly basis for 6–8 weeks to correct the 4 deformities, followed by bracing until school age (Figure 26–2). Surgical management may be necessary for residual deformity (ie, persistent equinus or dynamic inversion), a complex clubfoot, or a foot recalcitrant to nonoperative methods.

Chen C, Kaushal N, Scher DM, Doyle SM, Blanco JS, Dodwell ER: Clubfoot etiology: a meta-analysis and systematic review of observational and randomized trials. J Pediatr Orthop 2018;38(8):e462–e469 [PMID: 29917009].
Graf A, Wu KW, Smith PA, Kuo KN, Krzak J, Harris G: Comprehensive review of the functional outcome evaluation of clubfoot treatment: a preferred methodology. J Pediatr Orthop 2012; 27(1):93–104 [PMID: 19963172].
Miller NH et al: Does strict adherence to the Ponseti method improve isolated clubfoot treatment outcomes? A two-institution review. Clin Orthop Relat Res 2015:1–7. doi: 10.1007/s11999-015-4559-4 [PMID: 26394639].

Talipes Calcaneovalgus

▶ **Clinical Findings**

A. Symptoms and Signs

Talipes calcaneovalgus is characterized by excessive dorsiflexion at the ankle and eversion of the foot (Figure 26–3). This disorder can be associated with posteromedial bowing of the tibia and is due to intrauterine position and is often present at birth. The deformity occurs in 0.4–1.0 per 1000 live births.

▶ **Treatment**

Treatment consists of passive exercises, such as stretching the foot into plantar flexion. With or without treatment, the deformity usually resolves by age 3–6 months. In rare instances, it may be necessary to use plaster casts to help with manipulation and positioning. Complete correction is the rule.

"Calcaneovalgus Foot." Orthobullets, Lineage Medical Inc, 2 May 2018, www.orthobullets.com/pediatrics/4067/calcaneovalgus-foot.
Sankar WN, Weiss J, Skaggs DL: Orthopedic conditions in the newborn. J Am Acad Orthop Surg 2009;17(2):112–122 [PMID: 19202124].

Flatfoot

▶ **Clinical Findings**

A. Symptoms and Signs

Flatfoot is normal in infants. If the heel cord is of normal length, full dorsiflexion is possible when the heel is in the neutral position. If the heel cord is of normal length and

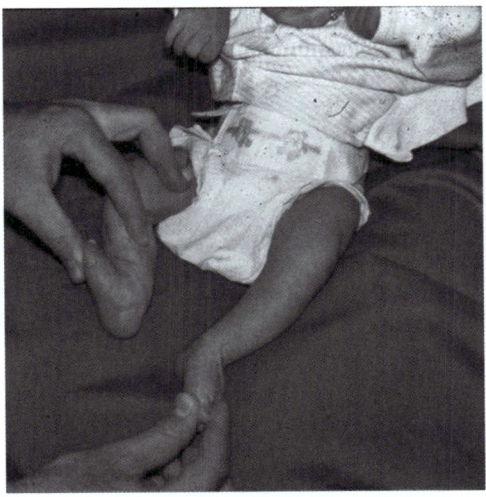

▲ **Figure 26–3.** Excessive dorsiflexion and eversion of the foot in talipes calcaneovalgus.

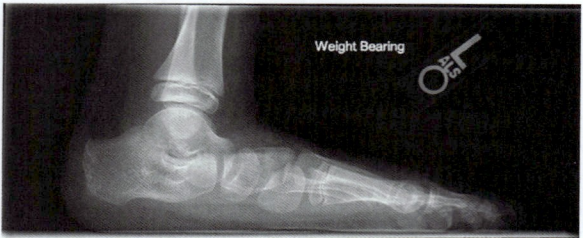

▲ **Figure 26–4.** Planovalgus foot deformity (flat foot).

a longitudinal arch is noted when the child is sitting in a non–weight-bearing position, a normal arch will generally develop.

Younger children who are male, obese, and have excessive joint laxity are more likely to be flatfooted. Around 15% of flatfeet do not resolve spontaneously (Figure 26–4). There is usually a familial incidence of flexible flatfeet in children who have no apparent arch. In any child with a shortened heel cord, pain, or stiffness of the foot, other causes of flatfoot such as tarsal coalition (congenital fusion of the tarsal bones) should be ruled out by a complete orthopedic examination, plain radiographs, and, sometimes, advanced imaging.

▶ **Treatment**

For an ordinary correctable flatfoot, no active treatment is indicated unless pain is present. In children who have leg pains attributable to flatfoot, a supportive shoe can be helpful. An orthotic that holds the heel in neutral position and supports the arch may relieve discomfort if more support is needed. An arch insert should not be prescribed unless passive correction of the arch is easily accomplished; otherwise, the skin over the medial side of the foot will be irritated. Surgical correction can be done; however, surgery has been found to only improve symptoms associated with shoe or brace wear such as pain, calluses, or skin breakdown, with limited improvement of the planovalgus deformity. Therefore, surgical correction should only be done in individuals with severe symptoms.

Bouchard M, Mosca VS: Flatfoot deformity in children and adolescents: surgical indications and management. J Am Acad Orthop Surg 2014;10:623–632 [PMID: 25281257].
Ford SE, Scannell BP: Pediatric flatfoot: pearls and pitfalls. Foot Ankle Clin 2017 Sep;22(3):643–656 [PMID: 28779814].

Cavus Foot

▶ **Clinical Findings**

A. Symptoms and Signs

Cavus foot consists of an unusually high longitudinal arch of the foot (Figure 26–5). It may be hereditary or associated with

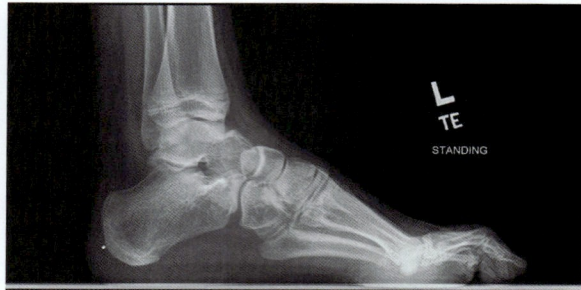

▲ **Figure 26–5.** Cavus foot.

neurologic conditions such as poliomyelitis, hereditary sensory motor neuropathies, tethered spinal cord, cerebral palsy, lipomeningocele, and diastematomyelia (congenital splitting of the spinal cord). Typically, there is an associated contracture of the toe extensors, producing a claw toe deformity in which the metatarsophalangeal joints are hyperextended and the interphalangeal joints are flexed. Cavus foot presents with diffuse and localized pain in the lower legs and is commonly associated with an inflexible foot deformity. Any child presenting with progressive cavus feet should receive a careful neurologic examination as well as radiographs and magnetic resonance imaging (MRI) of the spine and possible electromyography workup for neuromuscular disorder.

▶ **Treatment**

Conservative therapy, such as an orthotic to realign the foot, can be effective in milder cases. In moderate to severe cases, surgery may be necessary to lengthen the contracted extensor and flexor tendons and release the plantar fascia; occasionally, osteotomies are needed to correct the position of the medial column or hindfoot. If the deformity is secondary to a neurologic etiology, management of the neurologic condition is prioritized to prevent recurrence of deformity postoperatively.

Eleswarapu AS, Yamini B, Bielski RJ: Evaluating the cavus foot. Pediatr Ann 2016 Jun 1;45(6):e218–e222. doi: 10.3928/00904481-20160426-01 [PMID: 27294497].
Grice J, Willmontt J, Taylor H: Assessment and management of cavus foot deformity. Orthop Trauma 2016;30(1):68–74. doi: 10.1016/j.mporth.2016.02.001.

Bunions (Hallux Valgus)

▶ **Clinical Findings**

A. Symptoms and Signs

With a prevalence of 23%–35%, hallux valgus (bunion) is the most common forefoot deformity. The etiology is unknown. Adolescents may present with lateral deviation of the great toe associated with a prominence over the head of the first metatarsal. Around 60% of patients have a family history of this condition. The deformity is painful with shoe wear and almost always relieved by fitting shoes that are wide enough in the toe area (wide toe box). Since further growth tends to cause recurrence of the deformity, surgery should be avoided in the adolescent.

Treatment

Therapeutic treatments are aimed at correcting the muscular and weight-bearing forces that act on the joint. While conservative treatment provides symptomatic relief, it does not reverse the natural history, as these deformities will typically continue to progress until corrected surgically. A high percentage of these patients ultimately have surgery in adulthood due to a continued progression of the deformity through childhood and adolescence. Surgical treatment should be delayed until the patient is mature, due to the risk of recurrence of deformity. Surgery leads to satisfactory outcomes in 95% of patients.

Greene JD, Nicholson AD, Sanders JO, Cooperman DR, Liu RW: Analysis of serial radiographs of the foot to determine normative values for the growth of the first metatarsal to guide hemiepiphysiodesis for immature hallux valgus. J Pediatr Orthop 2017;37(5):338–343 [PMID: 26509315].

Sabah Y et al: Lateral hemiepiphysiodesis of the first metatarsal for juvenile hallux valgus. J Orthop Surg (Hong Kong) 2018;26(3):2309499018801135 [PMID: 30270740].

Wulker N, Mittag F: The treatment of hallux valgus. Dtsch Arztebl Int 2012;109(49):857–867; quiz 868 [PMID: 23267411].

GENU VARUM & GENU VALGUM

Clinical Findings

A. Symptoms and Signs

Genu varum (bowleg) is normal from infancy through 3 years of age. The alignment then changes to genu valgum (knock-knee, Figure 26–6) until about age 8 years, at which time adult alignment of 5–9 degrees of anatomic valgus is attained. If bowing persists beyond age 3, increases rather than decreases, occurs in only one leg, or if a patient is knock-kneed in association with short stature, the patient should be referred to an orthopedist. Pathologic genu varum is usually secondary to tibial rotation (Blount disease, proximal tibial epiphysial dysplasia, Figure 26–7), while pathologic genu valgum may be caused by skeletal dysplasia or rickets.

Treatment

Individuals with genu varum may be at a greater risk for future osteoarthritis due to possible changes in gait kinematics. Bracing may be appropriate. An osteotomy may be necessary for severe problems, such as occurs in Blount disease.

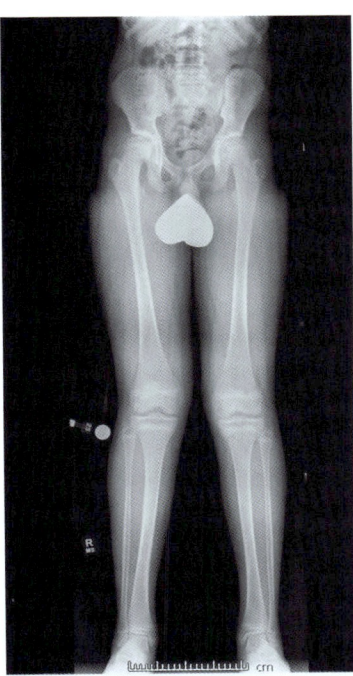

▲ **Figure 26–6.** Idiopathic genu valgum.

American Academy of Orthopaedic Surgeons: "Bowed Legs (Blount's Disease)–OrthoInfo AAOS." *OrthoInfo*, Feb 2015. orthoinfo. aaos.org/en/diseases–conditions/bowed-legs-blounts-disease/.

TIBIAL TORSION & FEMORAL ANTEVERSION (INTOEING)

Clinical Findings

A. Symptoms and Signs

"Intoeing" in small children is a common parental concern. Intoeing is usually due to either femoral anteversion or tibial torsion. Femoral anteversion is characterized by the presence of more internal rotation of the knees compared to the hips while tibial torsion refers to rotation of the leg between the knee and the ankle. These conditions usually do not cause any gait or ambulatory issues but may cause tripping, more commonly during running activities. Families will usually notice the intoeing later in the day, after school or activities, which is due to weakness of the hip external rotator musculature that is used to compensate for intoeing throughout the day. Femoral anteversion and tibial torsion are largely self-limiting, usually resolving spontaneously with further growth and development. Tibial torsion will continue to remodel up to 8–10 years of age in females and 10–12 in males, and femoral anteversion will continue to remodel another 2–4 years after this.

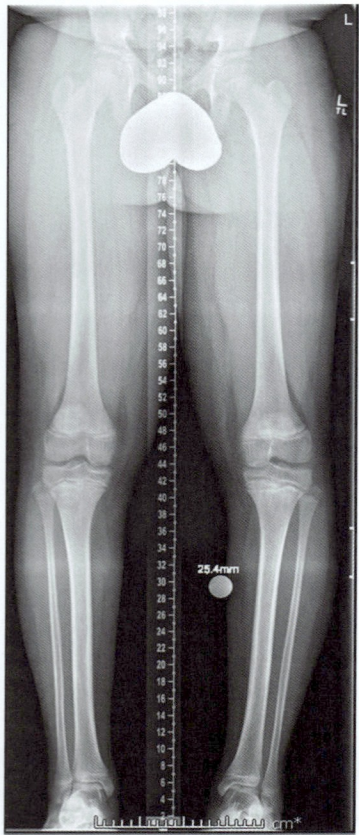

▲ **Figure 26–7.** Blount's disease with genu varum.

▶ **Treatment**

Treatment consists of education of patients and families as to the benign natural history of intoeing. Patients do not need an in-depth workup unless intoeing continues until 8–10 years of age and/or causes functional ambulatory issues. Physical therapy can be done to help improve hip and core strengthening. If there is a true bone rotational deformity, surgical treatment is required for correction, but it is usually only considered if the rotational deformity is symptomatic and is not generally performed until the patient is close to skeletal maturity.

Davids JR, Davis RB, Jameson LC, Westberry DE, Hardin JW: Surgical management of persistent intoeing gait due to increased internal tibial torsion in children. J Pediatr Orthop 2014;34(4):467–473 [PMID: 24531409].

Lincoln TL, Suen PW: Common rotational variations in children. J Am Acad Orthop Surg 2003;11:312 [PMID: 14565753].

Nourai MH, Fadaei B, Rizi AM: In-toeing and out-toeing gait conservative treatment; hip anteversion and retroversion: 10-year follow-up. J Res Med Sci 2015;20(11):1084–1087 [PMID: 26941813].

DEVELOPMENTAL DYSPLASIA OF THE HIP JOINT

▶ Clinical Findings

Developmental dysplasia of the hip (DDH) encompasses a spectrum of conditions where an abnormal relationship exists between the proximal femur and the acetabulum. In the most severe condition, the femoral head is not in contact with the acetabulum and is classified as a *dislocated hip*. In a *dislocatable hip*, the femoral head is within the acetabulum but can be dislocated with a provocative maneuver. A *subluxatable hip* is one in which the femoral head comes partially out of the joint with a provocative maneuver. *Acetabular dysplasia* is used to denote insufficient acetabular development and is a radiographic diagnosis. Congenital dislocation of the hip more commonly affects the left hip, occurring in approximately 1%–3% of newborns. At birth, both the acetabulum and femur are underdeveloped (Figure 26–8). The four major risk factors for DDH are first-born child, female gender, breech presentation, and family history of DDH.

A. Symptoms and Signs

Clinical diagnosis of dislocations in newborns is dependent on demonstrating the instability of the joint by placing the infant on his or her back and obtaining complete relaxation. The examiner's long finger is placed over the greater trochanter and the thumb over the inner side of the thigh. Both hips are flexed 90 degrees and then slowly abducted from the midline, one hip at a time. With gentle pressure, an attempt is made to lift the greater trochanter forward. A feeling of slipping as the head *relocates* is a sign of instability (Ortolani sign). When the joint is more stable, the deformity must be provoked by applying slight pressure with the thumb on the medial side of the thigh as the thigh is adducted, thus slipping

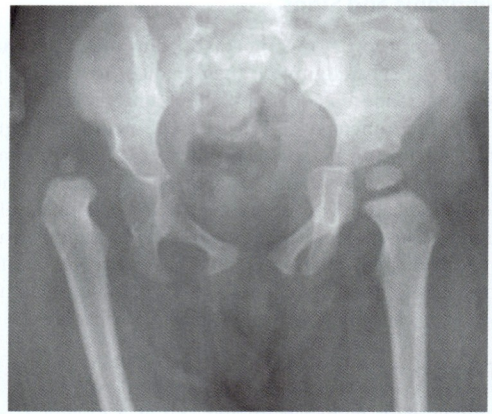

▲ **Figure 26–8.** Radiographic evidence of underdeveloped acetabulum and femur in developmental dysplasia of the hip.

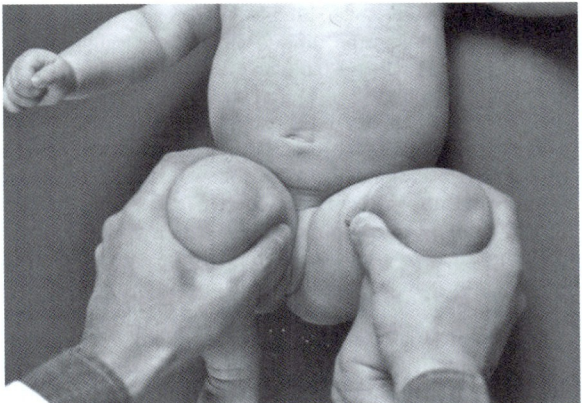

▲ **Figure 26–9.** Ortolani/Barlow examination technique.

the hip posteriorly and eliciting a palpable clunk as the hip *dislocates* (Barlow sign, Figure 26–9). Limited hip abduction of less than 60 degrees while the knee is in 90 degrees of flexion is believed to be the most sensitive sign for detecting a dysplastic hip.

The signs of instability become less evident after the first month of life. If the knees are at unequal heights when the hips and knees are flexed, the dislocated hip will be on the side with the lower knee (Galeazzi sign). When the child stands on the affected leg, a dip of the pelvis will be evident on the opposite side, due to weakness of the gluteus medius muscle (Trendelenburg sign), accounting for the unusual swaying gait.

B. Imaging Studies

Clinical signs of instability are more reliable than radiographs for diagnosing developmental dislocation of the hip in the newborn. Ultrasonography is most useful in newborns and can be helpful for screening high-risk infants, such as those with breech presentation or positive family history. Radiologic examination becomes more valuable after the first 6 weeks of life, with lateral displacement of the femoral head being the most reliable sign. In children with incomplete abduction during the first few months of life, a radiograph of the pelvis is indicated.

▶ Treatment

Dysplasia is progressive with growth unless the instability is corrected. If the dislocation is corrected in the first few weeks of life, the dysplasia can be completely reversible and a normal hip will more likely develop. If the dislocation or subluxation persists with age, the deformity will worsen until it is not completely reversible, especially after the walking age. For this reason, it is important to diagnose the deformity and institute treatment early.

A Pavlik harness, which maintains reduction by placing the hip in a flexed and abducted position, can be easily used

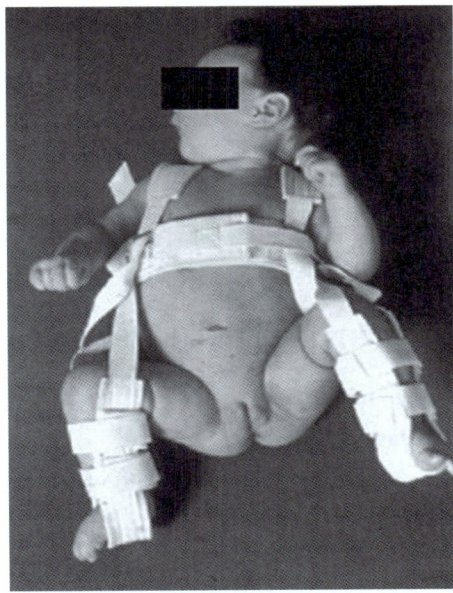

▲ **Figure 26–10.** A Pavlik harness used to treat developmental dysplasia of the hip.

to treat dislocation or dysplasia diagnosed in the first few weeks or months of life (Figure 26–10). To be safely treated in a Pavlik harness, hips must be manually reducible with only gentle manipulation. Treatment with a Pavlik harness in the face of a dislocated hip that does not reduce easily on clinical examination and with mild manipulation leads to Pavlik disease, which causes damage to the femoral head and acetabulum and can make relocation and reconstruction much more difficult. Forced abduction or reduction requiring extremes of motion for stability can lead to avascular necrosis of the femoral head and is contraindicated. An orthopedic surgeon with experience managing the problem is best to supervise treatment.

If a hip cannot be reduced and have a stable reduction with Pavlik treatment, a closed reduction with arthrogram is appropriate treatment. A hip spica cast is used after reduction. If the hip is not stable within a reasonable range of motion after closed reduction, open reduction is indicated.

Closed treatment is possible in the first year of life, but results are superior with early treatment (within the first 6 months of life). In patients older than 18 months, more aggressive surgeries to correct the deformities of the acetabulum and femur, as well as open reduction, are often necessary to create a more normal orientation and shape of the hip joint.

Murphy RF, Kim YJ: Surgical management of pediatric developmental dysplasia of the hip. J Am Acad Orthop Surg 2016 Sep;24(9):615–624 [PMID: 27509038].

Novais EN, Sanders J, Kestel LA, Carry PM, Meyers ML: Graf type-IV hips have a higher risk of residual acetabular dysplasia at 1 year of age following successful Pavlik harness treatment for developmental hip dysplasia. J Pediatr Orthop 2016;38(10):498–502 [PMID: 27662383].

Omeroglu H: Use of ultrasonography in developmental dysplasia of the hip. J Child Orthop 2014;8(2):105–113 [PMID: 24510434].

Wang TM, Wu KW, Shih SF, Huang SC, Kuo KN: Outcomes of open reduction for developmental dysplasia of the hip: does bilateral dysplasia have a poorer outcome? J Bone Joint Surg Am 2013;95(12):1081–1086 [PMID: 23783204].

SLIPPED CAPITAL FEMORAL EPIPHYSIS

▶ Clinical Findings

A. Symptoms and Signs

Slipped capital femoral epiphysis (SCFE) is caused by displacement of the proximal femoral epiphysis due to disruption of the growth plate (Figure 26–11). The head of the femur is usually displaced medially and posteriorly relative to the femoral neck. This condition is most commonly seen in adolescent, obese males. It occurs when stress increases across the proximal femoral physis (growth plate) or resistance to shear is reduced. Factors that can lead to this increase in stress or decrease in resistance include endocrine or renal disorders, obesity, coxa profunda (a deep acetabular socket), and femoral or acetabular retroversion. Retroversion of the femur occurs when the proximal femoral segment is angled posteriorly relative to the shaft of the femur. Acetabular retroversion refers to when the alignment of the opening of the acetabulum does not face the normal anterolateral direction but inclines more posterolaterally.

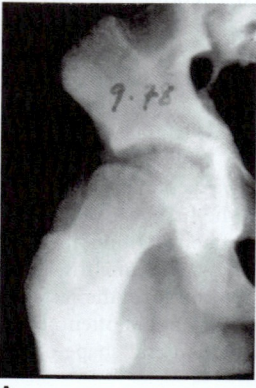 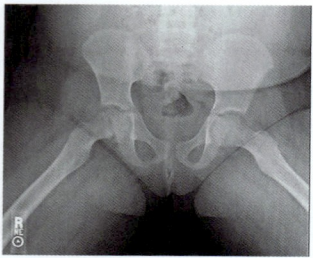

A　　　　　　　　　　**B**

▲ **Figure 26–11.** Radiographic evidence of slipped capital femoral epiphysis.

Clinically, SCFE is classified as stable or unstable. SCFE is considered stable if the child is able to bear weight on the affected extremity. In unstable SCFE, the child is unable to bear weight. An increased rate of avascular necrosis is correlated with the inability to bear weight.

Temporally, SCFE can be classified as acute or chronic. Acute SCFE occasionally occurs following a fall or direct trauma to the hip, with symptoms present for less than 3 weeks. More commonly, in a chronic SCFE, vague symptoms occur over a protracted period in an otherwise healthy child who presents with pain and limp. The pain can be referred into the thigh or the medial side of the knee, making examination of the hip joint important in any obese child complaining of knee pain. Physical examination consistently reveals a limitation of internal rotation of the hip. Appropriate diagnostic workup should include an AP and lateral pelvis radiograph.

▶ Treatment

Initial management consists of making the patient non-weight bearing on crutches and immediate referral to an orthopedic surgeon. Treatment is based on the same principles that govern treatment of any fracture of the femoral neck: the head of the femur is internally fixated in situ to the neck of the femur and the physeal injury allowed to heal. In situ fixation without closed reduction is considered the standard of care for SCFE treatment due to the high risk of avascular necrosis of the femoral head associated with attempted closed reduction (Figures 26–12 to 26–14).

For an SCFE that is significant in terms of displacement, specialized centers are beginning to perform open reduction through a surgical dislocation of the hip, but due to the risk of avascular necrosis of the femoral head, this should only be used by an orthopedic surgeon with experience in this procedure.

▶ Prognosis

The long-term prognosis is guarded because most of these patients continue to be overweight and overstress their hip joints. Follow-up studies have shown a high incidence of premature degenerative arthritis, even in those who do not develop avascular necrosis. The development of avascular necrosis almost guarantees a poor prognosis because new bone does not readily replace the dead bone at this late stage of skeletal development. About 30% of patients have bilateral involvement, which may occur as late as 1 or 2 years after the primary episode.

Kohno Y et al: Is the timing of surgery associated with avascular necrosis after unstable slipped capital femoral epiphysis? A multi-center study. J Orthop Sci 2017;22(1):112–115 [PMID: 27629912].

Novais EN, Millis MB: Slipped capital femoral epiphysis: prevalence, pathogenesis, and natural history. Clin Orthop Relat Res 2012;470(12):3432–3438 [PMID: 23054509].

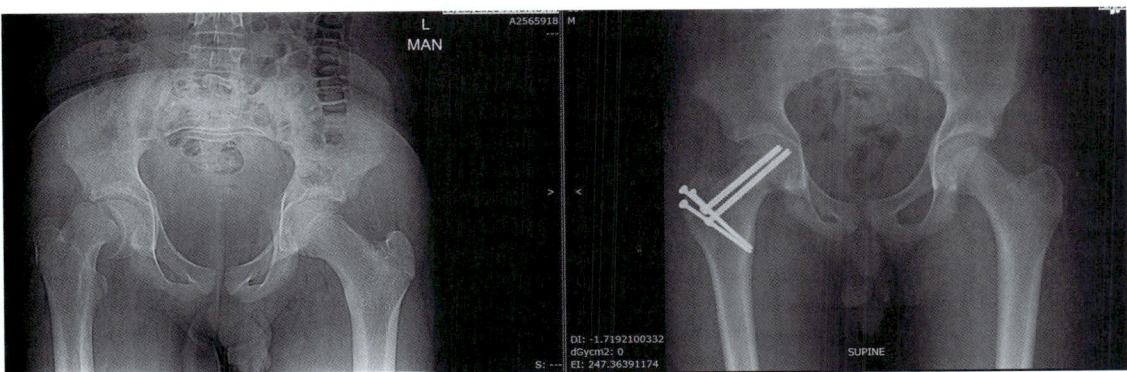

▲ **Figure 26–12.** Preoperative and postoperative comparison of slipped capital femoral epiphysis of the right femur s/p open reduction internal fixation of slipped capital femoral epiphysis through a surgical dislocation approach.

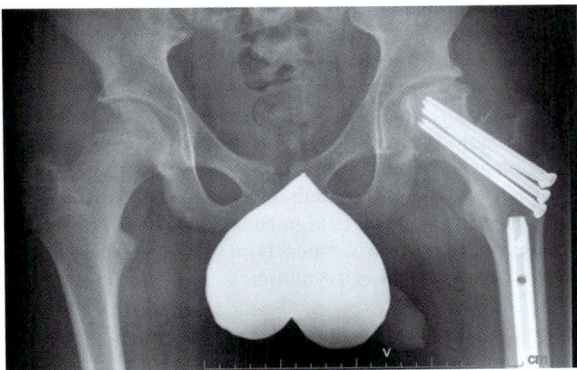

▲ **Figure 26–13.** Radiographic evidence of avascular necrosis after treatment of slipped capital femoral epiphysis with hardware/nails.

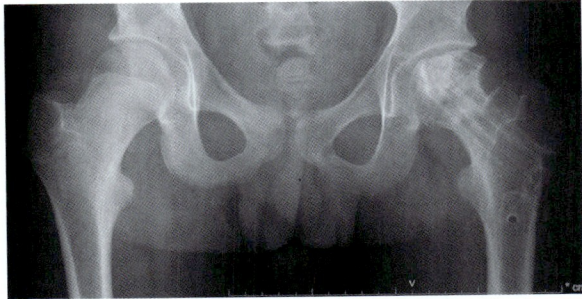

▲ **Figure 26–14.** Radiographic evidence of avascular necrosis after treatment of slipped capital femoral epiphysis without hardware/nails.

COMMON SPINE CONDITIONS

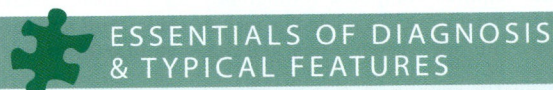

ESSENTIALS OF DIAGNOSIS & TYPICAL FEATURES

► Conditions most often present with a neck or back deformity.
► Treatment varies and is based on risk factors for progression.

BACK PAIN

► Clinical Findings

A. Symptoms and Signs

Back pain in a child may be the result of an acute traumatic event but could also be the only symptom of significant disease and warrants clinical investigation. Inflammation, infection, renal disease, or tumors can cause back pain in children, and sprain should not be accepted as a routine diagnosis. Spondylolysis, a stress injury or fracture that occurs in the lumbar spine along the facet joint, is a common cause of back pain in children and adolescents participating in sports (see Chapter 27). A thorough history and physical examination is warranted to elucidate the etiology of the back pain.

Gurd DP: Back pain in the young athlete. Sports Med Arthrosc Rev 2011;19:7–16 [PMID: 21293233].

TORTICOLLIS

▶ Clinical Findings

A. Symptoms and Signs

Injury to the sternocleidomastoid muscle during delivery or disease affecting the cervical spine in infancy, such as congenital vertebral anomalies, may cause torticollis. When contracture of the sternocleidomastoid muscle causes torticollis, the chin is rotated to the side opposite of the affected muscle, causing the head to tilt toward the side of the contracture (Figure 26–15). A mass felt in the midportion of the sternocleidomastoid muscle in a newborn is likely a hematoma or developmental fibroma, rather than a true tumor.

Acute torticollis may follow upper respiratory infection or mild trauma in children. Upper respiratory infections may lead to swelling in the upper cervical spine, particularly at the C1-C2 region. This swelling renders the C1-C2 articulation susceptible to rotatory subluxation, which commonly presents as torticollis. Rotatory subluxation of the upper cervical spine requires computed tomography for accurate assessment. Other causes of torticollis include spinal cord and cerebellar tumors, syringomyelia, and rheumatoid arthritis.

▶ Treatment

If torticollis in early infancy is left untreated, striking facial asymmetry can persist. Passive stretching is an effective treatment in up to 97% of cases. If the deformity does not correct with passive stretching during the first year of life, surgical release of the muscle origin and insertion can be an effective treatment option. For acquired torticollis in childhood, traction or a cervical collar usually results in resolution of the symptoms within 1 or 2 days.

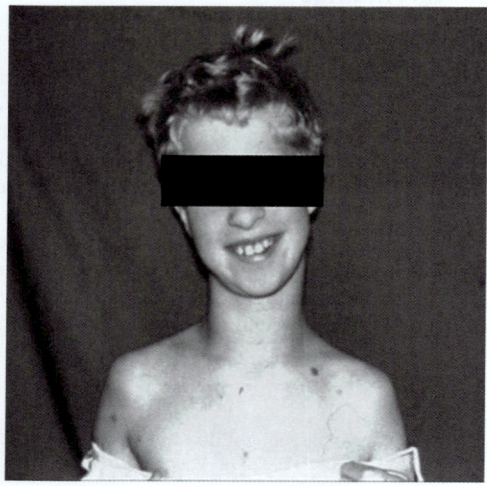

▲ **Figure 26–15.** Torticollis in a young male.

▶ Prognosis

Torticollis is occasionally associated with congenital deformities of the cervical spine. Radiographs of the spine are indicated in most cases when such anomalies are suspected. In addition, there is a 15%–20% incidence of associated hip dysplasia with torticollis.

Lee K, Chung E, Lee BH: A study on asymmetry in infants with congenital muscular torticollis according to head rotation. J Phys Ther Sci 2017;29(1):48–52 [PMID: 28210037].

Tomczak KK, Rosman NP: Torticollis. J Child Neurol 2013;28(3): 365–378 [PMID: 23271760].

SCOLIOSIS

Scoliosis is characterized by lateral curvature of the spine associated with rotation of the involved vertebrae and classified by its anatomic location in either the thoracic or lumbar spine. There are four main categories of scoliosis: idiopathic, congenital, neuromuscular (associated with a neurologic or muscular disease), and syndromic (associated with a known syndrome). Idiopathic scoliosis accounts for around 80% of cases. It is more common in girls and typically develops around 10–12 years of age but can occur earlier. There is a genetic component, but the etiology is multifactorial. Congenital scoliosis accounts for 5%–7% of cases and is a result of vertebral abnormalities due to a failure of formation or segmentation of the affected vertebrae. Cervical spine involvement is rare and is manifested most commonly as Klippel-Feil syndrome.

▶ Clinical Findings

A. Symptoms and Signs

Scoliosis in adolescents does not typically cause significant back pain. Deformity of the rib cage and asymmetry of the waistline are clinically evident for curvatures of 30 degrees or more. Lesser curves may be detected with the Adams Forward Bend test, which is designed to detect early abnormalities of rotation that may not be apparent when the patient is standing erect. Rotation of the spine may be measured with a scoliometer. Rotation is associated with a marked rib hump as the lateral curvature increases in severity.

B. Imaging

Radiographs taken of the entire spine in the standing position in both the posterior-anterior (PA) and lateral planes are the most valuable for diagnosis (Figure 26–16). Usually, a primary curve is evident with compensatory curvature to balance the body.

▶ Treatment

Treatment depends on the curve magnitude, skeletal maturity, and risk of progression, and specific management is

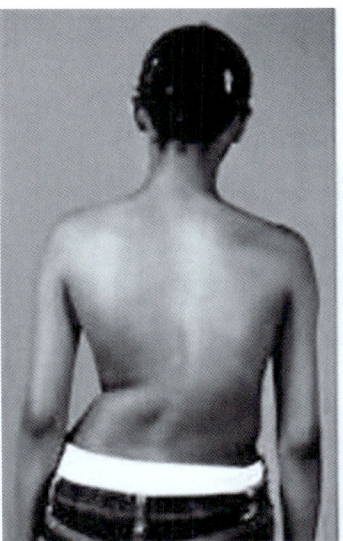
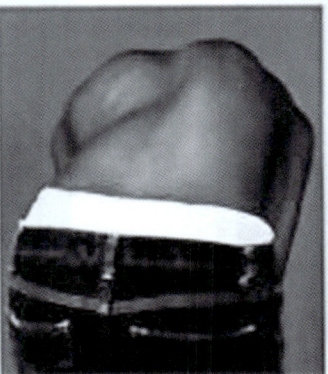
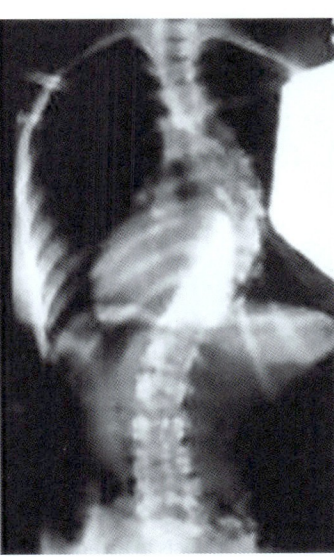

▲ **Figure 26–16.** Clinical and radiographic representation of scoliosis.

guided by the Cobb angle, measured on a standing PA x-ray of the spine. Curvatures of less than 20 degrees typically do not require treatment unless they show progression. Bracing is indicated for curvatures of 20–40 degrees in a skeletally immature child. Curvatures greater than 40 degrees are resistant to treatment by bracing. Thoracic curvatures greater than 70 degrees have been correlated with poor pulmonary function in adult life, leading treatment algorithms toward preventing progression to this extreme. Surgical correction is indicated for curvatures reaching a magnitude of 40–60 degrees as they are highly likely to continue to progress. Surgical intervention consists of spinal instrumentation and fusion. Spinal instrumentation (rods, screws, hooks, etc.) are applied to the region of the spine to be corrected and bone graft is added. Definitive spinal fusions should be delayed, if possible, in young children through the use of casting, bracing, and growth modulating surgeries such as growing rods, vertical expandable prosthetic titanium ribs (VEPTR), or magnetic expansion (MAGEC) rods to reduce anesthetic events and incisional complications.

▶ Prognosis

Compensated small curves that do not progress may cause minor deformities but are well tolerated throughout life. Early detection allows for simple brace treatment when indicated. Severe scoliosis may require correction by spinal fusion. Patients should be counseled about the genetic transmission of scoliosis and cautioned that their children's backs should be examined as part of routine physicals.

Erickson MA, Baulesh DM: Pathways that distinguish simple form complex scoliosis repair and their outcomes. Curr Opin Pediatr 2011;23(3):339–345 [PMID: 21508841]

Kim HJ: Cervical spine anomalies in children and adolescents. Curr Opin Pediatr 2013;25(1):72–77 [PMID: 23263023].

Xue X et al: Klippel-Feil syndrome in congenital scoliosis. Spine (Phila Pa 1976) 2014;39(23):E1353–E1358 [PMID: 25202932].

KYPHOSIS

▶ Clinical Findings

A. Symptoms and Signs

When looking at the sagittal view of a spine, there are two normal curves to be noticed. In the lumbar region, the normal curve with an anterior convexity is known as *lumbar lordosis*. In the thoracic region, a normal curve with a posterior convexity is called *kyphosis*. Excessive kyphosis is pathologic and known as *hyperkyphosis*. Clinically, a visible deformity may be visible on the back, exacerbated by the forward bend test (Figure 26–17). Kyphosis can often accompany scoliosis in which case the two conditions may share a common etiology. Additionally, excessive kyphosis can be caused by trauma and degenerative and inflammatory conditions. Congenital and developmental abnormalities, including Scheuermann disease (disorder characterized by three consecutive vertebrae with anterior wedging), are the most common cause of severe kyphosis. In congenital kyphosis, abnormal vertebrae arise from either a failure of segmentation or formation and commonly result in wedge-shaped vertebrae that cause severe kyphosis.

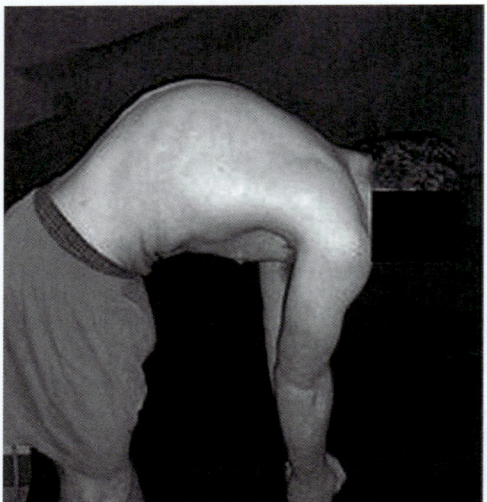

▲ **Figure 26–17.** Kyphosis in an adolescent.

B. Imaging

Standing radiographs taken in the lateral plane are necessary to quantify the severity of the angle of curve of the spine. The curve is typically measured across the thoracic region from T1 to T12. Normal values for this measurement fall in the 20- to 45-degree range; values in excess of 45 degrees are considered pathologic (Figure 26–18).

▶ Treatment

Treatment for kyphosis is similar to that of scoliosis. Mild forms of the deformity may undergo treatment with bracing. Indications for bracing and its effectiveness vary depending on etiology. Surgical intervention with spinal instrumentation and fusion may be indicated for more severe deformities. In patients who have congenital wedge-shaped vertebrae, vertebral column resection may be indicated.

Yaman O, Dalbayrak S: Kyphosis and review of the literature. Turk Neurosurg 2014;24(4):455–465 [PMID: 25050667].

SYNDROMES WITH MUSCULOSKELETAL INVOLVEMENT

ESSENTIALS OF DIAGNOSIS & TYPICAL FEATURES

► Many genetic syndromes include a musculoskeletal component or association.

► Resulting deformity can result in a lack of function.

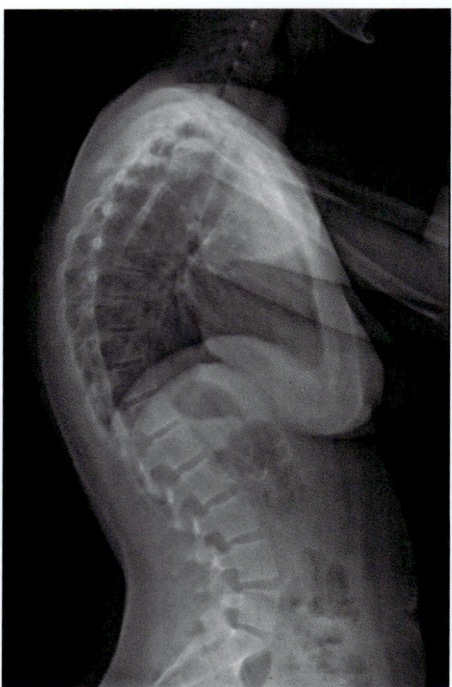

▲ **Figure 26–18.** Lateral radiograph showing severe kyphosis.

ARTHROGRYPOSIS MULTIPLEX CONGENITA (AMYOPLASIA CONGENITA)

▶ Clinical Findings

A. Symptoms and Signs

Arthrogryposis multiplex congenita (AMC) consists of incomplete fibrous ankylosis (usually bilateral) of many or all joints of the body. AMC affects both genders equally and occurs in approximately 1 in 2–3000 live births. Upper extremity contractures usually consist of adduction of the shoulders; extension of the elbows; flexion of the wrists; and stiff, straight fingers with poor muscle control of the thumbs. Common deformities of the lower extremities include dislocation of the hips, extension contractures of the knees, and severe club feet (Figure 26–19). The joints are fusiform, and the joint capsules are decreased in volume due to lack of movement during fetal development. Muscle development is poor and may be represented only by fibrous bands. The basic defect in AMC is attributed to an abnormality of muscle or lower motor neurons.

▶ Treatment

Passive mobilization of joints is the early treatment. Prolonged casting results in further stiffness and is not indicated. Removable splints combined with vigorous therapy

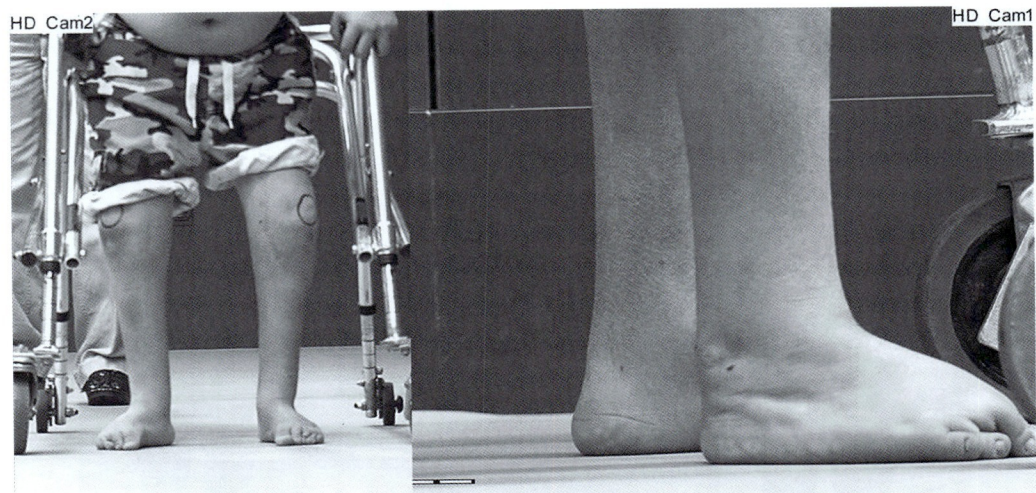

▲ **Figure 26–19.** A child with arthrogryposis with flexion contractures of the knees and severe club feet.

are the most effective conservative treatment; however, surgical release of the affected joints is often necessary. Clubfoot associated with arthrogryposis is very stiff and nearly always requires surgical correction. Knee surgery, including capsulotomy, osteotomy, and tendon lengthening, is used to correct deformities. In young children, a dislocated hip may be reduced operatively by a medial approach. Multiple operative hip procedures are contraindicated, as they may further stiffen the hip dislocation with consequent impairment of motion. Osteotomies are successful in treating some deformities by improving mechanical alignment to improve the function of a lower extremity. Affected children are often able to walk despite dislocations and contractures, but functional gait improves with treatment. The long-term prognosis for physical and vocational independence is guarded. These patients have normal intelligence, but they have such severe physical restrictions that gainful employment is hard to find.

Kalampokas E, Kalampokas T, Sofoudis C, Deligeoroglou E, Botsis D: Diagnosing arthrogryposis multiplex congenital: a review. ISRN Obstet Gynecol 2012;2012:264918 [PMID: 23050160].
Ma L, Yu X: Arthrogryposis multiplex congenital: classification, diagnosis, perioperative care, and anesthesia. Front Med 2017;11(1):48–52 [PMID: 28213879].

MARFAN SYNDROME

▶ Clinical Findings

A. Symptoms and Signs

Marfan syndrome is a connective tissue disorder characterized by unusually long fingers and toes (arachnodactyly); hypermobility of the joints; subluxation of the ocular lenses; other eye abnormalities, including cataract, coloboma, megalocornea, strabismus, and nystagmus; a high-arched palate; a strong tendency to scoliosis; pectus carinatum (an outward protrusion of the sternum); and thoracic aortic aneurysms due to weakness of the media layer (see Chapter 37) (Figures 26–20 to 26–22). Fibrillin-1 gene mutations are commonly associated with Marfan syndrome. Serum mucoproteins may be decreased, and urinary excretion of hydroxyproline increased. The phenotypic presentation is easily confused with homocystinuria, but the two diseases are differentiated by detecting homocysteine in the urine of patients with homocystinuria.

▶ Treatment

Treatment is usually supportive and includes management of blood pressure and restriction of physical activity. Scoliosis may require more vigorous treatment by bracing or spine fusion. The long-term prognosis has improved with better treatment of aortic aneurysms.

Dietz HC: Marfan syndrome. GeneReviews 2017; Internet: [PMID: 20301510].
Lebreiro A et al: Marfan syndrome clinical manifestations, pathophysiology and, new outlook on drug therapy. Rev Port Cardiol 2010;29(6):1021–1036 [PMID: 20964113].

SPRENGEL DEFORMITY

▶ Clinical Findings

A. Symptoms and Signs

Sprengel deformity is a congenital condition in which one or both scapulas are elevated and hypoplastic. The deformity

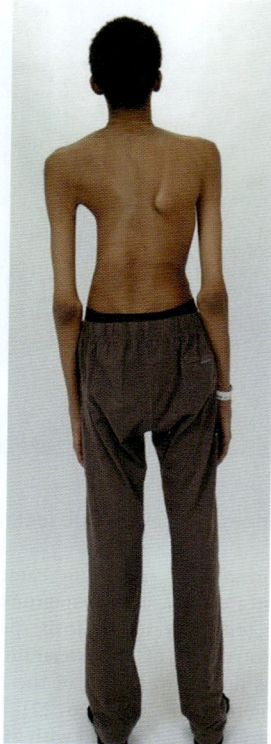

▲ **Figure 26–20.** Patient with Marfan syndrome with pectus carinatum and scoliosis: Posterior view.

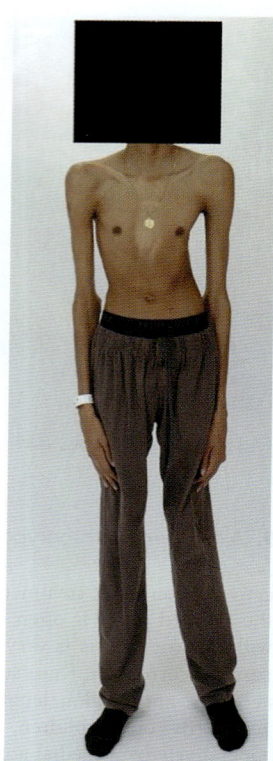

▲ **Figure 26–21.** Patient with Marfan syndrome with pectus carinatum and scoliosis: Anterior view.

prevents the arm from raising completely on the affected side, and torticollis may be an associated finding (Figures 26–23 to 26–25). The deformity occurs alone or in association with Klippel-Feil syndrome or scoliosis and rib abnormalities. If the deformity is functionally limiting, the scapula may be surgically relocated closer to the normal anatomic position. Surgical intervention improves cosmetic appearance and function.

Dhir R, Chin K, Lambert S: The congenital undescended scapula syndrome: Sprengel and the cleithrum: a case series and hypothesis. J Shoulder Elbow Surg 2018;27(2):252–259 [PMID: 28964675].

Harvey EJ, Bernstein M, Desy NM, Saran N, Ouellet JA: Sprengel deformity: pathogenesis and management. J Am Acad Orthop Surg 2012;20(3):177–186 [PMID: 22382290].

OSTEOGENESIS IMPERFECTA

▶ Clinical Findings

A. Symptoms and Signs

Osteogenesis imperfecta is a rare genetic connective tissue disease characterized by multiple and recurrent fractures.

The estimated incidence is 1 in 12,000–15,000. Clinical features of the disease lead to diagnosis in the majority of cases. There are several forms of osteogenesis imperfecta, designated types I–XII; types I–V are the result of autosomal dominant mutations and types VI–XII are autosomal recessive. Each type is associated with a mutation of a different gene, varying levels of severity, and a range of characteristic features. The severe fetal type (osteogenesis imperfecta congenita) is distinguished by multiple intrauterine or perinatal fractures. Moderately affected children have numerous fractures and exhibit dwarfism due to acquired bone deformities and growth retardation. Fractures begin to occur at different times and in variable patterns after the perinatal period, with fewer fractures and deformities relative to severe cases. Other physical characteristics of osteogenesis imperfecta include:

- Reduced cortical thickness in the shafts of the long bones
- Accessory skull bones that are completely surrounded by cranial sutures (wormian bones)
- Blue sclerae
- Thin skin

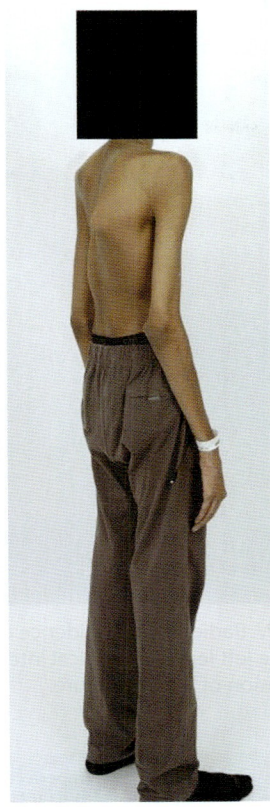

▲ **Figure 26–22.** Patient with Marfan syndrome with pectus carinatum and scoliosis: Posterolateral view.

- Hyperextensibility of ligaments
- Otosclerosis with significant hearing loss
- Hypoplastic and deformed teeth

An olecranon fracture in a child is rare and can be indicative of osteogenesis imperfecta. Affected patients are sometimes suspected of having suffered abuse. Conversely, osteogenesis imperfecta should be ruled out in cases of potential nonaccidental trauma. Cardiovascular and respiratory problems are the most common causes of morbidity and mortality in adulthood. Intelligence is not affected.

▶ **Treatment**

Surgical treatment involves deformity correction of the long bones. Multiple intramedullary rods have been used to decrease the incidence of fractures and prevent deformity from fracture malunion (Figures 26–26 and 26–27). Patients are often confined to wheelchairs during adulthood. Bisphosphonates have been shown to decrease the incidence of fractures.

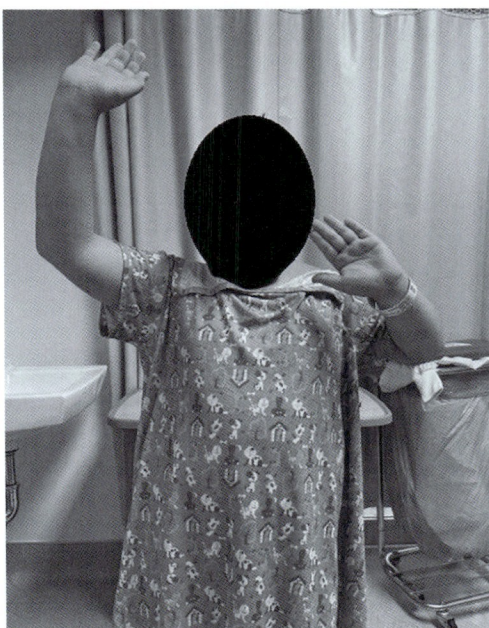

▲ **Figure 26–23.** Patient with Sprengel deformity affecting the left scapula: Frontal view.

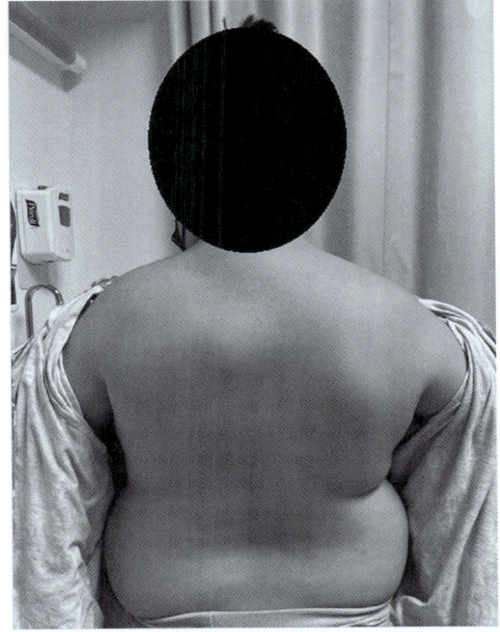

▲ **Figure 26–24.** Patient with Sprengel deformity affecting the left scapula: Posterior arms adducted view.

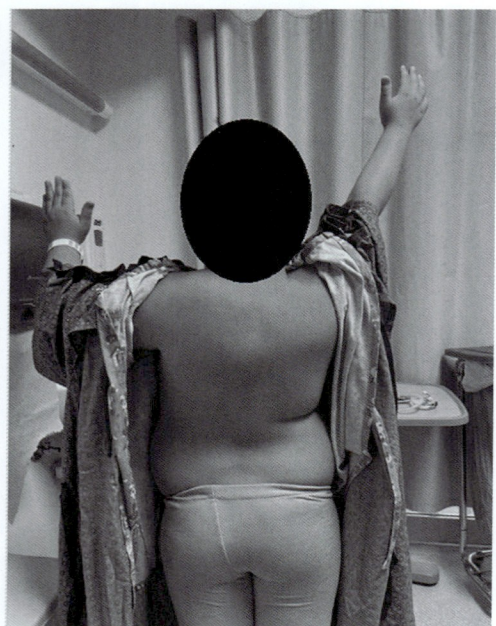

▲ **Figure 26–25.** Patient with Sprengel deformity affecting the left scapula: Posterior view.

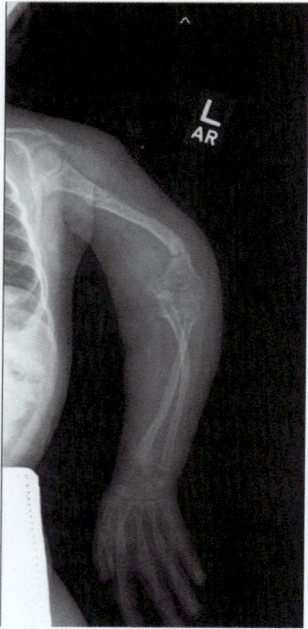

▲ **Figure 26–26.** Radiographic evidence of osteogenesis imperfecta of the left arm with healing osteotomies in the humerus and radial and ulnar deformities.

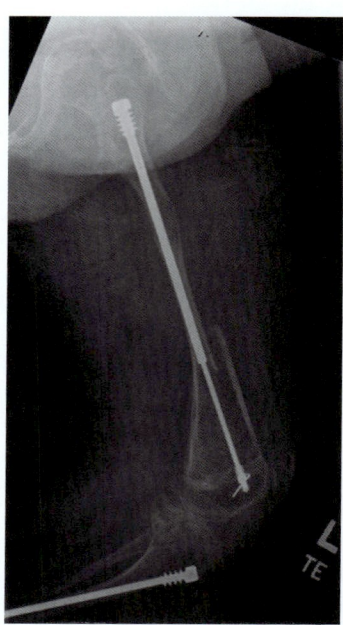

▲ **Figure 26–27.** Radiographic evidence of osteogenesis imperfecta of the left leg with surgical intervention with growing rod fixation of femur fracture.

Biggin A, Munns CF: Osteogenesis imperfecta: diagnosis and treatment. Curr Osteoporos Rep 2014;12(3):279–288 [PMID: 24964776].
Harrington J, Sochett E, Howard A: Update on the evaluation and treatment of osteogenesis imperfecta. Pediatr Clin North Am 2014;61(6):1243–1257 [PMID: 25439022].

ACHONDROPLASIA (CLASSIC CHONDRODYSTROPHY)

► Clinical Findings

A. Symptoms and Signs

Achondroplasia is the most common form of short-limbed dwarfism. The upper arms and thighs are proportionately shorter than the forearms and legs. Skeletal dysplasia is suspected based on abnormal stature, disproportion, dysmorphism, or deformity. Measurement of height is an excellent clinical screening tool. Findings frequently include bowing of the extremities, waddling gait, limitation of motion of major joints, relaxation of the ligaments, short stubby fingers of almost equal length, frontal bossing, midface hypoplasia, otolaryngeal system dysfunction, moderate hydrocephalus, depressed nasal bridge, and lumbar lordosis. Intelligence and

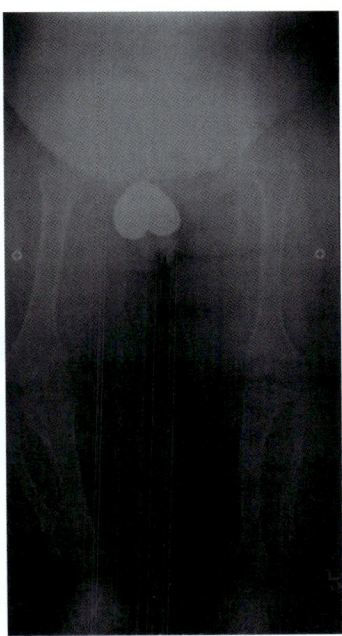

▲ **Figure 26–28.** Standing hips to ankles radiograph of a patient with achondroplasia.

sexual function are normal. While this disorder has an autosomal dominant transmission pattern, 80% of cases result from a random mutation in the fibroblast growth factor receptor-3 (*FGFR3*) gene.

B. Imaging

Radiographs demonstrate short, thick tubular bones and irregular epiphysial plates. The ends of the bones are thick, with broadening and cupping (Figure 26–28). Epiphysial ossification may be delayed. Due to diminished growth in the spinal pedicles, the spinal canal is narrowed (congenital stenosis) and a herniated disk in adulthood may lead to acute paraplegia.

▶ Treatment

Growth hormone is given to some children with bone dysplasia. Limb lengthening is possible to achieve a more normal proportion of extremities, but it is controversial.

Ornitz DM, Legeai-Mallet L: Achondroplasia: development, pathogenesis and therapy. Dev Dyn 2017;246(4):291–309 [PMID: 27987249].

Shirley ED, Ain MC: Achondroplasia: manifestations and treatment. J Am Acad Orthop Surg 2009;(17):231–241 [PMID: 19307672].

NEUROLOGIC DISORDERS INVOLVING THE MUSCULOSKELETAL SYSTEM

ESSENTIALS OF DIAGNOSIS & TYPICAL FEATURES

▶ A detailed birth history is important for diagnosis.

▶ The functional status of the patient should be assessed.

▶ Management should be geared toward maximizing function.

ORTHOPEDIC ASPECTS OF CEREBRAL PALSY

▶ Clinical Findings & Treatment

Cerebral palsy is defined as a nonprogressive brain injury with onset during the perinatal period. It usually causes difficulty with muscle control and can also affect cognitive and behavioral functioning. Evaluation and longitudinal care by a multidisciplinary team is recommended. Early physical therapy that facilitates completion of normal developmental patterns may be beneficial. Bracing and splinting are of questionable benefit, although ankle and foot orthoses (AFOs) or night splints may be useful in preventing equinus deformity of the ankle, the most common deformity found in this population, or adduction contractures of the hips. Orthopedic surgery is useful for treating joint contractures that interfere with function. Most orthopedic procedures are directed at tendon lengthening or bony stabilization by osteotomy or arthrodesis. Muscle transfers are effective in carefully selected patients.

Flexion and adduction of the hip due to hyperactivity of the adductors and flexors may produce a progressive neuromuscular dislocation of the hip (Figure 26–29). This can lead to pain and dysfunction, and treatment is difficult and generally unsatisfactory. Treatment can include abduction bracing, supplemented by release of the adductors and hip flexors, but this has been shown to only delay the need for osteotomy. Osteotomy of the femur and/or pelvis may be necessary to correct bony deformities of femoral anteversion, coxa valga, and acetabular dysplasia that are invariably present. Neuromuscular hip dysplasia should be followed every 6–12 months with anteroposterior pelvis radiographs. The Australian Hip Surveillance Guidelines for Children with Cerebral Palsy provide guidance on follow-up of patients with cerebral palsy, and the Pediatric Orthopaedic Society of North America is developing a protocol with indications for referral to orthopedic surgery.

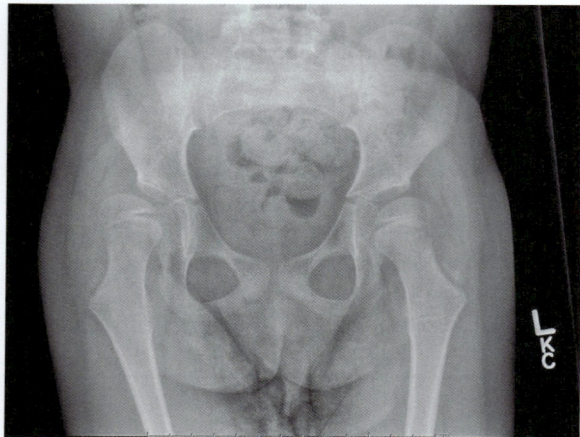

▲ Figure 26–29. Neuromuscular hip subluxation in a patient with spastic quadriplegic cerebral palsy.

Surgeons must examine patients on several occasions before any operative procedure as it is difficult to predict the surgical outcome in individuals with cerebral palsy. Follow-up care with a physical therapist can maximize the anticipated long-term gains.

Wynter M et al: Australian hip surveillance guidelines for children with cerebral palsy 2020. AusACPDM 2020. https://www .ausacpdm.org.au/wp-content/uploads/2020/12/200240-Hip-survey-A5-booklet-WEB.pdf.

ORTHOPEDIC ASPECTS OF MYELODYSPLASIA (SPINA BIFIDA)

▶ Clinical Findings & Treatment

The level of neurologic involvement in patients with myelodysplasia (spina bifida) determines the muscle imbalances that can produce deformity with growth. Involvement is often asymmetrical and tends to change during the first 12–18 months of life. Musculoskeletal problems may include congenital dislocation of the hip, arthrogryposis-type changes of the lower extremities, clubfoot, and congenital scoliosis and kyphosis. Spina bifida lesions occur most commonly at the L3–L4 level and tend to affect the hip joint, with progressive dislocation occurring during growth due to unopposed hip flexion and adduction forces. Foot deformities may occur in any direction depending on the muscle imbalance present and are complicated by the fact that sensation is generally absent. Spinal deformities develop in a high percentage of children, with scoliosis occurring in approximately 40%.

Patients with spina bifida should be examined early by an orthopedic surgeon. Ambulation may require long leg braces. In children who have a reasonable likelihood of walking,

operative treatment consists of reduction of the hip, alignment of the feet in the weight-bearing position, and stabilization of scoliosis. In children who lack active quadriceps function and extensor power of the knee, the likelihood of ambulation is greatly decreased. In such patients, aggressive surgery to the foot and hip region is usually not indicated, as it may result in stiffening of the joints and prevent sitting. Treatment of the child with spina bifida should be coordinated in a multidisciplinary clinic that includes medical specialists, therapists, social workers, and teachers.

▼ TRAUMA

 ESSENTIALS OF DIAGNOSIS & TYPICAL FEATURES

- ▶ Fall on outstretched hand (FOOSH) is the most common mechanism of orthopedic injury.
- ▶ Directed physical examination (eg, swelling, tenderness, deformity, instability) and radiographic examination are key for diagnosis.
- ▶ It is important to rule out physeal fracture.
- ▶ Early protected motion is indicated for sprains and strains.
- ▶ Reduction and immobilization are the basis for treatment of fractures.

SOFT TISSUE TRAUMA

Contusions are generally the result of tissue compression, with damage to blood vessels within the tissue and the formation of a hematoma. A sprain is the stretching of a ligament, and a strain is a stretch of a muscle or tendon (see also Chapter 27). Incomplete tearing of a ligament, with local pain and swelling but no joint instability, is considered a mild or moderate sprain. In a severe sprain, the ligament is completely disrupted, resulting in instability of the joint.

The initial treatment of any sprain consists of rest, ice, compression, and elevation. Brief splinting followed by early range of motion exercises of the affected joint protect against further injury and relieves swelling and pain. Nonsteroidal anti-inflammatory drugs (NSAIDs) are useful for pain. If more severe trauma results in complete tearing of a ligament, instability of the joint may be demonstrated by gross examination or by stress testing with radiographic documentation. Such deformity of the joint may cause persistent instability and result in other injuries. If instability is evident, surgical repair of the torn ligament may be indicated. If a muscle is torn at its tendinous insertion, it can be repaired surgically.

Contusions

▶ Clinical Findings

A. Symptoms and Signs

Muscle contusions with hematoma formation produce the familiar "charley horse" injury, which can last for weeks before complete pain resolution.

▶ Treatment

Treatment includes application of ice, compression, and rest. Exercise should be avoided for 5–7 days. Local heat may hasten healing once the acute phase of tenderness and swelling has passed.

Myositis Ossificans

▶ Clinical Findings

A. Symptoms and Signs

Myositis ossificans, ossification within muscle, occurs when sufficient trauma causes a hematoma that later heals in the manner of a fracture (Figure 26–30). Contusions of the quadriceps of the thigh or the triceps of the arm are the most common predisposing injuries. Disability is great, with local swelling, heat, and extreme pain with the slightest provocation of the adjacent joint.

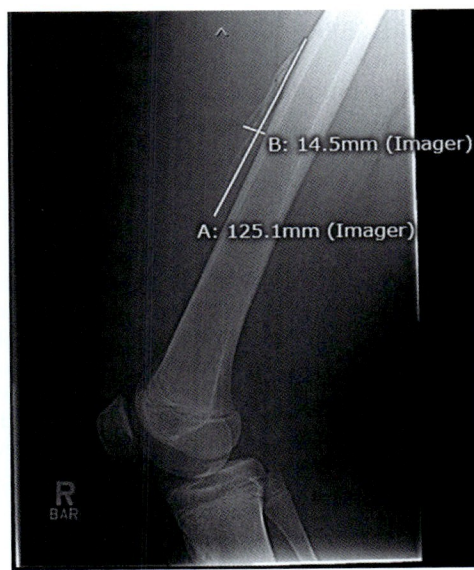

▲ **Figure 26–30.** Radiographic evidence of myositis ossificans on shaft of the right femur.

▶ Treatment and Prevention

The limb should be rested until the local reaction has subsided (5–7 days). When local heat and tenderness have decreased, gentle active exercises may be initiated. Passive stretching exercises are not indicated as they may stimulate the ossification reaction. Surgery to excise the ossification may restart the process and lead to an even more severe reaction and should not be attempted before 9 months to 1 year after injury.

If an extremity experiences a severe injury with a hematoma, it should be splinted, and further activity should be avoided until the acute reaction has subsided to reduce the risk of myositis ossificans formation.

Sferopoulos NK, Kotakidou R, Petropoulos AS: Myositis ossificans in children: a review. Eur J Orthop Surg Traumatol 2017;27(4): 491–502. doi: 10.1007/s00590-017-1932-x [PMID: 28275867].

TRAUMATIC SUBLUXATIONS & DISLOCATIONS

▶ Clinical Findings

Acromioclavicular Separation

A. Symptoms, Signs, and Treatment

Acromioclavicular (AC) separations involve partial or complete tearing of the ligament complex of the AC joint (Figure 26–31). They are among the most common shoulder injuries but vary significantly in severity (grade I–VI, with the latter the most severe) and treatment. Grade I–III acromioclavicular separations are most common and generally treated nonsurgically (including early physical therapy), while grades IV–VI are usually the result of high energy

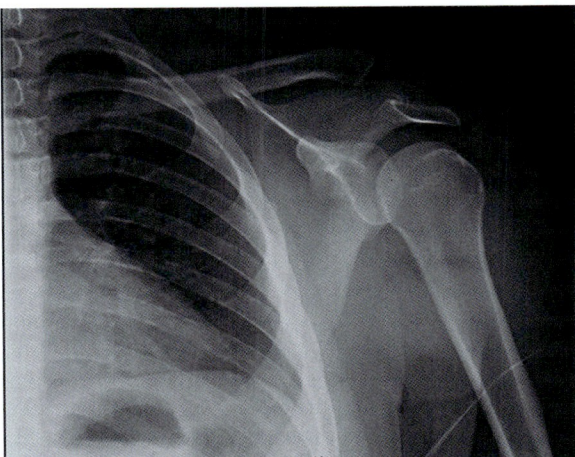

▲ **Figure 26–31.** Radiographic evidence of grade 2 acromioclavicular separation.

impacts and are treated surgically. The amount of displacement distinguishes grade III from higher grades. There is controversy about whether grade III AC separations should be treated surgically or nonsurgically.

Allemann F et al: Different treatment strategies for acromioclavicular dislocation injuries: a nationwide survey on open/minimally invasive and arthroscopic concepts. Eur J Med Res 2019;24(1):18 [PMID: 30904018].

Kraus N, Hann C, Gerhardt C, Scheibel M: Dynamic instability of the acromioclavicular joint: a new classification for acute AC joint separation. Obere Extremitat 2018;13(4):279–285 [PMID: 30546493].

Subluxation of the Radial Head (Nursemaid Elbow)

A. Symptoms, Signs, and Treatment

Infants may sustain subluxation of the radial head as a result of being lifted or pulled by the hand. The child presents with the elbow fully pronated and painful. The usual complaint is that the child's elbow will not bend. Radiographic findings are normal, but there is point tenderness over the radial head. A **subluxated** radial head (nursemaid's elbow) can be reduced by placing the elbow in full supination and slowly moving the arm from full extension to full flexion or by holding the elbow at a 90-degree angle of flexion, then slowly hyperpronating the wrist to complete reduction; a click may be palpated at the level of the radial head. Relief of pain is remarkable, as the child usually stops crying immediately. The elbow may be immobilized in a sling for comfort for a day. Occasionally, symptoms last for several days, requiring more prolonged immobilization. A pulled elbow may be a clue to non-accidental trauma. This should be considered during examination, especially if the problem is recurrent.

Bexkens R, Washburn FJ, Eygendaal D, Van Den Bekerom MP, Oh LS: Effectiveness of reduction maneuvers in the treatment of nursemaid's elbow: a systematic review and meta-analysis. Am J Emerg Med 2017;35(1):159–163 [PMID: 27836316].

Dislocation of the Patella

A. Symptoms and Signs

Complete patellar dislocations nearly always dislocate laterally. Pain is severe, and the patient will present with the knee slightly flexed and an obvious bony mass lateral to the knee joint associated with a flat area over the anterior knee. Radiologic examination, including sunrise views, confirms the diagnosis. When subluxation of the patella occurs, symptoms may be more subtle, and the patient will complain that the knee "gives out" or "jumps out of place."

Recurrent dislocations more commonly occur in individuals with hyperlaxity, especially adolescent girls. Factors that affect risk for recurrence include length of patellar tendon,

the depth of trochlear groove, and position of the patella in relation to the trochlear groove that is affected by axial and coronal boney alignment.

▶ Treatment of Dislocations

In contrast to fracture reduction, which may be safely postponed, most dislocations must be reduced immediately to minimize further joint damage. Dislocations can usually be reduced by gentle sustained traction. Radiographs should be obtained post-reduction to document congruency and assess for the presence of associated osteochondral fractures. Following reduction, the joint should be splinted for transportation of the patient. NSAIDs may be used along with ice for pain control and to reduce inflammation. Initial immobilization of the dislocated joint should be followed by graduated active exercises through a full range of motion. Vigorous passive manipulation of the joint by a therapist may be harmful, but muscle strengthening is key in long-term treatment.

Longo UG, Ciuffreda M, Locher J, Berton A, Salvatore G, Denaro V: Treatment of primary acute patellar dislocation: systematic review and quantitative synthesis of the literature. Clin J Sport Med 2017;27(6):511–523 [PMID: 28107220].

Nwachukwu BU, So C, Schairer WW, Green DW, Dodwell ER: Surgical versus conservative management of acute patellar dislocation in children and adolescents: a systematic review. Knee Surg Sports Traumotol Arthrsc 2016;24(3):760–767 [PMID: 26704809].

▼ FRACTURES

EPIPHYSEAL SEPARATIONS

▶ Clinical Findings

A. Symptoms and Signs

Epiphyseal separations (also referred to as epiphyseal fractures) are more common than ligamentous injuries in children since the ligaments of the joints are generally stronger than their associated growth plates. Radiographs should be taken whenever a dislocation is suspected to rule out epiphyseal fracture (Figure 26–32). Radiographs of the opposite extremity, especially for injuries around the elbow, are valuable for comparison. Fractures across the growth plate may produce bony bridges that will cause premature cessation of growth or angular deformities of the extremity. These bridges are due to trauma to the growth plate and can occur even with adequate reductions. Epiphyseal separations in a non-ambulatory child should be concerning for nonaccidental trauma.

▶ Treatment

Reduction of a fractured epiphysis should be done under anesthesia to align the growth plate with the least amount of force.

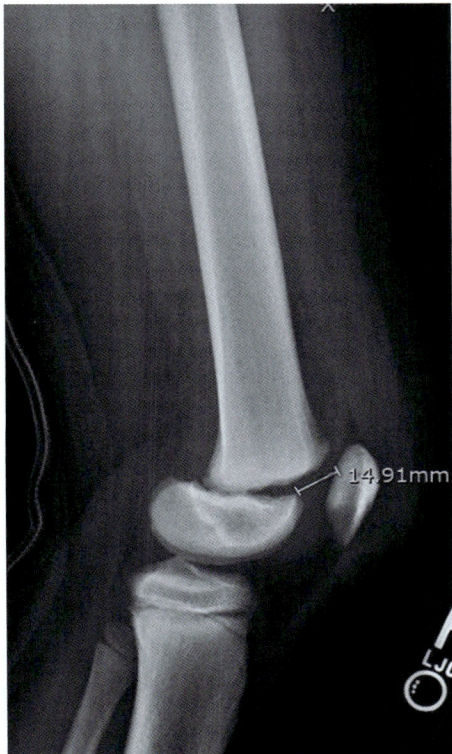

▲ **Figure 26–32.** Radiographic evidence of epiphyseal separation of the right femur in a displaced Salter-Harris type 1 fracture.

Epiphyseal fractures around the shoulder, wrist, and fingers can usually be treated by closed reduction, but fractures of the epiphyses around the elbow often require open reduction. In the lower extremity, accurate reduction of the epiphyseal plate is necessary to prevent joint deformity when a joint surface is involved. If angular deformities result, corrective osteotomy may be necessary. Multiple attempts at closed reduction are not recommended due to higher risk of physeal damage.

Dwek JR: The radiographic approach to child abuse. Clin Orthop Relat Res 2011;469:776–789 [PMID: 20544318].

TORUS (BUCKLE) FRACTURES

▶ Clinical Findings & Treatment

Torus fractures consist of "buckling" of the cortex due to compression of the bone (Figure 26–33). They are most common in the distal radius or ulna. Alignment is usually satisfactory, and simple immobilization for 3 weeks is sufficient. Soft bandage therapy and cast therapy are effective in preventing further angulation.

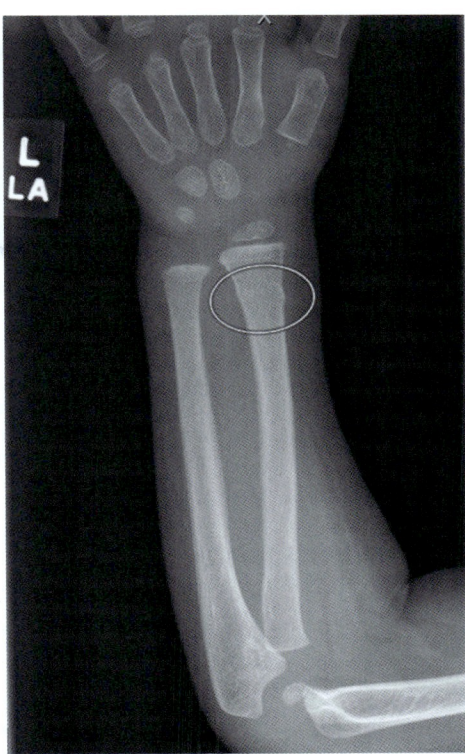

▲ **Figure 26–33.** Radiographic evidence of a buckle fracture of the distal radius. The circled area highlights the fractured area.

Jiang N, Cao ZH, Ma YF, Lin Z, Yu B: Management of pediatric forearm torus fractures: a systematic review and meta-analysis. Pediatr Emerg Care 2016;32(11):773–778 [PMID: 26555307].

GREENSTICK FRACTURES

▶ Clinical Findings & Treatment

Greenstick fractures involve frank disruption of the cortex on one side of the bone but no discernible cleavage plane on the opposite side. The term "greenstick" implies similarity to what happens when one tries to break a twig/stick from a live tree; commonly bark will break on one side of the stick, while remaining intact on the opposite side. Bone ends are not separated, making these fractures angulated but not displaced (Figure 26–34). Reduction is achieved by straightening the arm into normal alignment and maintaining alignment with a snugly fitting cast. It is necessary to obtain repeat radiographs of greenstick fractures in 7–10 days to make certain that the reduction has been maintained in the cast. A slight angular deformity can be

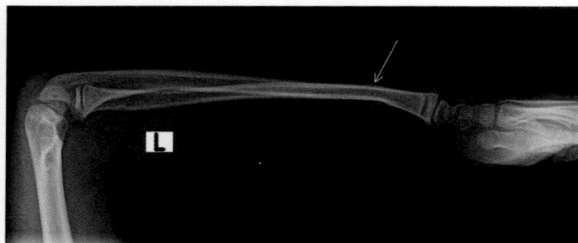

▲ **Figure 26–34.** Radiographic evidence of a greenstick fracture. The arrow points to the fractured area.

corrected by remodeling of the bone. The farther the fracture is from the growing end of the bone, the longer the time required for remodeling. The fracture can be considered healed when no tenderness is present, and a bony callus is seen on a radiograph.

SUPRACONDYLAR FRACTURES OF THE HUMERUS

▶ Clinical Findings

A. Symptoms and Signs

The condyles of the distal humerus form the proximal half of the elbow joint. There is a concavity in the posterior distal humerus that is present anatomically to accommodate the olecranon when the elbow reaches full extension. This anatomic accommodation, located in what is referred to as the supracondylar region of the humerus, also creates a thinner area of cortical bone that is more susceptible to injury/fracture (Figure 26–35). Supracondylar fractures tend to occur in children aged 3–6 years and are the most common elbow fracture in children. The proximity to the brachial artery creates a potential danger when dealing with these types of fractures. Absence of a distal pulse is a strong indicator of a secondary arterial injury. Swelling may be severe as these injuries are usually associated with a significant amount of trauma.

▶ Treatment

Most often, these fractures are treated by closed reduction and percutaneous pinning performed under general anesthesia. Complications associated with supracondylar fractures include Volkmann ischemic contracture of the forearm due to vascular compromise and cubitus varus (decreased carrying angle, "gunstock deformity") secondary to poor reduction. The "gunstock deformity" of the elbow may be somewhat unsightly but does not usually interfere with joint function.

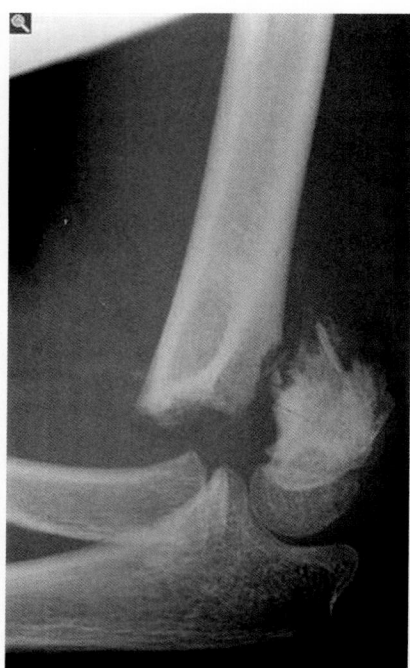

▲ **Figure 26–35.** Supracondylar fracture of the humerus.

Kumar V, Singh A: Fracture supracondylar humerus: a review. J Clin Diag Res 2016;10(12):RE01–RE06 [PMID: 28208961].

GENERAL COMMENTS ON OTHER FRACTURES IN CHILDREN

Reduction of fractures in children can usually be accomplished by simple traction and manipulation; open reduction is indicated if a satisfactory alignment is not obtained. Remodeling of the fracture callus generally produces an almost normal appearance of the bone over a matter of months (Figure 26–36). The younger the child, the more remodeling is possible. Angular deformities in the plane of joint motion remodel reliably while rotational malalignment does not remodel well.

There should be suspicion of child abuse whenever the age of a fracture does not match the history given or when the severity of the injury is more than the alleged accident would have produced. In suspected cases of abuse in which no fracture is present on the initial radiograph, a repeat radiograph 10 days later is indicated. Bleeding beneath the periosteum will be calcified by 7–10 days, and the radiographic appearance can be diagnostic of severe closed trauma characteristic of a battered child.

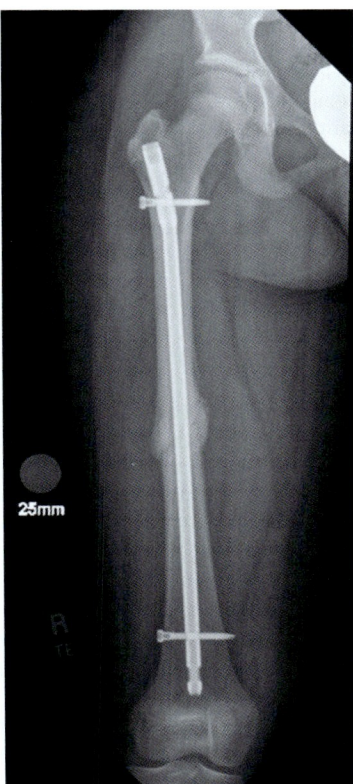

▲ **Figure 26–36.** Radiographic evidence of callus remodeling of a femur shaft fracture: postoperative radiograph s/p intramedullary nailing of femoral shaft fracture.

INFECTIONS OF THE BONES & JOINTS

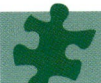

ESSENTIALS OF DIAGNOSIS & TYPICAL FEATURES

▶ Movement of the extremity causes pain, resulting in pseudoparalysis.

▶ Soft tissue swelling is usually present.

▶ Erythrocyte sedimentation rate (ESR) and C-reactive protein (CRP) are elevated in the majority of cases.

▶ Treatment consists of surgical drainage of abscess plus antibiotics.

▶ Antibiotic therapy alone may suffice for early osteomyelitis without abscess.

OSTEOMYELITIS

Osteomyelitis is an infectious process that usually starts in the spongy or medullary bone and extends into compact or cortical bone. Commonly preceded by trauma, the lower extremities are more likely to be affected. Osteomyelitis is most commonly caused by hematogenous spread of bacteria from other infected or colonized areas (eg, pyoderma or upper respiratory tract) but it may occur as a result of direct invasion from the outside (exogenous), through a penetrating wound (nail) or open fracture. *Staphylococcus aureus* is the most common infecting organism and tends to infect the metaphyses of growing bones. In the infant (< 1 year), there is direct vascular communication with the epiphysis across the growth plate, allowing bacterial spread from the metaphysis to the epiphysis and into the joint. In the older child, the growth plate provides an effective barrier, and the epiphysis is usually not infected. Infection spreads retrograde from the metaphysis into the diaphysis, and by rupture through the cortical bone, down along the diaphysis beneath the periosteum. Osteomyelitis often occurs around the knee joint in children age 7–10 years.

In hematogenous osteomyelitis, 85% of cases are due to *S aureus*. Streptococci (group B *Streptococcus* in neonates and young infants, *Streptococcus pyogenes* in older children) are a less common cause of osteomyelitis. *Pseudomonas aeruginosa* is common in cases of nail puncture wounds. Children with sickle cell anemia are especially prone to osteomyelitis caused by *Salmonella* species.

▶ Clinical Findings

A. Symptoms and Signs

Osteomyelitis may be subtle in infants, presenting as irritability, diarrhea, or failure to feed properly; temperature may be normal or slightly low; and white blood cell count may be normal or only slightly elevated. There may be pseudoparalysis of the involved limb. Manifestations are more striking in older children, with severe local tenderness and pain, refusal to bear weight, and, often, but not invariably, fever, tachycardia, and elevated white blood cell count, ESR, and CRP. Tenderness is most marked over the metaphysis of the bone where the process has its origin.

B. Laboratory Findings

Blood cultures are often positive early. The most important test is aspiration of pus or biopsy of involved bone for staining and cultures. Elevation of the ESR above 50 mm/h is typical for osteomyelitis. CRP is elevated earlier than the ESR.

C. Imaging

Osteomyelitis should be diagnosed clinically before significant plain radiographic findings are present.

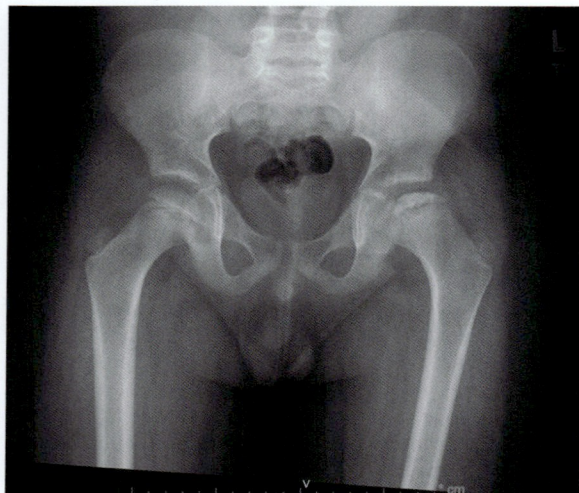

▲ **Figure 26–37.** A radiograph indicating osteomyelitis of the head of the left femur.

Plain film findings progress from nonspecific local swelling to elevation of the periosteum, with formation of new bone from the cambium layer of the periosteum occurring after 3–6 days. As infection becomes chronic, areas of cortical bone are isolated by pus spreading down the medullary canal, causing rarefaction and demineralization of the bone. Isolated pieces of cortex become ischemic and form sequestra (dead bone fragments). Bone scan is sensitive (before plain radiographic findings) but nonspecific and should be interpreted in the clinical context. MRI can demonstrate early edema and subperiosteal abscess and is helpful to confirm and localize disease prior to plain film changes (Figure 26–37).

▶ Treatment

A. Specific Measures

Intravenous antibiotics should be started as soon as the diagnosis of osteomyelitis is made and diagnostic specimens have been obtained. Transition to oral antibiotics occurs when tenderness, fever, white cell count, and CRP are all resolved/decreasing and is facilitated by a positive culture. Agents that cover *S aureus* and *S pyogenes* (eg, oxacillin, nafcillin, cefazolin, and clindamycin) are appropriate for most cases of hematogenous osteomyelitis. Alternative antistaphylococcal therapy (eg, vancomycin) may be needed if methicillin-resistant and clindamycin-resistant *S aureus* is suspected or isolated or in severe cases of hematogenous osteomyelitis pending culture and susceptibility results. Coverage for other pathogens is appropriate in specific circumstances (eg, group B *Streptococcus* in neonates and young infants, *P aeruginosa*

for nail puncture-associated osteomyelitis, *Salmonella* species in children with sickle cell anemia). Surgical debridement and broader antibiotic coverage (guided by cultures of infected bone) are often indicated for osteomyelitis resulting from penetrating injury. For specific recommendations, see Chapter 42.

Acute osteomyelitis is usually treated for a minimum of 4–6 weeks and until normalization of the physical examination and inflammatory markers. Chronic infections are treated for months. Following surgical debridement, *Pseudomonas* foot infections usually respond to 1–2 weeks of antibiotic treatment.

B. General Measures

Splinting minimizes pain and decreases spread of the infection through lymphatic channels. The splint should be removed periodically to allow the active use of adjacent joints and prevent stiffening and muscle atrophy. In chronic osteomyelitis, splinting may be necessary to guard against fracture of the weakened bone.

C. Surgical Measures

Aspiration of the metaphysis for culture and Gram stain is the most useful diagnostic measure. Surgical drainage is indicated if frank pus is aspirated from the bone or if there has not been a significant response within 24 hours. All devitalized soft tissue should be removed, and adequate exposure of the bone be obtained to permit free drainage. Bone damage is limited by surgical drainage, whereas failure to evacuate pus in acute cases may lead to widespread damage.

▶ Prognosis

When osteomyelitis is diagnosed in the early clinical stages and prompt antibiotic therapy is begun, the prognosis is excellent. If the process has been unattended for a week to 10 days, there is almost always some permanent loss of bone structure, as well as the possibility of future growth abnormality due to physeal injury.

Bouchoucha S et al: Epidemiology of acute hematogenous osteomyelitis in children: a prospective study over a 32 months period. Tunis Med 2012;90(6):473–480 [PMID: 22693089].

PYOGENIC (SEPTIC) ARTHRITIS

The source of pyogenic arthritis (septic arthritis) varies according to the child's age. Infantile pyogenic arthritis often develops from adjacent osteomyelitis. In older children, it usually presents as an isolated infection without bony involvement, although pyogenic arthritis may also secondarily affect adjacent bone. In teenagers with pyogenic arthritis, an underlying systemic disease or an organism that has an affinity for joints (eg, *Neisseria gonorrhoeae*) may be present.

The most frequent infecting organisms similarly vary with age: group B *Streptococcus* and *S aureus* in those younger than 4 months; *Haemophilus influenzae* B (if unimmunized), *Kingella kingae*, and *S aureus* in those aged 4 months to 4 years; and *S aureus* and *S pyogenes* in older children and adolescents. *Streptococcus pneumoniae* and *Neisseria meningitidis* are occasionally implicated, and *N gonorrhoeae* is a cause in adolescents.

The initial effusion of the joint rapidly becomes purulent in pyogenic arthritis. While a joint effusion may accompany osteomyelitis in the adjacent bone, a white cell count exceeding 50,000/μL in the joint fluid indicates a purulent infection involving the joint. The ESR is often above 50 mm/h, and the CRP is commonly elevated early.

▶ **Clinical Findings**

A. Symptoms and Signs

In older children, signs may be striking, with fever, malaise, vomiting, and restriction of motion, in addition to joint swelling, warmth, erythema, and/or tenderness. In infants, paralysis of the limb due to inflammatory pseudoparalysis may be evident. Infection of the hip joint in infants should be suspected if decreased abduction of the hip is present in an infant who is irritable or feeding poorly. A history of umbilical catheterization should alert the physician to the possibility of pyogenic arthritis of the hip.

B. Imaging

Early distention of the joint capsule is nonspecific and difficult to measure by plain radiograph. In infants with unrecognized pyogenic arthritis, dislocation of the joint structures may follow within a few days as a result of distention of the capsule by purulent effusion. Destruction of the joint space, resorption of epiphysial cartilage, and erosion of the adjacent bone of the metaphysis occur later. MRI and ultrasound imaging are useful adjuncts for detecting joint effusions. MRI is recommended if the clinical presentation does not fit the expected picture of septic arthritis and is beneficial to evaluate for associated bone or soft tissue infection.

▶ **Treatment**

Aspiration of the joint is the key to diagnosis and initial therapy. The need for aspiration is evaluated with the Kocher criteria that include fever, inability to bear weight, elevated WBC, ESR, and CRP (Table 26–1).

Surgical drainage, when intra-articular white cell count is greater than 30,000–50,000 cells/mm³, followed by the

Table 26–1. Kocher criteria to determine risk for pediatric septic joint.

Non–weight-bearing
ESR > 40 mm/h
Temperature > 101.3°F (38.5°C)
WBC > 12,000 cells/mm³
[a]CRP > 2.0 mg/dL

[a]CRP added by Caird et al; not part of the original Kocher Criteria.

appropriate antibiotic therapy provides the best treatment for pyogenic arthritis. Antibiotics should be selected based on the child's age and results of the Gram stain and culture of aspirated pus. Reasonable empiric therapy in infants and young children is an antistaphylococcal agent such as nafcillin or oxacillin plus a third-generation cephalosporin. An antistaphylococcal agent alone is usually adequate for children older than 5 years, unless gonococcal or meningococcal infection is suspected. Alternative antistaphylococcal therapy (eg, clindamycin or vancomycin) may be needed if methicillin-resistant *S aureus* is suspected or isolated.

▶ **Prognosis**

The prognosis for the patient with pyogenic arthritis is excellent if the joint is drained before damage to the articular cartilage has occurred. If infection is present for more than 24 hours, dissolution of the proteoglycans in the articular cartilage takes place, with subsequent arthrosis and fibrosis of the joint. Damage to the growth plate may occur, especially within the hip joint, where the epiphyseal plate is intracapsular.

Kocher MS, Zurakowski D, Kasser JR: Differentiating between septic arthritis and transient synovitis of the hip in children: an evidence-based clinical prediction algorithm. J Bone Joint Surg Am 1999;81(21):1662–1670 [PMID: 10608376].
Montgomery NI, Epps HR: Pediatric septic arthritis. Orthop Clin North Am 2017;48(2):209–216 [PMID: 28336043].

TRANSIENT (TOXIC) SYNOVITIS (VERSUS SEPTIC ARTHRITIS OF THE HIP)

▶ **Clinical Findings**

A. Symptoms and Signs

The most common cause of limping and hip pain in children in the United States is transient synovitis. This acute inflammatory reaction often follows an upper respiratory or gastrointestinal infection and is generally self-limited. Classically affecting children aged 3–10 years, it is more common in boys than girls. The hip joint experiences limitation of motion, particularly internal rotation, and radiographic changes are nonspecific, with some swelling apparent in the soft tissues around the joint.

It is important for the provider to differentiate between transient synovitis and septic arthritis despite similar early symptoms. Generally, toxic synovitis of the hip is not associated with elevation of the ESR, white blood cell count, or temperature above 38.3°C. In questionable cases, aspiration of the hip yields only yellowish fluid in transient synovitis rather than purulent fluid in pyogenic arthritis. Transient synovitis can also be distinguished from septic arthritis with a dynamic contrast enhanced MRI (DCE-MRI).

▶ Treatment

Rest and nonsteroidal anti-inflammatory medications are the preferred treatments for transient synovitis, whereas patients with septic arthritis of the hip are treated with operative drainage followed by antibiotic treatment. NSAIDs shorten the course of the transient synovitis, although even with no treatment, the disease usually runs its course in days. Radiographs should be obtained at 6 weeks after treatment, or earlier if either a persistent limp or pain is present, to evaluate for avascular necrosis of the femoral head, which can develop in a small percentage of patients.

Ryan DD: Differentiating transient synovitis of the hip from more urgent conditions. Pediatr Ann 2016;45(6):e209–e2013 [PMID: 27294495].

Whitelaw CC, Varacallo M: Transient synovitis. *StatPearls* 2019: Treasure Island, FL [PMID: 29083677].

Diskitis

Diskitis is pyogenic infectious spondylitis in children. Although many cases are culture-negative, *S aureus* is considered to be the most frequent etiologic pathogen. The typical clinical presentation includes avoidance of activity, back pain, and malaise over a several weeks to months duration. Younger children younger than 5 years may not be able to localize their complaints and commonly present with "abdominal" pain. Supportive treatment such as bracing and appropriate antibiotics is likely to lead to rapid relief of symptoms and signs without recurrence.

Early SD, Kay RM, Tolo VT: Childhood diskitis. J Am Acad Orthop Surg 2003;11:413–420 [PMID: 14686826].

Gouliouris T, Aliyu SH, Brown NM: Spondylodiscitis: update on diagnosis and management. J Antimicrob Chemother 2010;65:11–24 [PMID: 20876624].

VASCULAR LESIONS & AVASCULAR NECROSIS (OSTEOCHONDROSES)

ESSENTIALS OF DIAGNOSIS & TYPICAL FEATURES

▶ Diagnosis can be made by characteristic radiographic findings.
▶ Radiographic resolution lags behind symptomatic resolution.
▶ Treatment for most cases is supportive.

Rapid growth of the secondary ossification centers in the epiphyses in relation to their blood supply subject them to avascular necrosis. Osteochondrosis (degeneration of an ossification center) may affect various growth centers at different ages (Table 26–2).

In contrast to other body tissues that undergo infarction, bone removes necrotic tissue and replaces it with living bone through creeping substitution (a process in which necrotic bone is replaced by viable bone). The replacement of necrotic bone may be so complete that a normal bone results. Adequacy of replacement depends on the patient's age, the presence or absence of associated infection, the congruity of the involved joint, and other physiologic and mechanical factors. Even though the pathologic and radiographic features of avascular necrosis of the epiphyses are well known, the cause is not generally agreed upon. Necrosis may follow known causes such as trauma or infection, but idiopathic lesions usually develop during periods of rapid growth of the epiphyses.

Brewer P, Fernandes JA: Osteochondroses. Orthop Trauma 2016; 30(6):553–561.

Table 26–2. The osteochondroses.

Ossification Center	Eponym	Typical Age (y)
Capital femoral	Legg-Calvé-Perthes disease	4–8
Tarsal navicular	Köhler bone disease	6
Second metatarsal head	Freiberg disease	12–14
Vertebral ring	Scheuermann disease	13–16
Capitellum	Panner disease	9–11
Tibial tubercle	Osgood-Schlatter disease	11–13
Calcaneus	Sever disease	8–9

AVASCULAR NECROSIS OF THE PROXIMAL FEMUR (LEGG-CALVÉ-PERTHES DISEASE)

▶ Clinical Findings

A. Symptoms and Signs

The highest incidence of Legg-Calvé-Perthes disease occurs between 4 and 8 years of age and occurs when the vascular supply to the proximal femur is interrupted. Persistent pain is the most common symptom, and the patient may present with limp or limitation of motion.

B. Imaging

Radiographic findings correlate with progression of the disease and the extent of necrosis. Effusion of the joint associated with slight widening of the joint space and periarticular swelling are the early findings. Decreased bone density in and around the joint is apparent after a few weeks. The necrotic ossification center appears denser than the surrounding viable structures, and the femoral head is collapsed or narrowed (Figure 26–38). As replacement of the necrotic ossification center occurs, rarefaction of the bone begins in a patchwork fashion, producing alternating areas of rarefaction and relative density, referred to as "fragmentation" of the epiphysis. Widening of the femoral head may be associated with flattening, or coxa plana. If infarction has extended across the growth plate, a radiolucent lesion will be evident within the metaphysis. If the growth center of the femoral head has been damaged and normal growth arrested, shortening of the femoral neck results. Eventually, complete replacement of the epiphysis develops as living bone replaces necrotic bone by creeping substitution. The final shape of the head depends on the extent of the necrosis and collapse of weakened bone.

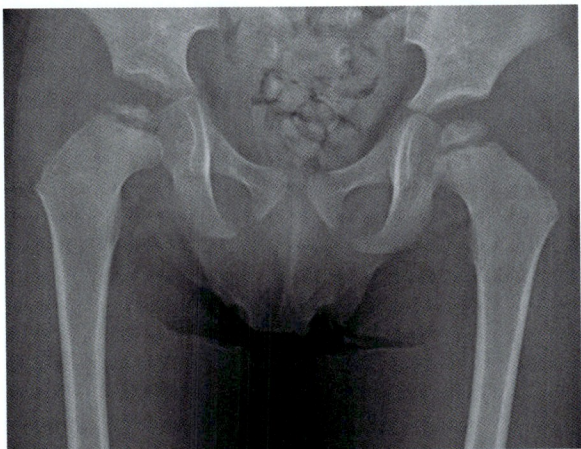

▲ **Figure 26–38.** Radiographic evidence of osteochondrosis of the right proximal femur.

Serial radiographs help to distinguish this disease from transient synovitis of the hip.

▶ Treatment

Protection of the joint by minimizing impact is the principal treatment. Nonoperative (casting) and surgical approaches are geared to promoting containment of the femoral head within the acetabulum and abduction of the hip.

▶ Prognosis

The prognosis for complete replacement of the necrotic femoral head in a child is excellent, but the functional result depends on the amount of deformity that has developed. Better outcomes are observed for patients with an onset of symptoms before the age of 6. Generally, a poorer prognosis is expected for patients who develop the disease late in childhood, those with more completed involvement of the epiphysial center, those with metaphyseal defects and those who have more complete involvement of the femoral head.

Chaudhry S, Phillips D, Feldman D: Legg-Calve-Perthes disease: an overview with recent literature. Bull Hosp Jt Dis 2014;72(1):18–27 [PMID: 25150324].

Kim HW, Herring JA: Pathophysiology, classifications, and natural history of Perthes disease. Orthop Clin N Am 2011;42:285–295 [PMID: 21742140].

▼ NEOPLASIA OF THE MUSCULOSKELETAL SYSTEM

 ESSENTIALS OF DIAGNOSIS & TYPICAL FEATURES

- ▶ Most lesions typically present with unresolving pain.
- ▶ Reassess *any* child with unresolved pain previously thought benign in origin.
- ▶ Radiographs are important for diagnosis.
- ▶ Refer any suspicious lesions for specialty evaluation.

The poor prognosis of malignant tumors arising in the bone or other tissues derived from the mesoderm makes neoplastic diseases of the musculoskeletal system a serious problem. Fortunately, few benign lesions undergo malignant transformation. Complaints about the knee should be investigated for tumor, although the usual causes of knee pain are traumatic, infectious, or developmental in origin.

Hashefi M: Ultrasound in the diagnosis of noninflammatory musculoskeletal conditions. Semin Ultrasound CT MR 2011; 32(2):74–90 [PMID: 21414544].

OSTEOCHONDROMA

▶ Clinical Findings

A. Symptoms and Signs

Osteochondroma is the most common benign bone tumor in children. It usually presents as a pain-free mass. When present, pain is caused by bursitis or tendinitis due to irritation by the tumor. Lesions may be single or multiple. Pathologically, the lesion is a bone mass capped with cartilage. These masses result from a developmental defect of the growth plate and tend to grow during childhood and adolescence in proportion to the child's growth. Males are more affected than females. Generally, the tumors are present on radiographs in the metaphyseal region of long bones and may be pedunculated or sessile (Figure 26–39). The cortex of the underlying bone "flows" into the base of the tumor.

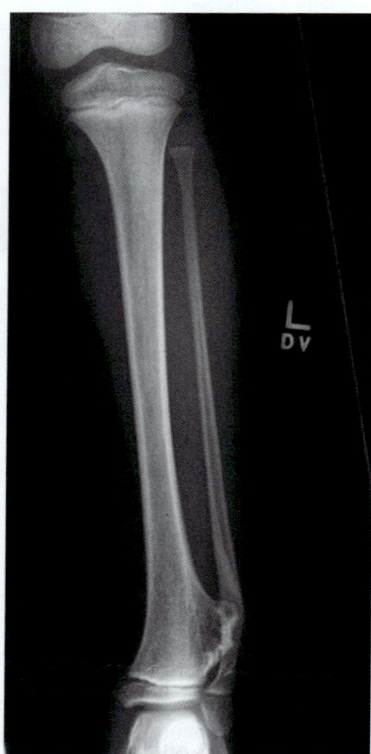

▲ **Figure 26–39.** Radiographic evidence of osteochondroma of the distal tibia.

▶ Treatment

An osteochondroma should be excised if it interferes with function, is frequently traumatized, or is large enough to be deforming. The prognosis is excellent. Malignant transformation is very rare.

OSTEOID OSTEOMA

▶ Clinical Findings

A. Symptoms and Signs

Osteoid osteoma is a benign bone-forming lesion of unclear etiology. It classically produces night pain that can be relieved by NSAIDs. There usually is tenderness over the lesion. An osteoid osteoma in the upper femur may cause referred pain to the knee. The radiographic lesion consists of a radiolucent nidus surrounded by dense osteosclerosis that may obscure the nidus (Figure 26–40). Bone scan shows intense uptake in the lesion. CT scans are confirmatory and delineate the nidus well.

▶ Treatment

Surgical excision or radiofrequency ablation of the nidus is curative and may be done using computed tomography imaging and a minimally invasive technique. The prognosis is

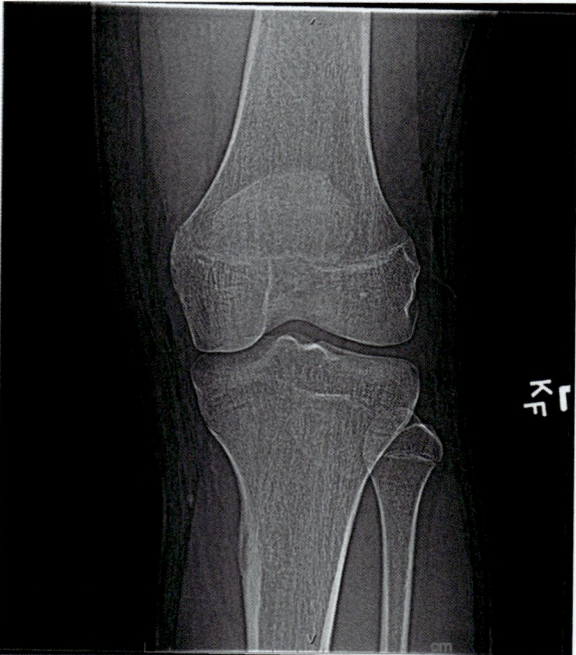

▲ **Figure 26–40.** Radiographic evidence of osteoid osteoma of the proximal tibia.

excellent, with no known cases of malignant transformation, although the lesion tends to recur if incompletely excised.

Noordin S et al: Osteoid osteoma: contemporary management. Orthop Rev (Pavia) 2018;10(3):7496 [PMID: 30370032].

ENCHONDROMA

▶ Clinical Findings & Treatment

Enchondroma (nest of benign cartilage within long bones) is usually a silent lesion unless it produces a pathologic fracture. On radiograph it is radiolucent, usually in a long bone (Figure 26–41). Speckled calcification may be present. The classic lesion looks as though someone dragged his or her fingernails through clay, making streaks in the bones. Enchondroma is treated by surgical curettage and bone grafting. The prognosis is excellent. Malignant transformation may occur but is very rare in childhood.

CHONDROBLASTOMA

▶ Clinical Findings & Treatment

The presenting complaint in chondroblastoma (benign chondral origin lesions typically in the epiphyses [joint ends] of long bones) is pain around a joint. This neoplasm

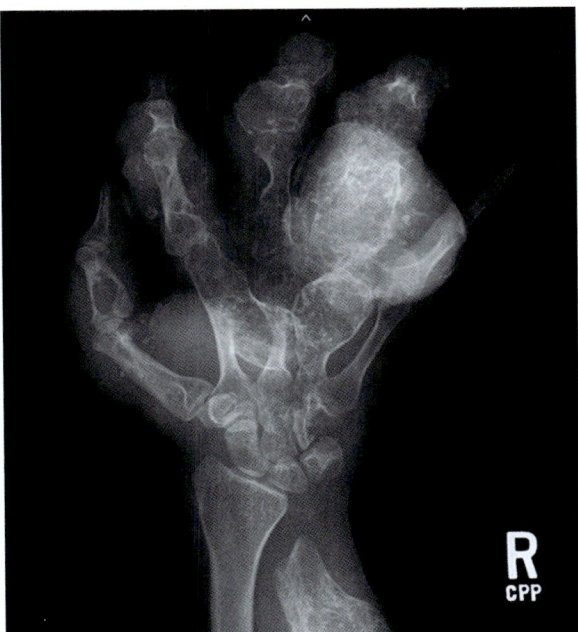

▲ **Figure 26–41.** Radiographic evidence of enchondromas involving multiple metacarpals and phalanges of the hand.

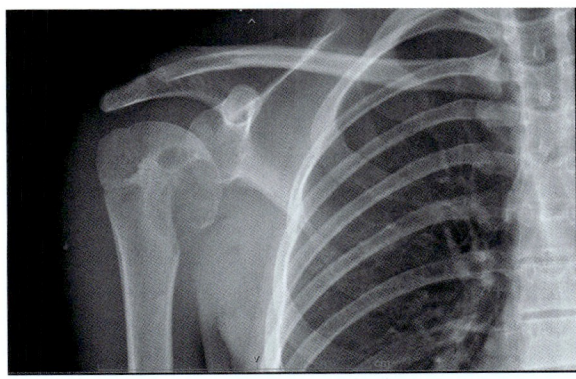

▲ **Figure 26–42.** Radiographic evidence of chondroblastoma of the head of the humerus.

may produce a pathologic fracture. On radiograph, the lesion is radiolucent and usually located in the epiphysis (Figure 26–42). With little to no reactive bone, calcification is unusual. The lesion is treated by surgical curettage and bone grafting. The prognosis is excellent if complete curettage is performed. There is no known malignant transformation.

Chen W, DiFrancesco LM: Chondroblastoma: an update. Arch Pathol Lab Med 2017;141(6):867–871 [PMID: 28557595].

NONOSSIFYING FIBROMA

▶ Clinical Findings & Treatment

Nonossifying fibroma, or benign cortical defect, is nearly always an incidental finding on radiograph. It is a radiolucent lesion eccentrically located in the metaphyseal region of the bone. Usually, a thin sclerotic border is evident. Multiple lesions may be present (Figure 26–43). The most frequent sites are the distal femur and proximal tibia. In general, no treatment is needed because these lesions heal as they ossify with maturation and growth. Rarely, pathologic fractures result from large lesions.

OSTEOSARCOMA

▶ Clinical Findings

A. Symptoms and Signs

Osteosarcoma is an aggressive form of cancer characterized by chromosomal instability. It is suspected that micro RNAs (noncoding, single-stranded molecules of RNA that regulate gene expression) play an important role. The presenting complaint is usually pain in a long bone; however, the patient may present with loss of function, mass, or limp. Pathologic fracture is uncommon. The malignant osseous

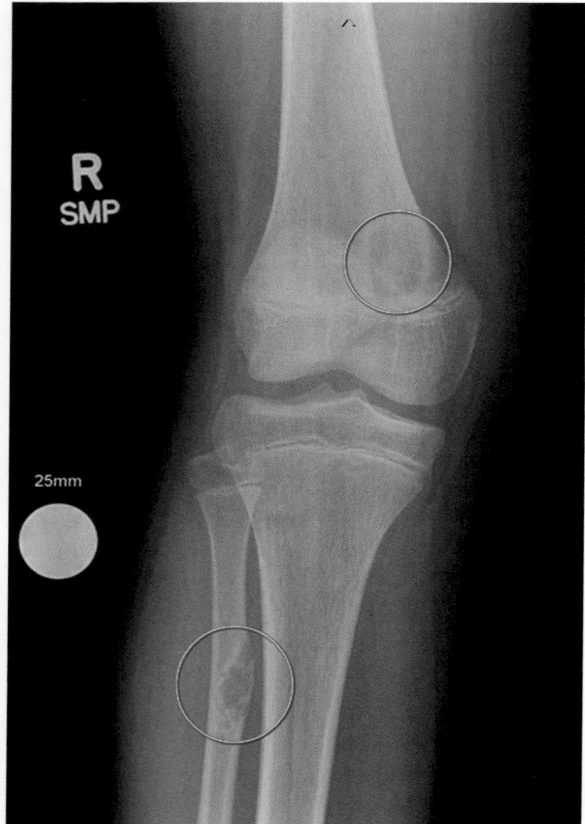

▲ **Figure 26–43.** Radiographic evidence of nonossifying fibroma on the distal femur and proximal fibula. Circles highlight the nonossifying fibromas.

tumor produces a destructive, expanding, and invasive lesion (Figure 26–44). A triangle may be adjacent to the tumor, produced by elevated periosteum and subsequent tumor ossification. The lesion may contain calcification and violates the cortex of the bone. Femur, tibia, humerus, and other long bones are the sites usually affected.

▶ **Treatment**

Surgical excision (limb salvage) or amputation is indicated based on the extent of the tumor. Adjuvant chemotherapy is routinely used prior to and after excision. The prognosis is improving, with greater than 65% long-term survival rates reported in modern series. Death usually occurs due to lung metastasis. Patients with osteosarcoma complicated by pathologic fracture have lower long-term survival rates than patients with osteosarcoma and no pathologic fracture.

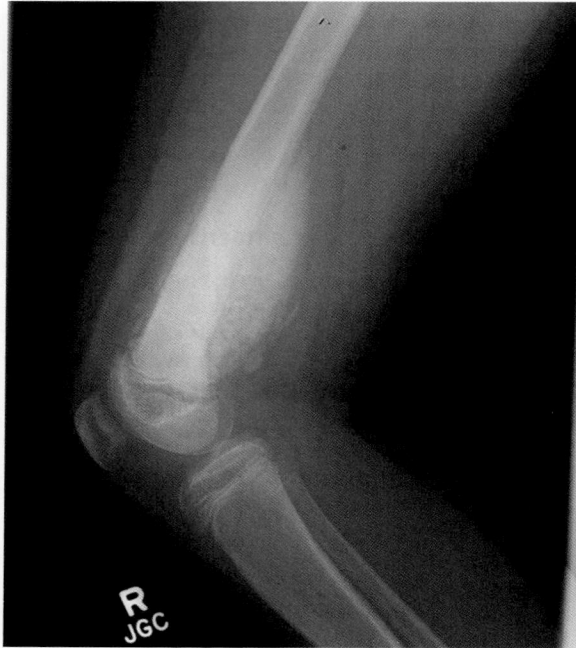

▲ **Figure 26–44.** Radiographic evidence of osteosarcoma of the distal femur.

Heare T, Hensley MA, Dell'Orfano S: Bone tumors: osteosarcoma and Ewing's sarcoma. Curr Opin Pediatr 2009;21(3):365–672 [PMID: 19421061].
Misaghi A Goldin A, Awad M, Kulidjian AA: Osteosarcoma: a comprehensive review. SICOT J 2018;4:12 [PMID: 29629690].

EWING SARCOMA

▶ **Clinical Findings**

A. Symptoms and Signs

Ewing sarcoma is a malignant tumor that usually presents with pain and tenderness. Fever and leukocytosis may also be present, and osteomyelitis is the main differential diagnosis. The lesion may be multicentric. It is radiolucent and destroys the cortex, frequently in the diaphyseal region (Figure 26–45). Reactive bone formation may occur around the lesion, seen as successive layers of the so-called onion skin layering.

▶ **Treatment**

Treatment is with multiagent chemotherapy, radiation, and surgical resection. Large tumor size, pelvic lesions, and inadequate response to chemotherapy portend a poor prognosis.

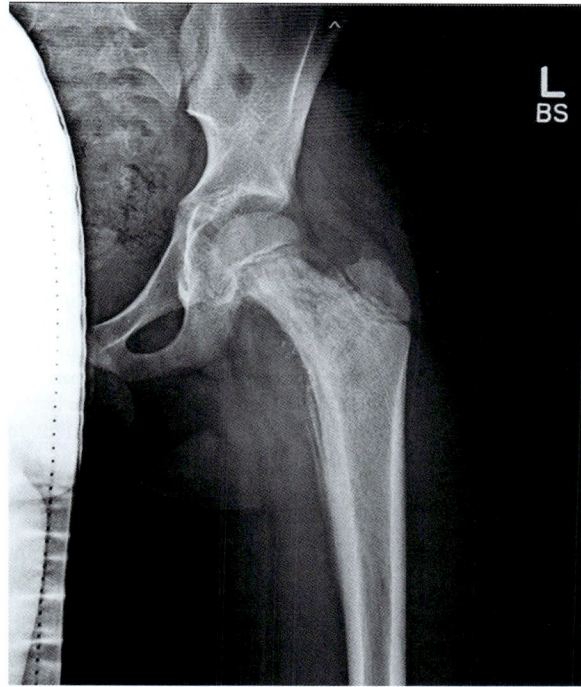

▲ **Figure 26–45.** Radiographic evidence of classic onion skin layering of an Ewing sarcoma of the proximal femur.

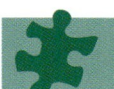

Parida L et al: Clinical management of Ewing sarcoma of the bones of the hands and feet: a retrospective single-institution review. J Pediatr Surg 2012;47(10):1806–1810 [PMID: 23084188].

MISCELLANEOUS DISEASES OF BONE & JOINT

ESSENTIALS OF DIAGNOSIS & TYPICAL FEATURES

▶ Malignant processes need to be ruled out.
▶ Obtain radiographs when indicated.
▶ Treatment is based on symptoms and location.

FIBROUS DYSPLASIA

Dysplastic fibrous tissue replacement of the medullary canal is accompanied by the formation of metaplastic bone in areas with fibrous dysplasia. Three forms of the disease are recognized: monostotic, polyostotic, and polyostotic with endocrine disturbances (precocious puberty in females, hyperthyroidism, and hyperadrenalism [Albright syndrome]).

▶ ### Clinical Findings

A. Symptoms and Signs

The lesion or lesions may be asymptomatic. If present, pain is probably due to pathologic fractures. In females, endocrine disturbances may be present in the polyostotic variety and are associated with café au lait spots.

B. Imaging

The lesion begins centrally within the medullary canal, usually of a long bone, and expands slowly (Figure 26–46). Pathologic fracture may occur (Figure 26–47). If metaplastic bone predominates, the contents of the lesion have the density of bone. The disease is often asymmetrical, and limb length disturbances may occur as a result of stimulation of epiphysial cartilage growth. Marked deformity of the bone may result; a severe varus deformity with rounding of the proximal femur (shepherd's crook deformity) is a classic feature of the disease.

▶ ### Treatment

If the lesion is small and asymptomatic, no treatment is needed. If the lesion is large and produces or threatens pathologic fracture, curettage and bone grafting are indicated. The prognosis is good, as malignant transformation is rare.

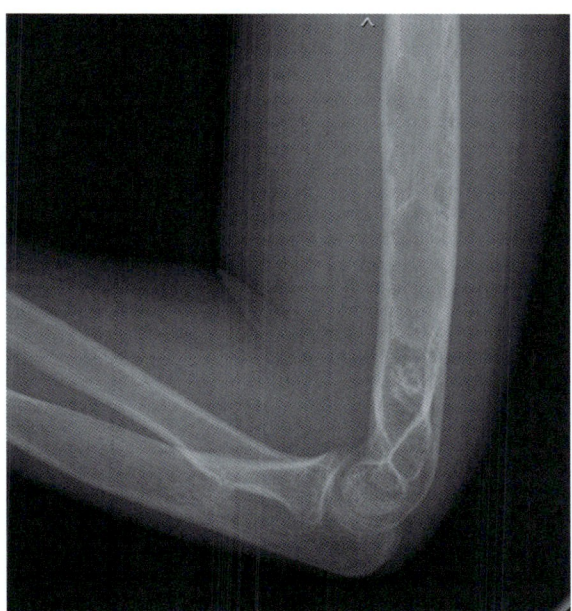

▲ **Figure 26–46.** Fibrous dysplasia of the distal humerus.

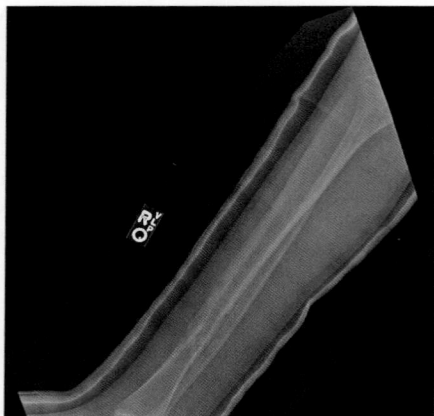

▲ Figure 26–47. Tibia fracture with fibrous dysplasia.

Boyce AM, Florenzano P, Castro L, Collins MT: Fibrous dysplasia/ McCune-Albright syndrome. In: GeneReviews (R), Adam MP et al (eds). 1993: Seattle, WA. Updated 2018 [PMID: 25719192].

BONE CYSTS, BAKER CYST, & GANGLIONS

▶ Clinical Findings

A. Symptoms and Signs

Unicameral Bone Cyst

Unicameral bone cysts occur in the metaphysis of a long bone, usually in the femur or humerus. A cyst begins in the medullary canal adjacent to the epiphysial cartilage. It probably results from a fault in endochondral ossification (the process where bone is formed from cartilaginous precursors). The cyst is considered active as long as it abuts onto the metaphyseal side of the epiphysial cartilage, and there is a risk of growth arrest with or without treatment. When a border of normal bone exists between the cyst and the epiphysial cartilage, the cyst is inactive. The lesion is usually identified when a pathologic fracture occurs, producing pain.

Laboratory findings are normal. Radiographically, the cyst is identified centrally within the medullary canal, producing expansion of the cortex and thinning over the widest portion of the cyst.

Aneurysmal Bone Cyst

Aneurysmal bone cyst is similar to unicameral bone cyst, except it contains blood rather than clear fluid. It usually occurs in a slightly eccentric position in a long bone, expanding the cortex of the bone but not breaking the cortex. Involvement of the flat bones of the pelvis is less common. Radiographically, the lesion appears somewhat wider than the width of the epiphysial cartilage, which can help distinguish it from a unicameral bone cyst. Chromosomal abnormalities have been associated with aneurysmal bone cysts. The lesion may appear aggressive histologically, and it is important to differentiate it from osteosarcoma or hemangioma.

Baker Cyst

A Baker cyst is a herniation of the synovium in the knee joint into the popliteal region. In children, the diagnosis may be made by aspiration of mucinous fluid. The cyst nearly always disappears with time.

Ganglion

A ganglion is a smooth, small cystic mass connected by a pedicle to the joint capsule, usually on the dorsum of the wrist. It may also occur in the tendon sheath over the flexor or extensor surfaces of the fingers. Ganglia may interfere with function or cause persistent pain.

▶ Treatment

Treatment of bone cysts and ganglion can be by curettage and bone grafting. Baker cysts usually require no surgical treatment. Ganglia can be excised if they cause symptoms.

Mascard E, Gomez-Brouchet A, Lambot K: Bone cysts: unicameral and aneurysmal bone cyst. Orthop Traumatol Surg Res 2015;101(1 Suppl):119–127 [PMID: 25579825].

Sports Medicine

Aubrey Armento, MD, CAQSM
Karin VanBaak, MD, CAQSM
Stephanie W. Mayer, MD

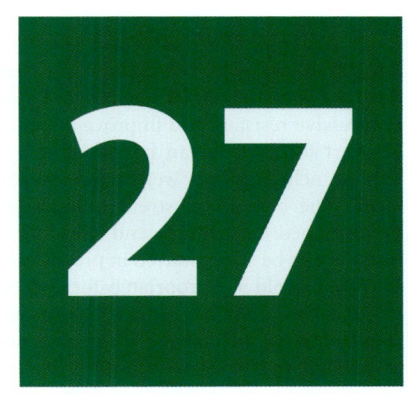

27

Sports medicine as a separate discipline has grown since the 1980s in response to an expanding body of knowledge in the areas of exercise physiology, biomechanics, and musculoskeletal medicine. As more children participate in recreational and competitive sports, pediatric health care providers are encountering more young athletes in their practice. Familiarity with the common medical and orthopedic issues faced by athletically active children and knowledge of which injuries necessitate referral to a sports medicine specialist are essential.

BASIC PRINCIPLES

Pediatric Injury Patterns

Although young athletes have injuries and issues similar to those of adults, there are many injuries that are unique to the pediatric and adolescent athlete. An understanding of the differences between adult and pediatric injury patterns is important to foster an appropriate index of suspicion for situations unique to pediatrics.

The anatomic components of a long bone are the diaphysis, metaphysis, and epiphysis. In the pediatric bone, the presence of cartilaginous growth plates and apophyses predispose children to unique injury patterns that are different from their adult counterparts. Open growth plates or physes and their various stages of development are important factors to consider when treating young athletes. The physes are located at the ends of the long bones and are the primary ossification centers where length is added to the immature skeleton. The physis is a weak link in the musculoskeletal complex and has a high risk of fracture, particularly during periods of rapid growth. The surrounding soft tissues, including ligaments and tendons, are relatively strong compared to the physis. Epiphyses are secondary centers of ossification that also contribute to long bone formation and, like the adjacent articular cartilage, are vulnerable to trauma.

Injuries that involve the epiphysis can lead to joint deformity. Apophyses are secondary centers of ossification that add contour but not length to the bone. The apophysis is the attachment site of the muscle-tendon unit and is vulnerable to both acute and chronic overuse traction injury, particularly during times of rapid growth. Unlike injuries to the physis and epiphysis, however, apophyseal injuries do not result in long-term growth disturbance. Recognizing injuries to growth centers is important because of the risk for partial or complete physeal arrest. Complications of growth plate injury can lead to limb length discrepancy or angular deformity.

FITNESS & CONDITIONING

Compared to children who are sedentary, physically active youth tend to develop greater agility and maintain better fitness throughout their lifetime. Young children and adolescents (6–17 years old) should participate in moderate to vigorous physical activity for 60 minutes or more each day. To improve overall fitness and reduce the risk of injury, children and adolescents should focus on three different components of exercise:

1. Integrative training, which includes developing fundamental skills and technique, learning proper movement mechanics, and aerobic and anaerobic conditioning

2. Neuromuscular conditioning, such as core strength exercises, agility, and plyometrics

3. Resistance (strength) training (progressive resistive loads in a variety of modalities)

Periodization is a training concept that emphasizes variations in the volume and intensity of training throughout the year in a conditioning program. Continuously varying the specific type and goals of training provides adequate recovery from each strenuous exercise session and avoids overtraining, burnout, and overuse injuries.

Strength Training

Strength is defined as the peak force that can be generated during a single maximal contraction. Strength training uses progressive resistance to improve an athlete's ability to resist or exert force. This can be achieved by a variety of techniques, including body weight, free weight, or machine resistance. The benefits of strength training include improved performance, endurance, and muscular strength. Strength training can be safely started in prepubescent athletes as early as 7–8 years old if appropriately focused on lighter resistance, increased repetitions, proper technique and mechanics, coordination, and building self-confidence. Children mature at varying paces, and strength training programs should be individualized to accommodate for these unique differences. All strength training regimens should be modified as needed to remain age-appropriate and pain-free. Sexual maturity rating (see Chapter 4) helps define readiness for progression to more strenuous programs. Power lifting and maximal weightlifting should be restricted to athletes who have reached or passed adult maturity. To prevent injuries, care should be taken to instruct children on the proper use of weight-training equipment at home. Children and adults with disabilities can benefit from weight-training programs modified to meet their specific needs.

Lobelo F, Muth ND, Hanson S, Nemeth BA; Council on Sports Medicine and Fitness; Section on Obesity: Physical activity assessment and counseling in pediatric clinical settings. Pediatrics Mar 2020;45(3):e20193992. doi: 10.1542/peds.2019-3992 [PMID: 32094289].

Stricker PR, Faigenbaum AD, McCambridge TM; Council on Sports Medicine and Fitness: Resistance training for children and adolescents. Pediatrics Jun 2020;145(6):e20201011. doi: 10.1542/peds.2020-1011 [PMID: 32457216].

SPORTS NUTRITION

Proper nutrition in young athletes focuses on maintaining an appropriate energy balance; creating healthy eating and hydration habits; and avoiding harmful food, drink, and supplement choices. Athletes should be encouraged to balance caloric intake with energy expenditure, ensure adequate carbohydrate intake to support exercise demands, prioritize healthy fats and proteins, and maintain proper hydration. Carbohydrates should compose 50%–60% of a young athlete's diet, with fat and protein making up 25%–30% and 15%–25%, respectively. Hydration can come mainly from water if the exercise lasts less than 1 hour, after which a carbohydrate-containing sports drink is appropriate. To avoid excessive caloric and sugar intake, sports drinks are not recommended at times other than prolonged exercise unless recommended by a registered dietitian. If the average athlete eats a well-balanced diet, nutritional supplementation is unnecessary unless specific nutritional deficiencies are identified by a health care professional. Similarly, energy drinks are not recommended in any youth younger than 18 years.

Pediatric practitioners should monitor young athletes for the Female (and Male) Athlete Triad. Originally defined as a syndrome comprising low energy availability, oligo- or amenorrhea, and low bone density, the more recently defined, expanded concept of relative energy deficiency in sport (REDs) raises awareness of negative effects on other body systems due to low energy availability and the possibility of this condition in males. The central tenant is that caloric intake that does not keep up with caloric expenditure can have negative effects on multiple physiologic systems. This condition should be considered in young athletes with menstrual irregularities (female athletes) or concern for hypogonadism (male athletes), bone health concerns, and poor recovery and performance. This condition may be seen in athletes with eating disorders and disordered eating or may occur due to unintentional underfueling. The primary intervention is focused on restoring adequate nutritional balance.

Committee on Nutrition and Council on Sports Medicine and Fitness: Sports drinks and energy drinks for children and adolescents: are they appropriate? Pediatrics 2011;127(6):1182–1189 [PMID: 21624882].

De Sousa MJ et al: 2014 female athlete triad coalition consensus statement on treatment and return to play of the female athlete triad. Br J Sports Med 2014;48(4):289–309 [PMID: 24463911].

Kleinman R (ed): *Pediatric Nutrition Handbook.* 6th ed. AAP; 2009.

Mountjoy M, et al. 2023 International Olympic Committee's (IOC) consensus statement on Relative Energy Deficiency in Sport (REDs). Br J Sports Med 2023 Sep;57(17):1073–1097. doi: 10.1136/bjsports-2023-106994. [PMID: 37752011].

PREPARTICIPATION PHYSICAL EVALUATION

The ultimate goal of the preparticipation physical evaluation (PPE) is to promote the health and safety of athletes. Its primary objectives are to screen for conditions that may be life threatening or disabling and for conditions that may predispose to injury or illness. Secondary objectives of the PPE include establishing a medical home, determining the general health of the individual, assessing fitness for specific sports, and counseling on injury prevention and health-related issues. The ideal timing of the examination is at least 6–8 weeks before training starts. This allows time to further evaluate, treat, or rehabilitate any identified problems.

Preparticipation History

The medical history is the most important part of the encounter, identifying 65%–77% of medical and musculoskeletal conditions. A standardized PPE form is included in the fifth edition of the PPE monograph that is the recommended standard for the preparticipation physical examination in the United States (Bernhardt and Roberts 2019; available from the American Academy of Pediatrics at https://www.aap.org/en/patient-care/preparticipation-physical-evaluation/). The history includes the following areas:

A. Cardiovascular History

Current American Heart Association (AHA) recommendations for cardiovascular screening, incorporated in the fifth edition PPE monograph, include the following screen:

Personal Medical History:

1. Chest pain or discomfort with exercise
2. Syncope or near syncope associated with exercise
3. Excessive shortness or breath or fatigue associated with exertion
4. History of heart murmur
5. History of elevated blood pressure

Family Medical History:

6. Premature death before age 50 years due to heart disease
7. Disability from heart disease in a close relative younger than 50 years
8. Knowledge of specific cardiac conditions: hypertrophic or dilated cardiomyopathy, long QT syndrome, other ion channelopathies, Marfan syndrome, or arrhythmias

Sudden cardiac arrest is the leading medical cause of sudden death in young athletes. Screening for congenital cardiovascular conditions with the history and physical examination may help identify potentially life-threatening cardiac conditions. However, there are currently no outcome-based studies that demonstrate the effectiveness of the PPE in preventing sudden cardiac death in athletes. In the United States, the most common causes of sudden cardiac death on the playing field are hypertrophic cardiomyopathy (HCM) and congenital coronary artery anomalies, with HCM accounting for one-third of sudden cardiac deaths in young athletes. Any athletes with cardiovascular symptoms require further evaluation before allowing them to participate in sports. Any activity restrictions or sports disqualification for an athlete should be made in consultation with a cardiologist.

The routine use of electrocardiogram (ECG) and echocardiography in the preparticipation cardiovascular screening in athletes remains a debated topic in sports medicine and sports cardiology. The AHA currently recommends against the routine use of ECG in asymptomatic athletes because of low sensitivity, high false-positive rate, limited resources, lack of trained physicians to interpret the ECG, and poor cost-effectiveness due to the low prevalence of disease.

B. History of Hypertension

The diagnosis of hypertension in children younger than 18 years is based on gender, age, and height and blood pressure measured on three separate occasions. Blood pressure measurements with values from 90% to 95% of gender, age, and height-based norms are considered prehypertension; values from 95% to 5 mm Hg above the 99% of norms are defined as stage 1 hypertension; and values greater than 5 mm Hg above the 99% of norms are defined as stage 2 hypertension. A history of hypertension requires investigation for secondary causes and end-organ damage. An athlete with hypertension who exercises may cause the blood pressure to rise even higher, increasing the risk for complications. Athletes with elevated blood pressure should be asked about the use of stimulants (ie, caffeine, nicotine, attention-deficit disorder medications) and a family history of hypertension.

Athletes with prehypertension are eligible to participate in sports. Counseling regarding lifestyle modifications should include healthy dietary changes, weight management, and daily physical activity. Those with stage 1 hypertension, in the absence of end-organ damage, may also participate in competitive sports but with appropriate subspecialist referral if the individual is symptomatic, has associated heart disease or structural abnormality, or has persistent elevated blood pressure on two additional occasions despite lifestyle modifications. Athletes who have stage 2 hypertension or end-organ damage should not be cleared to participate in competitive sports until their blood pressure is evaluated, treated, and under control.

C. Central Nervous System

A history of frequent or exertional headaches, seizure disorders, concussions or head injuries, recurrent stingers or burners, or cervical cord neurapraxia may affect an athlete's ability to participate in sports. These conditions require further evaluation, rehabilitation, or informed decision-making prior to clearance for sports participation. The fifth edition PPE monograph provides an updated review and recommendations on concussions in sports (see also section Concussion).

D. History of Chronic Diseases

Diseases such as reactive airway disease, exercise-induced asthma, diabetes, renal disease, liver disease, chronic infections, or hematologic diseases should be noted.

E. Surgical History

Surgical history may influence participation in certain sports. Full recovery with no long-term impact on athletic performance is required prior to clearance.

F. Infectious Mononucleosis

Possible occurrence of acute infectious mononucleosis in the last 4 weeks should be assessed. The risk for splenic rupture is highest within the first 3 weeks of illness and can occur in the absence of trauma. Therefore, physical activity should be avoided during the first 3–4 weeks after the infection starts. The athlete may return to play once clinical symptoms are resolved and risk for splenic rupture is assessed as minimal. The use of serial abdominal ultrasound to assess spleen size to aid in return-to-play decisions is not recommended. Parameters for spleen size based on ethnicity, sex, height, and weight have not yet been established, so determining when spleen size has normalized based on imaging is difficult.

G. Musculoskeletal Limitations and Prior Injuries

The physician should inquire about joints with limited range of motion, muscle weakness, and prior injuries that may affect future performance. Chronic pain or soreness long after activity may reflect overuse syndromes that require evaluation.

H. Menstrual History in Females

The presence of oligo- or amenorrhea should raise concern for possible underlying Female Athlete Triad/REDs (see section Sports Nutrition).

I. Nutritional Issues

The athlete should be assessed for risk factors for disordered eating or low energy availability, including the methods the athlete uses to maintain, gain, or lose weight.

J. Medication History

The use of prescription medications, over-the-counter medications, and supplements should be assessed. This may reveal problems omitted in the medical history, as well as provide data on medications whose side effects may necessitate activity modifications. Documenting drug use may provide the opportunity to explore the drawbacks of performance-enhancing compounds such as anabolic steroids, creatine, stimulants, and narcotics.

K. Mental Health

The fifth edition PPE monograph recommends screening young athletes for underlying mental health conditions. In addition to assessment of disordered eating characteristics, use of the Patient Health Questionnaire—4 as a screening tool for Depression and Anxiety is recommended.

Physical Examination

An example of a preparticipation physical examination form is endorsed in the fifth edition of the PPE monograph (https://services.aap.org/en/community/aap-councils/council-on-sports-medicine-and-fitness/preparticipation-physical-evaluation/). The examination should include routine vital signs, including seated blood pressure measurements obtained in the upper extremity. The cardiovascular

examination should include palpation of radial and femoral pulses, auscultation for murmurs while sitting and standing, and evaluation for physical stigmata of Marfan syndrome. Included is a quick guide that can be used to screen for musculoskeletal abnormalities (Table 27–1).

The examination should also address the skin (any contagious lesions such as herpes or impetigo?), vision (visual or retinal problems?), abdomen (hepatosplenomegaly?), genitourinary system (testicular abnormalities or hernias?), neurologic system (problems with coordination, gait, or mental processing?), and sexual maturity rating.

Recommendations for Participation

After completing the medical evaluation, the physician can make recommendations about sports clearance. The options include

- Cleared for all sports without restrictions
- Cleared for all sports without restrictions, with recommendations for further evaluation or treatment
- Not cleared: pending further evaluation, for any sports, or for certain sports

Table 27–2 is a composite of recommendations for sports participation organized by body system. Athletes with cardiac issues including syncope, aortic stenosis, arrhythmias, cardiomyopathies, congenital heart disease, Marfan syndrome, and Kawasaki disease should be evaluated by a cardiologist prior to clearance to participate in sports.

Bernhardt DT, Roberts WO: *Preparticipation Physical Evaluation.* 5th ed. American Academy of Pediatrics; 2019.
Bull MJ; Committee on Genetics: Health supervision for children with Down syndrome. Pediatrics 2011 Aug;128(2):393–406. 10.1542/peds.2011-1605 [PMID: 21788214].
Demorest RA, Washington RL; Council on Sports Medicine and Fitness: Athletic participation by children and adolescents who have systemic hypertension. Pediatrics 2010 Jun;125(6): 1287–1294. 10.1542/peds.2010-0658 [PMID: 20513738].
Evans N, Wingo B, Sasso E, Hicks A, Gorgey AS, Harness E: Exercise recommendations and considerations for persons with spinal cord injury. Arch Phys Med Rehabil 2015 Sep 1;96(9):1749–1750 [PMID: 26198424].
Gonzalez A, Mares AV, Espinoza DR: Common pulmonary conditions in sport. Clin Sports Med 2019 Oct 1;38(4):563–575 [PMID: 31472767].
Manuel C, Feinstein R: Sports participation for young athletes with medical conditions: seizure disorder, infections and single organs. Curr Probl Pediatr Adolesc Health Care 2018;48 (5–6):161–171 [PMID: 30017601].
Maron BJ et al: Eligibility and disqualification recommendations for competitive athletes with cardiovascular abnormalities: a scientific statement from the American Heart Association and American College of Cardiology. J Am Coll Cardiol 2015 Dec;66(21):2343–2349 [PMID: 26542655].
Peterson AR, Nash E, Anderson BJ: Infectious disease in contact sports. Sports Health 2019 Jan;11(1):47–58 [PMID: 30106670].

Table 27–1. The screening sports examination.[a]

General evaluation	Have patient stand in front of examiner; evaluate both front and back along with posture. Look at general body habitus. Look for asymmetry in muscle bulk, scars, or unusual postures. Watch how patient moves when instructed.
Neck evaluation	Evaluate ROM by having patient bend head forward (chin to chest), rotate from side to side, and laterally bend (ear to shoulder). Observe for asymmetry, lack of motion, or pain with movement.

Shoulder and upper extremity evaluation	Observe clavicles, shoulder position, scapular position, elbow position, and fingers.
	ROM screening:
	    Fully abduct arms with palms in jumping jack position.
	    Internally and externally rotate shoulder.
	    Flex and extend wrist, pronate and supinate wrist, flex and extend fingers.
	Do the following manual muscle testing:
	    Have patient shrug shoulders (testing trapezius).
	    Abduct to 90 degrees (testing deltoid).
	    Flex elbow (testing biceps).
	    Extend elbow over head (testing triceps).
	    Test wrist flexion and extension.
	    Have patient grasp fingers.

Back evaluation	General inspection to look for scoliosis or kyphosis.
	ROM screening:
	    Bend forward touching toes with knees straight (spine flexion and hamstring range).
	    Rotation, side bending, and spine extension.

Gait and lower extremity evaluation	General observation while walking. Have patient walk short distance normally (look at symmetry, heel-toe gait pattern, look at all joints involved in gait and leg lengths, any evidence of joint effusions or pain). Have patient toe-walk and heel-walk for short distance and check tandem walking (balance beam walking).

ROM, range of motion.
[a]If any abnormalities are found, a more focused evaluation is required.

Riddell MC et al: Exercise management in type 1 diabetes: a consensus statement. Lancet Diabetes Endocrinol 2017;5:377–390 [PMID: 28126459].

Schwellnus M et al: International Olympic Committee (IOC) consensus statement on acute respiratory illness in athletes part 1: acute respiratory infections. Br J Sports Med 2022;56:1066–1088 [PMID: 35863871].

Toldi J, Escobar J, Brown A: Cerebral palsy: sport and exercise considerations. Curr Sports Med Rep 2021 Jan 1;20(1):19–25 [PMID: 33395127].

Voet NB, van der Kooi EL, van Engelen BG, Geurts AC: Strength training and aerobic exercise training for muscle disease. Cochrane Database Syst Rev 2019 Dec 6;12(12):CD003907. doi: 10.1002/14651858.CD003907 [PMID: 31808555].

REHABILITATION OF SPORTS INJURIES

Participation in sports benefits children by promoting physical activity and acquisition of motor and social skills. All sports participation, however, carries an inherent risk of injury. Injuries are classified as either acute or chronic. Chronic injuries occur over time as a result of overuse, repetitive microtrauma, and inadequate repair of injured tissue. When the demands of exercise exceed the body's ability to recover, overuse injury may occur. Overuse injury accounts for up to 50% of all injuries in pediatric sports medicine. Risk factors for overuse injuries include year-round participation, participation on more than one team at a time, early specialization in one sport, poor mechanics, and training errors such as increasing exercise volume, load, frequency, or intensity too quickly. To avoid overuse injury, athletes should train with a regular variety of resistances, power, speed, agility, skills, and distance. Adequate periods of rest and recovery should be incorporated into every training regimen to ensure proper healing of stressed tissues.

Acute injuries or macrotrauma are one-time events that can cause alterations in biomechanics and physiology. Response to an acute injury occurs in predictable phases. The first week is characterized by an acute inflammatory response, resulting in the classical physical findings of local swelling, warmth, pain, and loss of function. The proliferative phase occurs over the next 2–4 weeks and involves repair and clean-up. Last, the maturation phase allows for repair and regeneration of the damaged tissues.

Table 27–2. Recommendations and considerations for participation in sports.

Disorders	Considerations and Recommendations	References
Cardiac		
Anticoagulation treatment	Need to avoid all contact/collision sports.	Maron et al (2015)
Hypertension	May participate: qualified yes. Those with hypertension > 5 mm Hg above 99th percentile for age, gender, and height should avoid heavy weightlifting and power lifting, bodybuilding, and high-static component sports.	Demorest et al (2010)
Endocrine		
Diabetes mellitus type 1	No restrictions to activity, and exercise should be encouraged. However, athletes are at risk for hypoglycemia and ketoacidosis, so ensure proper hydration and carbohydrate intake. As exercise enhances insulin sensitivity, the quantity and duration of aerobic and anaerobic exercise and intensity of practices and games need to be assessed. The insulin and carbohydrate needs before, during, and after exercise vary per individual and should be tailored based on duration and intensity of exercise, as guided by an endocrinologist.	Riddell et al (2017)
Eye		
Functionally one eyed	Defined as having best corrected visual acuity worse than 20/40 in the poorest seeing eye. Recommend that athletes with only one functional eye not participate in boxing or full contact martial arts. Otherwise, athletes should wear eye protection.	Manuel et al (2018)
Genitourinary		
One testicle	May participate, but athlete should wear protective cup in collision and contact sports.	Manuel et al (2018)
Solitary kidney	May participate: qualified yes; however, there is increased risk of possible loss of function of the single kidney in contact/collision sports.	Manuel et al (2018)
Hematologic		
Hemophilia	Avoid contact and collision sports.	
Sickle cell disease	May participate: qualified yes. If illness status permits, all sports may be played. However, any sport or activity that entails overexertion, overheating, dehydration, or chilling should be avoided. Participation at high altitude poses risk for sickle cell crisis.	Maron et al (2015)
Sickle cell trait	Currently, no recommendations for universal screening in athletes. However, the NCAA now requires screening for athletes if their sickle cell status is unknown. May participate: yes. Ensure acclimatization to extreme environment conditions (eg, altitude, heat, humidity) and adequate hydration during participation to reduce risk of heat illness and/or rhabdomyolysis.	Maron et al (2015)
Infectious disease		
Fever	May participate: no. Cardiopulmonary effort is increased while maximum exercise capacity is decreased during febrile illnesses. Risk of heat illness is also increased.	Manuel et al (2018)
Infectious mononucleosis	Splenic rupture is most important consideration. Risk of spleen rupture highest during first 3 wk of illness. No athletic participation during the first 3–4 wk after the infection starts. Too early a return to sports increases risk of splenic rupture or could cause EBV reactivation and relapse. If symptoms resolve by third week, light activities can be started during the fourth week with graded increases in intensity. Full contact activity participation may resume at week 5.	Manuel et al (2018)
Skin infections	Bacterial dermatoses (including impetigo, furuncles, cellulitis, folliculitis, and abscesses): Athletes with suspected MRSA infections should be cultured and treated accordingly with antibiotics. Abscesses should be treated with incision and drainage. Athlete may participate when no new lesions for 48 h, no moist or draining lesions, and has completed oral antibiotics for at least 72 h. Herpes gladiatorum: Athlete may participate when no new lesions for 72 h, all lesions are covered with a firm crust, and has been on oral antiviral treatment for 120 h. Molluscum contagiosum: Athletes must have lesions covered. Tinea: Oral or topical antifungal for at least 72 h (tinea corporis) and 14 days (tinea capitus).	Peterson et al (2019)

(Continued)

Table 27–2. Recommendations and considerations for participation in sports. (*Continued*)

Disorders	Considerations and Recommendations	References
Upper respiratory infections (including common cold)	Depends on symptoms and severity of illness. Generally, if mild illness and no systemic symptoms, breathing difficulties, chest pain/pressure/tightness, or moderate to severe cough, athletes can be cleared to continue exercise as tolerated. If moderate to severe illness and/or with symptoms noted above, exercise participation should be restricted and further evaluation may be necessary prior to gradual return to exercise once symptoms improve/resolve.	Schwellnus et al (2022)
Neurologic		
Epilepsy	Majority of sports are safe for those with adequate seizure control; contact sports are allowed with proper protection. Swimming and water sports should be supervised. Sports such as free climbing, hang gliding, and scuba are not recommended.	Manuel et al (2018)
Muscle disease or myopathy	Exercise as tolerated under supervision of a health care professional. Aerobic exercise and/or strength training may be acceptable, depending on specific muscle disease/myopathy and each individual's exercise tolerance.	Voet et al (2019)
Respiratory		
Asthma	No activity restrictions. Using an inhaled short-acting β_2-agonist 15–20 min before exercise is recommended to help prevent exercise-induced bronchoconstriction. For athletes with asthma symptoms unassociated with exercise or who have frequent use of β_2-agonists (> 2 times per week), a regular inhaled corticosteroid should be considered. Antidoping regulations need to be considered for athletes using β_2-agonists.	Gonzalez et al (2019)
Pneumothorax	Can occur spontaneously in sports, especially in young, tall males. Management is per standard guideline recommendations, including chest x-ray. Athlete may return to sports when there is evidence of radiographic resolution.	Gonzalez et al (2019)
Other		
Cerebral palsy	Exercise as tolerated under supervision of a health care professional.	Toldi et al (2021)
Down syndrome	10%–40% have atlantoaxial instability. Head or neck trauma in these patients may cause catastrophic spinal cord injury. Correlation of radiographic findings of atlantoaxial instability with neurologic abnormalities has not been well established. At present, there are no evidence-based guidelines for screening and activity restrictions. For management, see section Atlantoaxial Instability. 40%–50% of persons with Down syndrome have cardiac anomalies. Evaluation of underlying congenital heart disorders should be considered in this population.	Bull (2011)
Remote spinal cord injury or spina bifida	Full participation as tolerated under supervision of a health care professional. Modifications or accommodations may need to be made based on exercise/sport type and equipment needs. Be aware of thermoregulatory dysfunction, medications, and pressure areas.	Evans et al (2015)

AHA, American Heart Association; EBV, Epstein-Barr virus; ECG, electrocardiogram; LVEF, left ventricular ejection fraction; MRSA, methicillin-resistant *Staphylococcus aureus*; NCAA, National Collegiate Athletic Association.

The management of acute sports injuries focuses on optimizing healing and restoring function. The goals of immediate care are to minimize the effects of the injury by reducing pain and swelling, educate the athlete about the nature of the injury and how to treat it, and maintain the health and fitness of the rest of the body. The treatment for an acute injury is captured in the acronym PRICE:

Protect the injury from further damage (taping, splints, braces), Rest the area, Ice, Compression of the injury, and Elevation immediately. Nonsteroidal anti-inflammatory drugs (NSAIDs) may reduce the inflammatory response and reduce discomfort and can be used immediately after the injury. When safely and appropriately managed, therapeutic use of physical modalities, including early cold and later heat, hydrotherapy, massage, electrical stimulation, iontophoresis, and ultrasound, can enhance recovery in the acute phase.

The recovery phase can be lengthy and requires athlete participation. Physical therapy prescription is a common treatment modality. Initial treatment is focused on joint range of motion and flexibility. Range-of-motion exercises should follow a logical progression of starting with passive motion, then active assistive and finally active movement. Strength training can begin once normal joint range has been reestablished and active range of motion exercises are initiated. As the athlete approaches near-normal strength and is pain-free, the final maintenance phase can be introduced. During this phase, the athlete continues to build strength and work on endurance. The biomechanics of sport-specific activity need to be analyzed and retraining incorporated into the exercise program. Generalized cardiovascular conditioning should continue during the entire rehabilitation treatment. Typically, return-to-play guidelines after an injury include the attainment of full joint range of motion, nearly full and symmetric strength, full speed, and nearly full sport-specific agility and skill, all without pain.

Current evidence in injury prevention focuses on core stability training and dynamic warm-up. Core exercises emphasize isometric holds that activate the core and pelvis. They utilize light single limb movements to challenge endurance over protracted time periods. Dynamic warm-up programs concentrate on light movement involving controlled, full active range of motion of each joint prior to exercise. The aim is to initiate light perspiration and increase heart rate, peripheral circulation, and connective tissue suppleness through simple excitatory activity. In contrast to traditional static stretching regimens in which athletes hold a stretching position for a distinct period of time, an appropriate dynamic program will incorporate aerobic activity and moving stretches into sport-specific movement preparation. For example, athletes may work through a series of exercises such as side shuffle, high knee stepping, bear crawls, and double-leg hopping over cones three times. Static stretching is appropriate after exercise is complete.

Paterno M: Unique issues in the rehabilitation of the pediatric and adolescent athlete after musculoskeletal injury. Sports Med Arthrosc Rev 2016;24(4):178–183. doi:10.1097/JSA.0000000000000130 [PMID: 27811517].

COMMON SPORTS MEDICINE ISSUES & INJURIES

BONE STRESS INJURIES

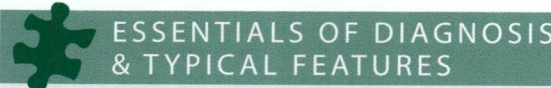

ESSENTIALS OF DIAGNOSIS & TYPICAL FEATURES

► Overuse injuries to the bone, commonly in the tibia and metatarsals.
► Often occur during periods of rapid increase in physical activity and/or in the setting of the Female or Male Athlete Triad.

Stress reactions and stress fractures of bone comprise a spectrum of severity collectively known as bone stress injuries. These are overuse injuries to the bone, with pathology ranging from bony edema with degradation of bony microarchitecture to frank fracture in the bony cortex. The most common locations for bone stress injuries are the posterior-medial tibia and the shaft of the metatarsals. Bone stress injuries occur with highest incidence in athletes who engage in repeated impact activities, such as distance running. Risk factors for bone stress injuries include overload in training, such as excessive total impact loading, lack of rest period, or increasing impact loading too quickly. Occurrence of a bone stress injury should raise concern for Female or Male Athlete Triad/REDs. Treatment of bone stress injuries mirrors treatment of a traumatic fracture of a certain bone. Some bone stress injuries, such as those at the femoral neck and anterior tibia, are more high risk for healing complications than others. Most bone stress injuries can be treated nonoperatively, but some may require operative intervention.

HEAD & NECK INJURIES

Head and neck injuries occur most commonly in contact and individual sports. Concussions most commonly occur in football, ice hockey, rugby, boxing, basketball, lacrosse, and soccer. As a general rule, treatment of head and neck injuries in young children should be more conservative because of their developing central nervous systems.

1. Concussion

ESSENTIALS OF DIAGNOSIS & TYPICAL FEATURES

► Symptoms appear after a traumatic blow causing sudden movement to the head.
► Common symptoms include headache, dizziness, light or noise sensitivity, balance issues, fatigue, fogginess, and concentration difficulties.
► Focal neurologic symptoms should raise concern for acute intracranial process and prompt more immediate workup.
► Efforts should be made to normalize activities of daily life as soon as possible by following a return to learn progression.
► Return to contact sports should take place only after the patient is back to baseline with no symptoms and has successfully completed the return-to-play protocol.

Concussion is a complex process that occurs when a direct blow to the body or head translates forces into the brain, causing a transient alteration of neurologic function. Even in the presence of neurologic symptoms, concussions are usually not associated with structural changes in brain tissue detectable by standard imaging studies. Instead, they may cause metabolic and vascular changes in cerebral tissues. Consequently, there are complex alterations in physiologic function, such as catecholamine surges and failure of cerebral blood flow autoregulation. Symptoms may appear and evolve over the first few hours after injury. Concussion should be suspected in any athlete with somatic, cognitive, or behavioral complaints listed in Table 27–3. Confusion, headache, visual disturbance, posttraumatic amnesia, and balance problems are common. Concussion does not have to involve loss of consciousness, but observers may notice physical signs, behavioral changes, or cognitive impairment. Diagnosis may be aided by the use of the Sport Concussion Assessment Tool v.3 (SCAT5) and the Child-SCAT5 (ages 5–12 years), which also include standardized patient handouts (available at: https://bjsm.bmj.com/content/51/11/851 and https://bjsm.bmj.com/content/bjsports/early/2017/04/26/bjsports-2017-097492childscat5.full.pdf).

Any athlete suspected of sustaining a concussion in a practice or competition should be immediately removed from play, and if a concussion is diagnosed, the athlete should not be permitted to return to sport on the day of injury. To monitor for deterioration, the athlete should not be left alone in the initial hours after injury. An athlete. Computed tomography (CT) should be considered during initial evaluation if the patient displays deteriorating or altered mental status, prolonged loss of consciousness, repeated vomiting, severe headache, signs of skull fracture, or focal neurologic deficit or if he/she experienced a severe mechanism of injury. CT imaging is rarely indicated beyond the first 24 hours after injury.

Table 27–3. Concussion: symptom checklist.

Headache
Confusion
Amnesia: classically anterograde
Dizziness
Balance problems
Nausea
Vomiting
Visual disturbances
Light sensitivity
Noise sensitivity
Ringing in the ears
Fatigue or excessive sleepiness
Sleep abnormalities
Memory problems
Concentration difficulties
Irritability
Behavioral changes

Symptoms associated with concussions usually follow a predictable pattern and most resolve within 1–4 weeks. Children and adolescents may have a longer recovery interval than adults. Acute management includes an early period of physical and cognitive rest (generally 1–2 days), the duration of which should be based on an individual's clinical condition. Return to school and light noncontact physical activity may be reasonable early during the recovery period if symptoms can be managed. In young athletes, interventions may include modified school attendance, decreased schoolwork, reduction in technological stimulation (television, internet, computer games, cellular phone), proper nutrition and hydration, and adequate rest and sleep. Before athletes are allowed to return to contact sports participation, symptoms should be resolved both at rest and during non-contact exercise without the aid of medication, and a graduated return-to-play protocol should be completed. Return to play is a six-step progression with each step lasting 24 hours: (1) when asymptomatic at rest for 24 hours, progress to (2) light aerobic exercise, followed by (3) sport-specific exercise and non-contact drills, then begin (4) full noncontact practice, followed by (5) full contact practice, and finally, (6) release to game play. If any symptoms recur during any of the steps, the athlete should not move to the next stage and should rest for 24 hours; thereafter, the athlete should restart at the previous step during which the athlete was asymptomatic. Commonly, it is recommended that an athlete follow up with a medical provider for clearance for return to contact or collision sports, and many states have passed legislation requiring medical assessment of concussed youth and medical clearance for return to play. Current expectations are that children should return to school prior to return to sport, and, in general, conservative return-to-play guidelines should be used in children. Concussion assessment tools, computerized testing, and symptom checklists are frequently helpful; additionally, neuropsychological testing may be useful for management decisions in complex cases but should not be used as the only source of clinical decision making.

Second impact syndrome is a controversial diagnosis primarily based on anecdotal reports. Advocates of this diagnosis endorse a rare but potentially deadly complication of repeated head injury, causing loss of vascular autoregulation, catecholamine surge, increased cerebral blood pressure, and subsequent malignant cerebral edema without intracranial hematoma. Consequences include massive brain swelling and herniation leading to seizure, coma, and, possibly, death. Others disagree about the existence of this diagnosis, suggesting instead that this phenomenon is actually the well-established condition of diffuse cerebral swelling, a known complication of head injury, particularly in younger individuals.

The long-term effects of concussions or contact/collision sports have yet to be established; specifically, a cause-and-effect relationship has not been proven between concussions and chronic traumatic encephalopathy (CTE).

The decision to retire an athlete from high risk or contact/collision sport is a sensitive and challenging one. There is currently little evidence to support a standardized approach to retirement decisions. However, considerations should include total number of concussions; increasing frequency; occurrence with serially less force; and prolonged, more severe, or permanent symptoms/signs.

Davis GA et al: SCAT5. Br J Sports Med 2017. https://bjsm.bmj.com/content/bjsports/early/2017/04/26/bjsports-2017-097506SCAT5.full.pdf.

Davis GA et al: The Child Sport Concussion Assessment Tool 5th Edition (Child SCAT5): background and rationale. Br J Sports Med 2017;51:859–861 [PMID: 28446452].

Harmon KG et al: American Medical Society for Sports Medicine position statement on concussion in sport. Br J Sports Med 2019; 53:213–225 [PMID: 3067819].

2. Atlantoaxial Instability

Atlantoaxial instability is common in children with Down syndrome because of hypotonia and ligamentous laxity, especially including the annular ligament of C1. Consequently, this condition causes increased mobility at C1 and C2. Most cases are asymptomatic. Lateral cervical neck films in flexion, extension, and neutral position evaluate the atlantodens interval (ADI). ADI is normally less than 2.5 mm, but up to 4.5 mm is acceptable in this population. Children with an ADI greater than 4.5 mm or who have neurologic symptoms with neck flexion or extension should be restricted from contact and collision activities, as well as any sport requiring excessive neck flexion or extension until evaluation by an orthopedic specialist.

Myśliwiec A et al: Atlanto-axial instability in people with Down's syndrome and its impact on the ability to perform sports activities—a review. J Hum Kinet 2015 Jan 12;48:17–24. doi: 10.1515/hukin-2015-0087 [PMID: 26834869].

3. Burners or Stingers

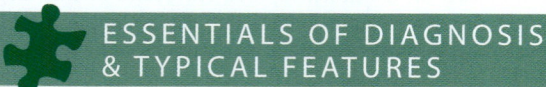

ESSENTIALS OF DIAGNOSIS & TYPICAL FEATURES

▶ Symptoms are unilateral, occurring on the same side as an injury to the neck and shoulder.

▶ Burning pain, numbness, or tingling in the shoulder and arm.

▶ Weakness may be present.

Burners or stingers are common injuries in contact sports, especially football. The two terms are used interchangeably to describe transient unilateral pain and paresthesias in the upper extremity. These cervical radiculopathies or brachial plexopathies typically occur when the head is laterally bent and the shoulder depressed, causing exacerbation of a degenerative cervical disk or stenosis, a compressive injury to a cervical nerve root on the symptomatic upper extremity, or a traction injury to the brachial plexus of the ipsilateral shoulder. Symptoms include immediate burning pain and paresthesias down one arm generally lasting only minutes. Unilateral weakness in the muscles of the upper arm also tends to resolve quickly but can persist for weeks. The most important part of the workup is a thorough neurologic assessment to differentiate this injury from a more serious brain or cervical spine injury. The key distinguishing feature of the stinger is its unilateral nature. If symptoms persist or include bilateral complaints, headache, change in mental status, or severe neck pain, further diagnostic evaluation including cervical spine radiographs with flexion/extension views, magnetic resonance imaging (MRI) scans, and electromyography (EMG) should be considered.

Treatment consists of removal from play and observation. The athlete can return to play once symptoms have resolved, neck and shoulder range of motion is pain-free, reflexes and strength are normal, and the Spurling test is negative. The Spurling test is performed by having the neck extended and rotated to the ipsilateral shoulder while applying an axial load. A positive test will reproduce pain or symptoms in the affected extremity. Restriction of same day return to play should be considered in athletes with a history of multiple stingers, particularly if sustained in the same season. Preventive strategies include wearing well-fitting protective gear, proper blocking and tackling techniques, and maintaining neck and shoulder strength. Long-term complications include permanent neurologic injury or repeated occurrence of stingers, which would necessitate further workup and possible lifetime exclusion from contact or collision sports.

Ahearn BM, Starr HM, Seiler JG: Traumatic brachial plexopathy in athletes: current concepts for diagnosis and management of stingers. J Am Acad Orthop Surg 2019;27(18):677–684 [PMID: 30741724].

SPINE INJURIES

Acute injury to the spine often results from an axial load injury. Patients present with focal tenderness of the thoracic or thoracolumbar spine. Evaluation includes plain radiography that may demonstrate anterior wedging of the thoracic vertebra, representing a compression fracture. When significant spinal tenderness or any neurologic abnormalities are present, radiographs are often followed by CT or MRI. Treatment of minor compression fractures includes pain control, bracing, rest from high-risk sports, and physical therapy. With appropriate rehabilitation, athletes can usually return to contact activity within 8 weeks.

1. Spondylolysis

ESSENTIALS OF DIAGNOSIS & TYPICAL FEATURES

▶ Bone stress injury to the pars interarticularis.
▶ Usually presents as low back pain with extension.

Spondylolysis is a repetitive overloading injury to the pars interarticularis of the vertebral complex, resulting in a bone stress injury. The pars interarticularis is the bony connection between the inferior and superior articulating facets. Injuries to the pars interarticularis, or pars defects, are present in 4%–6% of the population. In adolescent athletes, however, the incidence of spondylolysis in those presenting with lower back pain is close to 50%. As such, it should be high on the differential when evaluating lower back pain in this population. The incidence of pars defects in athletes such as gymnasts, dancers, divers, and wrestlers is significantly increased because of repetitive extension motions combined with rotation. Spondylolysis occurs at L5 in 85% of cases. The athlete presents with midline low back pain that is aggravated by back extension, such as arching the back in gymnastics. There may be palpable tenderness over the lower lumbar vertebrae, with pain on the single leg hyperextension test (Stork test). Evaluation includes anteroposterior (AP) and lateral radiographs of the lumbar spine. Although oblique radiographic views of the lumbar spine are helpful to look for the so-called "Scottie dog sign," they are falling out of favor because they do not significantly improve diagnostic accuracy and increase radiation exposure. Single-photon emission computed tomography (SPECT) scan, CT scan, and/or MRI can be useful to determine the presence of an active spondylotic lesion. MRI scans are moving into favor as they can show subtle bone marrow edema of early stress injuries and do not involve radiation exposure.

There is currently no gold standard for the treatment of spondylolysis. Management includes refraining from hyperextension and high-impact sporting activities and initiation of physical therapy. Athletes can cross-train with low-impact activity and neutral or flexion-based physical therapy while the lesion heals. Bracing is controversial; outcome studies show similar results regarding return to sports and bony healing whether or not braces are worn. It is important to note that clinical outcomes do not necessarily correlate with healed pars fracture versus bony nonunions (when the fractured bone fails to heal); satisfactory outcomes (asymptomatic patients who return to sport) can be achieved regardless of bony healing status. Typically, return to play is often delayed 8–12 weeks based on clinical signs of healing. Most symptomatic spondylolysis improves with rest and activity modifications (with or without radiologic evidence of healing). Once asymptomatic, an athlete can usually gradually return to sports without restrictions. Surgery is reserved for refractory cases that fail conservative measures.

2. Spondylolisthesis

ESSENTIALS OF DIAGNOSIS & TYPICAL FEATURES

▶ Bilateral pars interarticularis injury resulting in forward slippage of one vertebra over the one below it.
▶ Usually presents as low back pain with extension.
▶ Hyperlordosis or possible step-off of lumbar spine can occur.

When a bilateral pars defect occurs, slippage of one vertebra over another can lead to spondylolisthesis. Patients present with hyperlordosis, kyphosis, pain with hyperextension, and, in severe cases, a palpable step-off. A standing lateral radiograph is used to make the diagnosis and to monitor for any progression of slippage. These injuries are graded from 1 to 4 based on the percentage of slippage: grade 1 (0%–24%), grade 2 (25%–49%), grade 3 (50%–74%), and grade 4 (75%–100%).

Treatment is often symptom-based. Asymptomatic athletes with less than 25% slippage often have no restrictions and are followed on a routine basis for radiographic assessment. Management of symptomatic spondylolisthesis is similar to that of spondylolysis. Surgical intervention is considered for slippage greater than 50%, progressive spondylolisthesis, or intractable pain despite nonoperative treatment.

3. Disc Herniation

ESSENTIALS OF DIAGNOSIS & TYPICAL FEATURES

▶ Back pain worse with flexion and sitting.
▶ Radiculopathy can be present.
▶ Positive straight leg raise.

Discogenic back pain accounts for a small percentage of back injuries in children. These injuries are almost unheard of in preadolescence. Back pain can originate from disc bulging, disc herniation, or disc degeneration. Most injuries occur at L4–L5 and L5–S1 vertebrae. Not all disc bulges found on MRI are symptomatic. In adolescents, most disc herniations are central rather than posterolateral. Risk factors include heavy lifting, excessive or repetitive axial loading of the spine, rapid increases in training, or trauma. Symptoms include back pain, which may be increased with activities such as bending, sitting, and coughing. Although not as common as in adults, radicular symptoms of pain down the leg can also occur and are often associated with large disc herniations. Evaluation includes physical and neurologic examinations, including the straight leg test, sensory testing, and checking reflexes. Evaluation usually includes lumbar spine radiographs and an MRI, which is the imaging test of choice for diagnosing disc herniation.

Treatment usually is conservative, as most disc herniations, even if large, improve spontaneously. The athlete should rest for a short period, with avoidance of prolonged sitting, jumping, or hyperextension and hyperflexion of the spine, as these activities may increase pressure on the disc, leading to aggravation of symptoms. After a short period of rest, a structured physical therapy program should begin, focusing on core and pelvic stabilization, peripelvic flexibility, and sports-specific conditioning. If symptoms persist, a short course of oral steroids or epidural steroid injection may be indicated. Surgery is recommended for patients who fail conservative therapy, have significant or progressive radiculopathy, or who have progressive neurologic deficits.

Berger RG, Doyle SM: Spondylolysis 2019 update. Curr Opin Pediatr 2019; Feb;31(1):61–68. doi: 10.1097/MOP.0000000000000706 [PMID: 30531225].

Shimony N et al: Adolescent disc disease: risk factors and treatment success-related factors. World Neurosurg 2021 Apr;148:e314–e320. Epub 2021 Jan 4 [PMID: 33412329].

SHOULDER INJURIES

Acute injuries around the shoulder include contusions, fractures, sprains (or separations), and dislocations. The age of the patient affects the injury pattern, as younger patients are more likely to sustain fractures instead of sprains. Sprains (ligaments) and strains (muscle and tendon) are generally defined as low-grade soft tissue injuries that do not result in functional compromise of a structure.

1. Fracture of the Clavicle

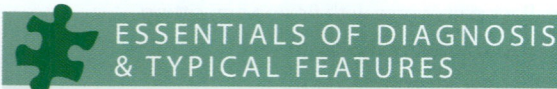

ESSENTIALS OF DIAGNOSIS & TYPICAL FEATURES

► Injury by fall on to the shoulder or outstretched hand.
► Severe pain in the shoulder.
► Tenderness, swelling, and/or deformity over the clavicle.

Clavicular fractures occur from a fall or direct trauma to the shoulder. Focal swelling, deformity, and tenderness are present over the clavicle. The diagnosis is made by radiographs of the clavicle; the fractures are most common in the middle third of the bone.

Initial treatment is focused on pain control and protection with a sling and swathe. Early range of motion is permitted based on pain level and displacement of the fracture. Progressive rehabilitation is important. Athletes cannot return to contact sports for 8–12 weeks. Absolute surgical indications for acute clavicular fractures include open fractures or neurovascular compromise. Fracture nonunion is unusual in young patients. However, there is recent evidence in the adult population recommending surgical stabilization for fractures that are very displaced or shortened. The role of acute surgical stabilization in the pediatric and adolescent population in regard to shortening is still being defined. Patients with recurrent fractures or nonunion typically will also require surgical fixation.

2. Fracture of the Proximal Humerus

ESSENTIALS OF DIAGNOSIS & TYPICAL FEATURES

► Injury with significant fall on outstretched arm.
► Severe pain in the proximal humerus.
► Tenderness, swelling, and/or deformity over the proximal humerus.

Fractures of the proximal humerus occur from a severe blow or fall on the shoulder. Pain and swelling are localized to the proximal humeral region. The fractures can include the physes or may be extraphyseal. A significant amount of displacement and angulation can be tolerated in this location, both physeal and extraphyseal, because of the young athlete's potential for remodeling and because of the intrinsic range of motion of the shoulder. Careful assessment of the brachial plexus and radial nerves is needed to rule out associated nerve damage.

Treatment consists of a sling and often a hanging arm cast to allow for gravity to reduce the fracture for 4–6 weeks followed by progressive rehabilitation with return to play at 8–12 weeks when bony healing, full range of motion, and strength have been achieved.

3. Acromioclavicular Separation

ESSENTIALS OF DIAGNOSIS & TYPICAL FEATURES

► Injury with fall onto the shoulder.
► Severe pain in the shoulder.
► Tenderness, swelling, and/or deformity over the acromioclavicular joint.

A fall on the point of the shoulder is the most common cause of acromioclavicular (AC) separation. Tearing of the AC joint capsule and possibly the coracoclavicular ligaments occurs. The injury is classified by the extent of the injuries to these ligaments. Athletes present with focal soft tissue swelling and tenderness over the AC joint. More severe injuries are associated with deformity. Patients have a positive cross-arm test, in which pain is localized to the AC joint. Radiographs are necessary to assess the degree of injury and to evaluate for a coexisting fracture or growth plate injury.

Treatment of low-grade AC injuries (grade I–III) is typically supportive, with rest and immobilization in a sling followed by progressive rehabilitation. Return to activity can be accomplished in 1–6 weeks depending on the severity of the injury and the persistence of symptoms. Full range of motion and full strength must be achieved prior to being cleared to return to sports. More severe injuries (grade IV–VI) may require surgical intervention.

4. Acute Traumatic Anterior Shoulder Instability (Anterior Shoulder Dislocation/Subluxation)

ESSENTIALS OF DIAGNOSIS & TYPICAL FEATURES

- ▶ Injury with an abducted and externally rotated arm.
- ▶ Squared-off shoulder on examination.
- ▶ Reduced range of motion of the shoulder.

Acute traumatic anterior shoulder instability occurs when significant force is applied to the abducted and externally rotated shoulder. Most often, the humeral head is dislocated in an anterior and inferior direction. The patient has severe pain and a mechanical block to motion. Some patients will spontaneously reduce within seconds or minutes of their injury. Most, however, require immediate closed reduction on the field or in the emergency room. Radiographs are helpful to confirm the position of the humeral head and to evaluate for coexisting fracture. MRI may be required for accurate visualization of fractures and soft tissue injury, including labral tears.

Initial treatment involves immobilization of the shoulder in a sling for comfort. Range-of-motion exercises and progressive rehabilitation are initiated as pain improves. Prolonged immobilization does not decrease the risk of recurrence and is discouraged. Return to play in-season can be considered with appropriate counseling regarding risk of re-injury and recurrent instability and when rehabilitation has achieved full range of motion and strength. A brace is often used when an athlete returns to sport in-season. Because of the high risk of recurrence in the adolescent population, options for treatment should be individualized, with consideration given to both nonoperative and surgical management. In cases of recurrent shoulder instability and/or labral tears, surgical intervention is often warranted.

5. Rotator Cuff Injury

ESSENTIALS OF DIAGNOSIS & TYPICAL FEATURES

- ▶ Injury can be acute or chronic.
- ▶ Pain is described as diffuse or anterior and lateral.
- ▶ Overhead activities exacerbate the pain.

Shoulder injuries are often a consequence of repetitive overuse and tissue failure. Rotator cuff tendonitis and bursitis are the most commonly observed rotator cuff injuries in youth sports. Rotator cuff tears, including traumatic tears, in children and adolescents are rare. Most commonly, rotator cuff injuries are overuse injuries and typically occur in sports requiring repetitive overhead motions. Muscle imbalances and injury can lead to entrapment of the supraspinatus tendon under the acromial arch, commonly referred to as subacromial impingement. Patients with nontraumatic shoulder instability due to ligamentous and capsular laxity (also known as multidirectional instability) are prone to overuse rotator cuff injury. These athletes present with chronic pain in the anterior and lateral shoulder, which is increased with overhead activities. Diagnostic workup includes plain radiographs to look for anatomic variability. Rehabilitation is geared toward reduction of inflammation and strengthening of the scapular stabilizers and rotator cuff muscles. A biomechanics evaluation can assist athletes in the recovery process by addressing muscular imbalances and compensation patterns. Surgery is rarely indicated.

6. Proximal Humeral Epiphysitis (Little League Shoulder)

ESSENTIALS OF DIAGNOSIS & TYPICAL FEATURES

- ▶ Participation in a throwing sport, particularly pitching.
- ▶ Pain in the lateral aspect of the humerus with throwing.
- ▶ Widening of the proximal humeral physis on radiographs.

Proximal humeral epiphysitis, or "Little League shoulder," is an overuse injury that occurs in children aged 11–14 years who play overhead sports such as baseball. The patient presents with activity-related pain in the lateral aspect of the proximal humerus. Examination often reveals tenderness over the proximal humerus. Absence of findings on examination does not preclude this diagnosis. The hallmark feature is pain with throwing. Radiographs show widening, sclerosis, and irregularity of the proximal humeral physis. Comparison views are often helpful.

Treatment consists of rest from throwing or other aggravating activity. Physical therapy is initiated during the rest period. Return to play can only be considered after a period of rest has significantly decreased the pain and the athlete has proceeded through a progressive throwing program. Healing can take several months. Signs of radiographic healing may lag behind the athlete's clinical progress, and normal radiographs are not necessarily required for return to play. Permanent sequelae such as fracture, growth arrest, or deformity is extremely rare but can occur in chronic cases that are not treated appropriately.

Bednar ED, Kay J, Memon M, Simunovic N, Purcell L, Ayeni OR: Diagnosis and Management of Little League Shoulder: a systematic review. Orthop J Sports Med 2021 Jul 29;9(7): 23259671211017563 [PMID: 34377716].

Zaremski JL, Galloza J, Sepulveda F, Vasilopoulos T, Micheo W, Herman DC: Recurrence and return to play after shoulder instability events in young and adolescent athletes: a systematic review and meta-analysis. Br J Sports Med 2017 Feb;51(3): 177–184. doi: 10.1136/bjsports-2016-096895. Epub 2016 Nov 10 [PMID: 27834676].

ELBOW INJURIES

Acute injuries to the elbow are quite common and often occur in athletes involved in throwing or overhead sports. Further, chronic overuse injuries are becoming more and more prevalent in young athletes. Risk factors leading to overuse elbow injury include single sport specialization, year-round participation, longer competitive seasons, insufficient rest, and poor biomechanics.

1. Medial Epicondyle Apophysitis (Little League Elbow)

ESSENTIALS OF DIAGNOSIS & TYPICAL FEATURES

► Children 9–12 years old who participate in a throwing sport.
► Pain over the medial epicondyle, especially with pitching and throwing.
► Tenderness and swelling of the medial elbow.

"Little League elbow" is a traction injury to the medial epicondylar apophysis, which develops in young overhead throwing athletes, particularly baseball pitchers, between the ages of 9 and 12 years. The biomechanical forces generated around the elbow during throwing, namely repetitive valgus stress, can result in shearing, inflammation, and abnormal bone development. The symptoms are primarily swelling, medial elbow pain, performance difficulties, and weakness. The pain localizes to the medial epicondyle, which may be tender to palpation, and worsens with valgus stress. Wrist flexion and forearm pronation may increase symptoms. The physician should inquire about the exposure to throwing, including pitch counts, the number of practices and games, and the duration of the season. Workup includes elbow radiographs, with comparison films of the unaffected side, to look for widening of the apophysis. Rarely, MRI is used to confirm the diagnosis.

Treatment includes complete rest from throwing activities and physical therapy. It is not uncommon for a player to be restricted from throwing for up to 6 weeks. Competition can be resumed once the player is asymptomatic and has progressed through a graduated, age-appropriate throwing program. The key approach to this injury is prevention. Children should be properly conditioned and coached in correct throwing biomechanics. Guidelines for Little League pitching limits in youth baseball have been developed (https://www.littleleague.org/playing-rules/pitch-count/).

2. Panner's Disease

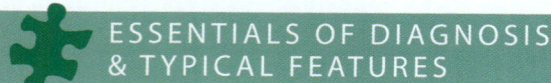

ESSENTIALS OF DIAGNOSIS & TYPICAL FEATURES

► Children 5–12 years old who participate in a throwing sport.
► Tenderness and swelling over the lateral elbow.
► Osteochondrosis of the capitellum.

Panner's disease refers to developmental osteochondrosis (degeneration of the ossification center) of the capitellum, the lower end of the humerus that articulates with the radius, as a result of overuse injury. This condition occurs in children aged 5–12 years who play sports that involve overhead throwing and in gymnasts. The repetitive lateral compressive forces from loading the elbow in these sports compromises the blood supply to the growing epiphysis and leads to degeneration of the ossification center. The child may have dull aching in the lateral elbow that worsens with throwing. Swelling and reduced elbow extension usually are present. Radiocapitellar compression test (with elbow fully extended, the arm is actively pronated and supinated) will also elicit pain. Radiographs show an abnormal, flattened capitellum, with fragmentation and areas of sclerosis. This should be distinguished from osteochondritis dissecans (OCD) of the capitellum, which typically occurs in older children (see section Osteochondritis Dissecans of the Elbow). Treatment is conservative, with rest, ice, splinting, and avoiding activities that load the elbow for 3–6 months. The child can return to play once symptoms resolve and there is evidence of healing on follow-up radiographs. The natural history is one of complete resolution of symptoms and, ultimately, normal ossification of the capitellum.

3. Ulnar Collateral Ligament Tear

ESSENTIALS OF DIAGNOSIS & TYPICAL FEATURES

► Sudden forceful tensile stress on the ligament from a fall or from valgus stress to elbow during overhead throwing.

► Feeling a pop or sensation of the elbow giving out.

► Medial elbow pain and tenderness distal to the medial epicondyle.

Once the medial epicondylar physis closes in a skeletally mature athlete, valgus forces are then transmitted to the ulnar collateral ligament, which can result in a sprain or tear. Patients present with medial elbow pain and are often unable to fully extend the elbow. Examination reveals tenderness just distal to the medial epicondyle, and there may be instability with valgus stressing. Treatment is often conservative, including rest, ice, and physical therapy directed at range of motion and strengthening. Surgical reconstruction may be suggested for those with persistent pain or instability and who desire to continue participating in overhead sports.

4. Osteochondritis Dissecans of the Elbow

ESSENTIALS OF DIAGNOSIS & TYPICAL FEATURES

► Adolescents who participate in a throwing sport.

► Pain over the lateral elbow, especially with pitching.

► Tenderness over the radiocapitellar joint and difficulty with full elbow extension.

Lateral elbow pain in a slightly older throwing athlete, usually aged 13–15 years, can be secondary to osteochondritis

dissecans (OCD), which is a more worrisome diagnosis than Panner's disease. Unlike Panner's disease, which is self-limiting, OCD lesions can lead to permanent destruction of the cartilage and bone. It is an injury to the subchondral bone, and its overlying articular cartilage can then become involved. Although it can involve different sites within the elbow, including the olecranon, radial head, or trochlea, it most commonly affects the capitellum. Repetitive valgus compressive forces can lead to avascular necrosis of the capitellum, which can ultimately result in the formation of loose bodies in the joint. The athlete presents with lateral pain, swelling, lack of full extension, and occasionally locking. Radiographs show lucency of the capitellum with surrounding sclerotic bone. MRI can more fully delineate the lesion and determine its stability.

A child with an OCD should be seen by either a sports medicine specialist or an orthopedic surgeon. Treatment is based on stability of the lesion and can be either conservative or surgical. For early or stable OCD lesions, particularly in skeletally immature individuals, management includes throwing activity restrictions and physical therapy. More advanced or unstable lesions or those with persistent symptoms despite conservative treatment may require surgical intervention.

5. Lateral Epicondylitis

Lateral epicondylitis (also known as "tennis elbow") is common in skeletally mature athletes participating in racquet sports. It is a tendinopathy of the extensor muscles in the forearm, which insert onto the lateral epicondyle causing lateral elbow pain. The pain is increased by wrist extension. Initial treatment is aimed at inflammation control, followed by stretching and strengthening of forearm muscles. Stroke mechanics may need to be altered, and a forearm brace can be used to decrease the forces in the extensor muscles.

Leahy I, Schorpion M, Ganley T: Common medial elbow injuries in the adolescent athlete. J Hand Ther 2015 Apr-Jun;28(2): 201–210; quiz 211. doi: 10.1016/j.jht.2015.01.003. Epub 2015 Jan 16 [PMID: 25840494].

HAND & WRIST INJURIES

The hand and wrist are the most common area of injury in children and account for a large proportion of emergency room visits. All hand and wrist injuries have the potential for serious long-term disability and require thorough evaluation, including neurovascular examination and evaluation of rotational or angular deformity or malalignment. Examples of complications include loss of range of motion, dysfunction, deformity, limb length discrepancy, and arthritis.

1. Distal Phalanx Injury

Tuft injuries require splinting for 3–6 weeks or until the patient is pain free. If there is significant displacement, a surgical K-wire can be used for reduction. Nail-bed injury often requires nail-bed suturing, splinting, and drainage of subungual hematomas. Patients with nail-bed injuries should be advised that nail regrowth may appear irregular or may not occur at all.

2. Distal Interphalangeal Injury

Mallet finger or extensor tendon avulsion occurs more commonly in ball-handling sports. The mechanism of injury is an axial load or forced flexion against an actively extending finger, causing avulsion fracture or rupture of the extensor digitorum tendon. Athletes present with a flexion contracture at the distal interphalangeal (DIP) joint and inability to actively extend the distal phalanx. Referral to an orthopedic surgeon is necessary. Conservative treatment consists of splinting in extension for 4 weeks for fractures and 6–8 weeks for tendon rupture. Surgery may be required if the initial fracture involves greater than 30% of the joint space or poor healing with loss of function occurs.

Jersey finger, or flexor tendon avulsion (tendon rupture with or without associated bony avulsion fracture), occurs in contact sports, particularly American football. The mechanism of injury is forced extension against an actively flexed finger. The fourth ("ring") finger is the most commonly injured digit. Athletes present with tenderness, swelling, and inability to flex at the DIP. The examiner can test the function of the flexor tendon by holding the proximal interphalangeal joint in extension while having the injured athlete attempt flexion at the DIP joint. The injured finger should be splinted in a comfortable position and immediately referred to an orthopedic surgeon, as definitive treatment is often surgical.

3. Thumb Injury

Gamekeeper's or skier's thumb is an injury to the ulnar collateral ligament from forced abduction of the thumb metacarpophalangeal (MCP) joint. It is a common skiing injury to those who fall while holding on to their ski poles. Patients will complain of pain over the medial aspect of the MCP joint and pain with apposition or pinching. If a radiograph shows an avulsed fragment that is displaced less than 2 mm or if there is no fragment, less than 35 degrees of joint space opening, or less than 15 degrees difference in joint space opening compared to the uninjured thumb with stress testing, a spica cast for 4–6 weeks is indicated. Surgery is required for more serious injuries.

4. Hand Fractures

All finger fractures should be assessed for growth plate involvement, rotation, angulation, and displacement. If stable and not displaced, these fractures typically can be splinted for 3–4 weeks and buddy-taped for immediate return to sports. However, spiral or oblique fractures of the middle phalanx, intra-articular fractures, and severely angulated physeal fractures are considered unstable and should be referred to an orthopedic surgeon.

Boxer's fracture is a neck fracture of the fourth or fifth metacarpal, typically caused by poor punching technique or punching into a hard surface. Less than 40 degrees of volar/dorsal angulation in the fourth or fifth metacarpals is acceptable. Assessment of displacement and rotational deformity by looking at the cascade of the fingers while the patient holds a loose fist is critical, as displaced or rotated fractures require reduction and fixation. Prior to definitive treatment with hand-based casting for 4 weeks, boxer's fractures may be temporarily immobilized with an ulnar gutter splint with the MCP joints flexed to 70 degrees.

5. Wrist Injury

Distal radial and ulnar fractures, which are common in children, must be ruled out when a patient presents with a swollen and painful wrist. Particular attention should be paid to the growth plates and the scaphoid bone. Typically, distal radius and ulna fractures require casting for 3–6 weeks in either a short or long arm cast, depending on the involvement of one or both bones and the severity of displacement or angulation. Torus, or buckle, fractures may be placed in a rigid wrist brace or short arm cast for 3–4 weeks.

Scaphoid fractures are caused by a force applied to a hyperextended wrist, most commonly a fall onto an outstretched hand. Despite normal radiographs, if there is tenderness of the scaphoid on examination, the patient should be immobilized for 10 days in a thumb spica splint and then reassessed both clinically and with follow-up radiographs. A nondisplaced scaphoid fracture requires at least 6 weeks of immobilization in a thumb spica cast. Nonunion can occur, particularly in fractures of the proximal pole of the scaphoid related to the poor blood supply of this area of the bone, requiring surgical treatment. Displaced fractures often require operative management.

Gymnast's wrist is chronic wrist pain due to repetitive overloading of the distal radial physis. Athletes complain of dorsal wrist pain, worsened with weight bearing on the affected upper extremity or active extension of the wrist. This overuse stress injury can cause long-term growth abnormalities or degenerative wrist joint changes, which may ultimately require surgical intervention. Athletes should be placed in a rigid wrist brace or short arm cast for 4 weeks with a period of relative rest and then gradual return to wrist loading once pain-free.

Zlotolow DA, Kozin SH: Hand and wrist injuries in the pediatric athlete. Clin Sports Med 2020 Apr;39(2):457–479. doi: 10.1016/j.csm.2020.01.001 [PMID: 32115094].

HIP INJURIES

Hip injuries in young children are rare, but sprains, strains, and avulsion fractures can occur. Athletes can be susceptible to overuse injuries involving the hip.

1. Hip Avulsion Fractures

ESSENTIALS OF DIAGNOSIS & TYPICAL FEATURES

► Fractures at apophyseal areas.

► Pain with weight bearing.

► Focal pain over the site of injury.

Avulsion fractures around the hip in adolescents occur at apophyseal regions such as the ischial tuberosity, anterior superior iliac spine, anterior inferior iliac spine, and iliac crest. The mechanism of injury is a forceful, unbalanced muscle contraction that causes avulsion of the muscle tendon insertion. The athlete presents with a history of an acute traumatic incident; often a "pop" is felt, and the athlete is immediately unable to bear weight. Range of motion of the hip is limited secondary to pain, and focal tenderness is present over the apophysis.

Treatment is usually conservative. Surgical management is reserved for significantly displaced fractures. The athlete is typically placed on crutches for the first couple of weeks for pain control and to normalize gait. After the acute phase, an athlete can progress to weight bearing as tolerated. The rehabilitation phase focuses on regaining motion, flexibility training and pelvic, and core strengthening. Progressive return to activity can occur when full range of motion, full strength, and sport-specific skills have been achieved.

2. Slipped Capital Femoral Epiphysis

ESSENTIALS OF DIAGNOSIS & TYPICAL FEATURES

► Pain in the hip or knee, or both.

► Loss of internal rotation of the hip.

► Radiographs in the frog-leg position show widening of the physis and epiphyseal displacement.

Slipped capital femoral epiphysis occurs in children aged 11–16 years and is associated with obesity and some endocrinopathies such as hypothyroidism. The physis is weakened during times of rapid growing and is susceptible to shearing failure either acutely secondary to a traumatic injury or insidiously from chronic overload. Patients complain of groin, thigh, or knee pain and often have a limp or, in unstable cases, they may not be able to bear weight. Examination shows painful range of motion of the hip,

limited internal rotation, and obligatory external rotation when the hip is flexed. Radiographs include AP and frog-leg lateral films, which demonstrate widening of the physis and epiphyseal displacement of the femoral head relative to the femoral neck.

Treatment consists of immediate non–weight-bearing and urgent referral to an orthopedic specialist for surgical stabilization. Failure to identify this injury can increase the chance of avascular necrosis resulting in early arthritis. Return to activity is progressive over months. (See also Chapter 26.)

3. Acetabular Labral Tears

Acetabular labral tears are an increasingly recognized cause of anterior hip and groin pain in athletes. The majority of hip labral tears occur as a result of an underlying anatomical abnormality such as femoroacetabular impingement (FAI) or hip dysplasia which cause the femoral head and acetabulum to abnormally contact each other during hip motion. Because of the activity level and range of motion requirements for sports, these injuries tend to present and be more symptomatic in the athletic population. Athletes with this injury typically do not report an acute traumatic event, and symptoms typically develop insidiously. Athletes often present with deep anterior hip or groin pain. Radiographic imaging generally shows no acute findings but will outline the bony structural aberrancies that may have caused the labral tear over time. An MRI is used to demonstrate the labral tear. Treatment typically starts conservatively and requires rest and physical therapy. Ultimately, treatment is tailored to the athlete's particular needs and symptoms. Arthroscopy to repair the tear and address any underlying structural issue that caused the tear is sometimes required.

4. Adductor Strain

An adductor strain or a groin pull is generally caused by forced abduction during running, falling, twisting, or tackling. Sports that require quick directional changes place athletes at risk for these types of injuries. There is often pain with hip adduction or flexion and tenderness over the adductor tendon or muscle belly. Treatment includes rest, ice, and protection (often with crutches), and physical therapy with strengthening of the muscle when it heals.

5. Hamstring Strain

ESSENTIALS OF DIAGNOSIS & TYPICAL FEATURES

► Mechanism is forced knee extension.

► Pain with tearing or popping sensation in the posterior leg.

► Pain with resisted knee extension.

Because the hamstring is a two-joint muscle, it is more susceptible to injury than other types of muscle, and hamstring strains are common in athletes. The majority occur in the muscle belly and can be treated successfully with nonoperative management. The mechanism of injury is forced extension of the knee or directional changes. Examination reveals pain on palpation of the muscle and, occasionally, a defect, as well as pain with resisted knee flexion.

Initial treatment is focused on minimizing swelling, bruising, and pain with ice and compression. In moderate and severe injuries, crutches may be needed for a short duration, with progression to weight bearing when the athlete can tolerate this activity. Eccentric strengthening is an important component of rehabilitation.

6. Quadriceps Contusion

Quadriceps contusion is caused by a direct injury to the muscle that causes bruising, swelling, and pain. The amount of damage is directly related to the amount of force. The anterior and lateral thigh regions are most commonly injured, often in contact sports such as football and lacrosse.

Treatment is rest, ice, and protection from repeat impact for the first 24 hours. The knee can be kept in a fully flexed position to tamponade any hematoma formation. Two to 3 days after the injury, range-of-motion exercises may begin in both flexion and extension. The athlete can return to full activity once range of motion and strength return and pain has abated. If the muscle remains firm on examination after 2 weeks, radiographs of the thigh should be obtained to rule out myositis ossificans, an abnormal deposition of calcium in the muscle in the area of trauma.

7. Hip Dislocation

ESSENTIALS OF DIAGNOSIS & TYPICAL FEATURES

▶ Posterior dislocation is most common.

▶ Presents with a flexed, adducted, and internally rotated leg.

▶ Hip pain is severe and is associated with inability to bear weight.

▶ This is an on-site emergency and must be treated quickly.

The hip joint has a high degree of inherent bony stability. Therefore, hip dislocations are rare and typically occur only in high energy or forceful injuries. Most hip dislocations occur in the posterior direction. Classically, these athletes present with an acutely painful hip with inability to move or weight bear on the limb following a major impact, and the hip is locked in flexion, adduction, and internal rotation. Hip dislocations in skeletally mature athletes are often associated with acetabular and femoral neck fractures. The preadolescent, skeletally immature competitor may have an isolated dislocation without fracture. Hip radiographs and advanced imaging such as a CT or MRI scan are needed to completely evaluate the injury.

This injury is an emergency. The athlete should be transported immediately to the nearest facility that has an orthopedic surgeon available. Severe bleeding, avascular necrosis, and nerve damage can result with delay in reduction. Closed reduction is usually successful. Once reduction has been established in an uncomplicated case, protected weight bearing on crutches for 6 weeks is recommended, followed by another 6 weeks of physical therapy with range-of-motion and strengthening exercises. An athlete may return gradually to competition after 3 months, when strength and motion are normal.

Surgery can be necessary if there is an associated fracture, labral tear, or loose body or in the case of unsuccessful closed reduction.

8. Pelvic Apophysitis

Pelvic apophysitis occurs in competitive adolescent athletes who typically are participating consistently, often year-round. Common locations are the ischial tuberosity and iliac crest. The athlete presents with pain over the apophysis and pain with resisted hip motion specific to the muscle insertion. Radiographs can show irregularity over the apophysis or may be normal. Treatment consists of relative rest, progressive rehabilitation focusing on flexibility, and pelvis and core stabilization.

9. Iliotibial Band Syndrome

ESSENTIALS OF DIAGNOSIS & TYPICAL FEATURES

▶ Overuse injury.

▶ Pain over lateral knee or hip.

▶ Positive Ober test.

Iliotibial (IT) band syndrome and associated trochanteric bursitis result when the bursa and IT band become inflamed because of repetitive friction from the underlying greater trochanter and lateral femoral condyle. This condition can cause pain when the hip or knee is flexed as a result of reduced flexibility of the IT band and gluteus medius tendons. The bursa normally allows for improved motion by reducing friction with motion, but, when it becomes inflamed, movement is painful and may be limited. Pain is reproduced with range of motion of the hip or knee. Patients may also have a positive Ober test which is used to measure flexibility of the IT band. The patient lies on his or her side with the affected leg on top. The examiner stabilizes the pelvis with one hand while the other hand moves the tested leg into knee flexion, hip abduction and extension and then lowers the leg into adduction until it stops via soft tissue stretch, posterior rotation of the pelvis, or both. The test is positive if the tested leg fails to adduct parallel to the table in a neutral position.

Initial treatment consists of modification of the offending activity followed by a stretching program targeting the IT band and hip abductors, along with core and pelvic stabilization. Soft tissue therapeutic ultrasound can be beneficial and corticosteroid injections may be used after conservative treatment has failed.

10. Femoral Neck Stress Fractures

Femoral neck stress fractures are generally the result of repetitive microtrauma. They commonly occur in running athletes who have rapidly increased their mileage. Athletes with this type of injury present with persistent pain in the groin, pain with hip range of motion, and a limp. Symptoms often initially occur only with sports, but as the fracture progresses, symptoms often develop with activities of daily living. Athletes with a history of previous stress fracture, disordered eating, or any disorder of calcium metabolism who present with groin pain should raise concern for this diagnosis. Special attention to the risk of stress fracture should be given to the female athlete with the triad of energy imbalance and possible disordered eating, amenorrhea or oligomenorrhea, and low bone density. Plain radiographs are often negative with lower-grade bone stress injuries, in which case MRI is indicated for definitive diagnosis.

Treatment is based on the type of fracture. A tension-sided fracture (on the superior aspect of the femoral neck) generally requires internal fixation to prevent completion of the fracture or displacement and reduce the risk of avascular necrosis. A compression-sided fracture (on the inferior aspect of the femoral neck) is less likely to become displaced; treatment is conservative and involves a period of 6 weeks on crutches.

Ferraro SL, Batty M, Heyworth BE, Cook DL, Miller PE, Novais EN: Acute Pelvic and hip apophyseal avulsion fractures in adolescents: a summary of 719 cases. J Pediatr Orthop 2023 Apr 1; 43(4):204–210 [PMID: 36727766].

Fukase N et al: outcomes and survivorship at a median of 8.9 years following hip arthroscopy in adolescents with femoroacetabular impingement: a matched comparative study with adults. J Bone Joint Surg Am 2022 May 18;104(10):902–909 [PMID: 35255011].

KNEE INJURIES

Injuries to the knee, which is stabilized by a complex system of ligaments, tendons, and menisci, are some of the most common sports-related conditions. Acute knee injuries occur during a traumatic incident. The mechanism of injury is an important historical feature, although many young patients have difficulty describing the details of the inciting event. Onset of rapid swelling after a traumatic event indicates the presence of a hemarthrosis and should raise concern for internal derangements such as fracture, rupture of the anterior cruciate ligament (ACL), meniscal tear, or patellar dislocation.

1. Anterior Knee Pain

The most common knee complaint in young athletes is anterior knee pain. This can be caused by multiple etiologies, including hip pathology as a possible source. The differential diagnosis of anterior knee pain is extensive and requires a thorough examination. The following are the most common knee diagnoses responsible for anterior knee pain.

A. Patellofemoral Overuse Syndrome

Patellofemoral overuse syndrome occurs during running and sports that involve repetitive stress in the lower extremity. The athlete presents with activity-related pain in the anterior knee. In young athletes, this condition is occasionally associated with swelling and crepitus of the knee joint. Evaluation of these injuries requires a "top-down" evaluation of the athlete's leg from the hip to the foot, as the causes of symptoms is typically multifactorial. Most athletes with this condition, regardless of level or physical condition, have hip/core weakness that results in altered knee biomechanics. A comprehensive evaluation of hip alignment and rotation, muscle development, tightness in the hamstrings and IT band, and foot mechanics is necessary to fully understand and treat the causes of this disorder. Athletes are often found to be overtraining and need to modify current activities. Addressing hip and pelvic stability is a mainstay of treatment. Stretching and strengthening of the hamstrings and quadriceps are recommended. The use of braces providing proprioceptive feedback during competition is controversial.

B. Patellar Tendonitis ("Jumper's Knee")

Patellar tendonitis is an overuse injury caused by repetitive loading of the quadriceps during running or jumping that is commonly seen in jumping sports such as basketball and volleyball. Tenderness is located directly over the patellar tendon at its insertion site at the inferior pole of the patella. Physical therapy, icing, and activity modification can help facilitate healing.

C. Osgood-Schlatter Disease (Tibial Tubercle Apophysitis)

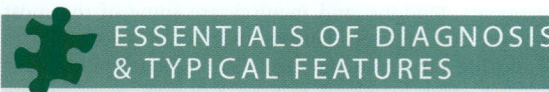

ESSENTIALS OF DIAGNOSIS & TYPICAL FEATURES

► Insidious onset of activity-related anterior knee pain in adolescents.

► Swelling and pain over the tibial tubercle.

► Progressive fragmentation of tibial tubercle apophysis.

Osgood-Schlatter disease is caused by recurrent traction on the tibial tubercle apophysis (growth plate), such as with jumping and running sports. Fragmentation and microfractures of the tibial tubercle occur during rapid growth. The condition occurs in the pre-teen and adolescent years and is most common in boys aged 12–15 years and girls aged 11–13 years. Pain is localized to the tibial tubercle and is aggravated by activities using eccentric quadriceps muscle movement. The pain can become so severe that routine activity must be curtailed. Radiographs typically demonstrate fragmentation or irregular ossification of the tibial tubercle.

Typically, the condition resolves spontaneously as the athlete reaches skeletal maturity. In the interim, pain control using NSAIDs is indicated. Physical therapy and stretching the hamstrings and application of ice after workouts are helpful.

D. Sinding-Larsen-Johansson Disease (Apophysitis of the Inferior Pole of the Patella)

Sinding-Larsen-Johansson disease involves a process similar to that of Osgood-Schlatter disease but occurs in younger athletes between ages 9 and 12 years. Traction from the patellar tendon on the inferior pole of the patella results in fragmentation of the inferior patella that is often obvious on a lateral knee radiograph. Treatment and prognosis are similar to those of Osgood-Schlatter disease.

► Treatment

The treatment of the knee disorders described above is generally similar. Control of pain and inflammation is essential, beginning with relative rest from offending activity and application of ice. Alignment problems and biomechanics across the anterior knee can be improved with an effective rehabilitation program that includes flexibility and strengthening. Quadriceps, pelvic, and core strengthening are all important components of this program. Orthotics can have

an impact on mechanics across the knee joint if they correct excessive pronation or supination. Knee bracing is controversial; the major benefits are proprioceptive feedback and patellar tracking. Return to activity is typically based on symptoms.

2. Posterior Knee Pain

Posterior knee pain often results from an injury to the gastrocnemius-soleus complex caused by overuse. Other causes include a Baker cyst (benign synovial fluid filled cyst in the posterior aspect of the knee), tibial stress fracture, or tendonitis of the hamstring. Treatment is rest, ice, and strengthening exercises after symptoms have improved. Intra-articular injuries such as meniscal tears and cartilage injuries can also cause posterior knee pain and should be considered if symptoms do not improve.

3. Meniscal Injuries

ESSENTIALS OF DIAGNOSIS & TYPICAL FEATURES

► Medial or lateral knee pain.

► Effusion and joint line tenderness.

► Feeling of locking or of the knee giving way.

► Positive McMurray, Apley, and Thessaly tests.

The meniscus of the knee cushions forces in the knee joint, increases nutrient supply to the cartilage, and stabilizes the knee. Most injuries are related to directional changes on a weight-bearing extremity. Medial meniscus injuries have a history of tibial rotation in a weight-bearing position. This injury happens frequently in ball-handling sports. Lateral meniscus injuries occur with tibial rotation with a flexed knee, as in exercises such as squatting or certain wrestling maneuvers. These injuries are uncommon in children younger than 10 years.

The athlete with such an injury has a history of knee pain, swelling, snapping, or locking and may report a feeling of the knee giving way. Physical examination often reveals effusion; joint line tenderness; and a positive McMurray hyperflexion-rotation test (pain elicited and click or catch felt along the joint line while the knee is maximally flexed and then rotated as it is extended), Apley test (pain elicited when an axial load is applied on the knee and the tibia is rotated with the patient in prone position and knee flexed to 90 degrees), and/or positive Thessaly test (joint line pain or a sense of knee locking or catching elicited when the patient stands on the injured leg with a slightly flexed knee and rotates his or her knee internally and externally three times). The diagnostic test of choice is MRI, although standard knee radiographs should be obtained initially. It is important to note that increased vascularity of the meniscus in the pediatric population often causes increased signal changes on MRI that can be confused with a tear. Therefore, an MRI diagnosis of a meniscal tear in a young athlete needs to be correlated with the clinical symptoms and examination.

Treatment of these injuries is typically surgical, although nonoperative management can be considered if the tear is minor and symptoms are minimal. Surgery can entail repairing the tear or removing the torn portion of the meniscus. Every attempt should be made to preserve the meniscal tissue in young athletes because of their favorable healing rates and the long-term concern over development of arthritis in meniscus-deficient patients. After meniscal repair, a period of crutch protection followed by physical therapy is required, with return to sports typically in 4–6 months. Patients undergoing meniscectomy (removal of torn tissue) can often return to sports 3–6 weeks after.

4. Medial & Lateral Collateral Ligament Injuries

ESSENTIALS OF DIAGNOSIS & TYPICAL FEATURES

- ▶ Pain on the medial or lateral portion of the knee.
- ▶ Tenderness along the ligament.
- ▶ Positive valgus or varus stress test at 0 and 30 degrees.

The medial collateral ligament (MCL) and lateral collateral ligament (LCL) are positioned along either side of the knee and act to stabilize the knee during varus and valgus stress. Medial injuries occur either with a blow to the lateral aspect of the knee, as seen in a football tackle, or with a noncontact rotational stress.

The athlete may feel an acute pop or pain along the medial or lateral aspect of the knee. The examination typically reveals a mild effusion and tenderness medially or laterally along the course of the ligament. In MCL injuries, a valgus stress test performed in 20–30 degrees of flexion reproduces pain and possibly instability. A varus stress test performed in 20–30 degrees of flexion reproduces pain and possible instability in LCL injuries. MCL and LCL injuries are graded on a scale of 1–3. Grade 1 injury represents a stretching injury. Grade 2 injury involves partial disruption of the ligament. Grade 3 injury is a complete disruption of the ligament. Radiographs are useful, especially in the skeletally immature athlete, to look for distal femoral or proximal tibial bone

injury. MRI scans are used if grade 2–3 injury or concomitant intra-articular derangement is suspected.

Treatment is generally conservative, including ice and elevation after initial injury. A protective brace is worn and full knee motion in the brace can be permitted within a few days. Weight bearing is allowed, and a strengthening program can be started as soon as tolerated. The athlete should use the brace until pain and range of motion have improved, with no subjective feelings of instability. Timing of return to sports is variable, depending on the severity of the tear and other associated injuries. Play can be resumed in 3–5 weeks in most isolated, low-grade MCL injuries.

5. Anterior Cruciate Ligament Injuries

ESSENTIALS OF DIAGNOSIS & TYPICAL FEATURES

- ▶ Pain and effusion of the knee.
- ▶ Pain along the lateral joint line.
- ▶ Positive Lachman test.

The anterior cruciate ligament (ACL) consists of two bundles that prevent anterior subluxation and rotation of the tibia. Most ACL injuries are noncontact and occur with deceleration, twisting, and cutting motions. ACL injuries can also occur with knee hyperextension or from a direct blow to the knee—typically on the lateral side—which causes an extreme valgus stress with both ACL and MCL disruption.

The athlete often reports hearing or feeling a "pop" followed by swelling that occurs within hours of the injury. The Lachman test (proximal tibia is pulled anteriorly with the knee in 30 degrees of flexion to assess the degree of excursion) is used to detect instability of the knee joint. Other knee structures should be examined to rule out concomitant injuries. Imaging includes plain radiographs and MRI. In skeletally immature athletes, a tibial spine avulsion is frequently seen on radiographs rather than a midsubstance ACL tear.

Initial treatment focuses on controlling swelling and pain. Physical therapy can be instituted early to assist in regaining range of motion and strength. Nonsurgical treatment includes bracing to enhance proprioception and control extension, strengthening, and restricting physical activity. Nonsurgical management can be complicated by continued instability and damage to meniscal and articular cartilage. Surgical reconstruction is typically indicated for young athletes in cutting sports and is also required for persistent instability. Surgery can be performed 2–6 weeks following the injury once swelling and motion of the knee have improved. Rehabilitation of the knee starts immediately after surgery. A structured ACL physical therapy protocol is initiated with the goals of building strength, muscle reeducation, endurance, agility, and coordination. Return to cutting and pivoting sports can be achieved by 9–12 months after surgery when criteria are met.

6. Posterior Cruciate Ligament Injuries

ESSENTIALS OF DIAGNOSIS & TYPICAL FEATURES

▶ Pain and swelling of the knee.
▶ Increased pain with knee flexion.
▶ Positive posterior drawer test.

The posterior cruciate ligament (PCL) runs from the medial femoral condyle to the posterior tibial plateau and has two bundles. Its main function is to prevent posterior tibial subluxation. Injury to the PCL is uncommon; it occurs when the individual falls on a flexed knee with the ankle in plantarflexion or with forced hyperflexion of the knee. PCL injuries are most commonly seen in American football and hockey.

The athlete presents with swelling and pain in the posterior and lateral knee. The posterior drawer test (the proximal tibia is pushed posteriorly with the patient supine and knee flexed to 90 degrees to assess for the degree of posterior excursion) is used to confirm the diagnosis and grade the injury based on the amount of translation. Grade 3 injuries are typically indicative that another ligament is injured in addition to the PCL. Diagnostic imaging includes plain radiographs and MRI.

Isolated ligamentous PCL injuries are remarkably well tolerated in athletes and can be treated nonoperatively with bracing and a progressive rehabilitation program. An exception is bony avulsions of the PCL off the femur or tibia, for which surgical fixation is generally recommended. Additionally, PCL injuries with injury to other structures are complex and often require surgical stabilization.

7. Osteochondritis Dissecans of the Knee

ESSENTIALS OF DIAGNOSIS & TYPICAL FEATURES

▶ Chronic pain and swelling of the knee in an adolescent.
▶ Most commonly occur in the medial femoral condyle.

OCD of the knee occurs most commonly in the lateral aspect of the medial femoral condyle. A typical presentation includes insidious onset of knee pain and swelling in an active adolescent, and mechanical symptoms such as locking and catching can be described. These lesions are typically identified initially on radiographs, and follow-up MRI is indicated to determine the stability of the lesion, including features that may indicate the osteochondral lesion could become a loose fragment within the joint. Stable lesions can be managed nonoperatively with immobilization, activity modification, and physical therapy for 3–6 months. Unstable lesions or stable lesions that do not respond to conservative treatment require operative intervention.

MacDonald J, Rodenberg R, Sweeney E: Acute knee injuries in children and adolescents: a review. JAMA Pediatr 2021;175(6):624–630. doi:10.1001/jamapediatrics.2020.6130 [PMID: 33749718].
Patel DR, Villalobos A: Evaluation and management of knee pain in young athletes: overuse injuries of the knee. Transl Pediatr 2017 Jul;6(3):190–198. doi: 10.21037/tp.2017.04.05 [PMID: 28795010].

FOOT & ANKLE INJURIES

The types of injuries commonly seen at the foot and ankle depend on the age group. Young children tend to have diaphyseal injuries, in contrast to rapidly growing older children who tend to have epiphyseal and apophyseal injuries. Skeletally mature adolescents are prone to adult-pattern ligamentous injury. Although fractures of the ankle are possible with inversion and eversion mechanisms, the most common acute injury involving the ankle is the lateral ankle sprain.

1. Ankle Sprain

ESSENTIALS OF DIAGNOSIS & TYPICAL FEATURES

▶ Mechanism is usually inversion and plantarflexion.
▶ Swelling and pain in the ankle over the injured ligament.
▶ Bruising over the ankle.

The ankle has three lateral ligaments (anterior talofibular, calcaneofibular, and posterior talofibular) and a medial deltoid ligament. Inversion of the foot generally damages the anterior talofibular ligament, whereas eversion injures the deltoid ligament. Tearing occurs when a ligament is overloaded. Lateral ankle sprains are far more common than medial ankle sprains because the deltoid ligament is stronger mechanically than the lateral ligaments. However, medial ankle sprains may have more severe complications, including syndesmotic tearing and instability of the ankle joint requiring surgical stabilization. High ankle sprains involve injury to the tibiofibular syndesmosis, a movable connection in which the adjacent tibia and fibula bones are bound together by ligamentous structures. High-ankle sprains occur most commonly with dorsiflexion and external rotation. Syndesmotic injuries involve longer healing times than low-grade medial or lateral ankle sprains.

Physical examination often reveals swelling, bruising, and pain. Injuries are graded as follows: grade 1 injury is a stretch without instability, grade 2 is a partial tear with some instability, and grade 3 is a total disruption of the ligament with instability of the joint. The syndesmotic squeeze test (pain in the distal syndesmosis above the ankle elicited with squeezing of the tibia and fibula) and Kleiger test (pain elicited with external rotation of the foot in dorsiflexion) are positive in high ankle sprains. Radiographs should be obtained when a bony injury is suspected and are especially important when evaluating skeletally immature athletes who are more prone to growth plate injury. Medial or excessive ankle swelling, tenderness over the malleoli or beyond ligament attachments, and bruising warrant radiographs to evaluate asymmetry and instability of the ankle. The Ottawa Ankle Rules are used to determine whether obtaining x-rays are necessary and appear to be reliable in patients older than 5 years.

A variety of other injuries should be considered when a patient presents with an apparent ankle sprain. Fifth metatarsal injuries, including avulsion, Jones, and diaphyseal fractures at the base of the metatarsal, can occur with an inversion mechanism, and present with swelling and tenderness over the base of the fifth metatarsal. Fractures of the tibial epiphysis, malleoli, fibula, talar dome, or calcaneus may also mimic an ankle sprain.

Appropriate treatment of ligamentous ankle injuries is imperative to ensure full recovery and should begin immediately after the injury. Nonoperative management is used for the vast majority of ankle sprains. Phase 1 care involves immediate compressive wrapping and icing to control swelling and inflammation. Protected weight bearing is encouraged as tolerated in the early phase of rehabilitation. Severe ankle sprains may benefit from a short period of treatment in a lower leg walking boot or cast. Phase 2 emphasizes range of motion and gradually increasing exercise and can begin when the athlete is able to ambulate without pain. Supervised physical therapy prescription may be beneficial. Phase 3 is designed to increase strength, improve proprioception, and incorporate more complex movement patterns and sport-specific agility and function. An appropriate rehabilitation program can be effective in returning athletes to activity within a few weeks, although up to 6 weeks may be required for return to full activity. To reduce risk of recurrent ankle sprain, the athlete should wear a protective brace for

3–4 months, continue phase 3 home exercises, and apply ice after exercising.

2. Sever's Disease

> ### ESSENTIALS OF DIAGNOSIS & TYPICAL FEATURES
>
> ► Activity-related heel pain in preadolescents.
> ► Pain localized to the calcaneal apophysis and Achilles insertion.
> ► Positive calcaneal squeeze test.

Sever's disease, or calcaneal apophysitis, occurs in athletes aged 8–12 years who are typically involved in high-impact activities such as gymnastics and soccer. Causes include overuse, improper footwear, and tightness in the calf musculature and Achilles tendon. Activity-related pain occurs about the heel and at the point of muscle tendon insertion onto the growth center of the calcaneus. Examination reveals focal tenderness over the calcaneal apophysis and a positive calcaneal squeeze test (tenderness elicited by forceful pressure on the lateral and medial heel).

Treatment is symptomatic and consists of reassurance and education, relative rest, heel cord stretching, eccentric calf strengthening, ice massage, heel cups (rubber or gel infused shoe inserts that provide heel lift and cushion), NSAIDs for pain control, and progression to activity as tolerated based on pain level. Activity restriction is not required. Refractory cases may benefit from brief immobilization and partial or total non–weightbearing in a walking boot or cast followed by supervised physical therapy.

3. Plantar Fasciitis

Plantar fasciitis is a common problem that occurs when the plantar fascia, a strong band of tissue that supports the arch of the foot, becomes irritated and inflamed in response to injury. It typically occurs in runners who log more than 30 miles per week and in athletes who have tight Achilles tendons or wear poorly fitting shoes. It is also common in people with cavus feet and in those who are overweight. Plantar fasciitis manifests as heel pain in the adolescent or older athlete. The pain is worse upon first standing up in the morning and taking a few steps. Differential diagnosis includes navicular or calcaneal stress fracture. A bone spur is often found on examination. Treatment involves local massage, stretching of the gastrocnemius-soleus-Achilles complex, NSAIDs, arch supports, and a focused rehabilitation program. Runners may need to cut back on their weekly mileage until these measures eliminate pain.

Gruskay JA, Brusalis CM, Heath MR, Fabricant PD: Pediatric and adolescent ankle instability: diagnosis and treatment options. Curr Opin Pediatr 2019 Feb;31(1):69–78. doi: 10.1097/MOP.0000000000000720 [PMID: 30531226].

Kaitlin MS, Dorgo S, Boyle JB: Growth plate injuries in children in sports: a review of Sever's disease. Strength Cond J 2017 Apr;39(2):59–68. doi: 10.1519/SSC.0000000000000295.

PREVENTION

Many sports-related injuries can be prevented by education, reducing dangerous behaviors, use of protective equipment, and proper training. Protective equipment should be properly fitted and maintained by an individual with training and instruction. Helmets should be used in football, baseball, hockey, bicycling, skiing, in-line skating, skateboarding, or any other sport with risk of head injury. Eye protection should be used in sports that have a high incidence of eye injuries. Proper protective padding should be used, including chest pads for catchers; shin guards in soccer; shoulder, arm, chest, and leg padding in hockey; and wrist and elbow protectors in skating. Other primary prevention strategies include inspecting playing fields for potential hazards, adapting rules to the developmental level of the participants, and matching opponents equally in skill level and size. Early recognition of injuries, proper treatment, and appropriate rehabilitation are also crucial to ensure safe sports participation.

Stracciolini A, Sugimoto D, Howell DR: Injury prevention in youth sports. Pediatr Ann 2017 Mar 1;46(3):e99–e105. doi: 10.3928/19382359-20170223-01 [PMID: 28287683].

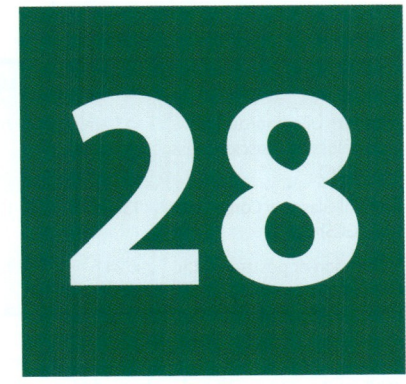

Rehabilitation Medicine

Cristina Sarmiento, MD
Pamela E. Wilson, MD
Aaron Powell, MD

28

Rehabilitation medicine is the multidisciplinary specialty focused on the diagnosis, functional optimization, and improvement of quality of life of individuals with congenital and acquired disabilities.

PEDIATRIC BRAIN INJURY

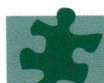

ESSENTIALS OF DIAGNOSIS & TYPICAL FEATURES

► Pediatric brain injury severity is classified using a variety of factors, including the Glasgow Coma Scale, duration of loss of consciousness, and duration of posttraumatic amnesia.

► Brain injury in young children has psychosocial implications throughout the developmental continuum.

Various estimates indicate that there are up to 500,000 pediatric traumatic brain injuries annually in the United States, resulting in 37,000–50,000 hospitalizations and 2000–3000 deaths annually. The cost of these injuries is significant, particularly when considering that survivors of pediatric brain injury may have long-term deficits with lifetime needs.

► Pathogenesis

Brain injury is classically divided into two categories based on the timing of the pathologic findings: primary and secondary injury.

Primary injury occurs at the time of trauma and is characterized by immediate mechanical disruptions such as parenchymal shearing, tearing, and bruising as well as initial neuronal death from cellular energy crises. Treatment of primary brain injury is prevention. This includes proper use of car seats; helmets; fencing around pools; and modification of playground equipment, for example, lower climbing heights and soft, energy absorbing wood chips or padding to dissipate forces during a fall.

Secondary injury occurs as a sequelae of primary injury hours to days after the initial insult. Continued metabolic stressors on neurons from neurochemical derangements and changes in intracranial and perfusion pressures from cerebral edema or hemorrhage are the main contributors to secondary injury. Mitigation of secondary injury focuses on monitoring and modulation of intracranial pressures and metabolic derangements (eg, as electrolyte abnormalities, hyper- or hypoglycemia, and hyperthermia). The complex biochemical cascades involved in secondary brain injury may represent potential future therapeutic targets.

► Clinical Findings

Classification & Assessment of Injury Severity

Traumatic brain injury is usually categorized as open or closed. *Open injuries* are the result of penetration of the skull by missile or sharp object or deformation of the skull with exposure of the underlying intracranial tissues. *Closed injuries* are the result of blunt trauma to the head, which causes movement (intracranial acceleration or deceleration and rotational forces) and compression of brain tissue. Brain contusions are referred to as *coup* (occurring at the site of injury) or *contra-coup* (occurring on the side of the brain opposite the injury). Rating the severity of injury and eventual outcomes is important in medical management.

A. Brain Injury Severity: Glasgow Coma Scale, Loss of Consciousness, and Posttraumatic Amnesia

The Glasgow Coma Scale (GCS), duration of loss of consciousness (LOC), and posttraumatic amnesia (PTA) are the most commonly used variables in assessing brain injury

Table 28–1. Brain injury severity.

Clinical Measure	Mild	Moderate	Severe
Length of coma/duration of loss of consciousness (LOC)	< 30 min	30 min to ~6 h	> 6 h
Initial Glasgow Coma Scale (GCS) score	13–15	9–12	3–8
Duration of posttraumatic amnesia	< 24 h	24 h–1 wk	> 1 wk

severity (Table 28–1). The GCS is the most frequently used system to assess the depth and duration of impaired consciousness in the acute setting. Duration of LOC is the length of time that it takes for an individual to regain his or her baseline level of awareness and responsiveness. PTA is the duration of time after injury during which new memories are not being made and retained. While brain injury severity can be assessed by any one of these factors, use of all three of these measures in conjunction with other factors such as clinical presentation and neuroimaging findings can improve prognostication of brain injury recovery.

B. Expected Stages of Recovery: Rancho Los Amigos Scale

The Rancho Los Amigos Levels of Cognitive Function (LCFS or "Rancho") is a helpful tool that describes the expected stages of recovery after brain injury. The scale has eight main levels of functioning ranging from "no response" to "purposeful, appropriate." Of note, Rancho Los Amigos level 4 is a significant level at which agitation in the patient is an expected clinical manifestation. The patient is expected to progress through this agitation phase, and providers should resist the temptation to treat the agitation unless there are safety concerns, as this treatment may slow recovery.

Common Sequelae of Brain Injury

Brain injury may result in deficits to cognition, sensory and motor function, emotional stability, social behavior, speed of mental processing, memory, speech, and language. Small intraparenchymal injuries, easily identified by computed tomographic (CT) or magnetic resonance imaging (MRI) scans, may not cause obvious signs or symptoms. Some brain injuries, most notably mild traumatic brain injury, also known as *concussion*, do not show changes on advanced imaging techniques. The following are common problems associated with brain injury.

A. Seizures

Seizures occurring in the first 24 hours after injury are referred to as *immediate seizures*. Those occurring during the first week are *early seizures*, and those starting more

than 1 week after injury are referred to as *late seizures*. Seizure prophylaxis with medications is recommended in the first week after brain injury in children at high risk for seizures and in very young children. Seizure prophylaxis is also recommended for 1 week after any penetrating brain trauma. Seizure prophylaxis is probably not effective for prevention of late-onset seizures; these may require long-term treatment.

B. Neuromotor Deficits/Movement Disorders

Neuromotor deficits after brain injury include movement disorders, spasticity, paralysis, and weakness. The type of disorder will be influenced by the areas damaged. The most common movement disorders are tremors and dystonia. These deficits can result in impaired ambulation or coordination, impaired ability to use upper extremities, and speech problems. Physical and occupational therapy are often prescribed for patients with movement disorders; a wide range of pharmacologic interventions for dystonia are also available (Table 28–2).

C. Communication Disorders

Language and communication disorders are common. Aphasia, difficulty in understanding and producing written and spoken language, is categorized as fluent, nonfluent, or global. Individuals with fluent aphasia or Wernicke-type disorder can produce speech but have little associated content. The nonfluent aphasias or Broca's type have a paucity of speech and may have word finding difficulties. Global aphasias are associated with extensive injuries and the most severe language disorders.

D. Paroxysmal Sympathetic Hyperactivity

Severe brain injuries may be associated with excessive sympathetic outflow, resulting in a constellation of symptoms known as paroxysmal sympathetic hyperactivity (PSH).

Table 28–2. Common medications for dystonia.

Medication	Mechanism of Action
Baclofen	$GABA_B$ receptor agonist
Clonazepam/diazepam	$GABA_A$ receptor agonist
Levetiracetam/valproic acid/oxcarbazepine	Antiepileptic: decrease neuro excitability
Trihexyphenidyl	Anticholinergic
Levodopa	Dopamine agonist
Phenobarbital	Barbiturate: nonspecific CNS depressant
Dantrolene	Skeletal muscle relaxant: post-synaptic acetylcholine inhibitor
Tetrabenazine	Vesicular monoamine transporter-2 inhibitor

This clinical presentation has many other names, including neurostorming, paroxysmal autonomic instability with dystonia, and diencephalic seizures. Symptoms of PSH are tachycardia, tachypnea, sweating, hyperthermia, hypertension, agitation, and posturing. Common medications used to treat PSH include dopamine agonists (eg, bromocriptine), β-blockers (eg, propranolol), and α-agonists (eg, clonidine).

E. Cognitive and Behavioral Deficits

After brain injury, cognitive and behavioral deficits are a frequent occurrence. Cognitive disorders depend on the location and severity of the injury. Damage to the frontal lobes can disrupt executive function and cause initiation delays. Neuropsychiatric sequelae are common, and depression, anxiety disorders, and posttraumatic stress disorders (PTSD) are present in one-third of those injured. Neuropsychological evaluation can facilitate development of accommodations in school and use of behavioral strategies.

F. Hypothalamic-Pituitary-Adrenal Axis Dysfunction

Dysfunction of the hypothalamic-pituitary-adrenal axis is common after head injury. The syndrome of inappropriate antidiuretic hormone secretion (SIADH) or diabetes insipidus (DI) from a posterior pituitary injury can result in significant electrolyte and osmolality imbalance. Amenorrhea that typically resolves spontaneously is common in females. Injury near the onset of puberty can complicate normal development, and endocrine status should be monitored closely.

G. Cranial Nerve Injuries

The most commonly injured cranial nerves are I, IV, VII, and VIII. Hyposmia or anosmia (cranial nerve I) can occur if the shearing forces at the cribriform plate disrupt the afferent olfactory nerves. Injury to the cranial nerve IV (trochlear) is common, as it has the longest intracranial length. Resulting superior oblique muscle palsy typically causes a head tilt and vertical diplopia. Facial nerve injuries (cranial nerve VII) are common, especially with temporal bone fractures. This impacts the ability to use the facial muscles, causes dryness in the eye and salivary glands, along with decreased taste in the anterior part of the tongue. The cochlear nerve (VIII) is also frequently damaged in temporal bone fractures and can result in vertigo and dizziness.

Developmental Considerations

The assumption that younger children will fare better than older children or adults after a brain injury is a myth. While a child has a significant amount of development and synaptic reorganization yet to occur, this does not guarantee an improved chance for functional recovery. Indeed, disruption of developmental processes, especially in very young infants

or neonates, may be catastrophic. These processes often cannot be recapitulated.

The mechanism of injury plays an important role in determining the severity of brain injury in very young children. Mechanisms associated with nonaccidental injury such as shaking often result in global diffuse damage. Weak neck musculature, large head-body mass ratio, immature blood-brain barrier, and high intracranial fluid-brain mass ratio all contribute to widespread damage.

During puberty, major hormonal changes have an impact on the outcome of brain injury. Behavioral problems may be pronounced in brain-injured adolescents. Precocious puberty and precocious development of sexual activity may occur in preadolescents and should be carefully monitored.

Careful consideration should be given to the developmental progress of the brain-injured child and adolescent. Delays can be anticipated after moderate and severe brain injuries related to abnormalities of cognition and behavior. Educational plans should include an individualized education program (IEP) to support the child with significant remediation and assistance during their school years. Programs should also include a 504 plan (Section 504 of the Rehabilitation Act and the Americans with Disabilities Act) that identifies accommodations necessary in regular school settings for students with lesser disabilities so that they may be educated with their peers.

▶ Treatment

The primary goal of rehabilitation after childhood brain injury is to maximize functional independence. Rehabilitative care can be divided into three phases: acute, subacute, and long term. The acute and subacute phases typically occur in the inpatient setting, while the long-term phase is an outpatient endeavor.

A. Acute Care

Therapy in the acute phase consists mainly of medical, surgical, and pharmacologic measures to decrease brain edema, treat increased intracranial pressure, and normalize laboratory values. Nutrition via parenteral nutrition or supplemental enteral feedings is essential for the healing process and is provided as soon as possible after brain injury, as this is associated with improved outcomes. Placement of a gastrostomy tube for supplemental enteral feeding is often performed in patients with severe brain injuries when recovery will be protracted and swallowing function is inadequate for safe oral feeding. Early mobilization, starting in the intensive care unit, has been shown to improve recovery time and decrease comorbidities in even the most acutely ill patients. It is important to consider rehabilitation early during hospitalization with appropriate consultation of rehabilitation medicine and therapy specialists, as earlier interventions are essential for the best outcomes.

B. Subacute Care

Therapy in the subacute phase is characterized by early, intensive participation in rehabilitative therapies with involvement of physical therapy, occupational therapy, speech-language specialists, and neuropsychologists to promote functional recovery. Nursing staff are a primary interface with the patient and often serve as educators for family-directed care. Pharmacologic approaches may be used to enhance arousal and focus in patients with traumatic brain injury to enable them to more fully participate in therapies or deal with subacute sequelae such as agitation. Most children are able to discharge home and often continue receiving outpatient therapies.

C. Long-Term Care

Long-term follow-up starts immediately after discharge. Annual multidisciplinary evaluation, including neuropsychological testing, is important as the child approaches school age so strategies to deal with deficits can be implemented to improve outcomes in the educational environment. Attention and arousal can be successfully addressed by utilizing behavioral techniques to reinforce desired behaviors and by identifying environmental situations that facilitate success. Gains made in the behavioral realm often have a positive impact on therapies designed to address physical issues.

D. Pharmacologic Management

Targeted pharmacologic intervention can be helpful for a variety of brain injury-related comorbidities throughout the stages of recovery (Table 28–3). Medication is often required for cognitive and behavioral issues. Attention deficit and fatigue may be amenable to treatment with stimulants such as methylphenidate and modafinil. Dopaminergic agents, such as amantadine, levodopa, and bromocriptine, can be useful in improving cognition, processing speed, and agitation. Antidepressants such as selective serotonin reuptake

Table 28–3. Common medications used for treatment of comorbidities occurring with brain injuries.

Symptom Targets	Medication	Mechanism of Action
Alertness and attention	Amantadine	Indirect dopaminergic agonist
	Methylphenidate	Dopaminergic and noradrenergic agonist
	Carbidopa/levodopa	Dopaminergic agonist
	Bromocriptine	Indirect dopaminergic agonist
Sympathetic storming	Propranolol	Central β-blocker
	Clonidine	α_2-adrenergic receptor agonist
	Opiates	Mu agonist
	Dantrolene	Depresses intrinsic mechanisms of excitation-contraction coupling in skeletal muscle
	Bromocriptine	Indirect dopaminergic agonist, sympatholytic
Hypertonicity	Baclofen	$GABA_B$ receptor agonist
	Benzodiazepine	$GABA_A$ receptor agonist
	Tizanidine	α_2-adrenergic receptor agonist
	Dantrolene	Skeletal muscle contraction coupling depressant
	Botulinum toxin	Intramuscular SNARE protein antagonist
Sleep promoter	Melatonin	Melatonin receptor type 1 A agonist
	Trazodone	Serotonin transporter and serotonin type 2 receptor antagonist
	Clonidine	α_2-adrenergic receptor agonist
	Quetiapine	Serotonin, dopamine, histamine, and adrenergic antagonist
Mood stabilizers	Selective serotonin reuptake inhibitors	Increase serotonin by blocking reuptake
	Serotonin-norepinephrine reuptake inhibitors	Increase serotonin and norepinephrine by blocking reuptake
	Atypical antipsychotics	Anti-dopaminergic (D2), mixed noradrenergic, cholinergic, and histaminergic antagonists

inhibitors can be helpful in treating depression and mood lability. Anticonvulsants can be used as mood stabilizers and in treating agitation and aggression; carbamazepine and valproic acid are typical agents for this purpose. Medications serve as a complement to environmental and therapeutic intervention, rather than a substitution.

▶ Prognosis & Outcomes

Poor pupillary reactivity, low blood pH, absence of deep tendon reflexes, and low GCS all correlate with poor outcome. Coalescing lesions noted on imaging and increased depth and duration of coma suggest more severe injury and poor functional recovery. Children younger than 1 year tend to have worse outcomes.

Functional outcome assessment is important for judging the efficacy of rehabilitation therapy. Global multidomain measures (eg, FIM/WeeFIM) are used to provide a functional "snapshot in time" of select functions—motor function and mobility, self-care, cognition, socialization, and communication. Simpler, single-domain functional assessment tools such as the Glasgow Outcome Scale (GOS) and its pediatric cousin, the Kings Outcome Scale for Childhood Head Injury (KOSCHI), may also be of use. Standardized measures of meaningful functional outcomes continue to be developed.

Outcomes associated with mild brain injury are often quite favorable. Most patients recover normal function within a short time. A small percentage develop persistent problems such as chronic headache, poor focusing ability, altered memory, and vestibular abnormalities which may last for many weeks or months. Differentiating between musculoskeletal and central nervous system (CNS) etiologies of persistent symptoms such as headache is important and can influence prognosis and care planning. Physical therapy can be quite useful in the management of persistent cervicogenic headaches or vestibular dysfunction. It is no longer standard of care for children to be placed on "brain rest" after experiencing mild traumatic brain injury. Evidence suggests that sequential and incremental return to school and to sports activity is important in the recovery process and should not be delayed after injury. Return to school should occur prior to complete return to sports, although noncontact activity can be quite helpful in recovery.

Cameron S et al: Early mobilization in the critical care unit: a review of adult and pediatric literature. J Crit Care 2015;30(4):664–672 [PMID: 25987293].

Capizzi A et al: Traumatic brain injury: an overview of epidemiology, pathophysiology, and medical management. Med Clin 2020;104(2):213–238 [PMID: 32035565].

Jafari AA et al: Paroxysmal sympathetic hyperactivity during traumatic brain injury. Clin Neurol Neurosurg 2022;212:107081 [PMID: 34861468].

Kochanek PM et al: Guidelines for the management of pediatric severe traumatic brain injury, third edition: update of the brain trauma foundation guidelines, executive summary. Pediatr Crit Care Med 2019;20(3):280–289 [PMID: 30830016].

SPINAL CORD INJURY

ESSENTIALS OF DIAGNOSIS & TYPICAL FEATURES

▶ Spinal cord injury (SCI) is an alteration in normal motor, sensory, or autonomic function secondary to spinal insult.

▶ Characterized as either complete (total loss of function) or incomplete (some preservation of function below the level of lesion).

Epidemiologic studies suggest that there will be about 18,000 new spinal cord injuries (SCIs) per year and that 20% will be in those younger than 20 years. Motor vehicle accidents are the leading cause of SCI in all ages. Falls are common causes in young children. Children from birth to 2 years tend to have high-level injuries to the cervical spine because of anatomical features of their spine, such as facets that tend to be shallower and oriented horizontally and a boney spine that is more flexible than the spinal cord. In addition, the head is disproportionately large, and the neck muscles are weak.

▶ Clinical Findings

A. Classification and Assessment of Injury Severity

SCI is classified using the International Standards for Neurological Classification of Spinal Cord Injury (ISNCSCI), formerly known as the American Spinal Injury Association (ASIA) classification system. This classification evaluates motor and sensory function, defines the neurologic level of the injury, and assesses the completeness of the deficit (how much motor or sensory signal is getting through to the lowest sacral segments as assessed by rectal and perianal examination). This assessment can be used to prognosticate functional return. The ISNCSCI classification is as follows:

1. **Class A**—complete SCI, with no motor or sensory function in the lowest sacral segments; portends the poorest prognosis, with significant recovery quite unlikely.

2. **Class B**—incomplete lesion, with preserved sensory function but no motor function in the sacral segments.

3. **Class C**—incomplete lesion in which some motor function below the injury level is preserved.

4. **Class D**—incomplete lesion in which more motor function below the injury level is preserved.

5. **Class E**—injury in which full motor and sensory function is preserved.

B. Clinical Patterns of Spinal Cord Injury

1. **Brown-Séquard injury**—The cord is hemisected causing motor paralysis, loss of proprioception and vibration on the ipsilateral side, and loss of pain and temperature sensation on the contralateral side.

2. **Central cord syndrome**—Injury to the central part of the cord results in greater weakness in the arms than the legs.

3. **Anterior cord syndrome**—Disruption of the anterior spinal artery causes motor deficits and loss of pain and temperature sensation. Proprioception and fine touch are spared.

4. **Conus medullaris syndrome**—Injury or tumor of the conus, the lower conical shaped end of the spinal cord, which can cause minimal motor impairment but significant sensory, bowel, and bladder abnormalities.

5. **Cauda equina syndrome**—Injury to the nerve roots produces flaccid bilateral weakness in the legs, sensory abnormalities in the perineum, and lower motor neuron (LMN) bowel and bladder dysfunction.

C. Imaging

The diagnosis and anatomic description of SCI is made mainly through imaging techniques. Initial studies should include radiographs of the entire spine (including cervical spine). MRI is required to evaluate soft tissues, and MRI with contrast will evaluate for infection, inflammation, or neoplasm of the cord. CT scans, including three-dimensional reconstructions, may be used to further define the injured elements.

▶ Treatment

A. Initial Management

The two primary precepts of SCI treatment are early identification and immediate stabilization of the spine to prevent further damage. The approach used to stabilize the spine is determined by the type of injury, location of injury, and underlying condition of the spinal cord and may include external traction devices, orthotics, or surgical internal stabilization. The benefit of methylprednisolone administration in acute SCI has recently come into question, and its administration is not considered standard of care.

B. Functional Expectations After Spinal Cord Injury

The lesions associated with SCI have a predictable impact on motor and sensory function. It is helpful to understand these concepts when discussing functional expectations with patients and families (Table 28–4).

Table 28–4. Functional expectations related to spinal cord injury.

Level of Injury and Key Muscle Function	Functional Skills
C1–C4 (no upper extremity function)	Dependent for all skills, can use voice-activated computer, mouth stick; can drive power wheelchair with technology devices such as sip and puff, chin drive, or head array
C5 (biceps function)	Can assist with ADLs, power wheelchair with joystick, push manual wheelchair short distances, use modified push rims
C6 (wrist extension)	More ADL skills; can push manual wheelchair indoors, perform level transfers; hand function augmented with adapted equipment
C7 (elbow extension)	ADLs independent; hand function augmented with adapted equipment; can push manual wheelchair indoor and outdoor
C8 (finger flexors)	ADLs independent; independent manual wheelchair skills; increased transfer skills
T1 (little finger abduction)	ADLs independent; independent fine motor ADLs such as shirt buttoning or using a key in a deadbolt lock
T2–T12 (chest, abdominal, and spinal extensors)	ADLs independent; independent manual wheelchair skills; improved transfer; standing with braces
L1 and L2 (hip flexors)	Standing and walking with long leg braces, KAFO, and RGO; swing-through gait; manual wheelchair main form of mobility
L3 (knee extension)	Home and limited community ambulation; long leg or short leg braces
L4 (ankle dorsiflexion)	Community ambulation with short leg braces, AFO
L5 (long toe extensors)	Community ambulation; may be slower than peers and have some endurance issues
S1 (ankle plantar flexors)	Community ambulation; some ability to run; increased endurance.

ADLs, activities of daily living; AFO, ankle-foot orthosis; KAFO, knee-ankle-foot orthosis; RGO, reciprocal gait orthosis.

C. Special Clinical Problems Associated With Spinal Cord Injury

1. Autonomic dysreflexia—This potentially life-threatening condition occurs approximately 2–4 weeks following spinal injuries above the T6 level. Noxious stimuli in the injured patient cause sympathetic vasoconstriction below the level of injury. Vasoconstriction produces hypertension and a compensatory, vagal-mediated bradycardia. Symptoms include hypertension, bradycardia, headaches, flushing, and diaphoresis. Systolic blood pressure of 20–30 mm Hg above baseline should be considered evidence of autonomic dysreflexia in those at risk. Treatment requires identification and relief of the underlying noxious stimuli. The patient should be placed in an upright position; restrictive clothing removed; bladder status evaluated, with catheterization or flushing of an indwelling catheter to relieve distension as indicated; bowel status assessed and stool evacuated as indicated; and skin examined for sores or ingrown nails. Blood pressure should be taken every 5 minutes until return to normotension. In refractory cases, a quick acting antihypertensive should be used. Nitropaste, a cutaneously administered nitroglycerin, is commonly used as it can be applied rapidly and wiped off as soon as the patient achieves normotension.

2. Hypercalcemia—Hypercalcemia, in response to immobilization, often occurs in male adolescents within the first 2 months of becoming paraplegic or tetraplegic. Patients complain of abdominal pain and malaise. Behavioral problems may occur. Initial treatment is focused on hydration and forced diuresis using fluids and furosemide to increase urinary excretion of calcium. In severe cases, especially in older children, calcitonin and etidronate may be required.

3. Thermoregulation problems—These are common in higher-level injuries due to impaired vasodilation/vasoconstriction below the injury level and usually result in a poikilothermic state where body temperature changes with that of the environment. Patients with an SCI above T6 are particularly susceptible to environmental temperature and at risk of hypothermia and hyperthermia.

4. Deep vein thrombosis—Thrombosis is a common complication of SCI, especially in postpubescent children. Deep vein thrombosis should be suspected in children with any unilateral extremity swelling, palpable cords in the calf muscles, fever, erythema, or leg pain. Diagnosis is confirmed by Doppler ultrasound, and full evaluation may require spiral CT scan if a pulmonary embolus is suspected. While all patients need to be assessed individually for their own venous thromboembolism risk factors, it is recommended that all adolescents with acute SCI be prophylactically anticoagulated with low-molecular-weight heparin for a minimum of 8 weeks, in conjunction with mechanical preventative measures (eg, elastic stockings, sequential compression devices) and early mobility. Younger children without other risk factors should receive mechanical prophylaxis.

5. Heterotopic ossification—This complication occurs in both spinal cord and traumatic brain injuries. Ectopic calcium deposits usually appear around joints in the first 6 months after injury. They may cause swelling, decreased range of motion, pain with motion, palpable firm masses, fever, elevated erythrocyte sedimentation rate, and abnormal triple phase bone scan. Nonsteroidal anti-inflammatory drugs or bisphosphonates such as etidronate should be started at the time of diagnosis. Surgical removal of ectopic deposits is controversial and usually performed only in cases of extreme loss of motion, pressure sores, or severe pain.

Eldahan KC et al: Autonomic dysreflexia after spinal cord injury: systemic pathophysiology and methods of management. Auton Neurosci 2018 Jan;209:59–70 [PMID: 28506502].

Powell A, Davidson L: Pediatric spinal cord injury: a review by organ system. Phys Med Rehabil Clin N Am 2015;26(1):109 [PMID: 25479784].

Prevention of Venous Thromboembolism in Individuals With Spinal Cord Injury: Clinical Practice Guidelines for Health Care Providers, 3rd ed: Consortium for Spinal Cord Medicine. Top Spinal Cord Inj Rehabil 2016;22(3):209–240 [PMID: 29339863].

Yue JK et al: Update on critical care for acute spinal cord injury in the setting of polytrauma. Neurosurg Focus 2017 Nov;43(5):E19 [PMID: 29088951].

BRACHIAL PLEXUS LESIONS

ESSENTIALS OF DIAGNOSIS & TYPICAL FEATURES

▶ Upper trunk (C5 and C6) is the most commonly injured area and results in the classic Erb's palsy.

▶ Injury to the lower trunk (C7–T1) produces Klumpke's palsy.

▶ Pan-plexus lesion involves all roots and results in flail arm.

▶ Pathogenesis

Brachial plexus lesions can be associated with delivery and are often associated with shoulder dystocia. The nerve injury can range from simple neuropraxia (stretch) to complete avulsion. Acquired brachial plexus lesions from sports, surgery, and accidents also involve stretches or injuries to the plexus.

Clinical Findings

Erb's palsy, described as the "waiter's tip posture," is characterized by shoulder weakness with internal rotation and adduction of the upper arm. The elbow is extended and the wrist flexed. There is good preservation of hand function. Klumpke's palsy is characterized by good shoulder function but decreased or absent hand function. Brachial plexus injuries may also cause Horner syndrome (unilateral miosis, ptosis, and facial anhidrosis) due to disruption of cervical sympathetic nerves. Physical examination should include inspection of the humerus and clavicle for fractures in babies. Potential injuries to the phrenic and facial nerves should be evaluated. The diagnosis of a brachial plexus lesion is primarily based on history and clinical examination; further diagnostic testing can confirm, localize, and classify the lesion. Electromyography is helpful 3–4 weeks after the injury and can be useful not only diagnostically but also for tracking recovery. MRI is used to visualize the plexus if there are inconsistencies in the clinical presentation.

Complications

The development of complications reflects the degree of nerve recovery. Severe injuries are at risk for shoulder contractures, muscle atrophy, osseous deformities, functional deficits, pain, and maladapted postures.

Treatment & Prognosis

Treatment will depend on the severity of the lesion. Many injuries will heal on their own and no interventions are needed. For persistent injuries, physical/occupational therapy is the major treatment and includes stretching, bracing, strengthening, electrical stimulation, and functional training. Surgical nerve reconstruction is indicated for children who have no spontaneous recovery of biceps function by 6–9 months. Secondary procedures to maximize function include muscle transfers and orthopedic interventions.

In general, injuries of the upper trunk do better than those of the lower trunk. The presence of Horner syndrome portends a poor recovery. Children in whom antigravity function returns within 2 months of injury will usually have good recovery of function. If antigravity function is delayed until 6 months, recovery will probably be limited. If antigravity function is absent at 6–9 months, there will be no recovery of function and surgery should be considered.

Chang KW et al: A systematic review of evaluation methods for neonatal brachial plexus palsy: a review. J Neurosurg Pediatr 2013;12(4):395 [PMID: 23930602].

Schmieg S, Nguyen JC, Pehnke M, Yum SW, Shah AS: Team approach: management of brachial plexus birth injury. JBJS Rev 2020 Jul;8(7):e1900200 [PMID: 32618739].

COMMON REHABILITATION PROBLEMS

ESSENTIALS OF DIAGNOSIS & TYPICAL FEATURES

▶ Neurogenic bladder may be caused by trauma or disease affecting central or peripheral nervous system connections and is characterized by postvoid residuals that exceed 20% of expected bladder volume.

▶ Neurogenic bowel may be caused by upper or lower motor neuron damage with loss of sensation and sphincter control, with or without reflexive bowel activity depending on injury.

▶ Spasticity is a velocity dependent increase in tone and loss of isolated muscle function.

1. Neurogenic Bladder

During the first year of life, the bladder is a reflex-driven system that empties spontaneously. After the first year, bladder control begins to develop, and most children achieve continence by age 5 years. Neurogenic bladder occurs when there is a disturbance in one or several of the urinary system's functions—low pressure storage, volitional complete emptying, and/or prevention of vesicoureteral reflux—caused by injury to either the central or peripheral nervous system. The diagnosis of neurogenic bladder requires a complete history and physical examination and often is missed because of lack of clinical suspicion.

Bladder volumes in children are estimated commonly by the Berger formula: age +2 = bladder capacity in ounces. Multiplying by 30 will convert this volume to milliliters. Establishing bladder volume will provide context as to whether a child is voiding adequately or whether his/her catheterization program is optimized. Postvoid residual volumes, ultrasound readings of the bladder immediately after spontaneous voids, are helpful in the acute setting to detect or characterize the presence of neurogenic bladder. If a patient voids yet retains more than 20% of his/her estimated bladder volume consistently, it is safe to assume that there are voiding deficits requiring evaluation and treatment. The upper tracts should be assessed, most commonly using renal ultrasound. Lower tract testing includes urinalysis, postvoid residuals, urodynamics, cystography, and cystoscopy. Common comorbidities of neurogenic bladder include urinary tract infections and hydronephrosis with ureteral reflux, with the potential to cause renal failure or death.

Treatment

Treatment is geared to the type of bladder dysfunction. The simplest method is timed voiding in which children are reminded verbally or use a cueing device (eg, watch with a timer) to void every 2–3 hours before bladder capacity is reached. The Credé and Valsalva maneuvers are used in some patients to assist in draining a flaccid bladder. There is a risk of provoking vesicoureteral reflux by increasing intravesicular pressure during these maneuvers in children with high-pressure neurogenic bladder systems. Therefore, characterization prior to intervention is essential.

Medications are often employed to treat neurogenic bladder. Anticholinergics (eg, oxybutynin, tolterodine, and hyoscyamine) are commonly used to reduce detrusor contractions, decrease the sense of urgency, and increase bladder capacity. Side effects include sleepiness, nausea, and constipation. Absorbent pads and diapers, external catheters, indwelling catheters, and intermittent catheterization are also used. A young child with a high-pressure bladder is at particular risk for reflux and may need medication, intermittent catheterization, or vesicostomy to prevent hydrostatic renal damage and infection. An older child may require reconstructive bladder surgery (bladder augmentation) to increase the capacity of the bladder or an intestinal conduit from bladder to skin surface (Mitrofanoff procedure) to relieve bladder distention and facilitate catheterization. If an incompetent urethral sphincter causes urinary leakage, injections, slings, or implants may be used to increase the urethral barrier. Recently, electrical stimulation of sacral roots has been used to initiate voiding. Biofeedback directed by a physical therapist has been shown to improve voiding continence.

2. Neurogenic Bowel

Control of bowel function depends on an intact autonomic (sympathetic and parasympathetic) and somatic nervous system. Upper motor neuron (UMN) bowel dysfunction results from damage above the conus medullaris. Affected patients usually have reflex bowel contractions of high amplitude, absence of sensation, and no voluntary sphincter control. Patients with lower motor neuron (LMN) bowel dysfunction have no voluntary sphincter control and no reflex contraction of the external anal sphincter (anocutaneous reflex); this has been described as a flaccid bowel. In general, establishing a bowel program, a specific set of practices to manually induce a bowel movement with the goal of "controlled incontinence," is easier in patients with UMN lesions.

▶ Treatment

Goals of treatment for patients with neurogenic bowel are to establish a predictable and reliable bowel habit and prevent incontinence and complications. Bowel movements should be scheduled to occur with meals, as the gastrocolic reflex can trigger defecation. Fiber intake and fluids are critical elements for maintaining a soft stool consistency. Laxative and stool softening medications are usually included in a comprehensive bowel program. Stool softeners and osmotic agents,

such as docusate and polyethylene glycol, respectively, retain stool water. Mineral oil is an acceptable stool softener in patients not at risk for pulmonary aspiration. Bulking agents such as fiber can help form the stool, limiting incontinence of stool with more liquid composition. Stimulants such as senna fruit extract or bisacodyl increase peristalsis. Suppositories and enemas are often used when other methods have not been successful or sufficient. In UMN bowel dysfunction, the retained colic reflex can be triggered using digital stimulation of the rectum, inciting peristalsis and transit of fecal matter manually. When conservative methods are ineffective, options may include surgical implantation of sacral nerve stimulators or techniques to facilitate antegrade flushing of the colon. For example, the ACE (antegrade continence enema) or Malone procedure approximates the appendix to the surface of the abdomen, providing a conduit for flushing.

3. Spasticity

Spasticity is a specific form of hypertonicity defined as a velocity-dependent increase in muscle tone and loss of isolated muscle function. Spasticity occurs when there is damage to the CNS from trauma or other injury. It is included in the UMN syndrome (hyperactive and exaggerated reflexes, increased tone, clonus, positive Babinski sign).

▶ Treatment

Treatment is goal-directed and influenced by the functional status of the patient. Options for therapy range from conservative to aggressive. Children should be positioned properly and have appropriate equipment to prevent nociceptive input and facilitate physical therapy. Physical therapy can reduce the long-term effects of spasticity by the use of stretching and range-of-motion exercises. Heat and/or cold treatments are useful in improving tone, but their effects are not long-lived. Casting of both upper and lower extremities can decrease tone and increase range of motion. Constraint-induced movement therapy, in which the functional upper extremity is physically constrained for set periods of time, can be used to try to improve function of the affected limb.

Pharmacologic support with medications can be effective. Baclofen (a direct γ-aminobutyric acid type B [GABA$_B$] agonist) is a first-line medication, which produces effects at the spinal cord level. Side effects are primarily sleepiness and weakness. Seizure threshold may be reduced by baclofen. Baclofen delivered directly to the CNS through an intrathecal pump has been used successfully in children with brain injury, cerebral palsy, and SCI. Diazepam, an allosteric modulator of postsynaptic GABA$_A$ receptors in both the brain and the spinal cord, can be effective, but its central CNS effects can cause drowsiness and dependence. Tizanidine is a newer agent and works at the α$_2$-adrenergic receptors presynaptically. It can cause dry mouth, sedation, and elevated liver enzymes. Dantrolene works peripherally on skeletal muscle by inhibiting excitation-contraction coupling and is a nice option as it is not sedating, but use can result in weakness or, rarely, hepatotoxicity.

Relief of focal spasticity can be achieved with chemodenervation techniques. Botulinum toxin can be injected in selected muscles to block acetylcholine release at the neuromuscular junction to decrease muscle tone. Botulinum toxin has also been used to treat sialorrhea, hyperhidrosis, and chronic pain. The effects are temporary, lasting only 3–6 months, and repeat injections are often needed. Technically more challenging, phenol injections denature proteins in both myelinated and unmyelinated fibers. The effects may last longer than botulinum toxin but carry a risk of sensory dysesthesia if mixed nerves (ie, motor and sensory) are injected.

Surgical options include orthopedic procedures geared toward improving function and ambulation and alleviating deformities produced over time by spasticity. Surgery can relieve contractures, which commonly occur in the lower extremities in the Achilles tendon, hamstrings, and hip adductors and in the upper extremities in the elbow, wrist, and finger flexors. Neurosurgical techniques such as selective dorsal rhizotomy, in which afferent sensory nerve fibers are sectioned, are used in a very select group of children to permanently alter spasticity patterns and improve ambulation. Identifying appropriate surgical candidates is important, as only patients who have a significant amount of volitional motor control and strength have good functional outcomes.

Berger RM, Maizels M, Moran GC, Conway JJ, Firlit CF: Bladder capacity (ounces) equals age (years) plus 2 predicts normal bladder capacity and aids in diagnosis of abnormal voiding patterns. J Urol 1983 Feb;129(2):347–349. doi: 10.1016/s0022-5347(17)52091-1 [PMID: 6834505].

McClugage SG et al: Review of tone management for the primary care provider. Pediatr Clin North Am 2021 Aug;68(4):929–944 [PMID: 34247718].

Wheeler TL et al: Translating promising strategies for bowel and bladder management in spinal cord injury. Exp Neurol 2018;306:169–176 [PMID: 29753647].

Rheumatic Diseases

Jennifer B. Soep, MD

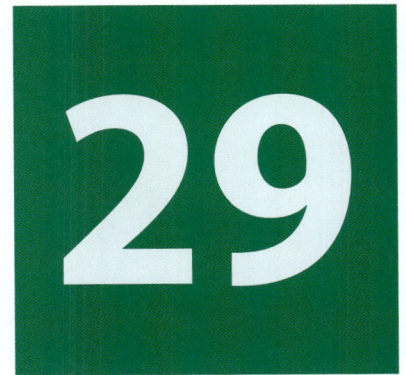

JUVENILE IDIOPATHIC ARTHRITIS

ESSENTIALS OF DIAGNOSIS & TYPICAL FEATURES

▶ Arthritis, involving pain, swelling, warmth, tenderness, morning stiffness, and/or decreased range of motion of one or more joints, lasting at least 6 weeks.

▶ May have associated systemic manifestations, including fever, rash, uveitis, serositis, anemia, and fatigue.

Juvenile idiopathic arthritis (JIA) is characterized by chronic arthritis in one or more joints for at least 6 weeks. There are six subtypes of JIA: (1) oligoarticular, (2) polyarticular, (3) systemic, (4) enthesitis associated, (5) psoriatic, and (6) undifferentiated. The exact cause of JIA is not known, but there is substantial evidence that it is an autoimmune process with genetic susceptibility factors.

▶ Clinical Findings

A. Symptoms and Signs

The most common type of JIA is the oligoarticular form, which constitutes approximately 40%–60% of patients and is characterized by arthritis of four or fewer joints. This type often affects medium to large joints. Because the arthritis is often asymmetrical, children may develop a leg-length discrepancy in which the involved leg may grow longer due to increased blood flow at the growth plates. Systemic features are uncommon except for inflammation in the eye. Approximately 20% of children with oligoarticular arthritis develop insidious, asymptomatic uveitis, which may cause blindness if untreated. The activity of the eye disease does not correlate

with that of the arthritis. Therefore, routine ophthalmologic screening with slit-lamp examination must be performed at 3-month intervals when the antinuclear antibody (ANA) test is positive, and at 6-month intervals if the ANA test is negative, for at least 4 years after the onset of arthritis, as this is the period of highest risk.

Polyarticular disease, which is defined as arthritis involving five or more joints, accounts for 20%–35% of JIA. Both large and small joints are involved, typically in a symmetrical pattern. Systemic features are not prominent, although low-grade fever, fatigue, rheumatoid nodules, and anemia may be present. This group is further divided into rheumatoid factor (RF)–positive and RF-negative disease. The former resembles adult rheumatoid arthritis with more chronic, destructive arthritis.

The systemic form comprises 10%–15% of patients with JIA. The arthritis can involve any number of joints and affects both large and small joints but may be absent at disease onset. One of the classic features is a high fever, often as high as 39°C–40°C, typically occurring one to two times per day. In between fever spikes, the temperature usually returns to normal or subnormal. Around 80%–90% of patients have a characteristic evanescent, salmon-pink macular rash that is most prominent on pressure areas and when fever is present (Figure 29–1). Other systemic features that may be present include hepatosplenomegaly, lymphadenopathy, leukocytosis, and serositis.

Enthesitis-associated arthritis is most common in males, older than 10 years, and is typically associated with lower extremity, large joint arthritis. The hallmark of this form is inflammation of tendinous insertions (enthesitis), such as the tibial tubercle or the heel. Low back pain and sacroiliitis are also commonly seen. This form of arthritis comprises approximately 5%–10% of patients with JIA.

There are two additional subtypes of JIA. Children with psoriatic arthritis may have typical psoriasis but may also present prior to the onset of the classic thick scaly plaques

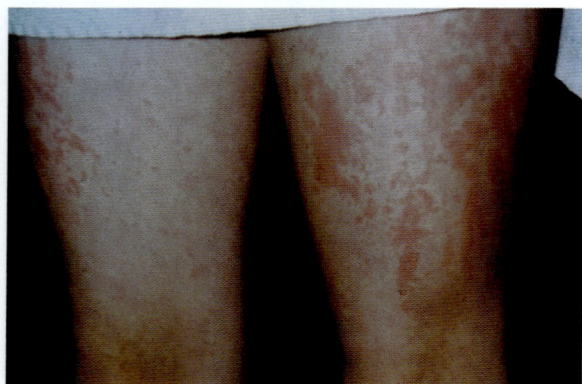

▲ **Figure 29–1.** Systemic JIA rash

and have more subtle changes such as nail pitting. Patients with psoriatic arthritis may also present with dactylitis or "sausage digit," which is painful swelling of an entire finger or toe. Undifferentiated JIA, comprising 10% of patients, includes children with chronic arthritis who do not meet criteria for any of the other subgroups or meet more than one criterion and therefore could be classified into multiple subgroups.

B. Laboratory Findings

There is no diagnostic test for JIA. A normal erythrocyte sedimentation rate (ESR) does not exclude the diagnosis of JIA. However, patients with systemic JIA typically have significantly elevated markers of inflammation, including ESR, C-reactive protein (CRP), white blood cell count, and platelets. RF is positive in about 5% of JIA patients, usually when the onset of polyarticular disease occurs after age 8 years. The anti-cyclic citrullinated peptide (anti-CCP) antibody has a high specificity for rheumatoid arthritis and may be detectable prior to the RF. While an ANA is not helpful in diagnosing JIA, ANAs are associated with an increased risk of uveitis in patients with oligoarticular disease and are also common in patients with the late-onset RF-positive form of the disease. Carriage of HLAB27 antigen is associated with an increased risk of developing enthesitis-associated arthritis.

Table 29–1 lists the general characteristics of joint fluid in various conditions. The main indication for joint aspiration and synovial fluid analysis is to rule out infection. A positive Gram stain or culture is the only definitive test for infection. A leukocyte count over 2000/μL suggests inflammation; this may be due to infection, rheumatologic diseases, leukemia, or reactive arthritis. A very low glucose concentration (< 40 mg/dL) and/or very high neutrophil count (> 60,000/μL) is highly suggestive of bacterial arthritis.

Table 29–1. Joint fluid analysis.

Disorder	Cells/μL	Glucose[a]
Trauma	More red cells than white cells; usually < 2000 white cells	Normal
Reactive arthritis	3000–10,000 white cells, mostly mononuclear cells	Normal
Juvenile idiopathic arthritis and other inflammatory arthritides	5000–60,000 white cells, mostly neutrophils	Usually normal or slightly low
Septic arthritis	> 60,000 white cells, > 90% neutrophils	Low to normal

[a]Normal value is ≥ 75% of the serum glucose value.

C. Imaging Studies

In the early stages of the disease, only soft tissue swelling, and possibly periarticular osteoporosis may be seen. Ultrasound is used to detect synovitis, tenosynovitis, and bony erosions without radiation and without requiring sedation. Magnetic resonance imaging (MRI) of involved joints may show early joint damage and, if obtained with gadolinium, can confirm the presence of synovitis. Later in the course of the disease, particularly in patients with RF-positive disease, plain films may demonstrate joint space narrowing due to cartilage thinning and/or erosive changes of the bone related to chronic inflammation on x-ray.

▶ Differential Diagnosis

Table 29–2 lists the most common causes of limb pain in childhood. JIA is a diagnosis of exclusion; therefore, it is important to rule out other causes of the clinical signs and symptoms prior to settling on this diagnosis. The differential diagnosis is often quite broad, including orthopedic conditions, infectious diseases, and malignancies. A few key features can help distinguish these different entities, including the timing of the pain and associated signs and symptoms. In inflammatory conditions, patients frequently have increased symptoms in the morning with associated stiffness, whereas patients with an orthopedic abnormality typically have increased symptoms later in the day and with activity. Growing pains, a common cause of leg pain in childhood, are characterized by poorly localized pain at night, which frequently wakes the child from sleep; no objective signs of inflammation; and no daytime symptoms. Patients with growing pains often ask to be massaged, which is not typical of those with arthritis.

It is particularly important to establish the diagnosis in the case of monoarticular arthritis. Bacterial arthritis is usually

Table 29–2. Differential diagnosis of limb pain in children.

Orthopedic
  Stress fracture
  Chondromalacia patellae
  Osgood-Schlatter disease
  Slipped capital femoral epiphysis
  Legg-Calvé-Perthes disease
  Hypermobility syndrome
Reactive arthritis
  IgA vasculitis
  Transient synovitis
  Rheumatic fever
  Poststreptococcal arthritis
Infections
  Bacterial
  Lyme arthritis
  Osteomyelitis
  Septic arthritis
  Discitis
  Viral (including parvovirus, Epstein-Barr virus, hepatitis B,
    dengue, chikungunya)
Rheumatologic
  Juvenile idiopathic arthritis
  Systemic lupus erythematosus
  Dermatomyositis
  Chronic nonbacterial osteomyelitis
Neoplastic/Hematologic
  Leukemia
  Lymphoma
  Neuroblastoma
  Osteoid osteoma
  Bone tumors (benign or malignant)
  Hemophilia
  Rhabdomyosarcoma
Pain syndromes
  Growing pains
  Fibromyalgia
  Complex regional pain syndrome

acute and monoarticular except for arthritis associated with gonorrhea, which may be associated with a migratory pattern and hemorrhagic pustules, usually on the distal extremities. Fever, leukocytosis, and increased ESR with an acute process in a single joint demand synovial fluid examination and culture to rule out an infection. Pain in the hip or lower extremity is a frequent symptom of childhood cancer, especially leukemia, neuroblastoma, and rhabdomyosarcoma. Radiographs of the affected site and examination of the blood smear for unusual cells and thrombocytopenia are necessary. An elevated lactate dehydrogenase value should also raise concern about an underlying neoplastic process. In doubtful cases, bone marrow examination or biopsies are indicated.

Reactive arthritis is joint pain and swelling triggered by an infection. The infection is nonarticular and can be either viral or bacterial. A preceding illness is identified in approximately half of cases. Patients often have acute onset of arthritis, and there may be a migratory pattern. The duration of symptoms is a very important distinction between reactive arthritides and JIA. Symptoms associated with reactive arthritis typically resolve within 4–6 weeks. In contrast, to meet criteria for chronic arthritis, symptoms must be present for at least 6 weeks.

The arthritis of rheumatic fever is migratory, transient, and often more painful than that of JIA. (see Chapter 20). In suspected cases, evidence of rheumatic carditis should be sought based on examination and electrocardiographic findings. Evidence of recent streptococcal infection is essential to the diagnosis. The fever pattern in rheumatic fever is low grade and persistent compared with the spiking fever that characterizes the systemic form of JIA. Lyme arthritis resembles oligoarticular JIA, but the former usually occurs as discrete, recurrent episodes of arthritis lasting 2–6 weeks and children should have a history of being in an endemic area. The typical bull's-eye rash, erythema chronicum migrans, is reported in approximately 70%–80% of patients, although it is resolved by the time the arthritis appears. For children suspected of having Lyme disease, testing for antibodies against *Borrelia burgdorferi* should be performed, with confirmatory testing by Western blot.

▶ **Treatment**

The objectives of therapy are to restore function, relieve pain, maintain joint motion, and prevent damage to cartilage and bone.

A. Nonsteroidal Anti-inflammatory Medications

Nonsteroidal anti-inflammatory drugs (NSAIDs) are frequently used for symptomatic relief. A wide range of agents is available, but only a few are approved for use in children, including naproxen (10 mg/kg per dose twice daily), ibuprofen (10 mg/kg per dose three to four times daily), and meloxicam (0.125–0.25 mg/kg once daily). NSAIDs are generally well tolerated in children, as long as they are taken with food and adequate hydration. The average time to symptomatic improvement is 1 month, but in some patients, a response is not seen for 8–12 weeks.

B. Disease-Modifying and Biologic Agents

Most patients with JIA require treatment with a disease-modifying medication, most commonly weekly methotrexate. Symptomatic response usually begins within 3–4 weeks. The low dosages used (5–10 mg/m^2/week or up to 1 mg/kg/week as a single dose with a maximum of 25 mg/week) are generally well tolerated. Potential side effects include nausea, vomiting, hair thinning, stomatitis, leukopenia, immunosuppression, and hepatotoxicity. A complete blood count and liver function tests should be obtained every 2–3 months. Several additional disease-modifying agents are available for use in patients with persistently active disease or those intolerant to methotrexate. Leflunomide is an antipyrimidine medication that is administered orally. Side effects may include diarrhea and alopecia. Biological-modifying medications that inhibit tumor necrosis factor, a cytokine known to play an important role in the pathogenesis of JIA, include etanercept, infliximab, and adalimumab. These drugs are generally quite effective in controlling disease and preventing cartilage and bone damage and have been associated with healing based on radiologic changes. However, they are very expensive and require parenteral administration. Anakinra and canakinumab, which block interleukin 1, and tocilizumab, which blocks interleukin 6, are particularly effective for systemic JIA. Additional targeted synthetic disease-modifying agents, including Janus kinase (JAK) inhibitors, are approved for use in polyarticular JIA. Other biologic agents, including rituximab and abatacept, have demonstrated efficacy in patients who have not responded to other treatments.

C. Corticosteroids

Local steroid joint injections may be helpful in patients who have arthritis in one or a few joints. Triamcinolone acetonide is a long-acting steroid that can be used for injections and is often associated with at least several months of disease control. Oral or parenteral steroids are reserved for children with severe involvement, primarily patients with systemic disease.

D. Uveitis

Inflammation of the uveal tract (uveitis or iridocyclitis) should be closely monitored by an ophthalmologist. Typically, treatment is initiated with corticosteroid eye drops to reduce inflammation as well as dilating agents to prevent scarring between the iris and the lens. In patients who fail topical treatments, methotrexate, cyclosporine, mycophenolate mofetil, and/or a tumor-necrosis factor inhibitor such as infliximab or adalimumab may be used.

E. Rehabilitation

Physical and occupational therapies are important to focus on range of motion, stretching, and strengthening. These exercises, as well as other modalities such as heat and water therapy, can help control pain, maintain, and restore function, and prevent deformity and disability. Young children with oligoarticular disease affecting asymmetrical lower extremity joints can develop a leg-length discrepancy, which may require treatment with a shoe lift on the shorter side.

▶ Prognosis

The course and prognosis for JIA is variable, depending on the subtype of disease. Children with persistent oligoarticular JIA have the highest rate of clinical remission, while patients with RF-positive disease are the least likely to achieve this status and are at highest risk for chronic, erosive arthritis that may continue into adulthood. The systemic features associated with systemic arthritis tend to remit within months to years. The prognosis in systemic disease is worse in patients with persistent systemic disease after 6 months, thrombocytosis, and more extensive arthritis. Patients with systemic JIA are at risk for macrophage activation syndrome, a severe, potentially fatal complication, with features of coagulopathy, pancytopenia, and liver dysfunction.

Mannion ML, Cron RQ: Therapeutic strategies for treating juvenile idiopathic arthritis. Curr Opin Pharmacol 2022;64:1022226 [PMID: 35461129].

McKenna D et al: Fifteen-minute guide to managing oligoarticular juvenile idiopathic arthritis. Arch Dis Child Educ Pract Ed 2022;107:175–181 [PMID: 34083213].

Thatayatikom A, Modica R, De Leucio A: Juvenile idiopathic arthritis. [Updated 2023 Jan 16]. In: StatPearls [Internet]. Treasure Island (FL): StatPearls Publishing; 2023 Jan [PMID: 32119492]. https://www.ncbi.nlm.nih.gov/books/NBK554605.

www.arthritis.org: Accessed May 21, 2023.

SYSTEMIC LUPUS ERYTHEMATOSUS

 ESSENTIALS OF DIAGNOSIS & TYPICAL FEATURES

▶ Multisystem inflammatory disease of the joints, serosal linings, skin, kidneys, blood, and central nervous system.

▶ Pathogenesis

Systemic lupus erythematosus (SLE) is the prototype of immune complex diseases; its pathogenesis is related to the formation of antibody–antigen complexes that exist in the circulation and deposit in the involved tissues. The spectrum of symptoms is due to tissue-specific autoantibodies as well as the damage to tissues by lymphocytes, neutrophils, and complement evoked by the deposition of immune complexes.

▶ Clinical Findings

A. Symptoms and Signs

Signs and symptoms depend on the organs affected by immune complex deposition. There are several established classification schemes and all require clinical and immunologic manifestations.

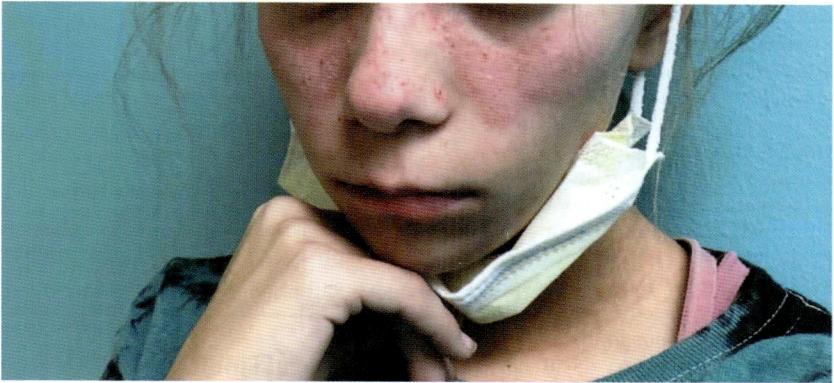

▲ **Figure 29–2.** SLE Malar rash

Clinical features include:

1. Skin manifestations—Acute and/or chronic cutaneous lupus (Figure 29–2), oral or nasal ulcers, nonscarring alopecia
2. Organ and musculoskeletal manifestations—Synovitis, serositis, nephritis, neurologic symptoms
3. Hematologic—Hemolytic anemia, leukopenia or lymphopenia and thrombocytopenia

Immunologic features include:

1. High ANA concentration
2. High anti-double-stranded DNA antibody concentration
3. Positive anti-Smith antibody
4. Positive anti-phospholipid antibodies
5. Low complement levels
6. Positive direct Coombs test

B. Laboratory Findings

Blood count abnormalities are common, including leukopenia, anemia, and thrombocytopenia. Approximately 15% of patients are Coombs test positive, and many patients develop anemia due to other causes, including chronic disease and blood loss. Patients with significant renal involvement may have electrolyte disturbances, elevated kidney function tests, and hypoalbuminemia. The ESR is frequently elevated during active disease. In contrast, many patients with active SLE have a normal CRP. When the CRP is elevated, it is important to investigate possible infectious causes, particularly bacterial infections. It is critical to monitor the urinalysis in patients with SLE for proteinuria and hematuria, as the renal disease may be otherwise clinically silent. In immune complex diseases, complement is consumed; therefore, levels of C3 and C4 are depressed with active disease.

The ANA test is positive in almost 100% of patients, usually at titers of 1:320 or above. In patients with suspected SLE, it is important to obtain a full ANA profile—including antibodies directed against double-stranded DNA, Smith, ribonucleic protein, and Sjögren-specific antibody A and B to better characterize their serologic markers of disease. Because approximately 50%–60% of pediatric SLE patients have antiphospholipid antibodies and are therefore at increased risk of thrombosis, it is important to screen all patients with SLE for these antibodies by checking partial thromboplastin time, anticardiolipin antibodies, antibeta-2 glycoprotein 1 antibodies, and lupus anticoagulant.

► Differential Diagnosis

Because there is such a wide spectrum of disease with SLE, the differential diagnosis is quite broad, including systemic JIA, mixed connective tissue disease (MCTD), rheumatic fever, vasculitis, malignancies, and bacterial and viral infections. A negative ANA test essentially excludes the diagnosis of SLE. Anti–double-stranded DNA and Smith antibodies are very specific for SLE.

► Treatment

The treatment of SLE should be tailored to the organ system involved so that toxicities may be minimized. Prednisone is a mainstay of treatment. Patients with severe, life-threatening, or organ-threatening disease are typically treated with intravenous pulse methylprednisolone, 30 mg/kg per dose (maximum of 1000 mg) daily for 3 days, and then switched to 2 mg/kg/day of prednisone. The dosage should be adjusted using clinical and laboratory parameters of disease activity, and the minimum amount of corticosteroid to control the disease should be used. Skin manifestations, arthritis, and fatigue are often managed by antimalarials such as hydroxychloroquine, 5 mg/kg/day orally. These medications may also prevent lupus from spreading to organs and reduce flares. Pleuritic pain or arthritis can often be managed with NSAIDs.

Most patients are also started on a steroid-sparing agent, such as mycophenolate mofetil, azathioprine, cyclophosphamide, or rituximab. Belimumab, a monoclonal antibody that blocks the biological activity of B-lymphocyte stimulator (BLyS), is a newer medication approved to treat lupus, including children aged 5 years and older. Patients who have evidence of antiphospholipid antibodies are often treated with a baby aspirin every day to help prevent thrombosis. Thrombotic events due to these antibodies require long-term anticoagulation.

The toxicities of the regimens must be carefully considered. Growth failure, osteoporosis, Cushing syndrome, adrenal suppression, infections, and aseptic bone necrosis are serious side effects of chronic use of prednisone. Cyclophosphamide can cause bone marrow suppression, bladder epithelial dysplasia, hemorrhagic cystitis, and sterility. Azathioprine has been associated with liver damage and bone marrow suppression. Rituximab can be associated with infusion reactions and can lead to long-term hypogammaglobulinemia. Retinal damage from hydroxychloroquine is generally not observed with recommended dosages, but patients should have routine visual field testing to screen for retinal toxicity.

▶ Prognosis

The disease has a natural waxing and waning cycle; it may flare at any time and spontaneous remission may rarely occur. The 5-year survival rate has improved from 51% in 1954 to 90% today. Factors that have contributed to improved prognosis include earlier diagnosis; more aggressive treatments with cytotoxic/immunosuppressive agents; pulse high-dose steroids; and advances in the treatment of hypertension, infections, and renal failure.

Aringer M et al: 2019 European League Against Rheumatism/American College of Rheumatology classification criteria for systemic lupus erythematosus. Ann Rheumat Dis 2019;78:1151–1159 [PMID: 31385462].

Charras A, Smith E, Hedrich C: Systemic lupus erythematosus in children and young people. Curr Rheumatol Rep 2021;23(20) [PMID: 33569643].

Trindade VC et al: An update on the management of childhood-onset systemic lupus erythematosus. Paediatr Drugs 2021;23(4):331–347 [PMID: 34244988].

www.lupus.org: Accessed May 21, 2023.

DERMATOMYOSITIS

ESSENTIALS OF DIAGNOSIS & TYPICAL FEATURES

- ▶ Pathognomonic skin rashes.
- ▶ Weakness of proximal muscles and occasionally of pharyngeal and laryngeal groups.
- ▶ Pathogenesis related to vasculopathy.

▶ Clinical Findings

A. Symptoms and Signs

The predominant symptom is proximal muscle weakness, particularly affecting pelvic and shoulder girdle muscles. Tenderness, stiffness, and swelling may be found. Pharyngeal involvement, manifested as voice changes and difficulty swallowing, is associated with an increased risk of aspiration. Intestinal vasculitis can be associated with ulceration and perforation of involved areas. Flexion contractures and muscle atrophy may produce significant residual deformities. Calcinosis may follow the inflammation in muscle and skin.

Several characteristic rashes are seen in dermatomyositis. Patients often have a heliotrope rash with a reddish-purple hue on the upper eyelids, along with a malar rash that may be accompanied by edema of the eyelids and face (Figure 29–3). Gottron papules are shiny, erythematous, scaly plaques on the extensor surfaces of the knuckles, elbows, and knees (Figure 29–4). Dilated nail-bed vessels are commonly seen with active disease. Thrombosis and dropout of periungual capillaries may identify patients with a more severe, chronic disease course.

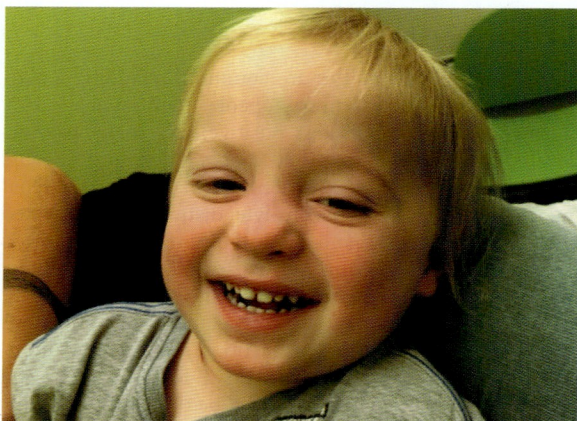

▲ **Figure 29–3.** Malar and heliotrope rash.

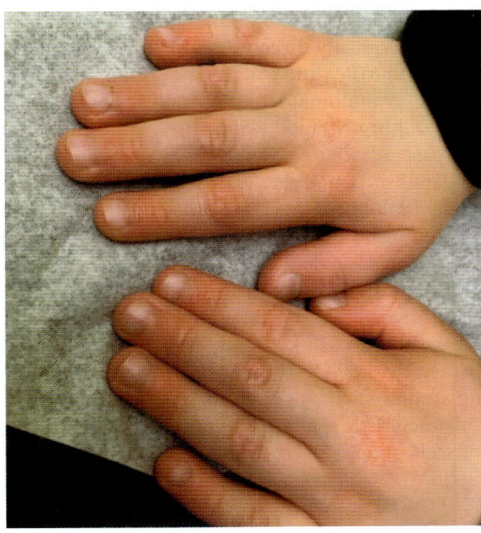

▲ **Figure 29–4.** Gottron papules on the hands.

B. Laboratory Findings/Imaging Studies/Special Tests

Determination of muscle enzyme levels, including aspartate aminotransferase, alanine aminotransferase, lactate dehydrogenase, creatine phosphokinase, and aldolase, is helpful in confirming the diagnosis, assessing disease activity, and monitoring the response to treatment. Even in the face of extensive muscle inflammation, the ESR and CRP may be normal. An MRI scan of the quadriceps muscle can be used in equivocal cases to confirm the presence of inflammatory myositis. Electromyography is useful to distinguish myopathic from neuropathic causes of muscle weakness. Muscle biopsy is indicated in cases of myositis without the pathognomonic rash. Myositis-specific antibodies can help determine the severity and prognosis of the disease.

▶ Treatment

Treatment is aimed at suppression of the inflammatory response and prevention of the loss of muscle function and joint range of motion. Acutely, it is very important to assess the adequacy of the ventilatory effort and swallowing and to rule out intestinal vasculitis. Corticosteroids are the initial therapy of choice. Treatment is usually initiated with prednisone, 2 mg/kg/day, and continued until signs and symptoms of active disease are controlled; the dosage is then gradually tapered. In severe cases, intravenous pulse methylprednisolone for 3 days is indicated. Therapy is guided by the physical examination findings and muscle enzyme values. Methotrexate is usually used concomitantly to achieve better control of the disease and minimize the steroid side effects. If patients continue to have active disease, additional steroid-sparing agents, such as mycophenolate mofetil, cyclosporine, intravenous immunoglobulin, and, in severe cases, rituximab or cyclophosphamide may be considered.

Hydroxychloroquine and intravenous immunoglobulin may be particularly helpful in managing the skin manifestations. As the rashes are photosensitive, sun protection is very important. Physical and occupational therapy should be initiated early in the course of disease. Initially, passive range-of-motion exercises are performed to prevent loss of motion. Later, once the muscle enzymes have normalized, a graduated program of stretching and strengthening exercises is introduced to restore normal strength and function.

▶ Prognosis

Patients may have a monocyclic, chronic or recurrent course. Factors that influence the outcome include the rapidity of symptom onset, extent of weakness, presence of cutaneous or gastrointestinal vasculitis, timeliness of diagnosis, initiation of therapy, and response to treatment. Dermatomyositis in children is not associated with cancer as it is in adults.

McCann LJ, Livermore P, Wilkinson MGL, Wedderburn LR: Juvenile dermatomyositis. Where are we now? Clin Exp Rheumatol 2022 Feb;40(2):394–403 [PMID: 35225221].

Wu Q et al: Juvenile dermatomyositis: advances in clinical presentation, myositis-specific antibodies and treatment. World J Pediatr 2020;16:31–43 [PMID: 31556011].

www.curejm.org: Accessed July 3, 2023.

VASCULITIS

ESSENTIALS OF DIAGNOSIS & TYPICAL FEATURES

▶ Cutaneous involvement with nonblanching, tender skin lesions.

▶ Frequent presence of systemic inflammation, particularly in the lungs and kidneys.

▶ Gold standard for diagnosis is demonstration of vasculitis on biopsy.

Vasculitides are a group of conditions that involve inflammation of blood vessels. They are classified by the size of the blood vessels affected (Table 29–3). The two most common forms of vasculitis in childhood—IgA vasculitis (previously known as Henoch-Schönlein purpura) and Kawasaki disease—are acute, self-limited forms of vasculitis. In contrast, there are idiopathic, chronic forms of vasculitis, such as granulomatosis with polyangiitis (GPA) and microscopic polyangiitis (MPA), which are rare in childhood.

Table 29–3. Classification of vasculitides by vessel size involved.

Large vessel
Takayasu arteritis
Giant cell arteritis
Medium vessel
Kawasaki disease
Granulomatosis with polyangiitis (previously called Wegener granulomatosis)
Polyarteritis nodosa
Eosinophilic granulomatosis with polyangiitis (previously called Churg-Strauss syndrome)
Small vessel
IgA vasculitis
Microscopic polyarteritis

► Clinical Findings

A. Symptoms and Signs

Signs and symptoms vary by disease, but most children with chronic vasculitis have persistent fever, fatigue, weight loss, and signs of pulmonary, renal, musculoskeletal, gastrointestinal, and/or skin inflammation.

Granulomatosis with polyangiitis (previously called Wegener granulomatosis) often causes nephritis and involves the lungs, manifesting as chronic cough, hemorrhage, and/or cavitating lesions. This form of vasculitis also frequently affects the upper respiratory tract, causing chronic otitis media, sinusitis, and/or inflammation of the trachea; saddle nose deformity may occur.

Children with polyarteritis nodosa (PAN) often present with skin lesions such as purpura, nodules or ulcers, and evidence of organ involvement with abdominal pain, testicular pain, hypertension, hematuria, and/or neurologic symptoms. MPA typically presents with pulmonary-renal syndrome with features of pulmonary hemorrhage and rapidly progressive kidney inflammation.

B. Laboratory Findings/Imaging Studies/Special Tests

Patients with vasculitis often have elevated inflammatory markers. If they have significant renal involvement, they will have elevated renal function tests and abnormal urinary sediment. Anemia is common, due to chronic disease and/or renal insufficiency. Low hemoglobin may also be an indicator of pulmonary hemorrhage in a patient with cough, hemoptysis, respiratory distress, and/or infiltrates on chest x-ray.

Antineutrophil cytoplasmic antibodies (ANCA) may be present in patients with small vessel vasculitis. Cytoplasmic ANCA (c-ANCA), which is usually directed against proteinase 3, is quite sensitive and specific for GPA and is positive in 80%–95% of patients. Perinuclear ANCA (p-ANCA) is typically directed against myeloperoxidase; is associated with MPA; and can also be seen in IgA vasculitis, eosinophilic granulomatosis with polyangiitis (previously known as Churg-Strauss syndrome), and inflammatory bowel disease.

The diagnosis is made based on a typical clinical presentation and laboratory findings. If the diagnosis remains uncertain, attempting to establish the diagnosis with a biopsy of involved tissue is warranted. A biopsy in patients with GPA typically demonstrates necrotizing granulomatous vasculitis. Biopsies of involved areas will confirm the presence of vasculitis in small vessels in patients with MPA and small and medium arteries in PAN. If a biopsy is not feasible, additional imaging studies such as an angiogram, which can demonstrate characteristic patterns of inflammation in affected blood vessels, should be considered.

► Treatment

The treatment of the various forms of chronic vasculitis is based on the severity of illness and the organs involved. Typically, corticosteroids are the initial therapy. Patients with severe disease are usually treated with intravenous pulse methylprednisolone, 30 mg/kg per dose (maximum of 1000 mg) daily for 3 days, and then switched to 2 mg/kg/day of prednisone. The dosage is then gradually tapered as tolerated based on clinical and laboratory markers of disease activity. Patients are usually treated with other immunosuppressant medications to gain and maintain control of the disease and minimize the steroid side effects. Standard treatment includes rituximab for induction therapy and cyclophosphamide may be added in severe cases. Maintenance therapy may consist of rituximab infusions every 6 months or can include methotrexate, azathioprine, or mycophenolate.

► Prognosis

Immunosuppressive medications have improved survival and remission rates for patients with chronic vasculitis. Conditions such as GPA had almost always been fatal. After introducing regimens that include high-dose steroids, rituximab and/or cyclophosphamide, patients with vasculitides have greatly improved outcomes, with 5-year survival ranging from 50% to 100%. Because relapses frequently occur when therapy is weaned or stopped, maintenance immunosuppression is commonly required.

Cannon L, Wu EY: Recent advances in pediatric vasculitis. Rheum Dis Clin North Am 2021 Nov;47(4):781–796 [PMID: 34635304].

Morishita KA et al: Consensus treatment plans for severe pediatric antineutrophil cytoplasmic antibody-associated vasculitis. Arthritis Care Res 2022 Sep;74(9):1550–1558 [PMID: 33675161].

Ozen S, Sag E: Childhood vasculitis. Rheumatology 2020;59 (Suppl 3):iii95–iii100 [PMID: 32348513].

RAYNAUD PHENOMENON

Raynaud phenomenon is an intermittent vasospastic disorder of the extremities. As much as 5%–10% of the adult population has this disorder, and onset in childhood is not uncommon. The classic triphasic presentation is cold-induced pallor, then cyanosis, followed by hyperemia, but incomplete forms are frequent. In adults older than 35 years who are ANA-positive, Raynaud phenomenon may be a harbinger of rheumatic disease. This progression is less common in childhood. Evaluation should include a detailed history with review of systems relevant to rheumatic disease. Examination of the cuticle edge, using an otoscope or a special microscope called a capillaroscope, is important to screen for dilated and/or tortuous capillaries that may suggest an underlying rheumatic disease such as lupus or scleroderma. In the absence of positive findings, Raynaud phenomenon is likely to be idiopathic.

Treatment involves education about keeping the extremities and core body warm and the role of stress, which may be a precipitant. In more symptomatic patients, treatment with vasodilators, such as calcium channel blockers, can be effective.

Choi E, Henkin S: Raynaud's phenomenon and related vasospastic disorders. Vasc Med 2021 Feb;26(1):56–70 [PMID: 33566754].
Esteireiro AS, Bicho A: Raynaud's phenomenon in paediatric age. BMJ Case Rep 2020 Jan 21;13(1):e233596 [PMID: 31969418].

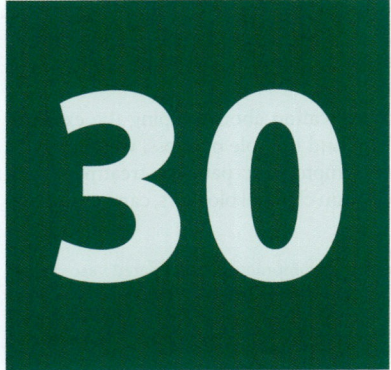

Hematologic Disorders

Christopher McKinney, MD

Rachelle Nuss, MD

Michael Wang, MD

NORMAL HEMATOLOGIC VALUES

The normal ranges for peripheral blood counts vary with age. Neonates have a hematocrit of 45%–65% accompanied by an increased reticulocyte count of 2%–8% in the first 24 hours. Within the first few days of life, erythrocyte production decreases as serum erythropoietin levels fall in response to increased tissue oxygenation, and the hemoglobin and hematocrit fall to a physiologic nadir around 10 g/dL and 30%, respectively, at 6–8 weeks of life. Thereafter, the normal values for hemoglobin and hematocrit gradually increase until adult values are reached after puberty with post-pubertal males having an average hemoglobin concentration about 1 g/dL higher than postpubertal females. Premature infants may have a more exaggerated and delayed hemoglobin nadir of 7–8 g/dL at 8–10 weeks. Anemia is defined as a hemoglobin concentration less than the 2.5th percentile for a normal population of the same gender and age.

Newborns have larger red cells than children and adults, with a mean corpuscular volume (MCV) at birth of more than 94 fL. The MCV subsequently falls to a nadir of 70–84 fL at about age 6 months. Thereafter, the normal MCV increases gradually until it reaches adult values after puberty.

The total white blood cell count (WBC) typically decreases with age. Lymphocytes are the predominant type of WBC in children between the ages of 1 and 6 years whereas neutrophils predominate at other ages. Previously referred to as benign ethnic neutropenia, patients with the Duffy null red cell phenotype (Fya-/Fyb-) have lower baseline absolute neutrophil counts (ANCs) with almost a quarter of patients having ANCs less than 2000/mcL. The Duffy null phenotype has a higher incidence (> 50%) in self-identified patients of African descent.

Normal values for the platelet count are 150,000–400,000/μL and vary little with age.

Merz L: Absolute neutrophil count by Duffy status among healthy black and African American adults. Blood Adv 2023;7:317–320 [PMID: 35994632].

BONE MARROW FAILURE

Failure of the marrow to produce adequate numbers of circulating blood cells may be congenital or acquired (eg, immune, medication, or toxin-associated) and may result in pancytopenia or single lineage cytopenias. Poor growth, comorbid congenital anomalies, and red cell macrocytosis should increase suspicion for an inherited bone marrow failure syndrome (IBMFS). Bone marrow failure caused by malignancy or other infiltrative disease is discussed in Chapter 31.

FANCONI ANEMIA

ESSENTIALS OF DIAGNOSIS & TYPICAL FEATURES

- ▶ Progressive pancytopenia.
- ▶ Macrocytosis.
- ▶ Multiple congenital anomalies in two-thirds.
- ▶ Increased chromosome breakage in peripheral blood lymphocytes.

General Considerations

Fanconi anemia is the most common IBMFS. It is a DNA repair disorder and cancer predisposition syndrome resulting from defects in the FA/BRCA pathway. Most commonly, inheritance is autosomal recessive, but X-linked and autosomal dominant forms do exist. Approximately 75%–90% of affected individuals develop bone marrow failure in the first 10 years of life.

Clinical Findings

A. Symptoms and Signs

Symptoms are determined by the type and severity of hematologic abnormality. Thrombocytopenia may cause purpura, petechiae, and bleeding; neutropenia may cause severe or recurrent infections; and anemia may cause weakness, fatigue, and pallor. Congenital anomalies are present in at least two-thirds of patients. The most common anomalies include abnormal pigmentation of the skin (generalized hyperpigmentation, café au lait or hypopigmented spots), short stature with delicate features, and skeletal malformations (hypoplasia, anomalies, or absence of the thumb and radius). More subtle anomalies are hypoplasia of the thenar eminence or a weak or absent radial pulse. Associated renal anomalies include aplasia, horseshoe kidney, and duplication of the collecting system. Other anomalies are microcephaly, microphthalmia, strabismus, ear anomalies, and hypogenitalism.

B. Laboratory Findings

Thrombocytopenia or leukopenia typically occurs first, followed over the course of months to years by anemia and progression to severe aplastic anemia. Macrocytosis is an important diagnostic clue and is virtually always present. It is usually associated with anisocytosis and an elevation in fetal hemoglobin levels. The bone marrow reveals hypoplasia or aplasia. The diagnosis is confirmed by demonstration of increased chromosome breakage and rearrangements in peripheral blood lymphocytes in response to stimulation with diepoxybutane or mitomycin c. Confirmatory genetic testing is also used to determine complementation type and genotype-phenotype correlations.

Differential Diagnosis

As some patients may not have classic physical dysmorphisms, Fanconi anemia must be distinguished from severe aplastic anemia and other causes of IBMFS. Thrombocytopenia absent radius (TAR) syndrome may also be confused due to the presence of severe thrombocytopenia with radial ray anomalies. Alternative constitutional causes of consideration include telomere biology disorders, Schwachman-Diamond syndrome, and congenital amegakaryocytic thrombocytopenia.

Complications

Complications are those related to thrombocytopenia and neutropenia. Endocrine dysfunction may include growth hormone deficiency, hypothyroidism, or impaired glucose metabolism. Persons with Fanconi anemia have a significantly increased risk of developing malignancies, especially acute nonlymphocytic leukemia (800-fold), head and neck cancers, genital cancers, and myelodysplastic syndromes related to defective DNA repair.

Treatment

Patients require specialized multidisciplinary care to monitor for complications and initiate early therapy. Bone marrow evaluations should be performed annually to assess for development of myelodysplasia or leukemias. Patients also should be screened routinely for other cancers. Patients with neutropenia who develop fever require prompt evaluation and parenteral broad-spectrum antibiotics. Transfusions are important, but should be used judiciously, especially in the management of thrombocytopenia, which frequently becomes refractory to platelet transfusions because of alloimmunization. Transfusions from family members should be discouraged because of the deleterious effect on the outcome of bone marrow transplantation. Historically, androgen therapy was used in patients to increase blood counts, but this was complicated by hepatotoxicity, hepatic adenomas, and masculinization. In the modern era, patients should be referred for allogeneic hematopoietic stem cell transplant at the first signs of bone marrow failure before significant transfusion needs arise. Clinical trials for autologous gene therapies are currently underway for certain subsets of patients with Fanconi anemia (eg, FANCA).

Prognosis

Many patients succumb to bleeding, infection, or malignancy in adolescence or early adulthood. Hematopoietic stem cell transplantation does not reduce the increased susceptibility for malignancy; 40% develop malignancy by 20 years posttransplant. Intensive posttransplant screening by subspecialists is required.

Martinez-Balsalobre E: Beyond current treatment of Fanconi anemia: what do advances in cell and gene-based approaches offer? Blood Rev 2023;60:101094 [PMID: 37142543].

Sroka I: Fanconi anemia clinical care guidelines. 5th Edition; Fanconi Anemia Research Fund 2020; https://www.fanconi.org/explore/clinical-care-guidelines.

ACQUIRED APLASTIC ANEMIA

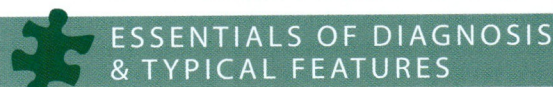

ESSENTIALS OF DIAGNOSIS & TYPICAL FEATURES

- ▶ Weakness and pallor.
- ▶ Petechiae, purpura, and bleeding.
- ▶ Frequent or severe infections.
- ▶ Pancytopenia with hypocellular bone marrow.

General Considerations

Acquired aplastic anemia is characterized by peripheral pancytopenia without an abnormal infiltrate or increased reticulin and a hypocellular bone marrow. Approximately 70% of cases in childhood are idiopathic and thought to be related to immune-mediated destruction of stem cells in the bone marrow. Other cases are secondary to idiosyncratic reactions to drugs such as nifedipine, sulfonamides, nonsteroidal anti-inflammatory drugs (NSAIDs), cytotoxic drugs, and anticonvulsants. Toxic causes include exposure to benzene, insecticides, and heavy metals. Infectious causes include viral hepatitis, infectious mononucleosis (Epstein-Barr virus [EBV]), and human immunodeficiency virus (HIV). In children with immune disorders, aplastic anemia has been associated with human parvovirus B19 infection.

Clinical Findings

A. Symptoms and Signs

Weakness, fatigue, and pallor result from anemia; petechiae, purpura, and bleeding occur due to thrombocytopenia; and fevers due to generalized or localized infections are associated with neutropenia. Hepatosplenomegaly and significant lymphadenopathy are unusual.

B. Laboratory Findings

The modified Camitta criteria are usually used for diagnosis and includes decreased bone marrow cellularity less than 25% and cytopenias in at least two peripheral blood cell lineages with ANC less than 500/μL, platelet count less than 20,000, or absolute reticulocyte count less than 60,000.

Differential Diagnosis

Exclusion of other acquired or constitutional causes of bone marrow failure is required. Myelodysplasia and leukemia can be ruled out through bone marrow examination and evaluation of cytogenetic and FISH studies. Patients should have additional screening for infectious etiologies (hepatitides, EBV, cytomegalovirus [CMV], HIV, parvovirus), nutritional deficiencies (eg, vitamin B_{12} or folate), autoimmune conditions, and paroxysmal nocturnal hemoglobinuria. Chromosome fragility testing and telomere length measurement is also usually performed to exclude potential IBMFS (eg, Fanconi anemia, telomere biology disorders). Genetic testing should be performed in patients with physical dysmorphism or other congenital anomalies.

Complications

Acquired aplastic anemia is characteristically complicated by infection and hemorrhage, which are the leading causes of death. Other complications are those associated with therapy.

Treatment

Comprehensive supportive care is essential. Febrile illnesses require prompt evaluation and usually parenteral antibiotics. Transfusion support with irradiated and leukodepleted red blood cells (RBCs) or platelets may be required. Platelets should be used sparingly because many patients eventually develop platelet alloantibodies and become refractory to transfusions.

Hematopoietic stem cell transplant is the treatment of choice for severe aplastic anemia when an HLA-identical sibling donor is available. Immunomodulation, usually with equine antithymocyte globulin and cyclosporine, is currently considered the standard of care upfront therapy for patients without an HLA-identical related donor. However, with improving transplant-related supportive care and increasing recognition of postimmunosuppressive therapy complications, such as relapse and development of myelodysplasia or leukemia, there is increasing interest in the use of alternative stem cell transplant donors in the upfront setting.

While thrombopoietin mimetics, for example eltrombopag, have augmented treatment response in adult patients, similar beneficial effects have not been noted in the pediatric population.

Prognosis

Sustained, complete remissions may be seen in 65%–80% of patients receiving immunosuppressive therapy. Children receiving early bone marrow transplant from an HLA-identical sibling have a long-term survival rate of greater than 90%. Matched unrelated donor and haploidentical transplant can be considered. Survivors are at an increased risk of myelodysplastic syndrome, acute leukemia, and other malignancies.

Groarke E et al: Eltrombopag added to immunosuppression for children with treatment-naïve severe aplastic anemia. Br J Hematol 2021;192:605–614 [PMID: 33410523].

Rogers Z et al: Immunosuppressive therapy for pediatric aplastic anemia: a North American Pediatric Aplastic Anemia Consortium study. Haematologica 2019;104:1974–1983 [PMID: 30948484].

Shimano K et al: Diagnostic work-up for severe aplastic anemia in children: consensus of the North American Pediatric Aplastic Anemia Consortium. Am J Hematol 2021;96:1491–1504 [PMID: 34342889].

ANEMIAS

APPROACH TO THE CHILD WITH ANEMIA

Anemia is a common finding, and identifying the cause is important. Even though anemia in childhood has many causes, the correct diagnosis can be established with a focused history and basic laboratory evaluation. Pertinent history should evaluate diet for nutritional deficiencies, growth and development, other chronic medical conditions, potential sources of blood loss or malabsorption, and signs and symptoms of hemolysis such as jaundice, gallbladder disease or splenomegaly. The child's ethnicity may suggest the possibility of hemoglobinopathies or deficiencies of red cell enzymes, such as glucose-6-phosphate dehydrogenase (G6PD). The patient's age is important because some causes of anemia are age related. For example, patients with iron deficiency anemia (IDA) and β-globin disorders present more commonly at ages 6–36 months than at other times in life.

The physical examination may also reveal clues to the cause of anemia. Poor growth may suggest chronic disease or hypothyroidism. Congenital anomalies may be associated with IBMFS. Other disorders may be suggested by the findings of petechiae or purpura (leukemia, aplastic anemia, hemolytic uremic syndrome), jaundice (hemolysis or liver disease), generalized lymphadenopathy (leukemia, juvenile rheumatoid arthritis, HIV infection), splenomegaly (leukemia, sickle hemoglobinopathy syndromes, hereditary spherocytosis, liver disease, hypersplenism), or evidence of chronic or recurrent infections.

The initial laboratory evaluation of the anemic child consists of a complete blood count (CBC) with differential, review of the peripheral blood smear, and a reticulocyte count.

The algorithm in Figure 30–1 uses limited laboratory information, together with the history and physical examination, to reach a specific diagnosis or to focus additional laboratory investigations on a limited diagnostic category (eg, microcytic anemia, bone marrow failure, pure red cell aplasia, or hemolytic disease). This diagnostic scheme depends principally on the MCV to determine whether the anemia is microcytic, normocytic, or macrocytic, according to the percentile curves of Dallman and Siimes (Figure 30–2).

Another key element of Figure 30–1 is the use of both the reticulocyte count and the peripheral blood smear to determine whether a normocytic or macrocytic anemia is due to hemolysis. Typically, hemolytic disease is associated with an elevated reticulocyte count, but some children with chronic hemolysis initially present during a period of a virus-induced aplasia when the reticulocyte count is not elevated. Thus, review of the peripheral blood smear for evidence of hemolysis (eg, spherocytes, red cell fragmentation, sickle forms) is important in the evaluation of children with normocytic anemias and low reticulocyte counts. When hemolysis is suggested, the correct diagnosis may be suspected by specific abnormalities of red cell morphology or by clues from the history or physical examination. Laboratory findings supporting

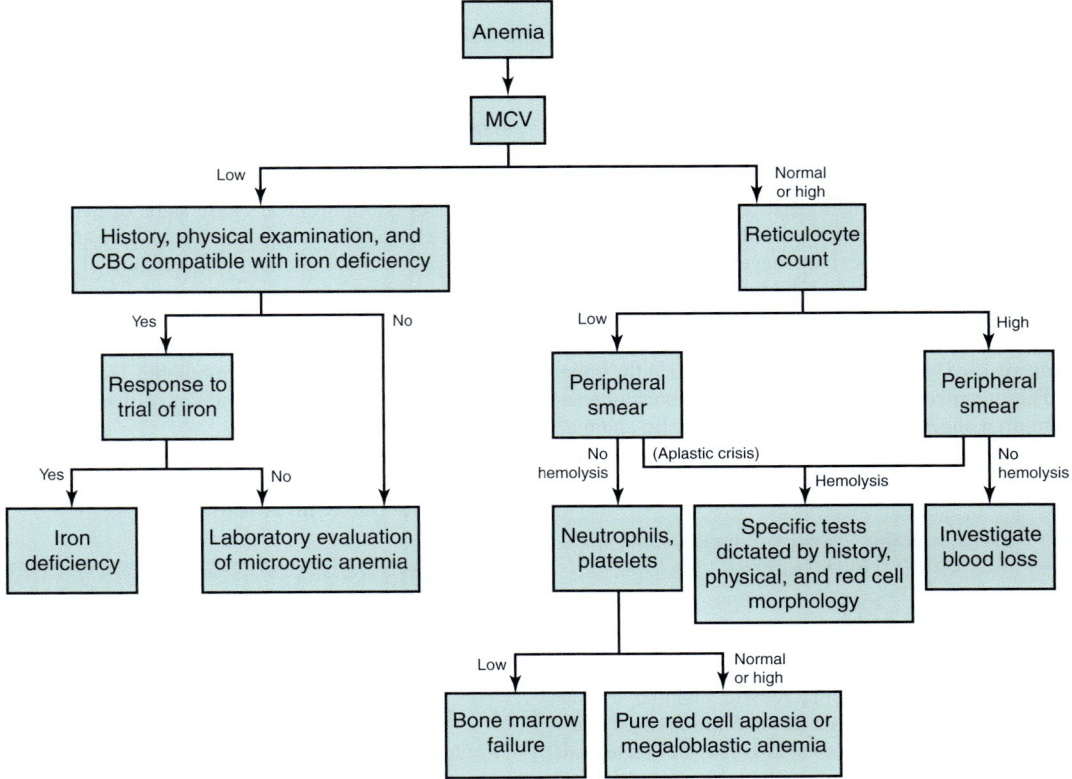

▲ **Figure 30–1.** Investigation of anemia.

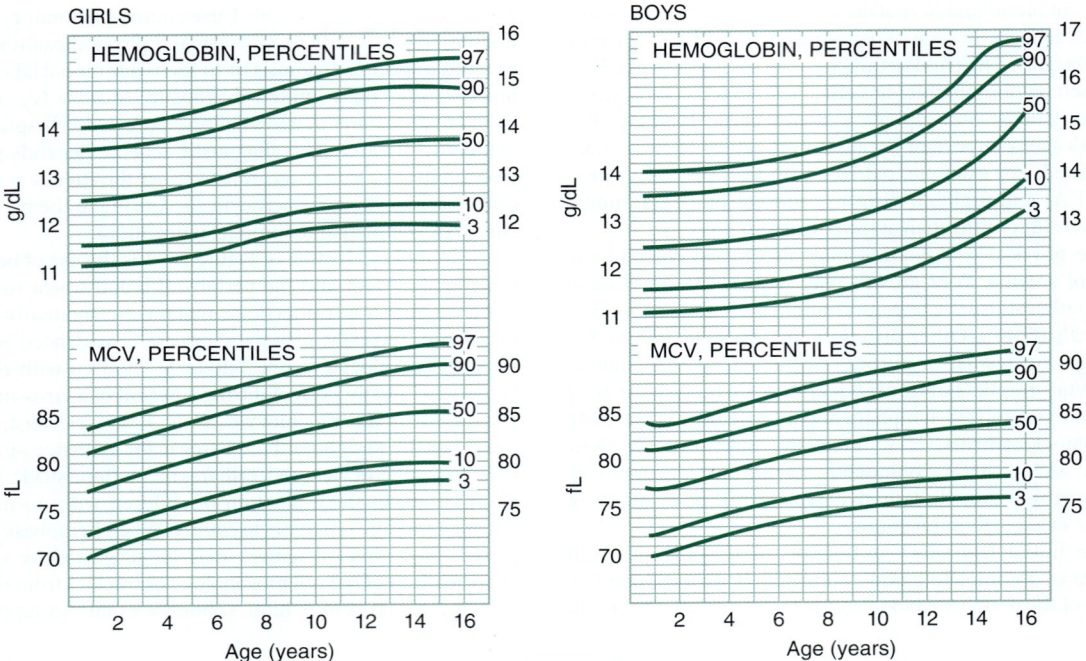

▲ **Figure 30–2.** Hemoglobin and red cell volume in infancy and childhood. (Reproduced with permission from Dallman PR, Siimes MA: Percentile curves for hemoglobin and red cell volume in infancy and childhood. J Pediatr 1979;94(1):26–31.)

a diagnosis of hemolytic anemia include increased lactate dehydrogenase or serum bilirubin, decreased serum haptoglobin, or presence of urobilinogen in the urine. Autoimmune hemolysis is usually excluded by a negative direct antiglobulin test (DAT). Review of blood counts and the peripheral blood smears of the mother and father may suggest genetic disorders such as hereditary spherocytosis. Children with normocytic or macrocytic anemias, with relatively low reticulocyte counts and no evidence of hemolysis on the blood smear, usually have anemias caused by inadequate erythropoiesis in the bone marrow. The presence of neutropenia or thrombocytopenia in such children suggests the possibility of aplastic anemia, malignancy, or severe folate or vitamin B_{12} deficiency, and usually dictates examination of the bone marrow.

Wood SK: Pediatric screening: development, anemia and lead. Prim Care 2019;46:69–84 [PMID: 30704661].

PURE RED CELL APLASIA

Pure red cell aplasia should be suspected in infants and children with normocytic or macrocytic anemia, a low reticulocyte count, and normal or elevated numbers of neutrophils and platelets. Pure red cell aplasia may be congenital (Diamond-Blackfan anemia), acquired, and transient (transient erythroblastopenia of childhood); a manifestation of a

systemic disease such as renal disease or hypothyroidism; or associated with malnutrition or mild deficiencies of folate or vitamin B_{12}. Examination of the peripheral blood smear in such cases is important because signs of hemolytic disease suggest chronic hemolysis complicated by an aplastic crisis due to parvovirus infection. Appreciation of this phenomenon is important because chronic hemolytic disease may not be diagnosed until the anemia is exacerbated by an episode of red cell aplasia (such as after parvovirus infection) and subsequent rapidly falling hemoglobin level. In such cases, cardiovascular compromise and congestive heart failure may develop quickly.

1. Congenital Hypoplastic Anemia (Diamond-Blackfan Anemia)

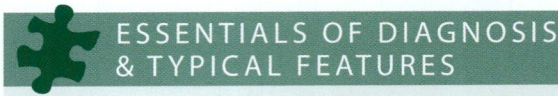

ESSENTIALS OF DIAGNOSIS & TYPICAL FEATURES

► Age: birth to 1 year.
► Macrocytic anemia with reticulocytopenia.
► Bone marrow with erythroid hypoplasia.
► Often short stature or congenital anomalies.

General Considerations

Diamond-Blackfan anemia is a relatively rare cause of anemia due to impaired erythroid maturation that usually presents before 1 year of age. Mutations of genes encoding ribosomal proteins are identified in 70%–80% of patients.

Clinical Findings

A. Symptoms and Signs

Signs and symptoms are those of chronic anemia, such as pallor and congestive heart failure. Jaundice, splenomegaly, or other evidence of hemolysis are usually absent. Short stature or other congenital anomalies are present in 50% of patients. A wide variety of anomalies have been described; craniofacial, renal, and cardiac anomalies are most common.

B. Laboratory Findings

Diamond-Blackfan anemia is characterized by severe macrocytic anemia and marked reticulocytopenia. The neutrophil count is usually normal or slightly decreased, and the platelet count is normal, elevated, or decreased. The bone marrow shows a marked decrease in erythroid precursors but is otherwise normal. In older children, fetal hemoglobin levels are usually increased.

Differential Diagnosis

Transient erythroblastopenia of childhood is the primary differential diagnosis (see section below). Other disorders associated with decreased red cell production such as transient aplasia due to parvovirus infection, renal failure, hypothyroidism, and the anemia of chronic disease should be considered.

Treatment

Patients usually receive repeated transfusions until 1 year of age to avoid steroid-related toxicities in the developing infant and to help facilitate growth. After one year, patients trial a course of oral corticosteroids. Eighty percent of patients respond to prednisone, 2 mg/kg/day, and many who respond subsequently tolerate significant tapering of the dose. Patients who are unresponsive to prednisone, unable to taper, or experience significant steroid-related toxicity, require chronic transfusion therapy and oral iron chelation therapy to prevent transfusion-related iron overload. Bone marrow transplant is an alternative definitive therapy that should be considered for transfusion-dependent patients who have HLA-identical siblings.

Prognosis

The prognosis for patients responsive to corticosteroids is generally good, particularly if remission is maintained with low doses of alternate-day prednisone. Unpredictable spontaneous remissions occur in up to 20% of patients.

Transfusion-dependent patients are at risk for developing cardiac or hepatic hemosiderosis. There is an increased risk for the development of myelodysplastic syndrome, acute myeloid leukemia (AML), and solid tumors.

Da Costa L et al: Diamond Blackfan anemia. Blood 2020;136:1262 [PMID: 32702755].

2. Transient Erythroblastopenia of Childhood

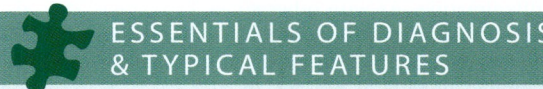

ESSENTIALS OF DIAGNOSIS & TYPICAL FEATURES

- ▶ Age: 6 months to 4 years.
- ▶ Normocytic anemia with reticulocytopenia.
- ▶ Absence of hepatosplenomegaly or lymphadenopathy.
- ▶ Erythroid precursors initially absent from bone marrow.

General Considerations

Transient erythroblastopenia of childhood is a relatively common cause of acquired anemia in early childhood. The disorder is suspected when a normocytic anemia is discovered during evaluation of pallor or when a CBC is obtained for another reason. Because the anemia is due to decreased red cell production, and thus develops slowly, the cardiovascular system has time to compensate. Therefore, children with hemoglobin levels as low as 4–5 g/dL may look remarkably well. The disorder is thought to be autoimmune in most cases because IgG from some patients has been shown to suppress erythropoiesis in vitro.

Clinical Findings

Pallor is the most common sign, and hepatosplenomegaly and lymphadenopathy are absent. The anemia is normocytic, and the peripheral blood smear shows no evidence of hemolysis. The platelet count is normal or elevated, and the neutrophil count is normal or, in some cases, decreased. Early in the course, no reticulocytes are identified. The Coombs test is negative, and there is no evidence of chronic renal disease, hypothyroidism, or other systemic disorder. Bone marrow examination is not usually required for diagnosis but shows severe erythroid hypoplasia initially; subsequently, erythroid hyperplasia develops along with reticulocytosis, and the anemia resolves.

Differential Diagnosis

Transient erythroblastopenia of childhood must be differentiated from Diamond-Blackfan anemia, particularly in infants younger than 1 year. In contrast to Diamond-Blackfan anemia, transient erythroblastopenia is not associated with macrocytosis, short stature, or congenital anomalies, or with evidence of fetal erythropoiesis prior to the phase of recovery. Transient erythroblastopenia is associated with normal levels of red cell adenosine deaminase, whereas adenosine deaminase levels are increased in Diamond-Blackfan anemia.

Other differential diagnoses include chronic disorders associated with decreased red cell production, such as renal failure, hypothyroidism, and other chronic states of infection or inflammation. As with other single cytopenias, the possibility of malignancy (ie, leukemia) should always be considered, particularly if fever, bone pain, hepatosplenomegaly, or lymphadenopathy is present. In such cases, examination of the bone marrow is generally diagnostic. Confusion may sometimes arise when the anemia of transient erythroblastopenia is first identified during the early phase of recovery when the reticulocyte count is high. In such cases, the disorder may be confused with the anemia of acute blood loss or with hemolytic disease. In contrast to hemolytic disorders, transient erythroblastopenia of childhood is not associated with jaundice or peripheral destruction of red cells.

▶ Treatment & Prognosis

By definition, this is a transient disorder. Some children require red cell transfusions if cardiovascular compromise is present. Resolution of the anemia is heralded by an increase in the reticulocyte count, which generally occurs within 4–8 weeks of diagnosis. Transient erythroblastopenia of childhood is not treated with corticosteroids because of its short course.

NUTRITIONAL ANEMIAS

B. Iron Deficiency Anemia

ESSENTIALS OF DIAGNOSIS & TYPICAL FEATURES

▶ Pallor and fatigue.

▶ Poor dietary intake of iron (especially ages 6–24 months).

▶ Chronic blood loss (especially adolescent females).

▶ Microcytic hypochromic anemia.

▶ General Considerations

Iron deficiency (ID) and iron deficiency anemia (IDA) are a worldwide concern. ID is defined as a state in which there is insufficient iron to maintain normal physiologic functions such that iron stores (serum ferritin or bone marrow iron content) are reduced. IDA is defined as a hemoglobin more than two standard deviations below normal for age and gender, which has developed as a consequence of ID.

Normal-term infants are born with sufficient iron stores to prevent ID for the first 4 months of life, whereas premature infants have reduced iron stores since iron is predominantly acquired in the last trimester. Thus, premature infants, as well as those with low birth weight, neonatal anemia, perinatal blood loss, or subsequent hemorrhage may have reduced iron stores. Breast milk is low in iron relative to cow's milk and fortified formulas, and without iron supplementation ID may develop in exclusively breast-fed children. Therefore, such children should receive 1 mg/kg/day of supplemental iron until 6 months of age when greater than one-half of intake is presumed to be iron-rich foods.

▶ Clinical Findings

A. Symptoms and Signs

Symptoms and signs vary with the severity of the deficiency. ID is usually asymptomatic. IDA may be associated with, pallor, fatigue, and irritability. A history of pica is common. It is controversial whether ID/IDA adversely affects long-term neurodevelopment and behavior. IDA is associated with increased lead absorption and subsequent neurotoxicity.

B. Laboratory Findings

According to the American Academy of Pediatrics (AAP) guidelines, screening for anemia should be performed at about 12 months of age with determination of hemoglobin concentration and an assessment of risk factors for ID/IDA. Risks include low socioeconomic status, prematurity or low birth weight, lead exposure, exclusive breast-feeding beyond 4 months of age without iron supplementation, weaning to whole milk or complementary foods that do not include iron, feeding problems, poor growth, and inadequate nutrition such as excessive milk intake. Classically, patients with ID have a microcytic anemia with decreased MCV, increased red cell distribution width, low serum ferritin and iron saturation, and increased total iron binding capacity. Laboratory values are usually interpreted holistically as a panel as no single measurement can determine iron status definitively.

▶ Differential Diagnosis

The differential diagnosis is that of microcytic, hypochromic anemia and includes thalassemia, lead toxicity, anemia of chronic inflammation, and sideroblastic anemias. One way to help differentiate IDA from thalassemia is evaluation of the Mentzer Index. The Mentzer Index is the ratio of the MCV to the RBC count. A Mentzer Index less than 13 is usually indicative of thalassemia. Additionally, the red cell distribution width is usually increased in patients with IDA and normal in patients with thalassemia trait.

Treatment

The AAP has published guidelines for routine iron intake for children. If a child has hemoglobin of 10–11 mg/dL at the 12-month screening visit, the child can be closely monitored or empirically treated with iron supplementation with a recheck of hemoglobin in 1 month. If a trial of therapeutic iron fails to correct the anemia and/or microcytosis, further evaluation is warranted with iron studies.

If a child is found to have ID/IDA, the recommended oral dose of elemental iron is 3 mg/kg/day for 3 months. Successful oral intake is preferred to avoid intravenous iron infusion or red cell transfusion. The dose for an adolescent is 65 mg/day. Absorption is augmented by concurrent vitamin C administration and inhibited by calcium-containing foods (eg, dairy), tea or coffee. Milk intake should be limited to 24 oz/day. Iron therapy results in an increased reticulocyte hemoglobin in 48 hours. The reticulocyte count will increase within 3–5 days and will be maximal between 5 and 7 days. The rate of hemoglobin rise is inversely related to the hemoglobin level at diagnosis and determined by whether the administered iron is in the ferrous or ferric state. Ferrous preparations are preferred. A rise in hemoglobin of 1 or more g/dL after 1 month of iron therapy indicates a good response. Treatment is continued for 3 months to replenish iron stores. If unresponsive, consider underlying cow's milk protein–induced colitis, inflammatory bowel disease, menorrhagia, or poor adherence. Parenteral iron is used as first-line treatment for children with chronic kidney disease and erythrocyte stimulants and may be indicated for those with celiac or inflammatory bowel disease. It can be considered for children not adherent or responsive to oral iron, but oral iron is preferred due to fewer potential complications and lower cost.

Mei Z et al: Physiologically based serum ferritin thresholds for iron deficiency in children and non-pregnant women: a US National Health and Nutrition Examination Surveys (NHANES) serial cross-sectional study. Lancet Haematol 2021;8:e572 [PMID: 34329578].

Parkin P et al: Association between serum ferritin and cognitive function in early childhood. J Pediatr 2020;217:189 [PMID: 31685227].

2. Megaloblastic Anemias

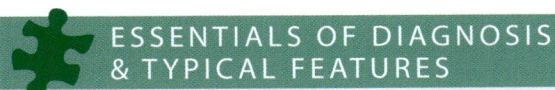

ESSENTIALS OF DIAGNOSIS & TYPICAL FEATURES

► Pallor and fatigue.

► Nutritional deficiency or intestinal malabsorption.

► Macrocytic anemia.

► Megaloblastic bone marrow changes.

General Considerations

Megaloblastic anemia occurs secondary to a disruption in DNA synthesis. It is a subset of macrocytic anemias and is characterized by large red cells with nuclear maturation arrest. Megaloblastic anemia can result from nutritional deficiencies (vitamin B_{12} or folate) or exposure to medications that interfere with DNA synthesis (eg, chemotherapeutics).

Vitamin B12 deficiency due to dietary insufficiency may occur in infants breast-fed by vegan mothers, or in children fed diets with little to no animal source foods. Intestinal malabsorption is the usual cause of vitamin B_{12} deficiency in children and occurs with Crohn disease, chronic pancreatitis, bacterial overgrowth of the small bowel, infection with the fish tapeworm (*Diphyllobothrium latum*), or after surgical resection of the terminal ileum. Deficiencies due to inborn errors of metabolism (transcobalamin II deficiency and methylmalonic aciduria) also have been described. Malabsorption of vitamin B_{12} due to deficiency of intrinsic factor (pernicious anemia) is rare in childhood.

Folate deficiency may be caused by inadequate dietary intake, malabsorption, increased folate requirements, or some combination of the three. Folate deficiency due to dietary deficiency alone is rare but occurs in severely malnourished infants and has been reported in infants fed with goat's milk not fortified with folate. Folate is absorbed in the jejunum, and deficiencies are encountered in malabsorptive syndromes such as celiac disease. Anticonvulsion medications (eg, phenytoin and phenobarbital) and cytotoxic drugs (eg, methotrexate) can also cause folate deficiency by interfering with folate absorption or metabolism. Finally, folate deficiency is more likely to develop in infants and children with increased requirements. This occurs during infancy because of rapid growth and in children with chronic hemolytic anemia. Premature infants are particularly susceptible to the development of the deficiency because of low body stores of folate.

Clinical Findings

A. Symptoms and Signs

Infants with megaloblastic anemia may show pallor and mild jaundice as a result of ineffective erythropoiesis. Classically, the tongue is smooth and beefy red. Infants with vitamin B_{12} deficiency may be irritable and poor feeders. Older children with vitamin B_{12} deficiency may complain of paresthesias, weakness, or an unsteady gait, and may show decreased vibratory sensation and proprioception on neurologic examination.

B. Laboratory Findings

The laboratory findings of megaloblastic anemia include an elevated MCV and mean corpuscular hemoglobin (MCH). The peripheral blood smear shows numerous macroovalocytes with anisocytosis and poikilocytosis. Neutrophils are large and have hypersegmented (more than five segments) nuclei. The white cell and platelet counts are normal with mild deficiencies but may be decreased in more severe cases. Examination of the bone marrow is not indicated, but typically shows erythroid hyperplasia with large erythroid and myeloid precursors. Nuclear maturation is delayed compared with cytoplasmic maturation. The serum indirect bilirubin concentration may be slightly elevated.

Children with vitamin B_{12} deficiency often, but not always, have a low serum vitamin B_{12} level. Decreased levels of serum vitamin B_{12} may also be found in about 30% of patients with folic acid deficiency. Normal vitamin B_{12} levels should not negate treatment if symptoms are present. The level of red cell folate is a better reflection of folate stores than is the serum folate level. Elevated serum levels of metabolic intermediates (methylmalonic acid and homocysteine) may have increased sensitivity than serum vitamin measurements. Elevated methylmalonic acid levels are consistent with vitamin B_{12} deficiency and generally decrease with treatment, whereas elevated levels of homocysteine occur with both vitamin B_{12} and folate deficiency as well as hypothyroidism.

▶ Differential Diagnosis

Most macrocytic anemias in pediatrics are not megaloblastic. Other causes of increased MCV include drug therapy (eg, anticonvulsants, anti-HIV nucleoside analogues), Down syndrome, an elevated reticulocyte count (hemolytic anemias), bone marrow failure syndromes (Fanconi anemia, Diamond-Blackfan anemia), liver disease, and hypothyroidism.

▶ Treatment

Treatment of vitamin B_{12} deficiency due to inadequate dietary intake is readily accomplished with high-dose oral supplementation that is as effective as parenteral treatment if absorption is normal. Folate deficiency is treated effectively with oral folic acid in most cases. Children at risk for the development of folic acid deficiencies, such as premature infants and those with chronic hemolysis, are often prescribed folic acid prophylactically.

Obeid R, Heil SG, Verhoeven MA, van den Heuvel EGHM, de Groot LCPGM, Eussen JPM: Vitamin B_{12} intake from animal foods, biomarkers, and health aspects. Front Nutr 2019;6:93. https://doi.org/:10.3389/fnut.2019.00093 [PMID: 31316992].

ANEMIA OF CHRONIC DISEASE

Anemia is a common manifestation of many chronic illnesses in children. In some instances, causes may be mixed. For example, children with chronic disorders involving intestinal malabsorption or blood loss may have anemia of chronic inflammation in combination with nutritional deficiencies of iron, folate, or vitamin B_{12}. In other settings, anemia is due to dysfunction of a single organ (eg, renal failure, hypothyroidism), and correction of the underlying abnormality resolves the anemia.

1. Anemia of Chronic Inflammation

Anemia is frequently associated with chronic infections or inflammatory diseases. The anemia is usually mild to moderate in severity, with a hemoglobin level of 8–12 g/dL. In general, the severity of the anemia corresponds to the severity of the underlying disorder, and there may be microcytosis, but not hypochromia. The reticulocyte count is inappropriately low. The anemia is thought to be due to inflammatory cytokines that inhibit erythropoiesis, and shunting of iron into, and impaired iron release from, reticuloendothelial cells. High levels of hepcidin, a peptide produced in the liver during infection or inflammation, reduce iron absorption by the duodenum and release from macrophages. Levels of erythropoietin are relatively low for the severity of the anemia. The serum iron concentration is low, but in contrast to ID, anemia of chronic inflammation is associated with an elevated serum ferritin level and not with an elevated iron-binding capacity. Serum inflammatory markers (erythrocyte sedimentation rate [ESR], C-reactive protein [CRP]) may be elevated. Treatment consists of correction of the underlying disorder, which, if controlled, generally results in improvement in hemoglobin level.

2. Anemia of Chronic Renal Failure

Severe normocytic anemia occurs in most forms of renal disease that have progressed to renal insufficiency. Although white cell and platelet production remain normal, the bone marrow shows significant hypoplasia of the erythroid series, and the reticulocyte count is low. The principal mechanism is deficiency of erythropoietin, a hormone produced in the kidney, but other factors may contribute to the anemia. Erythropoiesis-stimulating drugs and iron correct the anemia, largely eliminating the need for red cell transfusion.

3. Anemia of Hypothyroidism

Some patients with hypothyroidism develop significant anemia. Occasionally, anemia is detected before the diagnosis of the underlying disorder. A decreased growth velocity in an anemic child suggests hypothyroidism. The anemia is usually normocytic or macrocytic, but it is not megaloblastic, and hence not due to deficiencies of vitamin B_{12} or folate. Replacement therapy with thyroid hormone is usually effective in correcting the anemia.

Weiss G, Ganz T, Goodnugh LT: Anemia of inflammation. Blood 2019;133:40–50 [PMID: 6536698].

CONGENITAL HEMOLYTIC ANEMIAS: RED CELL MEMBRANE DEFECTS

The congenital hemolytic anemias are divided into three categories: defects of the red cell membrane, hemoglobinopathies, and disorders of red cell metabolism. Red cell membrane defects are secondary to mutations in genes that encode for cytoskeleton proteins, or transmembrane transporters and channels. Hereditary spherocytosis and elliptocytosis are the most common red cell membrane disorders. Abnormal red cell morphology (eg, spherocytes, elliptocytes) on peripheral blood smear may suggest the diagnosis. These disorders often, but not always, have an autosomal dominant inheritance, and family history is often suggestive. The hemolysis is due to the deleterious effect of the membrane abnormality on red cell deformability. Decreased cell deformability leads to entrapment of the abnormally shaped red cells in the spleen.

1. Hereditary Spherocytosis

ESSENTIALS OF DIAGNOSIS & TYPICAL FEATURES

▶ Anemia and jaundice

▶ Splenomegaly.

▶ Positive family history of anemia, jaundice, or gallstones in 75%.

▶ Spherocytosis with increased reticulocytes.

▶ Increased osmotic fragility.

▶ Negative DAT.

▶ General Considerations

Hereditary spherocytosis is the most common membrane disorder and the most common hereditary hemolytic anemia in people of Northern European background but occurs in all populations. The disorder is marked by mild to severe hemolysis, and potential splenomegaly, due to the inadequate vertical linkages between the cytoskeleton and lipid bilayer of the red cell membrane. In most persons, the disorder is mild to moderate because increased reticulocytosis partially compensates for hemolysis. The hallmark of hereditary spherocytosis is the presence of microspherocytes in the peripheral blood.

Hereditary spherocytosis is secondary to alteration of genes encoding for spectrin, band 3, ankyrin, or protein 4.2 of the red cell membrane; spectrin abnormalities are more often diagnosed in childhood and band 3 in adulthood. The vertical linkages in the membrane are impaired so that spherocytes form. These are poorly deformable, resulting in a shortened lifespan because they are trapped in the microcirculation of the spleen and engulfed by splenic macrophages.

▶ Clinical Findings

A. Symptoms and Signs

Extravascular hemolysis causes significant neonatal unconjugated hyperbilirubinemia. Splenomegaly develops in the majority and is often present by age 5 years. Jaundice is variably present and, in many patients, may be noted only during infection. Patients with significant chronic anemia may complain of pallor, fatigue, or malaise. Intermittent exacerbations of the anemia are caused by increased hemolysis, splenic sequestration, or aplastic crises, and may be associated with severe weakness, fatigue, fever, abdominal pain, or even heart failure.

B. Laboratory Findings

Most patients have mild chronic hemolysis with hemoglobin levels of 9–12 g/dL. In some cases, the hemolysis is fully compensated, and the hemoglobin level is in the normal range. Rare cases of severe disease require frequent transfusions. The anemia is usually normocytic and hyperchromic, and many patients have an elevated MCHC and RDW. The peripheral blood smear shows numerous microspherocytes and polychromasia. The reticulocyte count is elevated, often higher than might be expected for the degree of anemia. WBC and platelet counts are usually normal. Serum bilirubin usually shows an elevation in the unconjugated fraction. The DAT is negative. The osmotic fragility is increased, particularly after incubation at 37°C for 24 hours and confirms the diagnosis.

▶ Differential Diagnosis

Spherocytes are frequently present in persons with immune hemolysis. Thus, in the newborn, hereditary spherocytosis must be distinguished from hemolytic disease caused by ABO or other blood type incompatibilities. Older patients with autoimmune hemolytic anemia (AIHA) frequently present with jaundice, splenomegaly, and spherocytes on the peripheral blood smear. The DAT is positive in most cases of immune hemolysis and negative in hereditary spherocytosis. Occasionally, the diagnosis is confused in patients with splenomegaly from other causes, especially when hypersplenism increases red cell destruction and when some spherocytes are noted on the blood smear. In such cases, the true cause of the splenomegaly may be suggested by signs or symptoms of portal hypertension or by laboratory evidence of chronic liver disease. In contrast to children with hereditary spherocytosis, those with hypersplenism typically have some degree of thrombocytopenia or neutropenia.

▶ Complications

Severe jaundice may occur in the neonatal period and result in kernicterus if not controlled by phototherapy or exchange transfusion. Gallstones occur in 60%–70% of adults who have not undergone splenectomy and may form as early as age 5–10 years. Intermittent or persistent splenomegaly occurs in 10%–25% of patients.

► Treatment

Supportive measures include the administration of folic acid due to increased folate requirements due to red cell turnover. Acute hemolytic or aplastic crises caused by infection, often with human parvovirus, may be severe enough to require red cell transfusions. Laparoscopic splenectomy, if possible, may be indicated depending on clinical severity. Splenectomy increases survival of the red cells and results in complete correction of the hemolytic anemia in most cases. Except in unusually severe cases, the procedure should be postponed until the child is at least age 5 years because of the greater risk of postsplenectomy sepsis prior to this age (see section Splenectomy).

► Prognosis

Splenectomy eliminates signs and symptoms in all but the most severe cases. The abnormal red cell morphology and increased osmotic fragility persist without clinical consequence. Subtotal splenectomy (80%–90%) can be considered for children younger than 5 years, accepting that 50% will require subsequent surgery.

2. Hereditary Elliptocytosis

Hereditary elliptocytosis is a heterogeneous disorder that ranges in severity from an asymptomatic state with almost normal red cell morphology to about 10% having moderate to severe hemolytic anemia. It is hypothesized that this disorder improves survival from malaria. Most affected persons have numerous elliptocytes on the peripheral blood smear, but mild or no hemolysis. Those with hemolysis have an elevated reticulocyte count and may have jaundice and splenomegaly. This disorder is caused by weakened horizontal linkages in the red cell membrane skeleton due to either a defective spectrin dimer-dimer interaction or a defective spectrin-actin protein 4.1R junctional complex. Inheritance is autosomal dominant. Most patients are asymptomatic, no treatment is indicated. Patients with significant degrees of hemolytic anemia may benefit from folate supplementation or splenectomy but some degree of hemolysis persists postsplenectomy.

Some infants with hereditary elliptocytosis present in the neonatal period with moderate to marked hemolysis and significant hyperbilirubinemia. This disorder has been termed transient infantile pyknocytosis because such infants exhibit bizarre erythrocyte morphology with elliptocytes, microspherocytes, and red cell fragments. The MCV is low, and the anemia may be severe enough to require red cell transfusions. Typically, one parent has hereditary elliptocytosis, usually mild or asymptomatic. The infant's hemolysis gradually abates during the first year of life, and the erythrocyte morphology subsequently becomes more typical of hereditary elliptocytosis.

Lee GM: Preventing infections in children and adults with asplenia. Hematology Am Soc Hematol Educ Program 2020(1):328–335. doi: https://doi.org/10.1182/hematology.2020000117 [PMID: 33275684].

Risinger M, Kalfa TA: Red cell membrane disorders: structure meets function. Blood 2020;136:1250–6121. doi: https://DOI.ORG/10.1182/BLOOD.2019000946 [PMID: 32702754].

CONGENITAL HEMOLYTIC ANEMIAS: HEMOGLOBINOPATHIES

The hemoglobinopathies are an extremely heterogeneous group of congenital disorders that occur in all ethnic groups. The relatively high frequency of these genetic variants is related to the malaria protection afforded to heterozygous individuals. The hemoglobinopathies are generally classified into two major groups. The first, thalassemias, are due to imbalance between the α and β-globin chains that comprise hemoglobin. Defects in globin chain synthesis cause microcytic and hypochromic anemias. The second group of hemoglobinopathies consists of those caused by structural abnormalities of globin chains. The most important of these, hemoglobins S, C, and E, are all the result of point mutations and single amino acid substitutions in β-globin. Many, but not all, infants with hemoglobinopathies are identified by neonatal screening.

Figure 30–3 shows the normal developmental changes that occur in globin-chain production during gestation and the first year of life. At birth, the predominant hemoglobin is fetal (hemoglobin F), which is composed of two α-globin chains and two γ-globin chains. Subsequently, the production of γ-globin decreases, and β-globin increases so that adult hemoglobin (two α- and two β-globin chains) predominates after 2–4 months of age. Because α-globin chains are present in both fetal and adult hemoglobin, disorders of α-globin synthesis (α-thalassemia) are clinically manifest in the newborn as well as later in life. In contrast, patients with β-globin disorders such as β-thalassemia and sickle cell disease are generally asymptomatic during the first 3–4 months.

1. α-Thalassemia

ESSENTIALS OF DIAGNOSIS & TYPICAL FEATURES

► Predominately African, Mediterranean, Middle Eastern, Chinese, or Southeast Asian ancestry.

► Microcytic, hypochromic anemia of variable severity.

► Bart's hemoglobin (γ_4) detected on neonatal screening.

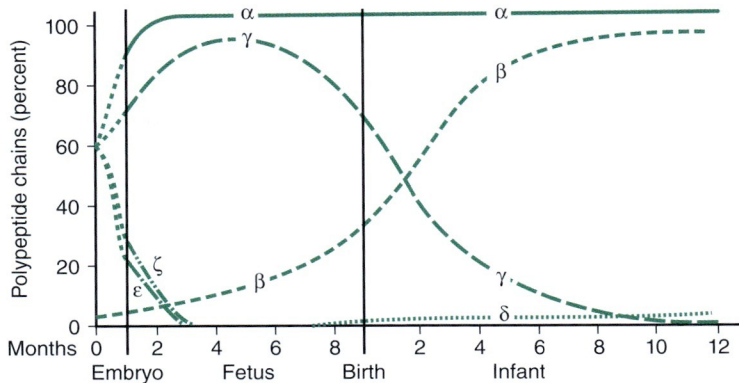

▲ **Figure 30–3.** Changes in hemoglobin polypeptide chains during human development. (Reproduced with permission from Miller DR, Baehner RL: *Blood Diseases of Infancy and Childhood.* 6th ed. Philadelphia, PA: Mosby; 1989.)

▶ General Considerations

Most of the α-thalassemia syndromes are the result of deletions of one or more of the four α-globin genes, a pair of two closely linked genes on each chromosome 16, although nondeletional mutations also occur. Excess non–α-globin chains damage the red cell membrane, causing ineffective erythropoiesis in the bone marrow and extravascular hemolysis. The variable severity of the α-thalassemia syndromes is generally related to the number of gene deletions (Table 30–1). The severity of the α-thalassemia syndromes varies among affected ethnic groups depending on whether the deletions are cis (α-thalassemia-1) or trans (α-thalassemia-2). In persons of African ancestry, α-thalassemia-2 is usually found; thus, in the African population, hemoglobin H disease and fetal hydrops do not occur. In contrast, Asians tend to have cis mutations (α-thalassemia-1) and Hemoglobin H and hydrops fetalis are more common.

▶ Clinical Findings

The clinical findings depend on the number of α-globin genes deleted. Table 30–1 summarizes the α-thalassemia syndromes. In general, the more affected genes, the more severe the phenotype. Persons with one α-globin gene deletion are silent carriers and are asymptomatic and have no hematologic abnormalities.

Persons with two α-globin gene deletions or α-thalassemia trait are typically asymptomatic. The MCV is usually less than 100 fL at birth. Hematologic studies in older infants and children show a normal or slightly decreased hemoglobin and elevated red cell count with a low MCV and a slightly hypochromic blood smear with some target cells. The hemoglobin electrophoresis at birth shows elevated Bart's hemoglobin (tetramer of gamma globin chains) but is normal later in life as γ-globin production falls dramatically after birth.

Persons with three α-gene deletions have hemoglobin H disease, a mild to moderately severe microcytic hemolytic anemia (hemoglobin level of 7–10 g/dL), and may develop

Table 30–1. The α-thalassemias.

Usual Genotypes[a]	α–Gene Deletions	Clinical Features	Hemoglobin Electrophoresis[b]	
			Birth	**>6 mo**
αα/αα	0	Normal	N	N
–α/αα	1	Silent carrier	0%–3% Hb Bart's	N
–/αα or –α/–α	2	α-Thal trait/minor	2%–10% Hb Bart's[c]	N
–/–α	3	Hb H disease	15%–30% Hb Bart's	Hb; H present
–/–	4	Fetal hydrops	> 75% Hb Bart's	–

[a]α indicates presence of α-globin gene; –α indicates deletion of α-globin gene.
[b]N = normal results, Hb = hemoglobin, Hb Bart's = γ_4, Hb H = β_4.
[c]The level of Hb Bart's does not directly correlate with the number of deleted α genes.

hepatosplenomegaly, pulmonary hypertension, leg ulcers, hemolytic episodes, and bony abnormalities caused by the expanded medullary space. The reticulocyte count is elevated, and the red cells show marked hypochromia and microcytosis with significant poikilocytosis and some basophilic stippling. Incubation of red cells with brilliant cresyl blue shows inclusion bodies formed by denatured hemoglobin H (β_4).

The deletion of all four α-globin genes causes severe intrauterine anemia and without intrauterine transfusions or stem cell transplant results in hydrops fetalis and fetal demise or neonatal death shortly after delivery. Extreme pallor and massive hepatosplenomegaly are present. With intrauterine transfusions and sophisticated prenatal support, there are a few transfusion-dependent survivors. Molecular analysis can be useful in diagnosis of the deletional and nondeletional α-thalassemias.

▶ Differential Diagnosis

α-Thalassemia trait (two-gene deletion) must be differentiated from other mild microcytic anemias, including IDA and β-thalassemia (see the next section). In contrast to children with ID, children with α-thalassemia trait have elevated red cell counts and normal or increased levels of ferritin and serum iron. In contrast to children with β-thalassemia, children with α-thalassemia trait have a normal hemoglobin electrophoresis after age 4–6 months and may have small amounts of Barts hemoglobin detected on newborn screen.

Children with hemoglobin H disease may have jaundice and splenomegaly, and the disorder must be differentiated from other hemolytic anemias. The key to the diagnosis is the decreased MCV and the marked hypochromia on the blood smear. With the exception of β-thalassemia, most other significant hemolytic disorders have a normal or elevated MCV and the RBCs are not hypochromic. Infants with hydrops fetalis due to severe α-thalassemia must be distinguished from those with hydrops due to other causes of anemia, such as alloimmunization or parvovirus.

▶ Complications

The principal complication of α-thalassemia trait is the needless administration of iron, given in the belief that a mild microcytic anemia is due to ID. Persons with hemoglobin H disease may have intermittent exacerbations of their anemia in response to oxidant stress or infection, which occasionally require blood transfusions. Splenomegaly may exacerbate the anemia. Women pregnant with hydropic α-thalassemia fetuses are subject to increased complications of pregnancy, particularly toxemia and postpartum hemorrhage.

▶ Treatment

Silent carriers and persons with α-thalassemia trait require no treatment. Those with hemoglobin H disease should receive supplemental folic acid and avoid the same oxidant drugs that cause hemolysis in persons with G6PD deficiency, as exposure to these drugs may exacerbate their anemia. The anemia may also be exacerbated during periods of infection and necessitate red cell transfusion. Hemoglobin H disease inherited with nondeletional mutations may be transfusion-dependent. Iron overload may occur independent of whether transfusions are given or not. Hypersplenism may develop later in childhood. Genetic counseling and prenatal diagnosis should be considered for all affected families.

Lal A, Vichinsky E: The clinical phenotypes of alpha thalassemia. Hematol Oncol Clin North Am 2023;37(2):327–339 [PMID: 36907606].

2. β-Thalassemia

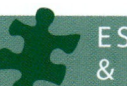

ESSENTIALS OF DIAGNOSIS & TYPICAL FEATURES

Non-transfusion dependent
- ▶ Normal neonatal screening test.
- ▶ Predominantly African, Mediterranean, Middle Eastern, or Asian ancestry.
- ▶ Mild to moderate microcytic, hypochromic anemia.
- ▶ Elevated level of hemoglobin F or A_2.

Transfusion-dependent
- ▶ Usually Mediterranean, Middle Eastern, or Asian ancestry.
- ▶ Generally homozygous or compound heterozygous for β-globin mutations that reduce hemoglobin A production to life-threatening levels or interfere with quality of life.
- ▶ Severe microcytic, hypochromic anemia.
- ▶ Marked hepatosplenomegaly, bony changes, and cardiac failure without chronic transfusion.

▶ General Considerations

Two β-globin genes are present, one on each chromosome 11. Excess non–β-globin chains damage the red cells, causing ineffective erythropoiesis and hemolysis. β-Thalassemias are complex since the mutations causing β-thalassemia are myriad, and the phenotype is not always predicted by the mutations. Thalassemias can be classified as transfusion-dependent or non-transfusion-dependent. Those with transfusion-dependent thalassemia require permanent or time-limited chronic transfusions to treat and prevent symptomatic anemia and suppress extramedullary hemato-poiesis and its complications. β-Thalassemia gene mutations may also interact with genes for structural β-globin variants, such as hemoglobin S and hemoglobin E to cause serious disease in compound heterozygous individuals. These disorders are discussed further in the sections dealing with sickle cell disease and hemoglobin E disorders.

▶ Clinical Findings

A. Symptoms and Signs

Persons with non–transfusion-dependent β-thalassemia may be asymptomatic with a normal physical examination or have mild-moderate anemia managed without transfusions. Persons with transfusion-dependent β-thalassemia are generally normal at birth but develop significant anemia during the first year of life. If the disorder is not identified and treated with blood transfusions, affected children grow poorly, develop massive hepatosplenomegaly and enlargement of the medullary space with thinning of the bony cortex, and may die of cardiac failure due to severe anemia. The skeletal changes (due to ineffective erythropoiesis and marrow hyperplasia) cause characteristic facial deformities (prominent forehead and maxilla) and predispose the child to pathologic fractures. Some children may only temporarily require blood transfusions and some adults may become transfusion-dependent later in life.

B. Laboratory Findings

Children with non–transfusion-dependent β-thalassemia have normal neonatal screening results but subsequently develop a decreased MCV with or without anemia of variable severity. The peripheral blood smear typically shows hypochromia, target cells, and sometimes basophilic stippling. Hemoglobin electrophoresis performed after 6–12 months of age is usually diagnostic when levels of hemoglobin A_2, hemoglobin F, or both are elevated. Transfusion-dependent β-thalassemia is suspected when hemoglobin A is absent on neonatal screening. Such infants are hematologically normal at birth, but they develop severe anemia after the first few months of life and become transfusion-dependent. The peripheral blood smear typically shows a severe hypochromic, microcytic anemia with marked anisocytosis and poikilocytosis. Target cells are prominent, and nucleated RBCs often exceed the number of circulating WBCs. The hemoglobin level usually falls to 5–6 g/dL or less, and the reticulocyte count is elevated. Platelet and WBC counts may be increased, and the serum unconjugated bilirubin level is elevated. Sixty-four to 89% of individuals with two β-thalassemia mutations are transfusion-dependent. α-Thalassemia deletions and mutations may occur with β-thalassemia mutations, thereby further complicating manifestations.

▶ Differential Diagnosis

Mild non–transfusion-dependent β-thalassemia must be differentiated from other causes of mild microcytic, hypochromic anemias, principally ID and α-thalassemia. In contrast to patients with IDA, those with mild non–transfusion-dependent β-thalassemia typically a decreased Mentzer Index less than 13. Generally, an elevated hemoglobin A_2 level is diagnostic; occasionally, the A_2 level may be lowered by coexistent ID.

Transfusion-dependent β-thalassemia is rarely confused with other disorders. Hemoglobin electrophoresis, DNA analysis and family studies readily distinguish it from hemoglobin E/β-thalassemia, which is the other increasingly important cause of transfusion-dependent thalassemia.

▶ Complications

The principal complication of non–transfusion-dependent β-thalassemia is the unnecessary use of iron therapy in a futile attempt to correct the microcytic anemia. Children with transfusion-dependent β-thalassemia who are inadequately transfused experience poor growth and recurrent infections and may have hepatosplenomegaly, thinning of the cortical bone, and pathologic fractures. Without red cell transfusions most children die within the first decade of life. The principal complication of transfusion-dependent β-thalassemia in nonchelated transfused children is hemosiderosis. Transfusion-related hemosiderosis requires chelation therapy to minimize cardiac, hepatic, and endocrine dysfunction. Nonadherence with chelation is associated with death from congestive heart failure, cardiac arrhythmias, or hepatic failure. Even with adequate transfusions, many patients develop splenomegaly and some degree of hypersplenism. Splenectomy increases the risk of thrombosis, pulmonary hypertension, and overwhelming sepsis.

▶ Treatment

Non–transfusion-dependent individuals may benefit from supplemental folic acid. Persons with transfusion-dependent β-thalassemia require transfusions temporarily or chronically. Red cell transfusion is generally targeted to maintain a nadir hemoglobin level of 9.5–10.5 g/dL. This approach increases well-being and growth, and fewer complications ensue. Maintenance of good health requires iron chelation. Small doses of supplemental ascorbic acid may enhance the efficacy of iron chelation. For the population with significant hemolysis and anemia who are clinically stable, close follow-up is indicated since they can become transfusion-dependent. The decision to initiate transfusions is dependent on symptoms and especially signs of anemia. Other indications are failure to thrive, especially in height, and development of splenomegaly or bone deformities.

The erythroid maturing agent, luspatercept has been approved for adult patients and has been shown to decrease annual transfused blood volumes in a subset of thalassemia patients.

Hematopoietic stem cell transplant is a curative therapeutic option for children who are transfusion-dependent if there is a matched related donor. Autologous gene therapy was recently approved in the United States using lentiviral insertion of an alternative beta globin gene with a T87Q amino acid substitution. Clinical trials of competing gene editing strategies have also shown promise in increasing hemoglobin concentration through fetal hemoglobin induction and inhibition of the gamma globin repressor BCL11a.

Frangoul H et al: CRISPR-Cas9 gene editing for sickle cell disease and beta thalassemia. New Engl J Med 2021;384(3):252–260 [PMID: 33283989].

Taher A et al: Beta thalassemias. New Engl J Med 2021;384(8): 727–743 [PMID: 33626255].

3. Sickle Cell Disease

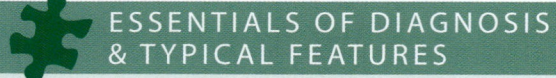

ESSENTIALS OF DIAGNOSIS & TYPICAL FEATURES

▶ Neonatal screening test usually with hemoglobins FS, FSC, or FSA (S > A).

▶ Predominantly African, Mediterranean, Middle Eastern, Indian, or Caribbean ancestry.

▶ Anemia, elevated reticulocyte count, usually jaundice.

▶ Recurrent episodes of musculoskeletal or abdominal pain.

▶ Often hepatomegaly and splenomegaly that resolves.

▶ Increased risk of bacterial sepsis.

▶ General Considerations

Sickle cell disease encompasses a family of disorders with manifestations secondary to the propensity of deoxygenated sickle hemoglobin (S) to polymerize. Sickle hemoglobin is a consequence of a change in the sixth chain of the β-globin whereby valine is substituted for glutamic acid. Polymerization of sickle hemoglobin distorts erythrocyte morphology; decreases red cell deformability; causes hemolysis and a marked reduction in red cell lifespan; increases blood viscosity; and predisposes to inflammation, coagulation activation, and episodes of vaso-occlusion. Sickle cell anemia, the most severe sickling disorder, is caused by homozygosity for

the sickle gene and is the most common form of sickle cell disease. Other clinically important sickling disorders are compound heterozygous conditions in which the sickle gene interacts with genes for hemoglobins C, E, D_{Punjab}, O_{Arab}, C_{Harlem}, or β-thalassemia.

Overall, sickle cell disease occurs in about 1 of every 400 African-American and 1 of every 1200 Hispanic-American infants. Eight percent of African Americans are heterozygous carriers of the sickle gene and thus have sickle cell trait.

▶ Clinical Findings

A. Symptoms and Signs

These are related to the hemolytic anemia, tissue ischemia, and organ dysfunction caused by vaso-occlusion. They are most severe in children with sickle cell (SS) anemia or sickle $β^0$-thalassemia. Physical findings are normal at birth, and symptoms are unusual before age 3–4 months because high levels of fetal hemoglobin inhibit sickling. A moderately severe hemolytic anemia may be present by age 1 year. This causes pallor, fatigue, and jaundice, and predisposes to the development of gallstones during childhood and adolescence. Intense congestion of the spleen with sickled cells may cause splenomegaly but usually results in functional asplenia as early as age 3 months in sickle cell anemia. This places children at great risk for overwhelming infection with encapsulated bacteria, particularly pneumococci. Up to 30% of patients experience one or more episodes of acute splenic sequestration, characterized by sudden enlargement of the spleen with pooling of red cells, acute exacerbation of anemia with a drop in hemoglobin by at least 2 g/dL, and, in severe cases, shock and death. Acute exacerbation of anemia also occurs with aplastic crises, usually caused by infection with human parvovirus B19 and other viruses.

Recurrent episodes of vaso-occlusion and tissue ischemia cause acute and chronic morbidity. Dactylitis, or hand-and-foot syndrome, which is the most common initial symptom of the disease, occurs in up to 50% of children with sickle cell anemia, not treated with hydroxyurea, before age 3 years. Recurrent episodes of abdominal and musculoskeletal pain may occur throughout life. Historically, overt strokes occurred in about 11% of children with sickle cell anemia and without chronic transfusion tended to be recurrent; recurrence is significantly reduced with chronic red cell transfusions. The acute chest syndrome, characterized by respiratory symptoms and a new acute pulmonary infiltrate, is caused by pulmonary infection, infarction, or fat embolism from ischemic bone marrow. All tissues are susceptible to damage from vaso-occlusion. Multiple organ dysfunction is common by adulthood in those with sickle cell anemia or sickle $β^0$-thalassemia. The common manifestations of sickle cell disease are listed in Table 30–2. Manifestations are generally less frequent in those with SC and S $β^+$-thalassemia.

Table 30–2. Common clinical manifestations of sickle cell disease.

	Acute	Chronic
Children	Bacterial sepsis or meningitis Splenic sequestration Aplastic crisis Vaso-occlusive events Dactylitis Bone infarction Acute chest syndrome Stroke Priapism	Functional asplenia Delayed growth and development Avascular necrosis of the hip Hyposthenuria Cholelithiasis
Adults	Bacterial sepsis[a] Aplastic crisis Vaso-occlusive events Bone infarction Acute chest syndrome Stroke Priapism Acute multiorgan failure syndrome	Leg ulcers Proliferative retinopathy Avascular necrosis of the hip Cholecystitis Chronic organ failure Liver Lung Kidney Decreased fertility

[a]Associated with significant mortality rate.

B. Laboratory Findings

Children with SS or Sβ⁰-thalassemia generally show a baseline hemoglobin level of 7–10 g/dL. The baseline reticulocyte count is elevated. The anemia is usually normocytic or macrocytic, and the peripheral blood smear typically shows the characteristic sickle cells as well as numerous target cells. Patients with sickle β-thalassemia have a low MCV and hypochromia. Those with sickle β⁺-thalassemia tend to have less hemolysis and anemia. Persons with sickle hemoglobin C disease have fewer sickle forms and more target cells, and the hemoglobin level may be normal or only slightly decreased because the rate of hemolysis is much less than in sickle cell anemia.

Most infants with sickle hemoglobinopathies born in the United States are identified by universal neonatal screening. Results indicative of possible sickle cell disease require prompt confirmation. Children with sickle cell anemia and with sickle β⁰-thalassemia have only hemoglobins S, F, and A₂. Persons with sickle β⁺-thalassemia have a preponderance of hemoglobin S with a lesser amount of hemoglobin A and elevated A₂. Persons with sickle hemoglobin C disease have about equal amounts of hemoglobins S and C although the quantity of S is greater than the C. The use of solubility tests to screen for the presence of sickle hemoglobin should be avoided because a positive result does not differentiate sickle cell trait from sickle cell disease. Solubility tests will not identify hemoglobin variants other than S. Hemoglobin

electrophoresis and HPLC and/or or DNA analysis is always necessary to accurately identify sickle cell disease.

▶ Differential Diagnosis

Hemoglobin electrophoresis and sometimes hematologic studies of the parents are generally sufficient to confirm sickle cell disease, although DNA testing is available. It is critical to determine whether the child with only F and S hemoglobins on newborn screening has sickle cell anemia, sickle β⁰-thalassemia, or is a compound heterozygote for sickle hemoglobin and pancellular hereditary persistence of fetal hemoglobin.

▶ Complications

Repeated tissue ischemia and infarction can cause damage to virtually every organ system. Table 30–2 lists the most significant complications. Patients who require frequent red cell transfusions are at risk of developing transfusion-related hemosiderosis and infections as well as red cell antibodies. Guidelines for routine evaluation for stroke risk with transcranial Doppler screening are available and if necessary red cell transfusion and possibly hydroxyurea has reduced the incidence of stroke. Silent infarct is a frequent complication occurring in up to 37% with severe disease by their teens.

▶ Treatment

The cornerstone of treatment is enrollment in a sickle cell program involving patient and family education, comprehensive outpatient care, and appropriate treatment of acute and chronic complications. Important to the success of such a program are psychosocial services, blood bank services, and the ready availability of baseline patient information in the setting in which acute illnesses are evaluated and treated.

Management of sickle cell anemia and sickle β⁰-thalassemia includes daily prophylactic penicillin, which should be initiated by age 2 months and continued to age 5 years. The routine use of penicillin prophylaxis in sickle hemoglobin C disease and sickle β⁺-thalassemia is controversial. Pneumococcal conjugate and polysaccharide vaccines should be administered to all children who have sickle cell disease. Other routine immunizations, including vaccination against *Haemophilus influenzae* and meningococcus, should be provided. All illnesses associated with fever greater than 38.5°C should be evaluated promptly, bacterial cultures performed, parenteral broad-spectrum antibiotics administered, and careful inpatient or outpatient observation conducted.

Treatment of painful vaso-occlusive episodes includes the maintenance of adequate hydration (with avoidance of overhydration), correction of acidosis if present, administration of adequate analgesia, maintenance of normal oxygen saturation, and the treatment of any associated infections.

Red cell transfusions play an important role in management. Transfusions are indicated to improve oxygen-carrying capacity during acute severe exacerbations of anemia, as occurs during episodes of splenic sequestration or aplastic crisis. Red cell transfusions are not indicated for the treatment of chronic steady-state anemia or for uncomplicated episodes of vaso-occlusive pain. Simple or partial exchange transfusion to reduce the percentage of circulating sickle cells is indicated for some acute events and may be lifesaving. These events include stroke, moderate to severe acute chest syndrome, and multiorgan failure. Transfusions administered prior to procedures or surgery that require general anesthesia reduce the risk of secondary complications. Some patients with severe complications may benefit from chronic transfusion therapy. The most common indications for transfusions are stroke or an abnormal transcranial Doppler assessment indicating an increased risk for stroke. Leukocyte-depleted red cells negative for C, E, and Kell antigens reduce the incidence of alloimmunization.

Successful hematopoietic stem cell transplant can cure sickle cell disease. Gene therapy is being evaluated as curative therapy. Daily administration of oral hydroxyurea increases levels of fetal hemoglobin, decreases hemolysis, and reduces the frequency of acute chest syndrome, hospitalization rates, and need for transfusions. The primary toxicity of hydroxyurea is neutropenia, so blood counts must be monitored regularly. Hydroxyurea is recommended for children and adolescents with sickle cell anemia and sickle β^0-thalassemia beginning at 9 months of age; efficacy in SC and β^+-thalassemia has not been formally studied. L-glutamine is also Food and Drug Administration (FDA) approved to reduce the frequency of vaso-occlusive events. There are two additional FDA-approved therapies: crizanlizumab and voxelotor. Crizanlizumab reduces the frequency of vaso-occlusive events. For most individuals, hemoglobin is raised by at least 1 g with voxelotor.

▶ Prognosis

Early identification by neonatal screening, combined with sickle cell comprehensive care that includes prescription of prophylactic penicillin, instruction on splenic palpation, and education on the need to urgently seek care when fever occurs, and routine screening for stroke risk, has markedly reduced morbidity and mortality in childhood. Most patients now live well into adulthood, with survival to 45–50 years, but eventually succumb to complications.

Brandow A et al: American Society of Hematology 2020 guidelines for sickle cell disease: management of acute and chronic pain. Blood Adv 2020;4(12):2656–2701 [PMID: 32559294].

Cisneros GS, Thein SL: Recent advances in the treatment of sickle cell disease. Front Physiol 2020;11:435. doi: https://doi.org/10.3389/fphys.2020.00435 [PMID: 32508672].

DeBaun M et al: American Society of Hematology 2020 guidelines for sickle cell disease: prevention, diagnosis, and treatment of cerebrovascular disease in children and adults. Blood Adv 2020;4(8):1554–1588 [PMID: 32298430].

Chou S et al: American Society of Hematology 2020 guidelines for sickle cell disease: transfusion support. Blood Adv 2020;4(2):327–355 [PMID: 31985807].

4. Sickle Cell Trait

Individuals who are heterozygous for the sickle gene have sickle cell trait; neonatal screening shows hemoglobin FAS (A > S). Adults typically have about 60% hemoglobin A and 40% hemoglobin S. No anemia or hemolysis is present, and the physical examination is normal. Persons with sickle cell trait are generally healthy with normal life expectancy despite a slight increased risk for pulmonary embolism, kidney disease, and exertional rhabdomyolysis.

However, sickle trait erythrocytes are capable of sickling, with acidemia and hypoxemia. Thus, the kidney may be affected with the most common manifestation of sickle trait being hyposthenuria. Transient painless hematuria, usually microscopic, affects about 4% of those with sickle trait and does not progress to significant renal dysfunction. Sickle cell trait is a risk factor for chronic kidney disease. Although renal medullary carcinoma is rare, the majority with this malignancy have sickle trait. The incidence of bacteriuria and pyelonephritis may be increased during pregnancy, but overall rates of maternal and infant morbidity and mortality are not affected by sickle cell trait.

Exertion at moderate altitudes rarely precipitates splenic infarction. In general, exercise tolerance seems to be normal; the incidence of sickle cell trait in black professional football players is similar to that of the general African-American population. The risk for exertional rhabdomyolysis is increased 1.5-fold.

There is no reason to restrict strenuous activity for individuals with sickle cell trait. As is true for all individuals performing strenuous activity, it is important to be conditioned, dress appropriately, have access to fluids, rest periodically, and perform moderate activity in extreme heat and humidity. Sickle cell trait is most significant for its genetic implications.

5. Hemoglobin C Disorders

Hemoglobin C can be detected by neonatal hemoglobinopathy screening. Two percent of African Americans are heterozygous for hemoglobin C and thus have hemoglobin C trait. They have no symptoms, anemia, or hemolysis, but the peripheral blood smear may show some target cells. Identification of persons with hemoglobin C trait is important for genetic counseling, particularly with regard to the possibility of sickle hemoglobin - C disease in offspring.

Persons with homozygous hemoglobin C have a mild microcytic hemolytic anemia and may develop splenomegaly.

The peripheral blood smear shows prominent target cells. As with other hemolytic anemias, potential complications of homozygous hemoglobin C include gallstones and aplastic crises.

6. Hemoglobin E Disorders

Hemoglobin E is the second most common hemoglobin variant worldwide, with a gene frequency up to 60% in northeast Thailand and Cambodia. Persons heterozygous for hemoglobin E show hemoglobin FAE by neonatal screening and are asymptomatic and usually not anemic, but they may have mild microcytosis. Individuals homozygous for hemoglobin E are also asymptomatic but may have mild anemia; the peripheral blood smear shows microcytosis and some target cells.

Compound heterozygotes for hemoglobin E and β^0-thalassemia are normal at birth and, like infants with homozygous E, show hemoglobin FE on neonatal screening. They subsequently develop mild to severe microcytic hypochromic anemia. Such children may exhibit jaundice, hepatosplenomegaly, and poor growth if the disorder is not recognized and treated appropriately. In some cases, the anemia becomes severe enough to require lifelong transfusion therapy. Even without regular transfusions, hemosiderosis may occur. In certain areas of the United States, hemoglobin E/β^0-thalassemia has become a more common cause of transfusion-dependent anemia than homozygous β-thalassemia.

7. Other Hemoglobinopathies

Hemoglobin variants are common. Heterozygous individuals, who are frequently identified during the course of neonatal screening programs, are generally asymptomatic and usually have no anemia or hemolysis. The principal significance of most hemoglobin variants is the potential for disease in compound heterozygous individuals who also inherit thalassemia or sickle hemoglobin. For example, children who are compound heterozygous for hemoglobins S and D_{Punjab} ($D_{Los\ Angeles}$) are symptomatic.

Reeves S et al: Health outcomes and services in children with sickle cell trait, sickle cell anemia, and normal hemoglobin. Blood Adv 2019;3:1574 [PMID: 31101648].

CONGENITAL HEMOLYTIC ANEMIAS: DISORDERS OF RED CELL METABOLISM

Erythrocytes depend on the anaerobic metabolism of glucose for the maintenance of adenosine triphosphate levels sufficient for homeostasis. Glycolysis also produces the 2,3-diphosphoglycerate (2,3-DPG) levels needed to modulate the oxygen affinity of hemoglobin. Glucose metabolism via the hexose monophosphate shunt is necessary to generate sufficient reduced nicotinamide adenine dinucleotide phosphate (NADPH) and reduced glutathione to protect red cells against oxidant damage. Congenital deficiencies of many glycolytic pathway enzymes have been associated with hemolytic anemias. In general, the morphologic abnormalities present on the peripheral blood smear are nonspecific, and the inheritance of these disorders is autosomal recessive or X-linked. Thus, the possibility of a red cell enzyme defect should be considered during the evaluation of a patient with a congenital hemolytic anemia in the following instances: when the peripheral blood smear does not show red cell morphology typical of membrane or hemoglobin defects (eg, spherocytes, sickle forms, target cells); when hemoglobin disorders are excluded by laboratory results and when family studies are inconsistent. The diagnosis is confirmed by finding a low level of the deficient enzyme and/or a consistent DNA mutation. The two most common disorders of erythrocyte metabolism are G6PD deficiency and pyruvate kinase deficiency.

1. Glucose-6-Phosphate Dehydrogenase Deficiency

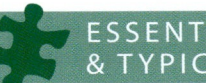

ESSENTIALS OF DIAGNOSIS & TYPICAL FEATURES

► Predominantly African, Mediterranean, or Asian ancestry.

► Neonatal hyperbilirubinemia.

► Generally sporadic hemolysis associated with infection or with ingestion of oxidant drugs or fava beans.

► X-linked inheritance but 50% sporadic.

► Rarely chronic nonspherocytic hemolytic anemia.

► General Considerations

Deficiency of glucose-6-phosphate dehydrogenase (G6PD) is the most common red cell enzyme defect to cause hemolytic anemia. The disorder has an X-linked recessive inheritance and occurs with a higher frequency among persons of African, Mediterranean, and Asian ancestry but is sporadic in at least 50% affected. Girls may be affected. In most instances, the deficiency is due to a missense mutation causing enzyme instability; thus, older red cells are more deficient than younger ones and are unable to generate sufficient nicotinamide adenine dinucleotide (NADH) to maintain the levels of reduced glutathione necessary to protect the red cells against oxidant stress. Most persons with G6PD deficiency do not have a chronic hemolytic anemia; instead, they have episodic hemolysis at times of exposure to the oxidant stress of infection or of certain drugs or food substances. The severity of the disorder varies among ethnic groups; G6PD deficiency in persons of African ancestry usually is less severe than in other ethnic groups.

▶ Clinical Findings

A. Symptoms and Signs

Neonates with G6PD deficiency may have significant unconjugated hyperbilirubinemia and require phototherapy or exchange transfusion to prevent kernicterus. Hemolytic episodes are often triggered by infection or by the ingestion of oxidant drugs such as antimalarial compounds, rasburicase, and sulfonamide antibiotics. Ingestion of fava beans may trigger hemolysis, especially in children of Mediterranean or Asian ancestry. Episodes of hemolysis are associated with pallor, jaundice, hemoglobinuria, and sometimes cardiovascular compromise.

B. Laboratory Findings

The hemoglobin concentration, reticulocyte count, and peripheral blood smear are usually normal in the absence of oxidant stress. Episodes of intravascular hemolysis are associated with a variable fall in hemoglobin. "Bite" cells or "blister" cells may be seen, along with a few spherocytes on blood smear. Hemoglobinuria is common, and the reticulocyte count increases within a few days. Heinz bodies may be demonstrated with appropriate stains. The diagnosis is confirmed by the finding of reduced levels of G6PD in erythrocytes. Because this enzyme is present in increased quantities in reticulocytes, the test is best performed at a time when the reticulocyte count is normal or near normal. DNA testing may be done at any time.

▶ Complications

Kernicterus is a risk for infants with significant neonatal hyperbilirubinemia. Episodes of acute hemolysis in older children may be life threatening. Rare G6PD variants are associated with chronic nonspherocytic hemolytic anemia; the clinical course of patients with such variants may be complicated by splenomegaly and by the formation of gallstones. Plasma free hemoglobin released from red cells may cause renal injury.

▶ Treatment

The most important treatment issue is avoidance of food (eg, fava beans) or drugs known to be associated with hemolysis. Most episodes of hemolysis are self-limited, but red cell transfusions may be lifesaving when signs and symptoms indicate cardiovascular compromise. Additional IV fluid hydration may be needed to prevent renal injury if hemolysis is brisk.

2. Pyruvate Kinase Deficiency

Pyruvate kinase deficiency is an autosomal recessive disorder resulting in deficiency of a glycolytic enzyme in RBCs. It is observed in all ethnic groups but is most common in northern Europeans. The deficiency is associated with a chronic nonspherocytic extravascular hemolytic anemia of varying severity. Approximately one-third of those affected present in the neonatal period with jaundice and hemolysis that require phototherapy or exchange transfusion. Occasionally, the disorder causes hydrops fetalis and neonatal death. The hemolysis may be so severe that chronic red cell transfusions are indicated but can be mild enough to go unnoticed for many years. Jaundice and splenomegaly frequently occur in the more severe cases. The diagnosis of pyruvate kinase deficiency is occasionally suggested by the presence of echinocytes on the peripheral blood smear, but these findings may be absent prior to splenectomy. The diagnosis depends on the demonstration of low levels of pyruvate kinase activity in red cells and/or associated DNA mutations.

Treatment of pyruvate kinase depends on the severity of the hemolysis. Blood transfusions may be required for significant anemia, and splenectomy may be beneficial. Although the procedure does not cure the disorder, it ameliorates the anemia and its symptoms. Characteristically, the reticulocyte count increases and echinocytes become more prevalent after splenectomy, despite the decreased hemolysis and increased hemoglobin level. Mitapivat, an allosteric activator of red cell pyruvate kinase enzyme, has recently been approved for use in patients with pyruvate kinase deficiency and has been shown to increase hemoglobin concentrations and decrease the degree of hemolysis.

Al-Samkari H et al: Mitapivat versus placebo for pyruvate kinase deficiency. New Engl J Med 2022;386(15):1432–1442 [PMID: 35417638].
Grace RF, Barcellini W: Management of pyruvate kinase deficiency in children and adults. Blood 2020;136:1241–1249. doi: 10.1182/blood.2019000945.Blood 2020 [PMID: 32732739].
Luzzatto L, Ally Mwashungi, Notaro R: Glucose-6-phosphate dehydrogenase deficiency. Blood 2020;136:1225–1240. doi: 10.1182/blood.2019000944 [PMID: 32702756].

ACQUIRED HEMOLYTIC ANEMIA

1. Autoimmune Hemolytic Anemia

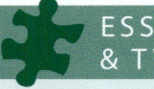

ESSENTIALS OF DIAGNOSIS & TYPICAL FEATURES

▶ Pallor, fatigue, jaundice, and dark urine.

▶ Splenomegaly.

▶ Positive DAT.

▶ Reticulocytosis and spherocytosis.

▶ General Considerations

Acquired autoimmune hemolytic anemia (AIHA) is rare during the first 4 months of life but is one of the more common causes of acute anemia after the first year. It may arise as a primary disorder or may complicate an infection (hepatitis, upper respiratory tract infections, EBV mononucleosis, or CMV infection); systemic lupus erythematosus and other autoimmune syndromes; immunodeficiency states, including autoimmune lymphoproliferative syndrome (ALPS); or, very rarely, malignancies. Drugs may induce antibody-associated hemolytic anemia, and recently third-generation cephalosporins, such as ceftriaxone, have become a common cause for this adverse event.

▶ Clinical Findings

A. Symptoms and Signs

The disease usually has an acute onset manifested by weakness, pallor, dark urine, and fatigue. Jaundice is a prominent finding, and splenomegaly is often present in the setting of extravascular hemolysis. Some cases have a more chronic, insidious onset. Clinical evidence of an underlying disease may be present.

B. Laboratory Findings

The anemia is normochromic and normocytic and may vary from mild to severe (hemoglobin concentration < 5 g/dL). The reticulocyte count and index are usually increased but occasionally are normal or low. Spherocytes and nucleated red cells may be seen on the peripheral blood smear. Although leukocytosis and elevated platelet counts are common, thrombocytopenia occasionally occurs. Other laboratory data observed with hemolysis are increased indirect and total bilirubin, lactic dehydrogenase, aspartate aminotransferase, and urinary urobilinogen. Intravascular hemolysis is indicated by hemoglobinemia, hemoglobinuria, and decreased levels of haptoglobin. Examination of bone marrow shows marked erythroid hyperplasia and hemophagocytosis but is seldom required for the diagnosis.

Serologic studies are helpful in defining pathophysiology, planning therapeutic strategies, and assessing prognosis (Table 30–3). In almost all cases, the DAT and indirect antiglobulin test (IAT) are positive. Rarely patients with AIHA may have a negative DAT due to the presence of IgG bound to RBCs with low affinity or below the level of detection of the assay, low affinity to an immature antigen found on reticulocytes, or IgA bound to RBCs not recognized by the Coombs reagent.

Further evaluation allows distinction into one of three syndromes. The presence of IgG and no or low level of C3 on the patient's RBCs, maximal in vitro antibody activity at 37°C, and either no antigen or an Rh-like specificity, which constitutes warm AIHA with mostly extravascular destruction by

Table 30–3. Classification of AIHA in children.

Syndrome	Warm AIHA	Cold AIHA	Paroxysmal Cold Hemoglobinuria
Specific antiglobulin test IgG Complement	Strongly positive. Negative or mildly positive.	Negative. Strongly positive.	Negative. Strongly positive.
Temperature at maximal reactivity (in vitro)	37°C.	4°C.	4°C.
Antigen specificity	**May be panagglutinin or may have an** Rh-like specificity.	I or i.	P.
Other		Clinically significant if agglutination occurs ≥ 30°C.	Positive biphasic hemolysin test.
Pathophysiology	Extravascular hemolysis, destruction by the RES (eg, spleen). Rarely an intravascular component early in the course.	Intravascular hemolysis (may have extravascular component).	Intravascular hemolysis (may have extravascular component).
Prognosis	May be more chronic (> 3 mo) with significant morbidity and mortality. May be associated with a primary disorder (lupus, immunodeficiency, etc).	Generally acute (< 3 mo). Good prognosis: often associated with infection.	Acute, self-limited. Associated with infection.
Therapy	Responds to RES blockade, including steroids (prednisone, 2 mg/kg/day), IVIG (1 g/kg/day for 2 days), or with specific indication, splenectomy.	May not respond to RES blockade. Severe cases may benefit from plasmapheresis.	Usually self-limited. Symptomatic management.

AIHA, autoimmune hemolytic anemia; IgG, immunoglobulin G; IVIG, intravenous immune globulin; RES, reticuloendothelial system.

the reticuloendothelial system. In contrast, the detection of complement alone on RBCs, optimal reactivity at 4°C, and I or i antigen specificity are diagnostic of cold AIHA with mostly intravascular and mild extravascular hemolysis. Cold agglutinins are relatively common (~10%) in normal individuals, but clinically significant cold (IgM) antibodies exhibit in vitro reactivity at 30°C or above.

Paroxysmal cold hemoglobinuria presents a third category of disease. The laboratory evaluation is identical to cold AIHA except for antigen specificity (P) and the exhibition of an in vitro hemolysis. Paroxysmal cold hemoglobinuria is almost always associated with significant infections, such as *Mycoplasma*, parvovirus, adenovirus, EBV, and CMV.

Differential Diagnosis

AIHA must be differentiated from other forms of congenital or acquired hemolytic anemias. The DAT discriminates antibody-mediated hemolysis from other causes, such as hereditary spherocytosis. The presence of other cytopenias and antibodies to platelets or neutrophils suggests an autoimmune (eg, lupus) syndrome, immunodeficiency (eg, ALPS, congenital immunodeficiency), or Evans syndrome (AIHA and ITP or other cytopenias associated with autoantibodies). Over half of patients diagnosed as Evans syndrome may have ALPS or other genetic immune dysregulation disorders.

Complications

The anemia may be very severe and result in cardiovascular collapse, requiring emergency management. The complications of an underlying disease, such as disseminated lupus erythematosus or an immunodeficiency state, may be present.

Treatment

Medical management of the underlying disease is important in symptomatic cases. Defining the clinical syndrome provides a useful guide to treatment. Most patients (50%–80%) with warm AIHA (in which hemolysis is mostly extravascular) respond to prednisone (2 mg/kg/day). After the initial treatment, the dose of corticosteroids may be decreased slowly. Patients may respond to 1 g of intravenous immune globulin (IVIG) per kilogram per day for 2 days, but fewer patients respond to IVIG than to prednisone. In severe cases, rituximab may be a successful alternative; however, this drug should be avoided in AIHA associated with ALPS. Although remission with splenectomy may be as high as 50%–60%, in warm AIHA, this strategy should be considered only for patients older than 5 years who are refractory or resistant to first-line therapies. Short- and long-term complications are now appreciated, and include infection with encapsulated organisms, increased risk for venous thromboembolism (VTE), and risk for portal and pulmonary arterial hypertension. In cases unresponsive to more conventional therapy, immunosuppressive agents such as mycophenolate, sirolimus, cyclosporine, tacrolimus, cyclophosphamide, azathioprine, or methotrexate may be tried alone or in combination with corticosteroids. The first four therapies, which produce less myelosuppression and risk for infection, may be helpful when hemolysis is associated with Evans syndrome or ALPS. Plasma exchange is not indicated for warm, IgG, autoantibody diseases. Transplantation, especially when hemolysis is secondary, has been used successfully in small numbers of cases.

Patients with cold AIHA and paroxysmal cold hemoglobinuria are less likely to respond to corticosteroids or IVIG. Because these syndromes are most apt to be associated with infections and have an acute, self-limited course, supportive care alone may be sufficient. Plasma exchange may be effective in severe cold autoimmune (IgM) hemolytic anemia because the offending antibody has an intravascular distribution. Rituximab, other immunosuppressive therapies, or complement inhibitors may be helpful in rare cases.

Supportive therapy is crucial. Patients with cold-reacting antibodies, particularly paroxysmal cold hemoglobinuria, should be kept in a warm environment. Transfusion may be necessary because of the complications of severe anemia but should be used only when there is no alternative. In most patients, cross-match compatible blood will not be found, and the least incompatible unit among the few tested will be transfused. Transfusion must be conducted carefully, beginning with a test dose (see section Transfusion Medicine). Identification of the patient's phenotype for minor red cell alloantigens may be helpful in avoiding alloimmunization or in providing appropriate transfusions if alloantibodies arise after initial transfusions. Patients with severe intravascular hemolysis will have associated disseminated intravascular coagulation (DIC), and heparin therapy should be considered in such cases.

Prognosis

The outlook for AIHA in childhood usually is good unless associated diseases are present (eg, likely to have a chronic course). In general, children with warm (IgG) AIHA are at greater risk for more severe and chronic disease with higher morbidity and mortality rates than those with cold AIHA. Hemolysis and positive antiglobulin tests may continue for months or years. Patients with cold AIHA or paroxysmal cold hemoglobinuria are more likely to have acute, self-limited disease (< 3 months). Paroxysmal cold hemoglobinuria is almost always associated with infection (eg, *Mycoplasma* infection, CMV, and EBV).

Berentsen S, Barcellini W: Autoimmune hemolytic anemias. New Engl J Med 2021;385:1407–1419 [PMID: 34614331].

Berentsen S et al: The choice of new treatments in autoimmune hemolytic anemia: how to pick from the basket? Front Immunol 2023;14:1180509 [PMID: 37168855].

Despotovic J, Kim O: Cold AIHA and the best treatment strategies. Hematology Am Soc Hematol Educ Program 2022;2022:90–95 [PMID: 36485161].

2. Nonimmune Acquired Hemolytic Anemia

Hepatic disease may alter the lipid composition of the red cell membrane. This usually results in the formation of target cells and is not associated with significant hemolysis.

Occasionally, hepatocellular damage is associated with the formation of spur cells and brisk hemolytic anemia. Renal disease may also be associated with significant hemolysis; hemolytic-uremic syndrome is one example. In this disorder, hemolysis is associated with the presence, on the peripheral blood smear, of echinocytes, helmet cells, fragmented red cells, and spherocytes.

A microangiopathic hemolytic anemia with fragmented red cells and some spherocytes may be observed in several conditions associated with intravascular coagulation and fibrin deposition within vessels. This occurs with DIC complicating severe infection but may also occur when the intravascular coagulation is localized, as with giant cavernous hemangiomas (Kasabach-Merritt syndrome). Fragmented red cells may also be seen with mechanical damage (eg, associated with artificial heart valves and devices).

POLYCYTHEMIA & METHEMOGLOBINEMIA

Polycythemia in children is defined as a hemoglobin or hematocrit greater than two standard deviations above the normal for age and is usually secondary to chronic hypoxemia. Hereditary polycythemia is rare. The most common cause of secondary polycythemia in children is cyanotic congenital heart disease, but it also occurs in chronic pulmonary disease such as cystic fibrosis. Persons living at extremely high altitudes, as well as some with methemoglobinemia, develop polycythemia. Polycythemia may occur in the neonatal period; it is particularly exaggerated in infants who are preterm or large for gestational age. It may occur in infants of diabetic mothers, in infants with trisomies 13, 18, or 21, or as a complication of congenital adrenal hyperplasia.

The disorder differs from polycythemia vera in that only RBCs are affected; the WBC and platelet counts are normal. There are usually no physical findings except for plethora and splenomegaly. Symptoms are generally limited to headache and lethargy.

ID may complicate polycythemia and aggravate the associated hyperviscosity. This complication of polycythemia should be suspected when the MCV falls below the normal range. Coagulation and bleeding abnormalities, including thrombocytopenia, mild consumption coagulopathy, and elevated fibrinolytic activity, have been described in severely polycythemic cardiac patients. Bleeding at surgery may be severe.

The ideal treatment of secondary polycythemia is correction of the underlying disorder. When this cannot be done, phlebotomy may be necessary to control symptoms. Iron sufficiency should be maintained. These measures help prevent the complications of thrombosis and hemorrhage.

METHEMOGLOBINEMIA

When heme iron is oxidized, it changes from the ferrous to the ferric state and methemoglobin is produced. Normally, methemoglobin is enzymatically reduced back to hemoglobin. Methemoglobin is unable to deliver oxygen to the tissues and causes a left shift in the oxygen dissociation curve. Cyanosis is seen with methemoglobin levels greater than 15%.

1. Hemoglobin M

This designation is given to several abnormal hemoglobins associated with methemoglobinemia due to amino acid substitutions in the globin chains. Hemoglobin M is transmitted in an autosomal dominant disorder. Hemoglobin electrophoresis at the usual pH will not always demonstrate the abnormal hemoglobin, and isoelectric focusing or DNA analysis may be needed. Affected individuals are cyanotic, but they have normal exercise tolerance and life expectancy. No treatment is indicated.

2. Congenital Methemoglobinemia Due to Enzyme Deficiencies

Congenital methemoglobinemia is caused most frequently by deficiency of the reducing enzyme cytochrome b5 reductase and is transmitted as an autosomal recessive trait. Affected individuals may have as much as 40% methemoglobin but usually have no symptoms, although a mild compensatory polycythemia may be present. Patients with diaphorase I deficiency respond to treatment with ascorbic acid and methylene blue (see the next section), but treatment is not usually indicated.

3. Acquired Methemoglobinemia

Nitrites and nitrates, chlorates, and quinines such as aniline dyes, sulfonamides, acetanilid, phenacetin, bismuth subnitrate, and potassium chlorate generate methemoglobin. The recreational use of volatile nitrites ("poppers") and cocaine may precipitate methemoglobinemia. Poisoning with a drug or chemical containing one of these substances should be suspected with sudden onset cyanosis. Methemoglobin levels in such cases may be extremely high and can produce anoxia, dyspnea, unconsciousness, circulatory failure, and death. Because of transiently deficient NADH methemoglobin reductase, newborns are more susceptible to drug- or chemical-induced methemoglobinemia, especially when exposed to lidocaine, benzocaine, or prilocaine. Infants with metabolic acidosis may also develop methemoglobinemia.

Children with acquired methemoglobinemia (other than those related to G6PD deficiency) respond dramatically to intravenous methylene blue. Ascorbic acid administered orally or intravenously also reduces methemoglobin, but the response is slower.

DISORDERS OF LEUKOCYTES

NEUTROPENIA

ESSENTIALS OF DIAGNOSIS & TYPICAL FEATURES

▶ Increased frequency of infections.

▶ Ulceration of oral mucosa and gingivitis.

▶ Decreased absolute neutrophil count, normal numbers of red cells and platelets.

General Considerations

Neutropenia is an ANC of less than 1500/μL in childhood, or less than 1100/μL between ages 1 month and 2 years. During the first few days of life, an ANC of less than 3500/μL may be considered neutropenia in term infants. Neutropenia results from absent or defective myeloid stem cells; ineffective or suppressed myeloid maturation; altered production of hematopoietic cytokines or chemokines or abnormalities in their receptors; decreased marrow release; increased neutrophil apoptosis; destruction or consumption; or, in pseudoneutropenia, from an increased neutrophil marginating pool (Table 30–4). A decrease in neutrophil mass diminishes delivery of these cells to areas where the balance favors bacterial proliferation and invasion.

The severity of neutropenia may be characterized by the level of peripheral neutrophils, the number and severity of infections, and the production of mature neutrophils in the marrow. Also important is whether the neutropenia is acute (< 3 months) or chronic (> 3 months). The most severe types of chronic neutropenia include reticular dysgenesis (congenital aleukocytosis), severe congenital neutropenia (severe neutropenia with maturation defect in the marrow progenitor cells associated with specific gene defects), Shwachman-Diamond syndrome (neutropenia with pancreatic insufficiency), neutropenia with immune deficiency states, cyclic neutropenia, and myelokathexis or dysgranulopoiesis.

The most common causes of acute neutropenia are viral infection or drugs, resulting in decreased neutrophil production in the marrow, increased peripheral turnover, or both. Severe bacterial infections may be associated with neutropenia. Although not commonly identified, neonatal alloimmune neutropenia can be severe and associated with infection. Autoimmune neutropenia occurs with chronic benign neutropenia of childhood, immunodeficiency syndromes, autoimmune disorders, or, in the newborn, as a result of passive transfer of antibody (alloimmune) from the mother to the fetus. Malignancies, osteopetrosis, marrow failure syndromes, and hypersplenism usually are not associated with isolated neutropenia.

Table 30–4. Classification of neutropenia in childhood.

Congenital neutropenia with abnormalities of stem cells or committed myeloid progenitor cells
Reticular dysgenesis
Chronic idiopathic neutropenia of childhood
Severe congenital neutropenias
Cyclic neutropenia
Shwachman-Diamond syndrome
WHIM syndrome
Glycogenosis Ib
Chédiak-Higashi syndrome
Cohen syndrome
Hermansky-Pudlak syndrome
Griscelli syndrome
Telomere biology disorders
Organic acidemias (eg, propionic, methylmalonic)
Osteopetrosis
Neutropenia with immunodeficiency disorders
Acquired neutropenias affecting stem cells
Malignancies (leukemia, lymphoma) and preleukemic disorders
Drugs, toxic substances, ionizing radiation
Aplastic anemia
Acquired neutropenias affecting committed myeloid progenitors or survival of mature neutrophils
Ineffective myelopoiesis (vitamin B_{12}, folate, and copper deficiency)
Infection
Immune (neonatal alloimmune or autoimmune, autoimmune, or chronic benign neutropenia)
Hypersplenism

Clinical Findings

A. Symptoms and Signs

Acute severe bacterial or fungal infection is the most significant complication of neutropenia. Although the risk is increased when the ANC is less than 500/μL, the actual susceptibility is variable and depends on the cause of neutropenia, marrow reserves, and other factors. The most common types of infection include septicemia, cellulitis, skin abscesses, pneumonia, and perirectal abscesses. In addition to local signs and symptoms, patients may have chills, fever, and malaise. Sinusitis, aphthous ulcers, gingivitis, and periodontal disease are also significant problems in chronic neutropenia. In most cases, the spleen and liver are not enlarged. *Staphylococcus aureus* and gram-negative bacteria are the most common pathogens.

B. Laboratory Findings

Neutrophils are absent or markedly reduced in the peripheral blood. In most forms of neutropenia or agranulocytosis, the monocytes and lymphocytes are normal, and the red cells and platelets are not affected. The bone marrow usually shows a normal erythroid series, with adequate megakaryocytes, but a marked reduction in the myeloid cells or a significant delay in maturation of this series may be noted at various stages of myeloid maturation. Total cellularity may be decreased.

In the evaluation of neutropenia (eg, persistent, intermittent, cyclic), attention should be paid to the duration and pattern of neutropenia, the types of infections and their frequency, and phenotypic abnormalities on physical examination. A careful family history and blood counts from the parents may be useful. If an acquired cause, such as viral infection or drug, is not obvious as an acute cause, no other primary disease is present, and the neutropenia is chronic, WBC counts, white cell differential, and platelet and reticulocyte counts should be completed two to three times weekly for 6–8 weeks to determine the pattern of neutropenia. Bone marrow aspiration and biopsy including cytogenetic analysis are most important to characterize the morphologic features of myelopoiesis. Other tests that aid in the diagnosis include measurement of neutrophil antibodies, immunoglobulin levels, antinuclear antibodies, and lymphocyte phenotyping to detect immunodeficiency states. Cytokines in plasma or produced by mononuclear cells can be measured directly. Some neutropenia disorders have abnormal neutrophil function, but severe neutropenia may preclude collection of sufficient cells to complete assays. Analysis for gene mutations noted above may help confirm the diagnosis of a severe neutropenia syndrome. Increased apoptosis in marrow precursors or circulating neutrophils is a general characteristic described in several congenital or genetic disorders.

▶ Treatment

Underlying disorders should be identified and treated or associated agents should be eliminated. Infections should be aggressively assessed and treated. Prophylactic antimicrobial therapy is not indicated for afebrile, asymptomatic patients but may be considered in rare cases with recurrent infections. Recombinant granulocyte-colony–stimulating factor (G-CSF) will increase neutrophil counts in most patients. G-CSF may be started at 3–5 mcg/kg/day subcutaneously or intravenously once a day, and the dose adjusted to keep the ANC between 500/μL and 10,000/μL. In a small number of patients, G-CSF therapy has been shown to be safe for mothers and not teratogenic. Some patients maintain adequate counts with G-CSF given every other day. Treatment will decrease infectious complications but may have little effect on periodontal disease. However, not all patients with neutropenia syndromes require G-CSF (eg, chronic benign neutropenia of childhood). Patients with cyclic neutropenia may have a milder clinical course as they grow older. Immunizations should be given if the adaptive immune system is normal. Hematopoietic stem cell transplant may be considered for patients with severe complications, especially those with severe congenital neutropenia refractory to G-CSF administration.

▶ Prognosis

The prognosis varies greatly with the cause and severity of the neutropenia. In severe cases with persistent agranulocytosis, the prognosis is poor in spite of antibiotic therapy, but G-CSF has the potential to prolong life expectancy. In mild or cyclic forms of neutropenia, symptoms may be minimal and the prognosis for normal life expectancy excellent. Chronic benign neutropenia of childhood resolves spontaneously in up to 90% of children by 5 years of age. Up to 50% of patients with Shwachman-Diamond syndrome may develop aplastic anemia, myelodysplasia, or leukemia during their lifetime. Patients with other SCNs also have a potential for leukemia, as do patients with neutropenia associated with some immune disorders. Hematopoietic stem cell transplant may be the only curative therapy for some disorders.

Connelly J, Walkovich K: Diagnosis and therapeutic decision-making for the neutropenic patient. Hematology Am Soc Hematol Educ Program 2021;2021(1):492–503 [PMID: 34889413].

Donadieu J, Bellanne-Chantelot C: Genetics of severe congenital neutropenia as a gateway to personalized therapy. Hematology Am Soc Hematol Educ Program 2022;2022:658–665 [PMID: 36485107].

McKinney C et al: Metabolic abnormalities in G6PC3-deficient human neutrophils result in severe functional defects. Blood Adv 2020;4(23):5888–5901 [PMID: 33259599].

NEUTROPHILIA

Neutrophilia is an increase in the ANC in the peripheral blood to greater than 7500–8500/μL for infants, children, and adults. To support the increased peripheral count, neutrophils may be mobilized from bone marrow storage or peripheral marginating pools. Neutrophilia occurs acutely in association with bacterial or viral infections, inflammatory diseases (eg, juvenile rheumatoid arthritis, inflammatory bowel disease, Kawasaki disease), surgical or functional asplenia, liver failure, diabetic ketoacidosis, azotemia, congenital disorders of neutrophil function (eg, chronic granulomatous disease, leukocyte adherence deficiency), and hemolysis. Drugs such as corticosteroids, lithium, and epinephrine increase the blood neutrophil count. Corticosteroids cause release of neutrophils from the marrow pool, inhibit egress from capillary beds, and postpone apoptotic cell death. Epinephrine causes release of the marginating pool. Acute neutrophilia has been reported after stress, such as from electric shock, trauma, burns, surgery, and emotional upset. Tumors involving the bone marrow, such as lymphomas, neuroblastomas, and rhabdomyosarcoma, may be associated with leukocytosis and the presence of immature myeloid cells in the peripheral blood. Infants with Down syndrome have defective regulation of proliferation and maturation of the myeloid series and may develop neutrophilia. At times this process may affect other cell lines and mimic myeloproliferative disorders or acute leukemia.

Neutrophilias must be distinguished from myeloproliferative disorders such as chronic myelogenous leukemia and juvenile chronic myelogenous leukemia. In general, abnormalities involving other cell lines, the appearance of immature cells on the blood smear, and the presence of hepatosplenomegaly are important differentiating characteristics.

DISORDERS OF NEUTROPHIL FUNCTION

Neutrophils play a key role in host defenses. Circulating in the laminar flow of blood vessels, they adhere to capillary vascular endothelium adjacent to sites of infection and inflammation. Moving between endothelial cells, the neutrophil migrates toward the offending agent. Contact with a microbe that is properly opsonized with complement or antibodies triggers ingestion, a process in which cytoplasmic streaming results in the formation of pseudopods that fuse around the invader, encasing it in a phagosome. During the ingestion phase, the oxidase enzyme system assembles in the phagosomal membrane and is activated, taking oxygen from the surrounding medium and reducing it to form toxic oxygen metabolites critical to microbicidal activity. Concurrently, granules from the two main classes (azurophil and specific) fuse and release their contents into the phagolysosome. The concentration of toxic oxygen metabolites (eg, hydrogen peroxide, hypochlorous acid, hydroxyl radical) and other compounds (eg, proteases, cationic proteins, cathepsins, defensins) increases dramatically, resulting in the death and dissolution of the microbe. Complex physiologic and biochemical processes support and control these functions. Defects in any of these processes may lead to inadequate neutrophil function and an increased risk of recurrent, unusual, or severe infections. Further discussion of specific neutrophil function defects (eg, chronic granulomatous disease or leukocyte adhesion deficiency) is presented in Chapter 33.

LYMPHOCYTOSIS

From the first week up to the fifth year of life, lymphocytes are the most numerous leukocytes in human blood. The ratio then reverses gradually to reach the adult pattern of neutrophil predominance. An absolute lymphocytosis in childhood is associated with acute or chronic viral infections, pertussis, syphilis, tuberculosis, and hyperthyroidism. Other noninfectious conditions, drugs, and hypersensitivity and serum sickness–like reactions cause lymphocytosis.

Fever, upper respiratory symptoms, gastrointestinal complaints, and rashes are clues in distinguishing infectious from noninfectious causes. The presence of enlarged liver, spleen, or lymph nodes is crucial to the differential diagnosis, which includes acute leukemia and lymphoma. Most cases of infectious mononucleosis are associated with hepatosplenomegaly or adenopathy. The absence of anemia and thrombocytopenia helps to differentiate these disorders. Evaluation of the morphology of lymphocytes on peripheral blood smear is crucial.

Infectious causes, particularly infectious mononucleosis, are associated with atypical features in the lymphocytes, such as basophilic cytoplasm, vacuoles, finer and less-dense chromatin, and an indented nucleus. These features are distinct from the characteristic morphology associated with lymphoblastic leukemia. Lymphocytosis in childhood is most commonly associated with infections and resolves with recovery from the primary disease.

EOSINOPHILIA

Eosinophilia in infants and children is an absolute eosinophil count greater than 300/μL. Marrow eosinophil production is stimulated by the cytokine IL-5. Allergies, particularly those associated with asthma and eczema, are the most common primary causes of eosinophilia in children. Eosinophilia also occurs in drug reactions, with tumors (Hodgkin and non-Hodgkin lymphomas and brain tumors), and with immunodeficiency and histiocytosis syndromes. Increased eosinophil counts are a prominent feature of many invasive parasitic infections. Gastrointestinal disorders such as chronic hepatitis, ulcerative colitis, Crohn disease, and milk precipitin disease may be associated with eosinophilia. Increased blood eosinophil counts have been identified in several families without association with any specific illness. Rare causes of eosinophilia include the hypereosinophilic syndrome, characterized by counts greater than 1500/μL and organ involvement and damage (hepatosplenomegaly, cardiomyopathy, pulmonary fibrosis, and central nervous system injury). This is a disorder of middle-aged adults and is rare in children. Eosinophilic leukemia has been described, but its existence as a distinct entity is very rare.

Eosinophils are sometimes the last type of mature myeloid cell to disappear after marrow ablative chemotherapy. Increased eosinophil counts are associated with graft-versus-host disease after bone marrow transplant, and elevations are sometimes documented during rejection episodes in patients who have solid organ grafts.

BLEEDING DISORDERS

Bleeding disorders may occur because of (1) quantitative or qualitative abnormalities of platelets, (2) quantitative or qualitative abnormalities in plasma procoagulant factors, (3) vascular abnormalities, or (4) accelerated fibrinolysis. The coagulation cascade and fibrinolytic system are shown in Figures 30–4 and 30–5.

The most critical aspect in evaluating the bleeding patient is obtaining detailed personal and family bleeding histories, including bleeding complications associated with birth and the perinatal period, dental interventions, minor procedures, surgeries, and trauma. Excessive mucosal bleeding is suggestive of a platelet disorder, von Willebrand disease (vWD), dysfibrinogenemia, or vasculitis. Bleeding into muscles and joints may be associated with a plasma procoagulant factor

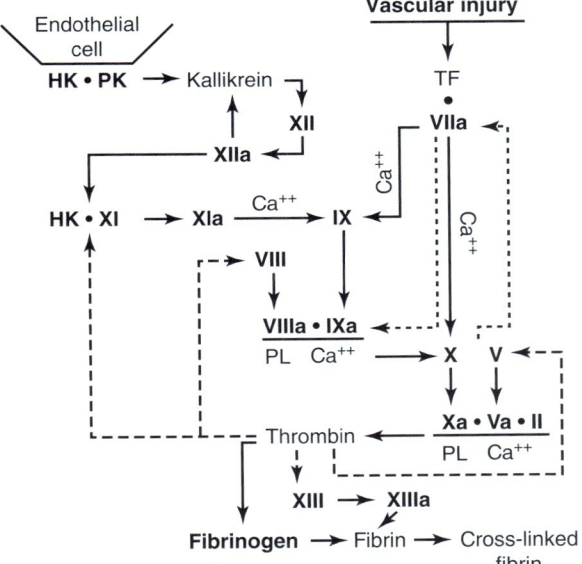

▲ **Figure 30–4.** The procoagulant system and formation of a fibrin clot. Vascular injury initiates the coagulation process by exposure of tissue factor (TF); the dashed lines indicate thrombin actions in addition to clotting of fibrinogen. The dotted lines associated with VIIa indicate the feedback activation of the VII-TF complex by Xa and IXa. Ca^{++}, calcium; HK, high-molecular-weight kininogen; PK, prekallikrein; PL, phospholipid. (Reproduced with permission from Goodnight SH, Hathaway WE: *Disorders of Hemostasis & Thrombosis: A Clinical Guide.* 2nd ed. New York, NY: McGraw Hill; 2001.)

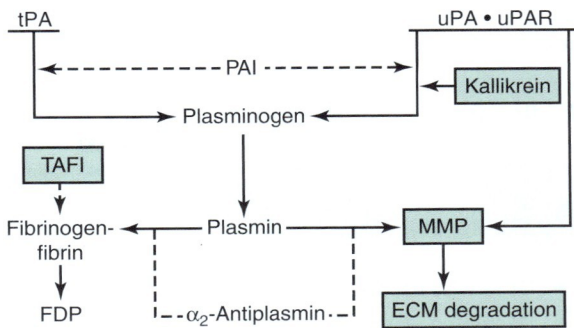

▲ **Figure 30–5.** The fibrinolytic system. Solid arrows indicate activation; dashed line arrows indicate inhibition. ECM, extracellular matrix; FDP, fibrinogen-fibrin degradation products; MMP, matrix metalloproteinases; PAI, plasminogen activator inhibitor; TAFI, thrombin activatable fibrinolysis inhibitor; tPA, tissue plasminogen activator; uPA, urokinase; uPAR, cellular urokinase receptor. (Reproduced with permission from Goodnight SH, Hathaway WE: *Disorders of Hemostasis & Thrombosis: A Clinical Guide.* 2nd ed. New York, NY: McGraw Hill; 2001.)

abnormality. In either scenario, the abnormality may be congenital or acquired. A thorough physical examination should be performed with special attention to the skin, oro- and nasopharynx, liver, spleen, and joints. Screening and diagnostic evaluation in patients with suspected bleeding disorders (Table 30–5).

Goodnight SH, Hathaway WE (eds): *Disorders of Hemostasis & Thrombosis: A Clinical Guide.* 2nd ed. New York, NY: McGraw Hill; 2001:41–51.

ABNORMALITIES OF PLATELET NUMBER OR FUNCTION

Thrombocytopenia in the pediatric age range is often immune-mediated (eg, ITP, neonatal auto- or alloimmune thrombocytopenia) but is also caused by consumptive coagulopathy (eg, DIC, Kasabach-Merritt phenomenon), acute leukemias, or rarer disorders such as Wiskott-Aldrich syndrome and type 2b vWD, and artifactually in automated cytometers

Table 30–5. Bleeding assessment.

Test	Assessment
Prothrombin time (PT)	Clotting function of factors X, VII, V, II, and fibrinogen
Activated partial thromboplastin time (aPTT)	Clotting function of high-molecular-weight kininogen, prekallikrein, and factors XII, XI, IX, VIII, X, V, II, and fibrinogen
Complete blood count (CBC)	Platelet size and number, anemia
Platelet function analyzer-100 (PFA-100) or whole blood platelet aggregometry	Platelet functional assessment
Fibrinogen and thrombin time	Clotting function of fibrinogen. Dysfibrinogenemia. Thrombin time measures the generation of fibrin from fibrinogen following conversion of prothrombin to thrombin, as well as the antithrombin effects of fibrin degradation products and heparin
Euglobulin lysis time (ELT)	Fibrinolysis. The ELT is shortened, assess hyperfibrinolysis due to congenital deficiency of the fibrinolytic inhibitors plasminogen activator inhibitor-1 and α_2-antiplasmin. In ill patients, measurement of fibrin degradation products may assist in the diagnosis of disseminated intravascular coagulation (DIC)

(eg, Bernard-Soulier syndrome), where giant forms may not be enumerated as platelets.

1. Idiopathic Thrombocytopenic Purpura

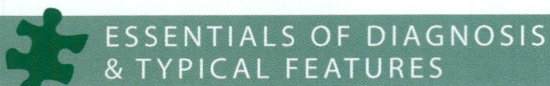

ESSENTIALS OF DIAGNOSIS & TYPICAL FEATURES

▶ Otherwise healthy child.
▶ Decreased platelet count.
▶ Petechiae, ecchymoses.

▶ General Considerations

Acute ITP is the most common bleeding disorder of childhood. It occurs most frequently in children aged 2–5 years and often follows infection with viruses. The thrombocytopenia results from clearance of circulating IgM- or IgG-coated platelets by the reticuloendothelial system. The spleen plays a predominant role in ITP by sequestering antibody-bound platelets. Most patients recover spontaneously within months. Chronic ITP (> 12 months duration) occurs in 10%–20% of affected patients.

▶ Clinical Findings

A. Symptoms and Signs

Onset of ITP is usually acute, with the appearance of multiple petechiae and ecchymoses. Epistaxis and gingival bleeding are common, while hematuria and hematochezia are less common. No other physical findings are usually present. Rarely, concurrent infection with EBV or CMV may cause hepatosplenomegaly or lymphadenopathy.

B. Laboratory Findings

The platelet count is markedly reduced (usually < 50,000/μL and often < 10,000/μL), and large platelets are present in the peripheral blood smear, suggesting accelerated new platelet production. The WBC count and differential are normal, and the hemoglobin concentration is preserved unless hemorrhage has been significant.

▶ Differential Diagnosis

Table 30–6 lists common causes of thrombocytopenia. ITP remains a diagnosis of exclusion. Family history or the finding of predominantly giant platelets on the peripheral blood smear is helpful in distinguishing ITP from hereditary thrombocytopenia. Bone marrow examination should be performed when the history is atypical (ie, the child is not otherwise healthy, or there is a family history of bleeding), if abnormalities other than purpura and petechiae are present on physical examination, or if other cell lines are abnormal on the CBC. Bone marrow examination prior to treatment with corticosteroids is usually not required.

▶ Complications

Life-threatening hemorrhagic complications like intracranial hemorrhage are rare and occur in less than 1% of patients even with very low platelet counts.

▶ Treatment

A. General Measures

Observation is recommended for most children in the absence of bleeding regardless of platelet count. NSAIDs such as aspirin, ibuprofen, and naproxen compromise platelet function and should be avoided. Bleeding precautions (eg, restriction from physical contact activities and use of helmets) should be observed. Platelet transfusion

Table 30–6. Common causes of thrombocytopenia.

Increased Turnover			Decreased Production	
Antibody-Mediated	Coagulopathy	Other	Congenital	Acquired
Idiopathic thrombocytopenic purpura	Disseminated intravascular coagulopathy	Hemolytic-uremic syndrome	Fanconi anemia Amegakaryocytic thrombocytopenia	Aplastic anemia
Infection	Sepsis	Thrombotic thrombocytopenic purpura	Wiskott-Aldrich syndrome	Leukemia and other malignancies
Immunologic diseases	Necrotizing enterocolitis Thrombosis Cavernous hemangioma	Hypersplenism Respiratory distress syndrome Wiskott-Aldrich syndrome	Thrombocytopenia with absent radii Metabolic disorders Osteopetrosis	Vitamin B_{12} and folate deficiencies Medications

should be avoided except in circumstances of life-threatening bleeding, in which case emergent splenectomy may be considered. In this setting, administration of corticosteroids and IVIG is also advisable. Bleeding assessment tools such as the Buchanan and Adix bleeding scale help the clinician organize and determine treatment.

B. Corticosteroids

Patients with clinically significant but non–life-threatening bleeding (ie, epistaxis, hematuria, and hematochezia) and those with a platelet count of less than 10,000/dL may benefit from treatment with corticosteroids. Prednisone 2–4 mg/kg/day (maximum of 120 mg/day) for 5–7 days is preferred as first-line therapy. Long-term use of corticosteroids should be avoided because of toxicity.

C. Intravenous Immunoglobulin

Intravenous immunoglobulin (IVIG) at a dose of 1 g/kg can be used for patients with severe, acute bleeding or life-threatening hemorrhage if a rapid increase in platelet count is needed. Responses are prompt and may last for several weeks. Platelets may be given simultaneously during life-threatening hemorrhage but are rapidly destroyed. Side effects of IVIG are common, including transient neurologic complications in one-third of patients (eg, headache, nausea, and aseptic meningitis) that mimic intracranial hemorrhage and necessitate radiologic evaluation.

D. Anti-Rh(D) Immunoglobulin

This polyclonal immunoglobulin binds to the D antigen on RBCs. The splenic clearance of anti-D–coated red cells interferes with removal of antibody-coated platelets, resulting in improvement in platelet count. This approach is effective only in Rh(+) patients with a functional spleen who are DAT negative. Significant hemolysis may occur in up to 5% of patients and fatal intravascular hemolysis has been reported leading to an FDA black box warning for its use.

E. Splenectomy

Many children with chronic ITP have platelet counts less than 30,000/μL. Corticosteroids, IVIG, and anti-D immunoglobulin are typically effective treatment for acute bleeding. Splenectomy produces a complete response in 70% and partial response in 20% of children with ITP, but it should be considered only after persistence of significant thrombocytopenia for more than 12 months and the failure of a preferred or alternative second-line therapy. Postoperatively, a reactive thrombocytosis may raise the platelet count to more than 1 million/μL, but it is not associated with thrombosis in children. However, thrombosis is recognized as a long-term potential postsplenectomy complication.

F. Rituximab (Anti-CD20 Monoclonal Antibody)

There have been no randomized trials for rituximab in children. The efficacy of treating childhood chronic ITP in several series and case studies has demonstrated response rates between 26% and 60%, but only 20%–30% remain in remission. Because of significant adverse events, this therapy is be reserved for refractory cases with significant bleeding or as an alternative to splenectomy.

G. Thrombopoietin mimetics

Thrombopoietin receptor agonists are the only FDA-approved second-line treatments in pediatric patients over 1 year of age with chronic ITP. Eltrombopag and romiplostim are the two currently available thrombopoietin receptor agonists. Phase III clinical trials show similar platelet response rates exceeding 70%. Preliminary data show adequate long-term safety profiles.

▶ Prognosis

Eighty percent of children with ITP will achieve a remission. Risk for chronic ITP is higher in females and patients older than 10 years at presentation. Older child- and adolescent-onset ITP may be associated with development of other autoimmune conditions.

Bennett CM: Predictors of remission in children with newly diagnosed immune thrombocytopenia: data from the Intercontinental Cooperative ITP Study Group Registry II participants. Pediatr Blood Cancer 2018;65(1) [PMID: 28792679].

Neunert CE: Evidence-based management of immune thrombocytopenia: ASH guideline update. Hematology Am Soc Hematol Educ Program 2018;2018(1):568–575 [PMID: 30504359].

Provan D: Updated international consensus report on the investigation and management of primary immune thrombocytoipenia. Blood Adv 2019;3(22):3280–3817 [PMID: 31770441].

2. Thrombocytopenia in the Newborn

Thrombocytopenia is one of the most common causes of neonatal hemorrhage and should be considered in any newborn with petechiae, purpura, or other significant bleeding. Defined by a platelet count of less than 150,000/μL, thrombocytopenia occurs in approximately 0.9% of unselected neonates; however, up to 80% of neonates in a newborn intensive care unit may experience thrombocytopenia; most of these cases are transient. Infection and DIC are the most common causes of thrombocytopenia in ill preterm and full-term newborns. In the healthy neonate, antibody-mediated thrombocytopenia (alloimmune or maternal autoimmune), viral syndromes, hyperviscosity, and major-vessel thrombosis are frequent causes of thrombocytopenia. Management is directed toward the underlying etiology. Other infants are affected in mothers with preeclampsia. Most of these cases resolve over several days to a few weeks without treatment, but some are severe enough to warrant platelet transfusions. More rarely, thrombocytopenia may be due to an inherited genetic cause (see Table 30–6).

A. Thrombocytopenia Associated With Platelet Alloantibodies (Fetal and Neonatal Alloimmune Thrombocytopenia [FNAIT])

FNAIT is the most common cause of thrombocytopenia in well, term infants, with a prevalence of 0.3–1 in 1000 pregnancies. Alloimmunization occurs when a platelet antigen of the infant from the father differs from that of the mother, and the mother is sensitized by fetal platelets that cross the placenta into the maternal circulation. In Caucasians, 80% are associated with HPA1a, and 10%–15% HPA5b. Bleeding can vary from minor skin effects to severe intracranial hemorrhage (1 in 11,000 neonates). Other platelet-specific alloantigens may be etiologic. Unlike in Rh incompatibility, 30%–40% of affected neonates are first-born. Thrombocytopenia is progressive over the course of gestation and worse with each subsequent pregnancy. The presence of antenatal maternal platelet antibodies on more than one occasion and their persistence into the third trimester is predictive of severe neonatal thrombocytopenia; a weak or undetectable antibody does not exclude thrombocytopenia. Intracranial hemorrhage occurs in 10%–30% of affected neonates as early as 20 weeks' gestation. Petechiae or other bleeding manifestations are usually present shortly after birth. The disease is self-limited, and the platelet count normalizes within 4 weeks.

If alloimmunization is associated with clinically significant bleeding, transfusion of HPA-selected irradiated platelets is preferred if immediately available; otherwise unselected platelets may be used. If platelets are unavailable, infuse IVIG 1 g/kg. The rise in platelets will occur in 24–72 hours. If thrombocytopenia is not severe (>30,000/µL) and bleeding is absent, observation alone may be appropriate.

Intracranial hemorrhage in a previous child secondary to alloimmune thrombocytopenia is a strong risk factor for severe fetal thrombocytopenia and hemorrhage in a subsequent pregnancy. Amniocentesis or chorionic villus sampling to obtain fetal DNA for platelet antigen typing is sometimes performed if the father is heterozygous for HPA1a. If alloimmunization has occurred with a previous pregnancy, irrespective of history of intracranial hemorrhage, screening cranial ultrasound for hemorrhage should begin at 20 weeks' gestation and be repeated regularly. If the fetal platelet count is less than 100,000/µL, the mother should be treated with weekly IVIG with or without corticosteroids. Delivery near term by elective cesarean section is recommended if the fetal platelet count is less than 50,000/µL.

B. Thrombocytopenia Associated With ITP in the Mother (Neonatal Autoimmune Thrombocytopenia)

Infants born to mothers with ITP or other autoimmune diseases (eg, antiphospholipid antibody syndrome or systemic lupus erythematosus) may develop thrombocytopenia because of transfer of antiplatelet IgG from the mother. Unfortunately, maternal and fetal platelet counts and maternal antiplatelet antibody levels are unreliable predictors of bleeding risk. Antenatal corticosteroid administration to the mother is considered if maternal platelet count falls below 50,000/µL, with or without a concomitant course of IVIG.

Most neonates with autoimmune thrombocytopenia do not develop clinically significant bleeding, and treatment is not often required. The risk of intracranial hemorrhage is 0.2%–1.5%. If diffuse petechiae or minor bleeding are evident, a 1- to 2-week course of oral prednisone, 2 mg/kg/day, may be helpful. If the platelet count remains consistently less than 20,000/µL or if severe hemorrhage develops, IVIG should be given (1 g/kg daily for 1–2 days). Platelet transfusions are indicated only for life-threatening bleeding and may be effective only after removal of antibody by exchange transfusion. The platelet nadir is typically between the fourth and sixth day of life and improves significantly by 1 month; full recovery may take 2–4 months. Platelet recovery may be delayed in breastfed infants because of transfer of IgG by milk.

C. Neonatal Thrombocytopenia Associated With Infections

Thrombocytopenia is commonly associated with severe generalized infections during the newborn period. Between 50% and 75% of neonates with bacterial sepsis are thrombocytopenic. Intrauterine infections such as rubella, syphilis, toxoplasmosis, HIV, CMV, herpes simplex (acquired intra- or postpartum), enteroviruses, and parvovirus are often associated with thrombocytopenia. In addition to specific treatment for some underlying diseases, platelet transfusions may be indicated in severe cases.

D. Kasabach-Merritt Phenomenon

A rare but important cause of thrombocytopenia in the newborn is Kasabach-Merritt phenomenon associated with kaposiform hemangioendotheliomas, a benign neoplasm with histopathology distinct from that of classic infantile hemangiomas or less often with tufted angioma. Intense platelet sequestration in the lesion results in thrombocytopenia and may rarely be associated with a DIC-like picture and hemolytic anemia. The bone marrow typically shows megakaryocytic hyperplasia in response to the thrombocytopenia. Corticosteroids and vincristine or steroids and sirolimus are treatment options if significant coagulopathy is present, a vital structure is compressed, or the lesion is cosmetically unacceptable. Depending on the site, embolization may be an option. Surgery is often avoided because of the high risk of hemorrhage.

Adams DM, Ricci KW: Vascular anomalies: diagnosis of complicated anomalies and new medical treatment options. Hematol Oncol Clin North Am 2019 Jun;33(3):455–470 doi: 10.1016/j.hoc.2019.01.011 [PMID: 31030813].

Lieberman L: Fetal and neonatal alloimmune thrombocytopenia: recommendations for evidence-based practice, an international approach. Br J Haematol 2019 May;185(3):549–562. doi: 10.1111/bjh.15813. Epub 2019 Mar 3 [PMID: 30828796].

3. Disorders of Platelet Function

Individuals with platelet function defects typically develop abnormal bruising and mucosal bleeding similar to that occurring in persons with thrombocytopenia. The PFA-100, which can evaluate platelet dysfunction and vWD, has replaced the template bleeding time in many institutions but is not unanimously endorsed. Platelet aggregometry is important for in vitro assessment of platelet function where available. It uses platelet activators, such as adenosine diphosphate, collagen, arachidonic acid, and ristocetin. Unfortunately, none of these screening tests of platelet function uniformly predicts clinical bleeding severity.

Platelet dysfunction may be inherited or acquired, the latter being more common. Acquired disorders of platelet function may occur secondary to uremia, cirrhosis, sepsis, myeloproliferative disorders, congenital heart disease, and viral infections. Many pharmacologic agents decrease platelet function. The most common offending agents in children are aspirin and other NSAIDs, synthetic penicillins, and valproic acid. In acquired platelet dysfunction, the PFA-100 closure time is prolonged with collagen-epinephrine, while normal with collagen-ADP.

The inherited disorders are due to defects in platelet-vessel interaction, platelet-platelet interaction, platelet granule content or release (including defects of signal transduction), thromboxane and arachidonic acid pathway, and platelet-procoagulant protein interaction. Individuals with hereditary platelet dysfunction have a prolonged bleeding time but may have normal platelet number and morphology by light microscopy. PFA-100 closure time is typically prolonged with both collagen-ADP and collagen-epinephrine.

Congenital causes of defective platelet-vessel wall interaction include Bernard-Soulier syndrome, which is characterized by increased platelet size and decreased platelet number. This autosomal recessive disorder is a deficiency or dysfunction of glycoprotein Ib-V-IX complex on the platelet surface resulting in impaired von Willebrand factor (vWF) binding, impairing platelet adhesion to the vascular endothelium.

Glanzmann thrombasthenia is an example of severe platelet-platelet dysfunction. In this autosomal recessive disorder, glycoprotein IIb-IIIa is deficient or dysfunctional. Platelets do not bind fibrinogen effectively and exhibit impaired aggregation. As in Bernard-Soulier syndrome, acute bleeding is treated with platelet transfusion and recombinant factor VIIa.

Disorders involving platelet granule content include storage pool disease and Quebec platelet disorder. In individuals with storage pool disease, platelet-dense granules lack adenosine diphosphate and adenosine triphosphate and are decreased in number by electron microscopy. These granules are also deficient in Hermansky-Pudlak, Chédiak-Higashi, and Wiskott-Aldrich syndromes. Whereas deficiency of a second granule class, α-granules, results in the gray platelet syndrome. Quebec platelet disorder is characterized by a normal platelet α-granule number, but with abnormal proteolysis of α-granule proteins and deficiency of platelet α-granule multimerin. α-Granule abnormality in this disorder also results in increased serum levels of urokinase-type plasminogen activator. Epinephrine-induced platelet aggregation is markedly impaired.

Platelet dysfunction has also been observed in other congenital syndromes, such as Down and Noonan syndromes, without a clear understanding of the molecular defect.

▶ **Treatment**

Acute bleeding in many individuals with acquired or selected congenital platelet function defects responds to therapy with desmopressin acetate, likely due to an induced release of vWF from endothelial stores and/or upregulated expression of glycoprotein Ib-V-IX on the platelet surface. If this therapy is ineffective or if the patient has Bernard-Soulier syndrome or Glanzmann syndrome, the mainstay of treatment for bleeding episodes is platelet transfusion, preferably with HLA type–specific platelets. Recombinant VIIa, which may be helpful in platelet transfusion-refractory patients, is FDA-approved for patients with Glanzmann syndrome.

Sharma R: Congenital disorders of platelet function and number. Pediatr Clin North Am 2018;65(3):561–578 [PMID: 29803283].

INHERITED BLEEDING DISORDERS

Table 30–7 lists normal values for coagulation factors. The more common factor deficiencies are discussed in this section. Individuals with bleeding disorders should avoid exposure to medications that inhibit platelet function. Participation in contact sports should be considered in the context of the severity of the bleeding disorder.

1. Factor VIII Deficiency (Hemophilia A)

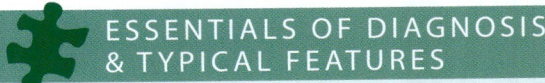

ESSENTIALS OF DIAGNOSIS & TYPICAL FEATURES

- ▶ Bruising, soft-tissue bleeding, hemarthrosis.
- ▶ Prolonged aPTT.
- ▶ Reduced factor VIII activity.

Table 30–7. Physiologic alterations in measurements of the hemostatic system.

Measurement	Normal Adults	Fetus (20 wk)	Preterm (25–32 wk)	Term Infant	Infant (6 mo)	Pregnancy (term)	Exercise (acute)	Aging (70–80 y)
Platelets								
Count μL/10³	250	107–297	293	332	–	260	↑18%–40%	225
Size (fL)	9.0	8.9	8.5	9.1	–	9.6	↑	–
Aggregation ADP	N	+	→	→	–	↑	↓15%	–
Collagen	N	→	→	→	–	N	↓60%	N
Ristocetin	N	–	↑	↑	–	–	↓10%	–
BT (min)	2–9	–	3.6±2	3.4±1.8	–	9.0±1.4	–	5–6
Procoagulant system								
PTT*	1	4.0	3	1.3	1.1	1.1	↓15%	→
PT*	1.00	2.3	1.3	1.1	1	0.95	N	–
TCT*	1	2.4	1.3	1.1	1	0.92	N	–
Fibrinogen, mg/dL	278 (0.61)	96 (50)	250 (100)	240 (150)	251 (160)	450 (100)	↓25%	↑15%
II, U/mL	1(0.7)	0.16 (0.10)	0.32 (0.18)	0.52 (0.25)	0.88 (0.6)	1.15 (0.68–1.9)	–	N
V, U/mL	1.0 (0.6)	0.32 (0.21)	0.80 (0.43)	1.00 (0.54)	0.91 (0.55)	0.85 (0.40–1.9)	N	N
VII, U/mL	1.0 (0.6)	0.27 (0.17)	0.37 (0.24)	0.57 (0.35)	0.87 (0.50)	1.17 (0.87–3.3)	↑200%	↑25%
VIIIc, U/mL	1.0 (0.6)	0.50 (0.23)	0.75 (0.40)	1.50 (0.55)	0.90 (0.50)	2.12 (0.8–6.0)	↑250%	1.50
vWF, U/mL	1.0 (0.6)	0.65 (0.40)	1.50 (0.90)	1.60 (0.84)	1.07 (0.60)	1.7	↑75%–200%	↑
IX, U/mL	1.0 (0.5)	0.10 (0.05)	0.22 (0.17)	0.35 (0.15)	0.86 (0.36)	0.81–2.15	↑25%	1.0–1.40
X, U/mL	1.0 (0.6)	0.19 (0.15)	0.38 (0.20)	0.45 (0.3)	0.78 (0.38)	1.30	–	N
XI, U/mL	1.0 (0.6)	0.13 (0.08)	0.2 (0.12)	0.42 (0.20)	0.86 (0.38)	0.7	–	N
XII, U/mL	1.0 (0.6)	0.15 (0.08)	0.22 (0.09)	0.44 (0.16)	0.77 (0.39)	1.3 (0.82)	–	↑16%
XIII, U/mL	1.04 (0.55)	0.30	0.4	0.61 (0.36)	1.04 (0.50)	0.96	–	N
PreK, U/mL	1.12 (0.06)	0.13 (0.08)	0.26 (0.14)	0.35 (0.16)	0.86 (0.56)	1.18	–	↑27%
HK, U/mL	0.92 (0.48)	0.15 (0.10)	0.28 (0.20)	0.64 (0.50)	0.82 (0.36)	1.6	–	↑32%

Anticoagulant system							
AT, U/mL	1.0	0.23	0.35	0.56	1.04	1.02	↑ 14%	N
α₂-MG, U/mL	1.05 (0.79)	0.18 (0.10)	—	1.39 (0.95)	1.91 (1.49)	1.53 (0.85)	—	—
C1IN, U/mL	1.01	—	—	0.72	1.41	—	—	—
PC, U/mL	1.0	0.10	0.29	0.50	0.59	0.99	N	N
Total PS, U/mL	1.0 (0.6)	0.15 (0.11)	0.17 (0.14)	0.24 (0.1)	0.87 (0.55)	0.89	—	N
Free, PS, U/mL	1.0 (0.5)	0.22 (0.13)	0.28 (0.19)	0.49 (0.33)	—	0.25	—	—
Heparin	1.01	0.10 (0.06)	0.25 (0.10)	0.49 (0.33)	0.97 (0.59)	—	—	↓ 15%
Cofactor II, U/mL	(0.73)							
TFPI, ng/mL	73	21	20.6	38	—	—	—	—
Fibrinolytic system							
Plasminogen, U/mL	1.0	0.20	0.35 (0.20)	0.37 (0.18)	0.90	1.39	↓ 10%	N
tPA, ng/mL	4.9	—	8.48	9.6	2.8	4.9	↑ 300%	N
α₂-AP, U/mL	1.0	1.0	0.74 (0.5)	0.83 (0.65)	1.11 (0.83)	0.95	N	N
PAI-1, U/mL	1.0	—	1.5	1.0	1.07	4.0	↓ 5%	N
Overall fibrinolysis	N	↑	↑	↓	—	→	→	→

Except as otherwise indicated values are mean ±2 standard deviation (SD) or values in parentheses are lower limits (−2 SD or lower range); +, positive or present; ↓, decreased; ↑, increased; N, normal or no change;* values as ratio or subject/mean of reference range; α2-MG, α2-macroglobulin; ADP, adenosine diphosphate; AT, antithrombin; BT, bleeding time; C1IN, C1 esterase inhibitor; HK, high-molecular-weight kininogen; PAI, plasminogen activator inhibitor; PC, protein C; PreK, prekallikrein; PS, protein S; PT, prothrombin time; PTT, partial thromboplastin time; TCT, thrombin clotting time; TFPI, tissue factor pathway inhibitor; tPA, tissue plasminogen activator; vWF, von Willebrand factor. Overall fibrinolysis is measured by euglobulin lysis time.

Reproduced with permission from Goodnight SH, Hathaway WE: *Disorders of Hemostasis & Thrombosis: A Clinical Guide.* 2nd ed. New York, NY: McGraw Hill; 2001.

General Considerations

Factor VIII (FVIII) activity is reported in units per milliliter, with 1 U/mL equal to 100% of the factor activity found in 1 mL of normal plasma. The normal range for FVIII activity is 0.50–1.50 U/mL (50%–150%). Hemophilia A occurs predominantly in males as an X-linked disorder. One-third of cases are due to a spontaneous mutation. The incidence of FVIII deficiency is 1:5000 male births.

Clinical Findings

A. Symptoms and Signs

Persons with hemophilia who have less than 1% FVIII activity have severe hemophilia A and have frequent spontaneous bleeding episodes involving skin, mucous membranes, joints, muscles, and viscera. In contrast, patients with mild hemophilia A (5%–40% FVIII activity) mainly bleed at times of trauma or surgery. Those with moderate hemophilia A (1% to < 5% FVIII activity) typically have intermediate bleeding manifestations but their treatment should be similar to patients with severe hemophilia. The most crippling aspects of FVIII deficiency are the development of recurrent hemarthroses that incites joint destruction, and the sequelae of intracranial hemorrhage.

B. Laboratory Findings

Individuals with hemophilia A have a prolonged activated partial thromboplastin time (aPTT), except in some cases of mild deficiency, where the partial thromboplastin time (PTT) is normal. The diagnosis is confirmed by a decreased FVIII activity with normal vWF activity. In two-thirds of families of people with hemophilia (PwH), female carriers may manifest symptomatic bleeding. Carriers of hemophilia can be diagnosed by DNA sequencing, and their bleeding severity by factor activity. In a male fetus or newborn with a family history of hemophilia A, cord blood sampling for FVIII activity is accurate.

Complications

Intracranial hemorrhage is the leading disease-related cause of death among persons with hemophilia. Most intracranial hemorrhages in moderate to severe deficiency are spontaneous and not associated with trauma. Hemarthroses begin early in childhood and, when recurrent, can result in joint destruction (ie, hemophilic arthropathy). Large intramuscular hematomas can lead to compartment syndrome with resultant neurologic compromise or pseudotumors. Although these complications are most common in severe hemophilia A, they may occur in individuals with moderate or mild disease. Neutralizing antibodies to FVIII, which are a potential serious complication after treatment with FVIII concentrate, develop in up to 30% of patients with severe hemophilia A, especially in patients with absent or large

deletions in the FVIII gene. Inhibitors may be desensitized with regular FVIII infusion (immune tolerance induction). The bispecific monoclonal antibody emicizumab, which is approved for all patients with hemophilia A, is the standard of care for prophylaxis in patients with an FVIII inhibitor. Therapy that bypasses the FVIII inhibitor with recombinant factor VIIa and/or FEIBA (factor eight inhibitor bypassing agent) is used to treat acute hemorrhage in patients with hemophilia A and a high-titer inhibitor. FEIBA is contraindicated for FVIII inhibitor patients using emicizumab.

In prior decades, therapy-related complications in hemophilia A have included factor-related infection with HIV, hepatitis B virus, and hepatitis C virus. Through stringent donor selection, implementation of sensitive screening assays, use of heat or chemical methods for viral inactivation, and development of recombinant products, the risk of these infections is effectively eliminated. Inactivation methods do not eradicate viruses lacking a lipid envelope; therefore, transmission of parvovirus and hepatitis A remains a concern with the use of plasma-derived products. Immunization with hepatitis A and hepatitis B vaccines is recommended for hemophilia patients.

Treatment

The general aim of management is to raise the FVIII activity to prevent or stop bleeding. Some patients with mild FVIII deficiency may respond to desmopressin via release of endothelial stores of FVIII and vWF into plasma; however, many patients still require administration of exogenous FVIII to achieve hemostasis. The in vivo half-life of infused standard half-life FVIII is 6–14 hours but varies among PwH. Non–life-threatening, non–limb-threatening hemorrhage is treated with 20–30 U/kg of FVIII, to achieve a plasma FVIII activity of 40%–60%. Joint hemarthrosis and life- or limb-threatening hemorrhage is treated with 50 U/kg of FVIII, targeting 100% FVIII activity. Subsequent doses are determined according to the site and extent of bleeding, and clinical response to FVIII infusion. In circumstances of poor clinical response, recent change in bleeding frequency, or comorbid illness, monitoring plasma FVIII activity is recommended. For most instances of non–life-threatening hemorrhage in experienced PwH with moderate or severe hemophilia A, treatment can be administered at home, provided adequate intravenous access and management with the hemophilia treatment center.

FVIII prophylaxis to prevent bleeding and arthropathy in severe and moderate hemophilia is the standard of care in pediatric and adult hemophilia. Extended half-life FVIII concentrates have decreased infusion frequency while maintaining low bleeding rates. In addition, multiple nonfactor replacement strategies (eg, emicizumab, Mim8, fitusiran, concizumab, marstacimab, serpinPC) are emerging that may replace FVIII for prophylaxis. Along with gene therapy, which is in phase 3 clinical trial(s), they look to reshape the lives and outcomes of PwH.

Prognosis

The development of innovative, safe, and effective therapies for hemophilia A has resulted in improved long-term survival in recent decades. In addition, comprehensive care managed through hemophilia treatment centers has greatly improved quality of life and level of function.

2. Factor IX Deficiency (Hemophilia B, Christmas Disease)

The mode of inheritance and clinical manifestations of factor IX (FIX) deficiency are the same as those of FVIII deficiency. Hemophilia B is 15%–20% as prevalent as hemophilia A. FIX deficiency is associated with a prolonged aPTT and normal prothrombin time (PT) and thrombin time; however, the aPTT is less sensitive to FIX deficiency than FVIII deficiency. Diagnosis of hemophilia B is made by assaying FIX activity, and severity is determined as with hemophilia A.

The treatment in hemophilia B is infusion of exogenous FIX. Unlike FVIII, about 50% of the administered dose of FIX distributes into the extravascular space. Therefore, 1 U/kg of plasma-derived or recombinant FIX concentrate is expected to increase plasma FIX activity by approximately 1%. FIX typically has a half-life of 18–22 hours in vivo. In contrast to severe FVIII deficiency, only 1%–3% of persons with FIX deficiency develop a FIX inhibitor, but those patients are at risk for anaphylaxis when receiving exogenous FIX. The prognosis for persons with FIX deficiency is comparable to that of patients with FVIII deficiency. Extended half-life factor concentrates have changed treatment of severe and moderate hemophilia B. Gene therapy is available using adeno-associated virus FIX gene addition. Nonfactor therapies (fitusiran, concizumab, marstacimab, serpin PC) are emerging as subcutaneously administered options for prophylaxis.

Croteau S: 2021 clinical trials update: innovations in hemophilia therapy. Am J Hematol 2021;96(1):128–144 [PMID: 33064330].
Srivastava A: WFH Guidelines for the management of hemophilia, 3rd Edition. Haemophilia 2020 Aug;26 Suppl 6:1–158 [PMID: 32744769].

3. Factor XI Deficiency (Hemophilia C)

Factor XI (FXI) deficiency is a genetic, autosomal coagulopathy, typically of mild to moderate clinical severity. Cases of FXI deficiency account for less than 5% of all persons living with hemophilia. Homozygous individuals generally bleed at surgery or following severe trauma and at hyperfibrinolytic sites but do not commonly have spontaneous hemarthroses. In contrast to FVIII and FIX deficiencies, FXI activity is less predictive of bleeding risk. Pathologic bleeding may be seen in heterozygous individuals with FXI activity as high as 60%. The aPTT is often considerably prolonged. In individuals with deficiency of both plasma and platelet-associated FXI, the PFA-100 may also be prolonged. Management consists of perioperative prophylaxis and episodic therapy for acute hemorrhage with infusion of fresh frozen plasma (FFP). Platelet transfusion may also be useful for acute hemorrhage in patients with deficiency of platelet-associated FXI. rFVIIa use is more common in severe FIX deficiency while antifibrinolytic therapy is used for all severities.

Lewandowska MD: Factor XI deficiency. Hematol Oncol Clin North Am. 2021 Dec;35(6):1157–1169 [PMID: 34535287].

4. Other Inherited Bleeding Disorders

Other hereditary single clotting factor deficiencies are rare and generally autosomal. Homozygous individuals with a deficiency or structural abnormality of prothrombin, factor V, VII, or X may have excessive bleeding.

Persons with dysfibrinogenemia (ie, structurally or functionally abnormal fibrinogen) may develop recurrent venous thromboembolic episodes or bleeding. Immunologic assay of fibrinogen is normal, but clotting assay may be low and the thrombin time prolonged. The PT and aPTT may be prolonged.

Afibrinogenemia resembles hemophilia clinically but has an autosomal recessive inheritance. Affected patients experience a variety of bleeding manifestations, including mucosal bleeding, ecchymoses, hematomas, hemarthroses, and intracranial hemorrhage, especially following trauma. Fatal umbilical cord hemorrhage has been reported. The PT, aPTT, and thrombin time are all prolonged. A severely reduced fibrinogen concentration in an otherwise well child is confirmatory of the diagnosis. As in dysfibrinogenemia, fibrinogen concentrates are used for perioperative prophylaxis and for acute hemorrhage.

Meiejer K: Diagnosis of rare bleeding disorders. Haemophilia 2021;3:60–65 [PMID: 32578312].

VON WILLEBRAND DISEASE

ESSENTIALS OF DIAGNOSIS & TYPICAL FEATURES

- ▶ Easy bruising and epistaxis from early childhood.
- ▶ Menorrhagia.
- ▶ Prolonged PFA-100 normal platelet count, absence of acquired platelet dysfunction.
- ▶ Reduced amount or abnormal activity of vWF.

General Considerations

von Willebrand disease (vWD) is the most common inherited bleeding disorder among Caucasians, with a prevalence as high as 1%. vWF is a multimeric plasma protein that binds FVIII and facilitates platelet adhesion to damaged endothelium. An estimated 70%–80% of all patients with vWD have type 1 vWD, caused by a partial quantitative deficiency of vWF. vWD type 2 involves a qualitative deficiency of (ie, dysfunctional) vWF, and vWD type 3 is characterized by a nearly complete deficiency of vWF. vWD is most often transmitted as an autosomal dominant trait, but it can be autosomal recessive. Acquired vWD is most often caused by the development of an antibody to vWF, or increased turnover of vWF in association with hypothyroidism, Wilms tumor, cardiac disease, renal disease, or systemic lupus erythematosus, and in individuals receiving valproic acid.

Clinical Findings

A. Symptoms and Signs

Mucocutaneous bleeding, increased bruising, and excessive epistaxis is often present. Prolonged bleeding occurs with trauma and surgery. Menorrhagia is often a presenting finding in females.

B. Laboratory Findings

PT is normal and aPTT is prolonged when FVIII is decreased. Prolongation of the PFA-100 is often present. Platelet number may be decreased in type 2b vWD. FVIII and vWF antigen are decreased in types 1 and 3 but may be normal in type 2 vWD. vWF activity (eg, ristocetin cofactor, collagen binding, GP1bM/R) is decreased in all types. Complete laboratory classification also requires vWF multimer or collagen binding assay, and measurement of vWF propeptide for VWD 1C. The diagnosis requires confirmatory laboratory testing.

Treatment

Desmopressin acetate can be given intravenously or subcutaneously to release vWF from endothelial stores in many patients with vWD types 1 and 2 to prevent or halt bleeding. In responding patients, the increase in vWF and FVIII in the plasma can be two- to fivefold. Because response to vWF is variable, FVIII and vWF activities are typically measured before, 30–60 minutes post, and 4 hours after desmopressin administration to document response. Desmopressin causes fluid retention that can result in hyponatremia; therefore, fluid restriction should be discussed. Because release of stored vWF is limited, tachyphylaxis often occurs after two to three administered doses of desmopressin.

If further therapy is indicated, vWF-replacement therapy (plasma-derived or recombinant VWF) is recommended. Such therapy is used in patients with type 1 or 2a vWD who exhibit suboptimal laboratory response to desmopressin, and for all individuals with type 2b or 3 vWD. Antifibrinolytic agents (eg, ε-aminocaproic acid and tranexamic acid) can help control mucosal bleeding. Oral or intrauterine contraceptive therapy may be helpful for menorrhagia.

Prognosis

With the availability of effective treatment and prophylaxis for bleeding, life expectancy in vWD is normal.

http://practical-hemostasis.com (Excellent Practical source for Laboratory Hemostasis). Accessed June 20, 2023.
James PD: ASH USTH NHF WFH 2021 guidelines on the diagnosis of von Willebrand disease. Blood Adv. 2021 Jan 12;5(1):280–300. doi: 10.1182/bloodadvances.2020003265 [PMID: 33570651].

ACQUIRED BLEEDING DISORDERS

1. Disseminated Intravascular Coagulation

ESSENTIALS OF DIAGNOSIS & TYPICAL FEATURES

► Presence of a disorder known to trigger DIC.
► Evidence for consumptive coagulopathy (prolonged aPTT, PT, or thrombin time; increase in FSPs [fibrin-fibrinogen split products] and D-dimer; decreased fibrinogen or platelets).

General Considerations

Disseminated intravascular coagulation (DIC) is an acquired coagulopathy characterized by tissue factor–mediated coagulation activation. DIC involves dysregulated, excessive thrombin generation, with consequent intravascular fibrin deposition and consumption of platelets and procoagulants. Microthrombi, composed of fibrin and platelets, produce tissue ischemia and end-organ damage. The fibrinolytic system is frequently activated in DIC, leading to plasmin-mediated destruction of fibrin and fibrinogen. These fibrin-fibrinogen degradation products (FDPs) exhibit anticoagulant and platelet-inhibitory functions. While DIC commonly accompanies severe infection, other conditions known to trigger DIC include endothelial damage (endotoxin, virus), tissue necrosis (burns), diffuse ischemic injury (shock, hypoxia, and acidosis), and systemic release of tissue procoagulants (certain cancers, placental disorders).

Clinical Findings

A. Symptoms and Signs

Signs of DIC may include (1) complications of shock, often including end-organ dysfunction; (2) diffuse bleeding tendency (eg, hematuria, melena, purpura, petechiae, persistent oozing from needle punctures or other invasive procedures); and (3) evidence of thrombosis (eg, small and large vessel thrombosis, purpura fulminans).

B. Laboratory Findings

Tests that are sensitive, easiest to perform, useful for monitoring, and reflect the hemostatic capacity of the patient are the PT, aPTT, platelet count, fibrinogen, and FDPs (including D-dimer). The PT and aPTT are typically prolonged, and the platelet count and fibrinogen concentration may be decreased. However, in children the fibrinogen level may be normal until late in the course. Levels of FSPs are increased. Elevated levels of D-dimer, a cross-linked fibrin degradation byproduct, may be helpful in monitoring the degree of activation of both coagulation and fibrinolysis. However, D-dimer is nonspecific and may be elevated in the context of a triggering event (eg, severe infection) without concomitant DIC. Often, physiologic inhibitors of coagulation, especially antithrombin III, protein C, and protein S are consumed, predisposing to thrombosis. The specific laboratory abnormalities in DIC may vary with the triggering event and the course of illness.

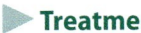 Differential Diagnosis

DIC can be difficult to distinguish from the coagulopathy of liver disease (ie, hepatic synthetic dysfunction), especially when the latter is associated with thrombocytopenia secondary to portal hypertension and hypersplenism. Generally, factor VII activity is decreased markedly in liver disease due to deficient synthesis of this protein, which has the shortest half-life among the procoagulant factors, but only mildly to moderately decreased in DIC (due to consumption). FVIII activity is often normal or even increased in liver disease but decreased in DIC.

▶ Treatment

A. Therapy for Underlying Disorder

The most important aspect of therapy in DIC is the identification and treatment of the triggering event. If the pathogenic process underlying DIC is reversed, often no other therapy is needed.

B. Replacement Therapy for Consumptive Coagulopathy

Replacement of consumed procoagulant factors with FFP, cryoprecipitate, unactivated prothrombin complex concentrates (PCCs), and platelets is warranted in the setting of DIC with hemorrhagic complications, or as periprocedural bleeding prophylaxis. Infusion of 10–15 mL/kg FFP typically raises procoagulant factor activities by approximately 10%–15%. Cryoprecipitate can also be given as a rich source

of fibrinogen, FVIII, vWF, and factor XIII; one bag of cryoprecipitate per 3 kg in infants or one bag of cryoprecipitate per 6 kg in older children typically raises plasma fibrinogen concentration by 75–100 mg/dL.

C. Anticoagulant Therapy for Coagulation Activation

Continuous intravenous infusion of unfractionated heparin is sometimes given to attenuate coagulation activation and consequent consumptive coagulopathy. The rationale for heparin therapy is to maximize the efficacy of, and minimize the need for, replacement of procoagulants and platelets; however, clinical evidence demonstrating benefit of heparin in DIC is lacking. Prophylactic doses of unfractionated heparin or low-molecular-weight heparin (LMWH) in critically ill and nonbleeding patients with DIC may be considered for prevention of VTE.

D. Specific Factor Concentrates

A nonrandomized pilot study of antithrombin concentrate in children with DIC and associated acquired antithrombin deficiency demonstrated favorable outcomes, suggesting that replacement of this consumed procoagulant may be beneficial. Protein C concentrate has also shown promise in two small pilot studies of meningococci-associated DIC with purpura fulminans.

2. Liver Disease

The liver is the major synthetic site of prothrombin, fibrinogen, high-molecular-weight kininogen, and factors V, VII, IX, X, XI, XII, and XIII. Plasminogen and the physiologic anticoagulants (antithrombin III, protein C, and protein S) are synthesized in the liver, as is α_2-antiplasmin, a regulator of fibrinolysis. Deficiency of factor V and the vitamin K–dependent factors (II, VII, IX, and X) is most often a result of decreased hepatic synthesis and is manifested by a prolonged PT and often a prolonged aPTT. Extravascular loss and increased consumption of clotting factors may also contribute to PT and aPTT prolongation. Fibrinogen production is often decreased, or an abnormal fibrinogen (dysfibrinogen) containing excess sialic acid residues may be synthesized, or both. Hypofibrinogenemia or dysfibrinogenemia is associated with prolongation of thrombin time and reptilase time. FSPs and D-dimers may be present because of increased fibrinolysis, particularly in the setting of chronic hepatitis or cirrhosis. Thrombocytopenia secondary to hypersplenism may occur. DIC and the coagulopathy of liver disease also mimic vitamin K deficiency; however, vitamin K deficiency has normal factor V activity. Treatment of acute bleeding in the setting of coagulopathy of liver disease consists of replacement with FFP or PCCs and platelets. Desmopressin may shorten the bleeding time and aPTT in patients with chronic liver disease, but its safety is not well established. Recombinant VIIa can be efficacious for life-threatening refractory hemorrhage.

3. Vitamin K Deficiency

The newborn period is characterized by physiologically depressed activity of the vitamin K–dependent factors (II, VII, IX, and X). If vitamin K is not administered at birth, a bleeding diathesis termed *vitamin K deficiency bleeding* (VKDB), may develop. Outside of the newborn period, vitamin K deficiency may occur because of inadequate intake, excess loss, inadequate formation of active metabolites, or competitive antagonism.

One of three patterns is seen in the neonatal period:

1. Early VKDB occurs within 24 hours of birth, most often manifested by cephalohematoma, intracranial hemorrhage, or intra-abdominal bleeding. Although occasionally idiopathic, it is most often associated with maternal ingestion of drugs that interfere with vitamin K metabolism (eg, warfarin, phenytoin, isoniazid, and rifampin). Early VKDB occurs in 6%–12% of neonates born to mothers who take these medications without receiving vitamin K supplementation. The disorder is life threatening.

2. Classic VKDB occurs at 24 hours to 7 days of age and usually is manifested as gastrointestinal, skin, or mucosal bleeding. Bleeding after circumcision may occur. Although occasionally associated with maternal drug usage, it most often occurs in well infants who do not receive vitamin K at birth and are solely breast-fed.

3. Late neonatal VKDB occurs on or after day 8. Manifestations include intracranial, gastrointestinal, or skin bleeding. This disorder is often associated with fat malabsorption (eg, in chronic diarrhea) or alterations in intestinal flora (eg, with prolonged antibiotic therapy). Like classic VKDB, late VKDB occurs almost exclusively in breast-fed infants.

The diagnosis of vitamin K deficiency is suspected based on the history, physical examination, and laboratory results. The PT is prolonged out of proportion to the aPTT (also prolonged). The thrombin time becomes prolonged late in the course. The platelet count is normal. This laboratory profile is similar to the coagulopathy of acute liver disease, but with normal fibrinogen level and absence of hepatic transaminase elevation. The diagnosis of vitamin K deficiency is confirmed by a demonstration of noncarboxylation of specific clotting factors in the absence of vitamin K in the plasma and by clinical and laboratory responses to vitamin K. Intravenous or subcutaneous treatment with vitamin K should be given immediately and not withheld while awaiting test results. In the setting of severe bleeding, additional acute treatment with FFP or PCCs may be indicated.

4. Uremia

Uremia is frequently associated with acquired platelet dysfunction. Bleeding occurs in approximately 50% of patients with chronic renal failure. The bleeding risk conferred by platelet dysfunction associated with metabolic imbalance may be compounded by decreased vWF activity and procoagulant deficiencies (eg, factors II, XII, XI, and IX) due to increased urinary losses of these proteins in some settings of renal insufficiency. In accordance with platelet dysfunction, uremic bleeding is typically characterized by purpura, epistaxis, menorrhagia, or gastrointestinal hemorrhage. Acute bleeding may be managed with infusion of desmopressin acetate, FVIII concentrates containing vWF, or cryoprecipitate with or without coadministration of FFP. Severe anemia increases the potential for bleeding; therefore, RBC transfusion may be required. Recombinant VIIa may be used in refractory bleeding.

Rajagopal R: Disseminated intravascular coagulation in paediatrics. Arch Dis Child 2017;102:187–193 [PMID: 27540263].
Shearer MJ: Vitamin K deficiency bleeding (VKDB) in early infancy. Blood Rev 2009;23:49–59 [PMID: 18804903].

VASCULAR ABNORMALITIES ASSOCIATED WITH BLEEDING

1. Immunoglobulin A Vasculitis (Henoch-Schönlein Purpura)

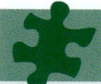

ESSENTIALS OF DIAGNOSIS & TYPICAL FEATURES

▶ Purpuric cutaneous rash.
▶ Migratory polyarthritis or polyarthralgia.
▶ Intermittent abdominal pain.
▶ Nephritis.

▶ General Considerations

Immunoglobulin A vasculitis, which is the most common type of small vessel vasculitis in children, primarily affects boys 2–7 years of age. Occurrence is highest in the spring and fall, and upper respiratory infection precedes the diagnosis in two-thirds of children.

Leukocytoclastic vasculitis in immunoglobulin A vasculitis principally involves the small vessels of the skin, gastrointestinal tract, and kidneys, with deposition of IgA immune complexes. The most common and earliest symptom is palpable purpura, which results from extravasation of erythrocytes into the tissue surrounding the involved venules. Antigens from group A β-hemolytic streptococci and other bacteria, viruses, drugs, foods, and insect bites have been proposed as inciting agents.

Clinical Findings

A. Symptoms and Signs

Skin involvement may start as urticaria; progress to maculopapules; and coalesce to a symmetrical, palpable purpuric rash distributed on the legs, buttocks, and elbows. New lesions may continue to appear for 2–4 weeks and may extend to involve the entire body. Two-thirds of patients develop migratory polyarthralgia or polyarthritis, primarily of the ankles and knees. Intermittent, sharp abdominal pain occurs in approximately 50% of patients, and hemorrhage and edema of the small intestine can often occur. Intussusception may develop. Approximately 25%–50% develop renal involvement in the second or third week of illness with either a nephritic or, less commonly, nephrotic picture, often with high blood pressure. Testicular torsion may also occur. Neurologic symptoms are possible due to small vessel vasculitis.

B. Laboratory Findings

The platelet count is normal or elevated, and other screening tests of hemostasis and platelet function are typically normal. Urinalysis frequently reveals hematuria, and sometimes proteinuria. Stool may be positive for occult blood. The antistreptolysin O (ASO) titer is often elevated and the throat culture positive for group A β-hemolytic streptococci. Serum IgA may be elevated.

Differential Diagnosis

The rash of septicemia (especially meningococcemia) may be similar to skin involvement in immunoglobulin A vasculitis, although the distribution tends to be more generalized. The possibility of trauma should be considered in any child presenting with purpura. Other vasculitides should also be considered. The lesions of thrombotic thrombocytopenic purpura (TTP) are not palpable.

Treatment

Generally, treatment is supportive. NSAIDs may be useful for arthritis. Corticosteroid therapy may provide symptomatic relief for severe gastrointestinal or joint manifestations but does not alter skin or renal manifestations. If culture for group A β-hemolytic streptococci is positive or if the ASO titer is elevated, a course of penicillin is warranted.

Prognosis

The prognosis for recovery is generally good, although symptoms frequently (25%–50%) recur over a period of several months. In patients who develop renal manifestations, microscopic hematuria may persist for years. Progressive renal failure occurs in fewer than 5% of patients with immunoglobulin A vasculitis, with an overall fatality rate of 3%.

Key NS: Vascular hemostasis. Haemophilia 2010 Jul;16(Suppl 5): 146 [PMID: 20590874].

Ozen S: European consensus-based recommendations for diagnosis and treatment of immunoglobulin A vasculitis—the SHARE initiative. Rheumatology (Oxford) 2019 Sep 1;58(9):1607–1616 [PMID: 30879080].

2. Collagen Disorders

Mild to life-threatening bleeding occurs with some types of Ehlers-Danlos syndrome, the most common inherited collagen disorder. Ehlers-Danlos syndrome is characterized by joint hypermobility, skin extensibility, and easy bruising. Coagulation abnormalities may sometimes be present, including platelet dysfunction and deficiencies of coagulation factors VIII, IX, XI, and XIII. However, bleeding and easy bruising, in most instances, relate to fragility of capillaries and compromised vascular integrity. Ehlers-Danlos syndrome types 4 and 6 are associated with at risk for aortic dissection and spontaneous rupture of aortic aneurysms. Surgery should be avoided for patients with Ehlers-Danlos syndrome, as should medications that induce platelet dysfunction.

Jesudas R: An update on the new classification of Ehlers-Danlos syndrome and review of the causes of bleeding in this population. Haemophilia 2019;25(4):558–566 [PMID: 31329366].

THROMBOTIC DISORDERS

General Considerations

Uncommon in children, thrombotic disorders are recognized with increasing frequency because of heightened physician awareness and improved survival in pediatric intensive care settings.

Clinical Findings

Initial evaluation of the child who has thrombosis includes an assessment for potential provoking factors, family history of thrombosis, and early cardiovascular or cerebrovascular disease.

A. Clinical Risk Factors

Clinical risk factors are present in more than 90% of children with acute VTE. These conditions include the presence of an indwelling vascular catheter, cardiac disease, infection, trauma, surgery, immobilization, collagen-vascular or chronic inflammatory disease, renal disease, sickle cell anemia, and malignancy. Prospective findings using serial radiologic evaluation as screening indicate that the risk of VTE is nearly 30% for short-term central venous catheters placed in the internal jugular veins. Retrospective data suggest that approximately 8% of children with cancer develop symptomatic VTE.

1. Inherited Thrombophilia (Hypercoagulable) States

A. PROTEIN C DEFICIENCY—Protein C is a vitamin K–dependent protein activated by thrombin bound to thrombomodulin, which inactivates activated factors V and VIII. In addition, activated protein C promotes fibrinolysis. Two phenotypes of hereditary protein C deficiency exist. Heterozygous individuals with autosomal dominant protein C deficiency often present with VTE as young adults, but the disorder may present during childhood or in later adulthood. In mild protein C deficiency, anticoagulant prophylaxis is typically limited to periods of increased prothrombotic risk. Homozygous or compound heterozygous protein C deficiency is rare and phenotypically severe. Affected children generally present within the first 12 hours of life with purpura fulminans (Figure 30–6) and/or VTE. Prompt protein C replacement by infusion of protein C concentrate or FFP every 6–12 hours, along with therapeutic heparin administration, is recommended. Subsequent management requires chronic therapeutic anticoagulation, often with protein C concentrate infusion. Recurrent VTE is common, especially during periods of subtherapeutic anticoagulation or in the presence of conditions associated with increased prothrombotic risk.

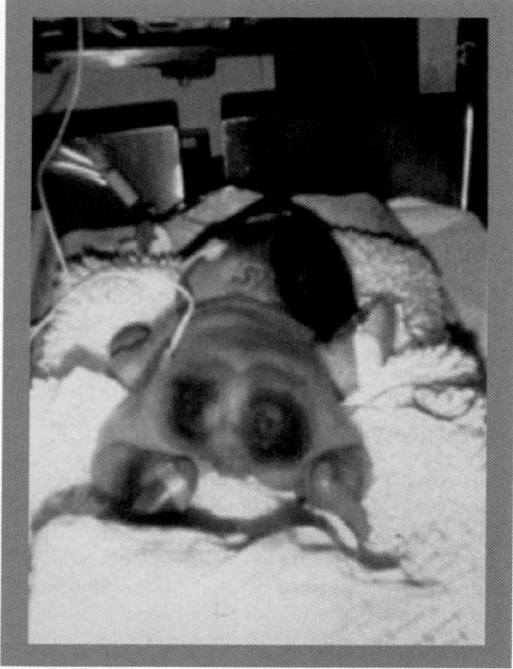

▲ **Figure 30–6.** Purpura fulminans in an infant with severe protein C deficiency.

B. PROTEIN S DEFICIENCY—Protein S is a cofactor for protein C. Neonates with homozygous protein S deficiency are similar to those with homozygous or compound heterozygous protein C deficiency. Lifelong anticoagulation therapy is indicated in homozygous/severe deficiency, or in heterozygous individuals who have experienced recurrent VTE. Efforts must be made to distinguish these conditions from acquired deficiency, which can be antibody-mediated or secondary to an increase in C4b-binding protein induced by inflammation.

C. ANTITHROMBIN DEFICIENCY—Antithrombin, which is the most important physiologic inhibitor of thrombin, also inhibits activated factors IX, X, XI, and XII. Antithrombin deficiency is transmitted in an autosomal dominant pattern and associated with VTE, typically with onset in adolescence or young adulthood. Therapy for acute VTE is therapeutic anticoagulation. The efficiency of heparin may be significantly diminished in the setting of severe antithrombin deficiency and may require supplementation with antithrombin concentrate. Patients with homozygous/severe deficiency or recurrent VTE are maintained on lifelong anticoagulation.

D. FACTOR V LEIDEN MUTATION—An amino acid substitution in the gene coding for factor V results in factor V Leiden, a factor V polymorphism that is resistant to inactivation by activated protein C. The most common cause of activated protein C resistance in Caucasians, factor V Leiden is present in approximately 5% of the Caucasian population, 20% of Caucasian adults with deep vein thrombosis (DVT), and 40%–60% of those with a family history of VTE. VTE occurs in both heterozygous and homozygous individuals. For heterozygous individuals, thrombosis is typically triggered by a clinical risk factor (or else develops in association with additional thrombophilia traits), whereas in homozygous people it can be spontaneous. Population studies suggest that the risk of incident VTE is increased two- to sevenfold in the setting of heterozygous factor V Leiden, 35-fold among heterozygous individuals taking the oral contraceptives, and 80-fold in those homozygous for factor V Leiden.

E. PROTHROMBIN MUTATION—The 20210 glutamine to alanine mutation in the prothrombin gene is a common polymorphism in Caucasians that enhances its activation to thrombin. In heterozygous form, this mutation is associated with a two- to threefold increased risk for incident VTE. This mutation also appears to modestly increase the risk for recurrent VTE.

F. OTHER INHERITED DISORDERS—Qualitative abnormalities of fibrinogen (dysfibrinogenemias) are usually inherited in an autosomal dominant manner. Most individuals with dysfibrinogenemia are asymptomatic. Some patients experience bleeding, while others develop venous or arterial thrombosis. The diagnosis is suggested by a prolonged thrombin time with a normal fibrinogen concentration. Hyperhomocysteinemia, which can be inherited or acquired, is associated with an increased risk for both arterial and venous thromboses. In children, it may be a risk factor for ischemic arterial stroke. Hyperhomocysteinemia is uncommon in the setting of dietary folate supplementation (as in the United States) and observed almost uniquely in cases of renal insufficiency or metabolic disease (eg, homocystinuria). Methylene tetrahydrofolate reductase receptor mutations do not appear to constitute a risk factor for thrombosis in US children unless homocysteine is elevated.

Lipoprotein(a) is a lipoprotein with homology to plasminogen. In vitro studies suggest that lipoprotein(a) may both promote atherosclerosis and inhibit fibrinolysis. Some evidence suggests that elevated plasma concentrations of lipoprotein(a) are associated with an increased risk of VTEs and recurrent ischemic arterial stroke in children.

Increased FVIII activity is a risk factor for incident VTE and is common among children with acute VTE. Most elevations in FVIII are acquired (acute phase reactant) but may also be inherited.

2. Acquired Disorders

A. ANTIPHOSPHOLIPID ANTIBODIES—The development of antiphospholipid antibodies is the most common form of acquired thrombophilia in children. Antiphospholipid antibodies, which include the lupus anticoagulant, anticardiolipin antibodies, and β_2-glycoprotein-1 antibodies (among others), can be present in acute childhood VTE. The lupus anticoagulant is detected in vitro by its inhibition of phospholipid-dependent coagulation assays (eg, aPTT, dilute Russell viper venom time, hexagonal phase phospholipid neutralization assay), whereas immunologic techniques (eg, enzyme-linked immunosorbent assays) are often used to detect anticardiolipin and β_2-glycoprotein-1 antibodies. While common in patients with autoimmune diseases such as systemic lupus erythematosus, antiphospholipid antibodies may also develop following certain drug exposures, infection, acute inflammation, and lymphoproliferative diseases. VTE and antiphospholipid antibodies may predate other signs of lupus. Viral illness is a common precipitant in children, and in many cases, the inciting infection may be asymptomatic.

When an antiphospholipid antibody persists for 12 weeks following an acute thrombotic event, the diagnosis of antiphospholipid syndrome (APS) is confirmed. Optimal duration of anticoagulation in this setting is unclear. Current pediatric treatment guidelines recommend a 3-month to lifelong course.

B. DEFICIENCIES OF INTRINSIC ANTICOAGULANTS— Acquired deficiencies of proteins C and S and antithrombin may be caused by specific antibodies (eg, protein S antibodies in varicella) or by excessive consumption, such as during sepsis, DIC, major-vessel or extensive VTE, and post–bone marrow transplant sinusoidal obstruction syndrome. Pilot studies in children have suggested a possible therapeutic role for antithrombin or protein C concentrates in sepsis-associated DIC (eg, meningococcemia) and severe posttransplant sinusoidal obstruction syndrome.

C. ACUTE PHASE REACTANTS—As part of the acute phase response, elevations in plasma fibrinogen concentration, plasma FVIII, vWF, and platelets may occur, all of which may contribute to an acquired prothrombotic state. Reactive thrombocytosis is rarely associated with VTEs in children when the platelet count is less than 1 million/μL.

B. Symptoms and Signs

Presenting features of thrombosis vary with the anatomic site, extent of vascular involvement, degree of vaso-occlusion, and the presence of end-organ dysfunction. The presentation of deep venous thrombosis of an upper or lower extremity is pain with acute or subacute extremity swelling, while pulmonary embolism commonly presents as dyspnea and pleuritic chest pain, and cerebral sinovenous thrombosis (CSVT) often includes severe or persistent headache, with or without neurologic deficit in otherwise well children. Arterial thrombosis of the lower extremity (eg, neonatal umbilical artery catheter–associated) as well as vasospasm without identified thrombosis, often manifests with diminished distal pulses and dusky discoloration of the limb.

C. Laboratory Findings

A comprehensive laboratory investigation for thrombophilia (ie, hypercoagulability) remains controversial with wide variation of practice. Recent trends favor thrombophilia testing in infants, children, and adolescents with unprovoked thrombosis, and in neonates/children with non–catheter-related thrombosis and stroke. There are insufficient data to recommend routine thrombophilia testing in neonates or children with catheter-related thrombosis. When indicated, thrombophilia testing can include: evaluation for intrinsic anticoagulant deficiency (proteins C and S and antithrombin), procoagulant factor excess (eg, FVIII), genetic mutations mediating enhanced procoagulant activity or reduced sensitivity to inactivation (factor V Leiden, prothrombin 20210 polymorphisms), biochemical mediators of endothelial damage (homocysteine), markers or regulators of fibrinolysis (eg, D-dimer, plasminogen activator inhibitor-1, and lipoprotein[a]), and antiphospholipid antibodies (DRVVT, Hex-PTT, anticardiolipin and anti-B2 GP1 antibodies). Interpretation of procoagulant factor and intrinsic anticoagulant levels should recognize the age-dependent normal values. Among VTE risk factors, antiphospholipid antibodies and elevated levels of homocysteine and lipoprotein(a) have also been demonstrated as risk factors for arterial thrombotic ischemic events.

D. Imaging

Appropriate radiologic imaging is essential for objective documentation of thrombosis and to delineate the type (venous vs arterial), degree of occlusion, and extent (proximal and distal termini) of thrombosis. Depending on site, typical imaging modalities include compression ultrasound with Doppler, computed tomographic (CT) venography, magnetic resonance venography, and conventional angiography.

▶ Treatment

Current guidelines for the treatment of first-episode VTE in children are largely based on adult experience and include therapeutic anticoagulation for at least 3 months. During the period of anticoagulation, bleeding precautions should be followed, as previously described (see section Treatment under Idiopathic Thrombocytopenic Purpura, earlier). Initial therapy for acute VTE uses continuous intravenous unfractionated heparin or subcutaneous injections of LMWH for at least 7 days, monitored by anti-Xa activity level to maintain safe and therapeutic anticoagulant levels of 0.3–0.7 or 0.5–1.0 IU/mL, respectively. Subsequent extended anticoagulant therapy is given with LMWH, daily oral warfarin, the latter agent monitored by the PT to maintain an international normalized ratio (INR) of 2.0–3.0, or a direct oral anticoagulant (DOAC). During warfarin treatment, the INR optimally should be within the therapeutic range before discontinuation of heparin. Warfarin pharmacokinetics are affected by acute illness, numerous medications, and changes in diet, and can necessitate frequent monitoring. In children, warfarin dose is determined by age and weight. LMWH offers the advantage of infrequent need for monitoring but is more expensive and difficult to administer than warfarin. Anatomic contributions to venous stasis (eg, mastoiditis or depressed skull fracture as risk factors for cerebral sinus venous thrombosis or congenital left iliac vein stenosis in DVT of proximal left lower extremity with May-Thurner anomaly) should be addressed to optimize response to anticoagulation. In cases of limb- or life-threatening VTEs, including massive proximal pulmonary embolus, and in cases of progressive VTE despite therapeutic anticoagulation, thrombolytic therapy (eg, tissue-type plasminogen activator) may be considered. In adolescent females, estrogen-containing contraceptives are relatively contraindicated in those with prior VTE if not using anticoagulation, particularly if an additional genetic cause for impairment of protein C pathway is disclosed.

DOACs (dabigatran, rivaroxaban, apixaban) are now first-line therapy for childhood and adult acute VTE and for extended anticoagulation.

▶ Prognosis

Recurrent VTE occurs in approximately 10% of children within 2 years. Persistent thrombosis is evident following completion of a standard therapeutic course of anticoagulation in up to 30% of children, with unclear clinical importance. Approximately one in four children with DVT

involving the extremities develop postthrombotic syndrome (PTS), a condition of venous insufficiency of varying severity characterized by chronic skin changes, edema, and dilated collateral superficial venous formation. PTS is often accompanied by functional limitation (pain with activities or at rest); less common are venous stasis ulcers and cellulitis. Complete veno-occlusion and elevated levels of FVIII and D-dimer at VTE diagnosis are negative prognostic factors for developing PTS among children with DVT affecting the limbs. The presence of homozygous anticoagulant deficiencies, multiple thrombophilia traits, or persistent antiphospholipid antibodies following VTE diagnosis has been associated with increased risk of recurrent VTE, leading to consideration of extended anticoagulation in these instances.

Monagle P: American Society of Hematology 2018 Guidelines for management of venous thromboembolism: treatment of pediatric venous thromboembolism. Blood Adv 2018 Nov 27;2(22):3292–3316 [PMID: 30482766].

Witmer C: Treatment of venous thromboembolism in pediatric patients. Blood 2020;135(5):335–343 [PMID: 31917400].

▼ SPLENIC ABNORMALITIES

SPLENOMEGALY & HYPERSPLENISM

The differential diagnosis of splenomegaly includes the categories of congestive splenomegaly, chronic infections, leukemia and lymphomas, hemolytic anemias, reticuloendothelioses, and storage diseases (Table 30–8).

Splenomegaly due to any cause may be associated with hypersplenism and the excessive destruction of circulating red cells, white cells, and platelets. The degree of cytopenia is variable and, when mild, requires no specific therapy. In other cases, the thrombocytopenia may cause life-threatening bleeding, particularly when the splenomegaly is secondary to portal hypertension and associated with esophageal varices or the consequence of a storage disease. In such cases, treatment with surgical splenectomy or with splenic embolization may be warranted. Although more commonly associated with acute enlargement, rupture of an enlarged spleen can be seen in more chronic conditions such as Gaucher disease.

Stirnemann J: A review of Gaucher disease pathophysiology, clinical presentation and treatments. Int J Mol Sci 2017;18(2) [PMID: 28218669].

ASPLENIA & SPLENECTOMY

Children who lack normal splenic function are at risk for sepsis, meningitis, and pneumonia due to encapsulated bacteria such as pneumococci, meningococcus, and *H influenzae*. Such infections are often fulminant and fatal because of

Table 30–8. Causes of chronic splenomegaly in children.

Cause	Associated Clinical Findings	Diagnostic Investigation
Congestive splenomegaly	History of umbilical vein catheter or neonatal omphalitis; signs of portal hypertension (varices, hemorrhoids, dilated abdominal wall veins); pancytopenia; history of hepatitis or jaundice	Complete blood count, platelet count, liver function tests, ultrasonography
Chronic infections	History of exposure to tuberculosis, histoplasmosis, coccidioidomycosis, other fungal disease; chronic sepsis (foreign body in bloodstream; subacute infective endocarditis)	Appropriate cultures and skin tests, i.e., blood cultures; PPD, fungal serology and antigen tests, chest film; HIV serology
Infectious mononucleosis	Fever, fatigue, pharyngitis, rash, adenopathy, hepatomegaly	Atypical lymphocytes on blood smear, monospot, EBV antibody titers
Leukemia, lymphoma, Hodgkin disease	Evidence of systemic involvement with fever, bleeding tendencies, hepatomegaly, and lymphadenopathy; pancytopenia	Blood smear, bone marrow examination, chest film, gallium scan, LDH, uric acid
Hemolytic anemia	Anemia, jaundice; family history of anemia, jaundice, and gallbladder disease in young adults	Reticulocyte count, Coombs test, blood smear, osmotic fragility test, hemoglobin electrophoresis
Reticuloendothelioses (histiocytosis X)	Chronic otitis media, seborrheic or petechial skin rashes, anemia, infections, lymphadenopathy, hepatomegaly, bone lesions	Skeletal radiographs for bone lesions; biopsy of bone, liver, bone marrow, or lymph node
Storages diseases	Family history of similar disorders, neurologic involvement, evidence of macular degeneration, hepatomegaly	Biopsy of liver or bone marrow in search for storage cells; specific enzyme measurements; genetic evaluation
Splenic cyst	Evidence of other infections (postinfectious cyst) or congenital anomalies; peculiar shape of spleen	Radionuclide scan, ultrasonography
Splenic hemangioma	Other hemangiomas, consumptive coagulopathy	Radionuclide scan, arteriography, platelet count, coagulation screen

EBV, Epstein-Barr virus; HIV, human immunodeficiency virus; LDH, lactic dehydrogenase; PPD, purified protein derivative.

inadequate antibody production and impaired phagocytosis of circulating bacteria.

Congenital asplenia is usually suspected when an infant is born with abnormalities of abdominal viscera and complex cyanotic congenital heart disease. Howell-Jolly bodies are usually present on the peripheral blood smear, and the absence of splenic tissue is confirmed by technetium radionuclide scanning. The prognosis depends on the underlying cardiac lesions, and many children die during the first few months. Prophylactic antibiotics, usually penicillin, and pneumococcal conjugate and subsequent pneumococcal polysaccharide, Hib, and meningococcal conjugate vaccines are recommended.

The risk of overwhelming sepsis following surgical splenectomy is related to the child's age and to the underlying disorder. Because the risk is highest when the procedure is performed earlier in life, splenectomy is usually postponed until after age 5 years. The risk of postsplenectomy sepsis is also greater in children with malignancies, thalassemias, and reticuloendothelioses than in children whose splenectomy is performed for ITP, hereditary spherocytosis, or trauma. Prior to splenectomy, children should be immunized against *Streptococcus pneumoniae*, *H influenzae*, and *Neisseria meningitidis*. Additional management should include penicillin

prophylaxis and prompt evaluation for fever 38.5°C or above or signs of severe infection.

Children with sickle cell anemia develop functional asplenia during the first year of life, and overwhelming sepsis is the leading cause of early deaths in this disease. Prophylactic penicillin reduces the incidence of sepsis by 84%.

Robinson CL: Advisory Committee on Immunization Practices recommended immunization schedule for children and adolescents aged 18 years or younger—United States, 2020. MMWR Morb Mortal Wkly Rep 2019;69(5):130–132 [PMID: 332027628].
Rubin LG: Care of the asplenic patient. New Engl J Med 2014; 371:349–356 [PMID: 25054718].

TRANSFUSION MEDICINE

DONOR SCREENING & BLOOD PROCESSING: RISK MANAGEMENT

Minimizing the risks of transfusion begins by screening volunteer donors with a universal donor questionnaire designed to protect the recipient from transmission of infectious agents as well as other risks of transfusions. The questions focus on identifying donors at higher risk for possible transmission of HIV, hepatitis, and other diseases. Positive responses may result in temporary or permanent deferral from donation. In 2023, the FDA released guidance eliminating mandatory donor deferrals of men who have sex with men.

Before blood components can be released for transfusion, donor blood is screened for hepatitis B surface antigen; antibodies to hepatitis B core antigen, hepatitis C, HIV-1 and 2, and human T-cell lymphotropic virus (HTLV) I and II; and a serologic test for syphilis. Screening donor blood for viral genome (nucleic acid amplification [NAAT] testing) is done for HIV, HCV, West Nile virus, and Zika virus.

Positive tests are repeated. If confirmed, the unit is destroyed and the donor notified and deferred from future donations. Many of the screening tests used are very sensitive and have a high false-positive rate. As a result, confirmatory tests have been developed to check the initial screening results and separate the false positives from the true positives. This allows donors with reactive screening tests on a specific donation to be reentered into the donor pool in the future if they meet specifications of an algorithm for further testing. Bacterial culture of apheresis or pooled platelet concentrates is included in the testing paradigm.

With these approaches, the risk of transmitting an infection with blood components has been minimized. The absolute risk of hepatitis C or HIV transmission from blood transfusion is less than 1:1–2 million and hepatitis B transmission less than 1:500,000. Recent addition of pathogen reduction techniques to blood components will provide an additional strategy to reduce transfusion-transmitted infections and reduce the expense of additional testing for emerging infectious agents associated with blood transfusion.

Primary CMV infections are significant complications of blood transfusion in transplant recipients, neonates, and immunodeficient individuals. Transmission of CMV can be avoided by using seronegative donors, apheresis platelet concentrates collected by techniques ensuring low numbers of residual white cells, or red cell or platelet products that are leukocyte-depleted by filtration (<5 million WBCs per packed red cell unit or apheresis platelet concentrate equivalent).

PRETRANSFUSION TESTING

Donated blood and recipient samples are tested for ABO and Rh(D) antigens and screened for auto- or alloantibodies in the plasma. The cross-match is required on any component that contains red cells. In the major cross-match, washed donor red cells are incubated with the serum from the patient, and reactivity or agglutination is detected and

graded after immediate centrifugation. The antiglobulin phase of the test is then performed; Coombs reagent, which will detect the presence of IgG or complement on the surface of the red cells, is added to the mixture, and reactivity evaluated. In the presence of a negative antibody screen in the recipient, a negative immediate spin cross-match test confirms the compatibility of the blood and antiglobulin phase is not required. Further testing is required if the antibody screen or the cross-match is positive, and blood should not be given until the nature of the reactivity is delineated. An incompatible cross-match is evaluated first with a DAT or Coombs test to detect IgG or complement on the surfaces of the recipient's red cells. The IAT is also used to determine the presence of antibodies that will coat red cells or activate complement, and additional studies are completed to define the antibody.

TRANSFUSION PRACTICE

General Rules

Several rules should be observed in administering any blood component:

1. Transfusion consent should be verified before administration of any blood product.
2. Before transfusion, the blood component should be inspected visually for any unusual characteristics, such as the presence of flocculent material, hemolysis, or clumping of cells, and mixed thoroughly.
3. The unit and the recipient should be identified properly.
4. The administration set includes a standard 170- to 260-μm filter. Under certain clinical circumstances, an additional microaggregate filter may be used to eliminate small aggregates of fibrin, white cells, and platelets that will not be removed by the standard filter.
5. The patient should be observed during the entire transfusion, more closely during the first 15 minutes. With the onset of any adverse symptoms or signs, the transfusion should be stopped, an evaluation initiated immediately, and the reaction reported promptly to the transfusion service. Untransfused components, blood samples from the patient, and appropriate paperwork should also be submitted to the transfusion service.
6. When cross-match–incompatible red cells or whole blood unit(s) must be given to the patient (as with AIHA), a test dose of 10% of the total volume (not to exceed 50 mL) should be administered over 15–20 minutes; the transfusion is then stopped and the patient observed. If no changes in vital signs or the patient's condition are noted, the remainder of the volume can be infused carefully.

7. Blood for exchange transfusion in the newborn period should be cross-matched with either the infant's or the mother's serum or plasma. If the exchange is for hemolysis, 1 unit of whole blood stored for less than 5–7 days will be adequate. If replacement of clotting factors is the goal, packed red cells reconstituted with ABO type-specific FFP may be considered. Based on posttransfusion platelet counts, additional platelet transfusion may be considered. Other problems to be anticipated are acid–base derangements, hyponatremia, hyperkalemia, hypocalcemia, hypoglycemia, hypothermia, and hypervolemia or hypovolemia.

Choice of Blood Component

Several principles should be considered when deciding on the need for blood transfusion. Indications for blood or blood components must be well defined, and the patient's medical condition, not just the laboratory results, should be the basis for the decision. Specific deficiencies exhibited by the patient (eg, oxygen-carrying capacity, thrombocytopenia) should be treated with appropriate blood components and the use of whole blood minimized. In general, very little is established about specific indications for blood component transfusion and outcomes. In recent years, the criteria have become more restrictive for transfusion of any component. A recent review evaluates what is known and presents fertile areas for investigation (see Josephson et al).

A. Whole Blood

In general, whole blood is rarely transfused in pediatric patients as specific blood components are preferred. The usual indication is for resuscitation in the setting of massive hemorrhage.

B. Packed Red Blood Cells

Packed red blood cell (PRBC) units are typically given to restore oxygen carrying capacity and prevent cardiopulmonary compromise in the setting of severe anemia or blood loss. The typical unit size is 200–250 mL and is transfused over 2–4 hours based on cardiovascular status. Transfusion of 10 mL/kg of PRBCs typically increases the patient's hemoglobin by about 2–3 g/dL.

C. Platelets

The decision to transfuse platelets depends on the patient's clinical condition, the status of plasma phase coagulation, the platelet count, the cause of the thrombocytopenia, and the functional capacity of the patient's platelets. In the face of decreased production, clinical bleeding, and platelet counts less than $10,000/\mu L$, the risk of severe, spontaneous bleeding is increased markedly. In the presence of these factors and in the absence heparin-induced thrombocytopenia, TTP, or antibody-mediated thrombocytopenia, transfusion may be considered. Under certain circumstances, especially with platelet dysfunction or treatment that inhibits the procoagulant system, transfusions at higher platelet counts may be necessary.

Transfused platelets are sequestered temporarily in the lungs and spleen before reaching their peak concentrations, 45–60 minutes after transfusion. A significant proportion of the transfused platelets never circulate but remain sequestered in the spleen. This phenomenon results in reduced recovery; under best conditions, only 60%–70% of the transfused platelets are accounted for in the peripheral platelet count increments used to measure response.

In addition to cessation of bleeding, two variables indicate the effectiveness of platelet transfusions. The first is platelet recovery, as measured by the maximum number of platelets circulating in response to transfusion. The practical measure is the platelet count at 1 hour after transfusion. In the absence of immune or drastic nonimmune factors that markedly decrease platelet recovery, one would expect a $7000/\mu L$ increment for each random donor unit and a 40,000–70,000/μL increment for each single-donor apheresis unit in a large child or adolescent. For infants and small children, 10 mL/kg of platelets will increase the platelet count by at least $50,000/\mu L$. The second variable is the survival of transfused platelets. If the recovery is greater than $50,000/\mu L$, transfused platelets will approach a normal half-life in the circulation. In the presence of increased platelet destruction, the lifespan may be shortened to a few days or a few hours. Frequent platelet transfusions may be required to maintain adequate hemostasis.

A particularly troublesome outcome in patients receiving long-term platelet transfusions is the development of a refractory state characterized by poor ($\leq 20\%$) recovery or no response to platelet transfusion (as measured at 1 hour). Most (70%–90%) of these refractory states result from the development of alloantibodies directed against HLA antigens on the platelet. Platelets have Class I HLA antigens, and the antibodies are primarily against HLA A or B determinants. A smaller proportion of these alloantibodies (<10%) may be directed against platelet-specific alloantigens. The most effective approach to prevent HLA sensitization is to use leukocyte-depleted components (< 5 million leukocytes per unit of packed red cells or per apheresis or 6–10 random donor unit concentrates). For the alloimmunized, refractory patient, the best approach is to provide HLA-matched platelets for transfusion. Platelet cross-matching procedures using HLA-matched or unmatched donors may be helpful in identifying platelet concentrates most likely to provide an adequate response.

D. Fresh Frozen Plasma

FFP contains greater than 80% of all procoagulant and anticoagulant plasma proteins. Primary indications for infusion of FFP include replacement of clotting factors in the bleeding patient with decreased liver production or increased consumption with INR greater than 1.5, warfarin reversal, treatment of TTP by providing a source of ADAMTS13, and treatment of bleeding in patients with congenital deficiencies of clotting factors if specific concentrates are not available. The usual dose is 10–15 mL/kg, which results in an increase in most clotting factor levels of 10%–20%.

E. Cryoprecipitate

Cryoprecipitate is produced by freezing fresh plasma to less than −65°C and then thawing for 18 hours at 4°C. After centrifugation, the final product contains concentrated amounts of FVIII, vWF, fibrinogen, fibronectin, and factor XIII. The main indications for cryoprecipitate administration are treatment of acquired or congenital deficiencies of fibrinogen or factor XIII. It can also be used for patients with FVIII deficiency or von Willebrand if factor-specific concentrates are not available. The usual dose is ½ pack/kg body weight that will increase FVIII levels by 80%–100% or fibrinogen by 200–250 mg/dL.

F. Granulocytes

With better supportive care over the past 20 years, the need for granulocytes in neutropenic patients with severe bacterial infections has decreased. Indications remain for severe bacterial or fungal infections unresponsive to vigorous medical therapy in either newborns or older children with bone marrow failure, or patients with neutrophil dysfunction. Mobilization schemes using G-CSF and steroids in donors result in granulocyte collections with at least 50 billion neutrophils. This may provide a better product for patients requiring granulocyte support.

G. Apheresis Products and Procedures

Apheresis equipment allows one or more blood components to be collected while the rest are returned to the donor. Apheresis platelet concentrates, which have as many platelets as 6–10 units of platelet concentrates from whole blood donations, are one example; granulocytes are another. Apheresis techniques can also be used to collect hematopoietic stem cells that have been mobilized into the blood by cytokines (eg, G-CSF) or mononuclear cells for immunotherapy. Stem cells are used for allogeneic or autologous bone marrow transplantation. Blood cell separators can be used for the collection of single-source plasma or removal of a blood component that is causing disease. Examples include red cell exchange in sickle cell disease and plasmapheresis in Goodpasture syndrome, Guillain-Barré syndrome, or other antibody-mediated disorders.

Adverse Effects

The noninfectious complications of blood transfusions are outlined in Table 30–9. Most complications present a significant risk to the recipient. Blood product modifications may

Table 30–9. Adverse events following transfusions.

Event	Pathophysiology	Signs and Symptoms	Management
Acute hemolytic transfusion reaction	Preformed alloantibodies (most commonly to ABO) and infrequently autoantibodies cause rapid intravascular hemolysis of transfused cells with activation of clotting (DIC), activation of inflammatory mediators, and acute renal failure.	Fever, chills, nausea, chest pain, back pain, pain at transfusion site, hypotension, dyspnea, oliguria, hemoglobinuria.	The risk of this type of reaction overall is low (1:70,000–1:30,000), but the mortality rate is high (up to 40%). Stop the transfusion; maintain renal output with intravenous fluids and diuretics (furosemide or mannitol); treat DIC with heparin; and institute other appropriate supportive measures.
Delayed hemolytic transfusion reaction	Formation of alloantibodies after transfusion and resultant destruction of transfused red cells, usually by extravascular hemolysis.	Jaundice, anemia. A small percentage may develop chronic hemolysis.	Detection, definition, and documentation (for future transfusions). Supportive care. Risk, < 5% of transfused patients may develop alloantibody; hemolysis, 1:11,000–1:2500.
Febrile reactions	Usually caused by leukoagglutinins in recipient, cytokines, or other biologically active compounds.	Fever. May also involve chills.	Supportive. Leukocyte-reduced products decrease reactions. Risk per transfusion, 1:100 transfusions.

(Continued)

Table 30–9. Adverse events following transfusions. (*Continued*)

Event	Pathophysiology	Signs and Symptoms	Management
Allergic reactions	Most causes not identified. In IgA deficient individuals, reaction occurs as a result of antibodies to IgA.	Itching, hives, and occasionally chills and fever. In severe reactions, may see signs of anaphylaxis: dyspnea, pulmonary edema.	Mild to moderate reactions: diphenhydramine. More severe reactions: epinephrine subcutaneously and steroids intravenously. Risk for mild to moderate allergic reactions, 1:100. Severe anaphylactic reactions, 1:50,000–1:20,000.
Transfusion-related acute lung injury	Acute lung injury occurring within 6 h after transfusion. Two sets of factors interact to produce the syndrome. Patient factors: infection, surgery, cytokine therapy. Blood component factors: lipids, antibodies, cytokines. Two groups of factors interact during transfusion to result in lung injury indistinguishable from ARDS.	Tachypnea, dyspnea, hypoxia. Diffuse interstitial markings. Cardiac evaluation normal.	May consider younger products: packed red blood cells ≤ 2 wk, platelets ≤ 3 days, washing components to prevent syndrome. Management: supportive care. Risk, 1:2000–1:3000 per transfusion. Current preventive procedures include avoiding donors at risk for alloimmunization: use of male-only FFP or white blood cell antibody-negative apheresis FFP or platelet products.
Transfusion-associated circulatory overload	Circulatory volume overload occurring within 6 hours of cessation of transfusion. Risk factors: age, history of heart failure, number of units transfused.	Acute respiratory distress, elevated brain natriuretic peptide, elevated central venous pressure, left heart failure, positive fluid balance, pulmonary edema.	Stop the transfusion; administer supplemental oxygen if needed; diuretics; ventilatory support.
Dilutional coagulopathy	Massive blood loss and transfusion with replacement with fluids or blood components and deficient clotting factors.	Bleeding.	Replacement of clotting factors or platelets with appropriate blood components.
Bacterial contamination	Contamination of units results in growth of bacteria or production of clinically significant levels of endotoxin.	Chills, high fever, hypotension, other symptoms of sepsis or endotoxemia.	Stop transfusion; make aggressive attempts to identify organism; provide vigorous support. Sepsis in 1:500,000–1:75,000.
Graft-versus-host disease	Lymphocytes from donor transfused in an immunocompromised host.	Syndrome can involve a variety of organs, usually skin, liver, gastrointestinal tract, and bone marrow.	Rare. Preventive management: irradiation (> 1500 cGy) of cellular blood components transfused to individuals with congenital or acquired immunodeficiency syndromes, intrauterine transfusion, very premature infants, and when donors are relatives of the recipient.
Iron overload	There is no physiologic mechanism to excrete excess iron. Target organs include liver, heart, and endocrine organs. In patients receiving red cell transfusions over long periods of time, there is an increase in iron burden.	Signs and symptoms of dysfunctional organs affected by the iron.	Significant risk with chronic transfusions. Treated with chronic administration of iron chelator such as deferoxamine given intravenously or Exjade given orally.

ARDS, adult respiratory distress syndrome; DIC, disseminated intravascular coagulation; FFP, fresh frozen plasma; IgA, immunoglobulin A.

decrease the risk of some of these adverse effects. Leukode-pletion of blood products can decrease febrile reactions and further decrease transmission of certain infectious agents. Irradiation of blood products should be performed in children < 1 year and immunocompromised individuals to prevent transfusion-associated graft versus host disease. Red cell containing products can be washed to remove additional plasma in patients with prior severe anaphylactic reactions.

Busch MP, Bloch EM, Kleinman S: Prevention of transfusion-transmitted infections. Blood 2019;133(17):1854–1864. doi: 10.1182/blood-2018-11-833996 [PMID: 30808637].

Jacquot C, Mo YD, Luban NLC: New approaches and trials in pediatric transfusion medicine. Hematol Oncol Clin North Am 2019;33(3):507–520. doi: 10.1016/j.hoc.2019.01.012 [PMID: 31030816].

Schulz WL et al: Blood utilization and transfusion reactions in pediatric patients transfused with conventional or pathogen reduced platelets. J Pediatr 2019 Jun;209:220–225. doi: 10.1016/j.peds.2019.01.046 [PMID: 30885645].

REFERENCES

Fung MK et al: *Technical Manual*. 19th ed. Bethesda, MD: AABB; 2017.

Goodnight SH, Hathaway WE (eds): *Disorders of Hemostasis and Thrombosis: A Clinical Guide*. 2nd ed. New York, NY: McGraw Hill; 2001.

Klein HG, Anstee DJ (eds): *Blood Transfusion in Clinical Medicine*. 12th ed. Hoboken, NJ: Wiley-Blackwell; 2014.

Petz L, Garratty G: *Immune Hemolytic Anemias*. 2nd ed. Philadelphia, PA: Churchill Livingstone; 2004.

Neoplastic Disease

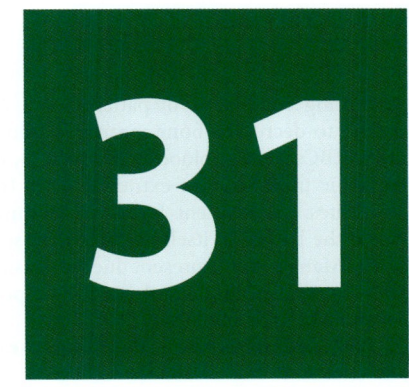

Kelly Maloney, MD

Jean M. Mulcahy Levy, MD

Timothy Price Garrington, MD

Vanessa Fabrizio, MD, MS

Rohini Chakravarthy, MD, MPH

Each year approximately 150 out of every 1 million children younger than 20 years are diagnosed with cancer. For children between the ages of 1 and 20 years, cancer is the fourth leading cause of death, behind unintentional injuries, homicides, and suicides. However, combined-modality therapy, including surgery, chemotherapy, and radiation therapy, has improved survival dramatically, such that the overall 5-year survival rate of pediatric malignancies is now greater than 80%. It is estimated that currently 1 in 570 adults will be a survivor of childhood cancer.

Because pediatric malignancies are rare, cooperative clinical trials have become the mainstay of treatment planning and therapeutic advances. The Children's Oncology Group (COG), representing the amalgamation of four prior pediatric cooperative groups (Children's Cancer Group, Pediatric Oncology Group, Intergroup Rhabdomyosarcoma Study Group, and the National Wilms Tumor Study Group), offers current therapeutic protocols and strives to answer important treatment questions. A child or adolescent newly diagnosed with cancer should be enrolled in a cooperative clinical trial whenever possible. Because many protocols are associated with significant toxicities, morbidity, and potential mortality, treatment of children with cancer should be supervised by a pediatric oncologist familiar with the hazards of treatment, preferably at a multidisciplinary pediatric cancer center.

Advances in molecular genetics, cell biology, and tumor immunology have contributed and are crucial to the continued understanding of pediatric malignancies and their treatment. Continued research into the biology of tumors will lead to the identification of targeted therapy for specific tumor types with, it is hoped, fewer systemic effects.

Research in supportive care areas, such as prevention and management of infection, pain, and emesis, has improved the survival and quality of life for children undergoing cancer treatment. Long-term studies of childhood cancer survivors are yielding information that provides a rationale for modifying future treatment regimens to decrease morbidity.

A guide for caring for childhood cancer survivors is now available to medical providers as well as families and details suggested examinations and late effects by type of chemotherapy received.

Cure Search: Children's Oncology Group: http://www.survivor-shipguidelines.org.

Seehuse DA, Baird D, Bode D: Primary care of adult survivors of childhood cancer. Am Fam Physician 2010 May 15;81(10): 1250–1255 [PMID: 20507049].

Signorelli C et al: The impact of long-term follow-up care for childhood cancer survivors: a systematic review. Crit Rev Oncol Hematol 2017 Jun;114:131–138 [PMID: 28477741].

▼ MAJOR PEDIATRIC NEOPLASTIC DISEASES

ACUTE LYMPHOBLASTIC LEUKEMIA

▶ General Considerations

Acute lymphoblastic leukemia (ALL) is the most common malignancy of childhood, accounting for about 25% of all cancer diagnoses in patients younger than 15 years. The worldwide incidence of ALL is about 1:25,000 children per year, including 3000 children per year in the United States. The peak age at onset is 4 years; 85% of patients are diagnosed between ages 2 and 10 years. Children with Down syndrome have a 10–20 times increase in the overall rate of leukemia.

ALL results from uncontrolled proliferation of immature lymphocytes. Its cause is unknown, and genetic factors may play a role. Leukemia is defined by the presence of more than 25% malignant hematopoietic cells (blasts) in the bone marrow aspirate. These blasts derive from B-cell precursors early in their development, called B-precursor ALL. Less commonly, lymphoblasts are of T-cell origin or of mature B-cell origin. Over 70% of children receiving aggressive combination chemotherapy and early presymptomatic treatment to the central nervous system (CNS) are now cured of ALL.

▶ Clinical Findings

A. Symptoms and Signs

Presenting complaints of patients with ALL include those related to decreased bone marrow production of red blood cells (RBCs), white blood cells (WBCs), or platelets and to leukemic infiltration of extramedullary (outside bone marrow) sites. Intermittent fevers are common as a result of either the leukemia itself or infections secondary to leukopenia. Many patients present due to bruising or pallor. About 25% of patients experience bone pain, especially in the pelvis, vertebral bodies, and legs.

Physical examination at diagnosis ranges from virtually normal to highly abnormal. Signs related to bone marrow infiltration by leukemia include pallor, petechiae, and purpura. Hepatomegaly and/or splenomegaly occur in over 60% of patients. Lymphadenopathy is common, either localized or generalized to cervical, axillary, and inguinal regions. The testes may occasionally be unilaterally or bilaterally enlarged secondary to leukemic infiltration. Superior vena cava syndrome is caused by mediastinal adenopathy compressing the superior vena cava. A prominent venous pattern develops over the upper chest from collateral vein enlargement. The neck may feel full from venous engorgement. The face may appear plethoric, and the periorbital area may be edematous. A mediastinal mass can cause tachypnea, orthopnea, and respiratory distress. Leukemic infiltration of cranial nerves may cause cranial nerve palsies with mild nuchal rigidity. The optic fundi may show exudates of leukemic infiltration and hemorrhage from thrombocytopenia. Anemia can cause a flow murmur, tachycardia, and, rarely, congestive heart failure.

B. Laboratory Findings

A complete blood count (CBC) with differential is the most useful initial test because 95% of patients with ALL have a decrease in at least one cell type (single cytopenia): neutropenia, thrombocytopenia, or anemia with most patients having a decrease in at least two blood cell lines. The WBC count is low or normal (= 10,000/µL) in 50% of patients, but the differential shows neutropenia (absolute neutrophil count < 1000/µL) along with a small percentage of blasts amid normal lymphocytes. In 30% of patients, the WBC count is between 10,000/µL and 50,000/µL; in 20% of patients, it is over 50,000/µL, occasionally higher than 300,000/µL. Blasts are usually readily identifiable on peripheral blood smears from patients with elevated WBC counts. Peripheral blood smears also show abnormalities in RBCs, such as teardrops. Most patients with ALL have decreased platelet counts (< 150,000/µL) and decreased hemoglobin (< 11 g/dL) at diagnosis. In approximately 1% of patients diagnosed with ALL, CBCs and peripheral blood smears are entirely normal, but patients have bone pain that leads to bone marrow examination. Serum chemistries, particularly uric acid and lactate dehydrogenase (LDH), are often elevated at diagnosis as a result of cell breakdown.

The diagnosis of ALL is made by bone marrow examination, which shows a homogeneous infiltration of leukemic blasts replacing normal marrow elements. Immunophenotyping and histochemical stains will distinguish ALL, either B- or T- cell and AML. About 5% of patients present with CNS leukemia, which is defined as a cerebrospinal fluid (CSF) WBC count greater than 5/µL with blasts present on cytocentrifuged specimen.

C. Imaging

Chest radiograph may show mediastinal widening or an anterior mediastinal mass and tracheal compression secondary to lymphadenopathy or thymic infiltration, especially in T-cell ALL. Abdominal ultrasound may show kidney enlargement from leukemic infiltration or uric acid nephropathy as well as intra-abdominal adenopathy. Plain radiographs of the long bones and spine may show demineralization, periosteal elevation, growth arrest lines, or compression of vertebral bodies. Although these findings may suggest leukemia, they are not diagnostic.

▶ Differential Diagnosis

The differential diagnosis, based on the history and physical examination, includes chronic infections by Epstein-Barr virus (EBV) and cytomegalovirus (CMV), causing lymphadenopathy, hepatosplenomegaly, fevers, and anemia. Prominent petechiae and purpura suggest a diagnosis of immune thrombocytopenic purpura. Significant pallor could be caused by transient erythroblastopenia of childhood, autoimmune hemolytic anemias, or aplastic anemia. Fevers and joint pains, with or without hepatosplenomegaly and lymphadenopathy, can suggest juvenile rheumatoid arthritis (JRA). The diagnosis of leukemia usually becomes straightforward once the CBC reveals multiple cytopenias and leukemic blasts. Serum LDH levels may help distinguish JRA from leukemia, as the LDH is usually normal in JRA. An elevated WBC count with lymphocytosis is typical of pertussis; however, in pertussis lymphocytes are mature and neutropenia is rarely associated.

▶ Treatment

A. Specific Therapy

Intensity of treatment is determined by specific prognostic features present at diagnosis, the patient's response to therapy, and specific biologic features of the leukemia cells. The majority of patients with ALL are enrolled in clinical trials designed by clinical groups and approved by the National Cancer Institute; the largest group is COG. The first month of therapy consists of induction, at the end of which over 95% of patients exhibit remission on bone marrow aspirates by morphology. The drugs most used in induction include oral prednisone or dexamethasone, intravenous vincristine, +/−daunorubicin, asparaginase, and intrathecal methotrexate.

Consolidation is the second phase of treatment, during which intrathecal chemotherapy along with continued systemic therapy and sometimes cranial radiation therapy are given to kill lymphoblasts "hiding" in the meninges. Several months of intensive chemotherapy follows consolidation, often referred to as intensification. This intensification has led to improved survival in pediatric ALL.

Maintenance therapy can include daily oral mercaptopurine, weekly oral methotrexate, and, often, pulses of intravenous vincristine and oral prednisone or dexamethasone. Intrathecal chemotherapy, either with methotrexate alone or combined with cytarabine and hydrocortisone, is usually given every 2–3 months.

Chemotherapy has significant potential side effects. Patients need to be monitored closely to prevent drug toxicities and to ensure early treatment of complications. The duration of treatment is now ~2 1/2 years in COG trials. Treatment for ALL is tailored to prognostic, or risk groups. An infant younger than 1 year at diagnosis would be considered very high risk and receive even more intensive chemotherapy (Table 31–1). Also important is the patient's response to treatment determined by minimal residual disease (MRD) monitoring. This risk-adapted treatment approach has significantly increased the cure rate among patients with less favorable prognostic features by allowing for early intensification while minimizing treatment-related toxicities in those with favorable features. Bone marrow relapse is usually heralded by an abnormal CBC, either during treatment or following completion of therapy.

The CNS and testes are sanctuary sites for leukemia, meaning that the chemotherapy has a harder time reaching the leukemic cells in these areas. Currently, about one-third of all ALL relapses are isolated to these sanctuary sites. Systemic chemotherapy does not penetrate these tissues as well as it penetrates other organs. Thus, presymptomatic

intrathecal chemotherapy is a critical part of ALL treatment, without which many more relapses would occur in the CNS, with or without bone marrow relapse. Most isolated CNS relapses are diagnosed in an asymptomatic child at the time of routine intrathecal injection when CSF cell count and differential show an elevated WBC with leukemic blasts. Occasionally, symptoms of CNS relapse develop headache, nausea and vomiting, irritability, nuchal rigidity, photophobia, changes in vision, and cranial nerve palsies. Currently, testicular relapse occurs in less than 5% of boys. The presentation of testicular relapse is usually unilateral painless testicular enlargement, without a distinct mass. Routine follow-up of boys both on and off treatment includes physical examination of the testes.

Hematopoietic stem cell transplantation (HSCT) is rarely used as initial treatment for ALL, because most patients are cured with chemotherapy alone. Patients whose blasts contain certain chromosomal abnormalities and patients with positive MRD at the end of the second or third month of therapy may have a better cure rate with early HSCT from a human leukocyte antigen (HLA)-DR–matched sibling donor, or a matched unrelated donor, than with intensive chemotherapy alone. HSCT and newer cellular therapies such as Car T cells are discussed later in this chapter.

Several years ago, imatinib, a tyrosine kinase inhibitor (TKI), directed against the Philadelphia chromosome (Ph+) protein product, was combined in a backbone of intensive chemotherapy for Ph+ ALL in pediatric patients. The results of this trial showed that the patients had an increased leukemia-free survival of 78% as compared to 50% in the past without imatinib. Ongoing trials for COG in Ph+ ALL are now incorporating newer TKIs within a chemotherapy backbone. Different than in adult Ph+ ALL, most pediatric patients with Ph+ ALL will not need to progress to HSCT. Two newer targeted agents are now used in relapsed ALL. Blinatumomab is a bispecific T-cell engager (BiTE) that brings the CD19 on a leukemia cell in direct contact with a T cell. Blinatumomab was found to improve outcome following relapse and was recently published. Another targeted agent, inotuzumab is an antibody-drug conjugate against CD22, also frequently found on the surface of the leukemia cells. This drug is also used in relapsed childhood ALL. Both of these drugs have now been moved to initial therapy in the COG studies for standard risk and high-risk B ALL, respectively. As more is understood about the biology of ALL, further therapy will likely include more of these targeted agents, in order to reduce late effects potentially while maintaining and improving leukemia-free survival.

B. Supportive Care

Tumor lysis syndrome, which consists of hyperkalemia, hyperuricemia, and hyperphosphatemia, should be anticipated when treatment is started. Maintaining brisk urine

Table 31–1. Risk group for B-cell ALL.

NCI Standard Risk	NCI High Risk	Infant ALL
1–9 y	≥ 10 y or > 1 y due to high WBC	Age < 1 y
Initial WBC < 50,000/μL	Initial WBC ≥ 50,000/ μL, regardless of age	Any WBC
No CNS leukemia	CNS leukemia	Could be negative or positive

output with intravenous fluids and treating with oral allopurinol are appropriate steps in managing tumor lysis syndrome. Rasburicase is indicated for severe tumor lysis syndrome with initial high uric acid values or high WBC at presentation. Serum levels of potassium, phosphorus, and uric acid should be monitored. If superior vena caval or superior mediastinal syndrome is present, general anesthesia is contraindicated temporarily and until there has been some decrease in the mass. If hyperleukocytosis (WBC count > 100,000/μL) is accompanied by hyperviscosity with symptoms of respiratory distress and/or mental status changes, leukapheresis may be indicated to rapidly reduce the number of circulating blasts and minimize the potential thrombotic or hemorrhagic CNS complications. Throughout the course of treatment, all transfused blood and platelet products should be irradiated to prevent graft-versus-host disease (GVHD) from the transfused lymphocytes. Whenever possible, blood products should be leuko-depleted to minimize CMV transmission, transfusion reactions, and sensitization to platelets.

Due to the immunocompromised state of the patient with ALL, bacterial, fungal, and viral infections are serious and can be life-threatening or fatal. During the course of treatment, fever (temperature = 38.3°C) and neutropenia (absolute neutrophil count < 500/μL) require prompt assessment, blood cultures from each lumen of a central line, and prompt treatment with empiric broad-spectrum antibiotics. Patients receiving ALL treatment must receive prophylaxis against *Pneumocystis jirovecii* (formerly *Pneumocystis carinii*). Trimethoprim-sulfamethoxazole given twice each day on 2 or 3 consecutive days per week is the drug of choice. Patients nonimmune to varicella are at risk for very serious—even fatal—infection. Such patients should receive varicella-zoster immune globulin (VZIG) within 72 hours after exposure and treatment with intravenous acyclovir for active infection.

▶ **Prognosis**

Cure rates depend on specific prognostic features present at diagnosis, biologic features of the leukemic blast, and the response to therapy. Two of the most important features are WBC count and age. Children aged 1–9 years whose diagnostic WBC count is less than 50,000/μL, standard risk ALL, have a leukemia-free survival of greater than 95%, while children 10 years or older have about an 88% chance of being cured the first time through therapy. MRD measurements are used to determine both the rapidity of response as well as the depth of remission attained at the end of induction (first 4–6 weeks of therapy). Patients with very low levels or no MRD at the end of induction will have a superior leukemia-free survival as compared to other patients with similar initial risk factors but a higher MRD level. On the flip side, by identifying patients with an increased risk of relapse at end induction, more intensified therapy can be delivered in order

to overcome this negative prognostic feature and increase their ultimate chance at staying leukemia free.

Certain chromosomal abnormalities present in the leukemic blasts at diagnosis influence prognosis. Patients with t(9;22), the Philadelphia chromosome, had a poor chance of cure in the past, but as discussed earlier in this chapter, they now have improved outcome with the incorporation of a directed TKI. Likewise, infants younger than 6 months with *11q23* rearrangements have a poor chance of cure with conventional chemotherapy. In contrast, patients whose blasts are hyperdiploid (containing > 50 chromosomes instead of the normal 46) with trisomies of chromosomes 4 and 10 and patients whose blasts have a t(12;21) and *ETV6-AML1* rearrangement have a greater chance of cure, approaching 95%–97% event-free survival (EFS), than do children without these characteristics.

Graff Z, Burke MJ, Gossai N. Novel therapies for pediatric acute lymphoblastic leukemia. Curr Opin Pediatr 2024 Feb 1;36(1): 64-70. [PMID: 37991046]

Hunger SP, Raety EA: How I treat relapsed acute lymphoblastic leukemia in the pediatric population. Blood 2020 Oct 15;136(16): 1803–1812. doi: 10.1182/blood.2019004043 [PMID: 32589723].

Inaba H, Mullighan CG: Pediatric acute lymphoblastic leukemia. Haematologica 2020 Nov 1;105(11):2524–2539. doi: 10.3324/haematol.2020.247031 [PMID: 33054110].

ACUTE MYELOID LEUKEMIA

▶ **General Considerations**

Approximately 500 new cases of AML occur per year in children and adolescents in the United States. Although AML accounts for only 25% of all leukemias in this age group, it is responsible for at least one-third of deaths from leukemia in children and teenagers. Congenital conditions associated with an increased risk of AML include Diamond-Blackfan anemia; neurofibromatosis (NF); Down; Wiskott-Aldrich, Kostmann, and Li-Fraumeni syndromes; and chromosomal instability syndromes such as Fanconi anemia. Acquired risk factors include exposure to ionizing radiation, cytotoxic chemotherapeutic agents, and benzenes. However, the vast majority of patients have no identifiable risk factors. Historically, the diagnosis of AML was based almost exclusively on morphology and immunohistochemical staining of the leukemic cells. Immunophenotypic, cytogenetic, and molecular analyses are increasingly important in confirming the diagnosis of AML and subclassifying it into biologically distinct subtypes that have therapeutic and prognostic implications. Recently the World Health Organization (WHO) classification was published to describe AML as AML with recurrent genetic abnormalities with a list of genetic abnormalities sufficient to diagnose AML and then AML not otherwise specified. Cytogenetic clonal abnormalities occur in 80% of patients with AML and are often predictive of outcome.

WHO classification of acute myeloid leukemia (AML) and related neoplasms.

AML with recurrent genetic abnormalities	AML with t(8;21)(q22;q22), RUNX1-RUNX1T1 AML with inv(16)(p13.1q22) or t(16;16) (p13.1;p22); CBFB-MYH11 Acute promyelocytic leukemia with t(15;17)(q22;q12);PML-RARA AML with t(9;11)(p22;q23)MLLT3-MLL AML with t(6;9)(p23;q34); DEK-NUP214 AML with inv(3)(q21q26.2) or t(3.3) (q21;q26.2); RPN1-EVI1 AML (megakaryoblastic) with t(1:22) (p13;q13); RBM15-MKL1 AML with mutated NPM1 AML with mutated CEBPA
AML with myelodysplasia-related changes	
Therapy-related myeloid neoplasms	
AML, not otherwise specified	AML with minimal differentiation AML without maturation AML with maturation Acute myelomonocytic leukemia Acute monoblastic and monocytic leukemia Acute erythroid leukemia Acute megakaryoblastic leukemia Acute basophilic leukemia Acute panmyelosis with myelofibrosis
Myeloid sarcoma	
Myeloid proliferation related to Down syndrome	Transient abnormal myelopoiesis Myeloid leukemia associated with Down syndrome

Data from Vardiman JW et al: The 2008 revision of the World Health Organization (WHO) classification of myeloid neoplasms and acute leukemia: rationale and important changes. Blood 2009 Jul 30;114(5):937–951.

Aggressive induction therapy currently results in a 75%–85% complete remission rate. However, long-term survival has improved only modestly to approximately 50%, despite the availability of several effective agents, improvements in supportive care, and increasingly intensive therapies.

▶ Clinical Findings

The clinical manifestations of AML commonly include anemia (44%), thrombocytopenia (33%), and neutropenia (69%). Symptoms may be few and innocuous or may be life threatening. The median hemoglobin value at diagnosis is 7 g/dL, and platelets usually number fewer than 50,000/μL. Frequently the absolute neutrophil count is under 1000/μL,

although the total WBC count is over 100,000/μL in 25% of patients at diagnosis.

Hyperleukocytosis may be associated with life-threatening complications. Venous stasis and sludging of blasts in small vessels cause hypoxia, hemorrhage, and infarction, most notably in the lung and CNS. This clinical picture is a medical emergency requiring rapid intervention, such as leukapheresis, to decrease the leukocyte count. CNS leukemia is present in 5%–15% of patients at diagnosis, a higher rate of initial involvement than in ALL. Certain subtypes, such as myelomonocytic and monocytic/monoblastic leukemia, have a higher likelihood of meningeal infiltration than do other subtypes. Additionally, clinically significant coagulopathy may be present at diagnosis in patients with these two subtypes as well as acute promyelocytic leukemia. This problem manifests as bleeding or an abnormal disseminated intravascular coagulation screen and should be at least partially corrected prior to initiation of treatment, which may transiently exacerbate the coagulopathy.

▶ Treatment

A. Specific Therapy

AML is less responsive to treatment than ALL and requires more intensive chemotherapy. Toxicities from therapy are common and likely to be life threatening; therefore, treatment should be undertaken only at a tertiary pediatric oncology center.

Current AML protocols rely on intensive administration of anthracyclines, cytarabine, and +/- etoposide for induction of remission. After remission is obtained, patients may undergo allogeneic bone marrow transplant while those without an appropriate related donor are treated with additional cycles of aggressive chemotherapy for a total of five cycles. Inv16 t(8;21), NPM1 mutations herald a more chemotherapy-responsive subtype of AML. In patients with a rapid response to induction chemotherapy, intensive chemotherapy alone may be curative in patients whose blasts harbor these cytogenetic abnormalities. Additional recognized genetic risk factors that carry a poor outcome for children with AML include monosomy 7, chromosomal rearrangements at 11q23, FLT3 internal tandem duplications (ITDs), and newer molecular subtypes. HSCT is recommended for all these patients, using either a related or unrelated donor. Trials with risk grouping are ongoing as more is understood about the varying biologic factors.

The biologic heterogeneity of AML is becoming increasingly important therapeutically. Acute promyelocytic leukemia, associated with t(15;17) demonstrated either cytogenetically or molecularly, is currently treated with all *trans*-retinoic acid, a differentiating therapy, and arsenic trioxide in addition to chemotherapy with high-dose cytarabine and daunorubicin when needed. All *trans*-retinoic acid leads to differentiation of promyelocytic leukemia cells and can induce remission, but cure requires conventional chemotherapy as well. This subtype has an increased EFS over other AML subtypes.

Another biologically distinct subtype of AML occurs in children with Down syndrome, almost exclusively acute megakaryoblastic leukemia. Using less intensive treatment, remission induction rate and overall survival of these children are dramatically superior to non–Down syndrome children with AML. It is important that children with Down syndrome receive appropriate treatment specifically designed to be less intensive due to their increased rate of toxicity with chemotherapeutic agents.

As with ALL, newer biologic agents with more specific targeting are available and undergoing clinical trials. One such group of agents called FLT3 inhibitors appear to be active against AML with Flt3 ITDs. Combining these agents with AML therapy has been useful in relapsed disease and is now being studied in upfront trials for pediatric patients. In addition, gemtuzumab ozogamicin, an antibody-drug conjugate directed against CD33 on AML cells, is used to treat AML, both upfront and in relapse.

B. Supportive Care

Tumor lysis syndrome occurs less often during induction treatment of AML (treatment outlined in section Acute Lymphoblastic Leukemia). Hyperleukocytosis (WBC > 100,000/µL) is a medical emergency and, in a symptomatic patient, requires rapid intervention to rapidly decrease the number of circulating blasts and thereby decrease hyperviscosity. Delaying transfusion of packed RBCs until the WBC can be decreased to below 100,000/µL avoids exacerbating hyperviscosity. It is also important to correct the coagulopathy commonly associated with APML and monocytic AML subtypes prior to beginning induction chemotherapy. Other supportive care measures are similar to ALL.

There is an increased risk for fever and neutropenia in patients being treated with AML as compared to AML and a higher risk of mortality associated with infection. These patients received prophylactic antibiotics with conversion to prompt initiation of broad-spectrum antibiotics with fever. Because of the high incidence of invasive fungal infections, patients should receive prophylactic antifungals with a low threshold to change to treatment doses. It must be stressed that the supportive care for this group of patients is as important as the leukemia-directed therapy and that this treatment should be carried out only at a tertiary pediatric cancer center.

▶ Prognosis

Published results from various centers show a 50%–60% survival rate at 5 years following first remission for patients who do not have matched sibling hematopoietic stem cell donors.

Patients with matched sibling donors fare slightly better, with 5-year survival rates of 60%–70% after allogeneic HSCT.

As treatment becomes more sophisticated, outcome is increasingly related to the subtype of AML. Currently, AML in patients with t(8;21), t(15;17), inv 16, or Down syndrome has the most favorable prognosis, with 70%–75% long-term survival using modern treatments, including chemotherapy alone. The least favorable outcome occurs in AML patients with monosomy 7 or 5, 7q, 5q–, 11q23 cytogenetic abnormalities, or FLT 3 mutations with ITD.

Cooper TM et al: Revised risk stratification criteria for children with newly diagnosed acute myeloid leukemia: a report from the Children's Oncology Group. Blood 2017;130:407–407.

Elgarten C, Aplenc R: Pediatric acute myeloid leukemia: updates on biology, risk stratification, and therapy. Curr Opin Pediatr. 2020 Feb;32(1):57–66. doi: 10.1097/MOP.0000000000000855 [PMID: 31815781].

Eryilmaz E, Canpolat C: Novel agents for the treatment of childhood leukemia: an update. Onco Targets Ther 2017 Jul 4;10: 3299–3306 [PMID: 28740405].

Getz KD et al: Four versus five chemotherapy courses in patients with low risk acute myeloid leukemia: a Children's Oncology Group report. J Clin Oncol 2017;35:10515–10515.

Klein K, de Haas V, Kapers GJL: Clinical challenges in de novo pediatric acute myeloid leukemia. Expert Rev Anticancer Ther 2018 Mar;18(3):277–293 [PMID: 29338495].

MYELOPROLIFERATIVE DISEASES

Myeloproliferative diseases in children are relatively rare. They are characterized by ineffective hematopoiesis that results in excessive peripheral blood counts. The three most important types are chronic myelogenous leukemia (CML), which accounts for less than 5% of the childhood leukemias, transient myeloproliferative disorder in children with Down syndrome, and juvenile myelomonocytic leukemia (JMML) (Table 31–2).

1. Chronic Myelogenous Leukemia

▶ General Considerations

Chronic myelogenous leukemia (CML) with translocation of chromosomes 9 and 22 (the Philadelphia chromosome, Ph+) is identical to adult Ph+CML. Translocation 9;22 results in the fusion of the *BCR* gene on chromosome 22 and the *ABL* gene on chromosome 9. The resulting fusion protein is a constitutively active tyrosine kinase that interacts with a variety of effector proteins and allows for deregulated cellular proliferation, decreased adherence of cells to the bone marrow extracellular matrix, and resistance to apoptosis. Without treatment, CML usually progresses within 3 years to an accelerated phase and then to a blast crisis. Ph+ cells have an increased susceptibility to the acquisition of additional molecular changes that lead to the accelerated and blast phases of disease.

Table 31–2. Comparison of JMML, CML, and TMD.

	CML	TMD	JMML
Age at onset	> 3 y	< 3 mo	< 2 y
Clinical presentation	Nonspecific constitutional complaints, massive splenomegaly, variable hepatomegaly	DS features, often no or few symptoms; or hepatosplenomegaly, respiratory symptoms	Abrupt onset; eczematoid skin rash, marked lymphadenopathy, bleeding tendency, moderate hepatosplenomegaly, fever
Chromosomal alterations	t(9;22)	Constitutional trisomy 21, but usually no other abnormality	Monosomy or del (7q) in 20% of patients
Laboratory features	Marked leukocytosis (> 100,000/μL), normal to elevated platelet count, decreased to absent leukocyte alkaline phosphatase, usually normal muramidase	Variable leukocytosis, normal to high platelet count, large platelets, myeloblasts	Moderate leukocytosis (> 10,000/μL), thrombocytopenia, monocytosis (> 1000/μL), elevated fetal hemoglobin, normal to diminished leukocyte alkaline phosphatase, elevated muramidase

CML, chronic myelogenous leukemia; DS, Down syndrome; JMML, juvenile myelomonocytic leukemia; TMD, transient myeloproliferative disorder.

▶ Clinical Findings

Patients with CML may present with nonspecific complaints similar to those of acute leukemia, including bone pain, fever, night sweats, and fatigue. However, patients can also be asymptomatic. Physical findings may include fever, pallor, ecchymoses, and hepatosplenomegaly. Anemia, thrombocytosis, and leukocytosis are frequent laboratory findings. The peripheral smear is usually diagnostic, with a characteristic predominance of myeloid cells in all stages of maturation, increased basophils and relatively few blasts but needs to be confirmed at a pediatric center with hematology/oncology expertise. Tumor lysis syndrome and leukostasis secondary to hyperleukocytosis are rare in CML, in contrast to acute leukemias.

▶ Treatment & Prognosis

TKIs are standard up-front therapy for CML, which were rationally designed based on the molecular mechanism of the pathogenesis of CML. Hydroxyurea can be added in the beginning for cytoreduction. There are a variety of TKIs to choose from for CML, all with different side effect profiles. Typically, imatinib and dasatinib are common choices for initial therapy. Bosutinib is a newer TKI for CML that may be important for young children with CML as it does not target PDGFR and other tyrosine kinases that affect growth.

2. Transient Myeloproliferative Disorder

Transient myeloproliferative disorder is unique to patients with trisomy 21 or mosaicism for trisomy 21. It is characterized by uncontrolled proliferation of blasts, usually of megakaryocytic origin, during early infancy and spontaneous resolution. The pathogenesis of this process is not well understood, although mutations in the *GATA1* gene have recently been implicated as initial events.

Although the true incidence is unknown, it is estimated to occur in up to 10% of patients with Down syndrome. Despite the fact that the process usually resolves by 3 months of age, organ infiltration may cause significant morbidity and mortality.

Patients can present with hydrops fetalis, pericardial or pleural effusions, or hepatic fibrosis. More frequently, they are asymptomatic or only minimally ill. Therefore, treatment is primarily supportive. Patients without symptoms are not treated, and those with organ dysfunction receive low doses of chemotherapy or leukapheresis (or both) to reduce peripheral blood blast counts. Although patients with transient myeloproliferative disorder have apparent resolution of the process, approximately 30% go on to develop acute megakaryoblastic leukemia within 3 years.

3. Juvenile Myelomonocytic Leukemia

Juvenile myelomonocytic leukemia (JMML) accounts for approximately one-third of the myelodysplastic and myeloproliferative disorders in childhood. Patients with neurofibromatosis type 1 (NF1) are at higher risk of JMML than the general population. It typically occurs in infants and very young children and is occasionally associated with monosomy 7 or a deletion of the long arm of chromosome 7.

Patients with JMML present similarly to those with other hematopoietic malignancies, with lymphadenopathy, hepatosplenomegaly, skin rash, or respiratory symptoms. Patients may have stigmata of NF1 with neurofibromas or café au lait spots. Laboratory findings include anemia, thrombocytopenia, leukocytosis with monocytosis, and elevated fetal hemoglobin.

The results of chemotherapy for children with JMML have been disappointing, with estimated survival rates of less than 30%. Approximately 40%–45% of patients are projected to survive long-term using HSCT, although optimizing conditioning regimens and donor selection may improve these results.

Hasle H: Myelodysplastic and myeloproliferative disorders of childhood. Hematology Am Soc Hematol Educ Program 2016 Dec 2;2016(1):598–604 [PMID: 27913534].

Hijiya N, Millot F, Suttorp M: Chronic myeloid leukemia in children: clinical findings, management, and unanswered questions. Pediatr Clin North Am 2014 Feb;62(1):107–119 [PMID: 25435115].

Hijiya N, Suttorp M: How I treat chronic myeloid leukemia in children and adolescents. Blood 2019 May 30;133(22):2374–2384 [PMID: 30917954].

Niemeyer CM: JMML genomics and decisions. Hematology Am Soc Hematol Educ Program 2018 Nov 30;2018(1):307–312 [PMID: 30504325].

Tunstall O et al: Guidelines for the investigation and management of transient leukaemia of Down syndrome. Br J Haematol 2018;182:200–211 [PMID: 29916557].

BRAIN TUMORS

▶ General Considerations

Brain tumors are the most common solid tumors of childhood, accounting for 1500–2000 new malignancies in children each year in the United States and for 25%–30% of all childhood cancers. Because pediatric brain tumors are rare, they are often misdiagnosed or diagnosed late; most pediatricians see no more than two children with brain tumors during their careers. In general, children with brain tumors have a better prognosis than adults.

Brain tumors in childhood are biologically and histologically heterogeneous, ranging from low-grade localized lesions to high-grade tumors with neuraxis dissemination. High-dose systemic chemotherapy is used frequently, especially in young children with high-grade tumors, to delay, decrease, or completely avoid cranial irradiation. Such intensive treatment may be accompanied by autologous HSCT or peripheral stem cell reconstitution.

The causes of most pediatric brain tumors are unknown, although some are associated with genetic predisposition syndromes such as optic gliomas in children with NF or subependymal giant cell astrocytomas with tuberous sclerosis. All children with gliomas and meningiomas should be screened for NF-1. In children with meningiomas, without the skin findings of NF1 or NF2, von Hippel-Lindau syndrome should be considered. Inherited germline mutations are possible in atypical teratoid/rhabdoid tumors (AT/RTs) and in choroid plexus carcinomas. The syndrome of constitutional mismatch repair deficiency (CMMRD) should be considered carefully in the child presenting with a glioma who has been previously diagnosed with leukemia/lymphoma. There are treatment implications in recognizing CMMRD as these patients require additional life-long screening and may have an improved response to immunotherapy. The risk of developing a brain tumor is also increased in children who received cranial irradiation for treatment of meningeal leukemia. Careful family histories should be taken in these tumors and genetic counseling considered if this is indicative of CMMRD, familial polyposis, or Li-Fraumeni syndrome (LFS).

▶ Clinical Findings

A. Symptoms and Signs

Clinical findings at presentation vary depending on the child's age and the tumor's location. Children younger than 2 years more commonly have infratentorial tumors. Children with such tumors usually present with nonspecific symptoms such as vomiting, unsteadiness, lethargy, and irritability. Signs may be surprisingly few or may include macrocephaly, ataxia, hyperreflexia, and cranial nerve palsies. Because the head can expand in young children, papilledema is often absent. Measuring head circumference and observing gait are essential. Eye findings and apparent visual disturbances such as difficulty tracking can occur in association with optic pathway tumors. These eye and visual changes have some potential for improvement with therapy, although permanent loss of vision may occur. These patients should be closely followed by ophthalmology for potential eye patching, eye muscle surgery, or specialty glasses with prisms to manage double vision and vision loss.

Older children more commonly have supratentorial tumors, which are associated with headache, visual symptoms, seizures, and focal neurologic deficits. Initial presenting features are often nonspecific. School failure and personality changes are common. Vaguely described visual disturbance is often present. Headaches are common, but they often will not be predominantly in the morning and may be confused with migraine. If neurologic symptoms are severe, persistent, or worsening with time, a magnetic resonance imaging (MRI) of the brain would be recommended. Focal neurologic deficits or the presence of any indications of increased intracranial pressure (ie, papilledema) should be investigated by an MRI or a computed tomography (CT) if MRI is not readily available.

Older children with infratentorial tumors characteristically present with symptoms and signs of hydrocephalus, which include progressively worsening morning headache and vomiting, gait unsteadiness, double vision, and papilledema. Cerebellar astrocytomas enlarge slowly and symptoms may worsen over several months. Morning vomiting may be the only symptom of posterior fossa ependymomas, which originate in the floor of the fourth ventricle near the vomiting center. Children with brainstem tumors may present with facial and extraocular muscle palsies, ataxia, and hemiparesis; hydrocephalus occurs in approximately 25% of these patients at diagnosis.

B. Imaging and Staging

In addition to the tumor biopsy, neuraxis imaging studies are obtained to determine whether dissemination has occurred. It is unusual for brain tumors in children and adolescents to disseminate outside the CNS.

MRI has become the preferred diagnostic study for pediatric brain tumors. MRI provides better definition of the tumor and delineates indolent gliomas that may not be seen on CT scan. In contrast, a CT scan can be done in less than 10 minutes—as opposed to the 30 minutes or more required for an MRI scan—and is still useful if an urgent diagnostic study is necessary or to detect calcification of a tumor. Both scans are generally done with and without contrast enhancement. Contrast enhances regions where the blood-brain barrier is disrupted. Postoperative scans to document the extent of tumor resection should be obtained within 48 hours after surgery to avoid postsurgical enhancement.

Imaging of the entire neuraxis and CSF cytologic examination should be part of the diagnostic evaluation for patients with tumors such as medulloblastoma, ependymoma, and pineal region tumors. Diagnosis of neuraxis drop metastases (tumor spread along the neuraxis) can be accomplished by gadolinium-enhanced MRI incorporating sagittal and axial views. MRI of the spine should be obtained preoperatively in all children with midline tumors of the fourth ventricle or cerebellum. A CSF sample for cytologic examination should be obtained during the diagnostic surgery or, if that is not possible, 7–10 days after the surgery. Lumbar CSF is preferred over ventricular CSF. Levels of biomarkers in the blood and CSF, such as human chorionic gonadotropin and α-fetoprotein, may be helpful in diagnosis and follow-up. Both human chorionic gonadotropin and α-fetoprotein should be obtained from the blood preoperatively for all pineal and suprasellar tumors, and if positive, the need for an operation should be discussed with a neuro-oncologist.

Except in emergencies, it is recommended that the neurosurgeon discuss staging and sample collection with an oncologist before surgery in a child newly presenting with a scan suggestive of brain tumor.

C. Classification

About 50% of pediatric brain tumors occur above the tentorium and 50% in the posterior fossa. In the very young child, posterior fossa tumors are more common. Most childhood brain tumors can be divided into two categories according to the cell of origin: (1) glial tumors, such as astrocytomas and ependymomas, or (2) embryonal tumors, such as medulloblastoma and AT/RT. Some tumors contain both glial and neural elements (eg, ganglioglioma). A group of less common

Table 31–3. Location and frequency of common pediatric brain tumors.

Location	Frequency of Occurrence (%)
Hemispheric	37
Low-grade astrocytoma	23
High-grade astrocytoma	11
Other	3
Posterior fossa	49
Medulloblastoma	15
Cerebellar astrocytoma	15
Brainstem glioma	15
Ependymoma	4
Midline	14
Craniopharyngioma	8
Chiasmal glioma	4
Pineal region tumor	2

CNS tumors does not fit into either category (ie, craniopharyngiomas, germ cell tumors, choroid plexus tumors, and meningiomas). Low- and high-grade tumors are found in most categories. Table 31–3 lists the locations and frequencies of the common pediatric brain tumors.

Astrocytoma is the most common brain tumor of childhood. Most are juvenile pilocytic astrocytoma (WHO grade I) found in the posterior fossa with a bland cellular morphology and few or no mitotic figures. Low-grade astrocytomas, especially those in the cerebellum may be curable by complete surgical excision alone. Upfront chemotherapy is effective alone in about 40%–50% of low-grade astrocytomas but many will need multiple treatment courses. The recent advent of targeted therapy for mutations common in these tumors offers the potential for better outcomes.

Medulloblastoma are the most common high-grade brain tumors in children and are now molecularly classified into four subgroups: WNT, SHH, Group 3, and Group 4. These tumors usually occur in the first decade of life, with a peak incidence between ages 5 and 10 years and a female-male ratio of 2.1:1.3. The tumors typically arise in the midline cerebellar vermis, with variable extension into the fourth ventricle. Neuroaxis dissemination at diagnosis affects from 10% to 46% of patients. Prognostic factors are outlined in Table 31–4. Determination of risk to date has largely used histology, age, and stage, but molecular classifications is increasingly used to determine therapy.

Brainstem tumors are third in frequency of occurrence in children. They are frequently of astrocytic origin and often are high grade. Children with tumors that diffusely infiltrate the brainstem and involve primarily the pons (diffuse

Table 31–4. Prognostic factors in children with medulloblastoma.

Factor	Favorable	Unfavorable
Extent of disease	Nondisseminated	Disseminated
Histologic features	Undifferentiated, desmoplastic	Large cell, anaplastic
Age	≥ 4 y	< 4 y
Molecular tumor characteristics	WNT, young patients with SHH	MYC, MYCN

intrinsic pontine gliomas [DIPG]) have a long-term survival rate of less than 5%. There has been considerable biologic discovery for DIPG from autopsy samples. The discovery that most DIPG have the histone mutation *H3 K27M* and that diffuse gliomas can occur anywhere in the midline has led to a change in their classification to diffuse midline glioma (DMG) with or without *H3 K27M*. It is hoped that the understanding of the mutational drivers in this tumor will result in improved therapy. Brainstem tumors that occur above or below the pons grow in an eccentric or cystic manner and do not have the K27M mutation have a somewhat better outcome. Exophytic tumors in this location may be amenable to surgery. Sometimes, brainstem tumors are treated without a tissue diagnosis although improved safety in the biopsy of brainstem tumors is increasing diagnostic sampling of these patients.

Other brain tumors such as ependymomas, germ cell tumors, choroid plexus tumors, and craniopharyngiomas are less common, and each is associated with unique diagnostic and therapeutic challenges.

▶ **Treatment**

A. Supportive Care

Dexamethasone should be started prior to initial surgery to help relieve symptoms with recommended dosages of 4 mg every 6 hours in those children greater than 4 years and 2 mg every 6 hours in those less than 4. Anticonvulsants should be started if the child has had a seizure or if the surgical approach is likely to induce seizures. Levetiracetam (Keppra) is now the preferred anticonvulsant as it does not induce liver enzymes or interact with chemotherapy. Because postoperative treatment of young children with high-grade brain tumors incorporates increasingly more intensive systemic chemotherapy, consideration should also be given to the use of prophylaxis for *Pneumocystis* infection. Dexamethasone potentially reduces the effectiveness of chemotherapy and should be discontinued as soon after surgery as possible.

Optimum care for the pediatric patient with a brain tumor requires a multidisciplinary team, including subspecialists in pediatric neurosurgery, neuro-oncology, neurology, endocrinology, neuropsychology, radiation therapy, and rehabilitation medicine, as well as highly specialized nurses, social workers, and staff in physical therapy, occupational therapy, and speech and language science.

B. Specific Therapy

The goal of treatment is to eradicate the tumor with the least short- and long-term morbidity. Long-term neuropsychological morbidity becomes an especially important issue related to deficits caused by the tumor itself and the sequelae of treatment. Maximal safe surgical resection is generally the preferred initial approach. Technologic advances in the operating microscope, the ultrasonic tissue aspirator, and the CO_2 laser (which is less commonly used in pediatric brain tumor surgery); the accuracy of computerized stereotactic resection; and the availability of intraoperative monitoring techniques such as evoked potentials and electrocorticography have increased the feasibility and safety of surgical resection of many pediatric brain tumors. Second-look surgery after chemotherapy is increasingly being used when tumors are incompletely resected at initial surgery.

Radiation therapy for pediatric brain tumors is in a state of evolution. For tumors with a high probability of dissemination (eg, medulloblastoma), craniospinal irradiation is still standard therapy in children older than 3 years. Attempts at elimination of craniospinal radiation for certain types of intracranial germ-cell tumors and further reduction of craniospinal radiation dosing in medulloblastoma have not been successful. In others (eg, ependymoma), craniospinal irradiation has been abandoned because dissemination at first relapse is rare. Conformal radiation and the use of three-dimensional treatment planning are now in routine. Proton beam radiation has become routine in some centers, although safety studies in comparison to photon radiation are lacking in childhood.

Chemotherapy is effective in treating low-grade and malignant astrocytomas and medulloblastomas. Intensive chemotherapy is effective in a minority of children AT/RTs. The utility of chemotherapy in ependymoma is being reexplored in national trials. A series of brain tumor protocols for children younger than 3 years involved intensive chemotherapy after tumor resection and delaying or omitting radiation therapy. Superior results seem to have been obtained in the very young with high-dose chemotherapy strategies with stem cell rescue often followed by conformal radiotherapy. Conformal techniques allow the delivery of radiation to strictly defined fields and may limit side effects.

Perhaps the most exciting development in pediatric neuro-oncology is the development of biologically and clinically relevant subclassifications in both medulloblastoma and ependymoma. This development will drive a new generation of targeted therapy aimed at these biologically defined groups. The consensus definition of four biologically defined entities in medulloblastoma, including the Wnt and SHH groups, is the best example of this. New studies based on this new-defined biology are ongoing.

In older children with malignant glioma, the current approach is surgical resection of the tumor and combined-modality treatment with irradiation and intensive chemotherapy. It has recently been realized there is considerable heterogeneity in pediatric high-grade gliomas. Some, such as the congenital tumors, may do well with relatively modest therapy. Others, such as epithelioid glioblastomas, may harbor *BRAF* mutations and may be targetable with specific agents. Generally, however, the prognosis is poor for children with high-grade gliomas, and there has been little progress in finding better chemotherapeutic agents and strategies for most children with these devastating tumors.

The treatment of low-grade astrocytomas with chemotherapy has likewise shown only disappointing progress. However, there are potentially exciting, targeted agents in ongoing, and completed but unreported, low-grade astrocytoma trials that have the potential to greatly improve outcomes for these patients.

▶ Prognosis

Despite improvements in surgery and radiation therapy, the outlook for cure remains poor for children with high-grade glial tumors. For children with high-grade gliomas, an early CCG study showed a 45% progression-free survival rate for children who received radiation therapy and chemotherapy, but this may have been due to the inclusion of low-grade patients. More recent studies would suggest survival rate of less than 10%. The major exception to this is congenital glioblastomas that appear to have a much more favorable prognosis. Biologic factors that may affect survival are being increasingly recognized. The prognosis for diffuse pontine gliomas remains very poor, with the standard therapy of radiation alone, being only palliative.

The 5- and even 10-year survival rate for low-grade astrocytomas of childhood is 60%–90%. However, prognosis depends on both site and grade and, as it is increasingly realized, on biology. A child with a pilocytic astrocytoma of the cerebellum has a considerably better prognosis than a child with a fibrillary astrocytoma of the cerebral cortex. For recurrent or progressive low-grade astrocytoma of childhood, relatively moderate chemotherapy may improve the likelihood of survival.

Conventional craniospinal irradiation for children with low-stage medulloblastoma results in survival rates of 60%–90%. Ten-year survival rates are lower (40%–60%). Chemotherapy allows a reduction in the craniospinal radiation dose while improving survival rates for average-risk patients (86% survival at 5 years on the most recent COG average-risk protocol). However, even reduced-dose craniospinal irradiation has an adverse effect on intellect, especially in children younger than 7 years. Five-year survival rates for high-risk medulloblastoma have been 25%–40%, but this may be improved with the introduction of more chemotherapy during radiation although this still awaits the reporting of formal trials.

The previously poor prognosis for children with AT/RTs seems improved by intensive multimodality therapy in a national study.

Major challenges remain in treating brain tumors in children younger than 3 years and in treating DMG K27M and malignant gliomas. Given the inadequate results for treatment of childhood brain tumors, reduction of therapy trials should be fully evaluated and considered in the context of recent treatment failures using reduced therapy regimens. The increasing emphasis is on the quality of life of survivors, not just the survival rate.

Buczkowicz P et al: Genomic analysis of diffuse intrinsic pontine gliomas identifies three molecular subgroups and recurrent activating ACVR1 mutations. Nat Genet 2014;46(5):451–456 [PMID: 24705254].

Chi SN et al: Intensive multimodality treatment for children with newly diagnosed CNS atypical teratoid rhabdoid tumor. J Clin Oncol 2009;20:385 [PMID: 19064966].

Gajjar A et al: COG Brain Tumor Committee: Children's Oncology Group's 2013 blueprint for research: central nervous system tumors. Pediatr Blood Cancer 2013 Jun;60(6):1022–1026 [PMID: 23255213].

Khatua S, Song A, Sridhar DC, Mack SC: Childhood medulloblastoma: current therapies, emerging molecular landscape and newer therapeutic insights. Curr Neuropharmacol 2018 Aug;16(7):1045–1058 [PMCID: PMC6120114].

Korshunov A et al: Molecular staging of intracranial ependymoma in children and adults. J Clin Oncol 2010;28:3182 [PMID: 20516456].

Macy ME et al: Clinical and molecular characteristics of congenital glioblastoma. Neuro Oncol 2012;14:931 [PMID: 22711608].

Northcott PA et al: Medulloblastoma comprises four distinct molecular variants. J Clin Oncol 2011;29:1408 [PMID: 20823417].

LYMPHOMAS & LYMPHOPROLIFERATIVE DISORDERS

The term *lymphoma* refers to a malignant proliferation of lymphoid cells, usually in association with and arising from lymphoid tissues (ie, lymph nodes, thymus, spleen). In contrast, the term *leukemia* refers to a malignancy arising from the bone marrow, which may include lymphoid cells. Because lymphomas can involve the bone marrow, the distinction between the two can be confusing. The diagnosis of lymphoma is a common one among childhood cancers, accounting for 10%–15% of all malignancies. The most common form is Hodgkin disease, which represents nearly one-half of all cases. The remaining subtypes, referred to collectively as non-Hodgkin lymphoma (NHL), are divided into four main groups: lymphoblastic lymphoma (LL), small noncleaved cell lymphoma, large B-cell lymphoma (LBCL), and anaplastic large cell lymphoma (ALCL).

In contrast to lymphomas, lymphoproliferative disorders (LPDs) are quite rare in the general population. Most are polyclonal, nonmalignant (though often life-threatening) accumulations of lymphocytes that occur when the immune system fails to control virally transformed lymphocytes. However, a malignant monoclonal proliferation can also arise. The posttransplant LPDs arise in patients who are immunosuppressed to prevent solid organ or bone marrow transplant rejection, particularly liver and heart transplant patients. Spontaneous LPDs occur in immunodeficient individuals and, less commonly, in immunocompetent persons.

1. Hodgkin Lymphoma

▶ General Considerations

Children with Hodgkin lymphoma have a better response to treatment than do adults, with 5- to 10-year overall survival rate of greater than 90% when all stages are evaluated. Although adult therapies are applicable, the management of Hodgkin lymphoma in children younger than 18 years frequently differs. Because excellent disease control can result from several different therapeutic approaches, selection of staging procedures (radiographic, surgical, or other procedures to determine additional locations of disease) and treatment are often based on the potential long-term toxicity associated with the intervention.

Although Hodgkin lymphoma represents 50% of the lymphomas of childhood, only 15% of all cases occur in children aged 16 years or younger. Children younger than 5 years account for 3% of childhood cases. There is a 4:1 male predominance in the first decade. Notably, in underdeveloped countries the age distribution is quite different, with a peak incidence in younger children.

Hodgkin disease is subdivided into four histologic groups, and the distribution in children parallels that in adults: nodular lymphocyte-predominant (10%–20%); nodular sclerosing (40%–60%) (increases with age); mixed cellularity (20%–40%); and lymphocyte-depleted (5%–10%). Prognosis is independent of subclassification, with appropriate therapy based on stage (see section Staging). Of note, nodular-lymphocyte predominant HL is treated differently than the other subtypes, which compromise classical HL.

▶ Clinical Findings

A. Symptoms and Signs

Children with Hodgkin lymphoma usually present with painless cervical adenopathy,. The lymph nodes often feel firmer than inflammatory nodes and have a rubbery texture. They may be discrete or matted together and are not fixed to surrounding tissue. The growth rate is variable and involved nodes may wax and wane in size over weeks to months (Figure 31–1).

As Hodgkin lymphoma nearly always arises in lymph nodes and spreads to contiguous nodal groups, a detailed

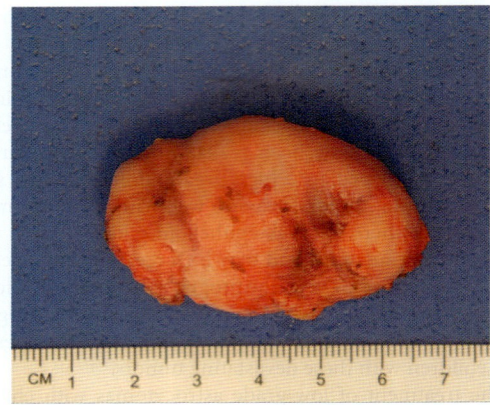

▲ **Figure 31–1.** Pathologic specimen showing an excised lymph node.

examination of all nodal sites is mandatory. Lymphadenopathy is common in children, so the decision to perform biopsy is often difficult or delayed for a prolonged period. Indications for consideration of early lymph node biopsy include lack of identifiable infection in the region drained by the enlarged node, a node greater than 2 cm in size, supraclavicular adenopathy or abnormal chest radiograph, and lymphadenopathy increasing in size after 2 weeks or failing to resolve within 4–8 weeks.

Constitutional symptoms occur in about one-third of children at presentation. Symptoms of fever greater than 38.0°C, weight loss of 10% in the previous 6 months, and drenching night sweats are defined by the Ann Arbor staging criteria as B symptoms. The A designation refers to the absence of these symptoms. B symptoms are of prognostic value, and more aggressive therapy is usually required for cure. Generalized pruritus and pain with alcohol ingestion may also occur.

One-half of patients have asymptomatic mediastinal disease (adenopathy or anterior mediastinal mass), although symptoms due to compression of vital structures in the thorax may occur. A chest radiograph should be obtained when lymphoma is being considered. The mediastinum must be evaluated thoroughly before any surgical procedure is undertaken to avoid airway obstruction or cardiovascular collapse during anesthesia and possible death. Splenomegaly or hepatomegaly is generally associated with advanced disease.

B. Laboratory Findings

The CBC is usually normal, although anemia, neutrophilia, eosinophilia, and thrombocytosis may be present. The erythrocyte sedimentation rate (ESR) and other acute-phase reactants are often elevated and can serve as markers of disease activity. Immunologic abnormalities occur, particularly in cell-mediated immunity, and anergy is common in patients with advanced-stage disease at diagnosis. Autoantibody phenomena such as hemolytic anemia and an idiopathic thrombocytopenic purpura–like picture have been reported.

C. Staging

Staging of Hodgkin lymphoma determines treatment and prognosis. The most common staging system is the Ann Arbor classification that describes extent of disease by I–IV and symptoms by an A or a B suffix (eg, stage IIIB). A systematic search for disease includes CT scan of the neck, chest, abdomen, and pelvis, as well as a positron emission tomography (PET) scan. Bone marrow aspirates and biopsies may not be required or performed as often bone marrow involvement can be determined by PET scan.

D. Pathologic Findings

The diagnosis of Hodgkin lymphoma requires the histologic presence of the Reed-Sternberg cell or its variants in tissue. Reed-Sternberg cells are germinal-center B cells that have undergone malignant transformation. Nearly 20% of these tumors in developed countries are positive for EBV. EBV has been linked to Hodgkin disease, and the large portion of Hodgkin patients with increased EBV titers suggests that EBV activation may contribute to the onset of Hodgkin lymphoma (Figure 31–2).

▶ Treatment & Prognosis

Treatment decisions are based on stage and presence of B symptoms, tumor bulk, and number of involved nodal regions. To achieve long-term disease-free survival while

minimizing treatment toxicity, Hodgkin disease is increasingly treated by chemotherapy and or immunotherapy alone—and less often by radiation therapy.

Several combinations of chemotherapeutic agents are effective, and treatment times are relatively short compared with pediatric oncology protocols for leukemia. Clinical trials have shown that only 9 weeks of therapy with AV-PC (Adriamycin [doxorubicin], vincristine, prednisone, and cyclophosphamide) is sufficient to induce a complete response in patients with low-risk Hodgkin lymphoma. Two additional drugs, bleomycin and etoposide, are currently added in the treatment of intermediate-risk patients for a total of 4–6 months of therapy for patients with intermediate-risk disease. The removal of involved field irradiation in patients with intermediate-risk Hodgkin lymphoma who respond early to chemotherapy has been shown to maintain excellent outcomes. Combined-modality therapy with chemotherapy and irradiation is used in advanced disease.

Current treatment gives an overall 5-year survival of 90%–95% to children with stages I and II Hodgkin lymphoma. Two-thirds of all relapses occur within 2 years after diagnosis, and relapse rarely occurs beyond 4 years. Although patients with advanced disease (stages III and IV) have slightly lower overall survival, more patients are becoming long-term survivors of Hodgkin disease. As a result, the risk of secondary malignancies, both leukemias and solid tumors, is becoming more apparent and is higher in patients receiving radiation therapy. Therefore, elucidating the optimal treatment strategy that minimizes such risk should be the goal of future studies.

Relapsed Hodgkin lymphoma remains responsive to treatment with chemotherapy and radiation therapy. Autologous HSCT after remission is achieved is used as consolidative

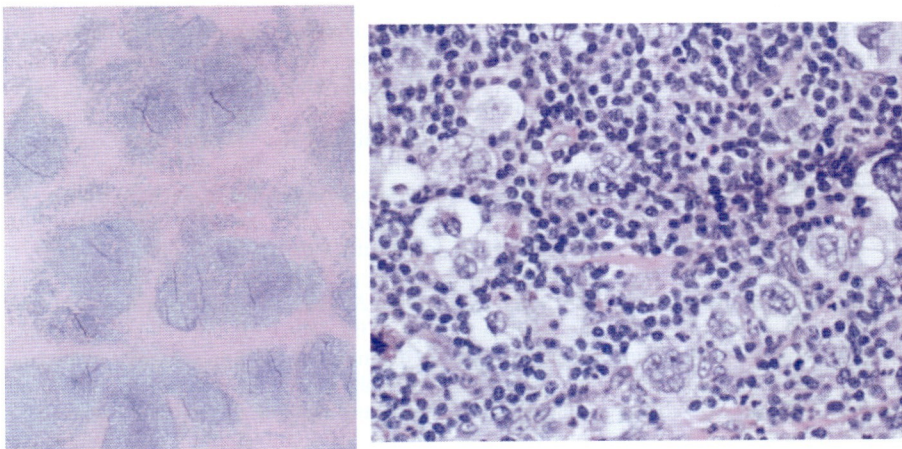

▲ **Figure 31–2.** Pathologic specimen at low power, showing classic nodules in the background. On the right, the large cells are the Reed Sternberg cells classic for Hodgkin lymphoma.

therapy to minimize the risk of subsequent relapse. Allogeneic HSCT is reserved for second or greater relapse as it carries increased risks of complications and may not offer added survival benefit.

Targeted immunotherapies have been incorporated into clinical trials for children with high-risk Hodgkin lymphoma, including antibody drug conjugates and checkpoint inhibitors. Brentuximab vedotin is an anti-CD30 murine/human chimeric monoclonal antibody linked to monomethyl auristatin E that targets CD30 which is highly expressed in Hodgkin lymphoma. Checkpoint inhibitors pembrolizumab and nivolumab that block PD-1 have recently been approved for recurrent Hodgkin lymphoma, as the tumor cells consistently express their target PDL-1 and PDL-2. Brentuximab and Nivolumab are now both used in up front high risk HD with excellent outcomes and minimal radiation therapy.

Friedman DL et al: Dose-intensive response-based chemotherapy and radiation therapy for children and adolescents with newly diagnosed intermediate-risk Hodgkin lymphoma: a report from the Children's Oncology Group Study AHOD0031. J Clin Oncol 2014;32:3561 [PMID: 25311218].
Kelly K: Hodgkin Lymphoma in children and adolescents: improving the therapeutic index. Blood 2015 Nov 26;126(22):2452–2458 [PMID: 26582374].
Mauz-Körholz C et al: Pediatric Hodgkin lymphoma. J Clin Oncol 2015 Sep 20;33(27):2975–2985. doi:10.1200/JCO.2014.59.4853. Epub 2015 Aug 24 [PMID: 26304892].
Younes A, Ansell SM: Novel agents in the treatment of Hodgkin lymphoma: biological basis and clinical results. Semin Hematol 2016 Jul;53(3):186–189 [PMID: 27496310].

2. Non-Hodgkin Lymphoma

General Considerations

Non-Hodgkin lymphomas (NHLs) are a diverse group of cancers accounting for 5%–10% of malignancies in children younger than 15 years. About 500 new cases arise per year in the United States. The incidence of NHLs increases with age. Children aged 15 years or younger account for only 3% of all cases of NHLs, and the disease is uncommon before age 5 years. There is a male predominance of approximately 3:1. In equatorial Africa, NHLs cause almost 50% of pediatric malignancies due to EBV and the associated Burkitt lymphoma (BL).

Most children who develop NHL are immunologically normal. However, children with congenital or acquired immune deficiencies (eg, Wiskott-Aldrich syndrome, severe combined immunodeficiency syndrome, X-linked lymphoproliferative syndrome, human immunodeficiency virus [HIV] infection, immunosuppressive therapy following solid-organ or marrow transplantation) have an increased risk of developing NHLs. Their risk is estimated to be 100–10,000 times that of age-matched control subjects.

Animal models suggest a viral contribution to the pathogenesis of NHL, and there is evidence of viral involvement in human NHL as well. In equatorial Africa, 95% of BLs contain DNA from the EBV. But in North America, less than 20% of Burkitt tumors contain the EBV genome. The role of other viruses (eg, human herpes viruses 6 and 8), disturbances in host immunologic defenses, chronic immunostimulation, and specific chromosomal rearrangements are potential triggers in the development of NHL.

Unlike adult NHL, virtually all childhood NHLs are rapidly proliferating, high-grade, diffuse malignancies. These tumors exhibit aggressive behavior but are usually very responsive to treatment. Nearly all pediatric NHLs are histologically classified into four main groups: LL, small noncleaved cell lymphoma (BL and Burkitt-like lymphoma [BLL]), LBCL, and ALCL. Immunophenotyping and cytogenetic features, in addition to clinical presentation, are increasingly important in the classification, pathogenesis, and treatment of NHLs. Comparisons of pediatric NHLs are summarized in Table 31–5.

Clinical Findings

A. Symptoms and Signs

Childhood NHLs can arise in any site of lymphoid tissue, including the lymph nodes, thymus, liver, and spleen. Common extralymphatic sites include bone, bone marrow, CNS, skin, and testes. Signs and symptoms at presentation are determined by the location of lesions and the degree of dissemination. Because NHL usually progresses very rapidly, the duration of symptoms is quite brief, from days to a few weeks. Nevertheless, children present with a limited number of syndromes, most of which correlate with cell type.

Children with LL often present with symptoms similar to ALL. For T-cell LL, symptoms of airway compression (cough, dyspnea, orthopnea) or superior vena cava obstruction (facial edema, chemosis, plethora, venous engorgement) are a result of mediastinal disease. *These symptoms are a true emergency necessitating rapid diagnosis and treatment.* Pleural or pericardial effusions may further compromise the patient's respiratory and cardiovascular status. CNS and bone marrow involvement are not common at diagnosis. When bone marrow contains more than 25% lymphoblasts, patients are diagnosed with ALL.

Most patients with BL and BLL present with abdominal disease. Abdominal pain, distention, a right lower quadrant mass, or intussusception in a child older than 5 years suggests the diagnosis of BL. Bone marrow involvement is common (~ 65% of patients). BL is the most rapidly proliferating tumor known and has a high rate of spontaneous cell death as it outgrows its blood supply. Consequently, children presenting with massive abdominal disease frequently have tumor lysis syndrome (hyperuricemia, hyperphosphatemia, and

Table 31–5. Comparison of pediatric non-Hodgkin lymphomas.

	Lymphoblastic Lymphoma	Small Noncleaved Cell Lymphoma (BL and BLL)	Large B-Cell Lymphoma	Anaplastic Large Cell Lymphoma
Incidence (%)	30–40	35–50	10–15	10–15
Histopathologic features	Indistinguishable from ALL lymphoblasts	Large nucleus with prominent nucleoli surrounded by very basophilic cytoplasm that contains lipid vacuoles	Large cells with cleaved or noncleaved nuclei	Large pleomorphic cells
Immunopheno-type	Immature T cell	B cell	B cell	T cell or null cell
Cytogenetic markers	Translocations involving chromosome 14q11 and chromosome 7; interstitial deletions of chromosome 1	t(8;14), t(8;22), t(2;8)	Many	t(2;5)
Clinical presentation	Intrathoracic tumor, mediastinal mass (50%–70%), lymphadenopathy above diaphragm (50%–80%)	Intra-abdominal tumor (90%), jaw involvement (10%–20% sporadic BL, 70% endemic BL), bone marrow involvement	Abdominal tumor most common; unusual sites: lung, face, brain, bone, testes, muscle	Lymphadenopathy, fever, weight loss, night sweats, extranodal sites including viscera and skin
Treatment	Similar to ALL therapy; 24 mo duration	Intensive administration of alkylating agents and methotrexate; CNS prophylaxis; 3–9 mo duration	Similar to therapy for BL/BLL	Similar to therapy for lymphoblastic lymphoma or BL/BLL

ALL, acute lymphoblastic leukemia; BL, Burkitt lymphoma; BLL, Burkitt-like lymphoma; CNS, central nervous system.

hyperkalemia). These abnormalities can be aggravated by tumor infiltration of the kidney or urinary obstruction by tumor. Although similar histologically, numerous differences exist between cases of BL occurring in endemic areas of equatorial Africa and the sporadic cases of North America (Table 31–6).

Table 31–6. Comparison of endemic and sporadic Burkitt lymphoma.

	Endemic	Sporadic
Incidence	10 per 100,000	0.9 per 100,000
Cytogenetics	Chromosome 8 breakpoint upstream of *c-myc* locus	Chromosome 8 breakpoint within *c-myc* locus
EBV association	≥ 95%	≤ 20%
Disease sites at presentation	Jaw (58%), abdomen (58%), CNS (19%), orbit (11%), marrow (7%)	Jaw (7%), abdomen (91%), CNS (14%), orbit (1%), marrow (20%)

CNS, central nervous system; EBV, Epstein-Barr virus.

Large cell lymphomas are similar clinically to the small noncleaved cell lymphomas, although unusual sites of involvement are quite common, particularly with ALCL. Skin lesions, focal neurologic deficits, and pleural or peritoneal effusions without an obvious associated mass are frequently seen. With improved diagnostic techniques, new categories of LBCLs including primary mediastinal B-cell lymphoma and gray zone lymphomas have been identified. The distinction is an important one as the approach to therapy differs significantly.

B. Diagnostic Evaluation

Diagnosis is made by biopsy of involved tissue with histology, immunophenotyping, and cytogenetic studies. If mediastinal disease is present, general anesthesia may need to be avoided if the airway or vena cava is significantly compromised by tumor. In these cases, samples of pleural or ascitic fluid, bone marrow, or peripheral nodes obtained under local anesthesia (in the presence of an anesthesiologist) may confirm the diagnosis. Major abdominal surgery and intestinal resection should be avoided in patients with an abdominal mass that is likely to be BL, as the tumor will regress rapidly with the initiation of chemotherapy. The rapid growth of these tumors and the associated life-threatening complications demand that further studies be done expeditiously so that specific therapy is not delayed.

After a thorough physical examination, a CBC, liver function tests, and a biochemical profile (electrolytes, calcium, phosphorus, uric acid, renal function) should be obtained. An elevated LDH reflects tumor burden and can serve as a marker of disease activity. Imaging studies should include a chest radiograph and CT scans of the neck, chest, abdomen and pelvis, and a PET scan. Bone marrow and CSF examinations are also essential.

▶ Treatment

A. Supportive Care

The management of life-threatening problems at presentation is critical. The most common complications are acute tumor lysis syndrome, superior vena cava syndrome, airway compromise, and cardiac tamponade. Patients with airway compromise require prompt initiation of specific therapy. Because of the risk of general anesthesia in these patients, it is occasionally necessary to initiate corticosteroids or low-dose emergency radiation therapy until the mass is small enough for a biopsy to be undertaken safely. Response to steroids and radiation therapy is usually prompt (12–24 hours).

Tumor lysis syndrome should be anticipated in all patients who have NHL with a large tumor burden. Maintaining a brisk urine output (> 5 mL/kg/h) with intravenous fluids and diuretics is the key to management. Allopurinol will reduce serum uric acid. Rasburicase is an effective intravenous alternative to allopurinol and is increasingly used for patients with high risk of tumor lysis based on tumor burden or in patients who do not have an optimal response to allopurinol. Renal dialysis is occasionally necessary to control metabolic abnormalities. Every attempt should be made to correct or minimize metabolic abnormalities before initiating chemotherapy; however, this period of stabilization should not exceed 24–48 hours.

B. Specific Therapy

Systemic chemotherapy is the mainstay of therapy for NHLs. Nearly all patients with NHL require intensive intrathecal chemotherapy for CNS prophylaxis. Surgical resection is not indicated unless the entire tumor can be resected safely, which is rare. Partial resection or debulking surgery has no role. Radiation therapy does not improve outcome, so its use is confined to exceptional circumstances.

Therapy for LL is generally based on treatment protocols designed for ALL and involves dose-intensive, multiagent chemotherapy. The duration of therapy is 2 years. Treatment of BL, BLL, and LCBL consists of alkylating agents and intermediate- to high-dose methotrexate administered intensively, but for a relatively short time as it produces the highest cure rates. Addition of rituximab (anti-CD20

monoclonal antibody) to the chemotherapy backbone has improved EFS and OS. Dose-adjusted EPOCH-R has demonstrated improved outcomes in adults with primary mediastinal B-cell lymphoma and gray zone lymphomas. Clinical trials utilizing this regimen are ongoing in children with these rare NHLs.

Additionally, oral small molecule inhibitors against the ALK oncogene are being explored as novel therapy for specific subsets of patients with ALCL. The ALK oncogene is activated by a 2;5 translocation leading to juxtaposition of NPM N-terminal region to the intracellular part of ALK and is the defining genetic lesions in ALK-positive ALCL. ALCL often express CD30 and studies are ongoing combining chemotherapy with brentuximab vedotin or ALK inhibitors.

▶ Prognosis

A major predictor of outcome in NHL is the extent of disease at diagnosis. Ninety percent of patients with localized disease can expect long-term, disease-free survival. Patients with extensive disease on both sides of the diaphragm, CNS involvement, or bone marrow involvement in addition to a primary site have a 70%–80% failure-free survival (FFS) rate. Relapses occur early in NHL; patients with LL rarely have recurrences after 30 months from diagnosis, whereas patients with BL and BLL very rarely have recurrences beyond 1 year. The cure rate for patients with relapsed T-cell lymphoblastic leukemia/lymphoma is particularly poor (3-year EFS rates < 20%). Patients who experience relapse may have a chance for cure by autologous or allogeneic HSCT.

Minard-Colin V et al: Rituximab for high risk, mature B-cell non-Hodgkin lymphoma in children. N Engl J Med 2020;382: 2207–2219 [PMID: 32492302].
Sandlund JT, Martin MG: Non-Hodgkin lymphoma across the pediatric and adolescent and young adult age spectrum. Hematology Am Soc Hematol Educ Program 2016 Dec 2;2016(1): 589–597 [PMID: 27913533].

3. Lymphoproliferative Disorders

Lymphoproliferative disorders (LPDs) can be thought of as a part of a continuum with lymphomas. Whereas LPDs represent inappropriate, often polyclonal proliferations of nonmalignant lymphocytes, lymphomas represent the development of malignant clones, sometimes arising from recognized LPDs.

A. Posttransplantation Lymphoproliferative Disorders

Posttransplantation lymphoproliferative disorders (PTLDs) arise in patients who have received substantial immunosuppressive medications for solid organ or bone marrow transplantation. In these patients, reactivation of latent EBV infection in B cells drives a polyclonal proliferation of these cells that is fatal if not halted. Occasionally a true lymphoma develops, often bearing a chromosomal translocation.

LPDs are an increasingly common and significant complication of transplantation. The incidence of PTLD ranges from approximately 2% to 15% of transplant recipients, depending on the organ transplanted and the immunosuppressive regimen.

Treatment of these disorders is a challenge for transplant physicians and oncologists. The initial treatment is reduction in immunosuppression, which allows the patient's own immune cells to destroy the virally transformed lymphocytes. However, this is only effective in approximately half of the patients. For those patients who do not respond to reduced immune suppression, chemotherapy of various regimens may succeed. The use of anti–B-cell antibodies, such as rituximab (anti-CD20), for the treatment of PTLDs has been promising in clinical trials. More recently, T-cell–based immune therapies, such as donor lymphocyte infusions and adoptive transfer of EBV-specific cytotoxic T lymphocytes, have also been explored as novel approaches.

B. Spontaneous Lymphoproliferative Disease

Immunodeficiencies in which LPDs occur include Bloom syndrome, Chédiak-Higashi syndrome, ataxia-telangiectasia, Wiskott-Aldrich syndrome, X-linked lymphoproliferative syndrome, congenital T-cell immunodeficiencies, and HIV infection. Treatment depends on the circumstances, but unlike PTLD, few therapeutic options are often available. Castleman disease is an LPD occurring in pediatric patients without any apparent immunodeficiency. The autoimmune lymphoproliferative syndrome (ALPS) is characterized by widespread lymphadenopathy with hepatosplenomegaly and autoimmune phenomena. ALPS results from mutations in the Fas ligand pathway that is critical in regulation of apoptosis.

Weintraub L et al: Identifying predictive factors for posttransplant lymphoproliferative disease in pediatric solid organ transplant recipients with Epstein-Barr virus viremia. J Pediatr Hematol Oncol 2014;36:e481 [PMID: 24878618].
Yang X, Miyawaki T, Kanegane H: Lymphoproliferative disorders in immunocompromised individuals and therapeutic antibodies for treatment. Immunotherapy 2013;5:415 [PMID: 23557424].

NEUROBLASTOMA

▶ General Considerations

Neuroblastoma arises from neural crest tissue of the sympathetic ganglia or adrenal medulla. It is composed of small, uniform cells with scant cytoplasm and hyperchromatic nuclei that may form a rosette pattern. It must be differentiated from other "small, round, blue cell" malignancies of childhood, such as Ewing sarcoma, rhabdomyosarcoma (RMS), peripheral neuroectodermal tumor (PNET), and NHL.

Neuroblastoma accounts for 7%–10% of pediatric malignancies and is the most common solid neoplasm outside the CNS. Fifty percent of neuroblastomas are diagnosed before age 2 years and 90% before age 5 years. It is a biologically diverse disease with clinical behavior that can range from spontaneous regression to relentless progression despite aggressive therapy. Historically, cure rates for patients with high-risk neuroblastoma were very poor. With promising recent advances, however, cure rates have been steadily improving, albeit at the price of significant toxicity from treatment.

▶ Clinical Findings

A. Symptoms and Signs

Clinical manifestations vary based on tumor location and neuroendocrine function of the tumor. Many children present with constitutional symptoms such as fever, weight loss, and irritability. Bone pain suggests metastatic disease, which is present in 60% of children older than 1 year at diagnosis. Physical examination may reveal a firm, fixed, irregularly shaped midline abdominal mass. Although most children have an abdominal primary tumor (40% adrenal gland, 25% paraspinal ganglion), neuroblastoma can arise wherever there is sympathetic nervous tissue. In the posterior mediastinum, the tumor is usually asymptomatic and discovered incidentally on a chest radiograph. Patients with cervical neuroblastoma present with a neck mass, sometimes misdiagnosed as infection. Horner syndrome (unilateral ptosis, myosis, and anhidrosis) or heterochromia iridis (differently colored irises) may accompany cervical neuroblastoma. Paraspinous tumors can extend through the spinal foramen, causing cord compression and leading to paresis, paralysis, or bowel/bladder dysfunction.

The most common sites of metastases are bone, bone marrow, lymph nodes, liver, and subcutaneous tissue. Neuroblastoma has a predilection for metastasis to the skull, particularly the sphenoid bone and retrobulbar tissue, causing periorbital ecchymosis ("raccoon eyes") and proptosis. Liver metastasis, particularly in the newborn, can lead to massive hepatomegaly. Skin metastases can appear as bluish or purplish subcutaneous nodules ("blueberry muffin baby") and can be associated with an erythematous flush followed by blanching when compressed, probably due to catecholamine release.

Neuroblastoma can have paraneoplastic manifestations, the most striking example being opsoclonus-myoclonus-ataxia (OMA) syndrome ("dancing eyes/dancing feet"). This phenomenon is characterized by rapid and chaotic eye movements, myoclonic jerking of the limbs and trunk, ataxia, and behavioral disturbances. This process, which often persists after treatment of the neuroblastoma is complete, is due to cross-reacting antineuronal autoantibodies. Treatment is with immunosuppression. Intractable, watery diarrhea can occur due to secretion of vasoactive intestinal peptide (VIP) by the tumor. Interestingly, both of these paraneoplastic syndromes, despite their morbidity, are associated with more favorable curative potential for the tumor itself.

B. Laboratory Findings

Anemia is present in 60% of children with neuroblastoma and can be due to chronic disease or marrow infiltration. Occasionally, thrombocytopenia is present, but thrombocytosis is a more common finding, even with metastatic disease in the marrow. Urinary catecholamines (vanillylmandelic acid [VMA] and homovanillic acid [HVA]) are elevated in at least 90% of patients at diagnosis and should be measured prior to surgery.

C. Imaging

Radiographs of the primary tumor may show stippled calcifications. Metastases to bone can appear irregular and lytic. Periosteal reaction and pathologic fractures may also be seen.

CT scanning shows extent of the primary tumor, effects on surrounding structures, and the presence of metastatic disease. Classically, in tumors originating from the adrenal gland, the kidney is displaced inferolaterally, which helps to differentiate neuroblastoma from Wilms tumor. MRI is useful in determining the presence of spinal cord involvement in tumors that invade neural foramina.

I-123-Metaiodobenzylguanidine (MIBG), a radiolabeled compound that localizes to adrenal tissue, is used to detect and quantify the degree of metastatic disease at diagnosis and to track response to treatment. PET-CT can be utilized in patients whose tumors are MIBG nonavid (8.7% of cases). MIBG and PET-CT scanning have supplanted technetium-99m bone scanning for evaluation of bone metastases in neuroblastoma (Figure 31–3).

D. Staging

Staging of neuroblastoma is usually performed according to the International Neuroblastoma Staging System (INSS) (Table 31–7), though a newer, International Neuroblastoma Risk Group (INRG) staging system that incorporates image-defined risk factors as part of the staging process is being used more commonly. Biopsy of the tumor is essential to confirm the diagnosis and determine the biologic characteristics

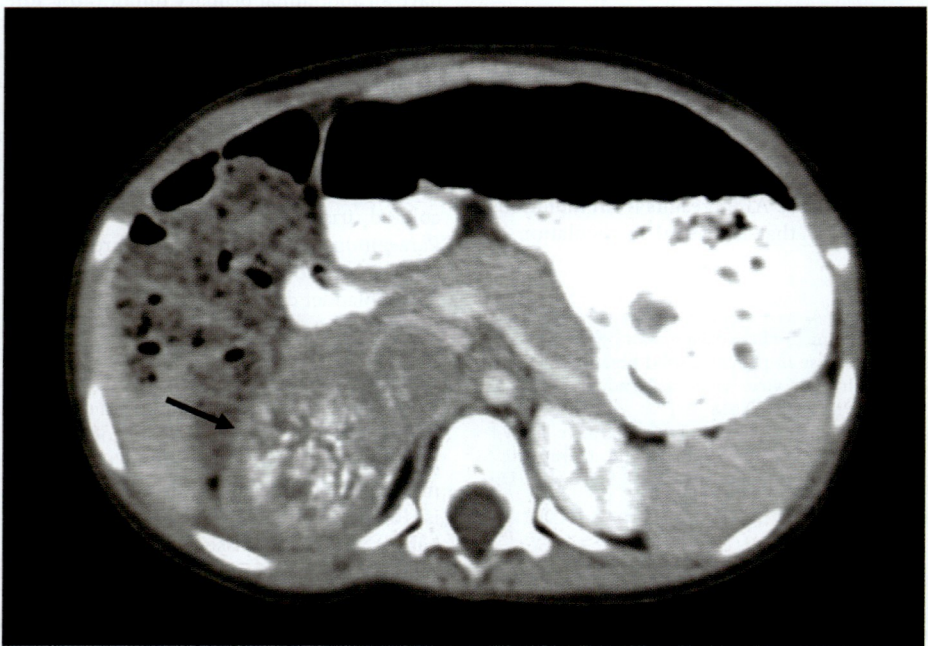

▲ **Figure 31–3.** CT of the abdomen of a 3-year-old girl shows a large right paraspinous mass (arrow) in the suprarenal area displacing the right kidney inferiorly. Calcifications are noted within the mass. Given these findings, neuroblastoma is the most likely diagnosis.

Table 31–7. International Neuroblastoma Staging System.

Stage	Description
1	Localized tumor with complete gross excision, with or without microscopic residual disease; representative ipsilateral lymph nodes negative for tumor microscopically.
2A	Localized tumor with incomplete gross excision; representative ipsilateral nonadherent lymph nodes negative for tumor microscopically.
2B	Localized tumor with or without complete gross excision, with ipsilateral nonadherent lymph nodes positive for tumor. Enlarged lymph nodes must be negative microscopically.
3	Unresectable unilateral tumor infiltrating across the midline, with or without regional lymph node involvement; or localized unilateral tumor with contralateral regional lymph node involvement; or midline tumor with bilateral extension by infiltration (unresectable) or by lymph node involvement. The midline is defined as the vertebral column. Tumors originating on one side and crossing the midline must infiltrate to or beyond the opposite side of the vertebral column.
4	Any primary tumor with dissemination to distant lymph nodes, bone, bone marrow, liver, skin, or other organs, except as defined for stage 4S.
4S	Localized primary tumor, as defined for stage 1, 2A, or 2B, with dissemination limited to skin, liver, or bone marrow, and limited to infants aged < 1 y. Marrow involvement should be < 10% of nucleated cells.

of the tumor. In addition, bilateral bone marrow aspirates and biopsies must be performed to evaluate for bone marrow involvement.

Tumors are classified as favorable or unfavorable based on histologic characteristics and the age of the patient at diagnosis, with younger age (< 18 months) being associated with a more favorable prognosis. Amplification of the *MYCN* protooncogene is a reliable marker of aggressive clinical behavior. Tumor cell DNA content is also predictive of outcome. Hyperdiploidy is a favorable finding, whereas diploid DNA content is associated with a worse outcome. Loss of heterozygosity at chromosome bands 1p36 and 11q23 also confers a worse prognosis.

▶ **Treatment & Prognosis**

Patients are treated according to a risk stratification system that takes into account INSS or INRG stage, patient age, *MYCN* status, histology, cytogenetic findings, and DNA index. Based on these factors, patients are classified as having low-, intermediate-, or high-risk disease.

For low-risk disease (INSS stages 1 and 2, with favorable biologic features), surgical resection of more than 50% of the tumor is usually sufficient for cure. Aggressive surgery to remove the entire tumor at the expense of surrounding normal structures is not necessary and can lead to unnecessary morbidity. Infants younger than 6 months with small adrenal masses consistent radiographically with neuroblastoma can be treated with close observation alone, even in the absence of a biopsy. Survival rates for patients with low-risk neuroblastoma are more than 98%. Infants younger than 1 year with INSS stage 4S disease may need little if any therapy, with the disease regressing spontaneously, although chemotherapy may be initiated because of bulky disease (generally massive hepatomegaly) causing mechanical complications. Survival rates with 4S disease are more than 90%.

With intermediate-risk neuroblastoma (subsets of patients with INSS stages 3 and 4 disease), the primary treatment approach is surgery combined with chemotherapy. The size or location of the tumor often makes primary resection impossible. Under these circumstances, a biopsy alone is performed to make a definitive diagnosis and evaluate biologic characteristics. Shrinkage of the tumor with chemotherapy often allows a second surgery with more complete tumor resection. Chemotherapeutic agents typically used include carboplatin, etoposide, cyclophosphamide, vincristine, and doxorubicin. The number of cycles used (usually 2–8) depends on multiple factors, including the age of the patient, the INSS stage, biologic features of the tumor, and response to treatment. Radiation therapy is rarely necessary. Survival rates for intermediate risk neuroblastoma are 90%–95%.

High-risk patients (the majority with INSS stages 3 and 4 disease, generally with older age and unfavorable tumor biology) require intensive, multimodal therapy including chemotherapy, surgery, autologous HSCT, irradiation, biologic therapy, and immunotherapy. Several cycles of intensive chemotherapy are followed by resection of as much of the tumor as possible. Following this induction phase, tandem (two sequential) autologous HSCTs are performed as consolidative therapy. Following the HSCTs, the site of the primary tumor and any areas with evidence of active disease prior to transplant are irradiated. At this point, patients have reached a state of MRD. To reduce the risk of recurrence, a maintenance phase follows. Patients receive immunotherapy with an antibody directed against the GD2 antigen expressed on the surface of the neuroblastoma cells together with GM-CSF to enhance immune-mediated cell killing. These treatments are alternated with treatments with 13-*cis*-retinoic acid, an agent that induces terminal differentiation of neuroblastoma cells. Results of recent studies incorporating all of these treatment modalities are encouraging, with 5-year EFS rates of 56% and overall survival rates of 73%. An ongoing COG treatment study is looking at the incorporation of therapeutic radioactive I-121-MIBG into the upfront treatment regimen. Also, use of targeted therapies, such as ALK inhibition in patients whose tumors express ALK mutations, is being investigated. Despite advancements, high-risk neuroblastoma remains a challenging disease, and much work remains to improve cure rates while minimizing the toxicity of treatment.

Maris JM: Recent advances in neuroblastoma. N Engl J Med 2010; 362:2202–2211 [PMID: 20558371].

Neuroblastoma—Patient Version: National Cancer Institute: http://www.cancer.gov/cancertopics/types/neuroblastoma.

Nuchtern JG et al: A prospective study of expectant observation as primary therapy for neuroblastoma in young infants: a Children's Oncology Group study. Ann Surg 2012;256:573–580 [PMID: 22964741].

Park J et al: Effect of tandem autologous stem cell transplant vs single transplant on event-free survival in patients with high-risk neuroblastoma: a randomized clinical trial. JAMA 2019 Aug 27;322(8):746–755 [PMID: 31454045].

PDQ Neuroblastoma Treatment (PDQ®)–Health Professional Version: National Cancer Institute: https://www.cancer.gov/types/neuroblastoma/hp/neuroblastoma-treatment-pdq. Updated April 07, 2023. Accessed June 27, 2023 [PMID: 26389190].

Tolbert VP, Matthay KK: Neuroblastoma: clinical and biological approach to risk stratification and treatment. Cell Tissue Res 2018 May;372(2):195–209 [PMID: 29572647].

WILMS TUMOR (NEPHROBLASTOMA)

▶ General Considerations

Approximately 460 new cases of Wilms tumor occur annually in the United States, representing 5%–6% of cancers in children younger than 15 years. After neuroblastoma, this is the second most common abdominal tumor in children. The majority of Wilms tumors are of sporadic occurrence. However, in a few children, Wilms tumor occurs in the setting of associated malformations or syndromes, including aniridia, hemihypertrophy, genitourinary (GU) malformations (eg, cryptorchidism, hypospadias, gonadal dysgenesis, pseudohermaphroditism, and horseshoe kidney), Beckwith-Wiedemann syndrome, Denys-Drash syndrome, and WAGR syndrome (Wilms tumor, aniridia, ambiguous genitalia, mental retardation).

The median age at diagnosis is related both to gender and laterality, with bilateral tumors presenting at a younger age than unilateral tumors, and males being diagnosed earlier than females. Wilms tumor occurs most commonly between ages 2 and 5 years; it is unusual after age 6 years. The mean age at diagnosis is 4 years.

▶ Clinical Findings

A. Symptoms and Signs

Most children with Wilms tumor present with increasing size of the abdomen or an asymptomatic abdominal mass incidentally discovered by a parent and/or health care provider. The mass is usually smooth and firm, well demarcated, and rarely crosses the midline, though it can extend inferiorly into the pelvis. About 25% of patients are hypertensive at presentation. Gross hematuria is an uncommon presentation, although microscopic hematuria occurs in approximately 25% of patients.

B. Laboratory Findings

The CBC is usually normal, but some patients have anemia secondary to hemorrhage into the tumor. Blood urea nitrogen and serum creatinine are usually normal. Urinalysis may show some blood or leukocytes.

C. Imaging and Staging

Ultrasonography or CT of the abdomen should establish the presence of an intrarenal mass. It is also essential to evaluate the contralateral kidney for presence and function as well as synchronous Wilms tumor. The inferior vena cava needs to be evaluated by ultrasonography with Doppler flow for the presence and extent of tumor propagation. The liver should be imaged for the presence of metastatic disease. Chest CT scan should be obtained to determine whether pulmonary metastases are present. Approximately 10% of patients will have metastatic disease at diagnosis. Of these, 80% will have pulmonary disease and 15% liver metastases. Bone and brain metastases are extremely uncommon and usually associated with the rarer, more aggressive renal tumor types, such as clear cell sarcoma or RT; hence, bone scans and brain imaging are not routinely performed. The clinical stage is ultimately decided at surgery and confirmed by the pathologist.

▶ Treatment & Prognosis

In the United States, treatment of Wilms tumor begins with surgical exploration of the abdomen via an anterior surgical approach to allow for inspection and palpation of the contralateral kidney. The liver and lymph nodes are inspected and suspicious areas biopsied or excised. En bloc resection of the tumor is performed. Every attempt is made to avoid tumor spillage at surgery as this may increase the staging and treatment. Because therapy is tailored to tumor stage, it is imperative that a surgeon familiar with the staging requirements perform the operation.

In addition to the staging, the histologic type has implications for therapy and prognosis. Favorable histology (FH; see later discussion) refers to the classic triphasic Wilms tumor and its variants. Unfavorable histology (UH) refers to the presence of diffuse anaplasia (extreme nuclear atypia) and is present in 5% of Wilms tumors. The finding of anaplasia correlates with *TP53* gene mutation within the tumor. Only a few small foci of anaplasia in a Wilms tumor portend a worse prognosis. Loss of heterozygosity of chromosomes 1p and 16q are adverse prognostic factors in those with FH. Following excision and pathologic examination, the patient is assigned a stage that defines further therapy.

Table 31–8. Treatment of Wilms tumor.

Stage/Histologic Subtype	Treatment
I–II FH and I UH	18 wk (dactinomycin and vincristine)
III–IV FH and II–IV focal anaplasia	24 wk (dactinomycin, vincristine, and doxorubicin) with radiation
II–IV UH (diffuse anaplasia)	24 wk (vincristine, doxorubicin, etoposide, and cyclophosphamide) with radiation

FH, favorable histology; UH, unfavorable histology.

Improvement in the treatment of Wilms tumor has resulted in an overall cure rate of approximately 90%. The National Wilms' Tumor Study Group's fourth study (NWTS-4) demonstrated that survival rates were improved by intensifying therapy during the initial treatment phase while shortening overall treatment duration (24 vs 60 weeks of treatment).

Table 31–8 provides an overview of the current treatment recommendations in NWTS-5. Patients with stage III or IV Wilms tumor require radiation therapy to the tumor bed and to sites of metastatic disease. Chemotherapy is optimally begun within 5 days after surgery, whereas radiation therapy should be started within 10 days. Stage V (bilateral Wilms tumor) disease dictates a different approach, consisting of possible bilateral renal biopsies followed by chemotherapy and second-look renal-sparing surgery. Radiation therapy may also be necessary.

Using these approaches, 4-year overall survival rates through NWTS-4 are as follows: stage I FH, 96%; stages II–IV FH, 82%–92%; stages I–III UH (diffuse anaplasia), 56%–70%; and stage IV UH, 17%. Patients with recurrent Wilms tumor have a salvage rate of approximately 50% with surgery, radiation therapy, and chemotherapy (singly or in combination). HSCT is also being explored as a way to improve the chances of survival after relapse.

Future Considerations

Although progress in the treatment of Wilms tumor has been extraordinary, important questions remain to be answered. Questions have been raised regarding the role of prenephrectomy chemotherapy in the treatment of Wilms tumor. Presurgical chemotherapy seems to decrease tumor rupture at resection but may unfavorably affect outcome by changing staging. Future studies will be directed at minimizing acute and long-term toxicities for those with low-risk disease and improving outcomes for those with high-risk and recurrent disease.

Aldrink JH et al: Update on Wilms tumor. J Pediatr Surg 2019 Mar;54(3):390–397 [PMID: 30270120].
Buckley KS: Pediatric genitourinary tumors. Curr Opin Oncol 2010;23(3):297 [PMID: 21460723].
Caldwell BT, Wilcox DT, Cost NG: Current management of pediatric urologic oncology. Adv Pediatr 2017 Aug;64(1):191–223 [PMID: 28688589].
Lopes RF, Lorenza A: Recent advanced in the management of Wilms' tumor. F1000Res 2017 May 12;6:670. doi:10.12688/f1000research.10760.1. eCollection 2017 [PMID: 28620463].
Oostveen RM, Pritchard-Jones K: Pharmacotherapeutic management of Wilms tumor: an update. Paediatr Drugs 2019 Feb;21(1):1–13 [PMID: 30604241].
PDQ Pediatric Treatment Editorial Board: Wilms tumor and other childhood kidney tumors treatment (PDQ®): Health Professional Version. In: PDQ Cancer Information Summaries [Internet]. Bethesda (MD): National Cancer Institute; 2002. https://www.ncbi.nlm.nih.gov/books/NBK65842/.
Sadak KT, Ritchey ML, Dome JS: Paediatric genitourinary cancers and late effects of treatment. Nat Rev Urol 2013 Jan;10(1):15–25 [PMID: 19657990].

BONE TUMORS

Primary malignant bone tumors are uncommon in childhood with only 650–700 new cases per year. Osteosarcoma accounts for 60% of cases and occurs mostly in adolescents and young adults. Ewing sarcoma is the second most common malignant tumor of bony origin and occurs in toddlers to young adults. Both tumors have a male predominance.

The cardinal signs of bone tumor are pain at the site of involvement, often following slight trauma, mass formation, and fracture through an area of cortical bone destruction.

1. Osteosarcoma

General Considerations

Although osteosarcoma is the sixth most common malignancy in childhood, it ranks third among adolescents and young adults. This peak occurrence during the adolescent growth spurt suggests a causal relationship between rapid bone growth and malignant transformation. Further evidence for this relationship is found in epidemiologic data showing patients with osteosarcoma to be taller than their peers, osteosarcoma occurring most frequently at sites where the greatest increase in length and size of bone occurs, and osteosarcoma occurring at an earlier age in girls than boys, corresponding to their earlier growth spurt. The metaphyses of long tubular bones are primarily affected. The distal femur accounts for more than 40% of cases, with the proximal tibia, proximal humerus, and mid and proximal femur following in frequency.

Clinical Findings

A. Symptoms and Signs

Pain over the involved area is the usual presenting symptom with or without an associated soft tissue mass. Patients generally have symptoms for several months prior to diagnosis.

Systemic symptoms (fever, weight loss) are rare. Laboratory evaluation may reveal elevated serum alkaline phosphatase or LDH levels.

B. Imaging and Staging

Radiographic findings show permeative ("moth-eaten" appearance) destruction of the normal bony trabecular pattern with indistinct margins. In addition, periosteal new bone formation and lifting of the bony cortex may create a Codman triangle. A soft tissue mass plus calcifications in a radial or sunburst pattern are frequently noted. MRI is more sensitive in defining the extent of the primary tumor and has mostly replaced CT scanning. The most common sites of metastases are the lung (≤ 20% of newly diagnosed cases) and the additional boney sites (10%). CT scan of the chest and bone scan are essential for detecting metastatic disease. PET-CT may be a consideration in monitoring response to therapy. Bone marrow aspirates and biopsies are not indicated.

Despite the rather characteristic radiographic appearance, a tissue sample is needed to confirm the diagnosis. Placement of the incision for biopsy is of critical importance. A misplaced incision could preclude a limb salvage procedure and necessitate amputation. The surgeon who will carry out the definitive surgical procedure should perform the biopsy. A staging system for osteosarcoma based on local tumor extent and presence or absence of distant metastasis has been proposed, but it has not been validated (Figure 31–4).

▶ Treatment & Prognosis

Historical studies showed that over 50% of patients receiving surgery alone developed pulmonary metastases within 6 months after surgery. This suggests the presence of micrometastatic disease at diagnosis. Adjuvant chemotherapy trials showed improved disease-free survival rates of 55%–85% in patients followed for 3–10 years.

Osteosarcomas are highly radioresistant lesions; for this reason, radiation therapy has no role in its primary management. Chemotherapy is often administered prior to definitive surgery (neoadjuvant chemotherapy). This permits an early attack on micrometastatic disease and may also shrink the tumor, facilitating a limb salvage procedure. Preoperative

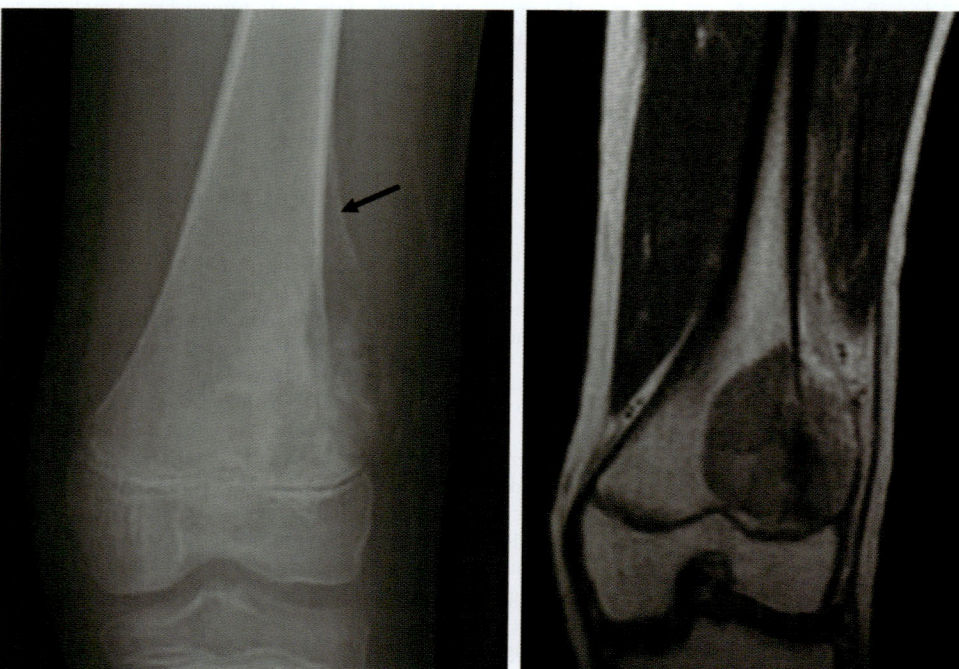

▲ **Figure 31–4.** The x-ray of the left knee (left) shows an aggressive lesion with bony destruction and formation of osteoid matrix in the distal left femoral metaphysis. There is associated periosteal reaction, forming the radiologic sign known as the Codman triangle (arrow). The MRI scan on the right shows the same lesion, outlining the extent of the tumor in the bone and surrounding soft tissues.

chemotherapy also makes detailed histologic evaluation of tumor response to the chemotherapy agents possible. If the histologic response is poor (> 10% viable tumor tissue), postoperative chemotherapy can be changed accordingly, but a recently completed COG Group study showed increased toxicity with no additional benefit. Chemotherapy may be administered intra-arterially or intravenously, although the benefits of intra-arterial chemotherapy (IAC) are disputed. Agents having efficacy in the treatment of osteosarcoma include doxorubicin, cisplatin, high-dose methotrexate, ifosfamide, and etoposide.

Definitive cure requires en bloc surgical resection of the tumor with a margin of uninvolved tissue. Amputation, limb salvage, and rotation plasty (Van Ness rotation) are equally effective in achieving local control of osteosarcoma. Contraindications to limb-sparing surgery include major involvement of the neurovascular bundle by tumor; immature skeletal age, particularly for lower extremity tumors; infection in the region of the tumor; inappropriate biopsy site; and extensive muscle involvement that would result in a poor functional outcome.

Postsurgical chemotherapy is generally continued until the patient has received 1 year of treatment. Relapses are unusual beyond 3 years, but late relapses do occur. Histologic response to neoadjuvant chemotherapy is an excellent predictor of outcome. Patients with localized disease having 90% or greater tumor necrosis have a 70%–75% long-term, disease-free survival rate. Other favorable prognostic factors include distal skeletal lesions, longer duration of symptoms, age older than 20 years, female gender, and near-diploid tumor DNA index. Patients with metastatic disease at diagnosis or multifocal bone lesions do not fair well, despite advances in chemotherapy and surgical techniques.

2. Ewing Sarcoma

▶ General Considerations

Ewing sarcoma accounts for only 30% of primary malignant bone tumors; fewer than 200 new cases occur each year in the United States. It is a disease primarily of white males, almost never affects blacks, and occurs mostly in the second decade of life. Ewing sarcoma is considered a "small, round, blue cell" malignancy. The differential diagnosis includes RMS, lymphoma, and neuroblastoma. Although most commonly a tumor of bone, it may also occur in soft tissue (extraosseous Ewing sarcoma or PNET).

▶ Clinical Findings

A. Symptoms and Signs

Pain at the site of the primary tumor is the most common presenting sign, with or without swelling and erythema. No specific laboratory findings are characteristic of Ewing

sarcoma, but an elevated LDH may be present and is of prognostic significance. Associated symptoms include fevers and weight loss.

B. Imaging and Staging

The radiographic appearance of Ewing sarcoma overlaps with osteosarcoma, although Ewing sarcoma usually involves the diaphyses of long bones. The central axial skeleton gives rise to 40% of Ewing tumors. Evaluation of a patient diagnosed as having Ewing sarcoma should include an MRI of the primary lesion to define the extent of local disease as precisely as possible. This is imperative for planning future surgical procedures or radiation therapy. Metastatic disease is present in 25% of patients at diagnosis. The lung (38%), bone (particularly the spine) (31%), and the bone marrow (11%) are the most common sites for metastasis. CT scan of the chest, bone scan, and bilateral bone marrow aspirates and biopsies are all essential to the staging workup. PET-CT may be considered to help monitor therapy response.

A biopsy is essential to establishing the diagnosis. Histologically, Ewing sarcoma consists of sheets of undifferentiated cells with hyperchromatic nuclei, well-defined cell borders, and scanty cytoplasm. Necrosis is common. Electron microscopy, immunocytochemistry, and cytogenetics may be necessary to confirm the diagnosis. A generous tissue biopsy specimen is often necessary for diagnosis but should not delay starting chemotherapy.

A consistent cytogenetic abnormality, t(11;22), has been identified in Ewing sarcoma and PNET and is present in 85%–90% of tumors. These tumors also express the protooncogene c-*myc*, which may be helpful in differentiating Ewing sarcoma from neuroblastoma, in which c-*myc* is not expressed.

▶ Treatment & Prognosis

Therapy usually commences with the administration of chemotherapy after biopsy and is followed by local control measures. Depending on many factors, including the primary site of the tumor and the response to chemotherapy, local control can be achieved by surgery, radiation therapy, or a combination of these methods. Following local control, chemotherapy continues for approximately 6 months. Effective treatment for Ewing sarcoma uses combinations of dactinomycin, vincristine, doxorubicin, cyclophosphamide, etoposide, and ifosfamide. Recent data showed that giving chemotherapy every 2 weeks, rather than every 3 weeks, improved the EFS for localized Ewing sarcoma.

Patients with small localized primary tumors have a 70%–75% long-term, disease-free survival rate. For patients with metastatic disease, survival is poor. Autologous HSCT may be considered as part of the treatment of these high-risk patients. Patients with pelvic tumors have an intermediate prognosis of around 50% long-term, disease-free survival.

Damon R et al: Treatment pathway of bone sarcoma in children, adolescents, and young adults. Cancer 2017;123(12):2206–2218 [PMID: 28323337].

Ewing Sarcoma and Undifferentiated Small Round Cell Sarcomas of Bone and Soft Tissue Treatment (PDQ®)-Health Professional Version: National Cancer Institute: https://www.cancer.gov/types/bone/hp/ewing-treatment-pdq. Updated June 14, 2023. Accessed June 27, 2023 [PMID: 26389480].

Geller DS, Gorlick R: Osteosarcoma: a review of diagnosis, management and treatment strategies. Clin Adv Hematol Oncol 2010;8(10):705 [PMID: 2137869].

Harrison DJ, Geller DS, Gill JD, Lewis VO, Gorlick R: Current and future therapeutic approaches for osteosarcoma. Expert Rev Anticancer Ther 2018 Jan;18(1):39–50 [PMID: 29210294].

Jackson TM, Bittman M, Granowetter L: Pediatric malignant bone tumors: a review and update on current challenges, and emerging drug targets. Curr Probl Pediatr Adolesc Health Care 2016 Jul;46(7):213–228 [PMID: 27265835].

Moore DD et al: Ewing sarcoma of bone. Cancer Treat Res 2014;162:93 [PMID: 25070232].

Osteosarcoma and Undifferentiated Pleomorphic Sarcoma of Bone Treatment (PDQ®)-Health Professional Version: National Cancer Institute: https://www.cancer.gov/types/bone/hp/osteosarcoma-treatment-pdq. Updated April 05, 2023. Accessed June 27, 2023[PMID: 26389179].

Womer R et al: Randomized controlled trial of interval-compressed chemotherapy for the treatment of localized Ewing sarcoma: a report from the Children's Oncology Group. J Clin Oncol 2012;30(33):41–48 [PMID: 23091096].

RHABDOMYOSARCOMA

► General Considerations

Rhabdomyosarcoma (RMS) is the most common soft tissue sarcoma of childhood and accounts for 10% of childhood solid tumors. The peak incidence is at age 2–5 years. A second, smaller peak is seen in adolescents with extremity tumors. Males are affected more commonly than females. Seventy percent of children with RMS are diagnosed before age 10 years.

RMS can occur anywhere in the body. When it imitates striated muscle and cross-striations are seen by light microscopy, the diagnosis is straightforward. Immunohistochemistry looking for expression of myogenic regulatory factors such as myoD and myogenin can support the diagnosis. Electron microscopy and chromosomal analysis are also helpful diagnostic tools. RMS is classified into subtypes based on pathologic features: embryonal RMS (ERMS), including the botryoid variant (so named because of its gross appearance similar to a bunch of grapes), makes up approximately 70% of childhood RMS. It tends to occur in the GU tract and the head and neck, particularly the orbit, and is typically seen in young children. Alveolar RMS (ARMS) makes up most of the remaining cases. It tends to occur in the trunk or extremities in older children and adolescents and has a worse prognosis than ERMS. Two characteristic chromosomal translocations, t(2;13) and t(1;13), are seen in 80% of cases of ARMS, leading to fusion of the FOXO1 transcription factor gene on chromosome 13 to the PAX3 or PAX7 gene on chromosome 2 or 1, respectively. Some studies suggest that patients with t(2;13) have a poorer outcome than patients with t(1;13), particularly when there is metastatic disease at diagnosis. Sclerosing/spindle cell RMS (SRMS) is a less common subtype that tends to occur in the paratesticular and head and neck regions and behaves similarly to ERMS. Pleomorphic RMS (PRMS) is rare and occurs mostly in adults.

In young children with RMS, the possibility that they may harbor an underlying cancer predisposition syndrome should be considered. Li-Fraumeni syndrome (LFS) is an inherited disorder most commonly due to mutation of the p53 tumor suppressor gene that results in a high risk of bone and soft tissue sarcomas, including RMS, in childhood as well as breast cancer and other malignant neoplasms in adulthood. RMS in children with LFS typically exhibits anaplasia. In a patient with RMS with anaplasia, LFS should be strongly considered as a predisposing cause. Patients with NF-1 are also predisposed to develop RMS, typically ERMS involving the GU tract.

► Clinical Findings

A. Symptoms and Signs

The presenting symptoms and signs of RMS result from disturbances of normal body function due to tumor growth (Table 31–9). For example, patients with orbital RMS present with proptosis, whereas patients with RMS of the bladder can present with hematuria, urinary obstruction, or a pelvic mass.

B. Staging

A CT and/or MRI scan should be obtained to determine the extent of the primary tumor and to assess regional lymph nodes. A CT scan of the chest is used to assess for pulmonary metastasis, the most common site of metastatic disease at diagnosis. A bone scan screens for bony metastases. PET-CT is another useful imaging modality when evaluating for metastatic disease, though its role in the management of RMS continues to be studied. Bilateral bone marrow biopsies and aspirates are obtained to look for bone marrow involvement. Additional studies may occasionally be warranted. For example, for parameningeal primary tumors, a lumbar puncture is performed to evaluate for CNS involvement. Also, sentinel node biopsy for extremity ARMS or biopsy of any suspicious lymph nodes is important for staging and treatment planning.

► Treatment

Optimal treatment of RMS is complex and requires combined modality therapy delivered by a multidisciplinary team, including oncologists, surgeons, and radiation oncologists. When feasible, the tumor should be completely excised with

Table 31–9. Characteristics of rhabdomyosarcoma.

Primary Site	Frequency (%)	Symptoms and Signs	Predominant Pathologic Subtype
Head and neck	35		Embryonal
Orbit	9	Proptosis	
Parameningeal	16	Cranial nerve palsies; aural or sinus obstruction with or without drainage	
Other	10	Painless, progressively enlarging mass	
Genitourinary	22		Embryonal (botryoid variant in bladder and vagina)
Bladder and prostate	13	Hematuria, urinary obstruction	
Vagina and uterus	2	Pelvic mass, vaginal discharge	
Paratesticular	7	Painless mass	
Extremities	18	Adolescents, swelling of affected body part	Alveolar (50%), undifferentiated
Other	25	Mass	Alveolar, undifferentiated

clear margins at diagnosis, but this is frequently not possible because of the site of origin and size of the tumor. When only partial tumor resection is feasible, the operative procedure is usually limited to biopsy and sampling of lymph nodes. Chemotherapy can often convert an inoperable tumor to a resectable one. Radiation therapy is effective for local tumor control with both microscopic and gross residual disease. Most patients end up receiving radiation, the exception being those with a localized tumor that has been completely resected. All patients with RMS receive chemotherapy, even when the tumor is fully resected at diagnosis. The exact regimen and duration of chemotherapy are determined by the histologic subtype, age at diagnosis, the primary site, the TNM (tumor-lymph node-metastasis) staging classification, and the grouping classification (disease extent after initial surgery). Based on these factors, patients are categorized into low risk, with an FFS of approximately 90%, intermediate risk, with an FFS of 60%–70%, and high risk, with an FFS of less than 20%.

The combination of vincristine, dactinomycin, and cyclophosphamide (VAC) has shown the greatest efficacy in the treatment of RMS. For low-risk patients, recent COG studies have focused on reducing the amount of cyclophosphamide to minimize late effects such as infertility and secondary cancers while maintaining high cure rates. For intermediate-risk patients, current studies are looking at incorporating irinotecan into treatment and adding a maintenance phase that includes cyclophosphamide and vinorelbine. High-risk (metastatic) RMS remains a major therapeutic challenge. For high-risk patients, several treatment strategies have been attempted. The most recent COG high-risk RMS study added several agents (irinotecan, ifosfamide, etoposide, doxorubicin) to standard VAC therapy. It also compressed the timing of some of the cycles from every 3 weeks to every 2 weeks.

Early results showed improvement in survival, but with longer follow-up most patients eventually relapsed, and survival rates were no better than what was seen historically. Clearly, new strategies are needed. A recent study treating patients with relapsed or refractory RMS with a combination of temsirolimus, vinorelbine, and cyclophosphamide showed promising results, prompting consideration of this drug combination for upfront treatment regimens. Agents targeting the insulin-like growth factor (IGF) pathway are also being investigated.

Childhood Rhabdomyosarcoma Treatment (PDQ®)–Health Professional Version: National Cancer Institute: https://www.cancer.gov/types/soft-tissue-sarcoma/hp/rhabdomyosarcoma-treatment-pdq. Updated January 10, 2023. Accessed June 27, 2023 [PMID: 26389243].

El Demellawy D, McGowan-Jordan J, de Nanassy J, Chernetsova E, Nasr A: Update on molecular findings in rhabdomyosarcoma. Pathology 2017;49(3):238–246 [PMID: 28256213].

Harrison DJ, Parisi MT, Shulkin BL: The role of 18F-FDG-PET/CT in pediatric sarcoma. Semin Nucl Med 2017;47(3):229–241 [PMID: 28417853].

Hawkins DS, Gupta AA, Rudzinski ER: What is new in the biology and treatment of pediatric rhabdomyosarcoma? Curr Opin Pediatr 2014;26(1):50 [PMID: 24326270].

Hayes-Jordan A, Andrassy R: Rhabdomyosarcoma in children. Curr Opin Pediatr 2009;21(3):373 [PMID: 19448544].

Malempati S, Hawkins DS: Rhabdomyosarcoma: review of the Children's Oncology Group (COG) soft-tissue sarcoma committee experience and rationale for current COG studies. Pediatr Blood Cancer 2012;59(1):5–10 [PMID: 22378628].

Martins AS, Olmos D, Missiaglia E, Shipley J: Targeting the insulin-like growth factor pathway in rhabdomyosarcomas: rationale and future perspectives. Sarcoma 2011;2011:209736 [PMID: 21437217].

Rudzinski ER, Anderson JR, Hawkins DS, Skapek SX, Parham DM, Teot LA: The World Health Organization classification of skeletal muscle tumors in pediatric rhabdomyosarcoma: a report from the Children's Oncology Group. Arch Pathol Lab Med 2015;139(10):1281–1287 [PMID: 25989287].

RETINOBLASTOMA

▶ General Considerations

Retinoblastoma is a neuroectodermal malignancy arising from embryonic retinal cells. It is rare, accounting for 3% of cases of childhood cancer. It is the most common intraocular tumor in children and causes 5% of cases of childhood blindness. In the United States, 200–300 new cases are diagnosed yearly. This is a malignancy of early childhood, with 90% of the tumors diagnosed before age 5 years. Retinoblastoma is the prototypic heritable cancer.

In almost all cases, retinoblastoma is caused by loss of function of *RB1*, a tumor suppressor gene located on the long arm of chromosome 13 (13q14). This gene encodes a protein that regulates progression through the cell cycle. When the gene is lost or inactivated, uncontrolled cell growth leads to tumor formation. Each cell carries two copies of *RB1*, one from each parent, and both copies must be lost or inactivated for tumor formation to occur.

Retinoblastoma exists in both a heritable and nonheritable form. The heritable form (30%–40% of cases) tends to have multiple tumors, is usually bilateral, and tends to occur at a younger age (median 14 months) while the nonheritable form is unilateral and tends to occur at an older median age (23 months). Based on these observations, Alfred Knudson proposed a "two-hit" hypothesis for retinoblastoma tumor development. He postulated that for a cell to become tumorigenic, it had to lose function of both copies of a tumor suppressor gene (later identified as *RB1*). In heritable cases, the first mutation is either inherited from a parent (10% of cases) or occurs very early in development (90% of cases), with the progeny of that cell all carrying the same mutation. In someone with germline loss of one allele, loss of function of the second *RB1* allele in a retinal cell is a likely event, occurring in 90% of persons who carry the germline mutation. Most will have multiple tumors and most will have bilateral disease. In nonheritable cases, both mutations must arise spontaneously in the same somatic cell, a much less likely event. Therefore, nonheritable cases are unilateral, single tumors. Because of the implications for both the patient and the patient's family, genetic counseling and *RB1* mutational analysis are essential for all patients diagnosed with retinoblastoma.

▶ Clinical Findings

A. Symptoms and Signs

Children with retinoblastoma in the United States generally come to medical attention while the tumor is still confined to the globe. Although sometimes present at birth, retinoblastoma is not usually detected until it has grown to a considerable size. Leukocoria (white pupillary reflex) is the most common sign (found in 60% of patients). Parents may note an unusual appearance of the eye or asymmetry of the eyes in a photograph. The differential diagnosis of leukocoria includes *Toxocara canis* granuloma, astrocytic hamartoma, retinopathy of prematurity, Coats disease, and persistent hyperplastic primary vitreous. Strabismus (in 20% of patients) is seen when the tumor involves the macula and central vision is lost. Rarely (in 7% of patients), a painful red eye with glaucoma, hyphemia, or proptosis is the initial manifestation. A single focus or multiple foci of tumor may be seen in one or both eyes at diagnosis.

B. Diagnostic Evaluation

Suspected retinoblastoma requires a detailed ophthalmologic examination under general anesthesia. An ophthalmologist makes the diagnosis based on the appearance of the tumor within the eye, without pathologic confirmation. A white to creamy pink mass protruding into the vitreous matter suggests the diagnosis. Intraocular calcifications and vitreous seeding are virtually pathognomonic findings. A CT scan of the orbits and MRI of the orbits and brain detect intraocular calcification, evaluate the optic nerve for tumor infiltration, and detect extraocular extension of tumor or involvement of the pineal gland (trilateral retinoblastoma). Metastatic disease to the marrow or meninges can be detected with bilateral bone marrow aspirates and biopsies and CSF cytology, respectively.

▶ Treatment

The first goal of treatment is prevention of metastatic disease. While cure rates for retinoblastoma confined to the orbit are excellent, survival rates decrease precipitously once the disease has spread beyond the orbit. An important secondary goal is preservation of the eye and of useful vision, and a third goal is prevention of late effects of therapy. Each eye is treated according to its potential for useful vision, and every attempt is made to preserve vision. The choice of therapy depends on the size, location, and number of intraocular lesions as well as if the disease is unilateral or bilateral.

Children with retinoblastoma confined to the retina (whether unilateral or bilateral) have an excellent prognosis, with 5-year survival rates greater than 95% in the United States. Small lesions may be amenable to local therapies such as cryotherapy or laser therapy, or, depending on the location, placement of a radioactive plaque outside of the globe to provide localized radiation therapy. Larger tumors may require use of systemic chemotherapy to shrink the tumors and allow local therapies to be used in conjunction. The most commonly used agents are vincristine, etoposide, and carboplatin

(VEC). For large intraocular tumors, a therapy that has been gaining in popularity is intra-arterial chemotherapy, where a catheter is threaded into the ophthalmic artery so that chemotherapy can be injected directly into the blood supply to the tumor. IAC is generally done in conjunction with other local therapies. Intravitreal injection of chemotherapy, usually melphalan, can be a particularly useful adjunctive therapy for treatment of vitreal tumor seeds. With use of these treatment modalities, many more eyes have been able to be saved and useful vision preserved.

Sometimes, enucleation of the eye is the best option. Absolute indications for enucleation include no salvageable vision, neovascular glaucoma, inability to examine the treated eye, suspicion of extraocular extension of tumor, and inability to control tumor growth with conservative treatment. Once the eye is removed, it is examined histopathologically to see if there are any high-risk features such as tumor invasion posterior to the lamina cribrosa of the optic nerve or extensive choroidal invasion by the tumor. In those situations, systemic chemotherapy is given to decrease risk of metastatic recurrence. Extraocular spread along the optic nerve or within the orbit requires treatment with systemic chemotherapy and external beam radiation. With proper treatment, cure rates remain good. With metastatic spread of disease outside of the orbit, however, cure rates are much poorer, with few patients cured of their disease. Treatment usually involves intensive chemotherapy followed by autologous HSCT. External beam irradiation was formerly a mainstay of therapy but now is used only in very select cases or with extraocular spread. Radiation leads to risk for significant late effects, including hypoplasia of the orbit and a greatly increased risk for secondary malignancies within the radiation field, particularly in patients with germline RB mutation.

Patients with the germline *RB1* mutation (heritable form) have a significant risk of developing second primary tumors. Osteosarcomas account for 40% of such tumors. The 30-year cumulative incidence for a second neoplasm is 35% in patients who received radiation therapy and 6% in those who did not receive radiation therapy. The risk continues to increase over time. Although radiation contributes to the risk, it is the presence of the retinoblastoma gene itself that is responsible for the development of nonocular tumors in these patients.

Dimaras H, Corson TW: Retinoblastoma, the visible CNS tumor: a review. J Neurosci Res 2019 Jan;97(1):29–44 [PMCID: PMC6034991].
Dimaras H et al: Retinoblastoma. Nat Rev Dis Primers 2015;1:1–22 [PMID: 27189421].
Lin P, O'Brien JM: Frontiers in the management of retinoblastoma. Am J Ophthalmol 2009;148(2):192 [PMID: 19477707].
Retinoblastoma Treatment (PDQ®)–Health Professional Version: National Cancer Institute: https://www.cancer.gov/types/retinoblastoma/hp/retinoblastoma-treatment-pdq. Updated April 11, 2023. Accessed June 27, 2023 [PMID: 26389442].

Sastre X et al: Proceedings of the consensus meetings from the International Retinoblastoma Staging Working Group on the pathology guidelines for the examination of enucleated eyes and evaluation of prognostic risk factors in retinoblastoma. Arch Pathol Lab Med 2009;133(8):1199 [PMID: 19653709].
Shields C et al: Targeted retinoblastoma management: when to use intravenous, intra-arterial, periocular, and intravitreal chemotherapy. Curr Opin Ophthalmol 2014;25(5):374–385 [PMID: 25014750].
Shinohara ET, DeWees T, Perkins SM: Subsequent malignancies and their effect on survival in patients with retinoblastoma. Pediatr Blood Cancer 2014;61:116–119 [PMID: 23918737].

HEPATIC TUMORS (SEE ALSO CHAPTER 22)

Two-thirds of liver masses found in childhood are malignant. Ninety percent of hepatic malignancies are either hepatoblastoma or hepatocellular carcinoma. Hepatoblastoma accounts for the vast majority of liver tumors in children younger than 5 years, hepatocellular carcinoma for the majority in children aged 15–19 years. The features of these hepatic malignancies are compared in Table 31–10. Of the benign tumors, 60% are hamartomas or vascular tumors such as hemangiomas. There is mounting evidence for a strong association between prematurity and the risk of hepatoblastoma.

Children with hepatic tumors usually come to medical attention because of an enlarging abdomen. Approximately 10% of hepatoblastomas are first discovered on routine examination. Anorexia, weight loss, vomiting, and abdominal pain are associated more commonly with hepatocellular carcinoma. Serum α-fetoprotein is often elevated and is an excellent marker for response to treatment.

Imaging studies should include abdominal ultrasound, CT scan, or MRI. Malignant tumors have a diffuse hyperechoic pattern on ultrasonography, whereas benign tumors are usually poorly echoic. Vascular lesions contain areas with varying degrees of echogenicity. Ultrasound is also useful for imaging the hepatic veins, portal veins, and inferior vena cava. CT scanning and, in particular, MRI are important for defining the extent of tumor within the liver. CT scanning of the chest should be obtained to evaluate for metastatic spread. Because bone marrow involvement is extremely rare, bone marrow aspirates and biopsies are not indicated.

The prognosis for children with hepatic malignancies depends on the tumor type and the resectability of the tumor. Complete resectability is essential for survival with both hepatoblastoma (HB) and hepatocellular carcinoma (HCC). Liver transplant should be considered if needed to achieve a complete resection. For HB, while ultimately surgical resection is key, chemotherapy is often effective in reducing tumor size and can used to make an unresectable tumor resectable. It can also help with management of metastatic disease. Following biopsy of the lesion, neoadjuvant chemotherapy is administered prior to attempting

Table 31–10. Comparison of hepatoblastoma and hepatocellular carcinoma in childhood.

	Hepatoblastoma	Hepatocellular Carcinoma
Median age at presentation	1 y (0–3 y)	12 y (5–18 y)
Male-female ratio	1.7:1	1.4:1
Associated conditions	Hemihypertrophy, Beckwith-Wiedemann syndrome, prematurity, Gardner syndrome	Hepatitis B virus infection, hereditary tyrosinemia, biliary cirrhosis, α_1-antitrypsin deficiency
Pathologic features	Fetal or embryonal cells; mesenchymal component (30%)	Large pleomorphic tumor cells and tumor giant cells
Solitary hepatic lesion	80%	20%–50%
Unique features at diagnosis	Osteopenia (20%–30%), isosexual precocity (3%)	Hemoperitoneum, polycythemia
Laboratory features		
Hyperbilirubinemia	5%	25%
Elevated AFP	> 90%	50%
Abnormal liver function tests	15%–30%	> 30%–50%

AFP, α-fetoprotein.

complete surgical resection. Monitoring the rate of decline of the α-fetoprotein levels can help indicate favorable versus poor responders to chemotherapy. Approximately 50%–60% of hepatoblastomas are fully resectable, following preoperative chemotherapy. Active agents in treating hepatoblastoma include cisplatin, carboplatin, doxorubicin, vincristine, 5-fluorouracil, irinotecan, ifosfamide, and etoposide. The current Pediatric Hepatic Malignancy International Therapeutic Trial (PHITT) risk stratifies hepatoblastoma patients according to how resectable the tumor is, the presence or absence of metastatic disease, age at diagnosis, and AFP level. Treatment may consist of surgery alone (very-low-risk group), surgery plus 2-6 cycles of cisplatin (low-risk group), surgery plus either 6 cycles of cisplatin or 6 cycles of C5VD (cisplatin, 5-FU, vincristine, and doxorubicin) (intermediate risk group), or intensive therapy involving surgery with multiagent chemotherapy including cisplatin, doxorubicin, carboplatin, etoposide, vincristine, and irinotecan (high risk group). HCC tends to be much less responsive to chemotherapy than HB and has a poorer prognosis as a result. As with HB, complete surgical resection is key to long-term cure and chemotherapy is primarily used to make an unresectable tumor resectable. The most commonly used chemotherapy agents for HCC include cisplatin, doxorubicin, gemcitabine, and oxaliplatin. Targeted agents such as sorafenib are also being studied. The current PHITT trial includes patients with HCC, looking at the efficacy of these agents for managing patients with both resectable and unresectable or metastatic disease.

Allen-Rhoades W, Whittle SB, Rainusso N: Pediatric solid tumors of infancy: an overview. Pediatr Rev 2018 Feb;39(2):57–67 [PMID: 29437125].

Childhood Liver Cancer Treatment (PDQ®)–Health Professional Version: National Cancer Institute: https://www.cancer.gov/types/liver/hp/child-liver-treatment-pdq. Updated April 07, 2023. Accessed June 27, 2023 [PMID: 26389232].

Czauderna P, Lopez-Terrada D, Hiyama E, Häberle B, Malogolowkin MH, Meyers RL: Hepatoblastoma state of the art: pathology, genetics, risk stratification and chemotherapy. Curr Opin Pediatr 2014 Feb;26(1):19–28 [PMID: 24322718].

Khaderi S, Guiteau J, Cotton RT, O'Mahony C, Rana A, Goss JA: Role of liver transplantation in the management of hepatoblastoma in the pediatric population. World J Transplant 2014;4(4):294 [PMID: 25540737].

Khan AS et al: Liver transplantation for malignant primary pediatric hepatic tumors. J Am Coll Surg 2017 Jul;225(1):103–113 [PMID: 28232059].

Trobaugh-Lotrario AD, Katzenstein HM: Chemotherapeutic approaches for newly diagnosed hepatoblastoma: past, present, and future strategies. Pediatr Blood Cancer 2012 Nov;59(5):809–812 [PMID: 22648979].

LANGERHANS CELL HISTIOCYTOSIS

▶ General Considerations

Langerhans cell histiocytosis (LCH) used to be called histiocytosis X, a name that highlighted its mysterious nature. It was long debated whether LCH was a dysregulation of the immune system or a neoplastic disorder. Our understanding of the biology of LCH has dramatically improved in recent years as we have learned more about the origin and genetics of the LCH cell. The discovery that most cases of LCH involve a V600E mutation of the *BRAF* gene or mutation of other genes in the RAS-RAF-MEK-ERK pathway has led us to view LCH as a neoplastic disorder, albeit one that does not typically behave in a malignant fashion. Studies on the origin of the LCH cell show that it is derived from a myeloid cell precursor rather than a mature Langerhans cell, placing it in the category of a myeloproliferative neoplasm. These discoveries have helped us to better understand the biology of LCH so that targeted treatments can be developed.

The distinctive pathologic feature of LCH is proliferation of abnormal histiocytes in an inflammatory background of eosinophils, neutrophils, macrophages, and lymphocytes. On light microscopy, the nuclei are deeply indented and elongated ("coffee bean–shaped"), and the cytoplasm is pale and abundant. Additional diagnostic characteristics include expression of CD1a, S-100, and CD207 (langerin), as detected by immunostaining, and the presence of Birbeck granules, recognizable by their tennis racquet appearance with electron microscopy.

▶ Clinical Findings

LCH can present as a wide spectrum of disease, ranging from an isolated bone lesion or chronic skin rash to a multisystem, life-threatening illness. Historically, LCH was classified into different descriptive categories, including eosinophilic granuloma (single or multiple lytic bone lesions, usually seen in older children and adolescents), Hand-Schüller-Christian disease (lytic bone lesions, exophthalmos, and diabetes insipidus [DI], typically in younger children), Letterer-Siwe disease (a severe, multisystem disorder involving the liver, spleen, lung, skin, and bone marrow, typically in infants aged < 2 years), and Hashimoto-Pritzker disease (also known as congenital self-healing reticulohistiocytosis, a cutaneous form of LCH in neonates that self-resolves during the first months of life). More recently, this terminology has been set aside in favor of a classification scheme based on site of disease, number of sites/organs involved, and the involvement of risk organs (bone marrow, liver, spleen), indicative of more aggressive disease, or CNS-risk lesions, indicative of an increased risk of development of neurodegenerative complications and DI.

The most common sites of disease are bone (80%), skin (33%), and the pituitary (25%). Bone lesions can be single or multiple and can occur anywhere in the skeleton, most commonly the skull. The lesions are usually painful. On plain film, a well-demarcated lytic bone lesion is seen. Vertebral lesions can present as vertebra plana. Lesions of the jaw can lead to loose or missing teeth. The skin rash can resemble seborrheic dermatitis, manifesting as a chronic rash resistant to treatment, or as a scattered papular rash. Involvement of the ear canal can lead to chronic ear drainage. Involvement of the pituitary most often manifests as DI. An MRI scan will show a thickened pituitary stalk and disappearance of the posterior pituitary bright spot on T1-weighted imaging, indicative of loss of vasopressin-containing granules. Other hormones produced by the anterior pituitary, such as growth hormone, can also be affected, leading to other endocrinopathies. Neurodegenerative LCH, manifested as neuromuscular, cognitive, and behavioral changes, is a rare but devastating complication of LCH. Liver, spleen, and bone marrow involvement are less common, though they indicate higher-risk disease. Lung involvement can be seen in young children with multisystem disease or in adults, usually associated with cigarette smoking. CT imaging of the lungs shows a reticulonodular pattern and bullae formation, with risk for spontaneous pneumothorax.

Diagnosis is confirmed by biopsy. Additional workup includes a CBC with differential, ESR, coagulation studies (PT/INR, PTT, fibrinogen), and liver and kidney function studies to screen for multisystem involvement. Measurement of urine osmolality from a first-morning void is a useful screen for DI. Chest x-ray (CXR) screens for pulmonary involvement, skeletal survey evaluates for multifocal bone involvement, and abdominal ultrasound assesses hepatosplenomegaly. PET-CT or technetium-99m bone scan can be used to evaluate extent of disease. PET-CT is particularly helpful in identifying active LCH lesions and monitoring response to therapy. Brain MRI should be obtained with suspicion of pituitary or CNS involvement.

▶ Treatment & Prognosis

Because LCH is a rare disorder with a wide clinical spectrum, it has been difficult to develop standardized diagnostic criteria and treatment regimens. The Histiocyte Society was founded in 1985 to advance knowledge of the disease and develop effective treatments through international collaboration. The society is currently supporting its fourth prospective trial, LCH-IV. The North American Consortium for Histiocytosis (NACHO) has also recently been formed to advance treatment for LCH refractory to standard treatments.

Treatment is based on the location and extent of disease. Isolated lytic bone lesions are generally treated with biopsy and curettage, which leads to healing and resolution of the lesion. Low-dose radiation is effective, though it is avoided in children due to concern for late effects. A study is underway to see if isolated skull lesions can be managed without biopsy and with observation alone if the lesion has a classic appearance by imaging. Isolated skin rashes can be observed and can resolve spontaneously or can be treated with topical steroids or nitrogen mustard. Young patients with isolated skin LCH need to be followed closely, since a significant percentage of them can progress to multisystem disease. Isolated lung LCH in adult smokers will often resolve with smoking cessation.

Multifocal bone disease, multisystem disease, disease involving CNS-risk sites (bones of the skull base and face, which have increased risk for development of DI or neurodegenerative LCH), disease involving risk organs, and disease that involves "special sites" (lesions that risk organ function and are not amenable to surgical treatment, such as vertebral lesions with soft tissue intraspinal extension) are all indications for systemic treatment. First-line treatment is usually with vinblastine and prednisone. The LCH-III study showed that treatment for 1 year led to reduced risk for disease recurrence compared with treatment for 6 months, so 1 year of treatment is currently the standard. LCH-IV is comparing 2 years of treatment with 1 year. Patients with multisystem disease with risk organ involvement also receive 6-mercaptopurine. For adolescent and young adult patients who may not tolerate the side effects of this regimen, single-agent treatment with cytarabine is effective and can be considered.

Multiple other options exist for disease that is recurrent or resistant to first-line treatments. A combination of vincristine and cytarabine is being studied as a second-line treatment in the LCH-IV study. Clofarabine or cladribine (2-Cda) used as single agents can be effective. Other effective agents include methotrexate and indomethacin. A combination of high-dose cytarabine and cladribine is being studied in patients with high-risk disease that fails first-line therapy, a patient population that has a particularly poor prognosis. Allogeneic bone marrow transplant may also be indicated in high-risk patients who fail other therapies.

The discovery of the role of *BRAF* mutations and the ERK pathway in the pathogenesis of LCH has led to the investigation of the use of kinase inhibitors such as vemurafenib (a BRAF kinase inhibitor) and trametinib (a MEK kinase inhibitor) in treatment of refractory disease. Early results are promising, and studies are ongoing.

In most cases, prognosis for LCH is excellent, though late effects can be problematic. If DI develops, it is usually permanent, requiring lifelong treatment. Late neurodegenerative changes can lead to severe disability or death. A major focus of current research is development of strategies to prevent these complications.

Allen CE, Ladisch S, McClain KL: How I treat Langerhans cell histiocytosis. Blood 2015;126(1):26–35 [PMID: 25827831].

Allen CE, Merad M, McClain KL: Langerhans-cell histiocytosis. N Engl J Med 2018;379:856–868 [PMID: 30157397].

Badalian-Very G et al: Recurrent *BRAF* mutations in Langerhans cell histiocytosis. Blood 2010;116(11):1919–1923 [PMID: 20519626].

Delprat C, Arico M: Blood spotlight on Langerhans cell histiocytosis. Blood 2014;124(6):867 [PMID: 24894775].

Emile J-F et al: Revised classification of histiocytoses and neoplasms of the macrophage-dendritic cell lineages. Blood 2016;127(22):2672–2681 [PMID: 26966089].

Haroche J et al: Dramatic efficacy of vemurafenib in both multisystemic and refractory Erdheim-Chester disease and Langerhans cell histiocytosis harboring the *BRAF* V600E mutation. Blood 2013;121(9):1495–1500 [PMID: 23258922].

Haupt R et al: Langerhans cell histiocytosis (LCH): guidelines for diagnosis, clinical work-up, and treatment for patients till the age of 18 years. Pediatr Blood Cancer 2013;60:175–184 [PMID: 23109216].

Langerhans Cell Histiocytosis Treatment (PDQ®)–Health Professional Version: National Cancer Institute: https://www.cancer.gov/types/langerhans/hp/langerhans-treatment-pdq. Updated April 19, 2023. Accessed June 27, 2023 [PMID: 26389240].

Monsereenusorn C, Rodriguez-Galindo C: Clinical characteristics and treatment of Langerhans cell histiocytosis. Hematol Oncol Clin N Am 2015;29:853–873 [PMID: 26461147].

Simko SJ et al: Clofarabine salvage therapy in refractory multifocal histiocytic disorders, including Langerhans cell histiocytosis, juvenile xanthogranuloma and Rosai-Dorfman disease. Pediatr Blood Cancer 2014 Mar;61(3):479–487. 2014;61:479–487 [PMID: 24106153].

Vaiselbuhh SR, Bryceson YT, Allen CE, Whitlock JA, Abla O: Updates on histiocytic disorders. Pediatr Blood Cancer 2014;61(7): 1329 [PMID: 24610771].

BLOOD & MARROW TRANSPLANT & CELLULAR THERAPEUTICS

GENERAL CONSIDERATIONS

Blood and marrow transplant (BMT) is considered standard therapy for a variety of pediatric disorders including, malignancies, hematologic disorders (bone marrow failure syndromes, aplastic anemia, and hemoglobinopathies), inborn errors of metabolism, and severe immunodeficiencies. Autologous transplantation, often referred to as "stem cell rescue," is infusion of the patient's own hematopoietic stem cells. This is restricted to the treatment of certain pediatric malignancies, including neuroblastoma, lymphoma, selected brain tumors, germ cell tumors, Ewing sarcoma and some other solid tumors. In contrast, allogeneic transplantation rescues hematopoiesis with stem cells from either a related family member or an unrelated individual from a volunteer bank. The selection of a suitable donor who matches the recipient most closely at key HLA loci, HLA-A, B, C, and DR, is critical, as disparities mediate graft rejection and GVHD. Every child expresses one set of paternal and one set of maternal HLA antigens. Thus, the probability of child fully matching another full sibling is one in four. When selecting a donor, a fully matched sibling is preferred, assuming not have the same underlying disease as the recipient. If a matched sibling is unavailable, alternative donor sources include a matched unrelated donor, umbilical cord blood, or a haploidentical (half-matched) family member, each with their own unique risk/benefit profile. Large worldwide registries of unrelated bone marrow and umbilical cord blood donors have been developed. Unfortunately, identification of a closely matched unrelated donor can be challenging, especially for underrepresented minorities, making haploidentical transplant an important option.

In most instances, high doses of chemotherapy and/or radiation are administered to the BMT patient for myeloablation prior to infusion of stem cells that rescue hematopoietic and lymphoid function. In patients with nonmalignant conditions, allogeneic donor stem cells replace the absent or defective hematopoietic or lymphoid elements of the recipient, curing the underlying disease. For children with oncologic disorders, high doses of chemotherapy and/or radiation are used to optimize tumor cell kill by overcoming cancer cell resistance. Additionally, in allogeneic BMT, the donor lymphoid cells may recognize the cancer as foreign and provide an immunologic attack on the malignancy, a concept known as graft-versus-leukemia (GVL).

BMT COMPLICATIONS

Supportive care during and after BMT after BMT includes management of chemotherapy side effects, nutritional support, prevention and treatment of infection, and the use of immunosuppressive medications to reduce the risk of GVHD in allogeneic BMT recipients. For the first several weeks, until the newly transplanted cells engraft, patients are most often pancytopenic and require frequent blood product support. These blood products should be leukocyte reduced to decrease the risk of CMV transmission and irradiated to prevent GVHD from residual lymphocytes that remain even in leukocyte-reduced blood products.

Patients are profoundly immunocompromised for many months following transplant. Infections from bacteria, viruses, fungi, and protozoa account for significant morbidity and mortality, and therefore routine prophylaxis and close surveillance are warranted. During profoundly neutropenic periods, patients often receive empiric coverage with broad-spectrum antibiotics to prevent bacteremia. Acyclovir prophylaxis is used to prevent the reactivation of herpes simplex virus that may occur early in up to 70% of seropositive patients as well as varicella zoster reactivation. Antifungal agents are routinely used to prevent infections from *Candida* and *Aspergillus* (Figure 31–5). Trimethoprim-sulfamethoxazole (or equivalent) is used to reduce the risk of *P jirovecii*

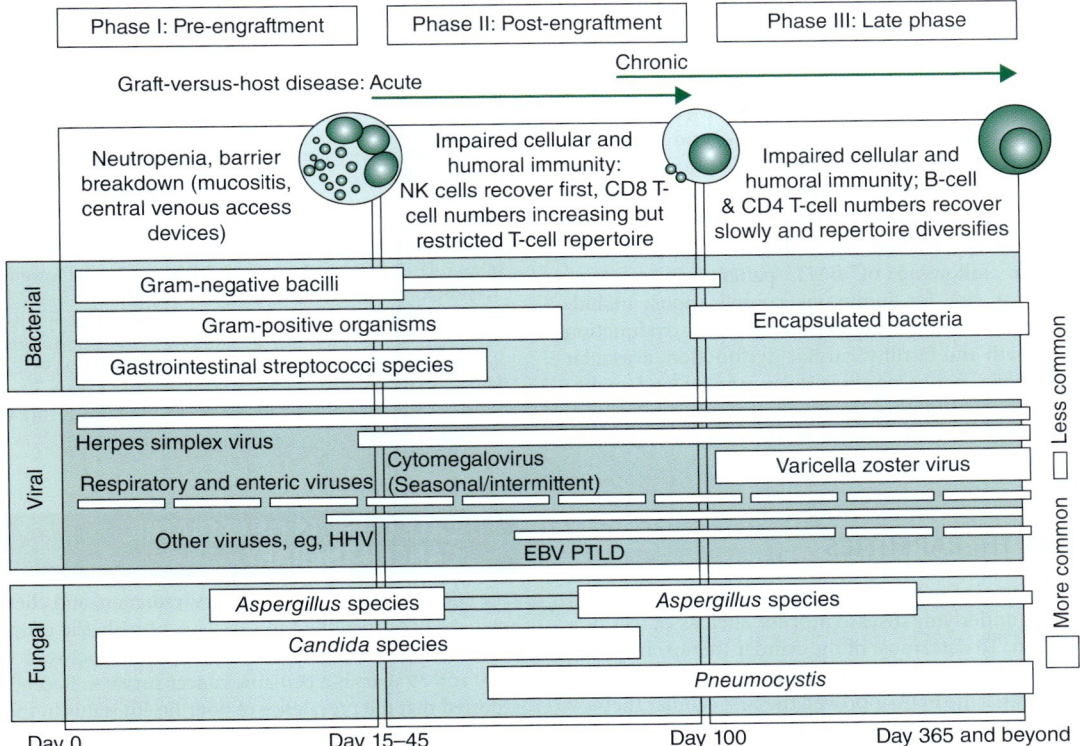

▲ **Figure 31–5.** Phases of opportunistic infections among allogeneic HCT recipients. EBV, Epstein-Barr virus; HHV6, human herpesvirus 6; PTLD, posttransplant lymphoproliferative disease. (Reproduced with permission from Tomblyn M, Chiller T, Einsele H et al: Guidelines for preventing infectious complications among hematopoietic cell transplantation recipients: a global perspective. Biol Blood Marrow Transplant. 2009;15(10):1143–1238.)

pneumonia. While transplant patients will frequently recover neutrophil function within the first few weeks, they remain very lymphopenic for many months, requiring ongoing infectious prophylaxis and prevention often through the first year or post-transplant. Despite prophylaxis, overwhelming illness from viral pathogens still occurs. CMV reactivation or de novo infection is relatively common and can result in retinitis, enteritis, and pneumonia. Treatment is usually successful if CMV infection is recognized early; therefore, routine surveillance is recommended. Common community-acquired viruses can also be life threatening, so prevention is critical. The use of frequent hand washing, contact restriction, and early treatment with available antiviral therapies, such as ribavirin and oseltamivir, can be lifesaving in this population.

GVHD occurs after allogeneic BMT when donor lymphocytes recognize the recipient tissues as foreign and mount an immunologic attack. Despite the use of immunosuppressive agents, anti–T-cell antibodies, and T-cell depletion of the donor graft, 20%–70% of allogeneic BMT patients experience some degree of acute GVHD. Factors influencing GVHD risk include the degree of HLA match, stem cell source, patient age, and donor sex. Acute GVHD generally occurs within the first 100 days after transplant but, on occasion, may occur later. It typically affects the the skin, GI tract, and or liver and presents with multiple organ systems; sclerotic skin, malabsorption, weight loss, keratoconjunctivitis sicca, oral mucositis, chronic lung disease, and cholestatic jaundice are common manifestations. Prevention and treatment of GVHD involves use of immunosuppressive agents. Patients on immunosuppressive treatment for GVHD have an increased and protracted risk of all types of infections.

Long-term follow-up of BMT patients is essential. Patients are at risk for numerous complications, including pulmonary disease, cataracts, endocrine dysfunction affecting growth and fertility, cardiac dysfunction, avascular necrosis of bone, neurocognitive delay, and second malignancies. Although BMT has many challenges, it represents an important advance in curative treatment for a variety of serious pediatric illnesses.

CELLULAR THERAPEUTICS

Cellular therapy is the transfusion of cells designed to treat or to cure an underlying disease process, such as cancer or a viral infection. To date, most of the cellular therapy has been administered to patients through clinical research trials. However, in 2017 the FDA approved the first cellular therapy known as CAR T cells for the treatment of pediatric ALL. This therapy involves the collection of the patient's own T cells, which are then genetically engineered to produce chimeric antigen receptors (CARs) expressed on the cell surface. These receptors allow the T cells to recognize an antigen on the tumor cells. In the case of pediatric ALL, this receptor

is CD19. After the T cells are engineered to express the CAR, they are expanded in the lab prior to infusion back into the patient. If successful, these T cells expand within the patient and eradicate any cells expressing the antigen the CAR T cells are designed to recognize. Development of CAR T cells against many other tumor antigens is ongoing. Similarly, T cells with activity against specific viruses such as CMV, EBV, and adenovirus can also be selected, and expanded ex vivo and then infused into a patient with a known infection. These viral-specific T cells can be obtained from third-party donor banks or, after BMT, can be collected from the stem cell donor. Currently, all administration of viral-specific T cells is done on clinical research trials.

Ardura MI: Overview of infections complicating pediatric hematopoietic cell transplantation. Infect Dis Clin North Am 2018 Mar;32(1):237–252 [PMID: 29406976].

Chow EJ et al: Late effects surveillance recommendations among survivors of childhood hematopoietic cell transplantation: a Children's Oncology Group report. Biol Blood Marrow Transplant 2016 May;22(5):782–795 [PMID: 26802323].

Malhi K, Lum LG, Schultz KR, Yankelevich M: Hematopoietic cell transplantation and cellular therapeutics in the treatment of childhood malignancies. Pediatr Clin North Am 2015 Feb;62(1):257–273 [PMID: 25435122].

Rocha V: Umbilical cord blood cells from unrelated donor as an alternative source of hematopoietic stem cells for transplantation in children and adults. Semin Hematol 2016 Oct;53(4): 237–245 [PMID: 27788761].

Rotz SJ, Bhatt NS, Hamilton BK, et al. International recommendations for screening and preventative practices for long-term survivors of transplantation and cellular therapy: a 2023 update. Bone Marrow Transplant. Published online February 27, 2024. doi:10.1038/s41409-023-02190-2

Sermer D, Brentjens R: CAR T-cell therapy: full speed ahead. Heamtol Oncol 2019 Jun;37(S1):95–100 [PMID: 31187533].

Shenoy S, Boelens JJ: Advances in unrelated and alternative donor hematopoietic cell transplantation for nonmalignant disorders. Curr Opin Pediatr 2015 Feb;27(1):9–17 [PMID: 25565572].

Weisdorf D: Can haploidentical transplantation meet all patients' needs? Best Pract Res Clin Haematol 2018 Dec;31(4):410–413 [PMID: 30466758].

LATE EFFECTS OF PEDIATRIC CANCER THERAPY

Late effects of treatment by surgery, radiation, and chemotherapy have been identified in survivors of pediatric cancer. Current estimates are that 1 in every 640 adults between the ages of 20 and 39 years is a pediatric cancer survivor. Recently it was reported that the prevalence of poor health status in this group is higher among adult survivors of pediatric cancer than siblings and increases rapidly with age, particularly among female survivors. One recent study found that 60% of survivors of pediatric cancer diagnosed between 1970 and 1986 have at least one chronic condition. Virtually any organ system can demonstrate sequelae related to previous cancer therapy. This has necessitated the creation of specialized oncology clinics whose function is to identify and provide treatment to these patients.

The Childhood Cancer Survivor Study, a pediatric multi-institutional collaborative project, was designed to investigate the various aspects of late effects of pediatric cancer therapy in a cohort of over 13,000 survivors of childhood cancer.

GROWTH COMPLICATIONS

Children who have received cranial irradiation are at highest risk of developing growth complications. Growth complications of cancer therapy in the pediatric survivor are generally secondary to direct damage to the pituitary gland, resulting in growth hormone deficiency. However, new evidence in children treated for ALL suggests that chemotherapy alone may result in an attenuation of linear growth without evidence of catch-up growth once therapy is discontinued. Up to 90% of patients who receive more than 30 Gy of radiation to the CNS will show evidence of growth hormone deficiency within two years. Approximately 50% of children receiving 24 Gy will have growth hormone problems. The effects of cranial irradiation appear to be age-related, with children younger than five years at the time of therapy being particularly vulnerable. These patients usually benefit from growth hormone therapy. Currently, there is no evidence that such therapy causes a recurrence of cancer.

Spinal irradiation inhibits vertebral body growth. In 30% of treated children, standing heights may be less than the fifth percentile. Asymmetrical exposure of the spine to radiation may result in scoliosis.

Growth should be monitored closely, particularly in young survivors of childhood cancer. Obesity may become an issue for selected survivors who are young at diagnosis and have received whole brain radiation. Follow-up studies should include height, weight, growth velocity, scoliosis examination, and, when indicated, growth hormone testing.

ENDOCRINE COMPLICATIONS

Thyroid dysfunction, manifesting as hypothyroidism, is common in children who received total body irradiation, cranial irradiation, or local radiation therapy to the neck and/or mediastinum. Particularly at risk are children with brain tumors who received more than 3000 cGy and those who received more than 4000 cGy to the neck region. The average time to develop thyroid dysfunction is 12 months after exposure, but the range is wide. Therefore, individuals at risk should be monitored yearly for at least seven years from the completion of therapy. Although signs and symptoms of hypothyroidism may be present, most patients will have a normal thyroxine level with an elevated thyroid-stimulating hormone level. These individuals should be given thyroid hormone replacement because persistent stimulation of the thyroid from an elevated thyroid-stimulating hormone level may predispose to thyroid nodules and carcinomas. In a recent report from the Childhood Cancer Survivor Study, thyroid cancer

occurred at 18 times the expected rate for the general population in pediatric cancer survivors who received radiation to the neck region. Hyperthyroidism, although rare, also occurs in patients who have received neck irradiation.

Precocious puberty, delayed puberty, and infertility are all potential consequences of cancer therapy. Precocious puberty, more common in girls, is usually a result of cranial irradiation causing premature activation of the hypothalamic-pituitary axis. This results in premature closure of the epiphysis and decreased adult height. Luteinizing hormone (LH) analogue and growth hormone are used to halt early puberty and facilitate continued growth.

Gonadal dysfunction in males is usually the result of radiation to the testes. Patients who receive testicular irradiation as part of their therapy for ALL, abdominal irradiation for Hodgkin disease, or total body irradiation for HSCT are at highest risk. Radiation damages both the germinal epithelium (producing azoospermia) and Leydig cells (causing low testosterone levels and delayed puberty). Alkylating agents such as ifosfamide and cyclophosphamide can also interfere with male gonadal function, resulting in oligospermia or azoospermia, low testosterone levels, and abnormal follicle-stimulating hormone (FSH) and LH levels. Determination of testicular size, semen analysis, and measurement of testosterone, FSH, and LH levels will help identify abnormalities in patients at risk. When therapy is expected to result in gonadal dysfunction, fertility counseling should be provided and pre-therapy sperm banking should be offered to males of reproductive age pretherapy sperm banking should be offered to pubertal males.

Exposure of the ovaries to abdominal radiation may result in delayed puberty with a resultant increase in FSH and LH and a decrease in estrogen. Girls receiving total body irradiation as preparation for HSCT and those receiving craniospinal irradiation are at particularly high risk for delayed puberty as well as diminished ovarian reserve. In patients at high risk for development of gonadal complications, a detailed menstrual history should be obtained, and LH, FSH, and estrogen levels should be monitored if indicated. When any female of reproductive age is expected to receive gonadotoxic therapy, appropriate fertility counseling should be provided including the options of oocyte or embryo cryopreservation.

No studies to date have confirmed an increased risk of spontaneous abortions, stillbirths, premature births, congenital malformations, or genetic diseases in the offspring of childhood cancer survivors. Women who have received abdominal irradiation may develop uterine vascular insufficiency or fibrosis of the abdominal and pelvic musculature or uterus, and their pregnancies should be considered high risk.

CARDIOPULMONARY COMPLICATIONS

Pulmonary dysfunction generally manifests as pulmonary fibrosis. Therapy-related factors known to cause pulmonary toxicities include certain chemotherapeutic agents, such as bleomycin, the nitrosoureas, and busulfan, as well as lung or total body irradiation. Pulmonary toxicity due to chemotherapy is related to the total cumulative dose received. Pulmonary function tests in patients with therapy-induced toxicity show restrictive lung disease, with decreased carbon monoxide diffusion and small lung volumes. Individuals exposed to these risk factors should be counseled to refrain from smoking and to give proper notification of the treatment history if they should require general anesthesia.

Cardiac complications usually result from exposure to anthracyclines (daunorubicin, doxorubicin, and mitoxantrone), which destroy myocytes and lead to inadequate myocardial growth as the child ages, and eventually result in congestive heart failure. The incidence of anthracycline cardiomyopathy increases in a dose-dependent fashion. A recent report indicates that survivors receiving cumulative doses larger than 360 mg/m^2 were more than 40 times more likely to die of cardiac disease. In a recent study, complications from these agents appeared 6–19 years following administration of the drugs. Pregnant women who have received anthracyclines should be followed closely for signs and symptoms of congestive heart failure, as peripartum cardiomyopathy has been reported.

Radiation therapy to the mediastinal region, which is a common component of therapy for Hodgkin disease, has been linked to an increased risk of coronary artery disease; chronic restrictive pericarditis may also occur in these patients.

Current recommendations include an echocardiogram and electrocardiogram every 1–5 years, depending on the age at therapy, total cumulative dose received, and presence or absence of mediastinal irradiation. Selective monitoring with various modalities is indicated for those who were treated with anthracyclines when they were younger than 4 years or received more than 500 mg/m^2 of these drugs. Biomarkers such as cardiac troponins and brain natriuretic peptides may be useful in assessing cardiotoxicity of anthracyclines.

RENAL COMPLICATIONS

Long-term renal side effects stem from therapy with cisplatin, alkylating agents (ifosfamide and cyclophosphamide), or pelvic irradiation. Patients who have received cisplatin may develop abnormal creatinine clearance, which may or may not be accompanied by abnormal serum creatinine levels, as well as persistent tubular dysfunction with hypomagnesemia. Alkylating agents can cause hemorrhagic cystitis, which may continue after chemotherapy has been terminated and has been associated with the development of bladder carcinoma. Ifosfamide can also cause Fanconi syndrome, which may result in clinical rickets if adequate phosphate replacement is not provided. Pelvic irradiation may result in abnormal bladder function with dribbling, frequency, and enuresis.

Patients seen in long-term follow-up who have received nephrotoxic agents should be monitored with urinalysis, appropriate electrolyte profiles, and blood pressure. Urine collection for creatinine clearance or renal ultrasound may be indicated in individuals with suspected renal toxicity.

NEUROPSYCHOLOGICAL COMPLICATIONS

Pediatric cancer survivors who have received cranial irradiation for ALL or brain tumors appear to be at greatest risk for neuropsychological sequelae. The severity of cranial irradiation effects varies among individual patients and depends on the dose and dose schedule, the size and location of the radiation field, the amount of time elapsed after treatment, the child's age at therapy, and the child's gender. Girls may be more susceptible than boys to CNS toxicity because of more rapid brain growth and development during childhood.

Auditory complications can be seen in childhood cancer survivors exposed to platinum-based chemotherapy and/or temporal or posterior fossa radiation. Difficulty hearing sounds, tinnitus, or hearing loss requiring an aid have been reported.

The main effects of CNS irradiation appear to be related to attention capacities, ability with nonverbal tasks and mathematics, and short-term memory. Recent studies support the association between treatment with high-dose systemic methotrexate, triple intrathecal chemotherapy, and, more recently, dexamethasone and more significant cognitive impairment.

Additionally, pediatric cancer patients have been reported as having more behavior problems and as being less socially competent than a sibling control group. Adolescent survivors of cancer demonstrate an increased sense of physical fragility and vulnerability manifested as hypochondriasis or phobic behaviors.

A recent report from Childhood Cancer Survivor Study noted that when compared to population norms, childhood cancer survivors and siblings report positive psychological health, good health-related quality of life, and life satisfaction. There are, however, subgroups that could be targeted for intervention.

SECOND MALIGNANCIES

Approximately 3%–12% of children receiving cancer treatment will develop a new cancer within 20 years of their first diagnosis. This is a 10-fold increased incidence when compared with age-matched control subjects. Particular risk factors include exposure to alkylating agents, epipodophyllotoxins (etoposide), and radiation therapy, primary diagnosis of retinoblastoma or Hodgkin disease, or the presence of an inherited genetic susceptibility syndrome (LFS or NF). In a recent report, the cumulative estimated incidence of second malignant neoplasms for the cohort of the Childhood Cancer Survivor Study was 3.2% at 20 years from diagnosis.

Second hematopoietic malignancies (acute myelogenous leukemia) occur as a result of therapy with epipodophyllotoxins or alkylating agents. The schedule of drug administration (etoposide) and the total dose may be related to the development of this secondary leukemia.

Children receiving radiation therapy are at risk for developing second malignancies, such as sarcomas, carcinomas, or brain tumors, in the field of radiation. A recent report examining the incidence of second neoplasms in a cohort of pediatric Hodgkin disease patients showed the cumulative risk of a second neoplasm to be as high as 8% at 15 years from diagnosis. The most common solid tumor was breast cancer (the majority located within the radiation field) followed by thyroid cancer. Girls aged 10–16 years when they received radiation therapy were at highest risk and had an actuarial incidence that approached 35% by age 40 years. Secondary gastrointestinal cancer is also increased in pediatric cancer survivors and is related to radiation exposure as well as to certain types of chemotherapeutic agents (procarbazine, platinum).

Bates JE et al: Therapy-related cardiac risk in childhood cancer survivors: an analysis of the Childhood Cancer Survivor Study. J Clin Oncol 2019 May 1;37(13):1090–1101 [PMID: 30860946].

Children's Oncology Group. Long-Term Follow-Up Guidelines for Survivors of Childhood, Adolescent and Young Adult Cancers, Version 6.0. Monrovia, CA: Children's Oncology Group; October 2023; Available on-line: www.survivorshipguidelines.org.

Fidler MM, Frobisher C, Hawkins MM, Nathan PC: Challenges and opportunities in the care of survivors of adolescent and young adult cancers. Pediatr Blood Cancer 2019 Jun;66(6):e27668 [PMID: 30815985].

Gibson TM et al: Temporal patterns in the risk of chronic health conditions in survivors of childhood cancer diagnosed 1970–99: a report from the Childhood Cancer Survivor Study cohort. Lancet Oncol 2018 Dec;19(12):1590–1601 [PMID: 30416076].

Green DM et al: Risk factors for obesity in adult survivors of childhood cancer: a report from the Childhood Cancer Survivor Study. J Clin Oncol 2012;30(3):246 [PMID: 22184380].

Henderson TO et al: Secondary gastrointestinal cancer in childhood cancer survivors: a cohort study. Ann Intern Med 2012;156(11):757 [PMID: 22665813].

Hudson MM et al: Approach for classification and severity grading of long-term and late-onset health events among childhood cancer survivors in the St. Jude lifetime cohort. Cancer Epidemiol Biomarkers Prev 2017 May;26(5):666–674 [PMID: 28035022].

Late Effects of Treatment for Childhood Cancer (PDQ®): Health Professional Version. PDQ Pediatric Treatment Editorial Board. PDQ Cancer Information Summaries [Internet]. Bethesda, MD: National Cancer Institute; 2002–2019 Jun 12 [PMID: 26389273].

Whelan K et al: Auditory complications in childhood cancer survivors: a report from the Childhood Cancer Survivor Study. Pediatr Blood Cancer 2011;57:126 [PMID: 21328523].

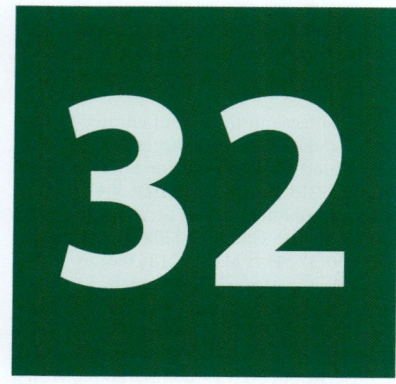

Pain Management & Pediatric Palliative & End-of-Life Care

Brian S. Greffe, MD   Nancy A. King, MSN, RN, CPNP
Sheryl J. Kent, PhD   Jeffrey L. Galinkin, MD

INTRODUCTION

Children experience pain to at least the same level as adults. Multiple studies have shown that neonates and infants perceive pain and have memory of these painful experiences. Frequently, children are under prescribed and under-dosed for opioid and nonopioid analgesics due to excessive concerns of respiratory depression and/or poor understanding of the need for pain medications in children. Few data are available to guide the dosing of many pain medications, and the majority of pain medications available on the market today are unlabeled for use in pediatric patients.

Birnie KA et al: Hospitalized children continue to report undertreated and preventable pain. Pain Res Manag 2014 Jul–Aug;19(4):198–204. Epub 2014 May 7 [PMID: 24809068].
Taddio A, Katz J: The effects of early pain experience in neonates on pain responses in infancy and childhood. Pediatr Drugs 2005;7:245–257 [PMID: 16118561].

PAIN ASSESSMENT

Standardizing pain measurements require the use of appropriate pain assessment tools. Typically, these tools are one of two types: observational/behavioral (measures a patient's reaction to pain) or self-report (patients quantify and describe pain). Self-report scales are standard of care in the assessment of pain, unless a patient is preverbal, cognitively impaired, or sedated. At most institutions, pain scales are stratified by age (Table 32–1) and are used throughout the institution from operating room to medical floor to clinic, creating a common language around a patient's pain. Pain assessment by scales has become the "5th vital sign" in hospital settings and is documented at least as frequently as heart rate and blood pressure at many pediatric centers around the world. There are many pain scales available, all of which have advantages and disadvantages (eg, Figures 32–1 and 32–2, and Table 32–1). For example, research has shown younger and school-age children prefer facial expression pain scales as it may be more difficult for them to understand numeric order and quantify pain, whereas older children and adolescents prefer numeric ratings. It is less important what type of scale is used, but that they are used on a consistent and continuous basis.

Special Populations

Noncommunicative patients such as neonates and children with cognitive impairment are often difficult to assess for pain, as are patients who are sedated. For these patients, using an appropriate observational/behavioral assessment tool (Table 32–2) on a frequent basis (every 1–2 hours) is essential to ensure adequate pain control. For these populations, increasing pain score trends are often a sign of discomfort. It is also critical to use validated pain assessment tools to minimize any unintentional racial bias, which has been documented in pain assessment and treatment.

Hoffman KM, Trawalter S, Axt JR, Oliver MN: Racial bias in pain assessment and treatment recommendations, and false beliefs about biological differences between blacks and whites. Proc Natl Aca Sci USA 2016;113(16):4296–4301 [PMID: 27044069].
Miro J, Huguet A: Evaluation of reliability, validity, and preference for a pediatric pain intensity scale: the Catalan version of the Faces Pain Scale–revised. Pain 2004;111:59–64 [PMID: 15327809].
von Baeyer CL et al: Three new datasets supporting use of the Numerical Rating Scale (NRS-11) for children's self-reports of pain intensity. Pain 2009;143:223–227 [PMID: 19359097].
von Baeyer CL, Spagrud LJ: Systematic review of observational (behavioral) measures for children and adolescents aged 3–18 years. Pain 2007;127:140–150 [PMID: 16996689].

ACUTE PAIN

▶ Definition Etiology

Acute pain is caused by an identifiable source such as a specific disease or injury. In most cases, it is self-limiting, and treatment reflects severity and type of injury. In children, the

Table 32–1. Pain scales—description and age-appropriate use.

Name of Scale	Type	Description	Age Group
Numeric	Self-report	Verbal 0–10 scale; 0 = no pain, 10 = worst pain you could ever imagine	Children who understand the concept of numbers, rank, and order; approximately > 8 y
Bieri and Wong-Baker scales	Self-report	Six faces that range from no pain to the worst pain you can imagine	Younger children who have difficulty with numeric scale; cognitive age 3–7 y
FLACC	Behavioral observer	Five categories: face, legs, activity, cry, and consolability; range of total score is 0.10; score ≤ 7 is severe pain. Figures 32–1 and 32–2 and Table 32–2	Nonverbal children > 1 y
CRIES, NIPS, PIPP	Behavioral observer	Rates a set of standard criteria and gives a score	Nonverbal infant < 1 y

CRIES, Crying Requires O2 saturation, Increased vital signs, Expression, and Sleeplessness; FLACC, Face, Legs, Activity, Crying, Consolability; NIPS, Neonatal Infant Pain Scale; PIPP, Premature Infant Pain Profile.

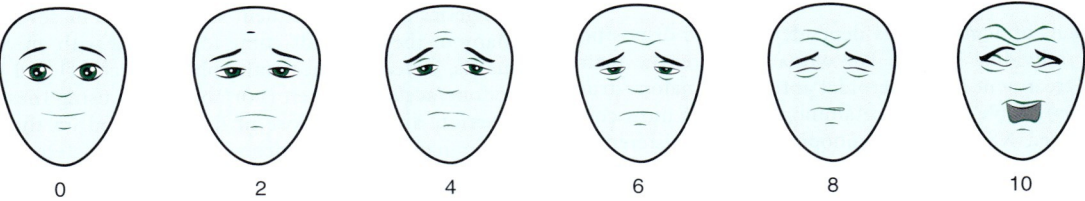

0	2	4	6	8	10

▲ **Figure 32–1.** Bieri Faces Pain Scale, revised. (Reproduced with permission from Hicks CL et al: The Faces Pain Scale–Revised: toward a common metric in pediatric pain measurement. Pain 2001 Aug;93(2):173–183.)

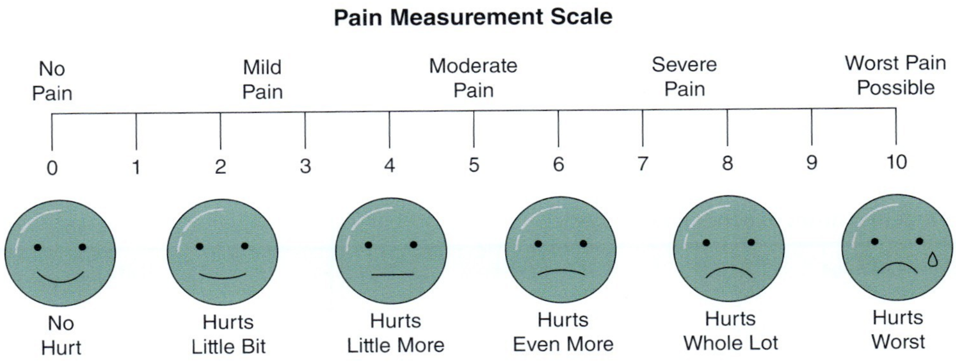

Pain Measurement Scale

No Pain		Mild Pain		Moderate Pain		Severe Pain		Worst Pain Possible
0	1	2	3	4	5	6	7	8	9	10

No Hurt	Hurts Little Bit	Hurts Little More	Hurts Even More	Hurts Whole Lot	Hurts Worst

▲ **Figure 32–2.** Horizontal pain measurement scale or pain assessment tool, vector. Visual pain chart or scale. (Used with permission from Oxy_gen/Shutterstock)

Table 32–2. FLACC pain assessment tool.

Categories	Score 0	Score 1	Score 2
Face	No particular expression or smile	Occasional grimace or frown, withdrawn, disinterested	Frequent to constant frown, clenched jaw, quivering chin
Legs	Normal position or relaxed	Uneasy, restless, tense	Kicking, or legs drawn up
Activity	Lying quietly, normal position, moves easily	Squirming, shifting back and forth, tense	Arched, rigid, or jerking
Cry	No cry (awake or asleep)	Moans or whimpers, occasional complaint	Crying steadily, screams or sobs, frequent complaints
Consolability	Content, relaxed	Reassured by occasional touching, hugging, or being talked to, distractible	Difficult to console or comfort

majority of acute pain is caused by trauma or, if in a hospital setting, an iatrogenic source such as surgery. Treatment focuses on addressing the underlying cause of the acute pain and interrupting the nociceptive signals.

▶ Treatment

Treatment of acute pain is dependent on the disposition of the individual patient. For outpatient care, the mainstay of treatment is nonsteroidal anti-inflammatory drugs (NSAIDs) (Table 32–3). Acetaminophen is the most commonly used NSAID. Acetaminophen is administered via the oral or rectal routes. Acetaminophen is more predictable in its effects as an oral dose. It has also been found that round-the-clock administration (oral 10–15 mg/kg, rectal 20 mg/kg) is better than PRN dosing for both minor pain and as an adjunct for major pain. The toxicity of acetaminophen is low in clinically used doses. However, the use of acetaminophen combined with many over-the-counter and prescription combination products has been a frequent cause of toxicity. Liver damage or failure can occur with doses exceeding 200 mg/kg/day. Other oral analgesics available in suspension are ibuprofen (10–15 mg/kg) and naproxen (10–20 mg/kg).

Motoyama EK, Davis PJ: *Smith's Anesthesia for Infants and Children.* 9th ed. St. Louis, MO: Mosby Elsevier; 2016.

Oral opioids can be added for short-term use and are recommended by the WHO in combination with non-opioid analgesics for the treatment of moderate to severe pain. Many of these opioids come formulated with an NSAID, that is, oxycodone/acetaminophen (Percocet) and hydrocodone/acetaminophen (Lortab). When using these combination drugs, the dose of drug is based on the opioid component. Other concomitantly administered similar NSAIDs should be discontinued. The most commonly used oral opioids are oxycodone, hydrocodone, morphine, and codeine. The use of codeine is least recommended due to its metabolism. Codeine is metabolized to morphine via the cytochrome P-450 2D4 isoenzyme. From 1% to 10% people (Asians 1%–2%, African Americans 1%–3%, Caucasians 5%–10%) are poor metabolizers as a result of a genetic polymorphism. Thus, patients with this defect get no effect from this drug. A very small percentage of patients (primarily from East Africa) are ultrarapid metabolizers. These patients convert 10–15 times the amount of parent drug to active compound that can result in clinical toxicity.

Table 32–3. Suggested doses of nonopioid analgesics.

Route		Dosage	Guidelines	Half-Life	Duration
Acetaminophen	PO		10–15 mg/kg/dose every 4–6 h, maximum dose 4000 mg/day	Neonates: 2–5 h	4 h
	PR		40 mg/kg loading dose, followed by 10–20 mg/kg/dose every 6 h	Adults: 2–3 h	
Ibuprofen	PO		4–10 mg/kg/dose every 6–8 h, maximum dose 40 mg/kg/day, no > 2400 mg/day	Children: 1–7 y: 1–2 h	6–8 h
				Adults: 2–4 h	
Ketorolac	IV		0.5 mg/kg/dose every 6 h, maximum of 30 mg/dose, maximum course of eight doses	Children: ~ 6 h	4–6 h
				Adults: ~ 5 h	

Morphine, oxycodone, and hydrocodone are all available as suspensions, are active as administered, and are metabolized by multiple routes.

Long-acting or extended-release preparations are available for morphine and oxycodone. These drugs are not recommended for acute pain management in children. They should be prescribed with great caution and only under close monitoring. Due to the high incidence of diversion and adulteration of these drugs for abuse, the Federal Drug Administration and manufactures of these products have worked together to develop abuse deterrent formulations of the extended-release products. When extended-release opioids are prescribed, it is prudent to administer an opioid risk assessment tool such as the CRAFFT assessment tool to assess the risk of potential opioid misuse (Box 32–1).

For severe pain not amenable to oral analgesics, an intravenous opioid can be titrated to effect; options for pain relief are dependent on severity and location of pain and age. Intravenous opioids used as bolus dose, continuous infusion, and as part of a patient-controlled analgesia (PCA) infusion have a long track record of both safe and efficacious use in children. Often, the NSAID ketorolac 0.5–1.0 mg/kg is used as an adjunct for severe pain. Side effects of ketorolac are the same as for adults: renal insufficiency, gastric irritability, and prolonged bleeding times due to decreased platelet adhesiveness. Patients with bleeding concerns should not receive ketorolac.

PCA pumps can be used in children as young as 6 years with proper instruction, frequent reminders, and coaching (Table 32–4). Morphine and hydromorphone are the most commonly used drugs for PCA management in the United States. Whenever PCA is used, it is imperative to assess patients frequently (at least hourly) to ensure adequate pain relief.

Andersson T et al: Drug-metabolizing enzymes: evidence for clinical utility of pharmacogenomic tests. Clin Pharmacol Ther 2005;78:559–581 [PMID: 16338273].
Berde CB, Sethna N: Analgesics for the treatment of pain in children. N Engl J Med 2002 Oct 3;347(14):1094–1103 [PMID: 12362012].
McCabe SE, West BT, Teter CJ, Cranford JA, Ross-Durow PL, Boyd CJ: Adolescent nonmedical users of prescription opioids: brief screening and substance use disorders. Addict Behav 2012 May;37(5):651–656 [PMID: 22366397].

CHRONIC PAIN MANAGEMENT

▶ Assessment

Chronic pain is pain that persists past the usual course of an acute illness or beyond the time that is expected for an acute injury, typically defined as 3 months. It is often associated with significant functional disability, challenges with academic, social, and emotional development, as well as with disruptions in family life, appetite, sleep, and participation in enjoyable activities. In children chronic pain has recently been recognized as a significant public health problem by the World Health Organization (WHO). It is estimated that chronic pain may affect as much as one-quarter to one-third of the pediatric population. The most common problems include headache, chronic abdominal pain, myofascial pain, fibromyalgia, juvenile rheumatoid arthritis, complex regional

Box 32–1. Opioid Risk Tool.

The CRAAFT assessment asks the following six "yes" or "no" questions:

- "Have you ever ridden in a car driven by someone (including yourself) who was high or had been using alcohol or drugs?"
- "Do you ever use alcohol or drugs to relax, feel better about yourself, or fit in?"
- "Do you ever use alcohol or drugs while you are by yourself (alone)?"
- "Do you forget things you did while using alcohol or drugs?"
- "Does your family or friends ever tell you that you should cut down on your drinking or drug use?"
- "Have you ever gotten into trouble while you were using alcohol or drugs?"

A score of 2 or higher on this scale for adolescents is associated with a higher risk of opioid misuse.

Table 32–4. PCA dosing recommendations.

	Morphine	Fentanyl	Hydromorphone
Solution	1 mg/mL	Solution 10 mcg/mL	0.1 mg/mL or 1 mg/mL
Initial dose	15–20 mcg/kg (max 1.5 mg)	0.25 mcg/kg	3–4 mcg/kg (max 0.3 mg)
Lockout time	8–10 min	8–10 min	8–10 min
Basal infusion	0–20 mcg/kg/h	0–1 mcg/kg/h	0–4 mcg/kg/h
Maximum starting dose (for nonopioid tolerant patients)	100 mcg/kg/h	1–2 mcg/kg/h	20 mcg/kg/h

pain syndrome, and pain associated with cancer. Chronic pain in children often has multiple other contributing factors, including psychological issues, psychosocial factors, sociologic factors, and family dynamics. For example, anxiety, depression, experience of stress, passive coping styles, and sleep difficulties, as well as depression, anxiety, and chronic pain in parents of youth with chronic pain, have all been identified as risk factors for the development and/or maintenance of pediatric chronic pain. Chronic pain prevalence rates generally increase in females and with age, and lower socioeconomic status is associated with higher chronic pain prevalence. Associating pain with a single physical cause can lead the physician to investigate the patient with repeated invasive testing, laboratory tests, and procedures and to over-prescribe medications. A multidimensional assessment to chronic pain using the biopsychosocial framework is optimal and encouraged by the WHO.

King S et al: The epidemiology of chronic pain in children and adolescents revisited: a systematic review. Pain 2011 Dec;152(12) 2729–2738 [PMID: 22078064].

McGrath PA, Ruskin DA: Caring for children with chronic pain: ethical considerations. Paediatr Anaesth 2007 Jun;17(6): 505–508 [PMID: 17498011].

McKillop HN, Banez GA: A broad consideration of risk factors in pediatric chronic pain: where to go from here? Children 2016;3(4):38 [PMID: 27916884].

Weisman SJ, Rusy LM: Pain management in infants and children. In: Motoyama EK, Davis PJ (eds): *Smith's Anesthesia for Infants and Children*. 9th ed. Mosby Elsevier; 2016.

World Health Organization: Guidelines on the management of chronic pain in children. Geneva: 2020.

▶ Treatment

A multidisciplinary team approach is standard of care for treating chronic pain in children. All children evaluated for chronic pain should be seen on their initial visit by all primary members of the team to establish a management strategy that focuses on pain reduction, increased function, and quality of life factors. Team members should include a pain physician, a pediatric psychologist and/or a psychiatrist, occupational and physical therapists (OT/PT), advanced pain nurses (APNs), and a social worker to fully utilize the biopsychosocial framework. The majority of pediatric chronic pain management programs in the United States base their approach on combined intensive rehabilitation and intensive psychotherapy relying minimally on invasive procedures and pharmacotherapy.

A. Tolerance, Dependence, and Addiction

Physiologic and psychological responses to opioids are similar between adults and children. A consensus paper by the American Academy of Pain Medicine, American Pain Society, and American Society of Addiction Medicine defined important differences between normal and pathologic responses to opioids. The definitions of tolerance dependence and addiction are listed as follows.

1. Tolerance—A state of adaptation in which exposure to a drug induces changes that result in a diminution of one or more of the drug's effects over time. Tolerance develops at different rates for different opioid effects; that is, tolerance to sleepiness and respiratory depression occurs earlier than that to constipation and analgesia.

2. Dependence—A state of adaptation that is manifested by a drug class-specific **withdrawal** syndrome that can be produced by abrupt cessation, rapid dose reduction, decreasing blood level of the drug, and/or administration of an antagonist.

3. Addiction—A primary, chronic, neurobiological disease, with genetic, psychosocial, and environmental factors influencing its development and manifestations. It is characterized by behaviors that include one or more of the following:

- Loss of **C**ontrol over the use of drug
- **C**raving and **C**ompulsive the use of drug
- Use despite adverse **C**onsequences

Addiction is rare when opioids are used appropriately for acute pain on both inpatient and outpatient settings. It should be emphasized that tolerance and dependence do not equal addiction.

Heit HA: Addiction, physical dependence, and tolerance: precise definitions to help clinicians evaluate and treat chronic pain patients. J Pain Palliat Care Pharmacother 2003;17:15–29 [PMID: 14640337].

B. Withdrawal

1. Recognition—Patients are at risk for experiencing withdrawal symptoms after 1 week of opioid treatment, and therefore should be monitored for signs of withdrawal after this duration of treatment. Signs of withdrawal in older children include agitation, irritability, dysphoria, tachycardia, tachypnea, nasal congestion, temperature instability, and feeding intolerance. In neonates with withdrawal (neonatal abstinence syndrome), common symptoms include neurologic excitability, breathing problems, including breathing rapidly, gastrointestinal dysfunction, and autonomic signs (increased sweating, nasal stuffiness, fever, mottling, poor weight gain).

2. Treatment

- Make a schedule/plan in conjunction with patient and family.
- Factor in duration of time on opioid.
- Consider switching to once-a-day opioid.

- Decrease the dose by 10%–25% every 1–2 days.
- Look for signs of withdrawal.
- Consider adding lorazepam 0.05–0.1 mg/kg every 6–8 hours to address anxiety, agitation, and restlessness.
- Consider adding clonidine patch 0.1 mg/day (changed every fifth day) to address physical symptoms of opioid withdrawal such as sweating, diarrhea, and abdominal cramps.

Richard J et al: A prospective evaluation of opioid weaning in opioid-dependent pediatric critical care patients. Anesth Analg 2006;102:1045–1050 [PMID: 16551896].

PEDIATRIC PALLIATIVE & END-OF-LIFE CARE

INTRODUCTION

It has been estimated that almost 55,000 children die each year in the United States. At least 50% of these children die during the newborn period or within the first year of life. Many of these children, particularly those older than 1 year, suffer from illnesses that are clearly life-limiting. Thousands more children are diagnosed with life-limiting illnesses, resulting in a chronic condition that may last for many years, even decades. Furthermore, children who are diagnosed with life-threatening illnesses that may be curable, such as cancer, continue to live with the potential of a recurrence of their malignancy for many years. The above populations are those where palliative and end-of-life care could play an important role during the illness of these patients.

It is estimated that over 8 million children worldwide need specialized palliative care. For example, the estimated need for pediatric palliative care ranges from 120 per 10,000 children (Zimbabwe) to 20 per 10,000 children (United Kingdom). Early data regarding the impact of palliative care programs on resource utilization support a trend toward fewer hospital admissions and shorter durations of admissions, but no change in utilization of emergency and outpatient care. Many children still die in a hospital setting, but those who have had involvement with pediatric palliative care have less aggressive end of life care.

Although commonly used interchangeably, *palliative care* and *end-of-life care* are not synonymous terms. Palliative care is a continuum of care that spans the duration of an illness. Palliative care aims to prevent, relieve, reduce, or soothe the symptoms produced by potential life-limiting illnesses or their treatments and to maintain the patient's quality of life along the entire continuum of treatment. Provision of palliative care does not imply imminent death, nor does it prohibit aggressive curative treatment modalities. Rather,

it acknowledges the uncertainty and potential for suffering inherent in a potentially life-limiting condition such as cancer. When it becomes clear that the chances for cure are poor or present an unreasonable cost to the child's quality of life, the goals of palliative care will shift toward end-of-life care where the focus will shift to promote quality of life while preparing for a comfortable and dignified end of life with increasingly less attention given to the treatment or cure of the disease itself. Understanding how a family defines quality of life and suffering for their child is imperative and provides a framework for decision-making between care provider and the family throughout treatment.

While a child is doing well with treatment, the primary focus will be on achieving cure or stabilization of the disease. Palliative care goals at this time focus on promoting quality of life in preparation for survivorship in the face of a potentially life-limiting illness. Some of these goals include helping a family come to terms with the diagnosis, addressing issues of treatment-related pain and distress, facilitating reintegration into the social realms of school and community, and promoting as much normalcy in the child's life as possible. Palliative care not only comprises support in the pain and symptom management of the disease but also addresses equally the psychosocial, emotional, and spiritual needs of the patient with a potential life-limiting illness and their family.

CHILDREN WHO MAY BENEFIT FROM PALLIATIVE CARE INTERVENTIONS

In a review by Himelstein et al, conditions that are appropriate for palliative care were divided into four groups as follows:

- Conditions for which curative treatment is possible but may fail such as advanced or progressive cancer and complex and severe congenital or acquired heart disease
- Conditions requiring intensive long-term treatment aimed at maintaining the quality of life such as HIV/AIDS, cystic fibrosis, and muscular dystrophy
- Progressive conditions in which treatment is exclusively palliative after diagnosis such as progressive metabolic disorders and certain chromosomal abnormalities
- Conditions involving severe, nonprogressive disability, causing extreme vulnerability to health complications such as severe cerebral palsy and anoxic brain injury

The United States Congress mandated in 2010 that palliative care will be covered concurrently with curative therapies for children with terminal conditions who are receiving Medicaid. Based on the *Patient Protection and Affordable Care Act*, a voluntary election to receive hospice care for a child does not constitute a waiver of any rights of the child to be provided with, or to have payments made for services that are related to the treatment of the child's condition. This significant milestone in pediatric palliative care should open the door to concurrent care being covered by private insurance companies in the future.

PAIN MANAGEMENT IN PEDIATRIC PALLIATIVE CARE

Optimal pain management is critical when providing pediatric palliative care. (See the section on Pain Management earlier for definitions and guidelines for treatment.) As end-of-life approaches, dosing of comfort medications may eventually exceed normally prescribed doses. The goal at all times must be to achieve and maintain comfort. When pain management at the end of life is provided with this goal at the forefront and in concert with careful ongoing assessment and documentation of the child's symptoms, there should be no reason to fear that this action is tantamount to euthanasia that is a conscious action intended to hasten death.

QUALITY-OF-LIFE ADJUNCTS & SYMPTOM MANAGEMENT IN PEDIATRIC PALLIATIVE CARE

When offering treatment to children with a life-limiting illness particularly at the end of life, certain non- pain symptoms and signs may develop more quickly in children when compared to the adult population. A thorough and complete history and physical examination should be obtained. It is critical to determine how much distress the symptom causes the child and how much it interferes with child and his/her family's routine when deciding upon treatment. Areas of management should include supportive treatment, including comfort medications, nursing care, and psychosocial support. Symptoms that commonly occur during disease progression and at the end of life in children with a life-limiting condition are listed in Table 32–5, with suggestions for management.

Complementary & Alternative Modalities

It is not unusual for families to seek complementary or alternative modalities (CAM) for their child when mainstream treatment has failed or is unavailable. Children with chronic conditions such as cancer, asthma, sickle cell disease, and epilepsy have a higher incidence of CAM usage compared to the general pediatric population (Post-White, 2009). The use of CAM in children is influenced primarily by parental use and acceptance of CAM. Culturally accepted beliefs and practices also play an important role. Most often, these treatments are aimed at improving physical or spiritual quality of life. Sometimes the goal is a desperate hope to find a treatment when other options have failed or an attempt to find something perceived as less toxic than mainstream treatments to induce remission, support the child's ability to fight the disease, or prolong life. Parents' report using CAM gives them a sense of control and hope. The most common modalities reported in pediatrics are prayer/meditation, relaxation techniques, massage, chiropractic care including acupuncture, and nutritional supplements (Post-White et al, 2009; Friedrichsdorf and Kohen, 2018).

Studies of the effectiveness of CAM use in children have been small, and the data are often conflicting. There is generally an acceptance for the lack of harm associated with mind-body techniques such as prayer, meditation, touch and sensory modalities, and relaxation. Hospice providers frequently incorporate relaxation and mind/body/spirit modalities into their programs. Acupuncture and acupressure are gaining more acceptance in the Western medical community and may be beneficial in some children for relief of pain, nausea, and other symptoms. Touch and sensory modalities such as massage, healing touch, and aromatherapy can induce a relaxation response in some children, which can be very helpful. The use of supplements including botanicals and vitamins has been of more concern due to the lack of dosing information for pediatrics, lack of standardization of some products, and the potential for serious drug interactions and toxicities. Treatments touted as alternative "cures" are likely not beneficial and can have very dangerous consequences. An increasing number of parents are considering the use of cannabinoids due to increased availability and purported claims of symptom relief (nausea, pain, anxiety) or as a cure for their child's condition. There are currently little data on dosing or efficacy for children. Cannabinoids are known to have the potential for interaction with many drugs; thus, all medications a child takes must be evaluated and the risks assessed (Treves et al, 2021). There are limited data on the use of cannabinoids in children with epilepsy that shows CBD is beneficial in decreasing seizure frequency in children with treatment-resistant epilepsy. Cannabis herbal extracts appear to induce a decrease seizure frequency, but the studies are either retrospective or small-scale observational studies. The two large randomized controlled studies assessing the efficacy of pharmaceutical-grade CBD in children with Dravet and Lennox-Gastaut syndromes showed similar efficacy to other anticonvulsants. The cost of CAM, particularly botanicals and alternative medicine treatments, can be prohibitive and the cost is rarely covered by insurance.

It is important for the health care provider to ask parents and adolescents about CAM usage and to be open to discussion with the family about modalities they are using or may wish to consider. Parents consistently have reported in studies their desire to inform and discuss CAM with their health care provider but may be reluctant to do so if they are unsure what response they will get from the provider. Providing families with clear information about the treatment they are considering or using and any contraindications is key. In some cases, recommendation of complementary techniques such as massage, mind-body modalities, and acupuncture/acupressure may be appropriate.

Table 32–5. Symptom management in pediatric palliative care.

Symptom	Etiology	Management
Nausea and vomiting	Chemotherapy, narcotics, metabolic	Diphenhydramine, hydroxyzine, 5-HT$_3$ inhibitors, prokinetic agents for GI motility
Anorexia	Cancer, pain, abnormal taste, GI alterations, metabolic changes, drugs, psychological factors	Treat underlying condition, exercise, dietary consultation, appetite stimulants (dronabinol, megestrol, steroid)
Constipation/diarrhea	Narcotics, chemotherapy, malabsorption, drug related	Laxatives (must be initiated whenever starting narcotics), loperamide for diarrhea, peripheral opioid antagonists (methylnaltrexone, alvimopan)
Dyspnea	Airway obstruction; decrease in functional lung tissue due to effusion, infection, metastases; impaired chest wall movement; anemia	Treatment of specific cause (surgery to alleviate obstruction, red blood cell transfusion, chemotherapy/radiation therapy for metastatic disease), nonpharmacologic management (reassurance, position of comfort, improvement of air circulation using electric fan, oxygen, and relaxation therapy), pharmacologic management with opioids given IV/SQ as continuous infusion, nebulized morphine in older patients, concomitant use of anxiolytics (lorazepam, midazolam) if agitation
Terminal respiratory congestion	Airway/oral secretions at the end of life, resulting in rattling, noisy, gurgling breath sounds	Repositioning, anticholinergics such as hyoscine IV/SQ/PO or transdermal scopolamine
Pressure sores	Direct tissue damage, tissue fragility, immobility, diminished response to pain or irritation	Prevention (avoidance of trauma, relieve pressure, good hygiene), treatment with local hygiene, debridement, use of appropriate wound dressings, antibiotics, analgesics
Bone pain	Bony metastases, leukemic infiltration of bone marrow	Palliative radiation, bone-seeking isotopes, bisphosphonates, chemotherapy, analgesics
Agitation	Present in conjunction with pain, dyspnea, terminal phase of illness	Benzodiazepines (midazolam), barbiturates to achieve complete sedation in terminal restlessness
Pruritus	Urticaria, postherpetic neuralgia, cholestasis, uremia, opioids	Antihistamines (cholestasis, uremia, opioids), 5-HT$_3$ receptor antagonists (cholestasis, opioids)
Hematologic	Marrow infiltration by malignant cells (leukemia) Coagulopathy Bleeding from erosive or ulcerative processes	Transfusions (red blood cells, platelets) to relieve symptoms, hemostatics (aminocaproic acid) Dark bath towel (black, burgundy, or dark purple) to help absorb and camouflage blood
Intractable pain	Various	Chronic pain team consult; consider palliative sedation in very selected cases

PSYCHOSOCIAL ASPECTS OF PEDIATRIC PALLIATIVE CARE

Pediatric palliative care is unique in that caregivers must be familiar with children's normal emotional and spiritual development. Working with a child at his or her level of development through the use of both oral and expressive communication techniques will allow the child to be more open with respect to hopes, dreams, and fears. A child's understanding of death will depend on his or her stage of development. Children understand death as a changed state by 3 years of age, universality (death happens to all living things) by 5–6 years of age, and personal mortality by 8–9 years of age. Table 32–6 shows a broad overview of children's concepts of death and offers some helpful interventions.

CHILDREN'S CONCEPT OF DEATH

As end-of-life approaches, psychosocial support is invaluable to the child and family. Children may need someone to talk to outside of the family unit who can respond to their questions and concerns openly and honestly. Parents may need guidance and support in initiating discussions with or responding to questions from their child about death and dying. Children and adolescents may have specific tasks they wish to complete before they die. Some want to have input into funeral and memorial service plans and disposition of their

Table 32–6. Children's concepts of death.

Age Group and Cognitive Development	Cognitive Understanding of Death	Response to Stress	Helpful Interventions
Infancy: Sense of self is directly related to having needs met	None	Lethargy, irritability, failure to thrive	Maintain routines Prompt response to physical and emotional caretaking needs Cuddling, holding, rocking
Toddler: Egocentric, concrete thinking; see objects and events in relationship to their usefulness to self	None but beginning to perceive implications of separation	Irritability, change in sleep-wake patterns, clinginess, regression, tantrums	Maintain routines Keep familiar people and objects at hand Prompt response to physical and emotional caretaking needs Accept need for increased physical and emotional comfort but continue to encourage acquisition of developmental skills
Preschool: Beginning to understand concept of time but limited sense of time permanence, curious, still quite concrete in thinking	View death as deliberately caused Magical thinking about causes of illness and death Death is not a permanent state	Oppositional behaviors, regression, sleep-wake changes, nightmares, somatic complaints Beginning to identify meaning and context of emotions	Simple, concrete explanations to questions—find out what it is they want to know Reassurance that death and illness are not the result of their thoughts or wishes Keep familiar people and objects at hand Play is a powerful tool to help children process events and emotions and as distraction from stressful situations
School age: Beginning of ability to apply logic; accept points of view other than their own	Death is seen in context of experience (pets, grandparents, what is seen on TV or in movies) Can understand that death is permanent	Oppositional behaviors, nightmares, sleep disruption, withdrawal, sadness Can verbally identify own feelings of fear, sadness, happiness	Ascertain how they perceive and understand what is happening and respond accordingly to their questions Acknowledge that feelings of sadness, fear, and anger are normal Allow age-appropriate control whenever possible Maintain as much normalcy in routine as possible Play is very important for expression of emotions and release of stress, amenable to directed play
Preadolescence and adolescence: Gaining mastery over themselves as individuals by exploring their own moral, ethical, and spiritual beliefs; increased reliance on peers for emotional support and information	Adult awareness of death but still may be highly experiential in understanding	Anger, withdrawal, sadness, depression, somatic complaints May have difficulty asking for emotional help	Set the tone for open, honest communication Allow the young person as much control as possible in decisions about his or her own health care Be willing to discuss and respect wishes and desires for disposition of belongings, funeral planning, what happens to his or her body Assist the young person in accomplishing important life tasks and activities that gives meaning to his or her existence or leaves behind a legacy

body. Parents often need support in making funeral arrangements, handling financial concerns, talking with siblings and other family members, and coping with their own grief.

It is important to recognize that grief is not an illness but a normal, multidimensional, unique, dynamic process presenting as pervasive distress due to a perceived loss. Once parents have accepted the reality of the loss of the child, they must then complete the other tasks of grief such as experiencing the pain of their loss and adjusting to an environment without their child in order to move on with their lives. Parents who lose a child are at high risk for complicated grief reactions such as absent grief, delayed grief, and prolonged or unresolved grief. Siblings are also at risk for complicated grief and require special attention (Morris et al,).

SPIRITUAL & CULTURAL SUPPORT

Health care decisions are often intertwined with a family's culture and belief system. Understanding the influences of a family's beliefs and culture allows the practitioner to provide sensitive, appropriate care, particularly at the end of life. Interaction with members of the family's faith and cultural communities can often be instrumental in helping both the care team and the community support of the family. Accommodation for specific prayers, rituals, or other activities may help facilitate procedures and discussions.

Families who speak a foreign language probably suffer from inadequate support the most. Every effort should be made to find and utilize a qualified interpreter, particularly for any discussion that involves delivering difficult news or making critical decisions. Many times, the role of interpreter is imposed upon a bilingual family member or friend who may not understand medical terminology well enough to translate clearly or who may deliberately translate the information inaccurately to protect the family.

The American Academy of Pediatrics has many resources listed on its website to help children, siblings, and parents at www.aap.org.

WITHDRAWAL OF MEDICAL LIFE SUPPORT

Medical technology has enabled many children with serious health conditions to enjoy a good quality of life. When technological support no longer enables a child's quality and enjoyment of life or there are no viable options to restore quality of life to the child, it may be appropriate to discontinue it. Feeding tubes, ventilators, dialysis, parenteral nutrition, and implanted cardiac pacemakers are examples of medical modalities that may need to be reevaluated when a child's condition deteriorates or in the case of a catastrophic injury.

There are five circumstances in which withdrawal of medical support and technology can be considered in children (Tournay, 2000). (See the following table.)

Brain death	All reversible causes excluded, meets established criteria for determination of brain death
Persistent vegetative state (PVS)	Child totally dependent for all cares, has no ability to interact meaningfully with his environment. Lack of cortical peaks in the somatosensory evoked potential may be helpful in making prognosis of PVS
Treatment will delay death without significantly relieving the suffering caused by the condition	No chance for cure, invasiveness of the treatment may prolong life but does not diminish or increases suffering
Child's life may be saved, but at the cost of physical and mental impairment that makes life intolerable for the child	Important to understand how child and family defines "intolerable life"
Additional treatment with potential benefit will cause further suffering	Burden of suffering outweighs the potential for benefit

Helping families identify and define what quality of life means to their child and to the family and what would be an intolerable life for the child is important. It is critical to present in a clear and understandable format the child's medical condition, test results, and treatments that have been tried, what the expectations are for the child's ability to survive or function and interact with his environment, and why it is believed that current or additional interventions will be futile or induce further suffering. These discussions should be conducted with sensitivity and without need for an immediate answer from the parents. It often takes several such discussions for families to come to a decision that they themselves will be able to live with and families should not be rushed into decision-making. The family may request additional testing or retesting to assure themselves they are making the right decision for their child. When feasible, these requests should be honored. Spiritual support may be very helpful to families during this process and should be offered.

Once the family has made the decision to withdraw support, it is helpful to explain what the anticipated course will be following withdrawal, what the child will likely look like during that time and what the plan of care will be to ensure comfort. Create a plan with the family for time and place of withdrawal, who they would like to be there with them, any specific requests for environment such as music, a favorite movie playing, or a book being read, and who they would like to perform the withdrawal. Offering the opportunity for rituals, prayer, or private time prior to or during the withdrawal is appropriate. If death is anticipated to happen quickly after withdrawal, any specific religious requirements for the body after death should be arranged in advance. In all cases of withdrawal, the family should be offered support during the process and after the death occurs.

ADVANCE CARE PLANNING

Advance care planning allows patients and families to make known their wishes about what to do in case of serious or life-threatening problems. Himelstein et al describe advance care planning as a four-step process. First, those individuals considered decision makers are identified and included in the process. Second, an assessment of the patient's and family's understanding of the illness and prognosis is made, and the impending death is described in terms that the child and family can understand. Third, based on their understanding of the illness and prognosis, the goals of care are determined regarding current and future intervention—curative, uncertain, or primarily focused on providing comfort. Finally, shared decisions about the current and future use or abandonment of life-sustaining techniques and aggressive medical interventions are made. In the event of a disagreement between parents or parents and their patient regarding these techniques or interventions, it may be prudent to involve the hospital's ethics committee in order to resolve these issues.

Some states permit parents to sign an advanced directive that asserts their decision not to have resuscitative attempts made in the event of a cardiac or respiratory arrest outside of the hospital. When an advanced directive is in place, emergency responders are not required to provide cardiopulmonary resuscitation (CPR) if called to the scene. Some school districts will respect an advanced directive on school property, many will not. If a child with an advanced directive in place wishes to go to school, a discussion between the medical team and school officials should be arranged to determine the best plan should the child have a cardiac or respiratory arrest at school.

Parents and, occasionally, the child may bring up the possibility of donating organs or body tissues after death. Although the tissues that may be donated by a child may be limited in some instances by the type of disease (eg, cancer), some parents find immense comfort in knowing their child was able to benefit another. If the parents have not discussed donation with the physician by the time of death and donation is possible, the physician should offer the opportunity to the family.

Autopsy is another subject many physicians find difficult to approach with a family, but it is an important option to discuss. In cases of anticipated death from natural causes, autopsies are generally not mandatory; however, information obtained from an autopsy may be useful for parental peace of mind or medical research. If death at home is to be followed by an autopsy, special arrangements for transporting and receiving the body will need to be made with the mortuary or the coroner.

REFERENCES

Amano K et al: Association between early palliative care referrals, inpatient hospice utilization, and aggressiveness of care at the end of life. J Palliat Med 2015 Mar;18(3):270–273 [PMID: 25210851].

Becker G, Blum HE: Novel opioid antagonists for opioid-induced bowel dysfunction and postoperative ileus. Lancet 2009;373:1198 [PMID: 19217656].

Conner SC: Estimating the global need for palliative care for children: a cross-sectional analysis. J Pain Symptom Manage 2017 Feb;53(2):171 [PMID: 27765706].

Friedrichsdorf SJ, Kohen DP: Integration of hypnosis into pediatric palliative care. Ann Palliat Med 2018 Jan;7(1):136–150. doi:10.21037/apm.2017.05.02 [PMID: 28866891].

Goldman A et al (eds): Oxford Textbook of Palliative Care for Children. Oxford University Press; 2006.

Hanny C: Complementary and alternative medicine use in pediatric hematology/oncology patients at the University of Mississippi Medical Center. J Altern Complement Med 2015 Nov 11;21:660–666.

Himelstein B et al: Pediatric palliative care. N Engl J Med 2004;350:1752 [PMID: 15103002].

Huntsman RJ, Tang-Wai R, Shackelford AE: Cannabis for pediatric epilepsy. J Clin Neurophysiol 2020 Jan;37(1):2–8. doi: 10.1097/WNP.0000000000000641 [PMID: 31895184].

ng T, Munson D, Klick J (eds): Pediatric palliative care. Pediatr Clin North Am 2007;54(5).

Kemppainen LM, Kemppainen TT, Reippainen JA, Salmennien ST, Vuolanto PH: Use of complementary and alternative medicine in Europe: health—related and sociodemographic determinants. Scand J Public Health 2018 Jun;46(4):448–455 [PMID: 28975853].

Knapp C, Thompson L: Factors associated with perceived barriers to pediatric palliative care: a survey of pediatricians in Florida and California. Palliat Med 2012;26(3):268–274 [PMID: 21680751].

Lindenfelser KJ, Hense C, McFerran K: Music therapy in pediatric palliative care: family-centered care to enhance quality of life. Am J Hosp Palliat Care 2012;29(3):219–226 [PMID: 22144660].

Morris S, Fletcher K, Goldstein R: The grief of parents after the death of a young child. J Clin Psychol Med Settings 2019 Sep;26(3):321–338 [PMID: 30488260].

October T et al: The parent perspective: "Being a good parent" when making critical decisions in the PICU. Pediatr Crit Care Med 2014;15:291–298 [PMID: 24583502].

O'Shea ER, Kanarek RB: Understanding pediatric palliative care: what it is and what it should be. J Pediatr Oncol Nurs 2013;(30)1:34–44 [PMID: 23372039].

Ott M: Mind-body therapies for the pediatric oncology patient: matching the right therapy with the right patient. J Pediatr Oncol Nurs 2006;223(5):254–257 [PMID: 16902078].

Pirie A: Pediatric palliative care communication: resources for the clinical nurse specialist. Clin Nurse Spec 2012;26(4):212–215 [PMID: 22678187].

Post-White J, Fitzgerald M, Hageness S, Sencer S: Complementary and alternative medicine use in children with cancer and general and specialty pediatrics. J Pediatr Oncol Nurs 2009;26(1):715 [PMID: 18936292].

Thompson LA et al: Pediatricians' perceptions of and preferred timing for pediatric palliative care. Pediatrics 2009;123:e777 [PMID: 19403469].

Tomlinson D et al: Chemotherapy versus supportive care alone in pediatric palliative care for cancer: comparing the preferences of parents and health care professionals. CMAJ 2011;183(17):E1252–E1258 [PMID: 22007121].

Tournay AE: Withdrawal of medical treatment in children. West J Med 2000;173:407–411 [PMID: 11112760].

Treves N et al: Efficacy and safety of medical cannabinoids in children: a systematic review and meta-analysis. Sci Rep 2021 Dec 6;11(1):23462. doi: 10.1038/s41598-021-02770-6 [PMID: 34873203].

Weaver MS et al: Establishing psychosocial palliative care standards for children and adolescents with cancer and their families: an integrative review. Palliat Med 2016 Mar;30(3):212–223 [PMID: 25921709].

Weigand D: In their own time: the family experience during the process of withdrawal of life-sustaining therapy. J Palliat Med 2008 Nov 8;11:1115–1121 [PMID: 18980452].

Widger K, Picot C: Parents' perceptions of the quality of pediatric and perinatal end-of-life care. Pediatr Nurs 2008;34(1):53–58 [PMID: 18361087].

Woodruff R (ed): *Palliative Medicine*. Oxford University Press; 2005.

Youngblut JM, Brooten D: Perinatal and pediatric issues in palliative and end-of-life care from the 2011 Summit on the Science of Compassion. Nurs Outlook 2012;60(6):343–350.

National Hospice and Palliative Care Organization (NHPCO)—Children's Project on Palliative/Hospice Services (ChiPPs): www.nhpco.org.

WHO Global Report on Traditional and Complementary Medicine, World Health Organization 2019 ISBN978-92-4-15.

Web Resources

Education on Palliative and End of Life Care (EPEC; adult focused): www.epec.net.

End of Life Nursing Education Consortium (ELNEC): http://www.aacn.nche.edu/elnec.

Initiative for Pediatric Palliative Care (IPPC): www.ippcweb.org.

Immunodeficiency

Jordan K. Abbott, MD, MA

Cullen M. Dutmer, MD

Pia J. Hauk, MD

INTRODUCTION

Immunodeficiency is a physiologic state in which the immune system succumbs to microbiologic exposures typically controlled by members of the nonimmunodeficient population. This state can be transient or persistent, in-born or acquired, and it can result from dysfunction of one or multiple components of the immune system. The infectious manifestations of immunodeficiency arise from a failure to prevent, clear, limit the spread, or suppress a microorganism that would typically be controlled in one of the modes of defense. Clinical manifestations therefore include infection with an unusual microorganism, greater extent of spread of an infection, persistent infection, recurrent infection, and the associated inflammatory consequences of these scenarios. Since infections in immunodeficiency are dependent on a relevant microbiologic exposure, it is possible that immunodeficiency can remain undiagnosed; however, careful consideration of associated features, family history, immunosuppressive medications, and laboratory findings can hasten the diagnosis and possibly prevent a severe infection or other complication. As a result, it is important that physicians be aware of clues that could lead to a prompt diagnosis.

The human immune system consists of the phylogenetically more primitive innate immune system and the adaptive immune system (Figure 33–1). To assist clinical categorization, immunodeficiencies are commonly divided into four main groups: antibody deficiencies, combined T- and B-cell immunodeficiencies, phagocyte disorders, and other deficiencies of innate immunity, which include complement deficiencies. Understanding the role each part of the immune system plays in host defense allows critical evaluation for possible immunodeficiency as the cause of recurrent infections and immune dysregulation, which can lead to associated autoimmunity and chronic inflammation.

The prevalence of primary immunodeficiency (PID) is currently unknown, particularly in the pediatric population;

however, significant advances have provided a more accurate understanding of parts of the PID picture. With the implementation of T-cell receptor rearrangement excision circle (TREC) newborn screening, the incidence of severe combined immunodeficiency disease (SCID) in newborns is estimated to be 1 in 50,000 births (Table 33–1). Likewise, the incidence of severely impaired or absent thymus activity is 1 in 50,000 births. Thus, the anticipated frequencies of two separate etiologies of severe T-cell deficiency are now more precisely known. The remainder of pediatric PID incidence or prevalence remains much less well understood. The scope of PID includes neutrophil, complement, B-cell, and T-cell deficiencies. In addition, several common chromosomal syndromes include a subset of patients with varying degrees of PID severity, including 10% of 22q11 deletion and most with trisomy 21. Including such patients, the landscape of PID includes many patients with syndromic immunodeficiency as well as rarer genetic defects that result in specific inborn errors of immunity. Combining all such patients, the prevalence in children is likely between 1 in 1000 and 1 in 10,000. PID patients are therefore not infrequently seen in the pediatric practice; although, any specific genetic etiology is rare.

IMMUNODEFICIENCY EVALUATION: PRIMARY CONSIDERATIONS

When evaluating for a possible PID, other conditions that increase susceptibility to infections must be considered, such as allergic rhinitis, asthma, cystic fibrosis, primary ciliary dyskinesia, foreign-body aspiration, and conditions that interfere with skin barrier function. Other common causes of secondary or acquired immunodeficiency include malnutrition, aging, protein loss (via gastroenteropathy, kidney disease, or lymphatic malformations), certain drugs (glucocorticoids, immunosuppressive medications, disease-modifying biologic drugs, chemotherapy); and other diseases associated with impaired immunity (bone marrow failure

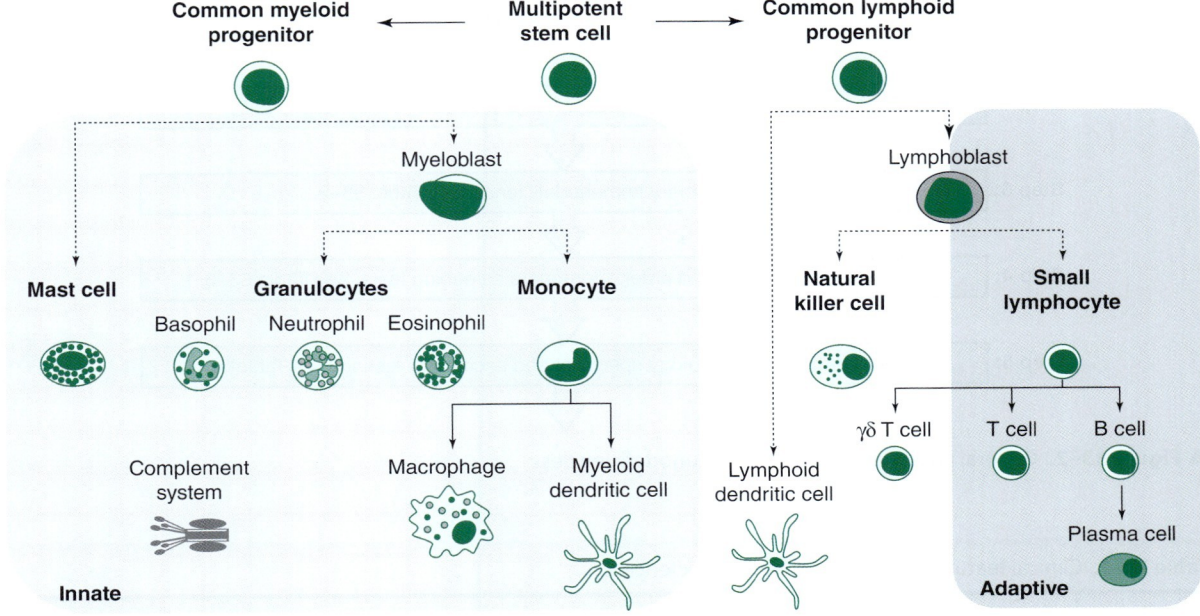

▲ **Figure 33-1.** Components of the human immune system.

and blood cell malignancies, and certain chronic infections, including AIDS). If a single site is involved, anatomic defects and foreign bodies may be present. Figure 33–2 outlines when PIDs should be considered.

Key clinical patterns can indicate the presence of a PID and the category of immune impairment. PID should be considered in patients with frequent, severe, or unusual infections. When the infection history suggests PID, the type of infections can help guide the initial workup. Antibody, complement, and phagocyte defects predispose mainly to bacterial infections, but diarrhea, superficial candidiasis, opportunistic infections, and severe herpesvirus infections are more characteristic of T-lymphocyte immunodeficiency. Location of infection can provide important clues. Additional features such as the presence of syndromic features, poor wound healing, immune dysregulation including autoimmunity or lymphoproliferative disease, age of disease onset, and failure to thrive can help further categorize the PID. Table 33–2 classifies PID into four main host immunity categories based on age of onset, infections with specific pathogens, affected organs, and other special features.

Initial laboratory investigation should be directed by the clinical presentation and the suspected category of host immunity impairment. If antibody deficiency is suspected, a complete blood cell (CBC) count with cell differential and measurement of quantitative immunoglobulins will identify most patients. If T-cell deficiency is suspected, lymphocyte phenotyping to quantify blood T cells, B cells, and natural killer (NK) cells should be sent. For phagocyte defects, testing of oxidative burst in stimulated granulocytes should be performed. For complement deficiency, testing of the function of the classical and alternative pathways should be performed. Table 33–3 summarizes the approach to laboratory evaluation of PID.

Table 33–1. Frequency of several pediatric diseases in the United States.

Diagnosis	Population Frequency[a,b]
Asthma	Prevalence: 1 in 12
Congenital heart disease	Incidence: 1 in 500
Trisomy 21	Incidence: 1 in 700
Juvenile idiopathic arthritis	Prevalence: 1 in 1000
Cystic fibrosis	Incidence: 1 in 3000
22q11 deletion syndrome	Incidence: 1 in 6000
Acute lymphoblastic leukemia	Incidence: 1 in 30000
Severe combined immunodeficiency	Incidence: 1 in 50000

[a]Incidence refers to cases per number of live births. [b]Prevalence refers to number of cases within the pediatric population of the United States at a given time.

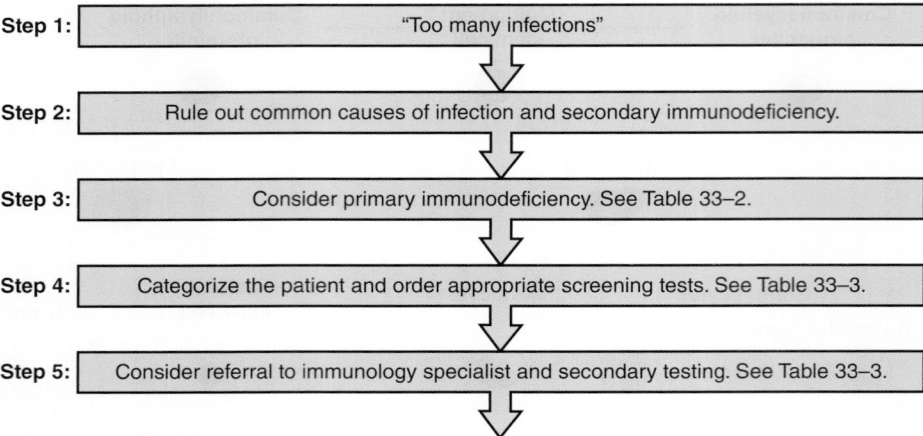

Step 1: "Too many infections"

Step 2: Rule out common causes of infection and secondary immunodeficiency.

Step 3: Consider primary immunodeficiency. See Table 33–2.

Step 4: Categorize the patient and order appropriate screening tests. See Table 33–3.

Step 5: Consider referral to immunology specialist and secondary testing. See Table 33–3.

▲ **Figure 33–2.** General approach to primary immunodeficiencies.

Table 33–2. Clinical features of primary immunodeficiencies.

Characteristic	Combined Deficiency (T- and B-Lymphocyte Defect)	Antibody Deficiency (B-Lymphocyte Defect)	Phagocyte Defect	Complement Defect
Age at onset of infections	Early onset, usually before 6 mo	Onset after maternal antibodies decline, usually after 3–6 mo; some later in childhood or adults	Early onset	Any age
Specific pathogens	**Bacteria:** *Streptococcus pneumoniae, Campylobacter fetus, Staphylococcus aureus, Haemophilus influenzae, Pseudomonas aeruginosa, Mycoplasma hominis, Ureaplasma urealyticum, Listeria monocytogenes, Salmonella* spp, enteric flora, atypical mycobacteria, and BCG **Viruses:** CMV, EBV, varicella, RSV, enterovirus, rotavirus **Fungi/protozoa:** *Candida albicans, Aspergillus fumigatus, Toxoplasma gondii* **Other:** *Pneumocystis carinii, Cryptosporidium*	**Bacteria:** *S pneumoniae, C fetus, H influenzae, P aeruginosa, U urealyticum, S aureus, M hominis* **Viruses:** Enteroviruses **Fungi/protozoa:** *Giardia lamblia*	**Bacteria:** *S aureus,* enteric flora, *Burkholderia* spp, *Aspergillus* spp, *P aeruginosa, Salmonella* spp, *Serratia* spp, *Nocardia asteroides, Klebsiella* spp, nontuberculous mycobacteria, and BCG **Viruses:** None **Fungi/protozoa:** *C albicans, A fumigatus*	**Bacteria:** *Neisseria meningitidis* and *gonorrhoeae, S pneumoniae, S aureus, P aeruginosa, H influenzae* **Viruses:** None **Fungi/protozoa:** None
Affected organs and infections	**General:** Failure to thrive **Infections:** Severe infections (meningitis, septicemia, sinopulmonary), recurrent candidiasis, protracted diarrhea	**Infections:** Recurrent sinopulmonary, pneumonia, meningitis **GI:** Chronic malabsorption, IBD-like symptoms **Other:** Arthritis	**Skin:** Dermatitis, abscesses, cellulitis **Lymph nodes:** Suppurative adenitis **Oral cavity:** Periodontitis, ulcers **Lungs:** Pneumonia, abscesses **Other:** Liver and brain abscesses, osteomyelitis	**Infections:** Meningitis, disseminated gonococcal infection, septicemia, pneumonia

(Continued)

Table 33–2. Clinical features of primary immunodeficiencies. (*Continued*)

Characteristic	Combined Deficiency (T- and B-Lymphocyte Defect)	Antibody Deficiency (B-Lymphocyte Defect)	Phagocyte Defect	Complement Defect
Special features	GVHD from maternal T cells or blood product transfusion Disseminated infection after BCG or live polio immunization Absent lymphoid tissue Absent thymic shadow on chest radiograph	Autoimmunity Lymphoreticular malignancy Postvaccination polio Chronic enteroviral encephalitis	Poor wound healing Pyloric and urethral stenosis, IBD	**Autoimmune disorders:** SLE, vasculitis, dermatomyositis,scleroderma, glomerulonephritis **Other:** Hereditary angioedema, aHUS

aHUS, atypical hemolytic uremic syndrome; BCG, bacillus Calmette-Guérin; CMV, cytomegalovirus; EBV, Epstein-Barr virus; GVHD, graft-versus-host disease; IBD, inflammatory bowel disease; RSV, respiratory syncytial virus; SLE, systemic lupus erythematosus.

Antibodies & Immunoglobulins

The initial laboratory screening for antibody deficiency includes the measurement of serum immunoglobulins: immunoglobulin G (IgG), immunoglobulin M (IgM), and immunoglobulin A (IgA), which have normal ranges that are significantly divergent depending on age. It is therefore essential to consult age-based reference ranges when evaluating immunoglobulin results. By default, naïve B cells produce IgM, and production of the other isotypes requires further B-cell differentiation. When IgM but no other isotypes are present, a problem in B-cell differentiation is likely. When all immunoglobulin isotypes are decreased, an earlier defect in B-cell development should be suspected. Normal IgG, IgM, and IgA, and increased immunoglobulin E (IgE) levels usually indicate atopy. Elevated immunoglobulin levels are often seen in autoimmunity.

Some patients may have normal immunoglobulin levels but fail to make protective antibodies. Assessing the immunologic response to vaccination is therefore recommended. Specific IgG antibodies to protein antigens (tetanus, diphtheria, rubella, mumps) and protein-conjugated polysaccharide

Table 33–3. Laboratory evaluation for primary immunodeficiency.

Suspected Defect	Screening Evaluation	Specialist Evaluation
B lymphocyte	• CBC with differential • Quantitative immunoglobulins	• T-cell, B-cell, and NK-cell enumeration • Extended phenotyping of B cells • IgG levels to immunization antigens • DNA analysis for specific genetic mutations
T lymphocyte	• CBC with differential • Quantitative immunoglobulins • T-cell, B-cell, and NK-cell enumeration	• Extended phenotyping of T cells • Lymphocyte proliferation to mitogens and antigens • Delayed-type hypersensitivity skin test • Cytotoxicity studies • ADA or PNP levels of RBC • DNA analysis for specific genetic mutations
Phagocyte	• CBC with differential	• DHR flow cytometry assay • Nitroblue tetrazolium reduction assay • Bactericidal assays • CD11/18 analysis • Chemotaxis assay
Complement	• CH50 • AH50	• Complement component levels • Complement component function • Complement antibodies

ADA, adenosine deaminase; CBC, complete blood cell count; CD, cluster of differentiation; DHR, dihydrorhodamine; NK, natural killer; PNP, purine nucleoside phosphorylase; RBC, red blood cell; WBC, white blood cell.
Adapted from Cunningham-Rundles C: Immune deficiency: office evaluation and treatment. Allergy Asthma Proc 2003 Nov–Dec;24(6):409–415.

antigens (*Streptococcus pneumoniae*, *Haemophilus influenzae*) can be measured after routine immunization. To test the response to pure polysaccharide vaccine, Pneumovax 23® or Typhim Vi® can be administered. The response to polysaccharide antigens develops during the second year of life, but protein-conjugated vaccines elicit an earlier response in immunocompetent children. The gold standard is comparison of pre- and postimmunization titers.

If an initial screen reveals very low concentrations of immunoglobulin isotypes, further studies are aimed at identifying the cause of immunoglobulin deficiency. Certain types of hypogammaglobulinemia are characterized by low levels of or absent B lymphocytes, such as X-linked Bruton agammaglobulinemia. Serum albumin should be measured in patients with hypogammaglobulinemia to exclude secondary deficiencies due to protein loss through bowel or kidneys. IgG or IgA subclass measurements may be abnormal in patients with varied immunodeficiency syndromes and malignancies, but they are rarely helpful in an initial evaluation.

T Lymphocytes

The initial laboratory screening for a T-lymphocyte deficiency includes a CBC with cell differential to evaluate for a decreased absolute lymphocyte count (< 1000/μL) and enumeration of absolute numbers of T cells and their subsets, B cells, and NK cells (see Table 33–3). T-cell function can be analyzed by in vitro lymphocyte proliferation. Borderline function must be interpreted based on clinical correlation. T-lymphocyte function is often also studied in vivo by delayed hypersensitivity skin tests to specific antigens, including *Candida albicans*, tetanus, or mumps, but a negative result is not helpful, as it may be due to young age, chronic illness, vitamin D deficiency, or poor test technique. T-lymphocyte deficiencies will often not manifest as skin-test anergy until the impairment is severe, for example, as in AIDS. It is important to evaluate a patient's specific antibody production because proper B-lymphocyte function and antibody production are dependent on adequate T-lymphocyte function. Therefore, most T-lymphocyte deficiencies manifest as combined T- and B-lymphocyte deficiencies.

Phagocyte Immunity

Phagocyte defects typically involve reduction in phagocyte numbers or defects in phagocyte function. The initial laboratory screening for phagocyte disorders should include a CBC and cell differential to look for neutropenia. A blood smear can detect Howell-Jolly bodies in erythrocytes, indicative of asplenia, and abnormalities in lysosomal granules in neutrophils. An abnormality of the neutrophil respiratory burst, which would lead to impaired neutrophil bactericidal activity, can be tested by flow cytometric analysis of stimulated neutrophils preloaded with dihydrorhodamine (DHR). Leukocyte adhesion molecules can be studied by flow cytometry. Assays to study neutrophil phagocytosis of bacteria and

phagocytic microbicidal activity are available in specialized laboratories. The clinical symptom pattern that suggests a possible defect of phagocytic cell function should dictate which tests are used.

Complement Pathways (Figure 33–3)

Testing for total hemolytic complement activity with the CH50 assay screens for most diseases of the complement system that increase susceptibility to infection. A normal CH50 titer depends on the ability of all 11 components of the classical pathway and membrane attack complex (MAC) to interact and then lyse antibody-coated sheep erythrocytes. Alternative complement pathway deficiencies are identified by subnormal lysis of rabbit erythrocytes in the AH50 assay. For both assays, the patient's serum must be separated and frozen at –70°C within 30–60 minutes after collection to prevent loss of activity. Measuring levels of individual components is not necessary when both CH50 and AH50 are normal. If both the CH50 and AH50 are low, a deficiency in their shared terminal pathway (C3, C5, C6, C7, C8, or C9) would be the most common explanation. If the CH50 is low but the AH50 is normal, the deficiency must affect C1, C4, or C2. If the AH50 is low but the CH50 is normal, a deficiency in factor D, factor B, or properdin should be suspected. Most quantitative deficiencies of complement components result from pathway activation and resultant consumption. It is therefore essential that complement activation be ruled out prior to diagnosing an inherited complement deficiency.

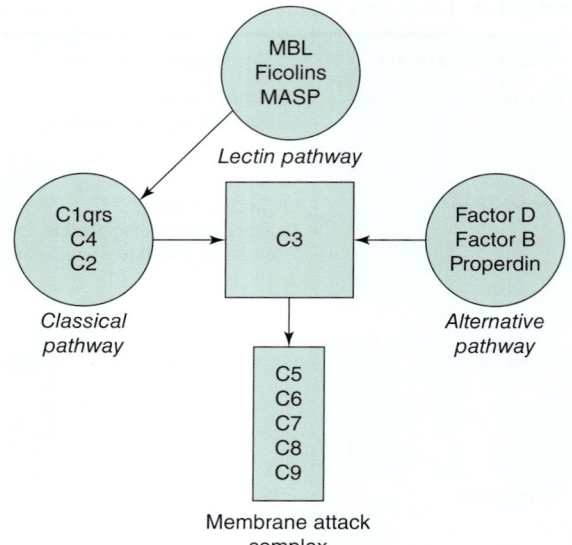

▲ **Figure 33–3.** Pathways of complement activation and the central functional role of C3. MASP, MBL-associated serine protease; MBL, mannose-binding lectin.

VACCINATION IN CHILDREN WITH IMMUNODEFICIENCY

Attenuated-live vaccines pose a risk of significant infection for certain patients with immunodeficiency. "Live" virus vaccines should not be administered to patients with a moderate to severe T-cell immunodeficiency. In the US, these vaccines include the oral Rotavirus vaccine, the measles, mumps, rubella (MMR) vaccine and certain formulations of varicella zoster virus (VZV) vaccines. The administration of these live-virus vaccines is contraindicated due to risk of disseminated or severe, persistent vaccine-strain induced viral disease and subsequent tissue invasion. For the same reason, live bacterial vaccines such as the oral typhoid (Ty21a) and the BCG vaccines are contraindicated in patients with congenital neutropenia and chronic granulomatous disease (CGD). Table 33–4 includes other relevant live vaccines.

The decision of whether a T-cell deficiency is severe enough to warrant avoiding live virus vaccines should be made with the consultation of a clinical immunologist. Many patients with the same disease state vary in the severity of T-cell deficiency, resulting in some able to receive live vaccines and others not. This is particularly true for diseases in which only a minority of patients do not have a severe T-cell defect, such as chromosome 22q11.2 deletion syndrome (22q11del) or Coloboma, Heart defect, Atresia choanae, Retardation of growth and development, Genital hypoplasia, Ear anomalies/deafness (CHARGE) syndrome. An immunologist will perform diagnostic testing to determine if there is adequate thymic T-cell output. These tests include the presence of recent thymic emigrant (RTE) T cells by flow cytometry, quantifying the number and type of T cells in the blood, and measuring the immune response to subcomponent vaccines with no potential for infection. In general, live virus vaccines can be administered when children have more than or equal to 400 CD4 T cells/μL and more than or equal to 200 CD8 T cells/μL of blood, predominance of naïve CD4 T cells, and protective IgG antibodies to tetanus after the third dose of the vaccine, which reflects T-cell–dependent specific antibody production. Administration of the first Rotavirus vaccine dose (RV1 or RV5) is recommended at age 2 months using all criteria outlined above with the exception for tetanus-specific IgG, which needs to be present prior to administration of the first doses of the MMR and VZV vaccines.

Nonlive vaccines are usually safe to administer in patients with immunodeficiency but may not be of benefit in patients with impaired antibody production exceptions include for the annual Influenza vaccine and SARS-CoV2-mRNA vaccine, human papilloma virus (HPV) vaccine and recombinant shingles vaccine due to the expected cellular immune response. Live and nonlive vaccines are usually also not recommended for patients on IgG replacement therapy who receive specific IgG antibodies for protection from a healthy plasma donor pool. Children with complement deficiencies and increased risk of infections with encapsulated bacteria as the result of anatomic or functional asplenia should be vaccinated early against infection with *Neisseria meningitidis* ACWY strains, starting at age 2 months, and will require additional vaccinations against Streptococcus pneumoniae if their initial vaccine series did not include the pneumococcal conjugate vaccine (PCV) 20. Following CDC guidelines for at-risk children age 2 years and older who have not yet received the 23-valent Streptococcus pneumoniae polysaccharide vaccine (PPSV23), PCV20 may be administered as early as 8 weeks after the last PCV vaccine (not PCV20) to complete their vaccination series. Alternatively, a dose of PPSV23 can be administered. Each initial vaccination with PPSV23 needs be followed by a second dose of PPSV23 or PCV20 at least 5 years later. Table 33–5 lists additional vaccines used in asplenic patients.

Table 33–4. Live vaccines that are contraindicated in most patients with a primary immunodeficiency.

- Rotavirus vaccine (oral)
- Measles, mumps, rubella (MMR combined vaccine)
- Varicella vaccine
- Intranasal influenza vaccine (FluMist®)
- Yellow fever vaccine
- Smallpox vaccine
- Adenovirus vaccine used by the military
- Live varicella zoster vaccine (VZV, Zostavax®) – no longer available in the US
- Oral polio vaccine – no longer available in the US
- Oral typhoid vaccine (Ty21a)
- Bacillus Calmette-Guerin (BCG) vaccine

Table 33–5. Vaccinations against encapsulated bacteria.

1. **Against *Streptococcus pneumoniae***
   - Primary pneumococcal conjugate vaccine (PCV) series with PCV15 or PCV20 according to childhood vaccination schedule
   - 23-valent pneumococcal polysaccharide vaccine (PPSV23) at age ≥ 2 y or PCV20 ≥ 8 weeks after primary PCV series with no PCV20
   - PPSV23 booster dose or PCV20 ≥ 5 y after the first dose of PPSV23
2. **Against *Haemophilus influenzae B (Hib)*:**
   - Primary HIB series and recommended boosters as per childhood vaccination schedule
3. **Against *meningococcal disease*:**
   - Primary series with MenACWY-CRM (Menveo®) starting at age 2 mo with initial booster 3 y after primary series, additional boosters every 5 y.
   - Age ≥ 10 years: Primary series of MenB-4C (Bexsero®) or MenB-FHbp (Trumenba®) vaccine.
   - Of note, while not Food and Drug Administration (FDA) approved for this age in the United States, Bexsero® is part of the infant immunization schedule in Great Britain (1st dose at age 2 mo and 2nd dose at age 4 mo). Dependent on exposure risk, early administration of Bexsero® may be considered.

Mustillo PJ et al: Clinical practice guidelines for the immunological management of chromosome 22q11.2 deletion syndrome and other defects in thymic development. J Clin Immunol 2023 Feb;43(2):247–270. doi: 10.1007/s10875-022-01418-y. Epub 2023 Jan 17 [PMID: 36648576].

Puck JM: Newborn screening for severe combined immunodeficiency and T-cell lymphopenia. Immunol Rev 2019 Jan;287(1):241–252. doi: 10.1111/imr.12729 [PMID: 30565242].

Sobh A, Bonilla FA: Vaccination in primary immunodeficiency disorders. J Allergy Clin Immunol Pract 2016 Nov–Dec;4(6):1066–1075. doi: 10.1016/j.jaip.2016.09.012 [PMID: 27836056].

Squire JD, Sher M: Asplenia and hyposplenism: an underrecognized immune deficiency. Immunol Allergy Clin North Am 2020 Aug;40(3):471–483. doi: 10.1016/j.iac.2020.03.006 [PMID: 32654693].

SEVERE COMBINED IMMUNODEFICIENCY DISEASES

ESSENTIALS OF DIAGNOSIS & TYPICAL FEATURES

- ► Onset in first year of life.
- ► Recurrent infections caused by bacteria, viruses, fungi, and opportunistic pathogens.
- ► Chronic diarrhea and failure to thrive.
- ► Absent lymphoid tissue.

► General Considerations

Severe combined immunodeficiency disease (SCID) is a group of rare immunologic disorders with the defining characteristic of severe deficiency of T-cell function and/or number. Due to the centrality of T cells in the immune system, the severity of T-cell deficit results in widespread immunologic dysfunction and broad susceptibility to infection. Left untreated, SCID uniformly results in death before the first year of life. The treatment approach varies depending on the underlying molecular defect, but for most patients with SCID, the optimal treatment is hematopoietic stem cell transplantation (HSCT). Transplant outcomes are favorable if performed within the first 3 months of life or if performed prior to the onset of SCID-associated chronic infections. Newborn screening of dried blood spots for evidence of T-cell deficiency occurs universally in the United States by quantifying T-cell receptor rearrangement excision circles (TRECs) that occur during normal T-cell development. Absent or reduced TRECs identify patients with SCID soon after birth. Suspected SCID is a medical emergency, and both the necessary steps to confirm the diagnosis and initiate treatment must be performed rapidly.

► Clinical Findings

A. Symptoms and Signs

SCID frequently presents with opportunistic, unusual, and persistent infection. Common organisms include but are not limited to *Pneumocystis jirovecii*, candidiasis, and cytomegalovirus. In the absence of an identified microorganism, SCID may present with any combination of the following: failure to thrive, chronic diarrhea, or unexplained chronic respiratory illness. Physical examination is notable for a lack of lymphoid tissue, including tonsils and lymph nodes. A chest radiograph usually demonstrates an absent thymic shadow.

B. Laboratory Findings

The characteristic feature of SCID is the deficiency in production of T cells by the host. Adequate production of T cells can be verified by quantifying TRECs in blood or by measuring the expression of CD31 on peripheral blood T cells. The presence of normal numbers of lymphocytes in a CBC or even normal numbers of CD3 T cells does not rule out SCID because of the possibility of either maternally derived T-cell populations or abnormally expanded endogenous T-cell populations with severely limited diversity. Associated laboratory findings can include decreases in numbers of NK cells and B cells, poor lymphocyte proliferative response to mitogens, and low immunoglobulin levels. Genetic testing should be pursued to confirm the diagnosis; although, treatment should not be delayed while awaiting results of genetic testing. Known genetic etiologies of SCID are listed in Table 33–6.

► Differential Diagnosis

The differential diagnosis of SCID must be carefully considered as misdiagnosis could potentially result in unwarranted HSCT. Infants born at a gestational age (GA) of less than 33 weeks and/or a birth weight of less than 800 g may present with an abnormal newborn screen for SCID related to transient T-cell lymphopenia, which usually normalizes when GA plus chronological age approaches full term. Disorders that result in either the abnormal loss or the compartmentalization of lymphatic fluid such as chylothorax, lymphangiectasia, gastroschisis, and omphalocele can result in the apparent absence of endogenously generated T cells even though they are being normally produced. HIV disease can result in severe deficiency of CD4 T cells and the same infections seen in SCID.

► Treatment

A variety of therapies are used in the treatment of SCID. These therapies include HSCT, gene therapy, thymus transplant, and enzyme replacement. Choice of therapy depends on the specific genetic defect, age at diagnosis, access to a suitable HSCT donor, and comorbidities. To optimize the

Table 33–6. Severe combined immunodeficiency classification.

	Genes Containing Defects	Likely Etiology	Characteristic Features
Defective T-cell development			
• Defective IL7R signaling	IL2RG, IL7RA, JAK3	IL-7 signaling is essential for T-cell development.	• IL2RG- and JAK3-deficiency have associated absence of NK cells and functional B-cell deficiency.
• Defective T-cell receptor (TCR) signaling	ZAP70, PTPRC, CD3D, CD3G, CD3E	TCR signaling is essential for T-cell development.	• ZAP70 has apparent deficiency of only CD8 T cells but CD4 T cells are also nonfunctional. • B cells are not affected.
• RAG-recombination defect	RAG1, RAG2	Functional TCR is not formed.	• Both B and T cells are deficient. NK cells are unaffected.
• NHEJ-recombination defect	LIG4, NHEJ1, DCLRE1C, PRKDC	Functional TCR is not formed.	• Both B and T cells are deficient. NK cells are unaffected. • Body wide sensitivity to radiation toxicity • Can be associated with microcephaly and other syndromic features
• Absent thymus function	22q11 deletion, CHARGE syndrome, FOXN1	Thymus is essential for T-cell development.	• B cell counts generally are not affected. • FOXN1 deficiency is associated with nail dysplasia.
Impaired T-cell survival			
• Impaired purine salvage	ADA, PNP	Toxic metabolites	• Varying degrees of B cell, T cell, and NK cell deficiency
• Dyskeratosis congenita (Hoyeraal-Hreidarsson syndrome)	DKC1, ACD (TPP1), TINF2, TERT, RTEL1	Telomere maintenance is severely defective.	• Associated intrauterine growth retardation (IUGR) and cerebellar hypoplasia
• Reticular dysgenesis	AK2	Possible cellular energy imbalance	• Associated with agranulocytosis and deficiency of all lymphocytes, but normal erythrocyte and platelet formation
• One-carbon pathway	TCN2, MTHFD1	Unclear	• Associated neurodegenerative defect • Megaloblastic anemia • Patients improve with adequate supplementation
• Ribosomal defect	RMRP	Unclear	• Associated with short-limb dwarfism
Impaired T-cell function			
• Ca²⁺-signaling defect	STIM1, ORAI1	Impaired T-cell activation, proliferation, and metabolism.	• Immunodeficiency, muscular hypotonia and anhydrotic ectodermal dysplasia, autoimmunity, and lymphoproliferative disease.

outcome of any chosen definitive therapy, concerted effort must be made to prevent clinical deterioration in the waiting period. Antimicrobial prophylaxis should be initiated with the aim of preventing pulmonary infection with *Pneumocystis*, as well as other fungal pathogens. Antiviral prophylaxis can be considered as well. Replacement immunoglobulin therapy should be initiated. Patients with suspected SCID should only be transfused with CMV-negative, irradiated blood products, and they should not receive any live vaccines. If the patient has received BCG vaccination, specific therapy should be considered. Isolation precautions should be initiated. Until more is known about CMV-transmission in CMV-positive mothers, breast-feeding should be discouraged. Additional precautions can be tailored based on the individual risk factor of the patient.

Currier R, Puck JM: SCID newborn screening: what we've learned. J Allergy Clin Immunol 2021 Feb;147(2):417–426. doi: 10.1016/j.jaci.2020.10.020 [PMID: 33551023].

SCID CLASSIFICATION

▶ Defective T-Cell Development

T cells develop in a multiple-stage process fostered by supporting cells and directive cytokines. Problems with the production or sensing of these developmental signals can result in a severe deficit of T-cell number.

Deficiency in the formation of a functionally rearranged T-cell receptor (TCR) or DNA repair mechanisms results in the absence of T cells, the latter also being associated with radiation sensitivity. Primary absence of the thymus prevents the development of mature T cells in severe presentations of 22q11 deletion syndrome, CHARGE syndrome, and deficiency of *FOXN1*.

▶ Impaired T-Cell Survival

Impaired T-cell survival is seen in deficiency of both adenosine deaminase (ADA) and purine nucleoside phosphorylase (PNP), as well as reticular dysgenesis and dyskeratosis congenita. ADA and PNP are components of purine salvage in lymphocytes, and loss of these enzymes results in buildup of toxic purine by-products. Dyskeratosis congenita results from abnormal telomere maintenance and results in survival defects in hematologic cells. Reticular dysgenesis is possibly the most severe form of combined immunodeficiency as a result of increased apoptosis of myeloid and lymphoid precursors. It is associated with sensorineural deafness. Defects in the one-carbon pathway can also result in severe deficiency of hematopoietic cells.

▶ Impaired T-Cell Function

Few syndromes have been identified where T cells mature normally despite a residual impairment in TCR signaling that results in susceptibility to infections typically seen in T-cell deficiency syndromes. In *STIM1* and *ORAI1* deficiency, defective mobilization of store-operated calcium channels results in inadequate activation of peripheral T cells despite normal numbers. In MHC class II deficiency, normal T cells are unable to respond to antigen because it is not presented by antigen presenting cells.

Omenn Syndrome

Omenn syndrome is a presentation of SCID caused by residual autoreactive T cells in the absence of T-cell immune competence. The syndrome can include severe rash, failure to thrive, splenomegaly, diarrhea, eosinophilia, and elevated IgE in association with typical infections seen in conventional SCID. T-cell numbers are elevated, but detailed phenotyping reveals most T cells to have a memory phenotype (CD45RO-positive). Omenn syndrome has been tied to mutations in genes known to cause conventional SCID, arising in part due to mutation-specific factors and partly due to the individual

susceptibility of the patient. A similar clinical presentation occurs in SCID patients who have engrafted maternal T cells.

ANTIBODY DEFICIENCY SYNDROMES

ESSENTIALS OF DIAGNOSIS & TYPICAL FEATURES

- ▶ Recurrent bacterial infections, typically due to encapsulated pyogenic bacteria.
- ▶ Low immunoglobulin levels.
- ▶ Inability to make specific antibodies to vaccine antigens or infections.

▶ General Considerations

Defective antibody-based immunity can be in-born or acquired from infection or medication. This chapter focuses on in-born errors in antibody production, as acquired forms generally fit the same classification scheme. Primarily antibody deficiencies (PAD) can be divided into (1) defects of B-cell development, (2) defects in Ig class switching, and (3) functional B-cell deficiency. Table 33–7 outlines primary antibody deficiency syndromes, laboratory findings, and genetic inheritance in these disorders.

▶ Clinical Findings

A. Symptoms and Signs

The range of infectious and inflammatory manifestations of PADs depends on the underlying defect, some of which are fairly limited to B-cell function/development and others which impair other immune cells, as well. As a result, some PADs can involve infections mainly attributable to non-B-cell defects; however, all PADs share a susceptibility to encapsulated bacterial infection as a result of defective antibody-based immunity. Pulmonary infection can be severe and chronic, resulting in bronchiectasis or other permanent lung damage. Severe pulmonary infections are generally preceded by chronic, recurrent middle ear and sinus infections. Additional infections can include bacteremia, bacterial meningitis, skin infection, and joint infection.

B. Laboratory Findings

The workup for PAD follows the classification scheme outlined in Table 33–7. Flow cytometry enumeration of B cells and B-cell subsets in peripheral blood reveals defects in B-cell development. Measurement of serum immunoglobulin levels reveals significant abnormalities in the production of one or multiple immunoglobulin isotypes as may be seen in class switching defects or CVID. Measurement of specific

Table 33–7. Antibody deficiency disorders.

	Genes Containing Defects	Likely Etiology	Characteristic Features
Defects in B-cell development			
• **Defect in developmental signal**	TCF3, IKZF1, LRRC8A	Commitment to B-cell lineage affected	• Peripheral B cells < 2% of lymphocyte count
• **Defect in pre–B-cell receptor (BCR)**	IGHM, IGLL1, CD79A, CD79B,	B-cell development requires functional pre-BCR.	• Peripheral B cells < 2% of lymphocyte count
• **Defect in pre-BCR downstream signaling**	BLNK, BTK	Pre-BCR signaling inadequate to support further development	• Peripheral B cells < 2% of lymphocyte count
• **Other**	CARD11	Unclear	• Variable developmental bottlenecks • Regulatory T-cell numbers reduced
Class-switching defects			
• **Defect in CD40L-CD40 interaction**	CD40L, CD40	CD40L signal initiates class switching	• Typically high IgM levels • No germinal centers • Susceptible to some typical T-cell deficiency-associated infections such as Pneumocystis jirovecii and cryptosporidial infection • Associated with biliary malignancy possibly from chronic infection
• **Defect in genomic rearrangement**	AICDA, UNG, INO80	Rearrangement of the IgH constant region is defective	• Normal B-cell numbers • Associated with significant autoimmunity • Large germinal center reactions because proliferative signaling remains intact
• **Varied**	IKBKG, IKBA	Unclear	• Usually associated with predominant T-cell abnormalities
Functional antibody deficiency			
• **Common variable immunodeficiency (CVID)**	Unknown	Heterogeneous	• Normal or low IgM, low IgG, low IgA, poor specific antibody production
• **Monogenetic syndromes previously characterized as CVID**	ICOS, CD19, TNFRSF13B, TNFRSF13C, CD20, CD81, CD225, NFKB1, NFKB2, IRF2BP2, MOGS, IKZF1	Impaired signaling through B-cell coreceptors	• Normal or low IgM, low IgG, low IgA, poor specific antibody production
• **Combined immunodeficiency syndromes**	CD21, CD27, PIK3R1, PIK3CD, LRBA	Impaired signaling through molecules present in B and T cells	• Normal or low IgM, low IgG, low IgA, poor specific antibody production • T-cell dysfunction
Selective immunoglobulin deficiencies			
• **IgG subclass deficiency**	IGHG1, IGHG2, IGHG3, IGHG4	Defects of isotype differentiation	• Decrease in one or more IgG isotypes
• **IgA deficiency**	IGAD1	Defect in IgA production	• Decrease or absent IgA
• **Specific antibody deficiency**	Unknown	Unclear	• Deficient antibody response to polysaccharide antigens

antibody production in response to vaccination reveals specific antibody deficiency, usually when applied to the unconjugated polysaccharide *S pneumoniae* vaccine. Finally, measurement of serum IgG subclass levels detects subclass deficiency. The role of genetic testing, in part, depends on the pattern of clinical and standard laboratory findings. When performed, genetic panel testing, exome, or even genome testing can help reveal the diagnosis.

▶ Differential Diagnosis

The differential diagnosis of antibody deficiency includes secondary causes of a decreased amount of immunoglobulin in the peripheral blood. Several medications are known to specifically decrease immunoglobulin levels in the blood. For some of these medications, the mechanism is idiosyncratic. For others, low immunoglobulin levels result from inhibition of normal B-cell development processes, such as in chronic prednisone use, or they result from direct effects on the B-cell compartment, such as with rituximab therapy. Additional secondary causes of low immunoglobulin include protein-losing states, malnutrition, and autoimmune conditions.

▶ Treatment

The primary intervention for preventing antibody-deficiency-associated infection is replacing deficient IgG, either by IV infusion or subcutaneously. There are no formulations of isolated IgM or IgA used in clinical practice. Some treatment centers advocate the use of prophylactic antibiotic therapy. In combined immunodeficiency or antibody deficiency syndromes with associated autoimmunity, immunosuppressive therapy or even HSCT may be required.

Antibody Deficiency Classification

▶ Defective B-Cell Development

B cells develop from precursors in the bone marrow in a process that is dependent on the generation of a functioning rearranged B-cell receptor (Figure 33–4). In the absence of the ability to transmit signals through a B-cell receptor, B cells do not continue development. Consistent with this model of B-cell development, congenital defects in several of the proteins essential for the formation and signaling of the B-cell receptor have been identified as causes of severe B-cell deficiency. Additional blocks in B-cell development have been identified prior to the expression of the B-cell receptor and later in development as cells approach the naïve B-cell stage.

Patients with defects in B-cell development are generally immunologically normal apart from a severe reduction of B cells in the blood and infections that result from their absence. Patients with early defects have little detectable lymphoid tissue, and upon physical examination, one may find an absence of tonsils or palpable lymph nodes. Patients with later defects may have palpable lymphoid tissue. In both groups, the spleen is generally normal in size.

▶ Class Switching Defects

Normal immunoglobulin isotype class switching occurs in germinal centers in response to antigenic and T-cell costimulatory signals, and the class switching defects involve severe dysfunction of this process. Defects in either T-cell surface CD40L or B-cell surface CD40 impair the initial step in the class-switching cascade, and as a result, no class switching occurs. Further downstream, defects in either AICDA or UNG impair class switching by preventing the formation of double-stranded breaks that are essential for the genomic rearrangement required to switch isotypes. Additional defects in class switching can be seen with genetic abnormalities in NF-κB and phosphatidylinositol 3-kinase (PI3K), but in either case, the class switching phenotype can be variable. Consultation of an immunologist will help determine where the class switching defect is located and direct clinical care.

Class switching presents with various associated features depending on the genetic cause. Defects in CD40L and CD40 can have risk of associated opportunistic infection with

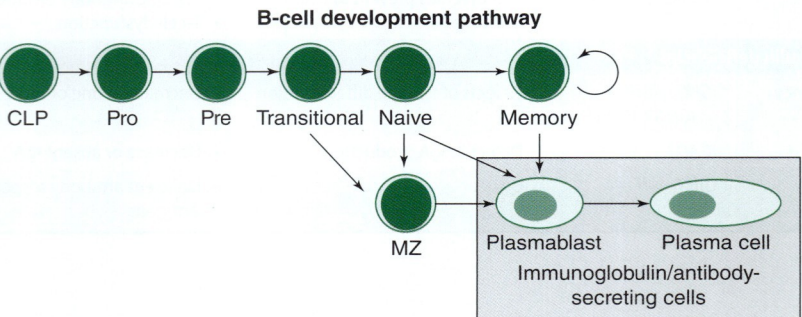

B-cell development pathway

CLP → Pro → Pre → Transitional → Naive → Memory

MZ

Plasmablast → Plasma cell

Immunoglobulin/antibody-secreting cells

▲ **Figure 33–4.** B-cell development. CLP, common lymphoid progenitor; MZ, marginal zone

Pneumocystis and *Cryptosporidium*, the latter increasing the risk for sclerosing cholangitis. Patients with defective AICDA can have associated autoimmunity, including immune thrombocytopenia (ITP), hemolytic anemia, autoimmune hepatitis, inflammatory bowel disease, arthritis, and interstitial lung disease. Both AICDA- and UNG-deficient patients suffer from lymphoid hyperplasia.

Functional Antibody Deficiency

CVID

CVID is defined by the combination of poor vaccine response and a decrease in blood levels of IgG in conjunction with a severe decrease in levels of either IgM or IgA, or a decrease of both (see Table 33–7). Associated cellular abnormalities can include reduced numbers of memory B-cell subsets in the blood, as well as mild T-cell lymphopenia. Patients have recurrent infections, most often of the sinus and pulmonary tract, but chronic gastrointestinal infections may manifest with recurrent diarrhea. Patients with CVID are at risk for developing bronchiectasis, autoimmune diseases (ITP, autoimmune hemolytic anemia, rheumatoid arthritis, and inflammatory bowel disease), and malignancies (especially gastric carcinoma and lymphoma).

Transient Hypogammaglobulinemia

Transient hypogammaglobulinemia represents a delay in the normal infant onset of immunoglobulin synthesis. The diagnosis is suspected in infants and young children with low levels of IgG and IgA (usually two standard deviations below normal for age), but normal levels of IgM and normal numbers of circulating B lymphocytes. Most affected children have normal specific antibody responses and T-lymphocyte function. Recovery occurs between 18 and 30 months of age, and the prognosis for affected children is excellent provided infections are treated promptly and appropriately. Affected infants typically do not suffer severe infections, and Ig replacement is rarely used; however, referral to a clinical immunologist is essential as in-born PADs can present in a similar fashion and require more aggressive management.

Monogenetic Causes of Functional Antibody Deficiency

Several monogenetic causes of functional antibody deficiency have been identified in scattered individuals that had previously been diagnosed with CVID. These syndromes encompass the range of phenotypes conventionally included in the broad category of CVID. Severe defects in the classic B-cell coreceptor complex, including CD19, CD21, CD81, and CD225, have been identified in individuals mainly with poor antibody response and infections that would be expected to follow. These defects presumably arise from an impaired germinal center reaction to foreign antigens in lymph nodes. Similar phenotypes were shown to result both with defects in other B-cell coreceptors such as BAFFR or TACI and with defects in molecules that signal through these receptors such as ICOS. Additional syndromes that include involvement of T-cell dysfunction as well as functional antibody deficiency have been identified in molecules that function in both cell types. These syndromes include, but are not limited to, CD27 deficiency, activated PI3K delta syndrome, and IL-21 deficiency. Additional combined immunodeficiency syndromes with both antibody deficiency and predominant features outside of antibody deficiency are discussed earlier in the chapter.

Selective Immunoglobulin Deficiencies

IgA or IgG subclass deficiency can be associated with both recurrent infections and other immune abnormalities; however, these deficiencies are often seen in the absence of any other identifiable immune abnormality. With an incidence of 1:700, isolated IgA deficiency is a common laboratory finding. Most patients with isolated IgA deficiency are asymptomatic, but associations also exist with inflammatory bowel disease, allergic disease, asthma, and autoimmune disorders (thyroiditis, arthritis, vitiligo, thrombocytopenia, and diabetes). Deficiency of IgG subclasses 2–4 can be identified in the absence of other laboratory immune abnormalities, whereas severe deficiency of IgG1 universally presents with an overall decrease in total IgG levels because it makes up the majority of IgG detectable in the blood. Deficiency of IgG2 can be seen in association with decreased IgA, and in that context, it is suggestive of an underlying functional antibody deficiency with a possibly identifiable genetic cause. IgG3 and IgG4 make up the smallest fraction of the total IgG pool, and in the absence of any other immune abnormality, deficiency of either of these IgG subclasses is generally not considered to cause increased susceptibility to infection. IgG replacement is not indicated in either IgA deficiency or IgG subclass deficiency when no other quantitative or functional immune abnormality has been identified. When other immune abnormalities are seen, antibody deficiency syndromes listed elsewhere in this chapter should be considered.

Smith T, Cunningham-Rundles C: Primary B-cell immunodeficiencies. Hum Immunol 2019 Jun;80(6):351–362. doi: 10.1016/j.humimm.2018.10.015. Epub 2018 Oct 22 [PMID: 30359632].

PHAGOCYTE DISORDERS

Phagocyte defects include abnormalities of both numbers (neutropenia) and function of polymorphonuclear neutrophils. Functional defects consist of impairments in adhesion, chemotaxis, bacterial killing, or, less often, of combinations of these.

1. Neutropenia

The presence of neutropenia should be considered when evaluating recurrent infections. The diagnosis and treatment of neutropenia is discussed in Chapter 30. Additionally, some PID syndromes are associated with neutropenia (eg, XLA).

2. Chronic Granulomatous Disease

ESSENTIALS OF DIAGNOSIS & TYPICAL FEATURES

▶ Recurrent infections with catalase-positive bacteria and fungi.

▶ XL and AR forms.

▶ Caused by abnormal phagocytosis-associated generation of microbicidal oxygen metabolites (respiratory burst) by neutrophils, monocytes, and macrophages.

▶ General Considerations

Chronic granulomatous disease (CGD) is caused by a defect in any of several genes encoding proteins in the enzyme complex nicotinamide adenine dinucleotide phosphate (NADPH) oxidase, which results in defective superoxide and hydrogen peroxide generation during ingestion of microbes. Most cases in the United States and Europe (probably 75%) are inherited as an XL recessive trait; however, in regions with widespread consanguineous mating, AR inheritance is seen with equal frequency.

▶ Clinical Findings

A. Symptoms and Signs

The typical clinical presentation is characterized by recurrent abscess formation in subcutaneous tissue, lymph nodes, lungs, and liver, and by pneumonia and eczematous and purulent skin rashes. Infecting organisms are typically catalase-positive bacteria, which can break down their own hydrogen peroxide and thus avoid death when captured in a CGD phagocytic vacuole. Aspergillosis is also common and a frequent cause of death. Granulomatous inflammation can narrow the outlet of the stomach or bladder in these patients, leading to vomiting or urinary obstruction.

B. Laboratory Findings

Patients typically present with serious infection, positive microbial cultures, and neutrophilia. The most common infecting organisms are *S aureus*, *Aspergillus* species, *Burkholderia cepacia*, and *Serratia marcescens*. (Culture of either of the last two should suggest this diagnosis.) Patients also present with granulomas of lymph nodes, skin, liver, and genitourinary tract. The diagnosis is confirmed by demonstrating lack of hydrogen peroxide production using the DHR flow cytometry assay or lack of superoxide production using the NBT test. Both tests can demonstrate carrier status of an XL mutation.

▶ Differential Diagnosis

The differential diagnosis includes other phagocyte abnormalities or deficiencies described in this section, as well as the rare neutrophil granule deficiency. Other immunodeficient states leading to severe bacterial or fungal infections should be considered.

▶ Treatment

Daily intake of an antimicrobial agent such as trimethoprim-sulfamethoxazole is indicated in all patients; an oral antifungal agent like itraconazole and regular subcutaneous injections of interferon-γ (IFN-γ) can greatly reduce the risk of severe infections. HSCT is the only curative option. Gastric or GU obstruction can be relieved by short-term steroid therapy.

3. Leukocyte Adhesion Defects Types I & II

ESSENTIALS OF DIAGNOSIS & TYPICAL FEATURES

▶ Recurrent serious infections.

▶ "Cold" abscesses (those without pus formation).

▶ Poor wound healing.

▶ Gingival or periodontal disease (or both).

▶ General Considerations

The ability of phagocytic cells to enter peripheral sites of infection is critical for effective host defense. In leukocyte adhesion deficiency (LAD), defects in proteins required for leukocyte adherence to and migration through blood vessel walls prevent these cells from arriving at the sites of infection. LAD I is an AR disease caused by mutations in the common chain of the β_2 integrin family (CD18) located on chromosome 21q22.3. These mutations result in impaired neutrophil migration, adherence, and antibody-dependent phagocytosis. LAD II is a rare AR disease caused by an inborn error in fucose metabolism that results in abnormal expression of leukocyte Sialyl-Lewis X (CD15s), which binds to selectins on the vessel endothelium. The resulting phenotype is similar to LAD I, with recurrent infections, lack of pus formation, poor wound healing, and periodontal disease. LAD II patients also have developmental delays, short stature, dysmorphic facies, and the Bombay (hh) blood group.

► Clinical Findings

A. Symptoms and Signs

Patients present with variably severe phenotypes, including recurrent serious infections, lack of pus formation, poor wound healing, and gingival and periodontal disease. The hallmark is little inflammation and absent neutrophils on histopathologic evaluation of infected sites (ie, "cold" abscesses), especially when concurrent with neutrophilia, and expression of poor adherence to vessel walls. The most severe phenotype manifests with infections in the neonatal period, including delayed separation of the umbilical cord with associated omphalitis.

B. Laboratory Findings

Laboratory evaluation often demonstrates a striking neutrophilia. Diagnosis of suspected cases is confirmed by flow cytometry analysis for CD18 (LAD I) or CD15s (LAD II).

► Treatment

Treatment includes aggressive antibiotic therapy. Fucose supplementation in LAD II has been reported with some success.

Marciano BE et al: Common severe infections in chronic granulomatous disease. Clin Infect Dis 2015;60:1176–1183 [PMID: 25537876].

DEFICIENCIES OF THE INNATE IMMUNE SYSTEM

► General Considerations

Deficiencies in the innate immune response comprise defects that are not the result of an impaired adaptive T- and B-cell response. Besides impaired neutrophil function, which is reviewed elsewhere in the book, they include deficiencies in complement function, defective recognition, and response to recognition of microbial molecular patterns, functional monocyte/macrophage deficiency, and innate cell deficiency including NK cell deficiency.

1. Complement Deficiencies

The complement system includes three interactive pathways of enzymatic reactions: classical, alternative, and lectin (see Figure 33–3). The pathways differ in how they are activated, but all three pathways converge by cleaving large amounts of C3 and proceeding down the common terminal pathway that ends in the formation of the MAC. The MAC punctures holes in microbial cell walls and cleaved C3 coats targeted microbes facilitating their removal and enhancing their immunogenicity.

► Complement Component Deficiencies

Deficiencies of individual complement components (C1–C9) can be grouped according to the pathway rendered inactive. Deficiencies of classic pathway proteins (C1, C2, or C4)

predispose to increased infections but are particularly associated with autoimmune disorders such as systemic lupus erythematosus. Deficiency of alternative pathway components (Factor D, Factor B, or Properdin) increase susceptibility to bacterial infection but do not predispose to autoimmunity. Lectin pathway deficiency results in pulmonary infections. Primary C3 deficiency presents with severe pyogenic infections and autoimmunity, since C3 is critical for opsonization in both the classic and alternative pathways. Deficiency of a terminal complement component in the MAC (C5, C6, C7, C8, and C9) or of properdin (an XL alternative pathway control protein) results in recurrent *N meningitidis* or disseminated gonococcal infection but no autoimmunity. Patients suspected of having a complement deficiency should be tested for function of the classical pathway (CH50), alternative pathway (AH50), and if possible, the lectin pathway. The combination of these results assists in locating the defect if one is present.

2. Pattern-Recognition Receptor Defects

Pattern-recognition receptor (PRR) defects include deficient toll-like receptor (TLR) signaling, defective intracellular signaling of viral nucleic acids, and defects of other receptors. TLRs and members of the interleukin-1 receptor (IL-1R) family signal through IL-1R–associated kinases (IRAK) 1 and 4 while using the adaptor molecule MyD88, leading to activation of NF-κB and inflammatory cytokine production. Patients with AR deficiencies in MyD88 and IRAK-4 are predisposed to severe bacterial infections that are not associated with a high fever or significant increase in C-reactive protein at the beginning of infection. Defects in intracellular virus sensing have been attributed to defects in TLR3, MDA5, DBR1, POLR3A, POLR3C, SAMD9, and SAMD9L. They result in variable susceptibility to viruses including HSV-1, rhinovirus, influenza, and varicella. Resulting infections are often limited only to the central nervous system, where there is no redundant defense against these viruses. Susceptibility to viral infection has resulted from impaired type I interferon (IFN) production and signaling after viral recognition by PRRs involving key players in this pathway (IRF7, IFNAR1, IFNAR1, STAT2, and IRF9). IFNAR2 and STAT2 deficiency have been associated with disseminated measles infection following live-virus vaccination, whereas the others were associated with varied viral infections.

3. Functional Monocyte/Macrophage Deficiency (Mendelian Susceptibility to Mycobacterial Disease)

IFN-γ is critical for macrophage activation and resistance to mycobacterial infections. Mutations that cause deficiency or reduced function of proteins that participate in IFN-γ signaling result in Mendelian susceptibility to mycobacterial disease (MSMD). To date, at least 14 genes are known to harbor such mutations in affected individuals: *JAK1, IL12B, IL12RB1, IL12RB2, IL23R, ISG15, TYK2, IRF8, SPPL2A,*

CYBB, IFNGR1, IFNGR2, STAT1, and *NEMO.* The infection susceptibility seen in patients with these mutations includes infection with typically nonpathogenic mycobacteria such as *Mycobacterium avium* complex or BCG, with some also demonstrating susceptibility to salmonellosis and candida infection. Treatment with supplemental IFN-γ is effective unless the IFN-γ receptor is not functional. Long-term mycobacterial prophylaxis should be considered in these individuals.

4. Innate-Cell Deficiency

Disseminated infection by nontuberculous mycobacteria, viruses (ie, HPV), and fungi were described in association with *GATA2* mutations or MonoMAC (sporadic monocytopenia and mycobacterial infection) syndrome. Patients usually become symptomatic during adulthood, but younger patients may also be affected. Patients typically present with low numbers and dysfunction of B lymphocytes and NK cells, monocytes, and dendritic cells. This is an autosomal-dominant inherited disease with an increased risk for malignancies, especially myelodysplasia and leukemia. Additional syndromes with predominant

NK-cell deficiency have been identified in patients with *MCM4* and *GINS1* deficiency.

Bucciol G et al: Lessons learned from the study of human inborn errors of innate immunity. J Allergy Clin Immun 2019;143:507–527 [PMID: 30075154].

Romano R, Giardino G, Cirillo E, Prencipe R, Pignata C: Complement system network in cell physiology and in human diseases. Int Rev Immunol 2020;1–12 [PMID: 33063546].

IMMUNE DYSREGULATION AND ADDITIONAL COMBINED IMMUNODEFICIENCY

Over the past two decades, PID has proven an insufficient term to describe the variability in immune dysregulation inborn errors of immunity can present with. Beyond infection susceptibility, the field of clinical immunology also encompasses diseases with profound propensity for auto-immunity/inflammation. Inborn errors of immunity (IEI) are now the accepted and widely used terminology to describe what was previously confined to PID. Diseases with unique infection susceptibility, immune dysregulation, or atopic patterns not otherwise described are outlined in Tables 33–8 to 33–10.

Table 33–8. Examples of immune dysregulation disorders.

	Genes Containing Defects	Characteristic Features
Regulatory T-cell defects	*FOXP3, IL2RA, IL2RB, CTLA4, LRBA, DEF6, STAT3, BACH2, FERMT1, IKZF1*	• Low and/or dysfunctional regulatory T cells • Immune dysregulation, polyendocrinopathy, enteropathy, X-linked (IPEX; *FOXP3*): multiorgan/system autoimmunity, eczema, lymphoproliferation • IPEX-like (*IL2RA, IL2RB, CTLA4, LRBA, DEF6, STAT3, BACH2, FERMT1, IKZF1*): similar to IPEX with varying degrees of hypogammaglobulinemia and infection susceptibility
Familial hemophagocytic lymphohistiocytosis (FHL)	*PRF1, UNC13D, STX11, STXBP2, FAAP24, SLC7A7, RHOG, LYST, RAB27, AP3B1, AP3D1, CEBPE*	• Decreased NK and CD8+ T-cell activities • Fever, hepatosplenomegaly, cytopenias, hemophagocytic lymphohistiocytosis (HLH) on bone marrow examination • HLH without albinism (*PRF1, UNC13D, STX11, STXBP2, FAAP24, SLC7A7, RHOG*) • HLH with partial albinism (*LYST, RAB27, AP3B1, AP3D1, CEBPE*) • Chediak-Higashi syndrome (*LYST*): giant lysosomes, neutropenia, bleeding tendency, neurological dysfunction
Autoimmune polyendocrinopathy with candidiasis and ectodermal dystrophy (APECED)	*AIRE*	• Autoimmunity, hypoparathyroidism, hypothyroidism, adrenal insufficiency, diabetes, gonadal dysfunction, dental enamel hypoplasia, alopecia, enteropathy, pernicious anemia, chronic mucocutaneous, candidiasis • Also called autoimmune polyglandular syndrome, type 1 (APS-1)
Autoimmune lymphoproliferative syndrome (ALPS)	*TNFRSF6 (FAS), TNFSF6 (FASL), CASP10, CASP8, FADD*	• Defective lymphocyte apoptosis, increased double-negative (CD4-CD8-) T cells • Lymphadenopathy, splenomegaly, autoimmune cytopenias, increased risk for lymphoma
X-linked lymphoproliferative disease (XLP)	*SH2D1A, XIAP*	• EBV susceptibility, splenomegaly, lymphadenopathy, HLH • SAP deficiency (XLP1; *SH2D1A*): hypogammaglobulinemia, aplastic anemia, risk for lymphoma • XIAP deficiency (XLP2; *XIAP*): colitis, hepatitis

Table 33–9. Examples of disorders with atopy/urticaria.

	Genes Containing Defects	Characteristic Features
Hyper IgE syndromes (HIES)	STAT3, IL6R, IL6ST, ZNF341, ERBB2IP, TGFBR1, TGFBR2, SPINK5, DOCK8, PGM3, CARD11	• Elevated IgE, eosinophilia, and eczema with varying degrees of allergies, asthma, and infection susceptibility • Job syndrome (STAT3) and similar phenotypes (ZNF341, IL6R, IL6ST): coarse facial features, "cold" abscesses, pneumatoceles, chronic mucocutaneous candidiasis, hyperextensible joints, scoliosis, bone fractures, retained primary teeth, coronary/cerebral aneurysms • Loeys-Dietz syndrome (TGFBR1, TGFBR2): hyperextensible joints, scoliosis, aortic aneurysms, eosinophilic esophagitis • Comel-Netherton syndrome (SPINK5): "bamboo" hair, congenital ichthyosis, failure to thrive • DOCK8 deficiency (DOCK8): low NK cells, low IgM, elevated IgA, cutaneous viral/fungal infections, increased risk for cancer • PGM3 deficiency (PGM3): autoimmunity, short stature, developmental delay, delayed CNS myelination
T-cell defects with associated congenital thrombocytopenia	WASP, WIPF1	• Elevated IgE and IgA, low IgM, poor T-cell function, thrombocytopenia • Wiskott-Aldrich syndrome (WASP): recurrent infections, bloody diarrhea, eczema, autoimmunity, lymphoma • WIP deficiency (WIPF1): similar to WAS
Inflammasomopathies with urticaria	NLRP3, NLRP12, PLCG2	• Non-pruritic urticaria • Muckle-Wells syndrome (NLRP3): sensorineural hearing loss, risk for amyloidosis • Familial cold autoinflammatory syndrome, type 1 (FCAS1; NLRP3) and type 2 (FCAS2; NLRP12): cold-induced urticaria/rash, arthritis, and fever • Neonatal onset multisystem inflammatory disease or chronic infantile neurologic cutaneous and articular syndrome (NOMID/CINCA; NLRP3): neonatal onset rash, meningitis, arthropathy, and fever • PLCγ2 associated antibody deficiency and immune dysregulation (PLAID; PLCG2): cold-induced urticaria, autoimmunity, atopy, and antibody deficiency • Autoinflammation, antibody deficiency, and immune dysregulation (APLAID; PLCG2): blistering skin disease, autoinflammation, autoimmunity, and antibody deficiency

Table 33–10. Examples of combined immunodeficiency diseases.

	Genes/Chromosomes Containing Defects	Characteristic Features
Thymic defects in congenital anomaly syndromes	22q11.2 deletion, TBX1, CHD7, SEMA3E, FOXN1, PAX1, 10p13-p14 deletion, 11q23 deletion	• Low/absent T cells; B and NK cells are less affected • DiGeorge syndrome (22q11.2 deletion / TBX1 / 10p13-p14 deletion): hypoparathyroidism, heart defects, velopharyngeal insufficiency, distinctive facies, intellectual disability • CHARGE syndrome (CHD7, SEMA3E): coloboma, heart defects, atresia choanae (choanal atresia), growth retardation, genital and ear abnormalities • FOXN1 deficiency (FOXN1): alopecia, nail dystrophy • Otofaciocervical syndrome, type 2 (PAX1): ear and shoulder girdle abnormalities, facial dysmorphism, vertebral anomalies, and intellectual disability • Jacobsen syndrome (11q23 deletion): Paris-Trousseau syndrome (a bleeding disorder), distinctive facial features, developmental delay, heart defects, short stature, skeletal abnormalities

(Continued)

Table 33–10. Examples of combined immunodeficiency diseases. (*Continued*)

	Genes/Chromosomes Containing Defects	Characteristic Features
Cartilage hair hypoplasia	*RMRP*	• Varying degrees of T-cell lymphopenia and hypogammaglobulinemia • Short-limbed dwarfism with metaphyseal dysostosis, sparse hair, autoimmunity, risk for bone marrow failure and cancer
Anhidrotic ectodermo-dysplasia with immunodeficiency (EDA-ID)	*IKBKG (NEMO), IKBKB, NFKBIA*	• Hypogammaglobulinemia, elevated IgM, poor T-cell activation • Anhidrotic ectodermal dysplasia, colitis, infections, conical teeth, alopecia
DNA repair defects	*ATM, NBS1, BLM, DNMT3B, ZBTB24, CDCA7, HELLS*	• Increased radiosensitivity and risk for cancer, hypogammaglobulinemia, variable T-cell lymphopenia/dysfunction, infections • Ataxia-telangiectasia (*ATM*): ataxia, telangiectasia, increased alpha fetoprotein • Nijmegen breakage syndrome (*NBS*): microcephaly, facial dysmorphism, short stature, intellectual disability • Bloom syndrome (*BLM*): short stature, narrow face, rash (sun-exposes areas), risk for bone marrow failure • Immunodeficiency with centromeric instability and facial anomalies (*ICF; DNMT3B, ZBTB24, CDCA7, HELLS*): developmental delay, macroglossia, cytopenias
Bare lymphocyte syndromes	*TAP1, TAP2, TAPBP, CIITA, RFX5, RFXAP, RFXANK*	• MHC class I deficiency (*TAP1, TAP2, TAPBP*): low CD8+ T cells, vasculitis, pyoderma gangrenosum • MHC class II deficiency (*CIITA, RFX5, RFXAP, RFXANK*): low CD4+ T cells, hypogammaglobulinemia, sinopulmonary and gastrointestinal infections, liver/biliary disease

Endocrine Disorders

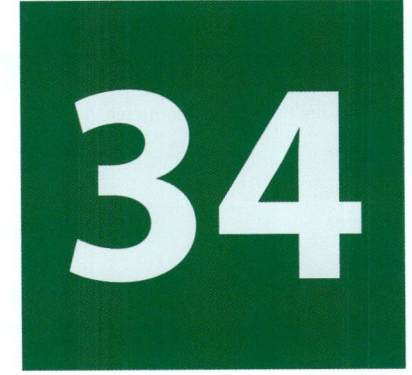

Sarah Bartz, MD

Christina Chambers, MD

Christine M. Chan, MD

Melanie Cree-Green, MD, PhD

Shanlee Davis, MD, PhD

Stephanie Hsu, MD, PhD

Animesh Sharma, MD

GENERAL CONCEPTS

The classic biology concept that *endocrine* effects are the result of substances secreted into the blood which act on distant target cells has been updated to account for additional ways in which hormonal effects occur. Specifically, *paracrine* systems involve the stimulation or inhibition of metabolic processes in neighboring cells (eg, within the pancreatic islets or cartilage). *Autocrine* hormone effects reflect the action of hormones on the same cells that produced them. The discoveries of local production of ghrelin, somatostatin, cholecystokinin, incretins, and many other hormones in the brain and gut support the concept of paracrine and autocrine processes in these tissues.

Another significant discovery in endocrine physiology was an appreciation of the role of specific hormone receptors in target tissues, without which the hormonal effects cannot occur. For example, in nephrogenic diabetes insipidus (DI), affected children have defective vasopressin or receptor function, and show the metabolic effects of DI despite more-than-adequate vasopressin secretion. Alternatively, ligand-independent activation of a hormone receptor leads to inappropriate effect without inappropriate hormone secretion. Examples of this phenomenon include McCune-Albright syndrome (precocious puberty and hyperthyroidism), testotoxicosis (familial male-limited precocious puberty), and hypercalciuric hypocalcemia.

HORMONE TYPES

Hormones typically fall into one of three classes based on chemistry: peptides and proteins, steroids, and amines. The peptide hormones include the releasing factors secreted by the hypothalamus; the hormones of the anterior and posterior pituitary gland; pancreatic islet cells; parathyroid glands, lung (angiotensin II), heart, and brain (atrial and brain natriuretic hormones); and local growth factors such as insulin-like growth factor 1 (IGF-1). Steroid hormones are secreted primarily by the adrenal cortex, gonads, and kidney (active vitamin D [1,25(OH)$_2$ D3]). The amine hormones are secreted by the adrenal medulla (epinephrine) and the thyroid gland (triiodothyronine [T$_3$] and thyroxine [T$_4$]).

Peptide hormones and epinephrine act through cell surface receptors. The metabolic effects of these hormones are usually stimulation or inhibition of the activity of preexisting enzymes or transport proteins (posttranslational effects). The steroid hormones, thyroid hormone, and active vitamin D, in contrast, act more slowly and bind to cytoplasmic receptors inside the target cell and subsequently to specific regions on nuclear DNA. Their metabolic effects are generally caused by stimulating or inhibiting the synthesis of new enzymes or transport proteins (transcriptional effects).

Metabolic processes that require rapid response, such as blood glucose or calcium homeostasis, are usually controlled by peptide hormones and epinephrine, while processes that respond more slowly, such as pubertal development and metabolic rate, are controlled by steroid hormones and thyroid hormone. The control of electrolyte homeostasis is intermediate and is regulated by a combination of peptide and steroid hormones (Table 34–1).

FEEDBACK CONTROL OF HORMONE SECRETION

Hormone secretion is regulated by feedback in response to changes in the internal environment. When the metabolic imbalance is corrected, stimulation of the hormone secretion ceases and may even be inhibited. Overcorrection of the imbalance stimulates secretion of counterbalancing hormone or hormones so that homeostasis is maintained within relatively narrow limits.

Hypothalamic-pituitary control of hormonal secretion is regulated by feedback. End-organ failure leads to decreased circulating concentrations of endocrine gland hormones and increased secretion of the respective hypothalamic releasing hormones and pituitary hormones (see

Table 34–1. Hormonal regulation of metabolic processes.

Rapid Response, Most Direct			
Metabolite or Other Parameter	**Stimulus**	**Endocrine Gland**	**Hormone**
Glucose	Hyperglycemia	Pancreatic beta cell	Insulin
Glucose	Hypoglycemia	Pancreatic alpha cell	Glucagon
Glucose	Hypoglycemia	Adrenal medulla	Epinephrine
Calcium	Hypercalcemia	Thyroid C cell	Calcitonin
Calcium	Hypocalcemia	Parathyroid	PTH
Sodium/plasma osmolality	Hypernatremia/hyperosmolality	Hypothalamus with posterior pituitary gland as reservoir	ADH
Plasma volume	Hypervolemia	Heart	ANH
Intermediate Response, Multiple Intermediaries			
Metabolite or Other Parameter	**Abnormality**	**Endocrine Gland**	**Hormone**
Sodium/potassium	Hyponatremia	Kidney	Renin (an enzyme)
	Hyperkalemia	Liver and others	Angiotensin I
	Hypovolemia	Lung	Angiotensin II
		Adrenal cortex	Aldosterone
Slow Response, Longer-Acting Processes			
Hypothalamic-Releasing Hormone	**Trophic Hormone (Pituitary Gland)**	**Endocrine Target Tissue**	**Endocrine Gland Hormone**
CRH	ACTH	Adrenal cortex	Cortisol
GHRH	GH	Liver and other tissues	IGF-1
GnRH	LH	Testis	Testosterone
GnRH	FSH/LH	Ovary	Estradiol/progesterone
TRH	TSH	Thyroid gland	T_4 and T_3

ACTH, adrenocorticotropic hormone; ADH, antidiuretic hormone; ANH, atrial natriuretic hormone; CRH, corticotropin-releasing hormone; FSH, follicle-stimulating hormone; GH, growth hormone; GHRH, growth hormone–releasing hormone; GnRH, gonadotropin-releasing hormone; IGF-1, insulin-like growth factor 1; LH, luteinizing hormone; PTH, parathyroid hormone; T_3, triiodothyronine; T_4, thyroxine; TRH, thyrotropin-releasing hormone; TSH, thyroid-stimulating hormone.

Table 34–1; Figure 34–1). If restoration of normal circulating concentration of hormones occurs, feedback inhibition at the pituitary and hypothalamus results in cessation of the previously stimulated secretion of hypothalamic and pituitary hormones and restoration of their circulating concentrations to normal.

Similarly, if there is autonomous endocrine gland hyperfunction (eg, McCune-Albright syndrome, Graves disease, or adrenal tumor), the specific hypothalamic releasing and pituitary hormones are suppressed (see Figure 34–1).

Bethin K, Fuqua JS: General concepts and physiology. In: Kappy MS, Allen DB, Geffner ME (eds): *Pediatric Practice-Endocrinology*. New York, NY: McGraw Hill; 2010:1–22.

DISTURBANCES OF GROWTH

Disturbances of growth and development are the most common problems evaluated by a pediatric endocrinologist. Deviations from the norm can be the first or only manifestation of an endocrine disorder. In evaluation of growth, height velocity is the most critical parameter. Height percentiles represent comparisons to a population and assume typical growth velocity. Therefore, a persistent increase or decrease in height percentiles between age 2 years and the onset of puberty indicates abnormal growth and always warrants evaluation. Similarly, substantial deviations from target (midparental) height may indicate underlying endocrine or skeletal disorders. It is more difficult to distinguish normal from abnormal growth in the

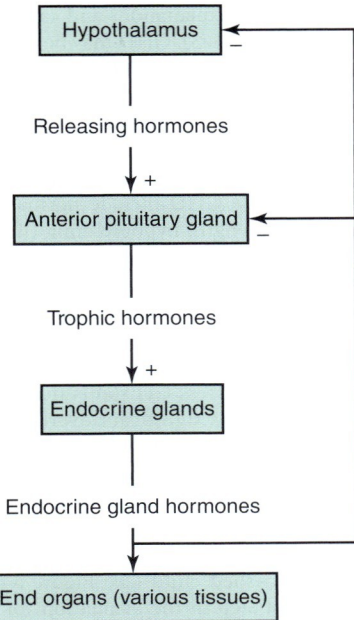

▲ **Figure 34–1.** General scheme of the hypothalamus-pituitary-endocrine gland axis. Releasing hormones synthesized in the hypothalamus are secreted into the hypophyseal portal circulation. Trophic hormones are secreted by the pituitary gland in response, and they in turn act on specific endocrine glands to stimulate the secretion of their respective hormones. The endocrine gland hormones exert their respective effects on various target tissues (end organs) and exert a negative feedback (feedback inhibition) on their own secretion by acting at the level of the pituitary and hypothalamus. This system is characteristic of those hormones listed in Table 34–1 (third level).

first 2 years of life. In addition, growth variations during the late childhood and early adolescent years require careful consideration due to the variable timing of the onset of puberty.

The National Center for Health Statistics provides standard cross-sectional growth charts for North American children and the World Health Organization (WHO) growth charts use an ethnically more diverse sample. Normal growth standards may vary with country of origin. Growth charts are available for some ethnic groups in North America and for some genetic syndromes with specific growth disturbance such as Turner or Down syndromes. Current treatment practices for patients with Turner and Down syndrome can cause children to grow differently than reflected in their specific growth charts.

TARGET HEIGHT & SKELETAL MATURATION

A child's height potential is determined largely by genetic factors. The target height of a child is calculated from the mean parental height plus 6.5 cm for boys or minus 6.5 cm for girls. This calculation helps identify a child's genetic growth potential. Most children achieve an adult height within 10 cm of the target height. Another parameter that determines growth potential is skeletal maturation or bone age. Beyond the neonatal period, bone age is evaluated by comparing a radiograph of the child's left hand and wrist with the standards of Greulich and Pyle. Delayed or advanced bone age is not diagnostic of any specific disease, but the extent of skeletal maturation allows determination of remaining growth potential as a percentage of total height and is used in the predication of adult height. However, it is important to remember that the bone age is a snapshot of a point in time, and bone age delay or advancement can change over time. For example, children with a previously delayed bone age may develop a bone age closer to their chronological age as they approach puberty.

SHORT STATURE

It is important to distinguish normal variants of growth (familial short stature and constitutional growth delay [CGD]) from pathologic conditions (Table 34–2). Pathologic short stature is more likely in children who have a low growth velocity or who are significantly short for their family. Children with chronic illness or nutritional deficiencies may have poor linear growth, and this can be associated with inadequate weight gain and low body mass index (BMI). In contrast, endocrine causes of short stature are usually associated with maintenance or increase in BMI percentiles.

1. Familial Short Stature & Constitutional Growth Delay

Children with familial short stature typically have normal birth weight and length. In the first 2 years of life, their linear growth velocity decelerates until they near their genetically determined percentile. Once the target percentile is reached, the child resumes normal linear growth parallel to the growth curve, usually between 2 and 3 years of age. Skeletal maturation and timing of puberty are consistent with chronologic age. The child grows along his/her own growth percentile, and the final height is short but appropriate for the family (Figure 34–2).

Children with constitutional growth delay (CGD) have a growth pattern similar to those with familial short stature with a decline in linear growth velocity between ages 2 and 3 years and then maintenance of a normal growth velocity prior to puberty. The difference is that children with CGD follow a growth percentile that is below what is expected based on parental heights, have a delay in skeletal maturation compared to chronologic age, and exhibit a delay in the onset

Table 34–2. Causes of short stature.

NORMAL
A. Familial short stature
B. Constitutional growth delay
PATHOLOGIC
C. Endocrine disturbances
1. Growth hormone (GH) deficiency
a. Hereditary
b. Idiopathic—with and without associated abnormalities of midline structures of the central nervous system
c. Acquired
d. Transient (eg, psychosocial short stature)
e. Organic—tumor, irradiation of the central nervous system, infection, or trauma
2. GH resistance/insulin-like growth factor 1 (IGF-1) deficiency
3. Hypothyroidism
4. Excess cortisol—Cushing disease and Cushing syndrome
5. Diabetes mellitus (poorly controlled)
6. Pseudohypoparathyroidism
7. Rickets
D. Intrauterine growth restriction
1. Intrinsic fetal abnormalities—chromosomal disorders
2. Syndromes (eg, Russell-Silver, Noonan, Bloom, de Lange, Cockayne)
3. Congenital infections
4. Placental abnormalities
5. Maternal abnormalities during pregnancy
E. Inborn errors of metabolism
F. Intrinsic diseases of bone
1. Defects of growth of tubular bones or spine (skeletal dysplasias)
2. Disorganized development of cartilage and fibrous components of the skeleton
G. Short stature associated with chromosomal defects
1. Autosomal (eg, Down syndrome, Prader-Willi syndrome)
2. Sex chromosomal (eg, Turner syndrome–XO)
H. Chronic systemic diseases, congenital defects, and cancers
I. Psychosocial short stature

of puberty. Late puberty often manifests as exaggerated short stature during the typical time of puberty. In these children, growth continues beyond the time the average child stops growing, and final height is appropriate for target height (Figure 34–3).

2. Growth Hormone Deficiency

Human growth hormone (GH) is produced by the anterior pituitary gland. Secretion is stimulated by growth hormone-releasing hormone (GHRH) and inhibited by somatostatin. GH is secreted in a pulsatile pattern and has direct growth-promoting and metabolic effects (Figure 34–4). GH also promotes growth indirectly by stimulating production of insulin-like growth factors, primarily IGF-1.

Growth hormone deficiency (GHD) is characterized by decreased growth velocity and delayed skeletal maturation

in the absence of other explanations and can be reversed by GH treatment. (Figure 34–5). GHD may be isolated or coexist with other pituitary hormone deficiencies. It may be congenital (septo-optic dysplasia or ectopic posterior pituitary), genetic (GH or GHRH gene mutation), or acquired (craniopharyngioma, germinoma, histiocytosis, or cranial irradiation). Idiopathic GHD is the most common deficiency state.

Features of infantile GHD include normal birth weight and slightly reduced length, hypoglycemia (if accompanied by adrenal insufficiency), micropenis (if accompanied by gonadotropin deficiency), and conjugated hyperbilirubinemia (if other pituitary hormone deficiencies present). In infantile GHD, growth abnormalities may not present until late in infancy or childhood.

Laboratory tests to assess GH status may be difficult to interpret because there is significant overlap in GH secretion between normal and GH-deficient children. GH secretion is pulsatile, so random samples for measurement of serum GH are of no value in the diagnosis of GHD outside of the first week of life. Serum concentrations of IGF-1 give reasonable estimations of GH secretion and action in the adequately nourished child (see Figure 34–4) and are often used as a first step in the evaluation for GHD. IGF-binding protein 3 (IGFBP-3) is a less sensitive marker of GH deficiency but may be useful in the underweight child or in children younger than 4 years, since it is less affected by age or nutritional status. Provocative studies using such agents as insulin arginine, levodopa, clonidine, or glucagon are traditionally done to clarify GH secretion, but are not physiologic and are often poorly reproducible, ultimately limiting their value in the clarification of GH secretion. The diagnosis of GHD is often a compilation of clinical and laboratory evidence. All patients diagnosed with GHD should have an MRI of the hypothalamus and pituitary gland to evaluate for tumors or structural abnormalities prior to starting therapy.

3. Small for Gestational Age/Intrauterine Growth Restriction

Small-for-gestational-age (SGA) infants have a birth weight that is below the 3rd percentile for the population's birth weight–gestational age relationship. SGA infants include constitutionally small infants and infants with intrauterine growth restriction (IUGR). Many children with mild SGA/IUGR and no intrinsic fetal abnormalities exhibit catch-up growth during the first 3 years, but 15%–20% remain short throughout life. Catch-up growth may also be inadequate in preterm SGA/IUGR infants with poor postnatal nutrition. Children who do not show catch-up growth may have normal growth velocity but follow a lower height percentile than expected for the family. In contrast to children with CGD, those with SGA/IUGR have skeletal maturation that corresponds to chronologic age or is only mildly delayed.

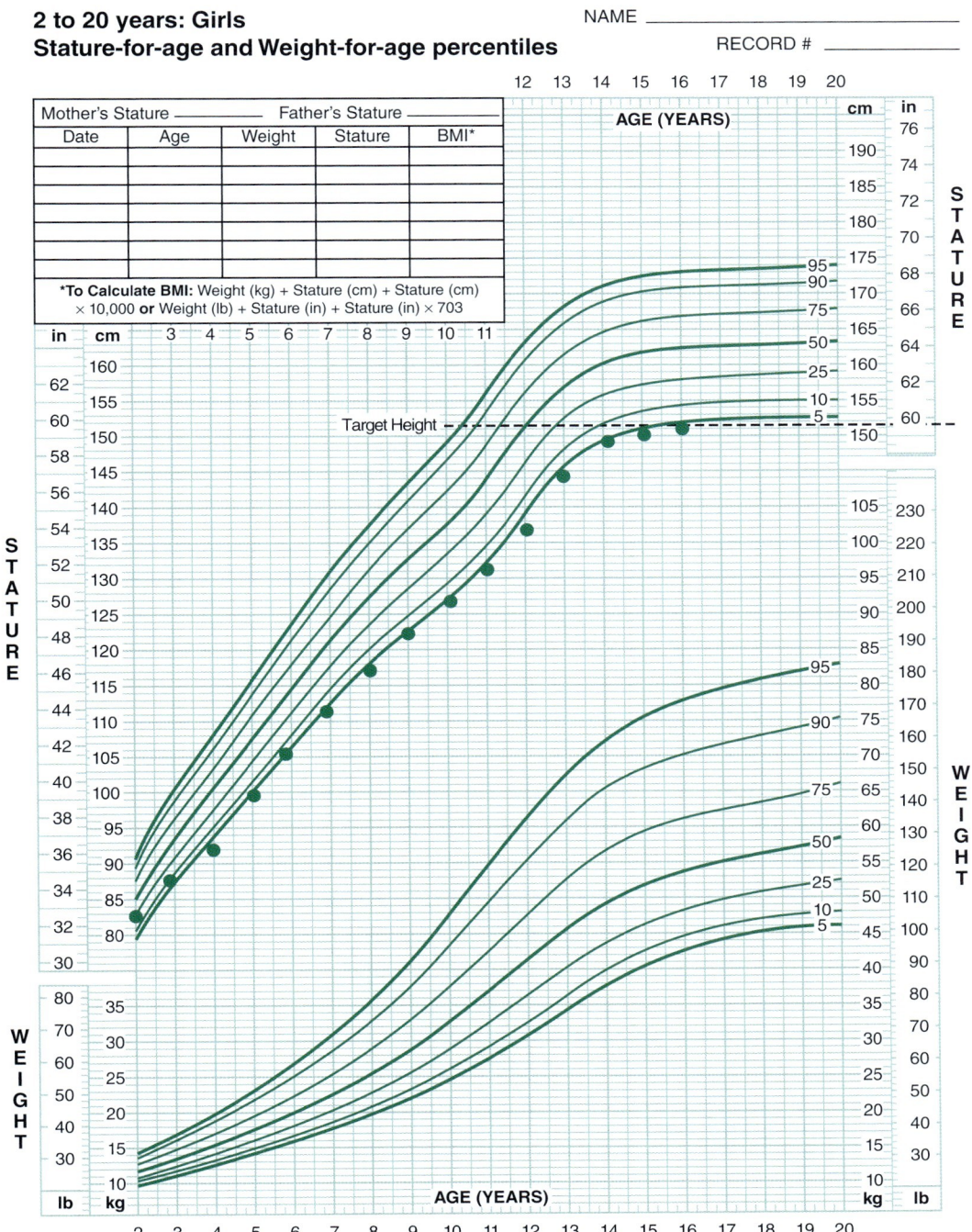

2 to 20 years: Girls
Stature-for-age and Weight-for-age percentiles

▲ **Figure 34–2.** Typical pattern of growth in a child with familial short stature. After attaining an appropriate percentile during the first 2 years of life, the child will have normal linear growth parallel to the growth curve. Skeletal maturation and the timing of puberty are consistent with chronologic age. The height percentile the child has been following is maintained, and final height is short but appropriate for the family.

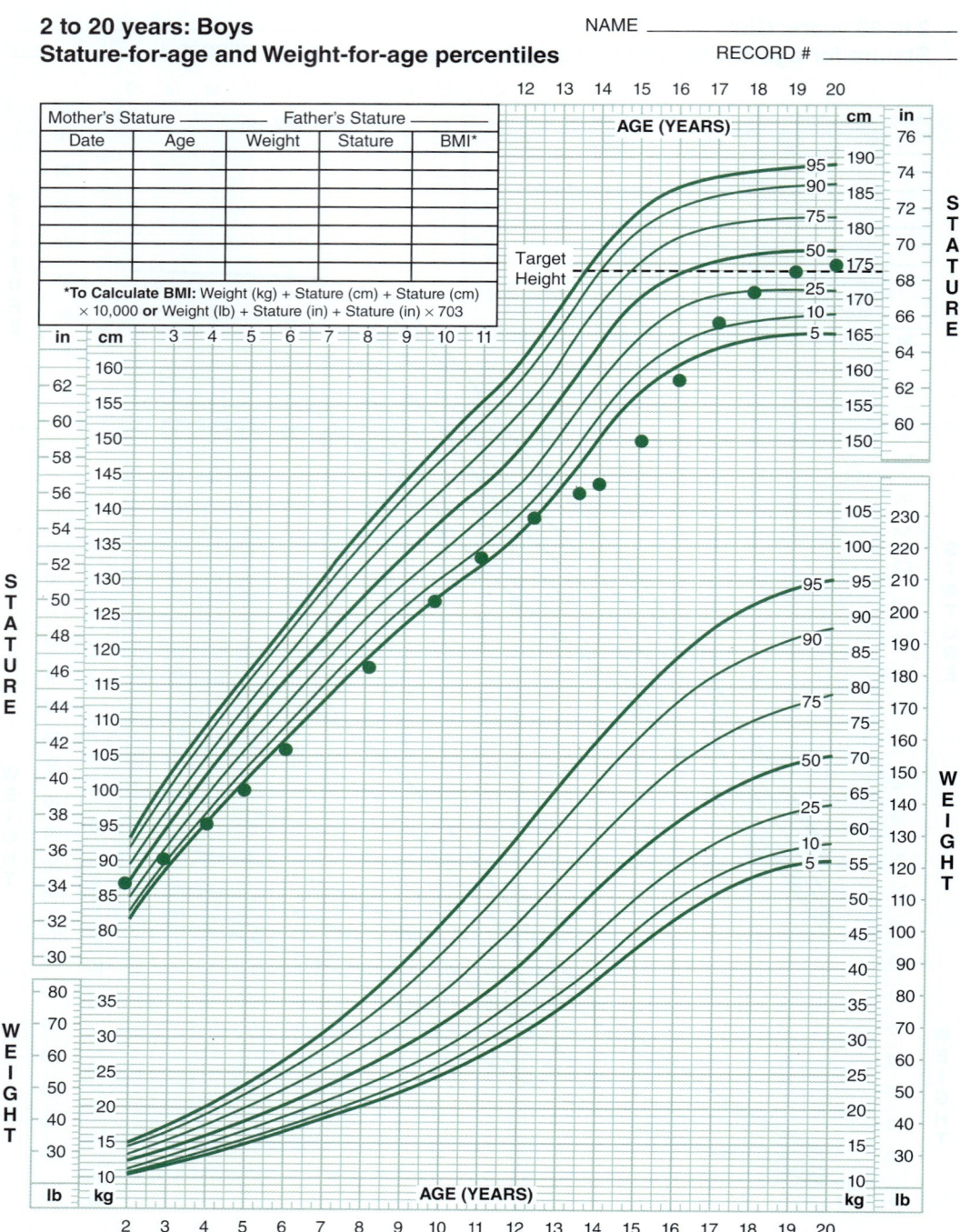

2 to 20 years: Boys
Stature-for-age and Weight-for-age percentiles

NAME _____

RECORD # _____

▲ **Figure 34–3.** Typical pattern of growth in a child with constitutional growth delay. Growth slows during the first 2 years of life, similarly to children with familial short stature. Subsequently the child will have normal linear growth parallel to the growth curve. However, skeletal maturation and the onset of puberty are delayed. Growth continues beyond the time the average child has stopped growing, and final height is appropriate for target height.

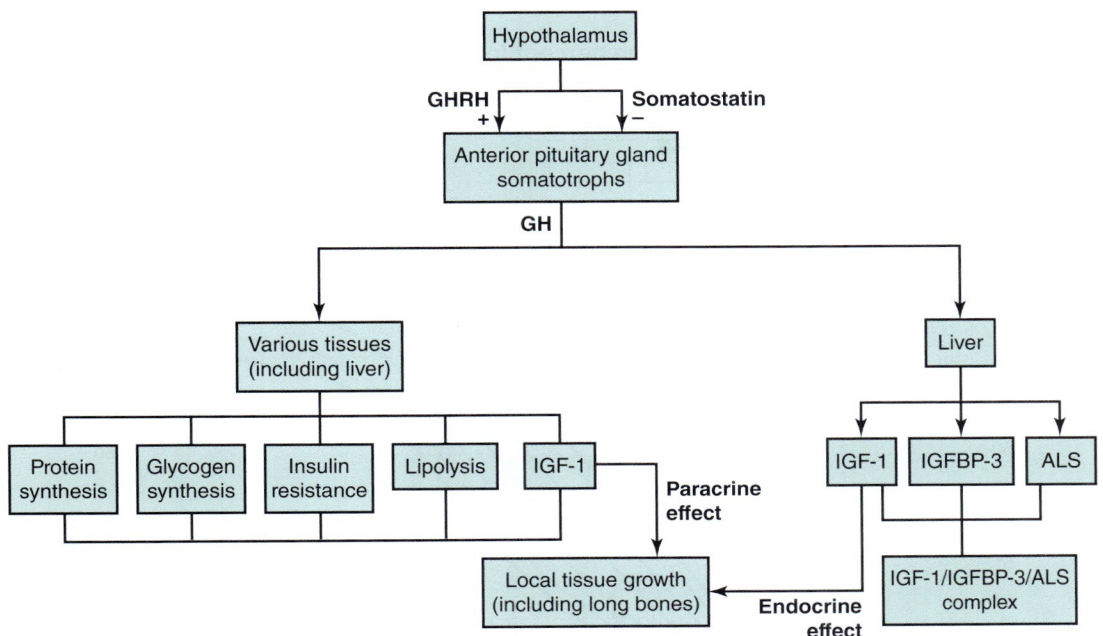

▲ **Figure 34–4.** The GHRH/GH/IGF-1 system. The effects of growth hormone (GH) on growth are partly due to its direct anabolic effects in the muscle, liver, and bone. In addition, GH stimulates many tissues to produce insulin-like growth factor 1 (IGF-1) locally, which stimulates the growth of the tissue itself (paracrine effect of IGF-1). The action of GH on the liver results in the secretion of IGF-1 (circulating IGF-1), which stimulates growth in other tissues (endocrine effect of IGF-1). The action of growth hormone on the liver also enhances the secretion of IGF-binding protein 3 (IGFBP-3) and acid-labile subunit (ALS), which form a high-molecular-weight complex with IGF-1. The function of this complex is to transport IGF-1 to its target tissues, but the complex also serves as a reservoir and possible inhibitor of IGF-1 action. In various chronic illnesses, the direct metabolic effects of GH are inhibited; the secretion of IGF-1 in response to GH is blunted, and in some cases IGFBP-3 synthesis is enhanced, resulting in marked inhibition in the growth of the child. GHRH, growth hormone-releasing hormone.

GH therapy for SGA/IUGR children with growth delay is approved by the US Food and Drug Administration (FDA) and appears to increase growth velocity and final adult height.

4. Disproportionate Short Stature

There are more than 200 sporadic and genetic skeletal dysplasias that may cause disproportionate short stature. Measurements of arm span and upper-to-lower body segment ratio are helpful in determining whether a child has normal body proportions. If disproportionate short stature is found, a skeletal survey may be useful to detect specific radiographic features characteristic of some disorders.

5. Short Stature Associated With Syndromes

Short stature is associated with many genetic syndromes, including Turner, Down, Noonan, and Prader-Willi. Girls with Turner syndrome often have many recognizable features (see Chapter 37), but short stature can be the only clinically obvious manifestation. Consequently, any girl with unexplained short stature for family warrants a chromosomal evaluation. Although girls with Turner syndrome are not usually GH-deficient, GH therapy can improve final height by an average of 6 cm. Duration of GH therapy is a significant predictor of long-term height gain; consequently, it is important that Turner syndrome be diagnosed early and GH started as soon as possible if the family desires to maximize height.

GH is approved for treatment of growth failure in Prader-Willi syndrome–associated GHD. GH improves growth, body composition, and physical activity. A few deaths have been reported in children with Prader-Willi syndrome receiving GH. These deaths occurred in very obese children, children with respiratory impairments, or possibly unidentified respiratory infections. The role of GH in these deaths is unknown,

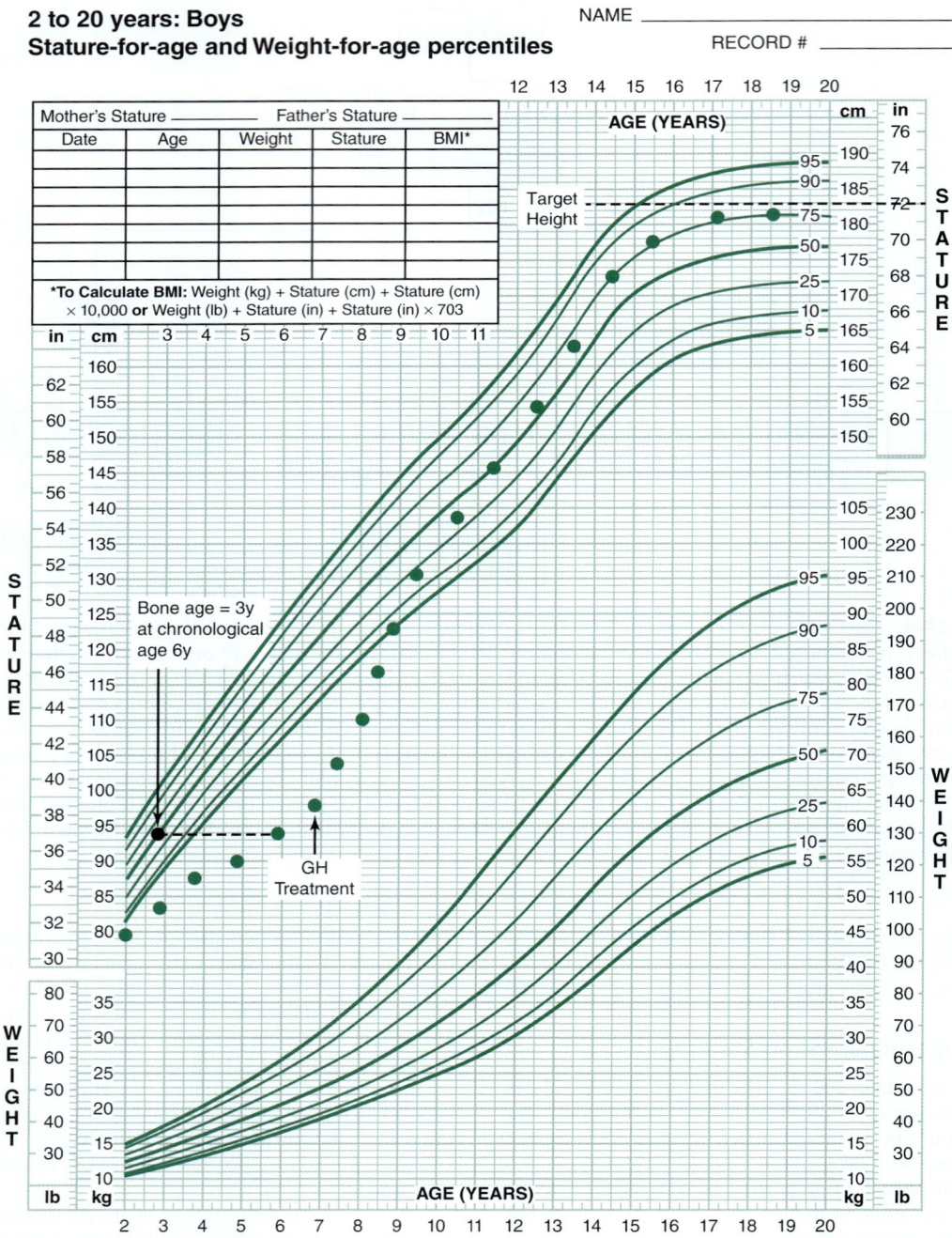

2 to 20 years: Boys
Stature-for-age and Weight-for-age percentiles

NAME _____

RECORD # _____

▲ **Figure 34–5.** Typical pattern of growth in a child with acquired growth hormone deficiency (GHD). Children with acquired GHD have an abnormal growth velocity and fail to maintain height percentile during childhood. Other phenotypic features (central adiposity and immaturity of facies) may be present. Children with congenital GHD will cross percentiles during the first 2 years of life, similarly to the pattern seen in familial short stature and constitutional delay, but will fail to attain a steady height percentile subsequently.

but it is recommended that all patients with Prader-Willi syndrome be evaluated for upper airway obstruction and sleep apnea prior to starting GH therapy.

6. Psychosocial Short Stature (Psychosocial Dwarfism)

Psychosocial short stature refers to growth impairment associated with emotional deprivation. Undernutrition probably contributes to growth slowing in some of these children. Other symptoms include unusual eating and drinking habits, bowel and bladder incontinence, social withdrawal, and delayed speech. GH secretion in children with psychosocial short stature is diminished, but GH therapy is usually not beneficial. A change in the psychological environment at home usually results in improved growth and improvement of GH secretion, personality, and eating behaviors.

▶ Clinical Evaluation

Laboratory investigation should be guided by the history and physical examination, including history of chronic illness and medications, birth weight and length, pattern of growth since birth, familial growth and puberty patterns, pubertal stage, dysmorphic features, body segment proportion, and psychological health. In a child with poor weight gain as the primary disturbance, a nutritional assessment is indicated. The following laboratory tests may be useful as guided by history and clinical judgment: (1) radiograph of left hand and wrist for bone age; (2) karyotype (girls) and/or Noonan syndrome testing; (3) thyroid function tests: T_4 and thyroid-stimulating hormone (TSH); (4) IGF-1 and/or IGFBP-3 in children younger than 4 years or in malnourished individuals; (5) complete blood count (to detect chronic anemia or leukocyte markers of infection); (6) erythrocyte sedimentation rate (often elevated in collagen-vascular disease, cancer, chronic infection, and inflammatory bowel disease); (7) urinalysis, blood urea nitrogen, and serum creatinine (occult renal disease); (8) serum electrolytes, calcium, and phosphorus (renal tubular disease and metabolic bone disease); and (9) stool examination for fat, or measurement of serum tissue transglutaminase (malabsorption or celiac disease).

▶ Growth Hormone Therapy

GH therapy is approved by the FDA in children with GHD; growth restriction associated with chronic renal failure; Turner, Prader-Willi, and Noonan syndromes; children born SGA who fail to demonstrate catch-up growth by age 2; and short stature *homeobox*-containing (SHOX) gene mutations. GH therapy has also been approved for children with idiopathic short stature whose current height is more than 2.25 standard deviations below the normal range for age. With GH treatment, final height may be 5–7 cm taller in this population. The role of GH for idiopathic short stature is unclear, especially due to the expense, long duration of treatment, and variability in height

outcomes. Side effects of recombinant GH are uncommon but include intracranial hypertension and slipped capital femoral epiphysis. With early diagnosis and treatment, children with GH deficiency reach normal or near-normal adult height. The recommended schedule for GH therapy is recombinant GH given subcutaneously 6 or 7 days per week with total weekly dose of 0.15–0.47 mg/kg. Duration of treatment depends on individual goals of therapy.

Altzoglou KS et al: Isolated growth hormone deficiency (GHD) in childhood and adolescence: recent advances. Endocr Rev 2014;35:376–432 [PMID: 24450934].
Cohen LE: Idiopathic short stature: a clinical review. JAMA 2014;311:1787–1796 [PMID: 24794372].
Loche S et al: Growth hormone treatment in non-growth hormone-deficient children. Ann Pediatr Endocrinol Metab 2014;19:1–7 [PMID: 24926456].
Rogol AD, Hayden GF: Etiologies and early diagnosis of short stature and growth failure in children and adolescents. J Pediatr 2014 May;164(5 Suppl):S1–14.e6 [PMID: 24731744].

TALL STATURE

Although growth disturbances are usually associated with short stature, potentially serious pathologic conditions may also be associated with tall stature and excessive growth (Table 34–3). Excessive GH secretion is rare, particularly in children, and generally associated with a functioning pituitary adenoma. GH excess leads to gigantism if the epiphyses are open and to acromegaly if the epiphyses are closed. The diagnosis is confirmed by finding elevated random GH and IGF-1 levels and failure of GH suppression during an oral glucose tolerance test. Precocious puberty can also cause tall stature for age or rapid growth but would be associated with early signs of puberty and an advanced bone age. Obese youth are also often tall for age, but they do not achieve a taller final height.

Davies JH, Cheetham T: Investigation and management of tall stature. Arch Dis Child 2014;99:772–777 [PMID: 24833789].

Table 34–3. Causes of tall stature.

A. Constitutional (familial)
B. Endocrine causes
  1. Growth hormone excess (pituitary gigantism)
  2. Precocious puberty
  3. Hypogonadism
C. Nonendocrine causes
  1. Klinefelter syndrome
  2. XYY males
  3. Marfan syndrome
  4. Cerebral gigantism (Sotos syndrome)
  5. Homocystinuria

DISORDERS OF THE POSTERIOR PITUITARY GLAND

The posterior pituitary (neurohypophysis) is an extension of the ventral hypothalamus. Its two principal hormones—oxytocin and arginine vasopressin—are synthesized in the supraoptic and paraventricular nuclei of the ventral hypothalamus. These peptide hormones are packaged in granules with specific neurophysins and transported via the axons to their storage site in the posterior pituitary. Vasopressin is essential for water balance; it acts primarily on the kidney to promote reabsorption of water from urine. Oxytocin is most active during parturition and breast feeding and is not discussed further here.

ARGININE VASOPRESSIN (ANTIDIURETIC HORMONE) PHYSIOLOGY

Vasopressin release is controlled primarily by serum osmolality and intravascular volume. Release is stimulated by minor increases in plasma osmolality (detected by osmoreceptors in the anterolateral hypothalamus) and large decreases in intravascular volume (detected by baroreceptors in the cardiac atria). Disorders of vasopressin release and action include: (1) central DI, (2) nephrogenic DI (see Chapter 24), and (3) the syndrome of inappropriate secretion of antidiuretic hormone (SIADH).

CENTRAL DIABETES INSIPIDUS

ESSENTIALS OF DIAGNOSIS & TYPICAL FEATURES

▶ Polydipsia, polyuria, nocturia, dehydration, and hypernatremia.

▶ Inability to concentrate urine after fluid restriction (urine specific gravity < 1.010; urine osmolality < 300 mOsm/kg).

▶ Plasma osmolality 300 > mOsm/kg with urine osmolality < 600 mOsm/kg.

▶ Low plasma vasopressin, antidiuretic response to exogenous vasopressin.

▶ General Considerations

Central DI is an inability to synthesize and release vasopressin. Without vasopressin, the kidneys cannot concentrate urine, causing excessive urinary water loss. Genetic causes of central DI are rare and include mutations in the vasopressin gene and the *WFS1* gene that causes DI, diabetes mellitus, optic atrophy, and deafness (Wolfram or DIDMOAD syndrome). The most common causes of pediatric central DI are midline defects (septo-optic dysplasia, holoprosencephaly); trauma (surgery, injury); infiltrative/neoplastic disease (tumors such as craniopharyngioma, germinoma, Langerhans cell histiocytosis, sarcoidosis); infectious (meningitis); and idiopathic.

▶ Clinical Findings

Onset of DI is characterized by polyuria, nocturia, enuresis, and intense thirst. Hypernatremia, hyperosmolality, and dehydration occur if insufficient fluid intake does not keep up with urinary losses. In infants, symptoms may also include failure to thrive, vomiting, constipation, and unexplained fevers. Some infants may present with severe dehydration, circulatory collapse, and seizures. Vasopressin deficiency may be masked in patients with panhypopituitarism due to the impaired excretion of free water associated with adrenocorticotropic hormone (ACTH) insufficiency; treatment with glucocorticoids may unmask DI in these patients.

DI is confirmed when serum hyperosmolality is associated with urine hypo-osmolarity. If the history indicates that the child can go through the night comfortably without drinking, outpatient testing is appropriate. Osmolality, sodium, and specific gravity of the first morning void are obtained after a period of fluid restriction. If symptoms suggest child cannot safely go through night without drinking or if outpatient testing results are unclear, the water deprivation test should be done in the hospital. See "Essentials" box for diagnostic criteria. Children with central DI should have a magnetic resonance imaging (MRI) of the head with contrast to look for tumors or infiltrative processes.

Primary polydipsia must be distinguished from DI. Children with primary polydipsia tend to have lower serum sodium levels and usually can concentrate their urine with overnight fluid deprivation. Some may have secondary nephrogenic DI due to dilution of the renal medullary interstitium and decreased renal concentrating ability, but this resolves with restriction of fluid intake.

▶ Treatment

Central DI is treated with oral or intranasal desmopressin acetate (DDAVP). The aim of therapy is to provide antidiuresis that allows uninterrupted sleep. Breakthrough urination should occur before the next dose. It is important to note that postsurgical DI can be associated with disruption of thirst mechanism, and for these patients, a prescribed volume of fluid intake may be necessary. Children hospitalized with acute-onset DI can be managed with intravenous or subcutaneous vasopressin. Due to the amount of antidiuresis, electrolytes should be closely monitored to avoid water intoxication. Infants with DI should not be treated with DDAVP since their primary source of nutrition is through liquid calories and this combination can result in hyponatremia. For this reason, infants are treated with breast milk or a formula with a low renal solute load and thiazide diuretic.

Di Iorgi N et al: Diabetes insipidus—diagnosis and management. Horm Res Paediatr 2012;77:69 [PMID: 22433947].

Rivkees SA et al: The management of central diabetes insipidus in infancy: desmopressin, low renal solute load formula, thiazide diuretics. J Pediatr Endocrinol Metab 2007;20:459 [PMID: 17550208].

Wise-Faberowski L et al: Perioperative management of diabetes insipidus in children. J Neurosurg Anesthesiol 2004;16:14 [PMID: 14676564].

THYROID GLAND

FETAL DEVELOPMENT OF THE THYROID

As early as the 10th week of gestation, the fetal thyroid synthesizes thyroid hormone, which appears in the fetal serum by the 11th week of gestation and progressively increases throughout gestation. The fetal pituitary-thyroid axis functions largely independently of the maternal pituitary-thyroid axis because maternal TSH cannot cross the placenta. However, maternal thyroid hormone can cross the placenta in limited amounts.

At birth, there is a TSH surge peaking at about 70 mU/L within 30 minutes. Thyroid hormone levels increase rapidly during the first days of life in response to this TSH surge. The TSH level decreases to childhood levels within a few weeks. This physiologic neonatal TSH surge can produce a false-positive newborn screen for hypothyroidism (ie, high TSH) if the blood sample for the screen is collected on the first day of life.

PHYSIOLOGY

Hypothalamic thyrotropin-releasing hormone (TRH) stimulates the anterior pituitary gland to release TSH. In turn, TSH stimulates the thyroid gland to synthesize and release T_4 and T_3 via a process regulated by negative feedback involving the hypothalamus, pituitary, and thyroid (see Figure 34–1).

T_4 is the predominant thyroid hormone secreted by the thyroid gland. Most circulating T_3 and T_4 are bound to thyroxine-binding globulin (TBG), albumin, and prealbumin. Less than 1% of thyroid hormone exists in the free form. T_4 is deiodinated in the tissues to T_3, which binds to nuclear thyroid hormone receptors in the cytoplasm and translocates to the nucleus, exerting its biologic effects by modifying gene expression. Causes of low T_4 include hypothyroidism (central or primary), prematurity, malnutrition, and severe illness.

Total T_4 is also low in situations that decrease TBG, such as familial TBG deficiency, cirrhosis, or renal failure and in patients receiving glucocorticoids or androgens. Since these effects primarily involve TBG, TSH and free T_4 (FT_4) levels remain in the normal range. Conversely, total T_3 and T_4 levels may be elevated in conditions associated with increased TBG levels (congenital TBG excess, pregnancy, estrogen therapy) and increased thyroid hormone binding to transport proteins. Again, patients are clinically euthyroid in this circumstance. A T_3 resin uptake (T3RU) can help differentiate between binding protein problems and true hypo- or hyperthyroidism.

HYPOTHYROIDISM (CONGENITAL & ACQUIRED)

ESSENTIALS OF DIAGNOSIS & TYPICAL FEATURES

▶ Growth impairment, decreased physical activity, weight gain, constipation, dry skin, cold intolerance, and delayed puberty.

▶ Untreated congenital hypothyroidism: thick tongue, large fontanels, poor muscle tone, hoarseness, umbilical hernia, jaundice, and intellectual impairment.

▶ T_4, FT_4, and T_3 resin uptake are low; TSH levels are elevated in primary hypothyroidism.

▶ General Considerations

Thyroid hormone deficiency may be congenital or acquired (Table 34–4). It can be due to defects in the thyroid gland (primary hypothyroidism) or in the hypothalamus or pituitary (central hypothyroidism).

Congenital hypothyroidism occurs in about 1:3000–1:4000 infants. Untreated, it causes severe neurocognitive impairment. Most cases are sporadic resulting from hypoplasia or aplasia of the thyroid gland or failure of the gland to migrate to its normal anatomic location (eg, lingual or sublingual thyroid gland). Other causes are listed in Table 34–4. In severe maternal iodine deficiency, both the fetus and the mother are T_4-deficient, with irreversible brain damage to the fetus. Acquired hypothyroidism, particularly if goiter is present, is usually a result of chronic lymphocytic (Hashimoto) thyroiditis.

▶ Clinical Findings

A. Symptoms and Signs

Even when the thyroid gland is completely absent, most newborns with congenital hypothyroidism appear normal. However, because congenital hypothyroidism is associated with intellectual impairment, thyroid testing is included in the newborn screen and treatment must be initiated as early as possible. Jaundice associated with an unconjugated hyperbilirubinemia may be present in newborns with congenital hypothyroidism.

Features of juvenile hypothyroidism include poor linear growth; delayed bone age and delayed dental eruption; skin

Table 34–4. Causes of hypothyroidism.

> **A. Congenital**
> 1. Aplasia, hypoplasia, or maldescent of thyroid
> 2. Inborn errors of thyroid hormone synthesis, secretion, or recycling
> 3. Maternal antibody-mediated (inhibit TSH binding to receptor)
> 4. TSH receptor defect
> 5. Thyroid hormone receptor defect
> 6. In utero exposures
>   a. Radioiodine therapy
>   b. Goitrogens (propylthiouracil, methimazole)
>   c. Iodine excess
> 7. Iodide deficiency
> **B. Acquired (juvenile hypothyroidism)**
> 1. Autoimmune (lymphocytic) thyroiditis
> 2. Thyroidectomy or radioiodine therapy
> 3. Irradiation to the thyroid
> 4. Thyrotropin deficiency
> 5. TRH deficiency due to hypothalamic injury or disease
> 6. Medications
>   a. Iodides
>   (1) Excess (eg, amiodarone)
>   (2) Deficiency
>   b. Lithium
>   c. Cobalt
> 7. Large hemangiomas
> 8. Idiopathic

TRH, thyrotropin-releasing hormone; TSH, thyroid-stimulating hormone.

changes (dry, thick, scaly, coarse, pale, cool, or sallow); hair changes (dry, coarse, or brittle) and hair loss; lateral thinning of the eyebrows; neurologic findings (hypotonia and a slow relaxation component of deep tendon reflexes); physical and mental sluggishness; nonpitting myxedema; constipation; cold temperature intolerance; bradycardia; delayed puberty; and occasional pseudopuberty (secondary to weak FSH activity of marked elevated TSH levels).

In hypothyroidism resulting from enzymatic defects or chronic lymphocytic thyroiditis, the thyroid gland may be enlarged. Thyroid enlargement in children is usually symmetrical, and the gland is moderately firm and not nodular. In chronic lymphocytic thyroiditis, however, the thyroid frequently has a cobblestone surface.

B. Laboratory Findings

In primary hypothyroidism, the total T_4 and FT_4 may be normal or decreased and the serum TSH is elevated. Circulating autoantibodies to thyroid peroxidase and/or thyroglobulin may be present. In central hypothyroidism, the TSH is low or inappropriately normal in the face of a low total T_4 and FT_4. Other pituitary deficiencies may be present, as central hypothyroidism may be associated with congenital or acquired disorders of the hypothalamus or pituitary gland.

C. Imaging

Thyroid imaging, while helpful in establishing the cause of congenital hypothyroidism, does not affect the treatment plan and is not necessary. Bone age is delayed. Cardiomegaly is common.

D. Screening Programs for Neonatal Hypothyroidism

All newborns should be screened for congenital hypothyroidism shortly after birth. Depending on the state, the newborn screen measures either the total T_4 or TSH level. Abnormal newborn screening results should be confirmed immediately with a venous T_4 and TSH level. Treatment should be started as soon as possible. Initiation of treatment in the first month of life and good medication adherence during infancy usually results in a normal neurocognitive outcome.

► Treatment

Synthetic T_4 or levothyroxine (75–100 mcg/m²/day) is the drug of choice for hypothyroidism. In neonates with congenital hypothyroidism, the recommended initial dose is 10–15 mcg/kg/day. Serum total T_4 or FT_4 concentrations are used to monitor the adequacy of initial therapy because the high neonatal TSH may not normalize for weeks. Subsequently, T_4 and TSH are monitored in combination.

Kaplowitz, P: Neonatal thyroid disease: testing and management. Pediatr Clin North Am 2019;66(2):343–352 [PMID: 30819341].

Léger J et al: European Society for Paediatric Endocrinology consensus guidelines on screening, diagnosis, and management of congenital hypothyroidism. J Clin Endocrinol Metab 2014;99(2):363–384 [PMID: 24446653].

van der Sluijs Veer L et al: Evaluation of cognitive and motor development in toddlers with congenital hypothyroidism diagnosed by neonatal screening. J Dev Behav Pediatr 2012;33:633–640 [PMID: 23027136].

THYROIDITIS

1. Chronic Lymphocytic Thyroiditis (Chronic Autoimmune Thyroiditis, Hashimoto Thyroiditis)

ESSENTIALS OF DIAGNOSIS & TYPICAL FEATURES

► Firm, freely movable, nontender, diffusely enlarged thyroid gland.

► Thyroid function is often normal but may be elevated or decreased depending on the stage of the disease.

General Considerations

Chronic lymphocytic thyroiditis is the most common cause of goiter and acquired hypothyroidism in childhood. It is more common in girls, and the incidence peaks during puberty. The disease is caused by an autoimmune attack on the thyroid. The following conditions are associated with increased risk for autoimmune (Hashimoto) thyroiditis: Down syndrome, Turner syndrome, celiac disease, vitiligo, alopecia, and type 1 diabetes.

Clinical Findings

A. Symptoms and Signs

The thyroid is characteristically enlarged, firm, freely movable, nontender, and symmetrical. It may be nodular. Onset is usually insidious. No local signs of inflammation or systemic infection are present. Most patients are euthyroid. Some patients are symptomatically hypothyroid, and few patients are symptomatically hyperthyroid.

A detailed family history may reveal the presence of multiple autoimmune diseases in family members. Individuals at a high risk based on a chromosomal disorder or other autoimmune disease benefit from careful monitoring of growth and development, routine screening, and a low threshold for measurement of thyroid function.

B. Laboratory Findings

Laboratory findings vary. Serum concentrations of TSH, T_4, and FT_4 are often normal. Some patients are hypothyroid with an elevated TSH and low thyroid hormone levels. A few patients are hyperthyroid early in the disease course (aka Hashitoxicosis) with a suppressed TSH and elevated thyroid hormone levels. Thyroid antibodies (antithyroglobulin, antithyroid peroxidase) are frequently elevated.

C. Imaging

Routine thyroid ultrasound is not indicated unless a focal nodule or mass is palpated. Thyroid uptake scan adds little unless the diagnosis is uncertain.

Treatment

Hypothyroidism commonly develops over time. Consequently, patients require lifelong surveillance. Children with documented hypothyroidism should receive thyroid hormone replacement.

2. Acute (Suppurative) Thyroiditis

Acute thyroiditis is rare. The most common causes are group A streptococci, pneumococci, *Staphylococcus aureus*, and anaerobes. Thyroid abscesses may form and are often left sided due to pyriform sinus fistula. The patient presents with fever and an enlarged, tender thyroid gland with associated erythema, hoarseness, and dysphagia. Thyroid function tests are typically normal. Patients have a leukocytosis, "left shift," and elevated erythrocyte sedimentation rate. Antibiotic therapy is required.

3. Subacute (Nonsuppurative) Thyroiditis

Subacute thyroiditis (de Quervain thyroiditis) is rare. It is thought to be caused by viral infection with mumps, influenza, echovirus, coxsackievirus, Epstein-Barr virus, or adenovirus. Presenting features are similar to acute thyroiditis—fever, malaise, sore throat, dysphagia, and thyroid pain. The thyroid is firm and enlarged. Sedimentation rate is elevated. In contrast to acute thyroiditis, the onset is generally insidious and serum thyroid hormone concentrations may be elevated.

HYPERTHYROIDISM

ESSENTIALS OF DIAGNOSIS & TYPICAL FEATURES

► Palpitations, nervousness, hyperactivity, excessive appetite, tremor, weight loss, fatigue, and heat intolerance.

► Goiter, tachycardia, exophthalmos, systolic hypertension, widened pulse pressure, weakness, and moist, warm skin.

► TSH is suppressed. Thyroid hormone levels (T_4, FT_4, T_3) and T_3 resin uptake (T_3RU) are elevated.

General Considerations

In children, most cases of hyperthyroidism are due to Graves disease, caused by antibodies directed at the TSH receptor that stimulate thyroid hormone production. Other causes include thyroiditis (acute, subacute, or chronic); autonomous functioning thyroid nodules; tumors producing TSH; McCune-Albright syndrome; exogenous thyroid hormone excess; and acute iodine exposure.

Clinical Findings

A. Symptoms and Signs

Hyperthyroidism is more common in females than males. In children, it most frequently occurs during adolescence. Symptoms include poor concentration, hyperactivity, fatigue, emotional lability, personality disturbance/unmasking of underlying psychosis, insomnia, weight loss (despite increased appetite), palpitations, heat intolerance, increased perspiration, increased stool frequency, polyuria, and irregular menses. Signs include tachycardia, systolic hypertension, increased pulse pressure, tremor, proximal muscle weakness, and moist, warm skin. Accelerated growth and development may occur. Thyroid storm is a rare condition characterized by fever, cardiac failure, emesis, and delirium that can result in coma or death. Most cases of Graves disease are associated with a diffuse firm goiter. A thyroid bruit and thrill may be present. Many cases are associated with exophthalmos.

B. Laboratory Findings

TSH is suppressed. T_4, FT_4, T_3 are elevated except in rare cases in which only the serum T_3 is elevated (T_3 thyrotoxicosis). The presence of thyroid-stimulating immunoglobulin (TSI) or thyroid eye disease confirms the diagnosis of Graves disease. TSH receptor-binding antibodies (TRAb) are usually elevated.

C. Imaging

Radioactive iodine uptake by the thyroid is increased in Graves disease, whereas in subacute and chronic thyroiditis it is decreased. An autonomous hyperfunctioning nodule takes up iodine and appears as a "hot nodule" while the surrounding tissue has decreased iodine uptake. In children with hyperthyroidism, bone age may be advanced. In infants, accelerated skeletal maturation may be associated with premature fusion of the cranial sutures. Long-standing hyperthyroidism causes osteoporosis.

▶ Treatment

A. General Measures

Strenuous physical activity should be avoided in untreated severe hyperthyroidism due to concern for cardiovascular instability.

B. Medical Treatment

1. β-Adrenergic blocking agents—These are adjuncts to therapy. They can rapidly ameliorate symptoms and are indicated in severe disease with tachycardia and hypertension. β_1-Specific agents such as atenolol are preferred because they are more cardioselective. Propranolol also decreases conversion of T_4 to active T_3, so is preferred in severe cases.

2. Antithyroid agents (methimazole)—Antithyroid agents are frequently used in the initial treatment of childhood hyperthyroidism. These drugs interfere with thyroid hormone synthesis, and usually take a few weeks to produce a clinical response. Adequate control is usually achieved within a few months. If medical therapy is unsuccessful, more definitive therapy, such as thyroidectomy or radioiodine ablation should be considered. Propylthiouracil (PTU) is rarely utilized because of reports of severe hepatotoxicity.

A. INITIAL DOSAGE—Methimazole is initiated at a dose of 10–60 mg/day (0.5–1 mg/kg/day) given once a day. Initial dosing is continued until FT_4 or T_4 have normalized and signs and symptoms have subsided.

B. MAINTENANCE—The optimal dose of antithyroid agent for maintenance treatment remains unclear. Recent studies suggest that 10–15 mg/day of methimazole provides adequate long-term control in most patients with a minimum of side effects. Treatment usually continues for 2 years with the goal of inducing remission. If thyroid hormone levels are well controlled at that point, a trial off medication could be considered.

C. TOXICITY—If vasculitis, arthralgia, arthritis, granulocytopenia, or hepatitis occur, the drug must be discontinued. Urticarial rash can sometimes be treated symptomatically.

3. Iodide—Large doses of iodide usually produce a rapid but short-lived blockade of thyroid hormone synthesis and release. This approach is recommended only for acute management of severely thyrotoxic patients or in preparation for thyroidectomy.

C. Radioactive Iodine Therapy

Radioactive iodine ablation of the thyroid is usually reserved for children with Graves disease who do not respond to antithyroid agents, develop adverse effects from the antithyroid agents, fail to achieve remission after several years of medical therapy, or have poor medication adherence. Antithyroid agents should be discontinued 4–7 days prior to radioiodine treatment to allow radioiodine uptake by the thyroid. [131]I is administered orally, concentrating in the thyroid and resulting in decreased thyroid activity. In the first 2 weeks following radioiodine treatment, hyperthyroidism may worsen as thyroid tissue is destroyed and thyroid hormone is released. Temporary therapy with a β-adrenergic antagonist or methimazole may be necessary. In most cases, hypothyroidism develops and thyroid hormone replacement is needed. Long-term follow-up studies have not shown any increased incidence of thyroid cancer, leukemia, infertility, or birth defects when ablative doses of ^{131}I were used.

D. Surgical Treatment

Subtotal and total thyroidectomies may also be considered in children with Graves disease. Surgery is indicated for extremely large goiters, goiters with a suspicious nodule, very young or pregnant patients, or patients refusing radioiodine ablation. Before surgery, a β-adrenergic blocking agent is given to treat symptoms, and antithyroid agents are given for several weeks to minimize the surgical risks associated with hyperthyroidism. Iodide (eg, Lugol solution, one drop every 8 hours, or saturated solution of potassium iodide, one to two drops three times per day) can be given for 1–2 weeks prior to surgery to reduce thyroid vascularity and inhibit release of thyroid hormone. Surgical complications include hypocalcemia due to hypoparathyroidism and recurrent laryngeal nerve damage. An experienced thyroid surgeon is crucial to good surgical outcome. After thyroidectomy, patients become hypothyroid and need thyroid hormone replacement.

Course & Prognosis

Partial remissions and exacerbations may continue for several years. Treatment with an antithyroid agent results in prolonged remissions in one-third to two-thirds of children.

Bauer AJ: Approach to the pediatric patient with Graves' disease: when is definitive therapy warranted? J Clin Endocrinol Metab 2011;96:580–588 [PMID: 21378220].
Rivkees SA: Pediatric Graves' disease: management in the post-propylthiouracil. Int J Pediatr Endocrinol 2014;2014(1):10 [PMID: 25089127].

Neonatal Graves Disease

Transient congenital hyperthyroidism (neonatal Graves disease) occurs in about 1% of infants born to mothers with Graves disease. It occurs when maternal TSH receptor antibodies cross the placenta and stimulate excess thyroid hormone production in the fetus and newborn. Neonatal Graves disease can be associated with irritability, IUGR, poor weight gain, flushing, jaundice, hepatosplenomegaly, and thrombocytopenia. Severe cases may result in cardiac failure and death. Hyperthyroidism may develop several days after birth. In high-risk neonates, TSH receptor antibody (TRAb) level should be obtained at birth and free T4 and TSH obtained day of life 3–5. Immediate management should focus on the cardiac manifestations. Temporary treatment may be necessary with iodide, antithyroid agents, β-adrenergic antagonists, or corticosteroids. Hyperthyroidism gradually resolves over 1–3 months as maternal antibodies decline. As TRAbs may still be present in the serum of previously hyperthyroid mothers after thyroidectomy or radioablation, neonatal Graves disease should be considered in all infants of mothers with a history of hyperthyroidism.

Léger J, Carel JC: Hyperthyroidism in childhood: causes, when, and how to treat. J Clin Res Pediatr Endocrinol 2013;5(Suppl 1):50–56 [PMID: 23154161].
van der Kaay et al: Management of neonates born to mothers with Graves' disease. Pediatrics 2016;137(4):e20151878 [PMID: 26980880].

THYROID CANCER

Thyroid cancer is rare in childhood. Children usually present with a thyroid nodule or an asymptomatic asymmetrical neck mass. Dysphagia and hoarseness are unusual symptoms. Thyroid function tests are usually normal. A "cold" nodule is often seen on a technetium or radioiodine uptake scan of the thyroid. Fine-needle aspiration biopsy of the nodule assists in the diagnosis.

The most common thyroid cancer is papillary thyroid cancer, a well-differentiated cancer arising from the thyroid follicular cell. Follicular thyroid cancer is another type of differentiated thyroid cancer. Treatment consists of total thyroidectomy and removal of involved lymph nodes, often followed by radioiodine ablation to destroy residual thyroid remnant and metastatic tissue left behind after surgery. Thyroid hormone replacement is started to suppress TSH stimulation of residual thyroid tissue and to treat the hypothyroidism that results from surgical removal of the thyroid gland. Since thyroid cancer in children is associated with a high recurrence rate, long-term follow-up is required.

Medullary thyroid cancer arises from the thyroid C cells, which secrete calcitonin, and is associated with elevated serum calcitonin levels. In children, medullary thyroid cancer is usually familial due to an inherited mutation in the RET proto-oncogene as seen in multiple endocrine neoplasia type 2 (MEN2). In affected families, all members should be screened for the mutation, and those identified with the mutation should be treated with prophylactic thyroidectomy in early childhood.

Chan et al: Pediatric thyroid cancer. Adv Pediatr 2017;64(1):171–190 [PMID: 28688588].
Francis GL et al: Management guidelines for children with thyroid nodules and differentiated thyroid cancer. Thyroid 2015;25(7):716–759 [PMID: 25900731].
Wells SA Jr et al: Revised American Thyroid Association guidelines for the management of medullary thyroid carcinoma. Thyroid 2015;25(6):567–610 [PMID: 25810047].

DISORDERS OF CALCIUM & PHOSPHORUS METABOLISM

Calcium plays an important role in virtually every cell. It is necessary for muscle function, neurotransmission, adenosine triphosphate (ATP) metabolism, and many other roles. Serum calcium concentration is tightly regulated by the coordinated actions of the parathyroid glands, kidney, liver, and small intestine. Low serum calcium concentrations, detected by calcium-sensing receptors on the surface of parathyroid cells, stimulate parathyroid hormone (PTH) release. PTH in turn promotes release of calcium and phosphorus from the bone, reabsorption of calcium from the renal tubule, excretion of phosphorus in the urine, and conversion of vitamin D from its inactive to active form. The first step in production of this active form of vitamin D, 1,25 dihydroxy vitamin D (calcitriol), occurs in the liver where dietary vitamin D is hydroxylated to 25-hydroxy vitamin D. The final step in formation of calcitriol is 1α-hydroxylation, which takes place in the kidney under control of PTH. Calcitriol then increases absorption of calcium from the intestines. The net effect of

PTH secretion is to increase serum calcium and decrease serum phosphate.

HYPOCALCEMIC DISORDERS

A normal serum calcium concentration varies with age. It is approximately 8.8–10.2 mg/dL in children and young adults. Preterm infants may be as low as 7 mg/dL. Fifty to sixty percent of calcium in the serum is protein-bound and metabolically inactive. Thus, measurement of ionized serum calcium, the metabolically active form, is helpful if serum proteins are low or in conditions such as acidosis that cause abnormal calcium binding to protein.

ESSENTIALS OF DIAGNOSIS & TYPICAL FEATURES

► Tetany with facial and extremity numbness, tingling, cramps, spontaneous muscle contractures, carpopedal spasm, positive Trousseau and Chvostek signs, loss of consciousness, and convulsions.

► Diarrhea, prolongation of electrical systole (QT interval), and laryngospasm.

► In hypoparathyroidism or pseudohypoparathyroidism (PHP): defective nails and teeth, cataracts, and ectopic calcification in the subcutaneous tissues and basal ganglia.

► General Considerations

Hypocalcemia results from an imbalance of calcium absorption, excretion, and distribution. Causes of hypocalcemia include the following:

- Nutritional calcium deficiency
- Hypoparathyroidism
- Vitamin D deficiency
- Hyperphosphatemia (eg, rhabdomyolysis, tumor lysis syndrome, etc)
- Activating mutation of calcium-sensing receptor (hypercalciuric hypocalcemia)
- Hypomagnesemia
- Hypoalbuminemia (eg, nephrotic syndrome)
- Drugs (eg, diuretics, chemotherapy, transfusion products)

Rickets is a disorder that results from decreased bone mineralization due to deficiencies of calcium and/or phosphate in patient's whose epiphyses have not yet fused. It is characterized by genu varum, prominent costochondral junctions (rachitic rosary), enlarged wrists, frontal bossing, craniotabes, and delayed closure of the fontanelles. Vitamin D deficiency, caused by lack of sunlight exposure or dietary deficiency, is the most common cause of rickets. High rates of occult vitamin D deficiency formed the basis for the 2008 recommendation by the American Academy of Pediatrics that breast-fed infants receive vitamin D supplementation of at least 400 IU/day. Familial hypophosphatemic rickets is due to abnormal renal phosphate loss related to abnormal fibroblast growth factor 23 (FGF23) regulation. Causes and features of the forms of rickets are outlined in Table 34–5.

Deficient PTH *secretion* may be due to deficient parathyroid tissue (DiGeorge syndrome), autoimmunity, or sometimes, magnesium deficiency. Decreased PTH *action* may be due to magnesium deficiency, vitamin D deficiency, or defects in the PTH receptor (eg, pseudohypoparathyroidism). Occasionally, PTH deficiency is idiopathic. Table 34–6 summarizes the clinical and laboratory characteristics of disorders of PTH secretion and action.

Autoimmune parathyroid destruction with subsequent hypoparathyroidism may be isolated or associated with other autoimmune disorders in the APECED (autoimmune polyendocrinopathy-candidiasis-ectodermal dystrophy, or APS-1) syndrome. Hypoparathyroidism may also be secondary to manipulation of the blood supply of the parathyroid glands or removal of the parathyroid glands during thyroidectomy. Autosomal dominant hypocalcemia, also called familial hypercalciuric hypocalcemia, is associated with a gain-of-function mutation in the calcium-sensing receptor, which causes a low serum PTH despite hypocalcemia, and excessive urinary loss of calcium. A family history of hypocalcemia may be the clue that differentiates this condition from other causes of hypocalcemia.

Transient neonatal hypoparathyroidism is caused both by a relative deficiency of PTH secretion and PTH action (see Table 34–6). The late form of transient neonatal hypoparathyroidism (after 2 weeks of age) occurs in infants receiving high-phosphate formulas (whole cow's milk is a well-known example) due to intestinal calcium-phosphate binding, resulting in decreased absorption of intestinal calcium.

► Clinical Findings

A. Symptoms and Signs

Prolonged hypocalcemia from any cause is associated with tetany, photophobia, blepharospasm, and diarrhea. Symptoms of tetany include numbness, muscle cramps, twitching of the extremities, carpopedal spasm, and laryngospasm. Tapping the face in front of the ear causes facial spasms (Chvostek sign), and inflation of a sphygmomanometer above systolic blood pressure causes a carpal spasm (Trousseau sign). Some patients with hypocalcemia exhibit bizarre behavior, irritability, loss of consciousness, and convulsions. Electrocardiogram may demonstrate prolonged QTc. Headache, vomiting, increased intracranial pressure, and papilledema may occur. In early infancy, respiratory distress may be a presenting finding.

Table 34–5. Hypocalcemia associated with rickets.

Condition	Pathogenesis	Disease States/ Inheritance	Clinical Features	Initial Biochemical Findings				
				Serum Calcium	Serum Phosphorus	Serum Alkaline Phosphatase	Other	
Vitamin D-deficiency rickets	Deficient dietary vitamin D, vitamin D malabsorption; other risk factors include dark skin and lack of sunlight exposure	May cluster in families due to shared risk factors	Characteristic skeletal changes appear early, poor growth, symptomatic hypocalcemia is a late finding	Normal until late in course	Low or normal	Elevated	Elevated PTH levels, low 25-OH vitamin D	
Vitamin D 1α-hydroxylase deficiency	Mutation in 1-hydroxylase enzyme required for synthesis of fully active 1,25-OH vitamin D	Autosomal recessive inheritance	Skeletal changes of rickets, symptomatic hypocalcemia	Low	Low or normal	Elevated	Elevated PTH, low 1,25-OH vitamin D	
Vitamin D resistance	Mutation in 1,25-OH vitamin D receptor	Autosomal recessive inheritance	Severe skeletal changes of rickets, total alopecia, symptomatic hypocalcemia	Low	Low or normal	Elevated	Elevated PTH, elevated 1,25-OH vitamin D	
Hypophosphatemic rickets	Excessive loss of phosphate in the urine. Decreased fibroblast growth factor 23 (FGF23) activity	X-linked dominant due to PHEX activation or autosomal dominant due to FGF23 mutations	Skeletal changes primarily in the lower extremities—genu varum or valgus, short stature	Normal or low	Very low	Usually high	Normal PTH levels initially, abnormally high urinary phosphate excretion	

Table 34–6. Hypocalcemia associated with disorders of parathyroid hormone secretion or action.

Condition	Pathogenesis	Inheritance Pattern	Clinical Features	Initial Biochemical Findings[a]			
				Serum Calcium	Serum Phosphorus	Serum Alkaline Phosphatase	Serum PTH
Acquired isolated hypoparathyroidism	Trauma, surgical destruction, iron overload, isolated autoimmune destruction	None known	Symptoms of hypocalcemia	Low	High	Normal or low	Low, low 1,25-OH vitamin D
Familial Isolated hypoparathyroidism	Mutations in GCMB, PTH gene, preproPTH gene	Autosomal recessive (GCMB, PTH gene) or Autosomal dominant (preproPTH gene)	Symptoms of hypocalcemia	Low	High	Normal or low	Low, low 1,25-OH vitamin D
DiGeorge syndrome	Deletion in chromosome 22	Majority represent new mutations	Symptoms of hypocalcemia, cardiac anomalies, immune disorder	Low	High	Normal or low	Low, low 1,25-OH vitamin D
APS type 1	Autoimmune destruction	Autosomal recessive	Mucocutaneous candidiasis, Addison disease; potential for autoimmune destruction in other endocrine glands	Low	High	Normal or low	Low, low 1,25-OH vitamin D
PHP type IA	Mutation in stimulatory G protein; resistance to PTH action	Autosomal dominant	AHO phenotype, short stature, variable hypocalcemia, may have resistance to other hormones using G protein signaling	Low or normal	Elevated or normal	Variable	Very elevated, low 1,25-OH vitamin D
PPHP	Mutation in stimulatory G protein	Autosomal dominant—frequently found within same families with PHP type IA	AHO phenotype, biochemical parameters are normal	Normal	Normal	Normal	Normal
Transient neonatal hypoparathyroidism—early	Deficiency in PTH secretion or action	Sporadic—associated with birth asphyxia, infants of diabetic mothers, or maternal hyperparathyroidism	Onset of symptoms of hypocalcemia within 2 wk of birth	Low	Normal or low	Normal or low	Normal or low, low 1,25-OH vitamin D
Transient neonatal hypoparathyroidism—late onset	Deficiency in PTH secretion or action	Sporadic—associated with infant formulas that have a high phosphate content	Onset of symptoms of hypocalcemia after 2 wk of age	Low	Normal or low	Normal or low	Normal or low, low 1,25-OH vitamin D
Familial hypercalciuric hypocalcemia	Gain of functional mutation of calcium-sensing receptor	Autosomal dominant	Symptoms of hypocalcemia, family history	Low	High	Normal or low	Low, low 1,25-OH vitamin D

AHO, Albright hereditary osteodystrophy; APS, autoimmune polyglandular syndrome; PHP, pseudohypoparathyroidism; PPHP, pseudo-pseudohypoparathyroidism; PTH, parathyroid hormone.

[a] Urinary calcium excretion (calcium-creatinine ratio) is low in all but familial hypercalciuric hypocalcemia.

B. Laboratory Findings

Tables 34–5 and 34–6 outline the specific laboratory findings in various causes of hypocalcemia. It is important to obtain the samples at the time of hypocalcemia. Critical diagnostic samples typically include serum calcium, phosphate, magnesium, intact PTH, 25-hydroxyvitamin D, 1,25-dihydroxyvitamin D. Measurement of urinary excretion of calcium (calcium-creatinine ratio) can also assist in the diagnosis of calcium disorders.

C. Imaging

Soft tissue and basal ganglia calcification may occur in idiopathic hypoparathyroidism and PHP. Various skeletal changes are associated with rickets, including cupped and irregular long bone metaphyses. Torsional deformities can result in genu varum. Accentuation of the costochondral junction gives the rachitic rosary appearance seen on the chest wall.

▶ Differential Diagnosis

Tables 34–5 and 34–6 outline the features of disorders associated with hypocalcemia. In individuals with hypoalbuminemia, the total serum calcium may be low and yet the functional serum ionized calcium is normal. Ionized calcium is the test of choice for hypocalcemia in patients with low serum albumin.

▶ Treatment

A. Acute or Severe Tetany

Symptomatic patients are treated acutely by infusion of IV calcium. Patients are at risk for tissue necrosis if extravasation occurs. Cardiac monitoring should be performed during calcium infusion. Rise in serum calcium is limited to about 2–3 hours after an intravenous calcium bolus infusion, therefore the bolus will need to be followed by oral or continuous calcium infusions if hypocalcemia persists. Given these risks and limitations of intravenous calcium, it is recommended to transition to oral calcium supplementation as soon as patient is no longer symptomatic.

B. Maintenance Management of Hypoparathyroidism or Chronic Hypocalcemia

The objective of treatment is to maintain the serum calcium and phosphate at near-normal levels without excess urinary calcium excretion.

1. Diet—Calcium supplementation should start at a dose of 50–75 mg/kg/day of elemental calcium divided in three to four doses. Supplemental calcium can often be discontinued in patients with rickets after vitamin D therapy has stabilized.

2. Vitamin D supplementation—Ergocalciferol (vitamin D_2) and cholecalciferol (vitamin D_3) are the most commonly used oral vitamin D preparations. Cholecalciferol is slightly more active than ergocalciferol. Calcitriol (1,25-dihydroxy vitamin D_3) supplementation is only recommended for impaired metabolism of dietary vitamin D to 25-OH vitamin D as seen in hepatic dysfunction, impaired metabolism to its active end product, 1,25-dihydroxy vitamin D, or impaired PTH function. Selection and dosage of vitamin D supplements varies with the underlying condition and the response to therapy.

3. Monitoring—Dosage of calcium and vitamin D must be tailored for each patient. Monitoring serum calcium, urine calcium, and serum alkaline phosphatase levels at 1- to 3-month intervals is necessary to ensure adequate therapy and to prevent hypercalcemia, hypercalciuria/nephrocalcinosis, and vitamin D toxicity.

The major goals of monitoring in vitamin D deficiency are to ensure: (1) maintenance of serum calcium and phosphorus concentrations within normal ranges, (2) normalization of alkaline phosphatase activity for age, (3) regression of skeletal changes, and (4) maintenance of an age-appropriate urine calcium-creatinine ratio. The urine calcium-creatinine ratio should be less than 0.8 in newborns, 0.3–0.6 in children, and less than 0.2 in adolescents (when using creatinine and calcium measured in mg/dL).

Clarke B et al: Epidemiology and diagnosis of hypoparathyroidism. J Clin Endocrinol Metab 2016 Jun;101(6):2284–2299 [PMID: 26943720].
Elder CJ, Bishop NJ: Rickets [Review]. Lancet 2014;383:1665–1676 [PMID: 24412049].
Shaw N: A practical approach to hypocalcaemia in children [Review]. Endocr Dev 2015;28:84–100 [PMID: 26138837].

HYPERCALCEMIC STATES

Hypercalcemia is defined as a serum calcium concentration greater than 11 mg/dL. Severe hypercalcemia is a concentration greater than 13.5 mg/dL.

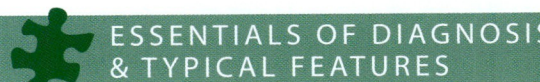

ESSENTIALS OF DIAGNOSIS & TYPICAL FEATURES

▶ Abdominal pain, polyuria, polydipsia, hypertension, nephrocalcinosis, failure to thrive, renal stones, intractable peptic ulcer, constipation, uremia, and pancreatitis.

▶ Bone pain or pathologic fractures, subperiosteal bone resorption, renal parenchymal calcification or stones, and osteitis fibrosa cystica.

▶ Impaired concentration, altered mental status, mood swings, and coma.

General Considerations

Hypercalcemia is less common in children than in adults and etiology varies by age. Table 34–7 summarizes the differential diagnosis of childhood hypercalcemia.

Hyperparathyroidism is rare in childhood and may be primary or secondary. The most common cause of primary hyperparathyroidism is due to a single parathyroid adenoma. Familial hyperparathyroidism may be an isolated disease, or it may be associated with MEN type 1 (MEN1) or rarely type 2A. Hypercalcemia of malignancy is associated with solid and hematologic malignancies and is due either to local destruction of bone by tumor or to ectopic secretion of PTH-related protein (PTHrP). Chronic renal disease with impaired phosphate excretion is the most common cause of secondary hyperparathyroidism.

Table 34–7. Hypercalcemic states.

A. Primary hyperparathyroidism
  1. Parathyroid hyperplasia
  2. Parathyroid adenoma
  3. Familial, including MEN types 1 and 2
  4. Ectopic PTH secretion
  5. Maternal hypoparathyroidism
B. Other hypercalcemic states resulting from increased intestinal or renal absorption of calcium
  1. Hypervitaminosis D (including idiopathic hypercalcemia of infancy)
  2. Familial hypocalciuric hypercalcemia
  3. Lithium therapy
  4. Sarcoidosis
  5. Phosphate depletion
  6. Aluminum intoxication
  7. Subcutaneous fat necrosis (due to vitamin D activation)
  8. Premature infant on human milk or standard formula
C. Other hypercalcemic states
  1. Hyperthyroidism
  2. Immobilization
  3. Lithium and Thiazides
  4. Vitamin A intoxication
  5. Adrenal insufficiency
  6. Hypophosphatasia
  7. Genetic syndromes
    a. William syndrome
    b. IMAGe syndrome
    c. Blue diaper syndrome
    d. Jansen metaphyseal chondrodysplasia
  8. Malignant neoplasms
    a. Ectopic PTH secretion or PTH-related protein (PTHRP)
    b. Prostaglandin-secreting tumors
    c. Tumors metastatic to bone
    d. Myeloma

MEN, multiple endocrine neoplasia; PTH, parathyroid hormone.

Clinical Findings

A. Symptoms and Signs

1. Due to hypercalcemia—Manifestations include hypotonicity and muscle weakness; apathy, mood swings, and bizarre behavior; nausea, vomiting, abdominal pain, constipation, and weight loss; hyperextensibility of joints; and hypertension, cardiac irregularities, bradycardia, and shortening of the QT interval. Coma rarely occurs. Calcium deposits occur in the cornea or conjunctiva (band keratopathy) and are detected by slit-lamp examination. Intractable peptic ulcer and pancreatitis occur in adults but rarely in children.

2. Due to increased calcium and phosphate excretion—Loss of renal concentration causes polyuria, polydipsia, and calcium phosphate deposition in renal parenchyma or as urinary calculi resulting in progressive renal damage.

3. Due to changes in the skeleton—Initial findings include bone pain, osteitis fibrosa cystica, subperiosteal bone absorption in the distal clavicles and phalanges, absence of lamina dura around the teeth, spontaneous fractures, and moth-eaten appearance of the skull on radiographs. Later, there is generalized demineralization.

B. Imaging

Bone changes may be subtle in children. Technetium sestamibi scintigraphy is preferred over conventional procedures (ultrasound, computed tomography [CT], and MRI) for localizing parathyroid tumors.

Treatment

A. Symptomatic

Initial management is vigorous hydration with normal saline to rehydrate the patient, dilute serum calcium concentration, and to promote urinary calcium excretion. Loop diuretic can increase urinary calcium excretion but may exacerbate intravascular volume contraction so should be used with caution. If response is inadequate, glucocorticoids or calcitonin may be used. Bisphosphonates, standard agents for the management of acute hypercalcemia in adults, are being used more often in refractory pediatric hypercalcemia.

B. Chronic

Treatment options vary with the underlying cause. Resection of parathyroid adenoma or subtotal removal of hyperplastic parathyroid glands is the preferred treatment. Postoperatively, hypocalcemia due to the rapid remineralization of chronically calcium-deprived bones may occur (hungry bone syndrome). A diet high in calcium and vitamin D is recommended immediately postoperatively and is continued until serum calcium concentrations are normal and stable. Treatment of secondary hyperparathyroidism from chronic renal disease is primarily directed at controlling serum phosphorus levels with phosphate binders and pharmacologic doses of calcitriol are used to suppress PTH secretion. Long-term therapy for hypercalcemia of malignancy is the treatment of the underlying disorder.

FAMILIAL HYPOCALCIURIC HYPERCALCEMIA (FAMILIAL BENIGN HYPERCALCEMIA)

Familial hypocalciuric hypercalcemia is characterized by slightly elevated serum calcium, low urine calcium, and normal (or slightly elevated) PTH. In most cases, the genetic defect is an inactivating mutation in the membrane-bound calcium-sensing receptor expressed on parathyroid and renal tubule cells. It is inherited as an autosomal dominant trait with high penetrance. There is a low rate of new mutations. Most patients are asymptomatic, and treatment is unnecessary. However, a severe form of symptomatic neonatal hyperparathyroidism may occur in infants homozygous for the receptor mutation.

HYPERVITAMINOSIS D

Vitamin D intoxication is almost always the result of ingestion of excessive amounts of vitamin D. Signs and symptoms of vitamin D–induced hypercalcemia are the same as those in other hypercalcemic conditions. Treatment depends on the severity of hypercalcemia and initial treatment is similar to other hypercalcemic states. However, due to the storage of vitamin D in the adipose tissue, several months of a low-calcium, low-vitamin D diet may also be required.

IMMOBILIZATION HYPERCALCEMIA

Abrupt immobilization, particularly in a rapidly growing adolescent, may cause hypercalcemia and hypercalciuria. Abnormalities often appear 1–3 weeks after immobilization. The mechanism is not fully understood but is thought to result from increased osteoclastic activity and reduced osteoblastic activity. Medical or dietary intervention may be required in severe cases.

HYPOPHOSPHATASIA

Hypophosphatasia is a rare autosomal recessive condition characterized by deficiency of alkaline phosphatase activity in serum, bone, and tissues, resulting from mutations in the gene for tissue-nonspecific isozyme of alkaline phosphatase (TNSALP). Enzyme deficiency leads to poor skeletal mineralization with clinical and radiographic features similar to rickets. Severity ranges from severe skeletal deformity and perinatal death to milder skeletal findings (including craniosynostosis), reduced bone mineral density, and motor delays. Serum calcium levels may be elevated. The diagnosis of hypophosphatasia is made by demonstrating elevated urinary phosphoethanolamine associated with low serum alkaline phosphatase. Enzyme-replacement therapy was approved in 2015 and shows promise for improved prognosis.

Belcher R et al: Characterization of hyperparathyroidism in youth and adolescents: a literature review. Int J Pediatr Otorhinolaryngol 2013 Mar;77(3):318–322 [PMID: 23313432].
Stokes V et al: Hypercalcemic disorders in children. J Bone Miner Res 2017 Nov;32(11):2157–2170 [PMID: 28914984].

GONADS (OVARIES & TESTES)

DEVELOPMENT

Sex development is a complex process beginning with the differentiation of the bipotential gonad into either a testis or ovary. In an infant with a Y chromosome, expression of the transcription factor SRY initiates a cascade of gene expression that directs the formation of testes. Without expression of SRY, ovaries develop; however, a 46,XX complement of chromosomes, in addition to several unique genes, is necessary for the development of normal ovaries. Secretion of testosterone and antimüllerian hormone (AMH) by the testes results in the development of male internal ducts (epididymis, seminal vesicle, and vas deferens) and regression of the müllerian ducts, which are the precursors of the female internal genital structures (fallopian tubes, uterus, and vagina) (Figure 34–6).

The external genitalia develop from sexually indifferent structures called the genital tubercle, the urethral folds, and

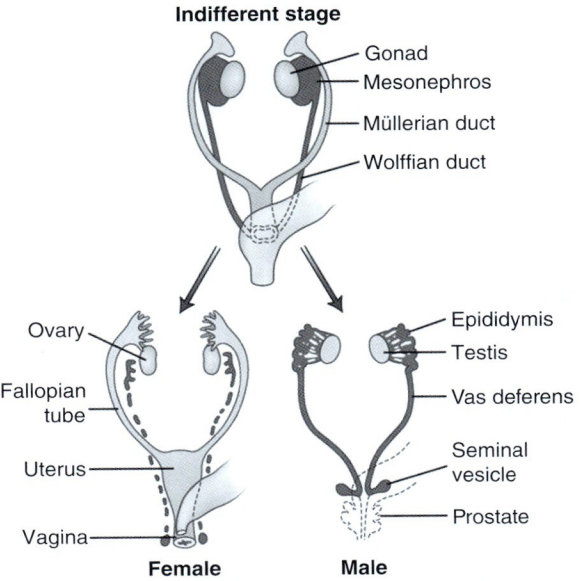

▲ **Figure 34–6.** Differentiation of internal reproductive ducts. (Reproduced with permission from Kronenberg H: *Williams Textbook of Endocrinology*, 11th ed. Philadelphia, PA: Saunders/Elsevier; 2008.)

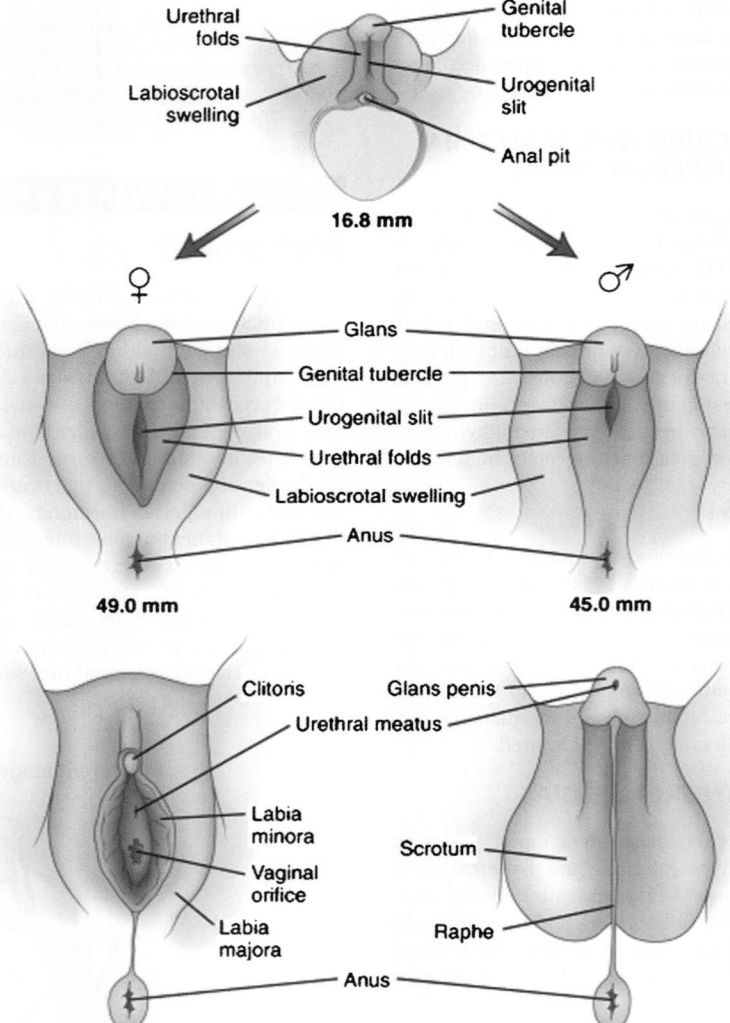

▲ **Figure 34–7.** Differentiation of external genitalia ducts. (Adapted from Spaulding MH: The development of the external genitalia in the human embryo. Contrib Embryol 1921;13:69–88.)

the labioscrotal swellings (Figure 34–7). Development of typical male external genitalia depends on an adequate circulating concentration of testosterone and its metabolite dihydrotestosterone (DHT). Sexual differentiation of the external genitalia is completed at about 12 weeks of gestation.

DIFFERENCES OF SEXUAL DEVELOPMENT

Differences of sex development (DSD) can arise from alterations in three main processes: gonadal differentiation, steroidogenesis, or androgen action. Many DSDs will be evident

in the newborn period, but some will not manifest until later with abnormal pubertal development. In disorders of gonadal differentiation, the testes or ovaries do not develop normally, which results in either ambiguous genitalia or sex reversal. As an example, individuals with 46,XY complete gonadal dysgenesis do not develop normal gonadal tissue (ie, have streak gonads), and this results in typical female internal and external reproductive structures. XY partial gonadal dysgenesis is associated with incomplete testes development and usually results in a phenotype of ambiguous genitalia. Mutations in genes important for gonadal differentiation have been demonstrated in many patients with both complete and partial gonadal dysgenesis. Mixed gonadal dysgenesis is usually due to the presence of both 45,XO and 46,XY cell lines in the same individual. There is typically a testis on one side and a streak gonad on the contralateral side. Ovotesticular DSD occurs when there is both ovarian and testicular tissue. Steroidogenesis refers to steroid hormone biosynthesis and depends on the function of multiple enzymes (Figure 34–8). Enzymatic defects in this pathway can result in increased or decreased androgen synthesis resulting in ambiguous genitalia.

Disorders of androgen action include the diagnosis of androgen insensitivity syndrome (AIS) that is caused by an inactivating mutation in the androgen receptor gene located on the proximal long arm of the X chromosome. In complete AIS (CAIS), there is no androgen action; thus, 46,XY affected individuals have normal appearing female external genitalia with a short vagina, absent müllerian structures and absence or rudimentary wolffian structures. Gonads are located either intra-abdominally or in the inguinal canal. Many of these individuals present when surgery for an inguinal hernia

reveals a testis in the hernia sack. With partial AIS (PAIS), the degree of virilization and ambiguity depends on the degree of abnormality in androgen binding.

Evaluation

On physical examination, dysmorphic features and other congenital anomalies should be noted. The genital examination should include measuring the width and length of the stretched phallus and noting the position of the urethral meatus as well as degree of labioscrotal fusion. The normal stretched penile length (SPL) is greater than 2.0 cm in term male infants. The labioscrotal and inguinal regions should be palpated for the presence of gonads. Since ovaries and streak gonads do not typically descend, the presence of a palpable gonad is suggestive of a 46,XY or 45X/46,XY karyotype. In all these infants, laboratory studies should be done within the first 24 hours of life and include a FISH for SRY/X-centromere, chromosomal analysis or microarray, electrolytes, LH, FSH, testosterone, and 17-hydroxyprogesterone. Additional laboratory evaluation is usually based on these results.

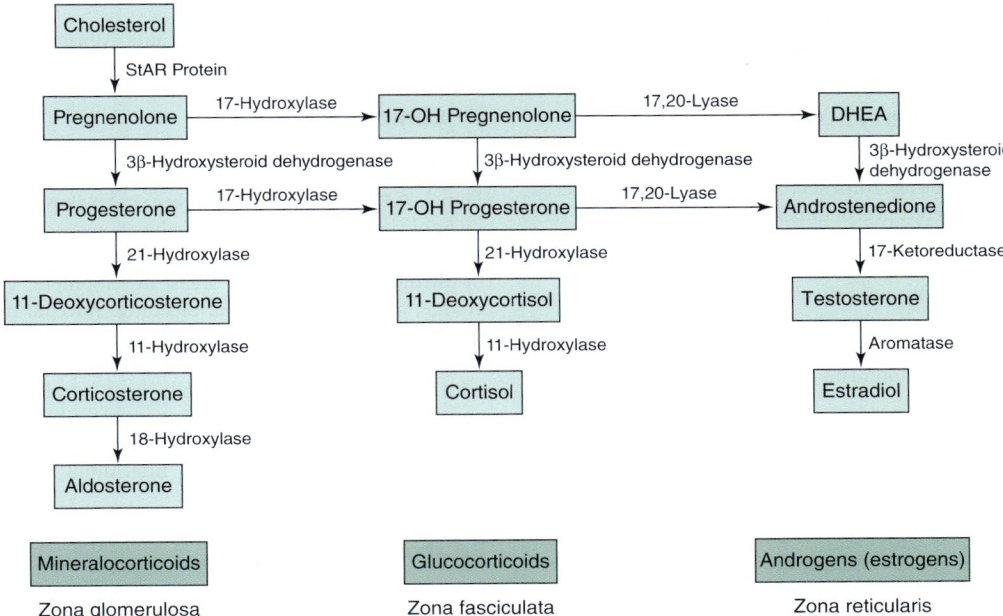

▲ **Figure 34–8.** The corticosteroid hormone synthetic pathway. The pathways illustrated are present in differing amounts in the steroid-producing tissues: adrenal glands, ovaries, and testes. In the adrenal glands, mineralocorticoids from the zona glomerulosa, glucocorticoids from the zona fasciculata, and androgens (and estrogens) from the zona reticularis are produced. The major adrenal androgen is androstenedione because the activity of 17-ketoreductase is relatively low. The adrenal gland does secrete some testosterone and estrogen, however. The pathways leading to the synthesis of mineralocorticoids and glucocorticoids are not present to any significant degree in the gonads; however, the testes and ovaries each produce both androgens and estrogens. Further metabolism of testosterone to dihydrotestosterone occurs in target tissues of the action of the enzyme 5α-reductase. DHEA, dehydroepiandrosterone.

A pelvic ultrasound can be helpful to evaluate for the presence of a uterus; however, ultrasound findings can be unreliable so should be done in an institution that has expertise in pediatric imaging. Many times, laparoscopic examination is necessary to delineate internal structures. It is important that gender assignment be avoided until expert evaluation by a multidisciplinary team is performed. Ideally this team includes pediatric specialists from endocrinology, urology, gynecology, genetics, psychology, and nursing. The team should develop a plan for diagnosis, gender assignment, and treatment options before making any recommendations. Open communications with the parents is essential and their participation in decision-making encouraged.

Arboleda VA, Sandberg DE, Vilain E: DSDs: genetics, underlying pathologies and psychosocial differentiation. Nat Rev Endocrinol 2014:10(10):603–615 [PMID: 25091731].
Lambert SM, Vilain EJ, Kolon TF: A practical approach to ambiguous genitalia in the newborn period. Urol Clin N Am 2010;37(2):195–205 [PMID: 20569798].
Ostrer H: Disorders of sex development (DSDs): an update. J Clin Endocrinol Metab 2014;99:1503–1509 [PMID: 24758178].

ABNORMALITIES IN FEMALE PUBERTAL DEVELOPMENT & OVARIAN FUNCTION

1. Precocious Puberty in Girls

Precocious puberty is defined as pubertal development occurring below the age limit set for normal onset of puberty. Puberty is considered precocious in girls if the onset of secondary sexual characteristics occurs before age 8 years in Caucasian girls and 7 years for African-American and Hispanic girls. Precocious puberty is more common in girls than in boys. Many girls showing signs of puberty between 6 and 8 years of age have a benign, slowly progressing form that requires no intervention. The age of pubertal onset may be advanced by obesity.

Central (gonadotropin-releasing hormone [GnRH]-dependent) precocious puberty (CPP) involves activation of the hypothalamic GnRH pulse generator, an increase in gonadotropin secretion, and a resultant increase in production of sex steroids (Table 34–8). The sequence of hormonal and physical events in central precocious puberty is identical to that of normal puberty. Central precocious puberty in girls is generally idiopathic but may be secondary to a central nervous system (CNS) abnormality that disrupts the prepubertal restraint on the GnRH pulse generator. Such CNS abnormalities include, but are not limited to, hypothalamic hamartomas, CNS tumors, cranial irradiation, hydrocephalus, and trauma. Peripheral precocious puberty (GnRH-independent) occurs independent of gonadotropin secretion. In girls, peripheral precocious puberty can be caused by ovarian or adrenal tumors, ovarian cysts, late-onset congenital

Table 34–8. Causes of precocious pubertal development.

A. **Central (GnRH-dependent) precocious puberty**
 1. Idiopathic
 2. Central nervous system abnormalities
   a. Acquired—abscess, chemotherapy, radiation, surgical trauma
   b. Congenital—arachnoid cyst, hydrocephalus, hypothalamic hamartoma, septo-optic dysplasia, suprasellar cyst
   c. Tumors—astrocytoma, craniopharyngioma, glioma
B. **Peripheral (GnRH-independent) precocious puberty**
 1. Congenital adrenal hyperplasia
 2. Adrenal tumors
 3. McCune-Albright syndrome
 4. Familial male-limited gonadotropin independent precocious puberty
 5. Gonadal tumors
 6. Exogenous estrogen—oral (contraceptive pills) or topical
 7. Ovarian cysts (females)
 8. HCG-secreting tumors (eg, hepatoblastomas, choriocarcinomas) (males)

GnRH, gonadotropin-releasing hormone; HCG, human chorionic gonadotropin.

adrenal hyperplasia (CAH), McCune-Albright syndrome, or exposure to exogenous estrogen.

▶ Clinical Findings

A. Symptoms and Signs

Female CPP usually starts with breast development, followed by pubic hair growth and menarche. However, the order may vary. Girls with ovarian cysts or tumors generally have signs of estrogen excess such as breast development, vaginal discharge, and possibly vaginal bleeding. Adrenal tumors and CAH produce signs of androgen excess that include pubic hair, axillary hair, acne, and increased body odor. Children with precocious puberty usually have accelerated growth and skeletal maturation and may temporarily be tall for age. However, because skeletal maturation advances at a more rapid rate than linear growth, final adult height may be compromised.

B. Laboratory Findings

If the bone age is advanced, further laboratory evaluation is warranted. In CPP, random FSH and LH concentrations may confirm the diagnosis. However, in early central puberty, gonadotropins are secreted overnight and may drop to prepubertal levels during the daytime. If random gonadotropins are in prepubertal range but clinical suspicion remains high for CPP, a GnRH stimulation test is needed to demonstrate a pubertal LH response indicative of CPP. In peripheral precocious puberty, the LH response to GnRH stimulation is suppressed by the autonomously secreted gonadal steroids (see Figure 34–1). In girls with an ovarian cyst or tumor, estradiol levels will be markedly elevated. In girls who present with pubic and/or axillary hair but no breast development, androgen levels (testosterone, androstenedione, dehydroepiandrosterone sulfate) and 17-hydroxyprogesterone should be measured.

C. Imaging

One of the first steps in evaluating a child with early pubertal development is obtaining a radiograph of the left hand and wrist to determine skeletal maturity (bone age). When a diagnosis of central precocious puberty is made, an MRI of the brain should be done to evaluate for CNS lesions. In girls whose laboratory tests suggest peripheral precocious puberty, an imaging of the ovaries and/or adrenal gland may be indicated.

▶ Treatment

Girls with CPP can be treated with GnRH analogues that downregulate pituitary GnRH receptors and thus decrease gonadotropin secretion. Currently, the two most common GnRH analogues used are (1) leuprolide, which is given as an intramuscular injection at 1-, 3-, or 6-month intervals or (2) histrelin subdermal implant, which is replaced annually. With treatment, physical changes of puberty regress or cease to progress and linear growth slows to a prepubertal rate. Projected final heights often increase as a result of slowing of skeletal maturation. After stopping therapy, pubertal progression resumes.

Treatment of peripheral precocious puberty is dependent on the underlying cause. In a girl with an ovarian cyst, intervention is generally not necessary, as the cyst usually regresses spontaneously. Serial ultrasounds are recommended to document this regression. Surgical resection and possibly chemotherapy are indicated for the rare adrenal or ovarian tumor. Regardless of the cause of precocious puberty or the medical therapy selected, attention to the psychological needs of the patient and family is essential.

2. Benign Variants of Precocious Puberty

Benign premature thelarche (breast development) occurs most commonly in girls younger than 2 years. Girls present with isolated breast development without other signs of puberty such as linear growth acceleration and pubic hair development. The breast development is typically present since birth and often waxes and wanes in size. It may be unilateral or bilateral. Treatment is parental reassurance regarding the self-limited nature of the condition. Observation of the child every few months is indicated. Onset of thelarche after age 36 months or in association with other signs of puberty requires evaluation.

Benign premature adrenarche (adrenal maturation) is manifested by early development of pubic hair, axillary hair, acne, and/or body odor. Benign premature adrenarche is characterized by normal linear growth and no or minimal bone age advancement. Laboratory tests will differentiate benign premature adrenarche from late-onset CAH and adrenal tumors. It is recognized that approximately 15% of girls with benign premature adrenarche will go on to develop polycystic ovary syndrome (PCOS).

Fuqua J: Treatment and outcomes of precocious puberty: an update. J Clin Endocrinol Metab 2013;98(6):2198–2207 [PMID: 23515450].
Latronico AC et al: Causes, diagnosis, and treatment of central precocious puberty. Lancet Diabetes Endocrinol 2016;4(3):265–274 [PMID: 26852255].
Utriainen P et al: Premature adrenarche—a common condition with variable presentation. Horm Res Paediatr 2015;83(4):221–231 [PMID: 25676474].

3. Delayed Puberty

Delayed puberty in girls should be evaluated if there are no pubertal signs by age 13 years or menarche by 15 years. Primary amenorrhea refers to the absence of menarche, and secondary amenorrhea refers to the absence of menses for at least 6 months after regular menses have been established. The most common cause of delayed puberty is CGD (Table 34–9). This growth pattern, characterized by short stature, normal growth velocity, and a delay in skeletal maturation, is described in detail earlier in this chapter. The timing of puberty in children with CGD is commensurate to the bone age, not the chronologic age. Girls may also have

Table 34–9. Causes of delayed puberty or amenorrhea.

A. **Constitutional growth delay**
B. **Hypogonadism**
   1. Primary ovarian insufficiency
     a. Gonadal dysgenesis (Turner syndrome, true gonadal dysgenesis)
     b. Premature ovarian failure
       (1) Autoimmune disease
       (2) Surgery, radiation, chemotherapy
     c. Galactosemia
   2. Central hypogonadism
     a. Hypothalamic or pituitary tumor, infection, irradiation
     b. Congenital hypopituitarism
     c. Kallmann syndrome (hypogonadism plus anosmia)
     d. Hyperprolactinemia, Cushing's syndrome, hypothyroidism
     e. Functional (chronic illness, undernutrition, exercise, hyperprolactinemia)
C. **Anatomic**
   1. Müllerian agenesis (Mayer-Rokitansky-Küster-Hauser syndrome)
   2. Complete androgen resistance

delayed puberty from any condition that delays growth and skeletal maturation, such as hypothyroidism and GHD.

Primary hypogonadism in girls refers to a primary abnormality of the ovaries. The most common diagnosis in this category is Turner syndrome, in which the lack of or an abnormal second X chromosome leads to early loss of oocytes and accelerated stromal fibrosis. Other types of primary ovarian insufficiency include 46,XY gonadal dysgenesis and 46,XX gonadal dysgenesis, galactosemia, autoimmune ovarian failure, radiation, and chemotherapy. Premutation carriers for fragile X syndrome are also at increased risk of premature ovarian failure.

Central hypogonadism refers to a hypothalamic or pituitary deficiency of GnRH or FSH/LH, respectively. Central hypogonadism can be functional (reversible), caused by stress, undernutrition, hyperprolactinemia, excessive exercise, or chronic illness. Permanent central hypogonadism is typically associated with conditions that cause multiple pituitary hormone deficiencies, such as congenital hypopituitarism, CNS tumors, or cranial irradiation. Isolated gonadotropin deficiency is rare but may occur in Kallmann syndrome, which is also characterized by hyposmia or anosmia. In either primary or central hypogonadism, signs of adrenarche are generally still present.

Clinical Evaluation

The history should ascertain whether and when puberty commenced, level of exercise, nutritional intake, stressors, sense of smell, symptoms of chronic illness, and family history of delayed puberty. Past growth records should be assessed to determine if height and weight velocity have been appropriate. Physical examination includes body proportions, breast and genital development, and stigmata of Turner syndrome. Pelvic examination or pelvic ultrasonography should be considered, especially in girls with primary amenorrhea.

A bone age radiograph should be obtained. If the bone age is lower than that consistent with pubertal onset (< 12 years in girls), evaluations should focus on finding the cause of the bone age delay. If short stature and normal growth velocity are present, CGD is likely. If growth rate is abnormal, evaluation for causes of growth delay is warranted. Measurement of FSH and LH may not be helpful in the setting of delayed bone age since prepubertal levels are normally low.

If the patient has attained a bone age of more than 12 years and there are minimal or no signs of puberty on physical examination, FSH and LH levels will distinguish between primary ovarian failure (elevated FSH/LH) and central hypogonadism (low FSH/LH). If gonadotropins are elevated, a karyotype should be performed to evaluate for Turner syndrome. Central hypogonadism is characterized by low gonadotropin levels, and evaluation is geared toward determining if the hypogonadism is functional or permanent. Laboratory tests should be directed toward identifying chronic disease and hyperprolactinemia. Cranial MRI may be helpful.

In girls with adequate breast development and amenorrhea, a progesterone challenge may be helpful to determine if sufficient estrogen is being produced and to evaluate for anatomical defects. Girls who are producing estrogen typically have a withdrawal bleed after 5–10 days of oral progesterone, whereas those who are estrogen-deficient or have an anatomical defect have little or no bleeding. The most common cause of amenorrhea in girls with sufficient estrogen is PCOS. Girls who are estrogen-deficient should be evaluated similarly to those who have delayed puberty.

Treatment

Replacement therapy in hypogonadal girls begins with estrogen alone at the lowest available dosage. Oral preparations such as estradiol or topical estrogen patches are used. Estrogen doses are gradually increased every 6 months and then 18–24 months later, progesterone is added either cyclically or continuously. Eventually, the patient may change over to an estrogen-progestin combined pill or patch if desired. Progesterone therapy is needed to counteract the effects of estrogen on the uterus, as unopposed estrogen promotes endometrial hyperplasia. Estrogen replacement will also stimulate growth rates but close growth plates. It is also necessary to promote bone mineralization and prevent osteoporosis.

Nelson LM: Clinical practice: primary ovarian insufficiency. N Engl J Med 2009;360:606 [PMID: 19196677].
Silvereira LF, Latronico AC: Approach to the patient with hypogonadotropic hypogonadism. J Clin Endocrinol Metab 2013;98: 1781–1788 [PMID: 23650335].
Villanueva C, Argente J: Pathology or normal variant: what constitutes a delay in puberty? Horm Res Paediatr 2014;82:213–221 [PMID: 25011467].

4. Secondary Amenorrhea

See discussion of amenorrhea in Chapter 4.

POLYCYSTIC OVARY SYNDROME

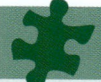 ESSENTIALS OF DIAGNOSIS & TYPICAL FEATURES

► Oligomenorrhea or amenorrhea and clinical or laboratory signs of hyperandrogenism.

► Diagnosis of exclusion and other causes of menstrual dysfunction or elevated androgens need to be ruled out.

► Increased risk of many comorbidities including type 2 diabetes, fatty liver disease, hypertension, depression, and obstructive sleep apnea.

1. General Considerations

Polycystic ovary syndrome (PCOS) is one of the most common menstrual disorders in women, estimated to affect 10%–15% of all reproductive age women. The underlying pathology of PCOS is not well understood. Many girls with PCOS will have a history of early adrenarche. The diagnosis cannot formally be made until at least 1 year post-menarche or with primary amenorrhea, due to the normal duration of time required for girls to establish regular menstrual cycles. Many girls with PCOS are obese, which contributes to an increased prevalence of the disease, but PCOS is also present in girls without obesity. Adolescents with PCOS typically present for cosmetic concerns such as cystic acne or menstrual irregularities. However, PCOS is associated with many comorbidities and it is important to provide comprehensive screening and care.

2. Clinical Findings

PCOS should be considered in adolescents who have (1) menstrual abnormalities including (a) oligomenorrhea of less than 8 menses a year 2 years following menarche, (b) severe oligomenorrhea: more than 90 days between cycle at least a year post-menarche, (c) primary amenorrhea, and (2) clinical signs and symptoms of hyperandrogenism such as hirsutism, cystic acne, androgenic alopecia, and/or biochemical hyperandrogenism. PCOS is a diagnosis of exclusion and other causes of irregular menses should be excluded. Causes of hyperandrogenism such as adrenal tumors, ovarian tumors, or CAH should be ruled out with laboratory testing. The physical examination should be comprehensive and assess for severity of acne, hirsutism as scored by the Ferriman-Gallwey scale, alopecia, acanthosis nigricans, skin tags, pilonidal cysts, hidradenitis, thyroid size, airway and tonsil size, liver size, peripheral edema, striea size, and color and clitoral enlargement. Ovarian ultrasound is not recommended for the diagnosis of PCOS until 8 years post-menarche due to the large variability of normal ovaries in adolescent girls. Uterine ultrasound can be used to determine structural abnormalities causing amenorrhea, thickness of the endometrium in cases of failure to initiate a menstrual bleed following a short course of medroxyprogesterone or to monitor for large cysts causing ovarian pain.

Once a diagnosis of PCOS is established, girls also need to be screened for associated co-morbidities. Adolescents with PCOS have an increased risk of developing insulin resistance and type 2 diabetes, and a 75-g 2-hour oral glucose tolerance should be performed, or alternatively a hemoglobin A_{1C} test at diagnosis and then every 1–2 years. Fasting lipids should be measured at diagnosis and then per American Academy of Pediatrics guidelines. Up to 50% of obese girls with PCOS have nonalcoholic fatty liver disease, and transaminases should be checked at diagnosis, and liver size assessed by examination. The risk of hypertension is increased, and blood pressure should be checked at every appointment with an appropriately sized cuff. If symptoms of obstructive sleep apnea are present, overnight polysomnography should be performed. All girls should be screened for anxiety and depression on a routine basis.

3. Treatment

The treatment for PCOS should be comprehensive, personalized for each individual, and ideally delivered via a coordinated multidisciplinary approach. All girls, even those of normal weight are encouraged to maintain a healthy lifestyle, with moderate to vigorous activity 3–5 days a week and a healthy diet. Monophasic combined oral contraceptives, with 30–35 mcg of estradiol and a third- or fourth-generation nonandrogenic progestin are used to regulate menses, decrease acne, hirsutism, and alopecia. Other methods of delivery including combined estradiol and progesterone patches or vaginal rings can also be used, although they are less reliable for contraception in individuals greater than 200 pounds. Long-acting implantable and uterine progestins can be utilized to prevent endometrial hyperplasia, although due to the risk of weight gain, multiple doses of injectable progesterone should be avoided. Cyclic oral progesterone, at a dose of 10 mg daily for 10 days can be utilized to initiate menses every 3 months in those that do not desire to take oral contraceptives. Metformin, at a dose of 1000 mg twice a day can be used to treat insulin resistance and hyperglycemia and can induce modest improvements in menstrual regularity. The extended-release form can be prescribed at 2000 mg once a day in those with gastric intolerance to the regular formulation. Typical acne treatments should be used, and for hirsutism treatments include spironolactone up to 200 mg/day, eflornithine cream, electrolysis, and laser hair treatment. Topical minoxidil can reduce androgenic alopecia, and alpha-hydroxy acid lotion can be used for acanthosis. Standard therapies for obstructive sleep apnea, hyperlipidemia, hypertension, and psychological disturbances should be utilized as needed. The use of weight loss medications such as topiramate, phentermine, or glucagon like receptor-1 agonist should be considered in older obese adolescents in conjunction with lifestyle therapies. Patients should be seen every 3–6 months, pending the complexity of their medical needs.

Teede HJ et al: Recommendations from the international evidence-based guideline for the assessment and management of polycystic ovary syndrome. Hum Reprod 2018;33:1602–1618 [PMID: 30052961].

Witchel SF et al: The diagnosis of polycystic ovary syndrome during adolescence. Horm Res Paediatr 2015;83:376–389 [PMID: 25833060].

ABNORMALITIES IN MALE PUBERTAL DEVELOPMENT & TESTICULAR FUNCTION

1. Precocious Puberty in Boys

Puberty is considered precocious in boys if secondary sexual characteristics appear before age 9 years and can be central (gonadotropin-dependent) or peripheral (gonadotropin-independent). While the frequency of central precocious puberty is much lower in boys than girls, boys are much more likely to have an associated CNS abnormality (see Table 34–8).

► Evaluation

History should include age at first onset of pubertal signs and the presence of CNS symptoms (eg headaches, polydipsia, vision changes). Appearance of pubic hair is the most common presenting sign of puberty in boys, followed by enlargement of the phallus, scrotal maturation, axillary hair, voice deepening, and increased growth velocity. On physical examination, testicular size differentiates central precocity, in which the testes enlarge (> 2 cm in the longitudinal axis or > 4 mL using Prader beads), from gonadotropin-independent causes, in which the testes usually remain much smaller than expected for the degree of virilization. Tumors of the testis are associated with either asymmetrical or unilateral testicular enlargement.

Laboratory evaluation for precocious puberty will frequently show elevated serum testosterone concentrations. Basal high-sensitivity serum LH and FSH concentrations will be in the pubertal range in boys with central precocious puberty but suppressed in peripheral precocity. GnRH-analogue (leuprolide) stimulation testing can also distinguish central from peripheral puberty but is often not needed in boys because increased testicular volume is usually a reliable physical sign of central puberty. In boys with peripheral precocious puberty caused by CAH, plasma adrenal androgens and 17-hydroxyprogesterone will be elevated. Serum β-HCG concentrations signify the presence of an HCG-producing tumor (eg, CNS dysgerminoma or hepatoma) in boys who present with precocious puberty and testicular enlargement but suppressed gonadotropins. Genetic testing may be helpful in diagnosing familial male-limited precocious puberty (which is due to mutations in the LH receptor).

A radiograph of the left hand to assess epiphyseal maturation (bone age) is useful in evaluating precocious puberty. In all boys with central precocious puberty, brain MRI should be obtained to evaluate for a CNS abnormality. If testing suggests peripheral precocious puberty and laboratory studies are not consistent with CAH, additional imaging may be useful to detect hepatic, adrenal, and testicular tumors.

► Treatment

Treatment of central precocious puberty in boys entails treatment of the underlying cause and the use of GnRH analogues. Boys with McCune-Albright syndrome or familial male-limited precocious puberty are treated with agents that block steroid synthesis (eg, ketoconazole) or with a combination of antiandrogens (eg, spironolactone) and aromatase inhibitors (eg, anastrozole or letrozole) that block the conversion of testosterone to estrogen.

2. Delayed Puberty

Boys should be evaluated for delayed puberty if they have no secondary sexual characteristics by 14 years of age or if more than 5 years have elapsed since the first signs of puberty without completion of genital growth.

By far the most common cause of delayed puberty in boys is CGD, a normal variant of growth. Pathologic hypogonadism in boys may be primary or central. Primary hypogonadism refers to testicular insufficiency and may be due to anorchia; Klinefelter syndrome (47,XXY) or other sex chromosome anomalies; enzymatic defects in testosterone synthesis; or inflammation or destruction of the testes following infection (eg, mumps), autoimmune disorders, radiation, medications (eg chemotherapies), trauma, or tumor. Central hypogonadism refers to deficiencies in pituitary and/or hypothalamic function and may be isolated (gonadotropin deficiency only) or accompany multiple pituitary hormone deficiencies. The etiologies of central hypogonadism in boys are the same as girls (see Table 34–9).

► Evaluation

The history should focus on when first signs of puberty appeared, growth pattern, symptoms of chronic illness, medications/supplements, history of excessive exercise, sense of smell, and family history of delayed puberty. Physical examination should include growth parameters, pubertal stage, and testicular location, size, and consistency. Testes less than 2 cm in length, or less than 4 mL using Prader beads, are prepubertal; symmetric testes more than 2.5 cm or more than 4 mL typically indicate onset of central puberty.

A radiograph of the left hand and wrist to assess bone age should be the first step in evaluating delayed puberty. If bone age is delayed relative to chronological age and growth velocity is normal for a prepubertal boy, CGD is the most likely diagnosis.

Laboratory evaluation may include measurement of LH and FSH levels (if bone age is > 12 years) with elevated gonadotropins indicating primary hypogonadism or testicular failure. Low gonadotropins are not specific but may suggest the possibility of central hypogonadism and warrant further evaluation to assess for pituitary hormone deficiencies, chronic disease, undernutrition, hyperprolactinemia, or CNS abnormalities. Inhibin B, a hormone made by Sertoli cells in the testes, may help differentiate between constitutional delay (normal concentrations) and idiopathic hypogonadotropic hypogonadism (lower concentrations), although there can be significant overlap in levels in these conditions.

► Treatment

Boys with delayed puberty who are troubled by their stature and/or prepubertal appearance may be offered a 4- to 6-month course of low-dose depot testosterone (50–100 mg/mo given intramuscularly) to promote virilization and possibly "jump-start" their endogenous development. In adolescent boys with permanent hypogonadism, testosterone treatment will need to be gradually increased over 3–4 years to adult dosing. Topical testosterone gel applied daily is an alternative to injections but often is too potent in commercially available concentrations to use in early puberty.

3. Gynecomastia

Gynecomastia is a common, self-limited condition that occurs in up to 75% of normal pubertal boys. Adolescent gynecomastia typically resolves within 2 years but may not completely resolve if the degree of gynecomastia is extreme (> 2 cm of tissue). Gynecomastia is more common in obese boys, possibly due to adipose aromatization of testosterone to estrogen. Gynecomastia may also occur in untreated male hypogonadism and as a side effect of some medications. Medical therapy using antiestrogens and/or aromatase inhibitors may be beneficial if initiated early when there is active stimulation of the mammary glands, but given that most pubertal gynecomastia will self-resolve, pharmacologic management is rarely pursued. Surgical intervention should be considered for prolonged and/or severe cases.

Harrington J, Palmert MR: An approach to the patient with delayed puberty. J Clin Endocrinol Metab 2022 Jun;107(6):1739–1750 [PMID: 35100608]

Hutson JM, Thorup J: Evaluation and management of the infant with cryptorchidism. Curr Opin Pediatr 2015 Aug;27(4):520–524 [PMID: 26087417].

Latronico AC et al: Causes, diagnosis, and treatment of central precocious puberty. Lancet Diabetes Endocrinol 2016 Mar;4(3):265–274. [PMID: 26852255].

▼ ADRENAL CORTEX

The adult adrenal cortex consists of three zones responsible for synthesis of distinct steroids from the precursor, cholesterol (see Figure 34–8):

- Outermost zona glomerulosa—mineralocorticoids
- Middle zona fasciculata—glucocorticoids
- Innermost zona reticularis—androgens

The predominant regulator of mineralocorticoid production and secretion is the volume- and sodium-sensitive renin-angiotensin-aldosterone system. Mineralocorticoids promote sodium retention and stimulate potassium excretion in the distal renal tubule.

Glucocorticoid production is under the control of pituitary (see Figure 34–1 and Table 34–1), which is in turn regulated by hypothalamic corticotropin-releasing hormone (CRH). ACTH concentration is greatest during the early morning hours with a smaller peak in the late afternoon and a nadir at night. The pattern of serum cortisol concentration

follows this pattern with a lag of a few hours. In the absence of cortisol feedback, there is dramatic CRH and ACTH hypersecretion.

Glucocorticoids are critical for gene expression in many cell types. Glucocorticoids also help maintain blood pressure by promoting peripheral vascular tone and sodium and water retention. In excess, glucocorticoids are both catabolic and antianabolic; they promote the release of amino acids from muscle and increase gluconeogenesis while decreasing incorporation of amino acids into muscle protein. They also antagonize insulin activity and facilitate lipolysis.

At the onset of puberty, production of androgens (dehydroepiandrosterone and androstenedione) increases and is an important contributor to pubertal development in both sexes. The adrenal gland is the major source of androgen in females.

ADRENOCORTICAL INSUFFICIENCY

Adrenal insufficiency may be primary—due to disorders of the adrenal gland itself, or central/secondary—due to disorders of CRH and/or ACTH secretion. Primary adrenal insufficiency impairs the production of all adrenal steroids, whereas secondary adrenal insufficiency should not affect production of mineralocorticoids or androgens as these are not regulated by ACTH. The causes of primary and secondary adrenal insufficiency are listed in Table 34–10.

▶ Clinical Findings

A. Symptoms and Signs

1. Acute symptoms (adrenal crisis)—Nausea, vomiting, abdominal pain; dehydration; fever (sometimes followed by hypothermia); weakness; hypoglycemia; hypotension and circulatory collapse; and confusion and coma. Acute illness, surgery, trauma, or hyperthermia may precipitate an adrenal

Table 34–10. Causes of adrenal insufficiency.

A. Primary adrenal insufficiency
a. Congenital adrenal hyperplasia (enzyme defect)
b. Addison disease (autoimmune)
c. Hemorrhage (Waterhouse-Friderichsen syndrome)
d. Tumor, calcification, or infection in the gland
e. X-linked adrenal hypoplasia congenita (DAX1 mutation or deletion)
f. Adrenoleukodystrophy
B. Secondary adrenal insufficiency
a. Congenital hypopituitarism secondary to transcription factor mutations or structural defects of the hypothalamus or pituitary; sometimes associated with other midline defects or optic nerve hypoplasia sequence
b. Congenital absence of transcription factors
c. Intracranial tumor
d. Surgery or radiation of the hypothalamus or pituitary gland

crisis in patients with adrenal insufficiency. Adrenal crisis can be life threatening.

2. Chronic symptoms—Fatigue, hypotension, weakness, weight loss or failure to gain weight, vomiting and dehydration, and recurrent hypoglycemia. Additionally, in primary adrenal insufficiency, salt craving and generalized hyperpigmentation are seen.

B. Laboratory Findings

1. Baseline Labs:

- Serum ACTH and renin are elevated in primary adrenal insufficiency but are not helpful in diagnosing central adrenal insufficiency.
- Serum morning fasting cortisol < 3 mcg/dL is highly suggestive of adrenal insufficiency, whereas > 10 mcg/dL is reassuring against adrenal insufficiency.
- Hypoglycemia and hyponatremia can be seen in both primary and central adrenal insufficiency; however only primary adrenal insufficiency will also have hyperkalemia.

2. ACTH (cosyntropin) stimulation test—Intravenous cosyntropin should stimulate functional adrenal glands to produce cortisol that can be measured in plasma within 1 hour. If primary adrenal insufficiency is suspected, a high-dose (250 mcg) of cosyntropin should be given, whereas a low-dose (1 mcg) of cosyntropin is used to evaluate for central adrenal insufficiency. Cortisol less than 18 mcg/dL 30 and 60 minutes after either high- or low-dose intravenous cosyntropin is consistent with adrenal insufficiency.

3. Glucagon stimulation test—Glucagon 0.05 mg/kg or 1 mg given subcutaneously or intravenously should stimulate functional adrenal glands secondary to counter-regulatory mechanisms. Cortisol less than 10 mcg/dL at 120 and 150 minutes is consistent with adrenal insufficiency.

▶ Differential Diagnosis

Acute adrenal insufficiency must be differentiated from sepsis, diabetic coma, CNS disturbances, dehydration, and acute poisoning. In the neonatal period, adrenal insufficiency may be clinically indistinguishable from respiratory distress, intracranial hemorrhage, or sepsis. Chronic adrenocortical insufficiency must be differentiated from anorexia nervosa, depression, neuromuscular disorders, salt-losing nephropathy, malignancy, and chronic debilitating infections.

▶ Treatment

A. Acute Insufficiency (Adrenal Crisis)

1. Hydrocortisone sodium succinate—Hydrocortisone sodium succinate (50 mg/m² intravenously over 2–5 minutes or intramuscularly) is given initially followed by 12.5 mg/m²

IV or oral every 4–6 hours until 24 hours after stabilization and resolution of the acute illness. Patients with known adrenal insufficiency should have intramuscular hydrocortisone 50 or 100 mg for home use in the case of an emergency or inability to tolerate enteral stress dosing.

2. Fluids and electrolytes—In primary adrenal insufficiency, 5%–10% glucose in normal saline, 10–20 mL/kg intravenously, is given over the first hour and repeated if necessary to reestablish vascular volume. Normal saline is continued thereafter at 1.5–2 times maintenance fluid requirements until volume and electrolytes have normalized. In central adrenal insufficiency, routine fluid management is generally adequate after initial restoration of vascular volume and institution of cortisol replacement.

3. Fludrocortisone—Stress doses of hydrocortisone provide adequate mineralocorticoid activity in the acute setting. When oral intake is tolerated, fludrocortisone should be started for primary adrenal insufficiency.

B. Maintenance Therapy

1. Glucocorticoids—A maintenance dosage of 6–10 mg/m²/day of hydrocortisone (or equivalent) is given orally in two or three divided doses. To prevent acute adrenal crises, the dose of hydrocortisone is increased to 30–50 mg/m²/day during intercurrent illnesses or other times of stress (fever, trauma, surgery, or systemic illness) should also be increased during significant diarrhea due to reduced absorption.

2. Mineralocorticoids—In primary adrenal insufficiency, oral fludrocortisone 0.05–0.15 mg daily as a single dose or in two divided doses is given. Periodic monitoring of blood pressure is recommended to avoid overdosing. Children should be given ready access to table salt. In infants, supplementation of breast milk or formula with 3–5 mEq Na⁺/kg/day is generally required until table foods are introduced.

Kirkgoz T, Guran T: Primary adrenal insufficiency in children: diagnosis and management. Best Pract Res Clin Endocrinol Metab 2018 Aug;32(4):397–424 [PMID: 30086866].

Patti G et al: Central adrenal insufficiency in children and adolescents. Best Pract Res Clin Endocrinol Metab 2018 Aug;32(4):425–444 [PMID: 30086867].

CONGENITAL ADRENAL HYPERPLASIAS

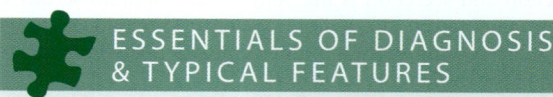

ESSENTIALS OF DIAGNOSIS & TYPICAL FEATURES

- ▶ Primary adrenal insufficiency.
- ▶ Genital virilization in females, with labial fusion, urogenital sinus, enlargement of the clitoris, or other evidence of androgen action in the most common form.

► Increased linear growth and advanced skeletal maturation.

► Elevation of plasma 17-hydroxyprogesterone concentrations in the most common form; may be associated with hyponatremia, hyperkalemia, and metabolic acidosis if mineralocorticoid deficiency included.

General Considerations

Autosomal recessive mutations in the enzymes of adrenal steroidogenesis cause impaired cortisol biosynthesis with increased ACTH secretion. ACTH excess subsequently results in adrenal hyperplasia with increased production of adrenal hormone precursors that are metabolized through the unblocked androgen pathway. Increased pigmentation, especially of the scrotum, labia majora, and nipples, is common due to excessive ACTH secretion. CAH is most commonly (> 90% of patients) the result of homozygous or compound heterozygous mutations in the cytochrome P-450 C21 (CYP21A2) gene causing 21-hydroxylase deficiency (see Figure 34–8). The defective gene is present in 1:250–1:100 people and the worldwide incidence of the disorder is 1:15,000. In its severe form, excess adrenal androgen production starting in the first trimester of fetal development causes virilization of the female fetus and life-threatening hypovolemic and hyponatremic

shock (adrenal crisis) in the newborn if untreated. There are other enzyme defects that less commonly result in CAH. The clinical syndromes associated with these defects are shown in Figure 34–8 and Table 34–11.

Prenatal genetic testing is available and newborn screening by measurement of serum 17-hydroxyprogesterone (17-OHP) is routine in all 50 US states and many countries worldwide.

Clinical Findings in 21-Hydroxylase Deficiency

A. Symptoms and Signs

1. Classic CAH in females—Virilization of the external genitalia varies from mild enlargement of the clitoris to complete fusion of the labioscrotal folds forming an empty scrotum, a penile urethra, a penile shaft, and clitoral enlargement sufficient to form a normal-sized glans (see Figure 34–7). Signs of adrenal insufficiency (salt loss) typically appear 5–14 days after birth. Without adequate treatment, virilization progresses with accelerated growth, pubic hair, acne, voice deepening, and advanced skeletal maturation with premature epiphyseal fusion resulting in a compromised adult height. Central precocious puberty may occur if treatment is not initiated. Other signs of primary adrenal insufficiency, including hyperpigmentation and adrenal crises, can also occur.

Table 34–11. Clinical and laboratory findings in adrenal enzyme defects resulting in congenital adrenal hyperplasia.

Enzyme Deficiency[a]	Elevated Plasma Metabolite	Plasma Androgens	Aldosterone	Hypertension	Salt Wasting	External Genitalia
StAR protein	–	↓↓↓	↓↓↓	–	+	Males: ambiguous Females: normal
3β-Hydroxysteroid dehydrogenase	17-OH pregnenolone (DHEA)	↑ (DHEA)	↓↓↓	–	+	Males: ambiguous Females: possibly virilized
17α-Hydroxylase/17–20 lyase	Progesterone	↓↓	(↑ DOC)	+	–	Males: ambiguous Females: normal, absent puberty
21-Hydroxylase[a]	17-OHP	↑↑	↓↓	–	+	Males: normal Females: virilized
11β-Hydroxylase	11-Deoxycortisol, DOC	↑↑	(↑ DOC)	+	–	Males: normal Females: virilized
P450 oxidoreductase	17-OHP (mild elevation)	↓↓	Normal or mildly elevated	+	–	Males: ambiguous Females: ambiguous

DHEA, dehydroepiandrosterone; DOC, deoxycorticosterone; 17-OHP, 17-hydroxyprogestrone.
[a]Children with "simple virilizing (non–salt-wasting)" forms of 21-hydroxylase deficiency congenital adrenal hyperplasia (CAH) may have normal aldosterone production and serum electrolytes, but some children have normal aldosterone production and serum electrolytes at the expense of elevated plasma renin activity and are, by definition, compensated salt-wasters. These children usually receive mineralocorticoid as well as glucocorticoid treatment. Children with 21-hydroxylase deficiency CAH should therefore have documented normal plasma renin activity in addition to normal serum electrolytes before they are considered non–salt-wasters.

2. Classic CAH in males—The male infant usually appears normal at birth and presents with salt-losing crisis in the first weeks of life if treatment is not initiated. Like females, progressive virilization and skeletal maturation occurs in the setting of inadequate treatment, sometimes leading to central precocious puberty. Testicular adrenal rest tumors develop in many males with CAH. These are often benign and asymptomatic but can result in impaired spermatogenesis and hypogonadism. Like in females, all other symptoms of primary adrenal insufficiency can occur. In some rare enzyme defects, ambiguous genitalia may be present due to impaired androgen production (see Table 34–11).

3. Nonclassic CAH—With mild 21-hydroxylase deficiency, affected individuals have a normal phenotype at birth but develop virilization during later childhood, adolescence, or early adulthood. This is included among the causes of gonadotropin-independent precocious puberty, hirsutism, and/or oligomenorrhea. Nonclassic CAH typically does not present with adrenal crisis.

B. Laboratory Findings

1. Blood—Hormonal studies are essential for accurate diagnosis. Findings characteristic of the enzyme deficiencies are shown in Table 34–11.

2. Genetic studies—Rapid assessment of sex chromosomes should be obtained in any newborn with ambiguous genitalia since 21-hydroxylase deficiency is the most common cause of ambiguity in females.

C. Imaging

Imaging is generally not required to make the diagnosis of CAH. Ultrasonography, CT scanning, and MRI may be useful in defining pelvic anatomy or to exclude an adrenal tumor.

▶ Treatment

A. Medical Treatment

1. Glucocorticoids—Supraphysiologic doses of hydrocortisone are often needed to suppress androgen excess in classic CAH. Maintenance doses of hydrocortisone 10–15 mg/m²/day in three divided doses with dosages adjusted to maintain normal growth rate and skeletal maturation. Serum 17-hydroxyprogesterone and androgens are usually measured to monitor therapy, however the normalization of these lab values often results in overtreatment. The goal is to use the smallest dose of glucocorticoid that will prevent adrenal crisis and virilization while allowing normal growth and development. Excessive glucocorticoids cause the undesirable side effects of Cushing syndrome. Nonclassic CAH may also benefit from glucocorticoid treatment if symptomatic; if not, treatment may not be needed.

2. Mineralocorticoids—In classic CAH, fludrocortisone, 0.05–0.15 mg/day, is given orally once a day or divided in two divided doses. Periodic monitoring of blood pressure, electrolytes and plasma renin activity are recommended to avoid overdosing. Salt supplements are often needed for infants.

B. Surgical Treatment

While early surgery for virilized females was routinely advised in the past, guidelines have evolved in recent years. A multidisciplinary team consultation including urology and/or gynecology should be arranged as soon as possible to inform shared decision-making, including surgical options.

▶ Course & Prognosis

The goal of treatment is to prevent adrenal crises and permit normal growth, development, and sexual maturation. If not adequately controlled, CAH results in sexual precocity and masculinization throughout childhood. If treatment is delayed or inadequate, androgens convert to estrogen resulting in rapid skeletal maturation, and true central precocious puberty may occur. Such children often exhibit tall stature and increased growth velocity in childhood, but their adult height is impaired due to premature epiphyseal fusion. Patient education stressing lifelong therapy is important to ensure adherence. Ongoing psychological evaluation and support is a critical component of care.

Speiser PW et al: Congenital adrenal hyperplasia due to steroid 21-hydroxylase deficiency: an endocrine society clinical practice guideline. J Clin Endocrinol Metab 2018;103(11):4043–4088 [PMID: 30272171].

ADRENOCORTICAL HYPERFUNCTION

ESSENTIALS OF DIAGNOSIS & TYPICAL FEATURES

▶ Truncal adiposity, thin extremities, moon facies, muscle wasting, weakness, plethora, easy bruising, purple striae, decreased growth rate, and delayed skeletal maturation.

▶ Hypertension, osteoporosis, and glycosuria.

▶ Elevated 24-hour urinary free cortisol, elevated midnight salivary cortisol, failed low-dose dexamethasone suppression test.

▶ General Considerations

Cushing syndrome may result from excessive autonomous secretion of adrenal steroids, excess pituitary ACTH secretion

(Cushing disease), ectopic ACTH or CRH secretion, or chronic exposure to exogenous glucocorticoids. In children younger than 12 years, Cushing syndrome is usually iatrogenic.

▶ Clinical Findings

A. Symptoms and Signs

1. Excess glucocorticoid—Adiposity, most marked on the face, neck, and trunk—a fat pad (buffalo hump) in the interscapular area is characteristic but not diagnostic; fatigue; plethoric facies; purplish striae; easy bruising; osteoporosis and back pain; hypertension and glucose intolerance; proximal muscle wasting and weakness; and impairment of growth and skeletal maturation.

2. Excess mineralocorticoid—Hypokalemia and mild hypernatremia, increased blood volume, edema, and hypertension.

3. Excess androgen—Hirsutism, acne, virilization, and menstrual irregularities.

B. Diagnosis of Cushing Syndrome

1. Salivary cortisol—Elevated salivary cortisol obtained at midnight is a specific and sensitive test for hypercortisolism.

2. 24-hour urinary-free cortisol excretion—Elevated 24-hour urinary-free cortisol/creatinine suggests Cushing Syndrome.

3. Low-dose (15 mcg/kg) dexamethasone suppression test—Dexamethasone (15 mcg/kg, max 1 mg) is given at midnight followed by measurement of fasting plasma cortisol and ACTH at 8 AM the following morning. Failure to suppress cortisol less than 1.8 ug/dL suggests Cushing syndrome.

C. Establishing the Cause of Cushing Syndrome

1. ACTH concentration—Decreased ACTH values (< 5 pg/mL) suggest an adrenal cause. Intermediate ACTH values (5–29 pg/mL) are indeterminant and warrant further investigation. Elevated ACTH values (> 29 pg/mL) suggest an ACTH-dependent (pituitary or ectopic) cause.

2. High-dose (8 mg) dexamethasone testing—High-dose dexamethasone testing may help to determine ACTH-dependent Cushing syndrome from ACTH-independent Cushing syndrome.

D. Imaging

Pituitary imaging may demonstrate a pituitary adenoma. Adrenal imaging by CT scan may demonstrate adenoma or bilateral hyperplasia. MRI and nuclear medicine studies of the adrenals may be useful in complex cases.

▶ Differential Diagnosis

Children with exogenous obesity accompanied by striae and hypertension are often suspected of having Cushing syndrome. However, children with Cushing syndrome have a poor growth velocity, relatively short stature, and delayed skeletal maturation, while those with exogenous obesity usually have a normal or slightly increased growth velocity, normal to tall stature, and advanced skeletal maturation. The color of the striae (purplish in Cushing syndrome, pink in obesity) and the distribution of the obesity may assist in differentiation. The urinary-free cortisol excretion may be mildly elevated in obesity, but midnight salivary cortisol is normal and cortisol secretion is suppressed by low-dose dexamethasone suppression test.

▶ Treatment

In cases of primary adrenal hyperfunction due to tumor, surgical removal is indicated. Glucocorticoids should be administered parenterally in pharmacologic doses during and after surgery until the patient is stable. Supplemental oral glucocorticoids, potassium, salt, and mineralocorticoids may be necessary until the suppressed contralateral adrenal gland recovers, sometimes over a period of several months. Similarly, pituitary adenomas and ectopic sources of ACTH or CRH are generally treated surgically.

Lodish et al: Cushing's syndrome in pediatrics: an update. Endocrinol Metab Clin North Am 2018 Jun;47(2):451–462 [PMID: 29754644].

PRIMARY HYPERALDOSTERONISM

Primary hyperaldosteronism may be caused by an adrenal adenoma or adrenal hyperplasia. It is characterized by paresthesias, tetany, weakness, periodic paralysis; nocturnal enuresis; hypokalemia, hypernatremia, metabolic alkalosis; hypertension; glucose intolerance; elevated plasma and urinary aldosterone; and suppressed plasma renin activity. Primary hyperaldosteronism is rare in pediatrics but can occur due to an adrenal tumor or autosomal dominant genetic causes. Imaging and genetic testing are warranted to evaluate the etiology and determine appropriate surgical or medical management.

Funder JW et al: The management of primary aldosteronism: case detection, diagnosis, and treatment: an Endocrine Society Clinical Practice Guideline. J Clin Endocrinol Metab 2016 May;101(5):1889–1916 [PMID: 26934393].

USES OF GLUCOCORTICOIDS & ADRENOCORTICOTROPIC HORMONE IN TREATMENT OF NONENDOCRINE DISEASES

Glucocorticoids are used for their anti-inflammatory and immunosuppressive properties in a variety of conditions. Pharmacologic doses are necessary to achieve these effects, and side effects are common. Numerous synthetic preparations possessing variable ratios of glucocorticoid to mineralocorticoid activity are available (Table 34–12).

Table 34–12. Potency equivalents for adrenocorticosteroids.

Adrenocorticosteroid	Trade Names	Potency/mg Compared With Cortisol (Glucocorticoid Effect)	Potency/mg Compared With Cortisol (Sodium-Retaining Effect)
Glucocorticoids			
Hydrocortisone (cortisol)	Cortef	1	1
Cortisone	Cortone Acetate	0.8	1
Prednisone	Meticorten, others	4–5	0.8
Methylprednisolone	Medrol, Meprolone	5–6	Minimal
Triamcinolone	Aristocort, Kenalog Kenacort, Atolone	5–6	Minimal
Dexamethasone	Decadron, others	25–40	Minimal
Betamethasone	Celestone	25	Minimal
Mineralocorticoid			
Fludrocortisone	Florinef	15–20	300–400

When the prolonged use of supraphysiologic doses of glucocorticoids is necessary, clinical manifestations of Cushing syndrome are common. Side effects may occur with the use of synthetic exogenous agents by any route, including inhalation and topical administration, or with the use of ACTH. Using the lowest effective dose and/or alternate-day therapy reduce the incidence and severity of some of the side effects (Table 34–13).

▶ **Tapering of Pharmacologic Doses of Steroids**

The prolonged use of pharmacologic doses of glucocorticoids causes suppression of ACTH secretion and consequent adrenal atrophy; the abrupt discontinuation of glucocorticoids may result in adrenal insufficiency. ACTH secretion generally does not restart until the administered steroid has been given in subphysiologic doses (< 6 mg/m²/day hydrocortisone equivalent orally) for several weeks.

If pharmacologic glucocorticoid therapy has been given for less than approximately 2 weeks, the drug can be discontinued abruptly because adrenal suppression will be short-lived. However, it is advisable to educate the patient and family about the signs and symptoms of adrenal insufficiency in case problems arise.

In longer treatment durations, stress dose precautions should be provided when therapeutic dosing decreases below approximately 30 mg/m²/day hydrocortisone equivalents. Although it is not unsafe from an adrenal insufficiency perspective to rapidly decrease glucocorticoid dosing to the physiologic range (8–10 mg/m²/day hydrocortisone or equivalent) without tapering, some patients may experience a steroid withdrawal syndrome, characterized by malaise, insomnia, fatigue, and loss of appetite. These symptoms may necessitate a two- or three-step decrease in dose to the physiologic range. Endogenous adrenal function will not resume until glucocorticoid dosing is below physiologic dosing and can take months to fully recover (highly correlated with the duration of suppression). There is no evidence to support any particular regimen of glucocorticoid tapering.

Stress dose precautions need to be continued until endogenous adrenal recovery has been documented. After basal physiologic adrenal function returns, the adrenal reserve or capacity to respond to stress and infection can be estimated by the low-dose ACTH stimulation test. Even if the results of testing are normal, careful monitoring and the use of stress doses of glucocorticoids should be considered during severe illnesses and surgery.

Borresen SW, Klose M, Glintborg D, Watt T, Andersen MS, Feldt-Rasmussen U. Approach to the patient with glucocorticoid-induced adrenal insufficiency. J Clin Endocrinol Metab. 2022 Jun 16; 107(7):2065–2086 [PMID: 35302603].

Wildi-Runge S et al: A search for variables predicting cortisol response to low-dose corticotropin stimulation following supraphysiological doses of glucocorticoids. J Pediatr 2013 Aug;163(2): 484–488 [PMID: 23414662].

ADRENAL MEDULLA PHEOCHROMOCYTOMA

Pheochromocytoma and paragangliomas are uncommon tumors, but up to 20% of reported cases occur in pediatric patients. These neuroendocrine tumors can be located wherever chromaffin tissue (adrenal medulla, sympathetic ganglia, or carotid body) is present. If it arises in the adrenal gland, it is referred to as a pheochromocytoma whereas

Table 34–13. Side effects of glucocorticoid use.

A. **Endocrine and metabolic effects**
   1. Hyperglycemia and glycosuria (chemical diabetes)
   2. Cushing syndrome
   3. Persistent suppression of pituitary-adrenal responsiveness to stress with resultant hypoadrenocorticism

B. **Effects on electrolytes and minerals**
   1. Marked retention of sodium and water, producing edema, increased blood volume, and hypertension (more common in endogenous hyperadrenal states)
   2. Potassium loss with symptoms of hypokalemia
   3. Hypocalcemia, tetany

C. **Effects on protein metabolism and skeletal maturation**
   1. Negative nitrogen balance, with loss of body protein and bone protein, resulting in osteoporosis, pathologic fractures, and aseptic bone necrosis
   2. Suppression of growth, retarded skeletal maturation
   3. Muscular weakness and wasting
   4. Osteoporosis
   5. Avascular necrosis

D. **Effects on the gastrointestinal tract**
   1. Excessive appetite and intake of food
   2. Activation or production of peptic ulcer
   3. Gastrointestinal bleeding from ulceration or from unknown cause (particularly in children with hepatic disease)
   4. Fatty liver with embolism, pancreatitis, nodular panniculitis

E. **Lowering of resistance to infectious agents; silent infection; decreased inflammatory reaction**
   1. Susceptibility to bacterial, viral, fungal, and parasitic infections
   2. Activation of tuberculosis; false-negative tuberculin reaction
   3. Reactivation and poor containment of herpesviruses

F. **Neuropsychiatric effects**
   1. Euphoria, excitability, psychotic behavior, and status epilepticus with electroencephalographic changes
   2. Increased intracranial pressure with pseudotumor cerebri syndrome

G. **Hematologic and vascular effects**
   1. Bleeding into the skin as a result of increased capillary fragility
   2. Thrombosis, thrombophlebitis, cerebral hemorrhage

H. **Miscellaneous effects**
   1. Myocarditis, pleuritis, and arteritis following abrupt cessation of therapy
   2. Cardiomegaly
   3. Nephrosclerosis, proteinuria
   4. Acne (in older children), hirsutism, amenorrhea, irregular menses
   5. Posterior subcapsular cataracts; glaucoma

extra-adrenal locations are called paragangliomas. Pheochromocytoma may be multiple, recurrent, and sometimes malignant. Genetic testing is indicated in pediatric cases including neurofibromatosis 1, MEN2, von Hippel-Lindau syndromes, and mutations of the succinate dehydrogenase genes.

The symptoms of pheochromocytoma are caused by excessive secretion of catecholamines (epinephrine and/or norepinephrine) that can be episodic: headache; sweating; palpitations, tachycardia, hypertension with postural hypotension; anxiety; tremor; dizziness; weakness; nausea, vomiting, diarrhea, weight loss; dilated pupils, blurred vision; abdominal and precordial pain. However, 10%–15% of patients with pheochromocytomas are asymptomatic. Unrecognized and untreated, pheochromocytoma can lead to fatal cardiovascular complications and stroke.

Biochemical testing is indicated for individuals with symptoms of catecholamine excess, adrenal masses incidentally found on imaging, and known genetic mutations associated with pheochromocytoma. Plasma-free metanephrines are the most sensitive and specific test; a level three times the normal range is strongly suggestive of hormonally active tumor, while normal range values exclude pheochromocytoma with high accuracy. Intermediate values require additional testing as medications and collection techniques can lead to false elevations. Plasma chromogranin A can also be measured to aid in the diagnosis of pheochromocytoma. After biochemical tests confirm catecholamine excess, MRI is used to localize the tumor and functional imaging is used to assess for extension and metastases. Surgical removal is the mainstay of treatment; however, massive release of catecholamines intraoperatively occurs if pretreatment with alpha- followed by beta-blockade is inadequate. Long-term prognosis following uncomplicated surgical resection of an isolated pheochromocytoma is generally good for nonmetastatic disease; however, there is a risk of recurrence that requires ongoing surveillance.

Jain A et al: Pheochromocytoma and paraganglioma—an update on diagnosis, evaluation, and management. Pediatr Nephrol 2020;35:581–594 [PMID: 30603807].

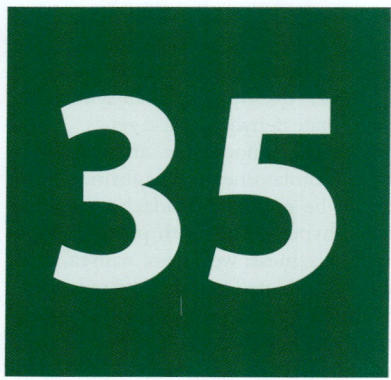

Diabetes Mellitus

Brigitte I. Frohnert, MD, PhD

Erin Cobry, MD

Marian Rewers, MD, PhD

ESSENTIALS OF DIAGNOSIS & TYPICAL FEATURES

► Polyuria (heavy diapers in infants), polydipsia, weight loss, and candidal infections.

► Hyperglycemia and glucosuria, often with dehydration and ketonemia/ketonuria at presentation.

► Diabetic ketoacidosis (DKA) can present as respiratory distress and/or severe nausea and vomiting.

Epidemiology & Description

Diabetes mellitus is defined by chronic hyperglycemia caused by defects in insulin secretion, insulin action, or a combination of the two.

A. Type 1 Diabetes

Type 1 diabetes (T1D) is characterized primarily by insulin deficiency. While it is the most common type of diabetes mellitus in people younger than 20 years, it can develop at any age and most cases are diagnosed after age 20. The classic presentation includes increased thirst (polydipsia), increased urination (polyuria), and weight loss; however, the patient may be overweight or even obese. T1D is further divided into T1a (autoimmune) (~ 95% of the cases) and T1b (idiopathic) diabetes. T1b is more common in individuals of African or Asian ancestry. In the United States, T1D affects an estimated 1.6 million people, including about 244,000 patients younger than 20. Incidence of T1D in youth is about 22 per 100,000 per year, with an annual increase of 2%–4% reported worldwide.

T1D incidence is the highest in children of European ancestry, followed by people of African American and Hispanic ancestry; rates are low in Asians and Native Americans. While most diagnoses occur in older school children, the distribution has shifted to include more infants and preschool age children. About 6% of siblings or offspring of persons with T1D also develop diabetes (compared to 0.2%–0.3% in the general population). However, fewer than 10% of children newly diagnosed with T1D have a parent or sibling with the disease.

B. Type 2 Diabetes

Type 2 diabetes (T2D) is characterized by resistance to the action of insulin. Insulin production may be high initially, but it gradually decreases leading to hyperglycemia. T2D has a heterogeneous phenotype and is diagnosed most often in persons older than 40 who are usually obese and initially not insulin dependent. T2D is rare before age 10; however, puberty is a time of heightened risk for development of T2D in susceptible individuals. Due to increased prevalence of excess weight in childhood, T2D has increased in frequency in older children. T2D is more common in youth of minoritized ethnic and racial groups, particularly the Native American and African American populations. Other risk factors include female sex, poor diet and sleep, and low socioeconomic status. The vast majority of the 29 million patients with diabetes in the United States have T2D, but only about 39,000 patients are younger than 20. Incidence of T2D between ages 10 and 20 in the United States is about 18 per 100,000 per year, with a peak at age 16 and has increased about 5% per year over the past two decades.

C. Monogenic Forms of Diabetes

Monogenic forms of diabetes can be diagnosed at any age and are caused by single gene defects affecting insulin signaling and secretion. The two major categories of monogenic diabetes are maturity-onset diabetes of the young (MODY) and neonatal diabetes. They account for 1%–4% of childhood diabetes but represent the majority of cases diagnosed before the ninth month of life. Neonatal diabetes is transient in about one-half of cases. MODY presents as a nonketotic and usually non–insulin-dependent diabetes in the absence of obesity or islet autoantibodies. A strong family history of early-onset diabetes is common as inheritance is autosomal dominant. The most common forms are due to mutations in glucokinase (*GCK*) or hepatic nuclear factor 1 or 4 genes (*HNF1A* and *HNF4A*). Glucokinase mutations rarely require medications, while other forms respond to oral hypoglycemic agents or insulin. Commercial and research-oriented genotyping services are available to aid correct diagnosis.

D. Diseases of the Exocrine Pancreas

Diseases that impact pancreatic function or loss of pancreatic mass due to damage or surgical removal can result in diabetes. The most common of these is cystic fibrosis (CF)–related diabetes (CFRD) that occurs in about 20% of adolescents with CF and is the most common comorbidity in CF, although it remains to be seen whether newer modulator therapies may alter this trend (for more information, see Chapter 19). The primary defect in CFRD is insulin insufficiency, exacerbated by insulin resistance especially in times of illness or with glucocorticoid therapy. Patients with CF should be screened annually by oral glucose tolerance test (OGTT) beginning by age 10. Other disorders in this category include hereditary hemochromatosis, chronic pancreatitis, and a variety of genetic disorders impacting pancreatic development.

ElSayed et al: 2. Classification and diagnosis of diabetes: standards of care in diabetes-2023. Diabetes Care 2023 Jan;46(Suppl 1): S19–S40 [PMID: 36507649]. https://diabetesjournals.org/care/issue/46/Supplement_1.

Libman I et al: ISPAD Clinical Practice Consensus Guidelines 2022: Definition, epidemiology, and classification of diabetes in children and adolescents. Pediatr Diabetes 2022 Dec;23(8):1160–1174 [PMID: 36537527]. https://www.ispad.org/page/ISPADGuidelines2022.

▶ Pathogenesis

A. Type 1 Diabetes

T1D is caused by a combination of genetic and environmental factors. Autoimmune destruction of the insulin-producing β-cells of the pancreatic islets begins months to years before onset of clinical symptoms and is marked by the presence of autoantibodies to islet cell autoantigens (insulin, GAD65, IA-2, and ZnT8) in the blood. Persistence of two or more islet autoantibodies is highly predictive of development of symptomatic diabetes and defines stage 1 T1D (Figure 35–1). Ongoing β-cell destruction proceeds over months or years, leading first to asymptomatic dysglycemia (stage 2) and later to symptomatic T1D (stage 3) when most β cells have been destroyed. Endogenous insulin production (measured by C-peptide levels) is usually low at diagnosis but may increase after initiation of insulin therapy ("honeymoon period") and persist for weeks or months until eventual total or near-complete loss of β-cell function.

B. Type 2 Diabetes

T2D has a strong genetic component, although the inherited defects vary in different families. T2D progresses differently in youth compared to adults with more rapid decline in β-cell

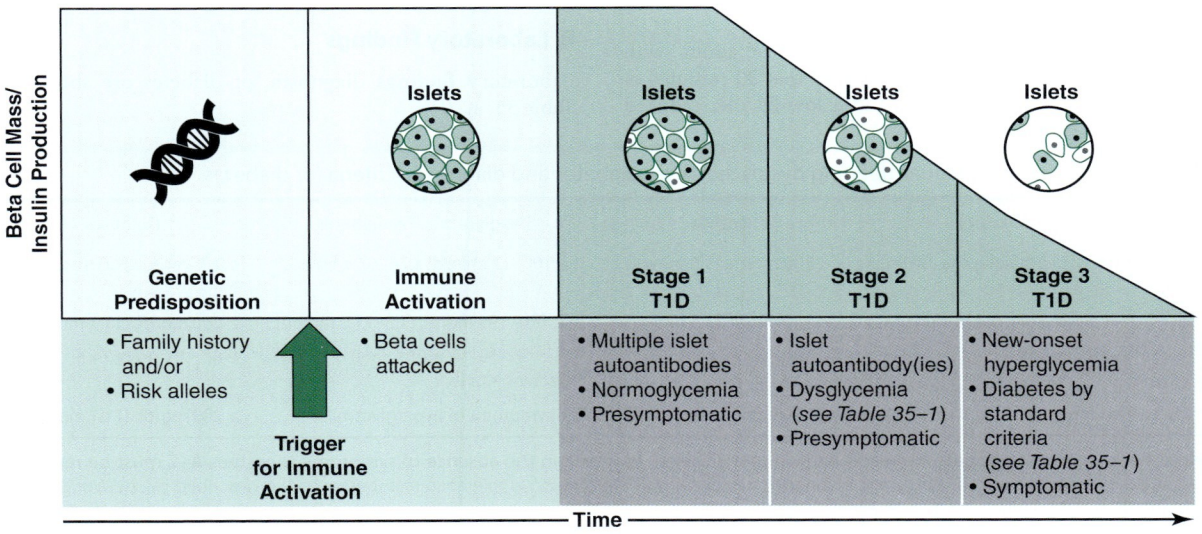

▲ **Figure 35–1.** Pathogenesis of type 1 diabetes (T1D) including staging.

function and greater risk for early complications. Excess weight, particularly central, and lack of exercise contribute to risk but are rarely sufficient alone to cause diabetes in youth.

Prevention

A. Type 1 Diabetes

Islet autoantibodies do not mediate β-cell destruction but offer a useful screening tool, as they are usually present for years prior to diagnosis. Intensive follow-up of individuals with multiple islet autoantibodies (stage 1 T1D) can reduce the severity of illness and risk of DKA upon progression to stage 3 T1D (see Figure 35–1). Antibody screening is not yet standard of care but is available in the research setting for children with a first- or second-degree relative with T1D (www.trialnet.org) or in the general population (www.askhealth.org or www.asktheexperts.org).

As β-cell damage is mediated by T lymphocytes, immunosuppression can slow down β-cell loss. Immunomodulation, including induction of tolerance to islet autoantigens, with or without immunosuppression, is an area of intensive research. In 2022, teplizumab (Tzield), became the first approved intervention available for individuals age 8 years and up with stage 2 T1D. Teplizumab is an anti-CD3 monoclonal antibody that can delay progression from stage 2 to 3 by a median two years. Investigation of teplizumab in younger children is ongoing. Treatment of individuals with early stage 3 T1D has demonstrated benefit in preserving residual β-cell function, but it is not currently approved for this indication. With the dawn of available interventions, identification of individuals with early-stage T1D through islet autoantibody screening is likely to play a significant role in efforts to modify disease progression in the future.

B. Type 2 Diabetes

The Diabetes Prevention Program study of adults with impaired glucose tolerance (IGT) found that 30 minutes of exercise per day (5 days/week) and a low-fat diet reduced the risk of diabetes by 58%. In adults, taking metformin also reduced the risk of T2D by 31%. There are less data in youth; however, a 12-month intensive behavior modification intervention resulted in reduced body mass index (BMI), plasma lipid concentrations, and insulin resistance in obese youth and improved the glycemic profile in youth with prediabetes.

Clinical Findings

A. Symptoms and Signs

Polyuria, polydipsia, and weight loss in a child are unique to diabetes. Other presenting complaints include enuresis, polyphagia, behavioral disturbance, poor growth, blurred vision, and candidal infections. Asymptomatic presentation is more frequent in T2D with up to half of cases identified via screening.

The frequency of diabetic ketoacidosis (DKA) in US children with newly diagnosed T1D is 40%–60% and has increased in the past 20 years. DKA is less common at presentation of T2D; however, rates of DKA at diagnosis of T2D increased from 3%–9% to 20% during the coronavirus-2019 (COVID-19) pandemic. Additionally, up to 2% of children with newly diagnosed T2D present with hyperosmolar hyperglycemic state (HHS). The clinical presentation of DKA includes abdominal pain, nausea, and vomiting that can mimic the flu, gastroenteritis or an acute abdomen. Patients are mildly to moderately dehydrated (5%–10%), may have Kussmaul respirations, and may become progressively somnolent and obtunded. Initial diagnosis can be done in a clinic through measurement of glucose and ketones in blood or urine. Identification of children at early-stage T1D using islet autoantibody screening followed by clinical monitoring has been shown to significantly reduce incidence of DKA at diagnosis.

B. Laboratory Findings

Laboratory findings diagnostic of diabetes are shown in Table 35–1.

Table 35–1. Laboratory values defining dysglycemia/prediabetes and diagnostic criteria for diabetes.

	Measure	Normal	Dysglycemia/Prediabetes	Diabetes
A.	Fasting plasma glucose (no intake for at least 8 h)	< 100 mg/dL (5.6 mmol/L)	IFG:100–125 mg/dL (5.6–6.9 mmol/L)	≥ 126 mg/dL (7.0 mmol/L)
B.	2-h plasma glucose during OGTT	< 140 mg/dL (7.8 mmol/L)	IGT: 140–199 mg/dL (7.8–11.0 mmol/L)	≥ 200 mg/dL (11.1 mmol/L)
C.	Hemoglobin A_{1C}[a]	< 5.7% (39 mmol/mol)	5.7–6.4% (39–47 mmol/mol) or ≥ 10% increase in HbA_{1C}[b]	≥ 6.5 (48 mmol/mol)
D.	Random plasma glucose (in patient with hyperglycemic crisis or classic symptoms of hyperglycemia):			≥ 200 mg/dL (11.1 mmol/L)

Note: For diagnosis of diabetes, any criteria A–D may be used; however, in the absence of symptoms, measures A–C must be repeated.
IFG, impaired fasting glucose; IGT, impaired glucose tolerance; OGTT, oral glucose tolerance test (performed as described by the World Health Organization [1.75 g glucose/kg up to a maximum of 75 g]).
[a]With laboratory method that is NGSP certified and standardized to the Diabetes Control and Complications Trial (DCCT) assay.
[b]Criteria for stage 2 T1D only, not used for defining prediabetes before T2D.

It should be noted that while hemoglobin A_{1C} (A_{1C}) can be used for diagnosis of diabetes, it is less sensitive than blood glucose-based criteria and may underestimate dysglycemia in young children whose progression to T1D can be especially rapid. Thus, a normal A_{1C} does not rule out a diagnosis of diabetes in a young child. Children with impaired fasting glucose (IFG) or IGT and no islet autoantibodies are at elevated risk of T2D and require careful follow-up and lifestyle modification with weight management.

▶ Differential Diagnosis

Blood glucose higher than 200 mg/dL (4.4 mmol/L) in a child is always abnormal and must be promptly and meticulously followed in consultation with a pediatric endocrinology service. If there are significant ketones in urine or blood, treatment is urgent. Conversely, if the presentation is mild and an outpatient diabetes education service is available, hospitalization is often not necessary.

Of note, not all hyperglycemia in children is diabetes; transient, "stress-" or steroid-induced hyperglycemia can occur with illness, trauma, or medications. In an asymptomatic well child, the diagnosis must not be based on a single blood glucose test or on a borderline result obtained using a glucose meter.

Differentiation between the types of diabetes can have important implications for management and education. Testing children for islet autoantibodies can be helpful to establish ongoing islet autoimmunity (T1D). The absence of the three most available autoantibodies (insulin, GAD, and IA-2) provides 80% negative predictive value, and other causes of hyperglycemia should be assessed. Monogenic diabetes should be considered in a child with an autosomal dominant family history of diabetes, presentation before 12 months of age, mild fasting hyperglycemia, a prolonged period of persistent insulin production ("honeymoon") after diagnosis, or associated conditions such as syndromic features, deafness, or optic atrophy. All children diagnosed with diabetes in the first 6 months of life should have genetic screening for neonatal diabetes.

If the A_{1C} is normal, home monitoring of blood glucose for several days, including fasting and 2-hour postprandial measurements, can be helpful to establish the glycemic profile. In children progressing to overt diabetes, hyperglycemia after meals is usually the initial abnormality, while fasting hyperglycemia develops later.

In an era of increasing prevalence of excess weight during childhood, it is important to note that T1D is still much more common than T2D in children, particularly in those who are younger than 10 or prepubertal, regardless of weight status. Factors supporting a diagnosis of T2D include a strong family history, higher-risk ethnic/racial status, increased central adiposity, and puberty. Acanthosis nigricans, a thickening and darkening of the skin over the posterior neck, armpits, or elbows, is a sign of insulin resistance and may increase suspicion for T2D; however, it is present in many children with excess weight and is not specific for the diagnosis of T2D.

▶ Treatment

Treatment of diabetes in youth should take a holistic approach to the child in the context of the family and environment and should include culturally sensitive and developmentally appropriate individualized care by a multidisciplinary diabetes team including a physician, diabetes educator, registered dietician, and psychologist or social worker.

A. General Principles for Diabetes Management

1. Treatment goals—Goals of therapy in diabetes include prevention of acute and long-term complications by reducing chronic hyperglycemia while maximizing quality of life. In T1D, these goals must be tempered by preventing frequent or prolonged hypoglycemia. The A_{1C} level reflects the average blood glucose concentrations over the previous 3 months. It should be noted that A_{1C} is higher in African Americans than in non-Hispanic white cohorts for the same mean glucose concentration. Time in range (TIR) indicates time spent with blood glucose levels between 70 and 180 mg/dL (3.9 and 10.0 mmol/L) and correlates well with A_{1C}. Each child should have targets individually determined to aim for the lowest achievable A_{1C} without severe or recurrent moderate hypoglycemia (Table 35–2)

Table 35–2. Blood glucose and CGM goals for children and adolescents.

	Most Children[a]	Higher Hypoglycemia Risk[b]
Target for A1c	< 7.0% (53 mmol/mol)	< 7.5% (58 mmol/mol)
Targets for CGM or Finger Stick Blood Glucose (most recent 14 days of data)		
Time in range: 70–180 mg/dL (3.9–10.0 mmol/L)	> 70%	> 60%
Time below range < 70 mg/dL (3.9 mmol/L)	< 4%	< 4%
Serious hypoglycemia < 54 mg/dL (3.0 mmol/L)	< 1%	< 1%

CGM, continuous glucose monitoring; HbA$_{1C}$, hemoglobin A$_{1C}$. Goals are for general reference only. ADA guidelines recommend all targets should be individualized to the patient.

[a]Lower A$_{1C}$ target of < 6.5% (48 mmol/mol) may be appropriate during the "honeymoon," those with access to advanced technology and those at low risk of hypoglycemia, such as patients with T2D especially when not on insulin.

[b]Higher hypoglycemia risk includes children without access to optimal diabetes care (analog insulin, CGM, pumps), inability to recognize and communicate symptoms of hypoglycemia, or history of severe hypoglycemic events.

Addressing excess weight and associated comorbidities is also a major focus in maximizing health outcomes (see Chapters 4 and 11).

2. Patient and family education—All caregivers need to learn about diabetes and the importance of daily management to prevent short- and long-term complications. Skills include how to perform home blood glucose monitoring, give insulin or other medications, and manage acute complications. The use of educational books and websites (see reference) can be helpful.

3. Psychosocial care—The diagnosis of diabetes brings on major life changes and relentless challenges. Meeting with a social worker or counselor may help with initial grief and stress responses as well as long-term adaptation. Diabetes in youth is associated with increased risk for depression, anxiety, disordered eating, and diabetes-related distress. People with socioeconomic stressors and excess weight are at higher risk for T2D. These are also risk factors for increased psychological stress, being bullied, depression, and other mental illness.

Routine assessment of diabetes-related knowledge, insulin adjustment skills, goal setting, problem-solving abilities, and self-care autonomy and competence are important, especially around later childhood, adolescence, and transition to adult care. Family functioning, including communication, parental involvement and support, and roles and responsibilities for self-care behaviors (with attention to developmentally appropriate expectations), should be assessed at every visit. Adolescents should be encouraged to assume increased responsibility for diabetes management, but with continued, mutually agreed-upon parental involvement and support. The transition to adult diabetes care should be planned between adolescents, their parents, and the diabetes team well in advance of the actual transfer.

4. Diet and exercise—A dietician is considered a crucial member of the diabetes team and should meet with the patient and family at least once per year, more often when working on weight management. At least 60 minutes of daily aerobic exercise is recommended for children with diabetes, with bone and muscle strength training at least 3 days/wk. Exercise fosters a sense of well-being; helps increase insulin sensitivity; and has a beneficial effect on weight, blood pressure, and high-density lipoprotein (HDL)-cholesterol levels.

Frohnert BI, Chase HP: A First Book for Understanding Diabetes. https://www.childrensdiabetesfoundation.org/books/.
Lindholm O et al; ISPAD Clinical Practice Consensus Guidelines 2022: Diabetes education in children and adolescents. Pediatr Diabetes 2022 Dec;23(8):1229–1242 [PMID: 36120721].
t1dtoolkit.org.

B. Treatment of Type 1 Diabetes

Children with diabetes should be evaluated by a diabetes provider every 3 months to assess glycemic pattern and factors contributing to above- or below-target glycemic trends, measure A_{1C} and TIR, adjust insulin dose according to growth and pubertal changes, and assess for short- and long-term complications and associated conditions.

1. Home blood glucose monitoring—Blood glucose levels should be monitored at least four times daily for safety and insulin management; however, 7–10 glucometer checks per day or the use of a continuous glucose monitor (CGM) is optimal (see A.1 Treatment goals). Glucose data can be downloaded from a device or by real-time wireless sharing to smart phone apps and "the cloud."

CGMs, which include a small metallic filament placed subcutaneously, measure interstitial glucose levels every 1–5 minutes, and can alarm for low and high glucose levels. Some CGMs can pair with an insulin pump and are used to automate insulin delivery (see section Automated Insulin Delivery Systems). As subcutaneous glucose levels can lag blood glucose levels by around 5–15 minutes, especially in times of rapid change, finger stick (glucometer) blood glucose tests are still recommended for hypoglycemic treatment and recovery monitoring.

2. Nutritional management—Nutritional management in children with T1D does not require a restrictive diet, just a healthy dietary regimen with avoidance of liquid carbohydrates. Insulin pump and multiple daily injection (MDI) therapy usually utilize carbohydrate counting in which the grams of carbohydrates to be eaten are counted and matched with a dose of insulin according to a prescribed ratio. This plan allows for the most freedom and flexibility in food choices but requires commitment and expert education. Carbohydrate counting may not be suitable for some families, and other strategies to match insulin to food intake can be used.

3. Insulin—Insulin has three key functions: (1) it allows glucose to pass into the cell for energy production; (2) it decreases the physiologic production of glucose, particularly in the liver; and (3) it turns off lipolysis and ketone production.

A. INSULIN TREATMENT OF NEW-ONSET TYPE 1 DIABETES—In children who present without DKA and who have adequate oral intake, the initial insulin dose can be administered subcutaneously. Typically, 0.2–0.3 U/kg of a long-acting insulin analog provides the "basal" level of insulin. A small amount of rapid-acting analog is used for glucose correction (to bring a high glucose down) and carbohydrate dosing (see Table 35–3 for list of insulin types). This usually suffices for the initial 12–24 hours until systematic diabetes education can be completed.

The initial daily dose of insulin is higher in the presence of ketosis, infection, obesity, or steroid treatment. It also varies

Table 35–3. Types of insulin and kinetics of action.[a]

Type of Insulin	Begins Working	Peak Effect	All Gone
Rapid-acting			
Insulin aspart (Fiasp)	5-10 min	60–70 min	3-5 h
Insulin aspart (NovoLog)	10–15 min	60–90 min	3–5 h
Insulin glulisine (Apidra)	10–15 min	40–90 min	3–5 h
Insulin lispro (Humalog, Admelog, Lyumjev)	10–15 min	60–90 min	3–5 h
Inhaled insulin (Afrezza)[b]	8–12 min	30–45 min	1.5–3 h
Short-acting			
Regular (Humulin R, Novolin R)	30–60 min	2–4 h	5-8 h
Intermediate-acting			
NPH (neutral protamine Hagedorn) (Humulin N, Novolin N)	1–2 h	4–12 h	8–18 h (usually ~ 12 h)
Long-acting			
Insulin degludec (Tresiba)	1–2 h	No peak	> 42 h
Insulin detemir (Levemir)	1–2 h	No peak	12–24 h
Insulin glargine (Lantus, Basaglar, Semglee)	1–2 h	No peak	18–26 h
Insulin glargine (Toujeo)	2–6 h	No peak	24–36 h
Premixed (available in various combinations)			
Humulin 70/30 or Novolin 70/30 (70% NPH/30% regular)	30 min	Dual peak	10–18 h
NovoLog Mix 70/30 (70% NPH/30% aspart) or Humalog Mix 75/25 (75% NPH/25% lispro) or Humalog Mix 50/50 (50% NPH/50% lispro)	15–30 min	Dual peak	10–18 h

[a]Insulin action may vary between individuals or within individual. All insulins listed given by subcutaneous injection, except nasal insulin (Afrezza)
[b]Not approved for those aged < 18 y. Avoid in patients with pulmonary disease

with age, pubertal status, and severity of onset. A total subcutaneous daily dose of 0.3–0.7 U/kg/day may suffice in prepubertal children, while pubertal or overweight children and those with initial A_{1C} greater than 12% (108 mmol/mol) commonly require 1.0–1.5 U/kg/day of insulin during the initial week of treatment. The dose is typically adjusted frequently during the first week starting at the low end of the estimated daily requirement and titrating up based on glucose levels.

The insulin dose peaks about 1 week after diagnosis and decreases slightly with the waning of glucotoxicity and voracious appetite. Approximately 3–6 weeks after diagnosis, most school-aged children and adolescents experience a partial remission or "honeymoon period." Temporary decreases in the insulin doses during this period are necessary to avoid recurrent or severe hypoglycemia. This remission tends to last longer in older children but is rarely complete and never permanent. Other types of diabetes should be considered in patients with persistently unusually low insulin requirements or negative islet autoantibody testing.

B. LONG-TERM INSULIN DOSAGE—The preferred treatment for youth with T1D is an intensive insulin regimen using an insulin pump or basal-bolus MDI. The latter usually consists of three to four injections (boluses) of rapid-acting analog before meals and snacks and one to two injections of long-acting analog insulin per day. (See Table 35–3 for description of insulin options.)

The dose of premeal rapid-acting insulin is calculated based on anticipated carbohydrate content of the meal or snack plus insulin to correct for high blood glucose, if needed. Sliding scales for dosing of rapid-acting insulin (based only on premeal blood glucose level) are helpful initially, while families learn carbohydrate counting. This shortcut assumes that the content of carbohydrates for a given meal or snack is similar from day to day and may lead to significant under- and overdosing in those with highly variable intake. Families who are unable to count carbohydrates can be taught to estimate carbohydrate intake for ongoing sliding scale regimens.

Children younger than 4 years usually need 0.5–2 units of rapid-acting insulin to cover mealtime or snack carbohydrate intake. Children aged 4–10 years may require up to 4 units of rapid-acting insulin, whereas 4–10 units of rapid-acting insulin are commonly used in older children. These estimates do not include correction for high blood glucose and will vary by the individual child.

Rapid-acting insulin is given 10–20 minutes before eating to account for delay in onset of insulin action. If slower human regular insulin is used, the injections should be given 30–60 minutes before meals—rarely a practical option. In young children who eat unpredictably, it may be necessary to wait until after the meal to decide on the appropriate dose of rapid-acting insulin, which is a compromise between avoiding hypoglycemia and tolerating hyperglycemia after meals.

A long-acting insulin is given once or twice a day to maintain basal insulin levels between meals. Daily adjustments in long-acting insulin dose are usually not needed. However, decreases should be made for heavy activity (eg, sports tournaments, hikes) or overnight events to avoid hypoglycemia.

In the past, most children would receive two injections per day of rapid-acting insulin and an intermediate-acting insulin (NPH), often mixed just before injection. About two-thirds of the total dosage would be given before breakfast and the remainder before dinner. This regimen has been shown to be inferior in achieving recommended A_{1C} levels and avoiding hypoglycemia and requires more restrictive eating schedules compared with the basal-bolus regimen described above.

C. Insulin pump treatment—Continuous subcutaneous insulin infusion (insulin pump) therapy is currently the best way to mimic the body's physiologic insulin profile. The standard insulin pump delivers rapid-acting insulin through a tiny tube placed subcutaneously (ie, insulin infusion set) using a variable programmed basal rate that can be adjusted according to the diurnal variation in insulin needs. Lower rates can be set for periods of vigorous activity. The user initiates bolus insulin doses before eating to cover carbohydrate intake as well as correct hyperglycemia. Most pumps can receive glucose data from a meter or CGM, but the child or caregiver must manually enter the amount of carbohydrates being consumed. The pump calculates the amount of insulin needed based on previously entered parameters that include insulin-to-carbohydrate ratios, insulin sensitivity (or correction) factors, glycemic targets, and duration of insulin action (typically set at 2–3 hours). The user must press a button to initiate the suggested bolus or override the suggestion.

Clinical trials have demonstrated lower A_{1C} levels and less severe hypoglycemia with pump therapy compared to MDI. Pump therapy can improve the quality of life in children who fear injections or who desire greater flexibility in their lifestyle, such as with irregular sleep schedules, sports, and irregular eating schedules or behaviors. Insulin pumps are the preferred method of insulin delivery in infants and preschoolers as they often have highly variable and frequent meals and snacks and require small doses of rapid-acting insulin.

The newer generation of insulin pumps can deliver as little as 0.025 U/h.

Infrequent blood glucose monitoring, not routinely changing pump infusion sets, not reacting to hyperglycemia, incorrect carbohydrate counting, or missing food boluses altogether can result in suboptimal pump use. A displaced or obstructed infusion set can cause failure of insulin delivery, which, if not recognized promptly, can lead to ketoacidosis within a few hours. Insulin pump treatment is more expensive than MDI and requires expert training before use.

D. Automated insulin delivery systems—The newest generation of insulin pumps use CGM sensor input to adjust insulin infusion using control algorithms. Systems known as hybrid closed-loop (HCL) or "Artificial Pancreas" systems react to both low and high predicted or actual glucose levels and automatically increase or decrease insulin delivery in response. Some HCL systems only adjust basal insulin delivery, while others additionally deliver automated correction boluses. These systems are associated with significantly higher rates of achieving glycemic targets (A_{1C} and TIR). All current HCL systems perform best when the user gives boluses before meals based on planned carbohydrate consumption.

4. Exercise—Hypoglycemia during exercise or in the 2–12 hours after exercise can be prevented using the following strategies:

1. Careful monitoring of blood glucose before, during, and after exercise.
2. Reducing the amount of injected insulin active during and after exercise. Strategies include reducing bolus dosing for meals within two hours of exercise, temporarily stopping or reducing the basal insulin infusion from an insulin pump or raising glycemic targets in HCL systems ("exercise mode").
3. Providing extra carbohydrates using snacks before the activity. Fifteen grams of glucose usually covers about 30–60 minutes of exercise. Sports drinks containing 5%–10% dextrose during exercise are also often helpful.

5. Sick day management—Families must be educated to check blood or urine ketone levels during any illness. Outside of an illness, ketones should be checked when a fasting blood/CGM glucose level is above 240 mg/dL (13.3 mmol/L), or a randomly measured glucose level is above 300 mg/dL (16.6 mmol/L) as this may indicate a lack of insulin and early development of ketones. The health care provider should be called in the presence of moderate or significant ketonuria or ketonemia (blood β-hydroxybutyrate > 1.0 mmol/L, by meter; moderate or large urine ketones). An additional 10%–20% of the total daily insulin dose is often necessary and should be given subcutaneously as rapid-acting analog or regular insulin every 2–3 hours until blood glucose normalizes, and ketones have cleared. During illnesses and ketosis, water is the oral fluid

of choice if glucose is more than 250 mg/dL (13.9 mmol/L). At lower levels of glycemia, sports drinks or other glucose-containing beverages may be used to raise blood glucose to a level high enough to safely allow insulin administration. Measuring and treating elevated ketones can prevent progression to DKA and allows most patients to be managed at home.

Cengiz E et al; ISPAD Clinical Practice Consensus Guidelines 2022: Insulin treatment in children and adolescents with diabetes. Pediatr Diabetes 2022 Dec;23(8):1277–1296 [PMID: 36537533].

Sherr JL et al; ISPAD Clinical Practice Consensus Guidelines 2022: Diabetes technologies: insulin delivery. Pediatr Diabetes 2022 Dec;23(8):1406–1431 [PMID: 36468192].

C. Treatment of Type 2 Diabetes

Treatment of T2D in children varies with the severity of the disease.

1. Lifestyle management—If the A_{1C} is still near normal, family-centered modification of lifestyle is the first line of therapy. Lifestyle interventions have mixed results in the pediatric population compared to adults, possibly reflecting the complex genetic, family and environmental context for T2D in youth. Interventions should emphasize eating a balanced diet, achieving, and maintaining a healthy weight, and regular exercise. Dietary intervention should be culturally appropriate and recognize limitations in family resources.

2. Medications—Pharmacologic therapy has been historically limited to two approved medications: metformin and insulin; however, in recent years, liraglutide, exenatide and semaglutide have been approved for youth with T2D.

With A1C less than 8.5% (69 mmol/mol) and no symptoms or ketosis, metformin is usually started at a dose of 500 mg daily and increased weekly to a maximum dose of 1000 mg twice daily. If target A1C of less than 7% (53 mmol/mol) is not achieved within 4 months on metformin alone, basal insulin should be considered (up to 1.5 U/kg/day).

If the initial presentation is more severe, with ketosis, A_{1C} 8.5% (69 mmol/mol) or greater, random blood glucose levels 250 mg/dL (13.9 mmol/L) or greater, or uncertainty regarding the distinction between T1D and T2D, initial treatment should include insulin. An initial basal insulin dose of 0.25–0.5 U/kg may be effective. Metformin can be initiated after ketosis has resolved. An attempt to wean insulin can be started after 2–6 weeks, once fasting and postprandial glucose levels have reached normal or near-normal levels. Many youth with T2D can be weaned off insulin and still achieve glycemic targets.

If glycemic targets are not met with metformin (with or without basal insulin), exenatide, liraglutide or semaglutide should be considered. These glucagon-like peptide-1 (GLP-1) agonist medications increase insulin production, reduce glucagon levels, delay gastric emptying, and decrease appetite. Personal or family history of medullary thyroid carcinoma or multiple endocrine neoplasia type 2 are contraindications for these medications. Like adults, youth may experience gastrointestinal side effects (nausea, vomiting and diarrhea), which can be minimized with low initial dose and gradual increase. Of note, both GLP-1 agonists improved weight loss in youth. Clinical trials are under way examining the safety and efficacy of additional pharmacologic therapies in youth. Those who do not reach glycemic targets on combination therapy with metformin, basal insulin, and GLP-1 agonist should be started on prandial insulin (MDI or insulin pump).

3. Home glucose monitoring—Home blood glucose monitoring is typically less frequent in youth who are treated with metformin or lifestyle alone (eg, first morning and 2-hour postprandial test on 3 days/week); however, those taking insulin may require more frequent testing depending on the dose and type of insulin used. CGMs are used less frequently in T2D than T1D but may be helpful even if used intermittently.

Arslanian S et al: Evaluation and management of youth-onset type 2 diabetes: a position statement by the American Diabetes Association. Diabetes Care 2018;41:2648–2668 [PMID: 30425094].

Nadeau KJ et al: Youth-onset type 2 diabetes consensus report: current status, challenges, and priorities. Diabetes Care 2016;39:1635–1642 [PMID: 27486237].

Shah A et al; ISPAD Clinical Practice Consensus Guidelines 2022: Type 2 diabetes in children and adolescents. Pediatr Diabetes 2022 Nov; 23(7) [PMID: 36250645].

QUALITY ASSESSMENT & OUTCOMES METRICS

Recommendations for the medical care of children and adolescents with diabetes and assessment of outcomes are summarized yearly in the American Diabetes Association's (ADA) position statement, the Standards of Medical Care in Diabetes, as well as the International Society for Pediatric and Adolescent Diabetes (ISPAD) Clinical Practice Consensus Guidelines.

In the seminal Diabetes Control and Complications Trial (DCCT) trial, A_{1C} values of 7% (53 mmol/mol), compared to 9% (75 mmol/mol), resulted in greater than 50% reductions in the eye, kidney, cardiovascular, and neurologic complications of T1D. Unfortunately, most US youth with T1D and almost half of youth with T2D are not meeting glycemic targets. In patients with access to comprehensive diabetes care with analog insulins, insulin pump technology and the ability to closely monitor glucose via frequent finger sticks or CGM, a target A1C of less than 7.0% (53 mmol/mol) is recommended. A goal of A_{1C} less than 7.5% (58 mmol/mol) may be more appropriate for those with resource limitations, a history of severe hypoglycemia, hypoglycemia unawareness, or an inability to articulate symptoms of hypoglycemia (eg, young children). A more stringent target of less than 6.5%

(48 mmol/mol) may be appropriate in selected patients, particularly those with residual β-cell function (eg, T2D, T1D in "honeymoon") if this can be achieved without significant hypoglycemia. CGM TIR is also a useful guide for diabetes management. Recommended goals for blood glucose and CGM values to reach A_{1C} targets are shown in Table 35–2.

de Bock M et al; ISPAD Clinical Practice Consensus Guidelines 2022: Glycemic targets and glucose monitoring for children, adolescents, and young people with diabetes. Pediatr Diabetes 2022 Dec;23(8):1270–1276 [PMID: 36537523]. https://www.ispad.org/page/ISPADGuidelines2022.

ElSayed et al; 14. Children and Adolescents: Standards of Care in Diabetes-2023. Diabetes Care 2023 Jan;46(Suppl 1):S230–S253 [PMID: 36507649]. https://diabetesjournals.org/care/issue/46/Supplement_1.

▶ Complications

A. Diabetic Ketoacidosis

Diabetic ketoacidosis (DKA) (see Table 35–4 for definition and findings) is unfortunately still a frequent acute complication in newly-diagnosed T1D, while in established T1D it occurs in those with missed insulin dosing or when insulin administration is insufficient in the context of increased needs (eg, infection, puberty). Repeated episodes of DKA are concerning and should trigger an assessment of barriers to care and adequacy of supervision/support.

Treatment of DKA is based on four physiologic principles: (1) restoration of fluid volume; (2) intravenous insulin infusion (insulin drip) to inhibit lipolysis and reestablish glucose utilization for energy production; (3) replacement of electrolytes; and (4) clearance of acidosis. Laboratory tests at the start of treatment should include venous blood pH, blood glucose, ketone level (blood or urine), and a basic metabolic panel. More severe cases may benefit from determination of blood osmolality, calcium, magnesium, and phosphorus levels. Serum glucose must be measured hourly while on an insulin drip. Electrolytes and venous pH levels should be assessed every two hours. Once venous pH is above 7.15, frequency of venous blood gas assessment can be decreased or eliminated. Monitoring blood β-hydroxybutyrate or urine ketones until resolution of ketosis can be helpful. Management and monitoring are based on severity of DKA (see Table 35–4).

1. Restoration of fluid volume—Severity of dehydration should be assessed on presentation. Initial treatment is with 10–20 mL/kg normal saline (0.9%), during the first hour (repeat in severely dehydrated patients during the second hour). The total volume of fluid in the first 4 hours of treatment should not exceed 20–40 mL/kg and subsequent fluid replacement should not exceed 1.5 times maintenance because of the danger of cerebral edema. As glucose levels drop, 5%–10% dextrose can be added to maintain mild hyperglycemia, allowing continued insulin infusion to resolve the ketoacidosis.

2. Inhibition of lipolysis and reestablishing glucose utilization for energy production—Insulin inhibits lipolysis and subsequent ketone formation and is thus a critical component of resolving acidosis. After the initial fluid bolus, regular insulin is given as a continuous infusion at a rate of 0.05–0.1 U/kg/h to achieve a decrease in blood glucose of approximately 100 mg/dL (5.6 mmol/L) per hour. An IV insulin bolus is not recommended in youth due to increased risk of brain edema. Insulin should be delayed if the patient is hypokalemic (see below). Intravenous insulin should be continued for at least 30 minutes after the initial subcutaneous injection of both a long- and short-acting insulin to prevent rebound ketosis.

3. Replacement of electrolytes—In patients with DKA, both sodium and potassium are depleted. Serum sodium concentrations should be corrected for the degree of hyperglycemia and is usually replaced adequately with rehydration fluids.

Although total body potassium is often depleted, serum potassium levels may be elevated initially because of cellular loss of potassium in the presence of acidosis. Potassium should not be added to IV fluids until the serum potassium level is known to be less than 5.5 mEq/L and urine output is confirmed.

If initial potassium is low (< 3.0 mEq/L), potassium replacement should be started at the time of initial fluid bolus and *before* initiation of insulin, as insulin will drive potassium from the blood into the cells, leading to potential life-threatening cardiac complications. Patients with potassium less than 3.0 mEq/L or greater than 6.0 mEq/L should have an electrocardiogram to assess for dysrhythmia.

4. Correction of acidosis—Acidosis corrects (clears) spontaneously as the fluid volume is restored and insulin facilitates aerobic glycolysis and inhibits ketogenesis. Bicarbonate is generally not recommended as it may increase the risk of cerebral edema.

5. Management of cerebral edema—Some degree of cerebral edema has been shown by computed tomography (CT) scan to commonly occur in DKA. Clinical symptoms are rare, unpredictable, and may be associated with increased risk of death. Cerebral edema may be related to the degree of dehydration, cerebral hypoperfusion, acidosis, decrease in serum sodium during treatment, and hyperventilation at the time of presentation. Neurologic monitoring should occur at least hourly during management of DKA. Early neurologic signs and symptoms may include headache, excessive drowsiness, and dilated pupils. Prompt initiation of therapy includes elevation of the head of the bed, mannitol (1 g/kg over 30 minutes), and fluid restriction. Hypertonic saline (3%) at 2.5–5 mL/kg over 10–15 minutes may be used as an alternative to mannitol or in addition to mannitol if there was no response

Table 35–4. Comparison of diabetic ketoacidosis (DKA) and hyperosmolar hyperglycemic state (HHS).

	DKA	HHS
Epidemiology	T1D, common • New onset • Known T1D with omission of insulin T2D, less common	T2D, rare
Primary defect	Absolute insulin deficiency or insufficient insulin for physiologic stress	Insulin resistance and relative insulin deficiency
Time course for onset	< 1 day	> 1 day
Signs/symptoms	Polyuria/polydipsia Dehydration: Moderate to severe Confusion, drowsiness Abdominal pain Nausea/vomiting Tachypnea/Kussmaul respiration Breath smells of acetone	Polyuria, ± polydipsia Dehydration: Severe to profound[a] Confusion, lethargy, seizure
Laboratory findings		
Glucose	> 200mg/dL[b] (11.1 mmol/L)	> 600 mg/dL (33.3 mmol/L)

Ketosis	Significant:
	  Blood: β-hydroxybutyrate ≥ 3 mmol/L
	  Urine: moderate to large
		Absent or mild:
		  Blood: β-hydroxybutyrate < 0.6 mmol/L
		  Urine: negative to trace

Acidosis	Present:
	  Mild: pH 7.2–7.29 / serum bicarbonate 10–17 mEq/L
	  Moderate: pH 7.1–7.19 / serum bicarbonate 5–9 mEq/L
	  Severe: pH < 7.1 / serum bicarbonate < 5 mEq/L
		Absent or mild[c]:
		  pH > 7.25
		  serum bicarbonate > 15 mEq/L

Osmolality	Moderate to severe[d] (300–320 mOsm/kg)	Severe (> 320 mOsm/kg)
Anion gap	Elevated	Normal to mild elevation
Potassium	Normal to elevated	Normal
Primary treatment	Insulin	Controlled rehydration

[a]Dehydration may be less evident due to preserved intravascular volume.
[b]Rarely, DKA can present with glucose < 200 mg/dL (11.1 mmol/L) in context of recent insulin dosing (after insulin deficiency), decreased caloric/carbohydrate intake, heavy alcohol consumption, chronic liver disease or recent use of sodium glucose cotransporter 2 (SGLT2) inhibitors.
[c]May have mild acidosis due to hypoperfusion, elevated lactate.
[d]A mixed presentation of DKA and HHS (DKA with glucose and osmolality levels meeting HHS criteria) must be managed with consideration for complications of both DKA and HHS.

to initial treatment. If cerebral edema is not recognized and treated early, over 50% of patients will die or have permanent brain damage.

Glaser N et al; ISPAD Clinical Practice Consensus Guidelines 2022: Diabetic ketoacidosis and the hyperglycemic hyperosmolar state. Pediatr Diabetes 2022 Nov;23(7):835–856 [PMID: 36250645].
Websites with useful protocols for DKA and HHS management: https://cpeg-gcep.net/content/dka-hhs-management-resources. http://www.bcchildrens.ca/health-professionals/clinical-resources/endocrinology-diabetes/dka-protocol.

B. Hyperosmolar Hyperglycemic State/ Hyperosmolar Hyperglycemic Nonketotic Syndrome

Hyperosmolar hyperglycemic state (HHS), also known as hyperosmolar hyperglycemic nonketotic syndrome (HHNS), is a rare but severe metabolic decompensation in an individual with some level of insulin production (see Table 35–4). HHS can often go unrecognized until a profound level of dehydration occurs, up to twice the fluid loss seen in DKA. Presentation frequently includes mental status changes ranging from combativeness to coma and seizures (noted in about 50% of cases); however, cerebral edema is quite rare.

Complications of HHS most often relate to thromboembolic events. Rhabdomyolysis may occur, resulting in muscle swelling (including compartment syndrome), kidney failure, and electrolyte disturbances including hypokalemia and hypocalcemia that may lead to cardiac arrhythmia or arrest. There are several reports of a malignant hyperthermia-like syndrome of unclear cause, and treatment with dantrolene should be initiated early if there is fever and elevated creatine kinase. Like reports in adults, HHS in the pediatric population is more common in obese, male African Americans. Adult literature describes HHS as a complication of T2D; however, in the pediatric population, it has been reported in individuals with both T1D and T2D.

Children with HHS should be managed in an intensive care unit with cardiac monitoring and hourly evaluation of serum glucose, vital signs, and hydration status as well as close monitoring of electrolytes, kidney function, osmolality, and creatine kinase (to evaluate for rhabdomyolysis). Cornerstones of care include restoration of fluid volume, avoidance of rapid decline in blood glucose, and replacement of electrolytes.

SEE RESOURCES IN ABOVE SECTION

Glaser N et al; ISPAD Clinical Practice Consensus Guidelines 2022: Diabetic ketoacidosis and the hyperglycemic hyperosmolar state. Pediatr Diabetes 2022 Nov;23(7):835–856 [PMID: 36250645]. Websites with useful protocols for DKA and HHS management: https://cpeg-gcep.net/content/dka-hhs-management-resources. http://www.bcchildrens.ca/health-professionals/clinical-resources/ endocrinology-diabetes/dka-protocol.

C. Hypoglycemia

An excess of insulin administration relative to current needs can result in hypoglycemia, the most common acute complication of T1D. Hypoglycemia is defined as a blood glucose level below 70 mg/dL (3.9 mmol/L). Clinically important or serious hypoglycemia is defined as blood glucose level below 54 mg/dL (3.0 mmol/L). Common symptoms of hypoglycemia are hunger, weakness, shakiness, tachycardia, sweating, drowsiness (at an unusual time), headache, irritability, and confusion. If low blood glucose is prolonged, loss of consciousness and seizures can occur; brain damage or death can occur in severe episodes. Severe hypoglycemic episodes (loss of consciousness or seizure) occur in patients with T1D at a rate of about 3–7 events per 100 patient-years

Children learn to recognize hypoglycemia at different ages but can often report "feeling funny" as young as age 4–5 years. School personnel, sports coaches, and babysitters must be trained to recognize and treat hypoglycemia. Consistency in daily routine, correct insulin dosage, regular glucose monitoring, controlled snacking, adherence to diabetes care plan and good education are all important in preventing severe hypoglycemia. The use of insulin analogs as well as technologies including insulin pumps, CGM, and HCL

systems that use CGM input to control insulin output (see section Treatment), have all helped to reduce the occurrence of hypoglycemia.

The treatment of mild hypoglycemia involves giving 5–15 g of rapidly-absorbed glucose (4 oz of juice; a sugar-containing soda drink, or milk) and waiting 10–15 minutes. If the glucose level is still below 70 mg/dL (3.9 mmol/L), the treatment is repeated. If the glucose level is above 70 mg/dL (3.9 mmol/L), solid foods containing 5–15 g carbohydrate may be given to prevent further hypoglycemia. Moderate hypoglycemia, in which the person is conscious but confused, can be treated by squeezing one-half tube of concentrated glucose (eg, Insta-Glucose or cake frosting) between the gums and lips and stroking the throat to encourage swallowing.

Families should have glucagon in the home, at school, activities, and in their travel pack to treat severe hypoglycemia. Injectable glucagon can be given either subcutaneously or intramuscular and dose is weight-based. A single dose of nasal glucagon (Baqsimi) is as effective as injected glucagon for resolution of hypoglycemia.

Some patients fail to recognize the symptoms of low blood glucose (hypoglycemic unawareness), often after a history of at least 10 years of diabetes or frequent hypoglycemic events. For these individuals, the use of CGM with hypoglycemia alarms or HCL systems should be considered.

Abraham MB et al; ISPAD Clinical Practice Consensus Guidelines 2022: Assessment and management of hypoglycemia in children and adolescents with diabetes. Pediatr Diabetes 2022 Dec;23(8):1322–1340 [PMID: 36537534].

D. Long-Term Complications

Table 35–5 summarizes screening guidelines for complications of both T1D and T2D, including details of timing and methods for assessment.

1. Hypertension—Elevated blood pressure is prevalent among youth with diabetes and strongly predicts micro- and macrovascular complications. Blood pressure should be evaluated at each clinic visit. If hypertension or high-normal blood pressure is confirmed, nondiabetic causes should first be excluded. (For details of evaluation and management, see Chapter 20 and reference below.)

2. Lipid abnormalities—Lipid profiles are generally favorable in children with T1D, but dyslipidemia is more common in children with T2D. Adequate glycemic management should be achieved in newly diagnosed patients prior to screening, but screening should not be delayed more than 1 year after diagnosis. Abnormal results from a random lipid panel should be confirmed with a fasting lipid panel. Initial therapy includes optimizing glycemic management, increasing physical activity, and decreasing saturated fat in the diet using a step 2 American Heart Association diet. Criteria for

Table 35–5. Checklist of recommended diabetes management in children and adolescents.

	Evaluation	Frequency	Assessment/Measure
Glycemic management	Hemoglobin A$_{1C}$ Glucose	Quarterly	See Table 35–2
	Glucose (glucometer or CGM download)	Quarterly	See Table 35–2
Cardiovascular risk	Blood pressure	Quarterly *If high normal or hypertension, confirm on 3 separate days.	Target: < 90th percentile for age, sex, and height or if ≥ 13 y <120/80 mm Hg
	Blood lipid panel (nonfasting)	T1D: Soon after diagnosis in those ≥ 2 y. If LDL ≤ 100 mg/dL, repeat at 9–11 y of age and every 3 y thereafter. T2D: At onset, then annually	LDL (target: < 100 mg/dL [2.6 mmol/L]) HDL (target: > 35 mg/dL [0.91 mmol/L]) Triglycerides (target: < 150 mg/dL [1.7 mmol/L])
	Smoking	Screen at diagnosis and follow-up visits	
Microvascular complications	Nephropathy (Urine microalbumin)	T1D: Annually after 2–5 y of diabetes (Starting age 11 y or puberty if earlier) T2D: At onset, then annually	Urinary ACR (nl: < 30 mg/g) First AM urine sample preferred, but random acceptable initially
	Retinopathy	T1D: Every 2–3 years after 2–5 y of diabetes (Starting age 11 y or puberty if earlier). T2D: At onset, then annually	Retinal photography or dilated ophthalmoscopy
	Neuropathy	T1D: Annually after 2–5 y of diabetes (age 11 y or puberty if earlier) T2D: At onset, then annually	Comprehensive foot examination: 10-g monofilament sensation, pinprick, vibration, pulses and ankle reflexes
Psychosocial	Psychosocial comorbidities	At diagnosis and routinely thereafter	Assess for depression, anxiety, poor diabetes adjustment, disordered eating, and family stresses impacting management
Autoimmune conditions (for T1D only)	Autoimmune thyroid disease	Screen at diagnosis Recheck TSH every 1–2 y if thyroid antibodies negative; more often if symptoms develop or antibodies are positive.	TSH (nl: 0.5–5.0 IU/mL) T$_4$ (nl: 4.5–10 mcg/dL) TPO Ab Antithyroglobulin Ab
	Celiac disease	Screen at diagnosis Repeat within 2 y after diagnosis and again at 5 y, sooner if symptoms or first-degree relative with celiac disease	IgA normal: tTG IgA Ab If IgA deficiency: tTG IgG and IgG-deamidated gliadin peptide Ab
	Addison disease	Quarterly: Assess for signs and symptoms of adrenal insufficiency. Consider lab evaluation if concerns.	21-hydroxylase Ab, plasma ACTH, fasting AM cortisol, electrolytes, plasma renin activity
Obesity-associated comorbidities (typically T2D)	Nonalcoholic fatty liver disease	At diagnosis of T2D and annually thereafter.	AST, ALT
	Sleep apnea	At diagnosis of T2D and routinely thereafter.	Assess for snoring, apnea, poor sleep quality, daytime sleepiness, morning headaches, and enuresis
	PCOS	For females at diagnosis of T2D and routinely thereafter	Assess for menstrual irregularities and signs/symptoms of hyperandrogenism

Ab, antibody; ACR, albumin/creatinine ratio; ACTH, adrenocorticotropic hormone; ALT, alanine aminotransferase; AST, aspartate aminotransferase; CGM, continuous glucose monitor; HDL, high-density lipoprotein; IgA, immunoglobulin A; IgG, immunoglobulin G; LDL, low-density lipoprotein; nl, normal range; PCOS, polycystic ovary syndrome; T$_4$, thyroxine; T1D, type 1 diabetes; T2D, type 2 diabetes; TPO, thyroid peroxidase autoantibodies; TSH, thyroid-stimulating hormone; tTG: tissue transglutaminase.

considering starting lipid-lowering therapy in T1D are age more than 10 years with persistent low-density lipoprotein (LDL) levels greater than 130 mg/dL (4.1 mmol/L) after 6 months of lifestyle changes. Statin therapy is recommended in youth with T2D with persistent LDL greater than 130 mg/dL (3.4 mmol/L). The treatment goals are LDL less than 100 mg/dL (2.6 mmol/L). Statins are teratogenic; therefore, prevention of unplanned pregnancies is critically important in post-pubertal girls.

For youth with T2D and hypertriglyceridemia (fasting triglycerides > 400 mg/dL [5.6 mmol/L] or nonfasting > 1000 mg/dL [11.3 mmol/L]), in addition to lifestyle modifications and promotion of weight loss, some studies have shown efficacy of omega-3 fatty acid supplementation at a dose of 2–4 g/day.

3. Nephropathy—Rapid decline of the glomerular filtration rate (GFR) is the first clinical manifestation of diabetic kidney disease and may be reversible with diligent glycemic and blood pressure management. Microalbuminuria is an early indication of renal damage, defined as urinary albumin excretion rate between 20 and 200 mcg/min, 30–300 mg/day or urinary albumin/creatinine ratio 2.5–25 mg/mmol in males and 3.5–25 mg/mmol in females. The diagnosis of microalbuminuria requires documentation of two out of three abnormal samples over a period of 3–6 months. When persistent microalbuminuria is confirmed and nondiabetic causes of renal disease are excluded, treatment with an angiotensin-converting enzyme (ACE) inhibitor should be started, even if the blood pressure is normal. Patients should be counseled about the importance of glycemic and blood pressure management and smoking cessation, if applicable.

4. Retinopathy—While less common in children, proliferative retinopathy does occur in adolescents with long duration and suboptimal management of diabetes (see Chapter 16 for discussion of treatment and prognosis).

5. Neuropathy—Annual comprehensive foot examination should include inspection; palpation of dorsalis pedis and posterior tibial pulses; evaluation of patellar and Achilles reflexes; and determination of proprioception, vibration, and monofilament sensation.

Bjornstad P et al; ISPAD Clinical Practice Consensus Guidelines 2022: Microvascular and macrovascular complications in children and adolescents with diabetes. Pediatr Diabetes 2022 Dec;23(8):1432–1450 [PMID: 36537531].

Flynn JT et al; Subcommittee on Screening and Management of High Blood Pressure in Children: Clinical practice guideline for screening and management of high blood pressure in children and adolescents. Pediatrics 2017 Sep;140(3):e20171904. doi: 10.1542/peds.2017-1904. Epub 2017 Aug 21 [PMID: 28827377].

ASSOCIATED AUTOIMMUNE DISEASES IN TYPE 1 DIABETES

Table 35–5 summarizes recommended screening for autoimmune diseases in T1D, including frequency and methods.

Thyroid Disease: While Hashimoto thyroiditis (associated with hypothyroidism) is the most common autoimmune thyroid disorder in individuals with T1D (17%–30%), Graves disease (hyperthyroidism) can also occur (~0.5%). Thyroid peroxidase autoantibody (TPO) is usually the first test to become abnormal in autoimmune thyroiditis. If autoantibodies are positive, screening with TSH is recommended every 6–12 months (for management, see Chapter 34).

Celiac Disease: Transglutaminase autoantibodies offer a sensitive and specific screening test for celiac disease affecting up to 10% of children with T1D with the highest risk in those diagnosed with T1D before age 5. Untreated celiac disease may lead to severe hypoglycemia (due to malabsorption), poor growth or weight gain, increased bone turnover, decreased bone mineralization, and other long-term complications (see Chapter 21 for further detail of diagnosis and management).

Addison Disease: The 21-hydroxylase autoantibody, a marker of increased risk of Addison disease, is present in approximately 2% of patients with T1D. Addison disease develops (usually slowly) in only about one-third of these antibody-positive individuals (see Chapter 34).

Other: Less common autoimmune disorders that occur more frequently in those with T1D than the general population include juvenile idiopathic arthritis, lupus, psoriasis, scleroderma, vitiligo, dermatomyositis, autoimmune hepatitis, autoimmune gastritis, pernicious anemia, alopecia, and myasthenia gravis.

Fröhlich-Reiterer E et al; ISPAD Clinical Practice Consensus Guidelines 2022: Other complications and associated conditions in children and adolescents with type 1 diabetes. Pediatr Diabetes 2022 Dec;23(8):1451–1467 [PMID: 36537532].

ASSOCIATED CONDITIONS WITH TYPE 2 DIABETES

At the time of diagnosis of T2D, comorbidities such as hypertension, dyslipidemia, nephropathy, and retinopathy may already be present and therefore should be evaluated within initial visits followed by ongoing screening (see Table 35–5). As T2D in youth frequently occurs in the setting of excess weight, hepatic steatosis, sleep apnea, and orthopedic complications should also be assessed (see Chapters 4 and 11). In female adolescents with T2D, assessment for polycystic ovary syndrome (PCOS) should also be considered (see Chapter 4).

▶ Prognosis

The long-term prognosis of children diagnosed with T1D has improved significantly over the past 20 years, primarily due to better management of blood glucose and blood pressure with medications and established screening guidelines. While life expectancy is now only slightly shorter compared to the general population, the risk of cardiovascular disease in later adulthood remains 4–10 times higher, especially in women. Adults with T2D diagnosed during childhood have a significantly higher prevalence of complications compared to those with T1D.

Modern diabetes management generally leads to excellent health outcomes. Tremendous progress in biotechnology—insulin analogs, insulin pumps, continuous glucose monitoring, as well as the HCL systems—has reduced the risk of acute and long-term complications. However, comprehensive, and continuing education of children and their families remains the foundation of a healthy and quality life with diabetes.

36

Inborn Errors of Metabolism

Janet A. Thomas, MD

Johan L. K. Van Hove, MD, PhD, MBA

Austin A. Larson, MD

Peter R. Baker II, MD

INTRODUCTION

Disorders in which single-gene defects cause clinically significant blocks in metabolic pathways are called *inborn errors of metabolism* (IEM). Once considered rare, the number of recognized IEM has increased dramatically, now recognized to affect 1:1500 children. Many of these disorders can be treated effectively. Even when treatment is not available, correct diagnosis permits parents to make informed decisions about future offspring.

Pathology in IEM usually results from accumulation of enzyme substrate behind a metabolic block or from deficiency of a reaction product. In some cases, the accumulated enzyme substrate is diffusible and has adverse effects on distant organs; in other cases, as in lysosomal storage diseases, the substrate primarily accumulates locally. The clinical manifestations of inborn errors vary widely with both mild and severe forms of virtually every disorder. Phenotypes vary from classic to more rare clinical presentations based on residual enzyme activity, which is in large part determined by specific mutations in a common gene.

One treatment strategy is to enhance the reduced enzyme activity. Gene replacement is a long-term goal. Previous problems with gene delivery to target organs and control of gene action made this clinically unavailable; however, numerous clinical research trials are now occurring and offer hope for success. Enzyme-replacement therapies using intravenously, intrathecally, or intraventricularly administered enzymes have been developed as effective strategies in many lysosomal storage disorders and more continue to be developed. Subcutaneous enzyme replacement therapy is also under development. Enzyme substitution therapy via subcutaneous injection with a modified bacterial enzyme is also now available for at least one disorder. Organ transplantation (liver, kidney, heart, or bone marrow) can provide a source of enzyme for some conditions. Pharmacologic doses of a cofactor such as a vitamin can sometimes be effective in restoring enzyme activity. Residual activity can be increased by pharmacologically promoting transcription (transcriptional upregulation) or by stabilizing the protein product through therapy with chaperones. Alternatively, some strategies are designed to cope with the consequences of enzyme deficiency. Strategies used to avoid substrate accumulation include restriction of precursor in the diet (eg, low-phenylalanine diet for phenylketonuria [PKU]), avoidance of catabolism (fasting or vomiting illnesses), inhibition of an enzyme in the synthesis of the precursor (eg, 2-(2-nitro-4-trifluoromethylbenzoyl)-1,3-cyclohexanedione [NTBC] therapy in tyrosinemia type I) (see section Hereditary Tyrosinemia), or removal of accumulated substrate pharmacologically (eg, glycine therapy for isovaleric acidemia) or by dialysis. An inadequately produced metabolite can also be supplemented (eg, glucose administration for glycogen storage disease [GSD] type I).

Inborn errors can manifest at any age, affect any organ system, and mimic many common pediatric problems. This chapter focuses on when to consider an IEM in the differential diagnosis of common pediatric problems. A few of the more important disorders are then discussed in detail.

DIAGNOSIS

SUSPECTING INBORN ERRORS OF METABOLISM

Inborn errors of metabolism (IEM) must be considered in the differential diagnosis of critically ill newborns, children with seizures, neurodegeneration, recurrent vomiting, Reye-like syndrome, parenchymal liver disease, cardiomyopathy, rhabdomyolysis, renal insufficiency, unexplained metabolic acidosis, hyperammonemia, or hypoglycemia. Intellectual disability, developmental delay, and poor growth are often present but offer little specificity. IEM should be suspected when (1) degree of illness appears out of proportion to history, (2) symptoms accompany changes in diet, (3) developmental regression occurs, (4) there are specific food preferences or aversions, or (5) the family has a history of parental consanguinity or problems suggestive of IEM such as intellectual disability or unexplained deaths in first- and second-degree relatives.

Physical findings associated with IEM include abnormally thin, wiry, or coarse hair; macular cherry-red spot; retinitis pigmentosa; optic atrophy; cataracts or corneal opacity; hepatosplenomegaly; thickened facial features; skeletal changes (including gibbus); and developmental regression, leukodystrophy, ataxia, or dystonia. Other features that may be important in the context of a suspicious history include microcephaly, rash, jaundice, and abnormal muscle tone. Of note, IEM have been misdiagnosed as more common clinical presentations including nonaccidental trauma (glutaric acidemia type 1 [GA1]) and poisoning (methylmalonic aciduria).

LABORATORY STUDIES

Laboratory studies are almost always needed for the diagnosis of IEM. Serum electrolytes and pH should be used to estimate anion gap and acid-base status. Urine ketones and blood glucose values are readily available at the bedside. Serum lactate, pyruvate, and ammonia levels are available in most hospitals, but care is needed in obtaining samples appropriately. Plasma amino acid, plasma acylcarnitine profile, and urine organic acid studies must be performed at specialized laboratories to ensure accurate analysis and interpretation. An increasing number of inborn errors are diagnosed with DNA sequencing, but interpretation of private variants or variants of uncertain significance can be problematic. Knowing the causative pathogenic variant in the family allows prenatal diagnosis to be done by molecular analysis. This can be done on any material that contains fetal DNA (eg, chorionic villi, amniotic cells, or fetal blood). Large-scale next-generation sequencing (whole-exome or whole-genome sequencing [WES or WGS]) has been very useful in identifying disorders with nonspecific symptoms that are not readily recognized by routine metabolite screening. Specific metabolite or enzyme assays are used for confirmation.

The physician should be familiar with what conditions a test can detect and when it can detect them. For example, urine organic acids may be normal in patients with medium-chain acyl-CoA dehydrogenase (MCAD) deficiency or biotinidase deficiency, and glycine may be elevated only in cerebrospinal fluid (CSF) in patients with nonketotic hyperglycinemia (NKH). A result that is normal in one physiologic state may be abnormal in another. For instance, ketone production (identified easily in urine) in a child who is hypoglycemic is expected. The absence of ketones in such a child would suggest a defect in fatty acid oxidation. Conversely, a newborn does not normally have the capacity to produce ketones. Neonatal ketosis suggests an organic acidemia.

Samples used to diagnose IEM may be obtained at autopsy. Samples must be obtained in a timely fashion and may be analyzed directly or stored frozen until analysis is justified by the postmortem examination, new clinical information, or developments in the field. Studies of other family members may help establish the diagnosis in a deceased patient.

COMMON CLINICAL SITUATIONS

1. Intellectual Disability

Biochemical screening for causes of intellectual disability has largely been supplanted by large next generation molecular panels populated with genes known to be associated with intellectual disability, developmental delay, or autism. When the indication is nonspecific, as in the case of most intellectual disability, broad molecular testing provides a higher yield than biochemical screening. Testing may be more targeted if physical examination, earlier laboratory testing, or imaging are suggestive of a specific diagnosis. Examples include urine screen for **glycosaminoglycans** if the examination suggests **mucopolysaccharidosis** or testing plasma for **very long chain fatty acids** if the examination suggests a peroxisomal disorder. Biochemical and enzymatic testing are more often used to resolve genetic variants of uncertain significance or to confirm molecular diagnoses.

2. Acute Presentation in the Neonate

Acute-onset IEM in the neonate is most often a result of disorders of energy metabolism and may be clinically indistinguishable from sepsis. Prominent symptoms include poor feeding, vomiting, altered mental status or muscle tone, jitteriness, seizures, and jaundice. Acidosis, alkalosis, or altered mental status out of proportion to systemic symptoms should increase suspicion of an IEM. Laboratory measurements should include electrolytes, ammonia, lactate, glucose, blood pH, urine ketones, and urine carbohydrate analysis. Amino acids in CSF should be measured if NKH is suspected. Plasma and urine amino acid, urine organic acid, and serum acylcarnitine analysis should be performed urgently. Neonatal cardiomyopathy or ventricular arrhythmias should be investigated with serum acylcarnitine analysis and carnitine levels. In parallel with biochemical testing, rapid WGS may also be done to aid in diagnosis of a very ill child.

3. Vomiting & Encephalopathy in the Infant or Older Child

Electrolytes, ammonia, and glucose should be measured and urinalysis performed in all patients with vomiting and encephalopathy, preferably before any treatment that may affect the results. Samples for plasma amino acids, serum acylcarnitine profile, and urine organic acid analysis should be obtained early. For a Reye-like syndrome presentation (ie, vomiting, encephalopathy, and hepatomegaly), amino acids, acylcarnitines, carnitine levels, and urine organic acids should be assessed immediately. Hypoglycemia with inappropriately low urine or quantitative serum ketones suggests the diagnosis of fatty acid oxidation or ketogenesis defects. If the results of the biochemical testing are highly suggestive or diagnostic of a specific disorder; enzymatic or molecular testing can confirm the diagnosis.

4. Hypoglycemia

Duration of fasting, presence or absence of hepatomegaly, and Kussmaul breathing provide clues to the differential diagnosis of hypoglycemia. Serum insulin, cortisol, and growth hormone should be obtained on presentation. Urine ketones, urine organic acids, plasma lactate, serum acylcarnitine profile, carnitine levels, ammonia, triglycerides, and uric acid should be measured. Ketonuria in a hypoglycemic or acidotic neonate suggests an organic acidemia. In the older child, inappropriately low urine ketone levels suggest an IEM of fatty acid oxidation. Assessment of ketone generation requires simultaneous measurements of quantitative serum 3-hydroxybutyrate, acetoacetate, and free fatty acids in relation to a sufficient duration of fasting and age. Metabolites obtained during the acute episode can be helpful and preclude a formal fasting test. Targeted molecular panels with genes known to be associated with hypoglycemia are useful to confirm a diagnosis.

5. Hyperammonemia

Symptoms of hyperammonemia may appear and progress rapidly or insidiously. Decreased appetite, irritability, and behavioral changes appear first with vomiting, ataxia, lethargy, seizures, and coma progressing as ammonia levels increase. Tachypnea and resulting respiratory alkalosis are characteristic in urea cycle defects (UCDs) and transient hyperammonemia of the newborn, while acidosis is characteristic of hyperammonemia associated with organic acidemias. Severe hyperammonemia may be due to urea cycle disorders, organic acidemias, or fatty acid oxidation disorders (FAODs). Hyperammonemia may also result from transient hyperammonemia of the newborn in the premature infant, portosystemic shunt, aortic coarctation, valproate toxicity, infection with urease splitting bacteria, and with some chemotherapeutic medications. IEM can usually be suggested by measuring quantitative plasma amino acids (eg, citrulline), plasma carnitine and acylcarnitine esters, and urine organic acids (including orotic acid).

6. Acidosis

IEM may cause chronic or acute acidosis at any age, with or without an increased anion gap. They should be considered when acidosis occurs with recurrent vomiting or hyperammonemia and when acidosis is out of proportion to the clinical status. Acidosis due to an IEM can be difficult to correct, while physiologic ketoacidosis in fasting is appropriate and corrects readily. The main causes of anion gap metabolic acidosis are lactic acidosis, ketoacidosis, methylmalonic aciduria or other organic acidurias, intoxication (ethanol, methanol, ethylene glycol, and salicylate), and uremia. Causes of nonanion gap metabolic acidosis include loss of base in diarrhea or renal tubular acidosis. If renal bicarbonate loss is found, a distinction must be made between isolated renal tubular acidosis and a more generalized renal tubular disorder or renal Fanconi syndrome by testing for renal losses of phosphorus and amino acids. IEM associated with renal Fanconi syndrome include cystinosis, tyrosinemia type I, carnitine palmitoyltransferase I, galactosemia, hereditary fructose intolerance (HFI), Lowe syndrome, lysinuric protein intolerance, and some mitochondrial diseases. Tests indicated for anion gap metabolic acidosis include urine organic acids, serum lactate and pyruvate, serum 3-hydroxybutyrate and acetoacetate, and plasma amino acids, in addition to a toxicology screen.

MANAGEMENT OF METABOLIC EMERGENCIES

Patients with severe acidosis, hypoglycemia, and hyperammonemia may be very ill; initially mild symptoms may worsen quickly, and coma and death may ensue within hours. With prompt and vigorous treatment, however, patients can recover completely, even from deep coma. All oral intake should be stopped. Sufficient glucose should be given intravenously to avoid or minimize catabolism in a patient with a known inborn error who is at risk for crisis. Most conditions respond favorably to glucose administration, although a few (eg, primary lactic acidosis due to pyruvate dehydrogenase deficiency) do not. After exclusion of FAODs, immediate institution of intravenous fat emulsions can provide crucial caloric input. Severe or increasing hyperammonemia should be treated pharmacologically or with dialysis (see section Disorders of the Urea Cycle), and severe acidosis should be treated with bicarbonate. More specific measures can be instituted when a diagnosis is established.

NEWBORN SCREENING

Criteria for screening newborns for a disorder include frequency, consequences if untreated, ability of therapy to mitigate consequences, ease and cost of testing, and availability and cost of treatment. With the availability of tandem mass spectrometry, newborn screening (NBS) has expanded greatly to include an ever-expanding group of core conditions and multiple secondary conditions screened by most states. Figure 36–1 provides a summary of the most common, time sensitive IEM targeted by NBS. In general, amino

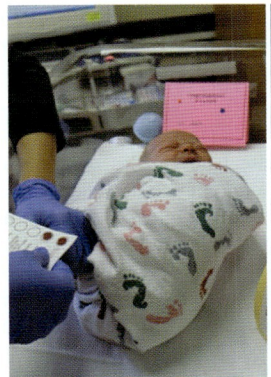

Primary Analyte	Primary Disease	Untreated	Treatment
Leu	MSUD	Sz, DD/ID	Anabolic therapy, Leu restricted diet
Phe	PKU	Sz, DD/ID	Phe restricted diet, sapropterin, pegvaliase
SA	HT1	ALF	NTBC, Tyr restricted diet, Liver Transplant
C0	CUD	ALF, CM	Carnitine
C3	MMA, PA	↑NH3, Acidosis, DD/ID	Anabolic therapy, Carnitine, Liver Transplant
C5	IVA	↑NH3, Acidosis, DD/ID	Anabolic therapy, Carnitine, Glycine
C5OH	Multiple	Acidosis	Anabolic therapy
C5DC	GA1	Basal Ganglia Stroke	Anabolic therapy, Carnitine, Arginine
C8	MCADD	↑NH3, ALF, Enceph	Anabolic therapy
C14:1	VLCADD	↑NH3, ALF, CM	Anabolic therapy, MCT
C16:1OH	LCHADD	ALF, CM	Anabolic therapy, MCT
C16, C18	CPT2, CACT	↑NH3, CM	Anabolic therapy, MCT
GALT	Galactosemia	ALF, Sepsis	Lactose/Galactose restricted diet
Biotinidase	Biotinidase Def	Sz, DD/ID	Biotin

▲ **Figure 36–1.** Primary analyte, disease target, untreated consequences, and basic therapies involved with the most common time-sensitive IEM on the modern newborn screen. Abbreviations: leucine (Leu); phenylalanine (Phe), succinylacetone (SA), galactose-1-phosphate uridylyltransferase (GALT), galactose-1-phosphate (Gal-1-P), maple syrup urine disease (MSUD), phenylketonuria (PKU), hereditary tyrosinemia type 1 (HT1), carnitine uptake deficiency (CUD), methylmalonic acidemia (MMA), propionic acidemia (PA), isovaleric acidemia (IVA), glutaric acidemia type 1 (GA1), medium chain/very long chain/long chain-3-hydroxy-acyl-CoA dehydrogenase deficiencies (MCADD, VLCADD, LCHADD), carnitine palmitoyl transferase deficiency type 2 (CPT2), carnitine acylcarnitine translocase deficiency (CACT), seizure (Sz), developmental delay (DD), intellectual disability (ID), acute live failure (ALF), cardiomyopathy (CM), hyperammonemia (↑NH3), encephalopathy (Enceph), 2-(2-nitro-4-trifluoromethylbenzoyl)-1,3-cyclohexanedione (NTBC), medium chain triglycerides (MCT). Note: Anabolic therapy includes avoidance of fasting and provision of calories (oral or intravenous) during illness. (Used with permission from Dr. Peter Baker.)

acidopathies, organic acidurias, and disorders of fatty acid oxidation are the disorders for which screening now occurs. Most states also screen for hypothyroidism, congenital adrenal hyperplasia, hemoglobinopathies, biotinidase deficiency, galactosemia, cystic fibrosis, severe combined immune deficiency, and spinal muscular atrophy (SMA), in addition to point-of-care screening for hearing loss and congenital heart disease. An increasing number of states have begun screening for some of the lysosomal and peroxisomal disorders, and a few states have begun screening for guanidinoacetate methyltransferase deficiency (GAMT). The Recommended Uniform Screening Panel (RUSP) provides guidance for the addition of new disorders to state NBS panels. Screening should occur for all infants between 24 and 48 hours of life or before hospital discharge.

Some screening tests measure a metabolite (eg, phenylalanine) that becomes abnormal with time and exposure to diet. In such instances, the disease cannot be detected reliably until intake of the substrate is established, typically around 24 hours of life. Other tests measure enzyme activity and can be performed at any time (eg, biotinidase deficiency). Transfusions may cause false-negative results in this instance, and exposure of the sample to heat may cause false-positive results. False positives also result from prematurity, parenteral nutrition, hyperbilirubinemia, and liver or renal disease. Technologic advances have extended the power of the NBS but have brought additional challenges. For example, although tandem mass spectrometry can detect many more disorders in the newborn period, consensus on efficacy of treatment for some conditions is still controversial.

Screening tests are not diagnostic, and diagnostic tests must be undertaken when an abnormal NBS result is obtained. Because false-negative results occur, a normal NBS does not rule out a condition, and some common disorders (eg, ornithine transcarbamylase [OTC] deficiency) are not detectable. The appropriate response to an abnormal NBS depends on the condition in question and the predictive value of the test. For example, when screening for galactosemia by enzyme assay, complete absence of enzyme activity is highly predictive of classic galactosemia. Failure to treat may rapidly lead to death. In this case, treatment must be initiated immediately while diagnostic studies are pending. In PKU, however, a diet restricted in phenylalanine is harmful to the infant whose screening test is a false-positive, while diet therapy produces an excellent outcome in the truly affected infant if treatment is established within the first weeks of life. Therefore, treatment for PKU should only be instituted when the diagnosis is confirmed. Physicians should review American College of Medical Genetics and Genomics recommendations, state laws, and regulations, and consult with their local metabolic center to arrive at appropriate strategies.

Ding S, Han L: Newborn screening for genetic disorders: current status and prospects for the future. Pediatr Investig 2022 Oct 24;6(4):291–298. doi: 10.1002/ped4.12343 [PMID: 36582269].

Kripps KA et al: Practical strategies to maintain anabolism by intravenous nutritional management in children with inborn metabolic diseases. Mol Genet Metab 2021 May 7;S1096-7192(21)00700-9 [PMID: 33985889].

Manickam K et al; ACMG Board of Directors: Exome and genome sequencing for pediatric patients with congenital anomalies or intellectual disability: an evidence-based clinical guideline of the American College of Medical Genetics and Genomics (ACMG). Genet Med 2021 Nov;23(11):2029–2037. doi: 10.1038/s41436-021-01242-6. Epub 2021 Jul 1 [PMID: 34211152].

Vergano SAS: Inborn errors of metabolism: becoming ready for rare. Pediatr Rev 2022 Jul 1;43(7):371–383. doi: 10.1542/pir.2022-005088 [PMID: 35773536].

DISORDERS OF CARBOHYDRATE METABOLISM

GLYCOGEN STORAGE DISEASES

ESSENTIALS OF DIAGNOSIS & TYPICAL FEATURES

► Types 0, I, III, VI, and IX manifest with hypoglycemia in infants.

► Types II, V, and VII manifest with rhabdomyolysis or muscle weakness.

► Types IV and IX manifest with hepatic cirrhosis.

Glycogen is a branched glucose polymer that found in the liver and muscle. Different enzyme defects affect its biosynthesis and degradation. The hepatic GSDs cause growth failure, hepatomegaly, and fasting hypoglycemia. Hepatic GSDs include glucose-6-phosphatase deficiency (type I), debrancher enzyme deficiency (type III), hepatic phosphorylase deficiency (type VI), and phosphorylase kinase deficiency (type IX), which normally regulates hepatic phosphorylase activity. Glycogen synthase deficiency (type 0) causes hypoglycemia, usually after about 12 hours of fasting, and can cause mild postprandial hyperglycemia and hyperlactatemia. There are two forms of glucose-6-phosphatase deficiency: type Ia, in which the catalytic glucose-6-phosphatase is deficient and there is pronounced lactic acidosis, hyperuricemia, hyperlipidemia, and hypoglycemia, and type Ib, in which the glucose-6-phosphate transporter is deficient and neutropenia and profound hypoglycemia occurs. GSD type IV, brancher enzyme deficiency, usually presents with progressive liver cirrhosis, as do some rare forms of phosphorylase kinase deficiency.

The myopathic GSDs affect skeletal and sometimes cardiac muscle. Skeletal myopathy with weakness or rhabdomyolysis may be seen in muscle phosphorylase deficiency (type V), phosphofructokinase deficiency (type VII), and acid maltase deficiency (type II; Pompe disease). The infantile form of Pompe disease also has hypertrophic cardiomyopathy and macroglossia.

► Diagnosis

Initial tests include glucose, lactate, triglycerides, cholesterol, uric acid, transaminases, and creatine kinase. Functional testing includes responsiveness of blood glucose and lactate to fasting; for myopathic forms, an ischemic or nonischemic exercise test is helpful. Most GSDs can now be diagnosed by molecular analysis, including next-generation panels. Other diagnostic studies include enzyme assays of leukocytes, fibroblasts, liver, or muscle.

► Treatment

Treatment is designed to prevent hypoglycemia and avoid secondary metabolite accumulation (eg, lactate in GSD type I). In GSD type I, the special diet must be strictly monitored with restriction of free sugars and measured amounts of uncooked cornstarch, which slowly releases glucose in the intestinal lumen. Good results have been reported following continuous nighttime carbohydrate feeding or uncooked cornstarch therapy. Late complications even after years of treatment include focal segmental glomerulosclerosis, hepatic adenoma or carcinoma, and gout. Enzyme-replacement therapy in Pompe disease corrects the cardiomyopathy, but the response in skeletal myopathy is variable depending on the presence or absence of "cross-reacting immunologic material" (CRIM). CRIM-positive patients have a more favorable response, due both to the presence of residual enzyme activity and the absence of an immune response to infused enzyme. Immunomodulation is used for all Pompe patients starting enzyme-replacement therapy and may be repeated for patients whose treatment response declines due to antibodies to the recombinant enzyme. In GSDs with intact gluconeogenesis (GSD III, VI, IX), a high-protein diet improves glucose control and reduces late complications. Gene therapies for many of these disorders are under development.

Kishnani PS et al: Diagnosis and management of glycogen storage disease type 1: a practice guideline of the American College of Medical Genetics and Genomics. Genet Med 2014;Nov 6. doi: 10.1038/gim.2014.128 [PMID: 25356975].

Marion RW, Paljevic E. The glycogen storage disorders. Pediatr Rev 2020 Jan;41(1):41–44. doi: 10.1542/pir.2018-0146. Erratum in: Pediatr Rev 2020 Feb;41(2):99 [PMID: 31894075].

Massese M, Tagliaferri F, Dionisi-Vici C, Maiorana A: Glycogen storage diseases with liver involvement: a literature review of GSD type 0, IV, VI, IX and XI. Orphanet J Rare Dis 2022 Jun 20;17(1):241. doi: 10.1186/s13023-022-02387-6 [PMID: 35725468].

Molares-Vila A, Corbalán-Rivas A, Carnero-Gregorio M, González-Cespón JL, Rodríguez-Cerdeira C: Biomarkers in glycogen storage diseases: an update. Int J Mol Sci 2021 Apr 22;22(9):4381. doi: 10.3390/ijms22094381 [PMID: 33922238].

Patient and parent support group website with useful information for families: http://www.agsdus.org.

Tarnopolsky MA: Metabolic myopathies. Continuum (Minneap Minn) 2022 Dec 1;28(6):1752–1777. doi: 10.1212/CON.0000000000001182 [PMID: 36537979].

Wright TLF, Umaña LA, Ramirez CM: Update on glycogen storage disease: primary hepatic involvement. Curr Opin Pediatr 2022 Oct 1;34(5):496–502. doi: 10.1097/MOP.0000000000001158. Epub 2022 Aug 3 [PMID: 35942643].

GALACTOSEMIA

ESSENTIALS OF DIAGNOSIS & TYPICAL FEATURES

► Severely deficient neonates present with vomiting, jaundice, and hepatomegaly on initiation of lactose-containing feedings.

► Renal Fanconi syndrome, cataracts of the ocular lens, hepatic cirrhosis, and sepsis occur in untreated children.

► Delayed, apraxic speech and ovarian failure occur frequently even with treatment. Developmental delay, tremor, and ataxia occur less frequently.

Classic galactosemia is caused by almost total deficiency of galactose-1-phosphate uridyltransferase (GALT). Accumulation of galactose-1-phosphate (Gal-1-P) and galactitol causes hepatic parenchymal disease and renal Fanconi syndrome. Onset of the severe disease is marked in the neonate by vomiting, jaundice (both direct and indirect), hepatomegaly, and rapid onset of liver insufficiency after initiation of milk feeding. Hepatic cirrhosis is progressive. Without treatment, death frequently occurs within 1 month, often from *Escherichia coli* sepsis. Cataracts usually develop within 2 months in untreated cases but generally reverse with treatment. With prompt institution of a galactose-free diet, the prognosis for survival without liver disease is excellent. Even when dietary restriction is instituted early, patients with galactosemia are at increased risk for speech and language deficits and ovarian failure. Some patients develop progressive intellectual disability, tremor, and ataxia. Milder variants of galactosemia with better prognosis exist. The disorder is autosomal recessive with an incidence of approximately 1:40,000 live births.

► Diagnosis

In infants receiving foods containing galactose, laboratory findings include liver dysfunction, particularly PT prolongation, together with proteinuria and aminoaciduria. Gal-1-P is elevated in red blood cells. When the diagnosis is suspected, GALT enzyme should be assayed in erythrocytes or *GALT*

sequencing pursued. Blood transfusions give false-negative results and sample deterioration confers false-positive results. NBS allows timely institution of treatment. Some patients identified on NBS have a genotype that results in sufficient residual activity (Duarte allele) and treatment is not always required.

► Treatment

A galactose-free (soy formula) diet should be instituted as soon as the diagnosis is made or suspected. Compliance with the diet can be monitored by following Gal-1-P levels in red blood cells or urinary galactitol levels. Appropriate diet management requires not only the exclusion of milk but also an understanding of the galactose content of foods. Avoidance of galactose should be lifelong with appropriate calcium and vitamin D replacement because of the need for restriction of dairy. DEXA scans are recommended for monitoring of bone health. All children should be monitored for appropriate development with special attention to speech and language development, and girls should routinely be screened for hypergonadotropic hypogonadism during adolescence.

Fridovich-Keil JL, Berry GT: Pathophysiology of long-term complications in classic galactosemia: what we do and do not know. Mol Genet Metab 2022 Sep–Oct;137(1–2):33–39. doi: 10.1016/j.ymgme.2022.07.005. Epub 2022 Jul 9 [PMID: 35882174].

Patient and parent support group website with useful information for families: http://www.galactosemia.org.

Succoio M, Sacchettini R, Rossi A, Parenti G, Ruoppolo M: Galactosemia: biochemistry, molecular genetics, newborn screening, and treatment. Biomolecules 2022 Jul 11;12(7):968. doi: 10.3390/biom12070968 [PMID: 35883524].

Welling L et al: International clinical guideline for the management of classical galactosemia: diagnosis, treatment, and follow-up. J Inherit Metab Dis 2017;40:171–176 [PMID: 27858262].

HEREDITARY FRUCTOSE INTOLERANCE

ESSENTIALS OF DIAGNOSIS & TYPICAL FEATURES

► Consider diagnosis in the setting of postprandial hypoglycemia and self-restriction of or aversion to sweets.

► Primary presentation outside of infancy includes poor growth and combined liver and kidney disease with lactic acidosis.

HFI is an autosomal recessive disorder in which deficient activity of fructose-1-phosphate aldolase (aldolase B) causes hypoglycemia and tissue accumulation of fructose-1-phosphate with fructose ingestion. This is genetically and clinically different from fructose malabsorption or "dietary fructose intolerance," which is similar to lactose intolerance. Onset of HFI is typically in infancy when solid foods are introduced, but the disorder may go undiagnosed for years despite recurrent vomiting symptoms. Conversely, symptoms may appear before solids are introduced due to the presence of fructose in some infant formulas. Other abnormalities include failure to thrive, vomiting, jaundice, hepatomegaly, acute liver failure, proteinuria, renal Fanconi syndrome, and acute renal failure. Hypoglycemia directly follows fructose ingestion (postprandial), and lactic acidosis, hypophosphatemia, and hyperuricemia may be significant. The untreated condition can progress to death from liver failure. Acute infusion of fructose may also result in death. Chronic liver disease, and more rarely chronic kidney disease, may occur despite adherence to dietary therapy.

▶ **Diagnosis**

The diagnosis is suggested by finding fructosuria or abnormally glycosylated transferrins in untreated patients. Although targeted testing of common mutations is available, diagnosis is best made by full sequencing of *ALDOB*, either as a single gene or as part of a broader genetic panel.

▶ **Treatment**

Treatment consists of strict dietary avoidance of fructose, sucrose, sorbitol, and related sugars. Vitamin supplementation is usually needed. Drugs and vitamins dispensed in a sucrose base should be avoided. Treatment monitoring can be done with transferrin glycosylation analysis. If diet compliance is poor, growth problems may occur. If the disorder is recognized early, the prospects for normal development and life expectancy are good. As affected individuals grow up, intentional avoidance of fructose-containing foods, and resultantly good dentition, are common.

Gaughan S et al (eds): Hereditary fructose intolerance. In: *GeneReviews®* [Internet]. Seattle, WA: University of Washington; 1993–2021. 2015 Dec 17 [updated 2021 Feb 18] [PMID: 26677512]. Patient and parent support group website with useful information for families: http://www.bu.edu/aldolase.

DISORDERS OF ENERGY METABOLISM

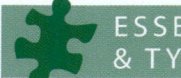

ESSENTIALS OF DIAGNOSIS & TYPICAL FEATURES

▶ Consider diagnosis in the setting of lactic acidosis, multisystem organ involvement (particularly brain, liver, eye, and/or muscle), or Leigh disease.

▶ Diagnosis is first accomplished through broad genomic testing combined with analysis of mitochondrial DNA.

Mitochondrial diseases comprise an array of hundreds of different genetic conditions with broadly varying ages of onset, rates of progression, and characteristic phenotypic features. The most common disorders are pyruvate dehydrogenase deficiency and deficiencies of respiratory chain components. Disorders of the Krebs cycle, which include deficiencies in fumarase, 2-ketoglutarate dehydrogenase, malate dehydrogenase, aconitase, and succinyl-CoA ligase, are rare. Patients with a defect in the pyruvate dehydrogenase complex (PDC) may have partial agenesis of the corpus callosum, cystic white matter lesions, or Leigh disease (characterized by injury of the basal ganglia, dentate nucleus, or periaqueductal gray matter). Recurrent altered mental status, recurrent ataxia, and recurrent lactic acidosis are frequently present in many disturbances of pyruvate metabolism. The most common genetic defect in PDC is in the X-linked $E_1\alpha$ component, with males carrying milder mutations presenting with Leigh disease and females carrying severe mutations leading to periventricular cystic brain lesions and presenting with epilepsy. The molecular heterogeneity is large, because defects in each of the subunits, the metabolism/transport of cofactors lipoate and thiamine, and the pyruvate transporter are described.

The respiratory chain disorders are frequent (1:5000) and involve a heterogeneous group of genetic defects that produce a variety of clinical syndromes (> 50) of varying severity and presentation (Table 36–1). The disorders can affect multiple organs.

Table 36–1. Clinical syndromes of mitochondrial diseases that present in childhood.

Leigh syndrome
Fatal infantile lactic acidosis and cardiomyopathy; isolated cardiomyopathy
Mitochondrial encephalomyopathy with lactic acidosis and stroke-like episodes (MELAS) (*MT-TL* m.3243A>G)
Myoclonic epilepsy and ragged red fibers (MERRF) (*MT-TK* m.8344A>G)
Progressive external ophthalmoplegia (PEO) or Kearns-Sayre syndrome (mtDNA deletion, *POLG1, TWNKLE, RRM2B*)
Alpers syndrome or hepatocerebral syndrome (*POLG, DGUOK*)
Leber hereditary optic neuropathy (LHON) (m.11778T>G, m.14484T>C, m.3460G>A, *OPA1*)
Myoneurogastrointestinal syndrome (MNGIE) (*TYMP*)
Neuropathy, ataxia, and retinitis pigmentosa (NARP) (*MT-ATP6/8* m.8993T>C and m.8993T>G)
Barth syndrome (*TAZ*)
Sensory ataxia, neuropathy, dysarthria, and ophthalmoparesis (SANDO) (*POLG, TWNKL*)
Myopathy, encephalomyopathy, reversible infantile myopathy
Leukoencephalopathy
Diabetes and deafness (*MT-TL* m.3243A>G)
Pearson syndrome (exocrine pancreatic and bone marrow failure) (mtDNA deletion)
Multisystem presentation

The following set of symptoms (not intended as comprehensive) can indicate a respiratory chain disorder:

1. General: Failure to thrive, fatigue
2. Brain: Progressive neurodegeneration, Leigh disease, myoclonic seizures, brain atrophy, movement disorders, cerebellar atrophy, stroke-like episodes, leukodystrophy
3. Eye: Optic neuropathy, retinitis pigmentosa, progressive external ophthalmoplegia
4. Ears: Sensorineural hearing loss
5. Muscle: Myopathy with decreased endurance or rhabdomyolysis
6. Kidney: Renal Fanconi syndrome, proteinuria (in coenzyme Q deficiency)
7. Endocrine: Diabetes mellitus, hypoparathyroidism
8. Intestinal: Pancreatic or liver insufficiency, intestinal pseudo-obstruction
9. Heart: Cardiomyopathy, conduction defects, arrhythmias

Respiratory chain disorders are among the more common causes of progressive neurodevelopmental problems in children. Fatigue is the most common symptom, and patients may present with nonspecific findings such as hypotonia, poor growth, or renal tubular acidosis, or with more specific features such as ophthalmoplegia or cardiomyopathy. Symptoms are often combined in recognizable clinical syndromes with ties to specific genetic causes (see Table 36–1). Thirteen of the more than 100 genes that impact function of the respiratory chain are part of the mitochondrial genome. Therefore, inheritance of defects in the respiratory chain may be strictly matrilineal (if encoded by mitochondrial DNA (mtDNA)) or may have Mendelian inheritance patterns (if encoded by nuclear DNA).

The genetic causes of mitochondrial disease are extremely heterogeneous, and over 300 different disease-causing genes have already been described. Mitochondrial biology is a complex system involving the maintenance of mtDNA and its transcription, mRNA processing, and translation machinery, the assembly of the complexes including cofactors, the import and processing of nuclear-encoded components, and the maintenance of the mitochondrial membrane and structural environment, with defects described at every step. Whereas some clinical presentations or biomarkers are specific to one gene, many clinical presentations (such as Leigh disease) have diverse genetic etiologies, complicating the diagnostic process. Identifying a specific genetic etiology of mitochondrial disease is important since some diseases have disease-modifying therapies available.

▶ Diagnosis

Biomarkers can aid in the recognition of mitochondrial disorders. In many, but not all, mitochondrial diseases, lactate is elevated in blood or CSF. In PDC deficiency, the lactate-pyruvate ratio is normal, whereas in respiratory chain disorders the ratio is often increased. Lactate is nonspecific and can be elevated in hypoxia, ischemia, congenital heart disease (including aortic coarctation), infection, physical exertion, or even sampling errors, which should be considered prior to a diagnostic evaluation for mitochondrial disease. Lactate elevations in CSF or on brain magnetic resonance spectroscopy (MRS) are more specific to mitochondrial disease than in blood. Large elevations of 3-methyl-glutaconic acid indicate a subset of mitochondrial disorders affecting the mitochondrial membrane. Elevation of thymidine specifically indicates thymidine kinase deficiency causing mitochondrial neurogastrointestinal encephalopathy (MNGIE). The protein biomarkers growth differentiation factor 15 (GDF15) and fibroblast growth factor 21 (FGF21) reflect the mitochondrial stress response and identify mitochondrial disorders in patients with a skeletal or ocular myopathy caused by mtDNA deletion, replication, or tRNA mutations.

Genetic testing is currently the preferred first-line evaluation for mitochondrial disease. Sometimes a clinical presentation is specific enough to allow for targeted genetic testing (eg, Alpers syndrome caused by mutations in POLG). Due to the large genetic heterogeneity, broad genetic testing using WES or WGS with mitochondrial DNA sequencing is effective. Several common mtDNA abnormalities (eg, mtDNA deletions, m.3243G>A) decrease in blood with age and require analysis in tissue (particularly muscle) to detect the genetic diagnosis. A multiomic approach is useful to resolve cases where sequencing has been unsuccessful. Further, in the case of nondiagnostic or uncertain genetic results with high clinical suspicion for mitochondrial disease, pathology and mitochondrial functional studies of patient's tissue are indicated. Classic pathologic features of mitochondrial disorders are the accumulation of mitochondria, which produces "ragged red fibers" in skeletal muscle biopsy, and abnormal mitochondrial shapes and inclusions inside mitochondria on electron microscopy. These changes are common in adults but only present in a minority of affected children. PDC deficiency can be diagnosed by enzyme assay in fibroblasts. Functional testing via respiratory chain enzyme assays, nondenaturing blue native gel assays, and analysis of assembly of complex I, in addition to measurement of specific protein levels by Western Blot in relevant tissues such as muscle, liver, or fibroblasts, remains important.

Diagnosis of mitochondrial disease is based on a convergence of clinical, biochemical, morphologic, enzymatic, and genetic data. Distinction of primary mitochondrial diseases from disorders with secondary mitochondrial dysfunction is important and correlation with genetic testing results is essential. The process of diagnosing a patient with mitochondrial disease can be time consuming and may require multiple studies to arrive at an accurate etiologic diagnosis. This is achievable in most patients with current technologies.

Treatment

A consensus statement on the treatment of mitochondrial diseases from the Mitochondrial Medicine Society has been published. Patients should first avoid situations that further compromise mitochondrial function. Medications that impair mitochondrial translation (eg, certain antibiotics) or mitochondrial replication (eg, AZT/zidovudine) or exhibit mitochondrial toxicity (eg, valproate and propofol) should be avoided where possible. Catabolism due to prolonged fasting should be avoided by provision of sufficient calories, intravenously if necessary. The best evidence for improvement in mitochondrial function for affected patients is with a regimen of regular exercise (eg, at least 20 minutes daily).

Disease-modifying therapies are available for certain specific mitochondrial diseases. A ketogenic diet is effective for most patients with PDC deficiency, particularly those with Leigh disease. High-dose coenzyme Q supplementation is effective for patients with coenzyme Q synthesis defects. A few conditions are responsive to riboflavin (*ACAD9*) or thiamine (*TPK, SLC19A3*). Stroke-like episodes, particularly in the mitochondrial encephalomyopathy, lactic acidosis, and stroke-like episodes (MELAS) syndrome, should be treated with intravenous arginine acutely, and either oral arginine or citrulline can be used for prevention of stroke-like episodes. Treatment with taurine has also been shown to reduce stroke-like episodes in MELAS caused by the m.3243G>A variant. Liver transplantation can treat mitochondrial diseases resulting from systemic accumulation of toxic metabolites, such as ETHF1-related disease and MNGIE. Few controlled studies exist for the clinical efficacy of dietary supplements, although many such as coenzyme Q, B-vitamins, lipoic acid, nicotinamide riboside, and others are often offered to patients with mitochondrial diseases. Multiple clinical trials are ongoing to evaluate new medications such as next-generation antioxidants, mitochondrial biogenesis upregulators, and molecular protectors. Referral to a mitochondrial care network center can help patients obtain accurate and timely diagnosis, access to clinical trials, and effective therapies for those few mitochondrial disorders that are amenable to disease-modifying therapies.

Alston CL, Stenton SL, Hudson G, Prokisch H, Taylor RW: The genetics of mitochondrial disease: dissecting mitochondrial pathology using multi-omics pipelines. J Pathol 2021;254(4):430–442 [PMID: 33586140].

Mitochondrial Care Network: www.mitonetwolrk.org.

Mitochondrial Medicine Society: Website with useful information for clinicians: http://www.mitosoc.org.

Parikh S et al: Diagnosis and management of mitochondrial disease: a consensus statement from the Mitochondrial Medicine Society. Genet Med 2015;17(9):689–701 [PMID: 25503498].

Patient and parent support group website with useful information for families: http://www.umdf.org.

DISORDERS OF AMINO ACID METABOLISM

DISORDERS OF THE UREA CYCLE

ESSENTIALS OF DIAGNOSIS & TYPICAL FEATURES

▸ Typical presentation is infantile encephalopathy; later onset presentations are common with cyclic vomiting or encephalopathy with illness or protein load.

▸ Diagnosis possibly suspected with hyperammonemia with minimal other laboratory findings, followed by analysis of amino acids and organic acids.

Ammonia is derived from the catabolism of amino acids and is converted to an amino group in urea by enzymes of the urea cycle. Patients with severe UCDs, often those enzymes early in the urea cycle such as OTC or argininosuccinic acid synthetase deficiency (citrullinemia type I) usually present in infancy with severe hyperammonemia, vomiting, and encephalopathy, which is rapidly fatal if untreated. Patients with milder genetic defects may present with vomiting, encephalopathy, or liver failure after increased protein ingestion or infection. Although late defects such as deficiency in argininosuccinic acid lyase (ASL or argininosuccinic aciduria) or arginase may cause hyperammonemia in infancy, the usual clinical course is chronic with intellectual disability without hyperammonemia. OTC deficiency is X-linked; the others are autosomal recessive. Age at onset of symptoms varies with residual enzyme activity, protein intake, growth, and stressors such as infection. Even within a family, patients with OTC deficiency may differ by decades in the age of symptom onset. Many female carriers of OTC deficiency have protein intolerance. Some develop migraine-like symptoms after protein loads, and others develop potentially fatal episodes of vomiting and encephalopathy after protein ingestion, infections, or in the postpartum period. Trichorrhexis nodosa can occur in patients with ASL deficiency. Arginase deficiency usually presents with spastic diplegia, cognitive problems and sometimes seizures. Citrullinemia type II due to citrin (transporter SLC25A13) deficiency presents in infancy as cholestasis and in adulthood as encephalopathic or psychiatric symptom episodes.

Diagnosis

Blood ammonia should be measured in any acutely ill newborn in whom a cause is not obvious and in any child with unexplained encephalopathy. Causes of severe neonatal hyperammonemia, in addition to UCD, include liver failure, portosystemic shunt, transient hyperammonemia of the neonate, and a variety of non-UCD metabolic disorders. In UCD, early hyperammonemia is associated with hyperventilation and respiratory alkalosis.

Plasma amino acids can reveal low or undetectable citrulline in carbamoyl phosphate synthetase and OTC deficiency and high citrulline in ASL deficiency and citrullinemia. Low arginine is present in most UCD, but very high in arginase deficiency. High glutamine is generally seen with hyperammonemia. Large amounts of argininosuccinic acid in urine are indicative of ASL deficiency. Urine orotic acid is increased in infants with OTC deficiency. In citrin deficiency, mild citrulline elevation are accompanied by elevated threonine, methionine, and triglycerides. Prenatal diagnosis is typically accomplished by gene sequencing.

▶ Treatment

During treatment of acute hyperammonemic crisis, protein intake should be temporarily stopped, and glucose and lipids should be given to reduce endogenous protein breakdown from catabolism. Careful administration of essential amino acids facilitates protein anabolism. Arginine is an essential amino acid for patients with UCD (except in arginase deficiency) and providing it (often intravenously) increases the excretion of waste nitrogen in citrullinemia type I and ASL deficiency. Sodium benzoate and phenylacetate are given intravenously to increase excretion of nitrogen as hippurate and phenylacetylglutamine. Hemodialysis or hemofiltration is indicated for severe or persistent hyperammonemia, as is often the case in the newborn. Peritoneal dialysis and exchange transfusion are ineffective. Long-term treatment includes low-protein diet, oral administration of arginine or citrulline, and sodium benzoate or sodium phenylbutyrate. Symptomatic heterozygous female carriers of OTC deficiency should also receive such treatment. Liver transplantation may be curative and is indicated for patients with severe disorders. Treatment with carbamylglutamate is effective for *N*-acetylglutamate synthase deficiency and mitochondrial carbonic anhydrase deficiency. Enzyme replacement therapy is available for arginase deficiency and normalizes arginine levels. Citrin deficiency is treated with a high-fat, high-protein, low-carbohydrate diet.

The outcome of UCDs depends on the genetic severity of the condition (residual activity) and both the severity and duration of hyperammonemic episodes that cause brain damage. Prolonged hyperammonemia causes permanent neurologic and intellectual impairments, with cortical atrophy and ventricular dilation seen on brain imaging. Rapid identification and urgent treatment of the initial hyperammonemic episode is critical in improving outcome, and hyperammonemia constitutes a metabolic emergency. In contrast, transient hyperammonemia due to shunting, however, generally has a favorable outcome even with high ammonia levels.

Ah Mew N, Simpson KL, Gropman AL, Lanpher BC, Chapman KA, Summar ML: Urea Cycle Disorders Overview. In: Adam MP et al (eds): *GeneReviews®* [Internet]. Seattle, WA: University of Washington; 1993–2021. 2003 Apr 29 [updated 2017 Jun 22] [PMID: 20301396].

Patient and parent support group website with useful information for families: http://www.nucdf.org.

Summar ML, Mew NA: Inborn errors of metabolism with hyperammonemia: urea cycle defects and related disorders. Pediatr Clin North Am 2018;65(2):231–246 [PMID: 29502911].

Urea Cycle Disorders Consortium: http://rarediseasesnetwork.epi.usf.edu/ucdc/about/index.htm.

PHENYLKETONURIA (PKU) & THE HYPERPHENYLALANINEMIAS

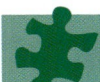 **ESSENTIALS OF DIAGNOSIS & TYPICAL FEATURES**

- ▶ Intellectual disability, hyperactivity, seizures, light complexion, and eczema characterize untreated patients.
- ▶ Newborn screening (NBS) for elevated plasma phenylalanine identifies most infants.
- ▶ Disorders of cofactor metabolism also produce elevated plasma phenylalanine level.
- ▶ Early diagnosis and treatment with phenylalanine-restricted diet prevent intellectual disability.

Probably the best-known disorder of amino acid metabolism is the classic form of phenylketonuria (PKU) caused by decreased activity of phenylalanine hydroxylase, the enzyme that converts phenylalanine to tyrosine. In classic PKU, there is little or no phenylalanine hydroxylase activity. In less severe hyperphenylalaninemia, there may be significant residual activity. Rare variants can be due to abnormalities of dihydropteridine reductase, biopterin synthesis, or *DNAJC12*.

PKU is an autosomal recessive condition, with an incidence in Caucasians of approximately 1:10,000 live births. On a normal neonatal diet, affected patients develop elevated phenylalanine levels (hyperphenylalaninemia). Patients with untreated PKU exhibit severe intellectual disability, hyperactivity, seizures, a light complexion, and eczema.

Success in preventing severe intellectual disability in children with PKU by restricting phenylalanine starting in early infancy led to NBS programs to detect the disease early. Because the outcome is best when treatment is begun in the first month of life, infants should be screened during the first few days by NBS. A second test is necessary when the NBS is done before 24 hours of age and should be completed by 7 days of age.

▶ Diagnosis & Treatment

The diagnosis of PKU is based on elevated plasma phenylalanine and elevated phenylalanine/tyrosine ratio in a child on a normal diet. The condition is differentiated from other causes of hyperphenylalaninemia by examining pterins in urine and dihydropteridine reductase activity in blood or via molecular testing. The diagnosis of hyperphenylalaninemia secondary to mutations in *DNAJC12* can only be made by molecular analysis. Determination of carrier status and prenatal diagnosis of PKU or pterin defects is possible using molecular methods.

A. Phenylalanine Hydroxylase Deficiency: Classic Phenylketonuria (PKU) and Hyperphenylalaninemia

In PKU, plasma phenylalanine levels are persistently elevated above 1200 μM (20 mg/dL) on a regular diet, with normal or low plasma levels of tyrosine, and normal pterins. Poor phenylalanine tolerance persists throughout life. Treatment to decrease phenylalanine levels is always indicated. Hyperphenylalaninemia is diagnosed in infants whose plasma phenylalanine levels are usually 240–1200 μM (4–20 mg/dL), and pterins are normal while receiving a normal protein intake. Treatment to reduce phenylalanine levels is indicated if phenylalanine levels consistently exceed 360 μM (6 mg/dL).

Treatment of all forms of PKU is aimed at maintaining phenylalanine levels less than 360 μM (6 mg/dL). Treatment can consist of dietary restriction of phenylalanine, increasing enzyme activity with pharmacologic doses of *R*-tetrahydrobiopterin (sapropterin dihydrochloride or BH_4), or enzyme substitution therapy with phenylalanine ammonia lyase.

Restricting dietary phenylalanine, while maintaining normal growth and development, is the most common therapy. This results in good outcomes if instituted in the first weeks of life and carefully maintained. Metabolic formulas deficient in phenylalanine are available but must be supplemented with normal milk and other foods to supply enough phenylalanine to permit normal growth and development. Plasma phenylalanine concentrations, growth, and development must be monitored frequently, which is best done in experienced clinics. Children with classic PKU who receive treatment effectively and promptly after birth will develop well physically and can be expected to have normal or near-normal intellectual development. Subtle changes in executive function may be apparent.

Patients who discontinued a phenylalanine-restricted diet after treatment for several years have developed subtle changes in intellect and behavior and risk neurologic damage; therefore, dietary therapy is lifelong. Counseling should be given during adolescence, particularly to girls about the risk of maternal PKU (see below). Women's diets should be monitored closely prior to conception and throughout pregnancy. Late treatment may still be of benefit in reversing behaviors such as hyperactivity, irritability, and distractibility, but it does not reverse intellectual disability.

Treatment with BH_4 results in improved phenylalanine tolerance in up to 50% of patients with a deficiency in phenylalanine hydroxylase. The best results and most frequent responsiveness are seen in patients with hyperphenylalaninemia. High doses of large neutral amino acids results in a moderate reduction in phenylalanine and is used as an adjunctive treatment in some adults with PKU. Treatment with subcutaneous administration of pegylated phenylalanine ammonia lyase has recently been approved for adults with PKU and is under study for younger ages.

B. Biopterin Defects: Dihydropteridine Reductase Deficiency and Defects in Biopterin Biosynthesis

In these patients, plasma phenylalanine levels vary. The pattern of pterin metabolites is abnormal; molecular testing is confirmatory. Clinical findings include myoclonus, tetraplegia, dystonia, oculogyric crises, and other movement disorders. Seizures and psychomotor regression occur even with diet therapy because the enzyme defect also causes neuronal deficiency of serotonin and dopamine. These deficiencies require treatment with levodopa-carbidopa, 5-hydroxytryptophan, and folinic acid. BH_4 may be added for some biopterin synthesis defects.

C. Tyrosinemia of the Newborn

Tyrosinemia of the newborn usually occurs in premature infants and is due to immaturity of 4-hydroxyphenylpyruvic acid oxidase, resulting in increased tyrosine and its precursor phenylalanine. Plasma phenylalanine levels are lower than those associated with PKU and are accompanied by marked hypertyrosinemia. The condition resolves spontaneously within 3 months, almost always without sequelae.

D. Maternal Phenylketonuria

High phenylalanine in pregnancy is teratogenic. Elevated maternal phenylalanine during pregnancy causes intellectual disability, microcephaly, growth retardation, and often congenital heart disease or other malformations in the offspring. The risk to the fetus is lessened considerably by maternal phenylalanine restriction with maintenance of phenylalanine levels below 360 μM (6 mg/dL) throughout pregnancy and optimally started before conception.

E. Hyperphenylalaninemia Due to DNAJC12 Mutations

Mild, non–BH_4-deficient hyperphenylalaninemia due to mutations in the gene *DNAJC12* is a recently reported autosomal recessive neurotransmitter disorder. *DNAJC12* functions as a co-chaperone to prevent the misfolding of proteins and interacts with neuronal phenylalanine, tyrosine, and tryptophan hydroxylases. The clinical phenotype is heterogeneous and ranges from normal to intellectual disability, autism spectrum disorder, hyperactivity, dystonia, and parkinsonism. Laboratory studies typically reveal mild, BH_4-responsive hyperphenylalaninemia (< 600 mmol/L) and low CSF homovanillic acid and 5-hydoxyindolacetic acid. Urine pterin profile and dihydropteridine reductase activity are normal. Some, but not all, patients may have an abnormal newborn screen suggestive of PKU. Therapy consists of BH_4 with L-dopa/carbidopa, with or without 5-hydroxytryptophan, and should be started as early as possible for best outcome. Subjective improvement in cognitive and motor function has been noted even with later therapy. All children with mild hyperphenylalaninemia and global developmental delay warrant targeted testing for *DNAJC12* mutations.

Patient and parent support group websites with useful information for families: http://www.pkunews.org, www.pkunetwork.org, and www.npkua.org.

Regier DS et al (eds): Phenylalanine hydroxylase deficiency. In: *GeneReviews*® [Internet]. Seattle, WA: University of Washington; 1993–2020. 2000 Jan 10 [updated 2017 Jan 5] [PMID: 20301677].

Thomas L, Olson A, Romani C: The impact of metabolic control on cognition, neurophysiology, and well-being in PKU: a systematic review and meta-analysis of the within-participant literature. Mol Genet Metab 2023 Jan;138(1):106969. doi: 10.1016/j.ymgme.2022.106969. Epub 2022 Dec 13 [PMID: 36599257].

van Spronsen FJ, Blau N, Harding C, Burlina A, Longo N, Bosch AM: Phenylketonuria. Nat Rev Dis Primers 2021 May 20;7(1):36. doi: 10.1038/s41572-021-00267-0 [PMID: 34017006].

HEREDITARY TYROSINEMIA

ESSENTIALS OF DIAGNOSIS & TYPICAL FEATURES

▶ Consider in a child presenting with liver disease with or without accompanying renal disease or bone disease.

▶ Elevated urinary succinylacetone is diagnostic of tyrosinemia, type 1.

Hereditary tyrosinemia type 1 (HT1) is an autosomal recessive condition caused by deficiency of fumarylacetoacetase (*FAH*). It presents with acute or progressive hepatic parenchymal damage, elevated α-fetoprotein, renal tubular dysfunction with generalized aminoaciduria, hypophosphatemic rickets, or neuronopathic crises. Patients may also have impaired cognition. Tyrosine and methionine are increased in blood and tyrosine metabolites and δ-aminolaevulinic acid are increased in urine. The key diagnostic metabolite is elevated succinylacetone in blood or urine. Liver failure may be rapidly fatal in infancy or more chronic, with a high incidence of liver cell carcinoma in untreated long-term survivors. Tyrosinemia type II (*TAT*) presents with corneal ulcers, palmar/plantar keratosis, neurologic dysfunction, and very high plasma tyrosine levels (> 600 μM). Patients with tyrosinemia type III (*HPD*) can have developmental delay and ataxia.

▶ Diagnosis

Similar clinical and biochemical findings of increased tyrosine and methionine may occur in other metabolic liver diseases like galactosemia, but increased succinylacetone occurs specifically in fumarylacetoacetase deficiency. An elevated level is detected in NBS. Mutation analysis is performed to confirm the diagnosis and also for prenatal diagnosis. Tyrosinemia types II and III are diagnosed by gene sequencing. Elevation of succinylacetone on NBS, resulting in a false positive for HT1, is seen in maleylacetoacetate isomerase deficiency. These individuals remain asymptomatic.

▶ Treatment

A diet low in phenylalanine and tyrosine ameliorates liver disease. Pharmacologic therapy to inhibit the upstream enzyme 4-hydroxyphenylpyruvate dehydrogenase using 2-(2-nitro-4-trifluoromethylbenzoyl)-1,3-cyclohexanedione (NTBC) decreases the production of toxic metabolites, maleylacetoacetate, and fumarylacetoacetate. It improves the liver disease and renal disease, prevents acute neuronopathic attacks, and greatly reduces the risk of hepatocellular carcinoma, but does not prevent neurocognitive dysfunction. Liver transplantation is effective therapy, and gene therapy is under development. Treatment following detection by NBS has an excellent outcome, but cognitive dysfunction is increasingly recognized. Tyrosinemia types II and III respond well to dietary tyrosine restriction. Maleylacetoacetate isomerase deficiency does not require treatment.

Chinsky JM et al: Diagnosis and treatment of tyrosinemia type 1: a US and Canadian consensus group review and recommendations. Genet Med 2017;19(12): Epub 2017 Aug 3 [PMID: 28771246].

King LS et al: Tyrosinemia Type I. 2006 Jul 24 [Updated 2017 May 25]. In: Adam MP, Feldman J, Mirzaa GM, et al., editors. *GeneReviews*® [Internet]. Seattle (WA): University of Washington, Seattle; 1993-2024. Available from: https://www.ncbi.nlm.nih.gov/books/NBK1515/.

MAPLE SYRUP URINE DISEASE (BRANCHED-CHAIN KETOACIDURIA)

ESSENTIALS OF DIAGNOSIS & TYPICAL FEATURES

▶ Typical presentation is infantile encephalopathy.

▶ Diagnosis is suspected with elevated plasma branched-chain amino acids plus alloisoleucine.

Maple syrup urine disease (MSUD) is due to deficiency of the enzyme complex that catalyzes the oxidative decarboxylation of the branched chain ketoacid derivatives of leucine, isoleucine, and valine, the essential branched chain amino acids (BCAAs). The complex is made up of three genetically distinct subunits. Accumulated ketoacids of leucine and isoleucine, which are converted to sotolone, cause the characteristic sweet odor. It is initially present in ear wax and, eventually, urine. Only leucine and its corresponding ketoacid have been implicated in causing neurologic dysfunction. Many variants of this disorder have been described, including mild, intermittent, and thiamine-dependent forms. All are autosomal recessive.

Patients with classic MSUD are normal at birth but, on day of life 2–3, develop irritability and feeding issues, and within 1 week progress to bicycling, opisthotonos, seizures, and coma, which is rapidly fatal. Nearly normal growth and development may be achieved if treatment is begun before day of life 10, which is facilitated by NBS, but psychological and psychiatric problems remain common in adults.

Diagnosis

Amino acid analysis shows marked elevation of BCAA including alloisoleucine, a diagnostic transamination product of the ketoacid of isoleucine. Urine organic acids demonstrate the characteristic ketoacids. The magnitude and consistency of metabolite changes are altered in mild and intermittent forms. A genetic testing panel that includes the multiple subunit genes can confirm the diagnosis and allows prenatal diagnosis by molecular analysis once the mutation is known.

Treatment

Dietary leucine restriction and avoidance of catabolism are the cornerstones of treatment. Infant formulas deficient in BCAA must be supplemented with normal foods to supply adequate BCAA to permit normal growth. Plasma levels of BCAA must be monitored frequently to deal with changing protein requirements. Acute episodes of metabolic decompensation must be aggressively treated to prevent catabolism and negative nitrogen balance. Very high leucine levels require hemodialysis. Liver transplantation corrects the disorder, and the MSUD-affected liver may then safely be used for an unaffected recipient in a "domino" transplant because an unaffected recipient has enough whole-body residual enzyme activity to metabolize BCAA.

Ewing CB et al: Metabolic control and "ideal" outcomes in liver transplantation for maple syrup urine disease. J Pediatr 2021;237:59–64 [PMID: 34153280]
Patient and parent support group website with useful information for families: http://www.msud-support.org.

Strauss KA, Puffenberger EG, Carson VJ: Maple syrup urine disease. In: Margaret AP (ed): *GeneReviews*® [Internet]. Seattle, WA: University of Washington; 1993–2020. 2006 Jan 30 [updated 2020 Apr 23] [PMID: 20301495].

HOMOCYSTINURIA

ESSENTIALS OF DIAGNOSIS & TYPICAL FEATURES

▶ Consider in a child of any age with a marfanoid habitus, dislocated lenses, or thrombosis.

▶ Diagnosis is suggested by elevated total homocysteine and methionine.

▶ NBS allows early diagnosis and treatment resulting in a normal outcome.

Homocystinuria (HCU) is most often due to deficiency of cystathionine β-synthase (CBS) but may also be due to remethylation defects such as deficiency of methylenetetrahydrofolate reductase (MTHFR) or defects in the biosynthesis of methyl-B_{12}, the coenzyme for methionine synthase. Classic HCU and most forms of inherited methyl-B_{12} deficiency are autosomal recessive. About 50% of patients with untreated CBS deficiency have intellectual disability, and most have arachnodactyly, osteoporosis, and a tendency to develop dislocated lenses and thromboembolism. Mild variants of CBS deficiency present with thromboembolism. Patients with severe remethylation defects usually exhibit failure to thrive and a variety of neurologic symptoms, including brain atrophy, microcephaly, hydrocephalus, and seizures in infancy and early childhood.

Diagnosis

Diagnosis is made by demonstrating elevated total serum homocysteine particularly in individuals who are not deficient in vitamin B_{12}. Plasma methionine levels are usually high in patients with CBS deficiency and often low in patients with inherited methyl-B_{12} deficiency. Cystathionine levels are low in CBS deficiency. In inherited methyl-B_{12} deficiency, megaloblastic anemia or hemolytic uremic syndrome may be present and an associated deficiency of adenosyl-B_{12} may cause methylmalonic aciduria. Mutation analysis confirms the diagnosis.

Treatment

About 50% of patients with CBS deficiency respond to large oral doses of pyridoxine. Patients also treated with dietary methionine restriction and oral betaine, which increases methylation of homocysteine to methionine and improves neurologic function. Early treatment prevents intellectual disability, lens dislocation, and thromboembolic manifestations, which justifies the screening of newborn infants, but dietary adherence is challenging. Studies with enzyme replacement therapy are ongoing. Intramuscular or subcutaneously administered pharmacologic doses of hydroxocobalamin are indicated in some patients with defects in cobalamin metabolism. In remethylation defects, methionine may be low, and early supplementation improves outcome.

Huemer M et al: Guidelines for diagnosis and management of the cobalamin-related remethylation disorders cblC, cblD, cblE, cblF, cblG, cblJ and MTHFR deficiency. J Inherit Metab Dis 2017;40(1):21–48 [PMID: 27905001].

Morris AA et al: Guidelines for the diagnosis and management of cystathionine beta-synthase deficiency. J Inherit Metab Dis 2017;40(1):49–74 [PMID: 27778219].

NONKETOTIC HYPERGLYCINEMIA

ESSENTIALS OF DIAGNOSIS & TYPICAL FEATURES

▶ Severely affected newborns present with apnea, hypotonia, lethargy, myoclonic seizures, and hiccups and develop severe mental and motor retardation.

▶ Mildly affected children have developmental delay, hyperactivity, mild chorea, and seizures.

▶ CSF glycine is elevated.

Inherited deficiency of protein subunits of the glycine cleavage enzyme causes classic nonketotic hyperglycinemia (NKH), and deficiency of the cofactor lipoate causes variant NKH. These defects and a defect in the glycine transporter *GLYT1* constitute the glycine encephalopathies. The pathophysiology is poorly understood but includes toxicity from excessive glycine accumulation in the brain, which could affect neurotransmission at the *N*-methyl-D-aspartate type of glutamate receptors. The severe form of classic NKH presents in the newborn as hypotonia, lethargy proceeding to coma, myoclonic seizures, and hiccups, with a burst suppression pattern on electroencephalogram (EEG). Respiratory depression may require ventilator assistance in the first 2 weeks, followed by spontaneous recovery. Patients develop severe intellectual disability and recalcitrant seizures. Some severely affected patients have a small corpus callosum or may develop hydrocephalus. All patients have restricted diffusion on magnetic resonance imaging (MRI) in the already myelinated long tracts at birth. Patients with an attenuated form present with treatable seizures, varying developmental delay, and chorea, and one-half of these may present later in infancy or in childhood. All forms of the condition are autosomal recessive. Lipoate disorders may have added optic neuropathy, white matter disease and cardiomyopathy. Glycine transporter defect causes severe spasticity and hyperekplexia.

▶ Diagnosis

NKH should be suspected in any neonate or infant with seizures, particularly those with burst suppression pattern on EEG. Diagnosis is confirmed by demonstrating a large increase in glycine in non-bloody CSF, with an abnormally high ratio of CSF glycine to plasma glycine, and recognition of the typical diffusion restriction pattern on brain MRI. Combined sequencing and exonic copy number analysis of *GLDC* and *AMT* is diagnostic in more than 98% of cases. Defects in biosynthesis of the cofactors lipoate or pyridoxal phosphate also present with epileptic encephalopathy with elevated CSF glycine. Prenatal diagnosis is possible by molecular analysis.

▶ Treatment

Treatment includes glycine reduction using high dose benzoate to conjugate with glycine, facilitating its removal. Ketogenic diet also reduces glycine levels. In patients with attenuated disease, glycine reduction treatment combined with dextromethorphan or ketamine (to block *N*-methyl-D-aspartate type of glutamate receptors) controls seizures and improves neurodevelopmental outcome. Treatment of severely affected patients improves wakefulness and seizure control but does not prevent severe intellectual disability. Clobazam is used as a first line antiepileptic medication.

NKH Crusaders: www.nkhcrusaaders.com.

Patient and parent support group website with useful information for families: http://www.nkh-network.org.

Van Hove JLK, Coughlin C II, Swanson M, Hennermann JB: Nonketotic hyperglycinemia. In: Adam MP (ed): *GeneReviews®* [Internet]. Seattle, WA: University of Washington; 1993–2021. 2002 Nov 14 [updated 2019 May 23] [PMID: 20301531].

ORGANIC ACIDEMIAS

ESSENTIALS OF DIAGNOSIS & TYPICAL FEATURES

▶ Consider in any child presenting with metabolic acidosis and ketosis in early infancy.

▶ Urine organic acid analysis is usually diagnostic.

Table 36–2. Clinical and laboratory features of organic acidemias.

Disorder	Enzyme Defect	Clinical and Laboratory Features
Isovaleric acidemia	Isovaleryl-CoA dehydrogenase	Acidosis and odor of sweaty feet in infancy, or growth retardation and episodes of vomiting, lethargy, and acidosis. Some forms mild. Persistent isovalerylglycine and intermittent 3-hydroxyisovaleric acid in urine.
3-Methylcrotonyl-CoA carboxylase deficiency	3-Methylcrotonyl-CoA carboxylase	Usually asymptomatic. Acidosis and feeding problems in infancy, or Reye-like episodes in older child. 3-Methylcrotonylglycine and 3-hydroxyisovaleric acid in urine.
Combined-carboxylase deficiency	Holocarboxylase synthetase	Hypotonia and lactic acidosis in infancy. 3-Hydroxyisovaleric acid in urine, often with small amounts of 3-hydroxypropionic and methylcitric acids. Often biotin responsive.
Biotinidase deficiency	Biotinidase	Alopecia, seborrheic rash, seizures, and ataxia in infancy or childhood. Urine organic acids as above. Always biotin responsive.
3-Hydroxy-3-methylglutaric acidemia	3-Hydroxy-3-methylglutaryl-CoA lyase	Hypoglycemia and acidosis in infancy; Reye-like episodes with nonketotic hypoglycemia or leukodystrophy in older children. 3-Hydroxy-3-methylglutaric, 3-methylglutaconic, and 3-hydroxyisovaleric acids in urine.
3-Ketothiolase deficiency	3-Ketothiolase	Episodes of vomiting, severe metabolic acidosis (hyperketosis), and encephalopathy. 2-Methyl-3-hydroxybutyric and 2-methylacetoacetic acids and tiglylglycine in urine, especially after isoleucine load.
Propionic acidemia	Propionyl-CoA carboxylase	Hyperammonemia and metabolic acidosis in infancy; ketotic hyperglycinemia syndrome later. 3-Hydroxypropionic and methylcitric acids in urine, with 3-hydroxy- and 3-ketovaleric acids during ketotic episodes.
Methylmalonic acidemia	Methylmalonyl-CoA mutase	Clinical features same as in propionic acidemia. Methylmalonic acid in urine, often with 3-hydroxypropionic and methylcitric acids.
	Defects in vitamin B_{12} biosynthesis	Clinical features same as above when adenosyl-B_{12} synthesis is decreased; early neurologic features prominent when accompanied by decreased synthesis of methyl-B_{12}. In latter instance, hypomethioninemia and homocystinuria accompany methylmalonic aciduria.
Pyroglutamic acidemia	Glutathione synthetase	Acidosis and hemolytic anemia in infancy; chronic acidosis later. Pyroglutamic acid in urine.
Glutaric acidemia type I	Glutaryl-CoA dehydrogenase	Progressive extrapyramidal movement disorder in childhood, with episodes of acidosis, vomiting, and encephalopathy. Risk window birth through 6 years. Glutaric acid and 3-hydroxyglutaric acid in serum and urine.
Glutaric acidemia type II	ETF:ubiquinone oxidoreductase (ETF dehydrogenase) and ETF	Hypoglycemia, acidosis, hyperammonemia, and odor of sweaty feet in infancy, often with polycystic and dysplastic kidneys. Severe neonatal onset is life limiting due to cardiac complications. Later onset may be with episodes of hypoketotic hypoglycemia, liver dysfunction, or slowly progressive skeletal myopathy. Glutaric, ethylmalonic, 3-hydroxyisovaleric, isovalerylglycine, and 2-hydroxyglutaric acids in urine, often with sarcosine in serum.
4-Hydroxybutyric acidemia	Succinic semialdehyde dehydrogenase	Seizures, ataxia, and developmental retardation. 4-Hydroxybutyric acid in urine.

CoA, coenzyme A; ETF, electron transfer flavoprotein.

Organic acidemias are disorders of metabolism in which nonamino, organic acids accumulate in serum and urine. These conditions are usually diagnosed by examining organic acids in urine in specialized laboratories. Table 36–2 lists the clinical features of organic acidemias, together with the urine organic acid patterns typical of each. Additional details about some of the more important organic acidemias are provided in the sections that follow.

PROPIONIC & METHYLMALONIC ACIDEMIA (KETOTIC HYPERGLYCINEMIAS)

The oxidation of valine, odd chain length fatty acids, methionine, isoleucine, and threonine (V.O.M.I.T) ultimately results in propionyl-CoA and methylmalonyl-CoA, which are metabolized to succinyl-CoA for entry into the tricarboxylic acid (Krebs) cycle. Gut bacteria also substantially contribute to propionyl-CoA production. Propionic acidemia (PA) is due to a defect in the biotin-dependent enzyme propionyl-CoA carboxylase. Methylmalonic acidemia (MMA) is due to a defect in the B12-dependent enzyme methylmalonyl-CoA mutase, in either the mutase apoenzyme or in the synthesis of its cofactor, adenosyl-B_{12}. Some disorders of vitamin B_{12} metabolism affect only the synthesis of adenosyl-B_{12} (Cbl A or B), whereas in others (Cbl C, D, F, J, X) the synthesis of methyl-B_{12} is also blocked leading to elevated homocysteine in addition to methylmalonic acid (see Homocystinuria).

Clinical symptoms vary according to the location and severity of the enzyme block. Children with severe blocks present with acute, life-threatening metabolic ketoacidosis, hyperammonemia, coma, and bone marrow depression in early infancy or with metabolic acidosis, vomiting, and failure to thrive during the first few months of life. Most patients with severe disease have mild or moderate intellectual disability. Other complications include pancreatitis, basal ganglia necrosis, cardiomyopathy (more in PA), and interstitial nephritis and chronic kidney disease (more in MMA). All forms of PA and MMA are autosomal recessive (except for X-linked Cbl X) and can be diagnosed *in utero* and through NBS.

▶ Diagnosis

Laboratory findings consist of increases in urinary organic acids derived from propionyl-CoA or methylmalonic acid (see Table 36–2) and elevated propionylcarnitine (C3, easily detected by the NBS). Hyperglycinemia and ketosis can be present, especially in acute illness. In some forms of abnormal vitamin B_{12} metabolism, homocysteine can be elevated. Confirmation is by molecular analysis and/or by assays in fibroblasts or lymphocytes (PA only).

▶ Treatment

Patients with enzymatic blocks in B_{12} metabolism usually respond to pharmacologic doses of vitamin B_{12} (hydroxocobalamin) given subcutaneously or intramuscularly. Vitamin B_{12} nonresponsive MMA and PA require amino acid restriction, strict prevention of catabolism, and carnitine supplementation to enhance C3 excretion. Intermittent metronidazole can help reduce the propionate load from the gut. In the acute setting, hemodialysis or hemofiltration may be needed. Liver transplant, or combined liver-renal transplantation, is an option in severe forms of these disorders.

Haijes HA, Jans JJM, Tas SY, Verhoeven-Duif NM, van Hasselt PM: Pathophysiology of propionic and methylmalonic acidemias. Part 1: complications. J Inherit Metab Dis 2019 Sep;42(5):730–744 [PMID: 31119747].

Haijes HA, van Hasselt PM, Jans JJM, Verhoeven-Duif NM: Pathophysiology of propionic and methylmalonic acidemias. Part 2: treatment strategies. J Inherit Metab Dis 2019 Sep;42(5):745–761 [PMID: 31119742].

Manoli I, Sloan JL, Venditti CP: Isolated methylmalonic acidemia. In: Pagon RA et al (eds): *GeneReviews®*. Seattle, WA: University of Washington; 2016 [updated 2022 Sep 8] [PMID: 20301409].

Sloan JL, Carrillo N, Adams D, Venditti CP: Disorders of intracellular cobalamin metabolism. In: Pagon RA et al (eds): *GeneReviews®*. Seattle, WA: University of Washington; 2008 [updated 2021 Dec 16] [PMID: 20301503].

CARBOXYLASE DEFICIENCY

Isolated pyruvate carboxylase deficiency presents with lactic acidosis and hyperammonemia in early infancy. Even if biochemically stabilized, the neurologic outcome in early onset disease is poor. Isolated 3-methylcrotonyl-CoA carboxylase (3MCC) deficiency is frequently recognized on NBS using acylcarnitine analysis. It is usually a benign condition that sometimes causes symptoms of acidosis. All carboxylases require biotin as a cofactor. Holocarboxylase synthetase covalently binds biotin to the apocarboxylases for pyruvate, 3-methylcrotonyl-CoA, and propionyl-CoA; biotinidase releases biotin from these proteins and from proteins in the diet. Recessively inherited deficiency of either enzyme causes deficiency of all three carboxylases (ie, multiple carboxylase deficiency). Patients with holocarboxylase synthetase deficiency present as neonates with hypotonia, skin problems, and severe acidosis. Those with biotinidase deficiency present later with ataxia, seizures, seborrhea, and alopecia. Untreated patients can develop intellectual disability, hearing loss, and optic nerve atrophy. Sequelae in most patients are preventable if treated early.

▶ Diagnosis

This diagnosis should be considered in patients with typical symptoms or in those with primary lactic acidosis. Urine organic acids are usually, but not always, abnormal (see Table 36–2). Diagnosis is made by enzyme assay of carboxylase activities and/or genetic testing. Biotinidase can be assayed in serum, and holocarboxylase synthetase in leukocytes or fibroblasts. Nearly all children with biotinidase deficiency are now diagnosed with NBS.

▶ Treatment

Isolated carboxylase deficiencies are often unresponsive to biotin supplementation. In biotinidase deficiency and holocarboxylase deficiencies, oral administration of pharmacologic doses of biotin reverses the organic aciduria within days and the clinical symptoms within days to weeks. Hearing loss can occur in patients with profound biotinidase deficiency despite treatment.

Donti TR, Blackburn PR, Atwal PS: Holocarboxylase synthetase deficiency pre and post newborn screening. Mol Genet Metab Rep 2016;7:40–44 [PMID: 27114915].

Wolf B: Biotinidase deficiency. In: Pagon RA et al (eds): *GeneReviews®*. Seattle, WA: University of Washington; 2016 [PMID: 20301497].

GLUTARIC ACIDEMIA TYPE I

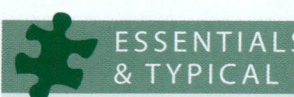

ESSENTIALS OF DIAGNOSIS
& TYPICAL FEATURES

▶ Suspect in children with acute basal ganglia necrosis, macrocephaly, subdural hemorrhage, and acute or progressive dystonia.

▶ Presymptomatic diagnosis by NBS and treatment reduces the incidence of acute encephalopathic crises.

Glutaric acidemia type I (GA1) occurs due to deficiency of glutaryl-CoA dehydrogenase. Patients have frontotemporal atrophy with enlarged sylvian fissures and macrocephaly. Sudden basal ganglia necrosis or chronic neuronal degeneration in the caudate and putamen cause an extrapyramidal movement disorder in childhood with dystonia and athetosis. Children with GA1 may present with retinal and/or subdural hemorrhages, possibly mistaken for child abuse. This is a disorder that primarily affects the central nervous system, and does not present with systemic acidosis, hypoglycemia, or primary end-organ damage elsewhere. Onset of basal ganglia necrosis has only been reported in the first 6 years of life, which represents the vulnerable period. The condition is autosomal recessive and prenatal diagnosis is possible.

▶ Diagnosis

GA1 should be suspected in patients with acute or progressive dystonia in the first 6 years of life. MRI of the brain is highly suggestive. The diagnosis is supported by finding glutaric, 3-hydroxyglutaric acid, and glutarylcarnitine (C5DC) in urine or serum or by finding two mutations in the *GCDH* gene. Demonstration of deficiency of glutaryl-CoA dehydrogenase in fibroblasts can confirm the diagnosis. Prenatal diagnosis is by mutation analysis, enzyme assay, or quantitative metabolite analysis in amniotic fluid. This condition is detected on the NBS.

▶ Treatment

Strict prevention of catabolism in fasting or illness is critically important. Supplementation with carnitine and a lysine-restricted diet reduce the risk of basal ganglia necrosis. Benefit of arginine supplementation is controversial. Early diagnosis does not prevent neurologic disease in all patients, but it reduces the risk, warranting NBS. Despite treatment, affected individuals may have deficiencies in speech and fine motor skills. Neurologic symptoms, once present, do not typically resolve. Symptomatic treatment of severe dystonia is important for affected patients.

Boy N et al: Proposed recommendations for diagnosing and managing individuals with glutaric aciduria type I: third revision. J Inherit Metab Dis 2023 May;46(3):482–519. doi: 10.1002/jimd.12566. [Epub 2022 Nov 17] [PMID: 36221165].

Boy N, et al: Subdural hematoma in glutaric aciduria type 1: high excreters are prone to incidental SDH despite newborn screening. J Inherit Metab Dis 2021 Nov;44(6):1343–1352 [PMID: 34515344].

Larson A, Goodman S: Glutaric acidemia type 1. In: Adam MP et al (eds): *GeneReviews®* [Internet]. Seattle, WA: University of Washington; 1993–2021. 2019 Sep 19 [PMID: 31536184].

DISORDERS OF FATTY ACID OXIDATION & CARNITINE

FATTY ACID OXIDATION DISORDERS

ESSENTIALS OF DIAGNOSIS
& TYPICAL FEATURES

▶ Obtain an acylcarnitine profile for children with hypoglycemia, rhabdomyolysis, hepatic encephalopathy, or cardiomyopathy to evaluate for a fatty acid oxidation defect.

▶ Early diagnosis and treatment can prevent morbidity and mortality in affected children, and avoidance of prolonged fasting is of paramount importance for long-term management.

Fatty acid oxidation disorders (FAODs) are disorders of the transport and catabolism of fatty acids in the mitochondria. In general, FAODs present with hypoketotic hypoglycemia and, depending on the specific disorder, may include hyperammonemia, hepatopathy, encephalopathy, and/or skeletal myopathy or cardiomyopathy. The long-chain defects, which include very-long-chain acyl-CoA dehydrogenase (VLCAD), long-chain 3-hydroxyacyl-CoA dehydrogenase (LCHAD), carnitine palmitoyltransferase deficiency I and II (CPT1, CPT2), and carnitine-acylcarnitine translocase (CACT) deficiency, cause episodic rhabdomyolysis, cardiomyopathy, and ventricular arrhythmias. Deficiencies of VLCAD and LCHAD also cause hepatic encephalopathy (Reye-like) episodes. Sudden infant death syndrome (SIDS) is a less common presentation. Symptoms specific to LCHAD deficiency include progressive liver cirrhosis, peripheral neuropathy, and pigmentary retinopathy and a higher-than-expected incidence of acute fatty liver of pregnancy (AFLP) and hemolysis, elevated liver enzymes, and low platelets (HELLP) syndrome during pregnancy in carrier mothers of affected infants.

Medium-chain acyl-CoA dehydrogenase deficiency (MCADD) is the most common FAOD, occurring in perhaps 1:9000 live births. Reye-like episodes, which historically have been largely caused by undiagnosed MCADD, may be fatal or cause residual neurologic damage. Similarly, SIDS occurrences are now thought to be in part because of undiagnosed MCADD and fasting in infancy. Episodes of hypoketotic hypoglycemia tend to become less frequent and severe with time. After the diagnosis is made (now by newborn screen) and treatment instituted, morbidity decreases and mortality is avoided.

Short-chain acyl-CoA dehydrogenase (SCAD) deficiency is characterized by the presence of ethylmalonic acid in the urine. Patients are generally asymptomatic, and this is increasingly considered a non-disease. Glutaric acidemia type II (GA2 or multiple acyl-CoA dehydrogenase deficiency) results from defects in the flavin-mediated transfer of electrons from fatty acid oxidation and some amino acid oxidation into the respiratory chain. Some patients with GA2 have a clinical presentation resembling MCADD. Patients with a severe neonatal presentation may also have renal cystic disease, dysmorphic features, and profound cardiomyopathy. The least affected patients can present with late-onset myopathy and be riboflavin responsive. Some develop cardiomyopathy or leukodystrophy. Deficiency of the ketogenic enzymes 3-hydroxymethylglutaryl-CoA synthase and lyase present with hypoketotic hypoglycemia. Disorders of cytoplasmic fatty acid metabolism are being increasingly recognized. Deficiency of lipin 1, a cytoplasmic triglyceride lipase, causes severe episodes of rhabdomyolysis starting at a very early age. These conditions are all autosomal recessive.

▶ Diagnosis

All FAOD have reduced ketogenesis in response to fasting. The analysis of acylcarnitine esters (via an acylcarnitine profile) is a first-line diagnostic test used in NBS because it reveals diagnostic metabolites regardless of clinical status. A typical pattern can be recognized for each disorder; for instance, MCADD is characterized by elevated octanoylcarnitine (C8). Some disorders have elevated acylglycine esters that can be identified in urine organic acid analysis or on specific quantitative acylglycine analysis. Further confirmation can be obtained from genetic testing or analysis of fatty acid oxidation in fibroblasts; enzyme assays are only rarely available.

▶ Treatment

Management of all FAOD involves avoidance of prolonged fasting (> 8–12 hours). This includes aggressive treatment of fasting associated with illness using glucose. Because fatty acid oxidation can be compromised by associated carnitine deficiency, young patients with MCADD usually receive oral carnitine when carnitine levels are low. Restriction of dietary long-chain fats is not necessary in MCADD but is required for severe VLCAD and LCHAD deficiencies. Medium-chain triglycerides or triheptanoin are a potential energy source for patients with long chain disorders, but not in MCADD. Other potential alternative fuel sources include protein and exogenous ketones. Peroxisome proliferator-activated receptor (PPAR) agonists like bezafibrate may be beneficial. Riboflavin may also be beneficial in some patients with GA2. Outcome in MCADD is excellent but is more guarded in patients with long chain disorders.

Anderson DR, et al: Clinical and biochemical outcomes of patients with medium-chain acyl-CoA dehydrogenase deficiency. Mol Genet Metab 2020 Jan;129(1):13–19 [PMID: 31836396].
Leslie ND, Saenz-Ayala S: Very long-chain acyl-coenzyme A dehydrogenase deficiency. 2009 May 28 [updated 2022 Jun 16]. In: Adam MP et al (eds): *GeneReviews*® [Internet]. Seattle, WA: University of Washington; 1993–2023 [PMID: 20301763].
Patient and parent support group website with useful information for families: http://www.fodsupport.org.
Prasun P, LoPiccolo MK, Ginevic I: Long-chain hydroxyacyl-CoA dehydrogenase deficiency/trifunctional protein deficiency. 2022 Sep 1. In: Adam MP et al (eds): *GeneReviews*® [Internet]. Seattle, WA: University of Washington; 1993–2023 [PMID: 36063482].

CARNITINE

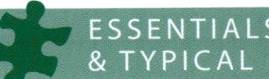

ESSENTIALS OF DIAGNOSIS & TYPICAL FEATURES

► Primary carnitine deficiency manifests as cardiac disease including cardiomyopathy and sudden death, as hypoketotic hypoglycemia, or as exercise intolerance.

► Treatment of primary carnitine deficiency with carnitine improves outcome and prognosis.

► There are many causes of secondary carnitine deficiency.

Carnitine is an essential nutrient found in highest concentration in red meat. Its primary function is to transport long-chain fatty acids into mitochondria for oxidation. Primary carnitine uptake deficiency (CUD) may manifest as hepatic encephalopathy (Reye-like syndrome), cardiomyopathy, or skeletal myopathy with hypotonia. These disorders are rare compared with secondary carnitine deficiency, which may be due to diet (vegan diet, intravenous alimentation, or ketogenic diet), renal losses, drug therapy (especially valproic acid), and other metabolic disorders (especially organic acidemias). The prognosis depends on the cause of the carnitine abnormality. CUD is one of the most treatable causes of dilated cardiomyopathy in children.

Free and esterified carnitine can be measured in blood. If carnitine insufficiency is suspected, the patient should be evaluated to rule out disorders that might cause secondary carnitine deficiency, like FAOD and organic acidemias. Oral or intravenous L-carnitine is used in carnitine deficiency in doses of 25–100 mg/kg/day or higher. Treatment is titrated to maintain normal plasma carnitine levels. Carnitine supplementation in patients with secondary deficiency may also augment excretion of accumulated metabolites, although supplementation may not prevent metabolic crises in such patients.

Crefcoeur LL et al: Clinical characteristics of primary carnitine deficiency: a structured review using a case-by-case approach. J Inherit Metab Dis 2022 May;45(3):386–405 [PMID: 34997761].

PURINE METABOLISM DISORDERS

ESSENTIALS OF DIAGNOSIS & TYPICAL FEATURES

► Lesch-Nyhan syndrome is classically described in boys with spasticity, dystonia, and self-mutilating behaviors.

► Urinary uric acid to creatinine ratio or urine purines are useful screening tests.

Hypoxanthine-guanine phosphoribosyl transferase (HPRT) deficiency (Lesch-Nyhan Syndrome or LNS) is the most well-known purine metabolism disorder. HPRT recycles the purine bases hypoxanthine and guanine to inosine monophosphate and guanosine monophosphate, respectively. In this X-linked disorder, complete deficiency is characterized by CNS dysfunction, purine wasting with compensatory increase in purine synthesis, and xanthine and hypoxanthine overproduction resulting in hyperuricemia and hyperuricosuria. Depending on the residual activity of the mutant enzyme, male hemizygous individuals may be severely disabled by choreoathetosis, dystonia, and self-mutilation (lip and finger biting), and they typically have gouty arthritis and urate ureterolithiasis. One of the first signs is a red/orange crystal in the diaper called "brick dust." Macrocytosis is often present but does not typically require treatment.

▶ Diagnosis

Diagnosis of LNS is made by demonstrating an elevated uric acid:creatinine ratio in urine, and/or by genetic analysis.

▶ Treatment

Hyperhydration and alkalinization are essential to prevent kidney stones and urate nephropathy. Allopurinol and probenecid may be given to reduce hyperuricemia and prevent gout but do not affect the neurologic status. Physical restraints are often more effective than neurologic medications for self-mutilation. Masseter Botox injection and oral barrier therapies help, but ultimately most patients require dental extraction to prevent self-harm.

Jinnah HA: *HPRT1* disorders. In: Adam MP et al (eds): *GeneReviews®* [Internet]. Seattle, WA: University of Washington; 1993–2023. 2000 Sept 25 [updated 2020 Aug 6] [PMID: 20301328].
Patient and parent support group websites with useful information for families: http://lndnet.ning.com and http://www.lesch-nyhan.org.

LYSOSOMAL DISEASES

ESSENTIALS OF DIAGNOSIS & TYPICAL FEATURES

► Lysosomal storage disorders may present clinically with multisystem involvement including hepatosplenomegaly, cardiac disease, and skeletal features, with or without neurologic involvement.

► Brain imaging, skeletal survey, and urinary mucopolysaccharide or oligosaccharide analyses may be helpful in initial screening studies; most diagnoses are made by enzyme assay followed by genetic confirmation.

► Therapy may be available for many of these previously untreatable disorders.

Lysosomes are cellular organelles in which complex macromolecules are degraded by specific acid hydrolases. Deficiency of a lysosomal enzyme causes its substrate to accumulate in the lysosomes, resulting in a characteristic clinical picture. These lysosomal storage disorders are classified as mucopolysaccharidoses, lipidoses, or oligosaccharidoses, depending on the nature of the stored material. Two additional disorders, cystinosis and Salla disease, are caused by defects in lysosomal proteins that normally transport material from the lysosome to the cytoplasm. Table 36–3 lists clinical and laboratory features of these conditions. Most are inherited as autosomal recessive traits, and all can be diagnosed in utero.

▶ Diagnosis

The diagnosis of mucopolysaccharidosis is suggested by certain clinical and radiologic features (see Table 36–3; Figure 36–2). Thickened soft tissue and characteristic facial features may be present. Multi-system signs can include corneal clouding, intellectual disability and neurobehavioral differences, hepatosplenomegaly, renal disease, and peripheral neuropathy, depending on the disorder. Radiographic findings can include dysostosis multiplex, manifesting with enlarged sella turcica; scaphocephaly; broad ribs; beaked vertebrae; gibus; and limited hand, shoulder, elbow, and knee extension.

Urine screening tests can detect increased mucopolysaccharides and oligosaccharides and further identify which specific species are present. Diagnosis must be confirmed by

Table 36–3. Clinical and laboratory features of lysosomal storage diseases.

Disorder	Enzyme Defect	Clinical and Laboratory Features	Available Therapies
I. Mucopolysaccharidoses			
Hurler syndrome	α-Iduronidase	Autosomal recessive. ID, hepatomegaly, umbilical hernia, coarse facies, corneal clouding, dorsolumbar gibbus, severe heart disease. Heparan sulfate and dermatan sulfate in urine.	HSCT ERT
Scheie syndrome	α-Iduronidase (incomplete)	Autosomal recessive. Corneal clouding, stiff joints, normal intellect. Clinical types intermediate between Hurler and Scheie common. Heparan sulfate and dermatan sulfate in urine.	ERT
Hunter syndrome	Sulfoiduronate sulfatase	X-linked recessive. Coarse facies, hepatomegaly, ID variable. Corneal clouding and gibbus not present. Heparan sulfate and dermatan sulfate in urine.	HSCT ERT
Sanfilippo syndrome: Type A Type B Type C Type D	Sulfamidase α-N-Acetylglucosaminidase Acetyl-CoA: α-glucosaminide-N-acetyltransferase α-N-acetylglucosamine-6-sulfatase	Autosomal recessive. Severe ID and hyperactivity, with comparatively mild skeletal changes, visceromegaly, and facial coarseness. Types cannot be differentiated clinically. Heparan sulfate in urine.	
Morquio syndrome	N-Acetylgalactosamine-6-sulfatase	Autosomal recessive. Severe skeletal changes, platyspondylisis, corneal clouding. Keratan sulfate in urine.	ERT
Maroteaux-Lamy syndrome	N-Acetylgalactosamine-4-sulfatase	Autosomal recessive. Coarse facies, growth retardation, dorsolumbar gibbus, corneal clouding, hepatosplenomegaly, normal intellect. Dermatan sulfate in urine.	HSCT ERT
B-Glucuronidase deficiency	β-Glucuronidase	Autosomal recessive. Variable ID, dorsolumbar gibbus, corneal clouding, and hepatosplenomegaly to mild facial coarseness, retardation, and loose joints. Hearing loss common. Dermatan sulfate or heparan sulfate in urine.	HSCT
II. Oligosaccharidoses			
Mannosidosis	α-Mannosidase	Autosomal recessive. Variable ID, coarse facies, short stature, skeletal changes, and hepatosplenomegaly to mild facial coarseness and loose joints. Hearing loss common. Abnormal oligosaccharides in urine.	HSCT
Fucosidosis	α-Fucosidase	Autosomal recessive. Variable ID, coarse facies, skeletal changes, hepatosplenomegaly, occasional angiokeratomas. Abnormal oligosaccharides in urine.	HSCT
I-cell disease (mucolipidosis II)	N-Acetylglucosaminyl phosphotransferase	Autosomal recessive; severe and mild forms known. Very short stature, ID, early facial coarsening, clear cornea, and stiffness of joints. Increased lysosomal enzymes in serum. Abnormal Sialyl oligosaccharides in urine.	HSCT
Sialidosis	Neuraminidase (sialidase)	Autosomal recessive. ID, coarse facies, skeletal dysplasia, myoclonic seizures, macular cherry-red spot. Abnormal Sialyl oligosaccharides in urine.	
III. Lipidoses			
Niemann-Pick disease	Sphingomyelinase	Autosomal recessive. Acute and chronic forms known. Acute neuronopathic form common in Eastern European Jewish ancestry. Accumulation of sphingomyelin in lysosomes of RE system and CNS. Hepatosplenomegaly, developmental retardation, macular cherry-red spot. Death by 1–4 y in severe type A; mild type B develops respiratory insufficiency usually in adulthood.	HSCT[a]

(Continued)

Table 36–3. Clinical and laboratory features of lysosomal storage diseases. (*Continued*)

Disorder	Enzyme Defect	Clinical and Laboratory Features	Available Therapies
Metachromatic leukodystrophy	Arylsulfatase A	Autosomal recessive. Late infantile form, with onset at 1–4 y, most common. Accumulation of sulfatide in white matter with central leukodystrophy and peripheral neuropathy. Gait disturbances (ataxia), motor incoordination, absent deep tendon reflexes, and dementia. Death usually in first decade.	HSCT[a]
Krabbe disease (globoid cell leukodystrophy)	Galactocerebroside α-galactosidase	Autosomal recessive. Globoid cells in white matter. Psychosine in blood. Onset at 3–6 mo with seizures, irritability, retardation, and leukodystrophy. Death by 1–2 y. Juvenile and adult forms are rare.	HSCT[a]
Fabry disease	α-Galactosidase A	X-linked recessive. Storage of trihexosylceramide in endothelial cells. Pain in extremities, angiokeratoma and (later) poor vision, hypertension, and renal failure.	ERT, CT
Farber disease	Ceramidase	Autosomal recessive. Storage of ceramide in tissues. Subcutaneous nodules, arthropathy with deformed and painful joints, and poor growth and development. Death within first year.	HSCT[a]
Gaucher disease	Glucocerebroside β-glucosidase	Autosomal recessive. Accumulation of glucocerebroside in lysosomes of RE system and CNS. Acute neuronopathic form: ID, hepatosplenomegaly, macular cherry-red spot, and Gaucher cells in bone marrow. Death by 1–2 y. Chronic form common in Eastern European Jewish ancestry. Hepatosplenomegaly and flask-shaped osteolytic bone lesions. Consistent with normal life expectancy.	ERT SIT
G$_{M1}$ gangliosidosis	G$_{M1}$ ganglioside β-galactosidase	Autosomal recessive. Accumulation of G$_{M1}$ ganglioside in lysosomes of RE system and CNS. Infantile form: abnormalities at birth with dysostosis multiplex, hepatosplenomegaly, macular cherry-red spot, and death by 2 y. Juvenile form: normal development to 1 y of age, then ataxia, weakness, dementia, and death by 4–5 y. Occasional inferior beaking of vertebral bodies of L1 and L2.	HSCT[a]
G$_{M2}$ gangliosidoses Tay-Sachs disease Sandhoff disease	β-N-Acetylhexosaminidase A β-N-Acetylhexosaminidase A and B	Autosomal recessive. Tay-Sachs disease common in Eastern European Jewish ancestry; Sandhoff disease is pan-ethnic. Clinical phenotypes are identical, with accumulation of G$_{M2}$ ganglioside in lysosomes of CNS. Onset at age 3–6 mo, with hypotonia, hyperacusis, ID, and macular cherry-red spot. Death by 2–3 y. Juvenile- and adult-onset forms of Tay-Sachs disease are rare.	
Wolman disease	Acid lipase	Autosomal recessive. Accumulation of cholesterol esters and triglycerides in lysosomes of reticuloendothelial system. Onset in infancy with gastrointestinal symptoms and hepatosplenomegaly, and death in the first year. Adrenals commonly enlarged and calcified.	HSCT ERT
Niemann-Pick disease type C	*NPC1* gene (95%), *NPC2* gene (5%)	Autosomal recessive. Blocked transport of lipids and cholesterol from late endosomes to lysosomes. Infantile cholestatic liver disease or later neurodegeneration with vertical supranuclear gaze palsy, ataxia, gelastic cataplexy, seizures, spasticity, and loss of speech. Some have splenomegaly.	SIT

CNS, central nervous system; CT, Chaperone therapy; ERT, enzyme-replacement therapy; HSCT, hematopoietic stem cell transplantation; ID, intellectual disability; RE, reticuloendothelial; SIT, substrate inhibition therapy.
[a]May be useful in selected patients.

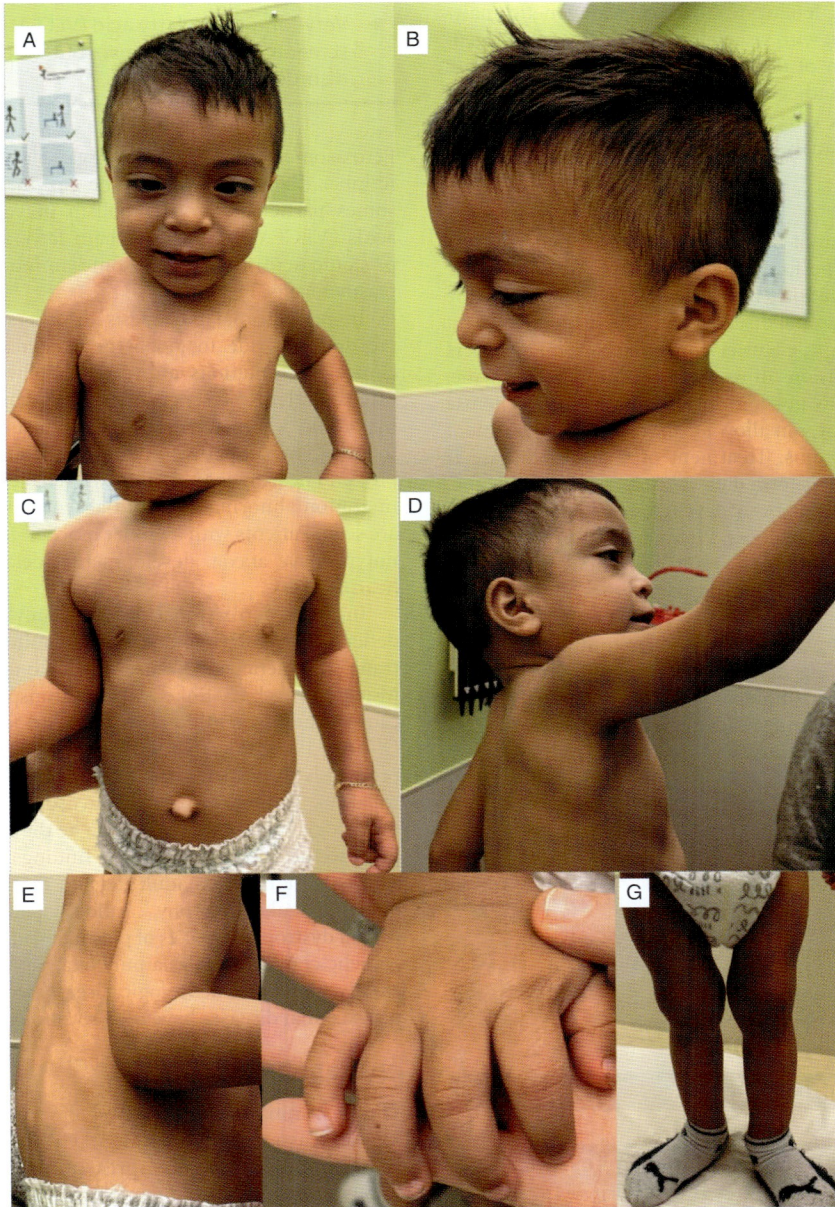

▲ **Figure 36–2.** Characteristic features of mucopolysaccharidosis in a 22-month-old boy with Maroteaux-Lamy syndrome (MPS type VI). Facial features include hypertelorism, strabismus, long broad philtrum, full cheeks, and thickened eyebrows (**A**), macrocephaly with frontal bossing and low-set ears (**B**), flared rib cage and umbilical hernia (**C**), limited range of motion at the shoulder (**D**), lumbar kyphosis with gibbus (**E**), contracture of the fingers (**F**), and genu valgum with pes valgo planus (**G**).

enzyme assays using leukocytes together with genetic analysis. Lipidoses present with visceral symptoms or neurodegeneration. The pattern of the leukodystrophy associated with many lipidoses can indicate a specific condition. Diagnosis is made by appropriate enzyme assays of peripheral leukocytes paired with genetic analysis.

Treatment

Most conditions cannot be treated effectively, but new avenues have given hope for many conditions. Hematopoietic stem cell transplantation (HSCT) can greatly improve the course of some lysosomal diseases and is first-line treatment in some, such as infantile Hurler syndrome. Several disorders are treated with infusions of recombinant modified enzyme. Infusions are typically given intravenously; however, the use of intrathecal infusion can allow for more effective treatment of neurologic symptoms. Treatment of Gaucher disease is very effective, and long-term data suggest excellent outcome. Similar treatments have been developed for Fabry disease, several mucopolysaccharidoses, Wolman disease, and Pompe disease (considered both a GSD and lysosomal storage disorder); substantial improvements in these conditions have been reported but with limitations. New avenues for treatment through substrate inhibition, chaperone therapy, and gene therapy are being developed. Treatment of cystinosis with cysteamine results in depletion of stored cystine, slowing complications including renal disease. Niemann-Pick C is being more effectively treated with cyclodextrin.

Huizing M, Gahl WA: Inherited disorders of lysosomal membrane transporters. Biochim Biophys Acta Biomembr 2020 Dec 1; 1862(12):183336 [PMID: 32389669].

McBride KL, Flanigan KM: Update in the mucopolysaccharidoses. Semin Pediatr Neurol 2021 Apr;37:100874 [PMID: 33892850].

Penon-Portmann M, Blair DR, Harmatz P: Current and new therapies for mucopolysaccharidoses. Pediatr Neonatol 2023 Feb; 64 (Suppl 1):S10–S17 [PMID: 36464587].

Platt FM et al: Lysosomal storage diseases. Nat Rev Dis Primers 2018 Oct 1;4(1):27 [PMID: 30275469].

PEROXISOMAL DISEASES

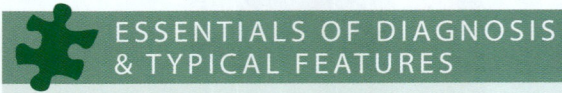

ESSENTIALS OF DIAGNOSIS & TYPICAL FEATURES

▶ Dysmorphic facial features, hypotonia, hearing loss, seizures, cataracts, retinopathy, liver disease, and renal disease are characteristic findings of severe peroxisomal disease.

▶ Change in behavior or school failure in a young boy may suggest X-linked adrenoleukodystrophy (X-ALD) and warrants a brain MRI with contrast.

▶ Very-long-chain fatty acid (VLCFA) analysis is a good screening test for most, but not all, peroxisomal disorders.

Peroxisomes are intracellular organelles that contain a large number (>70) of enzymes. The enzyme systems in peroxisomes participate in metabolism of very-long-chain fatty acids (VLCFAs), branched chain fatty acids (phytanic and pristanic acid), bile acids, some amino acids, oxalate, and plasmalogens.

In peroxisomal biogenesis disorders, multiple enzymes are deficient due to global peroxisomal dysfunction. The clinical presentations are termed Zellweger spectrum disorders. Patients present as neonates or infants with seizures, hypotonia, characteristic facies with a large forehead and fontanel, hepatopathy, feeding difficulties, retinal dystrophy, and hearing loss. At autopsy, renal cysts, brain neuronal migration abnormalities, and absent or empty peroxisomes are seen. Patients with a milder biochemical and clinical phenotype have ataxia, developmental delay, retinopathy, and hearing loss.

In other peroxisomal diseases, only a single enzyme is deficient. Primary hyperoxaluria (alanine-glyoxylate aminotransferase deficiency) causes renal stones and nephropathy. Mutations in the X-linked VLCFA transporter gene, *ABCD1*, cause either a rapidly progressive and fatal leukodystrophy (X-linked adrenoleukodystrophy (X-ALD)) or a slowly progressive spasticity and neuropathy (adrenomyeloneuropathy). Adrenal insufficiency usually accompanies both neurologic presentations and can be the presenting symptom prior to the onset of neurologic findings. Defective phytanic acid oxidation causes adult Refsum disease, with symptoms of ataxia, leukodystrophy, cardiomyopathy, neuropathy, and retinal dystrophy. Defects of plasmalogen synthesis cause rhizomelic chondrodysplasia punctata, with symptoms of skeletal dysplasia and neurologic disease. Except for X-ALD, all peroxisomal diseases have recessive inheritance.

Diagnosis

The best initial test for Zellweger spectrum disorders and X-ALD is assessment of fasting VLCFA levels in plasma. Measurements of phytanic acid, pristanic acid, pipecolic acid, bile acid intermediates, and plasmalogens are also appropriate for evaluation of some peroxisome disorders. Increasingly, peroxisomal disorders are identified with genetic testing. Many states now test for X-ALD with NBS.

Treatment

Treatment for most peroxisomal disorders is symptomatic and supportive. HSCT may be an effective treatment at the early stages of cerebral X-ALD, and close monitoring of at-risk males is necessary to determine optimal timing of HSCT.

Corticosteroid replacement is necessary for any patients with adrenal insufficiency. Avoidance of dietary sources of phytanic acid (mainly present in meat and dairy) is effective for adult Refsum disease. An RNA interference therapy for primary hyperoxaluria was recently approved.

Braverman NE et al: Peroxisome biogenesis disorders in the Zellweger spectrum: an overview of current diagnosis, clinical manifestations, and treatment guidelines. Mol Genet Metab 2016;117(3):313–321 [PMID: 26750748].

Engelen M et al: International recommendations for the diagnosis and management of patients with adrenoleukodystrophy: a consensus-based approach. Neurology 2022 99(21):940–951 [PMID: 36175155].

Patient and parent support group website with useful information for families: http://www.thegfpd.org.

CONGENITAL DISORDERS OF GLYCOSYLATION

ESSENTIALS OF DIAGNOSIS & TYPICAL FEATURES

► Analysis of glycosylation patterns of marker glycoproteins such as transferrin (N-linked glycosylation) and apolipoprotein C (O-linked glycosylation) is an initial screening test for these broad-spectrum, multisystem disorders.

Many proteins, especially extracellular and lysosomal proteins, require glycosylation for normal function. The congenital disorders of glycosylation (CDGs) are a family of over 170 different disorders that result from defects in the synthesis, modification or attachment of glycans (polysaccharides) to proteins and fats. The most common CDG is phosphomannomutase-2 deficiency (PMM2-CDG). Children with PMM2-CDG may present with diarrhea, developmental delay, abnormal subcutaneous fat distribution, inverted nipples, strabismus, progressive cerebellar hypoplasia, hepatopathy, nephrotic syndrome, cardiomyopathy and pericardial effusions, endocrine abnormalities, and peripheral neuropathy. Patients with phosphomannose isomerase deficiency (MPI-CDG) have a combination of hepatopathy, protein-losing enteropathy, and hyperinsulinemic hypoglycemia. Glycosylation defects are known to underlie syndromes such as multiple exostoses syndrome, Walker-Warburg syndrome, muscle-eye-brain disease, and dystroglycan-related muscular dystrophies.

Defects in the glycosylphosphatidylinositol anchor system cause neurologic symptoms such as epilepsy, hypotonia, brain abnormalities, and other organ dysfunction with elevated alkaline phosphatase (some patients) due to lack of anchoring of the enzyme to the endothelial cell wall.

Phosphoglucoisomerase deficiency (PGM1-CDG) causes both a GSD (type XIV) with hypoglycemia, but also congenital malformations such as cleft palate and liver, cardiac, and endocrine abnormalities. Finally, N-glycanase-1 (NGLY1) is the first described disorder of deglycosylation and presents with developmental delays, elevated transaminases, chorea, and alacrima.

► Diagnosis

Diagnosis may be suspected in the setting of altered function of glycosylated proteins such as thyroid-binding globulin and clotting factors (IX, XI, antithrombin III, and proteins C and S). Diagnosis is confirmed by finding patterns of abnormal glycosylation of selected proteins. Most diagnostic laboratories examine glycosylation patterns of serum transferrin to screen for N-linked CDGs and apoCIII for O-linked CDGs. In some cases, muscle biopsy with immunohistochemistry may be a diagnostic test. CDG diagnosis may be further confirmed by assaying enzyme activity in some cases. Increasingly, broad genetic testing is the initial diagnostic modality that suggests a CDG.

► Treatment

Treatment is mainly supportive for most CDGs, including monitoring and providing early treatment for expected clinical features. Mannose treatment may significantly improve symptoms for patients with MPI-CDG, and galactose treatment may be effective for patients with PGM1-CDG. Multiple other specific CDGs may respond to dietary supplementation of relevant rare sugars.

Boyer SW, Johnsen C, Morava E: Nutrition interventions in congenital disorders of glycosylation. Trends Mol Med 2022 Jun;28(6):463–481 [PMID: 35562242].

Ng BG, Freeze HH: Perspectives on glycosylation and its congenital disorders. Trends Genet 2018;34(6):466–476 [PMID: 29606283].

Sparks SE, Krasnewich DM: Congenital disorders of N-linked glycosylation and multiple pathway overview. *GeneReviews®* [Internet]. Seattle, WA: University of Washington; 2017. https://www.ncbi.nlm.nih.gov/books/NBK1332/.

SMITH-LEMLI-OPITZ SYNDROME & DISORDERS OF CHOLESTEROL SYNTHESIS

ESSENTIALS OF DIAGNOSIS & TYPICAL FEATURES

► Elevated 7- and 8-dehydrocholesterol in serum is diagnostic in Smith-Lemli-Opitz (SLO) syndrome, which presents with developmental delay and malformations.

► Cerebrotendinous xanthomatosis (CTX) presents with cataracts and progressive neurologic symptoms. Treatment with chenodeoxycholic acid (CDCA) can prevent some progression.

Several defects of cholesterol synthesis are associated with malformations and neurodevelopmental disability. Smith-Lemli-Opitz (SLO) syndrome (Chapter 37) is an autosomal recessive disorder caused by a deficiency of the enzyme 7-dehydrocholesterol Δ7-reductase. It is characterized by microcephaly, poor growth, intellectual disability, typical dysmorphic features of face and extremities (2,3-toe syndactyly), and, often, malformations of the heart and genitourinary system. Conradi-Hünermann syndrome is characterized by chondrodysplasia punctata and atrophic skin. Defects in the synthesis of bile acids from cholesterol usually cause cholestatic liver disease and failure to thrive. Cerebrotendinous xanthomatosis (CTX) manifests with progressive ataxia, spastic paraparesis, cataracts, cognitive decline, and, later, xanthomatous accumulations in the skin and tendons. Some patients with CTX may initially present with cholestatic liver disease or chronic diarrhea in infancy.

▶ Diagnosis

In SLO, elevated 7- and 8-dehydrocholesterol in serum or amniotic fluid is diagnostic. Serum cholesterol levels may be low or in the normal range. Enzymes of cholesterol synthesis may be assayed in cultured fibroblasts or amniocytes, and mutation analysis is possible. CTX is diagnosed by detecting elevated levels of bile alcohols in blood and urine as well as elevated cholestanol.

▶ Treatment

Although postnatal treatment does not resolve prenatal injury, supplementation with cholesterol in SLO may improve growth and behavior. CTX responds to treatment with chenodeoxycholic acid, which inhibits the formation of bile alcohols by suppressing the enzyme that converts cholesterol into bile acid precursors (7α-hydroxylase).

Bianca MLS et al: Expert opinion on diagnosing, treating and managing patients with cerebrotendinous xanthomatosis (CTX): a modified Delphi study. Orphanet J Rare Dis 2021 Aug 6; 16(1):353 [PMID: 34362411].

Nowaczyk MJM, Wassif CA: Smith-Lemli-Opitz syndrome. 1998 Nov 13 [updated 2020 Jan 30]. In: Adam MP et al (eds): *GeneReviews®* [Internet]. Seattle, WA: University of Washington, Seattle; 1993–2023 [PMID: 20301322].

Patient and parent support group website with useful information for families: http://www.smithlemliopitz.org.

DISORDERS OF BRAIN-SPECIFIC METABOLISM: NEUROTRANSMITTERS, AMINO ACIDS, & GLUCOSE TRANSPORT

ESSENTIALS OF DIAGNOSIS & TYPICAL FEATURES

► Consider in children with movement disorders, especially dystonia and oculogyric crises.

► Severe seizures, abnormal tone, ataxia, intellectual disability, and autonomic instability occur in severely affected infants.

► Mildly affected patients have dopa-responsive dystonia with diurnal variability.

► Deficient glucose transporter causes seizures and a movement disorder. Identifiable on CSF analysis and treatable with a ketogenic diet.

► Pyridoxine-dependent epilepsy causes neonatal seizures and developmental delays and can be effectively treated with pyridoxine and a lysine-restricted diet.

Abnormalities of neurotransmitter metabolism are increasingly recognized as causes of significant neurodevelopmental disabilities. These disorders impact the synthesis of the neurotransmitters, dopamine and serotonin. Affected patients may present with movement disorders (especially dystonia and oculogyric crises), seizures, abnormal tone, or intellectual disability, and may initially be diagnosed with cerebral palsy. Patients may be mildly affected (eg, dopa-responsive dystonia with diurnal variation and typical cognition) or severely affected (eg, intractable seizures with profound intellectual disability).

Pyridoxine-dependent epilepsy manifests as a seizure disorder in the neonatal or early infantile period that responds to high doses of pyridoxine. The disorder is caused by deficient activity of the enzyme α-amino adipic semialdehyde dehydrogenase, involved in lysine catabolism, resulting from mutations in *ALDH7A1*. Dietary lysine restriction aids in treatment. Pyridoxal-phosphate–responsive encephalopathy manifests as a severe seizure disorder in infancy that responds to pyridoxal-phosphate supplementation. This disorder is caused by mutations in *PNPO* encoding pyridoxamine oxidase, which is necessary for activation of pyridoxine.

Glut1 deficiency syndrome results from mutations in *SLC2A1*, the primary glucose transporter for the brain. It is autosomal dominant. The resultant CSF glucose deficiency causes seizures as well as dystonia and other movement disorders.

Diagnosis

Although some disorders can be diagnosed by examining plasma amino acids or urine organic acids (eg, 4-hydroxybutyric aciduria), in most cases, diagnosis requires analysis of CSF. Spinal fluid samples for neurotransmitter analysis, to detect disorders of dopamine and serotonin metabolism, require special collection and handling. Analysis of CSF shows elevated threonine and decreased pyridoxal-phosphate in pyridoxal-phosphate–responsive disease. Urine or plasma α-aminoadipic acid and piperideine-6-carboxylate are abnormal for children with pyridoxine-dependent seizures. Glut1 deficiency syndrome can be diagnosed by demonstrating low glucose and lactate in CSF compared to concurrent blood samples. All disorders can be diagnosed with genetic testing.

Treatment

Synthesis defects of dopamine and serotonin are usually treated with a combination of levodopa-carbidopa and 5-hydroxytryptophan (a serotonin precursor). Pyridoxine-dependent epilepsy is treated with pyridoxine in high doses and a lysine-restricted diet, whereas pyridoxal-phosphate–responsive encephalopathy requires pyridoxal-phosphate supplementation. Glut1 transporter deficiency syndrome is treatable with a ketogenic diet. For several conditions, such as pyridoxine-responsive seizures, pyridoxal-phosphate–responsive encephalopathy, or dopa-responsive dystonia, response to treatment may be dramatic.

Joerg K, et al. Glut1 deficiency syndrome (Glut1DS): state of the art in 2020 and recommendations of the international Glut1DS study group. Epilepsia Open 2020;5(3):354–365 [PMID: 32913944].
Patient and parent support group websites with useful information for families: http://www.pndassoc.org.
Tseng LA et al. Timing of therapy and neurodevelopmental outcomes in 18 families with pyridoxine-dependent epilepsy. Mol Genet Metab 2022 Apr;135(4):350–356 [PMID: 35279367].
Weissbach A et al: Relationship of genotype, phenotype, and treatment in dopa-responsive dystonia: MDSGene review. Mov Disord 2022 37(2):237–252 [PMID: 34908184].

CREATINE SYNTHESIS DISORDERS

ESSENTIALS OF DIAGNOSIS & TYPICAL FEATURES

- ► Consider in children with seizures, movement disorders, autistic features, and developmental delay, especially with severe expressive language delay.
- ► Early recognition and treatment of guanidinoacetate methyltransferase (GAMT) deficiency improves developmental outcomes.

Creatine is essential for storage and transmission of phosphate-bound energy in muscle and brain. The disorders arginine glycine amidinotransferase (AGAT) deficiency and guanidinoacetate methyltransferase (GAMT) deficiency are autosomal recessive, whereas creatine transporter deficiency (CTD) is X-linked. Patients demonstrate developmental delay, seizures, and severe expressive language delay. Patients may also show developmental regression and brain atrophy. Patients with GAMT deficiency have more severe seizures and an extrapyramidal movement disorder. The seizure disorder is milder in male CTD patients, but developmental delay is significant.

Diagnosis

Creatine and guanidinoacetate levels may be measured in blood or urine and are typically the initial diagnostic study. CTD is detected using the urine creatine:creatinine ratio. MRS may demonstrate decreased creatine concentration in the brain. Sequencing of *SLC6A8* (CTD), *GAMT*, and *AGAT* as part of neurodevelopmental genetic panels is standard. NBS for GAMT is available in some states.

Treatment

Treatment with oral creatine supplementation is partially successful in GAMT and AGAT deficiencies. Early treatment with combined arginine restriction and ornithine supplementation in GAMT deficiency can decrease guanidinoacetate concentrations and greatly improve the clinical course. Combined therapy using arginine, glycine, and creatine supplementation in CTD has been tried with no clear efficacy.

Fernandes-Pires G, Braissant O: Current and potential new treatment strategies for creatine deficiency syndromes. Mol Genet Metab 2022 Jan;135(1):15–26 [PMID: 34972654].

QUALITY INITIATIVES IN THE FIELD OF METABOLIC DISEASE

Expanded NBS has had a large impact on the field of metabolic disorders. Patients are being diagnosed earlier, which can dramatically reduce or eliminate sequelae. Modern NBS has also had unexpected consequences. For example, the clinical spectrum of many disorders is being expanded to include mildly affected or asymptomatic patients. Gradually, refined therapeutic approaches are being developed for mildly affected patients. For some patients on the milder end of a disease spectrum, therapy is not needed at all. In addition, NBS for several conditions may detect a disease in the mother of the screened infant such as maternal vitamin B_{12} deficiency and maternal CUD.

Limitations in diagnostic testing create difficulty in discriminating carriers of a single mutation for a recessive condition from patients affected with mild disease manifestations that may pose health risks (eg, VLCAD deficiency). The NBS may detect pseudodeficiency alleles that demonstrate biochemical and enzymatic abnormalities in the laboratory but do not result in clinical disease (eg, in Hurler and Pompe testing). These diagnostic challenges not only add to parental anxiety, but also potentially result in unnecessary medicalization for the child.

Continuous improvements in NBS have resulted in the addition of screening for several new conditions such as severe combined immunodeficiency (SCID) and peroxisomal and lysosomal disorders. Many more disorders will be considered candidates for NBS in coming years, while the future use of broad genetic testing as an adjunct to current metabolic testing will involve many years of optimization.

Careful consideration will need to be given to the risks and benefits of screening for new conditions. The U.S. Secretary for Health and Human Services' Advisory Committee on Heritable Disorders in Newborns and Children has established a rigorous process for review of any conditions nominated for NBS before recommending that a disorder be included for screening nationwide. There is still considerable variability in conditions screened and techniques used for screening between states, though the degree of variability has decreased with guidance from the federal government.

McCandless SE, Wright EJ:. Mandatory newborn screening in the United States: history, current status, and existential challenges. Birth Defects Res 2020;112(4):350–366.

Genetics & Dysmorphology

Aaina Kochhar, MD

Jessica Duis, MD

Margarita Saenz, MD

Naomi J. L. Meeks, MD

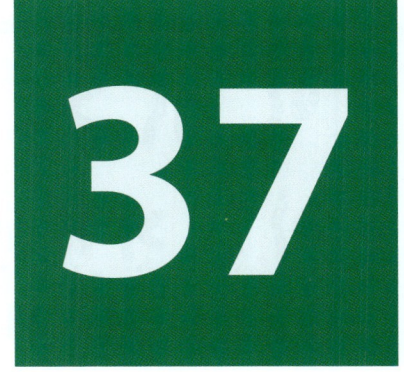

37

CYTOGENETICS

Cytogenetics is the study of genetics at the chromosome level. Chromosomal anomalies occur in 0.4% of all live births and are a common cause of intellectual disabilities and congenital anomalies. The prevalence of chromosomal anomalies is much higher among spontaneous abortions and stillbirths.

Chromosomes

Human chromosomes consist of DNA, specific proteins (histones) forming the backbone of the chromosome, and other chromatin structural and interactive proteins. Chromosomes contain most of the genetic information necessary for growth and differentiation. The nuclei of all normal human cells, with the exception of gametes, contain 46 chromosomes, consisting of 23 pairs (Figure 37–1). Of these, 22 pairs are called autosomes. They are numbered according to their size; chromosome 1 is the largest and chromosome 22 the smallest. In addition, there are two sex chromosomes: two X chromosomes in females and one X and one Y chromosome in males. The two members of a chromosome pair are called homologous chromosomes. One homolog of each chromosome pair is maternal in origin; the other is paternal. The egg and sperm each contain 23 chromosomes (haploid cells). During formation of the zygote, they fuse into a cell with 46 chromosomes (diploid cell).

Karyotype

A karyotype is the arrangement of chromosomes in homologous pairs in numerical order. There is a characteristic-banding pattern that is reproducible for each chromosome, allowing the chromosomes to be identified. High-resolution chromosome analysis is the study of elongated chromosomes and can detect smaller imbalances than routine chromosome analysis (see Figure 37–1). Although the bands can be visualized in greater detail, subtle chromosomal rearrangements less than 5 million base pairs (5 Mb) can still be missed.

Fluorescence in situ hybridization (FISH) is a technique that labels a known chromosome sequence with DNA probes attached to fluorescent dyes, thus enabling visualization of specific regions of chromosomes by fluorescent microscopy. FISH can detect submicroscopic structural rearrangements undetectable by classic cytogenetic techniques and can identify marker chromosomes.

Interphase FISH allows noncultured cells (lymphocytes, amniocytes) to be rapidly screened for numerical abnormalities such as trisomy 13, 18, or 21, and sex chromosome anomalies. However, because of the possible background or contamination of the signal, the abnormality must be confirmed by conventional chromosome analysis. Two hundred-cell FISH can be used to detect mosaicism.

Chromosomal Microarray Analysis or Array Comparative Genomic Hybridization

Chromosomal microarray (CMA) allows detection of small genetic imbalances in the genome. It is used to detect interstitial and submicroscopic imbalances, to characterize their size at the molecular level, and to define the breakpoints of translocations. This test has replaced high-resolution chromosomes as the first-line test in evaluating children with developmental delays and multiple congenital anomalies. The principle behind CMA is comparison of a patient's genome at hundreds of thousands of locations against a reference genome. Current CMAs are designed to screen the entire genome using single-nucleotide polymorphisms (SNPs), and these are particularly targeted toward known disease-causing regions. However, this technology is not able to detect very small deletions, duplications, or single-nucleotide changes. This technology can also identify cases of uniparental disomy (UPD) or loss of heterozygosity.

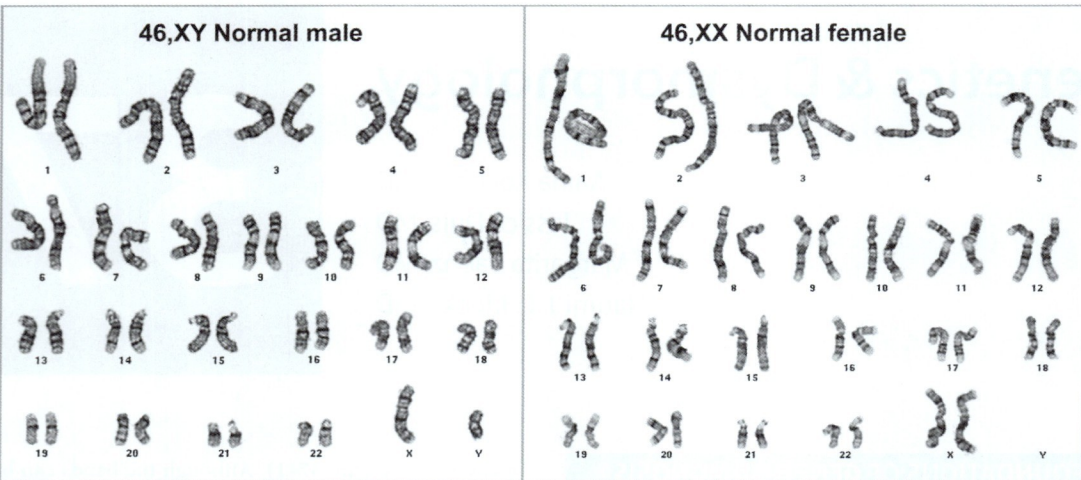

▲ Figure 37–1. Normal male and female human karyotype. (Reproduced with permission from Colorado Genetics Laboratory.)

Wiszneiwska J et al: Combined array CGH plus SNP genome analyses in a single assay for optimized clinical testing. Eur J Hum Genet 2014 Jan;22(1):79–87 [PMID: 23695279].

Chromosome Nomenclature

Visible under the microscope is a narrowing on the chromosome called the centromere, which separates the chromosome into two arms: p, for petite, refers to the short arm, and q, the letter following p, refers to the long arm. Each arm is further subdivided into numbered bands visible using different staining techniques. The use of named chromosome arms and bands provides a universal method of chromosome description. Common symbols include *del* (deletion), *dup* (duplication), *inv* (inversion), *ish* (in situ hybridization), *i* (isochromosome), *pat* (paternal origin), *mat* (maternal origin), and *r* (ring chromosome).

Chromosomal Abnormalities

There are two types of chromosomal anomalies: numerical and structural.

A. Abnormalities of Chromosomal Number

When a human cell has 23 chromosomes, such as human ova or sperm, it is in the haploid state (n). After conception, in cells other than the reproductive cells, 46 chromosomes are present in the diploid state (2n). Cells deviating from the multiple of the haploid number are called aneuploid, indicating an abnormal number of chromosomes. Trisomy, an example of aneuploidy, is the presence of three of a particular chromosome rather than two. It results from unequal

division, called nondisjunction, of chromosomes into daughter cells. Trisomies are the most common numerical chromosomal anomalies found in humans (eg, trisomy 21 [Down syndrome], trisomy 18, and trisomy 13). Monosomies, the presence of only one member of a chromosome pair, may be complete or partial. All complete autosomal monosomies appear to be lethal early in development and only survive in mosaic forms. Sex chromosome monosomy, however, can be viable (eg, Turner syndrome).

B. Abnormalities of Chromosomal Structure

Many different types of structural chromosomal anomalies exist. Figure 37–2 displays the formal nomenclature as well as the ideogram demonstrating chromosomal anomalies. In clinical context, the sign (+) or (–) *preceding* the chromosome number indicates increased or decreased number, respectively, of that whole chromosome in a cell. For example, 47, XY+21 designates a male with three copies of chromosome 21. The sign (+) or (–) *after* the chromosome number signifies extra material or missing material, respectively, on one of the arms of the chromosome. For example, 46, XX, 8q– denotes a deletion on the long arm of chromosome 8. Detailed nomenclature, such as 8q11, is required to further demonstrate a specific missing region.

1. Deletion (del) (see Figure 37–2A)—This refers to an absence of normal chromosomal material. It may be terminal (at the end of a chromosome) or interstitial (within a chromosome). The missing part is described using the code "del," followed by the number of the chromosome involved in parentheses, and a description of the missing region of that

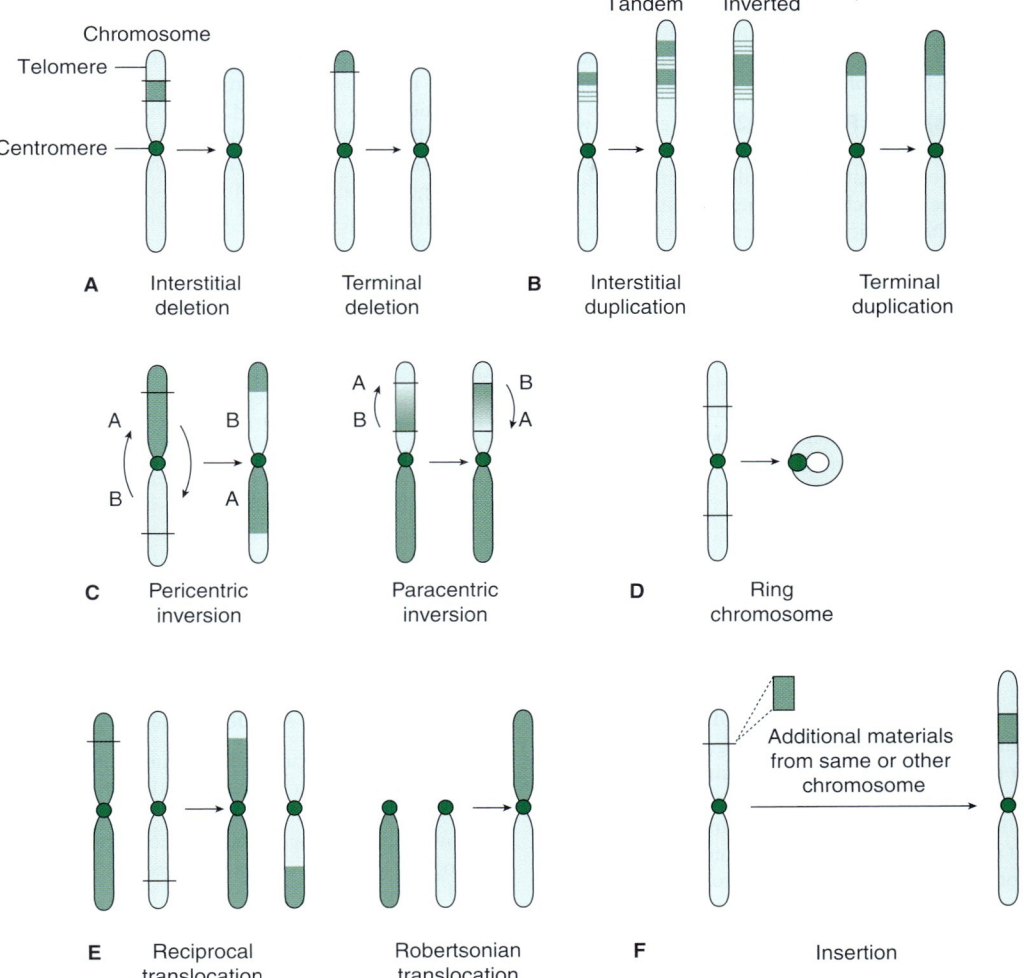

▲ **Figure 37–2.** Examples of structural chromosomal abnormalities: deletion, duplication, inversion, ring chromosome, translocation, and insertion.

chromosome, also in parentheses, for example, 46, XX, del(1) (p36.3). This chromosome nomenclature describes the loss of genetic material from band 36.3 of the short arm of chromosome 1, which results in 1p36.3 deletion syndrome.

2. Duplication (dup) (see Figure 37–2B)—An extra copy of a chromosomal segment can be in tandem (genetic material present in the original direction) or inverted (genetic material present in the opposite direction). A well-described duplication of chromosome 22q11 causes Cat eye syndrome, resulting in iris coloboma (see Chapter 16) and anal or ear anomalies.

3. Inversion (inv) (see Figure 37–2C)—In this anomaly, a rearranged section of a chromosome is inverted. It can be

paracentric (not involving the centromere) or pericentric (involving the centromere).

4. Ring chromosome (r) (see Figure 37–2D)—Deletion of the normal telomeres (and possibly other subtelomeric sequences) leads to subsequent fusion of both ends to form a circular chromosome. Ring chromosomal anomalies often cause growth delays and intellectual disability.

5. Translocation (trans) (see Figure 37–2E)—This interchromosomal rearrangement of genetic material may be balanced (the cell has a normal content of genetic material arranged in a structurally abnormal way) or unbalanced (the cell has gained or lost genetic material as a result of chromosomal interchange). Balanced translocations may further be described as reciprocal, the exchange of genetic material between two nonhomologous chromosomes, or Robertsonian, the fusion of two acrocentric chromosomes.

6. Insertion (ins) (see Figure 37–2F)—Breakage within a chromosome at two points and incorporation of another piece of chromosomal material is called an insertion. This may occur between two chromosomes or within the same chromosome. The clinical presentation or phenotype depends on the origin of the inserted materials as well as what material is disrupted.

C. Sex Chromosome Anomalies

Abnormalities involving sex chromosomes, including aneuploidy and mosaicism, are relatively common in the general population. The most common sex chromosome anomalies include 45,X (Turner syndrome), 47,XXX,47,XXY (Klinefelter syndrome), and 47,XYY.

D. Mosaicism

Mosaicism is the presence of two or more chromosome compositions in different cells of the same individual. For example, a patient may have some cells with 47 chromosomes and others with 46 chromosomes (46,XX/47,XX,+21 indicates mosaicism for trisomy 21; similarly, 45,X/46,XX/47,XXX indicates mosaicism for a monosomy and trisomy X). Mosaicism should be suspected if clinical signs are milder than expected, or if the patient's skin shows unusual pigmentation. The prognosis can be better for a patient with mosaicism than for one with a corresponding chromosomal abnormality without mosaicism. In general, the smaller the proportion of the abnormal cell line, the better the prognosis. In the same patient, however, the proportion of normal and abnormal cells in various tissues, such as skin, brain, internal organs, and peripheral blood, may be significantly different. Therefore, the prognosis for a patient with chromosomal mosaicism can seldom be assessed reliably based on the karyotype in peripheral blood cells alone.

E. Uniparental Disomy

Under normal circumstances, one member of each homologous pair of chromosomes is of maternal origin from the egg and the other is of paternal origin from the sperm (Figure 37–3A). In UPD, both copies of a particular chromosome pair originate from the same parent. If UPD is caused by an error in the first meiotic division, both homologous chromosomes of that parent will be present in the gamete—a phenomenon called heterodisomy (Figure 37–3B). If the disomy is caused by an error in the second meiotic division, two copies of the same chromosome will be present through the mechanism of rescue, duplication, and complementation (Figure 37–3C through 37–3E)—a phenomenon called

isodisomy. Isodisomy may also occur as a postfertilization error (Figure 37–3F).

UPD can cause a clinical phenotype due to imprinting, when it occurs in certain human chromosomes, including chromosomes 6, 7, 11, 14, 15. It has been found in patients with Prader-Willi, Angelman, and Beckwith-Wiedemann syndromes (BWS). On other chromosomes, by itself, it does not produce clinical features. It can, however, unmask an underlying autosomal recessive condition in the case of isodisomy.

F. Microdeletion and Microduplication Syndromes

Microdeletion and microduplication syndromes, also known as copy number variants (CNVs), result when there is a loss or gain of small regions of a chromosome. These may include one gene, multiple genes, or noncoding regions of the genome. Though high-resolution chromosomes can detect some CNVs, most are detected by FISH or CMA. These CNVs may be familial (passed on by a parent) or may occur de novo. Many CNVs are now known to be associated with specific syndromes. Generally, CNVs larger than 5–10 megabases (Mb) have some clinical impact. Some CNVs are classified as variants of uncertain significance (VUS) or may be benign changes. Therefore, parental studies are often required in interpreting the results of genetic testing.

G. Chromosomal Abnormalities in Cancer

Numerical and structural chromosomal abnormalities are often identified in hematopoietic and solid-tumor neoplasms. The sites of chromosome breaks coincide with the known loci of oncogenes and tumor suppressor genes. These cytogenetic abnormalities have been categorized as primary and secondary.

In primary abnormalities, their presence is necessary for initiation of the cancer; an example is 13q– in retinoblastoma (loss of q arm of chromosome 13). Secondary abnormalities appear de novo in somatic cells only after the cancer has developed, for example, the Philadelphia chromosome, t(9;22)(q34;q11), in acute and chronic myeloid leukemia. Primary and secondary chromosomal abnormalities are specific for particular neoplasms and can be used for diagnosis or prognosis. For example, the presence of the Philadelphia chromosome is a good prognostic sign in chronic myelogenous leukemia but indicates a poor prognosis in acute lymphoblastic leukemia.

MOLECULAR GENETICS

Advances in molecular biology have revolutionized human genetics, as they allow for the localization, isolation, and characterization of genes that encode protein sequences. Molecular genetics can help explain the complex underlying biology involved in many human diseases.

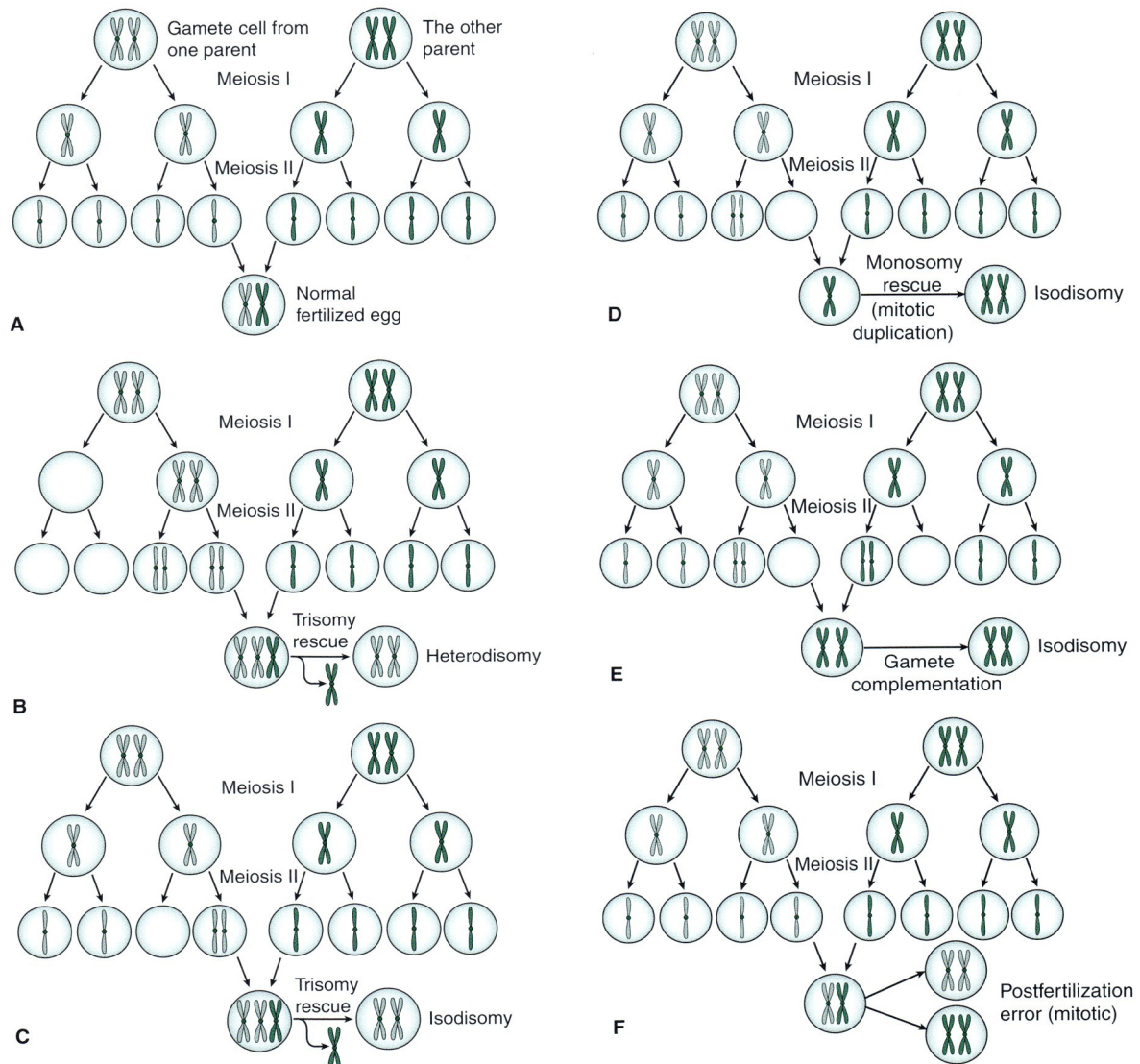

▲ **Figure 37–3.** The assortment of homologous chromosomes during normal gametogenesis and uniparental disomy. **A:** Fertilization of normal gametes. **B:** Heterodisomy by trisomy rescue. **C:** Isodisomy by trisomy rescue. **D:** Isodisomy by monosomy rescue (mitotic duplication). **E:** Gamete complementation. **F:** Postfertilization error.

Molecular diagnosis on a clinical basis can be achieved using many technologies. The **polymerase chain reaction** (PCR) replicates fragments of DNA between predetermined primers so that sufficient DNA is obtained for characterization or sequencing in the space of a few hours. **DNA sequencing** is the process of determining the nucleotide order of a given DNA fragment. **CMA** can also be used to look for small

deletions or duplications (as small as one exon) on the gene level. **Methylation** analysis can look for UPD or imprinting defects. **Next-generation sequencing** (NextGen or NGS) or massively parallel sequencing allows the sequencing of many genes quickly and accurately, and for less expense per gene than traditional DNA sequencing. This technology has allowed the screening of hundreds or thousands of genes at one time with targeted panel testing. This technology is also being used to perform **whole exome sequencing** (WES) or **whole genome sequencing** (WGS).

WES allows for sequencing of all known genes in the human genome, whereas WGS sequences all known coding and noncoding sequences. Difficulties in both WES and WGS involve limitations in the ability to interpret the results. Only about 25% of the genes contained within the human genome have a known function. Likewise, variations identified outside of coding regions of the genome (introns, regulatory regions) often have uncertain significance. Despite these limitations, WES or WGS performed in commercial laboratories has a meaningful diagnostic result in up to 40% of cases. NGS has changed the paradigm in clinical genetics. Rather than performing multiple single-gene tests, the current clinical practice is moving towards performing one or two screening tests and if testing is negative, moving toward WES or WGS to save time and limit costs. With improved technology, WES and WGS are now allowing for detection of sequence variants, CNVs, and information regarding trinucleotide repeats.

Variants may be classified as Pathogenic or Likely Pathogenic, Benign or Likely Benign, or of Uncertain Significance. Pathogenic and Likely Pathogenic variants are interpreted to mean disease-causing whereas benign and likely-benign are not. Variants of Uncertain Significance are variants for which there is not enough information published in the scientific literature to interpret the meaning. Parental testing, or re-evaluation of variants over time may result in reclassification.

Genetics & Its Clinical Applications

There are multiple reasons a patient may undergo genetic testing. It is important for families to receive genetic counseling prior to testing to understand how genetic testing results may impact the patient and other family members.

Patients are often referred for genetic testing if they present with specific features of a known condition, if they have clinical characteristics but an unknown cause for those characteristics, or because of a family history of a specific genetic condition. Genetic testing may confirm or identify a specific diagnosis, which can then be used to target specific treatments or interventions. Many families also feel a pressing need to know "why" a child has the condition they do, even in cases where a genetic diagnosis does not alter treatments and interventions. Other reasons for genetic testing include counseling about recurrence risks and testing for prenatal or preimplantation genetic diagnosis.

Confirmation of a specific diagnosis (such as 22q11.2 deletion syndrome) can result in additional recommendations for screening (laboratory and/or imaging studies) for additional medical complications. In other diagnoses, specific medical treatments are indicated, which do not impact the gene itself but are designed to minimize complications of the disorder. An example of this is Marfan syndrome (MFS) where

diagnosis leads to medical treatment to prevent complications related to Aortic root dilation and Aortic Aneurysms. In some inborn errors of metabolism, organ transplant can treat the disorder if the affected gene is expressed primarily in one organ (ie, liver transplantation for ornithine transcarbamylase deficiency). Finally, in rare genetic diagnoses, trials are underway to alter gene expression itself to ameliorate effects of the disease. An example of this is spinal muscular atrophy (SMA) where treatment to preserve a skipped exon in the gene has received Food and Drug Administration (FDA) approval.

On the forefront of clinical medicine are **Rapid WES or WGS**, in which new technology allows a fast turnaround time for these tests (3–14 days). Due to the cost, this is currently implemented primarily in critical care settings like neonatal intensive care units (NICUs) to quickly identify medically actionable diagnoses.

Advances in genetic testing have resulted in parents requesting testing for adult-onset disease, carrier status, and disease susceptibility in their children, which raises significant ethical and legal issues. The American College of Medical Genetics and Genomics and American Society of Human Genetics formed a consensus statement on the topic that educates families and health care providers on the potential negative impacts of such testing. The decision-making capacity of the minor undergoing testing should also be considered where applicable.

Personalized medicine (precision medicine) is an advancing field of medicine that offers increased precision and effectiveness than traditional medicine. As opposed to the current paradigm where genetic testing is performed due to the presence of specific clinical signs or to diagnose rare disease, precision genetic testing may be ordered preemptively to better understand an individual's health risks or response to interventions.

Anderson JA et al: Predictive genetic testing for adult-onset disorders in minors: a critical analysis of the arguments for and against the 2013 ACMG guidelines. Clin Genet 2015 Apr;87(4):301–310 [PMID: 25046648].

Eichinger et al: The full spectrum of ethical issues in pediatric genome-wide sequencing: a systematic qualitative review. BMC Pediatrics 2021;21:387 [PMID: 34488686].

Hammond SM et al: Systemic peptide-mediated oligonucleotide therapy improves long-term survival in spinal muscular atrophy. Proc Natl Acad Sci USA 2016 Sep 27;113(39):10962–10967 [PMID: 27621445].

Lionel AC et al: Improved diagnostic yield compared with targeted gene sequencing panels suggests a role for whole-genome sequencing as a first-tier genetic test. Genet Med 2018 Apr;20(4):435–443 [PMID: 28771251].

Richards S et al: Standards and guidelines for the interpretation of sequence variants: a joint consensus recommendation of the American College of Medical Genetics and Genomics and the Association for Molecular Pathology. Genet Med 2015 May;17(5):405–424 [PMID: 25741868].

Sadee et al: Pharmacogenomics: driving personalized medicine. Pharmacol Rev 2023 Jul; 75:789–814, July 2023 [PMID: 36927888].

PRINCIPLES OF INHERITED HUMAN DISORDERS

MENDELIAN INHERITANCE

Traditionally, autosomal single-gene disorders follow the principles explained by Gregor Mendel's observations. The inheritance of genetic traits through generations relies on segregation and independent assortment. **Segregation** is the process through which gene pairs are separated during gamete formation. **Independent assortment** refers to the segregation of different alleles independently.

Victor McKusick's catalog, *Mendelian Inheritance in Man*, lists more than 10,000 entries in which the mode of inheritance is presumed to be autosomal dominant, autosomal recessive, X-linked dominant, X-linked recessive, and Y-linked. Single genes at specific loci on one or a pair of chromosomes cause these disorders. An understanding of inheritance terminology is helpful in approaching Mendelian disorders. Analysis of the pedigree and the pattern of transmission in the family, identification of a specific condition, and knowledge of that condition's mode of inheritance usually allow for explanation of the inheritance pattern.

Terminology

The following terms are important in understanding heredity patterns:

1. Dominant and recessive—Concepts for dominant and recessive refer to the phenotypic expression of alleles and are not intrinsic characteristics of gene loci.

2. Genotype—Genotype means the genetic status, that is, the alleles an individual possesses.

3. Phenotype—Phenotype is the expression of an individual's genotype, including external and internal physical features, biochemical makeup, and physiologic expression. Phenotypic factors can be modified by the environment.

4. Pleiotropy—Pleiotropy refers to the phenomenon whereby a single mutant allele can have widespread effects or expression in different tissues or organ systems. In other words, an allele may produce more than one effect/impact on the phenotype. An example of the latter is the well-known genetic condition of MFS. MFS has multiple manifestations in different organ systems (skeletal, cardiac, ophthalmologic, etc) due to a single mutation within the fibrillin-1 (*FBN1*) gene.

5. Penetrance—Penetrance refers to the proportion of individuals with a particular genotype that express the same phenotype. Penetrance is a proportion that ranges between 0 and 1 (or 0% and 100%). When 100% of mutant individuals express the phenotype, penetrance is complete. If some mutant individuals do not express the phenotype, penetrance is said to be incomplete, or reduced. Dominant conditions with incomplete penetrance can be mistakenly interpreted by patients and caregivers as having "skipped" generations with unaffected, obligate gene carriers in a biological family.

6. Expressivity—Expressivity refers to the variability in degree of phenotypic expression seen in different individuals with the same mutant genotype. Expressivity may be extremely variable. Intrafamilial variability of expression may be due to factors such as epistasis, environment, genetic anticipation, nutritional status, and stochastic factors. Microdeletion and microduplication syndromes frequently demonstrate variable expressivity.

7. Genetic heterogeneity—Several different genetic mutations may produce phenotypes that are identical or similar enough to have been traditionally considered as one diagnosis, such as "intellectual disability".

8. Heterozygous—A cell or organism that has two nonidentical alleles at a corresponding genetic locus on homologous chromosomes is said to be heterozygous.

9. Homozygous—A cell or organism that has identical alleles at a locus is said to be homozygous. A cystic fibrosis patient with deltaF508 mutation on both alleles would be called homozygous for that mutation.

Hereditary Patterns

A. Autosomal Dominant Inheritance

Autosomal dominant inheritance has the following characteristics:

1. If a parent is affected, the risk for each offspring of inheriting the abnormal dominant gene is 50%, or 1:2. This is true whether the gene is penetrant or not in the parent.

2. Both males and females can pass on the abnormal gene to children of either sex, although the manifestations may vary according to sex.

3. Dominant inheritance is typically said to be vertical; that is, the condition passes from one generation to the next in a vertical fashion (Figure 37–4).

4. Explanations for a negative family history include the following:

   a. Nonpaternity/nonmaternity.

   b. Decreased penetrance or mild manifestations in one of the parents.

   c. Germline mosaicism (ie, mosaicism in the germ cell line of either parent). Germline mosaicism may mimic autosomal recessive inheritance because it leads to situations in which two children of completely normal parents are affected with a genetic disorder. Recurrence risks are in the range of 1%–3%.

   d. The abnormality present in the patient may be a phenocopy, or it may be a similar but genetically different abnormality with a different mode of inheritance.

   e. De novo mutation.

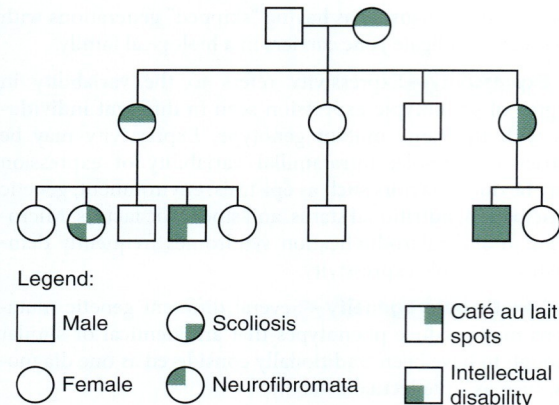

Legend:

☐ Male   ◐ Scoliosis   ◪ Café au lait spots

○ Female   ◐ Neurofibromata   ◪ Intellectual disability

▲ **Figure 37–4.** Autosomal dominant inheritance. Variable expressivity in neurofibromatosis type 1.

B. Autosomal Recessive Inheritance

Autosomal recessive inheritance also has some distinctive characteristics:

1. The recurrence risk for parents of an affected child is 25%, or 1:4 for each pregnancy. The gene carrier frequency in the general population is used to assess the risk of having

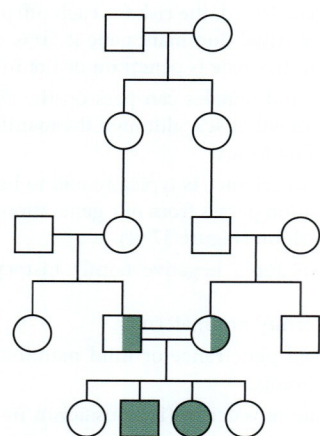

Legend:

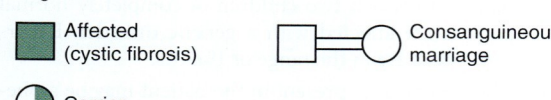

■ Affected (cystic fibrosis)   ☐—○ Consanguineous marriage

◐ Carrier

▲ **Figure 37–5.** Autosomal recessive inheritance: cystic fibrosis.

an affected child with a new partner, for unaffected siblings, and for the affected individuals themselves.

2. Parents are most often obligate carriers and are clinically unaffected.

3. Males and females are affected equally.

4. Inheritance is horizontal; siblings may be affected (Figure 37–5).

5. The family history is usually negative, apart from siblings.

6. In rare instances, a child with a recessive disorder may have inherited both copies of the abnormal gene from one parent and none from the other (UPD).

C. X-Linked Inheritance

When a gene for a specific disorder is on the X chromosome, the condition is said to be X-linked. Females may be either homozygous or heterozygous because they have two X chromosomes. Males have only one X chromosome and are hemizygous for any gene on their X chromosome. The severity of most X-linked disorders is generally greater in males than in females. One of the two X chromosomes in each cell is inactivated randomly. The clinical picture in females depends on the percentage of genetically altered versus normal alleles that are inactivated.

1. X-linked recessive inheritance—The following features are characteristic of X-linked recessive inheritance:

a. Males are affected, and heterozygous females are either not affected or have mild manifestations.

b. Inheritance is diagonal through the maternal side of the family (Figure 37–6A).

c. A female carrier has a 50% chance that each daughter will be a carrier and a 50% chance that each son will be affected.

d. All the daughters of an affected male are carriers and none of his sons is affected.

2. X-linked dominant inheritance—The X-linked dominant inheritance pattern is less common than the X-linked recessive type. Examples include incontinentia pigmenti and hypophosphatemic or vitamin D–resistant rickets. The following features are characteristic of X-linked dominant inheritance:

a. The heterozygous female is symptomatic, and the disease is twice as common in females because they have two X chromosomes that can have the mutation.

b. Clinical manifestations are more variable in females than in males.

c. The risk for the offspring of heterozygous females to be affected is 50% regardless of sex.

d. All daughters but none of the sons of affected males will have the disorder (Figure 37–6B).

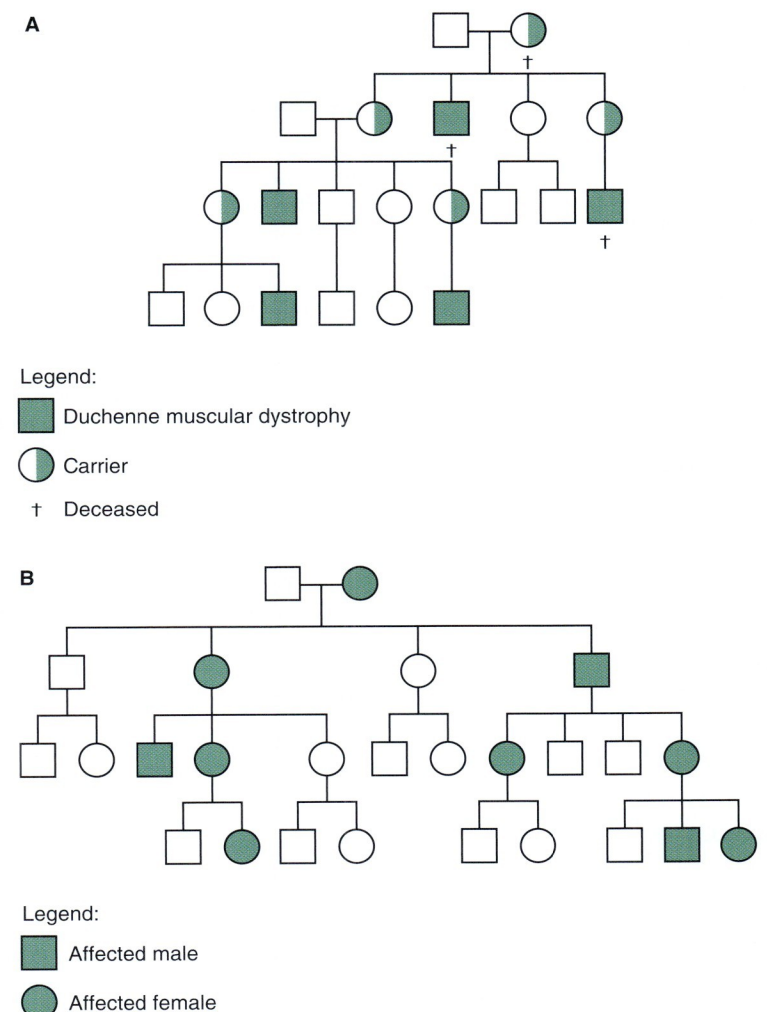

Legend:

■ Duchenne muscular dystrophy

◐ Carrier

† Deceased

Legend:

■ Affected male

● Affected female

▲ **Figure 37–6.** **A:** X-linked recessive inheritance. **B:** X-linked dominant inheritance.

MULTIFACTORIAL INHERITANCE

Many common attributes, such as height, are familial and are the result of the actions of multiple rather than single genes. Inheritance of these traits is described as **polygenic** or **multifactorial**. The latter term recognizes that environmental factors such as diet also contribute to these traits. Diagnostic clinical genetic testing for these conditions is not available.

Many disorders and congenital abnormalities that are clearly familial but do not segregate as Mendelian traits (eg, autosomal dominant, recessive) show polygenic inheritance. Often these conditions become manifest when thresholds of additive gene actions or contributing environmental factors are exceeded. Many common disorders ranging from hypertension, stroke, and alcoholism demonstrate multifactorial (polygenic) inheritance. Some common birth defects, including isolated congenital heart disease, cleft lip and palate, and neural tube defects, also demonstrate polygenic inheritance (Table 37–1).

NONMENDELIAN INHERITANCE

Epigenetic Regulation

Development is regulated by genes but is initiated and sustained by nongenetic processes. Epigenetic events are functionally relevant changes to the genome that are independent

Table 37–1. Empiric risks for some congenital disorders.

Anencephaly and spina bifida: incidence (average) 1:1000
One affected child: 2%–3%
Two affected children: 10%–12%
One affected parent: 4%–5%
Hydrocephalus: incidence 1:2000 newborns
Occasional X-linked recessive
Often associated with neural tube defect
Some environmental etiologies (eg, toxoplasmosis)
Recurrence risk, one affected child
Hydrocephalus: 1%
Some central nervous system abnormality: 3%
Nonsyndromic cleft lip and/or palate: incidence (average) 1:1000
One affected child: 2%–4%
One affected parent: 2%–4%
Two affected children: 10%
One affected parent, one affected child: 10%–20%
Nonsyndromic cleft palate: incidence 1:2000
One affected child: 2%
Two affected children: 6%–8%
One affected parent: 4%–6%
One affected parent, one affected child: 15%–20%
Congenital heart disease: incidence 8:1000
One affected child: 2%–3%
One affected parent, one affected child: 10%
Clubfoot: incidence 1:1000 (male:female = 2:1)
One affected child: 2%–3%
Congenital dislocated hip: incidence 1:1000
(female > male) with marked regional variation
One child affected: 2%–14%

of changes in the primary DNA sequence. Genetic imprinting and DNA methylation are examples of epigenetic processes that affect expression. Certain genes important in regulation of growth and differentiation are themselves regulated by chemical modification that occurs in specific patterns in gametes. Certain techniques developed to assist infertile couples (advanced reproductive technology) affect epigenetic marks in the fetus and placenta and may contribute to increased risk of adverse outcomes in the offspring conceived via these methods. It is unclear whether these epigenetic changes and adverse outcomes will have long-term effects on health and disease.

Mani S: Epigenetic changes and assisted reproductive technologies. Epigenetics 2020;15(1–2):12–25 [PMID: 31328632].

Imprinting

The parental origin of chromosome pairs affects which genes are transcribed and which are inactivated. The term *imprinting* refers to the process by which preferential transcription of certain genes takes place. Various chromosomes, particularly chromosome X, 15, 14, 11, 7, and 6, have imprinted regions where some genes are only read from one homolog (ie, either the maternal or paternal allele). Under typical circumstances, the gene on the other parental homolog is typically inactivated. Errors in imprinting may arise because of UPD (in which a copy from one parent is missing), chromosomal deletion causing loss of the gene normally transcribed, mutations in the imprinting genes that normally code for transcription, or inactivation of other genes downstream. A good example of how imprinting may affect human disease is BWS; the locus is located on chromosome band 11p15.

Cohen JL et al: Diagnosis and management of the phenotypic spectrum of twins with Beckwith-Wiedemann syndrome. Am J Med Genet A 2019 Jul;179(7):1139–1147 [PMID: 31067005].

Genetic Anticipation

Anticipation is a pattern of inheritance in which symptoms manifest at earlier ages and with increasing severity as traits are passed to subsequent generations. Associated repeat sequences of DNA at disease loci are not stable when passed through meiosis. Repeated DNA sequences, in particular triplets (eg, CGG and CAG), tend to increase their copy number. As these runs of triplets expand, they eventually affect the expression of genes and produce symptoms. Disorders undergoing triplet repeat expansion detected thus far produce primarily neurologic symptoms. Most conditions are progressive. The size of the triplet expansion is roughly correlated with the timing and severity of symptoms.

Examples include Huntington disease, Myotonic dystrophy, and Fragile X syndrome.

Mitochondrial Inheritance

Mitochondrial disorders can be caused by mutations in both nuclear and mitochondrial genes. Mitochondrial DNA (MtDNA) is double-stranded, 16,569 base pairs in length, circular, smaller than nuclear DNA, and is inherited maternally. MtDNA codes for 13 gene products involved in oxidative phosphorylation and electron transport.

MtDNA can sustain pathogenic point mutations, deletions, or duplications. However, there is a threshold effect depending on the heteroplasmy (cells contain both normal and abnormal mtDNA, Figure 37–7). Due to the difficulty in diagnosing mtDNA disorders, and the variability of the

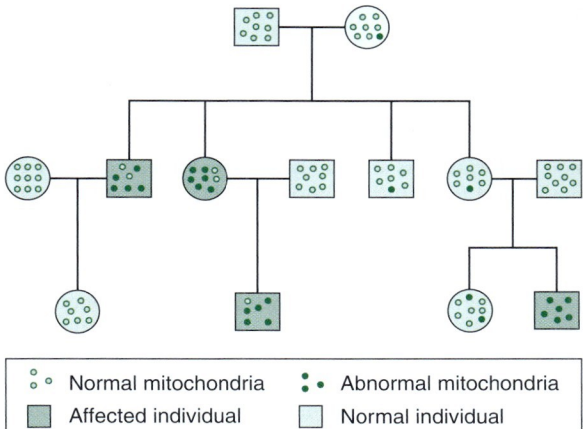

Normal mitochondria
Abnormal mitochondria
Affected individual
Normal individual

▲ **Figure 37–7.** Mitochondrial inheritance. Mutations are transmitted through the maternal line.

clinical course, it is often difficult to calculate specific recurrence risks. Further details are found in Chapter 36.

Dimmock DP, Lawlor MW: Presentation and diagnostic evaluation of mitochondrial disease. Pediatr Clin North Am 2017 Feb;64(1):161–171 doi: 10.1016/j.pcl.2016.08.011, Review [PMID: 27894442].
Rahman J: Mitochondrial medicine in the omics era. Lancet 2018 Jun 23;391(10139):2560–2574 [PMID: 29903433].

FAMILY HISTORY & PEDIGREE

Critical in the evaluation of a potential genetic condition is the construction of a family tree, also known as a pedigree. The pedigree is a valuable record of genetic and medical information, which has been widely reported as more efficient in diagram form than in list form.

While taking the family history, one may find information that is not relevant in elucidating the cause of the patients' problem but may indicate a risk for other important health concerns. Conditions unrelated to the chief complaint should be directed for follow-up care. Examples of the latter scenario include an overwhelming family history of early-onset breast and ovarian cancer, or multiple pregnancy losses noted in a pediatric genetic intake evaluation.

Bennett RL: Family health history: the first genetic test in precision medicine. Med Clin North Am 2019 Nov;103(6):957–966 [PMID: 31582006].
Bennett RL et al: Standardized human pedigree nomenclature: update and assessment of the recommendations of the National Society of genetic counselors. J Genet Couns 2008;17:424–433 [PMID: 18792771].

He D et al: IPED2X: a robust pedigree reconstruction algorithm for complicated pedigrees. J Bioinform Comput Biol 2014 Dec;12(6):1442007 [PMID: 25553812].

DYSMORPHOLOGY & HUMAN EMBRYOLOGY

The study of dysmorphology refers to aberrations in typical morphology that are observed in the population. Birth defects impact one in every 33 infants (3%) and are the leading cause of mortality accounting for 20% of all infant deaths. Environmental and genetic factors impact fetal morphology and growth and may influence heritability. Fetal malformations are commonly diagnosed prenatally during routine anatomic ultrasounds.

MECHANISMS

Developmental Biology

Cell proliferation, differentiation, migration, and programmed cell death (apoptosis) all contribute to embryonic structural formation. These processes are integral to typical growth and morphogenesis. Products of other genes establish regulatory pathways in which positive and negative signaling loops initiate and maintain cell differentiation with precise timing. Further understanding of these mechanisms may lead to interventions that could prevent birth defects or potentially provide treatment prenatally. A current intervention is fetal surgery for the treatment of neural tube defects.

Cellular Interactions

There is a hierarchy of gene expression during development. Morphogenesis begins with expression of genes encoding transcription factors. These proteins bind to DNA in undifferentiated embryonic cells and recruit them into developmental fields. From the blastocyst stage, unique factors secreted by surrounding cells establish a polarity that ultimately allows the inner cell mass and the embryonic tissues to differentiate. During gastrulation, cells rearrange themselves into three germ layers called the ectoderm, mesoderm, and endoderm. The endoderm becomes the central visceral core; the mesoderm becomes the kidneys, heart, vasculature, bone, and muscle; and the ectoderm becomes the skin and the central and peripheral nervous systems. Cell signaling proteins direct formation of the anterior-posterior, dorsal-ventral, and left-right axes.

Signaling proteins include growth factors and their receptors, cellular adhesion molecules, and extracellular matrix proteins that both provide structure and position signals to developing tissues. Genetic mutations that alter these pathways are associated with severe deformity and dysfunction.

Environmental Factors

The effects of exogenous agents during development are also mediated through genetically regulated pathways. At the cellular level, xenobiotics (compounds foreign to nature) cause birth defects either because they disrupt cell signaling and thereby misdirect morphogenesis, or because they are cytotoxic and lead to excessive cell death.

In general, drug receptors expressed in embryos and fetuses are the same molecules that mediate pharmacologic effects in adults. Over the counter, prescribed inhalants, and schedules I and II drugs that are pharmacologically active in mothers will be active across the placenta in the embryo and fetus. Exposure to agents achieving cytotoxic levels in adults is likely to be teratogenic. Abused substances such as alcohol that are toxic to adults are predictably toxic to embryos and fetuses.

Transplacental pharmacologic effects can be therapeutic. The potential for embryonic and fetal drug therapies during pregnancy is increasing. Folic acid supplementation can lower risks for birth defects such as spina bifida, and maternally administered corticosteroids can induce fetal synthesis and secretion of pulmonary surfactants prior to delivery.

Mechanical Factors

Much of embryonic development and all fetal growth occurs normally within the amniotic fluid. Loss or inadequate production of amniotic fluid can have disastrous effects, as can disruption of placental membranes.

Lung and kidney development are particularly sensitive to mechanical forces. Potter sequence results when there is oligohydramnios resulting in distinct facial features (flattened nose, recessed chin, prominent epicanthal folds, and low-set abnormal ears) and pulmonary hypoplasia. Constriction of the chest through malformation of the ribs, lack of surrounding amniotic fluid due to renal malformations, or lack of movement (fetal breathing) leads to varying degrees of pulmonary hypoplasia in which the lungs are smaller than normal and develop fewer alveoli. The presentation at birth is respiratory distress and may be lethal. This can be seen in conditions that cause renal malformations or agenesis such as Kallmann syndrome.

Uteropelvic junction (UPJ) obstruction causes obstruction of ureters or bladder outflow. As pressure within obstructed renal collecting systems increases, it distorts cell interactions and alters histogenesis. Developing kidneys exposed to increased internal pressures for long periods eventually become nonfunctional.

CLINICAL DYSMORPHOLOGY

An important task for the clinician presented with an infant with a birth defect is to determine whether the problem is isolated or part of a larger embryopathy (or syndrome).

Terminology

Classification of dysmorphic features strives to reflect mechanisms of abnormal development. Birth defects are referred to as **malformations** when they result from intrinsic alterations in genetic processes such as Dandy Walker malformation. **Deformations** are mainly structural defects caused by a mechanical force, such as positional clubfeet. The term **dysplasia** is used to denote abnormal development or growth of a group of tissues, organs, or cells, such as skeletal dysplasia. When physical forces interrupt or distort fetal tissue, their effects are termed **disruptions**, such as seen in amniotic bands. Those in which the chronological order of abnormal development is understood may be referred to as sequences, such as Pierre Robin sequence that describes jaw underdevelopment (retrognathia) resulting in displacement of the tongue and upper airway obstruction. However, not all birth defects and dysmorphic features result from a single mechanism; Prune Belly syndrome is caused by urinary tract malformations that result in over extension of the abdominal muscles.

Malformations classified by pattern include syndrome and association. **Syndromes** are defined as a cluster of malformations that occur in a recognizable pattern with a known genetic cause. Those malformations that are well known to co-occur but without known genetic cause are classified as **associations**, such as **VACTERL association**. Association should be used as a diagnosis of exclusion. When a unifying cause can be identified, such as a chromosomal anomaly or a pathogenic mutation of a single gene, a more precise diagnosis should replace "association."

Evaluation of the Dysmorphic Infant

History and physical examinations provide clues to diagnosis. The extent of an infant's abnormalities may not be immediately apparent, and often the role of genetics is to further define the extent of involvement and offer counseling and support to the family.

A. History

Pregnancy histories are a critical part of the history intake. Review of gestational age, pregnancy losses for the parents, intrauterine drug exposure, prenatal complications, and prenatal testing is important. Family histories may provide significant information to pinpoint a particular diagnosis and should not be overlooked. Environmental histories should include descriptions of parental habits and work settings. Targeted histories, based on the chief complaint, should be obtained with past medical and surgical histories, developmental history, and review of systems.

B. Physical Examination

Meticulous physical examination is crucial for accurate diagnosis in dysmorphic infants and children. The neonate's physical measurements, in particular growth parameters, may offer insight into a specific diagnosis. Photographs are helpful and should include a consistent method of measurement for reference.

C. Imaging and Laboratory Studies

A skeletal survey is useful in the evaluation of patients with suspected skeletal dysplasia. Magnetic resonance imaging (MRI), with or without angiogram, venogram, or spectroscopy, contributes to the diagnostic evaluation of individuals with neurologic symptoms. Computed tomography (CT) is useful for bony structure assessment such as evaluation of the skull sutures in suspected craniosynostosis. Ultrasonography offers a window to observe the brain and spine in neonates and provides imaging of the abdominal organs when concern exists for multiple malformations.

Benachi A, Sarnacki S: Prenatal counseling and the role of the Pediatric surgeon. Semin Pediatr Surg 2014 Oct;23(5):240–243 [PMID: 25459006].

Centers for Disease Control & Prevention: Data & Statistics on Birth Defects. https://www.cdc.gov/ncbddd/birthdefects/data.html.

Posey JE, Rosenfeld JA: Molecular diagnostic experience of whole-exome sequencing in adult patients. Genet Med 2016 Jul;18(7):678–685 [PMID: 26633545].

CHROMOSOMAL DISORDERS: ABNORMAL NUMBER

TRISOMIES

ESSENTIALS OF DIAGNOSIS & TYPICAL FEATURES

► Trisomy is the presence of three copies of a chromosome, rather than the normal two copies.

► Affected individuals have recognizable patterns of facial features, congenital anomalies and an increase in infant and neonatal mortality.

► Children that survive have cognitive and physical disabilities.

► Most trisomic embryos are lost early in pregnancy.

1. Trisomy 21

Down syndrome occurs in about 1:700 newborns and is characterized by distinctive facial features and generalized hypotonia. The affected newborn may have feeding problems, constipation, prolonged physiologic jaundice, and transient blood count abnormalities. Problems that may develop during childhood include thyroid dysfunction, visual issues, hearing loss, obstructive sleep apnea, celiac disease, and atlantooccipital instability. The degree of cognitive disability

is variable ranging from mild to severe. There is an increased incidence of transient myeloproliferative disorder, leukemia, and Alzheimer disease.

► Clinical Findings

The main physical findings include characteristic facies (upslanting palpebral fissures, flat nasal bridge, epicanthal folds, midface hypoplasia, flattened occiput), minor limb abnormalities, and generalized hypotonia. Up to 50% of children with Down syndrome have congenital heart disease, most often endocardial cushion defects or other septal defects. Anomalies of the gastrointestinal tract, including esophageal and duodenal atresias, are seen in about 15% of cases.

Health supervision guidelines for children with Down syndrome has been published by the American Academy of Pediatrics.

Marilyn Bull; Committee on Genetics: Clinical report: health supervision for children with Down syndrome. Pediatrics 2011;128:393–406 [PMID: 21788214].

2. Trisomy 18 Syndrome

The incidence of trisomy 18 syndrome is about 1:3500 live births. The incidence at conception, however, is much higher, with most trisomy 18 pregnancies resulting in spontaneous abortion. Trisomy 18 is characterized by severe prenatal and postnatal growth restriction, congenital heart disease, and high rates of neonatal and infant mortality. Those who survive are affected by profound intellectual disability, feeding dysfunction, and failure to thrive.

► Clinical Findings

Infants with trisomy 18 are small for gestational age and have characteristic facies (microcephaly, prominent occiput, small malformed ears, overlapping clenched fingers, and rocker-bottom heels). They can have congenital heart disease, often ventricular septal defect or patent ductus arteriosus, and undescended testes in males.

3. Trisomy 13 Syndrome

The newborn incidence of trisomy 13 is about 1 in 5000, although most trisomy 13 fetuses abort spontaneously in the first trimester. Mortality is high in neonates and infants with trisomy 13 due to complex and multiple congenital anomalies. Those who survive usually have feeding difficulties, failure to thrive, and profound intellectual disability.

► Clinical Findings

Newborns with trisomy 13 have dysmorphic facial features, scalp cutis aplasia, microcephaly, microphthalmia, brain malformations, congenital heart defects (most commonly ventricular septal defect and patent ductus arteriosus), cleft lip and/or palate, omphalocele, and postaxial polydactyly.

Treatment

A. Medical Therapy

Trisomy 21: Surgical intervention for cardiac and GI anomalies, developmental supports such as feeding therapy, physical, occupational, and speech therapies, screening for hearing loss, and screening for autoimmune disorders such as hypothyroidism and celiac disease are all indicated. The goal of treatment is to help affected children develop to their full potential. Parents' participation in support groups such as the local chapter of the National Down Syndrome Society should be encouraged. See the website: http://www.ndss.org/.

Trisomies 18 and 13: Due to the medically serious nature of these disorders, the traditional management approach has been to withhold technological support and surgery in the neonatal period and infancy. However, in the last decade, the care paradigm has shifted to include shared decision making between the family and the health care providers as a foundational principle. The extent of surgical, medical, and palliative care is decided on an individual basis.

A support group for families of children with trisomies 13 and 18 who survive beyond infancy is called SOFT. See the website: http://www.trisomy.org/.

Carey JC, Kosho T: Perspectives on the care and advances in the management of children with trisomy 13 and 18. Am J Med Genet Part C Semin Med Genet 2016 Sep;172(3):249–250 [PMID: 27643592].

B. Genetic Counseling

Trisomy arises from errors of nondisjunction. Most parents of trisomic infants have normal chromosomes. The risk of having a child affected with a trisomy increases with maternal age. The recurrence risk for trisomy in future pregnancies is equal to 1 per 100 plus the age-specific maternal risk.

If the child has a trisomy resulting from a translocation and the parent has an abnormal karyotype, the risks are increased depending on the type of translocation.

SEX CHROMOSOME ABNORMALITIES

1. Turner Syndrome (Monosomy X)

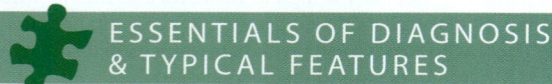

ESSENTIALS OF DIAGNOSIS & TYPICAL FEATURES

► Short stature, primary amenorrhea.
► Associated with coarctation of the aorta and genitourinary malformations.
► IQ is usually normal but learning disabilities are common.

The incidence of Turner syndrome is 1 per 2500 females. However, it is estimated that 95% of conceptuses with Turner syndrome are miscarried and only 5% are liveborn. The disorder is caused by a missing X or structurally abnormal X, leading to a single functional copy of the X chromosome instead of the normal two copies in women.

Clinical Findings

Newborns with Turner syndrome may have a short and webbed neck, edema of the hands and feet, and characteristic triangular facies. Other findings in older girls may include short stature, a shield chest with wide-set nipples, mixed conductive and sensorineural hearing loss, horseshoe kidneys, streak ovaries, amenorrhea, absence of development of secondary sex characteristics, and infertility. Some affected girls, particularly those with mosaicism, have only short stature and amenorrhea, without dysmorphic features. Cardiovascular anomalies including coarctation of the aorta, bicuspid aortic valve in the newborn period, and aortic root dilatation in the older girls and adult women can be seen. Learning disabilities are common, secondary to difficulties in perceptual motor integration.

Treatment

Hormonal treatments include growth hormone therapy for short stature and replacement therapy of both estrogen and progesterone to help with puberty and prevention of early onset osteoporosis. Surgical intervention for coarctation of the aorta with continued long term follow up with Cardiology is recommended. Speech therapy and academic support are given as needed. Treatment of infertility in women with Turner syndrome is complex and managed at specialized centers. Options for infertility treatment include oocyte donation, oocyte retrieval and cryopreservation, adoption, and using a gestational carrier. There are clinical practice guidelines for the care of girls and women with Turner syndrome from the proceedings of the 2016 Cincinnati International Turner Syndrome Meeting.

2. Klinefelter Syndrome (XXY)

ESSENTIALS OF DIAGNOSIS & TYPICAL FEATURES

► Tall stature with eunuchoid body habitus, prepubertal small testes, and male infertility.
► Variable degree of learning and cognitive difficulties.
► Diagnosis is rarely made before puberty.

The incidence of Klinefelter syndrome in the newborn population is roughly 1 per 1000, but it is about 1% among intellectual disabilities in males and about 3% among males seen at infertility clinics. Unlike Turner syndrome, Klinefelter syndrome is rarely the cause of spontaneous abortions. Prepubertal boys usually have a normal phenotype except for mild learning difficulties.

► Clinical Findings

The characteristic findings after puberty include small testicles with otherwise normal external genitalia, gynecomastia, diminished facial and body hair, tall, eunuchoid build and decreased muscle mass. IQ is borderline low to normal. The extra X chromosome affects testicular growth and affected males have low testosterone production leading to delayed, absent, or incomplete puberty, azoospermia, and infertility.

► Treatment

Males with Klinefelter syndrome require testosterone replacement therapy. Management of infertility in males with Klinefelter syndrome requires assisted reproductive techniques and/or adoption.

3. XYY Syndrome

Newborns with XYY syndrome in general are normal. Affected individuals may on occasion exhibit an abnormal behavior pattern from early childhood and may have mild intellectual disabilities. Fertility may be normal. Many older, adult males with an XYY karyotype are normal.

4. XXX Syndrome

The incidence of females with an XXX karyotype is approximately 1 per 1000. Females with XXX are phenotypically normal. However, they can be taller than expected and have lower intelligence quotients (IQs) than their typical siblings. Learning and behavioral issues are relatively common. This contrasts with individuals with XXXX, a much rarer condition causing more severe developmental issues, and a dysmorphic phenotype reminiscent of Down syndrome.

Jones KL: Smith's *Recognizable Patterns of Human Malformation.* 7th ed. Philadelphia, PA: Elsevier; 2013.

CHROMOSOME DELETION OR DUPLICATION DISORDERS

CMA is currently the gold standard for detection of microdeletions and microduplications including 1p36– syndrome, Wolf-Hirschhorn syndrome (4p–), and cri du chat syndrome (5p–) and DiGeorge syndrome (22q11.2 deletion).

1. Deletion 1p36 Syndrome

Typical features of 1p36 deletion syndrome include a large and late-closing anterior fontanel, microbrachycephaly, epicanthal folds, and low-set posteriorly rotated ears, developmental delay, intellectual disability, and hypotonia. Brain malformations, congenital heart defects, vision and hearing concerns, and genitourinary abnormalities are reported. Obesity is common.

2. Cri du Chat Syndrome

Also known as 5p– (deletion of terminal chromosome 5p), this disorder is characterized by unique facial features such as a broad nasal bridge and epicanthal folds, developmental delay, intellectual disability, growth retardation, and microcephaly. Patients have an unusual catlike cry. Malformations may include cardiac, genitourinary, and neurologic abnormalities.

Hypertension and spinal osteoarthritis occur in adults. Most patients have mild to moderate intellectual deficits.

3. Williams Syndrome

Williams syndrome is a contiguous gene disorder that deletes the gene for elastin and other neighboring genes at 7q11.2. It is characterized by short stature; congenital heart disease (supravalvular aortic or pulmonic stenosis); coarse, elfin-like facies with prominent lips; hypercalcemia or hypercalciuria in infancy; developmental delay; and neonatal irritability evolving into an overly friendly personality. Calcium restriction may be necessary in early childhood to prevent nephrocalcinosis. The hypercalcemia often resolves during the first year of life. The natural history includes progression of cardiac disease and predisposition to hypertension and spinal osteoarthritis in adults. Most patients have mild to moderate intellectual deficits. Duplication of chromosome 7q11.2 results in a syndrome that includes speech delay and features of autism spectrum disorders.

4. 22q11.2 Deletion Syndrome (Velocardiofacial Syndrome or DiGeorge Syndrome)

This condition was originally described in newborns presenting with cyanotic congenital heart disease, usually involving great vessel abnormalities; thymic hypoplasia leading to immunodeficiency; and hypocalcemia due to absent parathyroid glands. This phenotype is highly variable. Other characteristics have also been described including mild microcephaly, hypothyroidism, kidney and cervical spine malformations, palatal clefting, velopharyngeal insufficiency, speech and language delays, congenital heart disease (great vessel abnormalities, tetralogy of Fallot, and a variety of other cardiac abnormalities), psychiatric diagnoses such as attention-deficit hyperactivity disorder, anxiety, and psychoses, including schizophrenia in about 25% of cases. Duplication of the 22q11 region produces a mild and highly variable phenotype that ranges from developmental delays to functionally normal.

Oskarsdottir S et al: Updated clinical practice recommendations for managing children with 22q11.2 deletion syndrome. Genet Med 2023;25:100338 [PMID: 36729053].

MENDELIAN DISORDERS

AUTOSOMAL DOMINANT DISORDERS

Neurofibromatosis, MFS, achondroplasia, osteogenesis imperfecta, and craniosynostoses are among the most well-known autosomal dominant disorders. There are many other common autosomal dominant disorders, including Treacher Collins syndrome, Noonan syndrome, CHARGE syndrome, and Cornelia de Lange syndrome (CdLS).

1. Neurofibromatosis Type 1

Neurofibromatosis type 1 (NF1) is one of the most common autosomal dominant disorders, occurring in 1 per 3000 births, and is seen in all races and ethnic groups.

Neurofibromatosis type 2 (NF2), characterized by bilateral acoustic neuromas with minimal or no skin manifestations, is a different disease caused by a different gene.

The gene for NF1 is on the long arm of chromosome 17 and codes for a tumor suppresser factor. Approximately half of all NF cases are caused by new mutations. There is significant intra and interfamilial variability in affected individuals. Careful evaluation of the parents is necessary to provide accurate genetic counseling.

Café au lait spots, which are light brown macules, may be present at birth and are a hallmark of NF1. Affected individuals have more than six café au lait macules, along with axillary and inguinal freckling. In general, features of NF1 appear in an age dependent fashion.

Neurofibromas are benign tumors consisting of Schwann cells, nerve fibers, and fibroblasts. The incidence of Lisch nodules (benign iris hamartomas), which can be seen with a slit lamp, also increases with age. Affected individuals commonly have a large head, scoliosis, and a wide spectrum of developmental and learning problems.

Hyperpigmented macules can occur in other conditions such as McCune-Albright, Noonan, Leopard, and Bannayan-Riley-Ruvalcaba (BRR) syndromes that reflect the typical wide differential diagnosis for a single physical attribute. The genes for NF1, Noonan, and Leopard syndromes are molecules that control cell cycling through the RAS-MAPK signal transduction pathways; therefore, it is not surprising that some features can be shared.

Miller DT et al: Health supervision for children with neurofibromatosis type 1. Pediatrics 2019;143(5):e20190660 [PMID: 31010905].

2. Marfan Syndrome

ESSENTIALS OF DIAGNOSIS & TYPICAL FEATURES

► Skeletal abnormalities (Ghent criteria).
► Lens dislocation (ectopia lentis).
► Dilation of the aortic root.
► Dural ectasia.
► Positive family history in some cases.

► Clinical Findings

The diagnosis of Marfan syndrome (MFS) remains largely clinical and is based on the Ghent criteria. Children can present with a positive family history, suspicious skeletal findings, or ophthalmologic complications. Motor milestones are frequently delayed due to joint laxity. Adolescents are prone to spontaneous pneumothorax. Dysrhythmias may be present. Aortic root dilatation, leading to aortic aneurysm and dissection are fatal complications of MFS, leading to early morbidity and mortality.

The characteristic MFS patient has tall thin body habitus with long limbs, long and thin facies, deep set eyes with down-slanting palpebral fissures, malar flattening, and retrognathia. The palate is high arched, and dentition is often crowded. Mutations in the gene for fibrillin-1 (*FBN1*), an extracellular matrix protein, are causative.

► Differential Diagnosis

Homocystinuria should be excluded through metabolic testing in all individuals with marfanoid skeletal features. The differential diagnosis includes other connective tissue disorders including **Ehlers-Danlos syndrome** and **Loeys-Dietz syndrome**.

► Treatment

A. Medical Therapy

Medical treatment for patients with MFS includes surveillance for and appropriate management of ophthalmologic, orthopedic, and cardiac issues. Serial echocardiograms are indicated to diagnose and follow the degree of aortic root enlargement, which can be managed medically, or surgically in more severe cases. Prophylactic β-adrenergic blockade or angiotensin II receptor antagonists can slow the rate of aortic dilation and reduce the development of aortic complications.

B. Genetic Counseling

MFS is inherited in an autosomal dominant manner. Approximately 75% of individuals with MFS have an affected parent, and 25% have a de novo mutation in the *FBN1* gene.

Tinkle BT, Saal HM; Committee on Genetics: Health supervision for children with Marfan syndrome. Pediatrics 2013;132(4):e10 59–e1072 [PMID: 24081994].

3. Achondroplasia

Achondroplasia is the most common form of disproportionate short stature and is caused by a mutation in *FGFR3*.

Clinical Findings

Affected individuals have short limbed dwarfism, trident shaped hands, relative macrocephaly, and mid-face hypoplasia. The phenotype is apparent at birth. Children have hypotonia and delayed motor milestones in early childhood, but intelligence is normal. Additional complications include obstructive sleep apnea, kyphosis, and spinal stenosis.

Treatment

A. Medical Therapy

Bony overgrowth at the level of the foramen magnum may lead to progressive hydrocephalus and brainstem compression that may warrant neurosurgical intervention. Orthopedic intervention is necessary for spinal problems including severe lumbar lordosis and gibbus deformity. Adaptive modifications are required in daily life due to the short stature. A conjugated analog of C-type natriuretic peptide is approved by the FDA to help promote growth from age 5 years until growth plates close.

B. Genetic Counseling

Most cases (~ 90%) represent a new mutation. Two heterozygous parents with achondroplasia have a 25% risk of having a child homozygous for *FGFR3* mutations, which is a lethal disorder.

Savarirayan R, Tofts L, Irving M et al: Once-daily, subcutaneous vosoritide therapy in children with achondroplasia: a random-ized, double-blind, phase 3, placebo-controlled, multicenter trial. Lancet 2020 Sep 5;396(10252):684-692. [PMID: 32891212].

4. Osteogenesis Imperfecta

Osteogenesis imperfecta (OI), or brittle bone disease, is a relatively common disorder. More than 85% of cases are caused by dominant mutations affecting COL1A1 and COL1A2. Rarer forms of OI are caused by mutations in other genes and may be inherited as autosomal recessive.

Clinical Findings

The hallmark of OI is fractures with minimal or absent trauma. Affected individuals have short stature, frequent fractures, bowing of the extremities, and scoliosis. They also can have blue sclera, abnormal dentition (brown, translucent appearing teeth that break easily), and adult-onset hearing loss. Mildly affected individuals are relatively asymptomatic, while severely affected individuals often die in the perinatal period.

The four most common forms of OI are the following:

1. Classic nondeforming OI with blue sclera (previously OI type I)
2. Perinatal lethal OI (previously OI type II)
3. Progressively deforming OI (previously OI type III)
4. Common variable OI with normal sclera (previously OI type IV)

Treatment

A. Medical Therapy

Management includes orthopedic care, dental care, and physical and occupation therapy. Audiology assessments and hearing aids are provided as needed. Bisphosphonates are used for the treatment of moderate to severe forms of OI. They help in improving bone density and reducing the incidence of fractures.

B. Genetic Counseling

The milder forms of OI are often inherited as an autosomal dominant trait from an affected parent, while the more severe forms of OI generally result from new mutations.

5. Craniosynostosis Syndromes

The craniosynostosis syndromes are a group of disorders associated with premature fusion of cranial sutures and an abnormal skull shape. This class of autosomal dominant disorders is usually caused by mutations in *FGFR* genes.

Crouzon syndrome is the most common of these disorders and is associated with premature fusion of multiple sutures. Other craniosynostosis disorders have limb and craniofacial anomalies, and include Pfeiffer, Apert, Jackson-Weiss, and Saethre-Chotzen syndromes.

Affected individuals have abnormal skull shape, shallow orbits, widely spaced eyes, and midface narrowing. Children with craniosynostosis may require multiple-staged craniofacial and neurosurgical procedures but usually have normal intelligence.

6. CHARGE Syndrome

CHARGE syndrome is an autosomal dominant disorder associated with multiple congenital malformations. It is caused by mutations in the *CHD7* gene. The acronym CHARGE serves as a mnemonic for associated abnormalities that include Colobomas, congenital heart disease, choanal Atresia, growth Retardation, Genital abnormalities, and Ear abnormalities with deafness. Facial asymmetry is a common finding.

7. Noonan Syndrome

Noonan syndrome is a common autosomal dominant condition characterized by short stature, congenital heart disease, and mildly dysmorphic features. Birth weight is normal but feeding problems result in poor weight gain and failure to thrive. The congenital heart disease includes pulmonary stenosis and hypertrophic cardiomyopathy. Mild gross motor and speech delay are often present. About 25% of individuals with Noonan syndrome will have learning disability.

Noonan syndrome and Noonan-like disorders are caused by mutations in the RAS-mitogen-activated protein kinase (MAPK) pathway, and thus are often called as "RASopathies." Noonan syndrome is the most common of these disorders, usually caused by mutations in *PTPN11*. Other related disorders include cardiofaciocutaneous syndrome and Costello syndrome that have more distinctive facial features and more pronounced developmental delay. A genetic panel that screens for multiple genes in this pathway can help confirm a diagnosis.

Zenker M et al: Noonan syndrome: improving recognition and diagnosis. Arch Dis Child 2022;107:1073–1078 [PMID: 35246453].

AUTOSOMAL RECESSIVE DISORDERS

1. Cystic Fibrosis

The gene for cystic fibrosis, *CFTR*, is found on the long arm of chromosome 7. Approximately 1 in 22 people are carriers. Many different mutations have been identified; the most common mutation in the Caucasian population is known as Δ *F508*.

(For more details on clinical features and medical management of cystic fibrosis, see Chapters 19 and 22.)

2. Smith-Lemli-Opitz Syndrome

Smith-Lemli-Opitz syndrome is an inherited metabolic disorder in the final step of cholesterol biosynthetic pathway, resulting in low cholesterol levels and accumulation of the precursor 7-dehydrocholesterol (7-DHC). Cholesterol is a necessary precursor for sterol hormones and myelin and is an important component of cell membranes. Deficiency of cholesterol and accumulation of 7-DHC result in multisystemic effects.

▶ Clinical Findings

Patients with Smith-Lemli-Opitz syndrome present with a characteristic phenotype, including dysmorphic facial features (Figure 37–8), multiple congenital anomalies, hypotonia, growth failure, and intellectual disability. Mild cases may present with autism and 2–3 toe syndactyly. The diagnosis can be confirmed via a blood test looking for the presence of the precursor, 7-DHC. DNA sequencing of the *DHCR7* gene is also available.

▶ Treatment

Treatment with cholesterol can ameliorate the growth failure and lead to improvement in medical outcomes but is not curative.

3. Sensorineural Hearing Loss

Although there is marked genetic heterogeneity in causes of sensorineural hearing loss, including dominant, recessive, and X-linked patterns, nonsyndromic, recessively inherited hearing loss is the predominant form of severe inherited childhood deafness. Several hundred genes are known to cause hereditary hearing loss. The hearing loss may be

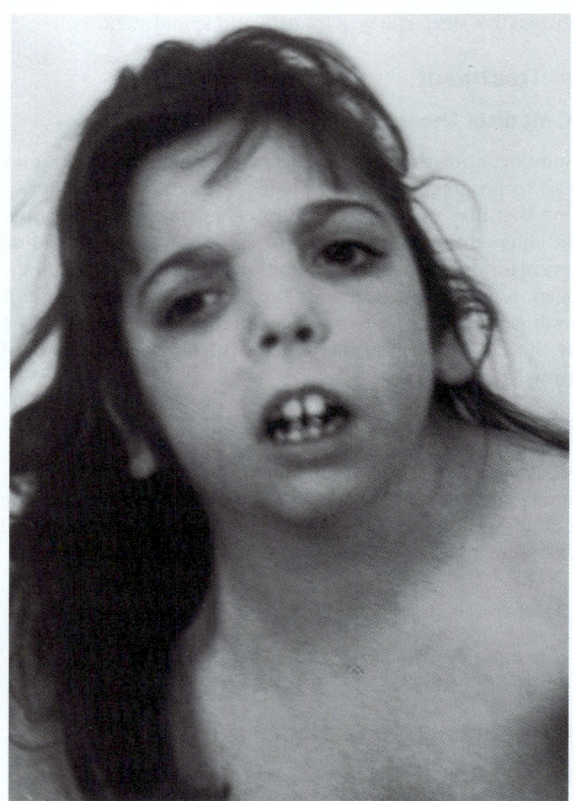

▲ **Figure 37–8.** Child with Smith-Lemli-Opitz syndrome, featuring bitemporal narrowing, upturned nares, ptosis, and small chin.

conductive, sensorineural, or a combination of both; syndromic or nonsyndromic; and prelingual or postlingual. The genetic forms of hearing loss are diagnosed by otologic, audiologic, and physical examination; family history; ancillary testing (such as petrous brain MRI to examine the inner ear and temporal bone); and molecular genetic testing. Panels screening for more than 100 genetic forms of hearing loss are available for many types of syndromic and nonsyndromic deafness.

Adam MP et al: Genetic Hearing Loss Overview—GeneReviews® NCBI Bookshelf (nih.gov), 2023.

4. Spinal Muscular Atrophy

Spinal muscular atrophy (SMA) is an autosomal recessive neuromuscular disorder in which anterior horn cells in the spinal cord degenerate. The mechanism for the loss of cells appears to involve apoptosis of neurons in the absence of the product of the *SMN1* (survival motor neuron) gene located on chromosome 5q. Loss of anterior horn cells leads to progressive atrophy of skeletal muscle. The disorder has an incidence of approximately 1 in 12,000, with most cases presenting in infancy. Carrier frequencies approach 1 in 40 in populations with European ancestry.

▶ Clinical Findings

Five clinical subtypes are recognized based on age of onset and rate of progression. SMA 0, which has prenatal onset, is the most devastating, with profound hypotonia and respiratory failure at birth. SMA I presents with mild weakness at birth but is clearly evident by 3 months and is accompanied by loss of reflexes and fasciculations in affected muscles. Progression of the disorder leads to eventual respiratory failure, usually by age 1 year. Symptoms of SMA II begin later, with weakness and decreased reflexes generally apparent by age 2 years. Children affected with SMA III begin to become weak as they approach adolescence. SMA IV presents with onset of muscle weakness in the second or third decades but with a normal lifespan.

Homozygous deletion of exon 7 of *SMN1* is detectable in approximately 95%–98% of cases of all types of SMA and confirms the diagnosis. The *SMN1* region on chromosome 5q is complex and variability in presentation of the disorder involves expression of up to three copies of the neighboring *SMN2* gene. More severe phenotypes have fewer *SMN2* copies. Approximately 2%–5% of patients affected with SMA will be compound heterozygotes in whom there is one copy of *SMN1* with exon 7 deleted and a second copy with a point mutation.

Prenatal diagnosis is available through genetic testing, but careful molecular analysis of the proband and demonstration of carrier status in parents is advised since, in addition to the problem of potential compound heterozygosity, 2% of cases

occur as a result of a de novo mutation in one *SMN1* allele. In this case, one of the parents is not a carrier and recurrence risks are low. Carrier testing is further complicated by a duplication of SMN1 in 4% of the population that results in there being two *SMN1* genes on one of their chromosomes. Hence, reproductive risk assessment, carrier testing, and prenatal diagnosis of SMA are best undertaken in the context of careful genetic counseling. In recent years, two different therapies (gene therapy and antisense oligonucleotide therapy) have achieved FDA approval for the treatment of SMA. Both require immediate treatment in affected individuals raising the potential benefit of newborn screening for SMA.

Schorling DC et al: Advances in treatment of spinal muscular atrophy—new phenotypes, new challenges, new implications for care. Neuromuscul Dis 2020:1–13 [PMID: 31707373].

X-LINKED DISORDERS

1. Duchenne & Becker Muscular Dystrophies

Duchenne muscular dystrophy (DMD) results from failure of synthesis of the muscle cytoskeletal protein dystrophin. The gene is located on the X chromosome, at position *Xp12*. Prevalence data are not available, but the incidence in Nova Scotia, Canada may be as high as 1/4700 live male births. The diagnosis should be suspected in a male with hypotonia, delayed motor milestones or abnormal gait. Elevated creatine kinase (CK) levels as part of screening workup for these symptoms suggests a diagnosis of muscular dystrophy. There are many different types of muscular dystrophies, but mutations in the Dystrophin gene lead to both DMD and Becker muscular dystrophy (BMD). In both DMD and BMD, progressive degeneration of skeletal and cardiac muscle occurs. Boys with DMD exhibit proximal muscle weakness and pseudohypertrophy of calf muscles by age 5–6 years. Without intervention, patients become nonambulatory by their early teens. Boys with DMD frequently die in their twenties of respiratory failure and cardiac dysfunction. The prognosis for BMD is more variable. Although corticosteroids are useful in maintaining strength, they do not slow progression of the disorder. Females with dystrophinopathies have an increased incidence of serious cardiovascular disease, including cardiomyopathy and arrhythmias.

The gene for dystrophin is very large and a common target for mutation. Large deletions or duplications can be detected in the gene for dystrophin in 65% of cases. Molecular analysis has largely replaced muscle biopsy for diagnostic purposes.

One-third of DMD cases presenting with a negative family history are likely to be new mutations. Germline mosaicism for mutations in the dystrophin gene occurs in approximately 15%–20% of families, which is among the highest rates for this otherwise rare phenomenon. Genetic counseling is recommended for families. Since mutations are now detected in the great majority of DMD cases, more accurate recurrence risk estimates and treatments in specific types of gene changes are now available. There are many therapeutic options under investigation, including gene therapies using CRISPR technology, antisense oligonucleotides, and exon skipping.

Echevarria L et al: Exon-skipping advances for Duchenne muscular dystrophy. Human Mol Genet 2019 Aug 1;27(R2):R163–R172 [PMID: 29771317].

2. Hemophilia

Hemophilia A is an X-linked, recessive, bleeding disorder caused by a deficiency in the activity of coagulation factor VIII. (See Chapter 30 for additional discussion.)

▼ NONMENDELIAN DISORDERS

DISORDERS OF IMPRINTING

1. Beckwith-Wiedemann Syndrome

The diagnosis of Beckwith-Wiedemann syndrome (BWS) may be suspected in individuals with macrosomia, macroglossia, lateralized overgrowth, omphalocele, embryonal tumors such as Wilms tumor, visceromegaly, cytomegaly of the fetal adrenal cortex, or anterior ear lobe creases and/or posterior helical ear pits. Other associated findings include hypertelorism, infantile hypoglycemia due to transient hyperinsulinemia, and multiple congenital anomalies (cleft palate and genitourinary anomalies).

Molecular testing may reveal one of several mechanisms impacting expression of the genes located on chromosome 11p15, for example, paternal UPD of this region. Mutations in the maternal copy of the CDKN1C gene are associated with BWS and may be a rare instance of recurrence risk in individuals with BWS by this mechanism. Most patients have methylation errors of DMR1 (differentially methylated region1, H19, 5%), and DMR2 (LIT1, 50%). H19 is a long noncoding RNA with a role in the negative regulation of cell proliferation. Isolated macroglossia or hemihyperplasia can be a mild form of BWS that may escape molecular diagnosis due to mosaicism. Children affected or suspected to have BWS should undergo tumor surveillance protocols, including serum AFP levels every 2–3 months until they reach age 4 and an abdominal ultrasound every 3 months until they reach age 8 to screen for hepatoblastoma and Wilms tumor. Recent literature confirms that molecular subtype correlates to overall tumor risk, but screening guidelines have not changed. An annual renal ultrasound should be performed between age 8 and mid-adolescence to identify those with medullary sponge kidney disease.

2. Prader-Willi Syndrome

Prader-Willi syndrome (PWS) results from lack of paternal expression of several imprinted genes, including SNRPN, located on chromosome 15q11. Clinical characteristics include severe hypotonia in infancy and poor feeding that progresses through multiple nutritional stages. In stage 3 (average age 8 years), individuals develop hyperphagia or an inability to achieve satiety. Characteristic features may include almond-shaped eyes, bitemporal narrowing, and small hands and feet. Obstructive sleep apnea is common, as are hypogonadotropic hypogonadism, and characteristic behaviors including behavioral rigidity, insistence on sameness, and obsessive-compulsive features. Growth hormone treatment is the only FDA-approved treatment for PWS and may offer benefits beyond linear growth. Obesity is the rule without environmental modifications. Genetic testing for PWS includes DNA methylation analysis, which can detect 99% of the cases that include paternally inherited deletions (~ 70%), maternal UPD (20%–30%), imprinting defects, imprinting center deletions, and unbalanced chromosome rearrangement.

3. Angelman Syndrome

Angelman syndrome (AS) results from absent maternal expression of the gene ubiquitin-protein ligase E3A gene, UBE3A, located at 15q11.2q13 in the PWS critical region. The classic phenotype includes developmental delay greatly impacting expressive language, intellectual disability, seizures, movement disorders, sleep disturbances, gastrointestinal concerns, and stereotypic behaviors including a characteristic excitable and happy demeanor.

DNA methylation analysis detects 80% of individuals with AS including those caused by a deletion of the maternal allele at 15q11 (~65%–75%), UPD of the paternal allele (3%–7%), and imprinting defects (3%). Mutations in UBE3A cause the disorder in about 11% of cases and require sequencing of the UBE3A gene.

Dagli AI, Mueller J, Williams CA: Angelman syndrome. 1998 Sep 15 [updated 2015 May 14]. In: Pagon RA et al (eds): GeneReviews® [Internet]. Seattle, WA: University of Washington; 1993–2017. https://www.ncbi.nlm.nih.gov/books/NBK1144/ [PMID: 20301323].

Driscoll DJ et al: Prader-Willi syndrome. 1998 Oct 6 [updated 2017 Dec 14]. In: Adam MP et al (eds): GeneReviews® [Internet]. Seattle, WA: University of Washington; 1993–2017. https://www.ncbi.nlm.nih.gov/books/NBK1330/.

DISORDERS ASSOCIATED WITH REPEAT EXPANSION

These disorders are caused by an expansion of the size of a tri (or tetra) nucleotide repeat (eg, CTG) from the lineage (maternal or paternal) in which it is more unstable and likely to expand.

1. Myotonic Dystrophy (Autosomal Dominant)

Myotonic dystrophy is an autosomal dominant condition characterized by muscle weakness and tonic muscle spasms (myotonia). Additional features include hypogonadism, frontal balding, cardiac conduction abnormalities, and cataracts. This disorder occurs when a CTG repeat in the *DMPK* gene on chromosome 19 expands to 50 or more copies. Normal individuals have from 5 to 35 CTG repeat copies. Individuals carrying 35–49 repeats are generally asymptomatic but repeat copies greater than 35 are meiotically unstable and tend to further expand when passed to subsequent generations.

CTG repeat sizes in the 100–1000 range usually develop Classic DM1 with muscle weakness and wasting, myotonia, cataracts, and often cardiac conduction abnormalities. Individuals with greater than 1000 copies often present as congenital DM1: infantile hypotonia, respiratory deficits, and intellectual disability. This occurs most frequently when the unstable repeats are passed through an affected mother. Therefore, an important component in the workup of the floppy or weak infant is a careful neurologic assessment of both parents for evidence of weakness or myotonia. Molecular testing that measures the number of CTG repeats is diagnostic clinically and prenatally. (See Chapter 25 for additional discussion.)

2. Friedreich Ataxia (Autosomal Recessive)

Symptoms of Friedreich ataxia (FA) include dysarthria, muscle weakness, lower limb spasticity, bladder dysfunction, and absent lower limb reflexes. Both motor and sensory findings begin in preadolescence and typically progress through the teenage years. The presentation can be variable. FA results from an abnormally expanded GAA repeat in intron 1 of *FXN*. Unaffected individuals typically carry 7–33 GAA repeats at this locus. Close to 96% of affected patients are homozygous for repeat expansions that exceed 66 copies. Point mutations in the gene also occur. Molecular diagnostic testing requires careful interpretation with respect to prognosis and reproductive risks. (See Chapter 25 for additional discussion.)

3. Fragile X Syndrome (X-Linked)

Fragile X syndrome, present in approximately 1 in 1000 males, has long been considered the most common cause of intellectual disability in males. The responsible gene is *FMR1*, which has unstable CGG repeats at the 5′ end. Normal individuals have up to 50 CGG repeats. Individuals with 51–200 CGG repeats have a premutation and may manifest symptoms including mild developmental disabilities and behavioral traits; premature ovarian failure in a subset of females; and a progressive, neurologic deterioration in older males called FXTAS (Fragile X-associated tremor-ataxia syndrome). Affected individuals with Fragile X syndrome (full mutation) have more than 200 CGG repeats and have hypermethylation of both the CGG expansion and an adjacent CpG island. This methylation turns off the *FMR1* gene. Molecular testing to determine the number of CGG trinucleotide repeats of more than 200 confirms the diagnosis of Fragile X syndrome.

▶ Clinical Features

Most males with Fragile X syndrome present with intellectual disabilities, oblong facies with large ears, and large testicles after puberty. Other physical signs include hyperextensible joints and mitral valve prolapse or aortic root dilation. Many affected individuals are hyperactive and meet the criteria for diagnosis of autism spectrum disorders. Other features may include hypotonia, seizures, GI concerns, sleeps disorders, and scoliosis.

Unlike other X-linked disorders where female heterozygotes are asymptomatic, females with a full mutation may exhibit a phenotype ranging from normal IQ to intellectual disability and may show behaviors along the autism spectrum.

Clinical expression of Fragile X differs in male and female offspring depends on which parent is transmitting the gene. The premutation can change into the full mutation only when passed through a female. Prenatal testing is available to pregnant women once an expanded *FMR1* allele is identified. (Management considerations for patients with Fragile X syndrome are described in Chapter 3.)

Hersh JH, Saul RA; Committee on Genetics: Health supervision for children with Fragile X syndrome. Pediatrics 2011 May;127(5):994–1006 [PMID: 21518720].

DISORDERS OF MULTIFACTORIAL INHERITANCE

Multifactorial inheritance is a type of hereditary pattern seen when there is more than one genetic factor involved and, sometimes, when there are also environmental factors and stochastic events participating in the causation and presentation of a condition. Examples include the following:

CLEFT LIP & CLEFT PALATE

 ESSENTIALS OF DIAGNOSIS & TYPICAL FEATURES

▶ Cleft lip is more common in males, cleft palate in females.

▶ Cleft lip and palate may be isolated defects (nonsyndromic) or associated with other anomalies as part of a genetic disorder (syndromic).

General Considerations

From a genetic standpoint, cleft lip with or without cleft palate is distinct from isolated cleft palate. The prevalence of facial clefting per 10,000 births is 10.2 in the United States, 12.1 in Western Europe, and 20.0 in Japan. Some in utero exposures may cause cleft lip and palate such as anti-seizure medications, acne drugs containing Accutane, and methotrexate.

Findings

A cleft lip may be unilateral or bilateral and complete or incomplete. It may occur with a cleft of the entire palate or just the primary (anterior and gingival ridge) or secondary (posterior) palate. An isolated cleft palate can involve only the soft palate or both the soft and hard palates. When the cleft palate is associated with micrognathia and glossoptosis, it is called the Pierre Robin sequence. Individuals with central clefts have increased association with other congenital anomalies or syndromes.

Differential Diagnosis

A facial cleft may occur in many different circumstances. It may be an isolated abnormality or part of a more generalized syndrome. Prognosis, management, and accurate determination of recurrence risks all depend on accurate diagnosis.

A. Nonsyndromic Cleft lip/Palate

Empiric recurrence risks for future pregnancies are in the range of 2%–3% because of nonpenetrance or the presence of other contributing genes.

B. Syndromic Cleft Lip/Palate

Cleft lip, with or without cleft palate, and isolated cleft palate may occur in a variety of syndromes that may be environmental, chromosomal, single gene, or of unknown origin (Table 37–2).

Complications

Problems associated with facial clefts include early feeding difficulties; airway challenges; recurrent serous otitis media; speech difficulties, articulation differences; and complex dental care.

A. Medical Therapy

Long-term management ideally should be provided through a multidisciplinary cleft palate clinic to include otolaryngologists, audiologists, social work, speech therapist, dentists, and genetic professionals.

B. Genetic Counseling

Genetic counseling depends on accurate diagnosis and the differentiation of syndromic from nonsyndromic clefts. A

Table 37–2. Syndromic isolated cleft palate (CP) and cleft lip with or without cleft palate (CL/CP).

Environmental
Maternal seizures, anticonvulsant usage (CL/CP or CP)
Fetal alcohol syndrome (CP)
Amniotic band syndrome (CL/CP)
Chromosomal
Trisomies 13 and 18 (CL/CP)
Wolf-Hirschhorn or 4p– syndrome (CL/CP)
Shprintzen or 22q11.2 deletion syndrome (CP)
Single-gene disorders
Treacher-Collins syndrome, AD (CP)
Stickler syndrome, AD (CP—particularly Pierre-Robin)
Smith-Lemli-Opitz, AR (CP)

AD, autosomal dominant; AR, autosomal recessive.

complete family history should be obtained. The choice of laboratory studies is guided by the history and physical examination and may include molecular and/or cytogenetic analysis. Clefts of both the lip and the palate can be detected on detailed prenatal ultrasound.

Basha M: Whole exome sequencing identifies mutation in 10% of patients with familial non-syndromic cleft lip and/or palate in genes mutated in well-known syndromes. J Med Genet 2018 Jul;55(7):449–458 [PMID: 29500247].

NEURAL TUBE DEFECTS

ESSENTIALS OF DIAGNOSIS & TYPICAL FEATURES

▶ Various defects, ranging from anencephaly to open or skin-covered lesions of the spinal cord, may occur in isolation or along with other congenital anomalies.

▶ Myelomeningocele is usually associated with hydrocephalus, Arnold-Chiari II malformation, neurogenic bladder and bowel, and congenital paralysis in the lower extremities.

▶ Anomalies of the central nervous system (CNS), heart, and kidneys may also be seen.

▶ MRI helps determine the extent of the anatomic defect in skin-covered lesions.

General Considerations

Neural tube defects comprise a variety of malformations, including anencephaly, encephalocele, spina bifida

(-myelomeningocele), sacral agenesis, and other spinal dysraphisms. Neural tube defects result from failure of closure of the neural tube, which normally occurs 18–28 days post fertilization. Hydrocephalus associated with the Arnold-Chiari type II malformation commonly occurs with myelomeningocele. Sacral agenesis, also called the caudal regression syndrome, occurs more frequently in infants of diabetic mothers.

▶ Clinical Findings

At birth, neural tube defects can present as an obvious open lesion, or as a more subtle skin-covered lesion. In the latter case, MRI should be conducted to better define the anatomic defect. The extent of neurologic deficit depends on the level of the lesion and may include clubfeet, dislocated hips, neurogenic bowel and bladder, and total flaccid paralysis below the level of the lesion. Hydrocephalus may be apparent prenatally or may develop after birth.

▶ Differential Diagnosis

Neural tube defects may occur in isolation or associated with other congenital anomalies. Maternal folic acid deficiency is the single most important risk factor for the development of NTDs. Other risk factors include history of maternal diabetes during pregnancy, prepregnancy obesity, or exposure to folic acid antagonists, for example valproate in the first trimester.

Any infant with dysmorphic features or other major anomalies in addition to a neural tube defect should be evaluated by a geneticist.

▶ Treatment

A. Neurosurgical Measures

Prenatal interventions including fetal surgery to correct an open neural tube defect are now much more common. Postnatally, neurosurgical closure should occur within 24–48 hours after birth to reduce risk of infection. Shunts are required in about 85% of cases of myelomeningocele.

B. Orthopedic Measures

Children with low lumbar and sacral lesions walk with minimal support, while those with high lumbar and thoracic lesions are rarely functional walkers. Orthopedic input is necessary to address foot deformities and scoliosis. Physical therapy services are indicated.

C. Urologic Measures

Neurogenic bladders require urologic consultations. Continence may be achieved using medications, clean intermittent catheterization, and a variety of urologic procedures. Renal function should be monitored regularly, and an ultrasound examination should be periodically repeated. Symptomatic infections should be treated.

Neurogenic bowel is managed with a combination of dietary modifications and medications. A surgical procedure called ACE (ante-grade continence enema) may be recommended for patients with severe constipation.

D. Genetic Counseling

Most isolated neural tube defects are polygenic, with a recurrence risk of 2%–3% in future pregnancies. A patient with spina bifida has a 5% chance of having an affected child. Prenatal diagnosis is possible with maternal serum screening and prenatal ultrasound.

Prophylactic folic acid can significantly lower the incidence and recurrence rate of neural tube defects if the intake of the folic acid starts at least 3 months prior to conception and continued for the first month of pregnancy.

▶ Special Issues & Prognosis

All children requiring multiple surgical procedures (ie, patients with spina bifida or urinary tract anomalies) have a significant risk for developing hypersensitivity type I (IgE-mediated) allergic reactions to latex. For this reason, nonlatex medical products are now routinely used when caring for patients with neural tube defects.

Most individuals with myelomeningocele are cognitively normal, but learning disabilities are common. Individuals with encephalocele or other CNS malformations have a much poorer intellectual prognosis. Individuals with neural tube defects have lifelong medical issues, requiring the input of a multidisciplinary medical team.

Family resources: https://www.spinabifidaassociation.org/.

COMMON RECOGNIZABLE DISORDERS WITH VARIABLE OR UNKNOWN CAUSE

There are several important and common human malformation syndromes. Illustrations of these syndromes are found in Smith's *Recognizable Patterns of Human Malformation.*

1. Arthrogryposis Multiplex

The term *arthrogryposis* describes multiple congenital contractures that affect two or more different areas of the body. Arthrogryposis is not a specific diagnosis, but rather a clinical finding, and it is a characteristic of more than 300 different disorders. Fetal akinesia and arthrogryposis are genetically heterogeneous, frequently involving in utero constraint, CNS malformation or injury, and neuromuscular disorders. Polyhydramnios is often present as a result of lack of fetal swallowing. Pulmonary hypoplasia also may be present, reflecting lack of fetal breathing. The initial workup includes brain imaging, consideration of metabolic disease, neurologic consultation, and in some cases, electrophysiologic studies and/or muscle biopsy. Rapid molecular analysis may be more cost effective and less invasive. Parental evaluation is important to determine if they also have symptoms demonstrating an inherited cause.

Family history review for findings such as muscle weakness or cramping, cataracts, and early-onset heart disease that indicate myotonic dystrophy is important. Distal arthrogryposis is primarily an autosomal dominant condition.

2. Goldenhar Syndrome

Goldenhar syndrome, also known as ocular-auriculo-vertebral (OAV) syndrome or craniofacial microsomia, is an association of multiple anomalies involving the head and neck. The classic phenotype includes hemifacial microsomia (one side of the face smaller than the other), and abnormalities of the pinna on the same side with associated deafness. Ear anomalies may be quite severe and include anotia and/or microtia. A characteristic benign fatty tumor in the outer eye, called an epibulbar dermoid, is frequently present, as are preauricular ear tags. Vertebral anomalies are common. The Arnold-Chiari type I malformation is a common associated anomaly. Cardiac anomalies and hydrocephalus are seen in more severe cases. Most patients with Goldenhar syndrome have typical intelligence. The cause is unknown, and some believe it is a blastocyst developmental field defect. Goldenhar syndrome is seen more frequently in infants of a diabetic mother. (See Craniofacial Microsomia Overview, GeneReviews, www.genereviews.org for an excellent discussion and differential diagnosis.)

3. Syndromic Short Stature

Short stature is an important component of numerous syndromes, or it may be an isolated finding. In the absence of nutritional deficiencies, endocrine abnormalities, evidence of skeletal dysplasia (disproportionate growth with abnormal skeletal films), or a positive family history, intrinsic short stature can be due to UPD. The phenotype of Russell-Silver syndrome—short stature with normal head growth, typical development, and minor dysmorphic features (especially fifth finger clinodactyly)—has been associated in some cases with maternal UPD7 and hypomethylation of *H19*, which is the opposite molecular mechanism seen in BWS. The diagnostic pearl for this condition is prenatal onset IUGR with spared head circumference. Short stature in girls may also be caused by Turner syndrome or a SHOX deletion.

4. VACTERL Association

VACTERL is sporadic and some of the defects may be life-threatening. The prognosis for typical development is good. The cause is unknown, but a high association with monozygotic twinning suggests a mechanism dating back to events perhaps as early as blastogenesis.

Careful examination and follow-up are important because numerous other syndromes have overlapping features.

Genetic consultation is warranted. No monogenic cause for VACTERL has been identified thus far.

ESSENTIALS OF DIAGNOSIS & TYPICAL FEATURES

VACTERL association is described by an acronym denoting the association of the following:

- ▶ Vertebral defects (segmentation anomalies).
- ▶ Imperforate anus.
- ▶ Cardiac malformation (most often ventricular septal defect).
- ▶ Tracheoesophageal fistula.
- ▶ Renal anomalies.
- ▶ Limb (most often radial ray) anomalies.

GENETIC EVALUATION OF THE CHILD WITH DEVELOPMENTAL DISABILITIES

Cognitive disabilities or developmental delays affect 8% of the general population. A Genetics consultation is recommended for the evaluation of any child with developmental delay. When evaluating a child with developmental delay, consider the following history, examination, and lab evaluations. (See Chapter 3 for additional information about developmental delay and intellectual disability.)

▶ History: Key Points

- Detailed pregnancy history (exposures, US abnormalities, growth restriction) and history regarding perinatal events.
- A full developmental history with age of onset and mode of presentation.
- Sex of the child: Females consider Rett syndrome. Males consider X-linked disorders.
- Feeding history and growth velocity. Many genetic disorders have feeding dysfunction and growth failure.
- Loss of skills or regression, which may indicate an underlying metabolic disorder.
- Involvement of other organ systems such as hearing loss, vision abnormalities, and organomegaly, which may provide diagnostic clues.
- Ethnicity: Certain neurometabolic disorders are more common in specific groups; for example, Tay Sachs disease in Ashkenazi Jewish populations.
- A three-generation family history can provide clues to suggest possible genetic etiologies, particularly if there is a history of consanguinity, which suggests recessive inheritance or a family pattern of other affected individuals.

▶ Evaluation: Key Points

- Anthropometric measurements, including height, weight, and head circumference.
- Attention to facial features and skeletal examination. Referral to a clinical geneticist is indicated whenever unusual features are encountered.
- Detailed physical examination, with attention to any hepatosplenomegaly, abnormal muscle tone, and skin findings such as hypo- or hyperpigmented spots.
- Neurologic, ophthalmologic, and audiologic consultation should be sought when indicated. Brain MRI should be requested in cases involving abnormal head size, seizures, and regression.
- Skeletal survey may be indicated when short stature and abnormal body proportions are noted.
- Genetic and metabolic testing based on relevant clinical scenario. Expanded Neurodevelopmental panels, whole exome and whole genome sequencing are being increasingly utilized as first tier tests in the evaluation of a child with developmental delay.

Interpretation & Follow-up

Clinical experience indicates that specific diagnoses can be made in approximately half of patients evaluated according to the protocol presented here. With specific diagnosis comes prognosis, ideas for management, and insight into recurrence risks.

Follow-up is important both for patients in whom diagnoses have been made and for those patients initially lacking a diagnosis. Genetic testing is advancing rapidly and can be translated into new diagnoses and better understanding with periodic review of clinical cases.

Manickam K et al: Exome and genome sequencing for pediatric patients with congenital anomalies or intellectual disability: an evidence-based clinical guidelines of the American College of Medical Genetics and Genomics: Genet Med 2021;23:2029–2037 [PMID: 34211152].
Moeschler JB, Scevell M; Committee on Genetics: Comprehensive evaluation of the child with intellectual disability or global developmental delay. Pediatrics 2014;134:e903 [PMID: 25157020].
Schaefer GB, Mendelsohn NJ; Professional Practice and Guidelines Committee: Clinical genetics evaluation in identifying the etiology of autism spectrum disorders: 2013 guideline revisions. Genet Med 2013 May;15(5):399–407 [PMID: 23519317].

Autism

Autism is a developmental disorder comprising abnormal function in three domains: language development, social development, and behavior. Many patients with autism also have cognitive disabilities and might be appropriately evaluated according to the recommendations above. However, given the enormous increase in prevalence of autism in the past decade (1 in 68 children per latest CDC report), it is worth discussing the genetic evaluation of autism separately.

Advances in molecular diagnosis, understanding of metabolic derangements, and technologies such as microarray and NGS, are allowing more patients with autism to be identified with specific genetic disorders. This allows more accurate genetic counseling for recurrence risk, as well as diagnosis-specific interventions, which may improve prognosis.

Recommendations for the genetic evaluation of a child with autism include the following:

1. Genetic referral if dysmorphic features or cutaneous abnormalities are present (ie, hypopigmented spots such as those seen in patients with **tuberous sclerosis**).
2. Laboratory testing to include the following:
   a. CMA.
   b. Molecular testing for **Fragile X syndrome**.
   c. Methylation testing for UPD15 if phenotype is suggestive of **AS**.
   d. Measurement of cholesterol and 7-DHC if syndactyly is present between the second and third toes to rule out a mild form of **Smith-Lemli-Opitz syndrome**.
   e. *MECP2* testing if clinical course is suggestive of **Rett syndrome** (ie, neurodegenerative course, progressive microcephaly, and seizures in a female patient).
   f. *PTEN* molecular testing if the head circumference is greater than two standard deviations above the mean, plus evidence of penile freckling, lipomatous lesions, or a strong family history of certain malignancies.
   g. Expanded neurodevelopmental panels if nonverbal autism, family history of autism, autism associated with dysmorphic facial features, and congenital anomalies are present.

Autism spectrum disorders are discussed in more detail in Chapter 3.

Christensen DL; CDC: Prevalence of autism spectrum disorder among children aged 8 years—autism and developmental disabilities monitoring network, 11 Sites, United States, 2010. MMWR Surveill Summ 2016 Apr 1;65(3):1–23. http://www.cdc.gov/mmwr [PMID: 27031587].

PERINATAL GENETICS

TERATOGENS

1. Drug Abuse & Fetal Alcohol Syndrome

Fetal alcohol syndrome (FAS) results from excessive exposure to alcohol during gestation and affects 30%–40% of offspring of mothers whose daily intake of alcohol exceeds 3 oz. Features of the syndrome include short stature, poor head growth (may be postnatal in onset), developmental delay, and midface hypoplasia characterized by a poorly developed philtrum, thin upper lip, narrow palpebral fissures, and short nose with anteverted nares. Facial findings may be subtle, but careful measurements and comparisons with standards are helpful. Structural abnormalities occur in half of affected children. Cardiac anomalies, genitourinary tract anomalies, and neural tube defects are commonly seen.

Alcohol exposure does not always result in classic FAS. In fact, facial and physical features are more related to the timing of exposure during fetal development and do not necessarily correlate with neurologic outcome. Alcohol-related neurodevelopmental disorder (ARND) describes the cognitive impairments linked to prenatal alcohol exposure including neurologic deficits such as poor motor skills and hand-eye coordination. Individuals with ARND may also have a complex pattern of behavioral and learning problems, including difficulties with memory, attention, and judgment. Diagnosis is based on maternal history and clinical findings.

Maternal abuse of psychoactive substances also is associated with increased risks for adverse perinatal outcomes including miscarriage, preterm delivery, growth restriction, and increased risk for injury to the developing CNS. Meth-amphetamine exposure also has been found in limited studies to cause impairment in executive function. Maternal abuse of inhalants, such as glue, appears to be associated with findings like those of FAS.

Careful evaluation for other syndromes and chromosomal disorders should be included in the workup of exposed infants. Fetal alcohol spectrum disorders are discussed in more detail in Chapter 3.

2. Maternal Anticonvulsant Effects

Anticonvulsant exposure during pregnancy is associated with adverse outcomes in approximately 10% of children born to women treated with these agents. A variable syndrome characterized by small head circumference, anteverted nares, cleft lip and palate and distal digital hypoplasia was first described in association with the maternal use of phenytoin, but also occurs with other anticonvulsants. Risks for spina bifida are increased especially in pregnancies exposed to valproic acid.

3. Retinoic Acid Embryopathy

Vitamin A and its analogues have considerable teratogenic potential. Developmental toxicity occurs in approximately one-third of pregnancies exposed in the first trimester to the synthetic retinoid, isotretinoin, commonly prescribed to treat acne. Exposure produces CNS malformation, especially of the posterior fossa; ear anomalies (often absence of pinnae); congenital heart disease (great vessel anomalies); and tracheoesophageal fistula. It is now recognized that vitamin A itself, when taken as active retinoic acid in doses exceeding 25,000 IU/day during pregnancy, can produce similar fetal anomalies. Maternal ingestion of large amounts of vitamin A taken as retinol during pregnancy, however, does not usually increase risks, because conversion of this precursor to active retinoic acid is internally regulated.

ASSISTED REPRODUCTION

Assisted reproductive technologies including in vitro fertilization (IVF) are now used in a significant number of pregnancies. Although healthy live births are accepted as the usual outcomes resulting from successful application of these procedures, the actual number of viable embryos is limited and questions about the risks of adverse effects continue to be raised. Increased rates of twinning, both monozygotic and dizygotic, are well recognized while the possibility of increased rates of birth defects remains controversial. Abnormal genetic imprinting appears to be associated with IVF. Evidence supports increased prevalence of BWS and AS among offspring of in vitro pregnancies.

PRENATAL DIAGNOSIS

Prenatal screening for birth defects is now routinely offered to pregnant women of all ages. Prenatal diagnosis introduces options for management.

Prenatal assessment of the fetus includes techniques that screen maternal blood, fetal imaging by ultrasound or MRI, fetal DNA analysis via maternal blood samples, and samples of fetal and placental tissues.

▶ Maternal Blood Analysis

Several options now exist to evaluate the fetus and pregnancy by obtaining a maternal blood sample. In the first trimester, measurements of PAPA (pregnancy-associated plasma protein A) and the free β-subunit of human chorionic gonadotropin (hCG) screen for trisomies 21 and 18. In the second-trimester maternal α-fetoprotein (AFP), hCG, unconjugated estradiol, and inhibin ("quad screen") combine to estimate risks for trisomies 21 and 18. Low estradiol levels can also predict cases of Smith-Lemli-Opitz syndrome. Noninvasive prenatal testing using NextGen sequencing, via maternal blood sample (also known as cell-free fetal DNA), can detect specific chromosome imbalances and typically tests for the presence of sex chromosomes as well as trisomies 13, 18, and 21. It is becoming more common to look for microdeletion and microduplication syndromes via this methodology. It is important to note that this testing is a screening test and diagnoses always need to be confirmed by a diagnostic method.

Amniocentesis and chorion villus sampling, followed by genetic analysis of fetal cells/tissue, are diagnostic tools used in pregnancy.

A. Amniocentesis

Amniocentesis samples fluid surrounding the fetus and is performed in the early second trimester (around 15–16 weeks' gestation). The cells obtained are cultured for cytogenetic, molecular, or metabolic analyses. AFP and other chemical markers can also be measured. This is a safe procedure with a complication rate (primarily for miscarriage) of less than 0.01% in experienced hands.

B. Chorionic Villus Sampling (Placental)

Chorionic villus sampling (CVS) is generally performed at 11–12 weeks' gestation. Tissue obtained by CVS provides DNA for molecular analysis. There is a slightly higher risk of miscarriage with CVS, as compared to amniocentesis (~ 1.5% of pregnancies that undergo CVS).

C. Fetal Blood and Tissue

Fetal blood can be sampled directly in late gestation through ultrasound-guided percutaneous umbilical blood sampling (PUBS). A wide range of biochemical and genetic diagnostic tests can be applied.

It is occasionally necessary to obtain biopsy specimens of fetal tissues such as liver or muscle for accurate prenatal diagnosis. These procedures are available in only a few perinatal centers.

D. Preimplantation Genetic Diagnosis

Pre-implantation genetic diagnosis following IVF is possible in human embryos by removing and analyzing blastocyst cells.

The use of this technology is limited to diagnosis of certain genetic diseases.

▶ Fetal Imaging

Fetal ultrasonography and MRI are widely available during pregnancy. Ultrasonography has joined maternal blood sampling as a screening technique for common chromosomal aneuploidies, neural tube defects, and other structural anomalies. Pregnancies with concerns for malformations require careful and frequent ultrasound examinations.

Beta J, Zhang W, Geris S, Kostiv V, Akolekar R: Procedure-related risk of miscarriage following chorionic villus sampling and amniocentesis. Ultrasound Obstet Gynecol 2019 Oct;54(4):452–457. Epub 2019 Sep 6 [PMID: 30977213].

Iwarsson E, Jacobsson B: Analysis of cell-free fetal DNA in maternal blood for detection of trisomy 21, 18 and 13 in a general pregnant population and in a high-risk population—a systematic review and meta-analysis. Acta Obstet Gynecol Scand 2017 Jan;96(1):7–18 [PMID: 27779757].

Liao GJ, Gronowski AM, Zhao Z: Non-invasive prenatal testing using cell-free fetal DNA in maternal circulation. Clin Chim Acta 2014 Jan 20;428:44–50 [PMID: 24482806].

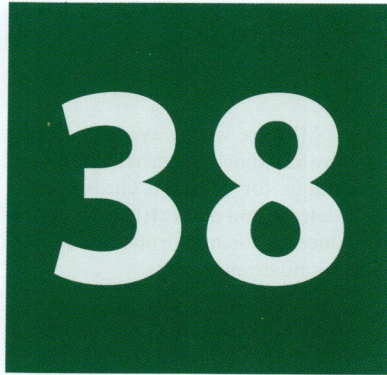

38

Allergic Disorders

Ronina A. Covar, MD

David M. Fleischer, MD

Christine Cho, MD

Mark Boguniewicz, MD

INTRODUCTION

Allergic disorders are among the most common problems seen by pediatricians and primary care physicians, affecting over 25% of the population in developed countries. According to the National Health and Nutrition Examination Survey, 54% of the population had positive test responses to one or more allergens. Data from the National Center for Health Statistics show that the prevalence of food (5.7%) and skin allergies (12%) has increased over the past decade. While the prevalence of respiratory allergies (10.1%) has been stable, it is still the highest among children. In children, asthma, allergic rhinitis, and atopic dermatitis have been accompanied by significant morbidity and school absenteeism, with adverse consequences for school performance and quality of life, as well as economic burden measured in billions of dollars. In this chapter, atopy refers to a genetically determined predisposition to develop IgE antibodies found in patients with asthma, allergic rhinitis, and atopic dermatitis.

ASTHMA

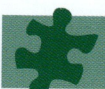

ESSENTIALS OF DIAGNOSIS & TYPICAL FEATURES

► The diagnosis of asthma is based on recurrent episodes of cough, wheezing, dyspnea, or chest tightness, with various triggers, most commonly respiratory infections, exercise, aeroallergens, cold air, and irritants. At least 80% of children with asthma have an allergic predisposition.

► Chronic airway inflammation, variable expiratory airflow limitation, and bronchial reactivity characterize the disease, but presentation is heterogeneous, and course over time, especially in children, is variable as well. The clinical course can be subtle for some children, but the risk of a severe, even life-threatening, asthma-related event is present.

► Assessment of severity can be challenging particularly if comorbidities and adverse effects of chronic disease and medications are present. Hence assessment of control is helpful when treatment changes are being made.

► The mainstay of asthma management involves targeting the inflammatory response and bronchoconstriction, avoidance of known triggers, identification of early warning signs, and creating an appropriate action plan. Regular assessment of response and control is necessary to prevent consequences of either poor disease control or medication side effects.

► Strategies using intermittent ICS with SABA at the onset of a respiratory illness or ICS-formoterol for rescue are now recommended.

► Biologic therapy can be helpful in reducing morbidity in a subgroup of children with asthma.

The Global Strategy for Asthma Management and Prevention (ginasthma.org) report gives a definition of asthma as "a heterogeneous disease, usually characterized by chronic airway inflammation. It is defined by the history of respiratory symptoms such as wheeze, shortness of breath, chest tightness, and cough, that vary over time and in intensity, together with variable expiratory limitation."

Asthma is the most common chronic disease of childhood, affecting 6.2 million children in the United States. While current prevalence rates for asthma have increased in the past decade, there has been an indication of a decrease in prevalence since 2011 (most recent estimate in children < 18 years is 8.4%). At least one-half of persons with current asthma reported having had an asthma attack in the past year. Gender, race, and socioeconomic disparities in the prevalence of asthma exist: (1) more boys than girls are affected in childhood; (2) higher percentage affected among black children compared to Hispanic and non-Hispanic white children; and (3) children belonging to poor families are more likely to be affected.

There is still a disproportionately higher health care utilization for asthma among children compared to adults affected by this disease. Hospitalizations and emergency department or urgent ambulatory or office visits, all indicators of asthma severity, impose significant costs to the health care system and to families, caretakers, schools, and parents' employers. About one-half of children with asthma report one or more asthma-related missed school days. Asthma remains a potentially life-threatening disease for children; among children, the population-based rate of asthma deaths per million was 2.8 in 2009, and the at-risk-based rate of asthma deaths per 10,000 children with asthma was 0.3. Similar to disparities in prevalence, morbidity and mortality rates for asthma are higher among minority and inner-city populations. The reasons for this may be related to a combination of more severe disease, poor access to health care, lack of asthma education, delay in use of appropriate controller therapy, and environmental factors (eg, irritants including smoke and air pollutants, and perennial allergen exposure).

Up to 80% of children with asthma develop symptoms before their fifth birthday. Atopy (personal or familial) is the strongest identifiable predisposing factor. Sensitization to inhalant allergens increases over time and is found in the majority of children with asthma. The principal allergens associated with asthma are perennial aeroallergens such as dust mite, animal dander, cockroach, and *Alternaria* (a soil mold). Rarely, foods may provoke isolated asthma symptoms.

About 40% of infants and young children who have wheezing with viral infections in the first few years of life will have continuing asthma through childhood. Viral infections (eg, respiratory syncytial virus [RSV], rhinovirus, parainfluenza and influenza viruses, metapneumovirus) are associated with wheezing episodes in young children. RSV may be the predominant pathogen of wheezing infants in the emergency room setting, but rhinovirus can be detected in the majority of older wheezing children. It is uncertain if these viruses contribute to the development of chronic asthma, independent of atopy. Severe RSV bronchiolitis in infancy has been linked to asthma and allergy in childhood. Although speculative, individuals with lower airway vulnerability to common respiratory viral pathogens may be at risk for persistent asthma.

Exposure to tobacco smoke is also a risk factor and a trigger for asthma. Other triggers include exercise, cold air, pollutants, strong chemical odors, and rapid changes in barometric pressure. Aspirin sensitivity is uncommon in children. Data suggest that microbiome may also play a role in the development of asthma and allergy. Psychological factors may precipitate asthma exacerbations and place the patient at high risk of the disease.

Pathologic features of asthma include shedding of airway epithelium, edema, mucus plug formation, mast cell activation, and collagen deposition beneath the basement membrane. The inflammatory cell infiltrate includes eosinophils, lymphocytes, and neutrophils, especially in fatal asthma exacerbations. Airway inflammation contributes to bronchial hyperresponsiveness, airflow limitation, and disease chronicity. Persistent airway inflammation can lead to airway wall remodeling and irreversible changes.

▶ **Clinical Findings**

A. Symptoms and Signs

The diagnosis of asthma in children, especially among preschool aged, is based largely on clinical judgment and an assessment of symptoms, activity limitation, and quality of life. For example, if a child with asthma refrains from participating in physical activities so as not to trigger asthma symptoms, their asthma would be inadequately controlled but not detected by the standard questions.

Wheezing is the most characteristic sign of asthma, although some children may have recurrent cough and shortness of breath. Complaints may include chest congestion and/or tightness prolonged cough, exercise intolerance, dyspnea, and recurrent bronchitis or pneumonia. Typically a combination of any of these symptoms is reported. Symptoms are often worse at night or in the early morning, and can vary over time and in severity. The symptoms are rated by viral illnesses/colds, allergens, weather or seasonal changes, cold air, emotions such as laughter or crying, irritants such as smoke, strong scents, or fumes, and exercise. Chest auscultation during forced expiration may reveal prolongation of the expiratory phase and wheezing. As the obstruction becomes more severe, wheezes become more high-pitched and breath sounds diminished. With severe obstruction, wheezes may not be heard because of poor air movement. Flaring of nostrils, intercostal and suprasternal retractions, and use of accessory muscles of respiration are signs of severe obstruction. Cyanosis of the lips and nail beds may be seen with underlying hypoxia. Tachycardia and pulsus paradoxus also occur. Agitation and lethargy may be signs of impending respiratory failure.

B. Laboratory Findings

Variable expiratory airflow limitation, bronchial hyperresponsiveness, and airway inflammation are key features of asthma. Documentation of all these components is not always necessary unless the presentation is rather atypical.

Assessment of airflow limitation in asthma can be done using spirometry, if possible, when the patient is not on treatment. The forced expiratory volume in 1 second (FEV_1) and FEV_1/FVC (forced vital capacity) can be measured and the raw values compared to reference or predicted values. Single measurements, especially if normal, may not be adequate in establishing a diagnosis, but serially they can be an important parameter to monitor asthma activity and treatment response. In children, FEV_1 may be normal, despite frequent symptoms. Spirometric measures of airflow limitation can be associated with symptom severity, likelihood of exacerbation, hospitalization, or respiratory compromise. Regular monitoring of prebronchodilator (and ideally postbronchodilator) FEV_1 can be used to track lung growth patterns over time. During acute asthma exacerbations, FEV_1 is diminished and the flow-volume curve shows a "scooping out" of the distal portion of the expiratory portion of the loop (Figure 38–1).

In addition to the importance placed on documentation of airflow limitation at any time during the diagnostic process, the GINA global strategy puts an emphasis on documenting excessive variability in lung function. This can be gleaned from any of the following:

- Bronchodilator reversibility (measured 10–15 minutes after 200–400 μg albuterol or equivalent): increase in FEV_1 greater than 12% predicted

- Excessive variability in twice-daily peak flow readings over 2 weeks: average daily diurnal PEF variability > 13% ([day's highest PEF minus day's lowest PEF]/mean of day's highest and lowest), averaged over 1 week

- Significant increase in lung function after 4 weeks of anti-inflammatory treatment (FEV_1 > 12% and 200 mL (or PEF > 20%)

- (+) Exercise challenge test: fall in FEV_1 greater than 12% predicted or PEF greater than 15%

- (+) Bronchoprovocation challenge test: fall in FEV_1 from baseline of ≥ 20% with standard doses of methacholine, or ≥ 15% with standardized hyperventilation, hypertonic saline, or mannitol challenge

- Excessive variation in lung function between visits: variation in FEV_1 of 12% or PEF of greater than 15% between visits (may include respiratory infections)

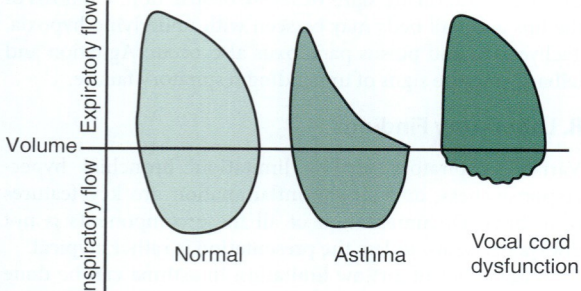

▲ **Figure 38–1.** Representative flow-volume loops in persons with normal lung function, asthma, and inducible laryngeal obstruction.

PEFR monitoring can be a simple and reproducible tool to assess asthma activity in children with moderate or severe asthma, a history of severe exacerbations, or poor perception of airflow limitation or worsening condition. Significant changes in PEFR may occur before symptoms become evident. In more severe cases, PEFR monitoring enables earlier recognition of suboptimal asthma control.

Lung function assessment using body box plethysmography to determine lung volume measurements can also be informative. The residual volume, functional residual capacity, and total lung capacity are usually increased in asthma (and may confer evidence of air trapping or hyperinflation), while the vital capacity is decreased. Reversal or significant improvement of these abnormalities in response to inhaled bronchodilator therapy or with anti-inflammatory therapy can be observed.

Infant pulmonary function can be measured in sedated children with compression techniques. The forced oscillation technique can be used to measure peripheral airway resistance even in younger children.

Bronchial hyperresponsiveness to various stimuli is a hallmark of asthma. These stimuli include inhaled pharmacologic agents such as histamine, methacholine, and mannitol, as well as physical stimuli such as exercise and cold air. Mannitol (Aridol) bronchoprovocation has been approved by the U.S. Food and Drug Administration (FDA) and is simpler and easier to administer in the office. It is available as a dry powder inhalation kit and takes less time to complete. Unlike methacholine and histamine challenges and similar to exercise challenge, it is considered an indirect challenge; that is, it simulates airway responses to specific physiologic situations, by creating an osmotic effect within the airway that subsequently leads to an inflammatory response. Airways may exhibit hyperresponsiveness or twitchiness even when baseline pulmonary function tests are normal. Giving increasing concentrations of a bronchoconstrictive agent to induce a decrease in lung function (usually a 20% drop in forced expiratory volume in 1 second [FEV_1] for histamine and methacholine and a 15% reduction for mannitol) and doing an exercise challenge are ways to determine airway responsiveness. Hyperresponsiveness in normal children younger than 5 years is greater than in older children. Bronchoprovocation challenges are not always available in a clinical setting, but they help to establish a diagnosis of asthma when the history, examination, and pulmonary function tests are not definitive.

Hypoxemia is present early with a normal or low Pco_2 level and respiratory alkalosis. Hypoxemia may be aggravated during treatment with a β_2-agonist due to ventilation-perfusion mismatch. Oxygen saturation less than 91% is indicative of significant obstruction. Respiratory acidosis and increasing CO_2 tension may ensue with further airflow obstruction and signal impending respiratory failure. Hypercapnia is usually not seen until the FEV_1 falls below 20% of predicted value.

Metabolic acidosis has also been noted in combination with respiratory acidosis in children with severe asthma and indicates imminent respiratory failure. Pao_2 less than 60 mm Hg despite oxygen therapy and $Paco_2$ over 60 mm Hg and rising more than 5 mm Hg/h are relative indications for mechanical ventilation in a child in status asthmaticus.

Pulsus paradoxus may be present with moderate or severe asthma exacerbation. In moderate asthma exacerbation in a child, this may be between 10 and 25 mm Hg, and in severe asthma exacerbation between 20 and 40 mm Hg. Absence of pulsus paradoxus in a child with severe asthma exacerbation may signal respiratory muscle fatigue.

Clumps of eosinophils on sputum smear and blood eosinophilia are findings in a subset of children with asthma. Their presence tends to reflect a specific phenotype and does not necessarily mean that allergic factors are involved. Leukocytosis is common in acute severe asthma without evidence of bacterial infection and may be more pronounced after epinephrine administration. Hematocrit can be elevated with dehydration during prolonged exacerbations or in severe chronic disease. Noninvasive measures of airway inflammation include exhaled nitric oxide concentrations, serum eosinophil cationic protein levels, serum total (and specific) IgE, and induced sputum. The National Asthma Education and Prevention Program: Expert Panel Report's (NAEPP EPR) recently released focused updates to the asthma management guidelines recommended fractional exhaled nitric oxide testing as an adjunct in the evaluation process to diagnose asthma when the diagnosis is uncertain using history, physical examination and other testing (eg, spirometry with bronchodilator). In addition, exhaled nitric oxide testing may be used as part of ongoing asthma monitoring and management strategy for patients with persistent allergic asthma when there is uncertainty in choosing, monitoring, or adjusting therapy using clinical assessment. It should not be used alone to assess asthma control, predict future exacerbations, assess asthma exacerbation severity, or predict the future development of asthma in preschool children.

C. Imaging

Evaluation of asthma usually does not need chest radiographs (posteroanterior and lateral views) since they often appear normal, although subtle and nonspecific findings of hyperinflation (flattening of the diaphragm), peribronchial thickening, prominence of the pulmonary arteries, and areas of patchy atelectasis may be present. Atelectasis may be misinterpreted as infiltrates of pneumonia. Some lung abnormalities, such as bronchiectasis, mosaic attenuation, tree in bud, or ground-glass opacities, which may point to a different diagnosis implicating an asthma masquerader, such as cystic fibrosis, allergic bronchopulmonary mycoses (aspergillosis), ciliary dyskinesias, immune deficiencies, constrictive bronchiolitis, hypersensitivity pneumonitis, or even aspiration, can be better appreciated with high-resolution computed tomography scans. It is primarily useful clinically in ruling out certain diagnoses in patients with difficult to manage asthma but radiation exposure should be considered when ordering HRCT, especially done serially. However, algorithms used in newer scanners allow for much reduced radiation exposure.

Allergy testing is discussed in section General Measures under Treatment, Chronic Asthma.

▶ Differential Diagnosis

Diseases that may be mistaken for asthma are often related to the patient's age (Table 38–1). Congenital abnormalities must be excluded in infants and young children. Asthma can be confused with croup, acute bronchiolitis, pneumonia, and pertussis. Immunodeficiency may be associated with cough and wheezing. Foreign bodies in the airway may cause dyspnea or wheezing of sudden onset, and on auscultation, wheezing may be unilateral. Asymmetry of the lungs secondary to air trapping may be seen on a chest radiograph, especially with forced expiration. Cystic fibrosis can be associated with or mistaken for asthma.

Inducible laryngeal obstruction (previously recognized as vocal cord dysfunction) is an important masquerader of asthma, although the two can coexist. It is characterized by the paradoxical closure of the vocal cords that can result in difficulty breathing commonly on inspiration, throat tightness, and even wheezing. In normal individuals, the vocal cords abduct during inspiration and may adduct slightly during expiration. Asthmatic patients may have narrowing of the glottis during expiration as a physiologic adaptation to airway obstruction. In contrast, patients with isolated inducible laryngeal obstruction typically show adduction of the anterior two-thirds of their vocal cords during inspiration, with a small diamond-shaped aperture posteriorly. Because this abnormal vocal cord pattern may be intermittently present, a normal examination does not exclude the diagnosis.

Table 38–1. Differential diagnosis of asthma in infants and children.

Viral bronchiolitis
Aspiration
Laryngotracheomalacia
Vascular rings
Airway stenosis or web
Enlarged lymph nodes
Mediastinal mass
Foreign body
Bronchopulmonary dysplasia
Obliterative bronchiolitis
Cystic fibrosis
Vocal cord dysfunction/Inducible laryngeal obstruction
Cardiovascular disease

Bronchial challenges preferably exercise can precipitate symptoms of inducible laryngeal obstruction. The flow-volume loop may provide additional clues to the diagnosis of inducible laryngeal obstruction. Truncation of the inspiratory portion can be demonstrated in most patients during an acute episode, and some patients continue to show this pattern even when they are asymptomatic (see Figure 38–1). Children and adolescents with inducible laryngeal obstruction tend to be overly competitive, primarily in athletics and scholastics. Treatment of isolated inducible laryngeal obstruction includes education regarding the condition, appropriate breathing exercises, and therapeutic continuous laryngoscopy. Biofeedback, psychotherapy, and even hypnosis have been effective for some patients.

▶ Conditions That May Increase Asthma Severity

Chronic hyperplastic sinusitis is frequently found in association with asthma. Upper airway inflammation has been shown to contribute to the pathogenesis of asthma, and asthma may improve after treatment of sinusitis. However, sinus surgery is usually not indicated for initial treatment of chronic mucosal disease associated with allergy. In older children, rarely, hyperplastic sinusitis and polyposis and severe refractory asthma can be associated with aspirin sensitivity, known as aspirin-exacerbated respiratory disease (AERD).

A significant correlation has been observed between nocturnal asthma and gastroesophageal reflux. Patients may not complain of burning epigastric pain or have other reflux symptoms—cough may be the only sign. For patients with poorly controlled asthma, particularly with a nocturnal component, investigation for gastroesophageal reflux may be warranted even in the absence of suggestive symptoms.

Population studies have demonstrated associations between obesity and asthma. Obesity has been linked not only to the development of asthma but also with asthma control and severity. What contributes to these associations or to what extent inflammation or physiologic impairment relates to both obesity and asthma is less established. It becomes difficult to determine if a child's trouble breathing is a result of obesity itself, its comorbidities (eg, gastroesophageal reflux or obstructive sleep apnea), and/or asthma. A management approach targeting weight reduction in obese children is encouraged to improve asthma control or its assessment.

The risk factors for death from asthma include psychological and sociologic factors. They are probably related to the consequences of illness denial, poor coping or self-management skills, as well as to nonadherence with prescribed therapy. Recent studies have shown that less than 50% of inhaled asthma medications are taken as prescribed and that compliance does not improve with increasing severity of illness. Moreover, children requiring hospitalization for asthma, or their caregivers, have often failed to institute appropriate home treatment.

▶ Complications

With acute asthma, complications are primarily related to hypoxemia and acidosis and can include generalized seizures. Pneumomediastinum or pneumothorax can be a complication in status asthmaticus. With chronic asthma, recent studies point to airway wall remodeling and loss of pulmonary function with persistent airway inflammation. Childhood asthma independent of any corticosteroid therapy has been shown to be associated with delayed maturation and slowing of prepubertal growth velocity.

▶ Treatment

A. Chronic Asthma

1. General measures—The NAEPP EPR and the GINA global strategy offer different management approaches. The NAEPP EPR released its focused updates to the asthma management guidelines in December 2020. Recommendations were based on Grading of Recommendations Assessment, Development and Evaluation (GRADE) approach which determined direction of recommendation and strength based on certainty of evidence, with review of relevant studies available by October 2018. There were six topic areas identified in 2015 after a needs assessment process from solicitation of public comments and these are covered in the updates: intermittent use of inhaled corticosteroids, use of long-acting muscarinic antagonists (LAMAs), fractional exhaled nitric oxide testing, indoor allergen mitigation, aeroallergen immunotherapy, and bronchial thermoplasty. Classification of asthma severity and control is still adopted from the NAEPP EPR 3 report (Tables 38–2 and 38–3), but the treatment table has been updated (Table 38–4).

GINA is updated about every 1–2 years based on new studies, with the most recent one from 2023. Their strategy is intended for broader application to an international base. Both guideline approaches include an assessment and regular monitoring of disease activity, education, and partnership to improve the child's and his/her family's knowledge and skills for self-management, identification, and management of triggers and conditions that may worsen asthma, and appropriate medications selected to address the patient's needs. The objective of asthma management is to attain the best possible symptom control and minimize risk of exacerbations, persistent airflow limitation, side effects of treatment, and asthma-related morbidity/mortality.

2. Assessment of severity and control—The NAEPP EPR3 stepwise approach is based on an assessment of severity and control. An assessment of asthma severity (ie, the intrinsic intensity of disease) is generally most accurate in patients not receiving controller therapy. Hence, assessing asthma severity directs the level of initial therapy. For those already on treatment, asthma severity can be classified according to the level of medication requirement to maintain adequate

Table 38–2. Assessing severity and initiating treatment for patients who are not currently taking long-term control medications.

Components of Severity		Intermittent	Classification of Asthma Severity		
			Persistent		
			Mild	**Moderate**	**Severe**
Impairment	Daytime symptoms	≤ 2 days/wk	> 2 days/wk but not daily	Daily	Throughout the day
	Nighttime awakenings				
	Age 0–4 y	0	1–2 ×/mo	3–4 ×/mo	> 1 ×/wk
	Age ≥ 5 y	≤ 2 ×/mo	3–4 ×/mo	> 1 ×/wk but not nightly	Often 7 ×/wk
	SABA use for symptoms (not prevention of EIB)	≤ 2 days/wk	> 2 days/wk but not daily, and not more than 1 × on any day	Daily	Several times per day
	Interference with normal activity	None	Minor limitation	Some limitation	Extremely limited
	Lung function	Normal FEV$_1$ between exacerbations			
	FEV$_1$% predicted				
	Age ≥ 5 y	> 80% predicted	≥ 80% predicted	60%–80% predicted	< 60% predicted
Normal FEV$_1$/FVC:	FEV$_1$/FVC ratio				
8 –19 y: 85	Age 5–11 y	> 85%	> 80%	75%–80%	< 75%
20–39 y: 80	Age ≥ 12 y	Normal	Normal	Reduced 5%	Reduced > 5%
Risk	Exacerbations requiring systemic corticosteroids				
	Age 0–4 y	0–1/y (see *Notes*)	≥ 2 exacerbations in 6 mo requiring systemic corticosteroids OR ≥ 4 wheezing episodes/year lasting > 1 day and risk factors for persistent asthma		
	Age ≥ 5 y	0–1/y (see *Notes*)	≥ 2/y (see *Notes*)		
		Consider severity and interval since last exacerbation. Frequency and severity may fluctuate over time for patients in any severity category. Relative annual risk of exacerbations may be related to FEV$_1$.			
Recommended step for initiating therapy		Step 1	Step 2	Age 0–4 y	
				Step 3	Step 3
				Age 5–11 y	
				Step 3, medium-dose ICS option	Step 3, medium-dose ICS option, OR step 4
				Age ≥ 12 y	
				Step 3	Step 4 or 5
				Consider a short course of systemic corticosteroids	
		In 2–6 wk, evaluate level of asthma control that is achieved and adjust therapy accordingly. If no clear benefit is observed within 4–6 wk, consider adjusting therapy or alternative diagnoses.			

EIB, exercise-induced bronchospasm; FEV1, forced expiratory volume in 1 second; FVC, forced vital capacity; ICS, inhaled corticosteroids; SABA, short-acting β2-agonist.

Notes:
- The stepwise approach is meant to assist, not replace, the clinical decision-making required to meet individual patient needs.
- Level of severity is determined by both impairment and risk. Assess impairment domain by patient's/caregiver's recall of previous 2–4 weeks. Symptom assessment for longer periods should reflect a global assessment such as inquiring whether a patient's asthma is better or worse since the last visit. Assign severity to the most severe category in which any feature occurs.
- At present, there are inadequate data to correspond frequencies of exacerbations with different levels of asthma severity. For treatment purposes, patients who had ≥ 2 exacerbations requiring oral systemic corticosteroids in the past 6 months, or ≥ 4 wheezing episodes in the past year, and who have risk factors for persistent asthma may be considered the same as patients who have persistent asthma, even in the absence of impairment levels consistent with persistent asthma.

Reproduced with permission from National Asthma Education and Prevention Program: Expert panel report 3 (EPR-3): guidelines for the diagnosis and management of asthma-summary report 2007. J Allergy Clin Immunol 2007; 120(5):S94–S138.

asthma control. The two general categories are intermittent and persistent asthma; the latter is further subdivided into mild, moderate, and severe (Table 38–2). In contrast, asthma control refers to the degree to which symptoms, ongoing functional impairments, and risk of adverse events are minimized and goals of therapy are met. Assessment of asthma control should be done at every visit as this is important in adjusting therapy. It is categorized as "well controlled," "not well controlled," and "very poorly controlled" (Table 38–3). Responsiveness to therapy is the ease with which asthma control is attained by treatment. It can also encompass monitoring for adverse effects related to medication use.

The NAEPP EPR3 classification of either asthma severity or control is based on the domains of current *impairment* and *risk*, recognizing that these domains may respond

Table 38–3. Assessing asthma control and adjusting therapy in children.

Components of Control		Classification of Asthma Control		
		Well Controlled	**Not Well Controlled**	**Very Poorly Controlled**
Impairment	Symptoms	≤ 2 days/wk but not more than once on each day	> 2 days/wk or multiple times on ≤ 2 days/wk	Throughout the day
	Nighttime awakenings			
	Age 0–4 y	≤ 1 × /mo	> 1 × /mo	> 1 × /wk
	Age 5–11 y	≤ 1 × /mo	≥ 2 × /mo	≥ 2 × /wk
	Age ≥ 12 y	≤ 2 × /mo	1–3 × /wk	≥ 4 × /wk
	SABA use for symptoms (not EIB pretreatment)	≤ 2 days/wk	> 2 days/wk	Several times per day
	Interference with normal activity	None	Some limitation	Extremely limited
	Lung function			
	Age 5–11 y			
	FEV$_1$% predicted or peak flow	> 80% predicted or personal best	60%–80% predicted or personal best	< 60% predicted or personal best
	FEV$_1$/FVC	> 80%	75%–80%	< 75%
	Age ≥ 12 y			
	FEV$_1$% predicted or peak flow	> 80% predicted or personal best	60%–80% predicted or personal best	< 60% predicted or personal best
	Validated questionnaires			
	Age ≥ 12 y			
	ATAQ	0	1–2	3–4
	ACQ	≤ 0.75[a]	≥ 1.5	N/A
	ACT	≥ 20	16–19	≤ 15
Risk	Exacerbations requiring systemic corticosteroids			
	Age 0–4 y	0–1 y	2–3/y	> 3/y
	Age ≥ 5 y	0–1 y	≥ 2/y (see *Notes*)	
	Consider severity and interval since last exacerbation.			
	Treatment-related adverse effects.	Medication side effects can vary in intensity from none to very troublesome and worrisome. The level of intensity does not correlate to specific levels of control but should be considered in the overall assessment of risk.		
	Reduction in lung growth or progressive loss of lung function.	Evaluation requires long-term follow-up care.		

(Continued)

Table 38–3. Assessing asthma control and adjusting therapy in children. (*Continued*)

Components of Control	Classification of Asthma Control		
	Well Controlled	**Not Well Controlled**	**Very Poorly Controlled**
Recommended action for treatment.	• Maintain current step. • Regular follow-up every 1–6 mo to maintain control. • Consider step-down if well controlled for at least 3 mo.	• Step up (1 step). • Reevaluate in 2–6 wk. • If no clear benefit in 4–6 wk, consider alternative diagnoses or adjusting therapy. • For side effects, consider alternative options.	• Consider short course of oral corticosteroids. • Step up (1–2 steps). • Reevaluate in 2 wk. • If no clear benefit in 4–6 wk, consider alternative diagnoses or adjusting therapy. • For side effects, consider alternative options.

EIB, exercise-induced bronchospasm; FEV1, forced expiratory volume in 1 second; FVC, forced vital capacity; SABA, short-acting β2-agonist.
Notes:

- The stepwise approach is meant to assist, not replace, the clinical decision-making required to meet individual patient needs.
- The level of control is based on the most severe impairment or risk category. Assess impairment domain by caregiver's recall of previous 2–4 weeks. Symptom assessment for longer periods should reflect a global assessment such as inquiring whether the patient's asthma is better or worse since the last visit.
- At present, there are inadequate data to correspond frequencies of exacerbations with different levels of asthma control. In general, more frequent and intense exacerbations (eg, requiring urgent, unscheduled care, hospitalization, or ICU admission) indicate poorer disease control. For treatment purposes, patients who had ≥ 2 exacerbations requiring oral systemic corticosteroids in the past year may be considered the same as patients who have not–well-controlled asthma, even in the absence of impairment levels consistent with not–well-controlled asthma.
- Validated questionnaires for the impairment domain (the questionnaires do not assess lung function or the risk domain):
  a. ATAQ = Asthma Therapy Assessment Questionnaire
  b. ACQ = Asthma Control Questionnaire
  c. ACT = Asthma Control Test
  d. Minimal Important Difference: 1.0 for ATAQ; 0.5 for the ACQ; not determined for ACT; ªACQ values of 0.76–1.40 are indeterminate regarding well-controlled asthma.
- Before step-up therapy:
  a. Review adherence to medications, inhaler technique, and environmental control.
  b. If alternative treatment option was used in a step, discontinue it and use preferred treatment for that step.

Reproduced with permission from National Asthma Education and Prevention Program: Expert panel report 3 (EPR-3): guidelines for the diagnosis and management of asthma-summary report 2007. J Allergy Clin Immunol 2007; 120(5):S94–S138.

differently to treatment. The level of asthma severity or control is established on the most severe component of impairment or risk. Generally, the assessment of impairment is symptom based, except for the use of lung function for school-aged children and youths. Impairment includes an assessment of the patient's recent symptom frequency and intensity and functional limitations (ie, daytime symptoms, nighttime awakenings, need for short-acting β$_2$-agonists [SABA] for quick relief, work or school days missed, ability to engage in normal or desired activities, and quality-of-life assessments) and airflow compromise preferably using spirometry. Numerous validated instruments and questionnaires for assessing health-related quality of life and asthma control have been developed. The Asthma Control Test (ACT, www.asthmacontrol.com), the Asthma Control Questionnaire (ACQ, www.qoltech.co.uk/Asthma1.htm), and the Asthma Therapy Assessment Questionnaire (ATAQ, www.ataqinstrument.com) for children 12 years of age and older and the Childhood ACT for children 4–11 years of age are examples of self-administered questionnaires that have been developed with the objective of addressing multiple aspects of asthma control such as frequency of daytime and nocturnal symptoms, use of reliever medications, functional status, and missed school or work. A five-item caregiver-administered instrument, the Test for Respiratory and Asthma Control in Kids (TRACK), has been validated as a tool to assess both impairment and risk presented in the NAEPP Expert Panel Report 3 (EPR3) guidelines in young children with recurrent wheezing or respiratory symptoms consistent with asthma.

Table 38–4. Stepwise approach for managing asthma in children and adolescents.

		STEP 1	STEP 2	STEP 3	STEP 4	STEP 5	STEP 6
Age 0–4 years	**PREFERRED**	PRN SABA and at the start of RTI: Add short course daily ICS*	Daily low-dose ICS and PRN SABA	Daily low-dose ICS-LABA and PRN SABA* or daily low-dose ICS + montelukast,* or daily medium-dose ICS, and PRN SABA	Daily medium-dose ICS-LABA and PRN SABA	Daily high-dose ICS-LABA and PRN SABA	Daily high-dose ICS-LABA + oral systemic corticosteroid and PRN SABA
	ALTERNATIVE		Daily montelukast* or Cromolyn,* and PRN SABA		Daily medium-dose ICS + montelukast* and PRN SABA	Daily high-dose ICS + montelukast* and PRN SABA	Daily high-dose ICS + montelukast* + oral systemic corticosteroid and PRN SABA
Age 5–11 years	**PREFERRED**	PRN SABA	Daily low-dose ICS and PRN SABA	Daily and PRN combination low-dose ICS-formoterol (SMART)	Daily and PRN combination medium-dose ICS-formoterol (SMART)	Daily high-dose ICS-LABA and PRN SABA	Daily high-dose ICS-LABA + oral systemic corticosteroid and PRN SABA
	ALTERNATIVE		Daily LTRA, or Cromolyn, or Nedocromil, or Theophylline,* and PRN SABA	Daily medium-dose ICS and PRN SABA or daily low-dose ICS-LABA, or daily low-dose ICS + LTRA,* or daily low-dose ICS +Theophylline,* and PRN SABA	Daily medium-dose ICS-LABA and PRN SABA or daily medium dose ICS + LTRA or daily medium-dose ICS + Theophylline,* and PRN SABA	Daily high-dose ICS + LTRA or daily high-dose ICS + Theophylline,* and PRN SABA	Daily high-dose ICS + LTRA + oral systemic corticosteroid or daily high-dose ICS + Theophylline* + oral systemic corticosteroid, and PRN SABA

Steps 2–4: Conditionally recommend the use of subcutaneous immunotherapy as an adjunct treatment to standard pharmacotherapy   Consider Omalizumab**

		STEP 1	STEP 2	STEP 3	STEP 4	STEP 5	STEP 6
Age ≥12 years	**PREFERRED**	PRN SABA	Daily low-dose ICS and PRN SABA or PRN concomitant ICS and SABA	Daily and PRN combination low-dose ICS-formoterol (SMART)	Daily and PRN combination medium-dose ICS-formoterol (SMART)	Daily medium-high-dose ICS-LABA + LAMA and PRN SABA	Daily high-dose ICS-LABA + oral systemic corticosteroids + PRN SABA
	ALTERNATIVE		Daily LTRA* and PRN SABA or Cromolyn, or Nedocromil, or Zileuton, or Theophylline,* and PRN SABA	Daily medium-dose ICS and PRN SABA or daily low-dose ICS LABA, or daily low-dose ICS + LAMA, or daily low-dose ICS + LTRA,* and PRN SABA or daily low-dose ICS + Theophylline* or Zileuton,* and PRN SABA	Daily medium-dose ICS-LABA or daily medium-dose ICS + LAMA, and PRN SABA or daily medium-dose ICS + LTRA,* or daily-medium-dose ICS + Theophylline,* or daily medium-dose ICS + Zileuton,* and PRN SABA	Daily medium-high-dose ICS-LABA or daily high-dose ICS + LTRA,* and PRN SABA	

*ICS, inhaled corticosteroids; LABA, long-acting β2-agonist; LAMA, long-acting muscarinic antagonist; LTRA, leukotriene-receptor antagonist; OCS: oral corticosteroids; SABA: short-acting β2-agonist.

In contrast to the NAEPP severity assessment based on clinical features present without controller therapy, GINA proposes a retrospective severity assessment, after at least 2 to 3 months of treatment required to control symptoms and exacerbations. This definition is suggested to be clinically useful for severe asthma to identify patients whose asthma is relatively refractory to conventional treatment with high-dose inhaled corticosteroid (ICS) and long-acting beta-agonist (LABA), who may benefit from additional treatment such as biologic therapy. Severe asthma should be distinguished from difficult-to-treat asthma stemming from inadequate or inappropriate treatment, or persistent problems with adherence, or comorbidities. Moderate asthma is controlled with Step 3 or Step 4 treatment, that is, with low- or medium-dose ICS–LABA. Mild asthma is asthma that is well controlled with low-intensity treatment, that is, as needed low-dose ICS–formoterol, or low-dose ICS plus as needed SABA. At the outset, GINA uses an assessment primarily based on presenting symptoms and risk for adverse outcomes (exacerbations, persistent airflow limitation, and long-term medication side effects) on which initial treatment recommendation options are proposed (2023 GINA Main Report, Global Initiative for Asthma. https://www.mhprofessional.com/gina). It emphasizes personalized asthma management by a continual cycle of *assessment, adjustment of treatment, and review.* Assessment includes confirmation of asthma diagnosis, if necessary; symptom control and modifiable factors, including lung function; comorbidities; inhaler technique and adherence; and patient/parent preferences and goals. Adjusting the patient's management including medications (down/up/between tracks), treatment of modifiable risk factors and comorbidities, using nonpharmacologic strategies, and education and skills training. Reviewing the parent/patient goals of treatment and satisfaction, factors affecting symptoms, risk of adverse outcomes, symptoms, exacerbations and side effects, arranging additional investigations, and readjusting treatment if warranted.

3. Risk assessment—"Risk" refers to an evaluation of the patient's likelihood of developing asthma exacerbations, reduced lung growth in children (or progressive decline in lung function in adults), or risk of untoward effects from medications. The GINA strategy also cites risk factors for the following poor asthma outcomes: exacerbations, persistent airflow limitation, and medication side effects). A major risk factor for exacerbations having uncontrolled asthma symptoms. In those with infrequent symptoms, the following are also considered potentially modifiable risk factors for flare-ups: excessive SABA use at least three 200-dose canister/year); inadequate inhaled corticosteroid (ICS) (from lack of prescription, poor adherence, or incorrect inhaler technique); low FEV_1, especially if less than 60% predicted or high bronchodilator reversibility; major psychological or socioeconomic problems; presence of smoking or allergen exposure

(if sensitized); having comorbidities (obesity, rhinosinusitis, confirmed food allergy); and presence of Type 2 inflammatory markers (blood eosinophilia or elevated exhaled nitric oxide). Considered major independent risk factors for flare-ups are history of intubation or ICU admission for asthma and one or more severe exacerbations in the last 12 months. Risk factors of asthma-related death include a history of near-fatal asthma requiring intubation and mechanical ventilation; hospitalization or emergency room visit for asthma in the past year; currently using or having recently stopped using oral corticosteroids; no current use of an inhaled corticosteroid; overuse of SABAs (especially use of > 1 canister of albuterol monthly); poor adherence with ICS–containing medications and/or poor adherence with (or lack of) written asthma action plan; history of psychiatric disease or psychosocial problems; food allergy in a patient with asthma; and presence of comorbidities such as pneumonia, diabetes, and arrhythmias (independently associated with an increased risk of death after hospitalization for an asthma exacerbation).

Risk factors for developing persistent airflow limitation are preterm birth (or low birth weight and greater infant weight gain), lack of ICS treatment; exposures to tobacco smoke, noxious chemicals, occupational exposures; low initial FEV_1; chronic mucus hypersecretion, and sputum or blood eosinophilia.

Frequent oral corticosteroid use, long-term high-dose and/or potent ICS, and intake of P450 inhibitors are risk factors for systemic medication side effects, while high-dose or potent ICS and poor inhaler technique are also risk factors for local side effects.

4. Education—Education is important and partnership with the child's family is a key component in the management to improve adherence and outcomes. The patient and family must understand the role of asthma triggers, the importance of disease activity even without obvious symptoms, how to use objective measures to gauge disease activity, and the importance of airway inflammation—and they must learn to recognize the warning signs of worsening asthma, allowing for early intervention. A stepwise care plan should be developed for all patients with asthma. Providing asthma action plans is currently a requirement that is tracked by many hospitals and others to document that educational instruction for chronic disease management has been given. Asthma action plans should be provided to school personnel and all those who care for children with asthma.

Because the degree of airflow limitation is poorly perceived by many patients, peak flow meters can aid in the assessment of airflow obstruction and day-to-day disease activity if used correctly and regularly, peak flow rates may provide early warning of worsening asthma. They are also helpful in monitoring the effects of medication changes. Spacer devices optimize delivery of medication from metered-dose inhalers (MDIs) to the lungs and, with inhaled steroids, minimize side effects. Large-volume spacers are preferred. Poor understanding by patients and families of proper device use can lead to inadequate delivery and treatment with inhaled medications, especially inhaled controllers. Short instructive videos for device use can be provided to educate families and other caregivers

https://www.childrenscolorado.org/conditions-and-advice/
conditions-and-symptoms/conditions/asthma/
https://www.nationaljewish.org/conditions/multimedia/
devices-to-inhale-medication.

5. Exposures—Patients should avoid exposure to tobacco smoke and allergens to which they are sensitized, exertion outdoors when levels of air pollution are high, β-blockers, and sulfite-containing foods. Patients with persistent asthma should be given the inactivated influenza vaccine yearly unless they have a contraindication.

For patients with persistent asthma, the clinician should use the patient's history to assess sensitivity to seasonal allergens and *Alternaria* mold and in vitro testing (either by skin or blood test) to assess sensitivity to perennial indoor allergens, to assess the significance of positive tests in the context of the patient's history, and to identify relevant allergen exposures. According to the asthma guidelines, indoor allergen mitigation strategies are to be implemented only in individuals with a history of exposure AND either sensitization OR symptoms upon exposure. For those with asthma who are exposed and allergic to a specific indoor aeroallergen using multiple strategies to reduce the allergen is recommended—using only one strategy often does not improve asthma outcomes.

For dust mite–allergic children, using allergen-impermeable pillow/mattress covers is recommended only as part of multicomponent intervention which should also include washing the sheets and blankets on the patient's bed weekly in hot water, keeping indoor humidity below 50%, minimizing the number of stuffed toys, and washing such toys weekly in hot water. Children allergic to furred animals or feathers should avoid indoor exposure to pets, especially for prolonged periods of time. If removal of the pet is not possible, the animal should be kept out of the bedroom with the door closed. Carpeting and upholstered furniture should be removed. While a high-efficiency particle-arresting filter unit in the bedroom may reduce allergen levels, symptoms may persist if the pet remains indoors. The NAEPP 2020 also highlights that integrated pest management in the home is recommended for individuals with asthma who have symptoms related to exposure to pests (cockroaches and rodents) and are allergic. For cockroach-allergic children, control measures need to be instituted when infestation is present in the home. Poison baits, boric acid, and traps are preferred to chemical agents, which can be irritating if inhaled by asthmatic

individuals. Indoor molds are especially prominent in humid or damp environments. Measures to control dampness or fungal growth in the home may be of benefit. Patients can reduce exposure to outdoor allergens by staying in an air-conditioned environment. Allergen immunotherapy may be useful for implicated aeroallergens that cannot be avoided. However, it should be administered only in facilities staffed and equipped to treat life-threatening reactions.

Patients should be treated for rhinitis, sinusitis, or gastroesophageal reflux if present. Treatment of upper respiratory tract symptoms is an integral part of asthma management. Intranasal corticosteroids are recommended to treat chronic rhinosinusitis in patients with persistent asthma because they reduce lower airway hyperresponsiveness and asthma symptoms. Intranasal cromolyn reduces asthma symptoms during the ragweed season but less so than intranasal corticosteroids. Treatment of rhinosinusitis includes medical measures to promote drainage and the use of antibiotics for acute bacterial infections (see Chapter 18). Medical management of gastroesophageal reflux includes avoiding eating or drinking 2 hours before bedtime, elevating the head of the bed with 6- to 8-in blocks, and using appropriate pharmacologic therapy.

6. Pharmacologic therapy—A revised stepwise approach to pharmacologic therapy, broken down by age categories, is recommended in the NAEPP EPR Focused Updates to the Asthma Management Guidelines (Table 38–4).

The choice of initial therapy is based on assessment of asthma severity. For patients who are already on controller therapy, treatment can be adjusted based on assessment of asthma control and responsiveness to therapy. The goals of therapy are to reduce the components of both impairment (eg, preventing chronic and troublesome symptoms, allowing infrequent need of quick-relief medications, maintaining "normal" lung function, maintaining normal activity levels including physical activity and school attendance, meeting families' expectations and satisfaction with asthma care) and risk (eg, preventing recurrent exacerbations, reduced lung growth, and medication adverse effects).

1. NAEPP 2020 Step 1 has *as needed* SABA as the preferred recommendation. For 0–4-year-old children, a short course of high-dose daily inhaled ICS with albuterol can be prescribed at the start of a respiratory tract illness.

2. NAEPP 2020 Step 2 therapy prefers daily low-dose ICS and as needed SABA. For adolescents and adults, *as needed* ICS and SABA is also a preferred option.

3. NAEPP 2020 Step 3 therapy is low-dose ICS-formoterol combination as a Single Maintenance And Reliever Therapy (low-dose SMART) for older children and adolescents. For younger children, daily *low-dose* ICS-LABA maintenance, or low-dose ICS and montelukast, or daily *medium*-dose ICS are preferred treatments.

4. NAEPP 2020 Step 4 therapy for older children and adolescents includes *medium*-dose ICS-formoterol as maintenance and reliever therapy (medium-dose SMART). For younger children recommended treatment is daily *medium*-dose ICS-LABA and as needed SABA.

5. NAEPP 2020 Step 5 therapy is daily high-dose ICS/LABA (and for adolescents, tiotropium can be added to medium- to high-dose ICS/LABA) and as needed SABA.

6. NAEPP 2020 Step 6 therapy is daily high-dose ICS/LABA plus oral systemic corticosteroid and as needed SABA.

7. Biologic therapy can be considered for NAEPP Steps 5 and 6 for children at least 6 years of age who meet therapy-specific criteria which are discussed in a later section.

The goals of asthma management are to achieve good symptom control, and to minimize future risk of asthma-related mortality, exacerbations, persistent airflow limitation, and side effects of treatment. The patient/parents' own goals should also be addressed. GINA 2023 offers five-step therapy options for children 6 years and older, and four-step options for younger children (0–5 years old), using different symptom assessment tools for these age groups. It does not distinguish between certain asthma severity groups recognized in the NAEPP guidelines, as the risk of adverse outcomes especially serious exacerbations occurs in any of the severity categories. Unfortunately, there is no consistent pattern of escalation in treatment across age groups and even across steps within an age group, which makes it challenging to tackle. The stepwise approach is meant to assist, not replace, the clinical decision-making required to meet individual patient needs. There are safety concerns raised with regular or frequent use of SABA related to occurrence of serious clinical outcomes such as severe exacerbations and even death. In addition, regular use of SABA even for 1–2 weeks is associated with decreased bronchoprotection, beta receptor downregulation, rebound hyperresponsiveness, decreased bronchodilator response, increased allergic response, and increased eosinophilic airway inflammation. ICS, on the other hand, reduces the risk of asthma deaths, hospitalization, and exacerbations; but adherence to daily ICS therapy especially in patients with infrequent symptoms is suboptimal. Because of this, GINA no longer recommends SABA-only treatment for step 1 in adolescents and adults.

For adolescents with asthma, there are two "tracks" specified in this stepwise approach for adolescents and adults based on **reliever therapy, and for whom M**aintenance **A**nd **R**eliever **T**herapy (**MART**) can be implemented (2023 GINA Main Report, Global Initiative for Asthma. https://www.mhprofessional.com/gina). Track 1 (preferred) using *as needed* low-dose ICS/formoterol and Track 2 (alternative) using *as needed* SABA or as needed ICS-SABA. Using Track 1, if they have infrequent symptoms (less than 4–5 days a week) and no risk factors for exacerbation, Track 1 recommends *as needed* low-dose ICS-formoterol (considered Steps 1 and 2). If they have symptoms most days, or waking once a week or more due to asthma, they are recommended to

be Step 3 which is low-dose maintenance and reliever ICS-formoterol (MART). If they have daily symptoms, or waking with asthma once at least once a week, and with low lung function, initial recommendation for Step 4 is medium-dose MART. A short course of oral corticosteroids may also be needed. Step 5 includes adding a LAMA; considering high-dose ICS-formoterol, and referring for phenotypic assessment ± biologic therapy.

Track 2 (now considered an alternative approach for adolescents and adults) uses as needed SABA or as needed ICS-SABA (dual or single inhalers) for reliever. Step 1 therapy is for adolescents with symptoms less than twice a month, recommendation is taking ICS whenever SABA is taken for rescue. If they have symptoms twice a month but less than 4–5 days a week, Step 2 is low-dose maintenance ICS. Step 3 (low-dose maintenance ICS-LABA) is for adolescents with symptoms most days, or waking with asthma at least once a week. Adolescents with daily symptoms or waking with asthma once a week or more and with low lung function, medium/high-dose maintenance ICS–LABA (Step 4). A short course of oral corticosteroids may also be needed. Step 5 includes adding a LAMA; considering high-dose ICS formoterol, and referring for phenotypic assessment ± biologic therapy.

For children aged 6–11 years, the relievers of choice are SABA and ICS formoterol for Steps 3 and 4. If they have symptoms less than twice a month, low-dose ICS is recommended to be taken whenever as needed SABA is taken (Step 1) (2023 GINA Main Report, Global Initiative for Asthma. https://www.mhprofessional.com/gina). Another Step 1 option is daily low-dose ICS and as needed SABA. If they are having symptoms twice a month or more, but less than daily, Step 2 treatment is daily low-dose ICS (alternatives are daily leukotriene receptor antagonist or low-dose ICS taken whenever SABA is taken). Step 3 therapy is for children having symptoms on most days, or waking with asthma once a week or more. There are three preferred options: low-dose ICS LABA; OR medium-dose ICS; OR very low-dose ICS–formoterol maintenance and reliever (MART). An alternative option is low-dose ICS and LTRA. For children having symptoms most days, or waking with asthma once a week or more, and with low lung function, preferred Step 4 options are medium-dose ICS–LABA; OR low-dose ICS–formoterol maintenance and reliever therapy (MART), and referring for expert advice. An alternative option is adding tiotropium or LTRA. A short course of oral corticosteroids may also be needed. Step 5 includes referring for phenotypic assessment ± biologic therapy; and higher-dose ICS-LABA. An alternative option is adding on low-dose oral corticosteroid.

For younger children (< 6 years old), SABA is the reliever of choice (2023 GINA Main Report, Global Initiative for Asthma. https://www.mhprofessional.com/gina). For patients with infrequent viral wheezing and no/few interval symptoms, Step 1 therapy is intermittent short course ICS at onset of viral illness and as needed SABA for rescue. If they have a symptom pattern which is not consistent with asthma but wheezing episodes requiring SABA occur frequently, for example, ≥ 3 per year, a diagnostic trial for 3 months of daily low-dose ICS (preferred Step 2) is recommended. Step 2 (preferred daily low dose ICS; alternative options are LTRA or intermittent short course ICS at onset of respiratory illness) is also recommended if these children have a symptom pattern that is consistent with asthma, and asthma symptoms are not well controlled or they have ≥ 3 exacerbations per year. For young children with an asthma diagnosis and whose asthma is not well controlled on low-dose ICS, before stepping up to doubling "low-dose" ICS (Step 3), it is important to check for alternative diagnosis, inhaler skills, adherence, and exposures. If their asthma is still not controlled on double ICS dose, their controller therapy should be continued and referral to a specialist is recommended (Step 4). Other options include adding an LTRA, increasing ICS frequency, or adding intermittent ICS.

Asthma medications are classified as long-term "controller" (preferably "maintenance") medications and reliever medications. The former includes anti-inflammatory agents (ICS and leukotriene modifiers), long-acting bronchodilators (LABAs and LAMAs), and biologics (omalizumab, mepolizumab, benralizumab, reslizumab, dupilumab, and tezepelumab). LABAs (salmeterol, formoterol, and vilanterol) are β-agonists, and they have been considered to be daily controller medications. In addition to SABAs, GINA 2023 and NAEPP 2020 recommend using combination ICS-formoterol as a rescue or reliever medication, in MART and SMART approach, respectively, as well. Bronchial thermoplasty has been an option for some adult patients with severe asthma, but the NAEPP 2020 focused updates recommend against this intervention in general (except for some individuals who may be willing to accept the risks after a shared decision-making) because benefits are small, risks are moderate, and long-term outcomes are uncertain.

1. Inhaled corticosteroids (ICS)—ICS are the most potent inhaled anti-inflammatory agents currently available. Although recommended as daily controller therapy, studies have shown their efficacy even for **intermittent** use in two different ways. The NAEPP 2020 now recommends a short course of ICS and albuterol at the onset of a respiratory tract illness in children 0–4 years old. As part of SMART (NAEPP 2020) or MART (GINA) approach, as needed low- or medium-dose ICS-formoterol can be used in children as part of Steps 3 or 4 therapy, respectively. Different ICS are not equivalent on a per puff or microgram basis (Table 38–5a and b). For most patients, low-dose ICS can provide adequate control, although some patients may need higher doses due to variable ICS responsiveness. High doses are associated with increased risk of local and systemic adverse effects. Early intervention with ICS can improve asthma control and prevent exacerbations during treatment, but they do not prevent the development of persistent asthma nor do they alter its natural history. Long-term ICS may be associated with early slowing of growth velocity in children, and although this can

impact the final adult height by a minimum degree, it is not a cumulative effect. Possible risks from ICS need to be weighed against the risks from undertreated asthma. The adverse effects from ICS are generally dose and duration dependent, so that greater risks for systemic adverse effects are expected with high doses. The various ICS are delivered in different devices such as MDI (beclomethasone, ciclesonide, fluticasone propionate, flunisolide, mometasone, and triamcinolone), dry powder inhaler (DPI) (fluticasone propionate [Diskus], fluticasone furoate [Ellipta], budesonide [Flexhaler], and mometasone [Twisthaler]), and nebulized aerosol suspensions (budesonide respules). Inhaled medications delivered in MDI now use the more ozone-friendly hydrofluoroalkane (HFA) propellant, which has replaced chlorofluorocarbons (CFC). See instructions for different device use at the following URL: https://www.nationaljewish.org/conditions/medications/inhaled-medication-asthma-inhaler-copd-inhaler/instructional-videos.

Only ICS has been shown to be effective in long-term clinical studies for infants. Nebulized budesonide is approved for children as young as 12 months. The suspension (available in quantities of 0.25 mg/2 mL, 0.5 mg/2 mL, and 1.0 mg/2 mL) is usually administered either once or twice daily in divided doses. For effective drug delivery, it is critical that the child has a mask secured on the face for the entire treatment, as blowing it in the face is not effective and yet a common practice by parents. Notably, this drug should not be given by ultrasonic nebulizer. Limited data suggest that ICS may be effective even in very young children when delivered by MDI with a spacer and mask. Low daily dose in μg (defined as a dose that has not been associated with adverse effects in trials that evaluated safety measures) for various ICS for children 5 years and younger is as follows: beclomethasone dipropionate (HFA) 100 μg; budesonide pMDI + spacer 200 μg; budesonide nebulized 500 μg; fluticasone propionate (HFA) 100 μg; and ciclesonide 160 μg.

2. Combination of inhaled steroid and long-acting bronchodilator—For school-aged children whose asthma is uncontrolled on low-dose ICS (ie, requiring Step 3 guidelines therapy), majority are likely to respond to a step-up combination therapy with a LABA bronchodilator (eg, salmeterol and formoterol), although some respond best either to an increased dose of ICS or to an addition of a leukotriene-receptor antagonist (LTRA). Salmeterol is available as an inhalation powder (one inhalation twice daily). It is also available combined with fluticasone (50 μg salmeterol with 100, 250, or 500 μg fluticasone or 14 μg salmeterol with 55, 113, and 232 μg fluticasone in a DPI and 21 μg salmeterol with 45, 115, or 230 μg fluticasone in an MDI). For children 12 years and older, one inhalation DPI or two inhalations MDI can be taken twice daily. (*Note:* The 100/50 fluticasone/salmeterol combination is approved in children aged 4 and older.) Salmeterol can also be used 30 minutes before exercise (but not in addition to regularly

Table 38-5a. NAEPP EPR 3 estimated comparative inhaled corticosteroid doses.

Drug	Low Daily Dose			Medium Daily Dose			High Daily Dose		
	0–4 y	5–11 y	≥12 y	0–4 y	5–11 y	≥12 y	0–4 y	5–11 y	≥12 y
Beclomethasone HFA, 40 or 80 mcg/puff	NA	80–160 mcg	80–240 mcg	NA	> 160–320 mcg	> 240–480 mcg	NA	> 320 mcg	> 480 mcg
Budesonide DPI 90, 80, or 200 mcg/inhalation	NA	180–400 mcg	180–600 mcg	NA	> 400–800 mcg	> 600–1200 mcg	NA	> 800 mcg	> 1200 mcg
Budesonide inhaled suspension for nebulization, 0.25-, 0.5-, and 1.0-mg dose	0.25–0.5 mg	0.5 mg	NA	> 0.5–1.0 mg	1.0 mg	NA	> 1.0 mg	2.0 mg	NA
Flunisolide, 250 mcg/puff	NA	500–750 mcg	500–1000 mcg	NA	1000–1250 mcg	> 1000–2000 mcg	NA	> 1250 mcg	> 2000 mcg
Flunisolide HFA, 80 mcg/puff	NA	160 mcg	320 mcg	NA	320 mcg	320–640 mcg	NA	≥640 mcg	> 640 mcg
Fluticasone HFA/MDI, 44, 110, or 220 mcg/puff	176 mcg	88–176 mcg	88–264 mcg	> 176–352 mcg	> 176–352 mcg	> 264–440 mcg	> 352 mcg	> 352 mcg	> 440 mcg
Fluticasone DPI, 50, 100, or 250 mcg/inhalation	NA	100–200 mcg	100–300 mcg	NA	> 200–400 mcg	> 300–500 mcg	NA	> 400 mcg	> 500 mcg
Mometasone DPI, 220 mcg/inhalation	NA	NA	220 mcg	NA	NA	440 mcg	NA	NA	> 440 mcg
Triamcinolone acetonide, 75 mcg/puff	NA	300–600 mcg	300–750 mcg	NA	> 600–900 mcg	> 750–1500 mcg	NA	> 900 mcg	> 1500 mcg

DPI, dry powder inhaler; HFA, hydrofluoroalkane; MDI, metered-dose inhaler; NA, not approved and no data available for this age group.

Reproduced with permission from National Asthma Education and Prevention Program: Expert panel report 3 (EPR-3): guidelines for the diagnosis and management of asthma-summary report 2007. J Allergy Clin Immunol 2007; 120(5):S94–S138.

Table 38–5b. GINA estimated comparative inhaled corticosteroid doses.

Drug	Low Daily Dose			Medium Daily Dose			High Daily Dose		
	0–5 y (age group with adequate safety and effectiveness data)	6–11 y	≥ 12 y	0–5 y	6–11 y	≥ 12 y	0–5 y	6–11 y	≥ 12 y
Beclomethasone dipropionate pMDI, standard particle, HFA	100 (ages ≥ 5 years)	100–200	200–500		> 200–400	> 500–1000		> 400	> 1000
Beclomethasone dipropionate (DPI or pMDI, extra fine particle, HFA)	50 (ages ≥ 5 years)	50–100	100–200		> 100–200	> 200–400		> 200	> 400
Budesonide DPI or pMDI, standard particle HFA		100–200	200–400		> 200–400	> 400–800		> 400	> 800
Budesonide nebules	500 (ages 1 year and older)	250–500			> 500–1000			> 1000	
Ciclesonide pMDI, extrafine particle, HFA	Not sufficiently studied in children ≤ 5 years	80	80–160		> 80–160	> 160–320		> 160	> 320
Fluticasone furoate (DPI)	Not sufficiently studied in children ≤ 5 years	50	100		50	100		NA	200
Fluticasone propionate DPI or pMDI, standard particle HFA	50 (ages 4 years and older)	50–100	100–250		> 100–200	> 250–500		> 200	> 500
Mometasone furoate DPI			Depends on DPI device			Depends on DPI device			Depends on DPI device
Mometasone furoate pMDI, standard particle HFA	100 (ages ≥ 5 years)	100	200–400		100	200–400		200	> 400

DPI, dry powder inhaler; HFA, hydrofluoroalkane; MDI, metered-dose inhaler; NA, not approved and no data available for this age group. Data from GINA.

used LABAs). Formoterol has a more rapid onset of action and is available singly either as a DPI (Aerolizer, 12 μg) or a nebulized solution approved only for chronic obstructive pulmonary disease (COPD, Performist); or combined with an inhaled steroid (formoterol fumarate, either 4.5 μg with budesonide [80 or 160 μg] or 5 μg with mometasone [100 or 200 μg], in an MDI). The combination product is approved for children 6 years and older, two inhalations twice daily. For long-term control, formoterol should be used in combination with an anti-inflammatory agent. It can be used for exercise-induced bronchospasm in patients 5 years and older, one inhalation at least 15 minutes before exercise (but not in addition to regularly used LABAs). An even longer-acting LABA, vilanterol, with a 24-hour activity, combined with fluticasone furoate (Breo) is approved for asthma in patients 18 years and older. A study, focused on the safety of LABAs in children 4–11 years of age, found that there was no excess risk of serious asthma-related event associated with fluticasone propionate-salmeterol combination compared to fluticasone alone. Similar findings were found in two other trials that enrolled adults and adolescents, that LABAs in fixed-dose combination with an ICS was not associated with the risk of serious asthma-related event comparable to the risk with the ICS alone. However, potential drug interactions between medications such as ritonavir-boosted nirmatrelvir (an anti-COVID–19 treatment) or itraconazole (a cytochrome P450 inhibitor used for treatment of allergic bronchopulmonary aspergillosis or fungal infection) and some LABAs such as salmeterol or vilanterol are recognized. To prevent asthma exacerbations or cardiovascular adverse effects, these LABAs should be discontinued if those medications are prescribed, by using formoterol for the duration of the nirmatelvir or itraconazole treatment. The NAEPP 2020 and GINA prefer ICS-LABA as maintenance therapy for at least Step 3. In addition, the SMART per NAEPP 2020 (or MART per GINA) approach using either low-dose or medium-dose ICS-formoterol as both maintenance and reliever treatment is now recommended as preferred Steps 3 and 4 therapy. The NAEPP 2020 specifies ICS-formoterol up to a total 8 puffs (36 μg formoterol) per day for children and 12 total puffs (54 μg formoterol) per day for adolescents and adults. Implementation guidelines for SMART therapy are available (Table 38–6). Randomized controlled clinical trials have found a 35%–51% relative risk reduction in exacerbations favoring SMART over daily ICS with quick relief SABA. ICS-formoterol should not be used as quick-relief therapy in individuals taking ICS-salmeterol as maintenance therapy. For mild asthma as preferred controller for Steps 1 and 2, GINA also recommends symptom driven (as needed) or before exercise use of low-dose ICS-formoterol for adults and adolescents, instead of SABA alone. This option using ICS-formoterol as reliever has been found to significantly reduce exacerbations and provide control at relatively low-maintenance ICS dose requirement.

3. Leukotriene antagonists—Montelukast and zafirlukast are LTRAs available in oral formulations. Montelukast is given once daily and has been approved for treatment of chronic asthma in children aged 1 year and older, as an alternative Step 2 monotherapy and add-on therapy for Steps 3–6. It is also indicated for seasonal allergic rhinitis in patients 2 years and older, and for perennial allergic rhinitis in patients 6 months and older. To date, no drug interactions have been noted. The dosage is 4 mg for children 1–5 years (oral granules are available for children aged 12–23 months), 5 mg for children aged 6–14 years, and 10 mg for those aged 15 years and older. The drug is given without regard to mealtimes, preferably in the evening. Zafirlukast is approved for

Table 38–6. Single maintenance and rescue treatment implementation considerations.

Age group	Budesonide-formoterol dose	Step 3		Step 4		Step 3 or 4
		Maintenance dose	As-needed dose	Maintenance dose	As-needed dose	Maximum total daily inhalations
Adults and adolescents aged ≥12 y	160/4.5 μg delivered dose	One inhalation twice daily or once daily	**One** *(to 6 on single occasion)* inhalation as needed	Two inhalations twice daily	**One** *(to 6 on single occasion)* inhalation as needed	12
Children 4-11 years	80/4.5 μg delivered dose	One inhalation once daily	**One** *(to 4 on single occasion)* inhalation as needed	One inhalation twice daily	**One** *(to 4 on single occasion)* inhalation as needed	8

There are no SMART studies with mometasone-formoterol, but if it were used, relevant formulations would be mometasone-formoterol 100/5 μg for adults and 50/5 μg for children, with the same dosing frequencies as shown.
The 200/5 μg formulation of mometasone-formoterol would not be suitable for SMART.
For beclomethasone-formoterol, the recommended maximum dose on any day is 8 inhalations.
Reddel HK, Bateman ED, Schatz M, Krishnan JA, Cloutier MM. A Practical Guide to Implementing SMART in Asthma Management. J Allergy Clin Immunol Pract. 2022 Jan;10(1S):S31-S38. doi: 10.1016/j.jaip.2021.10.011. Epub 2021 Oct 16. PMID: 34666208.

patients aged 5 years and older. The dose is 10 mg twice daily for those 5–11 years and 20 mg twice daily for those 12 years and older. It should be taken 1 hour before or 2 hours after meals. Zileuton is a 5-lipoxygenase inhibitor indicated for chronic treatment in children 12 years of age and older, available in regular 600 mg dose tablet four times a day or extended-release 600 mg dose tablet, two tablets twice a day. Patients need to have hepatic transaminase levels evaluated at initiation of therapy, then once a month for the first 3 months, every 2–3 months for the remainder of the first year, and periodically thereafter if receiving long-term zileuton therapy. Rare cases of Churg-Strauss syndrome have been reported in adult patients with severe asthma whose steroid dosage was being tapered during concomitant treatment with LTRAs (as well as ICS), but no causal link has been established. Both zafirlukast and zileuton are microsomal P-450 enzyme inhibitors that can inhibit the metabolism of drugs such as warfarin and theophylline. The FDA has requested that manufacturers include a precaution in the drug prescribing information (drug labeling) regarding neuropsychiatric events (agitation, aggression, anxiousness, dream abnormalities and hallucinations, depression, insomnia, irritability, restlessness, suicidal thinking and behavior, and tremor) based on postmarket reports of patients taking leukotriene-modifying agents. Of note, in a study of children with mild to moderate persistent asthma that looked at whether responses to an ICS and a LTRA were concordant for individuals or whether asthmatic patients who did not respond to one medication responded to the other, responses to fluticasone and montelukast were found to vary considerably. Children with low pulmonary function or high levels of markers associated with allergic inflammation responded better to the ICS.

Children with persistent asthma who remain uncontrolled on ICS monotherapy are more likely to respond to a combination treatment of an ICS and a LABA; however, some children respond best to a higher dose of ICS, or even a low-dose ICS plus montelukast. It has not yet been determined what clinical features would be helpful in selecting the most appropriate medication for any one patient.

4. Long-acting muscarinic antagonists—The LAMA, tiotropium (Spiriva Respimat [1.25 µg] has now been approved as once-daily maintenance treatment for asthma in patients 6 years and older, as an add-on therapy to ICS-LABA. The NAEPP 2020 recommends adding LAMA for patients at least 12 years of age whose asthma is not controlled with ICS-LABA (Step 5). A LAMA can be added to an ICS (as an alternative adjunct in Steps 3 and 4) only if a LABA cannot be used in certain individuals who are unable to tolerate or use the drug/device or have contraindication to LABA. GINA recommends tiotropium as an add-on therapy "other" controller option for Step 4 and "preferred" add-on controller option for Step 5 treatment for children 6 years and older. Tiotropium by mist inhaler (particularly at 5 µg daily dose) improves lung function and time to severe exacerbation.

5. Other treatment options—Biologics (Table 38–7): Anti-IgE (omalizumab) is a recombinant DNA-derived humanized IgG$_1$ monoclonal antibody that selectively binds to human IgE. It inhibits the binding of IgE to the high-affinity IgE receptor (FcεRI) on the surface of mast cells and basophils. Reduction in surface-bound IgE on FcεRI-bearing cells limits the degree of release of mediators of the allergic response. Treatment with omalizumab also reduces the number of FcεRI receptors on basophils in atopic patients. Omalizumab is now indicated for children as young as 6 years with moderate to severe persistent asthma who have a positive skin test or in vitro reactivity to a perennial aeroallergen with total serum IgE of 30–1300 IU/mL for children 6–11 years (30–700 IU/mL for adolescents), and whose symptoms are inadequately controlled with medium- to high-dose ICS. Omalizumab has been shown to decrease the incidence of asthma exacerbations and improve asthma control. Dosing is based on the patient's weight and serum IgE level and is given subcutaneously every 2–4 weeks. The FDA has ordered a black box warning on the label because of new reports of serious and life-threatening anaphylactic reactions (bronchospasm, hypotension, syncope, urticaria, and angioedema of the throat or tongue) in patients after treatment with omalizumab (Xolair®). Based on premarketing clinical trials in patients with asthma, anaphylaxis occurred in 0.1% of patients; in postmarketing spontaneous reports based on an estimated exposure of about 57,300 patients from June 2003 through December 2006, the frequency of anaphylaxis attributed to Xolair® use was estimated to be at least 0.2% of patients. From a case-control study, patients with a history of anaphylaxis from whatever cause were considered at increased risk of anaphylaxis with Xolair®, compared to those with no prior history of anaphylaxis. Although these reactions occurred within 2 hours of receiving an omalizumab subcutaneous injection, they also included reports of serious delayed reactions 2–24 hours or even longer after receiving the injections. Anaphylaxis occurred after any dose of omalizumab (including the first dose), even in patients with no allergic reaction to previous doses. Omalizumab-treated patients should be observed in the facility for an extended period after the drug is given, and medical providers who administer the injection should be prepared to manage life-threatening anaphylactic reactions. Patients who receive omalizumab should be fully informed about the signs and symptoms of anaphylaxis, their chance of developing delayed anaphylaxis following each injection, and how to treat it, including the use of auto-injectable epinephrine. Malignancy (eg, breast, nonmelanoma skin, prostate, melanoma, and parotid) was observed in 20 of 4127 (0.5%) Xolair-treated patients compared with 5 of 2236 (0.2%) control patients in clinical studies of adults and adolescents with asthma and other allergies. A more recent observational study of 5007 Xolair®-treated and 2829 non-Xolair®-treated patients with moderate to severe persistent allergic asthma followed for up

Table 38–7. Biologics for the treatment of severe asthma.

Name	Asthma age indication	Mechanism of action	Dose administration for asthma	Indications
Omalizumab	≥ 6 years	Prevents IgE from binding to its receptor	150–375 mg SQ every 2–4 weeks (dose by total serum IgE and body weight)	• Moderate to severe persistent asthma with sensitization to a perennial aeroallergen and total serum IgE: 30–700 kU/L in adolescents and 30–1200 kU/L in younger children • Chronic spontaneous urticaria (≥12 years) • Nasal polyposis (≥18 years)
Mepolizumab	≥ 6 years	Binds to IL5 ligand	40 mg SQ (6-11 years) 100 mg SQ ≥ 12 years	• Severe eosinophilic asthma, with blood eosinophil count ≥ 150 cells/microliter and at least 2 asthma exacerbations in the last year • EGPA (≥ 18 years) • Hypereosinophilic syndrome (≥ 18 years) • Chronic rhinosinusitis with nasal polyposis (≥ 18 years)
Dupilumab	≥ 6 years	Binds to IL4 receptor alpha	400 mg SQ loading dose, then 200 mg every 2 weeks OR 600 mg SQ loading dose, then 300 mg every 2 weeks	• Uncontrolled moderate to severe eosinophilic asthma (blood eosinophil count ≥ 150 cells/microliter and exhaled nitric oxide ≥ 25 ppb • Oral corticosteroid dependent asthma • Moderate to severe atopic dermatitis (≥ 6 months of age) • Chronic rhinosinusitis with nasal polyposis (≥ 18 years) • Eosinophilic esophagitis (≥ 1 year and at least 15 kg)
Benralizumab	≥ 12 years	Binds to IL-5 receptor	30 mg SQ monthly for 3 doses, then 30 mg every 8 weeks	• Severe eosinophilic asthma (blood eosinophil count (≥ 300 cells per microliter) and at least 2 asthma exacerbations in the previous year • Hyper eosinophilic syndrome
Tezepelumab	≥ 12 years	Blocks thymic stromal lymphopoietin, an epithelial cell-derived cytokine	210 mg SQ every 4 weeks	• Severe asthma without phenotypic or biomarker limitation
Reslizumab	≥ 18 years	IL5 antagonist	3 mg/kg IV every 4 weeks	• Severe eosinophilic asthma (blood eosinophil count (≥ 400 cells per microliter), and at least one asthma exacerbation in the previous year, and reduced lung function with FEV1 < 80% predicted

to 5 years showed similar incidence rates (per/1000 patient years) of primary malignancies among Xolair®-treated (12.3) and non-Xolair®-treated patients (13.0).

In addition to omalizumab, new biologics or immunomodulators directed against specific T2 airway inflammation have been studied to target the inflammatory component of asthma. The U.S. FDA has recommended approval of mepolizumab for children 6 years and older (Nucala, monoclonal antibody IgG1K, administered 100 mg subcutaneously every 4 weeks for patients 12 years and older and 40 mg subcutaneously every 4 weeks for children 6–11 years); reslizumab (Cinqair™, monoclonal antibody IgG4K, given 3 mg/kg intravenously monthly) for adult patients aged 18 years and

older; and benralizumab (Fasenra™, humanized monoclonal antibody directed against the alpha subunit of the IL-5 receptor, subcutaneous injection 30 mg every 4 weeks for the first 3 doses, then 30 mg every 8 weeks thereafter), for aged 12 years and older, as add-on maintenance treatment of patients with severe asthma and with an eosinophilic phenotype. Dupilumab, (Dupixent®) a monoclonal antibody directed against the IL4 receptor alpha, is the first FDA-approved biologic for asthma that can be self-administered subcutaneously every 2 weeks, for patients aged 6 years and older with eosinophilic moderate to severe asthma or oral corticosteroid-dependent asthma. Tezepelumab (Tezspire®), a human monoclonal antibody (IgG2λ) that blocks thymic stromal lymphopoietin (TSLP), has been approved for patients 12 years and older regardless of their eosinophilic phenotype. These drugs have been shown to be effective at reducing exacerbations, improving lung function and symptom control, and decreasing oral corticosteroid use. Some of them have also been approved for non-asthma conditions. A simple algorithm to direct specialists to biological therapy using available biomarkers is proposed, as shown in Figure 38–2.

Immunotherapy (discussed in more detail in section Immunotherapy) can be considered for children 5 years and older with allergic asthma. The NAEPP 2020 recommends subcutaneous (over sublingual) immunotherapy as an adjunct treatment to standard pharmacotherapy for individuals with mild-moderate allergic asthma who have demonstrated allergic sensitization and evidence of worsening asthma symptoms after exposure to relevant antigen(s). The GINA recommends adding house dust mite sublingual immunotherapy for adults and adolescents on Steps 2, 3, or 4 who are sensitized with allergic rhinitis and FEV_1 more than 70% predicted.

Chronic azithromycin therapy three times a week is presented as an option in GINA Step 5 for adult patients after being referred to a specialist. The recommendation is based on significant reduction in exacerbations in patients taking high-dose ICS-LABA and in patients with either eosinophilic or noneosinophilic asthma. Implementation tips include checking for evidence of atypical mycobacteria, ECG for prolonged QTc (before and after a month of treatment), and consideration of potential for developing antimicrobial resistance.

Theophylline is rarely used and is no longer mentioned in the GINA guidelines. Sustained-release theophylline, an alternative long-term control medication for older children, may have risks of adverse effects in infants, who frequently have febrile illnesses that increase theophylline concentrations. Hence, if theophylline is used, it requires monitoring of serum concentration to prevent numerous dose-related acute toxicities.

Oral corticosteroids (low dose) are only recommended as "other" controller option for Step 5 therapy in the GINA

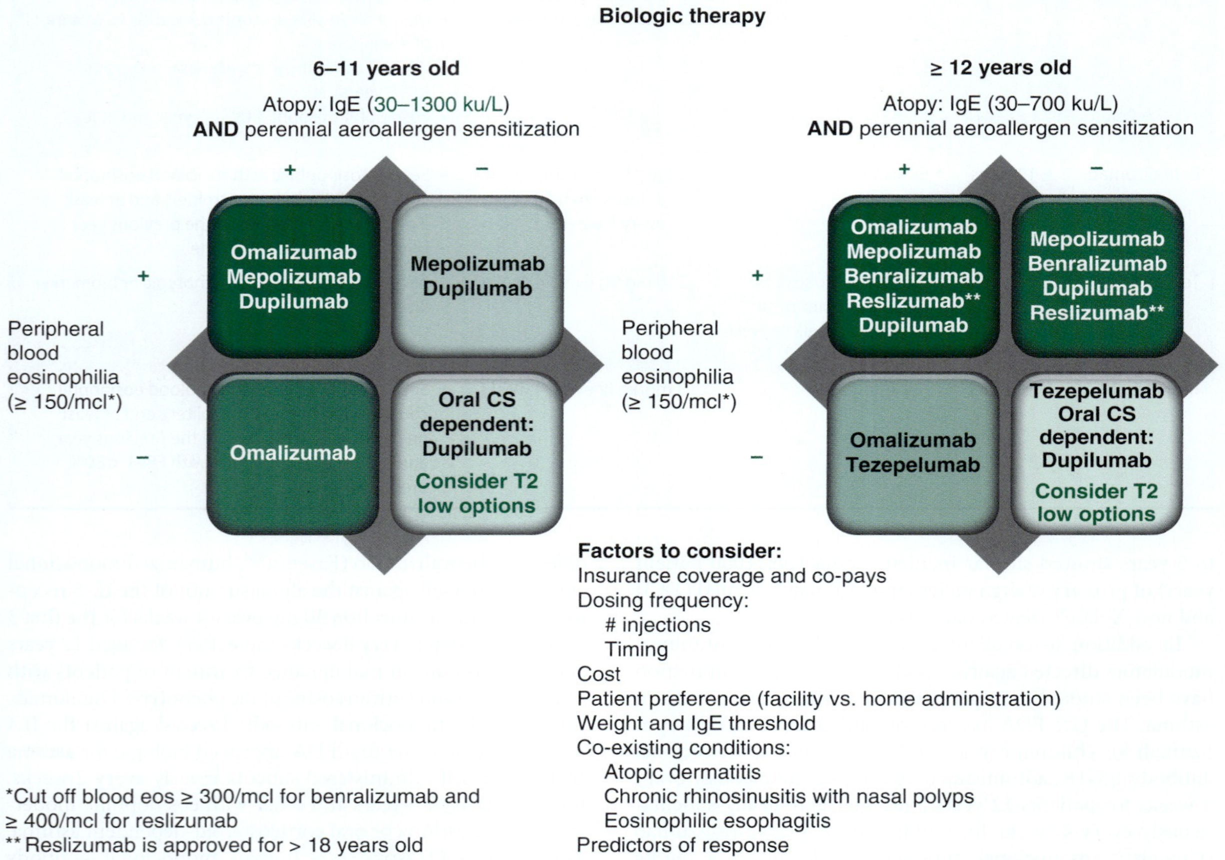

Biologic therapy

6–11 years old
Atopy: IgE (30–1300 ku/L)
AND perennial aeroallergen sensitization

≥ 12 years old
Atopy: IgE (30–700 ku/L)
AND perennial aeroallergen sensitization

Peripheral blood eosinophilia (≥ 150/mcl*)

+ / **–**

Omalizumab Mepolizumab Dupilumab

Mepolizumab Dupilumab

Omalizumab

Oral CS dependent: Dupilumab
Consider T2 low options

Omalizumab Mepolizumab Benralizumab Reslizumab** Dupilumab

Mepolizumab Benralizumab Dupilumab Reslizumab**

Omalizumab Tezepelumab

Tezepelumab Oral CS dependent: Dupilumab
Consider T2 low options

Factors to consider:
Insurance coverage and co-pays
Dosing frequency:
  # injections
  Timing
Cost
Patient preference (facility vs. home administration)
Weight and IgE threshold
Co-existing conditions:
  Atopic dermatitis
  Chronic rhinosinusitis with nasal polyps
  Eosinophilic esophagitis
Predictors of response

*Cut off blood eos ≥ 300/mcl for benralizumab and ≥ 400/mcl for reslizumab
** Reslizumab is approved for > 18 years old

▲ **Figure 38–2.** A simple algorithm to direct specialists to biological therapy using available biomarkers is proposed.

guidelines, because of adverse effects. They are recommended in NAEPP EPR Step 6 therapy.

6. Monitoring and management—Continual monitoring is necessary to ensure that control of asthma is achieved and sustained. Once control is established, gradual reduction in therapy is appropriate and may help determine the minimum amount of medication necessary to maintain control. Regular follow-up visits with the clinician are important to assess the degree of control and consider appropriate adjustments in therapy. At each step, patients should be instructed to avoid or control exposure to allergens, irritants, or other factors that contribute to asthma severity.

There are now digital intervention strategies (eg, electronic monitoring of maintenance and reliever medications and text/phone reminders) to enhance adherence, which have been shown to improve asthma control and reduce exacerbations.

Referral to an asthma specialist for consultation or co-management is recommended if there are difficulties in achieving or maintaining control. For children younger than 5 years, referral is recommended for moderate persistent asthma or if the patient requires Step 3 or 4 care and should be considered if the patient requires Step 2 care. For children 5 years and older, consultation with a specialist is recommended if the patient requires Step 4 care or higher and should be considered at Step 3. Referral is also recommended if allergen immunotherapy or a biologic is being considered.

Quick-relief medications include inhaled SABAs such as albuterol, levalbuterol, pirbuterol, or terbutaline, ICS-SABA (AirSupra™ single albuterol/budesonide inhaler now approved to treat bronchoconstriction in adults with acute asthma), and ICS-formoterol (see SMART). Albuterol can be given by nebulizer, 0.05 mg/kg (with a minimal dose of 0.63 mg and a maximum of 5 mg) in 2–3 mL saline (although it is also available in a 2.5 mg/3 mL single vial or 5 mg/mL concentrated solution) or by MDI (90 µg/actuation) or by breath-actuated DPI (Respiclick). It is better to use SABAs as needed rather than regularly. Increasing use, including more than one canister per month, may signify inadequate asthma control and the need to step up or revise controller therapy. Levalbuterol, the (R)-enantiomer of racemic albuterol, is available in solution for nebulization in patients aged 6–11 years, 0.31 mg every 8 hours, and in patients 12 years and older, 0.63–1.25 mg every 8 hours. It has recently become available in an HFA formulation for children 4 years and older, two inhalations (90 µg) every 4–6 hours as needed. Anticholinergic agents such as ipratropium, one to three puffs or 0.25–0.5 mg by nebulizer every 6 hours may provide additive benefit when used together with an inhaled SABA. Systemic corticosteroids such as prednisone, prednisolone, dexamethasone, and methylprednisolone can be given in single or divided doses for 3–10 days. There is no evidence that tapering the dose following a "burst" prevents relapse.

7. Exercise-induced bronchospasm—Exercise-induced bronchospasm should be anticipated in all asthma patients. It typically occurs during or minutes after vigorous activity, reaches its peak 5–10 minutes after stopping the activity, and usually resolves over the next 20–30 minutes. Participation in physical activity should be encouraged in children with asthma, although the choice of activity may need to be modified based on the severity of illness, presence of other triggers such as cold air, and, rarely, confounding factors such as osteoporosis. Poor endurance or exercise-induced bronchospasm can be an indication of poorly controlled persistent asthma. If symptoms occur during usual play activities, either initiation of or a step-up in long-term therapy is warranted. However, for those with exercise-induced bronchospasm as the only manifestation of asthma despite otherwise being "well-controlled," treatment immediately prior to vigorous activity or exercise is usually effective. SABAs, LTRAs, cromolyn, or nedocromil can be used before exercise. The combination of a SABA with either cromolyn or nedocromil is more effective than either drug alone. Salmeterol and formoterol may block exercise-induced bronchospasm for up to 12 hours (as discussed earlier). However, decreased duration of protection against exercise-induced bronchospasm can be expected with regular use. Montelukast may be effective for up to 24 hours. An extended warm-up period may induce a refractory state, allowing patients to exercise without a need for repeat medications.

B. Acute Asthma

1. General measures—The most effective strategy in managing asthma exacerbations involves early recognition of warning signs and early treatment. Exacerbations are acute or subacute worsening in symptoms and lung function from the baseline status. Patients with asthma should be provided a written action plan, which should incorporate their maintenance treatment regimen and reliever medications, when to use their reliever medications, and when to seek medical care. The child's green, yellow, and red zones based on symptoms (and PEFR for patients with poor symptom perception) with corresponding measures to take according to the state the patient is in should be included. PEFR cutoff values are conventionally set as more than 80% (green), 50%–80% (yellow), and less than 50% (red) of the child's personal best. Prompt communication with the clinician is indicated for children with severe symptoms or a drop in peak flow or with decreased response to SABAs or history of rapid deterioration. At such times, intensification of therapy may include a short course of oral corticosteroids, for patients with severe airflow limitation, or not responding to treatment over 48 hours, or needing frequent reliever treatments. The child should be removed from exposure to any irritants (smoke, fumes, or pollution) or allergens (aeroallergens or food) that could be contributing to the exacerbation.

2. Management at home—Early treatment of asthma exacerbations may prevent hospitalization and a life-threatening event. For children and adolescents (who are not on Steps 3 and 4 SMART), initial treatment should be with a SABA such as albuterol or levalbuterol; two to six puffs from an MDI can be given every 20 minutes up to three times, or a single treatment can be given by nebulizer (0.05 mg/kg [minimum dose, 1.25 mg; maximum, 2.5 mg] of 0.5% solution of albuterol in 2–3 mL saline; or 0.075 mg/kg [minimum dose, 1.25 mg; maximum, 5 mg] of levalbuterol). If the response is good as assessed by sustained symptom relief or improvement in PEFR to over 80% of the patient's best, the SABA can be continued every 3–4 hours for 24–48 hours. Patients should be advised to seek medical care once excessive doses of bronchodilator therapy are used or for prolonged periods (eg, > 12 puffs/day for > 24 hours). For children above 4 years old using the SMART/MART approach as Steps 3 and 4 therapy, ICS-formoterol (equivalent 4.5 μg delivered dose MDI; 1 to 4 puffs for children aged 4–11 and 1 to 6 puffs for >12 years old, at any one time) can be used as reliever treatment (maximum 8 puffs and 12 puffs daily, respectively). (see Table 38–6).

Doubling the dose of ICS is not proven sufficient to prevent worsening of exacerbations; and a recent study in children with mild persistent asthma also demonstrated lack of benefit of quintupling low-dose ICS as a yellow zone action plan. If the patient does not completely improve from the initial therapy or PEFR falls between 50% and 80% predicted or personal best, the SABA should be continued, an oral corticosteroid should be added, and the patient should contact the physician urgently. If the child experiences marked distress or if PEFR persists at 50% or less, the patient should repeat the SABA immediately and go to the ED or call 911 or another emergency number for assistance.

3. Management in the office or emergency department—Obtaining a history of symptom severity, maintenance and reliever medication use, presence of other symptoms of anaphylaxis, and risk factors for asthma-related exacerbations/mortality mentioned in the previous section should be done. Physical examination should focus on assessment of exacerbation severity including vital signs and respiratory effort, and presence of complicating factors such as pneumonia, atelectasis, pneumothorax, or alternative conditions (inducible laryngeal obstruction, inhaled foreign body especially in young children, aspiration, or pulmonary embolism). Functional assessment of the patient includes obtaining objective measures of airflow limitation with PEFR or FEV_1 and monitoring the patient's response to treatment; however, very severe exacerbations and respiratory distress may prevent the execution of lung function measurements using maximal expiratory maneuver. When possible flow-volume loops should be obtained to differentiate upper and lower airway obstruction, especially in patients with atypical presentation. Other tests should include oxygen saturation and if concerning then blood gases. Chest radiographs are not recommended routinely but should be considered to rule out pneumothorax, pneumomediastinum, pneumonia, or lobar atelectasis. If the initial FEV_1 or PEFR is over 40%, initial treatment can be with a SABA by inhaler (albuterol, four to eight puffs) or nebulizer (0.15 mg/kg of albuterol 0.5% solution; minimum dose, 2.5 mg), up to three doses in the first hour. Oxygen should be given to maintain oxygen saturation at greater than 90%. Oral corticosteroids (1–2 mg/kg/day in divided doses; maximum of 60 mg/day for children aged ≤ 12 years and 80 mg/day for those > 12 years) should be instituted if the patient responds poorly to therapy or if the patient has recently been on oral corticosteroids. Sensitivity to adrenergic drugs may improve after initiation of corticosteroids. For severe exacerbations or if the initial FEV_1 or PEFR is under 40%, initial treatment should be with a high-dose SABA plus ipratropium bromide, 1.5–3 mL every 20 minutes for three doses (each 3 mL vial contains 0.5 mg ipratropium bromide and 2.5 mg albuterol), then as needed by nebulizer. Continuous albuterol nebulized treatments (0.5 mg/kg/h for small and 10–15 mg/h for older children) can be administered for evidence of persistent obstruction. Oxygen should be given to maintain oxygen saturation at greater than 90% (about 93%–95%), and systemic corticosteroids should be administered. For patients with severe exacerbation having no response to initial aerosolized therapy, or for those who cannot cooperate with or who resist inhalation therapy, adjunctive therapies such as intravenous magnesium sulfate (25–75 mg/kg up to 2 g in children over 20 minutes) and heliox-driven albuterol nebulization should be considered. Epinephrine 1:1000 or terbutaline 1 mg/mL (both 0.01 mg/kg up to 0.3–0.5 mg) may be administered subcutaneously every 20 minutes for three doses, although the use of intravenous β_2-agonists is still unproven. For impending or ongoing respiratory arrest, patients should be intubated and ventilated with 100% oxygen, given intravenous corticosteroids, and admitted to an intensive care unit (ICU). Potential indications for ICU admission also include any FEV_1 or PEFR less than 25% of predicted that improves less than 10% after treatment or values that fluctuate widely. (See asthma [life-threatening] in Chapter 14.) Further treatment is based on clinical response and objective laboratory findings. Hospitalization should be considered strongly for any patient with a history of respiratory failure.

4. Hospital management—For patients who do not respond to outpatient and ED treatment, admission to the hospital becomes necessary for more aggressive care and support. The decision to hospitalize should also be based on the presence of risk factors for mortality from asthma, duration and severity of symptoms, severity of airflow limitation, course and severity of previous exacerbations, medication use at the time of the exacerbation, access to medical care, and home and psychosocial conditions. Fluids should be given at maintenance requirements unless the patient has poor oral intake secondary to respiratory distress or vomiting, because overhydration may contribute to pulmonary edema associated with high intrapleural pressures generated in severe asthma. Potassium requirements should be kept in mind because both corticosteroids and β_2-agonists can cause potassium loss. Moisturized oxygen should be titrated by oximetry to maintain oxygen saturation above 90%. Inhaled β_2-agonist should be continued by nebulization in single doses as needed or by continuous therapy, along with systemic corticosteroids (as discussed earlier). Ipratropium is no longer recommended during hospitalization. In addition, the role of methylxanthines in hospitalized children remains controversial. Antibiotics may be necessary to treat coexisting bacterial infection. Sedatives and anxiolytic agents are contraindicated in severely ill patients owing to their depressant effects on respiration. Chest physiotherapy is usually not recommended for acute exacerbations.

5. Patient discharge—Criteria for discharging patients home from the office or ED should include a sustained response of at least 1 hour to bronchodilator therapy with FEV_1 or PEFR greater than 70% of predicted or personal best and oxygen saturation greater than 90% in room air. Prior to discharge, the patient's or caregiver's ability to continue therapy and assess symptoms appropriately needs to be considered. Patients should be given an action plan for management of recurrent symptoms or exacerbations, and instructions about medications should be reviewed. The inhaled SABA as needed and oral corticosteroids should be continued, the latter for 3–10 days. Finally, the patient or caregiver should be instructed about the follow-up visit, recommended to happen within 2 days after an ED visit or hospitalization. Hospitalized patients should receive more intensive education prior to discharge. Referral to an asthma specialist should be considered for all children with severe exacerbations or multiple ED visits or hospitalizations.

▶ **Prognosis**

Since the 1970s, morbidity rates for asthma have increased, but mortality rates may have stabilized. Mortality statistics indicate that a high percentage of deaths have resulted from under-recognition of asthma severity and undertreatment, particularly in labile asthmatic patients and in asthmatic patients whose perception of pulmonary obstruction is poor. Long-term outcome studies suggest that children with mild symptoms generally outgrow their asthma, while patients with more severe symptoms, marked airway hyperresponsiveness, and a greater degree of atopy tend to have

persistent disease. Data from an unselected birth cohort from New Zealand showed more than one in four children had wheezing that persisted from childhood to adulthood or that relapsed after remission. Recent evidence suggests that early intervention with anti-inflammatory therapy does not alter the development of persistent asthma, and it is also unclear if such intervention or environmental control measures influence the natural history of childhood asthma. Nonetheless, the pediatrician or primary care provider together with the asthma specialist has the responsibility to optimize control and, it is hoped, reduce the severity of asthma in children. Interventions that can have long-term effects such as halting progression or inducing remission are necessary to decrease the public health burden of this common condition.

Resources for health care providers, patients, and families include the following:

- Asthma and Allergy Foundation of America
- 1233 20th St NW, Suite 402
- Washington, DC 20036; (800) 7-ASTHMA
- http://www.aafa.org/
- Asthma and Allergy Network/Mothers of Asthmatics
- 2751 Prosperity Avenue, Suite 150
- Fairfax, VA 22031; (800) 878-4403
- http://www.aanma.org/
- Asthma Device Training: http://www.thechildrenshospital.org/conditions/lung/asthmavideos.aspx
- Global Initiative for Asthma 2023 https://ginasthma.org/reports/. Accessed May 4, 2023.

Akinbami LJ, Simon AE, Rossen LM: Changing trends in asthma prevalence among children. Pediatrics 2016;137:2015–2354 [PMID: 26712860].

Centers for Disease Control and Prevention: National Center for Health Statistics. Health Data Interactive. Summary Health Statistics for U.S. Children: National Health Interview Survey, 2015. https://www.cdc.gov/nchs/fastats/asthma.htm. Accessed January 16, 2018.

Expert Panel Working Group of the National Heart, Lung, and Blood Institute (NHLBI) et al: 2020 Focused Updates to the Asthma Management Guidelines: A Report from the National Asthma Education and Prevention Program Coordinating Committee Expert Panel Working Group. J Allergy Clin Immunol 2020 Dec;146(6):1217–1270. doi: 10.1016/j.jaci.2020.10.003. Erratum in: J Allergy Clin Immunol 2021 Apr;147(4):1528–1530 [PMID: 33280709] [PMCID: PMC7924476].

National Asthma Education and Prevention Program: Expert Panel Report 3 (EPR 3): Guidelines for the Diagnosis and Management of Asthma—Summary Report 2007. J Allergy Clin Immunol 2007;120(5 Suppl):S94 [PMID: 17983880].

Reddel HK, Bateman ED, Schatz M, Krishnan JA, Cloutier MM: A Practical Guide to Implementing SMART in Asthma Management. J Allergy Clin Immunol Pract 2022 Jan;10(1S):S31-S38.

ALLERGIC RHINOCONJUNCTIVITIS

ESSENTIALS OF DIAGNOSIS & TYPICAL FEATURES

► Exposure to environmental allergens can affect primarily the nose and eyes, as they are major entry points, causing pruritus, mucus secretion or discharge, sneezing, irritation, and swelling.

► Although there is less threat of an acute major event, as seen with asthma and food- or drug-related reactions, the consequences of allergic rhinoconjunctivitis are certainly not trivial, especially when the symptoms occur chronically: sleep disturbance, poor school performance, uncontrolled asthma, sinusitis, and impaired quality of life.

► Similar to any allergic condition, avoidance of known triggers (determined from allergy skin testing or specific IgE antibody tests) is key. Pharmacologic chronic management can include systemic and topical antihistamines, mast cell stabilizers, topical corticosteroids, and LTRA.

► Immunotherapy, subcutaneous or oral, is recommended for more difficult to control disease.

Allergic rhinoconjunctivitis is the most common allergic disease and significantly affects quality of life as well as school performance and attendance. It frequently coexists with asthma, can impact asthma control, and is a risk factor for subsequent development of asthma. Over 80% of patients with asthma have rhinitis and 10%–40% of patients with rhinitis have asthma. About 80% of individuals with allergic rhinitis develop their symptoms before age 20 years. It is estimated that 13% of children have a physician diagnosis of allergic rhinitis. Prevalence of this disease increases during childhood, peaking at 15% in the post-adolescent years. Although allergic rhinoconjunctivitis is more common in boys during early childhood, there is little difference in incidence between the sexes after adolescence. Race and socioeconomic status are not considered to be important factors.

The pathologic changes in allergic rhinoconjunctivitis are chiefly hyperemia, edema, and increased serous and mucoid secretions caused by mediator release, all of which lead to variable degrees of nasal obstruction and conjunctival injection, nasal and ocular pruritus, or nasal and ocular discharge. Ocular allergies can occur in isolation, but more commonly, they are in conjunction with nasal symptoms. This process may involve other structures, including the sinuses and possibly the middle ear. Inhalant allergens are primarily responsible for symptoms, but food allergens can cause symptoms

as well. Children with allergic rhinitis seem to be more susceptible to—or at least may experience more symptoms from—upper respiratory infections, which, in turn, may aggravate the allergic rhinitis.

Allergic rhinoconjunctivitis has been classified according to temporal patterns, symptom frequency, and severity. Based on temporal pattern, it can be classified as perennial (usually caused by indoor allergens and year-round exposure to house dust mites, molds, cockroaches, and animal dander), or seasonal (hay fever most frequently caused by outdoor allergens such as pollens and molds), or episodic (from allergen exposure not usually encountered in the patient's home or environment such as visiting a home with pets not present in the child's home). The clinical limitation of this classification between seasonal or perennial allergic rhinitis occurs when polysensitized patients have both seasonal and perennial patterns. The classification of allergic rhinitis was revised by Allergic Rhinitis and its Impact on Asthma (ARIA) in 2001, based on symptom frequency. A major change was the introduction of the terms "intermittent" (ie, symptoms present < 4 days a week or for < 4 weeks) and "persistent" (ie, symptoms present > 4 days a week and for > 4 weeks). However, this classification has limitations in that some patients may have persistent symptoms with seasonal allergic rhinitis or intermittent symptoms with perennial allergic rhinitis. Severity classification is as follows: *mild* (ie, without impairment or disturbance of sleep, daily activities, leisure, sport, school, or work, or without troublesome symptoms) or *moderate-severe* (ie, presence of one or more of the aforementioned). The major pollen groups in the temperate zones include trees (late winter to early spring), grasses (late spring to early summer), and weeds (late summer to early fall), but seasons can vary significantly in different parts of the country. Mold spores also cause seasonal allergic rhinitis, principally in the summer and fall. Seasonal allergy symptoms may be aggravated by coincident exposure to perennial allergens.

► Clinical Findings

A. Symptoms and Signs

Patients may complain of itching of the nose, eyes, palate, or pharynx and loss of smell or taste. Nasal itching can cause paroxysmal sneezing and epistaxis. Repeated rubbing of the nose (so-called allergic salute) may lead to a horizontal crease across the lower third of the nose. Nasal obstruction is associated with mouth breathing, nasal speech, allergic salute, and snoring. Nasal turbinates may appear pale blue and swollen with dimpling or injected with minimal edema. Typically, clear and thin nasal secretions are increased, with anterior rhinorrhea, sniffling, postnasal drip, and congested cough. Nasal secretions often cause poor appetite, fatigue, and pharyngeal irritation. Conjunctival injection, tearing, periorbital edema, and infraorbital cyanosis (so-called allergic shiners) are frequently observed. Increased pharyngeal lymphoid tissue ("cobblestoning") from chronic drainage and enlarged tonsillar and adenoidal tissue may be present.

B. Laboratory Findings

Eosinophilia often can be demonstrated on smears of nasal secretions or blood. This is a frequent but nonspecific finding and may occur in nonallergic conditions. Although serum IgE may be elevated, measurement of total IgE is a poor screening tool owing to the wide overlap between atopic and nonatopic subjects. Skin testing to identify allergen-specific IgE is the most sensitive and specific test for inhalant allergies; alternatively, the Phadia ImmunoCAP assay, radioallergosorbent test (RAST), or other in vitro tests can be done for suspected allergens.

▶ Differential Diagnosis

Disorders that need to be differentiated from allergic rhinitis include infectious rhinosinusitis. Foreign bodies and structural abnormalities such as choanal atresia, marked septal deviation, nasal polyps, and adenoidal hypertrophy may cause chronic symptoms. Overuse of topical nasal decongestants may result in rhinitis medicamentosa (rebound congestion). The use of medications such as propranolol, clonidine, and some psychoactive drugs may cause nasal congestion. Illicit drugs such as cocaine can cause rhinorrhea. Spicy or hot foods may cause gustatory rhinitis. Nonallergic rhinitis with eosinophilia syndrome is usually not seen in young children. Vasomotor rhinitis is associated with persistent symptoms but without allergen exposure. Less common causes of symptoms that may be confused with allergic rhinitis include pregnancy, congenital syphilis, hypothyroidism, tumors, and cerebrospinal fluid rhinorrhea.

As in the differential diagnoses for allergic rhinitis, infectious conjunctivitis (secondary to viral, bacterial, or chlamydial etiology) can mimic allergic eye disorders. In this case, it typically develops in one eye first, and symptoms include stinging or burning sensation (rather than pruritus) with a foreign-body sensation and eye discharge (watery, mucoid, or purulent). Nasolacrimal duct obstruction, foreign body, blepharoconjunctivitis, dry eye, uveitis, and trauma are other masqueraders of ocular allergy.

The other conditions that comprise allergic eye diseases, presenting with bilateral conjunctivitis, include atopic keratoconjunctivitis, vernal conjunctivitis, and giant papillary conjunctivitis. Except for giant papillary conjunctivitis, the three (allergic conjunctivitis, atopic keratoconjunctivitis, and vernal conjunctivitis) are associated with allergic sensitization. Atopic keratoconjunctivitis and vernal conjunctivitis can cause vision impairment due to corneal damage including findings of conjunctivalization. Atopic keratoconjunctivitis is rarely seen before late adolescence, and it most commonly involves the lower tarsal conjunctiva. Ocular symptoms (itching, burning, and tearing) are more severe than in allergic conjunctivitis and persist all year round, with accompanying eyelid eczema with erythema and thick, dry scaling skin, which can extend to the periorbital skin and cheeks. Vernal conjunctivitis is characterized by giant papillae, described as cobblestoning, seen in the upper tarsal conjunctiva. It affects boys more often than girls, and patients of Asian and African descent are more predisposed. It affects individuals in temperate areas, with exacerbations in the spring and summer months. In addition to severe pruritus that can be exacerbated by exposure to irritants, light, or perspiration, other accompanying signs and symptoms include photophobia, foreign-body sensation, lacrimation, and presence of stringy or thick, ropey discharge, transient yellow-white points in the limbus (Trantas dots) and conjunctiva (Horner points), corneal "shield" ulcers, Dennie lines (prominent skin folds that extend in an arc form from the inner canthus beneath and parallel to the lower lid margin), and prominently long eyelashes. Giant papillary conjunctivitis is associated with exposure to foreign bodies such as contact lenses, ocular prostheses, and sutures. It is characterized by mild ocular itching, tearing, and mucoid discharge, especially on awakening. Trantas dots, limbal infiltration, bulbar injection, and edema may also be found. One eye condition, contact allergy, which can also involve the conjunctivae especially when associated with the use of topical medications, contact lens solutions, and preservatives, typically affects the eyelids.

▶ Complications

Sinusitis may accompany allergic rhinitis. Mucosal swelling of the sinus ostia can obstruct sinus drainage, interfering with normal sinus function, and predisposing to chronic mucosal disease. Symptoms of rhinosinusitis include nasal blockage/obstruction and/or nasal discharge/postnasal drip, facial pain/pressure, and/or reduction or loss of smell. The condition is considered acute if symptoms are less than 12 weeks and chronic when symptoms occur most days for at least 12 weeks. Rhinosinusitis can either be with (CRSwNP) or without nasal polyps (CRSsNP). Nasal polyps due to allergy are unusual in children, and other conditions such as cystic fibrosis or immunodeficiency should be considered if they are present. Unlike vision-threatening complications associated with atopic keratoconjunctivitis and vernal conjunctivitis, allergic conjunctivitis manifests primarily with significant pruritus and discomfort affecting the patient's quality of life.

▶ Treatment

A. General Measures

The value of identification and avoidance of causative allergens cannot be overstated. Reducing indoor allergens through environmental control measures as discussed in the section on asthma can be very effective. Nasal saline irrigation may be useful. For ocular allergies, cold compresses and lubrication are also important.

B. Pharmacologic Therapy

Evidence-based clinical practice guidelines such as the ARIA that include the pharmacologic management of allergic rhinitis have been developed. The ARIA initiative was initiated during a World Health Organization workshop in 1999 and updated in 2008. The ARIA 2010 revision was the first evidence-based guideline in allergy to follow the Grading of Recommendations, Assessment, Development, and Evaluation (GRADE) approach. The ARIA 2016 update, also used the GRADE methodology but focused only on three recommendations suggested by the ARIA panel members. A focused update on seasonal allergic rhinitis using GRADE was released in 2017. ARIA has developed a novel implementation strategy and communication technology system centered around the patient (adolescents and adults), MASK, which is freely available in Google Play and Apple Stores. It includes a medication list customized for each country, as well as VASs to assess rhinitis control and work productivity. Its most recent publication incorporates integrated care pathways and describes the process of next-generation guidelines for the treatment of allergic rhinitis. An algorithm, based on the Allergy Diary app from using a visual analogue scale, for initiating pharmacotherapy or stepping up or stepping down treatment based on control, is proposed (Figure 38–3).

The treatment of mild intermittent rhinitis includes oral or intranasal H_1-antihistamines and intranasal decongestants (for < 10 days and not to be repeated more than twice a month). Oral decongestants are not usually recommended in children. Options for moderate-severe intermittent rhinitis are oral or intranasal antihistamines, oral H_1-antihistamines and decongestants, intranasal corticosteroids, and cromones. The same medication options are available for persistent rhinitis, but a stepwise approach is proposed both for treatment of mild and moderate-severe persistent rhinitis. For mild persistent rhinitis, reassessment after 2–4 weeks is recommended and treatment should be continued, with a possible reduction in intranasal corticosteroids, even if the symptoms have abated. If, however, the patient has persistent mild symptoms while on H_1-antihistamines or cromones, an intranasal corticosteroid is appropriate. For moderate-severe persistent disease, use of intranasal corticosteroids as first-line therapy is recommended. For severe nasal congestion, either a short 1- to 2-week course of an oral corticosteroid or an intranasal decongestant for less than 10 days may be added. If the patient improves, the treatment should last for at least 3 months or until the pollen season is over. If the patient does not improve within 2–4 weeks despite adequate compliance and use of medications, comorbidities such as nasal polyps, sinusitis, and significant allergen exposure should be considered, as well as the possibility of misdiagnosis. Once these are ruled out, options include increasing the dose of the intranasal corticosteroid, combination therapy with an H_1-antihistamine (particularly if major symptoms are sneezing, itching, or rhinorrhea), ipratropium bromide (if major symptom is rhinorrhea), or an oral H_1-antihistamine and decongestant. Referral to a specialist may be considered if the treatment is not sufficient.

The 2016 ARIA update and the 2017 Seasonal Allergic Rhinitis (SAR) treatment update addressed several questions about comparative treatments for allergic rhinitis, based on new pieces of evidence, albeit obtained mostly from adult patients. The recommendations on these questions are mostly considered conditional, based on low to at best moderate certainty of evidence. One question is whether to use combination oral antihistamine and nasal steroid spray compared to nasal steroid spray alone for the treatment of allergic rhinitis. Either option is appropriate for seasonal allergic rhinitis, while nasal steroid spray alone may be adequate for perennial allergic rhinitis. The 2017 Seasonal Allergic Rhinitis (SAR) treatment update however concluded that in adolescent and adult patients, there is no clinical benefit of using a combination of an oral antihistamine and nasal corticosteroid compared with inhaled corticosteroid monotherapy. With regard to the use of nasal steroid with or without an intranasal antihistamine, either option for seasonal and perennial allergic rhinitis is also recommended. However, the combination of nasal steroid spray and intranasal antihistamine compared to intranasal antihistamine alone for seasonal rhinitis is favored. In addition, there seems to be a clinical benefit of using the combination of an intranasal antihistamine and nasal corticosteroid compared with nasal corticosteroid monotherapy based on symptom improvement for seasonal allergic rhinitis. The use of a nasal steroid spray is favored over an intranasal antihistamine for both seasonal and perennial allergic rhinitis (Table 38–8).

The preference of a LTRA versus an oral antihistamine or an intranasal corticosteroid was also evaluated. Based on the 2016 ARIA-focused update, either option is recommended for seasonal allergic rhinitis, while an oral antihistamine is suggested for perennial allergic rhinitis. According to the 2017 SAR Treatment update, in patients with SAR who are 15 years or older, intranasal corticosteroids have a greater clinical benefit over montelukast. Last, either intranasal or oral antihistamine for patients with seasonal or perennial allergic rhinitis can be used.

When a patient is already taking a nasal corticosteroid and is still symptomatic, the addition of an intranasal antihistamine, and not an oral antihistamine is preferred, although the rate of adverse effects with such combination is higher than with a nasal corticosteroid alone. With most of these, patient preferences, cost, and local availability are determinants of choice of medications. This systematic review and analysis report does not make any statements about oral antihistamines alone as initial treatment for SAR or about the treatment of perennial or mild seasonal allergic rhinitis. There is clearly a need for well-designed, nonbiased, appropriately powered pharmacotherapy studies, more so in

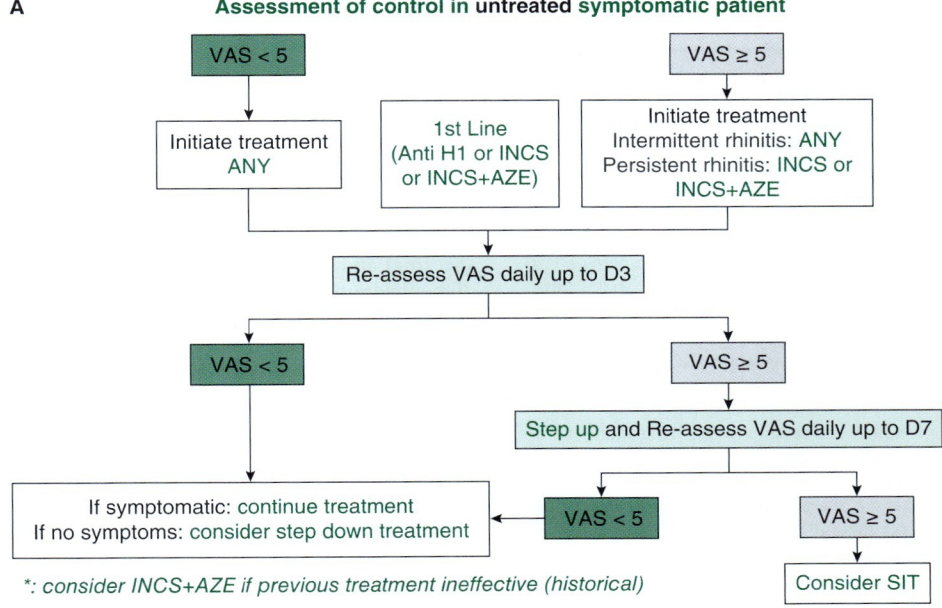

A   **Assessment of control in untreated symptomatic patient**

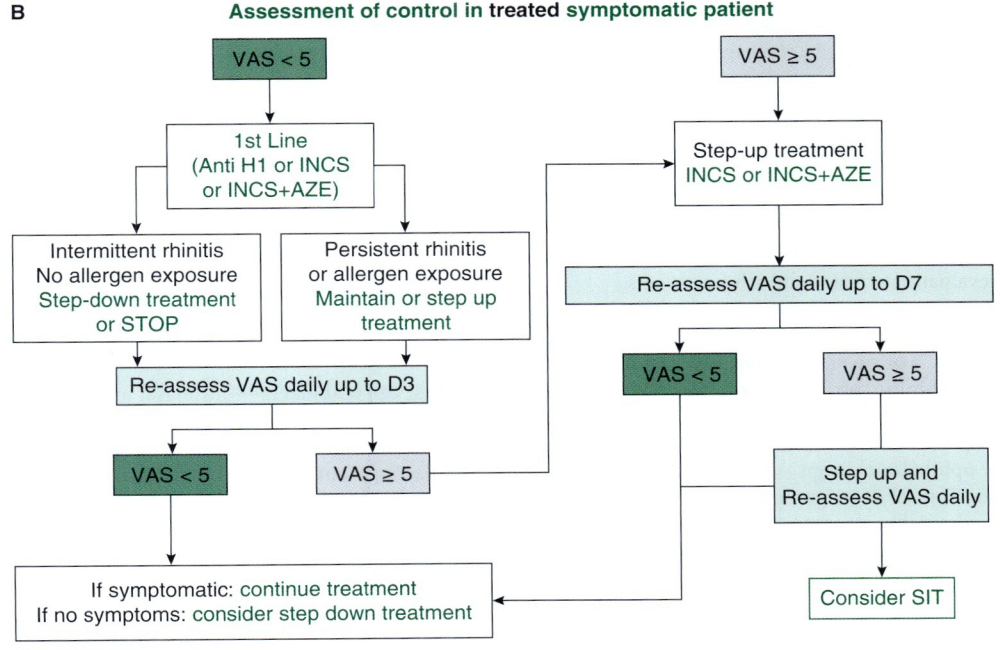

B   **Assessment of control in treated symptomatic patient**

Anti H1: Antihistamine
AZE: Azelastine
INCS: Intranasal corticosteroid
SIT: Subcutaneous immunotherapy

▲ **Figure 38–3.** Biologic therapy options for children and adolescents.

Table 38–8. Overall recommendations using GRADE.

ARIA 2016

1. In patients with seasonal allergic rhinitis, we suggest either a combination of intranasal corticosteroid + an oral antihistamine or intranasal corticosteroid alone, but the potential net benefit might not justify spending additional resources.
2. In patients with perennial allergic rhinitis, intranasal corticosteroids alone are recommended rather than a combination of an intranasal corticosteroid + an oral antihistamine.
3. In patients with seasonal allergic rhinitis, we suggest either a combination of an intranasal corticosteroid + an intranasal antihistamine or an intranasal corticosteroid alone, but the choice of treatment depends on patient preferences. At initiation of treatment (first 2 weeks), a combination of an intranasal corticosteroid + an intranasal antihistamine might act faster than an intranasal corticosteroid alone and might therefore be preferred by some patients. In settings in which the additional cost of combination therapy is not large, a combination therapy might be a reasonable choice.
4. In patients with perennial allergic rhinitis, we suggest either a combination of an intranasal corticosteroid + an intranasal antihistamine or an intranasal corticosteroid alone.

For all of these recommendations, the level of evidence was low or very low.

US practice parameters 2017

For initial treatment of nasal symptoms of seasonal allergic rhinitis in patients ≥ 12 years of age, clinicians:

- should routinely prescribe monotherapy with an intranasal corticosteroid rather than a combination of an intranasal corticosteroid and an oral H1-antihistamine or
- should recommend an intranasal corticosteroid over a leukotriene receptor antagonist (for ≥ 15 years of age).
- For moderate-to-severe symptoms, clinicians can recommend the combination of an intranasal corticosteroid and an intranasal antihistamine.

pediatrics, that include minimally important clinical differences when evaluating efficacy and adverse events.

For allergic rhinoconjunctivitis, topical nasal corticosteroids also reduce ocular symptoms, presumably through a naso-ocular reflex. For ocular allergies that persist or occur independent of rhinitis, pharmacologic treatment includes use of oral or topical antihistamines, topical decongestants, mast cell stabilizers, and anti-inflammatory agents. In general, topical ophthalmic drops should not be used with contact lenses. Topical decongestants relieve erythema, congestion, and edema but do not affect the allergic response. Combined therapy with an antihistamine and a vasoconstrictive agent is more effective than either agent alone. Topical medications with both antihistamine and mast cell blocking properties provide the most benefits that incorporate fast-acting symptom relief and anti-inflammatory action. Refrigerating ophthalmic drops before use can provide soothing relief as well. However, children can get wary of eye drops and prefer oral preparations. Avoiding contamination by preventing the applicator tip from touching the eye or eyelid

is important. Severe ocular allergy can be treated with topical, or rarely, oral corticosteroids. In such a case, a referral to an ophthalmologist is warranted, as these treatments can be associated with elevation of the intraocular pressure, viral infections, and cataract formation.

Allergen immunotherapy can be very effective in allergic rhinoconjunctivitis and may decrease the requirement for medications to control the symptoms in the long term.

1. Antihistamines—Antihistamines help control itching, sneezing, and rhinorrhea. Sedating antihistamines include diphenhydramine, chlorpheniramine, hydroxyzine, and clemastine. Sedating antihistamines may cause daytime somnolence and negatively affect school performance and other activities, especially driving. Second-generation antihistamines include loratadine, desloratadine, cetirizine, and fexofenadine. Cetirizine is approved for use in children aged 6–23 months (2.5 mg daily), 2–5 years (2.5–5.0 mg/day or 2.5 mg twice a day), and 6 years or older (5–10 mg/day). It is now available without a prescription. Loratadine is approved for use in children aged 2–5 years (5 mg/day) and 6 years or older (10 mg/day), and is available without prescription in tablet, rapidly disintegrating tablet, and liquid formulations. Desloratadine is approved for use in children aged 6–11 months (1 mg/day), 1–5 years (1.25 mg/day), and for 12 years and older (5 mg/day). Fexofenadine is approved for children aged 6–23 months (15 mg twice a day), 2–11 years (30 mg twice a day), and 12 years or older (60 mg twice a day or 180 mg once daily), and is also now available without a prescription. Levocetirizine (5 mg/day) is approved for children aged 6 years and older. Loratadine, fexofenadine, and cetirizine are available in combination with pseudoephedrine for patients aged 12 years or older, although regular use of these combination products is not recommended. Azelastine is available in nasal and ophthalmic formulations. Levocabastine and emedastine are available as ophthalmic preparations. They should not be used for treatment of contact lens-related irritation, and caution should be implemented with concomitant use of soft contact lenses.

2. Mast cell stabilizers—Intranasal ipratropium can be used as adjunctive therapy for rhinorrhea. Intranasal cromolyn may be used alone or in conjunction with oral antihistamines and decongestants. It is most effective when used prophylactically, one to two sprays per nostril, four times a day. This dose may be tapered if symptom control is achieved. Rarely, patients complain of nasal irritation or burning. Most patients find complying with four times–daily dosing difficult. Cromolyn is also available in an ophthalmic solution. It can be used to treat giant papillary and vernal conjunctivitis. Other ophthalmic mast cell stabilizers include lodoxamide 0.1% solution (can be used for vernal keratoconjunctivitis as well), one to two drops four times a day; nedocromil sodium 2%, one to two drops two times a day; and pemirolast potassium 0.1%, one to two drops four times a day.

3. Decongestants and vasoconstrictor agents—Nasal α-adrenergic agents help to relieve nasal congestion, and ophthalmic vasoconstrictors relieve ocular erythema, edema, and congestion. Topical nasal decongestants such as phenylephrine and oxymetazoline should not be used for more than 4 days for severe episodes because prolonged use may be associated with rhinitis medicamentosa, a condition of rebound nasal congestion. As with nasal decongestants, a rebound phenomenon (ie, conjunctivitis medicamentosa with hyperemia and stinging/burning) can occur with chronic use of ophthalmic vasoconstrictive agents such as naphazoline and tetrahydrozoline. Oral decongestants, including pseudoephedrine, phenylephrine, and phenylpropanolamine, are often combined with antihistamines or expectorants and cough suppressants in over-the-counter (OTC) cold medications, but there are no convincing data to support the use of oral decongestants for upper respiratory illnesses in children nor for regular use in patients with allergic rhinitis. They may cause insomnia, agitation, tachycardia, and, rarely, cardiac arrhythmias. Of note, the FDA has recommended the removal of phenylpropanolamine from all drug products due to a public health advisory concerning the risk of hemorrhagic stroke associated with its use.

4. Corticosteroids—Intranasal corticosteroid sprays are effective in controlling allergic rhinitis if used chronically. They are minimally absorbed in usual doses and are available in pressurized nasal inhalers and aqueous sprays. Mometasone and fluticasone furoate nasal sprays have been approved for use in children as young as age 2 years (one spray in each nostril once daily) and in children 12 years or older (two sprays/nostril once daily). Fluticasone propionate nasal spray is approved for children 4 years or older, and budesonide and triamcinolone nasal sprays are approved for those 6 years or older (one to two sprays/nostril once daily). Fluticasone propionate in an Optinose exhalation delivery system (Xhance®) is approved for the treatment of chronic rhinosinusitis with nasal polyps in patients 18 years of age or older. Flunisolide is approved for ages 6–14 years (one spray/nostril three times a day or two sprays/nostril twice a day). Ciclesonide is approved for seasonal allergic rhinitis in children 6 years and older and those with perennial allergic rhinitis for children 12 years and older, two sprays in each nostril once daily. Side effects include nasal irritation, soreness, and bleeding, although bleeding occurs commonly in patients with an allergic cause, if corticosteroids are used chronically. Rarely, these drugs can cause septal perforation. Excessive doses may produce systemic effects, especially if used together with orally inhaled steroids for asthma. Onset of action is within hours, although clinical benefit is usually not observed for a week or more. They may be effective alone or together with antihistamines. A combination nasal corticosteroid-antihistamine formulation spray has been found to be better than either agent alone in alleviating symptoms of moderate to severe seasonal allergic rhinitis.

Use of oral or topical (eg, loteprednol etabonate) corticosteroids for the treatment of ocular allergy should be worked out in conjunction with an ophthalmologist due to potential complications mentioned in the preceding section.

5. Other pharmacologic agents—Montelukast is approved for perennial allergic rhinitis in children aged 6 months and older (4 mg/day for ages 6–23 months) and seasonal allergic rhinitis in children 2 years and older in doses as discussed in section Pharmacologic Therapy under Treatment, Chronic Asthma. Oral antihistamines are also available in combination with a decongestant. Ketorolac, a nonsteroidal anti-inflammatory drug (NSAID), is available as an ophthalmic solution but should be avoided in patients with aspirin or NSAID sensitivity and should be used with caution in those with complicated eye surgeries, corneal denervation or epithelial defects, ocular surface diseases, diabetes mellitus, or rheumatoid arthritis. Combination ophthalmic preparations are available. Both antazoline and pheniramine are antihistamine/vasoconstrictor formulations. Olopatadine 0.1%, epinastine 0.05%, and ketotifen 0.025% ophthalmic solutions have antihistamine and mast cell-stabilizing actions and can be given to children older than 3 years as one drop twice a day (8 hours apart) for olopatadine and every 8–12 hours for ketotifen, respectively. Ketotifen fumarate 0.025% is now available as an OTC ophthalmic medication. Olopatadine 0.2% is the first once-daily ophthalmic medication available for the treatment of ocular pruritus associated with allergic conjunctivitis.

Biologic therapy (omalizumab, mepolizumab, and dupilumab) improves nasal symptoms and polyp size and has been approved for patients 18 years and older with CRSwNP.

C. Surgical Therapy

Surgical procedures, including turbinectomy, polypectomy, and functional endoscopic sinus surgery, are rarely indicated in allergic rhinitis or chronic hyperplastic sinusitis.

D. Immunotherapy

Allergen immunotherapy should be considered when symptoms are severe and due to unavoidable exposure to inhalant allergens, especially if symptomatic measures have failed. Immunotherapy is the only form of therapy that may alter the course of the disease. It should not be prescribed by sending the patient's serum to a laboratory where extracts based on in vitro tests are prepared for the patient (ie, the remote practice of allergy). Subcutaneous immunotherapy should be done in a facility where a physician prepared to treat anaphylaxis is present. Patients with concomitant asthma should not receive an injection if their asthma is not under good control (ie, peak flows preinjection are below 80% of personal best), and the patient should wait for

25–30 minutes after an injection before leaving the facility. Outcomes with single allergen immunotherapy show success rates of approximately 80%. The optimal duration of therapy is unknown, but data suggest that immunotherapy for 3–5 years may have lasting benefit.

Sublingual immunotherapy has been developed for treatment of allergic rhinitis caused by pollens in both adults and children and for allergic rhinitis caused by dust mites only in adults (in other countries). A recent specific SLIT practice parameter emphasized that this mode of immunotherapy may not be appropriate for patients with certain medical conditions, such as eosinophilic esophagitis and those that may hamper the patient's ability to deal with a systemic reaction or the treatment of the severe reaction.

There are no FDA-approved study indications for SLIT for oral allergy syndrome, food allergy, latex allergy, atopic dermatitis, or venom allergy. This mode of immunotherapy is attractive for pediatric patients because of convenience and ease. While there are off-label SLIT preparations (eg, liquid SCIT extract delivered sublingually, sublingual drops), there are only three FDA-approved sublingual immunotherapy tablets, all using a single allergen SLIT, as there are still no studies showing efficacy of multiple allergens in a mixture: Grastek, Ragwitek, and Oralair. Grastek may be prescribed for children (as young as 5 years) and adults who are allergic to timothy grass and cross-reactive pollens, while Ragwitek may be prescribed for persons 18 through 65 years of age who are allergic to ragweed pollen. Oralair is indicated for the treatment of grass pollen-induced allergic rhinitis with or without conjunctivitis, for any of five grass species: sweet vernal, orchard, perennial rye, timothy, and Kentucky blue grass, in patients 10–65 years old. They are recommended to be taken daily for about 12 weeks before and throughout the grass or ragweed pollens season, respectively, over a period of at least 3 years for sustained effects. Both timothy grass SLIT and 5-grass tablets have shown benefits beginning in the first year of treatment.

The first dose of SLIT should be in a supervised medical setting with much experience in the diagnosis and management of anaphylaxis, where patients can be observed closely for 30 minutes after taking the dose. Most systemic allergic reactions have been found to be with the first dose. Nevertheless, epinephrine should still be prescribed to patients receiving SLIT, and they should be trained when and how to use the device. Patients on SLIT should see an allergy specialist regularly for monitoring.

▶ Prognosis

Allergic rhinoconjunctivitis associated with sensitization to indoor allergens tends to be protracted unless specific allergens can be identified and eliminated from the environment. In seasonal allergic rhinoconjunctivitis, symptoms are usually most severe from adolescence through mid-adult life. After moving to a region devoid of problem allergens, patients may be symptom-free for several years, but they can develop new sensitivities to local aeroallergens.

Bousquet J et al: Next-generation Allergic Rhinitis and Its Impact on Asthma (ARIA) guidelines for allergic rhinitis based on Grading of Recommendations Assessment, Development and Evaluation (GRADE) and real-world evidence. J Allergy Clin Immunol 2020;145:70-80 [PMID: 31627910].

Brozek JL et al: Allergic Rhinitis and its Impact on Asthma (ARIA) guidelines—2016 revision. J Allergy Clin Immunol 2017 Oct; 140:950–958 [PMID: 28602936].

Cox L et al: Allergen immunotherapy: a practice parameter third update. J Allergy Clin Immunol 2011;127:S1 [PMID: 21122901].

Dykewicz MS et al: Treatment of seasonal allergic rhinitis: an evidence-based focused 2017 guideline update. Ann Allergy Asthma Immunol 2017 Dec;119(6):489–511.e41. doi: 10.1016/j.anai.2017.08.012 [Epub 2017 Nov 2] [PMID: 29103802].

Greenhawt M et al: Sublingual immunotherapy: a focused allergen immunotherapy practice parameter update. Ann Allergy Asthma Immunol 2017;118:276–282 [PMID: 28284533].

ATOPIC DERMATITIS

ESSENTIALS OF DIAGNOSIS & TYPICAL FEATURES

▶ Diagnosis of atopic dermatitis is based on the clinical features, including pruritus, a chronically relapsing course, and typical morphology and distribution of skin lesions.

▶ Patients with atopic dermatitis have increased susceptibility to infection or colonization with a variety of microbial organisms including *Staphylococcus aureus* and herpes simplex virus.

▶ Basics of skin care include avoidance of irritants and proven allergens along with appropriate skin hydration and use of a good-quality moisturizer.

▶ Topical corticosteroids are used as first-line therapy in patients requiring more than moisturizer; nonsteroidal treatments include crisaborole a topical phosphodiesterase 4 inhibitor approved in patients with mild-moderate atopic dermatitis 3 months or older and topical calcineurin inhibitors approved in patients 2 years or older for noncontinuous treatment, pimecrolimus cream for mild-moderate atopic dermatitis and tacrolimus ointment for moderate-severe atopic dermatitis.

▶ Biologic therapy approved for patients with moderate-to-severe atopic dermaincludes dupilumab, for ages 6 months and older and tralokinumab for 12 years and older.

▶ JAK inhibitors for patients 12 years and older include ruxolitinib cream for mild-moderate atopic dermatitis and abrocitinib and upadacitinib for oral treatment of moderate-severe atopic dermatitis.

Atopic dermatitis is a chronically relapsing inflammatory skin disease that typically presents in early childhood. Over one-third of patients with atopic dermatitis will develop asthma and/or allergic rhinitis. A subset of patients with atopic dermatitis has been shown to have mutations in the gene encoding filaggrin, a protein essential for normal epidermal barrier function. These patients have early-onset, more severe, and persistent disease. Mutations in filaggrin have also been associated with allergic sensitization as well as increased risk for asthma, but only in patients with atopic

dermatitis. Atopic dermatitis may result in significant morbidity, leading to school absenteeism, occupational disability, and emotional stress.

Clinical Findings

A. Symptoms and Signs

Atopic dermatitis has no pathognomonic skin lesions or laboratory parameters. Diagnosis is based on the clinical features, including pruritus, a chronically relapsing course, and typical morphology and distribution of the skin lesions (Figure 38–4). Acute atopic dermatitis is characterized by intensely pruritic, erythematous papules associated with excoriations, vesiculations, and serous exudate; subacute atopic dermatitis by erythematous, excoriated, scaling papules; and chronic atopic dermatitis by thickened skin with

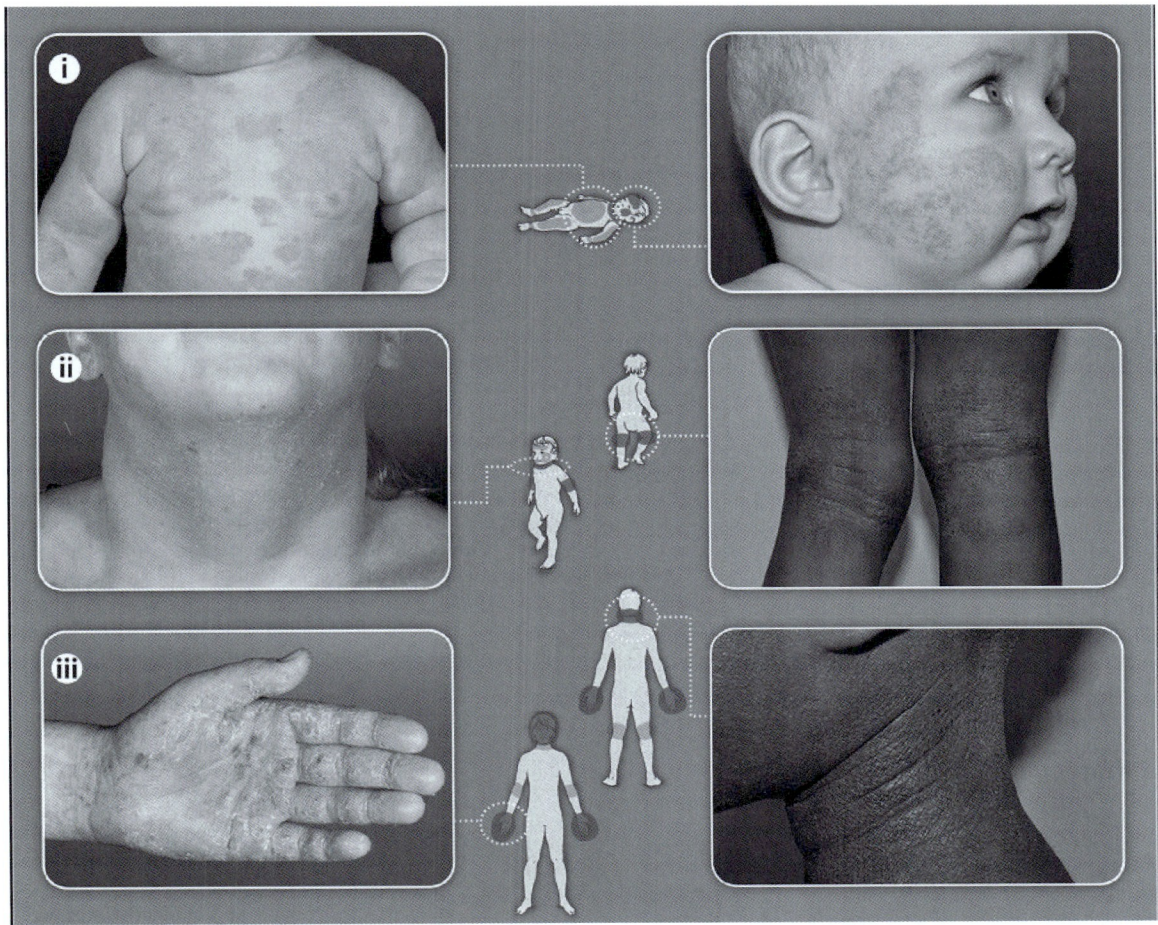

▲ Figure 38–4. Clinical presentation of atopic dermatitis in infants and children (Reproduced with permission from Langan SM, Irvine AD, Weidinger S: Atopic dermatitis. Lancet 2020 Aug 1;396(10247):345–360.)

accentuated markings (lichenification) and fibrotic papules. Patients with chronic atopic dermatitis may have all three types of lesions present concurrently. In skin of color, it may be difficult to appreciate erythema and associated inflammation. Patients usually have dry, xerotic skin. During infancy, atopic dermatitis involves primarily the face, scalp, and extensor surfaces of the extremities. The diaper area is usually spared. In older patients with long-standing disease, the flexural folds of the extremities are the predominant location of lesions, although this distribution can be seen even in infants.

B. Laboratory Findings

In patients with persistent disease despite appropriate treatment, consideration should be given for irritant, allergic, or infectious triggers. Elevated serum IgE levels can be demonstrated in 80%–85% of patients with atopic dermatitis but have little clinical utility, although they may be helpful in interpreting specific IgE tests. Identification of allergens involves taking a careful history and performing selective immediate hypersensitivity skin tests or in vitro tests when appropriate. Negative skin tests with proper controls have a high predictive value for ruling out a suspected allergen. Positive skin tests have a lower correlation with clinical symptoms in suspected food allergen–induced atopic dermatitis and should be confirmed with food challenges unless there is a coincidental history of anaphylaxis to the suspected food. Specific IgE levels determine probability of reaction, but not type of reaction or severity. Clinicians should avoid extensive testing, as results may reflect elevated total serum IgE with no clinical significance.

Exacerbation of atopic dermatitis can occur with exposure to aeroallergens such as house dust mites, and environmental control measures have been shown to result in clinical improvement. Patients can make specific IgE directed at *S aureus* toxins secreted on the skin. Peripheral blood eosinophilia is a common finding. Routine skin biopsy does not differentiate atopic dermatitis from other eczematous processes but may be helpful in atypical cases. Tests for the most common filaggrin gene mutations may identify patients who would be at increased risk for more severe, persistent atopic dermatitis and be more likely to develop allergic sensitizations and asthma. However, filaggrin gene mutations occur in individuals without atopic dermatitis.

▶ Differential Diagnosis

Scabies can present as a pruritic skin disease. However, distribution in the genital and axillary areas and the presence of linear lesions as well as skin scrapings may help to distinguish it from atopic dermatitis. Seborrheic dermatitis may be distinguished by a lack of significant pruritus, its predilection for the scalp (so-called cradle cap), and its coarse, yellowish scales. Allergic contact dermatitis may be suggested by the distribution of lesions with a greater demarcation of dermatitis than in atopic dermatitis. Allergic contact dermatitis superimposed on atopic dermatitis may appear as an acute flare of the underlying disease. Nummular eczema is characterized by coin-shaped plaques. Although unusual in children, mycosis fungoides or cutaneous T-cell lymphoma has been described and is diagnosed by skin biopsy. Eczematous rash has been reported in patients with human immunodeficiency virus (HIV) infection. Other disorders that may resemble atopic dermatitis include Wiskott-Aldrich syndrome, severe combined immunodeficiency disease, hyper-IgE syndrome, immunodeficiency with DOCK8 mutations, IPEX (immune dysregulation, polyendocrinopathy, enteropathy, X-linked) syndrome, zinc deficiency, phenylketonuria, and Letterer-Siwe disease (see Chapter 33).

▶ Complications

Ocular complications associated with atopic dermatitis can lead to significant morbidity. Atopic keratoconjunctivitis is always bilateral, and symptoms include itching, burning, tearing, and copious mucoid discharge. It is frequently associated with eyelid dermatitis and chronic blepharitis and may result in visual impairment from corneal scarring (see Chapter 16). Keratoconus in atopic dermatitis is believed to result from persistent rubbing of the eyes in patients with atopic dermatitis and allergic rhinitis. Anterior subcapsular cataracts may develop during adolescence or early adult life.

Patients with atopic dermatitis have increased susceptibility to infection or colonization with a variety of organisms. These include viral infections with herpes simplex, molluscum contagiosum, and human papillomavirus. Of note, even a history of atopic dermatitis is considered a contraindication for receiving smallpox (vaccinia) vaccine. Superimposed dermatophytosis may cause atopic dermatitis to flare. *S aureus* can be cultured from the skin of more than 90% of patients with atopic dermatitis, compared with only 5% of normal subjects. *S aureus* toxins can act as superantigens, contributing to persistent inflammation or exacerbations of atopic dermatitis. Community-acquired methicillin-resistant *S aureus* (MRSA) has become an increasing problem, especially in patients treated with frequent antibiotics. Although recurrent staphylococcal pustulosis can be a significant problem in atopic dermatitis, invasive *S aureus* infections occur rarely and should raise the possibility of an immunodeficiency.

Patients with atopic dermatitis often have nonspecific hand dermatitis. This is frequently irritant in nature and aggravated by repeated wetting.

Nutritional disturbances may result from unwarranted and extensive dietary restrictions imposed by providers or parents.

Poor academic performance and behavioral disturbances may be associated with uncontrolled itching, sleep loss, and poor self-image. Severe disease may lead to problems with social interactions and self-esteem.

▶ Treatment

A. General Measures

Avoidance of irritants such as detergents, chemicals, and abrasive materials as well as extremes of temperature and humidity is important. New clothing should be washed to reduce the content of formaldehyde and other chemicals. Because residual laundry detergent in clothing may be irritating, using a liquid rather than a powder detergent and adding an extra rinse cycle can be beneficial. Occlusive clothing should be avoided in favor of cotton or cotton blends. Temperature in the home should be controlled to minimize sweating. Swimming is usually well tolerated; however, patients should shower and use a mild cleanser to remove chemicals such as chlorine, and then apply a moisturizer. Sunlight may be beneficial in moderation, but nonsensitizing sunscreens should be used to avoid sunburn.

Avoidance of foods implicated in controlled challenges can lead to clinical improvement. Extensive elimination diets are almost never warranted. In addition, elimination of foods that a child is tolerating may result in immediate-type allergic reactions with future reintroduction. Environmental control measures (eg, dust mite–proof covers) in sensitized patients may improve atopic dermatitis.

Evaluation by a behavioral health clinician may be of benefit when dealing with a pruritic, relapsing disease. Relaxation, behavioral modification, or biofeedback training may help patients with habitual scratching. Patients with severe or disfiguring disease may require psychotherapy.

Clinicians should provide the patient and family with both general information and specific written skin care recommendations. The patient or parent should demonstrate an appropriate level of understanding to help ensure a good outcome. Educational pamphlets and a video about atopic dermatitis can be obtained from the National Eczema Association, a national nonprofit, patient-oriented organization, at: http://www.nationaleczema.org.

B. Hydration

Patients with atopic dermatitis have evaporative losses due to a defective skin barrier, so soaking the affected area or bathing for approximately 10 minutes in warm (not lukewarm) water, then applying an occlusive agent to retain the absorbed water, is an essential component of therapy. Oatmeal or baking soda added to the bath may feel soothing to certain patients but does not improve water absorption. Atopic dermatitis of the face or neck can be treated by applying a wet facecloth or towel to the involved area. The washcloth may be more readily accepted by a child if it is turned into a mask and also allows the older patient to remain functional (eg, reading during bath). Lesions limited to the hands or feet can be treated by soaking in a basin. Daily baths may be needed and increased to several times daily during flares of atopic dermatitis, while showers may be adequate for patients with mild disease. It is important to apply a topical moisturizer or medication within a few minutes after soaking the skin to prevent evaporation, which is both drying and irritating.

C. Moisturizers and Occlusives

An effective moisturizer combined with hydration therapy will help skin healing and can reduce the need for topical medications. Moisturizers are available as lotions, creams, and ointments. Lotions can be drying because of their evaporative effect, especially in a nonhumid climate. Preservatives and fragrances in lotions and creams may cause skin irritation. Moisturizers often need to be applied several times daily on a long-term basis and should be obtained in the largest size available. Crisco shortening can be substituted as an inexpensive alternative. Petroleum jelly (Vaseline) is an effective occlusive agent when used to seal in water after bathing. There are several topical nonsteroidal creams (eg, EpiCeram) approved as medical devices (thus, currently requiring prescriptions) for relief and management of signs and symptoms of dermatoses. Their potential benefits need to be weighed against their cost.

D. Corticosteroids

Corticosteroids reduce the inflammation and pruritus in atopic dermatitis. Topical corticosteroids can decrease *S aureus* colonization. Systemic corticosteroids, including oral prednisone, should be avoided in the management of this chronic relapsing disease as the rapid clinical improvement may be associated with an equally dramatic disease flaring following discontinuation. Topical corticosteroids are available in a variety of formulations and range in potency, ranging from extremely high- to low-potency preparations (see Table 15–2). Choice of a particular product depends on the severity and distribution of skin lesions. Patients need to be counseled regarding the potency of their corticosteroid preparation and its potential side effects. In general, the least potent agent that is effective should be used. However, choosing a preparation that is too weak may result in persistence or worsening of the atopic dermatitis. Side effects include thinning of the skin, telangiectasias, bruising, hypopigmentation, acne, and striae, although these occur infrequently when low- to medium-potency topical corticosteroids are used appropriately. In contrast, use of potent topical corticosteroids for prolonged periods—especially under occlusion—may result in atrophic changes or rarely systemic side effects. The face (especially the eyelids) and intertriginous areas are especially sensitive to corticosteroid side effects, and only low-potency preparations should be used routinely on these areas. Perioral dermatitis may occasionally be worsened by use of topical steroids. Because topical corticosteroids are commercially available in a variety of bases, including ointments, creams, lotions, oil, solutions, gels, foams, and even tape, there is no need to compound them. Ointments are most occlusive and, in general, provide better delivery of the medication while preventing evaporative losses. However, in a humid environment, creams may be better tolerated than ointments because the increased occlusion may cause itching or even folliculitis. Lotions, while easier to spread, can contribute to skin dryness and irritation. Solutions can be used on the scalp and hirsute areas, although they can sting or be irritating, especially to open lesions so an oil or foam base may be preferred. With clinical improvement, a less potent corticosteroid should be prescribed and the frequency of use decreased. Topical corticosteroids can be discontinued when inflammation resolves, but hydration and moisturizers need to be continued. In patients with a relapsing course, twice-weekly treatment to previously involved, clear or almost clear skin can be done as proactive therapy (off-label in the United States). Several topical steroids including alclometasone 0.05%, desonide 0.05% hydrogel, and fluticasone 0.05% cream have been approved in infants as young as 3 months of age for up to 28 days. Undertreatment remains a common problem due to caregiver concerns about potential side effects of topical corticosteroids along with inadequate prescription size.

E. Topical Calcineurin Inhibitors

Tacrolimus and pimecrolimus are nonsteroidal immunomodulatory agents that are available in topical formulations. Tacrolimus ointment—0.03% for children 2–15 years of age and 0.1% for older patients—is approved for twice-daily short-term and intermittent long-term use in moderate to severe atopic dermatitis. Pimecrolimus 1% cream is approved for patients 2 years of age or older who have mild to moderate atopic dermatitis. Local burning at the site of application has been the most common side effect, although this is usually a transient problem. As a precaution, patients should wear sunscreen with these medications. In Europe, tacrolimus ointment is approved as twice-weekly maintenance therapy for patients 2 years and older with a relapsing course after clearing up eczema with reevaluation of need for continued therapy after 12 months.

Although there is no evidence of a causal link between the use of topical calcineurin inhibitors and malignancy, in 2006, the FDA issued a boxed warning for these medications because of a lack of long-term safety data (see US package inserts for Elidel [Valeant] and Protopic [Leo]). In the United States, labeling states that these drugs are recommended as second-line treatment for short-term and noncontinuous chronic treatment and that their use in children younger than 2 years is currently not recommended. Long-term surveillance registries have been established for pediatric patients who had been treated with both topical tacrolimus and pimecrolimus.

F. PDE4 Inhibitors

Crisaborole 2% ointment has been approved in patients 3 months or older for mild to moderate atopic dermatitis. Reports of significant stinging or burning with application are common.

G. Systemic Biologics

Dupilumab is a fully human monoclonal antibody that blocks interleukin-4 receptor alpha through which both IL-4 and IL-13, two key type 2 cytokines, signal. It is approved for patients 6 months and older with moderate to severe atopic dermatitis not adequately controlled with topical medications or when those are not appropriate. In patients < 18 years, dosing is weight based by subcutaneous injection and for patients 60 kg or more, 600 mg initial dose, then 300 mg every 2 weeks, patients 30 kg to < 60 kg, 400 mg, then 200 mg every 2 weeks, 15 kg to < 30 kg, 600 mg, then 300 mg every 4 weeks. Patients 6 months to < 6 years 15 kg to < 30 kg receive 300 mg every 4 weeks without a loading dose, those 5 kg to < 15 kg, 200 mg every 4 weeks without a loading dose. Injections can be self-administered at home and currently, there is no requirement for any laboratory monitoring. For patients 2 years and older, dupilumab can also be administered by a pre-filled pen. Injection site reactions and conjunctivitis have been the most reported adverse events. Tralokinumab is a monoclonal antibody that targets IL-13, currently approved for moderate-to-severe atopic dermatitis in patients 12 years or older whose disease is not adequately controlled with topical prescription therapies or when those therapies are not advisable. The initial loading dose is 300 mg, followed by a 150 mg dose every 2 weeks by subcutaneous injection.

H. Janus Kinase (JAK) Inhibitors

A number of cytokines implicated in the pathophysiology of atopic dermatitis signal through the JAK-STAT pathway. JAK inhibitors are small molecules that act intracellularly. Topical ruxolitinib is a JAK 1/2 inhibitor approved for use in nonimmunocompromised patients 12 years and older with mild to moderate atopic dermatitis whose disease is not adequately controlled with topical prescription therapies or when those therapies are not advisable. It has an indication for short-term and noncontinuous chronic treatment applied twice daily up to 20% body surface area, no more than 60 g/wk. Laboratory monitoring is optional. Two oral JAK 1 inhibitors are approved in patients 12 years and older with moderate to severe atopic dermatitis when disease is not adequately controlled with other systemic therapies. Abrocitinib is dosed 100 mg QD and 200 mg QD if inadequate response after 12 weeks. Upadacitinib is dosed 15 mg once daily (patients weighing at least 40 kg) and may be increased to 30 mg once daily if an adequate response is not achieved. Patients treated with oral JAK inhibitors need to be educated on the boxed warning and have appropriate screening and laboratory monitoring performed.

I. Anti-Infective Therapy

Systemic antibiotic therapy may be important when treating atopic dermatitis secondarily infected with *S aureus*. For limited areas of involvement, a topical antibiotic such as mupirocin or retapamulin ointment may be effective. A first- or second-generation cephalosporin or semisynthetic penicillin is usually the first choice for oral therapy, as erythromycin-resistant organisms are common. Overuse may result in colonization by MRSA. Dilute bleach baths (6% sodium hypochlorite, ½ cup in a full tub of water) two times per week may be helpful for patients with atopic dermatitis, especially those with recurrent skin infections, although some patients find this treatment irritating.

Disseminated eczema herpeticum usually requires treatment with systemic antiviral. Patients with recurrent cutaneous herpetic lesions can be given prophylactic oral acyclovir or valacyclovir. Superficial dermatophytosis and *Malassezia sympodialis* infection can be treated with topical or (rarely) systemic antifungal agents.

J. Antipruritic Agents

Pruritus is usually the least well-tolerated symptom of atopic dermatitis. Oral antihistamines and anxiolytics may be effective owing to their tranquilizing and sedating effects and can be taken primarily at bedtime to avoid daytime somnolence. Nonsedating antihistamines may be helpful for associated allergic symptoms but are not usually effective in treating pruritus. Use of topical antihistamines and local anesthetics should be avoided because of potential sensitization.

K. Recalcitrant Disease

Erythrodermic patients may need to be hospitalized. Hospitalization may also be appropriate for those with severe disease failing outpatient management. Marked clinical improvement often occurs when the patient is removed from environmental allergens or stressors. In the hospital, adherence to therapy can be monitored, the patient and family can receive in-depth hands-on education, and controlled challenges can be conducted to help identify triggering factors.

Wet wrap therapy has been shown to be beneficial in severe atopic dermatitis. It can serve as an effective barrier against the persistent scratching that often undermines therapy. A layer of wet clothing (eg, pajamas, long underwear, tube socks) with dry layer on top (pajamas or a sweat suit, tube socks) over topical corticosteroid can be used for severely involved areas. Alternatively, wet gauze with a layer of dry gauze over it can be used and secured in place with an elastic bandage. Wet wraps can be removed when they dry out, usually after several hours, and are often best tolerated at bedtime. They should be considered an acute, not chronic intervention as overuse can result in chilling, skin maceration, or secondary infection.

Systemic immunosuppressive drugs including cyclosporine, methotrexate, mycophenolate, and azathioprine have been used in recalcitrant disease but are not approved for treatment of children with atopic dermatitis. Limited published data are available on use of cyclosporine in children treated with both continuous and intermittent therapy (5 mg/kg daily) for up to 1 year. Patients treated with this agent should have their dose titrated to the lowest effective dose after the disease is brought under control with appropriate monitoring, under the care of a specialist familiar with the drug. Ultraviolet light therapy approved for patients 12 years or older can be useful in a subset of patients under the supervision of a dermatologist.

L. Allergen Immunotherapy

Subcutaneous desensitization to dust mite allergen has been shown to improve atopic dermatitis in adult patients and sublingual desensitization in dust mite allergic children showed benefit in mild to moderate atopic dermatitis. A recent systematic review and meta-analysis found that allergen immunotherapy can improve atopic dermatitis severity and quality of life.

M. Experimental and Unproved Therapies

Treatment of atopic dermatitis with omalizumab and high-dose intravenous immunoglobulin has not shown consistent benefit. Although disturbances in the metabolism of essential fatty acids have been reported in patients with atopic dermatitis, controlled trials with fish oil and evening primrose have shown no clinical benefit.

N. Prevention

Studies of different hydrolyzed formulas, probiotics, and prebiotics have yielded inconsistent results. While preliminary studies suggested a beneficial effect with application of a moisturizer in high-risk infants from birth, recent large-scale studies did not show this benefit.

▶ Prognosis

While many children, especially those with mild disease will outgrow their atopic dermatitis, patients with filaggrin gene mutations are more likely to have more persistent and severe disease. In addition, these patients appear to be the ones at greater risk for developing asthma and allergic sensitizations.

AAAAI/ACAAI JTF Atopic Dermatitis Guideline Panel et al: Atopic dermatitis (eczema) guidelines: 2023 American Academy of Allergy, Asthma and Immunology/American College of Allergy, Asthma and Immunology Joint Task Force on Practice Parameters GRADE- and Institute of Medicine-based recommendations. Ann Allergy Asthma Immunol 2024;132:274 [PMID: 38108679].

Boguniewicz M et al: Atopic dermatitis yardstick update. Ann Allergy Asthma Immunol 2023;130:811 [PMID: 36931465].

URTICARIA & ANGIOEDEMA

ESSENTIALS OF DIAGNOSIS & TYPICAL FEATURES

▶ Urticaria and angioedema are caused by mast cell degranulation in the skin.

▶ The acute form (< 6 weeks duration) is most commonly caused by viral infections in children. Allergies to foods or drugs are other causes.

▶ Types of chronic urticaria (> 6 weeks duration) include chronic spontaneous urticaria, physical/inducible urticaria, and autoimmune urticaria.

▶ Testing is not indicated for chronic spontaneous urticaria.

▶ First-line treatment is the use of second-generation H₁-antihistamines, which can be given up to four times the standard dose.

▶ Omalizumab has been effective for antihistamine-refractory urticaria.

Table 38–9. Types/Causes of histamine-mediated urticaria/angioedema.

Acute Urticaria
  Infections
    Viral (picornavirus and many other common viruses, hepatitis A/B)
    Bacterial (*Mycoplasma*, *Helicobacter*, UTI)
    Parasitic (associated with eosinophilia)
  Allergies
    foods, food with exercise, drugs, latex, venoms
Chronic Urticaria
  Recurrent spontaneous
  Physical/Inducible
    Friction, radiation (solar), pressure, cold, heat, sweat (cholinergic), water, or vibration
  Autoimmunity

Urticaria and angioedema are common dermatologic conditions, with an incidence of 3%–6% in children. Urticarial lesions are arbitrarily designated as acute, lasting less than 6 weeks, or chronic, lasting more than 6 weeks. It is also classified by trigger: allergic, physical/inducible, infectious, autoimmune, or spontaneous/idiopathic. Note that bradykinin-mediated hereditary angioedema is discussed in the immunodeficiency chapter (see Chapter 33).

The pathophysiology of urticaria and angioedema involves the release of vasoactive mediators by dermal mast cells and basophils. Mast cell activation and degranulation can be triggered by different stimuli, allergic and nonallergic, such as cross-linking of Fc receptor-bound IgE by allergens or anti-FcεRI antibodies, complement anaphylatoxins (C3a, C5a), radiocontrast dyes, and physical stimuli.

Causes are identified more often in acute urticaria. Infections or the immune response to infections cause acute urticaria in the majority of pediatric patients, while allergic causes are less common. Allergic etiologies can be considered if the onset of urticaria was immediate after exposure and if exposure consistently causes symptoms. In chronic spontaneous urticaria, causes are not identified, although there can be exacerbating factors (infections, stress, heat, NSAIDs) Table 38–9.

Dermatographism is the most common form of physical/inducible urticaria, affecting up to 4% of the population and occurring at skin sites subjected to mechanical stimuli. Cold-induced urticaria or angioedema is triggered by decreased ambient temperature or as the skin is warmed following direct cold contact. Cholinergic urticaria occurs after increases in core body and skin temperatures, typically with bathing, exercise, or fever. The eruption appears as small punctate wheals surrounded by extensive areas of erythema. In pressure urticaria/angioedema, red, deep, painful swelling occurs immediately or 4–6 hours after the skin has been exposed to pressure.

▶ Clinical Findings

A. Symptoms and Signs

Urticaria manifests as wheals with reflex erythema that are pruritic. They resolve within 24 hours without any change to the skin. Angioedema is rapid erythematous or skin-colored swelling that is associated with burning or pain more than pruritus. Allergic etiologies, cold-induced, and cholinergic urticaria can be associated with anaphylaxis.

B. Diagnostic Evaluation

Testing is selected based on the history and physical findings. If the history is suggestive of an allergic etiology, then allergy testing can be performed. Specific tests for inducible urticarias, such as an ice cube test, pressure test, or intradermal injection of methacholine can be performed. In chronic spontaneous urticaria, evaluation has rarely been helpful in management; therefore, diagnostic tests should be limited. If by history, there is concern for underlying disease, a complete blood count, erythrocyte sedimentation rate, biochemistry panel, or antithyroid antibodies could be considered. If the history or appearance of the urticarial lesions suggests vasculitis, a skin biopsy for immunofluorescence is indicated.

▶ Differential Diagnosis

Urticarial lesions are usually easily recognized—the major dilemma is the etiologic diagnosis. Lesions of urticarial vasculitis typically last for more than 24 hours and are tender. Urticaria associated with serum sickness-like reaction and urticaria multiforme typically also have a longer duration. Urticaria Pigmentosa is associated with hyperpigmented macules and patches that urticate when scratched or rubbed (Darier Sign). "Papular urticaria" is a term used to characterize multiple papules from insect bites, found especially on the extremities, and is not true urticaria. Angioedema can be distinguished from other forms of edema because it is transient, asymmetrical, and nonpitting and does not occur predominantly in dependent areas. Hereditary angioedema is a rare autosomal dominant disorder caused by a quantitative or functional deficiency of C1-esterase inhibitor and characterized by episodic, frequently severe, nonpruritic angioedema of the skin, gastrointestinal tract, or upper respiratory tract (discussed in Chapter 33). Rare autoinflammatory disorders with urticaria or urticaria-vasculitic-like lesions include cold-induced autoinflammatory syndrome, Muckle-Wells syndrome, and Schnitzler syndrome. Melkersson-Rosenthal Syndrome is a rare disorder causing facial paralysis, facial edema (upper lip most commonly), and tongue folds and fissures.

Treatment

A. General Measures

The most effective treatment for allergic and inducible urticarias is identification and avoidance of the exacerbating factors or triggers. In the setting of chronic spontaneous urticaria, patients should be reassured that it is not from an allergy, there is no risk for anaphylaxis, it typically resolves over time, and treatment is directed at managing symptoms, as there is no "cure." Epinephrine autoinjectors should also be considered for those with severe cold-induced and cholinergic urticaria because of the risk of anaphylaxis.

B. First-line Pharmacologic Management

For the majority of patients, oral second-generation H_1-antihistamines are the mainstay of therapy. Antihistamines are more effective when given prophylactically rather than after lesions appear. Second-generation H_1-antihistamines (discussed previously under Allergic Rhinoconjunctivitis) are long acting, are non- or minimally sedating at usual dosing levels, and lack anticholinergic effects. If refractory at the recommended dose, second-line treatment is increasing the dose up to fourfold. Sedating first-generation antihistamines may be added in the evening if needed. There is conflicting evidence for the efficacy of adding H_2-antihistamines or montelukast.

For an acute, refractory exacerbation that is particularly angioedema-dominant, a short course of an oral corticosteroid can be considered.

C. Other Pharmacologic Agents

Third-line treatment for chronic spontaneous urticaria is the addition of omalizumab. Omalizumab has been demonstrated to be effective in antihistamine-resistant urticaria in a double-blind placebo-controlled trial and in case series in patients younger than 12 years. It obtained FDA approval for chronic urticaria in patients 12 years old or older in 2014. Dosing is 150 mg or 300 mg subcutaneously every 4 weeks. In the case of omalizumab failure, treatment with cyclosporine can be considered. Other biologic therapies for refractory urticaria/angioedema are currently being studied in clinical trials, including anti-IL-5, anti-IL-4Rα, anti-IL-17, anti-IL-1, anti-TSLP, and therapies targeting intracellular signaling pathways and surface inhibitory molecules.

Prognosis

Spontaneous remission of urticaria and angioedema is typical, but some patients have a prolonged course, especially those with inducible or autoimmune urticaria. Reassurance is important because this disorder can cause significant frustration. Periodic follow-up is indicated, particularly for patients with development of noncutaneous symptoms, to monitor for possible underlying cause.

Kolkhir P et al: Urticaria. Nat Rev Dis Primers 2022;8(1):61 [PMID: 36109590].
Maurer M et al: Biologics for the use in chronic spontaneous urticaria: when and which. J Allergy Clin Immunol Pract 2021;9(3):1067-1078 [PMID: 33685605].

ANAPHYLAXIS

ESSENTIALS OF DIAGNOSIS & TYPICAL FEATURES

► A clinical history of rapid onset of skin-mucosal tissue (urticaria, angioedema), respiratory compromise, hypotension, and/or GI symptoms after exposure to a common trigger is the key for proper diagnosis.

► Epinephrine is the treatment of choice for anaphylaxis, along with other secondary life-supportive measures.

► Prevention of future episodes of anaphylaxis by strict avoidance of known triggers, along with education regarding carrying and proper usage of an epinephrine autoinjector, is essential for patient management.

Considerations

Anaphylaxis is an acute life-threatening clinical syndrome that occurs when large quantities of inflammatory mediators are rapidly released from mast cells and basophils after exposure to an allergen in a previously sensitized patient. Anaphylactoid reactions mimic anaphylaxis but are not mediated by IgE antibodies; they may be mediated by anaphylatoxins such as C3a or C5a or through nonimmune mast cell degranulating agents. Idiopathic anaphylaxis has no recognized external cause. The clinical history is the most important tool in making the diagnosis of anaphylaxis.

Clinical Findings

A. Symptoms and Signs

The history is the most important tool to determine whether a patient has had anaphylaxis. The symptoms and signs of anaphylaxis depend on the organs affected. Onset typically occurs within minutes after exposure to the offending agent and can be short-lived, protracted, or biphasic, with recurrence after several hours despite treatment.

Anaphylaxis is highly likely when any one of the following three criteria is fulfilled:

1. Acute onset of an illness (minutes to several hours) with involvement of the skin, mucosal tissue, or both (eg, generalized hives, pruritus or flushing, swollen lips-tongue-uvula) *and at least one of the following*:
   a. Respiratory compromise (eg, dyspnea, wheeze, bronchospasm, stridor, reduced peak expiratory flow, hypoxemia)
   b. Reduced blood pressure or associated symptoms of end-organ dysfunction (eg, hypotonia [collapse], syncope, incontinence)

2. Two or more of the following that occur rapidly after exposure to a *likely* allergen for that patient (minutes to several hours):
   a. Involvement of the skin-mucosal tissue (eg, generalized urticaria, itch-flush, swollen lips-tongue-uvula)
   b. Respiratory compromise (eg, dyspnea, wheeze, bronchospasm, stridor, reduced PEFR, hypoxemia)
   c. Reduced blood pressure or associated symptoms (eg, hypotonia [collapse], syncope, incontinence)
   d. Persistent gastrointestinal symptoms (eg, crampy abdominal pain, vomiting)

3. Reduced blood pressure after exposure to a *known* allergen for that patient (minutes to several hours):
   a. Infants and children: low systolic blood pressure (age specific) or greater than 30% decrease in systolic pressure
   b. Low systolic blood pressure in children, defined as less than 70 mm Hg in those aged from 1 month to 1 year, less than (70 mm Hg + [2 × age]) in those 1–10 years of age, and less than 90 mm Hg in those 11–17 years

B. Laboratory Findings

An absence of laboratory findings does not rule out anaphylaxis. Tryptase released by mast cells can be measured in the serum within 3 hours of onset of the reaction and may be helpful when the diagnosis of anaphylaxis is in question. However, tryptase levels are often normal, particularly in individuals with food-induced anaphylaxis. Electrocardiographic abnormalities may include ST-wave depression, bundle branch block, and various arrhythmias. Arterial blood gases may show hypoxemia, hypercapnia, and acidosis. The chest radiograph may show hyperinflation.

Differential Diagnosis

Although shock may be the only sign of anaphylaxis, other diagnoses should be considered, especially in the setting of collapse without typical allergic findings. Other causes of shock along with cardiac arrhythmias must be assessed; respiratory failure associated with asthma may be confused with anaphylaxis. Mastocytosis, hereditary angioedema, scombroid fish poisoning, vasovagal reactions, inducible laryngeal obstruction, and anxiety attacks may cause symptoms mistaken for anaphylaxis.

Complications

Depending on the organs involved and the severity of the reaction, complications may vary from none to aspiration pneumonitis, acute tubular necrosis, bleeding diathesis, or sloughing of the intestinal mucosa. With irreversible shock, heart and brain damage can be terminal. Risk factors for fatal or near-fatal anaphylaxis include age (adolescents and young adults), reactions to peanut or tree nuts, associated asthma, strenuous exercise, and use of medications such as β-blockers.

Prevention

Strict avoidance of the causative agent is extremely important, and an effort to determine its cause should be made, beginning with a thorough history. Typically, there is a strong temporal relationship between exposure and onset of symptoms. With exercise-induced anaphylaxis, patients should be instructed to exercise with another person and to stop exercising at the first sign of symptoms. If prior ingestion of food has been implicated, eating within 4 hours—perhaps up to 12 hours—before exercise should be avoided. Patients with a history of anaphylaxis should carry epinephrine for self-administration, preferably in the form of an autoinjector (eg, Auvi-Q or EpiPen in 0.15- and 0.3-mg doses), and they and all caregivers should be instructed on its use. They should also carry an oral antihistamine such as diphenhydramine or cetirizine, preferably in liquid or chewable preparation to hasten absorption, but epinephrine should be considered as the first-line treatment of anaphylaxis. Patients with idiopathic anaphylaxis may require prolonged treatment with oral corticosteroids. Specific measures for dealing with food, drug, latex, and insect venom allergies as well as radio-contrast media reactions are discussed in the next sections.

Treatment

A. General Measures

Anaphylaxis is a medical emergency that requires rapid assessment and treatment. Exposure to the triggering agent should be discontinued. Airway patency should be maintained, and blood pressure and pulse monitored. Simultaneously and promptly, emergency medical services or a call for help to a resuscitation team should be made. The patient should be placed in a supine position with the legs elevated unless precluded by shortness of breath or emesis. Oxygen should be delivered by mask or nasal cannula with pulse oximetry monitoring. If the reaction is secondary to a sting or injection into an extremity, a tourniquet may be applied proximal to the site, briefly releasing it every 10–15 minutes.

B. Epinephrine

Epinephrine is the treatment of choice for anaphylaxis. Epinephrine 1:1000, 0.01 mg/kg to a maximum of 0.5 mg in adults and 0.3 mg in children, should be injected intramuscularly in the midanterolateral thigh without delay. This dose may be repeated at intervals of 5–15 minutes as necessary for controlling symptoms and maintaining blood pressure. There is no precisely established dosing regimen for intravenous epinephrine in anaphylaxis, but a 5–10 µg intravenous bolus for hypotension and 0.1–0.5 mg intravenously for cardiovascular collapse have been suggested.

C. Antihistamines

Diphenhydramine, an H_1-blocker, 1–2 mg/kg up to 50 mg, can be given orally, intramuscularly, or intravenously. Intravenous antihistamines should be infused over a period of 5–10 minutes to avoid inducing hypotension. Alternatively in young patients, cetirizine 0.25 mg/kg to a maximum dose of 10 mg could be given orally, as it was shown to have a longer duration of action and reduced sedation profile. Addition of ranitidine, an H_2-blocker, 1 mg/kg up to 50 mg intravenously, may be more effective than an H_1-blocker alone, especially for hypotension, but histamine blockers should be considered second-line treatment for anaphylaxis.

D. Fluids

Treatment of persistent hypotension despite epinephrine requires restoration of intravascular volume by fluid replacement, initially with a crystalloid solution, 20–30 mL/kg in the first hour.

E. Bronchodilators

Nebulized β_2-agonists such as albuterol 0.5% solution, 2.5 mg (0.5 mL) diluted in 2–3 mL saline, or levalbuterol, 0.63 mg or 1.25 mg, may be useful for reversing bronchospasm.

Intravenous methylxanthines are generally not recommended because they provide little benefit over inhaled β_2-agonists and may contribute to toxicity.

F. Corticosteroids

Although corticosteroids do not provide immediate benefit, when given early they may prevent protracted or biphasic anaphylaxis, although data are limited regarding this. Intravenous methylprednisolone, 50–100 mg (adult) or 1 mg/kg, maximum 50 mg (child), can be given every 4–6 hours. Oral prednisone, 1 mg/kg up to 50 mg, might be sufficient for less severe episodes. A single dose of oral steroids is sufficient if given; further doses of oral corticosteroids are not indicated for an acute episode of anaphylaxis.

G. Vasopressors

Hypotension refractory to epinephrine and fluids should be treated with intravenous vasopressors such as noradrenaline, vasopressin, or dopamine (see Chapter 14).

H. Observation

The necessity to call 911 and observe all patients in an acute care setting after epinephrine use in anaphylaxis has become a matter of debate, as most patients do not require further treatment after initial management of anaphylaxis with epinephrine and a H_1-blocker. Patients with severe anaphylaxis or those requiring more than 1 dose of epinephrine should have extended medical observation after the initial symptoms have subsided, because biphasic or protracted anaphylaxis can occur despite ongoing therapy. Biphasic reactions occur in 1%–20% of anaphylactic reactions, but no reliable clinical predictors have been identified. Observation periods should be individualized based on the severity of the initial reaction, but a reasonable time for observation is 2 hours up to 6 hours in most patients, with prolonged observation or admission possibly for severe or refractory symptoms.

Prognosis

Anaphylaxis can be fatal. The prognosis, however, is good when signs and symptoms are recognized promptly and treated aggressively, and the offending agent is subsequently avoided. Exercise-induced and idiopathic anaphylaxis may be recurrent. Because accidental exposure to the causative agent may occur, patients, parents, and caregivers must be prepared to recognize and treat anaphylaxis (have an anaphylaxis action plan and epinephrine readily available). Resources for anaphylaxis can be found by entering the term anaphylaxis in the search boxes at the websites for the national allergy and immunology academic societies: https://www.aaaai.org and https://acaai.org.

Special Considerations: Infant Anaphylaxis

The recognition, diagnosis, and management of anaphylaxis in infants/toddlers are associated with unique challenges given their nonverbal nature. Food allergy is the most common cause of anaphylaxis in this group. Guidance for the diagnosis and management of anaphylaxis in infants was published (see reference below). The FDA also approved an epinephrine autoinjector for infants and toddlers weighing between 7.5 and 15 kg (Auvi-Q 0.1 mg).

Cardona et al: World Allergy Organization anaphylaxis guidance 2020. World Allergy Organ J 2020;13:1–23 [PMID: 33204386].

Greenhawt et al: Guiding principles for the recognition, diagnosis, and management of infants with anaphylaxis: an expert panel consensus. J Allergy Clin Immunol Pract 2019;7:1148–1156 [PMID: 30737191].

Shaker et al: Anaphylaxis—a 2020 practice parameter update, systematic review, and Grading of Recommendations, Assessment, Development and Evaluation (GRADE) analysis. J Allergy Clin Immunol 2020 Apr;145(4):1082–1123 [PMID: 32001253].

ADVERSE REACTIONS TO DRUGS & BIOLOGICALS

ESSENTIALS OF DIAGNOSIS & TYPICAL FEATURES

▶ Allergic or hypersensitivity drug reactions are adverse reactions involving immune mechanisms, accounting for only 5%–10% of all adverse drug reactions.

▶ Less than 5% of children who are diagnosed or labeled with a drug allergy are actually allergic.

▶ Drug allergy labels are associated with adverse health outcomes and costs.

▶ While skin testing is available for penicillins, the majority of reactions to penicillins are mild delayed cutaneous reactions and do not require skin testing.

▶ Drug challenges can be performed for further evaluation of drug reactions. Desensitization causes temporary tolerance of the medication in patients who are allergic.

▶ Desensitizations are absolutely contraindicated with history of severe, delayed-type reactions such as serum sickness, severe cutaneous reactions (TEN/SJS), or drug reaction with eosinophilia and systemic symptoms (DRESS) syndrome.

Adverse drug reactions are any undesirable and unintended response elicited by a drug. Allergic or hypersensitivity drug reactions are adverse reactions involving immune mechanisms. Although hypersensitivity reactions account for only 5%–10% of all adverse drug reactions, they are the most serious, with 1:10,000 resulting in death. Other causes of adverse drug reactions include idiosyncratic reactions, overdosage, pharmacologic side effects, nonspecific release of pharmacologic effector molecules, and drug interactions. Clinicians can report adverse drug reactions and get updated information on drugs, vaccines, and biologics at the FDA's MedWatch website.

Immunopathologic reactions to antibiotics include type I (IgE-mediated) reactions, type II (cytotoxic) reactions such as drug-induced hemolytic anemia or thrombocytopenia, type III (immune complex) reactions such as serum sickness, and type IV (T-cell–mediated) reactions such as allergic contact dermatitis. Immunopathologic reactions not fitting into the types I–IV classification include interstitial nephritis, pneumonitis, hepatitis, eosinophilia, fixed-drug eruption, acute generalized exanthematous pustulosis (AGEP), Stevens-Johnson syndrome, exfoliative dermatitis, and maculopapular exanthemas. Serum sickness–like reactions resemble type III reactions, although immune complexes are not documented; β-lactams, especially cefaclor, and sulfonamides have been implicated most often.

1. Antibiotics

Antibiotics constitute the most frequent cause of allergic drug reactions. Amoxicillin, trimethoprim-sulfamethoxazole, and ampicillin are the most common causes of cutaneous drug reactions. In children, antibiotics commonly cause a rash only in the setting of particular infections, but this is not a true allergy to the medication, such as "amoxicillin rash." Infections alone also frequently cause different rashes, such as morbilliform, targetoid, or urticarial, that are blamed on the concomitant antibiotics.

The penicillins and other β-lactam antibiotics, including cephalosporins, carbacephems, carbapenems, and monobactams, share a common β-lactam ring structure and a marked propensity to couple to carrier proteins. Penicilloyl is the predominant allergenic metabolite of penicillin and is called the major determinant. The other penicillin metabolites are present in low concentrations and are referred to as minor determinants. Regarding cross-reactivity between penicillins and cephalosporins, the R-side chains of the penicillins and cephalosporins have been implicated in most allergic reactions to both of these medications.

Sulfonamide reactions are mediated presumably by a reactive metabolite (hydroxylamine) produced by cytochrome P-450 oxidative metabolism. Slow acetylators appear to be at increased risk. Other risk factors for drug reactions include previous exposure, previous reaction, age (20–49 years), route (parenteral), and dose of administration (high, intermittent). Atopy does not predispose to development of a reaction, but atopic individuals have more severe reactions.

2. Latex Allergy

Allergy to latex and rubber products was common among health care workers and children with spina bifida, but less so with the decreased use of latex equipment and gloves. The combination of atopy and frequent exposure seems to synergistically increase the risk of latex hypersensitivity.

3. Vaccines

Adverse effects of vaccines, such as large local reactions, fever, vasovagal response, panic attack, or rash are more common than allergic reactions to vaccines which are rare. Mumps-measles-rubella (MMR) and the influenza vaccines have been shown to be safe in egg-allergic patients (although rare reactions to gelatin or neomycin can occur). Large local reactions are not associated with a higher rate of systemic allergic reactions. Skin testing and vaccine challenge can be performed if an IgE-mediated allergy to the vaccine is suspected. While immediate reactions in adults have been reported to the SARS-CoV2 vaccines, the majority of these reactions have not been allergic, and booster doses have been tolerated.

4. Antiepileptic Drugs

Aromatic antiepileptic drugs (AEDs) have been most implicated in drug hypersensitivity reactions to AEDs, which can be severe. This class of medications is one of the most common causes of drug rash with eosinophilia and systemic symptoms (DRESS) syndrome in children.

5. Radiocontrast Media

Non-IgE-mediated anaphylactoid reactions may occur with radiocontrast media with up to a 30% reaction rate on re-exposure. Management involves using a low-molarity agent and premedication with prednisone, diphenhydramine, and, possibly, an H_2-blocker.

6. Anesthetics

Local anesthetics: Less than 1% of reactions to local anesthetics are IgE-mediated; most reactions are from toxic effects of the medication. Management involves selecting a local anesthetic from another class. Esters of benzoic acid include benzocaine and procaine; amides include lidocaine and mepivacaine. Alternatively, the patient can be skin-tested with the suspected agent, followed by a provocative challenge.

Perioperative anaphylaxis: While antibiotics are the most common allergen perioperatively, the most common anesthetic allergy is a neuromuscular blocking agent. Skin testing to nonirritating concentrations can be performed.

7. Aspirin & Other Nonsteroidal Anti-Inflammatory Drugs

As with antibiotics, NSAID allergy is often mislabeled because NSAIDs are used during infections that cause rash. Adverse reactions to aspirin and NSAIDs include urticaria and angioedema; rhinosinusitis, nasal polyps, and asthma (AERD); anaphylactoid reactions; and NSAID-related

hypersensitivity pneumonitis. All NSAIDs inhibiting cyclooxygenase (COX) cross-react with aspirin; patients with AERD and urticaria/angioedema will react to all except for selective COX-2 Inhibitors. Rarely patients will react to only one NSAID. No skin test or in vitro test is available to diagnose aspirin sensitivity; the gold standard is a drug challenge or oral provocation test. Aspirin desensitization can be performed to both diagnose and treat AERD.

8. Biological Agents

Biological medications may be associated with a variety of adverse reactions, including infusion reactions (fever, rigors/chills, flushing/pruritus, wheeze/dyspnea), rashes, increased risk of infections, neurologic defects, autoimmune syndromes, cardiovascular effects, and hypersensitivity reactions. Desensitization may be possible if there is no other good alternative in those patients who are allergic to these medications.

9. Adverse Reactions to Chemotherapeutic Agents

Several chemotherapeutic agents, including monoclonal antibodies, have been implicated in hypersensitivity reactions. Skin testing can be performed to platinum agents. Rapid desensitization to unrelated agents, including carboplatin, paclitaxel, peg-asparaginase, and rituximab, has been reported.

▶ Clinical Findings

A. Symptoms and Signs

Rash is the most common symptom of a hypersensitivity drug reaction in children. IgE-mediated reactions cause pruritus, erythema, urticaria, angioedema, bronchospasm, or anaphylaxis within 1 hour of the dose. Delayed reactions can occur hours to weeks after the onset of a medication. Serum sickness is characterized by fever, rash, lymphadenopathy, myalgias, and arthralgias. DRESS Syndrome can cause high fever, facial edema, morbilliform/confluent rash, lymphadenopathy, dyspnea/hypoxemia 2–8 weeks after drug initiation. It can progress even with withdrawal of the offending medication and can last for months.

B. Diagnostic Evaluations

Drug challenge is the gold standard for diagnosis of drug allergy. Drug challenge without skin testing is safe in children who have a history of benign rash with antibiotics. A recent meta-analysis found that for direct drug challenge (without skin testing), the incidence of any reaction was 5% and the risk of severe reaction was 0.036%. However, for severe reactions such as anaphylaxis or severe cutaneous adverse reactions, avoidance without challenge is reasonable. If anaphylaxis is suspected, a serum tryptase can be obtained within 2 hours of reaction onset. If the drug reaction was immediate and symptoms suggestive of an IgE-mediated etiology, skin testing can be considered with non-irritating concentrations, although predictive values are not known for most medications. Skin testing has been validated for penicillin allergy. Pre-Pen (penicilloyl-polylysine) and penicillin G or suspect penicillin, increases sensitivity to about 95%. Not using the minor determinant mixture, which is not commercially available, in skin testing can result in failure to predict potential anaphylactic reactions in up to 20% of those who test negative for both. Solid-phase in vitro immunoassays for IgE to penicillins are available for identification of IgE to penicilloyl but are considerably less sensitive than skin testing and the predictive values are not known. If skin testing is negative, drug provocation test should be performed for the final diagnosis.

For delayed reactions, skin testing is generally not indicated. Patch testing and/or delayed intradermal skin testing may be helpful in the evaluation of Allergic Contact Dermatitis and certain Severe Cutaneous Adverse Reactions. For benign cutaneous reactions to medications, particularly antibiotics, children are not likely to be allergic and should be able to tolerate the medication in the future or should be referred to undergo oral provocation testing to evaluate further.

DRESS syndrome is associated with hematologic abnormalities and HHV6 reactivation. Laboratory testing can reveal hepatic, renal, or cardiac involvement.

▶ Differential Diagnosis

Differential diagnosis for drug allergy includes other types of adverse drug reactions related to drug toxicity, drug interactions, idiosyncratic reactions, or pseudoallergic reactions. As infections commonly cause exanthems or urticaria, these are often confused with drug reactions when the patient is placed on antibiotics or NSAIDs.

▶ Treatment

A. General Measures

Withdrawal of the implicated drug is usually a central component of management. Acute IgE-mediated reactions such as anaphylaxis, urticaria, and angioedema are treated acutely (previous section Anaphylaxis). Drug-induced serum sickness can be suppressed by drug withdrawal, antihistamines, and corticosteroids. Contact allergy can be managed by avoidance and treatment with antihistamines and topical corticosteroids. Toxic epidermal necrolysis and Stevens-Johnson syndrome require immediate drug withdrawal and supportive care. Severe DRESS syndrome, particularly with pulmonary or renal involvement, is treated with systemic glucocorticoids.

B. Alternative Therapy

If possible, subsequent therapy should be with an alternative drug that has therapeutic actions similar to the drug in question but with no immunologic cross-reactivity.

C. Desensitization

For IgE-mediated drug allergies, administering gradually increasing doses of the drug either orally or parenterally over a period of hours to days may be considered if alternative therapy is not acceptable. This should be done only by a physician familiar with desensitization, typically in an intensive care setting. Of note, desensitization is only effective for the course of therapy for which the patient was desensitized, unless maintained on a chronic prophylactic dose of the medication as patients revert from a desensitized to an allergic state after the drug is discontinued. In addition, desensitization does not typically reduce or prevent non–IgE-mediated reactions. Patients with Stevens-Johnson syndrome, DRESS, or serum sickness should not be desensitized because of the high morbidity and mortality rate.

▶ Prognosis

The prognosis is good when drug allergens are identified early and avoided. Stevens-Johnson syndrome, toxic epidermal necrolysis, and DRESS syndrome are associated with a higher mortality rate.

Banerji A et al: Drug allergy practice parameter updates to incorporate into your clinical practice. J Allergy Clin Immunol Pract 2023;11(2)356–368 [PMID: 36563781].

FDAMedWatch: https://www.accessdata.fda.gov/scripts/medwatch/index.cfm?action=reporting.home. Accessed April 8, 2023.

Srisuwatchari W et al: The safety of the direct drug provocation test in beta-lactam hypersensitivity in children: a systematic review and meta-analysis. J Allergy Clin Immunol Pract 2023;11(2)506–518 [PMID: 36528293].

FOOD ALLERGY

ESSENTIALS OF DIAGNOSIS & TYPICAL FEATURES

▶ Diagnosis of food allergy is made by a clinical history consistent with an immune-mediated reaction to a food, either IgE- or non–IgE-mediated.

▶ Treatment for food allergy includes avoidance of that food and providing education on how to treat an allergic reaction after an accidental exposure; consultation with an allergist and with a dietitian is recommended.

▶ Food allergy treatment using oral immunotherapy is now available, and introduction of highly allergenic foods (eg, peanut, egg, milk) early into an infant's diet may prevent the development of allergy to those foods.

General Considerations

Food allergy is defined as an adverse health effect arising from a specific immune response that occurs reproducibly on exposure to a given food. Food allergy affects approximately 8%–10% of young children and 3%–4% of adults. The most common IgE-associated food allergens in children are milk egg, peanut, tree nuts, sesame seed, fish, and shellfish soy, and wheat. In older patients, peanut, tree nuts, fish, and shellfish, are most often involved in allergic reactions and are usually lifelong allergies. Food allergy can be caused by non–IgE-mediated mechanisms, in conditions such as food protein-induced enterocolitis (FPIES) or proctocolitis. It can also be caused by mixed IgE- and non–IgE-mediated mechanisms, as in eosinophilic esophagitis and gastroenteritis (Table 38–10).

Some adverse reactions diagnosed by patients or physicians as food allergy involve non–immune-mediated mechanisms, such as pharmacologic and metabolic mechanisms, reactions to food toxins, or intolerances (eg, lactose intolerance). These will not be covered in this chapter.

Clinical Findings

A. Symptoms and Signs

A thorough medical history is crucial to identifying symptoms associated with potential food allergy; a history of a temporal relationship between the ingestion of a suspected food and onset of a reaction—as well as the nature and duration of symptoms observed—is important in establishing the diagnosis. For all IgE-mediated reactions, reactions to foods occur within minutes and up to 2 hours after ingestion. Skin manifestations of an allergic reaction, including urticaria, flushing, facial angioedema are most common. In severe cases, angioedema of the tongue, uvula, pharynx, or upper airway can occur. Gastrointestinal symptoms include abdominal discomfort or pain, nausea, vomiting, and diarrhea. Children with food allergy may occasionally have isolated rhinoconjunctivitis or wheezing. Rarely, anaphylaxis to food may involve only cardiovascular collapse.

In patients with IgE antibodies to galactose-a-1,3-galactose (a-Gal), delayed anaphylaxis, urticaria, and angioedema can occur up to 4–6 hours after ingestion of mammalian meats. For non–IgE-mediated and mixed disorders, reactions can be delayed in onset for more than several hours, such as in FPIES, to possibly days later with onset of vomiting or an eczema flare after food exposure due to eosinophilic esophagitis or atopic dermatitis, respectively.

B. Laboratory Findings

Typically, fewer than 50% of histories of adverse reactions to foods will be confirmed as food allergy by blinded food challenge (although this percentage is much higher in food-induced anaphylaxis). Prick skin testing is useful to rule out a suspected food allergen because the predictive value is high for a properly performed negative test with an extract of good quality (negative predictive accuracy of > 95%). In contrast, the predictive value for a positive skin test is approximately 50%. Serum food-specific IgE tests have lower specificity and positive predictive values; therefore, doing serum IgE food panels is not recommended, with referral to an allergist preferred to obtain a detailed clinical history and selective testing, if necessary. A list of nonstandardized and unproven procedures for the diagnosis of food allergy includes the measurement of allergen-specific IgG, lymphocyte stimulation, cytotoxic assays, applied kinesiology, and provocation neutralization, to name a few.

The double-blind, placebo-controlled food challenge is considered the gold standard for diagnosing food allergy, except in severe reactions. If there is high suspicion of possible allergic reactivity to a food with a negative skin test or an undetectable serum IgE level (or both), a food challenge may be necessary to confirm the presence or absence of allergy. Even when multiple food allergies are suspected, most patients will test positive for only three or fewer foods on blinded challenge. Therefore, extensive elimination diets are almost never indicated, and an evaluation by an allergist is preferred before multiple foods are eliminated from the diet unnecessarily. If an elimination diet is started, it is recommended to consult with a dietitian experienced in food allergy to review proper avoidance of the food(s), but more importantly provide assurance that nutrition is still complete with the food(s) removed. Elimination diets and food challenges may be the only tools for evaluation of suspected non–IgE-mediated food reactions.

Table 38–10. Food allergy disorders.

IgE-mediated
 Gastrointestinal: Pollen-food allergy syndrome, immediate GI anaphylaxis
 Cutaneous: Urticaria, angioedema, morbilliform rashes, and flushing
 Respiratory: Acute rhinoconjunctivitis, acute wheezing
 Generalized: Anaphylactic shock
Mixed IgE- and non–IgE-mediated
 Gastrointestinal: Eosinophilic esophagitis/gastroenteritis/colitis
 Cutaneous: Atopic dermatitis
 Respiratory: Asthma
Non–IgE-mediated
 Gastrointestinal: Food protein-induced enterocolitis, proctocolitis, and enteropathy syndromes; celiac disease
 Cutaneous: Contact dermatitis, dermatitis herpetiformis
 Respiratory: Food-induced pulmonary hemosiderosis (Heiner syndrome)

Differential Diagnosis

Repeated vomiting in infancy may be due to pyloric stenosis or gastroesophageal reflux. With chronic gastrointestinal symptoms, enzyme deficiency (eg, lactase), cystic fibrosis, celiac disease, chronic intestinal infections, gastrointestinal malformations, and irritable bowel syndrome should be considered.

Treatment

Treatment consists of eliminating and avoiding foods that have been documented to cause allergic reactions. This involves educating the patient, parent/caregivers, and systems such as childcare and schools regarding hidden food allergens, the necessity for reading labels, and the signs and symptoms of food allergy and its appropriate management (anaphylaxis action plan; a copy of this plan can be obtained from the references). Consultation with a dietitian familiar with food allergy may be helpful. All patients with a history of IgE-mediated food allergy should carry self-injectable epinephrine (eg, Auvi-Q or Epipen) and a fast-acting antihistamine, have an anaphylaxis action plan, and consider wearing medical identification jewelry. Clinical trials of oral and epicutaneous immunotherapy, as well as studies using biologics such as anti-IgE monoclonal antibodies, e.g., omalizumab and ligelizumab) are under investigation as potential future treatments of food allergy, with recent FDA approval of a peanut oral immunotherapy product under the drug name Palforzia. Recent studies using food immunotherapy in toddlers have shown that earlier use of these treatments may be more efficacious than in older food-allergic children. However, diets containing extensively heated (baked) milk and egg are potential alternative approaches to food oral immunotherapy and are changing the previous standard of strict avoidance diets for patients with allergy to these foods.

Prognosis

The prognosis is good if the offending food can be identified and avoided. Unfortunately, accidental exposure to food allergens in severely allergic patients can result in death. Most children outgrow food allergies to milk, egg, wheat, and soy but not to peanut or tree nuts (only 20% and 10% of children may outgrow peanut and tree nut allergy, respectively). The natural history of food allergy can be followed by measuring food-specific IgE levels and performing food challenges when indicated. Approximately 3%–4% of children will have food allergy as adults. Resources for food-allergic patients include the Food Allergy Research & Education: www.foodallergy.org; the Food Allergy & Anaphylaxis Connection Team: www.foodallergyawareness.org; and the Consortium of Food Allergy Research: www.cofargroup.org.

Prevention

Recently, multiple randomized controlled trials (RCTs) and a meta-analysis have shown that there appears to be no benefit with respect to food allergy prevention in delaying the introduction of any major food allergen into an infant's diet.

Specific guidance and recommendations for the prevention of food allergy through nutritional means have recently been published.

Boyce JA et al: Guidelines for the diagnosis and management of food allergy in the United States: report of the NIAID-sponsored expert panel. J Allergy Clin Immunol 2010;126(Suppl 1): 158 [PMID: 21134576].

Fleischer DM et al: A consensus approach to the primary prevention of food allergy through nutrition: guidance from the American Academy of Allergy, Asthma, and Immunology; American College of Allergy, Asthma, and Immunology; and the Canadian Society for Allergy and Clinical Immunology. J Allergy Clin Immunol Pract 2021 Jan;9(1):22–43.e4. doi: 10.1016/j.jaip .2020.11.002. Epub 2020 Nov 26 [PMID: 33250376].

Fleischer DM et al: Effect of epicutaneous immunotherapy vs placebo on reaction to peanut protein ingestion among children with peanut allergy: the PEPITES randomized clinical trial. JAMA 2019;321(10):946–955 [PMID: 30794314].

Sampson HA et al: Food allergy: a practice parameter update—2014. J Allergy Clin Immunol 2014;134:1016–1025 [PMID: 25174862].

Jones SM et al: Efficacy and safety of oral immunotherapy in children aged 1-3 years with peanut allergy (the Immune Tolerance Network IMPACT trial): a randomised placebo-controlled study. Lancet 2022;399:359-371 [PMID 35065784].

INSECT ALLERGY

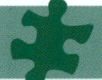

ESSENTIALS OF DIAGNOSIS & TYPICAL FEATURES

▶ Insect bites or stings can cause local or systemic reactions that can range from mild to fatal in susceptible individuals.

▶ Skin testing is indicated for children with systemic reactions to insect stings.

▶ Children who have had anaphylactic reactions to hymenoptera stings should have autoinjectable epinephrine and wear a medical alert bracelet.

▶ Patients who experience severe systemic reactions and have a positive skin test should receive venom immunotherapy.

Allergic reactions to insects include symptoms of respiratory allergy as a result of inhalation of particulate matter of insect origin, local cutaneous reactions to insect bites, and anaphylactic reactions to stings. The latter almost exclusively caused by Hymenoptera includes honeybees, yellow jackets, yellow hornets, white-faced hornets, wasps, and fire ants. Africanized honeybees, also known as killer bees, are a concern because of their aggressive behavior and excessive swarming, not because their venom is more toxic. Rarely, patients sensitized to reduviid bugs (also known as kissing bugs) may have episodes of nocturnal anaphylaxis. Lepidopterism refers to adverse effects secondary to contact with larval or adult butterflies and moths. Salivary gland antigens are responsible for immediate and delayed skin reactions in mosquito-sensitive patients.

▶ Clinical Findings

A. Symptoms and Signs

Insect bites or stings can cause local or systemic reactions ranging from mild to fatal responses in susceptible persons. Local cutaneous reactions include urticaria as well as papulovesicular eruptions and lesions that resemble delayed hypersensitivity reactions. Papular urticaria is almost always the result of insect bites, especially of mosquitoes, fleas, and bedbugs. Toxic systemic reactions consisting of gastrointestinal symptoms, headache, vertigo, syncope, convulsions, or fever can occur following multiple stings. These reactions result from histamine-like substances in the venom. In children with hypersensitivity to fire ant venom, sterile pustules occur at sting sites on a nonimmunologic basis due to the inherent toxicity of piperidine alkaloids in the venom. Mild systemic reactions include itching, flushing, and urticaria. Severe systemic reactions may include dyspnea, wheezing, chest tightness, hoarseness, fullness in the throat, hypotension, loss of consciousness, incontinence, nausea, vomiting, and abdominal pain. Delayed systemic reactions occur from 2 hours to 3 weeks following the sting and include serum sickness, peripheral neuritis, allergic vasculitis, and coagulation defects.

B. Laboratory Findings

Skin testing is indicated for children with systemic reactions to insect stings. Venoms of honeybee, yellow jacket, yellow hornet, white-faced hornet, and wasp are available for skin testing and treatment. Fire ant venom is not yet commercially available, but an extract made from fire ant bodies appears adequate to establish the presence of IgE antibodies in fire ant venom. Importantly, venom skin tests can be negative in patients with systemic allergic reactions, especially in the first few weeks after a sting, and the tests may need to be repeated. The presence of a positive skin test denotes prior sensitization but does not predict whether a reaction will occur with the patient's next sting, nor does it differentiate between local and systemic reactions. It is common for children who have had an allergic reaction to have positive skin tests for more than one venom. This might reflect sensitization from prior stings that did not result in an allergic reaction or cross-reactivity between closely related venoms. In vitro testing (compared with skin testing) has not substantially improved the ability to predict anaphylaxis. With in-vitro testing, there is a 15%–20% incidence of both false-positive and false-negative results. IgE to mosquito saliva antigen can be measured by in vitro assay.

▶ Complications

Secondary infection can complicate allergic reactions to insect bites or stings. Serum sickness, nephrotic syndrome, vasculitis, neuritis, and encephalopathy may be seen as late sequelae of reactions to stinging insects.

▶ Treatment

For cutaneous reactions caused by biting insects, symptomatic therapy includes cold compresses, antipruritics (including antihistamines), and, occasionally, potent topical corticosteroids. Treatment of stings includes careful removal of the stinger, if present, by flicking it away from the wound, not by grasping to prevent further envenomation. Topical application of monosodium glutamate, baking soda, or vinegar compresses is of questionable efficacy. Local reactions can be treated with ice, elevation of the affected extremity, oral antihistamines, and NSAIDs as well as potent topical corticosteroids. Large local reactions may require a short course of oral corticosteroids. Anaphylactic reactions following Hymenoptera stings should be managed as discussed above (see section Anaphylaxis). Children who have had severe or anaphylactic reactions to Hymenoptera stings—or their parents and caregivers—should be instructed in the use of autoinjectable epinephrine. Patients at risk for anaphylaxis from an insect sting should also wear a medical alert bracelet indicating their allergy. Children at risk from insect stings should avoid wearing bright-colored clothing and perfumes when outdoors and should wear long pants and shoes when walking in the grass. Patients who experience severe systemic reactions and have a positive skin test should receive venom immunotherapy. Venom immunotherapy is not indicated for children with only urticarial or local reactions.

▶ Prognosis

Children generally have milder reactions than adults after insect stings, and fatal reactions are extremely rare. Patients aged 3–16 years with reactions limited to the skin, such as urticaria and angioedema, appear to be at low risk for more severe reactions with subsequent stings.

Albuhairi S et al: A twenty-two-year experience with Hymenoptera venom immunotherapy in a US pediatric tertiary care center 1996–2018. Ann Allergy Asthma Immunol 2018;121:722.e1 [PMID: 30102964].

Golden DB et al: Stinging insect hypersensitivity: a practice parameter update 2016. Ann Allergy Asthma Immunol 2017;118:28 [PMID: 28007086].

39

Antimicrobial Therapy

Andrew S. Haynes, MD

Christine E. MacBrayne, PharmD, MSCS

Jason Child, PharmD

Sarah K. Parker, MD

PRINCIPLES OF ANTIMICROBIAL THERAPY

The discovery and rapid development of targeted antimicrobial agents, beginning in the 1930s, are among the most important scientific developments of 20th-century medicine. These drugs have changed the practice of medicine and remain one of medicine's most effective and widely used interventions. However, choosing an appropriate antimicrobial can be complex and difficult. Optimal antimicrobial use requires appreciation of the complicated interactions between host, organism, and drug. This decision-making process, summarized in Table 39–1, begins with an accurate working diagnosis, based on the patient's clinical history, physical examination, exposure history, and initial laboratory tests. From this foundation, the clinician must consider the most likely organism(s) and that organism's likely pattern of antimicrobial susceptibility. This information is considered in the context of numerous patient-specific factors, including age, immune status, relevant comorbidities, site of infection, prior antimicrobial exposure, the microbiology of the patient's prior infections, and the pace and severity of the illness. Unique exposures, based on environment, travel, diet, animal contact, or ill close contacts may suggest the likelihood of certain organisms. However, decisions of when not to use antimicrobials are equally important, as unnecessary or additional drugs and longer durations may harm patients. In addition to choosing an appropriate antimicrobial for treatment of a suspected or confirmed infection, antimicrobials are also often utilized to prevent infections (preexposure prophylaxis, post-exposure prophylaxis, or surgical/medical prophylaxis) and the same appreciation of the complicated interactions between host, organism, and drug should be utilized in these situations.

Once an appropriate initial antimicrobial is chosen, the clinician must consider the proper dose, route of administration, duration of therapy, and whether additional drugs are needed. Empiric therapy should be changed to definitive therapy as the clinical course evolves and additional laboratory data are available. Obtaining appropriate microbiologic specimens facilitates this transition. Antimicrobial susceptibility, antimicrobial families, and dosing recommendations are listed in Tables 39–2 to 39–4. The need to balance a treatment's efficacy with its potential toxicities and side effects makes this process even more complex.

CONCEPTS FOR JUDICIOUS USE OF ANTIMICROBIALS

Antimicrobials are the most prescribed class of medication for both adults and children. Over 25% of pediatric outpatient visits result in an antimicrobial prescription, and nearly 60% of pediatric inpatients receive antimicrobials. Much of this use (up to 40%–60%) is inappropriate. We not only overprescribe but also choose unnecessarily broad agents, which are often less effective. Overprescribing is problematic because, when the likelihood of benefit is low, more patients may experience harm from an antibiotic than benefit from it. Possible harms include gastrointestinal side effects, allergic reactions ranging from rashes to anaphylaxis, renal or hepatic toxicity, bone marrow suppression, prolonged QTc, and Stevens-Johnson syndrome, among others. Adverse drug reactions occur in approximately 30% of antibiotic courses, resulting in over 150,000 unplanned pediatric medical visits per year.

SUSCEPTIBILITY TESTING & DRUG DOSING PROPERTIES

When possible, cultures and other diagnostic material should be obtained prior to starting antimicrobial therapy. Identifying an etiologic agent helps to tailor therapy, choose appropriate treatment duration, and possibly even stop antimicrobials. This is especially important for complicated situations, such as when the patient has a serious infection, is at

Table 39–1. Steps in decision-making for use of antimicrobial agents.

Step	Action	Example
1	Determine presumptive diagnosis	Septic arthritis and osteomyelitis
2	Consider age, preexisting condition, antimicrobial penetration	Previously healthy 2-year-old child, bone and joint penetration desired
3	Consider common organisms (for age and site of infection)	*Staphylococcus aureus, Kingella kingae*
4	Consider organism susceptibility	Penicillin- or ampicillin-resistant; frequency of MRSA in community
5	Obtain proper cultures and gram stains if possible—especially if the organism or susceptibilities are unpredictable	Blood cultures, joint fluid, bone biopsy
6	Initiate empiric therapy based on above considerations, and guidelines if they exist	Cefazolin, add vancomycin to cefazolin if seriously ill or MRSA prevalent
7	Modify therapy based on culture results and patient response	*S aureus* isolated. Choose cefazolin or vancomycin based on susceptibility
8	Follow clinical response, consider laboratory responses	Interval physical examination, inflammatory markers
9	Change to oral therapy	Cephalexin if cefazolin susceptible, anti-MRSA drug if needed based on susceptibility. Change when afebrile, clinically improving, falling inflammatory markers, able to tolerate oral medications
10	Stop therapy	Clinically improved or well-treated minimal duration based on standard of care/guidelines

MRSA, methicillin-resistant *Staphylococcus aureus*.

risk for drug-resistant organisms, has failed prior treatment, had unusual exposures, or multiagent empiric therapy is anticipated.

For most bacteria, growth in culture remains the gold standard for identification and susceptibility testing. Although rapid molecular methods continue to improve, most antimicrobial susceptibility testing is still done by determining the minimum inhibitory concentration (MIC) for the organism-drug pair (eg, *Streptococcus pneumoniae* and penicillin) in a culture-based system. The MIC represents the amount of antibiotic (in mcg/mL) necessary to inhibit growth of the organism under specific laboratory conditions. The organism is then deemed susceptible, intermediate, or resistant based on widely accepted published breakpoints. Breakpoints are based on clinical trials and achievable drug concentrations in the serum, cerebral spinal fluid (CSF), or urine at recommended doses in healthy adults. Ultimately, the true test of therapeutic efficacy is patient response; for example, a patient may have a good clinical response to cephalexin for a urinary tract infection (UTI) with *Escherichia coli* reported to be cephalexin-resistant because cephalosporins are highly concentrated in urine. Conversely, patients who do not respond to seemingly appropriate therapy require reassessment, including reconsideration of the diagnosis, repeat cultures, and consideration of surgical debulking of the infection. Antimicrobial susceptibility testing, although an essential part of therapeutic decision-making, must be considered in context with drug concentrations at the site of infection, immune status, patient age, comorbid conditions, pharmacodynamics (PD), and patient clinical status.

PHARMACOKINETIC & PHARMACODYNAMIC CONCEPTS

Pharmacokinetics (PK) refers to what happens to a drug in the body (ie, its absorption, distribution, metabolism, and excretion), while pharmacodynamics (PD) refers to the effects a drug has on the body (ie, the relationship between a drug's concentrations and the response/effect). When considering efficacy of antibiotics, there are three PK/PD models used to predict cure (Figure 39–1). Common to all these concepts is that the concentration of drug at the site of the infection must exceed the MIC. An antibiotic's efficacy is then correlated with either time (the time that the MIC is exceeded, T > MIC), concentration (peak concentration over the MIC, peak/MIC), or a combination of both (described as the "area under the curve" [AUC] over the MIC, AUC/MIC) (see Figure 39–1). The T > MIC efficacy pattern applies to all β-lactam antibiotics (penicillins, cephalosporins, monobactams, and carbapenems) and means that the duration of antibiotic exposure is more important than achieving especially high antibiotic concentrations. T > MIC is calculated as the percentage of a 24-hour day that the drug concentration exceeds the MIC, with targets ranging from 30% to 40% to more than 90% depending on the severity and site of infection and the immune status of the host. For Peak/MIC-type antibiotics (eg, aminoglycosides, daptomycin), bacterial killing is more rapid and complete with higher antibiotic concentrations, and the duration of exposure is less important. Concentration-dependent drugs rapidly enter the microbe at high concentrations, and even when the drug is gone,

Table 39–2. Susceptibility of some common pathogenic microorganisms to various antimicrobial drugs.

Organism	Potentially Useful Antibiotics	
Bacteria		
	First choice examples	**Alternate choice examples**
Anaerobic bacteria[a]	Metronidazole, clindamycin	Penicillins with β-lactamase inhibitor, cefoxitin, carbapenems, tigecycline
Bartonella henselae	Azithromycin	Ciprofloxacin, clarithromycin, doxycycline, rifampin
Bordetella pertussis	Azithromycin	Clarithromycin, erythromycin, TMP/SMX
Campylobacter spp. (not fetus)	Azithromycin	Erythromycin, fluoroquinolones, doxycycline
Chlamydia/Chlamydophila spp.	Azithromycin, doxycycline	Clarithromycin, levofloxacin
Clostridium perfringens	Clindamycin, penicillin	Metronidazole, piperacillin/tazobactam, cephalosporins, doxycycline
Clostridioides difficile	Vancomycin (PO)	Fidaxomicin, metronidazole, fecal microbiota transplant
Corynebacterium diphtheriae	Erythromycin	Penicillin, clindamycin
Escherichia coli/Klebsiella spp.	Ampicillin/sulbactam, amoxicillin/ clavulanate, cephalosporins	Aminoglycosides, aztreonam, fluoroquinolones
ESBL (*E coli/Klebsiella*)	Meropenem	Ceftolozane/tazobactam, aminoglycosides, fluoroquinolones
KPC (*E coli/Klebsiella*)	Ceftazidime/avibactam	Colistin, aminoglycosides, tigecycline
Enterococcus faecalis	Ampicillin, vancomycin, (± gentamicin)	Daptomycin, linezolid, carbapenems
Enterococcus faecium	Vancomycin (± gentamicin)	Ampicillin, daptomycin, linezolid
Haemophilus influenzae	Amoxicillin/clavulanate, ampicillin (if β-lactamase−negative) [b], ceftriaxone	Fluoroquinolones, cefuroxime (not meningitis)
Kingella kingae	Cefazolin, cephalexin	Nafcillin
Listeria monocytogenes	Ampicillin	TMP/SMX, vancomycin
Moraxella catarrhalis	Amoxicillin/clavulanate	Cephalosporins (except for 1st generation), TMP/SMX, macrolides, fluoroquinolones
Mycoplasma spp.	Azithromycin	Clarithromycin, fluoroquinolones, tetracyclines
Neisseria gonorrhoeae	Ceftriaxone	Azithromycin
Neisseria meningitidis	Ceftriaxone	Ampicillin, penicillin
Nocardia asteroides	TMP/SMX (+ imipenem for severe infections)	Minocycline, linezolid + meropenem, imipenem + amikacin (combination therapy in severe disease)
Pasteurella multocida	Amoxicillin/clavulanate	Fluoroquinolones, cephalosporins, doxycycline, TMP/SMX
Pseudomonas aeruginosa	Cefepime	Ciprofloxacin, piperacillin/tazobactam, ceftazidime, aminoglycosides, meropenem
Salmonella spp.	Azithromycin, ceftriaxone	Ampicillin, fluoroquinolones, TMP/SMX
Shigella spp.	Fluoroquinolones	Azithromycin, ceftriaxone, TMP/SMX
Staphylococcus aureus (MSSA)	Cefazolin, cephalexin, nafcillin	Clindamycin, TMP/SMX, cefepime, ampicillin/sulbactam, amoxicillin/clavulanate
S aureus (MRSA)	Vancomycin	Clindamycin, daptomycin, linezolid, TMP/SMX, doxycycline, ceftaroline
Staphylococci (coagulase-negative)	Vancomycin	Cefazolin (if susceptible)[c], clindamycin, linezolid, TMP/SMX
Streptococci (groups A and B)	Penicillin, ampicillin, amoxicillin	Ceftriaxone, cefotaxime, clindamycin, levofloxacin, vancomycin

(Continued)

Table 39–2. Susceptibility of some common pathogenic microorganisms to various antimicrobial drugs. (*Continued*)

Organism	Potentially Useful Antibiotics	
Streptococci (viridans and anginosus groups)	Ceftriaxone, vancomycin	Penicillins, clindamycin, daptomycin
Streptococcus pneumoniae[d]	Ampicillin, amoxicillin, ceftriaxone	Penicillins, cephalosporins, vancomycin, levofloxacin, meropenem
Tick-borne illnesses		
Francisella tularensis (Tularemia)	Gentamicin (severe), ciprofloxacin (mild/moderate)	Doxycycline
Borrelia burgdorferi (Lyme) Borrelia hermsii (tick-borne relapsing fever)	Doxycycline, amoxicillin, ceftriaxone Doxycycline	Cefuroxime, azithromycin Penicillin, ceftriaxone
Anaplasmosis/Ehrlichiosis/Rocky Mountain spotted fever	Doxycycline	
Babesiosis	Atovaquone + azithromycin (any severity)	Clindamycin + quinine
Fungi		
Candida albicans Candida non-albicans	Fluconazole, echinocandins Echinocandins, fluconazole	Liposomal amphotericin B, azoles Azoles, liposomal amphotericin B
Aspergillus spp.	Voriconazole, isavuconazole	Posaconazole, liposomal amphotericin B, echinocandins
Dimorphic fungi	Liposomal amphotericin B	Itraconazole, voriconazole, posaconazole, fluconazole
Mucormycosis	Liposomal amphotericin B (± echinocandin)	Posaconazole, isavuconazole (azole + amphotericin combination therapy in severe disease)
Scedosporium	Voriconazole (± echinocandin)	Posaconazole
Pneumocystis jirovecii	TMP/SMX	Clindamycin + primaquine, atovaquone, pentamidine
Viruses		
Herpes simplex	Acyclovir, valacyclovir	Famciclovir. For resistant strains may use ganciclovir, cidofovir, foscarnet. For ophthalmic use—ganciclovir[e], trifluridine[e]
Human immunodeficiency virus		Refer to Chapter 41 for more details. Refer to https://hivinfo.nih.gov/ for current guidelines and dosing information
Influenza virus	Oseltamivir, baloxavir (aged ≥ 12 y)	Peramivir, zanamivir
Respiratory syncytial virus	Ribavirin[f]	
Varicella-zoster virus	Acyclovir, valacyclovir	Famciclovir. For resistant strains may use cidofovir, foscarnet.
Cytomegalovirus	Ganciclovir, valganciclovir	Foscarnet, cidofovir
Hepatitis B	Entecavir, tenofovir disoproxil fumarate, tenofovir alafenamide	Refer to Chapter 22
Hepatitis C	Direct-acting antiviral regimens now standard of care	Refer to Chapter 22

ESBL, extended-spectrum β-lactamase; KPC, *Klebsiella pneumoniae* carbapenemase; MRSA, methicillin-resistant *S aureus*; MSSA, methicillin-susceptible *S aureus*; PO, oral; TMP/SMX, trimethoprim/sulfamethoxazole.

[a]Species-dependent.

[b]Also applies to amoxicillin and related compounds.

[c]Only if the coagulase-negative *Staphylococcus* is also methicillin- or oxacillin-sensitive.

[d]Because of the possibility of *S pneumoniae* strains resistant to penicillin and cephalosporins, presumptive therapy for severe infections (eg, meningitis) should include vancomycin until susceptibility studies are available.

[e]Ophthalmic preparation.

[f]FDA approved for therapy of respiratory syncytial virus by aerosol, but clinical studies show variable efficacy.

Table 39–3. Guidelines for use of common antimicrobial agents in children age 1 month or older.[a]

Agent	Dose (mg/kg/day)[b]	Maximum Daily Dose	Interval (h)
Penicillin G (IV and short-acting intramuscular)	100,000–400,000 U/kg/day	24 million units	4–6
Penicillin VK (oral)	25–50	2000 mg	6–12
Ampicillin (IV)	100–400	12,000 mg	4–6
Amoxicillin (oral)	40–100	4000 mg	8–12
Ampicillin/sulbactam (IV)	100–400 (ampicillin)	12,000 mg	4–6
Amoxicillin/clavulanate (oral)	40–100 (amoxicillin)	Based on formulation and amoxicillin component 600–42.9-mg/5 mL suspension: 1000-mg 875–125-mg tablets: 875 mg	8–12 8
Piperacillin/tazobactam (IV)	240–300 (piperacillin)	16,000 mg	4–6
Nafcillin (IV)	150–200	12,000 mg	4–6
Oxacillin (IV)	100–200	12,000 mg	4–6
Dicloxacillin (oral)	25–100	2000 mg	6
Cefazolin (IV)	50–150	8000 mg	6–8
Cephalexin (oral)	25–150	4000 mg	6
Cefadroxil (oral)	30–150	2000 mg	8–12
Cefoxitin (IV)	80–160	12,000 mg	4–6
Cefuroxime (IV)	100–150	6000 mg	8
Cefuroxime axetil (oral)	30–100	1000 mg	12
Cefprozil (oral)	30	1000 mg	12
Cefpodoxime (oral)	10	400 mg	12
Cefdinir (oral)	14–25	600 mg	12–24
Cefotaxime (IV)	100–300	12,000 mg	6–8
Ceftazidime (IV)	100–150	6000 mg	8
Ceftazidime/avibactam (IV)	150 (ceftazidime)	6000 mg	8
Ceftriaxone (IV)	50–100	4000 mg/day (max 2000 mg in single dose)	12–24
Cefepime (IV)	100–150	6000 mg	8 (systemic)–12 (UTI)
Ceftolozane/tazobactam (IV)	60–120 (ceftolozane)	6000 mg	8
Ceftaroline (IV)	24–45	1800 mg	8 (preferred)–12
Aztreonam (IV)	90–300	12,000 mg	6–8
Meropenem (IV)	60–120	6000 mg	8
Ciprofloxacin (IV and oral)	20–30	1500 mg (IV/PO)	8–12
Levofloxacin (IV and oral)	< 5 y: 20 5–10 y: 14–16 > 10 y: 10	750 mg (IV/PO)	12 12 24
Gentamicin (IV)	3–7.5	Adjust based on concentrations (desired peak 8–12 mcg/mL for q8h dosing and 20–30 for q24h dosing and trough levels < 2 mcg/mL)	8
Tobramycin (IV)	3–7.5	Adjust based on concentrations (desired peak 8–12 mcg/mL for q8h dosing and 20–30 mcg/mL for q24h dosing and trough levels < 2 mcg/mL)	8

(Continued)

Table 39–3. Guidelines for use of common antimicrobial agents in children age 1 month or older.[a] (*Continued*)

Agent	Dose (mg/kg/day)[b]	Maximum Daily Dose	Interval (h)
Amikacin (IV)	15–22.5	Adjust based on concentrations (desired peak 20–35 mcg/mL for q8h dosing and trough < 10 mcg/mL)	8
Erythromycin (oral)	20–50	4000 mg	6–12
Azithromycin (IV and oral)	10 × 1 day, then 5	1000 mg	24
Clarithromycin (oral)	15	1000 mg	12
Metronidazole (IV and oral)	15–50	1500 mg	8 (once daily for appendicitis)
Clindamycin (IV and oral)	20–40	(IV) 2700 mg (PO) 1800 mg	6–8
Vancomycin (IV)	IV recommended starting dose 40–80 40–55 (as continuous infusion over 24 h)	(IV) 4000 mg	(IV) 6–8
Vancomycin (oral, only for *C difficile*)	(PO) 40	(PO) 2000 mg (recommend 500 mg/day but may use higher dose for complicated disease)	(PO) 6
Dalbavancin (IV)	18–22.5 12–15 followed by 6–7.5	1500 mg 1000 mg (Day 1) followed by 500 mg (on Day 8)	Once Two doses (7 days apart)
Linezolid (IV and oral)	< 12 y: 30 ≥ 12 y: 20	1200–1800 mg 1200 mg	8 12
TMP/SMX (IV and oral)	8–20 (TMP)	640 mg	6–12
Rifampin (IV and oral)	10–20	600 mg	12–24
Doxycycline (IV and oral)	2–4	200 mg	12
Tetracycline (oral)	25–50	2000 mg	6
Tigecycline (IV)	2.4	100 mg	12
Nitrofurantoin (oral)	5–7	400 mg	6
Nitazoxanide (oral)	1–3 y: 200 mg/day 4–11 y: 400 mg/day ≥ 12 y: 1000 mg/day	200 mg 400 mg 1000 mg	12
Albendazole (oral)	≤ 2 y 200 mg/day × 1 > 2 y 400 mg/day × 1	200 mg 400 mg	Once Once
Mebendazole (oral)	200 mg/day	200 mg	12
Acyclovir (IV and oral)	1 mo–3 mo: 60 > 3 mo: 30 All ages: 30 (or) All ages: 1500 mg/m²/day ≥ 2 y: 80 ≥ 12 y: 80 1–7 mo: 900 mg/m²/day 1–11 y: 60 ≥ 12 y: 60	 3200 mg 4000 mg N/A 1200 mg 800 mg	8 8 8 8 6–8 5 × daily 8 8 12
Valacyclovir (oral for HSV)	≥ 3 mo: 40–60 mg/kg/day	2000–3000 mg (max 1000 mg per dose)	8–12
Valacyclovir (oral for VZV)	≥ 3 mo: 40–60 mg/kg/day ≥ 12 y: 40–60 mg/kg/day	2000–3000 mg (max 1000 mg per dose) 1000–2000 mg (max 1000 mg per dose)	8–12 12–24

(*Continued*)

Table 39–3. Guidelines for use of common antimicrobial agents in children age 1 month or older.[a] (*Continued*)

Agent	Dose (mg/kg/day)[b]	Maximum Daily Dose	Interval (h)
Ganciclovir (IV)	5–10	Not applicable	12–24
Valganciclovir (oral)	15–36	1800 mg	12–24
Oseltamivir (oral)	3–6	150 mg	12–24
Baloxavir (oral)	≥ 12 y and ≥ 40 kg ≥ 80 kg	40 mg once 80 mg once	One-time dose
Peramivir (IV)	≤ 30 days: 6 ≤ 90 days: 8 ≤ 180 days: 10 ≤ 5 y: 12 > 5 y: 10	600 mg	24
Zanamivir (inhaled)	≥ 7 y ≥ 5 y	2 inhalations 2 inhalations	12 24
Remdesivir (IV)	> 3.5 kg Load: 5 mg/kg Maintenance: 2.5 mg/kg	200 mg 100 mg	24

Nystatin (oral)	Infants:
	  400,000–800,000 U/day
	Children:
	  2,000,000–4,000,000 U/day
			6

Fluconazole (IV and oral)	Oral: 3 Esophageal: 3–12 Systemic: 6–12	200mg 400mg 800mg	24
Voriconazole (IV and oral)	Pediatric: 18 Adult: 12 × 1 day then 8		12
Posaconazole (IV and oral)	IV: 7–10 DR tab: 7–10 Suspension: 12–20	IV: 300 mg DR tab: 300 mg Suspension: 800 mg	24 24 6–12
Isavuconazole (IV and oral)	6 months to < 1 y: 6 1–18 y: 10 Adult: 372 mg/dose		Load q8h × 6 doses followed by maintenance q24h
Micafungin (IV)	Prophylaxis: 1–2 Treatment: 3	50mg 150mg	24
Caspofungin (IV)	Loading dose: 70 mg/m²/day Maintenance dose: 50 mg/m²/day	Loading dose: 70mg Maintenance dose: 50mg	24
Anidulafungin (IV)	1.5–3	200	24
Amphotericin (IV)	0.5–1		24
Liposomal amphotericin (AmBisome) (IV)	3–10		24
Liposomal amphotericin (Abelcet) (IV)	3–5		24

DR, delayed release; IV, intravenous; PO, oral; TMP/SMX, trimethoprim/sulfamethoxazole; UTI, urinary tract infection.

[a]Neonatal dosing, due to its complexity, is not included here. Neonatal doses are generally based on a combination of weight, gestational age, and/or postnatal age. Please refer to a specific neonatal dosing reference for further guidance.

[b]Dosing ranges reflect the typical doses used for mild (low end) to severe (high end) infections.

Table 39–4. Empiric therapy for common clinical syndromes.[a]

Syndrome	Common Organisms (less common to consider)	Examples of Potentially Useful Empiric Antimicrobials (for specific bacteria, see Table 39–2)	Comments (relevant chapters/US guideline)
Fever in the normal newborn	Group B *Streptococcus* *Escherichia coli* *Enterococcus* (UTI) Other viral (enterovirus, parechovirus, RSV, rhinovirus) [*Meningococcus*] [HSV] [*Streptococcus pneumoniae*] [*Listeria* spp.]	IV: Age < 1 mo: • Ampicillin and gentamicin Age > 1 mo: • Ceftriaxone (± vancomycin)	Substitute cefotaxime (or alternative cephalosporin) for gentamicin if initial Gram stains (CSF, urine) concerning for gram-negative infection Consider HSV coverage (acyclovir) if clinical concern [see Newborn Infant and Infections: Bacterial and Spirochetal chapters]
Sepsis in previously healthy child	Neisseria meningitidis *Staphylococcus aureus* (MRSA or MSSA) GAS *S pneumoniae* [*Haemophilus influenzae* B]	IV: • Ceftriaxone or cefotaxime, and vancomycin	Consider protein synthesis inhibitor if toxic shock (clindamycin) Consider adding cefazolin if *Staphylococcus aureus* likely (better outcomes for MSSA than vancomycin) In many geographic areas, resistance to clindamycin among both MSSA and MRSA isolates is high. [see Infections: Bacterial and Spirochetal chapter]
Fever in patient with central venous access, not neutropenic	*Staphylococcus,* coagulase negative *S aureus* (MRSA or MSSA) Enteric gram negatives (particularly if GI compromise) *Enterococcus* spp. (particularly if GI compromise) [*Pseudomonas aeruginosa*] [Yeast]	IV: • Ceftriaxone or cefotaxime, and vancomycin	If recent history of resistant organism, add specific coverage GI/short gut patients higher risk for gram negatives If neutropenic, substitute cefepime for ceftriaxone/cefotaxime If high risk or not responding to antibiotics, consider coverage for yeast (fluconazole, micafungin) [see Infections: Bacterial and Spirochetal chapter]
Sepsis in a neutropenic child	*Pseudomonas aeruginosa* *Streptococcus viridans* *Staphylococcus,* coagulase negative *S aureus* (MRSA or MSSA) Enteric gram negatives [*Enterococcus* spp.] [Yeast]	IV: • Cefepime and vancomycin	If recent history of resistant organism, add specific coverage If high risk or not responding to antibiotics, consider coverage for yeast (micafungin) Consider adding ampicillin for *Enterococcus gallinarum* and *Enterococcus casseliflavus* or daptomycin for VRE depending on local epidemiology [see Infections: Bacterial and Spirochetal chapter]
Urinary tract infection/ pyelonephritis	*E coli* *Klebsiella* spp. *Enterococcus* spp. Other enteric gram negatives	Oral: • Cephalexin • Trimethoprim/sulfamethoxazole IV: • Ceftriaxone	Substitute amoxicillin/ampicillin for enterococcus [see Kidney and Urinary Tract and Infections: Bacterial and Spirochetal chapter, and US national guideline]
Acute suppurative otitis media	Virus *S pneumoniae* *H influenzae* *M catarrhalis*	Oral: • Amoxicillin (high dose) • Amoxicillin/clavulanic acid (if failed amoxicillin)	Antimicrobial therapy should be targeted toward *S pneumoniae*. As a large proportion of OM is viral, not all cases require treatment [see Ear, Nose and Throat and Infections: Bacterial and Spirochetal chapters, US national guideline]

(Continued)

Table 39–4. Empiric therapy for common clinical syndromes.[a] (*Continued*)

Syndrome	Common Organisms (less common to consider)	Examples of Potentially Useful Empiric Antimicrobials (for specific bacteria, see Table 39–2)	Comments (relevant chapters/US guideline)
Pharyngitis due to GAS	GAS	Oral: • Penicillin • Amoxicillin	Though other oral agents are active, they are broader than necessary and lead to resistance [see Ear, Nose and Throat and Infections: Bacterial and Spirochetal chapters, US national guideline]
Community-acquired pneumonia	Viruses *S pneumoniae* Mycoplasma [*S aureus* (MRSA or MSSA)] [GAS] [*H influenzae* (B or nontypable)] [*Moraxella catarrhalis*]	Oral: • Amoxicillin (high dose) • IV: • Ampicillin	Antimicrobial therapy should be targeted toward *S pneumoniae*. For sicker inpatients, consider *S aureus* coverage. Coverage of penicillin-resistant gram negatives (*H influenzae, M catarrhalis*) uncommonly needed. Though mycoplasma is common, it is not clear that directed therapy improves outcomes; if coverage desired, azithromycin is drug of choice, but it does not provide sufficient *S pneumoniae* coverage. In many geographic areas, resistance to clindamycin among both MSSA and MRSA isolates is high. [see Respiratory Tract and Mediastinum, and Infections: Bacterial and Spirochetal chapters, US national guideline]
Skin and soft tissue infection	*S aureus* (MRSA or MSSA) GAS	Oral: • Cephalexin • Clindamycin • TMP/SMX	May require drainage Consider other organisms if history of bite or trauma In many geographic areas, resistance to clindamycin among both MSSA and MRSA isolates is high. In many geographic areas, resistance to TMP/SMX among GAS isolates is high. [see Skin and Infections: Bacterial and Spirochetal chapters]
Acute suppurative adenitis	*S aureus* (MRSA or MSSA) GAS	Oral: • Cephalexin • Clindamycin IV: • Cefazolin • Clindamycin	May require drainage In many geographic areas, resistance to clindamycin among both MSSA and MRSA isolates is high. [see Ear, Nose and Throat and Infections: Bacterial and Spirochetal chapters]
Acute bacterial sinusitis	*S pneumoniae* *H influenzae* (B or nontypable) *M catarrhalis* *S aureus* (MRSA or MSSA) Anaerobic bacteria	Oral: • Amoxicillin (high dose) • Amoxicillin/clavulanic acid (high dose)	Therapy should be directed against *S pneumoniae* (amoxicillin); in severe sinusitis, expansion to other organisms reasonable. [see Ear, Nose and Throat and Infections: Bacterial and Spirochetal chapters, US national guideline]
Orbital cellulitis (sinusitis associated)	*S pneumoniae* *S anginosus/viridans* *H influenzae* (B or nontypable) *M catarrhalis* *S aureus* (MRSA or MSSA) Anaerobic bacteria	IV: • Ampicillin/sulbactam • Ceftriaxone + clindamycin	Consider addition of MRSA coverage (vancomycin) May require drainage In many geographic areas, resistance to clindamycin among both MSSA and MRSA isolates is high. [see Ear, Nose and Throat and Infections: Bacterial and Spirochetal chapters, US national guideline]

(Continued)

Table 39–4. Empiric therapy for common clinical syndromes.[a] (*Continued*)

Syndrome	Common Organisms (less common to consider)	Examples of Potentially Useful Empiric Antimicrobials (for specific bacteria, see Table 39–2)	Comments (relevant chapters/US guideline)
Acute suppurative mastoiditis	S pneumoniae GAS S aureus (MRSA or MSSA) [H influenzae (B or nontypable)] [Pseudomonas spp.]	IV: • Ampicillin/sulbactam • Ceftriaxone + clindamycin	May require drainage. In many geographic areas, resistance to clindamycin among both MSSA and MRSA isolates is high. [see Ear, Nose and Throat and Infections: Bacterial and Spirochetal chapters]
Brain abscess (sinusitis associated)	S anginosus/viridans S pneumoniae H influenzae (B or nontypable) M catarrhalis S aureus (MRSA or MSSA) Anaerobic bacteria	IV: • Vancomycin, ceftriaxone and metronidazole	May require drainage [see Ear, Nose and Throat and Infections: Bacterial and Spirochetal chapters]
Dental abscess	Polymicrobial mouth flora	Oral: • Penicillin • Clindamycin • Amoxicillin/clavulanic acid IV: • Ampicillin/sulbactam • Clindamycin	May require tooth extraction [see Oral Medicine and Dentistry and Infections: Bacterial and Spirochetal chapters]
Peritonsillar or para-pharyngeal abscess	GAS S aureus (MRSA or MSSA) S anginosus/viridans Other oral flora	IV: • Ampicillin/sulbactam • Ceftriaxone + clindamycin	May require drainage In many geographic areas, resistance to clindamycin among both MSSA and MRSA isolates is high. [see Ear, Nose and Throat and Infections: Bacterial and Spirochetal chapters]
Infected dog and cat bites	Pasteurella spp. S aureus (MRSA or MSSA) GAS [Capnocytophaga canimorsus]	Oral: • Amoxicillin/clavulanic acid (high dose) • Clindamycin + FLQ IV: • Ampicillin/sulbactam • Ceftriaxone + clindamycin	Consider rabies and tetanus prophylaxis May require suture removal and/or drainage In many geographic areas, resistance to clindamycin among both MSSA and MRSA isolates is high. [see Emergencies and Injuries and Infections: Bacterial and Spirochetal chapters, US national guideline]
Acute hematogenous musculoskeletal infection	S aureus (MRSA or MSSA) Kingella kingae GAS [S pneumoniae] [N meningitides] [Salmonella spp.]	Oral: • Cephalexin • Clindamycin IV: • Cefazolin • Clindamycin • Vancomycin	In many geographic areas, resistance to clindamycin among both MSSA and MRSA is high. [see Orthopedic and Infections: Bacterial and Spirochetal chapters]
Acute endocarditis	S viridans S aureus (MRSA or MSSA) HACEK organisms	IV: • Ceftriaxone + vancomycin + gentamicin	Assure multiple blood cultures prior to antibiotics. Alter empiric coverage based on risk factors.
Acute traveler's diarrhea	E coli Campylobacter Salmonella spp. Shigella spp. Others	Oral: • Azithromycin • Rifaximin • Ciprofloxacin • Cefixime	Choice of agent tailored to resistance in area of travel (see CDC travel website)

(Continued)

Table 39–4. Empiric therapy for common clinical syndromes.[a] (*Continued*)

Syndrome	Common Organisms (less common to consider)	Examples of Potentially Useful Empiric Antimicrobials (for specific bacteria, see Table 39–2)	Comments (relevant chapters/US guideline)
Acute appendicitis	E coli Bacteroides fragilis	IV: • Ceftriaxone + metronidazole	Both ceftriaxone and metronidazole can be dosed once daily for appendicitis
Liver abscess	S anginosus E coli Bacteroides fragilis Other GI flora [Entamoeba histolytica]	IV: • Ceftriaxone + metronidazole	May require drainage Consider E. histolytica if drainage with few PMNs, "anchovy paste" appearance, epidemiology supports [see Infections: Bacterial and Spirochetal chapters]

CDC, Centers for Disease Control and Prevention; CSF, cerebrospinal fluid; FLQ, fluoroquinolone; GAS, group A *Streptococcus*; GI, gastrointestinal; HACEK, (*Haemophilus, Aggregatibacter, Cardiobacterium, Eikenella,* and *Kingella*); HSV, herpes simplex virus; IV, intravenous; MRSA, methicillin-resistant *S aureus*; MSSA, methicillin-susceptible *S aureus*; OM, otitis media; PMN, polymorphonuclear neutrophils; RSV, respiratory syncytial virus; UTI, urinary tract infection.

Organisms [in brackets] are less likely, but need consideration in empiric choice of antimicrobials.

[a]Empiric therapy should always be tailored to specific risk factors and clinical clues on a case-by-case basis. Antimicrobial choices populated on right of table do not necessarily cover all microbes listed to left, rather they are meant as one potential option for empiric coverage. Local susceptibility patterns should always be considered in choice of empiric therapy. Antimicrobials should be adjusted to organism and susceptibility once known.

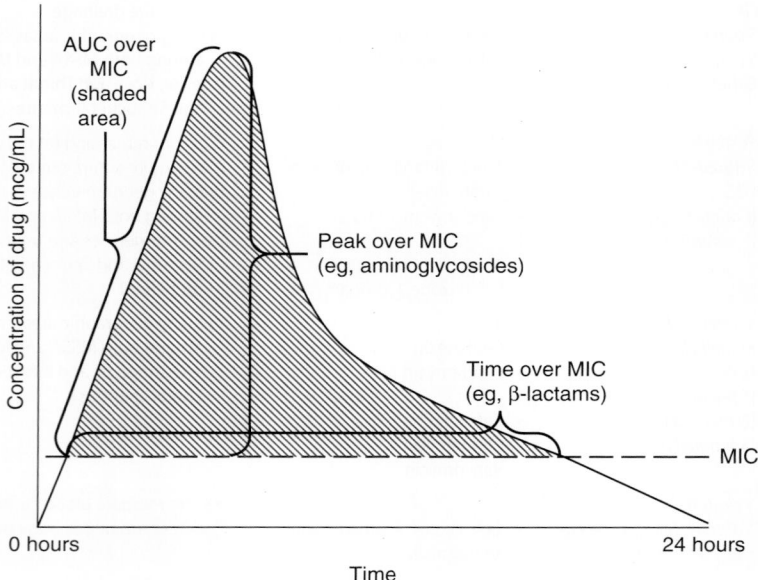

▲ **Figure 39–1.** Depiction of pharmacokinetic/pharmacodynamic parameters for antimicrobial efficacy. For β-lactams, efficacy is best correlated with the time antimicrobial concentrations exceed the organism's MIC at the site of infection (time over MIC). For concentration-dependent antibiotics (eg, aminoglycosides, daptomycin), the peak over MIC ratio best correlates with efficacy. For most other antibiotics, the total antibiotic exposure (quantified by the AUC over the MIC) best correlates with efficacy. AUC, area under the [concertation-time] curve; MIC, minimum inhibitory concentration.

the surviving microbes take hours to recover the ability to replicate, known as the postantibiotic effect (PAE), which allows for extended interval dosing. For most other drugs (clindamycin, tetracyclines, vancomycin, azithromycin, linezolid, metronidazole, trimethoprim/sulfamethoxazole [TMP/SMX], fluoroquinolones, etc), the AUC over the MIC is the best predictor of bacterial killing because it incorporates both the required time above MIC and PAE. In addition to antibiotic PK, other patient factors affect dosing, most notably organ dysfunction (especially the liver and kidney), concomitant medications, obesity, and age.

CHOICE OF ANTIMICROBIAL AGENTS

Recommendations for choosing antibiotics for specific conditions are based on the patient's age, diagnosis, site of infection, severity of illness, local antimicrobial susceptibility patterns, antimicrobial susceptibility of patient-specific bacterial isolates (historical and current), history of drug allergy, and potential drug interactions and side effects, as discussed above. Tables 39–2 to 39–4 provide further information, including dosing. Always consult the package insert for detailed prescribing information. Empiric and definitive therapies for many clinical entities are addressed throughout this textbook and in Table 39–4. Mechanisms of action and efficacy parameters are noted later and indicated in Figure 39–2.

SPECIFIC ANTIMICROBIAL AGENTS

β-LACTAM ANTIBIOTICS (STEP 1, FIGURE 39–2)

β-Lactam antimicrobials include the penicillins, cephalosporins, carbapenems, monobactams (step 1, Figure 39–2), and certain β-lactamase inhibitors (step 8, Figure 39–2). They are characterized by a four-member β-lactam ring, but otherwise they are structurally distinct, with differences in their ability to bind their target in the pathogen, the penicillin-binding proteins (PBPs). PBPs, originally named for their ability to bind penicillin experimentally, are functionally transpeptidase enzymes that are essential for bacterial cell wall synthesis. Bacteria have a large variety and number of PBPs, so the spectrum of β-lactam activity is related to the binding affinity to the key PBPs in a given bacterial isolate. Binding of PBPs by β-lactams prevents cross-linking of the peptidoglycan layer of the cell wall, resulting in bacterial death. Bacteria protect themselves from β-lactams mainly by (1) producing β-lactamases that hydrolyze the β-lactam ring, (2) altering the PBP to change the β-lactam–PBP-binding affinity, or (3) creating changes in porins or efflux pumps (step 9, Figure 39–2) to decrease the intracellular concentration of drug. There are many different types of β-lactamases that vary from very narrow penicillinases (such as that produced routinely by *Staphylococcus aureus*) to more sophisticated

and broad types produced by gram negatives, of which there are thousands. Among these are the inducible β-lactamases (IBL) that are chromosomally mediated but only become clinically apparent after β-lactam exposure. The most common IBL-producing organisms are certain *Enterobacter* and *Citrobacter* species, but there are many others. There are also the extended spectrum β-lactamases (ESBLs), which are primarily produced by *Klebsiella* species and *E coli*. These are of particular concern because the plasmids (see Figure 39–2) encoding them are transmissible between organisms and often harbor other types of resistance. Of increasing concern are the plasmids encoding carbapenem resistance because they often contain other types of resistance mutations and have the potential to lead to highly resistant infections that are untreatable with current drugs.

Although allergy to β-lactam antimicrobials is reported commonly by parents, this history is not highly predictive of an allergic reaction. Penicillin allergy is reported in up to 10% of the general population, but over 90% of those patients tolerate penicillin challenge without a reaction (suggesting either that the allergy has resolved or was never present). Because patients labeled with a penicillin allergy may receive inferior treatment strategies, confirming the details of the history is important. Patients unlikely to have a true allergy (eg family history alone, delayed onset [greater than 24 hours after first dose] or onset of isolated, nonprogressive symptoms [such as gastrointestinal symptoms or rash/hives alone]) should be "de-labeled," and those with a history consistent with a concerning reaction should be referred for allergy testing.

β-LACTAM: PENICILLINS

Penicillins & Aminopenicillins

Penicillins, amoxicillin, and ampicillin are the drugs of choice to treat infections with most streptococci (including group A *Streptococcus*, group B *Streptococcus*, and *S pneumoniae*), most enterococci, *Treponema pallidum*, *Neisseria meningitidis*, *Leptospira*, *Streptobacillus moniliformis* (rat-bite fever), *Actinomyces*, many oral anaerobes, and most *Clostridium* and *Bacillus* species. They are also used for prophylaxis in patients with rheumatic fever or asplenia. Amoxicillin and ampicillin are considered first line for community-acquired pneumonia and otitis media. They penetrate all tissues relatively well, and amoxicillin offers adequate oral bioavailability (it has the best bioavailability among β-lactams that, as a class, are generally poorly absorbed). More time above the MIC is achieved with higher, more frequent dosing; for example, amoxicillin dosed 90 mg/kg divided three times daily for *S pneumoniae* (with MIC of 1–2 mcg/mL) will achieve 7–8 hours of time over the MIC, while if divided only two times a day, it will exceed the MIC for only 5–6 hours.

The common β-lactamase inhibitors are themselves β-lactams in structure (including sulbactam, clavulanic acid,

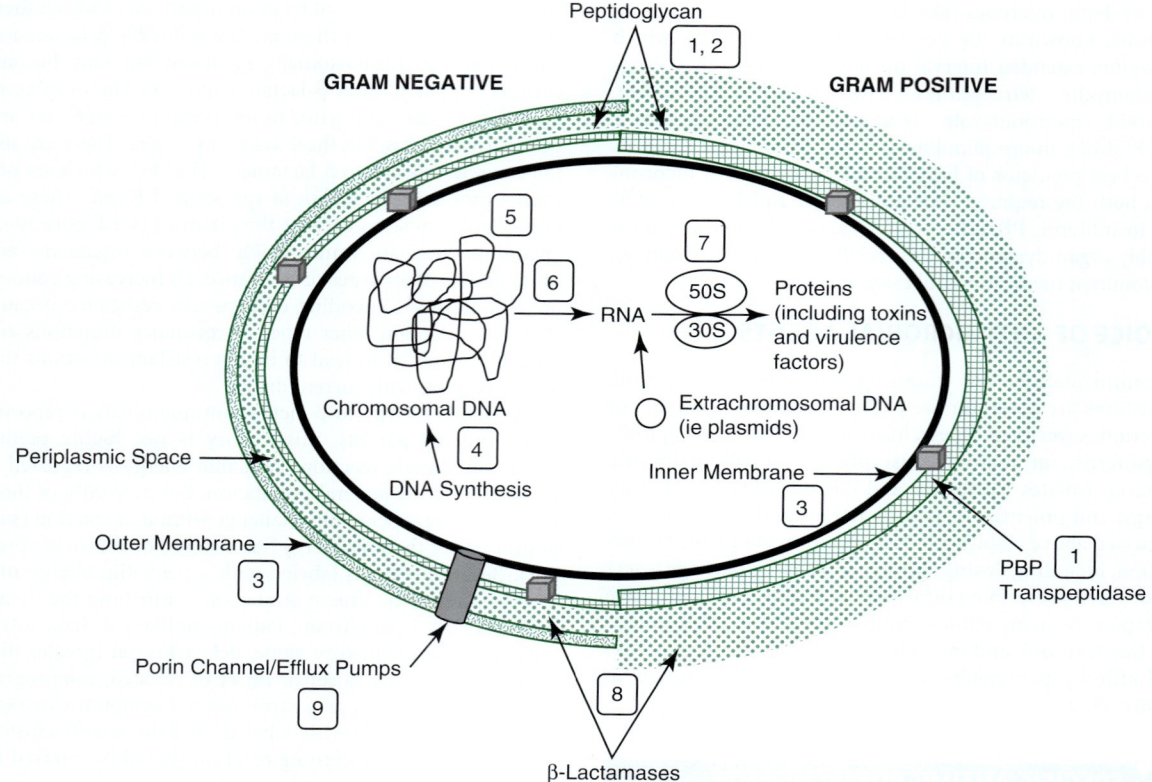

▲ **Figure 39–2.** Simple schematic of bacterial cell with antibiotic targets and resistance mechanisms. Antibiotic mechanisms of action include affecting cell wall and membrane synthesis/function (1, 2, 3), nucleic acid synthesis/function (4, 5, 6), or protein synthesis (7).

(1) All β-lactam antibiotics bind to the bacterial PBP, preventing enzymatic cross-linking necessary for cell wall maintenance.

(2) Glycopeptides (eg, vancomycin) inhibit peptidoglycan synthesis by preventing cross-linking at the terminal amino acids. Fosfomycin inhibits an early step in peptidoglycan synthesis.

(3) Daptomycin inserts into lipid-rich inner membrane of gram-positive bacteria leading to depolarization and cell death. Polymyxins cause membrane damage to both the inner and outer membranes.

(4) TMP/SMX inhibit two steps in the folate synthesis pathway, which then inhibits DNA biosynthesis.

(5) Fluoroquinolones target bacterial topoisomerases, inhibiting DNA replication and repair. Metronidazole and nitro-furantoin, after intracellular activation, produces active metabolites and free radicals that, in part, destabilize bacterial DNA.

(6) Rifamycins inhibit bacterial RNA polymerase, preventing RNA synthesis.

(7) Multiple antibiotics inhibit protein synthesis. At the 50S ribosomal subunit, oxazolidinones (eg linezolid) prevent initiation of protein synthesis, while both macrolides (eg, azithromycin) and lincosamides (eg, clindamycin) inhibit elongation of the peptide chain. At the 30S ribosomal subunit, tetracyclines inhibit peptide elongation by blocking transfer RNA (tRNA) binding, and aminoglycosides disrupt translational accuracy to impede peptide elongation.

(8) β-lactamases are enzymes that bind to and degrade β-lactam antibiotics with variable efficiency depending on the β-lactamase. Gram-positive bacteria secrete β-lactamases to the extracellular space, while Gram-negative bacteria secrete β-lactamases into the periplasmic space.

(9) Porins are transmembrane protein channels that allow antibiotic diffusion across the bacterial membrane, and mutations in porin-related genes can impair antibiotic influx and increase resistance. Efflux pumps, also transmembrane proteins, can actively export antibiotics from the cell, also leading to increased resistance.

and tazobactam, though not avibactam or vaborbactam), but they do not typically have antibacterial activity. Instead, they act as "decoys," binding bacterial β-lactamases so that their companion drug is free to bind the target PBP. They are available in combination with aminopenicillins in amoxicillin/clavulanic acid (oral) and ampicillin/sulbactam (IV), offering expanded activity to methicillin-susceptible *S aureus* (MSSA), *Moraxella catarrhalis*, *Klebsiella* spp., and β-lactamase–producing gram negatives (such as some *Haemophilus influenzae*, *E coli*) and anaerobes (such as *Bacteroides fragilis* and *Fusobacteria* spp.). This makes them useful for treating mixed infections, for example, dog bites or tonsillar and parapharyngeal abscesses, orbital cellulitis, step-down therapy for ruptured appendicitis, and refractory sinusitis and otitis media. Notably, they offer no advantage in the treatment of *S pneumoniae* or other streptococci, as these organisms do not produce β-lactamases. Piperacillin/tazobactam similarly expands coverage, including coverage for *Pseudomonas aeruginosa*. This drug has a niche in complex abdominal infections and hospital-associated pneumonia, but it should be used sparingly due to its broad spectrum. While penicillins and aminopenicillins penetrate most body tissues, the penetration of the β-lactamase inhibitors is poorly understood. Combinations of β-lactam with β-lactamase inhibitor are notorious for causing diarrhea, particularly amoxicillin/clavulanic acid, and care with dosing different formulations containing clavulanic acid is advised.

Penicillinase-Resistant Penicillins

The penicillinase-resistant penicillins were developed as anti-MSSA antibiotics to combat the narrow-spectrum β-lactamase (penicillinase) produced by nearly all MSSA. These drugs, which include nafcillin, oxacillin, methicillin, and dicloxacillin, offer structural protection from penicillinases to the β-lactam ring. They are associated with renal and hepatic toxicity, which limits their use. Drug fever, rashes, and neutropenia are also common. Methicillin is renally excreted, whereas oxacillin and nafcillin are excreted renally and through the biliary tract. Nafcillin is a venous irritant, making it difficult to maintain peripheral IV access; it also causes damage after extravasation, so it is best used with large vein or central lines. Because of their expense and side-effect profiles, these drugs have largely been supplanted by cefazolin (IV) and cephalexin (oral), but the IV forms retain a niche in the treatment of endocarditis and central nervous system (CNS) infections caused by MSSA.

β-LACTAM: CEPHALOSPORINS

Cephalosporins are often categorized in "generations," which is not a chemical relationship but rather represents similarity in antimicrobial spectra based on binding to various PBPs. All the resistance mechanisms mentioned above for β-lactams also apply to cephalosporins. Gram-negative organisms have an ever-expanding variety of β-lactamases, the most problematic of which in routine practice are the IBLs and ESBLs. No cephalosporins approved for use in the United States have activity against enterococci.

The first-generation cephalosporins include cefazolin (IV) and cephalexin (oral), which are mainly used to treat infections with MSSA or as empiric therapy for UTIs. They are highly effective treatments for SSTI (as they also have activity against group A streptococci), MSSA pneumonia, and in initial and oral step-down treatment of musculoskeletal infections in children. Because of its high concentration in urine, cephalexin is considered first line for UTIs and often achieves adequate killing in organisms deemed "resistant."

The second-generation cephalosporins include IV cefuroxime and oral cefprozil and cefuroxime. These have somewhat reduced, but acceptable, activity against gram-positive cocci, and greater activity against some gram-negative rods compared with first-generation cephalosporins, but not as much as the third-generation cephalosporins described below. They are active against *H influenzae* and *M catarrhalis*, including strains that produce β-lactamases capable of inactivating ampicillin. Cefoxitin and cefotetan, which are considered second-generation cephamycins, offer activity against anaerobes, making them potentially useful in the treatment of nonperforated appendicitis, cholangitis, and pelvic inflammatory disease; however, increasing resistance and short half-life (cefoxitin) are limitations.

Third-generation cephalosporins have substantially less activity against MSSA than first-generation cephalosporins, though notably increased activity against *S pneumoniae*. They also have increased activity against aerobic gram-negative bacteria that harbor narrow-spectrum β-lactamases. The most common intravenous forms are ceftriaxone and cefotaxime; due to production issues, availability of cefotaxime is currently limited. Ceftazidime provides similar coverage (though with inadequate *S pneumoniae* coverage) but provides some activity against *P aeruginosa*. These IV formulations have good CNS penetration. Oral third-generation options, including cefpodoxime, cefixime, and cefdinir, are limited by low serum concentrations and cannot be considered equivalent to IV formulations.

Cefepime is considered a fourth-generation cephalosporin. It retains considerable activity against MSSA while also being active against *P aeruginosa* and some other IBL producers, such as *Enterobacter* spp. It is a zwitterion and as such efficiently penetrates the gram-negative outer cell membrane. Despite its efficacy against IBL-producing organisms, cefepime is hydrolyzed by ESBLs so generally confers little advantage against ESBL-producing bacteria.

Ceftaroline is the only cephalosporin able to treat methicillin-resistant *S aureus* (MRSA) based on its ability to bind the PBP (PBP2a) in MRSA (encoded by *mecA*); it does not, however, have activity against *P aeruginosa*. Ceftaroline is approved in children, and perhaps has a place in children with invasive MRSA infections, particularly in patients with renal injury. CNS penetration may not be optimal.

There are now two cephalosporins combined with β-lactamase inhibitors, ceftazidime/avibactam and ceftolozane/tazobactam. These have activity against *P aeruginosa*, and variable coverage against many other highly resistant gram negatives.

With the exception of cephalexin, which has high oral bioavailability, other oral cephalosporins have poor serum concentrations and achieve adequate T > MIC for sufficient killing in only limited clinical scenarios. In general, they are poorly absorbed, highly protein bound, and often are given at ineffective long intervals. Though they should not be widely used, longer T > MIC is achieved in the middle ear and urine compared to other locations, improving likelihood of cure in those locations. For organisms susceptible to amoxicillin, oral cephalosporins are pharmacokinetically inferior and should be used only for patients with penicillin allergy. For example, high-dose amoxicillin is more effective than cefdinir for *S pneumoniae*.

β-LACTAM: MONOBACTAMS

Aztreonam is the only monobactam approved for use in the United States. Aztreonam is active against aerobic gram-negative rods, including *P aeruginosa*. Aztreonam has activity against *H influenzae* and *M catarrhalis*, including those that are β-lactamase producers. The most common uses of aztreonam are as an aerosol for therapy of *P aeruginosa* infection in patients with cystic fibrosis, and as an alternative therapy for severely β-lactam allergic patients, as there is little cross-reactivity between aztreonam and other β-lactams, except ceftazidime that shares a common side chain. Aztreonam also has a place in the treatment of certain carbapenem-resistant organisms, particularly in combination with avibactam, given that it is inherently stable against certain carbapenemases.

β-LACTAM: CARBAPENEMS

The carbapenems, including meropenem, ertapenem, doripenem, and imipenem, are broadly effective against gram-negative aerobes, most anaerobes, and many gram-positive organisms. They have some activity against MSSA (but not MRSA), *S pneumoniae*, *Enterococcus faecalis* (but not *Enterococcus faecium*), and various other gram positives. Except for ertapenem, they have good activity against *P aeruginosa* and retain activity against many multidrug-resistant gram negatives, including those with IBLs and ESBLs. Imipenem is available in combination with cilastatin, which inhibits the metabolism of imipenem in the kidneys resulting in high serum and urine concentrations. An increased frequency of seizures is encountered when CNS infections are treated with carbapenems, particularly imipenem; carbapenems also decrease valproic acid levels. Because carbapenems are active against so many species of bacteria, there is a strong temptation to use them as single-drug empiric therapy. However, overuse is linked to the development of multidrug resistance. Hospitals that use carbapenems heavily encounter resistance in many different species of gram-negative rods. This resistance can develop within days due to bacteria developing a porin/efflux resistance mechanism (step 9, Figure 39–2). Carbapenem use should therefore be reserved only for patients with confirmed (or at high risk for) infection due to highly resistant organisms. Bacteria with β-lactamases capable of attacking the carbapenems are spreading worldwide; organisms harboring these plasmids often have many resistance mechanisms and are susceptible to few (if any) remaining treatment options. To address some of these resistance mechanisms, meropenem is now available with a β-lactamase inhibitor, vaborbactam.

GLYCOPEPTIDE AGENTS (STEP 2, FIGURE 39–2)

Glycopeptides include vancomycin, telavancin, oritavancin, and dalbavancin. They are characterized by their large molecular size, which prevents them from penetrating the outer membrane of gram-negative organisms. Like the β-lactams, they also are active on the cell wall, inhibiting peptidoglycan synthesis by preventing cross-linking at the terminal amino acids (D-alanine). It is debated if their efficacy is most related to time over the MIC or AUC over MIC. Bacteria protect themselves mainly through (1) changing the terminal amino acid to D-lactate so that vancomycin cannot bind or (2) thickening the cell wall (vancomycin-intermediate and resistant *S aureus*) such that the glycopeptide cannot bind enough targets to prevent cross-linking. They have notable nephrotoxicity, and vancomycin is a common cause of drug-related acute kidney injury (AKI). Vancomycin flushing syndrome (flushing and itching with infusion), which is not an allergic response, can be mitigated with slower infusions (over 2 hours) and premedication with diphenhydramine (with or without hydrocortisone). All the glycopeptides have similar spectra of activity, including MRSA, coagulase negative staphylococci, ampicillin-resistant enterococci, and penicillin-resistant *S pneumoniae*. Oral vancomycin is not systemically absorbed but effectively kills *Clostridium difficile* in the GI tract and is more effective than metronidazole. The glycopeptides differ in dosing strategies, with telavancin dosed once daily, and both dalbavancin and oritavancin dosed once weekly. Dalbavancin has pediatric pharmacokinetic, safety, and efficacy data.

Efficacy of vancomycin requires sufficient drug exposure, and monitoring and dose adjustment are necessary given vancomycin's narrow therapeutic window and risk for drug-induced AKI. Vancomycin exposure can be monitored and adjusted with either trough-directed dosing or AUC/MIC-guided dosing. Current guidelines favor AUC/MIC-guided dosing (goal 400–600 mg*h/L), largely due to evidence that AUC/MIC-targeting results in less renal toxicity without an apparent loss in efficacy. However, measuring vancomycin AUC in clinical practice is practically difficult, requiring multiple blood draws and/or specialized PK software. Because of this, trough targeting is still widely used as a surrogate for AUC, though trough goals greater than 15 mcg/mL are associated with significantly increased nephrotoxicity in pediatrics without a clear clinical benefit. Both serum creatinine and vancomycin concentrations should be monitored closely in all patients receiving vancomycin. Continuous infusion can be used if sufficient concentrations are not achievable with every 6-hour dosing.

The empiric use of vancomycin has increased tremendously over the past decade. Thus, vancomycin-resistant enterococci (VRE) are now problematic, particularly in inpatient units, intensive care units, and oncology wards. Vancomycin-intermediate and vancomycin-resistant S aureus exist, which is of concern because of the inherent virulence of many S aureus strains. Vancomycin use should be monitored carefully in hospitals and intensive care units. Vancomycin should not be used empirically when an infection is mild or when other antimicrobial agents are likely to be effective, and it should be stopped promptly if infection is caused by organisms susceptible to other antimicrobials. Obtaining cultures prior to vancomycin initiation is required because there is no direct oral step-down therapy and susceptibilities to oral alternatives are not predictable.

DAPTOMYCIN (STEP 3, FIGURE 39–2)

Daptomycin is unique in being a lipopeptide that inserts into the lipid-rich cell inner membrane of gram-positive bacteria. This results in depolarization and cell death. It is unclear if efficacy correlates with the time that intracellular concentrations exceed the MIC or whether AUC over MIC is most important. Microbes protect themselves by changing the charge of their cell membranes, such that daptomycin cannot penetrate the inner membrane. Since daptomycin cannot penetrate the gram-negative outer cell membrane (envelope), it is only active against gram-positive organisms and has a clinical niche against MRSA and vancomycin-resistant E faecium. Daptomycin may insert itself into lipid layers of human cells, particularly muscle, causing creatinine phosphokinase (CPK) elevation. Due to the possibility of rhabdomyolysis, monitoring CPK is recommended. Daptomycin is a lipid-like molecule that is enveloped by pulmonary surfactant, rendering it inactive and not useful for lung infections.

TRIMETHOPRIM/SULFAMETHOXAZOLE (STEP 4, FIGURE 39–2)

Sulfonamides—the oldest class of antimicrobials—are usually used in a fixed combination with trimethoprim (TMP/SMX) for greater efficacy to inhibit two steps in the folate synthesis pathway (which then inhibits DNA biosynthesis, step 8, Figure 39–2). AUC over MIC correlates with efficacy. Resistance is usually related to alterations in the binding targets

or decreased drug concentrations due to efflux or decreased entry. TMP/SMX is particularly associated with drug hypersensitivity reactions and, more rarely, severe skin reactions such as Stevens-Johnson syndrome. It also may cause hematologic abnormalities that can be severe. It should not be used in patients with G6PD deficiency. TMP/SMX is most often used clinically to treat SSTIs caused by MRSA, UTIs, and susceptible strains of Haemophilus spp., Shigella spp., or Salmonella spp. TMP/SMX is a mainstay in prophylaxis and treatment of Pneumocystis jirovecii infection, and in treatment of Nocardia spp. and Stenotrophomonas maltophilia. As an intravenous formulation, it requires large volume infusion over 2 hours every 6–12 hours, so is rarely given via this route (especially given its high oral bioavailability). Pathogens with significant resistance include S pneumoniae and various gram negatives.

METRONIDAZOLE (STEP 5, FIGURE 39–2)

Metronidazole is a prodrug that is only converted to its active form by anaerobic bacteria and amoebic and other protozoal organisms. It is unclear if these active intermediates bind DNA, RNA, or essential proteins to cause microbial cell death. Effective killing is related to the AUC over MIC. It has a PAE and a long half-life so can be dosed less frequently than the currently recommended three times daily. When used IV for pediatric appendicitis, it often is dosed once daily, though it is still dosed three times daily orally for improved GI tolerance. Resistance mechanisms are not well investigated, but they likely relate to lack of conversion to active drug. It is most active against gram-negative and gram-positive anaerobic rods, such as Bacteroides, Fusobacterium, Clostridium, Prevotella, and Porphyromonas. Gram-positive anaerobic cocci such as Peptostreptococcus are often more susceptible to penicillin or to clindamycin. Metronidazole is the drug of choice for bacterial vaginosis and among the recommended options for C difficile enterocolitis. It is active against many parasites, including Giardia lamblia and Entamoeba histolytica. Metronidazole is highly bioavailable and has excellent tissue penetration, including to the CNS.

MACROLIDES (STEP 7, FIGURE 39–2)

The macrolide antimicrobials in common use include erythromycin, azithromycin, and clarithromycin. They inhibit protein synthesis by blocking RNA translation and assembly of the 50S ribosomal subunit. Efficacy is related to AUC over MIC. Microbes protect themselves by altering the macrolide binding site with methylation or through efflux of the drug. Because of ease of dosing and tolerability, azithromycin is the most prescribed macrolide worldwide and is one of the most commonly prescribed antimicrobials in the United States. This likely indicates overuse, as macrolides are rarely considered first-line agents in national treatment guidelines, and high rates of resistance exist among S pneumoniae, for which it is commonly prescribed. Gastrointestinal side effects are common with the macrolides, particularly with erythromycin, which is sometimes used as a promotility agent. Exposure to macrolides early in life is associated with infantile hypertrophic pyloric stenosis, though azithromycin is thought to pose a lower risk than erythromycin. They all prolong the QTc interval, a consideration in at-risk patients.

Azithromycin has a large volume of distribution and a long half-life; after a 5-day treatment course, intracellular drug persists for approximately 10 days. Azithromycin is used to treat *Campylobacter*, *Shigella*, and *Salmonella* infections, including typhoid fever resistant to ampicillin and TMP-SMX, so it is a reliable antibiotic for presumed bacterial traveler's diarrhea. All macrolides are active against many bacteria that are intrinsically resistant to cell wall–active antimicrobials, and they are effective for *Bordetella pertussis*, *Legionella pneumophila*, *Chlamydophila pneumoniae*, *Mycoplasma pneumoniae*, and *Chlamydia trachomatis* infections. Azithromycin and clarithromycin also have activity against some atypical mycobacteria. Resistance among other common pathogens, such as *S pneumoniae*, group A *Streptococcus*, *S aureus*, and *Haemophilus* spp., limits azithromycin efficacy for otitis media, sinusitis, and community-acquired pneumonia (except for *Mycoplasma*).

LINCOSAMIDES (STEP 7, FIGURE 39–2)

Clindamycin targets protein synthesis through inhibiting peptidyl transferase at the 50S ribosomal subunit. Its efficacy is related to the AUC over MIC. Resistance, which is mediated by methylation of the binding site, may be constitutive or may be induced. If inducible clindamycin resistance is present—detected using the D-test, a disk-diffusion-based test that uses erythromycin to induce and identify clindamycin resistance—an isolate is reported as resistant to clindamycin. Efflux of drug is another mechanism of resistance. Clindamycin is highly bioavailable and penetrates most body tissues, though should not be used to treat CNS or UTIs due to poor penetration to these spaces. Though clindamycin is not used to treat CNS bacterial infections, it may achieve sufficient CNS levels to treat CNS toxoplasmosis (given low parasiticidal concentrations), though it is not considered a first-line agent. It is active against many anaerobes and gram-positive aerobic organisms, including *S pneumoniae*, *S pyogenes*, and MRSA, though resistance is becoming more prevalent. It is not active against enterococci. Because of its unique spectrum of activity, it is often used to treat mixed aerobic gram-positive and anaerobic infections, such as sinusitis, dental, oral, and neck abscesses; pelvic inflammatory disease; and deep infections from pressure ulcers. Because it inhibits protein synthesis (and thus toxin production), it is often used as an adjunct to treat serious toxin-mediated diseases such as toxic shock syndrome. It also may be more active than β-lactams against nonreplicating bacteria that may be present in undrained abscesses. Clindamycin is associated with

C difficile–related pseudomembranous colitis in adults, but this relationship is uncommon in children, although diarrhea is a frequent side effect. Though clindamycin is an old drug, it is often more expensive than alternatives and has palatability issues.

OXAZOLIDINONES (STEP 7, FIGURE 39–2)

Linezolid, which was the first oxazolidinone in use, targets the 50S-ribosomal RNA subunit to prevent initiation of protein synthesis. Cross-resistance with other ribosomally active antimicrobials is uncommon, though a unique mutation of the binding site has made resistance increasingly common. Efficacy is related to AUC over MIC. Linezolid has broad gram-positive activity, including some anaerobes, but it is typically reserved for particular drug-resistant organisms (eg, VRE) when first-line agents are contraindicated (eg, for MRSA when vancomycin is avoided due to significant renal insufficiency) or when oral therapy is desired and no other oral options are available. It has minimal gram-negative activity. Linezolid comes in an IV formulation, but it is highly bioavailable and is usually used orally. Linezolid is safe and well tolerated in children, but neutropenia and thrombocytopenia are common and frequently dose limiting. A complete blood count should be monitored in patients at increased risk for these problems and in patients receiving therapy for 2 weeks or longer. Linezolid is an inhibitor of monoamine oxidase (MAO) and should not be used in patients taking MAO inhibitors. Tedizolid, a newer agent in this class, has a similar spectrum of activity, is less likely to cause neutropenia, and is approved for adolescents and adults.

TETRACYCLINES (STEP 7, FIGURE 39–2)

Tetracyclines, including doxycycline, minocycline, and tigecycline, interact with transfer RNA (tRNA) at the 30S ribosomal subunit to prevent protein synthesis. Resistance occurs when the microbe develops proteins that protect the tRNA target or when it encodes efflux pumps to decrease intracellular drug concentrations. Efficacy is related to AUC over MIC. Tetracyclines are broadly effective but are most commonly used against *B pertussis*, many species of *Rickettsia*, *Chlamydia/Chlamydophila*, and *Mycoplasma*. Doxycycline is also a first-line treatment option for *C trachomatis* in pelvic inflammatory disease and nongonococcal urethritis. Among tetracyclines, doxycycline is often preferred because it is better tolerated than tetracycline, its twice-daily administration is convenient, and it can be taken with food. Notable side effects of the tetracyclines are staining of permanent teeth, so long courses (longer than 21 days for doxycycline) are generally not given to children younger than 8 years if an alternative exists. However, a single course of a doxycycline, which causes less tooth discoloration than tetracycline, can be safely used in all age groups. Increased photosensitivity is a notable side effect, and minocycline (commonly used for acne) has a particular association with drug-induced hypersensitivity syndrome.

Doxycycline is used for therapy of Q fever and rickettsial infections (Rocky Mountain spotted fever, ehrlichiosis, anaplasmosis, rickettsial pox) and endemic and murine typhus. It is also a first line for treatment of *Borrelia* spp. (Lyme disease, relapsing fever). Doxycycline can also be used as an alternative to macrolides for *M pneumoniae* and *C pneumoniae* infections and for treatment of psittacosis, brucellosis, and *Pasteurella multocida* infection. Doxycycline also retains good activity against MRSA. While doxycycline can be used to treat neurologic Lyme disease, in part because *Borrelia* spp. have low MICs, doxycycline does not achieve sufficient CNS concentrations to treat most other bacterial CNS infections (eg, *S aureus*).

Tigecycline is a glycylcycline analogue of tetracycline that is active against many gram-negative aerobes, anaerobes, and gram-positive cocci including MRSA and enterococci. Tigecycline is not active against *P aeruginosa* but is useful against VRE and resistant gram negatives other than *P aeruginosa*. It is inferior to other agents for bacteremia when the organism is susceptible to alternative antibiotics. It is approved for children over 8 years.

AMINOGLYCOSIDES (STEP 7, FIGURE 39–2)

The aminoglycosides include gentamicin, tobramycin, amikacin, and streptomycin. They bind to the 30S subunit of ribosomal RNA to inhibit protein synthesis. A high peak above MIC is required for efficacy. Because microbes will not replicate for a long time after aminoglycoside exposure (PAE), aminoglycosides can be dosed once daily. However, once-daily dosing is still controversial in pediatrics due to faster clearance in children. Variation in dosing strategies exists due to lack of consensus. While efficacy is associated with an adequate peak to MIC ratio (with a goal peak of at least 8–10 times the MIC to achieve a longer PAE), toxicity is associated with a high trough. Renal toxicity is most common, followed by ototoxicity. Bacteria gain resistance either through bacterial enzymatic modification of the aminoglycoside to limit binding to its target or through changes in drug entry due to alterations in porin channels. Aminoglycosides are active against gram-negative bacteria. When used together with β-lactams and vancomycin, which damage cell walls against some gram positives, there is a synergistic effect such that aminoglycosides enter bacteria more efficiently. Synergy is described for group B streptococci, enterococci, staphylococci, and *Listeria monocytogenes*. All aminoglycosides are active against pseudomonas, but especially tobramycin. Amikacin is less susceptible to microbial modification, so organisms resistant to other aminoglycosides may remain susceptible to amikacin. Addition of an aminoglycoside to another active agent, such as for *P aeruginosa*, is generally considered to add more toxicity than benefit. However, this remains appropriate for empiric therapy in patients at risk for resistant gram-negative bacteria while awaiting speciation and susceptibilities. Tobramycin and amikacin are available as inhaled formulations, and though relative penetration to alveoli is not clear, they are used in patients with cystic fibrosis. As a group, the aminoglycosides do not penetrate CSF well; thus, treatment with a third-generation cephalosporin is preferred for most CNS infection. Aminoglycosides also are not active in acidic environments, rendering them less active in abscesses and bone.

Because of their renal toxicity and ototoxicity, creatinine and drug level monitoring are necessary. Drug concentrations are usually checked between the third and fourth doses, but sooner in children at high risk for renal impairment. For long-term therapy, drug concentrations and creatinine should be checked weekly and hearing screening should be considered, especially for those with elevated trough concentrations.

RIFAMYCINS (STEP 7, FIGURE 39–2)

Rifamycins include rifampin, rifabutin, rifaximin, and rifamycin B. They are the only antimicrobial inhibitors of RNA polymerase. They are active against a wide variety of organisms, including many mycobacteria. Resistance develops quickly (usually via a mutation in RNA polymerase) so they should not be used as monotherapy, except in select circumstances. Rifampin monotherapy is used as prophylaxis after exposure to *H influenzae* or *N meningitides*, as well as to treat latent *M tuberculosis* infection. It is also used as combination therapy to penetrate bacterial biofilms for patients with prosthetic material in place. Rifampin and rifabutin are used in combination therapy for active tuberculosis; rifabutin is often preferred in patients co-infected with human immunodeficiency virus (HIV) as rifampin decreases levels of some HIV medications. Most rifamycins, rifampin in particular, induce P450 enzymes, lowering the concentrations of many other drugs, including birth control, opiates (particularly methadone), immune-suppressive agents, HIV medications, some chemotherapy agents, and some anesthetics, and thus their possible benefit must be weighed against these drug-drug interactions. Rifamycins penetrate many tissue spaces and will turn body fluids such as tears, urine, and feces orange. This is an important side effect to warn patients about. Oral preparations of rifamycins are highly bioavailable. Rifaximin, because it is nonabsorbable, avoids drug interactions or side effects and is used for the treatment and prevention of traveler's diarrhea in people older than 12 years.

FLUOROQUINOLONES (STEP 5, FIGURE 39–2)

Fluoroquinolones include norfloxacin, ofloxacin, ciprofloxacin, levofloxacin, moxifloxacin, and gatifloxacin drops. They target bacterial topoisomerases, inhibiting DNA replication and repair. Efficacy is based on the AUC over MIC.

Levofloxacin and ciprofloxacin are active against *P aeruginosa*, with moxifloxacin having less systemic activity against *P aeruginosa*. In addition to gram-negative activity, levofloxacin has activity against some strains of MRSA, *S pneumoniae*, and *Enterococcus faecalis* (not *E faecium*). Fluoroquinolones are also active against many causes of atypical pneumonia, such as *Mycoplasma*, *Chlamydophila*, and *Legionella*. Ofloxacin and levofloxacin are used for treatment of some cases of *M tuberculosis* and some atypical mycobacterial infections. Due to activity against *N meningitides* and *Yersinia pestis*, ciprofloxacin is an option for prophylaxis of exposed persons. Fluoroquinolones are often active against *N gonorrhea* (though increasing resistance is described) and *C trachomatis*. They often are active against the common causes of traveler's diarrhea, though increasing resistance has removed them as first-line agents (in favor of azithromycin) in many geographic areas. Bacteria become resistant by mutating the targeted topoisomerases to avoid binding or by efflux of drug. This class of drugs is highly associated with bacterial resistance and secondary *C difficile* infection. When organisms acquire fluoroquinolone resistance genes by plasmid, these plasmids often also contain genes encoding resistance to other classes of antimicrobials. Fluoroquinolones also select for hypervirulent, superspreading strains of *C difficile* that endanger not only the patient receiving the fluoroquinolone but other patients on the same unit to whom the strain may spread. They have been associated with tendon rupture in adults, arthropathy in children, QTc interval prolongation, and numerous other side effects, which prompted labeling warnings about these side effects. Fluoroquinolones are highly bioavailable and generally should be used orally. One caveat is that they are inactivated by divalent cations, so they cannot be given with multivitamins, dairy-containing products, or infant formulas, making them difficult to administer to infants and children. Due to the issues mentioned above, fluoroquinolones should be used sparingly in pediatrics (and adults) and reserved for treatment of organisms resistant to other classes of drugs.

OTHER ANTIBIOTICS

While the above antibiotic classes encompass the most commonly used antibiotics, additional agents are used when antimicrobial resistance limits their use. This occurs most commonly among gram-negative bacteria, particularly ESBL-producing and carbapenem-resistant *Enterobacteriaceae*, which can harbor high levels of resistance to multiple antibiotic classes. Polymyxins (colistin and polymyxin B) are lipophilic antibiotics that disrupt the gram-negative outer cell membrane as well as the inner membrane of gram-positives (step 3, Figure 39–2). Given intravenously, they have a role in the treatment of highly resistant *P aeruginosa* and *Acinetobacter* spp. infections, though high rates of toxicity (particularly nephrotoxicity) limit their utility. Polymyxin B is generally favored over colistin due to slightly

fewer toxicities. Fosfomycin, which impairs cell wall synthesis through a different mechanism than β-lactams (step 2, Figure 39–2), also retains activity over most highly resistant *E coli*. Oral fosfomycin is highly effective (and commonly used in adults) for uncomplicated UTI, though IV formulations are required for systemic infections. Pediatric studies are ongoing, but fosfomycin is not approved for children. Nitrofurantoin, which like oral fosfomycin cannot be used for systemic infections, is among the first-line agents for simple cystitis but also may have activity for ESBL-producing organisms. While the polymyxins and fosfomycin play a role in treatment of highly resistant gram-negative infections, the newer β-lactam-β-lactamase combination agents discussed above (eg ceftazidime/avibactam, ceftolozane/tazobactam, meropenem/vaborbactam, etc) are often preferred due to similar or better efficacy with fewer toxicities. Aztreonam used in conjunction with avibactam (currently available only in combination with ceftazidime) is another highly effective option for resistant gram-negative infections, including most carbapenem-resistant isolates.

ANTIFUNGALS

The principles of antifungal therapy are similar to those of antibacterials, though there are fewer classes of agents. Amphotericin B is a polyene that interacts with ergosterol to disrupt the fungal cell membrane; ergosterol is not a component of mammalian cell membranes. Amphotericin B also inhibits fungal ATPase. It is available in deoxycholate or liposomal/lipid complex formulations; the latter has reduced side effects, including less renal toxicity. Lipid-based and conventional amphotericin are not interchangeable for dosing purposes. Its efficacy parameter is peak to MIC. Amphotericin is active against a broad range of yeasts and molds, with some rare but important exceptions. It is also a mainstay of treatment for some protozoal infections, for example, *Leishmania* spp.

The azoles, which are another important class of antifungals, include ketoconazole, fluconazole, itraconazole, voriconazole, posaconazole, and isavuconazole. The azole efficacy parameter is AUC over MIC. Azoles work through inhibition of the enzymes that convert lanosterol to ergosterol. Their spectra of activity, tissue penetration, side effects, drug interactions, and bioavailability vary, all of which should be considered when choosing an agent and route of administration. For some drugs, monitoring of serum concentrations is indicated.

The echinocandins (micafungin, caspofungin, anidulafungin) are a third class of antifungals for systemic use. These drugs, which have become a mainstay for the treatment of yeasts, work through inhibition of enzymes important to cell membrane integrity (β-(1-3)-D-glucan). They generally provide more rapid and reliable killing of yeasts (eg, *Candida* spp.) than of molds (eg, *Aspergillus* spp.), and have minimal activity against most molds, except *Aspergillus*. Echinocandins cannot be used reliably for CNS or UTIs due to poor

CSF and urine drug penetration. Their spectra of activity and side-effect profiles are similar.

Flucytosine is a less commonly used antifungal that inhibits fungal nucleic acid and protein synthesis. Its niche is only as an adjunctive agent for some fungal CNS infections. Flucytosine achieves high CNS penetration but develops resistance rapidly if used alone. Its use is severely limited due to cost and the common occurrence of neutropenia. Combination therapy remains controversial, though it can be considered in the situation of unknown/unpredictable susceptibilities or unclear tissue penetration. Additional detail on antifungals and some antiparasitics is available in Chapter 43, and limited information is included in Tables 39–2 and 39–3.

ANTIVIRALS

Antivirals are a complex group of agents that target various stages in the viral life cycle. This cycle occurs solely within a eukaryotic host cell, dependent on host cell machinery. Individual antiviral drugs may target viral entry into host cells, intracellular viral uncoating, integration, nucleic acid replication, assembly/packaging, and viral release from the host cell. Viral life cycles also vary, sometimes requiring infection of specific cell types, the presence of certain host proteins, and/or incorporation into host DNA. Many viruses, especially RNA viruses, develop resistant mutants quickly, making the development of antivirals challenging. Anti-HIV agents are discussed in Chapter 41; anti-influenza and anti-herpes (HSV, CMV, EBV) agents in Chapter 40; and anti-hepatitis virus agents in Chapter 22. Limited information is included in Tables 39–2 and 39–3.

REFERENCES

American Academy of Pediatrics. Committee on Infectious D, American Academy of Pediatrics. Committee on the Control of Infectious D: *Red book online*. 2021.

Bradley JS: *2019 Nelson's Pediatric Antimicrobial Therapy*. American Academy of Pediatrics; 2019.

The Sanford Guide to Antimicrobial Therapy. 50th ed. Sperryville, VA: Antimicrobial Therapy; 2020.

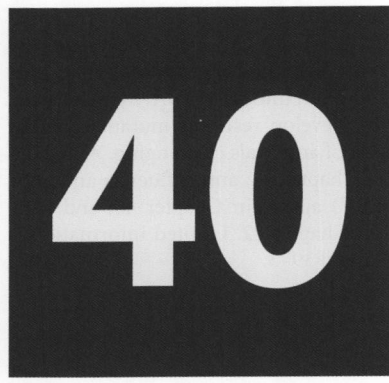

Infections: Viral & Rickettsial

Daniel Olson, MD, PhD

Edwin J. Asturias, MD

VIRAL INFECTIONS

Viruses cause most pediatric infections. Mixed viral or viral-bacterial infections of the respiratory and intestinal tracts are common, as is prolonged asymptomatic shedding of many viruses in childhood, especially in young children. Thus, the detection of a virus may be indicative of *infection*, but it may not always be the cause of a presenting *illness* or *disease*. Viruses are often a predisposing factor for bacterial respiratory infections (eg, otitis, sinusitis, and pneumonia). See Table 40–1 for an outline of viral illnesses described in this chapter.

The epidemiology of respiratory viruses is frequently changing, as is demonstrated by the recent emergence of SARS-CoV-2, and the impact that social distancing measures had not only on COVID-19 disease but many other respiratory viruses as well. As the world adapts to the post-pandemic phase of COVID-19 pandemic, previous and current patterns of seasonality, transmission, diagnosis, and even treatment and prevention may change significantly.

Many respiratory viruses and herpesviruses can now be detected within 24 hours through antigen or nucleic acid detection techniques. Polymerase chain reaction (PCR) amplification and sequencing of viral genes is leading to detection of previously unrecognized infections. It is now possible to detect multiple organisms causing the same syndrome (eg, respiratory, gastrointestinal, encephalitis/meningitis) within a single test system (multiplex assay). The available tests vary in format and turnaround time and can include both viral and bacterial etiologies. New diagnostic tests are challenging our previous paradigms of viral infections and their diagnosis more certain and complex brining along new therapeutic opportunities. Therefore, as a clinician and provider, it is critical to consult the microbiology laboratory for details regarding the optimal specimen collection, handling and shipping, and only laboratories with excellent quality-control procedures should be used. Table 40–2 lists diagnostic tests. The increasing availability of specific antiviral therapies increase the value of early diagnosis for some serious viral infections. Table 40–3 lists common causes of red rashes in children that should be considered in the differential diagnosis of certain viral illnesses.

RESPIRATORY INFECTIONS

Many viral infections can cause either upper or lower respiratory tract signs and symptoms, sometimes both in the same patient. Many so-called respiratory viruses can also produce distinct nonrespiratory disease (eg, enteritis, cystitis, or myocarditis caused by adenoviruses; parotitis caused by parainfluenza viruses). Respiratory viruses can cause disease in any area of the respiratory tree, although certain viruses tend to be closely associated with one anatomic area (eg, parainfluenza with croup, respiratory syncytial virus [RSV] with bronchiolitis) or with discrete seasonality (eg, influenza, RSV, parainfluenza), although that may change depending on large-scale public health interventions (during the COVID-19 pandemic). It is usually impossible on clinical grounds alone to be certain of the specific viral cause of an infection in a child. In immunocompromised patients, otherwise benign viruses can cause severe lower respiratory disease. The information provided by the virology laboratory is often important for epidemiologic, therapeutic, and preventive reasons. However, the ability to test for an expanding repertoire of viruses needs to be balanced with the increasing costs of such tests. Generally, testing should be limited to situations where it will likely change clinical management.

VIRUSES CAUSING THE COMMON COLD

The common cold syndrome (also called upper respiratory infection) is characterized by combinations of runny nose, nasal congestion, sore throat, conjunctivitis, cough, and sneezing. Low-grade fever may be present. Rhinoviruses, which are the most common cause (30%–40%), are present throughout the year, but are more prevalent in the colder months in temperate climates. Adenoviruses also cause colds in all seasons and epidemics are common. RSV, parainfluenza viruses, human metapneumovirus (hMPV), and influenza

Table 40–1. Outline of Chapter 40.

Topic
Respiratory Infections
- Viruses causing the common cold
- Adenoviruses
- Influenza
- Parainfluenza
- Respiratory Syncytial Virus (RSV)
- Human metapneumovirus (HMPV)
- Human Coronaviruses (HCoVs)
Infectious due to enteroviruses and parechoviruses
- Acute febrile illness
- Respiratory tract illness
- Rashes (including hand-foot-and-mouth)
- CNS illness
Infections due to herpesviruses
- Herpes simplex infections
- Varicella and herpes zoster
- Human Herpes Virus-6 (HHV-6, Roseola infantum)
- Cytomegalovirus (CMV)
- Epstein Barr Virus (EBV, infectious mononucleosis)
- Viral infections spread by insect vectors
- Encephalitis
- Dengue
- Chikungunya
- Zika
- Colorado Tick Fever
- Other important viruses in childhood
- Parvovirus B19 (erythema infectiosum)
- Measles (rubeola)
- Rubella
- Mumps
- Hantavirus
- Rabies
- Rickettsial Infections and Q Fever
- Human Ehrlichiosis and Anaplasma
- Rocky Mountain Spotted Fever
- Endemic Typhus (Murine Typhus)
- Q Fever

viruses cause the cold syndrome, typically during epidemics from late fall through winter. Multiple strains of coronaviruses account for 5%–10% of cold syndromes in winter. Often (25%–50%) more than one virus is detected during a common cold. Enteroviruses cause the "summer cold." The usual outcome of the common cold is morbidity continuing for 5–7 days. However, changes in the respiratory epithelium, local mucosal swelling, and altered local immunity may act as precursors to more severe bacterial illnesses, such as otitis media, sinusitis, and pneumonia. During and following a cold, the local microbiome changes and bacteria are found in normally sterile areas of the upper airway. Asthma attacks are frequently provoked by any of the viruses that cause the common cold. These "cold viruses" can also advance to lower respiratory tract infection in young children.

In 5%–10% of children, symptoms from these virus infections persist for more than 10 days. Overlap with the symptoms of bacterial sinusitis presents a difficult problem for clinicians, especially because colds can produce sinuses abnormalities on computed tomography (CT) scan. Some viruses, such as rhinoviruses, SARS-CoV-2, influenza, RSV, and metapneumovirus, can cause severe lower respiratory disease in immunologically or anatomically compromised children.

Supportive and symptomatic treatment are recommended which may include appropriate hydration, nasal suctioning/irrigation, honey (if cough and > 1 year), and analgesics/antipyretics. Over-the-counter (OTC) "cold" medications are generally not shown to be effective, and some may be associated with increased risk of side effects or toxicity, especially in younger children.

CDC: Common Cold Information for Parents: https://www.cdc.gov/antibiotic-use/community/for-patients/common-illnesses/colds.html.
Deckx L et al: Nasal decongestants in monotherapy for the common cold. Cochrane Database Syst Rev 2016; CD0096 [PMID: 27748955].

ADENOVIRUSES

ESSENTIALS OF DIAGNOSIS & TYPICAL FEATURES

► Year-round circulation; outbreaks in closed settings (day care, barracks).

► Multiple syndromes, depending on adenovirus type and host.

► URI with severe pharyngitis, conjunctivitis, tonsillitis, and cervical adenopathy.

► Pneumonia.

► Enteric adenoviruses cause mild diarrheal illnesses.

► Definitive diagnosis by antigen detection, PCR, or culture.

Table 40–2. Diagnostic tests for viral infections.

Agent	Rapid Antigen Detection (Specimen)	Tissue Culture Mean Days to Positive (Range)	Serology		PCR	Comments
			Acute	Paired		
Adenovirus	+ (Respiratory, eye, and enteric)	10 (1–21)	–	+	+	PCR of respiratory (most common) and serum. "Enteric" strains detected by culture on special cell line, antigen detection.
Arboviruses (general)	–	–	+	+	+	Acute serum (IgM) may diagnose many forms; these may be negative by day 7. May cross-react with other prior arbovirus infections; confirm by neutralization
Astrovirus	+ RL	–	–	–	+ RL	Diagnosis by electron microscopy
Calicivirus (norovirus)	+	–	–	–	+	PCR generally available for norovirus; present in RL for others
Chikungunya virus	–	–	+	+	+	
Colorado tick virus	On RBC	–	–	RL, CDC	+	IgM may become positive as late as 2–3 wk
Coronavirus	+	RL	+	+	+	Rapidly changing for SARS-Cov-2
Cytomegalo-virus	+	2 (2–28)	+	+	+	Diagnosis by presence of IgM antibody; rapid culture or PCR; low avidity antibody indicates recent infection
Dengue virus	+ (Days 1–6)	5 (RL)	+	+	+ (Days 1–5)	Serologic testing may cross-react with other flaviviruses (Zika), so PCR or NS1 antigen during acute disease is preferred
Enterovirus	–	3 (2–8) Coxsackie A; difficult to culture	–	+	+	PCR more sensitive than culture; poliovirus also isolated in cultures and detected by PCR
Epstein-Barr virus	–	–	+	+	+	Single serologic panel defines infection status; heterophil (monospot) antibodies less sensitive. PCR used primarily in immune compromised
Hantavirus	–	–	+	+	RL (blood, not lavage fluid)	Diagnosis by presence of IgM antibody
Herpes simplex virus	+	1 (1–5)	+	+	+	Serology rarely used for herpes simplex; IgM antibody used in selected cases
Human herpesvirus 6 and 7	–	2 (RL)	+	+	+	Roseola agent; type-specific serology available; PCR and serology may have low sensitivity

(Continued)

Table 40–2. Diagnostic tests for viral infections. (*Continued*)

Agent	Rapid Antigen Detection (Specimen)	Tissue Culture Mean Days to Positive (Range)	Serology		PCR	Comments
			Acute	Paired		
Human meta-pneumo-virus	+ (Respiratory secretions)	2	–	+	+	
Influenza virus	+ (Respiratory secretions)	2 (2–4)	–	+	+	Antigen detection 40%–90% sensitive (varies with virus strain) PCR preferable
Measles virus	+ (Respiratory secretions)	–	+	+	+	Difficult to grow; IgM serology or PCR diagnostic
Mumps virus	–	> 5	+	+	+	IgM ELISA antibody may allow single-specimen diagnosis
Parvovirus B19	–	–	+	ND	+	Erythema infectiosum agent; IgM serology is often diagnostic but may be positive for a prolonged period
Poliovirus	+ RL				+	
Parainfluenza virus	+ (Respiratory secretions)	5 (4–7)	–	+	+	Serology rarely helpful
Rabies virus	+ (Skin, conjunctiva, suspected animal source)	rarely used	+		CDC	Usually diagnosed by antigen detection
Respiratory syncytial virus	+ (Respiratory)	2 (1–5)	–	+ (rarely used)	+	Rapid antigen detection; 90% sensitive; PCR has excellent sensitivity
Rhinovirus	–	4 (2–7)	–	–	+	Too many strains to type serologically
Rotavirus	+ (Feces)	–	–	–	+	Rapid assay methods are usually reliable; can be positive in recent vaccinees
Rubella virus	–	> 10	+	+	+	Notify lab before culture; recommended that paired sera be tested simultaneously
Varicella-zoster virus	+ (Skin [vesicle] scraping, blood, CSF)	3 (3–21)	+	+	+	
West Nile virus	–	RL	+	+	+	IgM antibody usually detected by 1 wk; PCR is useful only on CSF
Zika virus	+	–	+	+	+	Serologic testing may cross-react with dengue virus, so PCR or NS1 antigen during acute disease is preferred

CSF, cerebrospinal fluid; ELISA, enzyme-linked immunosorbent assay; PCR, polymerase chain reaction; RBC, red blood cell. Plus signs signify commercially or widely available; minus signs signify not commercially available.
Note: Results from some commercial laboratories are unreliable. RL indicates research laboratory only; CDC: Specific antibody titers or PCR available by arrangement with individual research laboratories or the Centers for Disease Control and Prevention. ND: Not done.

Table 40–3. Some red rashes in children.

Condition	Incubation Period (day)	Prodrome	Rash	Laboratory Tests	Comments, Other Diagnostic Features
Adenovirus	4–5	URI; cough; fever	Morbilliform (may be petechial)	Normal; may see leukopenia or lymphocytosis	Upper or lower respiratory symptoms are prominent. No Koplik spots. No desquamation. Hemorrhagic conjunctivitis.
Dengue virus	4–7	Usually none	Erythema early on; maculopapular or urticarial in febrile phase	Leukopenia, thrombocytopenia, elevated transaminases; PCR	Rash has been described as "islands of white on a sea of red."
Drug allergy	Any time post-exposure	None, or fever alone, or with myalgia, pruritus	Macular, maculopapular, urticarial, or erythroderma, target lesions	Leukopenia, eosinophilia	Rash variable. Severe reactions may resemble measles, scarlet fever; Kawasaki disease; marked toxicity possible.
Enterovirus	2–7	Variable fever, chills, myalgia, sore throat	Variable; usually macular, maculo-papular on trunk or palms, soles; vesicles or petechiae also seen	PCR	Varied rashes may resemble those of many other infections. Pharyngeal or hand-foot-mouth vesicles may occur.
Ehrlichiosis (monocytic)	5–21	Fever; headache; flu-like; myalgia; GI symptoms	Variable; maculopapular, petechial, scarlatiniform, vasculitic	Leukopenia, thrombocytopenia, abnormal liver function. Serology for diagnosis; morulae in monocytes	Geographic distribution is a clue; seasonal; tick exposure; rash present in only 45%.
Erythema multiforme	—	Usually none or related to underlying cause	Discrete, red maculopapular lesions; symmetrical, distal, palms and soles; target lesions classic	Normal or eosinophilia	Reaction to drugs (especially sulfonamides), or infectious agents (*Mycoplasma*; herpes simplex virus). Urticaria, arthralgia also seen.
Infectious mononucleosis (EBV infection)	30–60	Fever, malaise	Macular, scarlatiniform, or urticarial in 5% to almost 100% who are on penicillins and related drugs (not a penicillin allergy)	Atypical lymphocytosis; heterophil antibodies; EBV-specific antibodies in an acute pattern EBV; abnormal liver function tests	Pharyngitis, lymphadenopathy, hepatosplenomegaly.
Juvenile rheumatoid arthritis (systemic; Still disease)	—	High fever, malaise	Evanescent salmon-pink macules, especially in pressure areas (prominent when fever is present)	Increased inflammatory markers; leukocytosis; thrombocytosis	Oligo- or polyarticular arthritis; asymptomatic anterior uveitis.
Kawasaki disease	Unknown	Fever, cervical adenopathy, irritability	Polymorphous (may be erythroderma) on trunk and extremities; red palms and soles, conjunctiva, lips, tongue, pharynx. Late desquamation is common. Some of these findings may be absent with atypical disease	Leukocytosis, thrombocytosis, elevated ESR or CRP; pyuria; decreased albumin; negative cultures and streptococcal serology; resting tachycardia	Swollen hands, feet; prolonged illness; uveitis; aseptic meningitis; no response to antibiotics. Vasculitis and aneurysms of coronary and other arteries occur (cardiac ultrasound).

	Incubation (days)	Prodrome/Symptoms	Rash	Laboratory	Comments
Leptospirosis	4–19	Fever (biphasic), myalgia, chills	Variable erythroderma	Leukocytosis; hematuria, proteinuria; hyperbilirubinemia	Conjunctivitis; hepatitis, aseptic meningitis may be seen. Rodent, dog contact.
Measles	9–14	Cough, rhinitis, conjunctivitis	Maculopapular; face to trunk; lasts 7–10 days; Koplik spots in mouth for 1–2 days	Leukopenia; anti-measles IgM	Toxic. Bright red rash becomes confluent, may desquamate. Fever falls after rash appears. Inadequate measles vaccination.
Parvovirus (erythema infectiosum)	10–17 (rash)	Mild (flu-like)	Maculopapular on cheeks ("slapped cheek"), forehead, chin; then down limbs, trunk, buttocks; may fade and reappear for several weeks	IgM-EIA; PCR	Purpuric stocking-glove rash is rare, but distinctive; aplastic crisis in patients with chronic hemolytic anemia. May cause arthritis or arthralgia.
Rocky Mountain spotted fever	3–12	Headache (retro-orbital); toxic; GI symptoms; high fever; flu-like	Onset 2–6 days after fever; palpable maculopapular on palms, soles, extremities, with spread centrally; petechial	Leukopenia; thrombocytopenia; hepatitis; CSF pleocytosis; serology positive at 7–10 days of rash; biopsy will give earlier diagnosis	Eastern seaboard and southeastern United States; April–September; tick exposure.
Roseola (HHV-6)	10–14	Fever (mean 4 days; 15 ≥ 6 days)	Pink, macular rash occurs at the end of febrile period; transient (only 20% get rash)	Normal; RT-PCR	Fever often high; disappears when rash develops; child appears well. Usually occurs in children 6 mo to 3 y of age. Seizures may complicate.
Rubella	14–21	Usually none	Mild maculopapular; rapid spread face to extremities; gone by day 4	Normal or leukopenia	Postauricular, occipital adenopathy common. Polyarthralgia in some older girls. Mild clinical illness. Inadequate rubella vaccination.
Staphylococcal scalded skin	Variable	Irritability, absent to low fever	Painful erythroderma, followed in 1–2 days by cracking around eyes, mouth; bullae with friction (Nikolsky sign)	Normal if only colonized by staphylococci; leukocytosis and sometimes bacteremia if infected	Normal pharynx. Look for focal staphylococcal infection. Usually occurs in infants.
Staphylococcal scarlet fever	1–7	Variable fever	Diffuse erythroderma; resembles streptococcal scarlet fever except eyes may be hyperemic and no "strawberry" tongue; pharynx spared	Leukocytosis is common because of infected focus	Focal infection usually present.
Stevens-Johnson syndrome	—	Pharyngitis, conjunctivitis, fever, malaise	Bullous erythema multiforme; may slough in large areas; hemorrhagic lips; purulent conjunctivitis	Leukocytosis	Classic precipitants are drugs (especially sulfonamides); Mycoplasma pneumoniae and herpes simplex infections. Pneumonitis and urethritis also seen.

(Continued)

Table 40–3. Some red rashes in children. (*Continued*)

Condition	Incubation Period (day)	Prodrome	Rash	Laboratory Tests	Comments, Other Diagnostic Features
Streptococcal scarlet fever	1–7	Fever, abdominal pain, headache, sore throat	Diffuse erythema, "sandpaper" texture; neck, axillae, inguinal areas; spreads to rest of body; desquamates 7–14 days; eyes not red	Leukocytosis; positive group A *Streptococcus* culture of throat or wound; positive streptococcal antigen test in pharynx	Strawberry tongue, red pharynx +/− exudate. Eyes, perioral and periorbital area, palms, and soles spared. Pastia lines. Cervical adenopathy. Usually occurs in children 2–10 y of age.
Toxic shock syndrome	Variable	Fever, myalgia, headache, diarrhea, vomiting	Nontender erythroderma; red eyes, palms, soles, pharynx, lips	Leukocytosis; abnormal liver enzymes and coagulation tests; proteinuria	*Staphylococcus aureus* infection; toxin-mediated multiorgan involvement. Swollen hands, feet. Hypotension or shock.
Zika virus	3–7	Variable	Common; erythema, macular, or maculopapular; conjunctivitis	Leukocytosis, thrombocytopenia, elevated transaminases; PCR	Rash is common and variable; often pruritic; petechiae are rare; conjunctivitis is common.

CRP, C-reactive protein; CSF, cerebrospinal fluid; EIA, enzyme immunoassay; ESR, erythrocyte sedimentation rate; GI, gastrointestinal; HHV-6, human herpesvirus 6; IFA, immunofluorescent assay; PCR, polymerase chain reaction; URI, upper respiratory infection.

There are more than 50 types of adenoviruses, which account for 5%–15% of all respiratory illnesses in childhood, usually pharyngitis or tracheitis, but also including 5% of childhood lower respiratory tract infections. Adenoviral infections, which are common early in life (most < 2 years old), occur 3–10 days after exposure to respiratory droplets or fomites. Enteric adenoviruses are an important cause of childhood diarrhea, most often in children younger than 4 years. Epidemic respiratory disease from adenoviruses occurs in winter and spring, especially in closed environments such as day care centers. Asymptomatic shedding from the respiratory or intestinal tract is common.

Specific Adenoviral Syndromes

A. Pharyngitis

Pharyngitis is the most common adenoviral disease. Fever and adenopathy are common. Tonsillitis may be exudative. Rhinitis and an influenza-like systemic illness may be present. Laryngotracheitis or bronchitis may accompany pharyngitis.

B. Pharyngoconjunctival Fever

Conjunctivitis may occur alone and be prolonged, but most often is associated with preauricular adenopathy, fever, pharyngitis, and cervical adenopathy. Foreign-body sensation in the eye and other symptoms last less than a week. Lower respiratory symptoms are uncommon. Epidemic keratoconjunctivitis is caused by certain adenovirus strains and may result in severe bilateral conjunctivitis, corneal opacities, and occasionally visual impairment. A foreign-body sensation, photophobia, and swelling of conjunctiva and eyelids are characteristic. Preauricular adenopathy and subconjunctival hemorrhage are common.

C. Pneumonia

Severe pneumonia may occur at any age. It is especially common in young children (< 3 years). Chest radiographs show bilateral peribronchial and patchy ground-glass interstitial infiltrates in the lower lobes. Symptoms persist for 2–4 weeks. Adenoviral pneumonia can be necrotizing and cause permanent lung damage, such as bronchiectasis and bronchiolitis obliterans. A pertussis-like syndrome with typical cough and lymphocytosis can occur with lower respiratory tract infection.

D. Gastrointestinal Disease

Enteric adenoviruses (types 40 and 41) cause 3%–5% of cases of short-lived diarrhea in afebrile children, especially in those younger than 4 years. Mesenteric lymphadenitis and abdominal pain may mimic appendicitis. Pharyngitis is often associated. Adenovirus-induced adenopathy may be a factor in appendicitis and intussusception.

E. Other Syndromes

Acute otitis media (in younger children) and a diffuse morbilliform (rarely petechial) rash may be present with various clinical presentations of adenovirus. Immunosuppressed patients, including neonates, may develop severe or fatal pulmonary or gastrointestinal infections or multisystem disease. Hemorrhagic cystitis can be a serious problem in immunocompromised children. Other rare complications that can occur in the immunocompetent child include encephalitis, hepatitis, and myocarditis. Adenoviruses have been implicated in the syndrome of idiopathic myocardiopathy.

▶ Laboratory & Diagnostic Studies

PCR of respiratory specimens, conjunctival, or stool specimens is rapid, sensitive, and the preferred diagnostic method for adenovirus infections. Diagnosis can also be made by culture, direct staining of respiratory or diarrheal specimens, and acute (during illness) and convalescent (post-illness) serology, though these are uncommon.

▶ Treatment

There is some evidence of successful treatment of immunocompromised patients with cidofovir, though risk of nephrotoxicity is high. Brincidofovir, a cidofovir derivative with good oral bioavailability and less nephrotoxicity, is under study. Intravenous immunoglobulin (IVIG) may be tried in immunocompromised patients with severe pneumonia. Adoptive T-cell transfer has shown promising results in hematopoietic stem cell transplant recipients.

Lion T: Adenovirus infections in immune competent and immunocompromised patients. Clin Microbiol Rev 2014;27:441 [PMID: 24982316].

INFLUENZA

ESSENTIALS OF DIAGNOSIS & TYPICAL FEATURES

- ▶ Seasonal: late fall through mid-spring.
- ▶ Fever, cough, pharyngitis, malaise, congestion.
- ▶ Pneumonia.
- ▶ Encephalitis.
- ▶ Detection of virus, viral antigens, or nucleic acid in respiratory secretions.

Symptomatic infections are common in children because they lack immunologic experience with influenza viruses. Infection rates in children are greater than in adults and are instrumental in initiating community outbreaks. Epidemics typically occur in fall and winter. Three main types of influenza viruses (A/H1N1, A/H3N2, B) cause most human epidemics, with antigenic drift ensuring a supply of susceptible hosts of all ages. In recent years, avian influenza A/H5N1 and A/H7N9 caused isolated human outbreaks in Asia that were associated with high rates of hospitalization and death, and H5N1 has caused global avian outbreaks. A swine-origin influenza A/H1N1 caused a human pandemic in 2009 and has since circulated with seasonal periodicity. Social distancing measures resulting from the COVID-19 pandemic resulted in dramatic decreases in influenza incidence and the possible extinction of influenza B Yamagata lineage.

Clinical Findings

Spread of influenza occurs by way of airborne respiratory secretions. The incubation period is 2–7 days.

A. Symptoms and Signs

Influenza infection in older children and adults produces a characteristic syndrome of sudden onset of high fever, severe myalgia, headache, and chills. These symptoms overshadow the associated coryza, pharyngitis, and cough. Usually absent are rash, marked conjunctivitis, adenopathy, exudative pharyngitis, and dehydrating enteritis. Fever, diarrhea, vomiting, and abdominal pain are common in young children. Infants may develop a sepsis-like illness and apnea. Chest examination is usually unremarkable. Less frequent clinical findings include croup, asthma exacerbation, myositis (especially calf muscles), myocarditis, parotitis, encephalopathy, nephritis, and a transient maculopapular rash. Acute illness lasts 2–5 days. Cough and fatigue may last several weeks. Viral shedding may persist for several weeks in young children.

B. Laboratory Findings

The leukocyte count is normal to low, with variable shift. Given difficulty in differentiating influenza from other common respiratory infections among children, laboratory testing or empiric treatment (if high community circulation) is recommended. PCR has the highest sensitivity and specificity (close to 100%) and has become the preferred test as the results can be available within several hours. Influenza virus can be cultured within 3–7 days from pharyngeal specimens, and some labs employ a rapid culture technique followed by viral antigen testing after 48 hours. A late diagnosis may be made with acute and convalescent serology, using hemagglutination inhibition assays.

C. Imaging

The chest radiograph is nonspecific; it may show hyperaeration, peribronchial thickening, diffuse interstitial infiltrates, or bronchopneumonia in severe cases. Pleural effusion is rare in uncomplicated influenza.

Complications & Sequelae

Lower respiratory tract symptoms are most common in children younger than 5 years. Hospitalization rates are highest in children younger than 2 years. Influenza can cause croup in these children. Secondary bacterial infections (classically staphylococcal) of the middle ear, sinuses, or lungs are common. Influenza can also cause viral or post-viral encephalitis, with cerebral symptoms much more prominent than those of the accompanying respiratory infection. Although the myositis is usually mild and resolves promptly, severe rhabdomyolysis and renal failure have been reported. Children with underlying obesity, cardiopulmonary, metabolic, neuromuscular, or immunosuppressive disease are at risk for severe disease.

Prevention

The trivalent and quadrivalent influenza vaccines are licensed as inactivated (IIV) or live attenuated (LAIV), are moderately protective, especially for severe disease (see Chapter 10), and are recommended annually for all individuals older than 6 months (first immunization requires two doses if ≤ 8 years). Influenza vaccination should occur before onset of influenza activity in the community, though immunity may wane during a single season. For egg-allergic children, the risk of anaphylaxis is generally no greater than background rates, though cell-based and recombinant influenza vaccines are available.

Prophylaxis with oseltamivir can be used in select cases for children older than 3 months. Inhaled zanamivir can also be used in children older than 5 years but avoid use in children with asthma or chronic pulmonary disease. Chemoprophylaxis may be considered during an epidemic for high-risk children who cannot be immunized or who have not yet developed immunity (about 6 weeks after primary vaccination or 2 weeks after a booster dose). For outbreak prophylaxis, therapy should be maintained for 2 weeks or more and for 1 week after the last case of influenza is diagnosed.

Treatment & Prognosis

Treatment consists of general support and management of pulmonary complications, especially bacterial superinfections. Antivirals are of benefit against seasonal influenza in immunocompetent hosts if begun within 48 hours of symptom onset and may be initiated later in severe (hospitalized) cases. In hospitalized children, early antiviral treatment shortens the duration of hospitalization. Treatment duration is typically 5 days and the doses are twice those used for prophylaxis. Peramivir is a neuraminidase inhibitor approved for IV administration.

Recovery is usually complete unless severe cardiopulmonary or neurologic damage has occurred. Fatal cases occur in very young infants, immunodeficient and anatomically compromised children, pregnant women, including the first 2 weeks postpartum, and obese individuals. Effective treatment or prophylaxis of influenza in children markedly reduces the incidence of acute otitis media and antibiotic usage during the flu season.

CDC: Influenza Antiviral Medications. https://www.cdc.gov/flu/professionals/antivirals/index.htm.

Grohskopf LA et al: Prevention and control of seasonal influenza with vaccines: recommendations of the Advisory Committee on Immunization Practices—United States, 2022-23 Influenza Season. https://www.cdc.gov/mmwr/volumes/71/rr/rr7101a1.htm.

PARAINFLUENZA

ESSENTIALS OF DIAGNOSIS & TYPICAL FEATURES

▶ Seasonality: fall and early winter

▶ Fever, nasal congestion, sore throat, cough.

▶ Croup and bronchiolitis.

▶ Detection of live virus, antigens, or nucleic acid in respiratory secretions.

Human parainfluenza viruses (HPIV) are the most important cause of croup in children. Four types of HPIV (1–4) are known. HPIV 1 and 2 cause most cases of croup, and infections occur during the first 5 years of life, usually during outbreaks in the fall. Most infants are infected with type 3 within the first 3 years of life, most often in the first year. HPIV 4 has year-round circulation and may be less pathogenic than other types.

▶ Clinical Findings

A. Symptoms and Signs

The incubation period is 2–7 days. Clinical disease has an acute onset that includes febrile upper respiratory infection (especially in older children with re-exposure), laryngitis, tracheobronchitis, croup, and bronchiolitis (second most common cause after RSV). Croup is characterized by a barking cough, inspiratory stridor, and hoarseness. HPIV can cause pneumonia in infants and immunodeficient children and causes particularly high mortality among stem cell recipients.

HPIV-induced respiratory syndromes are difficult to distinguish from those caused by other respiratory viruses. Viral croup must be distinguished from epiglottitis caused by *Haemophilus influenzae* type b (if unimmunized) or other bacterial infections causing upper airway obstruction (eg, peritonsillar abscess).

B. Laboratory Findings

Diagnosis is often based on clinical findings and testing is not recommended. These viruses can be identified by PCR (< 24 hours), rapid culture (48 hours), or direct immunofluorescence in respiratory secretions (< 3 hours).

▶ Treatment

No specific therapy or vaccine is available. Croup management is discussed in Chapter 19. Ribavirin is active in vitro and has been used in immunocompromised children, but its efficacy is unproven.

Frost HM et al: Epidemiology and clinical presentation of parainfluenza type 4 in children: a 3-year comparative study to parainfluenza types 1-3. J Clin Infect Dis 2014;209:695 [PMID: 24133181].

RESPIRATORY SYNCYTIAL VIRUS (RSV)

ESSENTIALS OF DIAGNOSIS & TYPICAL FEATURES

▶ Seasonality: late fall to early spring (January–February peak).

▶ Diffuse wheezing and tachypnea following upper respiratory symptoms in an infant (bronchiolitis).

▶ Hyperinflation on chest radiograph.

▶ Detection of RSV antigen or nucleic acid in nasal secretions.

▶ General Considerations

Respiratory syncytial virus (RSV) is the most important cause of lower respiratory tract illness in young children, accounting for more than 70% of cases of bronchiolitis and 40% of cases of pneumonia. RSV is very common in early childhood. Almost all children develop upper respiratory symptoms, and 20%–30% will manifest as lower respiratory infection. Outbreaks occur annually, and attack rates are high; 60% of children are infected in the first year of life, and 90% by age 2 years. During peak season (cold weather in temperate climates), the clinical diagnosis of RSV infection in infants with bronchiolitis is as accurate as most laboratory tests. As with influenza, social distancing practices resulting from the COVID-19 pandemic temporarily, but significantly reduced RSV transmission.

Despite the presence of serum antibody, reinfection is common. Two distinct genotypes can cocirculate or one may predominate in a community. Yearly shift in prevalence of these genotypes is a partial explanation for reinfection.

However, reinfection generally causes only upper respiratory symptoms in anatomically normal children. Immunosuppressed patients may develop progressive severe pneumonia. Children with congenital heart disease with increased pulmonary blood flow, children with chronic lung disease (eg, cystic fibrosis), and premature infants younger than 6 months (especially when they have chronic lung disease of prematurity) are also at higher risk for severe illness. No vaccine is available.

▶ Clinical Findings

A. Symptoms and Signs

Initial symptoms are those of upper respiratory infection. Low-grade fever may be present. The classic disease is bronchiolitis, characterized by diffuse wheezing, variable fever, cough, tachypnea, difficulty feeding, and in severe cases, cyanosis. Hyperinflation, crackles, prolonged expiration, wheezing, hypoxia, and retractions may be present. The liver and spleen may be palpable because of lung hyperinflation but are not enlarged. The disease usually lasts 3–7 days in previously healthy children. Fever is present for 2–4 days; it does not correlate with pulmonary symptoms and may be absent during the height of lung involvement.

Apnea, poor feeding, and lethargy may be presenting manifestations, especially in premature infants, in the first few months of life. Apnea usually resolves after a few days, often being replaced by obvious signs of bronchiolitis.

RSV infection in older children is more likely to cause tracheobronchitis or upper respiratory tract infection. Exceptions are immunocompromised children and those with severe chronic lung or heart disease, who may have especially severe or prolonged/primary infections and are subject to additional attacks of severe pneumonitis.

Although almost all cases of bronchiolitis are due to RSV during an epidemic, other respiratory pathogens such as parainfluenza, rhinovirus, *Mycoplasma/Chlamydia* pneumoniae, and especially hMPV cannot be excluded. Mixed infections with other viruses or bacteria can occur. Wheezing may be due to asthma, a foreign body, or other airway obstruction. Pertussis should also be considered in this age group, especially if cough is prominent and the infant is younger than 6 months. A markedly elevated leukocyte count should suggest bacterial superinfection (neutrophilia) or pertussis (lymphocytosis).

B. Laboratory Findings

Diagnostic testing is usually not necessary during RSV season. Real-time PCR, which may include multiplex panels of respiratory pathogens, has improved sensitivity, though it is also more expensive than traditional approaches such as antigen/ELISA testing (several hours) or rapid tissue culture (< 48 hours).

C. Imaging

Diffuse hyperinflation and peribronchiolar thickening are most common; atelectasis and patchy infiltrates also occur in uncomplicated infection, but pleural effusions are rare. Consolidation (usually subsegmental) occurs in 25% of children with lower respiratory tract disease.

▶ Complications

RSV commonly infects the middle ear. Symptomatic otitis media is the most common complication (10%–20%) and is more likely with secondary bacterial infection (usually due to pneumococcus or nontypable *H influenzae*). Bacterial pneumonia complicates only 0.5%–1% of hospitalized patients. Sudden exacerbations of fever and leukocytosis should suggest bacterial infection. Respiratory failure or apnea may require mechanical ventilation but occurs in less than 2% of hospitalized previously healthy full-term infants. Cardiac failure may occur as a complication of pulmonary disease or myocarditis. RSV commonly causes exacerbations of asthma. Nosocomial RSV infection is common and well-designed hospital programs to prevent nosocomial spread are imperative (see the next section).

▶ Prevention & Treatment

Oxygen therapy is only indicated in infants and children with oxyhemoglobin saturation less than 90%. Children who are very hypoxic or cannot feed because of respiratory distress must be hospitalized and given humidified oxygen as directed by oxygen saturation and given tube or intravenous feedings. Antibiotics, decongestants, and expectorants are of no value in routine infections. RSV-infected children should be kept in respiratory isolation. Cohorting ill infants in respiratory isolation during peak season (with or without rapid diagnostic attempts) and emphasizing good hand washing should decrease nosocomial transmission.

Clinicians should not administer albuterol (or salbutamol) or epinephrine to infants and young children with a diagnosis of bronchiolitis since this does not impact disease resolution, need for hospitalization, or length of stay. The use of systemic corticosteroids is also discouraged in RSV bronchiolitis unless there are complicating features such as asthma and chronic lung disease of prematurity.

Ribavirin is the only licensed antiviral therapy used for RSV infection. It is given by continuous aerosolization. It is rarely used in infants without significant anatomic or immunologic defects. At best, there is a very modest effect on disease severity in immunocompetent infants with no underlying anatomic abnormality. Even in high-risk infants, a favorable clinical response to ribavirin therapy was not demonstrated in several studies, although some data suggest that it might be more efficacious if initiated early in the illness.

Thus, ribavirin is only used in severely ill children who are immunologically or anatomically compromised and in those with severe cardiac disease.

Monthly intramuscular administration of humanized RSV monoclonal antibody is now recommended to prevent severe disease in selected high-risk patients during epidemic periods. Monthly administration should be considered during the RSV season for high-risk children (described in Chapter 10). Long-acting monoclonal antibodies (Nirsevimab) have been approved in the European Union (EU) for the prevention of respiratory syncytial virus (RSV) lower respiratory tract disease in newborns and infants during their first RSV season and is soon expected to be available in the United States. Use of passive immunization for immunocompromised children is logical but not established. RSV antibody is not effective for treatment of established infection. RSV vaccines are currently in advanced stages of development.

Prognosis

Although mild bronchiolitis does not produce long-term problems, 30%–40% of patients hospitalized with this infection will wheeze later in childhood, and RSV infection in infancy may be an important precursor to asthma. Chronic restrictive lung disease and bronchiolitis obliterans are rare sequelae.

AAP Practice Guideline: Updated guidance for palivizumab prophylaxis among infants and young children at increased risk of hospitalization for respiratory syncytial virus infection. Pediatrics 2014 Aug;134(2):e620–e638 [PMID: 25070304].

Hon KL, Leung AKC, Wong AHC, Dudi A, Leung KKY. Respiratory syncytial virus is the most common causative agent of viral bronchiolitis in young children: an updated review. Curr Pediatr Rev 2023;19(2):139–149. doi: 10.2174/1573396318666220810161945 [PMID: 35950255].

Ralston SL et al; American Academy of Pediatrics: Clinical practice guidelines: the diagnosis, management, and prevention of bronchiolitis. Pediatrics 2014 Nov;134(5):e1474–e1502 [PMID: 25349312].

HUMAN METAPNEUMOVIRUS (HMPV)

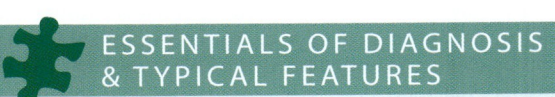

ESSENTIALS OF DIAGNOSIS & TYPICAL FEATURES

- ► Seasonality: late fall to early spring.
- ► Cough, coryza, sore throat.
- ► Bronchiolitis.
- ► Detection of nucleic acid in respiratory secretions.

General Considerations

Human metapneumovirus (hMPV) is a common agent of respiratory tract infections that is very similar to RSV in epidemiologic and clinical characteristics. Like RSV, parainfluenza, mumps, and measles, hMPV belongs to the paramyxovirus family. Humans are its only known reservoir. Seroepidemiologic surveys indicate that the virus has worldwide distribution. More than 90% of children contract hMPV infection by age 5 years, typically during late autumn through early spring outbreaks. hMPV accounts for 15%–25% of the cases of bronchiolitis and pneumonia in children younger than 2 years. Older children and adults can also develop symptomatic infection.

Clinical Findings

A. Symptoms and Signs

The most common symptoms are fever, cough, rhinorrhea, and sore throat. Bronchiolitis and pneumonia occur in 40%–70% of the children who acquire hMPV before the age of 2 years. Asymptomatic infection is uncommon. Other manifestations include otitis, conjunctivitis, diarrhea, and myalgia. Acute wheezing has been associated with hMPV in children of all ages, raising the possibility that this virus, like RSV, might trigger reactive airway disease.

B. Laboratory Findings

Diagnostic testing is usually not necessary. The preferred method of diagnosis is PCR performed on respiratory specimens. Rapid shell vial culture is an acceptable, albeit less sensitive. Antibody tests are used for epidemiologic studies.

C. Imaging

Lower respiratory tract infection frequently shows hyperinflation and patchy pneumonitis on chest radiographs.

Treatment & Prognosis

No antiviral therapy is available to treat hMPV. Ribavirin has in vitro activity against hMPV, but there are no data to support its therapeutic value. Children with lower respiratory tract disease may require hospitalization and ventilatory support, but less frequently than with RSV-associated bronchiolitis. Duration of hospitalization in hMPV is typically shorter than in RSV. Infection of immune-compromised children can lead to severe or fatal disease.

Esposito S, Masstrolia MV: Metapneumovirus infections and respiratory complications. Semin Respir Crit Care Med 2016;37:512 [PMID: 27486733].

Taylor S, Lopez P, Boria-Tabora C: Respiratory viruses and influenza-like illness: epidemiology and outcomes in children aged 6 months to 10 years in a multi-country population sample. J Infect 2017;29:74 [PMID: 27667752].

HUMAN CORONAVIRUSES

Human coronaviruses (HCoVs) are RNA viruses that can infect humans and various animals. They are transmitted via inoculation of the respiratory tract by droplets from the respiratory tract of infected individuals. The incubation period is 2–5 days for the nonsevere infections and potentially longer for severe acute respiratory syndromes. Infections from HCoVs, including strains OC43, NL63, HKU1, and 229E, manifest each year as the common cold and lower respiratory tract disease (LRTD). However, LRTD is more frequent and severe in immunocompromised children. Coinfections with other viruses occur in 10%–40% of HCoV infections. Severe acute respiratory syndrome (SARS) coronaviruses cause a variety of clinical manifestations, including severe disease.

▶ HCoV Clinical Syndromes

A. Upper and Lower Respiratory Tract Infection

HCoVs 229E, OC43, NL63, and HKU1 are the second most common cause of the common cold after rhinoviruses and manifest with rhinorrhea, sore throat, cough, and occasionally fever. HCoVs may also present as acute otitis media or trigger asthma exacerbations. HCoV NL63 is a common cause of croup. HCoV HKU1 also can present as acute gastroenteritis.

B. Severe Acute Respiratory Syndromes (SARS)

The three novel HCoVs causing severe symptoms are SARS-CoV, MERS-CoV, and SARS-CoV-2. SARS-CoV included moderate infectivity, caused epidemics in several countries, and had a case fatality rate of ~10%. The Middle Eastern Respiratory Syndrome (MERS)-CoV appeared in 2012 in Saudi Arabia, was less infectious, but more severe clinically with a case fatality rate of ~30%. It is endemic in the Middle East and acquired by close contact with camels, although human-to-human spread also occurs. HCoVs that cause severe disease disproportionally affect immune- or anatomically compromised adults and the elderly. Infected children are either asymptomatic or have typically milder symptoms that include fever, cough, myalgia, mild diarrhea, and abdominal pain.

The 2019 SARS-CoV-2 resulted in worldwide spread with the subsequent emergence of several novel variants associated with increased transmissibility, disease severity, and immune evasion. This virus can spread asymptomatically and prior to symptom onset, greatly expanding its transmissibility. High-risk populations are similar to those for other HCoVs.

Complications including multiorgan dysfunction and death can occur in children with comorbidities. SARS-CoV-2 infection is associated with Multisystem Inflammatory Syndrome in children (MIS-C), which is not completely understood immune-mediated complication that typically occurs 1-6 weeks following SARS-CoV-2 infection, and includes systemic inflammation, myocardial dysfunction, and multiorgan dysfunction.

▶ Laboratory & Diagnostic Studies

HCoVs, including the common seasonal HCoVs (229E, OC43, NL54, and HKU1), may be detected by PCR, including multiplex respiratory pathogen panels. Public health laboratories have added the capacity to diagnose novel coronaviruses causing severe disease, including the current pandemic SARS-CoV-2, by PCR.

Multiple diagnostic assays, including nucleic acid (PCR) and antigen, as well as antibodies from natural infection or vaccination, continue to be developed for detection of SARS-CoV-2 using a variety of sample types. The preferred diagnostic for acute SARS-CoV-2 infection includes PCR from a nasopharyngeal sample. Other specimen sources, such as nasal swab or saliva, may have decreased sensitivity, though sensitivity is generally higher in symptomatic patients (vs asymptomatic/exposed patients). Antigen tests have the advantage of being less costly, more rapid, and available for home testing, but are at risk of decreased sensitivity.

Post-acute SARS-CoV-2 infection may be diagnosed by serology though this may be difficult given prior infections and vaccinations. The gold standard serologic test includes the measuring titer of host-neutralizing antibodies against SARS-CoV-2, though this test is resource- and time-intensive. ELISA assays provide more immediate and less costly results but may have lower performance. For updated recommendations on diagnostic testing for SARS-CoV-2, see CDC Guidelines (see References).

▶ Treatment & Prevention

Most common HCoVs cause mild, self-limited disease, and treatment is supportive.

The management of COVID-19 in children is complicated and should be managed on a case-by-case basis given rapidly changing data on disease pathogenesis and complications. Primary considerations in treatment decisions include disease severity (hospitalization, oxygen requirements), risk factors (comorbidities, immunosuppression), and clinical trajectory. CDC, NIH, and the Pediatric Infectious Disease Society (PIDS) provide regular updated guidelines (see References).

Remdesivir has been the most commonly used antiviral medication for treatment of COVID-19, with relatively good safety. Thus, remdesivir may be considered (5 days) for cases of severe COVID-19 (hospitalized, on supplemental oxygen). Glucocorticoids have also demonstrated efficacy among adults with severe disease and may be considered in children with oxygen requirement. Convalescent plasma and monoclonal antibodies have shown some benefit in early trials and are undergoing further study for both treatment and prophylaxis. All these treatments need to be re-evaluated with each novel SARS-CoV-2 variant to ensure sustained efficacy, and updated recommendations can be found on the PIDS, CDC, and NIH websites.

Vaccines to prevent SARS-CoV-2 infection and COVID-19 demonstrate high efficacy and safety. mRNA vaccines (BNT162b2 and mRNA-1273) have shown improved efficacy/safety profile compared to adenovirus-vectored vaccine (Ad26.COV2.S), and have an emergency use authorization for children ≥ 6 months old. Number of vaccine doses, dosing interval, and boosters depend on age and host immune status, and continue to vary based on emerging evidence (see References for updated guidelines).

CDC: COVID-19 vaccination: https://www.cdc.gov/vaccines/covid-19/index.html.
CDC: Overview of testing for SARS-CoV-2 (COVID-19): https://www.cdc.gov/coronavirus/2019-ncov/hcp/testing-overview.html.
Chiotos et al: Multicenter interim guidance on use of antivirals for children with coronavirus disease 2019/severe acute respiratory syndrome coronavirus 2. J Pediatric Infect Dis Soc 2021 Jan;10(1):34–48.
NIH: Coronavirus Disease 19 (COVID-19) Treatment Guidelines: https://www.covid19treatmentguidelines.nih.gov/.
PIDS: https://pids.org/resources/covid-19-resources/.

INFECTIONS DUE TO ENTEROVIRUSES & PARECHOVIRUSES

ESSENTIALS OF DIAGNOSIS & TYPICAL FEATURES

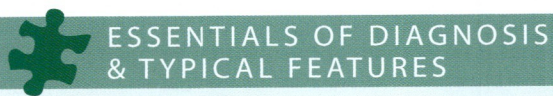

- ▶ Acute febrile illness with headache and sore throat.
- ▶ Summer-fall epidemics.
- ▶ Other common features: rash, nonexudative pharyngitis.
- ▶ Common cause of aseptic and viral meningitis.
- ▶ Complications: myocarditis, neurologic damage, life-threatening illness in newborns.

Enteroviruses (EV) are a major cause of acute febrile illness in young children. From the family of picornaviruses ("small"), antigenically they are divided into four groups: polioviruses (PV), coxsackieviruses A and B, and echoviruses. Their common RNA sequences and group antigens are the basis for diagnostic tests for enterovirus-specific nucleic acid and proteins. A PCR assay is available in many medical centers as a one-step test with results in a few hours. Cross-reactivity with rhinoviruses is common on the PCR respiratory panel. Viral cultures are more specific but take 2–5 days. PCR is now the diagnostic method of choice for meningoencephalitis and severe unexplained illness in neonates.

Human parechoviruses (PeV), also picornaviruses, are responsible for severe infections in young children including sepsis and meningoencephalitis. PeV genus is currently divided into six species (PeVA through F) of which PeVA infect humans with 19 types described.

Transmission of EV and PeV is fecal-oral or from upper respiratory secretions. Multiple enteroviruses circulate in the community at any one time; summer-fall outbreaks are common in temperate climates, but infections are seen year-round. After poliovirus, coxsackie B virus is most virulent, followed by echovirus. Neurologic, cardiac, and overwhelming neonatal infections are the most severe forms of illness.

ACUTE FEBRILE ILLNESS

Accompanied by nonspecific upper respiratory or enteric symptoms, the sudden onset of fever and irritability and poor feeding in infants or young children is often enteroviral, especially in late summer and fall. More than 90% of enteroviral infections are not distinctive. Occasionally a petechial rash is seen; more often a diffuse maculopapular or morbilliform eruption (often prominent on palms and soles) occurs on the second to fourth day of fever. Rapid recovery is the rule. More than one febrile enteroviral illness can occur in a patient in one season. The leukocyte count is usually normal. Infants, because of fever and irritability, may undergo an evaluation for sepsis or meningitis and be hospitalized. Approximately half of these infants have aseptic meningitis. Duration of illness is 4–5 days. PeV cause similar disease to echoviruses, ranging from asymptomatic or mild-to-severe illness predominantly in neonates and young children.

Abedi GR et al: Picornavirus etiology of acute infections among hospitalized infants. J Clin Virol 2019;116:39–43. doi: 10.1016/j.jcv.2019.04.005 [PMID: 31100674].

Tao L, Humphries RM, Banerjee R, Gaston DC. Re-emergence of parechovirus: 2017-2022 National trends of detection in cerebrospinal fluid. Open Forum Infect Dis 2023;10(3):ofad112. doi: 10.1093/ofid/ofad112 [PMID: 36968966].

RESPIRATORY TRACT ILLNESSES

1. Acute Febrile Pharyngitis

Sore throat, headache, myalgia, and abdominal discomfort lasting 3–4 days are common in older children. Vesicles or papules may be seen in the pharynx without exudate. Occasionally, enteroviruses are the cause of croup, bronchitis, or pneumonia. They may also exacerbate asthma as seen with the recent outbreaks of EV68.

2. Herpangina

Herpangina manifests as acute onset fever and posterior pharyngeal grayish-white vesicles that quickly form ulcers (< 20 in number), linearly along the posterior palate, uvula, and tonsillar pillars. Bilateral facial ulcers may also be seen. Dysphagia, drooling, vomiting, abdominal pain, and anorexia also occur and, rarely, parotitis or vaginal ulcers. Symptoms disappear in 4–5 days. Coxsackievirus A10 has been associated with a sporadic febrile pharyngitis, called acute lymphonodular pharyngitis, which is characterized by nonulcerative yellow-white posterior pharyngeal papules in the same distribution as herpangina. The duration is 1–2 weeks. Therapy is supportive.

Primary herpes simplex gingivostomatitis (ulcers are more prominent anteriorly, and gingivitis is present), aphthous stomatitis (fever absent, recurrent episodes, anterior lesions), trauma, hand-foot-and-mouth disease (see discussion in section Rashes [Including Hand-Foot-&-Mouth Disease]), and Vincent angina (painful gingivitis spreading from the gum line; older child; underlying dental disease) should be in the differential diagnosis.

3. Pleurodynia (Bornholm Disease, Epidemic Myalgia)

Caused by coxsackie B virus (epidemic form) or many nonpolio enteroviruses (sporadic form), pleurodynia is associated with an abrupt onset of unilateral or bilateral spasmodic pain over the lower ribs or upper abdomen. Associated symptoms include headache, fever, vomiting, myalgias, and abdominal and neck pain. Physical findings include fever, chest muscle tenderness, decreased thoracic excursion, and occasionally a friction rub. The chest radiograph is normal. Hematologic tests are not diagnostic. The illness generally lasts less than 1 week.

This is a disease of muscles, but the differential diagnosis includes bacterial pneumonia, bacterial and tuberculous effusion, and endemic fungal infections (all excluded radiographically and by auscultation), costochondritis (no fever or other symptoms), and a variety of abdominal problems, especially those causing diaphragmatic irritation. Epidemics of acute myalgia have also been reported due to HPeV type 3 in Japan in children and adults. Potent analgesic agents and chest splinting alleviate the pain.

Lugo D, Krogstad P: Enteroviruses in the early 21st century: new manifestations and challenges. Curr Opin Pediatr 2016 Feb;28(1):107–113. doi: 10.1097/MOP.0000000000000303 [PMID: 26709690].

RASHES (INCLUDING HAND-FOOT-&-MOUTH DISEASE)

The EV rash can be macular, maculopapular, urticarial, scarlatiniform, petechial, or vesiculo-pustular. One of the most characteristic is that of hand-foot-and-mouth disease (caused by coxsackieviruses, especially types A5, A10, and A16), in which vesicles or red papules are found on the pharyngeal pillars, tongue, oral mucosa, hands, and feet. Often, they appear near the nails and on the heels and may last up to 1–2 weeks. Associated fever, sore throat, and malaise are mild. The rash may appear when fever abates, simulating roseola.

Cardiac Involvement

Myocarditis and pericarditis can be caused by several nonpolio enteroviruses, particularly type B coxsackieviruses. Most commonly, upper respiratory symptoms are followed by substernal pain, dyspnea, and exercise intolerance. A friction rub or gallop may be detected. Echocardiogram will define ventricular dysfunction or pericardial effusion, and electrocardiography may show pericarditis or ventricular irritability. Creatine phosphokinase may be elevated, and troponin (hs-TnT) is highly sensitive for acute myocarditis. The disease may be mild or fatal; most children recover completely. In infants, other organs may be involved at the same time; in older patients, cardiac disease is usually the sole manifestation (see Chapter 20 for therapy). Enteroviral RNA is present in cardiac tissue in some cases of dilated cardiomyopathy or myocarditis; the significance of this finding is unknown. Epidemics of EV 71 in Asia, as well as sporadic cases in the United States, are associated with severe left ventricular dysfunction and pulmonary edema following typical mucocutaneous manifestations of enterovirus infection. Enterovirus 71 also can cause isolated severe neurologic disease or neurologic disease in combination with myocardial disease.

Gonzalez G, Carr MJ, Kobayashi M, Hanaoka N, Fujimoto T: Enterovirus-associated hand-foot and mouth disease and neurological complications in Japan and the rest of the world. Int J Mol Sci 2019 Oct 20;20(20):5201 [PMID: 31635198].

Tomatis Souverbielle C, Erdem G, Sánchez PJ. Update on non-polio enterovirus and parechovirus infections in neonates and young infants. Curr Opin Pediatr 2023. doi: 10.1097/MOP.0000000000001236 [PMID: 36876331].

Severe Neonatal Infection

Neonatal enteroviral infection is usually systemic and severe in otherwise normal newborns. Clinical manifestations include fever, rash, pneumonitis, aseptic meningitis, meningoencephalitis, viral sepsis, hepatitis with acute liver failure, gastroenteritis, myocarditis, pancreatitis, and myositis. Transplacental infections present within 1 week of birth as sepsis with cyanosis, dyspnea, and seizures. Nosocomial outbreaks are less common. The differential diagnosis includes bacterial and herpes simplex infections, necrotizing enterocolitis, other causes of heart or liver failure, and metabolic diseases. Diagnosis is suggested by the finding of cerebrospinal fluid (CSF) mononuclear pleocytosis and detection of EV RNA in stool or pharynx, and confirmed by PCR in CSF, blood, or urine. IVIG is often administered, but its value is still uncertain. Some investigational antivirals (eg, pleconaril, pocapavir) have shown promise. Passively acquired maternal antibody may protect newborns from severe disease. PeV infection of neonates are mostly due to PeVA3 infections, manifesting in sepsis-like disease and central nervous system (CNS) infection, with almost half of infected newborns requiring ICU management.

CENTRAL NERVOUS SYSTEM ILLNESSES

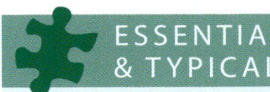

ESSENTIALS OF DIAGNOSIS & TYPICAL FEATURES

▶ Acute meningoencephalitis: headache, fever, meningismus.

▶ Asymmetrical, flaccid paralysis; muscle tenderness and hyperesthesia; intact sensation; late atrophy.

1. Poliomyelitis, Acute Flaccid Myelitis, & Acute Flaccid Paralysis

▶ General Considerations

Poliovirus infection is asymptomatic in 90%–95% of cases; presents as acute febrile illness in about 5% of cases or as aseptic meningitis, with or without paralysis, in 1%–3%. Polio has been eliminated from more than 99% of the world's population with the only endemic areas now in Pakistan and Afghanistan. Most older children and adults are now protected due to vaccination or previous silent infection.

Vaccine-associated paralytic polio (VAPP) and vaccine-derived polio viruses (VDPV) are a consequence of oral polio vaccine (OPV) that has mutated and reverted to neurovirulent. The latter has caused outbreaks of acute flaccid paralysis (AFP) like wild-type polio. Since 2000, inactivated poliovirus vaccine (IPV) has been the only polio vaccine in use in the United States, and since 2016, at least one dose of IPV along with bivalent OPV (types 1 and 3) and now novel OPV2 (nOPV2) is being given to children worldwide to prevent cVDPV (see Chapter 10). Other nonpolio EV can present as AFP, including EV71 in Asia and, since 2014, EV-68 in Europe and the United States as acute flaccid myelitis (AFM).

▶ Clinical Findings

A. Symptoms and Signs

The initial symptoms of polioviruses as well as other neurotropic enteroviruses (EV71 and EV68) are fever, myalgia, sore throat, and headache for 2–6 days. In less than 5% of infected children, symptom-free days are followed by recurrent fever and signs of aseptic meningitis: headache, nuchal rigidity, and nausea. Mild cases resolve completely. In 1%–2% of those infected, high fever, severe myalgia, and anxiety herald progression to loss of reflexes and subsequent acute flaccid asymmetrical paralysis. Proximal limb muscles are more often involved than distal, and lower limb involvement is more common than upper. Sensation remains intact, although hyperesthesia of skin overlying paralyzed muscles is common and pathognomonic.

Bulbar involvement affects swallowing, speech, and cardiorespiratory function and accounts for most deaths. Bladder distention and marked constipation characteristically accompany lower limb paralysis. Paralysis is usually complete by the time the temperature normalizes. Atrophy is usually apparent by 4–8 weeks. Most improvement of muscle paralysis occurs within 6 months.

B. Laboratory Findings

In patients with meningeal symptoms, the CSF shows a lymphocytic pleocytosis and a normal glucose with mildly elevated protein concentration. Poliovirus is easy to grow in cell culture and can be readily differentiated from other enteroviruses. It is rarely isolated from spinal fluid but is often present in the throat and stool for several weeks following infection. PCR is the method of choice for detection of polioviruses as well as other neurotropic enteroviruses.

▶ Differential Diagnosis

Aseptic meningitis due to poliovirus is indistinguishable from that due to other viruses. Paralytic disease in the United States is usually due to nonpolio enteroviruses (recently EV68). Polio and neurotropic EVs may resemble Guillain-Barré syndrome (minimal sensory loss, ascending symmetrical loss of function; minimal pleocytosis, high protein concentration in spinal fluid), polyneuritis (sensory loss), pseudoparalysis due to bone or joint problems (eg, trauma, infection), botulism, or tick paralysis. West Nile virus infection can present like AFP in children.

Complications

Complications are the result of permanent destruction of anterior horn cells and paralysis. Respiratory, pharyngeal, bladder, and bowel malfunction are most critical. Death is usually the consequence of respiratory dysfunction. Limbs injured near the time of infection (by intramuscular injections, prior excessive prior, or trauma) tend to be most severely involved and have the worst prognosis for recovery (provocation paralysis).

Treatment & Prognosis

Therapy is supportive. Investigational antivirals like pocapavir have demonstrated to be safe and accelerate poliovirus clearance but are not yet licensed for the treatment of polio or other enterovirus infections. Several potent antivirals are available to inhibit other positive-strand RNA viruses with a similar replication strategy. Bed rest, fever, and pain control (heat therapy is helpful), and careful attention to progression of weakness (particularly of respiratory muscles) are important. Early or late corticosteroid treatment has been associated with increased mortality in children infected with EV-71, so they are not recommended. No intramuscular injections should be given during the acute phase as they may lead to enhanced paralysis. Intubation or tracheostomy for secretion control and ventilation, enteral feeding and catheter drainage of the bladder may be needed. Disease is worse in adults and pregnant women. Post-polio muscular atrophy occurs in 30%–40% of paralyzed limbs 20–30 years later, characterized by increasing weakness and fasciculations in previously affected, partially recovered limbs. Fluoxetine has antiviral activity against EVD68 in vitro and has been used in cases of AFM in humans without proven benefit.

2. Nonpolio Viral Meningitis

Nonpolio enteroviruses cause over 80% of cases of aseptic meningitis at all ages, especially in the summer and fall. Nosocomial outbreaks also occur.

Clinical Findings

The usual EV incubation period is 4–6 days. Most EV infections are subclinical or not associated with central nervous system (CNS) symptoms; therefore, a history of a sick contact is unusual. Neonates may acquire infection from maternal blood, vaginal secretions, or feces at birth; occasionally the mother has had a febrile illness just prior to delivery.

A. Symptoms and Signs

Incidence is much greater in children younger than 1 year, and CSF pleocytosis is more frequent in very young children undergoing a septic work up during the summer and fall. Onset is usually acute with fever, marked irritability, and lethargy in infants. Older children also describe frontal headache, photophobia, and myalgia. Abdominal pain, diarrhea, and projectile vomiting may occur. The incidence of rash varies with the infecting strain. If rash occurs, it is usually seen after several days of illness and is diffuse, macular, or maculopapular, occasionally petechial, but not purpuric. Oropharyngeal vesicles and rash on the palms and soles suggest an enterovirus. The anterior fontanel may be full and meningismus present. The illness may be biphasic, with nonspecific symptoms and signs preceding those related to the CNS. In older children, meningeal signs are more frequent, but seizures are unusual. Focal neurologic findings, which are rare, should lead to a search for an alternative cause. Frank encephalitis, which is uncommon at any age, occurs most often in neonates. Because of the overall frequency of enteroviral disease in children, 5%–10% of all cases of encephalitis of proved viral origin are caused by enteroviruses. Enteroviruses tend to cause less severe encephalitis than other viruses. However, PeV CNS infections are associated with white matter injury and may manifest long-term sequelae including hypotonia and cerebral palsy.

EV71 infections that begin with typical mucocutaneous manifestations of enteroviruses can be complicated by severe brainstem encephalitis. Outbreaks of respiratory disease with meningitis and acute paralysis due to EV68 have occurred in western United States and Europe. Enterovirus 70 outbreaks are characterized by hemorrhagic conjunctivitis together with paralytic poliomyelitis.

B. Laboratory Findings

Blood leukocyte counts are often normal. The spinal fluid leukocyte count is 100–1000/μL with polymorphonuclear cells predominating early and shifting to mononuclear cells within 8–36 hours. In about 95% of cases, spinal fluid parameters include a total leukocyte count less than 3000/μL, protein less than 80 mg/dL, and glucose more than 60% of serum values. Marked deviation from any of these findings should prompt consideration of another diagnosis.

Culture of CSF may yield an enterovirus within a few days (< 70%), but EV PCR is the most useful diagnostic method in many centers (sensitivity > 90%) and can give an answer within few hours. PeV will be detected by most PCR methods but will be identified as "enterovirus." Virus may be detected even with no CSF pleocytosis. Detection of an enterovirus from throat or stool suggests, but does not prove, enteroviral meningitis. Vaccine-derived poliovirus present in feces in infants being evaluated for aseptic meningitis may confuse the diagnosis, but history of travel or exposure to OPV should help.

C. Imaging

Cerebral imaging is not often indicated; if done, it is usually normal. Subdural effusions, infarcts, edema, or focal abnormalities seen in bacterial meningitis are absent except for the rare case of focal encephalitis.

▶ Differential Diagnosis

Enteroviral infections account for up to 90% of the cases of aseptic meningitis in which an etiologic agent is identified, especially in the summer and fall. Other causative viruses are mosquito-borne (flavivirus, bunyavirus) and are part of the investigation of encephalitis, but many of them are more likely to cause isolated meningitis. Primary herpes simplex infection can cause aseptic meningitis in adolescents who have a genital herpes infection. In neonates, early herpes simplex meningoencephalitis may mimic enteroviral disease (see section Infections Due to Herpesviruses) and if suspected urgent antiviral therapy is recommended. Lymphocytic choriomeningitis virus causes meningitis in children in contact with rodents (pet or environmental exposure). Meningitis occurs in some patients at the time of infection with human immunodeficiency virus (HIV).

Other causes of aseptic meningitis that may resemble enteroviral infection include partially treated bacterial meningitis (recent antibiotic treatment, CSF parameters resembling those seen in bacterial disease and bacterial antigen sometimes present); bacterial para-meningeal foci such as brain abscess, subdural empyema, mastoiditis (predisposing factors, lower CSF glucose level, focal neurologic signs, and characteristic imaging); tumors or cysts (malignant cells on cytologic examination, higher protein or lower glucose levels in CSF); trauma (presence, without exception, of crenated red blood cells and fail to clear); tuberculous or fungal meningitis (see Chapters 42 and 43); cysticercosis; para and postinfectious encephalopathies (*M pneumoniae*, cat-scratch disease, influenza); leptospirosis; rickettsial diseases including Lyme; and acute demyelinating encephalomyelitis.

▶ Prevention & Treatment

No specific antiviral therapy exists. Infants are usually hospitalized, isolated, and treated with fluids and antipyretics. Moderately to severely ill infants are given empiric antibiotics for bacterial pathogens until cultures, or PCR, are negative. In children and infants at low risk of serious bacterial infection, antibiotics may be withheld, and the child observed until PCR results are available. The illness usually lasts less than 1 week. Strong analgesics may be needed. With clinical deterioration, repeat lumbar puncture, cerebral imaging, neurologic consultation, and more aggressive diagnostic

tests should be considered. Herpesvirus encephalitis is an important consideration in such cases, particularly in infants younger than 1 month, and often warrants empiric acyclovir until HSV infection can be ruled out.

▶ Prognosis

In general, enteroviral meningitis has no significant short-term neurologic or developmental sequelae. Developmental delay and cerebral palsy may follow severe neonatal infections. Unlike mumps, enterovirus infections rarely cause hearing loss.

Messacar K et al: Enterovirus D68 and acute flaccid myelitis-evaluating the evidence for causality. Lancet Infect Dis 2018 Aug;18(8):e239–e247 [PMID: 29482893].

Murphy OC et al; AFM working group: Acute flaccid myelitis: cause, diagnosis, and management. Lancet 2021 Jan 23; 397(10271): 334–346 [PMID: 33357469].

Tomatis Souverbielle C, Erdem G, Sánchez PJ: Update on non-polio enterovirus and parechovirus infections in neonates and young infants. Curr Opin Pediatr 2023. doi: 10.1097/MOP.0000000000001236 [PMID: 36876331].

▼ INFECTIONS DUE TO HERPESVIRUSES

HERPES SIMPLEX INFECTIONS

ESSENTIALS OF DIAGNOSIS & TYPICAL FEATURES

- ▶ Grouped vesicles on an erythematous base, typically in or around the mouth or genitals.
- ▶ Fever, malaise, and tender regional adenopathy common with primary infection.
- ▶ Recurrent episodes.

▶ General Considerations

There are two types of herpes simplex virus (HSV). Type 1 (HSV-1) causes most cases of oral, perioral, skin, and cerebral disease in children, while type 2 (HSV-2) is now equally as common as HSV-1 as cause of genital and congenital HSV infections. Latent infection is routinely established in sensory ganglia during primary infection. Recurrences, due to reactivation of latent HSV, may be spontaneous or induced by external events (eg, fever, menstruation, or sunlight) or immunosuppression. Transmission is by direct contact with infected secretions.

Primary infection with HSV-1 often occurs early in childhood by contact with infected oral secretions of playmates or caretakers, with a second peak of infection later in life as a sexually transmitted disease. Primary infection with HSV-1 is subclinical in 80% of cases and causes gingivostomatitis or genital disease in the remainder. HSV-2, which is mostly transmitted sexually, is also subclinical (65%) or produces mild, nonspecific symptoms. The source of primary infection is usually an asymptomatic excreter. Most previously infected individuals shed HSV at irregular intervals. At any one time (point prevalence), more than 5% of seropositive adults excrete HSV-1 in the saliva; the percentage is higher in recently infected children, and detection of viral DNA exceeds 12%. HSV-2 shedding in genital secretions occurs with a similar or higher point prevalence exceeding 15%, depending on the method of detection (viral isolation vs PCR) and the interval since the initial infection. A history of contact with clinically apparent HSV lesions is unusual. Infection with one type of HSV may prevent or attenuate clinically apparent infection with the other type, but individuals can be infected at different times with both HSV-1 and HSV-2.

▶ Clinical Findings

A. Symptoms and Signs

1. Gingivostomatitis—High fever, irritability, and drooling occur in infants. Multiple oral ulcers are seen on the tongue and on the buccal and gingival mucosa, occasionally extending to the pharynx. Pharyngeal ulcers may predominate in older children and adolescents. Diffusely swollen red gums that are friable, and bleed easily are typical. Cervical nodes are swollen and tender. Duration is 7–14 days. Herpangina, aphthous stomatitis, thrush, and Vincent angina should be excluded.

2. Vulvovaginitis or urethritis (see Chapter 44)—Genital herpes (especially HSV-2) in a prepubertal child should suggest sexual abuse. In sexually active adolescents, active vesicles or painful ulcers on the vulva, vagina, or penis and tender adenopathy are typical. Systemic symptoms (fever, flu-like illness, myalgia) are common with the initial episode. Painful urination is frequent, especially in females. Primary infection lasts 10–14 days before healing. Lesions may resemble trauma, syphilis (ulcers are painless), or chancroid (ulcers are painful and nodes are erythematous and fluctuant) in the adolescent, and bullous impetigo or severe chemical irritation in younger children.

3. Cutaneous infections—Direct inoculation onto cuts or abrasions may produce localized vesicles or ulcers. A deep HSV infection on the finger (herpetic whitlow) may be mistaken for a bacterial felon or paronychia; surgical drainage is of no value and is contraindicated. HSV infection of eczematous skin may result in disseminated viral infection characterized by fever and clusters of pruritic blisters, vesicles, and shallow ulcers (eczema herpeticum), which may be mistaken for impetigo or varicella.

4. Recurrent mucocutaneous infection—Recurrent oral shedding is asymptomatic. Recurrent perioral lesions (sometimes perinasal) often begin with a prodrome of tingling or burning limited to the vermillion border, followed by vesiculation, scabbing, and crusting around the lips over 3–5 days. Recurrent intraoral lesions are rare. Fever, adenopathy, and other symptoms are absent. Recurrent cutaneous herpes most closely resembles impetigo, but the latter is often outside the perinasal and perioral region, recurs infrequently in the same area of skin, responds to antibiotics, yields a positive result on Gram stain, and *Streptococcus pyogenes* or *Staphylococcus aureus* can be isolated. Recurrent genital disease is common after the initial infection with HSV-2. Recurrent infection is shorter (5–7 days) and milder (mean, four lesions) than primary infection and is not associated with systemic symptoms. Recurrent genital disease, which may also recur on the thighs and buttocks, is also preceded by a cutaneous sensory prodrome. Recurrence of HSV-1 in the genital region is much less frequent than are HSV-2 recurrences.

5. Keratoconjunctivitis—Keratoconjunctivitis may be part of a primary infection due to spread from infected saliva. Most cases are caused by reactivation of virus latent in the ciliary ganglion. Keratoconjunctivitis produces photophobia, pain, and conjunctival irritation. Dendritic corneal ulcers may be demonstrable with fluorescein staining. Stromal invasion may occur. Corticosteroids should never be used for unilateral keratitis without ophthalmologic consultation. Other causes of these symptoms include trauma, bacterial infections, and other viral infections (especially adenovirus if pharyngitis is present; bilateral involvement makes HSV unlikely) (see Chapter 16).

6. Encephalitis—Although unusual in infants outside the neonatal period, encephalitis may occur at any age, usually without cutaneous herpes lesions. In older children, HSV encephalitis (HSE) can follow a primary infection, but usually represents reactivation of latent virus. HSE is the most common cause of nonepidemic focal encephalitis in children older than 6 months. Diagnosis of HSE is critical because it is treatable with specific antivirals. Acute onset is associated with fever, headache, behavioral changes, and focal neurologic deficits, and/or focal seizures. Mononuclear pleocytosis is typically present along with an elevated protein concentration. In older children, hypodense areas with a medial and inferior temporal lobe predilection are seen on CT scan, especially after 3–5 days, but the findings in infants may be more diffuse. Magnetic resonance imaging (MRI) is more sensitive and can sometimes identify patients with HSE in whom the PCR is initially negative. The majority have imaging findings in the inferomedial temporal lobes. Periodic focal epileptiform discharges are seen on electroencephalograms but are not diagnostic of HSV infection. Viral cultures of CSF are rarely positive. The PCR assay to detect HSV DNA in CSF is a sensitive and specific rapid test. Without early antiviral therapy, the prognosis is poor. The differential diagnosis includes mosquito-borne and other viral encephalitis, para-infectious and postinfectious encephalopathy, brain abscess, acute demyelinating syndromes, and bacterial meningoencephalitis.

7. Neonatal infections—Infection is occasionally acquired by ascending spread prior to delivery (< 5% of cases), but most often occurs at the time of vaginal delivery from a mother with genital infection. Eight to fifteen percent of HSV-2–seropositive pregnant women at delivery have HSV-2 detected in the genital tract by PCR. In most cases, this results from reactivation of infection acquired in the distant past. Incidence of neonatal herpes is 1 in 1500–3000 births. HSV-1 has now become a common cause of neonatal HSV infection. Neonatal infection is rarely acquired from mothers with reactivation disease, whereas it is frequently acquired during delivery of mothers with current or recent primary infection. This is because transplacental acquired antibody is usually protective. Most cases of neonatal HSV infection are acquired from mothers with undiagnosed genital herpes who acquired the infection during the pregnancy—especially near term. Occasionally, the infection is acquired in the postpartum period from oral secretions of family members or hospital personnel. A history of genital herpes in the mother is often absent. Within a few days and up to 6 weeks (most often within 2–4 weeks), skin vesicles appear (especially at sites of trauma, such as where scalp monitors were placed). Some infants (45%) have infection limited to the skin, eye, or mouth. Other infants are acutely ill, presenting with jaundice, shock, bleeding, or respiratory distress (25%). Some infants appear well initially, but dissemination of the infection to the brain or other organs manifest during the ensuing week. HSV infection (and empiric therapy) should be strongly considered in newborns with the sepsis syndrome and negative bacterial cultures. A mononuclear pleocytosis in the CSF and suggestive skin lesions support this, although skin lesions may be absent at the time of presentation or may never develop. Some infected infants exhibit only neurologic symptoms at 2–3 weeks after delivery: apnea, lethargy, fever, poor feeding, or persistent seizures. The brain infection in these children is often diffuse and is best diagnosed by MRI. In contrast to HSE seen in older children, neonatal herpes is rarely hemorrhagic, and the medial temporal and inferior frontal lobes are typically spared. Skin lesions may resemble impetigo, bacterial scalp abscesses, or miliaria and may recur over weeks or months after recovery from the acute illness. Progressive culture-negative pneumonitis is another manifestation of neonatal HSV.

B. Laboratory Findings

Abnormalities in platelets, clotting factors, and liver function tests are often present in infants with multisystem disease.

Lymphocytic pleocytosis and elevated CSF protein indicates viral meningitis or encephalitis. Virus may be cultured from infected epithelial sites (vesicles, ulcers, or conjunctival scrapings). Viral cultures of CSF yield positive results in about 50% of neonatal cases but are uncommon in older children. HSV will be detected within 2 days by rapid tissue culture methods, but PCR is the preferred diagnostic method for all specimens. A positive test from skin, throat, eye, or stool of a newborn is diagnostic. Vaginal culture of the mother may offer circumstantial evidence for the diagnosis but may be negative.

Rapid diagnostic tests include immunofluorescent stains or ELISA to detect viral antigen in skin or mucosal scrapings. The PCR assay for HSV DNA is positive (> 95%) in the CSF when there is brain involvement. HSV DNA is often present in the blood of patients with multisystem disease. Typing of genital HSV isolates from adolescents has prognostic value, since HSV-1 genital infection recurs much less frequently than genital HSV-2 infection.

▶ Complications, Sequelae, & Prognosis

Gingivostomatitis may result in dehydration due to dysphagia; severe chronic oral disease and esophageal involvement may occur in immunosuppressed patients. Primary vulvovaginitis may be associated with aseptic meningitis, paresthesia, autonomic dysfunction due to neuritis (urinary retention, constipation), and secondary candida infection. HIV transmission is facilitated from individuals who are also seropositive for HSV infection, and HIV acquisition is enhanced in HSV-infected contacts. Extensive cutaneous disease (as in eczema) may be associated with dissemination and bacterial superinfection. Keratitis may result in corneal opacification. Untreated encephalitis is fatal in 70% of patients and causes severe damage in most of the remainder. Even with early acyclovir treatment, 20% of patients die and 40% are neurologically impaired.

Disseminated neonatal infection is fatal for 30%–40% of neonates despite therapy, and 20% of survivors are often impaired. Treated infants with CNS infection (30% of cases) have a 5% mortality and 45%–70% of survivors have neurological abnormalities; treated neonates with infection limited to skin, eye, and mouth survive mostly without sequelae.

▶ Treatment

A. Specific Measures

HSV is sensitive to existing antiviral therapy.

1. Topical antivirals—Antiviral agents are effective for corneal disease and include 1% trifluridine and 0.15% ganciclovir (1–2 drops five times daily). These agents should be used with the guidance of an ophthalmologist and concurrently with oral antiviral therapy.

2. Mucocutaneous HSV infections—These infections respond to administration of oral nucleoside analogues (acyclovir, valacyclovir, or famciclovir). The main indications are severe genital HSV infection in adolescents and severe gingivostomatitis in young children. Antiviral therapy is beneficial for primary disease when begun early. Recurrent disease rarely requires therapy. Frequent genital recurrences may be suppressed by oral administration of nucleoside analogues, but this approach should be used sparingly. Other forms of severe cutaneous disease, such as eczema herpeticum should be treated promptly with systemic parenteral acyclovir or valacyclovir to minimize complications and prevent progression to severe disease. Intravenous acyclovir may be required when disease is extensive in immunocompromised children (10–15 mg/kg or 500 mg/m^2 every 8 hours for 14–21 days). Oral acyclovir, which is available in suspension, is also used within 72–96 hours for severe primary gingivostomatitis in immunocompetent young children. Antiviral therapy does not alter the incidence or severity of subsequent recurrences of oral or genital infection. Development of resistance to antivirals, which is very rare after treating immunocompetent patients, occurs in immunocompromised patients who receive frequent and prolonged therapy.

3. Encephalitis—Treatment consists of intravenous high-dose acyclovir for 21 days.

4. Neonatal infection—Newborns receive high-dose intravenous acyclovir for 21 days (14 days if infection is limited to skin, eye, or mouth). Therapy should not be discontinued unless a repeat CSF HSV PCR assay is negative near the end of treatment. The outcome at 1 year is improved in infants that receive oral acyclovir (300 mg/m^2/dose three times daily) suppression therapy for 6 months after completion of IV therapy. Prematurity is associated frequent skin recurrences but no systemic or CNS recurrence after stopping suppressive therapy.

B. General Measures

1. Gingivostomatitis—Gingivostomatitis is treated with pain relief and temperature control measures. Maintaining hydration is important because of the long duration of illness (7–14 days). Topical anesthetic agents (eg, viscous lidocaine or an equal mixture of kaolin–attapulgite [Kaopectate], diphenhydramine, and viscous lidocaine) may be used as a mouthwash for older children who will not swallow it; ingested lidocaine may be toxic to infants or may lead to aspiration. Antiviral therapy is indicated in normal hosts with severe disease.

2. Genital infections—Genital infections may require pain relief, assistance with voiding (warm baths, topical anesthetics, rarely catheterization), and psychological support. Lesions should be kept clean; drying may shorten the duration of symptoms. Sexual contact should be avoided during the interval from prodrome to crusting stages. Because of the frequency of asymptomatic shedding, the only effective way to prevent sexual transmission is the use of condoms. Candida superinfection occurs in 10% of women with primary genital infections.

3. Cutaneous lesions—Skin lesions should be kept clean, dry, and covered, if possible, to prevent spread. Systemic analgesics may be helpful. Secondary bacterial infection is uncommon in patients with lesions on the mucosa or involving small areas, and with recurrences. Secondary infection should be considered and treated, if necessary, in patients with more extensive lesions.

4. Recurrent cutaneous disease—Recurrent disease is usually the cause of lesions. Sun block lip balm helps prevent labial recurrences that follow intense sun exposure. There is no evidence that the many popular topical or vitamin therapies are efficacious.

5. Keratoconjunctivitis—An ophthalmologist should be consulted regarding the use of cycloplegics, anti-inflammatory agents, local debridement, and other therapies.

6. Encephalitis—Extensive support will be required for obtunded or comatose patients. Rehabilitation and psychological support are often needed for survivors.

7. Neonatal infection—Infected infants should be isolated and given acyclovir. Cesarean delivery is indicated if the mother has obvious cervical or vaginal lesions, especially if these represent primary infection (35%–50% transmission rate). With infants born vaginally to mothers who have active lesions of recurrent genital herpes, appropriate cultures and PCR should be obtained at 24 hours after birth, and the infant evaluated thoroughly for possible HSV infection. If the results are positive or the infant has suggestive signs or symptoms preemptive therapy should be started. Treatment is given to infants whose PCR results are positive or who appear ill. Infants born to mothers with obvious primary genital herpes should also be evaluated but should then receive therapy before the culture or PCR results are known. For women with a history of genital herpes infection, but no genital lesions, vaginal delivery with peripartum cultures of maternal cervix is the standard. Clinical follow-up of the newborn is recommended when maternal PCR results are positive. Repeated cervical cultures or PCR during pregnancy are not useful.

A challenging problem is the newborn that presents with fever (or hypothermia) and a sepsis-like picture, especially in the first 3 weeks of life. This is further confounded in the late summer by the existence of circulating enteroviruses. These infants should be considered for empiric acyclovir therapy, pending results of PCR, given the poor outcome of disseminated herpes in the newborn. The index of suspicion is increased when there is a CSF pleocytosis, elevated hepatic transaminase levels, a very ill-appearing infant, rash, or respiratory distress.

Pinninti SG, Kimberlin DW: Neonatal herpes simplex virus infections. Semin Perinatol 2018 Apr;42(3):168–175 [PMID: 29544668].

VARICELLA & HERPES ZOSTER

ESSENTIALS OF DIAGNOSIS & TYPICAL FEATURES

► Varicella (chickenpox):
- Follows exposure to varicella or herpes zoster 10–21 days previously, no prior history of varicella.
- Widely scattered red macules and papules concentrated on the face and trunk, rapidly progressing to clear vesicles on an erythematous base, pustules, and then crusts, over 5–6 days.
- Variable fever and nonspecific systemic symptoms.

► Herpes zoster (shingles):
- History of varicella.
- Dermatomal paresthesia and pain prior to eruption (more common in older children).
- Dermatomal distribution of grouped vesicles on an erythematous base; often accompanied by pain.

► **General Considerations**

Primary infection with varicella-zoster virus results in varicella, which generally confers lifelong immunity, but the virus remains latent for life in sensory ganglia. Herpes zoster, which represents reactivation of this latent virus, occurs in 30% of individuals at some time in their life. The incidence of herpes zoster is highest in elderly individuals and in immunosuppressed patients, but herpes zoster also occurs in immunocompetent children. Spread of varicella from a close contact is mainly by respiratory droplets or aerosols (occasionally direct contact) from vesicles or pustules, with an 85% infection rate in susceptible persons. Over 95% of young adults with a history of varicella are immune, as is 90% of native-born Americans who are unaware of having had varicella. Many individuals from tropical or subtropical regions fail to develop varicella in their childhood and remain susceptible through early adulthood. Humans are the only reservoir.

► **Clinical Findings**

Exposure to varicella or herpes zoster has usually occurred 14–16 days previously (range, 10–21 days). Contact may not be recognized, since the index case of varicella is infectious 1–2 days before rash appears. A 1- to 3-day prodrome of fever, malaise, respiratory symptoms, and headache may occur, especially in older children. The unilateral, dermatomal vesicular rash and pain of herpes zoster is very distinctive. Pain before rash eruption of herpes zoster may last several days and be mistaken for other illnesses.

A. Symptoms and Signs

1. Varicella—Typical case presents with mild systemic symptoms followed by crops of red macules that rapidly become small vesicles with surrounding erythema (described as a "dew drop on a rose petal"), form pustules, become crusted, and then scab. Pruritus is often intense; scarring occurs, but it is not common. The rash appears predominantly on the trunk and face. Lesions occur in the scalp, and sometimes in the nose, mouth (where they are nonspecific ulcers), conjunctiva, and vagina. The magnitude of systemic symptoms usually parallels skin involvement. Up to five crops of lesions may be seen. New crops stop forming after 5–7 days. If varicella occurs in the first few months of life (except for the early postpartum period), it is often mild because of transplacental acquired maternal antibody. Once crusting begins, the patient is no longer contagious. A modified form of varicella occurs in about 15% of vaccinated children exposed to varicella, despite receiving a single dose of varicella vaccine. This is usually much milder than typical varicella, with fewer lesions that heal rapidly. Cases of modified varicella are contagious.

2. Herpes zoster (shingles)—Common risk factors for HZ are older age, immunosuppression, diabetes, infections, and mental stress. This eruption involves a single dermatome (thus unilateral and does not cross the midline), usually truncal or cranial; occasionally a contiguous dermatome is involved. In older children, this is preceded by neuropathic pain or itching in the same area (designated the "prodrome"). HZ ophthalmic, affecting the trigeminal nerve, is an ophthalmic emergency as it may be associated with corneal involvement. The closely grouped vesicles, which resemble a localized version of varicella or herpes simplex, often coalesce. Crusting occurs in 7–10 days. Postherpetic neuralgia is rare in children. Herpes zoster is a common problem in HIV-infected or other immunocompromised children and in children who had varicella in early infancy (< 1–2 years old) or whose mothers had varicella during pregnancy. Herpes zoster can occur infrequently in children who received the varicella vaccine.

B. Laboratory Findings

Leukocyte counts are normal or low. Leukocytosis suggests secondary bacterial infection. Vesicular fluid or a scab can be used to identify the virus using PCR as the method of choice. DFA assay is less sensitive. Serum aminotransferase levels may be modestly elevated during typical varicella.

C. Imaging

Varicella pneumonia classically produces numerous bilateral diffuse infiltrates, nodular densities and hyperinflation. This is very rare in immunocompetent children but is seen more frequently in adults and immunocompromised children.

Differential Diagnosis

Varicella is usually distinctive. Similar rashes include those of coxsackievirus infection (fewer lesions, lack of crusting), impetigo (fewer lesions, smaller area, no classic vesicles, positive Gram stain, perioral or peripheral lesions), papular urticaria (insect bite history, nonvesicular rash), scabies (burrows, no typical vesicles, failure to resolve), parapsoriasis (rare in children < 10 years, chronic or recurrent, often a history of prior varicella), rickettsial pox (eschar where the mite bites, smaller lesions, no crusting), dermatitis herpetiformis (chronic, urticaria, residual pigmentation), and folliculitis. Herpes zoster is sometimes confused with a linear eruption of herpes simplex or a contact dermatitis.

Complications & Sequelae

A. Varicella

Secondary bacterial infection with staphylococci or group A streptococci is most common, presenting as impetigo, cellulitis or necrotizing fasciitis, abscesses, scarlet fever, or sepsis. Bacterial superinfection occurs in 2%–3% of children with varicella. Before a vaccine became available, hospitalization rates associated with varicella were 1:750–1:1000 cases in children and 10-fold higher in adults.

Protracted vomiting or a change in sensorium suggests Reye syndrome or encephalitis. Because Reye syndrome usually occurs in patients who are also receiving salicylates, these should be avoided in patients with varicella. Encephalitis occurs in less than 0.1% of cases, usually in the first week of illness, and is usually limited to cerebellitis with ataxia, which resolves completely. Diffuse encephalitis can be severe.

Varicella pneumonia usually afflicts immunocompromised children (especially those receiving high doses of corticosteroids or chemotherapy) and adults. Cough, dyspnea, tachypnea, rales, and cyanosis occur several days after onset of rash. New lesions may erupt for an extended period, and varicella may be life-threatening in immunosuppressed patients. In addition to pneumonitis, their disease may be complicated by hepatitis and encephalitis. The acute illness in these children often begins with unexplained severe abdominal pain. Varicella exposure in varicella-naïve severely immunocompromised children must be evaluated immediately for postexposure prophylaxis (see Chapter 10).

Hemorrhagic varicella lesions may be seen without other complications. This is most often caused by autoimmune thrombocytopenia, but hemorrhagic lesions can occasionally represent idiopathic disseminated intravascular coagulation (purpura fulminans).

Congenital varicella syndrome occurs in 1%–2% of maternal VZV infection occurring in the first 20 weeks of pregnancy, and presents as fetal skin lesions, limb hypoplasia, neurologic abnormalities, and eye disorders. Neonates born to mothers who develop varicella from 5 days before to 2 days after delivery are at high risk for severe or fatal (5%) disease and must be given varicella-zoster immunoglobulin (VariZIG) and followed closely (see Chapter 10).

Unusual complications of varicella include optic neuritis, myocarditis, transverse myelitis, orchitis, and arthritis.

B. Herpes Zoster

Complications of herpes zoster include secondary bacterial infection, motor or cranial nerve paralysis, meningitis, encephalitis, keratitis and other ocular complications, and dissemination in immunosuppressed patients. These complications are rare in immunocompetent children. Postherpetic neuralgia occurs in immunocompromised children but is rare in immunocompetent children.

Prevention

Varicella-specific hyperimmune globulin is available for postexposure prevention of varicella in high-risk susceptible persons and should be administered within 10 days postexposure (see Chapter 10). In immunocompetent children, postexposure prophylaxis with acyclovir is effective when it is started at 7–9 days after exposure and is continued for 7 days, as is varicella vaccine when given within 3–5 days of the exposure.

Two doses of the live attenuated varicella vaccine provide close to 92% protection and are now part of routine childhood immunization. Catch-up immunization is recommended for all other susceptible children and adults.

Treatment

A. General Measures

Supportive measures include maintenance of hydration, administration of acetaminophen for discomfort, cool soaks or antipruritics for itching, and observance of general hygiene measures (keep nails trimmed and skin clean). Care must be taken to avoid overdosage with antihistaminic agents. Topical or systemic antibiotics may be needed for bacterial superinfection.

B. Specific Measures

Acyclovir is the preferred drug for varicella and herpes zoster infections. Recommended parenteral acyclovir dosage for severe disease is 10 mg/kg (500 mg/m^2) intravenously every 8 hours, each dose infused over 1 hour, for 7–10 days. Parenteral therapy should be started early in immunocompromised patients or high-risk infected neonates. Hyperimmune globulin is of no value for established disease. The effect of oral acyclovir (80 mg/kg/day, divided in four doses) on varicella in immunocompetent children is modestly beneficial and nontoxic, but only when administered within 24 hours after the onset of varicella. Valacyclovir may be preferable in children older than 2 years. Oral acyclovir should be used selectively in immunocompetent children: when a significant concomitant or underlying illness is present, or when the index case is a sibling or when the patient is an adolescent, both of which are associated with more severe disease. Valacyclovir and famciclovir are superior antiviral agents because of better absorption; only acyclovir is available as a pediatric suspension. Herpes zoster in an immunocompromised child should be treated with intravenous acyclovir when it is severe, but oral valacyclovir or famciclovir can be used when the nature of the underlying illness and the immune status support this decision.

► Prognosis

Except for secondary bacterial infections, serious complications are rare and recovery complete in immunocompetent hosts. Complications are common in severely immune compromised children unless treated promptly.

Blumental S, Lepage P: Management of varicella in neonates and infants. BMJ Paediatr Open 2019 May 30;3(1):E000433 [PMID: 31263790].

Leung J, Harpaz R: Impact of the maturing varicella vaccination program on varicella and related outcomes in the United States: 1994–2012. J Ped Infect Dis Soc 2016;5:395 [PMID: 26407276].

HUMAN HERPES VIRUS-6 (HHV-6, ROSEOLA INFANTUM)

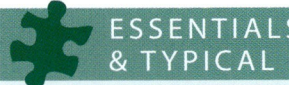

ESSENTIALS OF DIAGNOSIS & TYPICAL FEATURES

- ► High fever in a child aged 6–36 months.
- ► Minimal toxicity.
- ► Rose-pink maculopapular rash appears when fever subsides.

► General Considerations

Roseola infantum (also called exanthem subitum) is a benign illness caused by HHV-6 and rarely HHV-7. HHV-6 is a major cause of acute febrile illness in young children. Its significance is its common confusion with more serious causes of high fever and its role in inciting febrile seizures.

► Clinical Findings

The most prominent feature is the abrupt onset of fever, often reaching greater than 39.5°C, and lasting for 3–7 days (mean, 4 days: 15% ≥ 6 days) in an otherwise not critically-ill child. The fever then ceases abruptly, and a characteristic rash may appear. Roseola occurs predominantly in children aged 6 months to 3 years, with 90% of cases occurring before the second year. HHV-7 infection tends to occur somewhat later in childhood. These viruses are the most common recognized cause of fever and rash in this age group and are responsible for 20% of emergency department visits by children aged 6–12 months.

A. Symptoms and Signs

Mild lethargy and irritability may be present, but generally there is dissociation between other systemic symptoms and the febrile course. The pharynx, tonsils, and tympanic membranes may be injected. Conjunctivitis and pharyngeal exudate are notably absent. Diarrhea and vomiting occur in one-third of patients. Adenopathy of the head (especially postoccipital) and neck often occurs. The anterior fontanelle is bulging in one-quarter of HHV-6–infected infants. If rash appears (20%–30% incidence), it coincides with lysis of fever and begins on the trunk and spreads to the face, neck, and extremities. Rose-pink macules or maculo-papules, 2–3 mm in diameter, are nonpruritic, tend to coalesce, and disappear in 1–2 days without pigmentation or desquamation. Rash may occur without fever.

B. Laboratory Findings

Leukopenia and lymphocytopenia are present early. Laboratory evidence of hepatitis occurs in some patients, especially adults. Detection of HHV-6 and HHV-7 by PCR is available but rarely influences clinical management except in immunocompromised children. Some newly available multiplex CSF PCR includes HHV-6, but given the chromosomal integration of the virus, a positive result should be interpreted with caution in the presence of pleocytosis, especially in young infants.

► Differential Diagnosis

The initial high fever may require exclusion of serious bacterial infection. The relative well-being of most children and the typical course and rash soon clarify the diagnosis. These distinguish roseola from measles, rubella, adenoviruses, enteroviruses, drug reactions, and scarlet fever. In a child with febrile seizures, exclusion of bacterial meningitis is important. The CSF is normal in children with roseola. In children who receive antibiotics or other medication at the beginning of the fever, the rash may be attributed incorrectly to drug allergy.

► Complications & Sequelae

Febrile seizures occur in up to 10% of patients (even higher percentages in those with HHV-7 infections); especially if patients are younger than 24 months. There is evidence that HHV-6 can directly infect the CNS, causing meningoencephalitis. Multiorgan disease (pneumonia, hepatitis, bone marrow suppression, encephalitis) may occur in immunocompromised patients.

▶ Treatment & Prognosis

Fever is managed readily with acetaminophen and sponge baths. Fever control should be a major consideration in children with a history of febrile seizures. Roseola infantum is otherwise entirely benign. Systemic infection in immunocompromised children is treated with antiviral agents.

Green DA, Pereira M, Miko B, Radmard S, Whittier S, Thakur K: Clinical significance of human herpesvirus 6 positivity on the FILMARRAY meningitis/encephalitis panel. Clin Infect Dis 2018;67:1125–1128.

Mohammadpour Touserkani F, Gainza-Lein M, Jafarpour S, Brinegar K, Kapur K, Loddenkemper T: HHV-6 and seizure: a systematic review and meta-analysis. J Med Virol 2017;89(1):161–169 [PMID: 27272972].

CYTOMEGALOVIRUS (CMV)

ESSENTIALS OF DIAGNOSIS & TYPICAL FEATURES

- ▶ Primary infection:
  - Asymptomatic or minor illness in young children.
  - Mononucleosis-like syndrome without pharyngitis in adolescents.
- ▶ Congenital infection:
  - Leading cause of sensorineural hearing loss in children.
  - Saliva PCR is the preferred method for diagnosis of congenital CMV.
  - Majority of infants with congenital CMV are asymptomatic. Symptoms include: Intrauterine growth retardation, microcephaly with intracerebral calcifications and seizures, retinitis and encephalitis, hepatosplenomegaly with thrombocytopenia, "blueberry muffin" small purpuric spots rash.
- ▶ Immunocompromised hosts:
  - Retinitis and encephalitis.
  - Pneumonitis, enteritis, and hepatitis.
  - Bone marrow suppression.

▶ General Considerations

Cytomegalovirus (CMV) is a ubiquitous herpesvirus and the leading cause of congenital infections worldwide, affecting 3–6 per 1000 live born infants each year. It can be acquired in utero following maternal viremia or postpartum from birth canal secretions or maternal milk. Young children are infected by the saliva or urine from playmates; older individuals are infected by sexual partners (eg, from saliva, vaginal secretions, or semen). Transfused blood products and transplanted organs can be a source of CMV infection. Clinical illness is determined largely by the patient's immune competence. Immunocompetent individuals usually develop a mild self-limited illness, whereas immunocompromised children can develop severe, progressive, often multiorgan disease. In utero infection can be teratogenic.

1. In Utero Cytomegalovirus Infection

Approximately 0.5%–1.5% of children are born with CMV infections acquired during maternal viremia. CMV infection is asymptomatic in over 90% of these children, who are usually born to mothers who had experienced reactivation of latent CMV infection during the pregnancy. Infants with isolated sensorineural hearing loss but no apparent abnormalities can suggest congenital CMV disease and if confirmed are considered asymptomatic. Symptomatic infection occurs predominantly in infants born to mothers with primary CMV infection but can also result from reinfection during pregnancy. Even when exposed to a primary maternal infection, less than 50% of fetuses are infected, and in only 10% of those infants is the infection symptomatic at birth. Primary infection in the first half of pregnancy poses the greatest risk for spontaneous abortion and intrauterine fetal demise.

▶ Clinical Findings

A. Symptoms and Signs

Severely affected infants are born ill; they are often small for gestational age, limp, and lethargic. They feed poorly and have poor temperature control. Hepatosplenomegaly, jaundice, petechiae, seizures, and microcephaly are common. Characteristic signs are a distinctive chorioretinitis and periventricular calcification. A purpuric rash (named "blueberry muffin") like that seen with congenital rubella may be present in less than 5%, secondary to extramedullary hematopoiesis. Fatality rate is 10%–20%. Survivors usually have significant sequelae, especially mental retardation, neurologic deficits, retinopathy, and hearing loss. Isolated hepatosplenomegaly or thrombocytopenia may occur. Even mildly affected children may subsequently manifest cognitive impairment and psychomotor delay. Most infected infants (90%) are born to mothers with preexisting immunity who experienced reactivation of latent CMV or reinfection during pregnancy. These children have no clinical manifestations at birth, yet 10%–15% develop sensorineural hearing loss, which is often bilateral and may appear several years after birth.

B. Laboratory Findings

Diagnosis of congenital CMV requires detection of the virus within the first three weeks of life, as later testing does not differentiate intrauterine from perinatal or postnatal infection. The diagnosis is readily confirmed by CMV PCR from urine or saliva or using rapid culture methods combined with immunoassay. The presence in the infant of IgM-specific CMV antibodies suggests the diagnosis. In severely ill infants, anemia, thrombocytopenia, hyperbilirubinemia, and elevated aminotransferase levels are common. Lymphocytosis occurs occasionally. Pleocytosis and an elevated protein concentration are found in CSF. Some commercial ELISA kits are 90% sensitive and specific for these antibodies. Newborn screening for congenital CMV (using blood or saliva CMV PCR) is now more common with the goal of early identification of and intervention for affected infants. Hearing-targeted CMV screenings test only to infants who fail their newborn hearing screening, which is eightfold more common in CMV-infected infants. Retrospective diagnosis of congenital CMV following hearing loss identified later in infancy is difficult.

C. Imaging

Radiologic studies show microcephaly, periventricular calcifications, and ventricular dilation. Clinical guidelines recommend all infants receive a cranial ultrasound (CUS), followed by an MRI. MRI severity score is a better predictor of adverse neurologic sequelae than the presence of symptoms at birth. Long bone radiographs may show the "celery stalk" pattern characteristic of congenital viral infections. Interstitial pneumonia may be present.

▶ Differential Diagnosis

Congenital CMV infection should be considered in any seriously ill newborn after birth, especially once bacterial sepsis, metabolic disease, intracranial bleeding, and cardiac disease have been excluded. Other congenital infections to be considered in the differential diagnosis include toxoplasmosis (diffuse calcification of the CNS, specific type of retinitis, macrocephaly, serology), rubella (specific retinitis, cardiac lesions, eye abnormalities, serology), enteroviral infections (season, maternal illness, severe hepatitis), herpes simplex (skin lesions, severe hepatitis, pneumonitis), Zika virus (exposure, microcephaly), and syphilis (skin lesions, bone involvement, maternal and infant serology).

▶ Prevention & Treatment

Most children with symptoms at birth have significant neurologic, intellectual, visual, or auditory impairment. Interventions for congenital CMV consist of nonspecific standard management of sequelae (eg, antiepileptic drugs for seizures, physical therapy for gross motor delays). Transfusions are rarely required for anemia and thrombocytopenia. Intravenous ganciclovir has been recommended for children with severe, life- or sight-threatening disease, or if end-organ disease recurs or progresses. Guidelines recommend 6-month therapy with valganciclovir of infants with moderate-to-severe symptomatic CMV. The possible benefits of therapy must be balanced with the risks of adverse events, particularly neutropenia. Antiviral resistance is rarely a problem. Therapy must be started within the first month of life, as no proven benefit has been demonstrated after that age, or in neonates with asymptomatic CMV infection. Valganciclovir treatment trials are ongoing for children with asymptomatic infection and hearing loss at birth.

Recent developments in the diagnosis of primary CMV infection during pregnancy using anti-CMV IgM and low-avidity IgG assays followed by quantitative CMV PCR testing of the amniotic fluid at 20–24 weeks gestation have made possible the diagnosis of congenital CMV infection before birth. Many pregnant women elect to terminate gestation under these circumstances. Passive immunoprophylaxis with hyperimmune CMV IgG did not prevent development of congenital disease in a randomized placebo-controlled trial. Several candidate vaccines against CMV are currently in development.

2. Perinatal Cytomegalovirus Infection

CMV infection can be acquired from birth canal secretions or shortly after birth from breast milk. In some socioeconomic groups, 10%–20% of infants are infected at birth and excrete CMV for many months. Infection can also be acquired in the postnatal period from unscreened transfused blood products.

▶ Clinical Findings

A. Symptoms and Signs

Ninety percent of immunocompetent infants infected by their mothers at birth develop subclinical illness (ie, virus excretion only) or a minor illness within 1–3 months. The remainder develops an illness lasting several weeks characterized by hepatosplenomegaly, lymphadenopathy, and interstitial pneumonitis in various combinations. Very low birth weight and premature infants are at greater risk for severe disease. If they are born to CMV-negative mothers and subsequently receive CMV-containing blood or breast milk, they may develop severe infection and pneumonia after a 2- to 6-week incubation period.

B. Laboratory Findings

Lymphocytosis, atypical lymphocytes, anemia, and thrombocytopenia may be present, especially in premature infants. Liver function is abnormal. CMV is readily isolated from urine and saliva. Secretions obtained at bronchoscopy contain CMV and epithelial cells bearing CMV antigens. Serum levels of CMV antibody rise significantly.

C. Imaging

Chest radiographs may show a diffuse interstitial pneumonitis in severely affected infants.

▶ Differential Diagnosis

CMV infection should be considered as a cause of any prolonged illness in early infancy, especially if hepatosplenomegaly, lymphadenopathy, or atypical lymphocytosis is present. This must be distinguished from granulomatous or malignant diseases and from congenital infections (syphilis, toxoplasmosis, hepatitis B, HIV) not previously diagnosed. Other viruses (Epstein-Barr virus [EBV], HIV, adenovirus) can cause this syndrome. CMV is a recognized cause of viral pneumonia in this age group. Because asymptomatic CMV excretion is common in early infancy, care must be taken to establish the diagnosis and to rule out concomitant pathogens such as *Chlamydia* and RSV. Severe CMV infection in early infancy may indicate that the child has a congenital or acquired immune deficiency.

▶ Prevention & Treatment

The self-limited disease of normal infants requires no therapy. Severe pneumonitis in premature infants requires oxygen administration and often intubation. Very ill infants should receive ganciclovir. CMV infection acquired by transfusion can be prevented by excluding CMV-seropositive blood donors. Milk donors should also be screened for prior CMV infection. A common practice of freezing the milk prior to administration was shown to lack preventive effectiveness. It is likely that high-risk infants receiving large doses of IVIG for other reasons will be protected against severe CMV disease.

3. Cytomegalovirus Infection Acquired in Childhood & Adolescence

Young children are readily infected by playmates, especially because CMV continues to be excreted in saliva and urine for many months after infection. The cumulative annual incidence of CMV excretion by children in day care centers exceeds 75%. In fact, young children in a family are often the source of primary CMV infection of their mothers during subsequent pregnancies. An additional peak of CMV infection takes place when adolescents become sexually active. Sporadic acquisition of CMV occurs after blood transfusion and transplantation.

▶ Clinical Findings

A. Symptoms and Signs

Most young children who acquire CMV are asymptomatic or have a minor febrile illness, occasionally with adenopathy. They provide an important reservoir of virus shedders that facilitates spread of CMV. Occasionally a child may have prolonged fever with hepatosplenomegaly and adenopathy. Older children and adults, many of whom are infected during sexual activity, are more likely to be symptomatic and can present with a syndrome that mimics the infectious mononucleosis syndrome that follows EBV infection (1–2 weeks of fever, malaise, anorexia, splenomegaly, mild hepatitis, and some adenopathy; see the next section). This syndrome can also occur 2–4 weeks after transfusion of CMV-infected blood.

B. Laboratory Findings

In the CMV mononucleosis syndrome, lymphocytosis and atypical lymphocytes are common, as is a mild rise in aminotransferase levels. CMV is present in saliva and urine; CMV DNA can be uniformly detected in plasma or blood.

▶ Differential Diagnosis

In older children, CMV infection should be included as a possible cause of fever of unknown origin, especially when lymphocytosis and atypical lymphocytes are present. CMV infection is distinguished from EBV infection by the absence of pharyngitis, the relatively minor adenopathy, and the absence of serologic evidence of acute EBV infection. Mononucleosis syndromes also are caused by *Toxoplasma gondii*, rubella virus, adenovirus, hepatitis A virus, and HIV.

▶ Prevention

Screening of transfused blood or filtering blood (thus removing CMV-containing white blood cells) prevents cases related to this source.

4. Cytomegalovirus Infection in Immunocompromised Children

In addition to symptoms experienced during primary infection, immunocompromised hosts develop symptoms with reinfection or reactivation of latent CMV. This is clearly seen in children with acquired immunodeficiency syndrome (AIDS), after transplantation, or with congenital immunodeficiencies. However, in most immunocompromised patients, primary infection is more likely to cause severe symptoms than is reactivation or reinfection. The severity of the resulting disease is generally proportionate to the degree of immunosuppression.

▶ Clinical Findings

A. Symptoms and Signs

A mild febrile illness with myalgia, malaise, and arthralgia may occur, especially with reactivation disease. Severe disease often includes subacute onset of dyspnea and cyanosis as manifestations of interstitial pneumonitis. Auscultation reveals only coarse breath sounds and scattered rales. A rapid respiratory rate may precede clinical or radiographic evidence of pneumonia. Hepatitis without jaundice and hepatomegaly are common. Diarrhea, which can be severe, occurs with CMV colitis, and CMV can cause esophagitis with symptoms of odynophagia or dysphagia. These enteropathies are most common in AIDS, as is the presence of a retinitis that often progresses to blindness, encephalitis, and polyradiculitis.

B. Laboratory Findings

Neutropenia and thrombocytopenia are common. Atypical lymphocytosis is infrequent. Serum aminotransferase levels are often elevated. The stools may contain occult blood if enteropathy is present. CMV is readily isolated from saliva, urine, buffy coat, and bronchial secretions. Results are available in 48 hours. Interpretation of positive cultures is made difficult by asymptomatic shedding of CMV in saliva and urine in many immunocompromised patients. CMV disease correlates more closely with the presence of CMV in the blood or lung lavage fluid. Monitoring for the appearance of CMV DNA in plasma or CMV antigen in blood mononuclear cells is used as a guide to early antiviral ("preemptive") therapy.

C. Imaging

Bilateral interstitial pneumonitis may be present on chest radiographs.

▶ Differential Diagnosis

The initial febrile illness must be distinguished from treatable bacterial or fungal infection. Similarly, the pulmonary disease must be distinguished from intrapulmonary hemorrhage; drug-induced or radiation pneumonitis; pulmonary edema; and bacterial, fungal, parasitic, or other viral infections. CMV infection causes bilateral and interstitial abnormalities on chest radiographs, cough is nonproductive, chest pain is absent, and the patient is not usually toxic. *Pneumocystis jirovecii* infection may have a similar presentation. These patients may have polymicrobial disease. It is suspected that bacterial and fungal infections are enhanced by the neutropenia that can accompany CMV infection. Infection of the gastrointestinal tract is diagnosed by endoscopy. This will exclude candidal, adenoviral, and herpes simplex infections and allows tissue confirmation of CMV-induced mucosal ulcerations.

▶ Prevention & Treatment

Blood donors should be screened to exclude those with prior CMV infection, or blood should be filtered. Ideally, seronegative transplant recipients should receive organs from seronegative donors. Severe symptoms, most commonly pneumonitis, often respond to early therapy with intravenous ganciclovir for 14–21 days. Neutropenia is a frequent side effect of this therapy. Foscarnet and cidofovir are alternative therapeutic agents recommended for patients with

ganciclovir-resistant virus. Prophylactic use of oral or intravenous ganciclovir or foscarnet may prevent CMV infections in organ transplant recipients. Preemptive therapy can be used in transplant recipients by monitoring CMV in blood by PCR and instituting therapy when the results reach a certain threshold regardless of clinical signs or symptoms.

Pesch MH, Schleiss MR: Emerging concepts in congenital cytomegalovirus. Pediatrics 2022;150(2):e2021055896. doi: 10.1542/peds.2021-055896 [PMID: 35909155].
Ross SA, Kimberlin D: Clinical outcome and the role of antivirals in congenital cytomegalovirus infection. Antiviral Res 2021;5:105083 [PMID: 33964331].

EPSTEIN-BARR VIRUS (EBV)

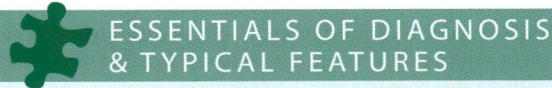

ESSENTIALS OF DIAGNOSIS & TYPICAL FEATURES

▶ Glandular fever (prolonged fever, exudative pharyngitis, enlarged lymph nodes).

▶ Hepatosplenomegaly.

▶ Atypical lymphocytosis.

▶ Heterophil antibodies.

▶ General Considerations

Epstein-Barr virus (EBV) is the most ubiquitous of human viruses, infecting at least 90% of adults worldwide. Infectious mononucleosis is the most characteristic syndrome produced by EBV infection. Young, infected children have either no symptoms or a mild nonspecific febrile illness. As the age of the host increases, EBV infection is more likely to produce the typical mononucleosis syndrome reaching 20%–25% of infected adolescents and 70% of university students. EBV is acquired by close contact from asymptomatic carriers (15%–20% of whom excrete the virus in saliva on any given day) and from recently ill patients, who excrete virus for many months. Young children are infected most via the oral route from saliva, but EBV can also spread through blood and semen during sexual contact, blood transfusions, and organ transplantations. EBV seroconversion peaks in children between 2 and 4 years and 14 and 18 years, and it increases with age.

▶ Clinical Findings

A. Symptoms and Signs

After an incubation period of 32–49 days, a 2- to 3-day prodrome of malaise and anorexia yields, abruptly or insidiously, to a febrile illness with temperatures exceeding 39°C. The major complaint is pharyngitis, which is often

(50%) exudative with transient petechiae. Lymph nodes are enlarged, firm, and mildly tender. Any area may be affected, but posterior and anterior cervical nodes are almost always enlarged. Splenomegaly is present in 50%–75% of patients. Hepatomegaly is common (30%), and the liver is frequently tender. Five percent of patients have a rash, which can be macular, scarlatiniform, or urticarial. Rash is almost universal in patients taking penicillin or ampicillin. Soft palate petechiae and eyelid edema are also observed. Median duration of acute illness is 18 days (range, 3–54 days).

B. Laboratory Findings

1. Peripheral blood—Leukopenia may occur early, but an atypical lymphocytosis (comprising over 10% of the total leukocytes at some time in the illness) is most notable. Absolute lymphocyte count less than 4000 mm³ has a 99% negative predictive value for infectious mononucleosis. Hematologic changes may not be seen until the third week of illness and may be entirely absent in some EBV syndromes (eg, neurologic).

2. Heterophile antibodies—These nonspecific antibodies appear in over 90% of older patients with mononucleosis, but in fewer than 50% of children younger than age 5 years. They may not be detectable until the second week of illness and may persist for up to 12 months after recovery. Rapid screening tests (slide agglutination) are usually positive if the titer is significant; a positive result strongly suggests but does not prove EBV infection.

3. Anti-EBV antibodies—Specific antibody titers have a 97% sensitivity and 94% specificity for diagnosis and are especially useful in children younger than 5 years. Acute EBV infection is established by detecting IgM antibody to the viral capsid antigen (VCA) or by detecting a fourfold or greater change of IgG anti-VCA titers (in normal hosts, IgG antibody peaks by the time symptoms appear; in immunocompromised hosts, the tempo of antibody production may be delayed). The absence of anti-EBV nuclear antigen (EBNA) antibodies, which are typically first detected at least 4 weeks after the start of symptoms, may also be used to diagnose acute infection in immunocompetent hosts. However, immunocompromised hosts may fail to develop anti-EBNA antibodies.

4. EBV PCR—EBV PCR is less useful than serology for diagnosis of acute EBV infection in immunocompetent hosts. Site-specific detection of EBV DNA is the method of choice for the diagnosis of CNS and ocular infections. Quantitative EBV PCR in peripheral blood mononuclear cells has been used to diagnose EBV-related lymphoproliferative disorders in transplant patients.

▶ Differential Diagnosis

Enlargement of only the anterior cervical lymph nodes, severe pharyngitis, neutrophilic leukocytosis, and the absence of splenomegaly suggest bacterial infection. Although a child with a positive throat culture result for *Streptococcus pyogenes* usually requires therapy, up to 10% of children with mononucleosis are asymptomatic streptococcal carriers. In this group, penicillin therapy is unnecessary and often causes a rash. Severe primary herpes simplex pharyngitis, occurring in adolescence, may also mimic infectious mononucleosis, although anterior mouth ulcerations should suggest the correct diagnosis. CMV mononucleosis is a close mimic except for minimal pharyngitis and less adenopathy; it is much less common. Serologic tests for EBV and CMV should clarify the correct diagnosis. The acute initial manifestation of HIV infection can be a mononucleosis-like syndrome. Adenoviruses are another cause of severe, often exudative pharyngitis. EBV infection should be considered in the differential diagnosis of any perplexing prolonged febrile illness. Similar illnesses that produce atypical lymphocytosis include rubella (pharyngitis not prominent, shorter illness, less adenopathy and splenomegaly), adenovirus (upper respiratory symptoms and cough, conjunctivitis, less adenopathy, fewer atypical lymphocytes), hepatitis A or B (more severe liver function abnormalities, no pharyngitis, no lymphadenopathy), and toxoplasmosis (negative heterophil test, less pharyngitis). Serum sickness-like drug reactions and leukemia (smear morphology is important) may be confused with infectious mononucleosis.

▶ Complications

Serious complications during the acute primary EBV infection occur in at least 1%. Complications include airway obstruction due to oropharyngeal inflammation, meningoencephalitis, hemolytic anemia, and thrombocytopenia. Splenic rupture is rare and usually follows significant trauma. Neurologic involvement can include aseptic meningitis, encephalitis, isolated neuropathy such as Bell palsy, and Guillain-Barré syndrome. Any of these may appear prior to or in the absence of the more typical signs and symptoms of infectious mononucleosis. Rare complications include myocarditis, pericarditis, and atypical pneumonia. Recurrence or persistence of acute EBV-associated symptoms for 6 months or longer characterizes chronic active EBV. This uncommon presentation is due to continuous viral replication and warrants specific antiviral therapy. Rarely EBV infection becomes a progressive lymphoproliferative disorder characterized by persistent fever, multiple organ involvement, neutropenia, or pancytopenia, and agammaglobulinemia. Hemophagocytosis is often present in the bone marrow. An X-linked genetic defect in immune response has been inferred for some patients (Duncan syndrome, X-linked lymphoproliferative disorder). Children with other congenital immunodeficiencies or chemotherapy-induced immunosuppression can also develop progressive EBV infection, EBV-associated lymphoproliferative disorder, lymphoma, and other malignancies.

Treatment & Prognosis

Bed rest may be necessary in severe cases. Acetaminophen controls high fever. Potential airway obstruction due to swollen pharyngeal lymphoid tissue responds rapidly to systemic corticosteroids. Corticosteroids may also be given for hematologic and neurologic complications, although no controlled trials have proven their efficacy in these conditions. Fever and pharyngitis disappear spontaneously by 10–14 days. Adenopathy and splenomegaly can persist several weeks longer. Some patients complain of fatigue, malaise, or lack of well-being for several months. Although corticosteroids may shorten the duration of illness by 12 hours, there is no evidence that its use decreases the course or severity of the disease. Patients may return to contact sports after 4 weeks if they have had resolution of symptoms and no splenomegaly. Acyclovir, valacyclovir, penciclovir, ganciclovir, and foscarnet are active against EBV and are indicated in the treatment of chronic active EBV. Antiviral therapy in the immunocompetent child has not proven efficacious.

Management of EBV-related lymphoproliferative disorders relies primarily on decreasing the immunosuppression whenever possible. Adjunctive therapy with acyclovir, ganciclovir, or another antiviral active against EBV as well as γ globulin has been used without scientific evidence of efficacy.

Dunmire SK, Verghese PS, Balfour HH Jr: Primary Epstein-Barr virus infection. J Clin Virol 2018; 102:84–92 [PMID: 29525635].
Marshall-Andon T, Heinz P: How to use … the Monospot and other heterophile antibody tests. Arch Dis Child Educ Pract Ed 2017;102(4):188–193 [PMID: 28130396].

VIRAL INFECTIONS SPREAD BY INSECT VECTORS

In the United States, mosquitoes are the most common insect vectors that spread viral infections (Table 40–4). Consequently, these infections—and others that are spread by ticks—tend to occur as summer-fall epidemics that coincide with the seasonal breeding and feeding habits of the vector, and the etiologic agent varies by region (see CDC references for maps). Other insect-borne viral infections are seen in international travelers. Thus, a careful travel and exposure history is critical for correct diagnostic workup.

ENCEPHALITIS

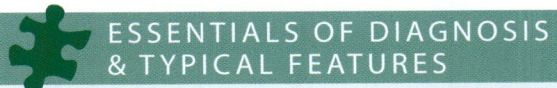

ESSENTIALS OF DIAGNOSIS & TYPICAL FEATURES

► Seasonality: summer and fall.
► Fever and headache.

► Change in mental status and/or behavior, with or without focal neurologic deficits.
► Mononuclear cell pleocytosis, elevated protein level, and normal glucose level.

Encephalitis is a common severe manifestation of many infections spread by insects (see Table 40–4). With many viral pathogens, the infection is often subclinical, or includes mild CNS disease such as meningitis. These infections have some distinguishing features in terms of subclinical infection rate, unique neurologic syndromes, associated systemic symptoms, and prognosis. The diagnosis is generally made clinically during recognized outbreaks and is confirmed by virus-specific serology or PCR. Prevention consists of control of mosquito vectors and precautions with proper clothing and insect repellents to minimize mosquito and tick bites. It is essential before making the diagnosis of arboviral encephalitis, which is not treatable, to exclude herpes encephalitis, which warrants specific antiviral therapy. Delay in administering this therapy may have dire consequences.

West Nile Virus Encephalitis

This flavivirus, primarily transmitted by *Culex* mosquitos, is the most important arbovirus infection in the United States. In 2003, there were more than 10,000 clinically apparent infections, more than 2900 nervous system infections, and 265 deaths in 47 states. In 2012, there was a resurgence to more than 5,000 reported cases, of which approximately half were neuroinvasive; 240 were fatal. Other years typically have 1,500–3,000 reported cases. The reservoir of West Nile virus includes more than 160 species of birds whose migration explains the extent of endemic disease. Epidemics occur in summer-fall. Approximately 20% of infected individuals develop West Nile fever, characterized by fever, headache, retro-orbital pain, nausea, vomiting, lymphadenopathy, and a maculopapular rash (20%–50%). Less than 1% of infected patients develop meningitis or encephalitis, but 10% of these cases are fatal. The major risk factors for severe disease are age older than 50 years and immune compromise. Symptomatic children usually manifest with West Nile fever and less than one-third will develop neuroinvasive disease, most likely limited to meningitis. Neurologic manifestations are most often those found with other meningoencephalitides, but some distinguishing features include polio-like acute flaccid paralysis, movement disorders (Parkinsonism, tremor, and myoclonus), brainstem symptoms, polyneuropathy, and optic neuritis. Muscle weakness, facial palsy, and hyporeflexia are common (20%). Recovery is slow and significant sequelae may persist in some severely affected patients. Diagnosis is best made by detecting IgM antibody (enzyme immunoassay) to the virus in CSF. This will be present by 5–6 days (95%) after onset. PCR is a specific diagnostic tool

Table 40–4. Some insect-borne viral diseases occurring in the United States or in returning US travelers.

Disease	Natural Reservoir (Vector)	Geographic Distribution	Incubation Period	Clinical Presentations	Laboratory Findings	Complications, Sequelae	Diagnosis, Therapy, Comments
Flaviviruses							
St. Louis encephalitis (SLE)	Birds (Culex mosquitoes)	Southern Canada, central and southern United States, Texas, Caribbean, South America	2–5 days (up to 3 wk)	Abrupt onset of fever, chills, headache, nausea, vomiting; may develop generalized weakness, seizures, coma, ataxia, cranial nerve palsies. Aseptic meningitis is common in children.	Modest leukocytosis, neutrophilia, elevated liver enzymes. CSF: 100–200 WBCs/μL; PMNs predominate early.	Mortality rate 2%–5% at age < 5 or > 50 y. Neurologic sequelae in 1%–20%.	~ 15 cases/y, < 2% symptomatic. (worse in elderly.) Therapy: supportive. Diagnosis: serology. Specific antibody often present within 5 days.
Dengue	Humans (Aedes mosquitoes) and nonhuman primates	Asia, Africa, Central and South America, Caribbean; observed in Texas/Mexico border area and Florida	4–7 days (range, 3–14 days)	Only 25% symptomatic. Fever, headache, myalgia, joint and bone pain, retroocular pain, nausea and vomiting; maculopapular or petechial rash in 50%, sparing palms and soles. Encephalitis in 5%–10% of children.	Leukopenia, thrombocytopenia. CSF: 100–500 mononuclear cells/μL if neurologic signs are present.	Hemorrhagic fever, shock syndrome, prolonged weakness, encephalitis.	High infection rate in endemic areas. Therapy: supportive. Diagnosis: RT-PCR or NS1 antigen first 5 days or IgM-EIA antibody by day 5. IgM and IgG may cross-react with other flaviviruses (Zika) so should be confirmed with neutralization testing. Vaccines available in endemic settings.
West Nile	Birds (Culex mosquitoes); small mammals	North Africa, Middle East, parts of Asia, Europe, continental United States	2–14 days	Abrupt onset of fever, headache, sore throat, myalgia, retroocular pain, conjunctivitis; 20%–50% with rash; adenopathy. Meningitis alone is most common in children. Encephalitis may be accompanied by muscle weakness, flaccid paralysis, or movement disorders.	Mild leukocytosis; 10%–15% lymphopenic or thrombocytopenic; CSF pleocytosis with < 500 cells; may be neutrophils early.	Mortality rate 10%, of those with CNS symptoms, but rare in children; weakness and myalgia may persist for an extended period.	Most important mosquito-borne encephalitis in the United States. (~ 150 cases reported each year.) Diagnosis: IgM-EIA serology; cross-reacts with St. Louis encephalitis; positive by 5–6 days after onset of CNS symptoms. Diagnosis by PCR is less sensitive. Therapy: supportive.
Japanese encephalitis	Birds, large mammals; reptiles (Culex mosquitos)	SE Asia; Australia	5–14 days	Onset with fever, cough, coryza, headache. Aseptic meningitis is common in children.	CSF: 10–100 lymphocytes/μL; atypical lymphocytes may be present; protein may reach 200 mg/dL.	Seizures are common in children; when encephalitis occurs, it can result in lasting motor, learning, and behavioral abnormalities.	Vaccination is an important consideration for children visiting or residing in endemic areas. IgM and IgG may cross-react with other flaviviruses (dengue, Zika), so should be confirmed with neutralization.

Disease	Reservoir/Transmission	Distribution	Incubation	Clinical Features	Laboratory Findings	Complications/Severe Disease	Diagnosis/Therapy
Zika	Humans (*Aedes* mosquitoes)	Asia, Africa, Central and South America, Caribbean; cases in Texas border area and Florida	3–7 days	Only 25% symptomatic. Maculopapular rash, fever, conjunctivitis, arthralgia. Congenital Zika syndrome with vertical transmission during pregnancy	Leukopenia, thrombocytopenia, elevated liver transaminases	Congenital Zika syndrome with many sequelae (eg, microcephaly, seizures, arthrogryposis, hearing and vision problems). Increased risk for Guillain Barré syndrome	High infection rate during epidemics. Therapy: supportive. Diagnosis: RT-PCR or NS1 antigen first 14 days and/or IgM-EIA antibody by day 5. IgM and IgG may cross-react with other flaviviruses (dengue, Japanese encephalitis), so should be confirmed with neutralization.
Powassan	Ticks, rodents	Northeast and upper midwestern United States; Russia, Canada	1–4 weeks	Fever, headache weakness, vomiting. Severe disease may include confusion, dysphasia, seizures, difficulty walking.	CSF: lymphocytic pleocytosis, normal or elevated protein, normal glucose	Severe disease: mortality rate of 10%; 50% with neurologic sequelae (hemiparalysis, memory problems, headaches)	IgM and neutralizing antibodies in serum and CSF. PCR or antigen testing of serum CSF, or tissue if early in the disease course.
Alpha toga viruses							
Chikungunya	Humans (*Aedes* mosquitoes)	Asia, Africa, Central and South America, Caribbean	3–7 days (range, 1–14 days)	Symptomatic in > 50%. Fever, headache, myalgia, conjunctivitis; arthralgia and/or arthritis in multiple joints, symmetric, mainly hands and feet; maculopapular rash in 30%–60%.	Leukopenia, thrombocytopenia, elevated creatinine and liver transaminases	Severe persistent arthralgia in adolescents and adults. Encephalitis, seizures, and bleeding in infants with risk of neurodevelopmental sequelae.	Therapy: supportive. Use NSAID for arthritis after dengue ruled out. Diagnosis: RT-PCR in first 7 days or IgM-EIA antibody after day 5 at CDC.
Eastern equine encephalitis	Birds (*Aedes, Coquillettidia, and Culex* mosquitoes)	Eastern seaboard United States, Caribbean, South America	2–5 days	Similar to that of St. Louis encephalitis, but more severe. Progresses rapidly in one-third to coma and death.	Leukocytosis with neutrophilia. CSF: 500–2000 WBCs/μL; PMNs predominate early.	Mortality rate 20%–50%; neurologic 50% of children.	< 10 cases/y usually (38 in 2019). Only 3%–10% of cases are symptomatic, but sequelae common in symptomatic young children. Therapy: supportive. Diagnosis: serology often positive in the first week. Equine deaths may signal an outbreak.

(Continued)

Table 40–4. Some insect-borne viral diseases occurring in the United States or in returning US travelers. (*Continued*)

Disease	Natural Reservoir (Vector)	Geographic Distribution	Incubation Period	Clinical Presentations	Laboratory Findings	Complications, Sequelae	Diagnosis, Therapy, Comments
Western equine encephalitis	Birds (mostly *Culex* mosquitoes)	Canada, Mexico, and United States west of Mississippi River	2–5 days	Similar to that of St. Louis encephalitis. Most infections are subclinical.	Variable white counts. CSF: 10–300 WBCs/μL.	Permanent brain damage, 10% overall; most severe in older adults.	No reported cases in the United States in recent years. Case/infection is 1:1000 for older adults and 1:1 for infants. Equine illness precedes human outbreaks. Diagnosis: IgM antibody in the first week. Therapy: supportive.
Venezuelan equine encephalitis	Horses (10 species of mosquitoes)	South and Central America, Texas	1–6 days	Similar to that of St. Louis encephalitis.	Lymphopenia, mild thrombocytopenia, abnormal liver function tests. CSF: 50–200 mononuclear cells/μL.	Severe disease more common in infants; 20% fatality rate for encephalitis.	Most infections do not cause encephalitis. No cases in the United States in recent years. Vaccination of horses will stop epidemic. Therapy: supportive. Diagnosis: IgM antibody (EIA).
Bunyavirus							
California encephalitis serogroup (LaCrosse, Jamestown Canyon, California)	Chipmunks and other small mammals (*Aedes* mosquitoes)	Northern and mid-central United States, southern Canada	3–7 days	Symptoms are similar to those of St. Louis encephalitis; sore throat and respiratory symptoms are common; focal neurologic signs in up to 25%. Seizures prominent. Prepubertal children are most likely to have severe disease. Can mimic herpes simplex encephalitis.	Variable white counts. CSF: 30–200 up to 600 WBCs/μL; variable PMNs; protein often normal.	Mortality rate < 2%. Seizures may occur during acute illness.	~ 75 cases/y in the United States, 5% symptomatic. > 10% with sequelae. Therapy: supportive. Diagnosis: serology. Up to 90% have specific IgM antibody in the first week; 25% of population in certain regions has IgG antibody.
Coltivirus							
Colorado tick fever	Small mammals (*Dermacentor andersoni* or wood tick)	Rocky Mountain region of United States and Canada	3–4 days (range, 2–14 days)	Fever, chills, myalgia, conjunctivitis, headache, retro-orbital pain; rash in < 10%. No respiratory symptoms. Biphasic fever in 50%.	Leukopenia (maximum at 4–6 days), mild thrombocytopenia.	Rare encephalitis, coagulopathy.	Patient may have no known tick bite. Acute illness lasts 7–10 days; prolonged fatigue in adults. Therapy: supportive. Diagnosis: serology, direct FA staining of red cells for viral antigen, PCR.

CNS, central nervous system; CSF, cerebrospinal fluid; EIA, enzyme immunoassay; FA, fluorescent antibody; NSAID, nonsteroidal anti-inflammatory drug; PCR, polymerase chain reaction; PMN, polymorphonuclear neutrophil; WBC, white blood cell.

but is less sensitive than antibody detection. Antibody rise in serum can also be used for diagnosis.

Treatment is supportive, although various antivirals and specific immunoglobulins are being studied. The infection is not spread between contacts, but can be spread by donated organs, blood, breast milk, and transplacental.

CDC: West Nile Virus Resources: https://www.cdc.gov/westnile/index.html.

Colpitts TM, Conway MJ, Montgomery RR, Fikrig E: West Nile virus: biology, transmission, and human infection. Clin Micro Rev 2012;25(4):635 [PMID: 20121004].

Gaensbauer JT, Lindsey NP, Messacar K, Staples JE, Fischer M: Neuroinvasive arboviral disease in the United States: 2003 to 2012. Pediatrics 2014;134(3):e642–e650 [PMID: 25113294].

DENGUE

ESSENTIALS OF DIAGNOSIS & TYPICAL FEATURES

▶ Travel or residence in an endemic area.

▶ First infection (first episode) is asymptomatic or may result in fever, rash, retro-orbital pain, severe myalgia, and/or arthralgia.

▶ Second infection with a different dengue serotype is more likely to result in severe dengue, which includes symptoms of plasma leakage, and may progress to dengue hemorrhagic fever (thrombocytopenia, bleeding) and dengue shock syndrome.

Dengue is one of the most common causes of fever in returning travelers and occurs throughout Latin America, the Caribbean, Southeast Asia, Oceania, and Africa; sporadic outbreaks occur occasionally in the southern United States, and dengue is hyperendemic (≥ 2 serotypes) in Puerto Rico. The spread of dengue requires the *Aedes* mosquito (present in the southern United States), which transmits virus from a reservoir of viremic humans in endemic areas. Most symptomatic patients have mild disease, especially young children, who may have a nonspecific fever and rash. Severity is a function of age, and prior infection with other serotypes of dengue virus significantly increases the risk for severe complications.

▶ Clinical Findings

A. Symptoms and Signs

Dengue fever begins abruptly 4–7 days after transmission (range, 3–14 days) with fever, chills, severe retro-orbital pain, severe muscle and joint pain ("breakbone fever"), nausea, and vomiting. Erythema of the face and torso may occur early.

After 3–4 days, a centrifugal maculopapular rash appears in half of the patients described as "islands of white in a sea of red." The rash can become petechial, and mild hemorrhagic signs (epistaxis, gingival bleeding, microscopic blood in stool or urine) may be noted. The illness lasts 3–7 days, although rarely fever may reappear for several additional days. Since there are four serotypes of dengue virus, multiple sequential infections can occur.

B. Laboratory Findings

In most symptomatic cases, mild leukopenia and thrombocytopenia occur. Liver transaminases are usually normal. Diagnosis during acute infection (≤ 5 days of symptoms) is usually made by detection of viral antigenemia (NS1 antigen) or RT-PCR (80%–90% sensitive, 95% specific). After 5 days, dengue may be diagnosed by detection of IgM-specific antibodies (70%–80% sensitive by day 6 and increases thereafter) or a rise in type-specific antibody during convalescent testing (10–14 days later). Any antibody test may cross-react with other flaviviruses (Zika). Neutralizing antibodies against dengue virus are the most accurate serologic method, but they are resource- and time-intensive, and they may also cross-react with other flaviviruses (eg, Zika). Therefore, early testing by RT-PCR or NS1 antigen is preferable.

▶ Differential Diagnosis

This diagnosis should be considered for any traveler to an endemic area who has symptoms suggestive of a systemic viral illness, although less than 1 in 1,000 travelers to these areas develops dengue. Often the areas visited have other endogenous pathogens circulating (eg, malaria, typhoid fever, leptospirosis, rickettsial diseases, other endemic alphaviruses and flaviviruses, and measles). Chikungunya has a similar geographic distribution and presents with fever and rash, but is more strongly associated with arthralgia/arthritis, which may persist for weeks to months. Zika is also clinically indistinguishable from dengue, EBV, influenza, enteroviruses, and acute HIV infection may produce a similar illness. Dengue is not associated with sore throat or cough. An illness that starts 2 weeks after the trip ends or that lasts longer than 2 weeks is probably not dengue.

▶ Complications

More common in endemic areas is the appearance of severe dengue, which typically occurs at the time of defervescence (day 3–7) and may include respiratory distress, circulatory shock (dengue septic shock), severe bleeding (dengue hemorrhagic fever), and end-organ damage. Severe dengue typically occurs during a second dengue episode because of preexisting, non-neutralizing antibodies enhancing virus uptake into cells and leading to increased viremia and cytokine response (antibody-dependent enhancement). Warning signs for severe dengue that may be seen during the acute febrile phase of illness include abdominal pain, persistent vomiting, clinical fluid accumulation (eg, pleural effusion, ascites), mucosal bleeding, altered mental status, hepatomegaly, and hemoconcentration (hematocrit > 20% higher than baseline) with concurrent thrombocytopenia (< 100,000 cells/μL).

Prevention

Prevention of dengue fever involves avoiding high-risk areas and using conventional mosquito avoidance measures. The *Aedes* mosquito vector is a daytime feeder. Several dengue vaccines are under development, and one licensed vaccine (CYD-TDV) demonstrated 60% efficacy in clinical trials, though it is only available for individuals with known seropositivity, given its association with increased risk of subsequent severe dengue disease in children without prior immunity. No vaccines are currently recommended for travelers and other vaccines are currently in clinical trials, though one other vaccine is now licensed outside of the United States (TAK-003).

Treatment

Dengue fever is treated by oral rehydration and antipyretics, avoiding nonsteroidal anti-inflammatory agents that affect platelet function. Recovery is complete without sequelae. The hemorrhagic syndrome and shock require prompt fluid therapy with plasma expanders and isotonic saline along with close ICU monitoring.

Guzman MG, Harris E: Dengue. Lancet 2015;385(9966):453–465 [PMID: 25230594].

Simmons CP, Farrar JJ, van Vinh Chau N, Wills B: Dengue. N Engl J Med 2012;366(15):14–23 [PMID: 22494122].

CHIKUNGUNYA

ESSENTIALS OF DIAGNOSIS & TYPICAL FEATURES

► Same mosquito vector and geographic distribution as dengue and Zika viruses.

► Acute symptoms are similar to dengue and Zika (fever, rash, headache), but arthralgia and arthritis can be more severe and persistent.

► Perinatal can be severe and include bleeding and/or neurological disease, resulting in neurodevelopmental sequelae.

Chikungunya has been endemic in Africa and Asia for decades but emerged in the Americas for the first time in 2013–2014, leading to a widespread epidemic that included transmission within the southern United States. Chikungunya is transmitted by *Aedes* mosquitos and has a similar geographic distribution and acute clinical presentation to dengue and Zika.

Clinical Findings

A. Symptoms and Signs

After a 3–7-day incubation period (maximum 14 days), high-grade fever appears suddenly and lasts 3–5 days. Symptoms may include headache (15%) and a diffuse maculopapular rash (30%–60%). Myalgia, arthralgia, and arthritis are more common in adults (87%–99%) than in children (30%–50%) and can be debilitating. Young children and infants, especially those perinatally infected, are more likely to have neurologic symptoms (seizure, encephalitis), bleeding, and multiorgan failure.

B. Laboratory Findings

Leukopenia, thrombocytopenia, and elevated transaminases may be seen, especially in young infants. Elevated creatinine is also observed. In the first 5–7 days of infection, RT-PCR is the preferred diagnostic test. Chikungunya IgM antibodies appear around day 5, lasting for 1–3 months and sometimes longer in individuals with persistent joint disease; IgG antibodies appear by 2 weeks and persist for years. They do not cross-react with flaviviruses but may with other alphaviruses.

Differential Diagnosis

Chikungunya is clinically indistinguishable from dengue and Zika acutely, which all demonstrate similar geographic distribution. Chikungunya is less likely than dengue to result in bleeding and shock (except in young infants). Other infections with similar clinical presentations include parvovirus, rubella, measles, leptospirosis, malaria, typhoid, *Rickettsia*, and influenza. A febrile illness that starts 2 weeks after the trip ends or that lasts longer than 2 weeks is probably not chikungunya.

Complications

Chronic musculoskeletal symptoms (arthritis, arthralgia, and tenosynovitis), though less common in children, may persist or relapse for months or even years following infection and can be severely debilitating. Individuals with encephalitis, which are typically neonates or young infants, may have long-term neurodevelopmental sequelae including hearing and vision impairment as well as cerebral disorders (eg, attention deficit hyperactivity disorder).

Prevention & Treatment

Prevention includes avoiding high-risk areas and using conventional mosquito avoidance measures. Treatment involves supportive care, including fluids and acetaminophen or non-steroidal anti-inflammatory drugs (NSAIDs) for fever and pain, though NSAIDS should be avoided if dengue is a possibility or if the patient has thrombocytopenia or bleeding. Chronic symptoms may be treated with NSAIDs, physical therapy, and other immune modulators if severe. Vaccines are under development.

Ritz N et al: Chikungunya in children. Pediatr Infect Dis J 2015; 34(7):789–791 [PMID: 26069950].
Weaver SC, Lecuit M: Chikungunya virus and the global spread of a mosquito-borne disease. N Engl J Med 2015;372(13): 1231–1239 [PMID: 25806915].

ZIKA

ESSENTIALS OF DIAGNOSIS & TYPICAL FEATURES

▶ Transmitted by *Aedes* mosquitos (same vector as dengue and chikungunya), sexual intercourse, and vertically (mother-to-child) during pregnancy.

▶ Acute symptoms are usually mild and similar to dengue and chikungunya (rash, fever, conjunctivitis).

▶ Vertical transmission during pregnancy may result in congenital Zika syndrome.

Zika virus has been endemic in Africa and Asia for decades but recently emerged in the Americas in 2015–2016 and resulted in a widespread epidemic, including endemic cases in the southern United States. Zika can be transmitted by *Aedes* mosquitos and sexually. Though most Zika infections are asymptomatic or benign, infection during pregnancy can result in vertical transmission and lead to severe neurodevelopmental sequelae in the infant, known as congenital Zika syndrome. Diagnosis is made difficult by similar geographic distribution and clinical presentation to dengue and chikungunya, as well as cross-reactivity of serologic testing with other flaviviruses such as dengue.

▶ Clinical Findings

A. Symptoms and Signs

After a 3- to 7-day incubation period, most acute Zika infections are asymptomatic (up to 75%) or mild. Symptoms are like dengue and chikungunya and include maculopapular rash, low-grade fever, nonpurulent conjunctivitis, and arthralgia. Most infections resolve within 2–7 days.

Maternal infection during pregnancy, which may be symptomatic or subclinical, can result in vertical transmission and lead to congenital Zika syndrome (see Complications).

B. Laboratory Findings

Leukopenia, thrombocytopenia, and elevated liver transaminases may be seen during acute infection. In the first 14 days of infection, RT-PCR of blood or urine is usually obtained first, but a negative result does not rule out infection. IgM antibodies against Zika appear around day 4 and usually last around 3 months. Early testing by RT-PCR is preferable as Zika antibodies may cross-react with other flaviviruses (eg, dengue), making serologic diagnosis more difficult. Infants exposed in utero should undergo extensive diagnostic evaluation for infection according to the latest guidelines, which may include placental and umbilical cord tissue assessment by RT-PCR. Congenitally exposed infants should also undergo neurodevelopment, ophthalmologic, and audiometric evaluation.

C. Radiologic Findings

Radiologic imaging of the fetus or neonate with congenital Zika syndrome may demonstrate growth restriction, intracranial calcifications, ventriculomegaly, reduced brain volume, and other abnormalities.

▶ Differential Diagnosis

Acutely, Zika is clinically indistinguishable from dengue and chikungunya, which are both transmitted by the same *Aedes* mosquito vectors. Unlike dengue, Zika does not lead to hemorrhage or shock. Unlike chikungunya, Zika does not usually lead to severe or persistent musculoskeletal symptoms. Other infections with similar acute presentations include parvovirus, rubella, measles, leptospirosis, malaria, typhoid, rickettsia, and influenza. Rubella, cytomegalovirus, toxoplasmosis, and other congenital infections should be considered in infants undergoing evaluation for congenital Zika syndrome. A febrile illness that starts 2 weeks after the trip ends or that lasts longer than 2 weeks is probably not Zika.

▶ Complications

Infants affected with congenital Zika syndrome may be small for gestational age and demonstrate neurodevelopmental sequelae, including microcephaly, seizures, irritability, spasticity, feeding difficulty, arthrogryposis, ocular findings, and sensorineural hearing loss. Additional sequelae may be described as more data become available and affected infants are followed into childhood, but preliminary data suggests 1%–13% of congenital infections result in congenital Zika syndrome, with higher risk in the first trimester (but risk persists into the third trimester). There is an increased risk of Guillain-Barré syndrome following Zika infection.

Prevention and Treatment

Prevention, which is particularly important for pregnant women and those intending to conceive, involves avoiding high-risk areas, using conventional mosquito avoidance measures, and using a barrier method for sex with potentially infected individuals (Zika virus persists in the genital tract for weeks). Acute disease is treated with supportive care. Multiple vaccines are in clinical trials.

Adebanjo T: Update: Interim guidance for the diagnosis, evaluation, and management of infants with possible congenital Zika virus infection—United States, October 2017. MMWR Morb Mortal Wkly Rep 2017;66:1089–1099 [PMID: 29049277].
Muss D et al: Zika virus. Clin Microbial Rev 2016;29(3):487–524 [PMID: 27029595].
Read JS et al: Symptomatic Zika virus infection in infants, children, and adolescents living in Puerto Rico. JAMA Pediatr 2018 Jul 1; 172(7):686–693 [PMID: 29813148].

COLORADO TICK FEVER

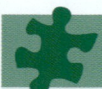

ESSENTIALS OF DIAGNOSIS & TYPICAL FEATURES

► Summer seasonality.
► Travel in endemic area; tick bite.
► Fever, chills, headache, retro-orbital pain, myalgia.
► Biphasic fever curve.
► Leukopenia early in the illness.

Colorado tick fever is endemic in the high plains and mountains of the central and northern Rocky Mountains and northern Pacific coast of the United States. The reservoir of the virus consists of squirrels and chipmunks. Many hundreds of cases of Colorado tick fever occur each year in visitors or laborers entering this region, primarily from May through July.

Clinical Findings

A. Symptoms and Signs

After a 3- to 4-day incubation period (maximum, 14 days), fever begins suddenly together with chills, lethargy, headache, ocular pain, myalgia, abdominal pain, nausea, and vomiting. Conjunctivitis may be present. A nondistinctive maculopapular rash occurs in 5%–10% of patients. The illness lasts 7–10 days, and half of patients have a biphasic fever curve with several afebrile days in the midst of the illness.

B. Laboratory Findings

Leukopenia is characteristic early in the illness. Platelets are modestly decreased. Specific ELISA testing is available, but 2–3 weeks may elapse before seroconversion. Fluorescent antibody staining will detect virus-infected erythrocytes during the illness and for weeks after recovery. RT-PCR is available in some areas and will be positive within the first week of illness.

► Differential Diagnosis

Early findings, especially if rash is present, may suggest enterovirus, measles, or rubella infection. Enteric fever may be an early consideration because of the presence of leukopenia and thrombocytopenia. A history of tick bite, information about local risk, and the biphasic fever pattern will help with the diagnosis. Because of the wilderness exposure, diseases such as leptospirosis, borreliosis, tularemia, ehrlichiosis, and Rocky Mountain spotted fever will be considerations.

► Complications

Meningoencephalitis occurs in 3%–7% of patients. Cardiac and pulmonary complications are rare.

► Prevention & Treatment

Prevention involves avoiding endemic areas and using conventional means to avoid tick bite. Therapy is supportive. Do not use analgesics that modify platelet function.

CDC: Colorado Tick Fever. https://www.cdc.gov/coloradotickfever/index.html.
Yendell SJ et al: Colorado tick fever in the United States, 2002–2012. Vector Borne Zoonotic Dis 2015 May;15(5):311–316 [PMID: 25988440].

OTHER IMPORTANT VIRAL INFECTIONS IN CHILDHOOD

See section Infections Due to Herpesviruses for a discussion of varicella and roseola, the two other major childhood exanthems.

ERYTHEMA INFECTIOSUM

ESSENTIALS OF DIAGNOSIS & TYPICAL FEATURES

► Fever and rash with "slapped-cheek" appearance, followed by a symmetrical, full-body reticular and maculopapular rash.
► Arthritis in older children.
► Profound anemia in patients with impaired erythrocyte production.
► Nonimmune hydrops fetalis following infection of pregnant women.

General Considerations

Human parvoviruses B19 are small DNA viruses causing erythema infectiosum, a benign exanthematous illness of school-aged children also known as the fifth disease. Spread is respiratory, occurring in winter-spring epidemics. A nonspecific mild flu-like illness may occur during the viremia at 7–10 days; the characteristic rash occurring at 10–17 days represents an immune response. The patient is viremic and contagious prior to—but not after—the onset of rash.

Approximately half of infected individuals have a subclinical illness. Most cases (60%) occur in children between ages 5 and 15 years, with an additional 40% occurring later in life. Forty percent of adults are seronegative. The secondary attack rate in a school or household setting is 50% among susceptible children and 20%–30% among susceptible adults.

Clinical Findings

Owing to the nonspecific nature of the exanthem and the many subclinical cases, a history of contact with an infected individual is often absent or unreliable. Recognition of the illness is easier during outbreaks. HB19v is responsible for 5%–10% of fever-rash illness presenting in children and adolescents.

A. Symptoms and Signs

Typically, the first sign of illness is the rash, which begins as raised, fiery red maculopapular lesions on the cheeks that coalesce to give a "slapped-cheek" appearance. The lesions are warm, nontender, and sometimes pruritic. They may be scattered on the forehead, chin, and postauricular areas, but the circumoral region is spared. Within 1–2 days, similar lesions appear on the proximal extensor surfaces of the extremities and spread distally in a symmetrical fashion. Palms and soles are usually spared. The trunk, neck, and buttocks are also commonly involved. Central clearing of confluent lesions produces a characteristic lace-like pattern. The rash fades in days to several weeks, but frequently reappears in response to local irritation, heat (bathing), sunlight, and stress. Nearly 50% of infected children have some rash remaining (or recurring) for 10 days. Fine desquamation may be present. Mild low-grade fever, malaise, myalgia, sore throat, and coryza occur in up to 50% of children. These symptoms appear for 2–3 days followed by a week-long asymptomatic phase before the rashes appear.

Purpuric stocking-glove rashes, neurologic disease, and severe disorders resembling hemolytic-uremic syndrome have also been described in association with parvovirus B19.

B. Laboratory Findings

A mild leukopenia occurs early in some patients, followed by leukocytosis and lymphocytosis. Specific IgM and IgG serum antibody tests are available, but care must be used in choosing a reliable laboratory. IgM antibody is present in 90% of patients at the time of the rash. PCR is often definitive, but parvovirus DNA may be detectable in blood for prolonged periods. Extremely high hB19V loads are observed in patients who develop aplastic crisis.

Differential Diagnosis

In children immunized against measles and rubella, parvovirus B19 is the most frequent agent of morbilliform and rubelliform rashes. The characteristic rash and the mild nature of the illness distinguish erythema infectiosum from other childhood exanthems. It lacks the prodromal symptoms of measles and the lymphadenopathy of rubella. Systemic symptoms and pharyngitis are more prominent with enteroviral infections and scarlet fever.

Complications & Sequelae

A. Arthritis

Arthritis is more common in older patients, girls more than boys, beginning with late adolescence. Approximately 10% of older children have severe joint symptoms. Pain and stiffness occur symmetrically in the peripheral joints. Arthritis usually follows the rash and may persist for 2–6 weeks but resolves without permanent damage.

B. Aplastic Crisis and Other Hematologic Abnormalities

Parvovirus B19 may cause reticulocytopenia for approximately 1 week during the illness. This goes unnoticed in individuals with a normal erythrocyte half-life but results in severe anemia in patients with chronic hemolytic anemia.

Pure red cell aplasia, leukopenia, pancytopenia, idiopathic thrombocytopenic purpura, and a hemophagocytic syndrome have been described. Patients with HIV infection and other immunosuppressive illnesses may develop prolonged anemia or pancytopenia. Patients with hemolytic anemia and aplastic crisis, or with immunosuppression, may be contagious and should be isolated while in the hospital. One of every three children with sickle cell disease (SCD) are positive for hB19v and seroprevalence increases with age. HB19v infections in SCD children are characterized persistent positive IgM up to a year and have a significantly higher red blood cell transfusion volume during infection.

C. Other End-Organ Infections

Parvovirus has been associated with neurologic syndromes, hepatitis, and suppression of bone marrow lineages. It is implicated as a cause of myocarditis.

D. In Utero Infections

Infection of susceptible pregnant women may produce fetal infection with hydrops fetalis. Fetal death occurs in about 6% of cases, most often in the first 20 weeks. This rate of fetal loss is higher than expected in typical pregnancies. Congenital anomalies have not been associated with parvovirus B19 infection during pregnancy.

▶ Treatment & Prognosis

Erythema infectiosum is a benign illness for immunocompetent individuals. Patients with aplastic crisis may require blood transfusions. This complication can rarely be prevented by quarantine measures because acute hB19v infection in contacts is often unrecognized and is most contagious prior to the rash. Routine screening for parvovirus immunity in low-risk pregnancies is not recommended. Pregnant women who are exposed to, at higher risk (day care workers) or who develop symptoms of hB19v infection should be tested with serology (IgM and IgG) for susceptibility to (nonimmune) or evidence of current infection. Susceptible pregnant women should then be followed up as 1.5% of women of childbearing age are infected during pregnancy. If maternal infection occurs, serial ultrasounds should be performed every 1–2 weeks, up to 12 weeks after infection for evidence of hydrops and distress. In utero transfusion or early delivery may salvage some fetuses. The risk of fetal death among exposed pregnant women of unknown serologic status is less than 2.5%.

High-dose IVIG has stopped viremia and led to marrow recovery in some cases of prolonged aplasia. Its role in immunocompetent patients and pregnant women is unknown. Intrauterine transfusion is the standard treatment for severe fetal anemia and is associated with a significant improvement in survival.

Ganaie SS, Qiu J: Recent advances in replication and infection of human parvovirus B19. Front Cell Infect Microbiol 2018 Jun 5; 8:166 [PMID: 29922597].

Qiu J, Soderland-Venemo M, Young NS: Human parvoviruses. Clin Microbiol Rev 2017;30:43 [PMID: 27806994].

MEASLES (RUBEOLA)

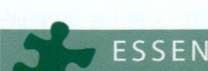

ESSENTIALS OF DIAGNOSIS & TYPICAL FEATURES

► Exposure to measles 9–14 days previously.

► Prodrome (2–3 days) of fever, cough, conjunctivitis, and coryza.

► Koplik spots (few to many small white papules on a diffusely red base on the buccal mucosa) 1–2 days prior to and after onset of rash.

► Maculopapular rash spreading from the face and hairline to the trunk over 3 days and later becoming confluent.

► Leukopenia.

▶ General Considerations

Measles is one of the most contagious infectious diseases of childhood that presents as a febrile exanthema. The attack rate in susceptible individuals is extremely high; spread is via respiratory droplets. Considered eliminated from the United States in 2000, frequent outbreaks have occurred recently (including 1000 cases in the first half of 2019), mainly due to accumulation of susceptible individuals, low vaccination coverage, increasing vaccine hesitancy, and importation. It is recommended that all children receive two doses of measles vaccine prior to primary or secondary school entry (see Chapter 10). Morbidity and mortality rates in the developing world are substantial because of underlying malnutrition and secondary infections. Because humans are the sole reservoir of measles, there is the potential to eliminate this disease worldwide.

▶ Clinical Findings

A history of contact with a suspected case may be absent because airborne spread is efficient, and patients are contagious during the prodrome. Contact with an imported case may not be recognized. In temperate climates, epidemic measles is a winter-spring disease. Because measles is uncommon in the United States, a high index of suspicion is required during outbreaks.

A. Symptoms and Signs

After 2–3 days of a prodrome of sneezing, eyelid edema, tearing, copious coryza, photophobia, and harsh cough, high fever and lethargy become prominent. Koplik spots are white macular lesions on the buccal mucosa, typically opposite the lower molars that appear in the first 2–4 days of the illness. A discrete maculopapular rash begins when the respiratory symptoms and fever are maximal and spreads quickly from the face to the trunk, coalescing to a bright red. As it spreads to the extremities, the rash fades turning coppery from the face and is completely gone within 6 days; fine desquamation may occur. Diarrhea can occur in young children and lead to hospitalization; persistent fever and cough may signal pneumonia. Measles should be considered in any child with febrile rash illness, especially if recently traveled internationally or exposed to a person with febrile rash illness. Suspected measles cases should be reported to local health department within 24 hours.

B. Laboratory Findings

Lymphopenia is characteristic. The diagnosis is usually made by PCR testing of oropharyngeal secretions (or urine), which is extremely sensitive and specific and can detect infection up to 5 days before symptoms. Measles may be diagnosed serologically by IgM detection in serum at ≥ 3 days after the onset of rash (false negative may occur early in infection), or significant rise in IgG antibody between acute and convalescent samples.

C. Imaging

Chest radiographs often show hyperinflation, perihilar infiltrates, or parenchymal patchy, fluffy densities. Secondary consolidation or effusion may be visible.

► Differential Diagnosis

Table 40–2 lists other illnesses that may resemble measles.

► Complications & Sequelae

A. Respiratory Complications

These occur in up to 15% of patients. Bacterial superinfection of the lungs, middle ear, sinus, and cervical nodes are most common. Fever that persists after the third or fourth day of rash and/or leukocytosis suggests such a complication. Bronchospasm, severe croup, and progressive viral pneumonia or bronchiolitis (in infants) also occur. Immunosuppressed patients are at much greater risk for fatal pneumonia than are immunocompetent patients.

B. Cerebral Complications

Encephalitis occurs in 1 in 2000 cases. Onset is usually within a week after appearance of rash. Symptoms include combativeness, ataxia, vomiting, seizures, and coma. Lymphocytic pleocytosis and a mildly elevated protein concentration are usual CSF findings, but the fluid may be normal. Forty percent of patients so affected die or have severe neurologic sequelae.

Subacute sclerosing panencephalitis (SSPE) is a slow measles virus infection of the brain that becomes symptomatic years later in about 1 in 100,000 previously infected children. This progressive cerebral deterioration is associated with myoclonic jerks and a typical electroencephalographic pattern. It is fatal in 6–12 months. High titers of measles antibody are present in serum and CSF.

C. Other Complications

These include hemorrhagic measles (severe disease with multiorgan bleeding, fever, and cerebral symptoms), thrombocytopenia, appendicitis, keratitis, myocarditis, and premature delivery or stillbirth. Mild liver function test elevation is detected in up to 50% of cases in young adults; jaundice may also occur. Measles causes transient immunosuppression; thus, reactivation or progression of tuberculosis (including transient cutaneous anergy) can occur in children.

► Prevention

The current two-dose active vaccination strategy provides more than 97% protection. Vaccine should not be withheld for concurrent mild acute illness, tuberculosis or positive tuberculin skin test, breast-feeding, or exposure to an immunodeficient contact. The vaccine is recommended for HIV-infected children without severe HIV complications, with CD4 cells more than or equal to 15%, and preferably receiving antiretroviral therapy.

► Treatment & Prognosis

Vaccination prevents the disease in susceptible exposed individuals if given within 72 hours (see Chapter 10). Immunoglobulin (0.25 mL/kg intramuscularly; 0.5 mL/kg if immunocompromised) will prevent or modify measles if given within 6 days. Suspected cases should be diagnosed promptly and reported to the local health department.

Recovery generally occurs 7–10 days after onset of symptoms. Therapy is supportive: eye care, cough relief (avoid opioid suppressants in infants), and fever reduction (acetaminophen, lukewarm baths; avoid salicylates). Secondary bacterial infections should be treated promptly; antimicrobial prophylaxis is not indicated. Ribavirin is active in vitro and may be useful in infected immunocompromised children. In malnourished children, vitamin A supplementation should be given to avoid blindness and decrease mortality.

Hübschen JM, Gouandjika-Vasilache I, Dina J. Measles. Lancet 2022; 399(10325):678–690. doi: 10.1016/S0140-6736(21)02004-3 [PMID: 35093206].

Peart Akindele N. Updates in the epidemiology, approaches to vaccine coverage and current outbreaks of measles. Infect Dis Clin North Am 2022 Mar;36(1):39–48. doi: 10.1016/j.idc.2021.11.010 [PMID: 35168713].

RUBELLA

ESSENTIALS OF DIAGNOSIS & TYPICAL FEATURES

- ► No previous rubella vaccination.
- ► Fever with postauricular and occipital adenopathy.
- ► Maculopapular rash from face to rest of the body.
- ► Congenital infection: growth retardation; cataracts, retinopathy; purpuric rash ("blueberry muffin") at birth; jaundice, thrombocytopenia; deafness, congenital heart defects.

► General Considerations

Rubella is an RNA virus in the genus Rubivirus and its infection is typically asymptomatic (> 80% subclinical) or results in mild symptoms, making disease diagnosis and surveillance challenging. When symptomatic, a mild, self-limited exanthema appears. Infection during pregnancy leads to teratogenicity and miscarriage. Rubella virus is transmitted through respiratory droplets and direct contact, replicating in the nasopharynx. Patients are infectious 5 days before until 5 days after the rash. Endemic rubella is absent in the United States and the Americas, and congenital rubella in infants born to unimmunized women and the occasional woman who is reinfected in pregnancy, is now very rare. Sporadic cases occur in migrants to the United States from Asia and Africa.

► Clinical Findings

The incubation period is 14–21 days. The nondistinctive signs may make exposure history unreliable. A history of immunization makes rubella unlikely but still possible. Congenital rubella usually follows placental infection during viraemia.

A. Symptoms and Signs

1. Infection in children—Young children may only have an erythematous rash with discrete maculopapules beginning on the face and spreading to the trunk and extremities within 24 hours. The rash fades from the face to extremities by the third day. Scarlatiniform, morbilliform, and erythema infectiosum-like rash variants may occur. Enanthema is usually absent. Older patients often have a nonspecific prodrome of low-grade fever, ocular pain, sore throat, and myalgia. Post-auricular and suboccipital adenopathy (sometimes generalized) is characteristic.

2. Congenital Rubella Syndrome (CRS)—More than 85% of women infected in the first trimester of pregnancy (25% near the end of the second trimester) deliver an affected infant; congenital disease occurs in less than 5% of women infected later in pregnancy. Later infections can result in isolated defects, such as deafness. The main manifestations include growth retardation (50%–85%), cardiac anomalies (pulmonary artery stenosis, patent ductus arteriosus, ventricular septal defects), ocular anomalies (cataracts, microphthalmia, glaucoma, retinitis), sensorineural hearing loss (> 50%), cerebral disorders (chronic encephalitis, developmental delay), hematologic disorders (thrombocytopenia, extramedullary "blueberry muffin" hematopoiesis, lymphopenia), and others (hepatitis, osteomyelitis, immune disorders, malabsorption, diabetes).

B. Laboratory Findings

Leukopenia is common, and platelet counts may be low. Congenital infection is associated with low platelet counts, abnormal liver function tests, hemolytic anemia, and CSF pleocytosis in the newborn period. Virus may be isolated from oral secretions or urine from 1 week before to 2 weeks after onset of rash. Children with congenital infection are infectious for months. PCR is very sensitive. Serologic immunoassay diagnosis is best made by demonstrating a four-fold rise in antibody titer between specimens drawn 1–2 weeks apart. The first should be drawn promptly, because titers increase rapidly after onset of rash; both specimens must be tested simultaneously by a single laboratory. Rubella IgM is present in 50% of patients at the onset of the rash but reach their peak by days after rash onset and decline rapidly until becoming undetectable by 8 weeks after infection. Because the decision to terminate a pregnancy is usually based on serologic results, testing must be done carefully. The positive predictive value of IgG seroconversion and IgM to assess primary maternal rubella virus infection is very low.

C. Imaging

Pneumonitis and bone metaphyseal longitudinal lucencies may be present in radiographs of children with congenital infection.

► Differential Diagnosis

Rubella may resemble infections due to measles, enterovirus, adenovirus, EBV, roseola, parvovirus, and *T gondii*. Drug reactions may also mimic rubella. Because public health implications are great, sporadic suspected cases should be confirmed serologically or virologically. Congenital rubella must be differentiated from congenital CMV infection, toxoplasmosis, Zika, and syphilis.

► Complications & Sequelae

A. Arthralgia and Arthritis

Joint signs and symptoms are more common in adolescent girls and adult women affecting20% who develop transient polyarthralgia or polyarthritis (fingers, knees, wrists) lasting a few days to weeks. Frank arthritis resembling acute rheumatoid arthritis occurs in a small percentage of patients.

B. Encephalitis and Other Neurological Sequelae

With an incidence of about 1:6000, this is a para-infectious encephalitis associated with a low mortality rate. A syndrome resembling SSPE (see section Measles) has also been described in congenital rubella. During the rubella epidemic of the 1960s, 8%–13% of children with CRS developed autism compared to the background rate of about 1 new case per 5000 children.

C. Rubella in Pregnancy

Infection in the mother as in older children is self-limited and not severe.

► Prevention

Rubella is one of the infections that could be eradicated through vaccination (see Chapter 10). Standard prenatal care should include rubella antibody testing. Seropositive mothers are at no risk; seronegative mothers are vaccinated after delivery.

A pregnant woman possibly exposed to rubella should be tested immediately; if seropositive, she is considered protected and without risk to the fetus. If she is seronegative, a second specimen should be drawn in 4 weeks, and both specimens should be tested simultaneously. Seroconversion in the first trimester is associated with high fetal risk; such women require counseling regarding therapeutic abortion.

When pregnancy termination is not an option, some experts recommend intramuscular administration of immunoglobulin (up to 0.55 mL/kg IM) within 72 hours after exposure to prevent infection. Only very small fractions of IgG are transferred to the fetus in early pregnancy and the efficacy of this practice is unknown.

▶ Treatment & Prognosis

Symptomatic therapy is sufficient. Arthritis may improve with administration of anti-inflammatory agents. The prognosis is poor in congenitally infected infants, in whom most defects are irreversible or progressive. The severe cognitive defects in these infants seem to correlate closely with the degree of growth failure.

Gordon-Lipkin E, Hoon A, Pardo CA: Prenatal cytomegalovirus, rubella, and Zika virus infections associated with developmental disabilities: past, present, and future. Dev Med Child Neurol 2021;63(2):135–143 [PMID: 33084055].

Winter AK, Moss WJ: Rubella. Lancet 2022;399(10332):1336–1346. doi: 10.1016/S0140-6736(21)02691-X [PMID: 35367004].

INFECTIONS DUE TO OTHER VIRUSES

HANTAVIRUS CARDIOPULMONARY SYNDROME

ESSENTIALS OF DIAGNOSIS & TYPICAL FEATURES

▶ Influenza-like prodrome for 3–7 days (fever, myalgia, headache, cough).

▶ Rapid onset of unexplained pulmonary edema and myocardiopathy.

▶ Residence or travel in endemic area; exposure to aerosols from mouse droppings or secretions.

▶ General Considerations

Hantaviruses are RNA viruses that typically cause chronic asymptomatic infection in rodents, but can infect humans through contact with rodent urine, saliva, or feces. Two types of illnesses are known to humans: (1) hantavirus pulmonary syndrome (HPS) or cardiopulmonary syndrome, prevalent in North and South America, and (2) hemorrhagic fever with renal syndrome, predominant to Asia and Northern Europe.

▶ Clinical Findings

Hantavirus cardiopulmonary syndrome (HPS) has been confirmed in more than 34 states and Canada that have the appropriate rodent reservoirs. In the United States, HPS most often caused by Sin Nombre Virus with a mortality rate of up to 35%. Epidemics occur when environmental conditions favor large increases in the rodent population and increased prevalence of virus.

A. Symptoms and Signs

After an incubation period of 1–3 weeks, onset is sudden, with a nonspecific virus-like prodrome: fever; back, hip, and leg pain; chills; headache; and nausea and vomiting. HPS diagnosis is difficult in children because of its rare occurrence and its similar presentation to other viral illnesses. Abdominal pain may be present. Sore throat, conjunctivitis, rash, and adenopathy are absent, and respiratory symptoms may be limited to a dry cough. After 3–7 days, dyspnea, tachypnea, and evidence of a pulmonary capillary leak syndrome appear. This often progresses rapidly over hours. Hypotension from hypoxemia and myocardial dysfunction is common, which is different from septic shock. Copious, amber-colored, nonpurulent secretions are common. Decreased cardiac output due to myocardiopathy and elevated systemic vascular resistance distinguish this disease from early bacterial sepsis.

B. Laboratory Findings

The hemogram shows leukocytosis with a prominent left shift and immunoblasts, thrombocytopenia, and hemoconcentration. Lactate dehydrogenase (LDH) is elevated, as are liver function tests; serum albumin is low. Creatinine is elevated in some patients, and proteinuria is common. Lactic acidosis and low venous bicarbonate are poor prognostic signs. A serum IgM ELISA test is positive early in the illness. Otherwise, the diagnosis is made by PCR or specific staining of tissue at autopsy.

C. Imaging

Initial chest radiographs are normal, progressing to bilateral interstitial infiltrates with the typical butterfly pattern of acute pulmonary edema, bibasilar airspace disease, or both. Significant pleural effusions are often present.

D. Differential Diagnosis

In some geographic areas, plague and tularemia may be possibilities. Infections with viral respiratory pathogens and

Mycoplasma have a slower progression, do not elevate the LDH, and do not cause the hematologic changes seen in this syndrome. Q fever, psittacosis, toxin exposure, legionellosis, and fungal infections are possibilities, but the history, tempo of the illness, and blood findings, as well as the exposure history, should be distinguishing features. HPS is a consideration in previously healthy persons from a rural area or potential exposure to wild rodents, who have a febrile illness associated with unexplained pulmonary edema.

E. Treatment and Prognosis

There is no established antiviral therapy. Management should concentrate on oxygen therapy and mechanical ventilation as required. Venoarterial extracorporeal membrane oxygenation can provide short-term support for selected patients. Highest hematocrit (hemoconcentration) and high creatinine are poor prognosis factors in children. Younger children have a shorter time between symptom onset and death compared to adolescents or adults (2 vs. 5 days). The strains of virus present in North America are not spread by person-to-person contact. No isolation is required. Guidelines are available for reduction of exposure to the infectious agent.

Thorp L, Fullerton L, Whitesell A, Dehority W. Hantavirus pulmonary syndrome: 1993-2018. Pediatrics 2023;151(4):e2022059352. doi: 10.1542/peds.2022-059352 [PMID: 36855865].

MUMPS

ESSENTIALS OF DIAGNOSIS & TYPICAL FEATURES

- ▶ No prior mumps immunization or waning vaccine immunity.
- ▶ Parotid gland swelling.
- ▶ Aseptic meningitis with or without parotitis.

▶ General Considerations

Mumps virus, a paramyxovirus, is spread by the respiratory route and attacks almost all nonprotected children (asymptomatically in 30%–40% of cases). As a result of prior clinical or subclinical infection, or childhood immunization, 95% of adults are immune, although immunity can wane in late adolescence. When the number of unprotected rises, epidemics (5833 cases in 2016 and 3176 at mid-2017) can occur, which are aborted by reimmunization of the at-risk population, especially college students. Infected patients are infectious from 2 days prior to 5 days after the onset of parotitis. The incubation period is 14–21 days. In an adequately immunized

individual, parotitis is usually due to another cause. Two doses of the vaccine are 88% (range: 66%–95%) effective at protecting against mumps; one dose is 78% effective (range: 49%–92%). However, an outbreak in Guam occurred even when most children had two doses of vaccine, likely spread by crowding.

▶ Clinical Findings

A. Symptoms and Signs

1. Salivary gland disease—After a prodrome of fever, severe headache, arthralgia, and anorexia, tender swelling of parotid glands occurs (70%–80% bilateral). The ear is displaced upward and outward; the mandibular angle is obliterated. Parotid stimulation with sour foods may be quite painful. The orifice of the Stensen duct may be red and swollen; yellow secretions may be expressed, but pus is absent. Parotid swelling dissipates after 1 week.

2. Meningoencephalitis—Once the most common cause of aseptic meningitis, mumps meningitis was manifested by severe headache, vomiting, and/or asymptomatic mononuclear pleocytosis. Fewer than 10% of patients had clinical meningitis or encephalitis. Parotitis is present in only half of the cases of mumps meningoencephalitis. Although neck stiffness, nausea, and vomiting can occur, encephalitic symptoms are rare (1:4000 cases of mumps); recovery in 3–10 days is the rule.

3. Pancreatitis—Epigastric abdominal pain may represent transient pancreatitis. Because salivary gland disease may elevate serum amylase, specific markers of pancreatic function (lipase, amylase isoenzymes) are required for assessing pancreatic involvement.

4. Orchitis, oophoritis—Involvement of the gonads is associated with fever, local tenderness, and swelling and is second to parotitis as presentation of mumps in adolescents. Epididymitis is usually present. Most often unilateral, it resolves in 1–2 weeks. Although one-third of infected testes atrophy, bilateral involvement and sterility are rare.

5. Other—Thyroiditis, mastitis (especially in adolescent females), arthritis, and presternal edema (occasionally with dysphagia or hoarseness) may be seen.

B. Laboratory Findings

Peripheral blood leukocyte count is usually normal. CSF may contain a modest number of cells (~ 250 cells/µL, predominantly lymphocytes), with mildly elevated protein and normal to slightly decreased glucose. Viral PCR or culture of saliva, throat, urine, or spinal fluid may be positive for at least 1 week after onset. Paired sera assayed by ELISA or a single positive IgM antibody test may be used for diagnosis.

Differential Diagnosis

A history of contact with a child with parotitis is not proof of mumps exposure. Mumps parotitis may resemble cervical adenitis (the jaw angle may be obliterated, but the ear does not usually protrude; the Stensen duct orifice is normal; leukocytosis and neutrophilia are observed), bacterial parotitis (pus in the Stensen duct, toxicity, exquisite tenderness), recurrent parotitis (idiopathic or associated with calculi), tumors or leukemia, and tooth infections. Many viruses, including parainfluenza, enteroviruses, EBV, CMV, and influenza, can cause parotitis. Parotid swelling in HIV infection is less painful and tends to be bilateral and chronic but may occur.

Unless parotitis is present, mumps meningitis resembles that caused by enteroviruses or early bacterial infection. An elevated amylase level may be useful clue in this situation. Isolated pancreatitis is not distinguishable from many other causes of epigastric pain and vomiting. Mumps is a classic cause of orchitis, but torsion, bacterial or chlamydial epididymitis, *Mycoplasma* infection, other viral infections, hematomas, hernias, and tumors must also be considered.

Complications

The major neurologic complication is nerve deafness (usually unilateral) which can result in inability to hear high tones. Although rare, occurring in less than 0.1% of cases of mumps, it may occur without meningitis. Aqueductal stenosis and hydrocephalus (especially following congenital infection), myocarditis, transverse myelitis, and facial paralysis are other rare complications.

Treatment & Prognosis

Treatment is supportive and includes provision of fluids, analgesics, and scrotal support for orchitis. Systemic corticosteroids have been used for orchitis, but their value is anecdotal.

Su SB, Chang HL, Chen AK: Current status of mumps virus infection: epidemiology, pathogenesis, and vaccine. Int J Environ Res Public Health 2020;17(5):1686 [PMID: 32150969].

RABIES

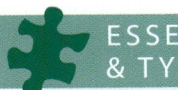

ESSENTIALS OF DIAGNOSIS & TYPICAL FEATURES

▶ History of animal bite 10 days to 1 year (usually < 90 days) previously.

▶ Paresthesias or hyperesthesia in bite area.

▶ Progressive limb and facial weakness in some patients (dumb rabies; 30%).

▶ Irritability followed by fever, confusion, combativeness, and muscle spasms (especially pharyngeal with swallowing) in all patients (furious rabies).

▶ Rabies nucleic acid (RT-PCR) or antigen detected in corneal scrapings or tissue obtained by brain or skin biopsy; Negri bodies seen in brain tissue.

General Considerations

Rabies is an acute progressive CNS viral zoonotic infection. It remains a serious public health problem wherever animal immunization is not widely practiced or when humans play or work in areas with sylvan rabies. Infection is almost invariably fatal and will occur in 40% after rabid animal bites. Any warm-blooded animal may be infected, but susceptibility and transmissibility vary with different species. Dogs are the most common source of human rabies deaths worldwide responsible for an estimated 60,000 annual cases globally. Bats are the most common source of domestically acquired rabies in the United States implicated in 31 (81.6%) of 38 human infections since 2000. Most rabid dogs and cats are usually clinically ill within 10 days after becoming contagious (the standard quarantine period for suspect animals). Rodents rarely transmit infection. Animal vaccines are very effective when properly administered, but a single inoculation may fail to produce immunity in up to 20% of dogs.

The risk is assessed according to the type of animal (high-risk animals include bats, raccoons, skunks, and foxes), wound extent and location (infection more common after head or hand bites, or if wounds have extensive salivary contamination and are not quickly and thoroughly cleaned), geographic area (urban rabies is rare to nonexistent in the United States; rural rabies is frequent in other countries), and animal vaccination history (risk low if documented). Most rabies in the United States is caused by bats yet a history of bat bite is often not obtained especially in young children. Aerosolized virus in caves inhabited by bats has caused infection.

Clinical Findings

A. Symptoms and Signs

Most cases occur within 3–12 weeks of exposure and may present with vague symptoms. Paresthesia at the bite site is usually the first symptom. Nonspecific anxiety, excitability, or depression follows, then muscle spasms, drooling, hydrophobia, delirium, and lethargy. Swallowing or even the sensation of air blown on the face may cause pharyngeal spasms. Seizures, fever, cranial nerve palsies, coma, and death follow within 7–14 days after onset. In a minority of patients, the spastic components are initially absent, and the symptoms are primarily flaccid paralysis and cranial nerve defects. The furious components appear subsequently.

B. Laboratory Findings

Leukocytosis is common. CSF is usually normal but may show elevation of protein and mononuclear cell pleocytosis. Cerebral imaging and electroencephalography are not diagnostic. Infection in an animal may be determined by PCR or fluorescent antibody test to examine brain tissue for antigen. Rabies virus is excreted in the saliva of infected humans, but the diagnosis is usually made by nucleic acid (RT-PCR) or antigen detection in scrapings or tissue samples of richly innervated epithelium, such as the cornea or the hairline of the neck. Classic Negri cytoplasmic inclusion bodies in brain tissue are not always present. Seroconversion measured by neutralizing antibody occurs after 7–10 days. Clinical recovery has been associated with detection of neutralizing antibody and clearance of infectious rabies virus in the CNS.

▶ Differential Diagnosis

Failure to elicit the bite history in areas where rabies is rare may delay diagnosis. Other disorders to be considered include parainfectious encephalopathy; encephalitis due to herpes simplex, mosquito-borne viruses, or other causes of viral encephalitis or acute paralysis. However, classic furious rabies is not readily confused with these alternative diagnoses.

▶ Prevention

See Chapter 10 for information regarding vaccination and postexposure prophylaxis. Rabies immunoglobulin and diploid cell vaccine have made prophylaxis more effective and minimally toxic. Because rabies is almost always fatal, presumed exposures must be managed carefully.

▶ Treatment & Prognosis

Survival is very rare, but it has been reported in a very small number of patients receiving meticulous intensive care and protocols that focus on the altered CNS metabolic state (eg, Milwaukee protocol). Early diagnosis is important for the protection and postexposure prophylaxis of patient contacts.

Blackburn D, et al: Human Rabies - Texas, 2021. MMWR Morb Mortal Wkly Rep 2022;71(49):1547–1549. doi: 10.15585/mmwr.mm7149a2 [PMID: 36480462].

Liu C, Cahill JD: Epidemiology of rabies and current US vaccine guidelines. R I Med J (2013) 2020;103(6):51–53 [PMID: 32752569].

▼ RICKETTSIAL INFECTIONS & Q FEVER

Rickettsiae are pleomorphic, gram-negative coccobacilli that are obligate intracellular parasites. Rickettsial diseases are often included in the differential diagnosis of febrile rashes. Severe headache, myalgia, and pulmonary symptoms are prominent manifestations. The endothelium is the primary target tissue, and the ensuing vasculitis is responsible for severe illness.

All rickettsioses are transmitted by arthropod contact (ticks, fleas, lice—depending on the disease), either by bite or by contamination of skin breaks with vector feces. Except Rocky Mountain spotted fever and murine typhus, all other rickettsial diseases have a characteristic eschar at the bite site, called the *tache noire*. Evidence of arthropod contact by history or physical examination may be lacking, especially in young children. The geographic distribution of the vector is often the primary determinant for suspicion of these infections. Therapy often must be empiric. Many new broad-spectrum antimicrobials are inactive against these cell wall-deficient organisms; tetracyclines are usually effective.

Q fever, which is not a rickettsiae, is included here because it was long classified as such and, like rickettsiae, is an obligate intracellular bacterium. It is not transmitted by an insect vector and is not characterized by rash.

HUMAN EHRLICHIOSIS & ANAPLASMOSIS

ESSENTIALS OF DIAGNOSIS & TYPICAL FEATURES

- ▶ Residing or travel in endemic area when ticks are active.
- ▶ Tick bite noted (~ 75%).
- ▶ Fever, headache, rash (~ 67%), gastrointestinal symptoms.
- ▶ Leukopenia, thrombocytopenia, elevated serum transaminases, hypoalbuminemia.
- ▶ Definitive diagnosis by specific serology.

In children, the major agent of North American human ehrlichiosis is *Ehrlichia chaffeensis*. The reservoir hosts are probably wild rodents, deer, and sheep; ticks are the vectors. Most cases caused by this agent are reported in the south-central, southeastern, and middle Atlantic states (Arkansas, Missouri, Oklahoma, Kentucky, Tennessee, and North Carolina are high-prevalence areas). Almost all cases occur between March and October, when ticks are active.

A second ehrlichiosis syndrome, seen in the upper Midwest and Northeast (Rhode Island, Connecticut, Wisconsin, Minnesota, and New York are high-prevalence areas), is caused by *Anaplasma phagocytophilum* and *Ehrlichia ewingii*. Anaplasmosis also occurs in the western United States.

E chaffeensis has a predilection for mononuclear cells, whereas *A phagocytophilum* and *E ewingii* infect and produce intracytoplasmic inclusions in granulocytes. Hence, diseases caused by these agents are referred to as human monocytic ehrlichiosis or human granulocytic ehrlichiosis, respectively. Ehrlichiosis, Lyme disease, and babesiosis share some tick vectors; thus, dual infections can occur and should be considered in patients who fail to respond to therapy.

▶ Clinical Findings

In approximately 75% of patients, a history of tick bite can be elicited. Most of the remaining patients report having been in a tick-infested area. The usual incubation period is 5–21 days.

A. Symptoms and Signs

Fever is universally present, and headache is common (less so in children). Gastrointestinal symptoms (abdominal pain, anorexia, nausea, and vomiting) are reported in most pediatric patients. Distal limb edema may occur. Chills, photophobia, conjunctivitis, and myalgia occur in more than half of patients. Rash occurs in ~ 50% of children with monocytic ehrlichiosis and is much less common in granulocytic ehrlichiosis. Rash may be erythematous, macular, papular, petechial, scarlatiniform, or vasculitic. Meningitis occurs, and altered mental status is common. Interstitial pneumonitis, acute respiratory distress syndrome, and renal failure occur in severe cases. Physical examination reveals rash (not usually palms and soles), mild adenopathy, and hepatomegaly. In children without a rash, infection may present as a fever of unknown origin.

B. Laboratory Findings

Laboratory abnormalities include leukopenia with left shift, lymphopenia, thrombocytopenia, elevated aminotransferase and LDH levels. Hypoalbuminemia and hyponatremia are common. Disseminated intravascular coagulation can occur. Anemia occurs in one-third of patients. CSF pleocytosis (mononuclear cells and increased protein) is common. The definitive diagnosis can be made by PCR or serologically, either by a single high titer or a fourfold rise in titer during acute and convalescent samples. The CDC uses an immunofluorescent antibody test to distinguish between the etiologic agents. Intracytoplasmic inclusions (morulae) may occasionally be observed in mononuclear cells in monocytic ehrlichiosis and are usually observed in polymorphonuclear cells from the peripheral blood or bone marrow in granulocytic ehrlichiosis. PCR may be negative after 48 hours if patient is on appropriate antibiotics.

▶ Differential Diagnosis

In regions where these infections exist, ehrlichiosis should be included in the differential diagnosis of children who present during tick season with fever, leukopenia or thrombocytopenia (or both), increased serum transaminase levels, and

rash. The differential diagnosis includes septic or toxic shock, other rickettsial infections (especially Rocky Mountain spotted fever), Colorado tick fever, leptospirosis, Lyme borreliosis, relapsing fever, EBV, CMV, viral hepatitis and other viral infections, Kawasaki disease, systemic lupus erythematosus, and leukemia.

▶ Treatment & Prognosis

Asymptomatic or clinically mild and undiagnosed infections are common in some endemic areas. The disease may last several weeks if untreated. One-quarter of hospitalized children require intensive care. Meningoencephalitis and persisting neurologic deficits occur in 5%–10% of patients. Doxycycline for 7–10 days is the treatment of choice. Delay in initiation of doxycycline has been associated with more severe ehrlichiosis leading to critical care, therefore children with suspected disease must be treated preemptively. Response to therapy should be evident in 24–48 hours. Immune compromise and asplenia are risk factors for severe disease. Deaths are uncommon in children.

Sanchez E, Vannier E, Wormser GP: Diagnosis, treatment and prevention of Lyme disease, human granulocytic anaplasmosis and babesiosis. JAMA 2016;315:1767 [PMID: 27115378].

Schultz GE, Buckingham SC, Marshall GS: Human monocytic ehrlichiosis in children. Pediatr Infect Dis J 2007;26:475 [PMID: 17529862].

ROCKY MOUNTAIN SPOTTED FEVER

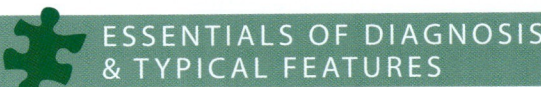

ESSENTIALS OF DIAGNOSIS & TYPICAL FEATURES

- ▶ Residing or travel in endemic area with ticks; tick bite reported for 50% only.
- ▶ Fever, rash (palms and soles), gastrointestinal symptoms, headache.
- ▶ Thrombocytopenia, hyponatremia, hypoalbuminemia.
- ▶ Begin treatment with doxycycline based on clinical suspicion.

Rickettsia rickettsii causes one of many similar tick-borne illnesses characterized by fever and rash that occur worldwide. Most are named after their geographic area. Dogs and rodents, as well as large mammals, are reservoirs of *R rickettsii*.

Rocky Mountain spotted fever is the most severe rickettsial infection and the number of cases has risen in the last two decades (~ 2000 cases per year) in the United States. It occurs predominantly along the eastern seaboard; in the southeastern states; and in Arkansas, Missouri, and Oklahoma. It is much less common in the west. Most cases occur in children exposed in rural areas from April to September. Infection can be acquired from dog ticks.

Clinical Findings

A. Symptoms and Signs

RMSF can be difficult to diagnose due to the nonspecific signs and symptoms. History of tick bites, travel to an endemic area, and exposures are useful. After the incubation period of 3–12 days (mean, 7 days), there is high fever (> 40°C), usually of abrupt onset, myalgia, severe and persistent headache (retro-orbital), toxicity, photophobia, vomiting, abdominal pain, and diarrhea. A rash occurs in more than 95% of patients and appears 2–6 days after fever onset as macules and papules; most characteristic (65%) is involvement of the palms, soles, and extremities; the face is spared. The rash becomes petechial and spreads centrally from the extremities. The rash reflects infection of endothelial cells, which also causes vascular leak and resulting edema, hypovolemia, and hypotension. Conjunctivitis, splenomegaly, pneumonitis, meningismus, and confusion may occur.

B. Laboratory Findings

Laboratory findings reflect diffuse vasculitis: thrombocytopenia, hyponatremia, early mild leukopenia, proteinuria, mildly abnormal liver function tests, hypoalbuminemia, and hematuria. Cerebrospinal fluid pleocytosis and protein elevation are common, with hypoglycorrhachia present in 20%. The "starry sky" sign in MRI (multifocal, punctate diffusion restricting or T2 hyperintense lesions) is universally seen in children with meningoencephalitis. Serologic diagnosis is achieved with indirect fluorescent or latex agglutination antibody methods, but generally is informative only 7–10 days after onset of the illness. Polymerase chain reaction (PCR) amplification can be done from whole blood and skin biopsies during the first week of the illness. A negative result does not rule out the diagnosis, and treatment should not be withheld due to a negative test.

Differential Diagnosis

The differential diagnosis includes meningococcemia, measles, meningococcal meningitis, staphylococcal sepsis, EBV infection, enteroviral infection, leptospirosis, Colorado tick fever, scarlet fever, murine typhus, Kawasaki disease, and ehrlichiosis.

Treatment & Prognosis

To be effective, therapy for Rocky Mountain spotted fever must be started early, frequently based on a high clinical suspicion prior to rash onset in endemic areas. Atypical presentations,

such as the absence of pathognomonic rash, can lead to delay in appropriate therapy. Rash is rarely present during the first day of diagnosis and in 50% within 3 days of onset of fever. Doxycycline is the treatment of choice for children, regardless of age, and should be continued for 10 days and at least 2–3 days after resolution of fever for a full day.

Complications and death result from severe vasculitis, especially in the brain, heart, and lungs. Current case fatality rate is 0.5% but clinical reviews report mortality rates of 5%–7%. Children under 10 years old represent the highest number of reported deaths. Persistent neurologic deficits occur in 10%–15% of children who recover. Delay in therapy is an important determinant of sequelae and mortality.

Because tick attachment lasting 6 hours or longer is associated with transmission of the pathogen, frequent tick removal is a preventive measure.

Biggs HM et al: Diagnosis and management of tickborne rickettsial diseases: rocky mountain spotted fever and other spotted fever group rickettsioses, ehrlichioses, and anaplasmosis - United States. MMWR Recomm Rep 2016;65(2):1–44. doi: 10.15585/mmwr .rr6502a1 [PMID: 27172113].

Mukkada S, Buckingham SC: Recognition and prompt treatment for tick-born infection in children. Infect Dis Clin North Am 2015;29:539 [PMID: 26188606].

ENDEMIC TYPHUS (MURINE TYPHUS)

ESSENTIALS OF DIAGNOSIS & TYPICAL FEATURES

- ▶ Residing in endemic area.
- ▶ Fever for 10–14 days.
- ▶ Headache, chills, myalgia.
- ▶ Maculopapular rash spreading from trunk to extremities (not on palms and soles) 3–7 days after fever onset.
- ▶ Definitive diagnosis by serology.

Endemic typhus (murine typhus) is caused by the bacterium *Rickettsia typhi* in the southern United States, mainly in Texas, California, and Hawaii. The disease is transmitted by fleas from infected rodents or inhalation of rodent feces. Domestic cats, dogs, and opossums may play a role in the transmission of suburban cases. The incubation period is 6–14 days. Headache, myalgia and arthralgia, and chills slowly worsen. Fever may last 10–14 days. After 3–7 days, a rash appears. Truncal macules and papules spread to the extremities; the rash is rarely petechial and resolves in less than 5 days. The location of the rash in typhus, with sparing of the palms and soles, helps distinguish the disease from Rocky Mountain spotted fever. Rash may be absent in 20%–40% of patients. Hepatomegaly may be present. Intestinal and respiratory symptoms may occur. Mild thrombocytopenia and elevated liver enzymes may be present. Prolonged neurologic symptoms can occur. During the COVID-19 pandemic, murine typhus can mimic Multisystem inflammatory syndrome in children (MIS-C) secondary to SARS-CoV2. PCR is most sensitive on samples from blood, plasma, or tissue taken during the first week of illness, but prior to the start of therapy. Fluorescent antibody and ELISA tests are also available. Clinicians in endemic areas should consider early treatment when presented with a child with protracted fever, rash, and headache. Doxycycline is the drug of choice, which should be continued for 3 days after evidence of clinical improvement.

Liddel PW, Sparks MJ: Murine typhus: endemic *Rickettsia* in southwest Texas. Clin Lab Sci 2012;25(2):81 [PMID: 20120614].
Tsioutis C: Clinical and laboratory characteristics, epidemiology, and outcomes of murine typhus: a systematic review. Acta Trop 2017 Feb;166:16–24 [PMID: 27983969].

Q FEVER

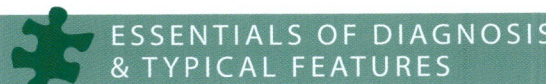

ESSENTIALS OF DIAGNOSIS & TYPICAL FEATURES

- ▶ Exposure to farm animals (sheep, goats, cattle) and pets.
- ▶ Flu-like illness (fever, severe headache, myalgia).
- ▶ Cough; atypical pneumonia.
- ▶ Hepatomegaly and hepatitis.
- ▶ Diagnosis by serology.

Coxiella burnetii is transmitted by inhalation rather than by an arthropod bite. Q fever is also distinguished from rickettsial diseases by the infrequent occurrence of cutaneous manifestations and by the prominence of pulmonary disease. The birth tissues and excreta of domestic animals and of some rodents are major infectious sources. The organisms may be carried long distances in fine particle aerosols. Unpasteurized milk from infected animals may also transmit disease.

▶ Clinical Findings

A. Symptoms and Signs

Most patients have a self-limited flu-like syndrome of chills, fever, severe headache, and myalgia of abrupt onset occurring 10–25 days after exposure. Abdominal pain, vomiting, chest pain, and dry cough are prominent in children. Examination of the chest may yield few findings, as in other atypical pneumonias. Hepatosplenomegaly is common. The illness lasts 1–4 weeks and frequently is associated with weight loss. Only about 50% of infected patients develop significant symptoms.

B. Laboratory Findings

Leukopenia with left shift is characteristic. Thrombocytopenia is unusual, which is another distinction from rickettsial diseases. Aminotransferase and γ-glutamyl transferase levels are elevated, but significant bilirubin elevation is unusual. Diagnosis is made by positive PCR from blood during the first week of illness, but prior to the start of therapy, or serologic response (fourfold rise or single high titer in ELISA, IFA, or CF antibody assay) to the phase II organism. Chronic infection is indicated by antibody against the phase I organism. IgM ELISA tests are available.

C. Imaging

Pneumonitis occurs in 50% of patients. Multiple segmental infiltrates are common, but the radiographic appearance is not pathognomonic. Consolidation and pleural effusion are rare.

▶ Differential Diagnosis

In the appropriate epidemiologic setting, Q fever should be considered in evaluating causes of atypical pneumonias, such as *M pneumoniae*, viruses, *Legionella*, and *C pneumoniae*. It should also be included among the causes of mild to moderate hepatitis without rash or adenopathy in children with exposure to farm animals.

▶ Treatment & Prognosis

Illness typically lasts 1–2 weeks without therapy. The course of the uncomplicated illness is shortened with doxycycline. Therapy is continued for several days after the patient becomes afebrile (usually 10–14 days). Quinolones are also effective. Chronic Q fever occurs in less than 5% of acutely infected patients. *C burnetii* is also one of the causes of "culture-negative" endocarditis. Coxiella endocarditis often occurs in the setting of valve abnormalities and is difficult to treat; mortality approaches 50%. Combination doxycycline and hydroxychloroquine are recommended for Q fever endocarditis or osteomyelitis in children. Adjunctive therapies, such as such as interferon gamma, has produced mixed outcomes. Other complications as myocarditis or granulomatous hepatitis, and meningoencephalitis are rare.

Cherry CC, Kersh GJ: Pediatric Q Fever. Curr Infect Dis Rep 2020;22(4):10.1007/s11908-020-0719-0. doi: 10.1007/s11908-020-0719-0 [PMID: 34135692].
Eldin C, Melenotte C, Mediannikov O: From Q fever to *Coxiella burnetii* infection: a paradigm change. Clin Micro Rev 2017;30:115 [PMID: 27856520].

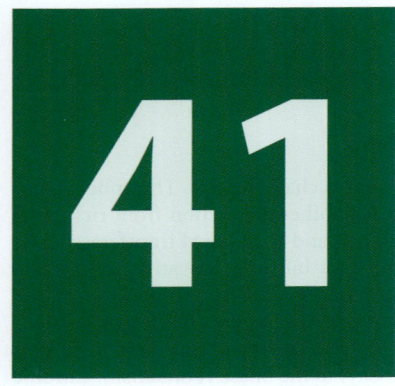

41 Human Immunodeficiency Virus Infection

Christiana Smith, MD, MSc

Elizabeth J. McFarland, MD

PATHOGENESIS & EPIDEMIOLOGY

ESSENTIALS OF DIAGNOSIS & TYPICAL FEATURES

- ▶ Human immunodeficiency virus (HIV) causes progressive destruction of CD4 T lymphocytes, ultimately leading to acquired immunodeficiency syndrome (AIDS).

- ▶ Perinatal transmission of HIV has declined worldwide due to antiretroviral treatment (ART) but persists in regions lacking ART access.

- ▶ In the United States, adolescents and young adults are at ongoing risk of HIV acquisition, particularly young men of color who have sex with other men.

▶ Pathogenesis & Transmission

Human immunodeficiency virus (HIV) is a retrovirus that can be found in blood, semen, preseminal fluids, rectal fluids, vaginal fluids, and breast milk of persons living with HIV, with transmission occurring via sexual contact, sharing contaminated needles, and perinatal routes (in utero, peripartum, breast-feeding). Infection resulting from accidental needle sticks or, rarely, mucosal exposure to blood may occur, mainly in health care settings.

At the time of initial infection, HIV migrates to regional lymph nodes, replicates, and spreads to lymphoid tissues throughout the body. Based on nonhuman primate models, replicating virus disseminates by 48 hours postinfection. Approximately 2 weeks after exposure, a high level of virus is detected in the bloodstream (Figure 41–1). In adults without therapy, the level of viremia declines concurrent with the appearance of an HIV-specific host immune response, and plasma viremia usually reaches a steady-state level about 6 months after primary infection. An asymptomatic period usually follows, lasting from 1 year to more than 12 years. However, ongoing viremia and immune activation causes injury to the immune system and other organs.

Infants with peripartum and in utero HIV infection have viremia that rises steeply after birth, reaching a peak at 1–2 months of age. In contrast with adults, infants have a gradual decline in plasma viremia that extends to age 4–5 years. Without treatment, up to 50% of infants will have rapid disease progression to acquired immunodeficiency syndrome (AIDS) or death by age 2 years.

HIV integrates its nucleic acid into the DNA of cells of the immune system. HIV infection, in the absence of treatment, causes progressive immune incompetence with a hallmark loss of CD4 T-lymphocyte numbers, ultimately leading to conditions that meet the definition of AIDS and, eventually, death. AIDS is diagnosed when an individual living with HIV develops any of the stage 3 opportunistic illnesses or other conditions listed in Table 41–1 or a CD4 T-lymphocyte count below the threshold for stage 3 in Table 41–2.

Antiretroviral treatment (ART) inhibits viral replication and permits immune reconstitution. Cells with latent HIV infection persist and viral replication recurs if ART is interrupted; thus, treatment must be lifelong. Even with effective viral suppression, ongoing immune activation can result in end-organ (eg, cardiovascular and central nervous system) damage consistent with premature aging. Nevertheless, HIV infection, once considered a terminal disease, is now a chronic condition for people with access to treatment.

▶ Epidemiology

The Joint United Nations Programme on HIV/AIDS (UNAIDS) estimated in 2022 that of 38.4 million

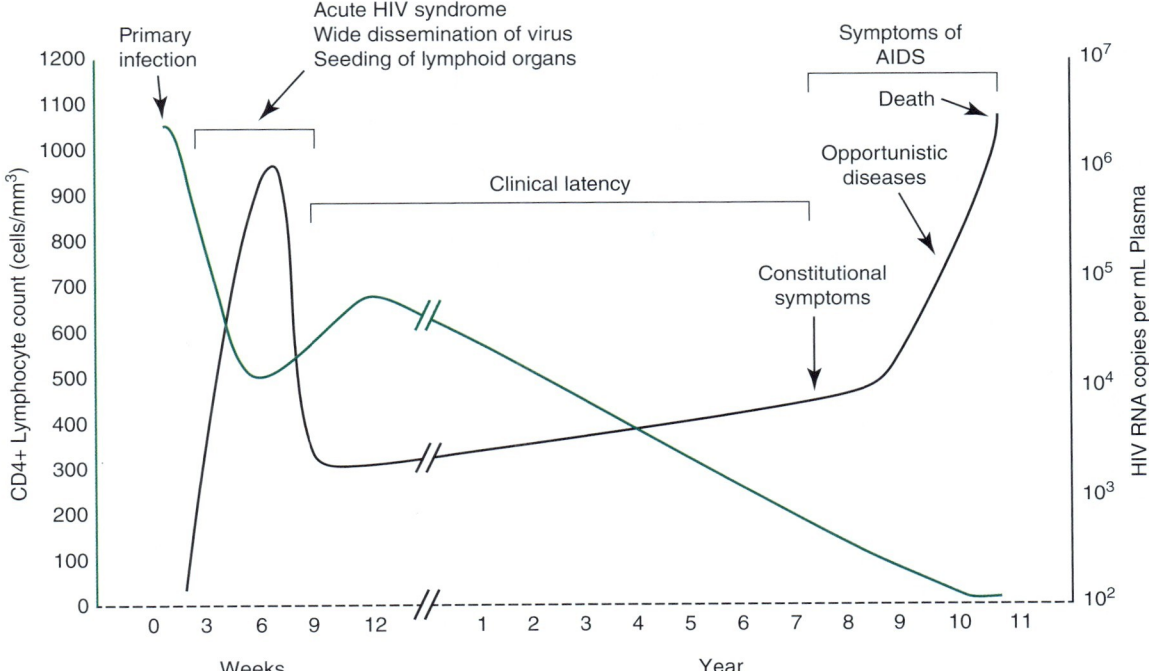

▲ **Figure 41–1.** Typical course of HIV infection without treatment. Soon after acute infection, there is a rapid rise in viral load and decline in the number of CD4 T lymphocytes in peripheral blood. As an immune response to HIV develops, the viral load decreases and there is a period of clinical latency. The CD4 T-lymphocyte count continues to decline until the person living with HIV becomes at risk of opportunistic disease and acquired immunodeficiency syndrome. (Reproduced from Wikimedia Commons/Sigve https://commons.wikimedia.org/w/index.php?curid=15383502.)

people living with HIV worldwide, 2.7 million are children aged 0–19 years (https://data.unicef.org/topic/hivaids/global-regional-trends/). Nearly 90% of these children live in low- and middle-income countries, primarily in sub-Saharan Africa. Perinatal infections continue to occur in resource-limited settings (160,000 new infections in children < 5 years in 2021); although access to preventive measures is improving, approximately 81% of all pregnant women living with HIV received recommended treatment in 2021. Worldwide, the annual number of new HIV infections has decreased by 52% since 2010 among children aged 0–9, but by only 40% among adolescents aged 10–19, who are more likely to acquire HIV through sexual contact or injecting drug use. An estimated 110,000 children and adolescents died from AIDS-related causes in 2021.

In the United States, there were 1447 children living with diagnosed HIV infection in 2020 (https://www.cdc.gov/hiv/pdf/library/reports/surveillance/cdc-hiv-surveillance-report-2020-updated-vol-33.pdf). Perinatal acquisition of HIV is rare in the United States, with only 32 infections reported in 2019.

Black/African American children made up approximately 14% of the US population younger than 13 years in 2020 but accounted for 56% of new HIV diagnoses in this age group. Adolescents and young adults aged 13–24 years accounted for 20% (6135) of the 30,635 new HIV infections in the United States in 2020. The primary HIV exposure type was male-to-male sexual contact, with highest incidence among young African American and Hispanic men.

Bekker LG, Beyrer C, Mgodi N, Lewin SR, Delany-Moretlwe S, Taiwo B, Masters MC, Lazarus JV. HIV infection. Nat Rev Dis Primers. 2023 Aug 17;9(1):42. doi: 10.1038/s41572-023-00452-3. Erratum in: Nat Rev Dis Primers. 2023 Sep 11;9(1):48. [PMID: 37591865].

Knapp KM: Prevention of mother-to-child human immunodeficiency virus transmission in resource-limited countries. Pediatr Clin North Am 2022;69(1):1–18. doi: 10.1016/j.pcl.2021.08.007 [PMID: 34794668].

Vijayan KKV, Karthigeyan KP, Tripathi SP, Hanna LE: Pathophysiology of CD4+ T-cell depletion in HIV-1 and HIV-2 infections. Front Immunol 2017;8:580. doi:10.3389/fimmu.2017.00580 [PMID: 28588579].

Table 41–1. HIV-related symptoms in children.

Mild Symptoms	Severe (Stage 3-defining) Opportunistic Illnesses and Other Conditions
Having two or more of the following conditions: Lymphadenopathy Hepatomegaly Splenomegaly Dermatitis Parotitis Recurrent or persistent upper respiratory infection, sinusitis, or otitis media	Bacterial infections, multiple or recurrent[a] Candidiasis of bronchi, trachea, or lungs Candidiasis of esophagus Cervical cancer, invasive[b] Coccidioidomycosis, disseminated or extrapulmonary Cryptococcosis, extrapulmonary Cryptosporidiosis, chronic intestinal (> 1 mo duration) Cytomegalovirus disease (other than liver, spleen, or nodes) with onset > age 1 mo Cytomegalovirus retinitis (with loss of vision) Encephalopathy attributed to HIV
Moderate Symptoms	Herpes simplex virus: chronic oral lesions (> 1 mo), or bronchitis, pneumonitis, or esophagitis (onset at > age 1 mo)
Anemia, neutropenia, thrombocytopenia Bacterial meningitis, pneumonia, sepsis (single episode) Candidiasis, oropharyngeal, persisting > 2 mo, in a child > 6 mo of age Cardiomyopathy Cytomegalovirus infection with onset < age 1 mo Diarrhea, recurrent or chronic Hepatitis Herpes simplex virus stomatitis (> 2 episodes in 1 y), bronchitis, pneumonitis, esophagitis at < 1 mo of age Herpes zoster, two or more episodes or more than one dermatome Leiomyosarcoma Lymphoid interstitial pneumonia Nephropathy Nocardiosis Persistent fever (lasting > 1 mo) Toxoplasmosis with onset < age 1 mo Varicella, complicated	Histoplasmosis, disseminated or extrapulmonary Isosporiasis, chronic intestinal (> 1 mo duration) Kaposi sarcoma Lymphoma: Burkitt, immunoblastic, or primary lesion in brain *Mycobacterium avium* complex or *Mycobacterium kansasii*, disseminated or extrapulmonary *Mycobacterium tuberculosis of any site, pulmonary,*[b] *disseminated, extrapulmonary* Mycobacterium, other species or unidentified, disseminated or extrapulmonary *Pneumocystis jirovecii* pneumonia Pneumonia, recurrent[b] Progressive multifocal leukoencephalopathy *Salmonella* septicemia, recurrent Toxoplasmosis of the brain with onset > age 1 mo Wasting syndrome

[a]Only among children younger than 6 years.
[b]Only among adults, adolescents, and children older than or equal to 6 years.
Adapted from Centers for Disease Control and Prevention (CDC): Revised surveillance case definition for HIV infection—United States, 2014, MMWR Recomm Rep 2014 Apr 11;63(RR-03):1–10.

Table 41–2. HIV infection stage based on age-specific CD4 T-lymphocyte counts and percentages of total lymphocytes.

	Age of Child					
	< 1 y		1–5 y		≥ 6 y	
Stage	Cells/μL	%	Cells/μL	%	Cells/μL	%
1	≥ 1500	≥ 34	≥ 1000	≥ 30	≥ 500	≥ 26
2	750–1499	26–33	500–999	22–29	200–499	14–25
3	< 750	< 26	< 500	< 22	< 200	< 14

Reproduced from Terms, Definitions, and Calculations Used in CDC HIV Surveillance Publications. Centers for Disease Control and Prevention. National Center for HIV/AIDS, Viral Hepatitis, STD and TB Prevention.

PREVENTION

ESSENTIALS OF DIAGNOSIS & TYPICAL FEATURES

► Prevention of perinatal transmission is highly successful with timely use of antiretroviral (ARV) drugs during pregnancy and breast-feeding.

► Prevention of sexual transmission can be accomplished through integrated biomedical and behavioral interventions, including ARV drugs for pre- and postexposure prophylaxis (PrEP and PEP, respectively) and condom use.

► Application of universal precautions (assumes all blood or bloody secretions are potentially infectious) prevents horizontal environmental transmission.

► Prevention of Perinatal HIV Transmission

Identification of pregnant women with HIV is key to implementing timely prevention techniques. Routine pregnancy care should include HIV testing early in gestation for all pregnant women and repeat testing in the third trimester for women with ongoing risk for HIV acquisition or if HIV seroprevalence is high (≥ 1/1000) among women delivering at the facility. For women presenting in labor with unknown HIV status, testing should be performed using assays that yield results within 60 minutes or less, allowing for ARVs to be initiated for the mother during labor and/or for the infant immediately postpartum.

Maternal ART started before or early in pregnancy, in combination with infant ARV prophylaxis for 2–6 weeks postpartum, can reduce the risk of transmission from 25%–40% to less than 1%. Even if the diagnosis of HIV is late, ARV medications given to women in labor and/or to infants as late as 48 hours postpartum, though less effective, still reduce transmission. The choice of ART during pregnancy is complex, and guidelines are updated frequently by the U.S. Department of Health and Human Services (HHS) (https://clinicalinfo.hiv.gov/en/guidelines/perinatal/). In addition, a consult line is available 24/7 for questions about prevention of perinatal HIV transmission (http://nccc.ucsf.edu/clinician-consultation/perinatal-hiv-aids/, 888-448-8765). Elective C-section prior to labor will reduce transmission risk for women who have plasma viral load greater than or equal to 1000 copies/mL.

Infants with perinatal HIV exposure typically receive ARV prophylaxis for 2–6 weeks. For infants born to women on ART with viral suppression during pregnancy, monotherapy with zidovudine or nevirapine is sufficient; for infants

at higher risk of transmission, empiric treatment with three ARVs is recommended (details of regimens are found at https://clinicalinfo.hiv.gov/en/guidelines/pediatric-arv/antiretroviral-management-newborns-perinatal-hiv-exposure-or-hiv-infection). During the period of ARV prophylaxis, some infants have reversible anemia or neutropenia that is usually not clinically significant.

In resource-limited settings, breast-feeding increases survival and is recommended for the first 12–24 months of life. In the United States and other high-income countries, breast-feeding has historically been discouraged for women living with HIV due to an ongoing risk of HIV transmission. However, maternal ART with viral suppression or extended ARV prophylaxis given to the infant for the duration of breast-feeding reduces HIV transmission during breast-feeding to less than 1%. Current HHS guidelines recommend counseling on infant feeding options and supporting women with well-controlled HIV to breast-feed if they choose to do so. In this scenario, attention to maternal adherence to ART and frequent monitoring of the mother for detectable plasma virus and of the infant for transmission are recommended.

► Prevention of Sexual Transmission

For individuals at risk of HIV acquisition through sexual contact, prevention interventions include combination ARV PrEP and PEP, barrier protection (male and female condoms), and behavioral risk reduction, all discussed in more detail in Chapter 44. The Centers for Disease Control and Prevention (CDC) has extensive HIV prevention guidance for clinicians (https://www.cdc.gov/hiv/clinicians/prevention/index.html) and the general public (https://www.cdc.gov/hiv/risk/index.html), and it publishes a compendium of evidence-based behavioral interventions to promote safer sex practices (https://www.cdc.gov/hiv/research/interventionresearch/compendium/index.html).

A high priority for HIV prevention is improving rates of diagnosis and treatment of people living with HIV since treatment leading to viral suppression prevents transmission to others. Large studies of partners discordant for HIV demonstrate that there is effectively no risk of sexual transmission of HIV when the partner living with HIV takes ART and has durable viral suppression, leading to the concept of Undetectable = Untransmittable (U=U) (https://www.niaid.nih.gov/diseases-conditions/treatment-prevention; https://www.cdc.gov/hiv/risk/art/index.html).

► Prevention Through Universal Precautions

Very rarely, HIV transmission occurs via exposure of nonintact skin or mucous membranes to blood or bloody secretions containing HIV or percutaneous exposure to objects contaminated with bloody secretions. Saliva, tears, urine, and stool are not infectious if they do not contain gross blood. Casual contact poses no risk. Universal precautions for blood exposure prevents transmission of HIV and other bloodborne pathogens in schools, day care centers, and similar venues. Thus, there is no legal requirement that individuals disclose a diagnosis of HIV to such settings.

Cardenas MD et al: Prevention of the vertical transmission of HIV; a recap of the journey so far. Viruses 2023;15(4):840. doi:10.3390/v15040849 [PMID: 37112830].
National Clinicians Consultation Center PrEPline: http://nccc.ucsf.edu/clinician-consultation/prep-pre-exposure-prophylaxis/.
Straub DM, Mullins TLK: Nonoccupational postexposure prophylaxis and preexposure prophylaxis for human immunodeficiency virus prevention in adolescents and young adults. Adv Pediatr 2019;66:245–261 [PMID: 31230697].

LABORATORY DIAGNOSIS OF HIV

ESSENTIALS OF DIAGNOSIS & TYPICAL FEATURES

► HIV antibody/antigen testing is the primary test used for diagnosis of established infection after loss of perinatally acquired maternal antibody.

► HIV nucleic acid testing is an important test for diagnosis during acute infection.

► In perinatally HIV-exposed infants, HIV infection can be diagnosed or excluded with HIV nucleic acid testing by age 3–4 months.

► Early diagnosis and treatment within a few weeks of birth reduce mortality.

Laboratory Diagnosis Without Perinatal Exposure

Tests for diagnosis of HIV infection include combination antigen/antibody tests, antibody-only tests, and nucleic acid tests (NATs) that detect HIV RNA and/or DNA. The current diagnostic algorithm in health care settings uses initial tests that detect HIV-1 and HIV-2 antibody and HIV-1 p24 antigen. These tests are more sensitive for acute/early infection than antibody-only tests because antigen can be detected earlier in acute infection than antibodies (Figure 41–2). After a positive screening test, an antibody-only confirmatory test is performed on the same sample. If this antibody-only test detects the presence of antibodies, infection with HIV-1 or HIV-2 is confirmed. If the initial test, which detects both HIV antigen and anti-HIV antibody, is reactive and the confirmatory test that detects only antibody is nonreactive, HIV

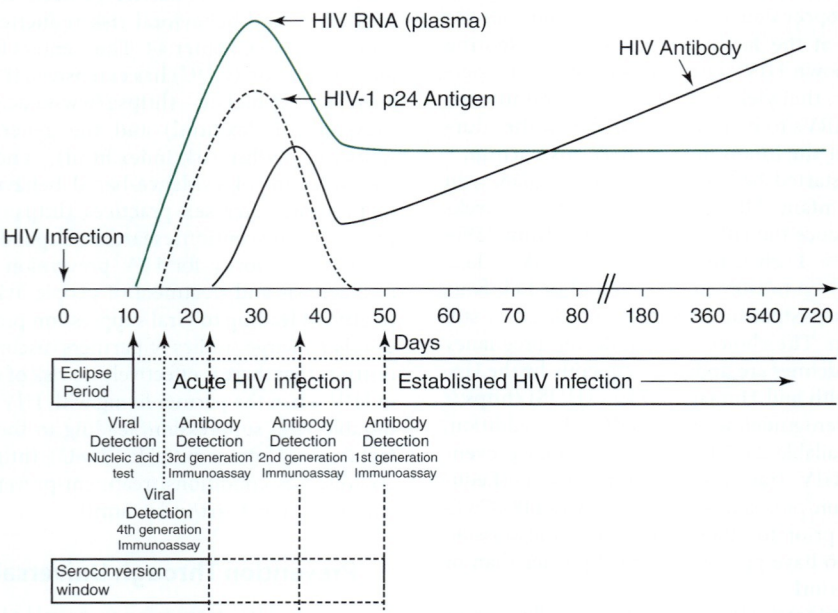

▲ **Figure 41–2.** Sequence of appearance of laboratory markers for HIV infection. Laboratory markers detected during acute HIV infection are shown by time of appearance. Units are not noted on the vertical axis because they differ for the various laboratory markers. (Reproduced from Branson BM, Owen SM, Wesolowski LG, et al: Laboratory Testing for the Diagnosis of HIV Infection Updated Recommendations. Centers for Disease Control and Prevention. National Center for HIV/AIDS, Viral Hepatitis, STD and TB Prevention.)

NAT testing is indicated to distinguish acute infection (with detectable antigen prior to antibodies) from a false positive screening test. If acute HIV infection (within the last 2 weeks) is suspected, HIV NAT should be sent simultaneously with antibody/antigen testing. Alternative HIV diagnostic tests, such as point of care and self-testing, for use in a range of settings (clinics, community-based or field locations, home testing) are described at https://www.cdc.gov/hiv/testing/index.html.

Laboratory Diagnosis for Infants with Perinatal HIV-Exposure

Infants born to mothers with HIV have passively transferred maternal HIV antibodies regardless of the infants' infection status. Therefore, it is necessary to use HIV NAT to identify infants younger than 24 months with HIV acquisition. A recommended schedule of HIV NAT testing for infants is outlined in Table 41–3.

Perinatal HIV infection can be "presumptively" excluded by two negative HIV NATs one obtained at age 2 weeks or older and another at 4 weeks or older, or by one negative HIV NAT at age 8 weeks or older. Definitive evidence of absence of infection, if no breast-feeding, is defined by two negative HIV NATs, one obtained at age 1 month or older and another at age 4 months or older. Breast-fed infants may acquire HIV at any time until they are fully weaned, and virus may not be detected until several weeks or months after exposure. Therefore, breast milk-exposed infants should be tested serially while breast-feeding and at 6 weeks, 3 months, and 6 months after their last exposure. Passively transferred maternal antibodies are undetectable by age 24 months, so HIV antibody tests are used for diagnosis of children with identification of perinatal exposure after age 24 months.

Centers for Disease Control and Prevention; Association of Public Health Laboratories: Laboratory testing for the diagnosis of HIV infection: updated recommendations. Published June 27, 2014. http://dx.doi.org/10.15620/cdc.23447. Accessed April 22, 2023.
Centers for Disease Control and Prevention: 2018 Quick Reference Guide: recommended laboratory HIV testing algorithm for serum or plasma specimens. https://stacks.cdc.gov/view/cdc/50872. Accessed April 22, 2023.
Panel on Antiretroviral Therapy and Medical Management of Children Living With HIV: Guidelines for the use of antiretroviral agents in pediatric HIV infection. https://clinicalinfo.hiv.gov/en/guidelines/pediatric-arv. Accessed April 22, 2023. Diagnosis of HIV Infection in Infants and Children, pp. C18–C38.

INFANTS WITH PERINATAL HIV EXPOSURE

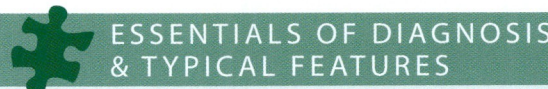

ESSENTIALS OF DIAGNOSIS & TYPICAL FEATURES

► Infants with HIV are typically asymptomatic at birth.
► Prophylaxis with medications can prevent development of *Pneumocystis jirovecii* infection.

Clinical Findings

Newborns with HIV rarely have symptoms or physical examination findings at birth or in the first months of life.

Table 41–3. Laboratory diagnostic schedule for infants exposed to perinatal HIV.[a]

Age	Infant at Low Risk (ARV Single-Drug Prophylaxis)	Infant at High Risk (ARV Combination Prophylaxis)	Infants Who Are Breast-fed[e]
Birth	Optional nucleic acid test[b]	Nucleic acid test[c]	Nucleic acid test
2–3 wk	Nucleic acid test	Nucleic acid test[c]	Nucleic acid test
4–8 wk	Nucleic acid test	Nucleic acid test[c]	Nucleic acid test
8–12 wk		Nucleic acid test[d]	Nucleic acid test
4–6 mo	Nucleic acid test	Nucleic acid test	Nucleic acid test

[a]Definitive infection requires two positives on two samples obtained on different dates.
[b]Some clinicians do not obtain birth testing in low-risk infants since in utero transmission is unlikely, and therefore birth testing is low yield and does not contribute to excluding HIV infection.
[c]For infants at high risk of HIV acquisition, either plasma HIV RNA or cell-associated DNA nucleic acid tests (NATs) may be used, although the sensitivity of plasma HIV RNA NAT or plasma HIV RNA/DNA NAT can be reduced by the use of combination ARV prophylaxis. In contrast, HIV proviral DNA NAT from whole blood detects cell-associated virus and is less affected by ARV prophylaxis.
[d]NAT at 2–6 weeks after cessation of combination ARV allows for earlier detection of HIV in infants at high risk of infection, particularly given the concern that combination ARV prophylaxis may reduce the sensitivity of diagnostic testing.
[e]If breast-feeding continues beyond 6 months of age, NAT should be performed every 3 months thereafter. NAT should also be performed 4–6 weeks, 3 months, and 6 months after cessation of breast-feeding.

However, 30%–80% of infants with HIV develop symptoms or signs within the first year of life. Hepatomegaly, splenomegaly, lymphadenopathy, parotitis, and recurrent respiratory tract infections are signs associated with slow progression. Infants with rapid progression may experience failure to thrive, neurodevelopmental delay, severe and/or recurrent bacterial infections, progressive neurologic disease, anemia, and fever. Opportunistic infections, including PCP, cytomegalovirus (CMV) end-organ disease, and candidal infections may be observed in the first year of life in infants with HIV.

Infants exposed to HIV but uninfected (HEU) are generally healthy, but a number of studies have demonstrated higher morbidity and mortality compared with HIV-unexposed infants. In particular, HEU infants are at higher risk of infections in the first 2 years of life, especially respiratory viral infections. In low- and middle-income countries, HEU infants are more likely to die from these infections, whereas in the United States, HEU infants are hospitalized more often but have similar mortality as HIV-unexposed infants. Alterations in growth, neurocognitive development, immune function, and end-organ parameters have also been reported in this population.

Several ARVs used in pregnant women can cross the placenta, which can provide PrEP to the fetus, but this also raises concern about potential teratogenicity. Thus far, no consistently observed increased risk of birth defects has been identified among infants exposed to ARV in utero, although there are too few known fetal exposures to draw conclusions for newer ARVs. The benefit of prenatal and postnatal treatment to prevent HIV transmission outweighs the potential risk, including for ART initiation in the first trimester, but ongoing studies are important to elucidate the effects of in utero and perinatal HIV and ARV exposure and to identify the safest regimens.

Prophylaxis Against *Pneumocystis jirovecii*

Infants with HIV have a high risk of *Pneumocystis jirovecii* pneumonia (PCP), with the peak incidence at age 2–6 months. Thus, prophylaxis for PCP is given to infants born to mothers with HIV beginning at age 4–6 weeks and continuing until HIV acquisition has been excluded or until age 12 months for infants found to be infected with HIV. PCP prophylaxis is not required if HIV is presumptively excluded (see Laboratory Diagnosis).

Chadwick EG, Ezeanolue EE; the Committee on Pediatric AIDS: Evaluation and management of the infant exposed to HIV in the United States. Pediatrics 2020;146(5):e2020029058. doi: 10.1542/peds.2020-029058 [PMID: 33077537].
du Toit LDV et al: Immune and metabolic alternations in children with perinatal HIV exposure. Viruses 2023;15(2):279. doi: 10.3390/v15020279 [PMID: 36851493].

ACUTE HIV IN ADOLESCENTS

ESSENTIALS OF DIAGNOSIS & TYPICAL FEATURES

- ▶ Adolescent transmission occurs primarily through sexual contact and less commonly via contaminated needles.
- ▶ Common symptoms of acute HIV, such as fever, pharyngitis, headache, diarrhea, oral ulcers, and rash, mimic other acute viral syndromes.
- ▶ Individuals living with HIV may be asymptomatic for years but have ongoing, active viral replication with end-organ damage and potential to transmit HIV.

Among adolescents and adults with acute HIV infection, symptoms of *acute retroviral syndrome* such as fever, pharyngitis, headache, diarrhea, oral ulcers, and rash beginning 2–4 weeks after exposure occur in 30%–90% (Chapter 44). Assessment for HIV exposure risk and consideration of HIV testing is appropriate for adolescents presenting with these symptoms, although not all individuals with acute HIV will seek medical attention. Adolescents may be asymptomatic for several years after HIV acquisition but during that time will have disease progression and the potential to transmit HIV to their sexual partners, hence the CDC recommendation to test all sexually active adolescents.

Chang JJ, Ashcraft AM: Human immunodeficiency virus in adolescents: risk, prevention, screening, and treatment. Prim Care 2020 Jun;47(2):351–365 [PMID: 32423719]. https://www-clinicalkey-com.proxy.hsl.ucdenver.edu/nursing/#!/content/playContent/1-s2.0-S0095454320300130?returnurl=null&referrer=null.
Crowell TA et al; RV254/SEARCH010 Study Group: Acute retroviral syndrome is associated with high viral burden, CD4 depletion, and immune activation in systemic and tissue compartments. Clin Infect Dis 2018 May 1566(10):1540–1549. doi:org/10.1093/cid/cix1063 [PMID: 29228130].

PROGRESSIVE HIV DISEASE

ESSENTIALS OF DIAGNOSIS & TYPICAL FEATURES

- ▶ Ongoing viral replication leads to cellular and humoral immunodeficiency and end-organ pathology.
- ▶ CD4 T-lymphocyte count and clinical events determine disease stage and indication for prophylaxis of opportunistic infections.

▶ As immunodeficiency progresses, patients are at risk for bacteremia, infections by pathogens such as *Mycobacterium tuberculosis*, and opportunistic infections such as *P jirovecii*, CMV, and *Mycobacterium avium* complex (MAC) infection.

▶ Patients with progressive HIV disease are also at risk for encephalopathy, nephropathy, hepatitis, cardiomyopathy, chronic diarrhea, and pulmonary disease.

▶ Individuals with HIV have higher rates of non-Hodgkin lymphoma and cervical and anal neoplasia.

A. Clinical Findings

1. Disease staging—HIV progression is staged by absolute CD4 T-lymphocyte counts and percentages and clinical events. CD4 T-lymphocyte counts are used to direct initiation of prophylaxis for selected opportunistic infections and, when considered together with viral load, predict risk of disease progression and mortality in the absence of ART (https://clinicalinfo.hiv.gov/en/guidelines/pediatric-arv/appendix-c-supplemental-information?view=full). The CDC three-stage classification of progressively severe immune suppression for adults, adolescents, and children is found in Tables 41–1 and 41–2 (https://www.cdc.gov/mmwr/preview/mmwrhtml/rr6303a1.htm). AIDS is defined as stage 3 based on age-adjusted CD4 T-lymphocyte parameters (see Table 41–2) and/or having one or more of the severe conditions listed in Table 41–1. The WHO four-stage system based on clinical events is used widely outside the United States (WHO Consolidated Guidelines on Antiretroviral Drugs for Treatment and Preventing HIV, Annex 10, found at https://www.who.int/hiv/pub/arv/arv-2016/en/).

2. Infections related to immunodeficiency—Rates of invasive bacterial infections, particularly due to *Streptococcus pneumoniae*, *Haemophilus influenzae* type b (Hib), and *Neisseria meningitidis*, are higher in people living with HIV even without severe immunosuppression and after initiating ART. Infections with *M tuberculosis* are a major cause of morbidity, so children with HIV and their family members should have annual TB testing if there is potential for *M tuberculosis* exposure.

Late-stage immunodeficiency is accompanied by susceptibility to a variety of opportunistic pathogens. Pneumonia caused by *P jirovecii* is a common AIDS-defining diagnosis in children with unrecognized HIV who, therefore, are not receiving PCP prophylaxis (see Chapter 43). Persistent candida oral thrush and esophagitis can occur. A variety of diarrheal pathogens that cause mild, self-limited symptoms in healthy persons may result in severe, chronic diarrhea in persons with HIV, including some not routinely included in syndromic molecular stool panels such as *Microsporidia*, *Cyclospora*, and *Isospora belli*. Chronic parvovirus infection manifested by anemia can occur.

With very low CD4-lymphocyte counts, cytomegalovirus (CMV) and *Mycobacterium avium* complex (MAC) may result in disseminated disease with multiorgan involvement. In late-stage disease, prophylactic measures are recommended to prevent selected opportunistic infections such as CMV and MAC (https://clinicalinfo.hiv.gov/en/guidelines/pediatric-opportunistic-infection/summary?view=full).

3. Organ system disease—HIV directly affects multiple organ systems and produces disease manifestations that include encephalopathy, pneumonitis, hepatitis, diarrhea, hematologic suppression, nephropathy, and cardiomyopathy. Most of these manifestations are most severe among children with rapid HIV disease progression. By contrast, lymphoid interstitial pneumonitis (LIP) occurs in untreated children with slow progression. It may be asymptomatic or associated with dry cough, dyspnea or wheezing on exertion, and parotid gland enlargement. Children with HIV, on average, have lower than normal neuropsychological functioning. Studies are evaluating how ongoing inflammation and immune activation in people with HIV might contribute to organ pathology and premature aging, particularly related to cardiovascular and neurologic complications.

4. Malignancy—Children and adolescents with HIV are at increased risk of malignancy. The most commonly occurring tumors are non-Hodgkin lymphomas and cervical/anal neoplasia related to human papillomavirus. Kaposi sarcoma, a skin and mucous membrane malignancy associated with advanced HIV in adults, is rare in children.

B. Laboratory Findings

The hallmark of HIV disease progression is a decline in the absolute number and percentage of CD4 T lymphocytes and an increasing percentage of CD8 T lymphocytes. The CD4 T-lymphocyte values are predictive of the child's risk of opportunistic infections. Healthy infants and children have CD4 T-lymphocyte numbers that are much higher than in adults; these gradually decline to adult levels by age 5–6 years. Hence, age-adjusted values must be used when assessing a child's absolute CD4 T-lymphocyte count (see Table 41–2). CD4 T-lymphocyte percentage, which is less variable with age, is used when CD4 T-lymphocyte count is not available.

Hypergammaglobulinemia of IgG, IgA, and IgM is characteristic in untreated HIV. Hematologic suppression and liver enzyme elevation abnormalities are common due to effects of HIV disease or ART. Cerebrospinal fluid (CSF) may either be normal or may be associated with elevated protein and a mononuclear pleocytosis; HIV NAT may be positive in CSF.

C. Differential Diagnosis

HIV infection should be in the differential diagnosis for children being evaluated for immunodeficiency. Depending on the degree of immunosuppression, the presentation in HIV infection may be similar to that of B-cell (eg, hypogammaglobinemia), T-cell, or combined immunodeficiencies (eg, severe combined immunodeficiency) (see Chapter 33). HIV infection should also be considered in the evaluation of individuals with failure to thrive, developmental delay, chronic lung disease, and *M tuberculosis* infection. HIV infection presenting with generalized lymphadenopathy or hepatosplenomegaly may resemble infections with viruses (eg, Epstein-Barr virus or CMV) or malignancy. Acute HIV is in the differential diagnosis for acute viral syndrome (eg, mononucleosis, flu-like illness) in adolescents.

Flynn PM, Abrams EJ: Growing up with perinatal HIV. AIDS 2019, 15 Mar;33(4):597–603. doi: 10.1097/QAD.0000000000002092 [PMID: 30531318].

Githinji L, Zar HJ: Respiratory complications in children and adolescents with human immunodeficiency virus. Pediatr Clin North Am 2021;68(1):131–145 [PMID: 33228928]. https://www-clinicalkey-com.proxy.hsl.ucdenver.edu/nursing/#!/content/playContent/1-s2.0-S0031395520301383?returnurl=null& referrer=null.

Panel on Opportunistic Infections in HIV-Exposed and HIV-Infected Children: Guidelines for the Prevention and Treatment of Opportunistic Infections in HIV-Exposed and HIV-Infected Children. Department of Health and Human Services. https://clinicalinfo.hiv.gov/en/guidelines/pediatric-opportunistic-infection. Accessed April 22, 2023.

TREATMENT

A. Antiretroviral Treatment

ESSENTIALS OF DIAGNOSIS & TYPICAL FEATURES

▶ ART suppresses viral replication and forestalls immunodeficiency.

▶ Early initiation of ART is recommended for all people living with HIV.

▶ Combinations of ARV drugs are required to avoid induction of viral drug resistance.

▶ ART is lifelong due to inability to eradicate latent virus.

▶ Adherence support is critical for durable viral suppression.

▶ Complications of ART may include dyslipidemia, weight gain, central nervous symptoms, decreased bone mineralization, renal dysfunction, and lactic acidosis.

1. Principles of HIV treatment—Studies in infants, children, and adults support initiation of ART early after diagnosis to prevent HIV progression. Current US and WHO guidelines recommend rapid initiation of ART for all individuals with HIV regardless of clinical, immunologic, or virologic status. The goal of ART is suppression of viral replication (plasma virus < 20–75 copies/mL), resulting in an increase in CD4 T-lymphocyte count and reconstitution of immune function (or maintenance if baseline parameters are within normal limits). HIV has a high spontaneous mutation rate allowing emergence of drug resistance with single-drug treatment; therefore, combination regimens, including at least two drugs with different mechanisms of action, are standard. Latent HIV persists in long-lived resting cells, the so-called viral reservoir, and cessation of ART results in resumption of viremia. Therefore, treatment for HIV with currently available modalities must be lifelong.

Strict adherence to the prescribed treatment is critical. A wide range of issues may impact adherence, including pill burden, dosing frequency, and tolerability, as well as psychosocial factors such as developmental stage, mental health of child and caregiver, HIV knowledge, and beliefs about treatment. Programs and services that enhance adherence are essential adjuncts of any HIV treatment regimen.

2. Antiretroviral medications—There are numerous ARV medications approved by the US Food and Drug Administration (FDA) that are categorized into five different drug classes. Many of the drugs have indications for older children, but pharmacokinetic data and administration forms appropriate for infants and toddlers are more limited. The drug classes, mechanism of action of each class, and common adverse effects are described in Table 41–4. Guidelines for the treatment of HIV developed by a US working group of pediatric HIV specialists are published and updated frequently at: https://clinicalinfo.hiv.gov/en/guidelines/pediatric-arv/regimens-recommended-initial-therapy-antiretroviral-naive-children and WHO recommendations are found at: https://apps.who.int/iris/bitstream/handle/10665/325892/WHO-CDS-HIV-19.15-eng.pdf?ua=1. Each medication has specific toxicities that are described in detail in the Guidelines for Use of ARV in Pediatric HIV Infection (found at https://clinicalinfo.hiv.gov/en/guidelines/pediatric-arv/overview-0?view=full).

B. Other Treatment Considerations

ESSENTIALS OF DIAGNOSIS & TYPICAL FEATURES

▶ Inactivated vaccines are recommended, and some require additional doses.

▶ Selected live attenuated vaccines (LAVs) are recommended in the absence of severe immunosuppression.

▶ Higher rates of mental health disorders indicate the need for psychosocial support.

Table 41–4. Antiretroviral drug class and mechanism of action.

Drug Class	Selected Antiretroviral Drugs	Mechanism of Action	Common Side Effects
Nucleoside/nucleotide reverse transcriptase inhibitors (NRTIs)	Abacavir,[a] emtricitabine,[a] lamivudine,[a] tenofovir alafenamide,[a] tenofovir disoproxil fumarate,[a] zidovudine[a]	Chain termination during reverse transcription of HIV DNA	Anemia, neutropenia, hypersensitivity reaction (abacavir), renal impairment and reduced bone mineral toxicity (tenofovir disoproxil fumarate), hyperlipidemia and excess weight gain (tenofovir alafenamide), lactic acidosis (rare but serious)
Non-nucleoside reverse transcriptase inhibitors (NNRTIs)	Doravirine, efavirenz,[a] etravirine,[a] nevirapine,[a] rilpivirine[b]	Inhibition of viral reverse transcriptase to prevent transcription of HIV RNA to DNA	Rash, elevation of liver enzymes, sleep disturbances, depression, hypersensitivity reaction (nevirapine)
Integrase inhibitor (INSTIs, IIs)	Bictegravir,[a] cabotegravir,[b] dolutegravir,[a] elvitegravir,[a,c] raltegravir[a]	Prevention of integration of HIV DNA in host genome	Nausea, headaches, dizziness, sleep disturbances, depression
Protease inhibitors (PIs)	Atazanavir,[a,c] darunavir,[a,c] lopinavir[a,c]	Inhibition of viral protease resulting in production of noninfectious virions	Nausea, vomiting, diarrhea, dyslipidemia, elevation of liver enzymes, hyperglycemia, QT and PR interval prolongation, hyperbilirubinemia (atazanavir)
Viral entry inhibitors	Fostemsavir	Inhibition of viral envelope attachment	Nausea, vomiting, diarrhea, dizziness, rash, elevation of liver enzymes, QT interval prolongation (fostemsavir)
	Ibalizumab[b]	Inhibition of CD4 postattachment	
	Maraviroc[a]	Blocking of CCR5 co-receptor	

[a]Pediatric dosing established; youngest age and lowest weight for initiating use varies by medication as recommended at https://clinicalinfo.hiv.gov/en/guidelines/pediatric-arv/overview-0?view=full.
[b]Long-acting formulation available.
[c]Co-administered with a pharmacokinetic enhancer, either cobicistat or ritonavir.

1. Immunizations—Inactivated vaccines are recommended, as they are safe and generally immunogenic in children with HIV. Children with HIV have higher rates of disease from pneumococcus, Hib, and meningococcus; therefore, recommendations for high-risk groups for these vaccines apply. Generally, LAVs are not recommended for children with severe immunosuppression (see definition in Table 41–5). However, for children without severe immunosuppression, rotavirus, measles-mumps-rubella, and varicella-zoster virus LAVs are recommended. Vaccine responses are more robust with higher CD4 T-lymphocyte counts and suppressed plasma virus. Therefore, for children who were immunized prior to establishment of effective ART, reimmunization should be considered. Vaccination recommendations specific to children living with HIV are provided in Table 41–5 (CDC guidance for vaccines indicated for children based on medical indications https://www.cdc.gov/vaccines/schedules/hcp/imz/child-indications.html).

2. Psychosocial support and mental health—Evaluation and support for psychosocial needs of HIV-affected families is imperative. As with other chronic illnesses, living with HIV affects all family members, and HIV also carries significant social stigma. Emotional concerns and financial needs, which are more prominent than medical needs at many stages of the disease process, influence the family's ability to adhere to a medical treatment regimen. Adolescents and children with perinatal HIV often (over 60% in some studies) have comorbid mental health conditions including attention-deficit/hyperactivity disorder, depression, and other behavioral health concerns. For adolescents, depression is a risk factor for HIV acquisition and for poor viral suppression on ART. Care coordinated by an interdisciplinary team familiar with HIV disease and its comorbidities, newest therapies, and community resources is ideal.

Lauenzi CA et al: How do psychosocial interventions for adolescents and young people living with HIV improve adherence and viral load? A realist review. J Adolesc Health 2022;71(3):254–269. doi: 10.1016/j.jadohealth.2022.03.0202 [PMID: 35606252].

Table 41–5. Special recommendations for vaccination of children with HIV.[a,b] (*Continued*)

Vaccine	Recommendation
Hepatitis B vaccine	• Test for serum hepatitis B surface antibody (anti-HepBs) after usual primary series; if < 10 mIU/mL, repeat the three-dose series and retest for anti-HepBs at 1–2 mo after 3rd dose. If still < 10 mIU/mL, child is considered at risk for Hep B acquisition. • A booster dose may be considered for those with ongoing Hep B exposure if annual testing identifies anti-HepBs < 10 mIU/mL.
Rotavirus vaccine	• Usual regimen if no severe immunosuppression. Not recommended if severe immunosuppression.[c]
Haemophilus influenzae type b (Hib) conjugate vaccine	• Additional doses if primary series not received prior to 12 mo. • Catchup regimen at and after 12 mo: Age 12–59 mo with ≤ 1 dose before age 12 mo, give 2 additional doses, 8 wk apart; if ≤ 2 doses before 12 mo, give 1 additional dose. • Age > 5–18 y, and no prior Hib vaccine, administer 1 dose.
Pneumococcal conjugate vaccine (PCV20) and pneumococcal polysaccharide vaccine 23 valent (PPSV23)	• Usual regimen of PCV for primary series and catchup prior to age 2 y. Either PCV15 or PCV20 can be used when PCV is indicated. • Catchup regimen: Age 2–5 y, administer 1 dose if any incomplete schedule of 3 doses; administer 2 doses separated by 8 wk if < 3 doses previously. If completed PCV series but has not received PPSV23 or PCV20, administer 1 dose of PCV20 or PPSV23 at least 8 weeks after most recent PCV dose. If PPSV23 is used, administer 1 dose of PCV20 or dose 2 of PPSV23 at least 5 years after dose 1. Age 6–18 y, administer 1 dose of PCV15 or PCV20 if no prior doses of PCV. If PCV15 is used and no prior receipt of PPSV23, administer 1 dose of PPSV23 at least 8 weeks after PCV15. When both PCV15 and PPSV23 are indicated, administer all doses of PCV15 first. PCV15 and PPSV23 should not be administered during the same visit. Administer 1 dose of PCV20 or PPSV23 at least 8 weeks after most recent PCV dose, if either of the following are true: 1) received PCV before age 6 years but has not received PPSV23 or PCV20; 2) received PCV13 at or after age 6 years. If PPSV23 is used, administer 1 dose of PCV20 or dose 2 of PPSV23 at least 5 years after dose 1. If received 1 dose of PCV13 and 1 dose PPSV23 at or after age 6 years, administer 1 dose of PCV20 or 1 dose PPSV23 at least 8 weeks after the PCV13 and at least 5 years after the PPSV23. Please refer to the mobile app to determine the optimal timing and choice of pneumococcal vaccines: www.cdc.gov/vaccines/vpd/pneumo/hcp/pneumoapp.html.
Influenza vaccine	• Usual regimen, inactivated influenza vaccine; live attenuated influenza vaccine not recommended.
Measles, mumps, rubella vaccine (MMR)	• Usual regimen recommended if no severe immunosuppression. Not recommended if severe immunosuppression.[c] • If immunized prior to ART, repeat the two-dose series after starting ART when CD4 percentage has been ≥ 15% and, for children ≥ 5 y, CD4 ≥ 15% and ≥ 200 lymphocytes/μL, for ≥ 6 mo.
Varicella-zoster vaccine (VAR)	• Usual regimen if no severe immunosuppression. Not recommended if severe immunosuppression.[c]
Measles, mumps, rubella, varicella vaccine (MMRV)	• Not recommended; no safety or efficacy data for children living with HIV.
Meningococcal conjugate vaccine (MenACWY)[d]	• Primary series initiated in infancy. • Catchup. Age > 2 y without prior dose, 2-dose series at least 8 wk apart Age ≥ 2 y with 1 prior dose of MenACWY should receive a second if at least 8 wk elapsed and then booster doses at intervals based on age. • Booster dose of MenACWY-CRM or MenACWY-D.[e] Age < 7 y at previous dose, booster dose at 3 y after last dose. Age ≥ 7 y at previous dose, booster dose at 5 y after last dose. For all ages after first booster dose, boosters repeated every 5 y thereafter.
Human papilloma vaccine (HPV)	• Three-dose schedule is recommended irrespective of age of first dose.
Yellow Fever vaccine	• May be given to children with stage 1 HIV and considered for children with stage 2 HIV.

(Continued)

Table 41–5. Special recommendations for vaccination of children with HIV.[a,b] *(Continued)*

Vaccine	Recommendation
Bacillus Calmette-Guérin (BCG)	• Not recommended.
Oral polio	• Not recommended. Inactivated polio vaccine can be used.
Live oral typhoid vaccine	• Not recommended. Capsular polysaccharide typhoid vaccine can be used.

[a]Limited to vaccines for which recommendations differ for children living with HIV. Recommendations for vaccines for tetanus, diphtheria, pertussis, inactivated polio, hepatitis A, and meningococcus B do not differ from routine guidelines.
[b]Recommendations from: Wodi AP, Ault K, Hunter P, McNally V, Szilagyi PG, Bernstein H; Advisory Committee on Immunization Practices recommended immunization schedule for children and adolescents aged 18 years or younger—United States, 2021. MMWR Morb Moral Wkly Rep 2021:70-189-192. doi: http://dx.doi.org/10.15585/mmwr.mm7006a1; Recommended Child and Adolescent Immunization Schedule by Medical Indication, United States, 2021, Table 3, https://www.cdc.gov/vaccines/schedules/hcp/imz/child-indications.html; Panel on Opportunistic Infections in HIV-Exposed and HIV-Infected Children. Guidelines for the Prevention and Treatment of Opportunistic Infections in HIV-Exposed and HIV-Infected Children. Department of Health and Human Services. Available at https://clinicalinfo.hiv.gov/en/guidelines/pediatric-opportunistic-infection/figure-1-recommended-immunization-schedule-children?view=full. Accessed (May 1, 2023) [C1-C4, Figure 1, JJ1-JJ6]; Mbaeyi SA et al: Meningococcal vaccination: recommendations of the Advisory Committee on Immunization Practices, United States, 2020. MMWR Recomm Rep 2020:69(Nov RR-9):1–41. doi: http://dx.doi.org/10.15585/mmwr.rr6909a1, available at https://www.cdc.gov/mmwr/volumes/69/rr/rr6909a1.htm#T3_down; Schillie S et al: Prevention of hepatitis B virus infection in the United States: recommendations of the Advisory Committee on Immunization Practices. MMWR Recomm Rep 2018;67(No. RR-1):1–31. doi: http://dx.doi.org/10.15585/mmwr.rr6701a1, available at https://www.cdc.gov/mmwr/volumes/67/rr/rr6701a1.htm.
[c]Severe immunosuppression defined as CD4 T-lymphocyte percentage < 15% for any age or CD4 T-lymphocyte count < 200/μL for individuals older than or equal to 5 years.
[d]For detailed recommendations see https://www.cdc.gov/mmwr/volumes/69/rr/rr6909a1.htm#T3_down.
[e]MenACWY-D should be given after all PCV13 doses completed and should be given before or concurrent with DTaP. Booster doses administered to children aged < 15 years, repeated booster doses, and booster doses administered at an interval of < 4 years are not licensed in the United States and are considered off-label.

PUBLIC HEALTH GOALS

The US HIV National Strategic Plan lays out the roadmap for the Ending the HIV Epidemic (EHE) initiative, with the goal to reduce the annual number of new HIV infections by 90% by 2030 (https://www.hiv.gov/federal-response/national-hiv-aids-strategy/national-hiv-aids-strategy-2022-2025/) and an emphasis on the continuum of care (https://www.hiv.gov/federal-response/policies-issues/hiv-aids-care-continuum/). The UNAIDS 2030 targets are that 95% of those living with HIV know their diagnosis, 95% of those diagnosed are on ART, and 95% of those on ART have viral suppression. The UNAIDS plan emphasizes integrating HIV services with other support services to reduce barriers to care (interactive website at https://aidstargets2025.unaids.org/).

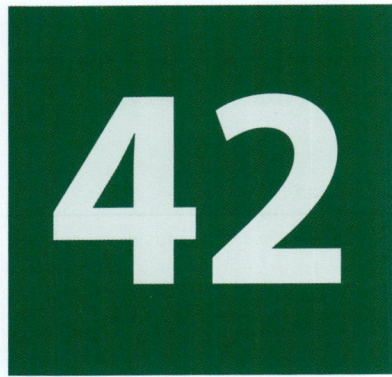

42

Infections: Bacterial & Spirochetal

Hai Nguyen-Tran, MD

Yosuke Nomura, MD

James Gaensbauer, MD, MScPH

BACTERIAL INFECTIONS

GROUP A STREPTOCOCCAL INFECTIONS

ESSENTIALS OF DIAGNOSIS & TYPICAL FEATURES

▶ Streptococcal pharyngitis:
- Sore throat, purulent tonsillitis, tender cervical adenopathy, fever, and absence of viral respiratory symptoms.
- Throat culture or rapid antigen detection test positive for group A streptococci (GAS).

▶ Impetigo:
- Rapidly spreading, highly infectious vesicopustular skin rash.
- Erythematous denuded areas and honey-colored crusts.
- GAS are grown in culture in most (not all) cases.

▶ General Considerations

Group A streptococci (GAS) are common gram-positive bacteria producing a wide variety of clinical illnesses, including acute pharyngitis, impetigo, cellulitis, and scarlet fever. GAS can also cause pneumonia, septic arthritis, osteomyelitis, meningitis, and other less common infections. GAS infections may also produce postinfectious sequelae (rheumatic fever and poststreptococcal glomerulonephritis [PSGN]).

Almost all GAS are β-hemolytic. These organisms may be carried without symptoms on the skin and in the pharynx, rectum, and vagina. GAS are sensitive to penicillin. Resistance to erythromycin is common in some countries and has increased in the United States.

▶ Prevention

GAS pharyngitis usually occurs after contact with respiratory secretions of a person infected with GAS. Crowding facilitates spread of GAS and outbreaks of pharyngitis and impetigo occur. Prompt recognition and institution of antibiotics may decrease spread. Treatment with antibiotics prevents acute rheumatic fever.

▶ Clinical Findings

A. Symptoms and Signs

1. Ear/nose/throat infections

A. INFANCY AND EARLY CHILDHOOD (AGE < 3 YEARS)— The onset is insidious, with mild symptoms (low-grade fever, serous nasal discharge, and pallor). Otitis media is common. Exudative pharyngitis and cervical adenitis are uncommon in this age group.

B. CHILDHOOD TYPE—Classic GAS pharyngitis presents with the sudden onset of fever, sore throat, headache, malaise, abdominal pain, and often vomiting. On examination, tonsillar exudate and tender anterior cervical adenopathy are usually noted. Petechiae are frequently seen on the soft palate.

2. Scarlet fever—In scarlet fever, the skin is diffusely erythematous and appears sunburned and roughened (sandpaper rash); most intense in the axillae, groin, and on the abdomen and trunk. It blanches except in the skin folds, which do not blanch and are pigmented (Pastia sign). The rash usually appears 24 hours after the onset of fever and rapidly spreads over the next 1–2 days. Desquamation begins on the face at the end of the first week and becomes generalized by the third week. Early in the infection, there is circumoral pallor and the surface of the tongue is coated white, with the papillae enlarged and bright red (white strawberry tongue). Subsequently desquamation occurs, and the tongue appears

beefy red (strawberry tongue). Petechiae may be seen on any mucosal surfaces.

3. Impetigo—Streptococcal impetigo begins as a papule that vesiculates and then breaks, leaving a denuded area covered by a honey-colored crust. Both *Staphylococcus aureus* and GAS are isolated in some cases. The lesions spread readily and diffusely. Local lymph nodes may become swollen and inflamed. Although the child often lacks systemic symptoms, a high fever and toxicity may be present. If flaccid bullae are noted, the disease is called bullous impetigo and is caused by an epidermolytic toxin-producing strain of *S aureus*.

4. Cellulitis—The portal of entry is often an insect bite or superficial abrasion. A diffuse, rapidly spreading cellulitis occurs that involves the subcutaneous tissues and extends along the lymphatic pathways with only minimal local suppuration. Local acute lymphadenitis occurs. The child is usually acutely ill, with fever and malaise. In erysipelas, the involved area is bright red, swollen, warm, and very tender with well-demarcated borders. The infection may extend rapidly from the lymphatics to the bloodstream.

Streptococcal perianal cellulitis is an entity peculiar to young children. Pain with defecation often leads to constipation, which may be the presenting complaint. The child is afebrile and otherwise well. Perianal erythema, tenderness, and painful rectal examination are the only abnormal physical findings. Scant rectal bleeding with defecation may occur. A perianal swab culture usually yields heavy growth of GAS. A variant of this syndrome is streptococcal vaginitis in prepubertal girls. Symptoms are dysuria and pain. Marked erythema and tenderness of the introitus and blood-tinged discharge are seen.

5. Necrotizing skin and soft tissue infection—This dangerous disease is reported sporadically and may occur as a complication of varicella infection. GAS is the most common cause of necrotizing skin and soft tissue infection in children, followed by *S aureus*. The disease is characterized by extensive necrosis of superficial fasciae, undermining of surrounding tissue, and usually systemic toxicity. Initially the skin overlying the infection is tender and pale red without distinct borders, resembling cellulitis. Blisters or bullae may appear. The color deepens to a distinct purple or in some cases becomes pale. Tenderness out of proportion to the clinical appearance, skin anesthesia (due to infarction of superficial nerves), or "woody" induration suggest necrotizing fasciitis. Involved areas may develop mild to massive edema.

6. Group A streptococcal infections in newborn nurseries—GAS epidemics occur occasionally in nurseries. The organism may be introduced into the nursery from the vaginal tract of a mother or from the throat or nose of a mother or a staff member. The organism then spreads from infant to infant. The umbilical stump is colonized while the infant is in the nursery. Most often, a colonized infant develops a chronic oozing omphalitis days later. The organism may spread from the infant to other family members. Serious and even fatal infections may develop, including sepsis, meningitis, empyema, septic arthritis, and peritonitis.

7. Streptococcal sepsis—Sepsis frequently occurs in conjunction with a focal source of infection, but can also manifest as isolated bacteremia. Scarletiniform rash may or may not be present. Prostration and shock result in high mortality rates. Pharyngitis is uncommon as an antecedent illness. Underlying disease is a predisposing factor.

8. Streptococcal toxic shock syndrome (STSS)—Toxic shock syndrome (TSS) can be caused by GAS and is typically more severe than *S aureus*–associated toxic shock; multiorgan system involvement is a prominent part of the illness. The diagnostic criteria include (1) isolation of GAS from a normally sterile site, (2) hypotension or shock, and (3) at least two of the following: renal impairment (creatinine more than two times the upper limit of normal for age), thrombocytopenia ($< 100,000/mm^3$) or coagulopathy, liver involvement (transaminases or bilirubin $\geq$ two times normal), acute respiratory distress syndrome, erythematous macular rash, or soft tissue necrosis (myositis, necrotizing fasciitis, gangrene). In cases that otherwise meet clinical criteria, isolation of GAS from a nonsterile site (throat, wound, or vagina) is indicative of a "probable case."

B. Laboratory Findings

Leukocytosis with a marked shift to the left is seen early. β-Hemolytic streptococci are cultured from the throat or site of infection. For suspected GAS pharyngitis, the throat should be swabbed and the specimen sent for GAS testing (rapid antigen detection tests and/or culture for GAS) because the clinical features of some viral infections may overlap with the clinical features of GAS. In children and adolescents, negative rapid antigen tests should be backed up by a culture. Patients with positive rapid strep antigen tests do not need a confirmation by throat culture, since the specificities of antigen tests are high. The Food and Drug Administration (FDA) has approved nucleic acid amplification tests (NAATs) for the detection of GAS from throat swab specimens. NAATs have similar sensitivity and specificity to culture, and offer the advantage of rapidly available results. The organism may be cultured from the skin and by needle aspiration from subcutaneous tissues and other involved sites such as infected nodes. Occasionally blood cultures are positive.

Antistreptolysin O (ASO) titers rise about 150 units within 2 weeks after acute infection. Elevated ASO and anti-DNase B titers may be useful in documenting prior throat infections in cases of acute rheumatic fever and poststreptococcal glomerulonephritis (PSGN), although they may remain elevated for several months and even years after the original infection.

Proteinuria, cylindruria, and minimal hematuria may be seen early in children with streptococcal infection.

Differential Diagnosis

Streptococcal infection in early childhood must be differentiated from adenovirus and other respiratory virus infections. The pharyngitis in herpangina (coxsackievirus A) is vesicular or ulcerative. Herpes simplex also causes ulcerative lesions, which most commonly involve the anterior pharynx, tongue, and gums. In infectious mononucleosis, the pharyngitis is also exudative, but splenomegaly and generalized adenopathy are typical, and laboratory findings are often diagnostic (atypical lymphocytes, a positive heterophile, or other serologic test for mononucleosis). Uncomplicated streptococcal pharyngitis improves within 24–48 hours if penicillin is given and by 72–96 hours without antimicrobials.

Arcanobacterium hemolyticum may cause pharyngitis with scarlatina-like or maculopapular truncal rash. In diphtheria, systemic symptoms, vomiting, and fever are less marked; pharyngeal pseudomembrane is confluent and adherent; the throat is less red; and cervical adenopathy is prominent. Pharyngeal tularemia causes white rather than yellow exudate; there is little erythema; and cultures for β-hemolytic streptococci are negative. A history of exposure to rabbits and a failure to respond to antimicrobials may suggest the diagnosis. Oral gonococcal infection may also cause pharyngitis with tonsillar exudate.

Scarlet fever must be differentiated from other exanthematous diseases, erythema due to sunburn, drug reactions, Kawasaki disease, TSS, and staphylococcal scalded skin syndrome (see also Table 40–3).

Complications

Suppurative complications of GAS infections include sinusitis, otitis, mastoiditis, cervical lymphadenitis, pneumonia, empyema, septic arthritis, sepsis, and meningitis. Spread of streptococcal infection from the throat to other sites—principally the skin (impetigo) and vagina—is common and should be considered in every instance of chronic vaginal discharge or chronic skin infection, such as that complicating childhood eczema. Both acute rheumatic fever and PSGN are nonsuppurative complications of GAS infections.

A. Acute Rheumatic Fever (See Chapter 20)

B. Acute Glomerulonephritis

PSGN can follow streptococcal infections of either the pharynx or the skin—in contrast to rheumatic fever, which follows pharyngeal infection. PSGN may occur at any age. The risk is higher in school-aged children and members of indigenous populations. In most reports of PSGN, males predominate by a ratio of 2:1. Rheumatic fever occurs with equal frequency in both sexes. Certain GAS strains are associated with PSGN (nephritogenic types).

The median period between infection and the development of glomerulonephritis is 10 days. In contrast, acute rheumatic fever occurs after a median of 18 days.

C. Poststreptococcal Reactive Arthritis

Following an episode of GAS pharyngitis, reactive arthritis develops in some patients. This reactive arthritis is believed to be due to immune complex deposition and is seen 1–2 weeks following the acute infection. Patients with poststreptococcal reactive arthritis do not have the full constellation of clinical and laboratory criteria needed to fulfill the Jones criteria for a diagnosis of acute rheumatic fever.

Treatment

A. Specific Measures

Treatment is directed toward both eradication of acute infection and prevention of rheumatic fever. In patients with pharyngitis, antibiotics should be started early to relieve symptoms and should be continued for 10 days to prevent rheumatic fever. Although early therapy has not been shown to prevent PSGN, it seems advisable to treat impetigo promptly in sibling contacts of patients with PSGN. Although topical therapy for limited impetigo with antimicrobial ointments (especially mupirocin) is possible, it does not eradicate pharyngeal carriage and is less practical for extensive disease.

1. Penicillin—For GAS pharyngitis, the following regimens can be used. Except for penicillin-allergic patients, penicillin V (phenoxymethyl penicillin) is the drug of choice. Penicillin resistance has never been documented. For children weighing less than 27 kg, the regimen is 250 mg, given orally two or three times a day for 10 days. For children or adults weighting more than 27 kg, 500 mg two or three times a day is recommended. Giving penicillin V twice daily is as effective as more frequent oral administration. Alternatively, amoxicillin 50 mg/kg/day as a single daily dose (maximum 1000 mg) can be used. Another alternative for treatment of pharyngitis and impetigo is a single dose of penicillin G benzathine given intramuscularly (600,000 units for children weighing ≤ 27 kg and 1.2 million units for children weighing > 27 kg). Intramuscular delivery ensures compliance, but is painful. Parenteral therapy is indicated if vomiting is present. Mild cellulitis due to GAS may be treated orally or intramuscularly. For severe or invasive GAS infections intravenous antibiotics are indicated.

GAS cellulitis requiring hospitalization can be treated with aqueous penicillin G or cefazolin until there is marked improvement. Penicillin V or cephalexin may then be given orally to complete a 10-day course.

2. Other antibiotics—Cephalexin and azithromycin are other effective oral antimicrobials. Clindamycin is also effective, but resistance is occasionally present. For penicillin-allergic patients with pharyngitis or impetigo, azithromycin or clindamycin may be used. Patients with immediate, anaphylactic hypersensitivity to penicillin should not receive cephalosporins, because up to 15% will also be allergic to cephalosporins. Macrolide resistance rates vary and may be high in some areas of the world. In general, macrolide resistance rates in most of the United States are 5%–8%. In most studies, bacteriologic failures after cephalosporin therapy are less frequent than failures following penicillin. However, there are few conclusive data on the ability of these agents to prevent rheumatic fever. Therefore, penicillin remains the agent of choice for nonallergic patients. Many strains are resistant to tetracycline. Neither sulfonamides nor trimethoprim-sulfamethoxazole (TMP-SMX) is effective in the treatment of streptococcal infections.

For serious infections requiring intravenous therapy, aqueous penicillin G is the drug of choice. Cefazolin, clindamycin, and vancomycin are alternatives in penicillin-allergic pediatric patients. Clindamycin should not be used alone empirically for severe, suspected GAS infections because a small percentage of isolates in the United States are resistant.

3. Serious GAS disease—Serious GAS infections, such as pneumonia, osteomyelitis, septic arthritis, sepsis, endocarditis, meningitis, and STSS, require parenteral penicillin G as the drug of choice. Clindamycin, a protein synthesis inhibitor, is advocated by many experts for STSS or necrotizing fasciitis as a second agent along with penicillin G to inhibit toxin production. Necrotizing skin and soft tissue infection requires prompt surgical debridement. In STSS, volume status and blood pressure should be monitored and patients evaluated for a focus of infection, if not readily apparent. Intravenous immunoglobulin (in addition to antibiotics) has been added in severe cases.

4. Treatment failure—Even when compliance is perfect, organisms will be found in cultures in 5%–35% of children after cessation of therapy. Reculture is indicated only in patients with relapse or recrudescence of pharyngitis or those with a personal or family history of rheumatic fever. Repeat treatment at least once with an oral cephalosporin or clindamycin is indicated in patients with recurrent culture-positive pharyngitis.

5. Prevention of recurrences in patients with previous rheumatic fever (see Chapter 20)

6. Poststreptococcal reactive arthritis—In contrast to rheumatic fever, nonsteroidal agents may not dramatically improve joint symptoms. However, like patients with rheumatic fever, some patients with poststreptococcal reactive arthritis have developed carditis several weeks to months after their arthritis symptoms began. Patients should be monitored for development of carditis for the next 1–2 years. Some experts recommend antibiotic prophylaxis of these patients (same prophylaxis prevention regimens as for acute rheumatic fever) for 1–2 years and monitoring for signs of carditis (see Chapter 20). If carditis does not develop, prophylaxis can be discontinued. If carditis develops, the patient should be considered to have acute rheumatic fever and prophylaxis continued.

B. General Measures

Acetaminophen or ibuprofen is useful for pain or fever. Local treatment of impetigo may promote earlier healing. Crusts should first be soaked off. Areas beneath the crusts should then be washed with soap daily.

C. Treatment of Complications

Acute cervical lymphadenitis may require incision and drainage. Treatment of necrotizing fasciitis requires emergency surgical debridement followed by high-dose parenteral antibiotics appropriate to the organisms cultured.

D. Treatment of Carriers

Identification and treatment of GAS carriers are difficult. There are no established clinical or serologic criteria for differentiating carriers from the truly infected. Up to 20% of school-aged children in some studies are asymptomatic pharyngeal carriers of GAS. Streptococcal carriers are individuals who do not mount an immune response to the organism and are therefore believed to be at low risk for nonsuppurative sequelae. Some children receive multiple courses of antimicrobials, with persistence of GAS in the throat, leading to a "streptococcal neurosis" on the part of families.

In certain circumstances, eradication of carriage may be desirable: (1) when a family member has a history of rheumatic fever; (2) when an episode of STSS or necrotizing fasciitis has occurred in a household contact; (3) multiple, recurring, documented episodes of GAS in family members despite adequate therapy; and (4) during an outbreak of rheumatic fever or GAS-associated glomerulonephritis. Clindamycin (20–30 mg/kg/day, given orally in three divided doses; maximum dose 300 mg) or a combination of rifampin (20 mg/kg/day, given orally for 4 days) and penicillin in standard dosage given orally has been used to attempt eradication of carriage.

▶ Prognosis

Death is rare except in infants or young children with sepsis, necrotizing infection, or pneumonia. The febrile course is shortened, and complications are eliminated by early and adequate treatment with penicillin.

Centers for Disease Control and Prevention: https://www.cdc.gov/groupastrep/index.html. Accessed May 9, 2023.

Shulman ST et al: Clinical practice guideline for the diagnosis and management of group A streptococcal pharyngitis: 2012 update by the Infectious Diseases Society of America. Clin Infect Dis 2012;55(10):1279–1282. http://cid.oxfordjournals.org/content/early/2012/09/06/cid.cis629.full [PMID: 22965026].

GROUP B STREPTOCOCCAL INFECTIONS

ESSENTIALS OF DIAGNOSIS & TYPICAL FEATURES

▶ Early-onset disease:
  • Newborn younger than 7 days, with rapidly progressing overwhelming sepsis, with or without meningitis.
  • Pneumonia with respiratory failure is frequent; chest radiograph resembles that seen in hyaline membrane disease.
  • Blood or cerebrospinal fluid (CSF) cultures growing group B streptococci (GBS).
▶ Late-onset disease:
  • Meningitis, sepsis, or other focal infection in a child aged 7–89 days with blood or CSF cultures growing GBS.

▶ Prevention

Many women of childbearing age possess type-specific circulating antibody to the polysaccharide antigens of group B *Streptococcus* (GBS). These antibodies are transferred to the newborn via the placental circulation. In contrast, women delivering infants who develop either early- or late-onset GBS disease rarely have detectable antibody in their sera. There is no licensed vaccine for GBS disease prevention, but vaccines are being studied for pregnant women.

▶ Recommendations for Prevention of Perinatal GBS Disease

1. Caregivers for pregnant women are referred to the American College of Obstetricians and Gynecologists (ACOG) guidelines for screening of pregnant women for GBS and use of intrapartum antibiotic prophylaxis (IAP)—see https://www.acog.org/clinical/clinical-guidance/committee-opinion/articles/2020/02/prevention-of-group-b-streptococcal-early-onset-disease-in-newborns.

2. Indications for IAP to prevent early-onset group B streptococcal (GBS) disease are given in Table 42–1.

3. Risk assessment for early-onset GBS infection for infants born ≥ 35 weeks' gestation.

4. Risk assessment for early-onset GBS infection for infants born ≤ 34 weeks' gestation.

▶ Clinical Findings

The incidence of perinatal GBS disease has declined dramatically since screening of pregnant mothers and provision of IAP began. Although most patients with GBS disease are infants younger than 3 months, cases are seen in infants aged 4–5 months. Serious GBS infection also occurs in women with puerperal sepsis, immunocompromised patients, patients with cirrhosis and spontaneous peritonitis, and diabetic patients with cellulitis. Two distinct clinical syndromes distinguished by differing perinatal event and age at onset occur in infants.

A. Early-Onset Disease

"Early-onset" disease is observed in newborns younger than 7 days. Risk factors for early-onset disease include maternal GBS colonization, gestational age less than 37 weeks, rupture of membranes more than 18 hours prior to presentation, young maternal age, history of a previous infant with invasive GBS disease, African-American or Hispanic ethnicity, and low or absent maternal GBS anticapsular antibodies. The onset of symptoms in the majority of these infants is in the first 48 hours of life, and most are ill within 6 hours. Respiratory abnormalities, irritability, lethargy, temperature instability, or poor perfusion may be presenting signs. Sepsis, shock, meningitis, and pneumonia are the most common clinical presentations. Although premature infants are at increased risk for the disease, most infants with early-onset infections are full term. Newborns with early-onset infection acquire GBS in utero as an ascending infection or during passage through the birth canal.

B. Late-Onset Disease

"Late-onset" disease occurs in infants between ages 7 and 89 days (median age at onset is about 4 weeks). Maternal obstetric complications are not usually associated with late-onset disease. However, young maternal age and prematurity remain risk factors. Late-onset disease is not prevented by IAP. The most common presentation of late-onset disease is bacteremia without focus, and compared to early-onset disease, with a higher proportion presenting with meningitis. Pneumonia, septic arthritis and osteomyelitis, otitis media, ethmoiditis, conjunctivitis, cellulitis (particularly of the face or submandibular area), lymphadenitis, breast abscess, empyema, and impetigo have also been described. The exact mode of transmission of the organisms is not well defined.

C. Laboratory Findings

Culture of GBS from a normally sterile site such as blood, pleural fluid, or CSF provides proof of diagnosis.

Table 42–1. Indications for intrapartum antibiotic prophylaxis to prevent neonatal group B streptococcal early-onset disease.

Intrapartum GBS Prophylaxis Indicated	Intrapartum GBS Prophylaxis Not Indicated
Maternal history • Previous neonate with invasive GBS disease	• Colonization with GBS during a previous pregnancy (unless colonization status in current pregnancy is unknown at onset of labor at term)
Current pregnancy • Positive GBS culture obtained at 36 0/7 weeks of gestation or more during current pregnancy (unless a cesarean birth is performed before onset of labor for a woman with intact amniotic membranes) • GBS bacteriuria during any trimester of the current pregnancy	• Negative vaginal–rectal GBS culture obtained at 36 0/7 weeks of gestation or more during the current pregnancy • Cesarean birth performed before onset of labor on a woman with intact amniotic membranes, regardless of GBS colonization status or gestational age

Intrapartum
• Unknown GBS status at the onset of labor (culture not done or results unknown) and any of the following:
  • Birth at less than 37 0/7 weeks of gestation
  • Amniotic membrane rupture 18 hours or more Intrapartum temperature 100.4°F (38.0°C) or higher[a]
  • Intrapartum NAAT result positive for GBS
  • Intrapartum NAAT result negative but risk factors develop (ie, less than 37 0/7 weeks of gestation, amniotic membrane rupture 18 hours or more, or maternal temperature 100.4°F (38.0°C) or higher
• Known GBS-positive status in a previous pregnancy
	• Negative vaginal–rectal GBS culture obtained at 36 0/7 weeks of gestation or more during the current pregnancy, regardless of intrapartum risk factors
	• Unknown GBS status at onset of labor, NAAT result negative and no intrapartum risk factors present (ie, less than 37 0/7 weeks of gestation, amniotic membrane rupture 18 hours or more, or maternal temperature 100.4°F (38°C) or higher

Abbreviations: GBS, group B *Streptococcus*: NAAT, nucleic acid amplification test.
[a]If intra-amniotic infection is suspected, broad-spectrum antibiotic therapy that includes an agent known to be active against GBS should replace GBS prophylaxis.
Modified from Verani JR, McGee L, Schrag SJ, et al: Prevention of perinatal group B streptococcal disease -revised guidelines from CDC, 2010. MMWR Recomm Rep. 2010 Nov 19;59(RR-10):1–36.

Treatment

Intravenous ampicillin and an aminoglycoside are the initial regimens of choice for newborns up to 7 days of age with presumptive invasive GBS disease. In a critically ill newborn, particularly in those with very low birth weight, empirical addition of broader-spectrum therapy should be considered. For late-onset disease in previously healthy infants in the community, empirical therapy consists of ampicillin and ceftazidime in infants 8–28 days of age and ceftriaxone alone in infants 29–90 days of age as long as the infant is not critically ill, and there is no evidence of meningitis. Vancomycin should be added to empiric coverage if there is evidence of meningitis, or if the infant is critically ill.

Penicillin G can be used alone once GBS is identified and clinical and microbiologic responses have occurred. Ampicillin is an acceptable alternative therapy. GBS is less susceptible than other streptococci to beta-lactam antibiotics, and high doses are recommended, especially for meningitis.

A second lumbar puncture after 24–48 hours of therapy is recommended by some experts to assess efficacy. Duration of therapy is 2 weeks for uncomplicated meningitis; at least

4 weeks for osteomyelitis, cerebritis, ventriculitis, or endocarditis, and 10 days for bacteremia. Therapy does not eradicate carriage of the organism.

Although streptococci have been universally susceptible to penicillins, increased minimum inhibitory concentrations (MICs) have been observed in some isolates. Resistance of isolates to clindamycin and erythromycin has increased significantly worldwide.

Infants diagnosed with GBS infection who are part of a multiple birth (twins, triplets, etc.) define a risk for acquisition of invasive GBS disease in their siblings, who should be closely monitored and if signs of illness occur, promptly evaluated and treated for possible systemic infection.

Prognosis

Mortality is correlated with gestational age—in EOD, case fatality was 2.1% in term and 19.2% in preterm infants and in LOD, 3.4% in term and 7.8% in preterm infants. Rates of recurrence of GBS disease range from 0.5% to 3%, and parents should be counseled on this possibility even after effective treatment.

https://www.acog.org/clinical/clinical-guidance/committee-opinion/articles/2020/02/prevention-of-group-b-streptococcal-early-onset-disease-in-newborns.

Prevention of group B streptococcal early-onset disease in newborns. ACOG Committee Opinion No. 797. American College of Obstetricians and Gynecologists. Obstet Gynecol 2020;135:e51–e72.

Puopolo KM, Lynfield R, Cummings JJ; Committee on Fetus and Newborn and Committee on Infectious Diseases: Management of infants at risk for group B streptococcal disease. Pediatrics Aug 2019;144(2):e20191881. doi: https://doi.org/10.1542/peds.2019-1881.

OTHER STREPTOCOCCAL & ENTEROCOCCAL INFECTIONS

▶ General Considerations

Streptococci of groups other than A and B are part of the normal flora of humans and can occasionally cause disease. Group C or G organisms occasionally produce pharyngitis, but without risk of subsequent rheumatic fever. AGN may occasionally occur. *Enterococcus* species are normal inhabitants of the gastrointestinal tract and may produce urinary tract infections, meningitis, sepsis in the newborn, and endocarditis.

Nosocomial infections caused by *Enterococcus* are frequent in neonatal and oncology units and in patients with central venous catheters. Nonhemolytic aerobic streptococci and β-hemolytic streptococci, which are normal mouth flora, are involved in the production of dental plaque and probably dental caries, and are the most common cause of subacute infective endocarditis. Finally, there are numerous anaerobic and microaerophilic streptococci, normal flora of the mouth, skin, and gastrointestinal tract, which alone or in combination with other bacteria may cause sinusitis, dental abscesses, brain abscesses, and intraabdominal or lung abscesses.

▶ Prevention

Streptococci (other than group A or B) are common normal flora in humans. Some disease caused by these organisms can be prevented by maintaining good oral hygiene. Spread of vancomycin-resistant enterococcal strains can be limited by good infection-control practices in healthcare environments and by antimicrobial stewardship.

▶ Treatment

A. Enterococcal Infections

Enterococcus faecalis and *Enterococcus faecium* are the most common and most important strains causing human infections. In general, *E faecalis* is more susceptible to antibiotics than *E faecium*, but antibiotic resistance is commonly seen with both species. Invasive enterococcal infections should be treated with ampicillin if the isolate is susceptible or vancomycin in combination with gentamicin. Gentamicin should be discontinued if susceptibility testing demonstrates high-level resistance to gentamicin. Isolates that are resistant to both ampicillin and vancomycin necessitate other therapeutic options.

1. Infections with ampicillin-susceptible enterococci— Lower urinary tract infections can be treated with oral amoxicillin. Pyelonephritis should be treated intravenously with ampicillin. Sepsis or meningitis in the newborn should be treated intravenously with a combination of ampicillin and gentamicin. Peak serum gentamicin levels of 3–5 mcg/mL are adequate as gentamicin is functioning as a synergistic agent. Consult the American Heart Association guidelines for treatment recommendations for infective endocarditis.

2. Infections with ampicillin-resistant or vancomycin-resistant enterococci—Ampicillin-resistant enterococci are often susceptible to vancomycin. Vancomycin-resistant enterococci are usually also resistant to ampicillin. Linezolid is the only agent approved for use in children for vancomycin-resistant *E faecium* infections. Daptomycin and tigecycline have been used off-label for vancomycin-resistant enterococci; quinupristin-dalfopristin has been used to treat vancomycin-resistant *E faecium* but is not effective against *E faecalis*. Isolates resistant to linezolid, daptomycin, and quinupristin-dalfopristin have been reported. Infectious disease consultation is recommended when use of these drugs is entertained or when vancomycin-resistant enterococcal infections are identified.

B. Viridans Streptococci Infections (Subacute Infective Endocarditis)

It is important to determine the penicillin sensitivity of the infecting strain as early as possible in the treatment of viridans streptococcal endocarditis. Resistant organisms are most commonly seen in patients receiving penicillin prophylaxis for rheumatic heart disease. Treatment of endocarditis varies depending on whether the patient has native valves or prosthetic valves/material and whether the organism is penicillin susceptible. Refer to the American Heart Association Guidelines on Infective Endocarditis for a complete discussion and recommendations.

C. Other Viridans Streptococci–Related Infections

Viridans streptococci are normal flora of the gastrointestinal tract, respiratory tract, and the mouth. In many cases, isolation of viridans streptococci from a blood culture is considered to be a "contaminant" in the absence of signs or symptoms of endocarditis or other invasive disease. However, in children who are immunocompromised, have congenital or acquired valvular heart disease, or who have indwelling lines, viridans streptococci may cause serious morbidity. About one-third of bacteremias in patients with malignancies may be due to bacteria from the *Streptococcus* viridans group. Mucositis and gastrointestinal toxicity from chemotherapy are risk factors for developing disease. Even in children with normal immune systems, viridans streptococci sometimes cause serious infections. For example, viridans streptococci isolated from an abdominal abscess after rupture of the appendix represents a true pathogen. *Streptococcus anginosus*, a member of the *Streptococcus* viridans group, can cause intracranial abscess (often as a complication of sinusitis) and abdominal abscesses. In patients with risk factors or signs/symptoms for subacute endocarditis, isolation of one of the members of the *Streptococcus* viridans group should prompt consideration and evaluation for possible endocarditis (see previous section).

Increasing prevalence of penicillin resistance has been seen in isolates of the streptococci viridans group. Penicillin resistance varies with geographic region, institution, and the populations tested, but ranges from 30% to 70% in oncology patients. Cephalosporin resistance is also relatively common. Therefore, it is important to obtain antibiotic susceptibilities to the organism to select effective therapy. Vancomycin, linezolid, and quinupristin-dalfopristin remain effective against most isolates.

Baltimore RS et al: Infective endocarditis in childhood: 2015 update: a scientific statement from the American Heart Association. Circulation 2015;132(15):1487–1515 [PMID: 26373317]. http://circ.ahajournals.org/content/132/15/1487.
Centers for Disease Control and Prevention: http://www.cdc.gov/hai/organisms/vre/vre.html. Accessed May 11, 2023.

PNEUMOCOCCAL INFECTIONS

ESSENTIALS OF DIAGNOSIS & TYPICAL FEATURES

► Bacteremia:
  • High fever (> 39.4°C).
  • Leukocytosis (> 15,000/μL).
► Pneumonia:
  • Fever, leukocytosis, and tachypnea.
  • Localized chest pain.
  • Localized or diffuse rales. Chest radiograph may show lobar infiltrate (with effusion).
► Meningitis:
  • Fever, leukocytosis.
  • Bulging fontanelle, neck stiffness.
  • Irritability and lethargy.
► All types:
  • Diagnosis confirmed by cultures of blood, CSF, pleural fluid, or other body fluid.

General Considerations

Sepsis, sinusitis, otitis media, pneumonitis, meningitis, osteomyelitis, cellulitis, arthritis, vaginitis, and peritonitis are part of the spectrum of pneumococcal infection.

The incidence of all pneumococcal disease phenotypes, including the invasive conditions of sepsis, pneumonia, and meningitis has decreased since incorporation of the pneumococcal conjugate vaccine into the infant vaccine schedule; however, sporadic cases still occur. Pneumococcal meningitis, sometimes recurrent, may complicate serious head trauma, particularly if there is persistent leakage of CSF.

Children with sickle cell disease, other hemoglobinopathies, congenital or acquired asplenia, and some immunoglobulin and complement deficiencies, and patients receiving biologic modifiers inhibiting B-cell and complement function, are unusually susceptible to pneumococcal sepsis and meningitis. They often have a catastrophic illness with shock and disseminated intravascular coagulation (DIC). The spleen is important in the control of pneumococcal infection. Autosplenectomy may explain why children with sickle cell disease are at increased risk of developing serious pneumococcal infections. Children with cochlear implants are at higher risk for pneumococcal meningitis.

S pneumoniae rarely causes serious disease in the neonate. However, occasionally pneumonia, sepsis, or meningitis may occur and clinically is similar to GBS infection.

Prevention

Two pneumococcal vaccines are licensed for use in children in the United States: 13-valent pneumococcal conjugate vaccine (PCV13) and 23-valent pneumococcal polysaccharide vaccine (PPSV23). PCV13 was licensed in 2010 (replacing the 7-valent pneumococcal vaccine). It contains antigens from 13 pneumococcal serotypes and is currently recommended for routine use in the infant and childhood immunization schedule. In 2023, ACIP recommended PCV15 or PCV20 for pneumococcal conjugate vaccination. These vaccines and indications for use are discussed in detail in Chapter 10.

Clinical Findings

A. Symptoms and Signs

In pneumococcal sepsis, fever usually appears abruptly, often accompanied by chills. There may be no respiratory symptoms. In infants and young children with pneumonia, fever, and tachypnea without auscultatory changes are the usual presenting signs. Respiratory distress is manifested by nasal flaring, chest retractions, and tachypnea. Abdominal pain is common. *Streptococcus pneumoniae* is a common cause of acute otitis media (AOM) and is the organism responsible for most cases of acute bacterial pneumonia in children. In older children, the adult form of pneumococcal pneumonia with signs of lobar consolidation may occur, but sputum is rarely bloody. Effusions are common, although frank empyema is less common. Abscesses also occasionally occur. Inspiratory pain (from pleural involvement) is sometimes present, but is less common in children. With involvement of the right hemidiaphragm, pain may be referred to the right lower quadrant, suggesting appendicitis. Vomiting is common at onset but seldom persists. Convulsions are relatively common at onset in infants.

Meningitis is characterized by fever, irritability or severe lethargy, convulsions, and neck stiffness. The most important sign in very young infants is a tense, bulging anterior fontanelle. In older children, fever, chills, headache, and vomiting are common. Classic signs are nuchal rigidity associated with positive Brudzinski and Kernig signs.

B. Laboratory Findings

With invasive disease leukocytosis is often pronounced (20,000–45,000/μL), with 80%–90% polymorphonuclear neutrophils. Levels of C-reactive protein and procalcitonin are typically very elevated. Neutropenia may be seen early in very serious infections. The presence of pneumococci in the nasopharynx is not a helpful finding, because up to 40% of healthy children carry pneumococci in the upper respiratory tract. A large number of organisms are seen on Gram-stained smears of endotracheal aspirates from patients with pneumonia. A positive blood culture in the setting of a lobar pneumonia is considered diagnostic. The CSF usually shows an elevated white blood cell (WBC) count of several thousand, chiefly polymorphonuclear neutrophils, with decreased glucose and elevated protein levels. Gram-positive diplococci may be seen on some (but not all) stained smears of CSF sediment. Isolation of S pneumoniae from a normally sterile site (eg, blood, CSF, joint fluid, middle ear fluid) or from a suppurative focus confirms the diagnosis. The diagnosis can also be confirmed using polymerase chain reaction (PCR)—often in the context of multiplex-PCR assays of positive blood culture or CSF samples. Chest radiographs frequently reveal lobar consolidation and may also demonstrate complications such as pleural effusions or empyema.

▶ Differential Diagnosis

There are many causes of high fever and leukocytosis in young infants other than invasive pneumococcal disease. The differential diagnosis includes viral infection, urinary tract infection, and unrecognized focal infection elsewhere in the body.

Though pneumococcus is the most common cause of severe pneumonia, other etiologies, such as S aureus or Klebsiella pneumoniae, should be considered until there is microbiological confirmation. Milder cases of pneumonia are frequently caused by viruses, particularly in the absence of lobar consolidation. Pneumonia caused by Mycoplasma pneumoniae may result in a similar illness to pneumococcal

disease, though onset is typically more insidious, with infrequent chills, low-grade fever, prominent headache and malaise, cough, and, often, striking radiographic changes. Marked leukocytosis (> 18,000/μL) is unusual.

Children with primary pulmonary tuberculosis (TB) are not toxic, and radiographs show a primary focus associated with hilar adenopathy, often with pleural involvement. Miliary TB presents a classic radiographic appearance.

Pneumococcal meningitis is diagnosed by lumbar puncture. Without a Gram-stain, PCR or culture confirmation from CSF, pneumococcal meningitis is not distinguishable from other types of acute bacterial meningitis.

▶ Complications

Complications of sepsis include meningitis and osteomyelitis; complications of pneumonia include empyema, parapneumonic effusion, and, rarely, lung abscess. Mastoiditis, subdural empyema, and brain abscess may follow untreated pneumococcal AOM. Both pneumococcal meningitis and peritonitis are more likely to occur independently without coexisting pneumonia. Shock, DIC, and Waterhouse-Friderichsen syndrome resembling meningococcemia are occasionally seen in pneumococcal sepsis, particularly in asplenic patients. Hemolytic-uremic syndrome (HUS) may occur as a complication of pneumococcal pneumonia.

▶ Treatment

A. Specific Measures

All S pneumoniae isolated from normally sterile sites should be tested for antimicrobial susceptibility. The term "nonsusceptible" is used to describe both intermediate and resistant isolates. Antimicrobial susceptibility breakpoints for S pneumoniae to penicillin and ceftriaxone are based on whether the patient has meningitis and the drug route (Table 42–2). Therapy of meningitis, empyema, osteomyelitis, and endocarditis due to nonsusceptible S pneumoniae is challenging because penetration of antimicrobials to these sites is limited. For empiric therapy of serious or life-threatening infections pending susceptibility test results, vancomycin and ceftriaxone are recommended.

1. Bacteremia—Prior to routine childhood immunization with conjugated pneumococcal vaccine, 3%–5% of blood cultures in patients aged younger than 2 years yielded S pneumoniae. Some children with positive blood cultures were well-appearing; such "occult bacteremias" were often managed with oral antibiotics. This clinical scenario has largely disappeared with pneumococcal conjugate vaccination. All children with blood cultures that grow pneumococci should be reexamined as soon as possible. The child who has a focal infection, such as meningitis, or who appears septic should be admitted to the hospital to receive parenteral antimicrobials. If the child is afebrile and appears well or mildly ill,

Table 42–2. Penicillin breakpoints (minimum inhibitory concentrations [MIC]) for *streptococcus pneumoniae* by susceptibility category—clinical and laboratory standards institute, 2008.

Drug	Clinical Syndrome and Drug Route	Susceptibility Category MIC (mcg/mL)		
		Susceptible	Intermediate	Resistant
Penicillin	Meningitis, intravenous penicillin	≤ 0.06	None[a]	≥ 0.12
	Nonmeningitis, intravenous penicillin	≤ 2	4	≥ 8
	Nonmeningitis, oral penicillin	≤ 0.06	0.12–1	≥ 2
Cefotaxime or ceftriaxone	Meningitis, intravenous cefotaxime or ceftriaxone	≤ 0.5	1	≥ 2
	Nonmeningitis, intravenous cefotaxime or ceftriaxone	≤ 1	2	≥ 4

[a]There is no intermediate category for meningitis.
Reproduced from Centers for Disease Control and Prevention (CDC): Effects of new penicillin susceptibility breakpoints for Streptococcus pneumoniae—United States, 2006–2007. MMWR Morb Mortal Wkly Rep 2008 Dec 19;57(50):1353–1355.

outpatient management is appropriate. Severely ill or immunocompromised children, in whom invasive infection with *S pneumoniae* is suspected, should be empirically treated with vancomycin (in addition to other appropriate antibiotics to cover other suspected pathogens). If meningitis is also suspected, use ceftriaxone in addition to vancomycin until the susceptibilities of the organism are known.

2. Pneumonia—For infants (≥ 1 month of age) with susceptible organisms, appropriate regimens include ampicillin if susceptible to penicillin or ceftriaxone if resistant to penicillin. If susceptibilities are not known and the patient is severely ill or immunocompromised, vancomycin should be used as part of the regimen to provide coverage for penicillin- or cephalosporin-resistant pneumococcus. Once results of susceptibility testing are available, the regimen can be tailored. Mild pneumonia may be treated with amoxicillin (80–90 mg/kg/day) for 7–10 days. Oral cephalosporins are alternatives for penicillin-allergic patients, but many (eg, cefdinir) have unfavorable pharmacokinetics for severe infection. Alternative regimens for penicillin and cephalosporin allergies include levofloxacin.

3. Otitis media—Current American Academy of Pediatrics guidelines recommend oral amoxicillin (80–90 mg/kg/day, divided in two doses) as first-line therapy. Children under 6 months, children 6 months to 23 months with bilateral disease, and children with severe disease require treatment. Young children and those with severe disease require 10 days of treatment; shorter courses (5–7 days) may be adequate for older children with mild or moderate otitis. Intramuscular administration of ceftriaxone may be required for refractory cases of presumed pneumococcal AOM.

4. Meningitis—Until bacteriologic confirmation and susceptibility testing are completed, patients should receive vancomycin and ceftriaxone. Patients with serious hypersensitivity to β-lactam antibiotics (eg, penicillins, cephalosporins) can be treated with a combination of vancomycin (see previous

dosage) and levofloxacin or meropenem. These regimens provide additional gram-negative coverage until culture and susceptibility results are obtained. Dexamethasone, 0.6 mg/kg/day, in four divided doses for 2–4 days may be considered for adjunctive therapy for pneumococcal meningitis. If started, it should be given prior to or concurrently with antibiotic therapy. A repeat lumbar puncture at 24–48 hours should be considered to ensure sterility of the CSF if resistant pneumococci were initially isolated or if the patient is not demonstrating expected improvement after 24–48 hours on therapy.

If the isolate is penicillin-susceptible, aqueous penicillin G can be administered. Alternatively, use of ceftriaxone is an acceptable alternative therapy for penicillin- and cephalosporin-susceptible isolates. Consult an infectious disease specialist or the *Red Book* (American Academy of Pediatrics, 2021) for a complete discussion of pneumococcal meningitis and for therapeutic options for isolates that are nonsusceptible to penicillin or cephalosporins.

▶ **Prognosis**

In children, case fatality rates of less than 1% should be achieved except for meningitis, where rates of 5%–20% still prevail. The presence of large numbers of organisms without a prominent CSF inflammatory response or meningitis due to a penicillin-resistant strain indicates a poor prognosis. Serious neurologic sequelae, particularly hearing loss, are frequent following pneumococcal meningitis.

Bradley JS et al: The management of community-acquired pneumonia in infants and children older than 3 months of age: clinical practice guidelines by the Pediatric Infectious Diseases Society and the Infectious Diseases Society of America. Clin Infect Dis 2011 Oct;53(7):617–630 [PMID: 21890766].
Lieberthal AS et al: Clinical practice guideline: The diagnosis and management of acute otitis media. Pediatrics Mar 2013;131(3):e964–e999. doi: https://doi.org/10.1542/peds.2012-3488.

Streptococcus pneumoniae (Pneumococcal) infections. In: Kimberlin DW, Brady MT, Jackson MA, Long SS (eds): *Red Book: 2021–2024 Report of the Committee on Infectious Diseases.* 32nd ed. Elk Grove Village, IL: American Academy of Pediatrics; 2021:717–727.

STAPHYLOCOCCAL INFECTIONS

ESSENTIALS OF DIAGNOSIS & TYPICAL FEATURES

► Purulent skin and soft tissue infections
  • Boils, furuncles, cellulitis
  • Leukocytosis (> 15,000/μL)
► Musculoskeletal infections
  • Localized pain and swelling
  • Fever
  • Abnormal MRI, possible positive blood culture
► Disseminated or severe infections:
  • Fever, septic shock, organ dysfunction, disseminated lesions, positive blood cultures
  • Toxin-mediated disease causing toxic shock syndrome, localized source of infection
  • Severe pneumonia with cavitation, abscesses, and empyema
  • Endocarditis and endovascular infections, particularly with indwelling lines and foreign material

► General Considerations

Staphylococcal infections are common in childhood and range from mild localized infections to overwhelming systemic infections. Diseases caused by staphylococci include, but are not limited to, furuncles, carbuncles, scalded skin syndrome, osteomyelitis, pyomyositis, septic arthritis, pneumonia, bacteremia, endocarditis, meningitis, and toxic shock syndrome (TSS). Staphylococci are the major cause of skin, soft tissue, bone and joint infections, and are an uncommon but important cause of bacterial pneumonia. Staphylococci are frequent colonizers of the nasopharynx, and a common route of entry to the body is through disruptions in the skin.

S aureus, which is the most common pathogenic species, often produces coagulase. Staphylococci that do not produce this enzyme are termed *coagulase-negative staphylococci.* They rarely cause disease except in compromised hosts, the newborn, or patients with indwelling lines.

Most strains of S aureus elaborate β-lactamase that confers penicillin resistance. This can be overcome by the use of a cephalosporin or a penicillinase-resistant penicillin, such as oxacillin, nafcillin, cloxacillin, or dicloxacillin. Methicillin-resistant S aureus (MRSA) are resistant in vivo to all of these penicillinase-resistant penicillins and cephalosporins. MRSA has dramatically increased in prevalence globally as both a health care-associated and a community-associated pathogen. Health care-associated infections are likely to be multidrug resistant. Community-associated MRSA are most often susceptible to clindamycin and/or TMP-SMX, but resistance rates to these agents vary widely geographically. MRSA strains with intermediate susceptibility to vancomycin occur, and vancomycin-resistant strains have been isolated.

S aureus produces a variety of exotoxins that contribute to specific disease manifestations. The exfoliatin toxin is largely responsible for bullous impetigo and scalded skin syndrome. Enterotoxin causes staphylococcal food poisoning. The exotoxin most commonly associated with TSS has been termed TSST-1. Panton-Valentine leukocidin (PVL) is an exotoxin produced by some isolates of methicillin-susceptible S aureus (MSSA) and MRSA. PVL is a virulence factor that causes leukocyte destruction and tissue necrosis. PVL-producing S aureus strains are often community-acquired and have most commonly produced boils and abscesses. However, they also have been associated with severe cellulitis, osteomyelitis, and deaths from necrotizing pneumonia.

► Prevention

Patients with recurrent skin infections with S aureus should practice good skin hygiene to try to prevent recurrences. Weekly baths with bleach (1 tsp per gallon or ¼ cup per ½ tub [~20 gal]) or chlorhexidine 4% may decrease skin contamination. Household eradication regimens include treatment of the patient and family with intranasal antibiotics (eg, mupirocin) and hot water washing of clothes and linens. Keeping fingernails short, good skin hygiene, not sharing towels or other personal items, and use of a clean towel daily may also help prevent recurrences. Preoperative skin hygiene and perioperative antibiotic prophylaxis are important measures to prevent staphylococcal surgical site infections.

► Clinical Findings

A. Symptoms and Signs

1. Staphylococcal skin diseases—Dermal infection with S aureus causes pustules, furuncles, carbuncles, or cellulitis. Skin lesions can be seen anywhere on the body but are commonly seen on the buttocks in infants and young children. Factors that facilitate transmission include crowding, compromised skin (eg, eczema), participation on contact sports teams, day care attendance, bare skin contact with surfaces used by others (exercise mats, sauna benches), and sharing towels or other personal items.

S aureus are often found along with streptococci in impetigo. If the strains produce exfoliatin, localized lesions become bullous (bullous impetigo).

Scalded skin syndrome is a toxin-mediated illness caused by exfoliative toxins A and B produced by certain strains of *S aureus*. The initial infection may begin at any site but occurs most frequently in the nasopharynx, a site that is frequently colonized by *S aureus*. Skin erythema, often beginning around the nose and mouth, is accompanied by fever and irritability. The involved skin becomes tender to touch. A day or so later, exfoliation begins, usually around the mouth. The inside of the mouth is red, and a peeling rash is present around the lips, often in a radial pattern. Generalized, painful peeling may follow, involving the limbs and trunk but often sparing the feet. If erythematous but unpeeled skin is rubbed, superficial epidermal layers separate from deeper ones and slough (Nikolsky sign). Generally, if secondary infection does not occur, there is healing without scarring. In the newborn (*Ritter disease)* exfoliation may be fulminant.

2. Osteomyelitis and septic arthritis—(See Chapter 26.)

3. Staphylococcal pneumonia—Staphylococcal pneumonia is often a severe respiratory and systemic illness. In the lungs, the organism is necrotizing, producing bronchoalveolar destruction. Pneumatoceles, pyopneumothorax, and empyema are frequently encountered. Rapid progression is characteristic. Purulent pericarditis occurs by direct extension in about 10% of cases, with or without empyema. Staphylococcal pneumonias are frequently encountered in the setting of an influenza infection, or in the context of a multifocal or disseminated staphylococcal infection associated with endovascular infection and persistent bacteremia.

Staphylococcal pneumonia can also occur in newborns. Infection with coagulase-negative *Staphylococcus* is most common, but infection with *S aureus* is more likely to result in a fulminant course. Most staphylococcal lung infections in newborns occur in susceptible infants with indwelling catheters and endotracheal tubes, and are often part of a systemic infectious process.

4. Staphylococcal food poisoning—Staphylococcal food poisoning is a result of ingestion of preformed enterotoxin produced by staphylococci growing in undercooked or improperly stored food. The disease is characterized by vomiting, prostration, and diarrhea occurring 2–6 hours after ingestion of contaminated foods.

5. Endocarditis and endovascular infection—Although the presence of a damaged or artificial heart valve or endocardium in children with congenital or rheumatic heart disease predisposes to endocarditis, *S aureus* may also produce infection of normal heart valves. A major risk factor for pediatric staphylococcal endocarditis is the presence of intravascular foreign bodies, including indwelling central catheters and prosthetic material used for repair of congenital heart disease. Infection usually begins in an extracardiac focus, often the skin or a catheter insertion site.

The presenting symptoms in staphylococcal endocarditis are fever, weight loss, weakness, muscle pain or diffuse skeletal pain, poor feeding, pallor, and cardiac decompensation. Signs include splenomegaly, cardiomegaly, petechiae, hematuria, and a new or changing murmur. The course of *S aureus* endocarditis is rapid, although subacute disease occurs occasionally. Peripheral septic embolization and uncontrollable cardiac failure are common, even when optimal antibiotic therapy is administered and may be indications for surgical intervention.

Septic thrombophlebitis can occur in the setting of localized primary infections such as osteomyelitis. Patients often progress to septic shock, respiratory failure, and multiorgan dysfunction due to persistent bacteremia and disseminated embolic foci. Imaging studies to identify infected thromboses should be considered in the presence of severe illness and persistent bacteremia.

6. Toxic shock syndrome—TSS most commonly occurs in menstruating females using tampons, but menstrual-associated TSS can occur without tampon use and TSS can arise from focal staphylococcal infection. The primary site may be relatively innocuous. TSS is characterized by fever, blanching erythroderma, diarrhea, vomiting, myalgia, prostration, hypotension, and multiorgan dysfunction. Additional clinical features include sudden onset; conjunctival suffusion; mucosal hyperemia; desquamation of skin on the palms, soles, fingers, and toes (during convalescence), DIC in severe cases; renal and hepatic functional abnormalities; and myolysis. The mortality rate with early treatment is now less than 1%. Recurrences during subsequent menstrual periods are not unusual, occurring in as many as 60% of untreated women who continue to use tampons.

7. Coagulase-negative staphylococcal infections—Localized and systemic coagulase-negative staphylococcal infections occur primarily in immunocompromised patients, high-risk (especially premature) newborns, and patients with intravascular foreign bodies. Coagulase-negative staphylococci are the most common nosocomial pathogen in hospitalized low-birth-weight neonates in the United States. Additional risk factors in these patients include intravenous administration of lipid emulsions and indwelling central venous catheters. Coagulase-negative staphylococci are a common cause of bacteremia and sepsis in patients with artificial heart valves, patches or conduits, ventriculoperitoneal shunts, or a central venous catheters, often necessitating removal of the foreign material and protracted antibiotic therapy. Coagulase-negative staphylococci are also normal skin flora and are thus a common cause of blood culture contamination.

B. Laboratory Findings

Moderate leukocytosis (15,000–20,000/μL) with a shift to the left is occasionally found, although normal counts are common, particularly in infants, and leukopenia (< 5000/μL) can occur in severe cases. Markers of inflammation, including the

C-reactive protein, procalcitonin, and sedimentation rate are frequently elevated except in localized mild infections. Blood cultures are frequently positive in systemic staphylococcal disease and should always be obtained when it is suspected. Similarly, pus from sites of infection should always be aspirated or obtained surgically, examined with Gram stain, and cultured. This is particularly important when MRSA is a possible pathogen.

▶ Differential Diagnosis

Staphylococcal skin disease takes many forms. Bullous impetigo must be differentiated from chemical or thermal burns, drug reactions, and, in the very young, from the various congenital epidermolytic syndromes or herpes simplex infections. Staphylococcal scalded skin syndrome may resemble scarlet fever, Kawasaki disease, Stevens-Johnson syndrome, erythema multiforme, and other drug reactions. A skin biopsy may be critical in establishing the diagnosis.

Severe, rapidly progressing pneumonia with formation of abscesses, pneumatoceles, and empyemas is typical of *S aureus* infection and group A *Streptococcus* (GAS), but may occasionally be produced by pneumococci, *Klebsiella pneumoniae* and *Haemophilus influenzae*.

Staphylococcal food poisoning often occurs in clusters associated with a single food source. It is differentiated from other common-source gastroenteritis syndromes (*Salmonella*, *Clostridium perfringens*, and *Vibrio parahaemolyticus*) by the short incubation period (2–6 hours), the prominence of vomiting (as opposed to diarrhea). Food poisoning from *Bacillus cereus* can result in a vomiting illness clinically indistinguishable from *S aureus*. Scromboid poisoning may look similar but will present with flushing or a rash.

Neonatal infections with *S aureus* and coagulase-negative staphylococci can resemble infections with streptococci and a variety of gram-negative organisms. Umbilical and respiratory tract colonization occurs with many pathogenic organisms (GBS, *Escherichia coli*, and *Klebsiella*), and both skin and systemic infections occur with virtually all of these organisms.

TSS must be differentiated from Rocky Mountain spotted fever, leptospirosis, Kawasaki disease, multisystem inflammatory syndrome associated with COVID-19, drug reactions, adenovirus, and measles (see Table 40–2).

▶ Treatment

A. General Considerations

The incidence of community-acquired MRSA isolates varies geographically. For empiric coverage of potentially life-threatening infections with suspected *S aureus* (in which susceptibilities are not known), initial therapy should include vancomycin in combination with either nafcillin or oxacillin (in addition to appropriate antibiotic therapy for other suspected pathogens). Antibiotic therapy can then be adjusted based on identification of the organism and susceptibility results.

Currently, most community-acquired MRSA strains are susceptible to TMP-SMX, and many are susceptible to clindamycin. Knowledge of local MRSA susceptibility patterns is useful in guiding empiric therapy. Less serious infections in nontoxic patients may be initially treated using TMP-SMX or clindamycin, while awaiting cultures and susceptibility data, if community MRSA resistance to these agents is low.

For MSSA strains, a β-lactamase–resistant penicillin is the drug of choice (oxacillin or nafcillin). In serious systemic disease, in osteomyelitis, and in the treatment of large abscesses, intravenous therapy is indicated initially with cefazolin or nafcillin. In serious or life-threatening illness, consultation with an infectious disease physician is recommended.

Many cephalosporins are active against MSSA. The first-generation cephalosporins cefazolin or cephalexin are preferred over broader subsequent generations.

Newer antistaphylococcal antibiotics with activity against MRSA include daptomycin, linezolid, and ceftaroline; these drugs should be used for severe infections under the guidance of infectious disease specialists. Rifampin is used occasionally for adjunctive treatment of persistent staphylococcal infections, particularly in the presence of foreign material, but it should never be used as monotherapy.

1. Skin infections—Treatment of skin and soft tissue infections depends, in part, on the extent of the lesion, immunocompetence of the host, and the toxicity of the patient. Afebrile, well-appearing patients with small abscesses may do well with incision and drainage (with or without the addition of oral antimicrobials). More serious infections or infections in immunocompromised patients should be treated more aggressively. Hospitalization and intravenous antibiotics may be required. Culture and susceptibility testing will help guide therapy.

For milder infections, selection of empiric antimicrobials depends on local rates of MRSA and local susceptibilities. β-Lactam antibiotics, such as penicillins and cephalosporins, can no longer be depended on as single agents for the majority of cases in communities with high MRSA rates, but may be considered as initial treatment in milder infections where good follow-up can be ensured. TMP-SMX or clindamycin (depending on local susceptibility patterns) may be used for empiric staphylococcal coverage. However, GAS may be resistant to TMP-SMX, and not all MSSA or MRSA will be covered by clindamycin.

2. Osteomyelitis and septic arthritis—Treatment should be begun intravenously, with antibiotics selected to cover the most likely organisms (staphylococci in hematogenous osteomyelitis; meningococci, pneumococci, *Kingella kingae*, staphylococci in children aged < 3 years with septic arthritis; staphylococci and gonococci in older children with septic arthritis). Knowledge of local MRSA rates will help guide empiric therapy. Antibiotic levels should be kept high at all times.

Clinical studies support the use of intravenous treatment for osteomyelitis until fever and local symptoms and signs and inflammatory markers are subsiding—usually at least 3–5 days—followed by oral therapy.

Nafcillin or cefazolin can be used for intravenous therapy of MSSA strains. Clindamycin is an alternative agent if the organism is susceptible, and the patient does not have a severe or life-threatening infection or ongoing bacteremia. Cephalexin 100–150 mg/kg/day in four divided doses can be used when the patient is ready for oral therapy; good compliance with oral therapy is essential.

Vancomycin can be used initially for MRSA osteomyelitis, while awaiting susceptibilities. Antibiotic regimens for MRSA osteomyelitis should be based on susceptibility results; isolates may be susceptible to clindamycin or linezolid.

The C-reactive protein (in the first or second week after therapy is started) and the erythrocyte sedimentation rate (ESR) (usually measured weekly) are good indicators of response to therapy. Duration of therapy is typically 3–4 weeks for septic arthritis and uncomplicated courses of acute osteomyelitis. Surgical drainage of osteomyelitis or septic arthritis is often required (see Chapter 26).

3. Staphylococcal pneumonia—For MSSA pneumonia, nafcillin or cefazolin are the usual drugs of choice. Vancomycin can be used empirically until results of cultures and susceptibility tests are obtained if community or hospital MRSA rates are high. In sicker patients, vancomycin plus nafcillin can be used (in addition to coverage of other pathogens) until the etiologic agent and susceptibilities are established. Linezolid has been reported to be as efficacious as vancomycin for the treatment of resistant gram-positive pneumonia and soft tissue infections.

Empyema and pyopneumothorax require drainage. The choice of chest tube versus thoracoscopic drainage depends on local institutional practice.

4. Staphylococcal food poisoning—Therapy is supportive and usually not required except in severe cases or for small infants with marked dehydration.

5. Staphylococcal endocarditis—The treatment of staphylococcal endocarditis depends on whether the patient has a prosthetic valve or material in the heart and on the susceptibilities of the organism. Please see the American Heart Association's Guidelines on Infective Endocarditis: Diagnosis and Management, and consult an infectious disease physician for this serious and sometimes complicated problem. High-dose, prolonged parenteral treatment is indicated.

Occasionally, medical treatment fails. Signs of treatment failure are: (1) recurrent fever without apparent treatable other cause (eg, thrombophlebitis, respiratory or urinary tract infection, drug fever), (2) persistently positive blood cultures, (3) intractable and progressive congestive heart failure, and (4) recurrent (septic) embolization. In such circumstances—particularly (2), (3), and (4)—evaluation for valve replacement becomes necessary.

6. Toxic shock syndrome—Treatment consists of vigorous fluid resuscitation, maintaining perfusion pressure with inotropic agents, prompt drainage of a focus of infection (or removal of tampons or foreign bodies), and intravenous antibiotics.

A β-lactam antibiotic (cefazolin or nafcillin) is used for empiric therapy. Vancomycin may be added for severe cases because TSS can be challenging to discriminate from staphylococcal sepsis. Many experts also add clindamycin, which is a protein synthesis inhibitor that may limit toxin production. Clindamycin should not be used empirically as a single agent until susceptibilities are known. Intravenous immunoglobulin has been used as adjunctive therapy for severe disease.

7. Vancomycin-resistant *S aureus* infections (VRSA)—Reports of VRSA isolates are rare but are likely to increase in frequency. Such isolates are sometimes susceptible to clindamycin or TMP-SMX. If not, therapeutic options include linezolid, ceftaroline, or daptomycin, assuming the strain is susceptible to these agents. Consultation with an infectious disease specialist is recommended.

8. Coagulase-negative staphylococcal infections—Coagulase-negative staphylococci are frequently resistant to penicillins and cephalosporins. Bacteremia and other serious coagulase-negative staphylococcal infections are treated initially with vancomycin until susceptibility results can guide subsequent therapy. Coagulase-negative staphylococci are uncommonly resistant to vancomycin. Many drugs used for MRSA are also effective against these pathogens.

Baltimore RS: Infective endocarditis in childhood: 2015 update: a scientific statement from the American Heart Association. Circulation 2015 Oct 13;132(15):1487–1515. doi: 10.1161/CIR.0000000000000298 [PMID: 26373317].

Woods CR et al: Clinical Practice Guideline by the Pediatric Infectious Diseases Society and the Infectious Diseases Society of America: 2021 Guideline on Diagnosis and Management of Acute Hematogenous Osteomyelitis in Pediatrics. J Pediatric Infect Dis Soc 2021 Sep 23;10(8):801–844. doi: 10.1093/jpids/piab027 [PMID: 34350458].

MENINGOCOCCAL INFECTIONS

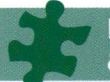

ESSENTIALS OF DIAGNOSIS & TYPICAL FEATURES

- ▶ Meningitis
  - Fever, headache, vomiting, convulsions, shock
- ▶ Meningococcemia
  - Fever, severe shock, petechial or purpuric skin rash
- ▶ Diagnosis confirmed by culture or PCR
- ▶ High attack rate for contacts, importance of chemoprophylaxis

General Considerations

Meningococci (*Neisseria meningitidis*) may be carried asymptomatically in the upper respiratory tract. Less than 1% of carriers develop disease. Meningitis and sepsis are the two most common forms of illness, but septic arthritis, pericarditis, pneumonia, chronic meningococcemia, otitis media, conjunctivitis, and vaginitis also occur. Meningococcal cases in the United States are rare; currently there are an estimated 300–400 cases annually. The highest attack rate for meningococcal meningitis is in the first year of life, with a secondary peak among adolescents and young adults including outbreaks that occur in college dorms and military barracks.

Meningococci are gram-negative organisms containing endotoxin in their cell walls that cause capillary vascular injury and leak, as well as DIC. Meningococci are classified serologically into groups: A, B, C, Y, and W are the groups most commonly implicated in systemic disease. B, C, and Y are the most common in the United States, and as a result of widespread vaccination against serotypes ACYW, nearly half of cases in the United States are caused by serotype B. *N meningitidis* is generally susceptible to penicillin but recent reports of beta-lactamase producing serotype Y strains mean that treatment with a third-generation cephalosporin should be used until penicillin susceptibility is demonstrated.

Complement deficiency, particularly late pathway components, increases susceptibility to meningococcal infection. Patients with invasive disease should be assessed for complement defects. Anatomic or functional asplenia, monoclonal anticomplement antibody treatment, and uncontrolled human immunodeficiency virus (HIV) infection are associated with increased susceptibility.

Prevention

A. Chemoprophylaxis

Close contacts are at increased risk for developing meningococcal infection and should be given chemoprophylaxis within 24 hours of identification of the source case. The secondary attack rate among household members is about 500–800 times the attack rate in the general population. Exposed contacts should be notified promptly. If they are febrile, they should be fully evaluated and treated empirically. Hospital personnel are not at increased risk unless they have had contact with a patient's oral secretions.

High-risk contacts are defined as:

- All household contacts (especially children < 2 years of age)
- Persons with child care or preschool contact with the index patient at any time in the 7 days prior to illness onset

- Persons with direct exposure to index patient's secretions (sharing of drinks, straws, cigarettes, toothbrushes, eating utensils, kissing) during the 7 days prior to illness onset
- Persons who have performed mouth-to-mouth resuscitation or performed unprotected endotracheal intubation of the index patient during the 7 days prior to illness onset
- Persons who have slept in the same dwelling as the index patient within 7 days of illness onset
- Passengers who were seated directly next to the index patient on a flight of more than 8 hours duration

The most commonly used agent for meningococcal chemoprophylaxis is oral rifampin given twice daily for 2 days (600 mg for adults; 10 mg/kg for children *older* than 1 month [maximum dosage 600 mg] and 5 mg/kg for infants *younger* than 1 month). Rifampin should not be given to pregnant women. Instead, intramuscular ceftriaxone is the preferred agent: 125 mg given as a single dose if the patient is younger than 15 years; 250 mg given if the patient is aged 15 years or older. Ciprofloxacin (20 mg/kg as a single dose, maximum dose 500 mg) effectively eradicates nasopharyngeal carriage in adults and children but is not recommended in pregnant women or in communities where fluoroquinolone-resistant strains of *N meningitidis* have been identified. Throat cultures to identify carriers are not useful.

B. Vaccine

Several types of vaccines are currently licensed in the United States for meningococcal disease prevention; 2-quadrivalent meningococcal conjugate vaccines that cover serogroups A, C, Y, and W are available in the United States. Two serogroup B vaccines are licensed for ages 10–25 years. (See Chapter 10 for a discussion on meningococcal vaccines.)

Clinical Findings

A. Symptoms and Signs

Many children with clinical meningococcemia also have meningitis, and some have other foci of infection. All children with suspected meningococcemia should have a lumbar puncture.

1. Meningococcemia—A prodrome of upper respiratory infection is followed by high fever, headache, nausea, marked toxicity, and hypotension. Purpura, petechiae, and occasionally bright pink, tender macules or papules over the extremities, and trunk are seen. The rash usually progresses rapidly. Occasional cases lack rash. Fulminant meningococcemia is characterized by DIC, massive skin and mucosal hemorrhages, and shock. This syndrome also may be caused by *H influenzae*, *S pneumoniae*, or other bacteria. Chronic meningococcemia is a rare condition characterized by periodic bouts of fever, arthralgia or arthritis, and recurrent petechiae. Splenomegaly often is present. Patients may be free of symptoms between bouts. Chronic meningococcemia occurs primarily in adults and mimics Henoch-Schönlein purpura.

2. Meningitis—In many children, meningococcemia is followed within a few hours to several days by symptoms and signs of acute purulent meningitis, with severe headache, stiff neck, nausea, vomiting, and stupor. Children with meningitis generally fare better than children with meningococcemia alone, probably because they survived the infection long enough to develop clinical signs of meningitis.

B. Laboratory Findings

The peripheral WBC count may be either low or elevated. Thrombocytopenia may be present with or without DIC. If petechial or hemorrhagic lesions are present, meningococci can sometimes be seen microscopically in tissue fluid expressed from a punctured lesion. CSF is generally cloudy and contains more than 1000 WBCs/μL, predominantly polymorphonuclear neutrophils, and gram-negative intracellular diplococci. A total hemolytic complement assay may reveal absence of late components as an underlying cause; because acute infection can consume complement proteins, testing for complement deficiency should be delayed several weeks after recovery. PCR assays with high sensitivity and specificity are available to detect *N meningitidis* in blood and CSF, and can be useful in cases where antibiotics were initiated before any cultures were obtained.

▶ Differential Diagnosis

The skin lesions of *H influenzae* or pneumococci, enterovirus infection, endocarditis, leptospirosis, Rocky Mountain spotted fever, other rickettsial diseases, Henoch-Schönlein purpura, and blood dyscrasias may be similar to meningococcemia. Severe *S aureus* sepsis in some patients can present with purpura. Chronic meningococcemia presents similarly to the acute arthritis-dermatitis syndrome caused by chronic gonococcemia.

▶ Complications

Meningitis may lead to permanent central nervous system (CNS) damage, with deafness, convulsions, paralysis, or impaired intellectual function. Hydrocephalus may develop and require a ventriculoperitoneal shunt. Subdural collections of fluid are common but usually resolve spontaneously. Extensive skin necrosis, loss of digits or extremities, intestinal hemorrhage, and late adrenal insufficiency may complicate fulminant meningococcemia.

▶ Treatment

Blood cultures should be obtained for all children with fever and purpura or other signs of meningococcemia, and antibiotics should be administered immediately as an emergency procedure.

Children with meningococcemia or meningococcal meningitis should be treated as though shock were imminent even if their initial vital signs are stable. If hypotension is present, supportive measures should be aggressive, because the prognosis is grave in such situations. Treatment should be started emergently in an intensive care setting and not be delayed while transporting the patient. Shock may worsen following antimicrobial therapy due to endotoxin release. To minimize the risk of nosocomial transmission, patients should be placed in respiratory isolation for the first 24 hours of antibiotic treatment.

A. Specific Measures

Antibiotics should be initiated promptly. Because other bacteria, such as *S pneumoniae*, *S aureus*, or other gram-negative organisms, can cause identical syndromes, initial therapy should be broad. Vancomycin and cefotaxime or ceftriaxone are preferred initial coverage. Once *N meningitidis* has been isolated, penicillin G, cefotaxime, or ceftriaxone intravenously for 7 days are the drugs of choice.

B. General Measures

Blood cultures should be drawn prior to initiation of antibiotic therapy; however, antibiotic therapy should not be delayed to obtain a lumbar puncture as prompt treatment portends better outcomes due to the aggressive nature of this infection. Supportive care includes early and aggressive fluid resuscitation and vasopressor initiation. For management of DIC, see Chapter 30.

▶ Prognosis

Unfavorable prognostic features include shock, DIC, and extensive skin lesions. The case fatality rate in fulminant meningococcemia is over 30%. In uncomplicated meningococcal meningitis, the fatality rate is much lower (10%–20%). An invasive meningococcal infection may be the first indication of an underlying immunodeficiency, particularly defects in terminal complement function.

Centers for Disease Control and Prevention (CDC): Meningococcal Disease: Technical and Clinical Information. https://www.cdc.gov/meningococcal/clinical-info.html. Accessed May 22, 2023.

Meningococcal Infections. In: Kimberlin DW, Brady MT, Jackson MA, Long SS (eds): *Red Book: 2021–2024 Report of the Committee on Infectious Diseases*. 32nd ed. Elk Grove Village, IL: American Academy of Pediatrics; 2021:519–532.

GONOCOCCAL INFECTIONS

ESSENTIALS OF DIAGNOSIS & TYPICAL FEATURES

► Neonatal
  • Purulent, edematous, sometimes hemorrhagic conjunctivitis with intracellular gram-negative diplococci in 2- to 4-day-old infants
► Sexually transmitted infection
  • Purulent urethral discharge with intracellular gram-negative diplococci on direct microscopic smear in male patients (usually adolescents) (see Chapter 44)
  • Vulvitis, vaginitis, risk of ascending infection to upper genital tract, pelvic inflammatory disease
► Disseminated disease
  • Fever, arthritis (often polyarticular) or tenosynovitis, and maculopapular peripheral rash that may be vesiculopustular or hemorrhagic
► Diagnosis
  • Positive culture of blood, pharyngeal, or genital secretions; Nucleic Acid Amplification Test on urine or genital secretions

► General Considerations

Neisseria gonorrhoeae is a gram-negative diplococcus. The cell wall of *N gonorrhoeae* contains endotoxin, which is liberated when the organism dies and stimulates the production of a cellular exudate. The incubation period is short, usually 2–5 days.

Reported cases of gonorrhea exceeded 710,000 in the United States in 2021 and have continued to increase since reaching historic lows in 2009. Gonococcal disease in children may be transmitted sexually or nonsexually. Prepubertal gonococcal infection outside the neonatal period should be considered presumptive evidence of sexual contact or child abuse. Prepubertal girls usually manifest gonococcal vulvovaginitis without cervicitis because of the neutral to alkaline pH of the vagina and thin vaginal mucosa.

In the adolescent or adult, the workup of every case of gonorrhea should include a careful inquiry into the patient's sexual practices and relevant diagnostic tests obtained. Efforts should be made to identify and provide treatment to all sexual contacts. Programs of expedited partner treatment where prescriptions are provided without first examining the sexual contact increase successful treatment. Young women are at risk for serious health consequences including infertility due to gonococcal infection.

► Clinical Findings

A. Symptoms and Signs

1. Asymptomatic gonorrhea—The ratio of asymptomatic to symptomatic gonorrheal infections in adolescents and adults is approximately 3–4:1 in women and 0.5–1:1 in men. Asymptomatic infections are as infectious as symptomatic ones.

2. Uncomplicated genital gonorrhea

A. MALE WITH URETHRITIS/EPIDIDYMITIS—Urethral discharge, often copious, is sometimes painful and bloody and may be white, yellow, or green. There may be associated dysuria. Epididymitis may present with acute scrotal swelling or pain. The patient usually is afebrile.

B. PREPUBERTAL FEMALE WITH VAGINITIS—The only clinical findings initially may be dysuria and polymorphonuclear neutrophils in the urine. Vulvitis characterized by erythema, edema, and excoriation accompanied by a purulent discharge may follow.

C. POSTPUBERTAL FEMALE WITH CERVICITIS—Symptomatic disease is characterized by a purulent, foul-smelling vaginal discharge, dysuria, and occasionally dyspareunia. Fever and abdominal pain are absent. The cervix is frequently hyperemic and tender when touched.

D. RECTAL GONORRHEA—Rectal gonorrhea often is asymptomatic. There may be purulent discharge, edema, and pain during evacuation.

3. Pharyngeal gonorrhea—Pharyngeal infection usually is asymptomatic. There may be some sore throat and, rarely, acute exudative tonsillitis with bilateral cervical lymphadenopathy and fever.

4. Neonatal Conjunctivitis (ophthalmia neonatorum)—Copious, usually purulent exudate is characteristic of gonococcal conjunctivitis. Newborns acquire infection in the perinatal period through exposure to the infected cervix; cases can occur after both vaginal and cesarean section. Infants are symptomatic on days 2–4 of life. Perinatal gonococcal infections can be complicated by sepsis, arthritis, and meningitis. Conjunctivitis can also occur in the adolescents; infection typically is spread from infected genital secretions by the fingers.

5. Pelvic inflammatory disease (salpingitis)—The interval between initiation of genital infection and its ascent to the uterine tubes is variable and may range from days to months. Menses frequently are the initiating factor. With the onset of a menstrual period, gonococci invade the endometrium, causing transient endometritis. Subsequently salpingitis may occur, resulting in pyosalpinx or hydrosalpinx. Rarely infection progresses to peritonitis or perihepatitis. Gonococcal salpingitis occurs in an acute, subacute, or chronic form.

All three forms have in common tenderness on gentle movement of the cervix and adnexal tenderness during pelvic examination.

Gonococci or *Chlamydia trachomatis* are the cause of about 50% of cases of pelvic inflammatory disease. A mixed infection caused by enteric bacilli, *Bacteroides fragilis*, or other anaerobes occurs in the other 50%.

6. Gonococcal perihepatitis (Fitz-Hugh-Curtis syndrome)— Typically the patient presents with right upper quadrant tenderness in association with signs of acute or subacute salpingitis. Pain may be pleuritic and referred to the shoulder. Hepatic friction rub is a valuable but inconstant sign.

7. Disseminated gonorrhea— Dissemination follows asymptomatic more often than symptomatic genital infection, often from gonococcal pharyngitis or anorectal gonorrhea. The most common form of disseminated gonorrhea is the triad of polyarthralgia, tenosynovitis, and dermatitis (also referred to as arthritis-dermatitis syndrome), although patients may not present with all three. Septic arthritis is less common, and gonococcal endocarditis and meningitis are rare.

A. ARTHRITIS-DERMATITIS SYNDROME— Disease usually begins with the simultaneous onset of low-grade fever, polyarthralgia, and malaise. After a day or so, joint symptoms become acute. Swelling, redness, and tenderness occur, frequently over the wrists, ankles, and knees but also in the fingers, feet, and other peripheral joints. The arthralgia may be migratory. Skin lesions may be noted at the same time. Discrete, tender, maculopapular lesions 5–8 mm in diameter appear that may become vesicular, pustular, and then hemorrhagic. They are few in number and noted on the fingers, palms, feet, and other distal surfaces. In patients with this form of the disease, blood cultures are often positive, but joint fluid rarely yields organisms. Skin lesions often are positive by Gram stain but rarely by culture. Genital, rectal, and pharyngeal cultures must be performed.

B. SEPTIC ARTHRITIS— In this less common form of disseminated gonorrhea, fever is often absent. Arthritis evolves in one or more joints. Dermatitis usually does not occur. Systemic symptoms are minimal. Blood cultures are negative, but joint aspirates may yield gonococci on smear and culture. Genital, rectal, and pharyngeal cultures must be performed.

B. Laboratory Findings

Demonstration of gram-negative, kidney-shaped diplococci in smears of urethral exudate in males is presumptive evidence of gonorrhea. Positive culture confirms the diagnosis. Negative smears do not rule out gonorrhea. Gram-stained smears of cervical or vaginal discharge in girls are more difficult to interpret because of normal gram-negative flora, but they may be useful when technical personnel are experienced. NAAT on urine or genital specimens enable detection of

N gonorrhoeae and *C trachomatis*. These tests have excellent sensitivity and have replaced culture in many laboratories, although culture and antibiotic susceptibility testing should still be performed in cases of suspected or documented treatment failure. All children or adolescents with a suspected or established diagnosis of gonorrhea should have serologic tests for syphilis and HIV.

If cultures are obtained, use of a selective media (eg, Thayer-Martin agar) is needed to suppress normal flora. In cases of possible sexual assault, notify the laboratory that definite speciation is needed, because nongonococcal *Neisseria* species can grow on the selective media.

▶ Differential Diagnosis

Urethritis in the male may be gonococcal or nongonococcal (NGU). NGU is a syndrome characterized by discharge (rarely painful), mild dysuria, and a subacute course. The discharge is usually scant or moderate and nonpurulent. *C trachomatis* is the most common cause of NGU. *C trachomatis* has been shown to cause epididymitis in males and salpingitis in females.

Vulvovaginitis in a prepubertal female may be due to infection caused by miscellaneous bacteria, including *Shigella*, GAS, *Candida*, and herpes simplex. Discharges may be caused by trichomonads, *Enterobius vermicularis* (pinworm), candidiasis or foreign bodies. Symptom-free discharge (leukorrhea) normally accompanies rising estrogen levels.

Cervicitis in a postpubertal female, alone or in association with urethritis and involvement of Skene and Bartholin glands, may be due to infection caused by *C trachomatis*, *Candida*, herpes simplex, *Trichomonas*, or inflammation caused by foreign bodies (usually some form of contraceptive device). Leukorrhea may be associated with birth control pills.

Salpingitis may be due to infection with other organisms. The symptoms must be differentiated from those of appendicitis, urinary tract infection, ectopic pregnancy, endometriosis, or ovarian cysts or torsion.

Disseminated gonorrhea presents a differential diagnosis that includes meningococcemia, acute rheumatic fever, Henoch-Schönlein purpura, juvenile idiopathic arthritis, lupus erythematosus, leptospirosis, secondary syphilis, certain viral infections (particularly rubella, but also enteroviruses and parvovirus), serum sickness, type B hepatitis (in the prodromal phase), infective endocarditis.

▶ Prevention

Prevention of gonorrhea is principally a matter of patient education, condom use, and identification and treatment of contacts. Providers should maintain a low threshold for routine screening for STIs, including gonorrhea, among adolescent patients in primary care.

Gonococcal conjunctivitis in newborns is prevented by universal prophylactic treatment with erythromycin 0.5% ointment after delivery.

▶ Treatment

N gonorrhoeae infections resistant to tetracyclines, penicillins, and fluoroquinolones are common.

A. Uncomplicated Urogenital, Pharyngeal, or Rectal Gonococcal Infections

Ceftriaxone (500 mg intramuscularly in a single dose; 1 g for patients > 150 kg) is recommended. If ceftriaxone cannot be used, cefixime 800 mg orally in a single dose or gentamicin 240 mg IM plus azithromycin 2 g orally as a single dose may be used, with the exception of pharyngeal infection for which ceftriaxone is the only reliable treatment. For chlamydia coinfection or when chlamydia has not been ruled out, doxycycline (100 mg orally twice daily for 7 days) should be used in addition to ceftriaxone.

A test-of-cure is not recommended for asymptomatic individuals who have received one of the recommended regimens for gonococcal urogenital or rectal infection. However, patients treated for pharyngeal infection should be retested 14 days after completing treatment. Patients with incomplete response or rapid recurrence (3–5 days) after treatment should have culture obtained to determine if there is antimicrobial resistance. Because of high rates of reinfection, retesting after 3 months is recommended for all patients treated for gonococcal infection.

B. Disseminated Gonorrhea

The recommended regimen is ceftriaxone (1 g intramuscularly or intravenously once daily). Alternative regimens include cefotaxime (1 g intravenously every 8 hours) or ceftizoxime (1 g intravenously every 8 hours). Oral therapy may follow parenteral therapy 24–48 hours after improvement if testing demonstrates susceptibility to cefixime. Duration of treatment is 7–14 days depending on clinical response.

C. Pelvic Inflammatory Disease

Treatment regimens include ceftriaxone plus metronidazole plus doxycycline, or doxycycline plus either cefoxitin or cefotetan. Parenteral treatment is given until the patient is clinically improved; then doxycycline and metronidazole are administered by mouth to complete 14 days of therapy. Alternative regimens include: (1) clindamycin plus gentamicin or (2) ampicillin-sulbactam plus doxycycline until the patient improves clinically. When tubo-ovarian abscess is present, either clindamycin or metronidazole should be used in addition to doxycycline for at least 14 days to provide better anaerobic coverage. In women with mild to moderate PID, an intramuscular plus oral regimen can be considered—see the CDC 2021 STI Treatment Guidelines for further details.

D. Neonatal Gonococcal Conjunctivitis

Infants with ophthalmia neonatorum due to gonorrhea should be treated with a single dose of ceftriaxone (25–50 mg/kg IM, not to exceed 250 mg). Newborns born to mothers with untreated gonococcal infection should be tested for gonococcus at exposed sites and treated presumptively with the same regimen.

Gonococcal infections. In: Kimberlin DW, Brady MT, Jackson MA, Long SS (eds): *Red Book: 2021–2024 Report of the Committee on Infectious Diseases*. 32nd ed. Itasca, IL: American Academy of Pediatrics; 2021:338–344.

Workowski KA et al. Sexually transmitted infections treatment guidelines, 2021. MMWR Recomm Rep 2021;70:1–187. doi: 10.15585/mmwr.rr7004a1. [PMID: 34292926].

BOTULISM

ESSENTIALS OF DIAGNOSIS & TYPICAL FEATURES

▶ Infant
  • Hypotonia, poor feeding, constipation, weak cry, poor gag reflex
  • Progression to respiratory failure
▶ Foodborne and wound botulism
▶ Difficulty in swallowing and speaking within 12–36 hours after ingestion of toxin-contaminated food.
  • Contaminated traumatic wounds or black tar heroin injection
  • Diplopia; dilated, unreactive pupils, blurry vision
  • Descending paralysis
  • Potential progression to respiratory failure
▶ Diagnosis by clinical findings and identification of toxin in blood, stool, or implicated food
▶ Empiric treatment before confirmatory testing to avoid delays

▶ General Considerations

Botulism is a paralytic disease caused by *Clostridium botulinum*, an anaerobic, gram-positive, spore-forming bacillus normally found in soil. The organism produces an extremely potent neurotoxin that prevents acetylcholine release from cholinergic fibers at neuromuscular junctions. Of the seven types of toxin (A–G), types A, B, and E cause most human diseases.

Food-borne botulism usually results from ingestion of toxin-containing food. Preformed toxin is absorbed from the gut and produces paralysis. Home-prepared or preserved foods are commonly implicated sources in the United States, but outbreaks in commercial foods also occur. Virtually any food will support the growth of *C botulinum* spores and the food may not appear or taste spoiled. The toxin is heat-labile, but the spores are heat-resistant. Inadequate heating during processing (temperature < 115°C) allows the spores to survive.

Infant botulism occurs in infants younger than 12 months. The toxin is produced by ingested *C botulinum* spores that germinate and produce toxin in the gastrointestinal tract.

Most cases of wound botulism occur in persons who inject drugs.

Clinical Findings

A. Symptoms and Signs

The incubation period for food-borne botulism may range from 2 hours to 12 days. The initial symptoms are lethargy and headache. These are followed by double vision, dilated pupils, ptosis, and within a few hours, difficulty with swallowing and speech. The mucous membranes often are very dry. Descending skeletal muscle paralysis may be seen. Death usually results from respiratory failure.

Botulism patients present with a "classic triad": (1) afebrile; (2) symmetrical, flaccid, descending paralysis with prominent bulbar palsies; and (3) clear sensorium. Recognition of this triad is important in making the clinical diagnosis. Botulism is caused by a toxin; thus, there is no fever unless secondary infection (eg, aspiration pneumonia) occurs. Common bulbar palsies seen include dysphonia, dysphagia, dysarthria, and diplopia (four "Ds").

Infant botulism is seen in infants younger than 12 months (peak onset 2–8 months). Infants younger than 2 weeks rarely develop botulism. The initial symptoms are usually constipation and progressive, often severe, hypotonia. Clinical findings include loss of facial expression, constipation, weak suck and cry, pooled oral secretions, cranial nerve deficits, generalized weakness. Feeding difficulties are common. Apnea and respiratory failure are the most severe symptoms.

B. Laboratory Findings

The diagnosis is made by demonstration of *C botulinum* toxin in stool, gastric aspirate or vomitus, or serum. Serum and stool samples can be sent for toxin confirmation (done by toxin neutralization mouse bioassay at CDC or state health departments). In infant botulism, serum assays for *C botulinum* toxin are usually negative. The tests take time, and therapy should not be withheld awaiting testing results. Foods that are suspected to be contaminated should be kept refrigerated and given to public health personnel for testing. Laboratory findings, including CSF examination, are usually normal.

Differential Diagnosis

Guillain-Barré syndrome is characterized by ascending paralysis, parasthesias, and elevated CSF protein without pleocytosis.

Other illnesses that should be considered include poliomyelitis, acute flaccid myelitis, post-diphtheritic polyneuritis, certain chemical intoxications, tick paralysis, and myasthenia gravis. The history and elevated CSF protein characterize post-diphtheritic polyneuritis. Tick paralysis presents with a flaccid ascending motor paralysis. An attached tick should be sought. Myasthenia gravis usually occurs in adolescent girls. It is characterized by ocular and bulbar symptoms, normal pupils, fluctuating weakness, absence of other neurologic signs, and clinical response to cholinesterase inhibitors.

Complications

Difficulty in swallowing leads to aspiration pneumonia. Serious respiratory paralysis may be fatal despite assisted ventilation and intensive supportive measures.

Treatment

A. General Measures

Patients with suspected botulism should be hospitalized and monitored closely for signs of impending respiratory failure and inability to manage secretions. General and supportive therapy consists of bed rest, ventilatory support (if necessary), fluid therapy, and enteral or parenteral nutrition. Aminoglycosides and clindamycin may exacerbate neuromuscular blockage and should be avoided.

B. Specific Measures

Early treatment of botulism with antitoxin is essential. The type of antitoxin treatment recommended differs depending on the type of botulism. Treatment should begin as soon as the clinical diagnosis is suspected (prior to microbiologic or toxin confirmation). Contact your state health department's emergency 24-hour telephone number immediately when a case of botulism is suspected to assist in therapeutic decisions and to help obtain treatment product.

For treatment of suspected infant botulism, intravenous human botulism immunoglobulin (BabyBIG) is approved by the US FDA. BabyBIG contains neutralizing antibodies against types A and B toxin. BabyBIG is not indicated for use in any form of botulism other than infant botulism. To obtain BabyBIG (in any state), contact the California Department of Public Health (24-hour telephone number: 510-231-7600; www.infantbotulism.org/). Antimicrobial agents are not recommended to treat infant botulism, except when bacterial complications occur (ie, pneumonia, line infection, etc.).

For non-infant botulism, patients should be treated with heptavalent botulinum antitoxin (HBAT). HBAT is an equine-derived antitoxin that contains antibodies to all seven botulinum toxin types (A through G). The treatment protocol (available from the CDC) includes detailed instructions for intravenous administration of antitoxin. State health departments can assist practitioners in obtaining the antitoxin; if state health department officials are unavailable, the CDC (770-488-7100) can be contacted for help in obtaining the product and for consultation. In addition, epidemic assistance, and laboratory testing services are available from the CDC through state health departments. For wound botulism, penicillin or metronidazole can be considered, once HBAT has been given. Surgical debridement of involved tissue is recommended.

► Prevention

Infant botulism is acquired by ingestion of botulism spores that then sporulate into *C botulinum* organisms that form botulinum toxin. Honey can contain botulism spores so it is recommended that honey not be consumed by infants younger than 12 months, though a definitive causative relationship has not been proven.

Food-borne botulism is acquired by ingesting preformed botulism toxin in food. In the United States, food-borne botulism is most commonly seen with ingestion of home-canned foods. Persons who eat home-canned foods should consider boiling foods for at least 10 minutes or heating to 80°F for 30 minutes (can destroy potential toxin). Safe food handling practices include keeping foods either refrigerated (< 45°F) or hot (> 185°F), and disposing of any cracked jars or bulging/dented cans.

► Prognosis

The mortality rate has declined substantially in recent years and currently is about 3%–5%. The prospect for full recovery is good but may take weeks to months depending on the severity of the initial illness.

Botulism and infant botulism. In: Kimberlin DW, Brady MT, Jackson MA, Long SS, (eds): *Red Book: 2021–2024 Report of the Committee on Infectious Diseases*. 32nd ed. Itasca, IL: American Academy of Pediatrics; 2021;266–269.

Rao AK et al: Clinical Guidelines for Diagnosis and Treatment of Botulism, 2021. MMWR Recomm Rep 2021;70(No. RR-2):1–30. doi: http://dx.doi.org/10.15585/mmwr.rr7002a1externalicon.

Centers for Disease Control and Prevention (CDC): Botulism. https://www.cdc.gov/botulism. Accessed June 8, 2021.

Chatham-Stephens K et al: Clinical features of foodborne and wound botulism: a systematic review of the literature, 1932–2015. Clin Infect Dis 2017 Dec 27;66(Suppl_1):S11–S16 [PMID: 29293923].

Infant Botulism Diagnosis and Treatment Program. California Department of Public Health. Available at: www.https://www.infantbotulism.org. Accessed June 8, 2021.

TETANUS

ESSENTIALS OF DIAGNOSIS & TYPICAL FEATURES

► Nonimmunized or partially immunized patient.

► History of skin wound.

► Spasms of jaw muscles (trismus).

► Stiffness of neck, back, and abdominal muscles, with hyperirritability and hyperreflexia.

► Episodic, generalized muscle contractions.

► Diagnosis is based on clinical findings and the immunization history.

► General Considerations

Tetanus is caused by *Clostridium tetani*, an anaerobic, gram-positive bacillus that produces a potent neurotoxin. In unimmunized or incompletely immunized individuals, infection follows contamination of a wound by soil-containing clostridial spores from animal manure. The toxin reaches the CNS by retrograde axon transport, is bound to cerebral gangliosides, and increases reflex excitability in neurons of the spinal cord by blocking function of inhibitory synapses. Intense muscle spasms result. Two-thirds of cases in the United States follow minor puncture wounds of the hands or feet. In many cases, no history of a wound can be obtained. IV drug use and diabetes may be risk factors (in individuals who are not tetanus-immune). In the newborn, usually in underdeveloped countries, infection generally results from contamination of the umbilical cord. The incubation period typically is 3–21 days, but in neonatal tetanus, the period is typically shorter, ranging from 4 to 14 days. In the United States, cases in young children are due to inadequate immunization.

► Prevention

A. Tetanus Toxoid

Active immunization with tetanus toxoid prevents tetanus. Immunity is almost always achieved after the third dose of vaccine. Tetanus immunoglobulin (TIG) is an additional agent used to prevent tetanus in persons with a tetanus-prone wound who have received less than three doses of tetanus toxoid or in immunocompromised patients who do not make sufficient antibody (ie, HIV infection; see Chapter 10). A tetanus toxoid booster at the time of injury is needed if none has been given in the past 10 years—or within 5 years for heavily contaminated wounds. Nearly all cases of tetanus

(99%) in the United States are in nonimmunized or incompletely immunized individuals. Many adolescents and adults lack protective antibody.

B. Wound Care and Prophylaxis for Tetanus-Prone Wounds

Wounds that are contaminated with soil, debris, feces, or saliva are at increased risk for tetanus. Puncture wounds, crush injuries, avulsions, frostbite, burns, or other wounds that contain devitalized tissue are also at increased risk of infection with *C tetani*. All wounds should be adequately cleaned, foreign material removed, and debrided if necrotic or devitalized tissue or residual foreign matter is present. The decision to use tetanus toxoid–containing vaccine, human TIG, or both depends on the type of injury and the tetanus immunization status of the patient (see Chapter 10; Table 10–5). TIG should be used in children with fewer than three previous tetanus toxoid immunizations (DPT, DTaP, DT, Td, Tdap) who have tetanus-prone wounds or are immune compromised, including those with HIV, who have tetanus-prone wounds, regardless of their immunization history. When TIG is indicated for wound prophylaxis 250 units are given intramuscularly regardless of age. If tetanus immunization is incomplete, a dose of age-appropriate vaccine should be given. When both are indicated, tetanus toxoid and TIG should be administered concurrently at different sites using different syringes.

▶ Clinical Findings

A. Symptoms and Signs

The first symptom often is mild pain at the site of the wound, followed by hypertonicity and spasm of the regional muscles. Characteristically, difficulty in opening the mouth (trismus) is evident within 48 hours. In newborns, the first signs are irritability and inability to nurse. The infant may then develop stiffness of the jaw and neck, increasing dysphagia, and generalized hyperreflexia with rigidity and spasms of all muscles of the abdomen and back (opisthotonos). The facial distortion resembles a grimace (risus sardonicus). Difficulty in swallowing and convulsions triggered by minimal stimuli such as sound, light, or movement may occur. Individual spasms may last for seconds or minutes. Recurrent spasms are seen several times each hour, or they may be almost continuous. In most cases, the temperature is normal or only mildly elevated. A high or subnormal temperature is a bad prognostic sign. Patients are fully conscious and lucid. A profound circulatory disturbance associated with sympathetic overactivity (elevated blood pressure, tachycardia, arrhythmia) may occur on the second to fourth day, which may contribute to the mortality rate.

B. Laboratory Findings

The diagnosis is made on clinical grounds. The CSF is normal with the exception of mild elevation of opening pressure. Serum muscle enzymes may be elevated. Anaerobic culture and microscopic examination of pus from the wound can be helpful, but *C tetani* is difficult to grow.

▶ Differential Diagnosis

Poliomyelitis is characterized by asymmetrical flaccid paralysis in an incompletely immunized child. The history of an animal bite and the absence of trismus may suggest rabies. Local infections of the throat and jaw should be easily recognized. Bacterial meningitis, phenothiazine reactions, decerebrate posturing, narcotic withdrawal, spondylitis, and hypocalcemic tetany may be confused with tetanus.

▶ Complications

Complications include sepsis, malnutrition, pneumonia, atelectasis, asphyxial spasms, decubitus ulcers, and fractures of the spine due to intense contractions. They can be prevented in part by skilled supportive care.

▶ Treatment of Tetanus

A. Specific Measures

Human TIG in a single dose 500 units, intramuscularly, is given to children and adults. Infiltration of part of the TIG dose around the wound is recommended. If TIG is indicated, but not available, intravenous immunoglobulin in a dose of 200–400 mg/kg intravenously can be infused over several hours (although it is not licensed for this indication; see package insert for infusion instructions). In countries where TIG or immunoglobulins are not available, equine tetanus antitoxin may be available. Surgical debridement of wounds is indicated, but more extensive surgery or amputation to eliminate the site of infection is not necessary. Antibiotics are given in an attempt to decrease the bacterial load and subsequent toxin production: oral or intravenous metronidazole for 7–10 days is the preferred agent. Parenteral penicillin G is an alternative regimen. An age-appropriate tetanus toxoid containing vaccine should be administered in a different limb from the TIG administration site.

B. General Measures

Treatment of tetanus is usually best accomplished in an intensive care unit. The patient is kept in a quiet room with minimal stimulation. Control of spasms and prevention of hypoxic episodes are crucial. Benzodiazepines and neuromuscular blocking agents can be used to help control spasms and provide some sedation. Magnesium sulfate may be used to manage autonomic dysfunction. Mechanical ventilation and muscle paralysis are necessary in severe cases. Nasogastric or intravenous feedings should be used to limit stimulation of feedings and prevent aspiration.

Prognosis

The fatality rate in newborns, injection drug users, and patients with diabetes is high. The overall mortality rate in the United States is 6%. The fatality rate depends on the quality of supportive care, the patient's age, and the patient's vaccination history. Many deaths are due to pneumonia or respiratory failure. If the patient survives 1 week, recovery is likely. Complete recovery may take months.

Centers for Disease Control and Prevention (CDC): Clinical Information. http://www.cdc.gov/tetanus/clinicians.html. Accessed May 24, 2023.

Centers for Disease Control and Prevention (CDC): Tetanus. http://www.cdc.gov/vaccines/pubs/pinkbook/tetanus.html. Accessed May 24, 2023.

GAS GANGRENE

ESSENTIALS OF DIAGNOSIS & TYPICAL FEATURES

- ► Contamination of a wound with soil or feces.
- ► Massive edema, skin discoloration, bleb formation, and pain in an area of trauma.
- ► Serosanguineous exudate from wound.
- ► Crepitation of subcutaneous tissue.
- ► Rapid progression of signs and symptoms.
- ► Clostridia cultured or seen on stained smears.

General Considerations

Gas gangrene (clostridial myonecrosis) is a necrotizing infection that follows trauma or surgery and is caused by several anaerobic, gram-positive, spore-forming bacilli of the genus *Clostridium*. Occasionally the source is the gastrointestinal tract, and muscles are hematogenously seeded. The spores are found in soil, feces, and vaginal secretions. In devitalized tissue, the spores germinate into vegetative bacilli that proliferate and produce toxins, causing thrombosis, hemolysis, and tissue necrosis. *C perfringens*, the species causing approximately 80% of cases of gas gangrene, produces at least eight toxins. The areas involved most often are the extremities, abdomen, and uterus. *Clostridium septicum* may also cause myonecrosis and causes septicemia in patients with neutropenia. Nonclostridial infections with gas formation can mimic clostridial infections and are more common. Neutropenia is a risk factor for this severe infection.

Prevention

Gas gangrene can be prevented by the adequate cleansing and debridement of all wounds. It is essential that foreign bodies and dead tissue be removed. A clean wound does not provide a suitable anaerobic environment for the growth of clostridial species.

Clinical Findings

A. Symptoms and Signs

The onset of gas gangrene usually is sudden, often 1 day after trauma or surgery, but can be delayed up to 20 days. Pain is intense and may seem out of proportion to the degree of trauma. There may be swelling and skin around the wound may become discolored (pale, red, or purple), with hemorrhagic bullae, serosanguineous exudate, and crepitus may be observed in subcutaneous tissues. The absence of fever or crepitus does not rule out the diagnosis. Systemic illness appears early and progresses rapidly to intravascular hemolysis, jaundice, shock, toxic delirium, and renal failure.

B. Laboratory Findings

Isolation of the organism requires anaerobic cultures. The wound exudate, soft tissue, muscle, and blood can be cultured. Gram-stained smears may demonstrate many gram-positive rods and few inflammatory cells. Two FDA-approved devices that use matrix-assisted laser desorption/ionization-time-of-flight (MALDI-TOF) have an approved indication to identify *C perfringens*.

C. Imaging

Radiographs may demonstrate gas in tissues, but this is a late finding and is also seen in infections with other gas-forming organisms or may be due to air introduced into tissues during trauma or surgery.

D. Operative Findings

Direct visualization of the muscle at surgery may be necessary to diagnose gas gangrene. Early, the muscle is pale and edematous and does not contract normally; later, the muscle may be frankly gangrenous.

Differential Diagnosis

Gangrene and cellulitis caused by other organisms and clostridial cellulitis (not myonecrosis) must be distinguished. Necrotizing fasciitis may resemble gas gangrene.

Treatment

A. Specific Measures

Penicillin G plus clindamycin is the recommended treatment. Metronidazole, meropenem, ertapenem, and chloramphenicol are alternatives for penicillin-allergic patients.

B. Surgical Measures

Surgery should be prompt and extensive, with removal of all necrotic tissue. Compartment syndromes can occur even if there are few cutaneous findings. Checking compartment pressures in patients with severe pain and any signs of compartment syndrome is prudent.

C. Hyperbaric Oxygen

Hyperbaric oxygen therapy is controversial, but good outcomes have been reported in nonrandomized studies using hyperbaric oxygen in combination with surgery and antibiotics.

▶ Prognosis

Clostridial myonecrosis is fatal if untreated. With early diagnosis, antibiotics, and surgery, the mortality rate is 20%–60%. Involvement of the abdominal wall, leukopenia, intravascular hemolysis, renal failure, and shock are ominous prognostic signs.

Stevens DL et al: Practice guidelines for the diagnosis and management of skin and soft tissue infections: 2014 update by the Infectious Diseases Society of America. Clin Infect Dis 2014;59:e10 [PMID: 24973422].

DIPHTHERIA

ESSENTIALS OF DIAGNOSIS & TYPICAL FEATURES

- ▶ Gray, adherent pseudomembrane, most often in the pharynx but also in the nasopharynx or trachea.
- ▶ Sore throat, serosanguineous nasal discharge, hoarseness, and fever in a nonimmunized child.
- ▶ Peripheral neuritis or myocarditis.
- ▶ Positive culture.
- ▶ Treatment should not be withheld pending culture results.

▶ General Considerations

Diphtheria is an acute infection of the upper respiratory tract or skin caused by toxin-producing *Corynebacterium diphtheriae*. Diphtheria in the United States is rare. However, significant numbers of elderly adults and unimmunized children are susceptible to infection. Diphtheria still occurs in epidemics in countries where immunization is not universal. Unimmunized travelers to these areas may acquire the disease.

Corynebacteria are gram-positive, club-shaped rods with a beaded appearance on Gram stain. The capacity to produce exotoxin is conferred by a lysogenic bacteriophage and is not present in all strains of *C diphtheriae*. In immunized communities, infection probably occurs through spread of the phage among carriers of susceptible *C diphtheriae* rather than through spread of phage-containing bacteria themselves. Diphtheria toxin kills susceptible cells by irreversible inhibition of protein synthesis.

The toxin is absorbed into the mucous membranes and causes destruction of epithelium and a superficial inflammatory response. The necrotic epithelium becomes embedded in exuded fibrin with WBCs and RBCs (red blood cells), forming a grayish pseudomembrane over the tonsils, pharynx, or larynx. Any attempt to remove the membrane exposes and tears the capillaries, resulting in bleeding. The diphtheria bacilli within the membrane continue to produce toxin, which is absorbed and may result in toxic injury to the heart muscle, liver, kidneys, and adrenals, and is sometimes accompanied by hemorrhage. The toxin also produces neuritis, resulting in paralysis of the soft palate, eye muscles, or extremities. Death may result from respiratory obstruction or toxemia and circulatory collapse. The patient may succumb after a somewhat longer time as a result of cardiac damage. The incubation period is 2–5 days.

▶ Clinical Findings

A. Symptoms and Signs

1. Pharyngeal diphtheria—Early manifestations of diphtheritic pharyngitis are mild sore throat, moderate fever, and malaise, followed fairly rapidly by prostration and circulatory collapse. The pulse is more rapid than the fever would seem to justify. A pharyngeal membrane forms and may spread into the nasopharynx or the trachea, producing respiratory obstruction. The membrane is tenacious and gray, and is surrounded by a narrow zone of erythema and a broader zone of edema. The cervical lymph nodes become swollen, which is associated with brawny edema of the neck (so-called bull neck). Laryngeal diphtheria presents with stridor, which can progress to airway obstruction.

2. Other forms—Cutaneous, vaginal, and wound diphtheria cases account for up to one-third and are characterized by ulcerative lesions with membrane formation.

B. Laboratory Findings

Diagnosis requires culture of *C diphtheriae* obtained from the nose, throat, or skin lesions present. Specialized culture media is required so laboratory personnel should be notified if diphtheria is suspected. A toxigenicity test should be performed to differentiate toxigenic from nontoxigenic strains of *C diphtheriae*. New non–culture-based methods such as PCR or MALDI-TOF mass spectroscopy can be useful as cultures may be negative in individuals who have received antibiotics. The WBC count usually is normal, but hemolytic anemia and thrombocytopenia are frequent.

Differential Diagnosis

Pharyngeal diphtheria resembles pharyngitis secondary to β-hemolytic *Streptococcus*, Epstein-Barr virus, or other viral respiratory pathogens. A nasal foreign body or purulent sinusitis may mimic nasal diphtheria. Other causes of laryngeal obstruction include epiglottitis and viral croup. Guillain-Barré syndrome, poliomyelitis, or acute poisoning may mimic the neuropathy of diphtheria.

Complications

A. Myocarditis

Diphtheritic myocarditis is characterized by a rapid, thready pulse; indistinct heart sounds, ST-T-wave changes, conduction abnormalities, dysrhythmias, or cardiac failure; hepatomegaly; and fluid retention. Myocardial dysfunction may occur from 2 to 40 days after the onset of pharyngitis.

B. Polyneuritis

Neuritis of the palatal and pharyngeal nerves occurs during the first or second week. Nasal speech and regurgitation of food through the nose are seen. Diplopia and strabismus occur during the third week or later. Neuritis may also involve peripheral nerves supplying the intercostal muscles, diaphragm, and other muscle groups. Generalized paresis usually occurs after the fourth week.

C. Bronchopneumonia

Secondary pneumonia is common in fatal cases.

Prevention

A. Immunization

Immunization with diphtheria toxoid combined with pertussis and tetanus toxoids (DTaP) should be used routinely for infants and children (see Chapter 10).

B. Care of Exposed Susceptibles

Children exposed to diphtheria should be examined, and nose and throat cultures obtained. Immunized asymptomatic individuals who have not received a diphtheria toxoid booster within 5 years and inadequately immunized individuals all should receive a diphtheria toxoid vaccine. Regardless of immunization status, close contacts should receive either erythromycin orally (40–50 mg/kg/day in four divided doses) for 7–10 days or a single dose of benzathine penicillin G intramuscularly (600,000 units for children weighing

< 30 kg, and 1.2 million units for children weighing ≥ 30 kg and for adults) and be closely observed.

Treatment

A. Specific Measures

1. Antitoxin—Suspected diphtheria should be reported promptly to the Centers for Disease Control Emergency Center (770-488-7100) so diphtheria antitoxin can be obtained. Diphtheria antitoxin is no longer commercially available. To be effective, diphtheria antitoxin should be administered within 48 hours of symptom onset (see Chapter 9).

2. Antibiotics—Acceptable regimens include erythromycin given parenterally or orally, aqueous penicillin G intravenously, or procaine penicillin G intramuscularly. Treatment should be given for 14 days.

B. General Measures

Patients should receive a diphtheria toxoid–containing vaccine during convalescence as infection does not confer immunity. Observation of patients in the hospital for 10–14 days is usually required. All patients must be strictly isolated for 1–7 days until respiratory secretions are noncontagious. Isolation may be discontinued when two successive nose and throat cultures at 24-hour intervals are negative. These cultures should be taken at least 24 hours after completion of antibiotic treatment.

C. Treatment of Carriers

All carriers should receive either erythromycin for 10–14 days or a single dose of benzathine penicillin G (600,000 units for children weighing < 30 kg, and 1.2 million units for children weighing ≥ 30 kg or for adults), and they must be quarantined. Before release from quarantine carriers must have two negative cultures of both the nose and the throat taken 24 hours apart and obtained at least 24 hours after the cessation of antibiotic therapy. If follow-up cultures remain positive, they should receive another 10 day course of erythromycin.

Prognosis

Mortality varies from 3% to 10% and is particularly high in the presence of early myocarditis. Neuritis is reversible. Diphtheria is fatal if an intact airway and adequate respiration cannot be maintained. Permanent heart damage from myocarditis occurs rarely.

Diphtheria. In: Kimberlin DW, Brady MT, Jackson MA, Long SS, (eds): *Red Book: 2021–2024 Report of the Committee on Infectious Diseases.* 32nd ed. Itasca, IL: American Academy of Pediatrics; 2021:304–307.

Centers for Disease Control and Prevention (CDC): Diphtheria. http://www.cdc.gov/diphtheria/clinicians.html. Accessed May 27, 2023.

INFECTIONS DUE TO ENTEROBACTERIACEAE

▶ General Considerations

Enterobacteriaceae are a family of gram-negative bacilli that are normal flora in the gastrointestinal tract of people and animals that contaminate water and soil. They cause gastroenteritis, urinary tract infections, neonatal sepsis and meningitis, and opportunistic infections. *Escherichia coli* is the organism in this family that most commonly causes infection in children, but *Klebsiella, Morganella, Enterobacter, Serratia, Proteus*, and other genera are also important, particularly in hospitalized persons or immune compromised hosts. *Shigella* and *Salmonella* are discussed in separate sections.

Some *E coli* strains cause diarrhea by several distinct mechanisms. Enteropathogenic *E coli* (EPEC) strains cause a characteristic histologic injury in the small bowel through adherence and effacement. Enteroaggregative *E coli* (EAEC) adheres to the small and large bowel and causes diarrhea through enterotoxin and cytotoxin production. Enterotoxigenic *E coli* (ETEC) adheres to enterocytes and secretes one or more plasmid-encoded enterotoxins. One of these, heat-labile toxin, resembles cholera toxin in structure, function, and mechanism of action. Enteroinvasive *E coli* (EIEC) are very similar to *Shigella* in their pathogenetic mechanisms. Shigella-toxin producing *E coli* (STEC) cause hemorrhagic colitis and hemolytic uremic syndrome (HUS). The STEC serotype is O157:H7 and is particularly virulent, although several other serotypes cause the same syndrome. These strains elaborate one of several cytotoxins, closely related to Shiga toxin produced by *Shigella dysenteriae*. Outbreaks of HUS associated with STEC have followed consumption of inadequately cooked ground beef, unpasteurized dairy, fruit juice, various uncooked vegetables, flour, and contaminated water. The common source for STEC in all of these foods and water is contamination with feces of cattle or several other animals. Person-to-person spread including spread in day care centers by the fecal-oral route has been reported. It is estimated that STEC causes over 265,000 illnesses in the United States each year. Eighty percent of *E coli* strains causing neonatal meningitis possess a specific capsular polysaccharide (K1 antigen), which alone or in association with specific somatic antigens confers virulence.

Among Enterobacteriaceae, *Klebsiella* may cause a bronchopneumonia with cavity formation. *Klebsiella, Enterobacter*, and *Serratia* are often hospital-acquired opportunists associated with antibiotic usage, debilitated states, and chronic respiratory conditions. They frequently cause urinary tract infection or sepsis. Many of these infections are difficult to treat because of antibiotic resistance including infections caused by extended-spectrum β-lactamase (ESBL) pathogens and carbapenem-resistant Enterobacterales (CRE). Antibiotic susceptibility tests are necessary given limited options for therapy.

▶ Clinical Findings

A. Symptoms and Signs

1. *E coli* gastroenteritis—*E coli* may cause diarrhea of varying types and severity. EPEC and EAEC often causes watery diarrhea, though EAEC can occasionally cause bloody diarrhea. ETEC usually produce mild, self-limiting illness without significant fever or systemic toxicity, often known as traveler's diarrhea. However, diarrhea may be severe in newborns and infants, and occasionally an older child or adult will have a cholera-like syndrome. EIEC strains, which cause a shigellosis-like illness, characterized by fever, systemic symptoms, blood and mucus in the stool, are uncommon in the United States. STEC strains cause hemorrhagic colitis. Diarrhea initially is watery and fever usually is absent. Abdominal pain and cramping occur; diarrhea progresses to blood streaking or grossly bloody stools. HUS typically occurs 1–2 weeks after the onset of diarrhea with a rate of 15% in children with O157:H7, and is characterized by microangiopathic hemolytic anemia, thrombocytopenia, and renal failure (see Chapter 24).

2. Neonatal sepsis—Findings include jaundice, hepatosplenomegaly, fever, temperature lability, apneic spells, irritability, and poor feeding. Respiratory distress develops when pneumonia occurs; it may appear indistinguishable from respiratory distress syndrome in preterm infants. Meningitis is associated with bacteremia in 25%–40% of cases. Other metastatic foci of infection may be present, including pneumonia and pyelonephritis. Sepsis may lead to severe metabolic acidosis, shock, DIC, and death.

3. Neonatal meningitis—Findings include high fever, full fontanelles, vomiting, coma, convulsions, paresis or paralyses, poor or absent Moro reflex, opisthotonos, and occasionally hypertonia or hypotonia. Sepsis coexists or precedes meningitis in most cases. CSF usually shows a cell count of over 1000 WBC/μL, mostly polymorphonuclear neutrophils, and bacteria on Gram stain. CSF glucose concentration is low (usually less than half that of blood), and the protein is elevated above the levels normally seen in newborns and premature infants (> 150 mg/dL).

4. Acute urinary tract infection—Symptoms include dysuria, increased urinary frequency, and fever in the older child. Nonspecific symptoms such as anorexia, vomiting, irritability, failure to thrive, and unexplained fever are seen in children younger than age 2 years. Young infants may present with jaundice. As many as 1%–3% of school-aged girls and 0.5% of boys have asymptomatic bacteriuria. Screening for and treatment of asymptomatic bacteriuria is not recommended.

B. Laboratory Findings

Because *E coli* are normal flora in the stool, a positive stool culture is not useful for determining the etiology of an illness. Multiplex PCR tests are available to rapidly diagnose STEC and other enteropathogens. Rapid immunologic assays such as enzyme immunoassays (EIA) and immunochromatographic assays are available to detect Shiga toxin. Blood cultures are positive in neonatal sepsis. Cultures of CSF and urine should also be obtained in neonatal sepsis. The diagnosis of urinary tract infections is discussed in Chapter 24.

► Differential Diagnosis

The clinical picture of *E coli* infection may resemble that of other enteric infections such as salmonellosis, shigellosis, or viral gastroenteritis. Neonatal sepsis and meningitis caused by *E coli* can be differentiated from other causes of neonatal infection by culture.

► Treatment

A. Specific Measures

1. *E coli* gastroenteritis—Gastroenteritis seldom requires antimicrobial treatment. Fluid and electrolyte therapy, preferably given orally, may be required to avoid dehydration. Antibiotics are generally not recommended because of potential selection for resistant organisms, risks and side effects of antibiotics, and because diarrhea caused by *E coli* will typically resolve spontaneously. Traveler's diarrhea may be treated with azithromycin in children and with fluoroquinolones in adults, although resistance to these drugs is increasing. The risk of HUS is not proven to be increased by antimicrobial therapy of STEC cases, but most experts recommend against antimicrobial treatment of suspected cases because some studies found an increased risk after antibiotics.

2. *E coli* sepsis and pneumonia—The drugs of choice are ampicillin, ceftriaxone, and gentamicin (specific dosing vary by age, weight, and co-morbidities). Initial therapy often includes at least two drugs until microbial etiology is established and susceptibility testing is completed. Third-generation cephalosporins are frequently utilized, because they are less toxic and require less monitoring than aminoglycosides. Treatment is continued for 10–14 days.

3. *E coli* meningitis—Third-generation cephalosporins such as ceftriaxone are given for a minimum of 3 weeks. Ampicillin is also effective for susceptible strains. Data supporting use of intrathecal and intraventricular medications are limited.

4. Acute urinary tract infection—(See Chapter 24.)

► Prognosis

Death due to gastroenteritis leading to dehydration can be prevented by early fluid and electrolyte therapy. Effective treatment has reduced mortality from neonatal sepsis with meningitis to 10%–20%; however, many survivors have some degree of residual disability. Most children with recurrent urinary tract infections do well if they have no underlying anatomic defects. The mortality rate in opportunistic infections usually depends on the severity of infection and the underlying immune compromising condition.

Centers for Disease Control and Prevention (CDC): *Escherichia coli*. http://www.cdc.gov/ecoli/. Accessed May 10, 2023.

Mody RK et al: Postdiarrheal hemolytic uremic syndrome in the United States children: clinical spectrum and predictors of in-hospital death. J Pediatr 2015 Apr;166(4):1022–1029. doi: 10.1016/j.jpeds.2014.12.064. Epub 2015 Feb 4 [PMID: 25661408].

Shane AL et al: 2017 Infectious Diseases Society of America clinical practice guidelines for the diagnosis and management of infectious diarrhea. Clin Infect Dis 2017;65(12):1963–1973 [PMID: 29194529].

Tamma PD et al: Infectious Diseases Society of America Guidance on the Treatment of Antimicrobial-Resistant Gram-Negative Infections: Version 1.0. https://www.idsociety.org/practice-guideline/amr-guidance/. Accessed May 10, 2023

PSEUDOMONAS INFECTIONS

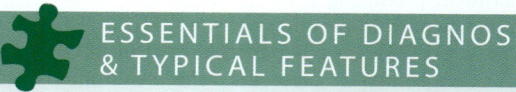

ESSENTIALS OF DIAGNOSIS & TYPICAL FEATURES

► Opportunistic and nosocomial infection.
► Immunocompromised hosts, cystic fibrosis, burns.
► Confirmed by cultures.

► General Considerations

Pseudomonas aeruginosa is an aerobic gram-negative rod with versatile metabolic requirements. The organism may grow in distilled water and in commonly used disinfectants, complicating infection control in medical facilities. *P aeruginosa* is both invasive and destructive to tissue as well as toxigenic due to secreted exotoxins, all factors that contribute to virulence. Other genera previously classified as *Pseudomonas* frequently cause nosocomial infections and infections in immunocompromised children. These include *Stenotrophomonas maltophilia* and *Burkholderia cepacia*.

P aeruginosa is an important cause of infection in children with cystic fibrosis, neoplastic disease, neutropenia, or extensive burns and in those receiving antibiotic therapy. *P aeruginosa* infects the tracheobronchial tree of nearly all patients with cystic fibrosis. Mucoid exopolysaccharide, an exuberant capsule, is characteristically overproduced by isolates from patients with cystic fibrosis. Although bacteremia seldom occurs, patients with cystic fibrosis can succumb to chronic lung infection with *P aeruginosa*.

Infections can occur in various locations including the urinary and respiratory tracts, ears, mastoids, paranasal sinuses, eyes, skin, meninges, and bones. *Pseudomonas* pneumonia is a common nosocomial infection in patients receiving assisted ventilation. *P aeruginosa* is a frequent cause of malignant external otitis media and of chronic suppurative otitis media. Outbreaks of vesiculopustular skin rash have been associated with exposure to contaminated water in whirlpool baths and hot tubs. Osteomyelitis of the calcaneus or other foot bones, which occurs after punctures such as stepping on a nail, is commonly due to *P aeruginosa*.

Sepsis can also be caused by *P aeruginosa* and may be accompanied by characteristic peripheral lesions called ecthyma gangrenosum. Ecthyma gangrenosum also may occur by direct invasion through intact skin in the groin, axilla, or other skinfolds. *P aeruginosa* is an infrequent cause of sepsis in previously healthy infants and may be the initial sign of underlying medical problems.

▶ Clinical Findings

The clinical findings depend on the site of infection and the patient's underlying disease. Sepsis with these organisms resembles gram-negative sepsis with other organisms, although the presence of ecthyma gangrenosum suggests the etiologic diagnosis. The diagnosis is made by culture. *Pseudomonas* infection should be suspected in neonates and neutropenic patients with clinical sepsis. A severe necrotizing pneumonia occurs in patients on ventilators.

Patients with cystic fibrosis have a persistent bronchitis that progresses to bronchiectasis and ultimately to respiratory failure. During exacerbations of illness, cough and sputum production increase along with low-grade fever, malaise, and diminished energy.

The purulent aural drainage without fever in patients with chronic suppurative otitis media is not distinguishable from that due to other causes.

▶ Prevention

A. Infections in Debilitated Patients

Colonization of extensive second- and third-degree burns by *P aeruginosa* can lead to fatal septicemia. Aggressive debridement and topical treatment with 0.5% silver nitrate solution, 10% mafenide cream, or silver sulfadiazine will greatly inhibit *P aeruginosa* contamination of burns. (See Chapter 12 for a discussion of burn wound infections and prevention.)

B. Nosocomial Infections

Faucet aerators, communal soap dispensers, disinfectants, improperly cleaned inhalation therapy equipment, infant incubators, and many other sources that usually are associated with wet or humid conditions all have been associated with *Pseudomonas* epidemics. Patient-to-patient transmission by hospital staff carrying *Pseudomonas* on their hands occurs when hand hygiene is inadequate. Careful maintenance of equipment and enforcement of infection control procedures are essential to minimize nosocomial transmission.

C. Patients with Cystic Fibrosis

Chronic infection of the lower respiratory tract occurs in nearly all patients with cystic fibrosis. The infecting organism is seldom cleared from the respiratory tract, even with intensive antimicrobial therapy, and the resultant injury to the lung eventually leads to pulmonary insufficiency.

▶ Treatment

P aeruginosa is inherently resistant to many antimicrobials and may develop resistance during therapy. Antibiotics effective against *Pseudomonas* include the aminoglycosides, ureidopenicillins (piperacillin), β-lactamase inhibitor with a ureidopenicillin (piperacillin-tazobactam), expanded-spectrum cephalosporins (ceftazidime and cefepime), monobactams (aztreonam), carbapenems (doripenem, meropenem), and fluoroquinolones (ciprofloxacin, levofloxacin). Aminoglycosides (gentamicin, tobramycin) may be used as an adjunct to the drugs listed above, but not as monotherapy except in the case of urinary tract infections. Colistin and polymyxin have been used in children with extensive drug resistance. Several next-generation treatments have shown promise with multidrug-resistant *P aeruginosa* infections, including imipenem-cilastatin-relibactam, ceftazidime-avibactam, ceftolozane-tazobactam, and cefiderocol, although pediatric data are limited. Antimicrobial susceptibility patterns vary regionally and within facilities, driven in part by institutional practice, and resistance tends to appear as new drugs become heavily used. Treatment of infections is best guided by clinical response and susceptibility tests.

Several antibiotic classes can generally be used as monotherapy for most pseudomonas infections if the isolate is susceptible. Cefepime is widely utilized in pediatric patients, particularly those who are immunocompromised or critically ill. Levofloxacin or ciprofloxacin are also common choices when there is beta-lactam allergy or resistance; the fluoroquinolones also have the advantage of highly bioavailable oral formulations. Meropenem and piperacillin-tazobactam have the disadvantage of very broad activity. Coverage with two antipseudomonal antibiotics is standard practice for the treatment of pulmonary exacerbations in patients with cystic fibrosis. Aerosolized antipseudomonal antibiotics, tobramycin and aztreonam, have been very useful adjunctive therapy for these patients.

Pseudomonas osteomyelitis due to punctures requires thorough surgical debridement and antimicrobial therapy. *Pseudomonas* folliculitis does not require antibiotic therapy.

Chronic suppurative otitis media may be treated with topical ofloxacin or ciprofloxacin and aural toilet. Failure of treatment with conservative measures may necessitate oral or parenteral antibiotic therapy guided by culture results. Swimmer's ear may be caused by *P aeruginosa* and responds well to topical drying agents (alcohol–vinegar mix) and cleansing.

► Prognosis

Because debilitated patients are most frequently affected, the mortality rate is high. These infections may have a protracted course, and eradication of the organisms may be difficult.

Tamma PD et al: Infectious Diseases Society of America 2022 guidance on the treatment of extended-spectrum β-lactamase producing enterobacterales (ESBL-E), carbapenem-resistant enterobacterales (CRE), and *Pseudomonas aeruginosa* with difficult-to-treat resistance (DTR-*P. aeruginosa*). Clin Infect Dis 2022 Aug 25;75(2):187–212. doi: 10.1093/cid/ciac268.

Wuyts L et al: Juvenile ecthyma gangrenosum caused by *Pseudomonas aeruginosa* revealing an underlying neutropenia: case report and review of the literature. J Eur Acad Dermatol Venereol 2019 Jan 11. https://doi.org/10.1111/jdv.15420.

Yahav D et al: New β-lactam-β-lactamase inhibitor combinations. Clin Microbiol Rev 2020;34:E00115-20. doi: 10.1128/CMR.00115-20.

SALMONELLA GASTROENTERITIS

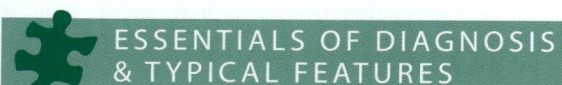

ESSENTIALS OF DIAGNOSIS & TYPICAL FEATURES

► Nausea, vomiting, headache.

► Fever, diarrhea, abdominal pain.

► Culture or PCR of organism from stool or blood.

► General Considerations

Salmonellae are gram-negative rods that frequently cause food-borne gastroenteritis and occasionally bacteremia, infection of bone, meninges, and other foci. Over 2600 serovars of *Salmonella enterica* are recognized and nomenclature typically refers to specific serovars which are not italicized, for example, *Salmonella typhimurium*. It is estimated that more than 1.35 million cases occur yearly in the United States.

Salmonellae are able to penetrate the mucin layer of the small bowel, attach to and penetrate epithelial cells, and multiply in the submucosa. Infection results in fever, vomiting, and watery diarrhea; the diarrhea occasionally includes mucus and polymorphonuclear neutrophils in the stool. Salmonella infections in childhood occur in two major forms: (1) gastroenteritis (including food poisoning), which may be complicated by sepsis and focal suppurative complications; and (2) enteric fever (see section Typhoid Fever & Paratyphoid Fever). Although the incidence of typhoid fever has decreased in the United States, *Salmonella* gastroenteritis remains common. The highest attack rates occur in children younger than 5 years.

Salmonellae are widespread in nature, infecting domestic and wild animals. Fowl and reptiles have a particularly high carriage rate. Outbreaks have been associated with petting zoos, pet reptiles, and backyard chickens. Numerous foods, especially milk, eggs, and poultry, are associated with outbreaks.

Because salmonellae are susceptible to gastric acidity, elderly patients, infants, and those taking antacids or H_2-blocking drugs are at increased risk for infection. Most cases of *Salmonella* meningitis (80%) and bacteremia occur in infancy. Newborns may acquire the infection from their mothers during delivery.

► Clinical Findings

A. Symptoms and Signs

There is a very wide range of severity of infection. Infants usually develop fever, vomiting, and diarrhea. Older children may complain of headache, nausea, and abdominal pain. Stools are often watery or may contain mucus and, in some instances, blood, suggesting shigellosis. Drowsiness and disorientation may occur in association with meningismus. Convulsions occur less frequently than with shigellosis. Splenomegaly occasionally occurs. In the usual case, diarrhea is moderate and subsides after 4–7 days, but it may be protracted.

B. Laboratory Findings

Diagnosis is made by isolation in culture or by PCR of the organism from stool, blood, or, in some cases from urine, CSF, or pus from a suppurative lesion. The WBC count usually shows a polymorphonuclear leukocytosis but may show leukopenia. *Salmonella* isolates should be reported to public health authorities for epidemiologic purposes.

Differential Diagnosis

In staphylococcal food poisoning, the incubation period is shorter (2–4 hours) than in *Salmonella* food poisoning (6–48 hours), fever is absent, and vomiting rather than diarrhea is the main symptom. In shigellosis, many polymorphonuclear leukocytes usually are seen on a stained smear of stool, and the peripheral WBC count is more likely to show a marked left shift, although some cases of salmonellosis are indistinguishable from shigellosis. *Campylobacter* gastroenteritis commonly resembles salmonellosis. Culture or PCR of stool is necessary to distinguish the causes of bacterial gastroenteritis.

Complications

Unlike most causes of infectious diarrhea, salmonellosis is frequently accompanied by bacteremia, especially in infants, who are also susceptible to developing meningitis. Septicemia with extraintestinal infection is seen, most commonly with *Salmonella choleraesuis*, but also with *S enterica*, *S typhimurium*, and *S paratyphi* serotypes. The organism may spread to any tissue and may cause arthritis, osteomyelitis, cholecystitis, endocarditis, meningitis, pericarditis, pneumonia, or pyelonephritis. Patients with sickle cell anemia or other hemoglobinopathies have a predilection for the development of osteomyelitis. Severe dehydration and shock are more likely to occur with shigellosis but may occur with *Salmonella* gastroenteritis.

Treatment

A. Specific Measures

In uncomplicated *Salmonella* gastroenteritis, antibiotic treatment does not shorten the course of the clinical illness and may prolong convalescent carriage of the organism. Colitis or secretory diarrhea due to *Salmonella* may improve with antibiotic therapy. In more severe cases, treatment should be initiated with ceftriaxone followed by a transition to azithromycin.

Because of the higher risk of sepsis and focal disease, antibiotic treatment is recommended in infants younger than 3 months; in severely ill children; and in children with sickle cell disease or hemoglobinopathies, malignancy, HIV infection, or on immunosuppressive treatments. Infants younger than 3 months with positive stool cultures or suspected salmonellosis sepsis should be admitted to the hospital, evaluated for focal infection including cultures of blood and CSF, and given treatment intravenously. A third-generation cephalosporin is usually recommended due to frequent resistance

to ampicillin and TMP-SMX. Older patients developing bacteremia during the course of gastroenteritis should receive parenteral treatment initially, and a careful search should be made for additional foci of infection. After signs and symptoms subside, these patients should receive oral medication selected based on susceptibilities. Parenteral and oral treatment should last a total of 7–10 days. Longer treatment is indicated for specific complications (eg, ~4–6 weeks for meningitis or osteomyelitis). If susceptibility tests indicate resistance to ampicillin/amoxicillin, third-generation cephalosporins, TMP-SMX, fluoroquinolones, or azithromycin may be used.

B. Treatment of the Carrier State

About one-half of patients may have positive stool cultures after 4 weeks. Infants tend to remain convalescent carriers for up to 1 year. Antibiotic treatment of carriers is not effective.

C. General Measures

Careful attention must be given to maintaining fluid and electrolyte balance, especially in infants.

Prevention

Measures for the prevention of *Salmonella* infections include good hand hygiene after handling birds or reptiles, thorough cooking of food derived from contaminated sources, adequate refrigeration, control of infection among domestic animals, and meticulous meat and poultry inspections. Raw and undercooked fresh eggs should be avoided. Food handlers and child care workers with salmonellosis should be cleared (eg, need for negative stool cultures) before resuming work. Asymptomatic children, who have recovered from *Salmonella* infection, do not need school or day care exclusion.

Prognosis

In gastroenteritis, the prognosis is good. In sepsis with focal suppurative complications, the prognosis is more guarded. The case fatality rate of *Salmonella* meningitis is high in infants and there is a risk of relapse if treatment is not continued for at least 4 weeks.

Centers for Disease Control and Prevention (CDC): *Salmonella* infection (salmonellosis). http://www.cdc.gov/salmonella/. Accessed May 10, 2023.

Shane AL et al: 2017 Infectious Diseases Society of America clinical practice guidelines for the diagnosis and management of infectious diarrhea. Clin Infect Dis 2017 Dec 15;65(12):e45–e80 [PMID: 29053792].

Wen SC et al: Non-typhoidal *Salmonella* infections in children: review of literature and recommendations for management. J Paediatr Child Health 2017 Oct;53(10):936–941. doi: 10.1111/jpc.13585 [PMID: 28556448].

TYPHOID FEVER & PARATYPHOID FEVER

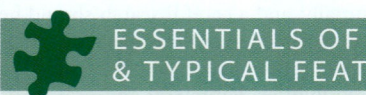

ESSENTIALS OF DIAGNOSIS & TYPICAL FEATURES

▶ Insidious or acute onset of headache, anorexia, vomiting, constipation or diarrhea, ileus, and high fever.

▶ Meningismus, splenomegaly, and rose spots.

▶ Leukopenia; positive blood, stool, bone marrow, and urine cultures.

▶ Fever in the returning traveler.

▶ General Considerations

Typhoid fever is caused by the gram-negative bacillus *S enterica* serotypes Typhi and Paratyphi. The incubation period is generally 7–14 days. The organism enters the body through the walls of the intestinal tract and, following a transient bacteremia, multiplies in the reticuloendothelial cells of the liver and spleen. Persistent bacteremia and symptoms then follow. Reinfection of the intestine occurs as organisms are excreted in the bile. Bacterial emboli produce the characteristic skin lesions (rose spots). Typhoid fever is transmitted by the fecal-oral route and by contamination of food or water. Unlike other *Salmonella* species, there are no animal reservoirs of typhoid; each case is the result of direct or indirect contact with the bacteria or with an individual who is actively infected or a chronic carrier.

It is estimated that there are 11–21 million cases a year of typhoid fever worldwide with nearly 6000 cases estimated to affect those in the United States, mainly among American travelers.

▶ Clinical Findings

A. Symptoms and Signs

Typhoid fever is frequently encountered as an undifferentiated febrile illness in recent travelers from low- and middle-income countries. In children, the onset of typhoid fever usually is sudden rather than insidious, with malaise, headache, cough, crampy abdominal pain and distention, and sometimes constipation, followed within 48 hours by diarrhea, high fever, and toxemia. An encephalopathy may be seen with irritability, confusion, delirium, and stupor. Vomiting and meningismus may be prominent in infants and young children.

During the prodromal stage, physical findings may be absent, but abdominal distention and tenderness, meningismus, mild hepatomegaly, and splenomegaly may be present. The typical typhoidal rash (rose spots) is present in 10%–15%

of children. A small number (< 20) appear during the second week of the disease and may erupt in crops for the succeeding 10–14 days. Rose spots are erythematous maculopapular lesions 2–3 mm in diameter that blanch on pressure. They are found principally on the trunk and chest, and they generally disappear within 3–4 days.

B. Laboratory Findings

Typhoid bacilli can be isolated from many sites, including blood, stool, urine, bile, and bone marrow. Blood cultures are positive in 60% of cases in children, particularly if obtained early in the illness. Most patients will have negative cultures (including stool) by the end of a 6-week period. Leukocytosis may occur early, but leukopenia is common in the second week. Proteinuria, mild elevation of liver enzymes, thrombocytopenia, and DIC are common.

▶ Differential Diagnosis

Typhoid and paratyphoid fevers must be distinguished from other serious prolonged fevers, including brucellosis, tularemia, TB, vasculitis, lymphoma, mononucleosis, and Kawasaki disease, or causes of fever in returning travelers (particularly malaria).

▶ Complications

The most serious complications of typhoid fever are gastrointestinal hemorrhage and perforation (commonly in the terminal ileum or cecum). They occur in 10%–15% of hospitalized patients and occur toward the end of the second week or during the third week of the disease.

Bacterial pneumonia, meningitis, septic arthritis, abscesses, and osteomyelitis are uncommon complications, particularly if specific treatment is given promptly. Shock and electrolyte disturbances may lead to death.

About 1%–6% of patients become chronic typhoid carriers, which is defined as excretion of typhoid bacilli for more than a year, though carriage is often lifelong. Adults with underlying biliary or urinary tract disease are much more likely than children to become chronic carriers.

▶ Treatment

A. Specific Measures

Third-generation cephalosporins, such as ceftriaxone, azithromycin, or a fluoroquinolone are used for presumptive therapy (weight and age-based dosing). Antimicrobial susceptibility testing and local experience are used to direct subsequent therapy. Typical courses of treatment are 7–10 days. Alternative regimens for susceptible strains include: TMP-SMX, amoxicillin, and ampicillin. These regimens generally require longer durations (~14 days) than azithromycin or fluoroquinolone-based regimens. Aminoglycosides and first- and second-generation cephalosporins are clinically ineffective regardless of in vitro susceptibility results. Patients may remain febrile for 3–5 days even with appropriate therapy. The carrier state can be treated with a prolonged course of a fluoroquinolone which can achieve high levels in the biliary system. Multidrug-resistant and extensively drug-resistant *S enterica* serotype Typhi isolates are a global problem and cases in the United States are reported. These cases are more difficult to treat.

B. General Measures

General support of the patient is exceedingly important, as are careful observation with particular regard to evidence of intestinal bleeding or perforation. Blood transfusions may be needed even in the absence of frank hemorrhage.

▶ Prevention

Typhoid vaccine should be considered for foreign travel to endemic areas (see Chapter 10).

▶ Prognosis

With early antibiotic therapy, the prognosis is excellent, and the mortality rate is less than 1%. Relapse occurs within 4 weeks in 10%–20% of patients despite appropriate antibiotic treatment.

Centers for Disease Control and Prevention. Information for Healthcare Professionals and Laboratories. Available at: https://www.cdc.gov/salmonella/general/technical.html. Accessed May 10, 2023.

Salmonella infections. In: Kimberlin DW, Brady MT, Jackson MA, Long SS, (eds): *Red Book: 2021–2024 Report of the Committee on Infectious Diseases*. 32nd ed. Itasca, IL: American Academy of Pediatrics; 2021;655–663.

SHIGELLOSIS (BACILLARY DYSENTERY)

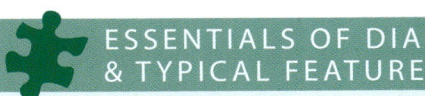

ESSENTIALS OF DIAGNOSIS & TYPICAL FEATURES

▶ Cramps and bloody diarrhea.

▶ High fever, malaise, convulsions.

▶ Pus and blood in diarrheal stools examined microscopically.

▶ Diagnosis confirmed by stool culture.

▶ General Considerations

Shigellae are nonmotile gram-negative rods of the family Enterobacteriaceae that are closely related to *E coli*.

The genus *Shigella* is divided into four species: *Shigella dysenteriae*, *Shigella flexneri*, *Shigella boydii*, and *Shigella sonnei*. An estimated 450,000 cases of *Shigella* diarrhea occur every year in the United States. *S sonnei* followed by *S flexneri* are the most common isolates. *S dysenteriae*, which causes the most severe diarrhea of all species and the greatest number of extraintestinal complications, accounts for less than 1% of all *Shigella* infections in the United States.

Shigellosis may be a serious disease, particularly in young children. In older children and adults, the disease tends to be self-limited and milder. *Shigella* is usually transmitted by the fecal-oral route. Food- and water-borne outbreaks also occur. The disease is very communicable—as few as 200 bacteria can produce illness in an adult volunteer. The secondary attack rate in families is high, and shigellosis is a serious problem in day care centers and those living in crowded conditions. *Shigella* organisms produce disease by invading the colonic mucosa, causing mucosal ulcerations and microabscesses.

▶ Clinical Findings

A. Symptoms and Signs

The incubation period of shigellosis is usually 1–3 days. Onset is abrupt, with abdominal cramps, urgency, tenesmus, chills, fever, malaise, and diarrhea. Hallucinations and seizures sometimes accompany high fever. In severe forms, blood and mucus are seen in stools. In older children, the disease may be mild and characterized by watery diarrhea without blood. In young children, higher fever is common. Rarely there is rectal prolapse. Symptoms generally last 3–7 days.

B. Laboratory Findings

The total WBC count varies, but often there is a marked left shift. The stool may contain gross blood and mucus, and many neutrophils are seen if mucus from the stool is examined microscopically. Stool cultures are usually positive; however, they may be negative because the organism is somewhat fragile and present in small numbers late in the disease. Multiplex PCR tests are available for rapid diagnosis of *Shigella* and other enteropathogens.

▶ Differential Diagnosis

Usually children with viral gastroenteritis are not as febrile or toxic as those with shigellosis, and the stool does not contain gross blood or neutrophils. Intestinal infections caused by *Salmonella* or *Campylobacter* are differentiated by culture or PCR. Grossly bloody stools in a patient without fever or stool leukocytes suggest *E coli* O157:H7 infection. Amebic dysentery is diagnosed by PCR, antigen detection or microscopic examination of fresh stools or sigmoidoscopy specimens. Intussusception is characterized by an abdominal mass with so-called currant jelly stools without leukocytes, and by absence of initial fever. Mild shigellosis is not distinguishable clinically from other forms of infectious diarrhea.

Complications

Dehydration, acidosis, shock, and renal failure are the major complications. In some cases, a chronic form of dysentery occurs, characterized by mucoid stools and poor nutrition. Bacteremia and metastatic infections are rare but serious complications. Seizures, particularly associated with high fever, are common. Fulminating fatal dysentery and HUS occur rarely. Reactive arthritis may follow *Shigella* infection in patients with HLA-B27 genotype.

Treatment

A. Specific Measures

Milder infections may not require antibiotic treatment. Treatment is recommended for those with severe disease or in immunocompromised individuals. Azithromycin is usually effective, as is ciprofloxacin, though the latter should not be used routinely in children. Parenteral ceftriaxone is an option for severe infections. Antibiotic resistance in *Shigella* is an increasing problem and thus antimicrobial susceptibility testing should be done to guide therapy. Successful treatment reduces the duration of fever, cramping, and diarrhea and terminates fecal excretion of *Shigella*.

B. General Measures

In severe cases, immediate rehydration is critical. A mild form of chronic malabsorption syndrome may supervene and require prolonged dietary control. Zinc and vitamin A supplementation may aid recovery in populations at risk of deficiency. Antimotility agents such as loperamide may increase rates of complication and should be avoided.

Prognosis

The prognosis is excellent if treated promptly by adequate fluid therapy. The mortality rate is high in very young, malnourished infants who do not receive fluid and electrolyte therapy. Convalescent fecal excretion of *Shigella* lasts 1–4 weeks in patients not receiving antimicrobial therapy. Long-term carriers are rare.

Centers for Disease Control and Prevention (CDC): Shigellosis. www.cdc.gov/shigella/index.html. Accessed May 10, 2023.

Puzari M et al: Emergence of antibiotic resistant *Shigella* species: a matter of concern. J Infect Public Health 2018 Jul–Aug;11(4):451–454. doi: 10.1016/j.jiph.2017.09.025 [PMID: 29066021].

Shane AL et al: 2017 Infectious Diseases Society of America clinical practice guidelines for the diagnosis and management of infectious diarrhea. Clin Infect Dis 2017 Dec 15;65(12):e45–e80 [PMID: 29053792].

CHOLERA

ESSENTIALS OF DIAGNOSIS & TYPICAL FEATURES

► Sudden onset of severe watery diarrhea.

► Persistent vomiting without nausea or fever.

► Extreme and rapid dehydration and electrolyte loss, with rapid development of vascular collapse.

► Contact with a case of cholera or with shellfish, or the presence of cholera in the community.

► Diagnosis confirmed by stool culture or PCR.

General Considerations

Cholera is an acute diarrheal disease caused by the gram-negative organism *Vibrio cholerae*. It is transmitted by contaminated water or food, especially contaminated shellfish. Epidemics are common in impoverished areas where hygiene and safe water supply are limited. Individuals with mild illness and young children may play an important role in transmission of the infection.

Asymptomatic infection is far more common than clinical disease. In endemic areas, rising titers of vibriocidal antibody are seen with increasing age. Infection occurs in individuals with low titers. The age-specific attack rate is highest in children younger than 5 years and declines with age. Cholera is unusual in infancy.

Cholera toxin is a protein enterotoxin that is responsible for symptoms. Cholera toxin binds to a regulatory subunit of adenylyl cyclase in enterocytes, causing increased cyclic adenosine monophosphate and an outpouring of NaCl and water into the lumen of the small bowel.

The incubation period is short, usually 1–2 days. Duration of diarrhea is prolonged in adults and children with severe malnutrition.

Cholera is endemic in India and southern and Southeast Asia and in parts of Africa. Pandemics worldwide have occurred, leading to millions of deaths. Cholera in the United States occurs after foreign travel or rarely as a result of consumption of contaminated seafood, particularly from the Gulf Coast.

V cholerae is a natural inhabitant of shellfish and copepods in estuarine environments. Seasonal multiplication of *V cholerae* may provide a source of outbreaks in endemic areas.

Clinical Findings

A. Symptoms and Signs

Many patients infected with *V cholerae* have mild disease, though up to 10% will have severe symptoms. During severe cholera, there is a sudden onset of massive, frequent, watery stools, generally light gray in color and containing some mucus (so-called rice-water stools). Vomiting may be projectile and is not accompanied by nausea. Within 2–3 hours, the tremendous loss of fluids results in life-threatening dehydration, metabolic acidosis, and electrolyte derangement, with marked weakness. This can lead to renal failure and irreversible peripheral vascular collapse. The illness lasts 1–7 days and is shortened by appropriate antibiotic therapy.

B. Laboratory Findings

Markedly elevated hemoglobin (20 g/dL) and marked acidosis, hypochloremia, and hypokalemia are seen. Culture confirmation requires specific media and takes 16–18 hours for a presumptive diagnosis and 36–48 hours for a definitive bacteriologic diagnosis. PCR assays are available in high-resource settings.

▶ Prevention

Cholera vaccines are available outside of the United States. They provide 50%–75% efficacy with protection lasting 2–3 years depending on the vaccine. A live-attenuated oral cholera vaccine was approved in the United States in 2016 for those 2–64 years of age traveling to cholera endemic areas, but as of December 2020 the vaccine has been unavailable. Tourists visiting endemic areas are at little risk if they exercise caution in what they eat and drink and practice good hand hygiene. In endemic areas, all water must be boiled, shellfish should be thoroughly cooked, food and drink protected from flies, and sanitary precautions observed. Foods should be promptly refrigerated whenever possible after meals. Simple filtration of water is highly effective in reducing cases. All patients with cholera should be isolated.

Chemoprophylaxis (eg, tetracycline for 5 days) may limit secondary cases in a household or institutional setting, but there is currently insufficient data to support this practice.

▶ Treatment

Replacement and maintenance of fluids and electrolytes hydration are the most important aspects of cholera treatment. Lactated Ringers (if available; normal saline is alternative) solution should be administered intravenously in large amounts to restore blood volume and urine output and to prevent irreversible shock. Moderate dehydration and acidosis can be corrected by oral therapy alone, because the active glucose transport system of the small bowel is normally functional. The optimal composition of the oral solution is described in Table 45–5.

In addition to fluid and electrolyte replacement, antibiotic treatment can also shorten the duration and decrease severity and should be used for severe cases. First-line treatment for children in the United States is doxycycline. Azithromycin or ciprofloxacin as a single dose (specific dosing vary by age, weight, and co-morbidities) are alternatives.

▶ Prognosis

With early and rapid replacement of fluids and electrolytes, the case fatality rate is 1%–2% in children. If significant symptoms appear and no treatment is given, the mortality rate is over 50%.

Centers for Disease Control and Prevention: Cholera—*Vibrio cholerae* infection. www.cdc.gov/cholera/index.html. Accessed May 10, 2023.
Deen J et al: Epidemiology of Cholera. *Vaccine* 2020 Feb 29; 38(Suppl 1):A31–A40. doi: https://doi.org/10.1016/j.vaccine.2019.07.078.

CAMPYLOBACTER INFECTION

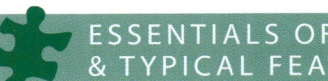

ESSENTIALS OF DIAGNOSIS & TYPICAL FEATURES

▶ Fever, vomiting, abdominal pain, diarrhea.
▶ Definitive diagnosis by stool culture or PCR.

▶ General Considerations

Campylobacter species are small gram-negative, curved or spiral bacilli that are commensals or pathogens in many animals. Thera are over 20 species with *Campylobacter jejuni* and *Campylobacter coli* most frequently causing acute gastroenteritis in humans. In the United States *C jejuni* affects an estimated 1.5 million people annually and is more common than *Salmonella* or *Shigella*. *Campylobacter fetus* causes bacteremia and meningitis in immunocompromised patients. *C fetus* may also cause maternal fever, abortion, stillbirth, and severe neonatal infection.

Campylobacter colonizes domestic and wild animals, especially poultry. Numerous cases have been associated with sick puppies or other animal contacts. Contaminated food and water, undercooked poultry, and person-to-person spread by the fecal-oral route are common routes of transmission. Newborns may acquire the organism from their mothers at delivery. *Campylobacter* is a major cause of diarrhea in travelers to low- and middle-income countries.

▶ Clinical Findings

A. Symptoms and Signs

C jejuni enteritis can be mild or severe. In low-income countries, asymptomatic stool carriage is common. The incubation period is usually 2–5 days. The disease usually begins with sudden onset of high fever, malaise, headache, abdominal cramps, nausea, and vomiting. Diarrhea follows and may be watery or bile stained, mucoid, and bloody. The illness is self-limiting, lasting 2–7 days, but relapses may occur. Without antimicrobial treatment, the organism remains in the stool for ~2–3 weeks but can last up to 7 weeks. Immune compromised patients may suffer prolonged or relapsing disease or complications due to bacteremia.

B. Laboratory Findings

The peripheral WBC count generally is elevated, with many band forms. Microscopic examination of stool reveals erythrocytes and leukocytes. Diarrheal disease associated with fever or severe abdominal pain should prompt testing for other pathogens including *Campylobacter*. Isolation of *C jejuni* from stool is not difficult but requires selective agar and incubation conditions. Multiplex PCR tests are available for rapid diagnosis of *Campylobacter* and other enteropathogens.

► Differential Diagnosis

Campylobacter enteritis may resemble viral gastroenteritis, salmonellosis, shigellosis, amebiasis, or other infectious diarrheas. Because it also mimics ulcerative colitis, Crohn disease, intussusception, and appendicitis, mistaken diagnosis can lead to unnecessary diagnostic testing or surgery.

► Complications

The most common complication is dehydration. Other uncommon complications include erythema nodosum, convulsions, reactive arthritis, bacteremia, urinary tract infection, and cholecystitis. *Campylobacter* is the most commonly identified cause of Guillain-Barré syndrome (estimated to occur in 1 in 1000 cases), which typically follows *C jejuni* infection by 1–3 weeks.

► Treatment

Treatment of fluid and electrolyte disturbances is important and in milder cases is the only required intervention. Antimicrobial therapy given early in the course of the illness will shorten the duration of symptoms. Treatment with azithromycin once daily for 3 days terminates fecal excretion and may limit spread in households. Ciprofloxacin may be used; but fluoroquinolone-resistant *C jejuni* are common worldwide, particularly in low- and middle-income countries.

► Prevention

Hand washing and adherence to basic food sanitation practices help prevent disease, particularly after contact with raw poultry. Adequate cooking of poultry is also important.

► Prognosis

Generally, most individuals improve and recover, particularly if dehydration is treated promptly.

Centers for Disease Control and Prevention (CDC): *Campylobacter* (Campylobacteriosis). Available at: https://www.cdc.gov/campylobacter/index.html. Accessed May 10, 2023.

Shane AL et al: 2017 Infectious Diseases Society of America clinical practice guidelines for the diagnosis and management of infectious diarrhea. Clin Infect Dis 2017 Dec 15;65(12):e45–e80 [PMID: 29053792].

TULAREMIA

ESSENTIALS OF DIAGNOSIS & TYPICAL FEATURES

► A cutaneous or mucous membrane lesion at the site of inoculation and regional lymph node enlargement.

► Sudden onset of fever, chills, and prostration.

► History of contact with infected animals, principally wild rabbits, or tick or deer fly exposure.

► Positive culture, PCR, or immunofluorescent staining of samples from mucocutaneous ulcer or regional lymph nodes.

► High serum antibody titer.

► General Considerations

Tularemia is caused by *Francisella tularensis*, a gram-negative organism usually acquired directly from infected animals (particularly rabbits and other large rodents) or by the bite of an infected tick (dog tick, wood tick, lone star tick) or deer fly. Occasionally infection is acquired from infected domestic dogs or cats; by contamination of the skin or mucous membranes with infected blood or tissues; by inhalation of aerosolized infected material; or by ingestion of contaminated meat or water. Aerosols containing *F tularensis* from cultures in a laboratory may be highly infectious. The incubation period is short, usually 3–7 days, but may vary from 2 to 25 days. Approximately 200 cases are reported in the United States each year.

► Prevention

Children should be protected from insect bites, especially those of ticks and deer flies, by the use of proper clothing and repellents. The dressing and handling of rabbits and similar game should be performed with great care and using rubber gloves. Care should be taken to avoid mowing over dead animals. If contact occurs, thorough washing with soap and water is indicated. Microbiology laboratory personnel should be notified and take appropriate precautions whenever *F tularensis* is suspected.

Clinical Findings

A. Symptoms and Signs

Several clinical types of tularemia occur in children. Sixty percent of infections are of the ulceroglandular form that starts as a relatively nonpainful, reddened papule that may be pruritic and quickly ulcerates. Soon, the regional lymph nodes become large and tender. Fluctuance quickly follows. There may be marked systemic symptoms, including high fever, chills, weakness, and vomiting. Pneumonitis occasionally accompanies the ulceroglandular form or may be seen as the sole manifestation of infection (pneumonic form). A detectable skin lesion may be absent, and localized lymphoid enlargement may exist alone (glandular form). Oculoglandular and oropharyngeal forms also occur. The latter is characterized by tonsillitis, often with membrane formation, cervical adenopathy, and high fever. In the absence of a primary ulcer or localized lymphadenitis, a prolonged febrile disease reminiscent of typhoid fever can occur (typhoidal form). Meningitis is rare but may occur in disseminated disease. Splenomegaly is common in all forms.

B. Laboratory Findings

F tularensis can be recovered from ulcers, regional lymph nodes, blood, and sputum of patients with the pneumonic form. However, the organism grows only on an enriched medium (blood-cystine-glucose agar). Laboratory handling is dangerous owing to the risk of airborne transmission to laboratory personnel. PCR or immunofluorescent staining of biopsy material or aspirates of involved lymph nodes is diagnostic.

The WBC count is not remarkable. The diagnosis is typically confirmed with serologic testing. Antibodies are usually present during the second week of illness. In the absence of a positive culture, a tube agglutination antibody titer of 1:160 or greater or a microagglutination titer of 1:128 or greater is presumptively positive for tularemia. Confirmation of disease may also be established by demonstration of a fourfold antibody titer rise between acute and convalescent serum samples, which is particularly useful when initial serologies are obtained in the first week of illness.

Differential Diagnosis

The typhoidal form of tularemia may mimic typhoid, brucellosis, miliary TB, Rocky Mountain spotted fever, and mononucleosis. Pneumonic tularemia resembles atypical pneumonia. The ulceroglandular type of tularemia resembles pyoderma caused by staphylococci or streptococci, plague, anthrax, and cat-scratch fever. The oropharyngeal type must be distinguished from streptococcal or diphtheritic pharyngitis, mononucleosis, herpangina, or other viral pharyngitides.

Treatment

A. Specific Measures

Historically, streptomycin was the drug of choice. However, gentamicin (5 mg/kg/day) is efficacious, more available, and familiar to clinicians. A 10-day course is usually sufficient, although more severe infections may need longer therapy. Ciprofloxacin also can be used in patients with less severe disease. Doxycycline is often effective but is a bacteriostatic agent and is associated with higher relapse rates.

B. General Measures

Antipyretics and analgesics may be given as necessary. Skin lesions are best left open. Glandular lesions occasionally require incision and drainage.

Prognosis

The prognosis is excellent in most cases of tularemia that are recognized early and treated appropriately.

Centers for Disease Control (CDC) and Prevention: Tularemia. http://www.cdc.gov/tularemia/clinicians/index.html. Accessed July 9, 2021.

Imbimbo C et al: Tularemia in Children and Adolescents. Pediatr Infect Dis J 2020 Dec;39(12):e435–e438. doi: 10.1097/INF.0000000000002932.

PLAGUE

ESSENTIALS OF DIAGNOSIS & TYPICAL FEATURES

▶ Sudden onset of fever, chills, and prostration.

▶ Regional lymphadenitis with suppuration of nodes (bubonic form).

▶ Hemorrhage into skin and mucous membranes and shock (septicemia).

▶ Cough, dyspnea, cyanosis, and hemoptysis (pneumonia).

▶ History of exposure to infected animals, flea bites.

▶ Diagnosis is confirmed by positive culture, PCR, or immunofluorescent staining of culture material.

General Considerations

Plague is an extremely serious acute infection caused by a gram-negative coccobacillus, *Yersinia pestis*. It is a disease of rodents that is transmitted to humans by flea bites. Plague bacilli have been isolated from ground squirrels, prairie dogs, and other wild rodents in many of the western and south-western states in the United States. Most cases have come from New Mexico, Arizona, Colorado, and California. Direct contact with rodents, rabbits, or domestic dogs and cats provides exposure to fleas infected with plague bacilli. Most cases occur from June through September. Human plague in the United States appears to occur in cycles that reflect cycles in wild animal reservoirs. On average, seven cases per year are reported in the United States.

Prevention

Proper disposal of household and commercial wastes and control of rats and other animals are basic elements of plague prevention. Flea control in pet animals is also important. Children vacationing in remote areas should be warned not to handle dead or dying animals. Domestic cats that roam freely in suburban areas may contact infected wild animals and acquire infected fleas.

All persons exposed to plague in the previous 6 days (via personal contact with an infected person, contact with plague-infected animals or exposure to infected tissues) should be given antimicrobial prophylaxis or be instructed to report fever or other symptoms to their physician. Persons who have close personal contact (< 2 m) with a person with pneumonic plague should receive antimicrobial prophylaxis with doxycycline or a fluoroquinolone for 7 days from the last exposure. Patients on prophylaxis should still seek prompt medical care for onset of fever or other illness.

Clinical Findings

A. Symptoms and Signs

Plague assumes several clinical forms; the two most common are bubonic and septicemic. Pneumonic plague is uncommon.

1. Bubonic plague—After an incubation period of 2–8 days, there is the sudden onset of high fever, chills, headache, vomiting, and marked delirium or clouding of consciousness. A less severe form also exists, with a less precipitous onset, but with progression over several days to severe symptoms. Although the flea bite is rarely seen, the regional lymph node/s, usually inguinal and unilateral, is/are painful and tender, 1–5 cm in diameter. The node usually suppurates and drains spontaneously after 1 week. Bacilli may overwhelm regional lymph nodes and enter the circulation to produce septicemia. Plague bacilli produce endotoxin that causes vascular necrosis that can result in widely disseminated hemorrhage in skin, mucous membranes, liver, and spleen. Myocarditis and circulatory collapse may result from damage by the endotoxin. Plague meningitis or pneumonia may occur following bacteremic spread from an infected lymph node.

2. Septicemic plague—Plague may present as septicemia without evidence of lymphadenopathy. In some series, 25% of cases are initially septicemic. Septicemic plague carries a worse prognosis than bubonic plague, largely because it is not recognized and treated early. Patients may present with a nonspecific febrile illness characterized by fever, myalgia, chills, and anorexia. Septicemic plague may be complicated by secondary seeding of the lung causing plague pneumonia. Necrosis of distal body parts such as the fingers, toes, and nose tip may occur.

3. Primary pneumonic plague—Inhalation of *Y pestis* bacilli causes primary plague pneumonia. This form of plague is transmitted from human to human and to humans from cats or dogs with pneumonic plague and would be the form of plague most likely seen after aerosolized release of *Y pestis* in a bioterrorism incident. After an incubation of 1–6 days, the patient develops fever; cough; shortness of breath; and bloody, watery, or purulent sputum. Gastrointestinal symptoms are sometimes prominent. Because the initial focus of infection is the lung, buboes are usually absent; occasionally cervical buboes may be seen.

B. Laboratory Findings

Aspirate from a bubo contains bipolar-staining gram-negative bacilli. Pus, sputum, and blood all yield the organism. Rapid diagnosis can be made with fluorescent antibody detection or PCR on clinical specimens (available through state health departments). Confirmation is made by culture or serologic testing. Cultures are usually positive within 48 hours. Paired acute and convalescent sera may be tested for a fourfold antibody rise. Automated bacterial identification systems have been known to misidentify *Y pestis* and are unreliable.

Differential Diagnosis

The septic phase of the disease may be confused with illnesses such as meningococcemia, sepsis caused by other bacteria, and rickettsioses. The bubonic form resembles tularemia, anthrax, cat-scratch fever, lymphadenitis, and cellulitis.

Treatment

A. Specific Measures

2021 guidance from the Centers for Disease Control and Prevention recommends dual therapy for moderate or severe disease, bubonic plague with large buboes and bioterrorism pneumonic forms. Treatment options depend on the type of infection and pregnancy status, but generally include aminoglycosides (gentamicin, streptomycin), fluoroquinolones (ciprofloxacin, moxifloxacin, or levofloxacin), or doxycycline. Single-drug treatment with one of these agents is recommended for milder disease. Chloramphenicol or a fluroquinolone (moxifloxacin or levofloxacin) should be used for meningitis.

Every effort should be made to effect resolution of buboes without surgery. Pus from draining lymph nodes is infectious.

B. General Measures

State health officials should be notified immediately about suspected cases of plague. Pneumonic plague is highly infectious, and droplet isolation is required until the patient has been on effective antimicrobial therapy for 48 hours. Laboratory personnel should be notified if suspicion for plague exists to exercise precaution and prevent occupational acquisition.

▶ Prognosis

The mortality rate in untreated bubonic plague is about 50%. The mortality rate for pneumonic and septicemic plague is higher, possibly due to delays in diagnosis. With timely treatment, mortality rates are less than 20% in the general population.

Centers for Disease Control and Prevention (CDC): Plague. http://www.cdc.gov/plague/healthcare/clinicians.html. Accessed May 27, 2023.

Kugeler KJ et al: Epidemiology of human plague in the United States, 1900–2012. Emerg Infect Dis 2015 Jan;21(1):16–22 [PMID: 25529546].

Nelson CA et al: Antimicrobial Treatment and Prophylaxis of Plague: Recommendations for Naturally Acquired Infections and Bioterrorism Response. MMWR Recomm Rep 2021;70 (No. RR-3):1–27. DOI: http://dx.doi.org/10.15585/mmwr.rr7003a1.

INVASIVE *HAEMOPHILUS INFLUENZAE* INFECTIONS

ESSENTIALS OF DIAGNOSIS & TYPICAL FEATURES

▶ Purulent meningitis in children younger than 4 years with direct smears of CSF showing gram-negative pleomorphic rods.

▶ Acute epiglottitis: high fever, drooling, dysphagia, aphonia, and stridor.

▶ Septic arthritis: fever, local redness, swelling, heat, and pain with active or passive motion of the involved joint in a child 4 months to 4 years of age.

▶ Cellulitis: sudden onset of fever and distinctive cellulitis in an infant, often involving the cheek or periorbital area.

▶ In all cases, a positive culture from the blood, CSF, or aspirated pus confirms the diagnosis.

▶ General Considerations

H influenzae is classified by its polysaccharide capsule into six serotypes (a–f), and those without a polysaccharide capsule are considered nontypeable. *H influenzae* type b (Hib) was a common cause of invasive disease, such as meningitis, bacteremia, epiglottitis, septic arthritis, periorbital and facial cellulitis, pneumonia, and pericarditis, but is now uncommon because of widespread immunization in early infancy. The 99% reduction in incidence seen in many parts of the United States is due to high rates of vaccine coverage and reduced nasopharyngeal carriage after vaccination. Currently other types, particularly type a and nontypeable *H influenza*, cause the majority of invasive disease. Non–type b serotypes may cause meningitis, bacteremia and other diseases previously caused by Hib.

Unencapsulated, nontypeable *H influenzae* frequently colonize the mucous membranes and cause otitis media, sinusitis, bronchitis, and pneumonia in children and adults. Unencapsulated, nontypeable *H influenzae* also cause invasive disease. Neonatal sepsis that is similar to early-onset GBS occurs, especially in preterm and low-birth-weight infants. Obstetric complications of chorioamnionitis and bacteremia are usually the source of neonatal cases. Beta-lactamase production resulting in ampicillin resistance occurs in 25%–40% of nontypeable *H influenzae*. β-lactamase-negative, ampicillin-resistant (BLNAR) *H influenzae* has emerged in some regions of the globe, though less so in the United States. Thus for severe infections, determination of susceptibility should not be based on beta-lactamase production alone.

Among children younger than 5 years, American Indian and Alaska Native children have a five times greater rate of invasive *H influenzae* disease than other races. Children with sickle cell disease, HIV infection, immunoglobulin and early complement deficiency, functional or anatomic asplenia, and immunocompromise due to chemotherapy are also at increased risk.

▶ Prevention

Several carbohydrate protein conjugate Hib vaccines are currently available (see Chapter 10). The risk of invasive Hib disease is highest in unimmunized, or partially immunized, household contacts of a Hib patient when the contact is younger than 4 years. The following situations require rifampin chemoprophylaxis of all household contacts (except pregnant women) to eradicate potential nasopharyngeal colonization with Hib and limit risk of invasive disease: (1) families where at least one household contact is younger than 4 years and either unimmunized or incompletely immunized against Hib; (2) an immunocompromised child (of any age or immunization status) resides in the household; or (3) a child younger than 12 months resides in the home and has not received the primary series of the Hib vaccine. Preschool and day care center contacts may need prophylaxis if more than one case has occurred in the center in the previous 60 days (discuss with state health officials). The index case also needs chemoprophylaxis if treated with an antibiotic regimen *other than* ceftriaxone or cefotaxime (both are effective in eradication of Hib from the nasopharynx) and if the patient is younger than 2 years or resides in a household with a household contact at risk of disease (as described above). Household contacts and index cases older than 1 month who need chemoprophylaxis should be given rifampin, 20 mg/kg per dose (maximum adult dose, 600 mg) orally, once daily for 4 successive days. Infants who are younger than 1 month should be given oral rifampin (10 mg/kg per dose once daily for 4 days). Rifampin should not be used in pregnant females. Chemoprophylaxis may be considered for household contacts of children with invasive disease caused by *H influenzae* type a. For other strains, including nontypeable *H influenzae*, chemoprophylaxis is generally not recommended because secondary cases are rare.

Clinical Findings

A. Symptoms and Signs of Hib and Non–Type B Invasive Disease

1. Meningitis—Infants usually present with fever, irritability, lethargy, poor feeding with or without vomiting, and a high-pitched cry.

2. Acute epiglottitis—The most useful clinical finding in the early diagnosis of *Haemophilus* epiglottitis is evidence of dysphagia, characterized by a refusal to eat or swallow saliva and by drooling. This finding, plus the presence of a high fever in a toxic child should strongly suggest the diagnosis and lead to prompt intubation. Stridor is a late sign (see Chapter 19).

3. Septic arthritis—In the prevaccine era, Hib was a common cause of septic arthritis in children younger than 4 years in the United States.

4. Cellulitis—Cellulitis due to *Hib* occurred almost exclusively in children between the ages of 3 months and 4 years but is now uncommon. The cheek or periorbital (preseptal) area was often involved.

B. Laboratory Findings

The WBC count in Hib infections may be high or normal with a shift to the left. A positive culture of blood, CSF, aspirated pus, or fluid from the involved site proves the diagnosis. In untreated meningitis, CSF smear may show the characteristic pleomorphic gram-negative rods. Hib may be identified in CSF as a component of a multiplex PCR assay.

C. Imaging

A lateral view of the neck may suggest the diagnosis in suspected acute epiglottitis, but misinterpretation is common. Intubation should not be delayed to obtain radiographs.

Differential Diagnosis

A. Meningitis

Meningitis must be differentiated from head injury, brain abscess, tumor, lead encephalopathy, and other forms of meningoencephalitis, including mycobacterial, viral, fungal, and other bacterial agents.

B. Acute Epiglottitis

In croup caused by viral agents (parainfluenza 1, 2, and 3, respiratory syncytial virus, influenza A, adenovirus), the child has more definite upper respiratory symptoms, cough, hoarseness, slower progression of obstructive signs, and lower fever. Spasmodic croup usually occurs at night in a child with a history of previous attacks. Sudden onset of choking and paroxysmal coughing suggests foreign-body aspiration. Retropharyngeal abscess may have to be differentiated from epiglottitis.

C. Septic Arthritis

Differential diagnosis includes acute osteomyelitis, prepatellar bursitis, cellulitis, rheumatic fever, and fractures and sprains.

D. Cellulitis

Erysipelas, streptococcal cellulitis, insect bites, and trauma (including popsicle panniculitis or other types of freezing injury) may mimic Hib cellulitis. Periorbital cellulitis must be differentiated from paranasal sinus disease without cellulitis, allergic inflammatory disease of the lids, conjunctivitis, and herpes zoster infection.

Complications

A. Meningitis (See Chapter 25)

B. Acute Epiglottitis

The disease may rapidly progress to complete airway obstruction with complications owing to hypoxia (see Chapter 19). Mediastinal emphysema and pneumothorax may occur.

C. Septic Arthritis

Septic arthritis may result in rapid destruction of cartilage and ankylosis if diagnosis and treatment are delayed. Even with early treatment, the incidence of residual damage and disability after septic arthritis in weight-bearing joints may be as high as 25%.

D. Cellulitis

Bacteremia from a cutaneous source may lead to meningitis or pyarthrosis.

Treatment

All patients with bacteremic or potentially bacteremic *H influenzae* diseases require hospitalization for treatment. The drug of choice in hospitalized patients is a third-generation cephalosporin (ceftriaxone or cefotaxime) until the sensitivity of the organism is known. Meropenem is an alternative choice. Persons with invasive Hib disease should be in droplet isolation for 24 hours after initiation of parenteral antibiotic therapy.

A. Meningitis

Therapy is begun as soon as bacterial meningitis is suspected. Empiric intravenous therapy recommended for meningitis (until organism identified) is vancomycin in combination with ceftriaxone. Once the organism has been identified as *H influenzae* and the susceptibilities are known, the antibiotic regimen can be tailored accordingly. Therapy should be given intravenously for the entire course. Duration of therapy is 10 days for uncomplicated meningitis. Longer treatment is reserved for children who respond slowly or have complications.

Dexamethasone given immediately after diagnosis and continued for up to 4 days may reduce the incidence of hearing loss in children with Hib meningitis; the dosage is 0.6 mg/kg/day in four divided doses for 2–4 days. Starting dexamethasone more than 6 hours after antibiotics have been initiated is unlikely to provide benefits.

Repeated lumbar punctures are usually not necessary in Hib meningitis. They should be obtained in the following circumstances: unsatisfactory or questionable clinical response, seizure occurring after several days of therapy, if the neurologic examination is abnormal or difficult to evaluate, or prolonged (7 days) or recurrent fever.

B. Acute Epiglottitis (See Chapter 19)

C. Septic Arthritis

Initial therapy should include an effective antistaphylococcal antibiotic and cefotaxime or ceftriaxone until identification of the organism is made and susceptibilities are known, at which time therapy for Hib is continued. If improved following initial intravenous therapy, the patient can be transitioned to oral therapy based on susceptibilities (eg, amoxicillin or amoxicillin/clavulanate). Antibiotics should be administered to complete a 3- to 4-week course (longer if complications or signs and symptoms are unresolved). Drainage of infected joint fluid is an essential part of treatment. In joints other than the hip, this can often be accomplished by one or more needle aspirations. In hip infections—and in arthritis of other joints when treatment is delayed or clinical response is slow—surgical drainage is advised.

D. Cellulitis, Including Orbital Cellulitis

Initial therapy for orbital cellulitis should be broad spectrum antibiotics, and regimens frequently include ceftriaxone. Therapy is given parenterally for at least 3–7 days followed by oral treatment. The total antibiotic course will vary with the severity of the infection, response to therapy, the presence of an abscess, and whether drainage was performed. A minimum course of 21 days is reasonable in uncomplicated cases without abscess and good therapeutic response, assuming all signs of orbital cellulitis have completely resolved. In cases with severe ethmoid sinusitis and evidence of boney destruction at least a 4-week treatment course is advisable. Complicated cases may require longer treatment courses.

Prognosis

The case fatality rate for invasive *H influenzae* is 15% but may be higher depending on the serotype. Young infants and older adults have the highest mortality rate. Hearing loss or other neurologic sequelae develop in 15%–30% of patients with Hib meningitis. Patients with Hib meningitis should have their hearing checked during the course of the illness or shortly after recovery. Children in whom invasive Hib infection develops despite appropriate immunization should have tests to investigate immune function and to rule out HIV. Deaths from epiglottitis are associated with bacteremia and the rapid development of airway obstruction. The prognosis for the other diseases requiring hospitalization is good with the early institution of adequate antibiotic therapy.

Haemophilus influenzae infections. In: Kimberlin DW, Brady MT, Jackson MA, Long SS, (eds): *Red Book: 2021–2024 Report of the Committee on Infectious Diseases.* 32nd ed. Itasca, IL: American Academy of Pediatrics; 2021:345–354.

BORDETELLA PERTUSSIS (WHOOPING COUGH)

ESSENTIALS OF DIAGNOSIS & TYPICAL FEATURES

► Prodromal catarrhal stage (1–3 weeks) characterized by mild cough and coryza, but without fever.

► Persistent staccato, paroxysmal cough ending with a high-pitched inspiratory "whoop" during paroxysmal stage.

► Convalescent stage with slowly resolving cough over weeks to months.

► Leukocytosis with absolute lymphocytosis.

► Diagnosis confirmed by PCR of nasopharyngeal secretions.

General Considerations

Pertussis is an acute, highly communicable infection of the respiratory tract caused by *Bordetella pertussis* where the organism attaches to the ciliated respiratory epithelium. Disease is due to several bacterial toxins, including pertussis toxin that is the most potent. Children usually acquire the disease from symptomatic family contacts who have mild respiratory illness, not recognized as pertussis. Asymptomatic carriage of *B pertussis* has not been demonstrated. Infectivity is greatest during the catarrhal and early paroxysmal cough stage (communicable period from onset to 3 weeks after start of paroxysmal cough).

In the United States, approximately 18,000–20,000 cases per year are reported, though many cases go unreported. Pertussis is most severe in the very young with a case fatality rate of approximately 1% in infants younger than 6 months.

The duration of immunity following natural pertussis is not known but is not lifelong. Reinfections are usually mild. Immunity following vaccination wanes in 5–10 years; thus, the majority of young adults in the United States are susceptible to pertussis infection, and disease is probably common but unrecognized. Decreased efficacy of acellular vaccines (now standard in the United States) compared to whole-cell vaccines and low rates of immunization due to vaccine hesitancy in some communities have contributed significantly to pertussis epidemics in the United States.

Bordetella parapertussis and *Bordetella holmesii* cause a similar but milder syndrome.

Clinical Findings

A. Symptoms and Signs

The onset of pertussis is insidious, with catarrhal upper respiratory tract symptoms (rhinitis, sneezing, and an irritating cough). Fever above 38.3 is unusual and suggests an alternative diagnosis. After about 2 weeks, cough becomes paroxysmal, characterized by repeated forceful coughing ending with a loud inspiration (the whoop). Infants and adults with severe pertussis, as well as patients with milder pertussis, may lack the characteristic whoop. Vomiting commonly follows a paroxysm. Coughing may be accompanied by cyanosis, sweating, prostration, and exhaustion. Coughing fits occur more frequently at night. This stage lasts for 2–4 weeks, with gradual improvement. Paroxysmal coughing may continue for some months and wane during the convalescent stage, but may worsen with intercurrent viral respiratory infection. Infants with pertussis frequently present with choking, apnea and bradycardia, poor feeding, and failure to thrive, whereas paroxysms and whoop are generally not present. In adults, older children, and partially immunized individuals, symptoms may consist only of irritating cough lasting 1–2 weeks. Clinical pertussis is milder in immunized children.

B. Laboratory Findings

WBC counts of 20,000–30,000/μL with 70%–80% lymphocytes typically appear near the end of the catarrhal stage. Severe pulmonary hypertension and hyperleukocytosis (> 70,000/μL) are associated with severe disease and death in young children with pertussis. Many older children and adults with mild infections never demonstrate lymphocytosis.

The preferred method of diagnosis in most centers is identification of *B pertussis* by PCR from nasopharyngeal specimens. The organism may be found in the respiratory tract in diminishing numbers beginning in the catarrhal stage and ending about 2 weeks after the beginning of the paroxysmal stage. After several weeks of symptoms, PCR testing is frequently negative. Culture requires specialized media, careful attention to specimen collection and transport, and is now unavailable in many labs.

The chest radiograph reveals thickened bronchi and sometimes shows a "shaggy" heart border.

Differential Diagnosis

In the catarrhal phase, pertussis is difficult to discriminate from viral causes of upper respiratory infection. The differential diagnosis of pertussis includes viral and bacterial (particularly *M pneumoniae*) causes of pneumonia. The absence of fever in pertussis differentiates this disease from most other bacterial infections. Cystic fibrosis and foreign-body aspiration may be considerations with chronic cough. Adenoviruses and respiratory syncytial virus may cause paroxysmal coughing with an associated elevation of lymphocytes in the peripheral blood, mimicking pertussis. *Bordetella parapertussis* can also cause similar symptoms as *B pertussis* and can be diagnosed and differentiated from *B pertussis* via PCR assays.

Complications

Bronchopneumonia due to superinfection is the most common serious complication. It is characterized by abrupt clinical deterioration during the paroxysmal stage, accompanied by high fever and sometimes a striking leukemoid reaction with a shift to predominantly polymorphonuclear neutrophils. Intercurrent viral respiratory infection is also a common complication and may provoke worsening or recurrence of paroxysmal coughing. Otitis media is common. Residual bronchiectasis is an infrequent but serious complication. Apnea and sudden death may occur during a particularly severe paroxysm. Rib fractures may occur due to the force of coughing. Epistaxis and subconjunctival hemorrhage also occur. Seizures and encephalopathy may occur though in 1%–2% and < 1% of cases, respectively. The encephalopathy frequently is fatal.

Treatment

A. Specific Measures

Antibiotics may ameliorate early infections (ie, in the catarrhal phase) but have no effect on clinical symptoms in the paroxysmal stage. Thus, treatment should be initiated as quickly as possible and should not wait for confirmatory testing in cases where the diagnosis is strongly suspected. Azithromycin for 5 days (specific dosing age dependent) is the drug of choice because it promptly terminates respiratory tract carriage of *B pertussis*. Erythromycin given four times daily for 14 days is acceptable but not preferred. Erythromycin has been associated with pyloric stenosis in infants younger than 1 month, and azithromycin is preferred in this age. The risk of pyloric stenosis after azithromycin treatment is likely less, but cases have occurred. Parents of infants younger than 1 month who require treatment with azithromycin should be informed of this risk and counseled on the signs of pyloric stenosis. Resistance to macrolides has been rarely reported. TMP-SMX may also be used for macrolide-intolerant patients.

B. General Measures

Nutritional support during the paroxysmal phase is important. Frequent small feedings, tube feeding, or parenteral fluid supplementation may be needed. Minimizing stimuli that trigger paroxysms is optimal for controlling cough. There are no adequate clinical trials that identify an effective treatment for cough paroxysms.

C. Treatment of Complications

Respiratory insufficiency due to pneumonia or other pulmonary complications should be treated with oxygen and assisted ventilation if necessary. Convulsions are treated with appropriate supportive care and anticonvulsants. Bacterial pneumonia or otitis media will require additional antibiotics. Infants with an extremely high WBC count (> 70,000/μL) are at high risk of severe disease and death. They may require additional management, such as use of extracorporeal membrane oxygenation (ECMO).

Prevention

Active immunization (see Chapter 10) with DTaP (diphtheria, tetanus, and acellular pertussis) vaccine should be given in early infancy. The occurrence and increased recognition of disease in adolescents and adults contribute to the increasing number of cases. A booster dose of Tdap vaccine for adolescents, ideally between the ages of 11 and 12 years, is recommended. Subsequent booster doses of Tdap are recommended for adults aged 18–60 years to replace Td boosters, including when administered for tetanus prophylaxis. Immunization of pregnant women in the last trimester prior to 36 weeks gestation, new mothers, care givers of infants younger than 6 months, and health care workers of young children is also recommended.

Chemoprophylaxis with azithromycin should be strongly considered for exposed family, household, and childcare contacts who are within 21 days since the onset of cough in the index case, even if they are vaccinated. Chemoprophylaxis in health care settings and schools may be considered depending on specific circumstances as determined by infection control or public health services. Hospitalized children with pertussis should be isolated because of the great risk of transmission to patients and staff.

Prognosis

The prognosis for patients with pertussis has improved in recent years because of excellent supportive care, treatment of complications, attention to nutrition, and modern intensive care. However, the disease is still very serious in infants younger than 1 year; most deaths occur in this age group. Children with encephalopathy have a poor prognosis.

Centers for Disease Control and Prevention (CDC): Pertussis (Whooping Cough). https://www.cdc.gov/pertussis/index.html. Accessed May 10, 2023.

Lumbreras AM et al: Antenatal vaccination to decrease pertussis in infants: safety, effectiveness, timing, and implementation. J Matern Fetal Neonatal Med 2019 May;32(9):1541–1546. doi: 10.1080/14767058.2017.1406475 [PMID: 29199493].

McGirr A, Fisman DN: Duration of pertussis immunity after DTaP immunization: a meta-analysis. Pediatrics 2015;135(2):331 [PMID: 25560446].

Pertussis (Whooping Cough). In: Kimberlin DW, Brady MT, Jackson MA, Long SS, (eds): *Red Book: 2021–2024 Report of the Committee on Infectious Diseases*. 32nd ed. Itasca, IL: American Academy of Pediatrics; 2021;578–589.

LISTERIOSIS

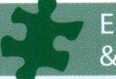

ESSENTIALS OF DIAGNOSIS & TYPICAL FEATURES

► Early-onset neonatal disease:
  • Signs of sepsis a few hours after birth in an infant born with fetal distress and hepatosplenomegaly; maternal fever.
► Late-onset neonatal disease:
  • Meningitis, sometimes with monocytosis in the CSF and peripheral blood.
  • Onset at age 8–30 days.
► Immunosuppressed patients:
  • Fever and meningitis.

General Considerations

Listeria monocytogenes is a gram-positive, non–spore-forming aerobic rod distributed widely in animals and in food, dust, and soil. It causes systemic infections in newborn infants and immunosuppressed older children. In pregnant women, infection is relatively mild, with fever, aches, and chills, but is accompanied by bacteremia and sometimes results in intrauterine or perinatal infection with grave consequences for the fetus or newborn. Pregnant women are particularly susceptible to listeriosis, and 20% of affected pregnancies end in stillbirth or neonatal death. In the United States, pregnant Hispanic women are 24 times more likely to contract listeriosis than the general population. Outbreaks of listeriosis have been associated with multiple foods, particularly unpasteurized dairy products including homemade Mexican-style cheese and prepared meats. Though cases have decreased since the adoption of strict regulations for ready-to-eat foods, outbreaks continue to occur in the United States.

Clinical Findings

A. Symptoms and Signs

In the early neonatal infection, symptoms of listeriosis usually appear on the first day of life and always by the third day. Fetal distress is common, and infants frequently have signs of severe disease at birth. Respiratory distress, diarrhea, and fever occur. On examination, hepatosplenomegaly and a papular rash are found. A history of maternal fever is common. Meningitis may accompany the septic course. The late neonatal form occurs after 7 days until as late as 5 weeks. Meningitis is common, characterized by irritability, fever, and poor feeding.

Listeria infections are rare in older children and usually are associated with immunodeficiency including cancer chemotherapy and treatment with tumor necrosis factor-α inhibitors. Signs and symptoms are those of meningitis or meningoencephalitis, often with insidious onset.

B. Laboratory Findings

In all patients except those receiving white cell depressant drugs, the WBC count is elevated, with 10%–20% monocytes. The characteristic CSF cell count in meningitis is high (> 500/μL) with a predominance of polymorphonuclear neutrophils, though monocytes may predominate in up to 30% of cases. *Listeria* are typically gram-positive rods, though they can be gram variable, and may be mistaken for "diphtheroids." Gram-stained smears of CSF are frequently negative. The chief pathologic feature in severe neonatal sepsis is miliary granulomatosis with microabscesses in the liver, spleen, CNS, lung, and bowel.

Culture results are frequently positive from multiple sites, including blood from the infant and the mother. Listeria can also be diagnosed in blood and CSF by PCR, often as a component of a multiplex assay.

Differential Diagnosis

Early-onset neonatal disease resembles hemolytic disease of the newborn, GBS sepsis or severe cytomegalovirus infection or toxoplasmosis. Late-onset disease must be differentiated from meningitis due to parechovirus, enterovirus, GBS, and gram-negative enteric bacteria.

Treatment

Ampicillin is the drug of choice in most cases of listeriosis. Gentamicin has a synergistic effect with ampicillin and should be given in serious infections and to patients with immune deficits; doses depend on age and birth weight. If ampicillin cannot be used, TMP-SMX or fluoroquinolones are effective and achieve adequate levels in the CNS. Meropenem and linezolid are also active and may be used in certain scenarios. Vancomycin may be substituted for ampicillin when empirically treating meningitis but is not preferred over ampicillin. Cephalosporins are not active. Treatment of severe disease should continue for at least 2 weeks; meningitis is treated for 3–4 weeks.

Controversy exists about the need for empiric *Listeria* coverage for a febrile neonate. Risk factors for listeria such as severe disease, maternal illness, maternal risk factors (eg, exposure to unpasteurized cheese), early (day of life 1) onset of infection, or suspected meningitis should be considered when making decisions when a cephalosporin might be used as a single drug.

Prevention

Immunosuppressed, pregnant, and elderly patients can decrease the risk of *Listeria* infection by avoiding soft unpasteurized cheeses, by thoroughly reheating or avoiding delicatessen and ready-to-eat foods, by avoiding raw meat and milk, and by thoroughly washing fresh vegetables.

Prognosis

The mortality rate of listeriosis is 15%–20%, with higher rates seen in high risk groups such as neonates and immunocompromised individuals Meningitis in older infants has a good prognosis.

Centers for Disease Control and Prevention (CDC): Listeriosis. http://www.cdc.gov/listeria/index.html. Accessed May 10, 2023.

Charlier C et al: Clinical features and prognostic factors of listeriosis: the MONOAISA national prospective cohort study. Lancet Infect Dis 2017;17(5):510–519 [PMID: 28139432].

Listeria monocytogenes Infections (Listeriosis). In: Kimberlin DW, Brady MT, Jackson MA, Long SS, (eds): *Red Book: 2021–2024 Report of the Committee on Infectious Diseases.* 32nd ed. Itasca, IL: American Academy of Pediatrics; 2021;478–482.

TUBERCULOSIS

ESSENTIALS OF DIAGNOSIS & TYPICAL FEATURES

► All types: positive tuberculin test or interferon-γ release assay (IGRA) in patient or members of household, suggestive chest radiograph, history of contact, and demonstration of organism by stain and culture.

► Pulmonary: fatigue, irritability, weight loss, with or without fever and cough.

► Glandular: chronic cervical adenitis.

► Miliary: classic snowstorm appearance of chest radiograph.

► Meningitis: fever and manifestations of meningeal irritation and increased intracranial pressure, with characteristic CSF.

General Considerations

Tuberculosis (TB) is a granulomatous disease caused by *Mycobacterium tuberculosis* (MTb). It is a leading cause of death throughout the world. Children younger than 5 years are most susceptible with highest risk in the first year of life. Primary infection occurs via the lungs with subsequent lymphohematogenous dissemination to extrapulmonary sites, including lymph nodes, the brain and meninges, bones and joints, kidneys, intestine, larynx, eyes, and skin. A greater proportion of pediatric TB disease is extrapulmonary compared to adults. Though TB is rare in many US communities, outbreaks in children occur, particularly in schools. Exposure to an infected adult is the most important risk factor for a pediatric patient. Groups at highest risk of TB infection are those who were born or lived in TB endemic countries and, to a lesser extent, US-born children with family members from endemic countries. Additional epidemiologic risk factors may include exposure to foreign-born persons, prisoners, residents of nursing homes, impoverished individuals, migrant workers, and health care providers. Rates of TB in American Indians, Asian, Hawaiian and Pacific Islanders, and Hispanic people are substantially greater than in Caucasians. Nationally about 9% of cases have resistance to at least one drug (drug-resistant [DR] TB) and 1% if the TB cases are multiple drug resistant (MDR TB). HIV infection and other immune compromising diseases are important risk factors for both development and spread of disease and thus diagnosis of *M tuberculosis* in a child is an indication for HIV testing.

An important distinction is the difference between TB infection (TBI) and disease. In infection, there are no clinical or radiographic signs of active disease. This scenario has previously been termed latent tuberculosis infection, though the current terminology drops the term "latent" as it is biologically inaccurate. TBI may affect up to one-quarter of the world population and approximately 13 million persons in the United States. TBI may progress (quickly in the very young, and often after decades of infection in older children and adults) to symptomatic disease that requires aggressive multidrug therapy.

Of note, *Mycobacterium bovis* infection is clinically identical to *M tuberculosis*, though extrapulmonary disease (particularly gastrointestinal) is more common with *M bovis*. *M bovis* may be acquired from unpasteurized dairy products obtained outside the United States.

► Clinical Findings

A. Symptoms and Signs

1. Tuberculosis Infection (TBI)—By definition, there are no symptoms or signs in TBI, and diagnosis occurs in the context of a positive skin or blood test on TB screening.

2. Pulmonary—(See Chapter 19.)

3. Miliary—This manifestation of disseminated disease is common in young children and can be rapidly progressive. Affected children have fever, weight loss, or failure to thrive, and can become systemically unwell. Diagnosis is suggested by the classic "millet seed" appearance of lung fields on radiograph, although early in the course the chest radiograph may show only subtle abnormalities. Other tissues may be infected to produce osteomyelitis, arthritis, meningitis, tuberculomas of the brain, enteritis, or infection of the kidneys and liver.

4. Meningitis—Symptoms include fever, vomiting, headache, lethargy, and irritability, with signs of meningeal irritation and increased intracranial pressure, cranial nerve palsies, convulsions, and coma. The presentation of TB meningitis is typically subacute.

5. Lymphatic—Enlarged cervical lymph nodes usually present in a subacute manner. Involved nodes may become fixed to the overlying skin, suppurate, and drain.

6. Additional extrapulmonary sites—In addition to the meninges and lymphatic system, infection can occur in other sites (e.g., abdomen, joints, skin, kidney, eye) and symptoms depend on location of disease.

B. Laboratory Findings

For decades, the tuberculin skin test (TST) has been the standard diagnostic tool for TB. However, the skin test has a number of disadvantages: Placement of TST can be difficult, measurement of induration can be subjective, it requires two health care visits to complete, the amount of induration that indicates a positive reaction varies with the epidemiologic risk and immune status of the patient, and both false-positive and false-negative results occur. False-positive reactions are most common in children previously vaccinated with bacille Calmette-Guerin (BCG), though exposure to nontuberculous mycobacteria (NTM) can also lead to TST positivity. Approximately 75% of positive TSTs in BCG-vaccinated individuals (children and adults) may be due to the BCG rather than TBI. This has significant implications for screening populations from TB endemic countries where the majority of children receive BCG. False-negative reactions are also a concern, occurring in malnourished patients, those with overwhelming disease, and in 10% of children with isolated pulmonary disease. Temporary suppression of tuberculin reactivity may be seen with viral infections (eg, measles, influenza, varicella, and mumps), after live virus immunization, and during corticosteroid or other immunosuppressive drug therapy. For these reasons, a negative TST does not exclude the diagnosis of TB.

Interferon-gamma release assays (IGRAs) measure in vitro release of interferon-γ from blood lymphocytes in response to TB-specific antigens. These assays, which have much higher specificity for MTb, are unaffected by antigens from BCG and the majority of NTM. IGRAs are done on blood obtained by venipuncture and require only a single visit. These tests are preferred in adults and BCG-immunized children older than 2 years. IGRAs are reported as positive, negative, or indeterminate.

Definitive diagnosis of TB disease requires microbiologic or molecular identification of *M tuberculosis*. However, children have pauci-bacillary disease and at young age are less able to produce sputa, even with induction. Cultures of pooled early morning gastric aspirates from 3 successive days will yield *M tuberculosis* in about 40% of cases, but smears on gastric specimens are usually negative. Biopsy may be necessary to establish the diagnosis, but it may be difficult to justify invasive tests in mildly ill or asymptomatic children. Therapy should not be delayed in suspected cases. The CSF in tuberculous meningitis shows slight to moderate pleocytosis (50–300 WBCs/μL, predominantly lymphocytes), decreased glucose, and increased protein.

Acid-fast bacilli can be demonstrated on microscopy from patient samples. Culture for definitive identification and susceptibilities remains a mainstay of laboratory diagnosis, though nucleic amplification tests (NAATs) including the Xpert MTB/RIF are increasingly available and are able to rapidly identify *Mtb* genes associated with antimicrobial susceptibilities directly from patient samples. Current World Health Organization (WHO) guidelines recommend utilization of Xpert testing on all sputa tested for TB. NAATs are increasingly available for testing of nonsputum samples including cerebrospinal fluid, tissue, pleural fluid and even stool, though the lower sensitivity for these samples means that negative tests cannot be relied upon to rule out infection.

C. Imaging

Chest radiograph should be obtained in all children with suspicion of TB at any site or with a positive TB test. Segmental consolidation with some volume loss and hilar adenopathy are common findings in children. Paratracheal adenopathy is a classic presentation. Pleural effusion also occurs with primary infection. Cavities and apical disease are unusual in children but are common in adolescents and adults. Computed tomography (CT) scanning more clearly demonstrates pathology in questionable cases but is unnecessary in the majority of cases.

▶ Differential Diagnosis

Pulmonary TB must be differentiated from fungal, parasitic, mycoplasmal, and bacterial pneumonias; lung abscess; foreign-body aspiration; lipoid pneumonia; sarcoidosis; and mediastinal cancer. Cervical lymphadenitis is most likely due to streptococcal or staphylococcal infections. Cat-scratch fever and infection with atypical mycobacteria may need to be distinguished from tuberculous lymphadenitis. Viral meningoencephalitis, head trauma (child abuse), lead poisoning, brain abscess, acute bacterial meningitis, brain tumor, and disseminated fungal infections must be excluded in tuberculous meningitis. A positive TST or IGRA in the patient or family contacts is frequently valuable in suggesting the diagnosis of TB. A negative TST or IGRA does not exclude TB.

▶ Prevention

A. BCG Vaccine

BCG vaccines are live-attenuated strains of *M bovis*. Although neonatal and childhood administration of BCG is carried out in countries with a high prevalence of TB, protective efficacy varies greatly with vaccine potency and method of delivery. BCG protects infants and toddlers against disseminated TB and meningitis but does not protect against pulmonary TB later in childhood or adolescence. In the United States where rates of TB are low among US-born children, BCG vaccination is not recommended, in part because of challenges posed by potential false positive TST reactions in BCG-vaccinated children.

B. TBI Treatment and Window Prophylaxis

Children with TBI should be treated to prevent future development of TB disease. Traditionally, treatment with 9 months of isoniazid (9H) has been utilized, but shorter regimens of daily rifampin weight-based dosing for 4 months or once-weekly isoniazid/rifapentine (weight-based dosing ranges) for 3 months are now preferred by many experts. These regimens have equal efficacy and better completion rates compared to 9H. Because it can take up to 8 weeks for IGRA or skin tests to convert after infection and disease can progress quickly in young children, exposed asymptomatic children younger than 5 years should receive treatment as for TBI until repeat testing can be performed at least 8 weeks after the last exposure (window prophylaxis). If follow-up testing is positive, they can simply complete the TBI treatment.

C. Other Measures

Prevention of TB in children requires identification and treatment of infectious adult cases in a community or within a household. Because children are not generally contagious, a pediatric case indicates an active adult case, often a family member in the household. Contact tracing through public health agencies and TB screening of high-risk individuals are the most effective ways to prevent pediatric TB cases. Routine TB testing is not recommended for children without risk factors who reside in communities with a low incidence of TB. Children with travel or immigration from a country with a high incidence of infection should be tested on entry to the United States or on presentation to health care providers.

▶ Treatment

A. Specific Measures

Most children with suspected TB disease do not require hospitalization. If the infecting organism has not been isolated from the presumed source (and therefore susceptibility testing is unavailable), reasonable attempts should be made to obtain using morning gastric aspirates, sputum, bronchoscopy, thoracentesis, or biopsy when appropriate. Unfortunately, cultures are frequently negative in children, and the risk of these procedures must be weighed against the yield.

Directly observed administration of all doses of antituberculosis therapy by a trained health care professional is essential to ensure compliance with therapy.

Most regimens for TB disease infection begin with four drug therapy for the first 2 months. For example, children with active pulmonary disease receive isoniazid, rifampin, pyrazinamide, and ethambutol in single daily oral doses for 2 months, followed by isoniazid plus rifampin (either in a daily or thrice-weekly regimen) for 4 months. For more severe disease, such as miliary or CNS infection, higher doses of drugs are used, and the duration of the two-drug continuation phase is increased to 10 months or more. The duration of therapy is prolonged in immunocompromised children and if drug resistance necessitates alternative regimens. Such patients should be managed in consultation with a TB specialist. TB meningitis is often treated with additional IV medications to achieve better CSF penetration, including levofloxacin, linezolid, and amikacin.

Drugs to treat TB are generally better tolerated in children than adults. Clinically significant hepatotoxicity is rare, and routine monitoring of liver function tests in otherwise healthy children is generally not required. Peripheral neuropathy associated with pyridoxine deficiency is rare in children, so it is not necessary to add pyridoxine unless significant malnutrition coexists or if the child is strictly breastfed. Rifampin causes an orange color of urine and secretions, which is benign but may stain contact lenses or clothes. Rifampin alters the kinetics of many medications including some anticonvulsants and oral contraceptives.

Optic neuritis is the major side effect of ethambutol in adults; thus, there has been concern with use in children too young to screen for color discrimination. However, optic neuritis is rare and usually occurs in adults receiving more than the recommended dosage of 25 mg/kg/day. Since documentation of optic neuritis in children is lacking despite considerable worldwide experience, many four-drug regimens for children now include ethambutol.

B. Chemotherapy for Drug-Resistant Tuberculosis

The incidence of drug resistance is increasing transmission of MDR and extensively drug-resistant (XDR) strains to contacts has occurred in some epidemics. Traditionally, four to six first- and second-line medications including parenteral formulations have been required and often require more prolonged courses of therapy. However, recent advances in oral MDR treatments for adults and children such as bedaquiline and delaminid are likely to shorten MDR courses and may avoid parenteral drugs. Consultation with a TB expert is recommended for all cases of TB, but particularly for MDR-TB and XDR-TB.

C. General Measures

Corticosteroids may be used for suppressing inflammatory reactions in meningeal, pleural, and pericardial TB and for the relief of bronchial obstruction due to hilar adenopathy. Prednisone is given orally over 4–6 weeks with a taper. The use of corticosteroids may mask progression of disease. Accordingly, the clinician needs to be sure that an effective regimen is being used.

▶ Prognosis

If bacteria are sensitive and treatment is completed, most children are cured with minimal sequelae. Repeat treatment is more difficult and less successful. Without treatment, the mortality rate in both miliary TB and tuberculous meningitis is almost 100%. In the latter form, about two-thirds of patients receiving treatment survive, but there may be a high incidence of neurologic abnormalities among survivors if treatment is started late.

Centers for Disease Control and Prevention (CDC): Tuberculosis (TB). https://www.cdc.gov/tb/default.htm. Accessed May 10, 2023.

Lewinsohn DM et al: Official ATS/CDC/IDSA clinical practice guidelines: diagnosis of tuberculosis in adults and children. Clin Infect Dis 2017;64(2):e1–e33 [PMID: 27932390].

Nahid P et al: Official ATS/CDC/ERS/IDSA clinical practice guidelines: treatment of drug-resistant tuberculosis. Am J Respir Crit Care Med 2019;200(10):e93–e142 [PMID: 31729908].

Nahid P et al: Official ATS/CDC/IDSA clinical practice guidelines: treatment of drug susceptible tuberculosis. Clin Infect Dis 2016;63(1 Oct):e147 [PMID: 31729908].

Sterling TR et al: Guidelines for the treatment of latent tuberculosis infection: recommendations from the National Tuberculosis Controllers Association and CDC, 2020. MMWR Recomm Rep 2020;69(No. RR-1):1–11. doi: http://dx.doi.org/10.15585/mmwr.rr6901a1.

INFECTIONS WITH NONTUBERCULOUS MYCOBACTERIA

ESSENTIALS OF DIAGNOSIS & TYPICAL FEATURES

▶ Chronic unilateral cervical lymphadenitis.

▶ Granulomas of the skin.

▶ Chronic bone lesion with draining sinus (chronic osteomyelitis).

▶ TST of <10 mm, negative interferon-gamma release assay, chest radiograph, and negative history of contact with TB.

▶ Diagnosis by positive culture.

▶ Disseminated infection in immunocompromised patients, particularly with AIDS.

▶ General Considerations

Nearly 200 species of acid-fast mycobacteria other than *M tuberculosis* (nontuberculous mycobacteria, NTM) may cause subclinical infections and occasionally clinical disease resembling TB. Strains of NTM are common in soil, food, and water. Organisms enter the host by small abrasions in skin, oral mucosa, or gastrointestinal mucosa. NTM can be hospital-acquired. Outbreaks have been associated with health care facilities, tattoo parlors, and spas.

Mycobacterium avium complex (MAC), *Mycobacterium kansasii, Mycobacterium fortuitum, Mycobacterium abscessus, Mycobacterium marinum*, and *Mycobacterium chelonae*

are most commonly encountered. *M fortuitum, M abscessus, M smegmatis,* and *M chelonae* are "rapid growers" requiring 3–7 days for recovery in culture, whereas other mycobacteria require up to several weeks. After inoculation they form colonies closely resembling *M tuberculosis* morphologically.

▶ Clinical Findings

A. Symptoms and Signs

1. Lymphadenitis—In children, the most common form of infection due to NTM is cervical lymphadenitis. In the United States MAC is the most common organism. A submandibular or cervical node swells slowly and is firm and initially somewhat tender. A purplish hue in the overlying skin is commonly noted. Low-grade fever may occur. Over time, the node may suppurate and drain chronically. Nodes in other areas of the head and neck and elsewhere are sometimes involved. Chronic intermittent drainage is common, but in many cases spontaneous healing occurs after 4–12 months.

2. Pulmonary disease—In the western United States, pulmonary disease is usually due to *M kansasii* or MAC. In the eastern United States and in other countries, disease is usually caused by MAC. Immune deficiency, particularly deficiency of cellular immunity, is commonly present. Presentation is clinically indistinguishable from that of TB. Adolescents with cystic fibrosis may be infected with NTM with resulting fever and declining pulmonary function.

3. Swimming pool granuloma—This is commonly due to *M marinum*. A solitary chronic granulomatous lesion with satellite lesions develops after minor trauma in infected swimming pools or other aquatic sources, such as home aquariums.

4. Chronic osteomyelitis—Osteomyelitis is caused by MAC, *M kansasii, M fortuitum*, or other rapid growers. Findings include swelling and pain over a distal extremity, radiolucent defects in bone, and fever.

5. Disseminated infection—Disseminated infection occurs most often, though not exclusively, in children with immune deficiency. Children are ill, with fever and hepatosplenomegaly, and organisms are demonstrated in bone lesions, blood culture, lymph nodes, or liver. Chest radiographs are usually normal. Prior to antiretroviral therapy 60%–80% of patients with AIDS acquired disseminated MAC infection. Infection usually indicates severe immune dysfunction and is associated with CD4 lymphocyte counts less than 50/μL.

B. Laboratory Findings

In most cases, there is a negative or small reaction to TST (< 10 mm); larger reactions may be seen particularly with *M marinum* infection. IGRA tests are commonly negative although *M marinum, M kansasii*, and *M szulgai* may cause cross-reactions. The chest radiograph is negative, and there is no history of contact with a case of TB. Needle aspiration of the node excludes bacterial infection and may yield acid-fast bacilli on stain or culture. Cultures of any normally sterile body site may yield MAC in immunocompromised patients with disseminated disease and blood cultures are frequently positive in these cases. Nucleic acid amplification tests and matrix assisted laser desorption ionization-time of flight mass spectrometry (MALDI-TOF) are increasingly useful for categorization and speciation of NTMs.

Differential Diagnosis

See section on differential diagnosis in the previous discussion of TB and in Chapter 19.

Treatment

A. Specific Measures

Medical therapy for NTM can be complex and it is prudent to obtain expert consultation for complicated, refractory or severe infections. The usual treatment of lymphadenitis is complete surgical excision after which antimicrobial therapy may be unnecessary. Cases can be successfully treated nonsurgically as well. A typical regimen for cervical adenopathy involves multiple months of clarithromycin or azithromycin, ethambutol, and/or rifampin or rifabutin. Susceptibility testing is useful to optimize therapy. More locally invasive or disseminated disease often requires a combination of three or more active drugs. A macrolide is typically a backbone of treatment, with addition of TMP-SMX, a rifamycin (eg, rifampin), ethambutol, an aminoglycoside (eg, amikacin), doxycycline, a fluoroquinolone (eg, ciprofloxacin), linezolid, or a carbapenem (eg, meropenem), depending on the infecting species and susceptibility patterns from culture. When *M tuberculosis* cannot be excluded, it is sometimes necessary to add a macrolide to typical four-drug MTb treatment regimens.

B. General Measures

Isolation of the patient is usually not necessary. General supportive care is indicated for the child with disseminated disease.

Prognosis

The prognosis is good for patients with localized disease, although fatalities occur in immunocompromised patients with disseminated disease.

Centers for Disease Control and Prevention. Hospital Acquired Infections: Non-tuberculous Mycobacteria. Available at: https://www.cdc.gov/hai/organisms/nontuberculous-mycobacteria.html. Accessed May 16, 2023.

Gallois Y et al: Nontuberculous mycobacterial lymphadenitis in children: what management strategy? Int J Pediatr Otorhinolaryngol 2019 Jul;122:196–202. doi: 10.1016/j.ijporl.2019.04.012 [PMID: 31039497].

LEGIONELLA INFECTION

ESSENTIALS OF DIAGNOSIS & TYPICAL FEATURES

▶ Severe progressive pneumonia in an immunocompromised child.

▶ Hospital-acquired infection can be due to contaminated water supply.

▶ Positive culture or urine antigen assay in suspected patients.

General Considerations

Legionella pneumophila is a ubiquitous gram-negative bacillus that causes two distinct clinical syndromes: Legionnaires disease and Pontiac fever. *L pneumophila* causes most infections, though many other *Legionella* species can be pathogenic. *Legionella* is present in many natural water sources as well as domestic water supplies and fountains. In water, *Legionella* can reside inside amoebas, which may protect the organism from chlorination. Infection is thought to be acquired by inhalation of a contaminated aerosol. Contaminated cooling towers and heat exchangers have been implicated in several large institutional outbreaks, including health care facilities. Person-to-person transmission is extremely rare.

Legionella infection is rare in children, except in children with compromised cell-mediated immunity (cell-mediated immunity required to activate macrophages to kill the intracellular bacteria), and neonates, particularly premature infants. In adults, risk factors include smoking, underlying cardiopulmonary or renal disease, alcoholism, and diabetes. Significant epidemiologic risk factors include travel (especially cruise ship) or a stay in a health care facility.

Clinical Findings

A. Symptoms and Signs

Legionella can cause both community- and hospital-acquired pneumonia, often characterized by abrupt onset of fever, chills, anorexia, and headache. Pulmonary symptoms appear within 2–3 days and progress rapidly. The cough is nonproductive early and purulent sputum occurs late. Hemoptysis, diarrhea, and neurologic signs (including lethargy, irritability, tremors, and delirium) are seen. Pontiac fever is a milder, self-limited flu-like illness not associated with pneumonia. In neonates infection can cause sepsis and cardiorespiratory failure.

B. Laboratory Findings

The WBC count is usually elevated with neutrophilia in Legionnaires disease. Chest radiographs show rapidly progressive patchy consolidation. Cavitation and large pleural effusions are uncommon. *Legionella* take up Gram stain poorly so may not be observed during the initial microscopic examination of respiratory specimens. Cultures from sputum, tracheal aspirates, or bronchoscopic specimens are considered the gold-standard for diagnosis but require specialized media and can take > 5 days to grow. Direct fluorescent antibody staining of sputum or other respiratory specimens is 95% specific but is only 25%–75% sensitive. A false-positive test can be seen in patients with tularemia. PCR detection of respiratory secretions for *Legionella* is available at some centers and is highly sensitive and specific. Urine antigen tests for *Legionella* antigen are rapid and highly specific but only detect *L pneumophila* serotype 1, which is the most common community-acquired *L pneumophila* infection. A positive urine antigen in a patient with pneumonia is strong evidence for *L pneumophila* infection.

Differential Diagnosis

Legionnaires disease is usually a rapidly progressive pneumonia in a patient who appears very ill with unremitting fevers, particularly those who have been hospitalized or who are immunodeficient. Both typical and atypical bacterial pathogens associated with pneumonia should be considered such as *Streptococcus pneumoniae* and *Chlamydophila pneumoniae*.

Complications

Hematogenous dissemination may result in extrapulmonary foci of infection, including the pericardium, myocardium, and kidneys. *Legionella* may cause culture-negative endocarditis.

Treatment

Children with *Legionella* infection should be treated with levofloxacin (specific dosing varies by age and co-morbidities) or azithromycin. Immunocompromised children should receive levofloxacin. Doxycycline and TMP-SMX are alternative agents. Duration of therapy is 5–10 days if azithromycin is used; for other antibiotics a 14- to 21-day course. Oral therapy may be substituted for intravenous therapy as the patient's condition improves. Pontiac fever does not require antibiotic treatment.

Prevention

Ensuring proper disinfectant (eg, monochloramine rather than chlorine) and water temperature maintenance of building and municipal water systems is essential. Regular cleaning, attention to pH, and proper disinfectants in hot tubs are important. Any single case of *Legionella* acquired in a health care setting should prompt a thorough investigation to identify a potential source.

Prognosis

For Legionanaires disease, mortality rate is high (5%–25%) if untreated and higher for immunocompromised patients (approaching 80%). Otherwise, the mortality rate is less than 5% in normal hosts with early appropriate therapy. Malaise, problems with memory, and fatigue are common after recovery.

Centers for Disease Control and Prevention: *Legionella.* http://www.cdc.gov/legionella/clinicians.html. Accessed May 16, 2023.
Herwaldt LA et al: *Legionella*: a reemerging pathogen. Curr Opin Infect Dis 2018 Aug;31(4):325–333.

CHLAMYDOPHILA & CHLAMYDIA INFECTIONS (PSITTACOSIS, C PNEUMONIAE, & C TRACHOMATIS)

ESSENTIALS OF DIAGNOSIS & TYPICAL FEATURES

▶ Psittacosis:
- Fever, cough, malaise, chills, headache.
- Diffuse rales; no consolidation.
- Long-lasting radiographic findings of bronchopneumonia.
- Exposure to infected birds (ornithosis).

▶ Neonatal *Chlamydia* conjunctivitis:
- Watery, mucopurulent, to blood-tinged discharge and conjunctival injection presenting from a few days of life until 16 weeks of age.
- May be associated with *Chlamydia* pneumonia.
- Identification of *Chlamydia* conjunctivitis or pneumonia in a neonate should prompt evaluation and treatment of the mother and her sexual partner.

General Considerations

New taxonomic studies distinguish the genera *Chlamydophila* (*C psittaci, C pneumoniae*) and *Chlamydia* (*C trachomatis*) within the family Chlamydiaceae.

Psittacosis is a rare but potentially severe pulmonary infection caused by *Chlamydophila psittaci*, transmitted to humans from psittacine birds (parrots, parakeets, cockatoos, and budgerigars), as well as other avian species (eg, turkeys). Infections are rare in children, and human-to-human spread rarely occurs. The incubation period is 5–14 days. The bird from which the disease was transmitted may not be ill.

C pneumoniae (formerly *Chlamydia pneumoniae*) may cause atypical pneumonia similar to that due to *M pneumoniae*. Transmission is by respiratory spread. Lower respiratory tract infection due to *C pneumoniae* is uncommon in infants and young children and is most common in the second decade. *C pneumoniae* has been associated with acute chest syndrome in children with sickle cell disease.

C trachomatis causes urogenital infections including asymptomatic infections, lymphogranuloma venereum, nongonococcal urethritis, epididymitis, cervicitis, and pelvic inflammatory disease. Serovars D–K (and L1, L2, L3 in lymphogranuloma venereum) are responsible for most of these infections. Sexually transmitted urogenital infections caused by *C trachomatis* are discussed in Chapter 44. In infants born to infected mothers, *C trachomatis* infection can be acquired through exposure in the birth canal, causing neonatal conjunctivitis and/or pneumonia. The risk of acquisition for a baby born vaginally to an infected mother is approximately 50%.

Trachoma is a rare disease in the United States but is a major cause of disability in low-income countries. Trachoma is caused by certain *C trachomatis* serovars (A–C) that cause chronic keratoconjunctivitis that results in inflammation and neovascularization of the cornea, leading to corneal scarring and blindness.

▶ Clinical Findings

A. Symptoms and Signs

1. *C psittaci* pneumonia—The disease is extremely variable but tends to be mild in children. The onset is rapid or insidious, with fever, chills, headache, backache, malaise, myalgia, and dry cough. Signs include pneumonitis, altered percussion notes and breathe sounds, and rales, but pulmonary findings may be absent early. Dyspnea and cyanosis may occur later. Splenomegaly, epistaxis, prostration, and meningismus are occasionally seen. Delirium, constipation or diarrhea, and abdominal distress may occur.

2. *C pneumoniae* pneumonia—Clinically, *C pneumoniae* infection is similar to *M pneumoniae* infection. Most patients have mild upper respiratory symptoms. Lower respiratory tract infection is characterized by fever, sore throat, cough, and bilateral pulmonary findings and infiltrates. Many infections are mild and self-limited.

3. *C trachomatis* neonatal conjunctivitis and pneumonia—Neonatal conjunctivitis caused by *C trachomatis* can occur from a few days until 12–16 weeks after birth but is most common at 5–10 days (in contrast to gonococcal ophthalmia neonatorum which typically occurs before 5 days) (see Chapter 16). There may be mild to moderate swelling of the lids and watery or mucopurulent discharge. A pseudomembrane may be present, the conjunctivae may be friable, and there may be some bloody discharge. Pneumonia may occur in babies with or without neonatal conjunctivitis. Pneumonia is most commonly seen between 2 and 12 weeks of age. Most babies are afebrile, tachypneic, and have a staccato cough.

4. *C trachomatis* trachoma—Trachoma is seen in developing countries where poor hygienic conditions exist. It is the most common cause of acquired blindness worldwide. The peak incidence of trachoma is seen at 4–6 years of age, with scarring and eventual blindness occurring in adulthood. Infections occur from direct contact with infected secretions (eye, nose, throat) or by direct contact with contaminated objects (secretions on towels, washcloths, handkerchiefs).

B. Laboratory Findings

1. *C psittaci*—In psittacosis, the WBC count is normal or decreased, often with a left shift. Proteinuria is common. Hepatitis is common in severe infections. *C psittaci* can be present in the blood and sputum during the first 2 weeks of illness, but submitting cultures can represent a hazard to laboratory workers and should generally be avoided. Serologic testing is challenging and may be affected by antimicrobial treatment and cross-react with other chlamydial species. Acute and convalescent titers may help confirm infection but are impractical for therapeutic decisions; empiric treatment in the right clinical and exposure setting is common.

2. *C pneumoniae*—Eosinophilia is sometimes present. PCR-based diagnosis from respiratory samples, which is increasingly available as part of a multiplex PCR platform, is rapidly replacing culture and serologic diagnostic methods.

3. *C trachomatis*—NAATs have largely replaced direct immunostaining methods for the diagnosis of chlamydia infections in children. In countries where trachoma occurs, the diagnosis is often made clinically.

C. Imaging

The radiographic findings in psittacosis are those of central pneumonia that later becomes widespread or migratory. Psittacosis is indistinguishable from viral pneumonias by radiograph. Signs of pneumonitis may appear on radiograph in the absence of clinical suspicion of pulmonary involvement. Pneumonia from *C pneumoniae* produces variable radiographic findings including bilateral interstitial infiltrates or a unilateral subsegmental infiltrate. In neonatal pneumonia due to *C trachomatis*, infiltrates, and often hyperinflation, are seen.

▶ Differential Diagnosis

Psittacosis can be differentiated from viral or mycoplasmal pneumonias only by the history of contact with potentially infected birds. In severe or prolonged cases with extrapulmonary involvement the differential diagnosis is broad, including typhoid fever, brucellosis, and rheumatic fever.

C pneumoniae pneumonia is not distinguishable clinically from *Mycoplasma* or viral pneumonia.

C trachomatis conjunctivitis must be differentiated from gonococcal conjunctivitis, chemical conjunctivitis, or viral conjunctivitis. Gonococcal conjunctivitis is often severe, with purulent drainage. PCR and culture of conjunctival discharge can provide the diagnosis of gonococcal conjunctivitis.

Complications

Complications of psittacosis include myocarditis, endocarditis, hepatitis, pancreatitis, and secondary bacterial pneumonia. *C pneumoniae* infection may be prolonged or may recur. Trachoma caused by *C trachomatis* can lead to blindness.

Treatment

Psittacosis—Doxycycline is the preferred treatment and should be used for all critically ill children regardless of age. Alternatively, erythromycin or azithromycin may be used, though treatment failures with macrolides have been described.

    Chlamydophila pneumonia—Many suspected atypical pneumonias are treated empirically. *C pneumoniae* responds to macrolides (eg, azithromycin). Doxycycline for 10–14 days is an alternative.

    Neonatal conjunctivitis or pneumonia—Systemic antibiotic therapy is required for neonatal chlamydia infections, even when the only manifestation is conjunctivitis. Although the current consensus recommendation is a 10-day course of erythromycin base or ethylsuccinate (weight-based dosing), treatment with azithromycin (weight-based dosing for 3 days) appears effective and may increase compliance with treatment. Treatment failures are not uncommon and repeat treatment courses may be necessary. Both erythromycin and azithromycin are associated with an increased risk of pyloric stenosis in infants and parents should be counseled to recognize the symptoms of this condition. The diagnosis of an infant with chlamydial conjunctivitis and/or pneumonia should prompt evaluation and treatment of the mother and her sexual partner for *Chlamydia* and other sexually transmitted diseases (see Chapter 44). Screening for *Neisseria gonorrhoeae* should also be performed and treated if positive.

    Trachoma is treated with a single dose of oral azithromycin (weight-based dosing).

Prevention

Bird cages should be cleaned regularly, particularly when the bird is sick. *C psittaci* is susceptible to a 1:100 dilution of household bleach. Sick birds should be evaluated by a veterinarian and treated with antimicrobials. *C pneumoniae* is transmitted person to person by infected respiratory tract secretions. Prevention involves avoidance of known infected persons, using good hand hygiene, and encouraging good respiratory hygiene (covering mouth with coughing, disposing of tissues contaminated with respiratory secretions).

    The diagnosis and treatment of genital *Chlamydophila* (chlamydial) infections in pregnant women and their sexual partners is the most effective way to prevent neonatal conjunctivitis and pneumonia (see Chapter 44). Application of ocular prophylactic antibiotic after birth reduces gonococcal infection, but it is not effective at preventing *C trachomatis* infection. Because trachoma is highly contagious, the WHO recommends community or regional mass treatment when the prevalence of trachoma among children exceeds 10%.

Centers for Disease Control and Prevention: Psittacosis. http://www.cdc.gov/pneumonia/atypical/psittacosis.html. Accessed May 16, 2023.

Pickering LK: American Academy of Pediatrics: Chlamydial infections. *Red Book: 2021–2024 Report of the Committee on Infectious Diseases.* 32nd ed. Elk Grove Village, IL: American Academy of Pediatrics; 2021:256–266.

Zikic A et al: Treatment of neonatal chlamydial conjunctivitis: a systematic review and meta-analysis. J Pediatric Infect Dis Soc 2018 Aug 17;7(3):e107–e115 [PMID: 30007329].

CAT-SCRATCH DISEASE

ESSENTIALS OF DIAGNOSIS & TYPICAL FEATURES

► History of a cat scratch or cat contact.

► Primary lesion (papule, pustule, or conjunctivitis) at site of inoculation.

► Acute or subacute regional lymphadenopathy.

► Biopsy of node or papule showing histopathologic findings consistent with cat-scratch disease and occasionally characteristic bacilli on Warthin-Starry stain.

► Positive cat-scratch serology (antibody to *Bartonella henselae*).

General Considerations

The causative agent of cat-scratch disease is *Bartonella henselae*, a gram-negative bacillus that also causes bacillary angiomatosis. It is estimated that more than 20,000 cases per year occur in the United States, the majority of which are in the southeast. Children 5–9 years old have the highest incidence. Cat-scratch disease is usually a benign, self-limited form of lymphadenitis. Patients often report a cat scratch, bite (less common), or contact with a cat or kitten. The organism is transmitted among cats by fleas, and kittens are more likely to be bacteremic. Occasionally dogs can be infected and transmit disease.

Clinical Findings

A. Symptoms and Signs

About 50% of patients with cat-scratch disease develop a primary lesion at the site of the wound. The lesion usually is a papule or pustule that appears 7–10 days after injury and is located most often on the arm or hand (50%), head or leg (30%), or trunk or neck (10%). The lesion may be conjunctival (10%). Regional lymphadenopathy appears 10–50 days later and may be accompanied by mild malaise, fatigue, headache, and fever. Multiple sites are seen in about 10% of cases. Involved nodes may be hard or soft and 1–6 cm in diameter. They are usually tender, warm, and erythematous and 10%–20% suppurate. Lymphadenopathy usually resolves in about 2 months but may persist for up to 8 months.

Unusual manifestations include erythema nodosum, thrombocytopenic purpura, conjunctivitis (Parinaud oculoglandular syndrome), parotid swelling, pneumonia, osteolytic lesions, mesenteric and mediastinal adenitis, neuroretinitis, peripheral neuritis, hepatitis, granulomata of the liver and spleen, and encephalopathy. Bartonella can also cause a subacute endocarditis.

Immunocompetent patients may uncommonly develop a systemic form of cat-scratch disease. These patients have prolonged fever, fatigue, and malaise. Lymphadenopathy may be present. Hepatosplenomegaly or low-density hepatic or splenic lesions visualized by ultrasound or CT scan are seen in some patients.

Infection in immunocompromised individuals may take the form of bacillary angiomatosis, presenting as vascular tumors of the skin and subcutaneous tissues. Immunocompromised patients may also have bacteremia or infection of the liver (peliosis hepatis).

B. Laboratory Findings

Serologic evidence of *Bartonella* infection by indirect immunofluorescent antibody with IgG titer of more than 1:256 is strongly suggestive of recent infection. A positive IgM antibody is sometimes positive. Aspirated samples from infected lymph nodes can be tested for *Bartonella* by PCR and are increasingly available. *Bartonella* is rarely isolated in culture.

Histopathologic examination of involved tissue may show pyogenic granulomas or bacillary forms demonstrated by Warthin-Starry silver stain (bacillary forms on stain are not specific for cat scratch disease). Later in the course necrotizing granulomas may be seen. In patients with CNS involvement, the CSF is usually normal but may show a slight pleocytosis and modest elevation of protein.

▶ Differential Diagnosis

Cat-scratch disease must be distinguished from pyogenic adenitis, TB (typical and atypical), tularemia, brucellosis, lymphoma, primary toxoplasmosis, infectious mononucleosis, lymphogranuloma venereum, and fungal infections.

▶ Treatment

Treatment of cat-scratch disease adenopathy is not always required because the disease typically resolves without therapy treatment. If antibiotics are given, a 5-day course of azithromycin is typically used. In cases of nodal suppuration, needle aspiration under local anesthesia relieves the pain. Excision of the involved node is indicated in cases of chronic adenitis.

Immunocompromised patients with evidence of infection should be treated with antibiotics: long-term therapy (months) of these patients with azithromycin or doxycycline often is needed to prevent relapses. Immunocompetent patients with more severe disease or evidence of systemic infection (eg, hepatic or splenic lesions) should also be treated with antibiotics.

▶ Prevention

Cat-scratch disease can be largely prevented by avoiding cat scratches or bites, especially by kittens. Flea control of animals will reduce cat-to-cat transmission.

▶ Prognosis

The prognosis is good if complications do not occur.

Bartonella henselae (Cat-Scratch Disease). In: Kimberlin DW, Brady MT, Jackson MA, Long SS (eds): *Red Book: 2021–2024 Report of the Committee on Infectious Diseases.* 32nd ed. Elk Grove Village, IL: American Academy of Pediatrics; 2021:226–229.
Centers for Disease Control and Prevention: Bartonella. http://www.cdc.gov/bartonella/clinicians/index.html. Accessed May 16, 2023.

▼ SPIROCHETAL INFECTIONS

SYPHILIS

ESSENTIALS OF DIAGNOSIS & TYPICAL FEATURES

▶ Congenital:
- Undiagnosed or undertreated maternal syphilis
- Newborn: hepatosplenomegaly, characteristic radiographic bone changes, anemia, increased nucleated red cells, thrombocytopenia, abnormal spinal fluid, jaundice, edema.
- Young infant (3–12 weeks): snuffles, maculopapular skin rash, mucocutaneous lesions, pseudoparalysis (in addition to radiographic bone changes).
- Children: stigmata of early congenital syphilis, Hutchinson teeth, sensorineural hearing loss, interstitial keratitis, saber shins, gummas of nose and palate.

▶ Acquired:
- Chancre of genitals, lip, or anus in child or adolescent.
- Pleomorphic rash, adenopathy, systemic symptoms.
- History of sexual contact and a positive serologic test.

General Considerations

Syphilis is a chronic, generalized infectious disease caused by a spirochete, *Treponema pallidum*. In the acquired form, the disease is transmitted by sexual contact. Primary syphilis is characterized by the presence of an indurated painless chancre, which heals in 7–10 days. A secondary eruption involving the skin and mucous membranes appears in 4–6 weeks. After a long latency period, late lesions of tertiary syphilis involve the eyes, skin, bones, viscera, CNS, and cardiovascular system.

Congenital syphilis results from transplacental infection. Infection may result in stillbirth or produce illness in the newborn, in early infancy, or later in childhood. Syphilis occurring in the newborn and young infant is comparable to secondary disease in the adult but is more severe and may be life threatening. Late congenital syphilis (developing in childhood) is comparable to tertiary disease.

The incidence of all forms of syphilis is increasing over the last decade in the United States, particularly among men who have sex with men. In 2021, there were over 2000 cases of congenital syphilis and approximately 176,000 total reported cases.

Prevention

A serologic test for syphilis should be performed at the initiation of prenatal care and should be repeated at 28 weeks gestation and at delivery in women at increased risk for syphilis. Adequate treatment of mothers with secondary syphilis before the last month of pregnancy reduces the incidence of congenital syphilis from 90% to less than 2%. Reducing the number of sexual partners and use of condoms can reduce transmission of syphilis, particularly among men who have sex with men.

Clinical Findings

A. Symptoms and Signs

1. Congenital syphilis

A. NEWBORNS—Most newborns with congenital syphilis are asymptomatic. If infection is not detected and treated, symptoms develop within weeks to months. When clinical signs are present, they usually consist of jaundice, anemia with or without thrombocytopenia, increase in nucleated red blood cells, hepatosplenomegaly, and edema. Overt signs of meningitis (bulging fontanelle or opisthotonos) may be present, but subclinical infection with CSF abnormalities is more common.

B. YOUNG INFANTS (3–12 WEEKS)—The infant may appear normal for the first few weeks of life only to develop mucocutaneous lesions and pseudoparalysis of the arms or legs. Shotty lymphadenopathy may be felt. Hepatomegaly is universal, with splenomegaly in 50% of patients. Other signs of

disease similar to those seen in the newborn may be present. Anemia can be the only presenting manifestation of congenital syphilis in this age group. "Snuffles" (syphilitic rhinitis), characterized by a profuse mucopurulent discharge, is present in 15%–25% of patients. A syphilitic rash is common on the palms and soles but may occur anywhere on the body. The rash consists of bright red, raised maculopapular lesions that gradually fade. Occasionally the rash is vesicular or bullous. Moist lesions occur at the mucocutaneous junctions (nose, mouth, anus, and genitals) and lead to fissuring and bleeding.

C. CHILDREN—Syphilis in later childhood may present with characteristic facial features such as rhagades (scars) around the mouth or nose, a depressed bridge of the nose (saddle nose), and a high forehead (secondary to mild hydrocephalus associated with low-grade meningitis and frontal periostitis). The permanent upper central incisors may be peg-shaped with a central notch (Hutchinson teeth), and the cusps of the sixth-year molars may have a lobulated mulberry appearance. Bilateral interstitial keratitis (at age 6–12 years) is characterized by photophobia, increased lacrimation, and vascularization of the cornea associated with exudation. Sensorineural hearing loss (at age 8–10 years), interstitial keratitis, and Hutchinson teeth comprise Hutchinson triad. Chorioretinitis and optic atrophy may also be seen. Meningovascular syphilis (at age 2–10 years) is usually slowly progressive, with intellectual disability, spasticity, abnormal pupillary response, speech defects, and abnormal CSF. Thickening of the periosteum of the anterior tibias produces saber shins. A bilateral effusion in the knee joints may occur but is not associated with sequelae. Soft inflammatory growths called gummas may develop in the nasal septum, palate, long bones, and subcutaneous tissues.

2. Acquired syphilis

The primary chancre of the genitals, mouth, or anus may occur from genital, anal, or oral sexual contact. If the chancre is missed, the first manifestations of secondary syphilis may be a disseminated pleomorphic rash which is prominent on palms and soles, fever, adenopathy, headache, and malaise, and hepatitis. Latent syphilis, by definition, lacks any clinical manifestations. Tertiary syphilis may manifest with multiple gummas, aortitis or central nervous system disease. Central nervous system infiltration including neurosyphilis, ocular syphilis, and otosyphilis can occur at any stage of syphilis.

B. Laboratory Findings

1. Darkfield microscopy

Treponemes can be seen in scrapings from a chancre and from moist lesions, but darkfield examinations are not often available.

2. Serologic tests for syphilis

There are two general types of serologic tests for syphilis: treponemal and nontreponemal. The two nontreponemal tests, Venereal Disease

Research Laboratory (VDRL), and the rapid plasma reagin (RPR), are useful for screening and may be quantitated to follow disease activity and adequacy of therapy. False-positive nontreponemal tests can occur in patient with measles, hepatitis, mononucleosis, lymphoma, TB, endocarditis, pregnancy, autoimmune diseases, and intravenous drug abuse. When evaluating a newborn for potential syphilis, umbilical cord blood specimens should not be used for nontreponemal tests: a false-positive test may result from Wharton jelly contamination of the sample. Conversely, a false-negative test may be seen in the setting where maternal infection occurred late in pregnancy.

Positive nontreponemal tests should be confirmed with a more specific treponemal test such as the fluorescent treponemal antibody absorbed (FTA-ABS) test or the *T pallidum* particle agglutination (TP-PA) test. False-positive FTA-ABS tests are uncommon except with other spirochetal diseases such as leptospirosis, rat bite fever, and Lyme disease.

One or two weeks after the onset of primary syphilis (chancre), the FTA-ABS test becomes positive. The nontreponemal tests usually turns positive a few days later. By the time the secondary stage has been reached, virtually all patients show both positive FTA-ABS and positive nontreponemal tests. During latent and tertiary syphilis, the VDRL may become negative, but the FTA-ABS test usually remains positive. The quantitative VDRL or RPR should be used to follow up treated cases (see following discussion).

Enzyme immunoassay (EIA) tests specific for *T pallidum* are available in many laboratories and are replacing FTA-ABS and TP-PA tests. As these are rapid, inexpensive tests with greater specificity, a "reverse" screening strategy is used by some laboratories. The initial screen is done with EIA test followed by the RPR or VDRL, if positive. If results are discordant, a third treponemal test such as the FTA-ABS or TP-PA may serve as a tie-breaker. If the second treponemal test is positive, this indicates either current syphilis infection or previously treated infection. If the second treponemal test is negative and the person is considered low risk, then it is reasonable to consider the initial EIA a false-positive result. In an individual at high risk for syphilis infection, consider repeating the tests in 2–4 weeks.

For evaluation of possible neurosyphilis, the CSF should be examined for cell count, glucose, protein, and a CSF VDRL. A negative CSF VDRL does not rule out neurosyphilis.

C. Imaging

Radiographic abnormalities are present in 90% of infants with symptoms of congenital syphilis and in 20% of asymptomatic infants. Metaphyseal lucent bands, periostitis, and a widened zone of provisional calcification may be present. Bilateral symmetrical osteomyelitis with pathologic fractures of the medial tibial metaphyses (Wimberger sign) is almost pathognomonic.

▶ Differential Diagnosis

A. Congenital Syphilis

1. Newborns—Sepsis, congestive heart failure, congenital rubella, toxoplasmosis, disseminated herpes simplex, cytomegalovirus infection, and hemolytic disease of the newborn have to be differentiated.

2. Young infants—Injury to the brachial plexus, poliomyelitis, acute osteomyelitis, and septic arthritis must be differentiated from pseudoparalysis.

3. Children—Interstitial keratitis and bone lesions of TB are distinguished by positive tuberculin reaction and chest radiograph. Arthritis associated with syphilis is unaccompanied by systemic signs, and joints are nontender. Mental retardation, spasticity, and hyperactivity due to syphilis is determined by strongly positive serologic tests.

B. Acquired Syphilis

Herpes genitalis, traumatic lesions, and other venereal diseases must be differentiated from primary chancres.

▶ Treatment

A. Specific Measures

Penicillin is the drug of choice for *T pallidum* infection. If the patient is allergic to penicillin, desensitization should be attempted, especially in neurosyphilis, congenital syphilis, syphilis during pregnancy, and with HIV infection. Azithromycin, ceftriaxone, or one of the tetracyclines are alternative agents but close monitoring to demonstrate clinical and laboratory improvement is essential for nonpenicillin regimens.

1. Congenital syphilis

A. INITIAL EVALUATION AND TREATMENT—Newborns should not be discharged from the hospital until the mother's serologic status for syphilis has been determined. Infants born to seropositive mothers require careful examination and quantitative nontreponemal syphilis testing. The same quantitative nontreponemal test used in evaluating the mother should be used in the infant so the titers can be compared. Maternal records regarding any prior diagnosis of syphilis, treatment, and follow-up titers should be reviewed. Infants should be further evaluated for congenital syphilis in any of the following circumstances:

- The infant's titer is at least fourfold greater than the maternal titer.
- Signs of syphilis are found on examination.
- Maternal syphilis was not treated, inadequately treated, treatment completed less than 4 weeks prior to delivery, treated with a nonpenicillin regimen during pregnancy or adequately treated but without the appropriate decrease in maternal nontreponemal titers after treatment.

The complete evaluation of an infant for possible congenital syphilis includes complete blood count, liver function tests, long bone radiographs, CSF examination (cell counts, glucose, and protein), CSF VDRL, and quantitative serologic tests. In addition, the placenta and umbilical cord, if available, should be examined pathologically using fluorescent treponemal antibody. If clinically indicated, ophthalmologic examination, auditory brainstem response, chest radiograph, and cranial ultrasound may be done.

Treatment for congenital syphilis is indicated for infants with consistent physical signs, umbilical cord or placenta positive by DFA-TP staining or darkfield examination, abnormal radiographs, elevated CSF protein or cell counts, reactive CSF VDRL, or serum quantitative nontreponemal titer that is more than fourfold higher than the maternal titer (using same test). Newborns with proven or highly probable congenital syphilis should receive (1) aqueous crystalline penicillin G, 50,000 U/kg per dose intravenously every 12 hours (if < 1 week old) or (2) every 8 hours (if 1–4 weeks old) for 10 days. Procaine penicillin G, 50,000 U/kg in a single daily intramuscular dose for 10 days is an alternative if compliance is ensured. All infants diagnosed after age 4 weeks should receive 50,000 U/kg per dose aqueous crystalline penicillin intravenously every 4–6 hours for 10 days.

Additionally, the same treatment should be given to infants whose mothers have inadequately treated syphilis, whose mothers received treatment less than 1 month before delivery, whose mothers have undocumented or inadequate serologic response to therapy, whose mother's partner was recently diagnosed with syphilis, and whose mothers were given nonpenicillin drugs to treat syphilis. If the infant is asymptomatic, has a normal physical examination, normal CSF parameters, nonreactive CSF VDRL, normal bone films, quantitative nontreponemal titer less than fourfold of the mother's titer, and good follow-up is certain, some experts would give a single dose of penicillin G benzathine, 50,000 U/kg intramuscularly. If there is any abnormality in the preceding evaluation or if the CSF testing is not interpretable, the full 10 days of intravenous penicillin should be given. Close clinical and serologic follow-up is necessary.

Asymptomatic, seropositive infants with normal physical examinations born to mothers who received adequate syphilis treatment (completed > 4 weeks prior to delivery) and whose mothers have an appropriate serologic response (fourfold or greater decrease in titer) to treatment may be at lower risk for congenital syphilis. Some experts believe complete laboratory and radiographic evaluation in these infants (CSF and long bone films) is not necessary. Infants who meet the preceding criteria, who have nontreponemal titers less than fourfold higher than maternal titers, and for whom follow-ups are certain can be given benzathine penicillin G, 50,000 U/kg intramuscularly in a single dose. Infants should be followed with quantitative serologic tests and physical examinations until the nontreponemal serologic test is negative. Rising titers or clinical signs require a full evaluation (including CSF studies and long bone radiographs) and institution of intravenous penicillin therapy, even if previously treated.

B. FOLLOW-UP FOR CONGENITAL SYPHILIS—Children treated for congenital syphilis need both physical examinations and quantitative VDRL or RPR tests performed every 2–3 months until the tests become nonreactive. Repeat CSF examination, including a CSF VDRL test every 6 months until normal, is indicated for infants with an initial positive CSF VDRL reaction or with abnormal cell counts or protein in the CSF. A reactive CSF VDRL test or abnormal CSF indices at the 6-month interval is an indication for retreatment. Serum titers decline with treatment and are usually negative by 6 months. Repeat treatment is indicated for children with rising titers or stable serum titers that do not decline. Children born to mothers with a reactive nontreponemal test but who themselves had a nonreactive nontreponemal test should still be retested at 3 months to rule out incubating syphilis.

2. Acquired syphilis of less than 1 year's duration—Benzathine penicillin G (50,000 U/kg, given intramuscularly, to a maximum of 2.4 million units) is given to adolescents with primary, secondary, or latent disease of less than 1 year's duration. All children with recently diagnosed or suspected syphilis should have a CSF examination (with CSF VDRL) prior to commencing therapy, to exclude neurosyphilis. Adolescents and adults need a CSF examination if clinical signs or symptoms suggest neurologic involvement or if they are HIV infected.

3. Syphilis of more than 1 year's duration (late latent disease)—Syphilis of more than 1 year's duration (without evidence of neurosyphilis) requires weekly intramuscular benzathine penicillin G therapy for 3 weeks. CSF examination and VDRL test should be done on all children and patients with coexisting HIV infection, or neurologic or ophthalmic symptoms, or evidence of active tertiary syphilis. In addition, patients who have failed treatment or who were previously treated with an agent other than penicillin need a CSF examination and CSF VDRL.

4. Neurosyphilis—Aqueous crystalline penicillin G is recommended, 50,000 U/kg/dose every 4 hours, given intravenously for 10–14 days. The maximum adult dose is 4 million units per dose. Some experts recommend following this regimen with an intramuscular course of benzathine G penicillin, 50,000 U/kg given once a week for 3 consecutive weeks, to a maximum dose of 2.4 million units.

B. General Measures

Penicillin treatment of early congenital, primary, or secondary syphilis may result in a dramatic systemic febrile illness termed the Jarisch-Herxheimer reaction. Treatment is symptomatic, with careful follow-up.

Prognosis

Severe disease, if undiagnosed, may be fatal in the newborn. Complete cure can be expected if the young infant is given penicillin. Serologic reversal usually occurs within 1 year. Treatment of primary syphilis with penicillin is curative. Permanent neurologic sequelae may occur in meningovascular syphilis.

Centers for Disease Control and Prevention: Sexually Transmitted Diseases: Syphilis https://www.cdc.gov/std/syphilis/default.htm. Accessed May 28, 2023.

Workowski KA et al: Sexually Transmitted Infections Treatment Guidelines, 2021. MMWR Recomm Rep. 2021 Jul 23;70(4):1–187. doi: 10.15585/mmwr.rr7004a1 [PMID: 34292926].

Syphilis. In: Kimberlin DW, Brady MT, Jackson MA, Long SS (eds): *Red Book: 2021–2024 Report of the Committee on Infectious Diseases.* 32nd ed. Itasca, IL: American Academy of Pediatrics; 2021:729–744.

RELAPSING FEVER

ESSENTIALS OF DIAGNOSIS & TYPICAL FEATURES

► Episodes of relapsing fever, chills, malaise.

► Occasional rash, arthritis, cough, hepatosplenomegaly, conjunctivitis.

► Diagnosis confirmed by direct microscopic identification of spirochetes in smears of peripheral blood.

General Considerations

Relapsing fever is a vector-borne disease caused by spirochetes of the genus *Borrelia*. There are two forms: Epidemic relapsing fever is transmitted to humans by body lice (*Pediculus humanus*) and endemic relapsing fever by soft-bodied ticks (genus *Ornithodoros*). Tick-borne relapsing fever, most commonly due to *Borrelia hermsii*, is endemic in the western United States, and infection is commonly associated with tick exposure in mountain cabins. Transmission usually takes place during the warm months, though winter cases occur in warmer climates and in cabins that have been heated. *Ornithodoros* (soft) ticks are nocturnal feeders and remain attached for only 5–20 minutes. Consequently, the patient seldom remembers a tick bite. As the adaptive immune system begins to produce antibodies, *B hermsii* uses genetic recombination to modify its surface antigens, resulting in relapse. Louse-borne relapsing fever, caused by *B recurrentis*, was a cause of significant mortality in the early 20th century and World War I and remains a major health problem among displaced and refugee populations. A recently described species, *B miyamotoi* found in a similar geographic distribution

as Lyme disease, causes a febrile illness that may be relapsing in some patients.

Clinical Findings

A. Symptoms and Signs

The incubation period is 2–18 days. The attack is sudden, with high fever, chills, sweats, tachycardia, nausea and vomiting, headache, myalgia, and arthralgia. Febrile episodes classically last 3 days and end abruptly and dramatically (chill phase, flush phase). If untreated, relapses typically occur at ~1-week intervals. The relapses duplicate the initial attack but become progressively less severe. In louse-borne relapsing fever, there is usually a single relapse, though more can occur (1–5). In tick-borne infection, 2–10 relapses occur.

Hepatomegaly, splenomegaly, pneumonitis, meningitis, and myocarditis may appear later in the course of the disease. An erythematous rash may be seen over the trunk and extremities, and petechiae may be present. Jaundice, iritis, conjunctivitis, and cranial nerve palsies occur more commonly during relapses.

In *B miyamotoi* infection, fever, headache, malaise, and arthralgias are common. Rash is rarely seen. Relapses have been described in a few cases, but this does not appear to be as consistent an observation as with *B hermsii*.

B. Laboratory Findings

During febrile episodes, the patient's urine contains protein, casts, and occasionally erythrocytes; a marked polymorphonuclear leukocytosis is present; about 25% of patients have a false-positive serologic test for syphilis. Spirochetes can be found in the peripheral blood by direct microscopy in approximately 70% of cases by darkfield examination or by Wright, Giemsa, or acridine orange staining of thick and thin smears (Figure 42–1). Spirochetes are not found during afebrile periods. Immunofluorescent antibody (or enzyme-linked immunosorbent assay [ELISA] confirmed by Western blot) can help establish the diagnosis serologically. However, high titers of *B hermsii* can cross-react with *Borrelia burgdorferi* (the agent in Lyme disease) or *Leptospira*. Serologic testing is available at laboratories in many western U.S. state health departments or through the CDC.

Differential Diagnosis

Relapsing fever may be confused with malaria, leptospirosis, dengue, typhus, rat-bite fever, Colorado tick fever, Rocky Mountain spotted fever, and collagen-vascular disease.

Complications

Complications include facial paralysis, iridocyclitis, optic atrophy, hypochromic anemia, pneumonia, nephritis, myocarditis, endocarditis, and seizures. CNS involvement occurs in 10%–30% of patients.

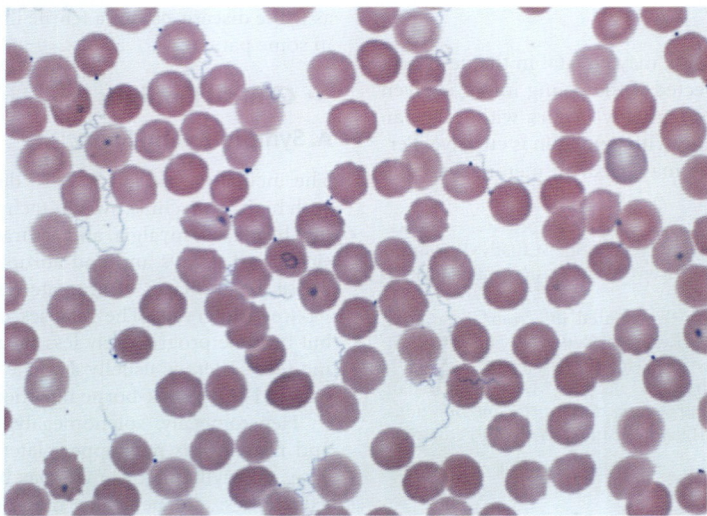

▲ **Figure 42–1.** Wright-stained peripheral blood smear showing spirochetes in a patient with relapsing fever (1000x magnification). Photo courtesy of Drs. Mark Lovell and Sarah Jung.

▶ Treatment

Doxycycline is the treatment of choice for children with tick-borne relapsing fever, regardless of age. Severe disease has also been successfully treated with initial use of IV ceftriaxone or IV penicillin G. Louse-borne relapsing fever is most commonly treated with tetracycline or erythromycin.

Severely ill patients should be hospitalized. Patients may experience a Jarisch-Herxheimer reaction (usually noted in the first few hours after commencing antibiotics).

▶ Prevention

Measures that decrease exposures to soft ticks and body lice will prevent most cases. Soft-bodied ticks often are found in rodent burrows or nests, so rodent (the tick reservoir host) control, particularly in mountain cabins, is important.

The mortality rate in treated cases of relapsing fever is very low, except in debilitated or very young children. With treatment, the initial attack is shortened and relapses are prevented.

Centers for Disease Control: Relapsing fever. http://www.cdc.gov/relapsing-fever/. Accessed May 15, 2023.

Cutler S et al: A new Borrelia on the block: Borrelia miyamotoi—a human health risk? Euro Surveill 2019 May 2;24(18):1800170. doi: 10.2807/1560-7917.ES.2019.24.18.1800170.

Warrell DA: Louse-borne relapsing fever (*Borrelia recurrentis* infection). Epidemiol Infect 2019 Jan;147:e106 [PMID: 30869050].

LEPTOSPIROSIS

 ESSENTIALS OF DIAGNOSIS & TYPICAL FEATURES

- ▶ Classic course is biphasic lasting 2–3 weeks.
- ▶ Initial phase: high fever, headache, myalgia, and conjunctivitis.
- ▶ Apparent recovery for 2–3 days.
- ▶ Return of fever associated with meningitis.
- ▶ Jaundice, hemorrhages, and renal insufficiency (severe cases).
- ▶ Rising titers, positive leptospiral agglutination assay.

▶ General Considerations

Leptospirosis is a zoonosis caused by many antigenically distinct, but morphologically similar, spirochetes. The organism enters through the abraded skin, eye, or respiratory tract after exposure to infectious animal urine or contaminated water or soil. A variety of animals (eg, dogs, rats, and cattle) may serve as reservoirs for pathogenic *Leptospira*, and severe disease may be caused by many different serogroups.

Leptospirosis occurs throughout the world and is endemic in tropical and subtropical climates. Leptospirosis is an important consideration in returning travelers with a febrile illness, particularly if there is a history of fresh-water exposure. In the United States, leptospirosis usually occurs after contact with infected dogs. Sewer workers, farmers, slaughterhouse workers, animal handlers, and soldiers are at risk for occupational exposure. The highest US rates of leptospirosis infection occur in Hawaii. Approximately one million case are reported worldwide annually; however, it is likely underreported given its nonspecific clinical symptoms and challenges in diagnosis.

Clinical Findings

A. Symptoms and Signs

Leptospirosis is classically defined by a biphasic illness with the initial manifestations associated with active disseminated spirochetal infection, and the second phase due to immune-mediated pathology.

1. Initial septic phase—The incubation period is typically 5–14 days. Patients present with nonspecific symptoms including: chills, fever, headache, myalgia (especially lumbar area and calves), photophobia, cervical lymphadenopathy, and pharyngitis. Conjunctival suffusion is often a pathognomonic symptom but does not occur in all patients. The initial leptospiremic phase lasts for 3–7 days.

2. Phase of apparent recovery—Symptoms typically (but not always) subside for 2–3 days.

3. Immune-mediated phase—Fever reappears and is associated with headache, muscular pain, tenderness in the abdomen and back, and nausea and vomiting. Conjunctivitis and uveitis are common. Lung, heart, and joint involvements occasionally occur. These manifestations are due to extensive vasculitis.

A. CNS INVOLVEMENT—The CNS is involved in 50%–90% of cases in the form of an aseptic meningitis.

B. RENAL AND HEPATIC INVOLVEMENT (WEIL SYNDROME)—In about 50% of cases, the kidneys or liver is affected. Gross hematuria and oliguria or anuria is sometimes seen. Jaundice may be associated with an enlarged and tender liver.

C. GALLBLADDER INVOLVEMENT—Leptospirosis may cause acalculous cholecystitis in children, demonstrable by abdominal ultrasound as a dilated, nonfunctioning gallbladder.

D. HEMORRHAGE—Petechiae, ecchymoses, and gastrointestinal bleeding may be severe.

E. RASH—A rash is seen in 10%–30% of cases. It may be maculopapular and generalized or may be petechial or purpuric. Erythema nodosum, peripheral desquamation, and gangrenous areas are sometimes reported.

B. Laboratory Findings

Leptospires are present in the blood and CSF only during the first 10 days of illness. They appear in the urine during the second week, where they may persist for 30 days or longer. Culture is difficult and requires specialized media and conditions but organisms can be identified by PCR of blood, CSF, or tissue. Elevated WBC, liver function tests, serum creatine kinase, and ESR may be seen. CSF shows moderate pleocytosis ($< 500/\mu L$), predominantly mononuclear cells, increased protein (50–100 mg/dL), and normal glucose. Urine often shows microscopic pyuria, hematuria, and, less often, moderate proteinuria (or greater).

Serum antibodies measured by enzyme immunoassay may be demonstrated during or after the second week of illness. The confirmatory test is a microscopic agglutination test performed at the CDC. Leptospiral agglutinins generally reach peak levels by the third to fourth week. Fourfold or greater titer rise in acute and convalescent specimens is diagnostic.

Differential Diagnosis

During the prodrome, malaria, typhoid fever, murine typhus, rheumatoid arthritis, brucellosis, and influenza may be suspected. Later, depending on the organ systems involved, a variety of other diseases need to be distinguished, including encephalitis, viral or tuberculous meningitis, viral hepatitis, glomerulonephritis, viral or bacterial pneumonia, rheumatic fever, subacute infective endocarditis, acute surgical abdomen, MIS-C, and Kawasaki disease (see Table 40–3).

Treatment

A. Specific Measures

Targeted and early treatment can help shorten duration of symptoms and improve outcomes for severe cases. Aqueous penicillin G intravenously for 7–10 days should be given when the diagnosis is suspected in severe cases. Alternative agents include parenteral ceftriaxone or doxycycline. A Jarisch-Herxheimer reaction may occur. Oral doxycycline may be used for mildly ill patients.

B. General Measures

Symptomatic and supportive care, in addition to antibiotics, is indicated. Renal failure may require dialysis.

Prevention

Preventive measures for endemic exposure include avoidance of contaminated water and soil—particularly with mucous membranes or nonintact skin, rodent control, immunization of dogs and other domestic animals, and avoidance of contact with animal urine.

Prognosis

There are usually no permanent sequelae associated with CNS infection, although headache may persist. The mortality rate is 5%–15% in severe illness.

Centers for Disease Control and Prevention: Leptospirosis. http://www.cdc.gov/leptospirosis/infection/index.html. Accessed May 19, 2023.

Haake DA et al: Leptospirosis in humans. Curr Top Microbiol Immunol 2015;387:65–97 [PMID: 25388133].

Leptospirosis. In: Kimberlin DW, Brady MT, Jackson MA, Long SS (eds): *Red Book: 2021–2024 Report of the Committee on Infectious Diseases*. 32nd ed. Elk Grove Village, IL: American Academy of Pediatrics; 2021;475–477.

Levett PN: Leptospirosis. Clin Microbiol Rev 2001;14(2):296–326 [PMID: 11292640].

LYME DISEASE

ESSENTIALS OF DIAGNOSIS & TYPICAL FEATURES

▶ Early localized disease: characteristic skin lesion (erythema migrans [EM]) 3–30 days after tick bite.

▶ Early disseminated: multiple EM, constitutional symptoms, cranial nerve palsies, meningitis.

▶ Late disease: arthritis, usually pauciarticular, occurring about 4 weeks after appearance of skin lesion.

▶ Residence or travel in an endemic area during the late spring to early fall.

▶ Positive serologic screening test with confirmatory immunoblot.

General Considerations

Lyme disease is a subacute or chronic spirochetal infection caused by *Borrelia burgdorferi* that is transmitted by an infected deer tick (*Ixodes* species). The most prominent endemic areas in the United States include the Northeast and upper Midwest. It is estimated that more than 450,000 cases per year occur in the United States. Knowledge of the local epidemiology is important as Lyme disease is common in certain areas of the United States, but very rare in others. Most cases with rash are recognized in spring and summer, when most tick bites occur; however, because the incubation period for joint and neurologic disease may be months, cases may present at any time. *Ixodes* ticks are very small, and their bite is often unrecognized.

Clinical Findings

A. Symptoms and Signs

1. Early localized disease: Erythema migrans (EM), the most characteristic feature of Lyme disease, is recognized in 60%–80% of patients. Between 3 and 30 days after the bite, a ring of erythema develops at the site and spreads over days. It may attain a diameter of 20 cm. The center of the lesion may clear, remain red, or become raised. Mild tenderness may occur. Most patients are otherwise asymptomatic, but mild constitutional symptoms may occur. Untreated, the rash lasts days to 3 weeks.

2. Early disseminated disease: Multiple satellite EM lesions, urticaria, or diffuse erythema may occur. Fever, headache, myalgias, and constitutional symptoms are more common than in localized disease. Neurologic manifestations, which develop in up to 20% of untreated patients, commonly include Bell palsy, aseptic meningitis, or polyradiculitis, alone or in various combinations. Peripheral neuritis, Guillain-Barré syndrome, encephalitis, ataxia, chorea, and other cranial neuropathies are less common. Seizures suggest another diagnosis. Untreated, the neurologic symptoms are usually self-limited but may be chronic or permanent. Self-limited heart block or myocardial dysfunction occurs in less than 5% of patients.

3. Late disease: In up to 50% of untreated patients, arthritis develops several weeks to months after the bite. Recurrent attacks of migratory, monoarticular, or pauciarticular arthritis involving the knees (90%) and other large joints occur. Fever is common and pain is often less pronounced than swelling. Each attack lasts for days to a few weeks. Complete resolution between attacks is typical. Chronic arthritis develops in less than 10% of patients, more often in those with the DR4 haplotype. Neurologic manifestations of late disease are uncommon.

Although fatigue and nonspecific neurologic symptoms may be prolonged in a few patients, Lyme disease is not a cause of chronic fatigue syndrome. Persistence of symptoms of fatigue, myalgia, and arthralgia for greater than 6 months are termed posttreatment Lyme disease syndrome, but there is no evidence that chronic Lyme infection exists, nor is there any evidence of benefit from antibiotic therapy in patients properly treated for Lyme disease.

B. Laboratory Findings

Most patients with only rash have normal laboratory tests. Children with arthritis may have moderately elevated ESRs and WBC counts. Joint fluid may show up to 100,000 cells with a polymorphonuclear predominance, normal glucose, and elevated protein and immune complexes; Gram stain and culture are negative. In patients with CNS involvement, the CSF may show lymphocytic pleocytosis and elevated protein; cultures and stains are negative. Papilledema may be present on fundoscopic examination. Abnormal nerve conduction may be present with peripheral neuropathy. Electrocardiogram (ECG) may show carditis in early disseminated disease.

C. Diagnosis

Local epidemiology, history of travel to endemic areas, physical examination, and laboratory features are important to consider. Serologic diagnosis of Lyme disease is based on a two-test approach: an antibody screen (IgM and/or IgG) with an immunoblot to confirm a positive or indeterminate screening test. Antibodies may not be detectable until several weeks after infection has occurred; therefore, serologic testing in children with a typical acute EM rash is not recommended; treatment is recommended based on clinical diagnosis. Therapy early in disease may blunt antibody titers. Serologic testing of patients with nonspecific complaints from low prevalence areas may result in falsely positive tests, particularly when ordered through "Lyme specialty" labs. Sera from patients with syphilis, HIV, and leptospirosis may give false-positive results. Diagnosis of CNS disease requires objective abnormalities of the neurologic examination, laboratory or radiographic studies, and consistent positive serology.

▶ Differential Diagnosis

EM rash may resemble pityriasis, erythema multiforme, a drug eruption, or erythema nodosum. Southern tick-associated rash illness (STARI) is an uncommon condition associated with a bite from the lone-star tick (*Amblyomma americanum*), which can result in a rash and clinical syndrome indistinguishable from acute Lyme infection. Lyme cases with more severe manifestations (especially hematologic or hepatic abnormalities) or those that persist after appropriate treatment may represent co-infection with Anaplasma, Babesia or *Borrelia miyamotoi*. The arthritis may resemble juvenile rheumatoid arthritis, reactive arthritis, septic arthritis, rheumatic fever, poststreptococcal arthritis/acute rheumatic fever, systemic lupus erythematosus, and Henoch-Schönlein purpura. The neurologic signs may suggest idiopathic Bell palsy, viral or parainfectious meningitis or meningoencephalitis, lead poisoning, and psychosomatic illness.

▶ Treatment

Antimicrobial therapy is beneficial in most cases of Lyme disease. It is most effective if started early. Prolonged treatment is important for all forms. Relapses occur in some patients on all regimens.

A. Rash, Early Infections

Doxycycline for 10 days or amoxicillin for 14 days are the currently recommended treatments (weight-based dosing).

Azithromycin or cefuroxime are used in children who cannot tolerate doxycycline or amoxicillin.

B. Arthritis

The amoxicillin or doxycycline regimen (same dosage as for the rash) should be used, but treatment should continue for 4 weeks. Parenteral ceftriaxone is used for recurrent arthritis.

C. Bell Palsy

Doxycycline for 2 weeks is preferred.

D. Other Neurologic Disease or Cardiac Disease

Parenteral therapy with 14 days of ceftriaxone was traditionally used for meningitis, but recent evidence demonstrates that doxycycline orally for the same duration is equally effective. Both ceftriaxone and oral doxycycline are effective for Lyme carditis.

▶ Prevention

Prevention consists of avoidance of endemic areas or if in these areas wearing long sleeves and pants, frequent checks for ticks, and application of tick repellents. Ticks are attached for a minimum of 36–48 hours before transmission of Lyme disease occurs. Ticks should be removed with a tweezer by pulling gently without twisting or excessive squeezing of the tick. Permethrin sprayed on clothing decreases tick attachment. Repellents containing high concentrations of N,N-Diethyl-meta-toluamide (DEET) are also effective. Prophylactic antibiotics may be effective for tick bites in areas of high endemicity when the tick can be identified as *Ixodes scapularis*, has been attached for more than 36 hours (based on exposure or tick engorgement), and prophylaxis can be started within 72 hours of tick removal. There is no current Lyme vaccine.

Centers for Disease Control and Prevention (CDC): Lyme disease. http://www.cdc.gov/lyme/. Accessed May 19, 2023.

Halperin JJ: Chronic Lyme disease: misconceptions and challenges for patient management. Infect Drug Resist 2015 May 15;8:119–128 [PMID: 26028977].

Lopez SMC, Campfield BT, Nowalk AJ: Oral management for pediatric Lyme meningitis. J Pediatric Infect Dis Soc 2019 Jul 1;8(3):272–275 [PMID: 30169816].

Lyme Disease (Lyme Borreliosis, Borrelia burgdorferi sensu lato Infection). In: Kimberlin DW, Brady MT, Jackson MA, Long SS (eds): *Red Book: 2021–2024 Report of the Committee on Infectious Diseases*. 32nd ed. Elk Grove Village, IL: American Academy of Pediatrics; 2021;482–489.

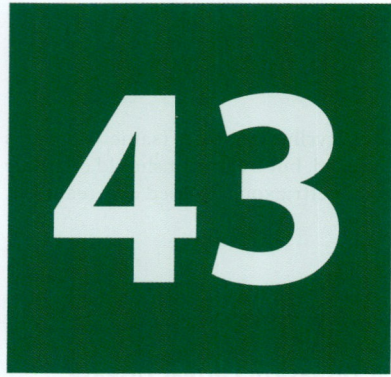

Infections: Parasitic & Mycotic

James Gaensbauer, MD, MScPH

Monika Jelic, MD

Juri Boguniewicz, MD

PARASITIC INFECTIONS

The parasites that cause human disease represent a diverse, highly evolved, and complex group of organisms. Parasitic diseases are a major cause of global pediatric morbidity and mortality, with the heaviest disease burden occurring in low- and middle-income countries. Though less common in industrialized nations, parasites represent an important class of pathogens to recognize, as both endemic and imported cases are frequently encountered in pediatric practice. Given the complexity of this category of pathogens, a framework to organize human parasites according to their major biologic classification and predominant site (intestinal vs blood/tissue) of human interaction can be useful (Table 43–1). Additionally, understanding which parasitic organisms are associated with specific clinical presentations can help focus the diagnostic process (Table 43–2).

Selection of Patients for Evaluation

The incidence of parasitic infections varies greatly with geographic area. Children who have traveled or lived in areas where parasitic infections are endemic are at risk for infection with a variety of intestinal and tissue parasites. Children who have resided only in developed countries are usually free of tissue parasites (with few exceptions, eg, *Toxocara*, *Toxoplasma*). Searching for intestinal parasites is expensive for the patient and time-consuming for the laboratory; more than 90% of ova and parasite (O&P) examinations performed in the United States are negative. A frequent misperception is that intestinal helminths are common causes of diarrhea; with rare exception (eg, Trichuris dysentery syndrome) they are not. Parasitic diarrhea is almost exclusively caused by protozoa (*Giardia, Cryptosporidium, Entamoeba*) that are now commonly diagnosed with molecular methods. Moreover, it may also be cost-effective to empirically treat symptomatic US immigrants with albendazole for common intestinal parasites and to investigate only those whose symptoms persist.

Immunodeficient children are very susceptible to protozoal intestinal infections and multiple opportunistic pathogens are often identified. Thus, the threshold for evaluation should be low for these children.

Specimen Processing

Many laboratories now use polymerase chain reaction (PCR)–based diagnostic assays for stool pathogens that have fewer specimen handling challenges. Practitioners should contact the laboratory for proper collection procedures for diagnostic testing that requires microscopy and/or a fresh sample to visualize viable parasites. Many laboratories will reject formed stool samples submitted to detect parasites as the etiology of a diarrheal illness. The US Centers for Disease Control and Prevention (CDC) provides an online resource (http://dpd.cdc.gov/dpdx) to assist in the laboratory diagnosis of common parasitic diseases, including specimen collection and processing.

Eosinophilia & Parasitic Infections

Although certain parasites commonly cause eosinophilia, in high-income countries other causes are much more common. These include allergies, drugs, and other infections. Nor do all parasitic infections result in eosinophilia. Eosinophilia due to parasitic infection is most common when multicellular organisms are migrating through host tissues (eg, lymphatic filariasis, hookworm). The unicellular protozoa (eg, malaria, leishmaniasis) rarely cause eosinophilia, even when infection is severe or invasive (eg, amebic liver abscess). Likewise, eosinophilia is uncommon with parasites residing exclusively in the lumen of the intestinal tract.

The most common parasitic infection in the United States that causes significant eosinophilia with negative stool examination is toxocariasis. Trichinosis, which is a rare parasitic infection in the United States, causes marked eosinophilia. Strongyloidiasis is a cause of eosinophilia that may be difficult to diagnose with stool examinations. The differential

Table 43–1. Framework for conceptualization of human parasitic infections and examples of representative organisms.[a]

Parasite Class	Prominent Site of Involvement	
	Intestinal	Tissue/Blood
Protozoa	*Entamoeba* *Giardia* *Cryptosporidium*	Malaria *Leishmania* *Naegleria* *Toxoplasma*
Platyhelminthes (flatworms)		
Cestodes (tapeworms)	*Taenia* (ingested larvae) *Diphyllobothrium*	*Taenia*/cysticercosis (ingested eggs) *Echinococcus*
Trematodes (flukes)		*Schistosoma* *Fasciola* *Clonorchis*
Nematodes (roundworms)	*Ascaris* Hookworms *Strongyloides* *Trichuris*	*Trichinella* *Dracunculus* *Angiostrongylus* *Filaria*

[a]Not all organisms listed are described in the chapter.

diagnosis of eosinophilia is broad for patients who have been in developing countries (see Table 43–2).

Centers for Disease Control and Prevention: DPDx—Laboratory Identification of Parasites of Public Health Concern: https://www.cdc.gov/dpdx/index.html. Accessed April 10, 2023.

Pisarki K: The global burden of disease of zoonotic parasitic diseases: top 5 contenders for priority consideration. Trop Med Infect Dis 2019 Mar;4(1):44. doi:10.3390/tropicalmed4010044 [PMID: 30832380].

PROTOZOAL INFECTIONS

SYSTEMIC INFECTIONS

1. Malaria

ESSENTIALS OF DIAGNOSIS & TYPICAL FEATURES

▶ Residence in or travel to an endemic area (fever in the returning traveler).

▶ Paroxysms of fever, chills, and intense sweating.

▶ Headache, myalgias, cough, abdominal pain, nausea, vomiting, and diarrhea.

▶ Splenomegaly, anemia.

▶ Can progress to coma, seizures.

▶ Malaria parasites in peripheral blood smear.

▶ General Considerations

Malaria causes more than 500,000 deaths each year, over 75% of which occur in children younger than 5 years of age. Global efforts toward malaria prevention and treatment have led to declining mortality and morbidity. Approximately 2000 imported cases are diagnosed in the United States each year. Human malaria is caused by five *Plasmodium* species—*vivax* (most common), *falciparum* (most virulent), *ovale* (similar to *P vivax*), *malariae*, and *knowlesi* (a primate parasite that causes a cause falciparum-like malaria in humans).

The female *Anopheles* mosquito transmits the parasite. Infected mosquitoes inoculate sporozoites into the bloodstream of a susceptible host, resulting in infection of hepatocytes. In the hepatic phase, the sporozoites mature into schizonts, which rupture and release merozoites into the circulation. These infect and rupture red blood cells (RBCs) in the erythrocytic phase, as they mature from trophozoites to schizonts and release additional merozoites. In early stages of infection, asynchronous cycles of erythrocyte hemolysis commonly cause daily fevers. Eventually if untreated, synchronous cycles of hemolysis occur when parasites rupture infected erythrocytes at more regular 48- or 72-hour intervals, depending on the infecting species. A small percentage of trophozoites mature into the sexual form (gametocytes) that are taken up in a mosquito blood-meal, thus completing the cycle. Two species, *P vivax* and *P ovale*, can remain dormant in liver cells (hypnozoites) leading to recrudescence, months and even years after the acute infection.

Disease severity in malaria is closely linked with prior immunity. Thus, in areas where transmission is stable and frequent, older children and adults will generally develop milder illness with infection, though complete protective immunity rarely occurs. On the other hand, younger children, persons without prior exposure (eg, foreign travelers), or individuals living in areas where transmission is intermittent are at increased risk of severe disease. Additionally, young children, pregnant women, and persons with certain immune dysfunctions (eg, asplenia) are at higher risk of severe disease regardless of prior exposure.

▶ Clinical Findings

A. Symptoms and Signs

Clinical manifestations vary according to infecting species and host immunity. The most common manifestations of acute malaria in children include fever, chills, malaise, body aches, and headache. Nausea, vomiting, and abdominal pain are common. Infants commonly present with recurrent fever,

Table 43–2. Signs and symptoms of parasitic infection.

Sign/Symptom	Agent[a]	Comments[b]
Abdominal pain	*Anisakis*	Shortly after raw fish ingestion.
	Ascaris	Heavy infection may obstruct bowel, biliary tract.
	Clonorchis	Heavy, early infection. Hepatomegaly later.
	Entamoeba histolytica	Hematochezia, variable fever, diarrhea.
	Fasciola hepatica	Diarrhea, vomiting.
	Hookworm	Iron deficiency anemia with heavy infection.
	Strongyloides	Eosinophilia, pruritus. May resemble peptic disease.
	Trichinella	Myalgia, periorbital edema, eosinophilia.
	Trichuris	Diarrhea, dysentery with heavy infection.
Cough	*Ascaris*	Wheezing, eosinophilia during migration phase.
	Paragonimus westermani	Hemoptysis; chronic. May mimic tuberculosis.
	Strongyloides	Wheezing, pruritus, eosinophilia during migration or dissemination.
	Toxocara	Affects ages 1–5 y; hepatosplenomegaly; eosinophilia.
	Tropical eosinophilia	Pulmonary infiltrates, eosinophilia.
Diarrhea	*Blastocystis*	Unclear significance as a diarrheal pathogen, immunodeficiency may be a risk factor.
	Cyclospora	Watery; severe in immunosuppressed individuals.
	Cryptosporidium	Watery; chronic in immunosuppressed individuals.
	Dientamoeba fragilis	Only with heavy infection.
	E histolytica	Hematochezia, variable fever; no eosinophilia.
	Giardia	Afebrile, chronic; anorexia.
	Schistosoma	Chronic; hepatosplenomegaly (some types).
	Strongyloides	Abdominal pain; eosinophilia.
	Trichinella	Myalgia, periorbital edema, eosinophilia.
	Trichuris	With heavy infection.
Dysentery	*Balantidium coli*	Swine contact.
	E histolytica	Few to no leukocytes in stool; fever; hematochezia.
	Schistosoma	During acute infection.
	Trichuris	With heavy infection.
Dysuria	*Enterobius*	Usually girls with worms in urethra, bladder; nocturnal, perianal pruritus.
	Schistosoma (*S haematobium*)	Hematuria. Exclude bacteriuria, stones (some types).
Headache (and other cerebral symptoms)	*Angiostrongylus*	Eosinophilic meningitis.
	Baylisascaris procyonis	Eosinophilic meningitis.
	Gnathostoma	Eosinophilic meningitis.
	Naegleria	Freshwater swimming; rapidly progressive meningoencephalitis.
	Plasmodium	Fever, chills, jaundice, splenomegaly. Cerebral ischemia (with *P falciparum*).
	Taenia solium	Cysticercosis. Focal seizures, deficits; hydrocephalus, aseptic meningitis.
	Toxoplasma	Meningoencephalitis (especially in infants and the immunosuppressed); focal lesions in immunosuppressed; hydrocephalus in infants.
	Trypanosoma	African forms. Chronic lethargy (sleeping sickness).
Pruritus	*Ancylostoma braziliense*	Creeping eruption; dermal serpiginous burrow.
	Enterobius	Perianal, nocturnal.
	Filaria	Variable; seen in many filarial diseases; eosinophilia.
	Hookworm	Local at penetration site in heavy exposure.
	Strongyloides	Diffuse with migration; may be recurrent.
	Trypanosoma	African forms; one of many nonspecific symptoms.
Rash	Hookworm	Pruritic, papulovesicular rash at site of penetration.
	Schistosoma	Maculopapular rash at site of penetration.
	Strongyloides	Pruritic rash at site of penetration.
	Toxoplasma	Maculopapular rash seen with congenital and sometimes acquired infection.

(Continued)

Table 43–2. Signs and symptoms of parasitic infection. (*Continued*)

Sign/Symptom	Agent[a]	Comments[b]
Anemia	*Diphyllobothrium* Hookworm *Leishmania donovani* *Plasmodium* *Trichuris*	Megaloblastic due to vitamin B_{12} deficiency; rare. Iron deficiency. Fever, hepatosplenomegaly, leukopenia (kala-azar). Hemolysis. Heavy infection; due to iron loss.
Eosinophilia	*Angiostrongylus* *Baylisascaris procyonis* *Fasciola* *Gnathostoma* *Filaria* *Onchocerca* *Schistosoma* *Strongyloides* *Toxocara* *Trichinella* *T solium* (cysticercosis)	Eosinophilic meningitis. Eosinophilic meningitis. Abdominal pain. Eosinophilic meningitis. Microfilariae in blood; lymphadenopathy; tropical pulmonary eosinophilia (cough, wheezing, weight loss) Skin nodules, keratitis. Chronic; intestinal or genitourinary symptoms. Abdominal pain, diarrhea. Hepatosplenomegaly, cough; affects ages 1–5 y. Myalgia, periorbital edema. Eosinophils in CSF.
Hematuria	*Schistosoma*	*S haematobium*. Bladder, urethral granulomas. Exclude stones.
Hemoptysis	*P westermani*	Lung fluke. Variable chest pain; chronic.
Hepatomegaly	*Clonorchis* *Echinococcus* *E histolytica* *L donovani* *Schistosoma* (not *haematobium*) *Toxocara*	Heavy infection. Tenderness early; cirrhosis late. Chronic; cysts. Toxic hepatitis or abscess. No eosinophilia. Splenomegaly, fever, pancytopenia. Chronic; hepatic fibrosis, splenomegaly (some types). Splenomegaly, eosinophilia, cough; no adenopathy.
Splenomegaly	*L donovani* *Plasmodium* *Schistosoma* (not *haematobium*) *Toxocara* *Toxoplasma*	Hepatomegaly, fever, anemia. Fever, chills, jaundice, headache. Hepatomegaly. Eosinophilia, hepatomegaly. Lymphadenopathy, other symptoms.
Lymphadenopathy	*Filaria* *L donovani* *Schistosoma* *Toxoplasma* *Trypanosoma*	Inguinal typical; chronic. Hepatosplenomegaly, pancytopenia, fever. Acute infection; fever, rash, arthralgia, hepatosplenomegaly. Cervical common; may involve single group of nodes; splenomegaly. Localized near bite or generalized; hepatosplenomegaly (Chagas disease); generalized (especially posterior cervical) in African forms.

[a]Not all organisms listed are described in the chapter.
[b]Symptoms usually related to degree of infestation. Infestation with small numbers of organisms is often asymptomatic.

irritability, poor feeding, vomiting, jaundice, and splenomegaly. Rash is usually absent, which helps distinguish malaria from some viral infections in patients presenting with similar symptoms. In the classic descriptions of malaria, cyclic patterns of fever specific to the infecting species were noted. These patterns can take many days to develop, are affected by numerous factors including prior immunity, multiple species infection and treatment, and are rarely useful diagnostically in current practice.

The clinician must be vigilant in monitoring patients with malaria for signs and symptoms of complicated or severe infection, including severe anemia and cerebral malaria, described later.

Infection during pregnancy often causes intrauterine growth restriction or premature delivery and can result in spontaneous abortion and stillbirth, but rarely true fetal infection.

Physical examination in patients with uncomplicated cases may show only mild splenomegaly and mild pallor.

B. Laboratory Findings

Because the manifestations of malaria overlap with a number of other common conditions, the diagnosis should always be confirmed with laboratory testing. The diagnosis relies on detection of one or more of the five human plasmodia in thick and thin blood smears. Three separate sets of thick and thin smears separated by 12–24 hours in a 72-hour period are recommended to rule out malaria infection. Thick smears are most sensitive for detection of small numbers of malaria parasites; thin smears allow identification of species and semiquantitative determination of percentage of parasitemia.

Most acute infections are caused by *P vivax*, *P ovale*, or *P falciparum*, although 5%–7% are due to multiple species. Identification of the *Plasmodium* species relies on morphologic criteria and requires an experienced observer. Bench aids to assist in the identification of *Plasmodium* species can be found at https://www.cdc.gov/dpdx/Malaria/index.html. A US Food and Drug Administration (FDA)–approved antigen detection test is available and approved for rapid diagnostic testing of malaria. This test should be used in conjunction with microscopic examination to confirm diagnosis, look for mixed infection, and quantitate degree of parasitemia. The rapid antigen test has poor sensitivity for low levels of parasitemia. Up-to-date information on rapid diagnostic testing for malaria can be found athttps://www.cdc.gov/malaria/diagnosis_treatment/diagnosis.html. Alternative techniques of similar or higher diagnostic accuracy for *P falciparum* include DNA hybridization and PCR, which are only available in research and reference laboratories and at CDC and some health departments.

Determining the degree of parasitemia (% of visualized erythrocytes that are infected) from thin smears is important because high levels (> 5%), most often seen in *P falciparum* malaria, are associated with increased morbidity and mortality and require hospitalization. Measurement over time (12–24 hours) can also be used to monitor treatment responses; the parasite burden should decrease during the first 24–48 hours of therapy.

Hemolytic anemia and thrombocytopenia are common; the incidence of leukocytosis is variable. In severe cases, metabolic acidosis, hypoglycemia, and azotemia may occur. The pathogenesis of cerebral malaria is microvascular obstruction. Cerebrospinal fluid (CSF) analysis is typically normal.

▶ Differential Diagnosis

Clinical features may not reliably distinguish malaria from other infections in children, so a high index of suspicion in patients with exposure in endemic areas is necessary. The differential diagnosis of fever in a returning traveler should be based on diseases endemic to the region of travel (see Chapter 45; Travel Medicine). Autochthonous infections such as respiratory viral infections should also be considered. Though CSF is typically normal in cerebral malaria, any child with suspected cerebral malaria should undergo lumbar puncture to exclude bacterial meningitis.

▶ Complications & Sequelae

Severe complications, which occur most often in *P falciparum* and *P knowlesi* infection, result from hemolysis, microvascular obstruction, and tissue ischemia. The most common complications of malaria in children are cerebral malaria, respiratory distress, severe anemia, and/or hypoglycemia. Cerebral malaria, which is the most serious and life-threatening complication in children, may progress to seizures, coma, and death. Approximately 20% of children with cerebral malaria die and 10% have long-term neurologic sequelae. Signs of severe malaria in children include altered mental status, seizures, respiratory distress, hypoglycemia, acidosis, end-organ failure, extreme pallor, and parasitemia greater than 5%.

▶ Prevention

There are many strategies to prevent malaria transmission in a community. The most effective is the widespread use of bed nets impregnated with long-acting insecticide, as the majority of *Anopheles* bites occur from dusk to dawn. Mosquito larva control and indoor insecticide spraying are also widespread.

Strategies for personal protection against malaria (particularly for travelers to endemic areas) include the use of bed nets, proper clothing, insect repellent, and malaria chemoprophylaxis. Chemoprophylaxis is discussed in detail in Chapter 45. No drug regimen guarantees protection against malaria. If fever develops within 1 year (particularly within 3 months) after travel to an endemic area, the possibility of malaria should be considered.

In the past several years, significant progress has been made in the development of an effective malaria vaccine. The World Health Organization (WHO) approved a recombinant protein vaccine (RTS,S) against *P falciparum* in October 2021 for children in Sub-Sahara Africa and other endemic areas with high transmission. There has also been interest in using monoclonal antibodies to provide immune protection against malaria, especially in those unable to mount an immune response to vaccination.

▶ Treatment

Choice of antimalarial treatment depends on the immune status of the person, plasmodium species, degree of parasitemia, and resistance patterns in the geographical region of acquisition. A description of the recommended antimalarial drugs available in the United States with updated treatment guidelines is available at https://www.cdc.gov/malaria/diagnosis_treatment/treatment.html. Atovaquone/proguanil and the artemisinin combination artemether/lumefantrine are first-line therapies for uncomplicated malaria. For severe malaria, intravenous artesunate is the preferred treatment but must always be followed by an oral combination drug when the patient improves in order to prevent resistance;

quinidine has been taken off the market in the United States. In 2020, the US FDA approved IV artesunate for the treatment of severe malaria in children. Common treatments for infections with *P vivax* and *P ovale* include chloroquine plus either primaquine or tafenoquine, which can eradicate liver stage malaria with a single dose. The CDC provides 24-hour telephone malaria hotline consultation for providers at (770) 488-7788. In cases in which IV artesunate delivery may be delayed more than a few hours, clinicians may consider initiating treatment with an oral drug (eg, artemether-lumefantrine) if the patient can tolerate it.

Treatment for malaria includes a variety of supportive strategies in addition to the antimalarial drugs. In the United States, it is most common to hospitalize nonimmune pediatric patients infected with *P falciparum* and *P knowlesi* until a decrease in parasitemia is demonstrated, indicating that treatment is effective and severe complications are unlikely to occur. Patients with signs of severe malaria (parasitemia > 5%, cerebral malaria, acidosis, hypoglycemia, shock) require intensive care and parenteral treatment. Hydration and treatment of hypoglycemia are of utmost importance. Anemia, seizures, pulmonary edema, and renal failure require conventional supportive management. Corticosteroids are contraindicated for cerebral malaria because of increased mortality. Exchange transfusion is no longer recommended for the treatment of severe malaria.

Partially immune patients with uncomplicated *P falciparum* and *P knowlesi* infection and nonimmune persons infected with *P vivax*, *P ovale*, or *P malariae* can receive outpatient treatment if follow-up is reliable.

Centers for Disease Control and Prevention: *CDC Yellow Book 2020:* Health Information for International Travel. New York: Oxford University Press; 2020. https://wwwnc.cdc.gov/travel/page/yellowbook-home. Accessed April 18, 2023.

Centers for Disease Control and Prevention. DPDx Malaria. https://www.cdc.gov/dpdx/malaria/index.html. Accessed April 7, 2023.

Chandramohan D et al: Seasonal malaria vaccination with or without seasonal malaria chemoprevention. N Engl J Med 2021;385:1005–1017. doi:10.1056/NEJMoa2026330 [PMID: 34432975].

Esu EB et al: Intermittent preventive treatment for malaria in infants. Cochrane Database Syst Rev 2021;(7). doi:10.1002/14651858.CD011525 [PMID: 34273901].

2. Babesiosis

Babesia microti (most common in the United States), *Babesia divergens* and *Babesia duncani* are malaria-like protozoa that infect humans bitten by infected nymphal-stage *Ixodes scapularis* (deer tick). After inoculation, the protozoa penetrate erythrocytes and start an asynchronous cycle that causes hemolysis. In the United States, the majority of cases occur in the Northeast and upper Midwest from May to October. Babesiosis can also be transmitted via blood transfusions and organ transplantation.

▶ **Clinical Findings**

A. Symptoms and Signs

The incubation period is 1–4 weeks after tick bite or 1–9 weeks after blood transfusion. The tick bite may go unnoticed as *Ixodes* nymphs are about the size of a poppy seed. Approximately half of infected children are asymptomatic. Symptoms are nonspecific and most commonly include sustained or cyclic high fever, rigors, and sweats. Physical examination findings are usually minimal but may include hepatosplenomegaly and jaundice. The disease is usually self-limited, causing symptoms for 1–2 weeks with fatigue that may persist for months. Severe cases have been described in asplenic patients, immunocompromised hosts, and elderly patients with comorbidities. Because *Babesia*, *Borrelia burgdorferi*, and *Anaplasma phagocytophilum* share a common vector, physicians should consider the possibility of coinfection in patients diagnosed with any of these pathogens. As many as 50% of babesiosis cases may have *B burgdorferi* (Lyme) coinfection.

B. Laboratory Findings

Anemia, thrombocytopenia, and evidence of intravascular hemolysis. Definitive diagnosis is made by identifying parasites in blood by microscopic evaluation of thin or thick blood smears or by PCR amplification of DNA in blood samples. *Babesia* parasites are intraerythrocytic organisms that resemble *P falciparum* ring forms. The tetrad form, if visualized, is pathognomonic. Specific serologic tests are also available through the CDC, although a single serology does not discriminate current from past infection.

▶ **Treatment**

Azithromycin (10 mg/kg up to 500 mg on the first day, followed by 5 mg/kg up to 250 mg/day) in combination with atovaquone (20 mg/kg, up to 750 mg, twice a day) for 7–10 days is the treatment of choice for mild-to-moderate disease. For severely ill patients, clindamycin (10 mg/kg, up to 600 mg, every 8 hours) in combination with quinine (8 mg/kg, up to 650 mg, every 8 hours) is standard of care. Longer courses of treatment may be needed in immunocompromised patients. Partial or complete RBC exchange transfusion is indicated for persons with severe babesiosis, as indicated by high-grade parasitemia (≥ 10%); significant hemolysis; or renal, hepatic, or pulmonary compromise.

Centers for Disease Control and Prevention. Parasites—Babesiosis. https://www.cdc.gov/parasites/babesiosis/index.html. Accessed April 7, 2023.

Krause PJ et al: Clinical practice guidelines by the Infectious Diseases Society of America (IDSA): 2020 Guideline on diagnosis and management of babesiosis. Clin Infect Dis 2020;72(2):e49–e64. doi:10.1093/cid/ciaa1216 [PMID: 33252652].

3. Toxoplasmosis

▶ General Considerations

T gondii is a worldwide parasite of animals and birds. Felines, the definitive hosts, excrete oocysts in their feces. Ingested mature oocysts or tissue cysts lead to tachyzoite invasion of intestinal cells. Intracellular replication of the tachyzoites causes cell lysis and spread of the infection to adjacent cells or to other tissues via the bloodstream. In chronic infection, *T gondii* appears as bradyzoite-containing tissue cysts that do not trigger an inflammatory reaction. In immunocompromised hosts, tachyzoites are released from cysts and begin a new cycle of infection.

The two major routes of *Toxoplasma* transmission to humans are oral and congenital. Oral infection occurs after ingestion of cysts from food, water, or soil contaminated with cat feces or from ingestion of undercooked meat or other food products that contain cysts. Oocysts survive up to 18 months in moist soil but survival is limited in dry, very cold, or very hot conditions and at high altitude, which probably accounts for the lower incidence of toxoplasmosis in these regions. In the United States, less than 1% of cattle and 25% of sheep and pigs are infected with toxoplasmosis. In humans, depending on geographic area, seropositivity increases with age from 0% to 10% in children younger than 10 years to 3%–70% in adults.

Congenital transmission occurs during acute infection of pregnant women. Rarely, fetal infection has been documented in immunocompromised mothers with reactivation of latent toxoplasmosis. Treatment during pregnancy decreases transmission by 60%.

▶ Clinical Findings

Clinical toxoplasmosis can be divided into four groups: (1) congenital infection, (2) infection acquired in the immunocompetent host, (3) infection acquired or reactivated in the immunocompromised host, and (4) ocular disease.

A. Congenital Toxoplasmosis

Congenital toxoplasmosis is discussed in further detail in Chapter 2.

B. Acquired *Toxoplasma* Infection in the Immunocompetent Host

Typically, acquired infection in the immunocompetent host is asymptomatic. About 10%–20% of patients develop an infectious mononucleosis-like syndrome with non-suppurative lymphadenopathy and/or a flu-like illness. Recovery typically occurs without any specific antiparasitic treatment, although lymph node enlargement may persist or wax and wane for a few months to 1 or more years.

C. Acute Toxoplasmosis in the Immunocompromised Host

Patients infected with human immunodeficiency virus (HIV), and those with lymphoma, leukemia, or transplantation, are at high risk for developing severe disease (most commonly CNS disease, but also chorioretinitis, myocarditis, or pneumonitis) following acute infection or reactivation. *Toxoplasma* encephalitis is a common cause of mass lesions in the brain in those living with untreated HIV/AIDS.

D. Ocular Toxoplasmosis

Ocular toxoplasmosis is an important cause of chorioretinitis in the United States. In children, it results most often from reactivation of congenital infection but can also follow acquired infection. Congenitally infected individuals are usually asymptomatic until the second or third decade of life when rupture of tissue cysts and the release of bradyzoites and tachyzoites into the retina causes symptoms. Typically, ocular toxoplasmosis presents as focal necrotizing retinochoroiditis often associated with a preexistent chorioretinal scar, and variable involvement of the vitreous, retinal blood vessels, optic nerve, and anterior segment of the eye.

E. Diagnostic Findings

Toxoplasmosis is diagnosed most commonly by serologic tests, but results must be interpreted carefully, particularly in the evaluation of congenital toxoplasmosis. Active infection can also be diagnosed by PCR of blood or body fluids; by visualization of tachyzoites in histologic sections or cytology preparations, cysts in placenta or fetal tissues; or by characteristic lymph node histology. Immunoglobulin G (IgG) antibodies become detectable 1–2 weeks after infection and persist for life. Immunoglobulin M (IgM) antibodies appear earlier and decline faster than IgG antibodies but can last for 12–18 months after acute infection; they are used to help separate remote infection from one that is potentially more recent. Isolated IgM antibodies with negative IgG may represent a false positive result. A single positive titer determination is nondiagnostic and may indicate past infection; IgG seroconversion or a fourfold increase in titer from paired samples drawn at least 3 weeks apart are diagnostic for recent infection. Absence of both serum IgG and IgM in an immunocompetent individual virtually rules out the diagnosis of toxoplasmosis. In the immunocompromised host, serologic tests are not as sensitive, and active infection is documented by PCR or finding tachyzoites by histologic examination. PCR cannot distinguish between acute acquired infection or reactivation.

The diagnosis of toxoplasmosis in the older child with visual complaints is usually made by finding *T gondii* IgG or IgM antibodies in the serum in the presence of a typical eye lesion. The diagnosis can be confirmed by detecting *T gondii* DNA by PCR in the aqueous humor, though this is rarely performed.

Congenital infection is confirmed by histologic or molecular identification of trophozoites in amniotic fluid, placenta, or infant tissue. Infant blood, CSF, and amniotic fluid specimens should be assayed by PCR. More often, diagnosis is established using a combination of serologic testing of mother and baby and clinical findings. Evaluation of a newborn should include *Toxoplasma*-specific IgG, IgM, immunoglobulin A (IgA), and immunoglobulin E (IgE) of the newborn and mother in coordination with an experienced reference lab. A congenital infection is confirmed serologically by detecting persistent or increasing newborn IgG antibody levels compared to the mother, persistently positive IgG antibodies beyond the first year of life, and/or a positive *T gondii*–specific IgM or IgA antibody test in the infant. In addition, the child should have thorough ophthalmologic, auditory, and neurologic evaluation; a lumbar puncture; and computed tomographic (CT) scan of the head (to detect CNS calcifications).

Differential Diagnosis

Congenital toxoplasmosis must be differentiated from infection with cytomegalovirus, rubella, herpes simplex, and syphilis. Acquired infection in immune competent host can mimic infectious mononucleosis, as well as other viral or bacterial infections including acute HIV, tularemia and cat scratch disease. Lymphoproliferative disorders may cause a similar presentation.

Prevention

Primary prevention of toxoplasmosis in pregnant women (and immunocompromised patients) is an essential public health goal. Effective strategies to prevent food-borne transmission of toxoplasmosis include adequate cooking or prolonged freezing of meat, and avoidance of unpasteurized milk and uncooked mollusks, particularly during pregnancy. Pregnant women and immunocompromised patients should not purchase a new kitten and should avoid changing cat litter; if unavoidable, gloves and hand-hygiene are essential and litter should be changed daily because oocysts require 48–72 hours to sporulate and become infectious. Though maternal treatment can prevent congenital transmission, implementation of serologic screening of pregnant women is challenging. Screening and prophylaxis against reactivation is important for seropositive patients undergoing immunosuppression such as stem cell transplant recipients.

Treatment

The most common medications to treat toxoplasmosis are pyrimethamine (given with leucovorin [folinic acid] to limit bone marrow toxicity) and sulfadiazine. Acute toxoplasmosis in the immunocompetent host does not require specific therapy, unless the infection occurs during pregnancy. In primary maternal infection during the first 18 weeks of pregnancy, spiramycin is recommended to attempt to prevent fetal infection. Spiramycin does not cross the placenta, so does not treat fetal infection once established. If fetal infection has been documented or if primary maternal infection occurs after the first 18 weeks of pregnancy, pyrimethamine, sulfadiazine, and leucovorin are recommended. Pyrimethamine is teratogenic and should not be used before 18 weeks of gestation.

Treatment of toxoplasmic chorioretinitis consists of oral pyrimethamine (loading dose 1 mg/kg once every 12 hours for 2 days followed by 1 mg/kg daily) plus sulfadiazine (loading dose 75 mg/kg followed 12 hours later by 50 mg/kg every 12 hours), given with leucovorin (10–20 mg/dose daily). In addition, corticosteroids (prednisone 1 mg/kg daily) are given when lesions threaten vision but should be started 48–72 hours after *Toxoplasma* treatment. The duration of additional therapy should be guided by frequent ophthalmologic examinations. Pyrimethamine can cause gastrointestinal upset, leukopenia, thrombocytopenia, and rarely, agranulocytosis; weekly complete blood counts should be checked while on therapy.

A year of treatment is recommended for congenitally infected infants. Children treated with pyrimethamine (loading dose 2 mg/kg daily for 2 days followed by 1 mg/kg daily for 6 months followed by 1 mg/kg every other day for 6 months) plus sulfadiazine (100 mg/kg divided twice daily for 12 months) plus leucovorin (10 mg three times a week) have better neurodevelopmental and visual outcomes than historical controls. While on therapy, infants should be monitored for bone marrow toxicity.

Bollani L et al: Congenital toxoplasmosis: the state of the art. Front Pediatr 2022 Jul;10. doi:10.3389/fped.2022.894573 [PMID: 35874584].

Centers for Disease Control and Prevention. Parasites—Toxoplasmosis (Toxoplasma infection). https://www.cdc.gov/parasites/toxoplasmosis/. Accessed April 9, 2023.

Dunay IR et al: Treatment of toxoplasmosis: historical perspective, animal models and current clinical practice. Clin Microbiol Rev 2018 Sep;31(4). doi: 10.1128/CMR.00057-17 [PMID: 30209035].

Schwenk HT et al: Toxoplasmosis in pediatric hematopoietic stem cell transplantation patients. Transplant Cell Ther 2021 Apr;27(4): 292–300. doi:10.1016/j.jtct.2020.11.003 [PMID: 33840441].

GASTROINTESTINAL INFECTIONS

1. Amebiasis

ESSENTIALS OF DIAGNOSIS & TYPICAL FEATURES

► Acute dysentery: diarrhea with blood and mucus, abdominal pain, tenesmus.

► Chronic non-dysenteric diarrhea.

► Hepatic abscess.

► Amebas or cysts in stool or abscesses.

► Positive ameba PCR in stool.

► Serologic evidence of amebic infection.

► General Considerations

Infection with *Entamoeba histolytica* occurs worldwide but has a particularly high prevalence in areas with poor sanitation and socioeconomic conditions. In the United States, most infections are seen in travelers to, and emigrants from, endemic areas, but can occur without travel exposure. The majority of infections are asymptomatic (> 90%), but tissue invasion can result in amebic colitis, hepatic abscess, and hematogenous spread to other organs. Transmission is usually fecal-oral. Two *Entamoeba* species, *E dispar* and *E moshkovskii*, are morphologically indistinguishable from *E histolytica* and are much more commonly encountered in stool samples. Infections with these species cause minimal (*E moshkovskii*) or no human disease (*E dispar*).

► Clinical Findings

A. Symptoms and Signs

Patients with intestinal amebiasis can have asymptomatic cyst passage (> 90%), or be symptomatic with acute amebic proctocolitis, chronic non-dysenteric colitis, or ameboma.

Patients with acute amebic colitis typically have a 1- to 2-week history of loose stools containing blood and mucus, abdominal pain, and tenesmus. A minority of patients are febrile or dehydrated. Abdominal examination is notable for lower abdominal tenderness.

Fulminant colitis is an unusual complication of amebic dysentery that is associated with a grave prognosis (> 50% mortality), and is characterized by severe bloody diarrhea, fever, and diffuse abdominal pain and may mimic inflammatory bowel disease. Children younger than 2 years are at increased risk for fulminant colitis. An ameboma is a localized amebic infection, usually in the cecum or ascending colon, which presents as a painful abdominal mass.

Intestinal amebiasis can be complicated by intestinal perforation, toxic megacolon, and peritonitis. Perianal ulcers, a less common complication, are painful, punched-out lesions that usually respond to medical therapy.

Patients with amebic liver abscess, the most common form of extraintestinal amebiasis, typically present with acute fever and right upper quadrant tenderness (see also Chapter 22). The pain may be dull, pleuritic, or referred to the right shoulder. The liver feels normal on examination in most patients. Some patients have a subacute presentation lasting 2 weeks to 6 months with hepatomegaly, anemia, and weight loss. Jaundice and diarrhea are uncommon. Intestinal tract infection tends to be absent in those with extraintestinal disease. Amebic liver abscess should be considered in the differential for children with fever of unknown origin who have been in endemic areas.

The most common complication of amebic liver abscess is pleuropulmonary amebiasis due to rupture of a right liver lobe abscess. Lung abscesses may also occur from hematogenous spread. Rupture of hepatic abscesses can lead to peritonitis and more rarely to pericarditis. Amebic brain or spinal cord abscess is an infrequent manifestation.

B. Diagnostic Findings

Acute amebic colitis must be differentiated from bacterial (eg, *Salmonella* spp., *Shigella* spp., *Escherichia coli* spp., *Campylobacter* spp.), parasitic (eg, *Balantidium coli*), and non-infectious (eg, inflammatory bowel disease, diverticulitis, ischemic colitis) causes of dysentery. Amebic liver abscess must be distinguished from an echinococcal hydatid cyst and abscesses caused by enteric bacteria. Occult blood in stool is present in virtually all cases of amebic colitis and can be used as an inexpensive screening test. Fecal leukocytes are uncommon.

Intestinal amebiasis has been traditionally diagnosed by detecting trophozoites or cysts on stool examination or mucosal biopsy. However, *E histolytica* is morphologically identical to nonpathogenic *E dispar* and *E moshkovskii*, and the majority of amebas diagnosed by microscopy are not *E histolytica*. Multiplex stool pathogen PCR panel can confirm the diagnosis. Colonoscopy and biopsy are most helpful when stool studies are nondiagnostic and other intestinal pathology (eg, Crohn's) are possible. Barium studies are contraindicated for patients with suspected acute amebic colitis due to risk of perforation.

Diagnosis of extra-intestinal *E histolytica* infection often relies on serum specific antibody detection as stool testing is often negative. Enzyme-linked immunosorbent assays (ELISAs) are positive in approximately 95% of patients with extraintestinal amebiasis. However, these antibodies persist for years, and a positive result does not distinguish between acute and past infection. Ultrasonographic examination and CT are sensitive techniques to detect hepatic abscesses that are used to guide fine-needle aspiration for definitive diagnosis. The classic appearance of drainage from a hepatic amebic abscess is described as "anchovy paste."

▶ Prevention & Treatment

Travelers to endemic areas should drink bottled or boiled water and eat cooked or peeled vegetables and fruits to prevent enteric infection.

Treatment of amebic infection is complex because different agents are required for eradicating the parasite from the bowel or tissue. Whether treatment of asymptomatic cyst passers is indicated is unclear though it is offered to decrease risk of spreading to family members and development of invasive disease. Asymptomatic *E histolytica* cyst excreters may be treated with paromomycin or iodoquinol, nonabsorbable intraluminal amebicides. Metronidazole and tinidazole are not effective against cysts. Corticosteroids and anti-motility agents should be avoided as they can worsen symptoms.

Patients with symptomatic intestinal amebiasis or extraintestinal disease require treatment with an absorbable agent, such as metronidazole or tinidazole, followed by an intraluminal agent, even if the stool examination is negative. Tinidazole is more effective than metronidazole and is well tolerated in children. Metronidazole and paromomycin should not be given concurrently, because the diarrhea that is a common side effect of paromomycin may make it difficult to assess response to therapy. In most patients with amebic liver abscess, aspiration is unnecessary and does not speed recovery. Drainage may be considered when response to medical therapy is inadequate or there is a risk of rupture. Follow up stool examination should be performed after treatment.

American Academy of Pediatrics Committee on Infectious Diseases. Amebiasis. In: Kimberlin DW et al (eds): Red Book: 2021 Report of the Committee on Infectious Diseases. 32nd ed. Elk Grove Village, IL: American Academy of Pediatrics; 2021:190–193.
Gonzales MLM et al: Antiamoebic drugs for treating amoebic colitis. Cochrane Database Syst Rev 2019 Jan 9;1:CD006085. doi:10.1002/14651858.CD006085.pub3 [PMID: 30624763].

2. Giardiasis

ESSENTIALS OF DIAGNOSIS & TYPICAL FEATURES

- ▶ Chronic relapsing diarrhea, flatulence, bloating, anorexia, poor weight gain.
- ▶ Absence of fever or hematochezia.
- ▶ Detection of trophozoites, cysts, or *Giardia* antigens in stool, or positive stool PCR.

▶ General Considerations

Giardiasis, caused by *Giardia duodenalis*, is the most common intestinal protozoal infection in children in the United States and in most of the world. The infection is classically associated with drinking contaminated water, either in rural areas or in areas with faulty purification systems. Even ostensibly clean urban water supplies and pristine mountain streams can be contaminated intermittently, and infection has been acquired in swimming pools. Fecal-oral contamination allows person-to-person spread. Day care centers are a major source of infection. Food-borne outbreaks also occur. Giardiasis may occur at any age, although infection is rare in neonates. High rates of transmission occur among men who have sex with men. Domestic animals are rare sources of human infection.

▶ Clinical Findings

A. Symptoms and Signs

Giardia infection results in either asymptomatic cyst passage, acute self-limited diarrhea, or a chronic syndrome of diarrhea, malabsorption, and weight loss. Acute diarrhea occurs 1–2 weeks after infection and is characterized by abrupt onset of diarrhea with greasy, malodorous stools, malaise, flatulence, bloating, and nausea. Fever and vomiting are unusual. The disease has a protracted course (> 1 week) and frequently leads to weight loss. Chronic diarrhea frequently leads to malabsorption, steatorrhea, micronutrient deficiencies, and disaccharidase depletion. Lactose intolerance, which develops in 20%–40% of patients can persist for several weeks after treatment and needs to be differentiated from relapsing giardiasis or reinfection.

B. Laboratory Findings

Increasingly, the diagnosis of giardiasis in the United States is made by stool PCR, often in the context of a multiplex stool pathogen panel. Though these assays are sensitive and specific for *Giardia*, identification of multiple pathogens in a stool sample can present challenges in determining the etiologic cause of diarrhea, particularly in patients exposed in poor income countries where carriage of *Giardia* is extremely common. Alternative methods of diagnosis include *Giardia* antigen detection by means of ELISAs, nonenzymatic immunoassays, and direct fluorescence antibody tests. In areas without access to PCR or antigen tests, the diagnosis of giardiasis can be made by finding the parasite in stool. Examining up to three daily stool specimens increases sensitivity. For O&P examination, a fresh stool provides the best results. Liquid stools have the highest yield of mobile trophozoites, which are more readily identified on wet mounts. With semi-formed stools or those that cannot immediately be examined, the examiner should look for cysts in fresh or fixed specimens, preferably using a concentration technique.

▶ **Prevention**

The prevention of giardiasis requires proper treatment of water supplies and interruption of person-to-person transmission. Where water might be contaminated, travelers, campers, and hikers should use methods to make water safe for drinking. Boiling is the most reliable method; the necessary time of boiling (1–3 minute at sea level) will depend on the altitude. Chemical disinfection with iodine or chlorine and filtration are alternative methods of water treatment.

Interrupting fecal-oral transmission requires strict hand washing. Outbreaks of diarrhea in day care centers might be particularly difficult to eradicate. Reinforcing hand washing and treating the disease in both symptomatic and asymptomatic carriers may be necessary.

▶ **Treatment**

Metronidazole, tinidazole, and nitazoxanide are the traditional drugs of choice for treatment of giardiasis. A recent meta-analysis concluded that single dose tinidazole (50 mg/kg; max 2 g) should be the preferred treatment based on both better efficacy and convenience compared to other treatments. There are fewer data on the use of tinidazole in children younger than 3 years. When given at 5 mg/kg (up to 250 mg) three times a day for 5–7 days, metronidazole has 80%–95% efficacy. Nitazoxanide (100 mg [5 mL] every 12 hours for children 12–47 months of age, 200 mg every 12 hours for 4- to 11-year-olds, and 500 mg every 12 hours for children 12 years or older) is available in liquid formulation and requires only 3 days of treatment but is costly. For patients who do not respond to therapy or are reinfected, switching to another drug may be advisable. In cases of repeated treatment failure paromomycin or albendazole may be effective.

Centers for Disease Control and Prevention. Parasites—Giardia. https://www.cdc.gov/parasites/giardia/. Accessed April 10, 2023.
Ordonez Mena JM et al: Comparative efficacy of drugs for treating giardiasis: a systematic update of the literature and network meta-analysis of randomized clinical trials. J Antimicrob Chemother 2018;73(3):596. doi:10.1093/jac/dkx430 [PMID: 29186570].

3. Cryptosporidiosis

The intracellular protozoa cryptosporidia are the leading cause of recreational water-associated diarrheal outbreaks in the United States. Cryptosporidia may also cause severe and devastating diarrhea in immunocompromised patients, including those with untreated acquired immunodeficiency syndrome (AIDS). This ubiquitous parasite infects and reproduces in the epithelial cell lining of the digestive and respiratory tracts of humans and most other vertebrate animals. Humans acquire the infection from contaminated drinking water, recreational water sources (including swimming pools, fountains, and lake water), or from close contact with infected humans or animals. Petting zoos and day care centers have been other sources of *cryptosporidia* outbreaks. Most human infections are caused by *Cryptosporidium parvum* or *Cryptosporidium hominis*.

▶ **Clinical Findings**

A. Symptoms and Signs

Immunocompetent persons infected with *Cryptosporidium* usually develop self-limited diarrhea (2–26 days) with or without abdominal cramps. Diarrhea can be mild and intermittent or continuous, watery, and voluminous. Low-grade fever, nausea, vomiting, loss of appetite, and malaise may accompany the diarrhea. Children younger than 2 years are more susceptible to infection than older children. Immunocompromised patients (either cellular or humoral deficiency) tend to develop a severe, prolonged, chronic diarrhea that, despite treatment, can result in severe malnutrition and subside only after the immunodeficiency is corrected. Other clinical manifestations associated with cryptosporidiosis in immunocompromised hosts include cholecystitis, pancreatitis, hepatitis, biliary tree involvement, and respiratory symptoms.

B. Laboratory Findings

Though visualization of oocysts in concentrated stool samples is diagnostic, multiplex stool pathogen PCR panels have largely replaced diagnostic microscopy and are highly sensitive and specific. Alternate tests include direct immuno-fluorescent antibody (DFA) of stool.

▶ **Prevention & Treatment**

Prevention of *Cryptosporidium* infection is limited by oocyst resistance to some of the standard water purification procedures (including chlorine) and common disinfectants. Enteric precautions are recommended for infected persons. Boiled or bottled drinking water may be considered for patients at high risk for developing chronic infection (eg, inadequately treated patients with AIDS). *Cryptosporidium*-infected persons should avoid swimming pools.

Many infections in immunocompetent individuals are self-limited; thus treatment is supportive and primarily directed at prevention of dehydration. Severe or prolonged cases in immunocompetent patients and some patients with immunodeficiencies respond to treatment with nitazoxanide, antidiarrheal agents, and hydration. Immunocompromised patients usually require more intense supportive care with parenteral nutrition in addition to hydration and nonspecific antidiarrheal agents. Recommended doses of nitazoxanide are 100 mg (5 mL) every 12 hours for children 12–47 months of age, 200 mg every 12 hours for 4- to 11-year-olds, and 500 mg every 12 hours for children 12 years or older for three days. Immunocompromised patients often require a longer duration of nitazoxanide therapy, typically at least 2 weeks. For patients with advanced AIDS, antiparasitic therapy alone has not proven efficacious. Institution of effective antiretroviral therapy results in elimination of symptomatic cryptosporidiosis.

Centers for Disease Control and Prevention. Parasites—Cryptosporidium (also known as "Crypto"). https://www.cdc.gov/parasites/crypto/index.html. Accessed April 11, 2023.

La Hoz RM et al: Intestinal parasites including *Cryptosporidium*, *Cyclospora*, *Giardia*, and *Microsporidia*, *Entamoeba histolytica*, *Strongyloides*, schistosomiasis, and *Echinococcus*: guidelines from the American Society of Transplantation Infectious Diseases Community of Practice. Clin Transplant 2019;33(9):e13618. Epub 2019 Jun 23 [PMID: 31145496].

Love MS et al: Emerging treatment options for cryptosporidiosis. Curr Opin Infect Dis 2021 Oct 1;34(5):455–462. doi:10.1097/QCO.0000000000000761 [PMID: 34261904].

4. Cyclosporiasis

Cyclospora spp. are ubiquitous parasites, but *Cyclospora cayetanensis* is the only species known to infect humans. Cyclosporiasis is seen in three main epidemiologic settings: sporadic cases in endemic areas, travelers to endemic areas, and in food- or water-borne outbreaks in nonendemic areas, particularly in relation to importation of fresh produce. In the immunocompetent host, diarrhea usually lasts 10–25 days, but may relapse. The infection can be unusually severe in immunocompromised patients, especially those with inadequately treated HIV/AIDS. Diagnosis is based on finding oocysts in stool or biopsy specimens stained with acid-fast stain. PCR of stool is available at the CDC and as a component of multiplex assays. Treatment is trimethoprim-sulfamethoxazole for 7 days; no other medication has proven effective.

Casillas S et al: Notes from the field: multiple cyclosporiasis outbreaks—United States, 2018. MMWR Morb Mortal Wkly Rep 2018 Oct 5;67(39):1101–1102 [PMID: 30286055].

Centers for Disease Control and Prevention. Parasites—Cyclosporiasis (Cyclospora infection). https://www.cdc.gov/parasites/cyclosporiasis/index.html. Accessed April 24, 2023.

5. Free-Living Amebas

ESSENTIALS OF DIAGNOSIS & TYPICAL FEATURES

► Primary amebic meningoencephalitis: fever, headache, stiff neck, acute mental deterioration, fatal infection.

► Swimming in warm, freshwater in an endemic area.

► Granulomatous amebic encephalitis: insidious onset of focal neurologic deficits.

► Amebic keratitis: pain, photophobia, conjunctivitis, blurred vision.

► General Considerations

Infections with free-living amebas are uncommon. *Naegleria* species, *Acanthamoeba* species, and *Balamuthia* amoebas have been associated with human disease, primarily infections of the central nervous system. They exist as motile, infectious trophozoites and non-infectious cysts.

Primary amebic meningoencephalitis (PAM), caused by *Naegleria fowleri*, occurs mostly in children and young adults. Patients present with abrupt fever, headache, nausea, and vomiting and disturbances in smell and taste, signs of meningeal irritation, and decreased mental status a few days to 2 weeks after exposure. Infection is often associated with swimming in warm freshwater lakes and using contaminated tap water for nasal irrigation. CNS invasion occurs after nasal inoculation of *N fowleri*, which travel along the olfactory nerves via the cribriform plate to the brain. The disease is rapidly progressive and nearly universally fatal within a week of symptom onset.

Granulomatous amebic encephalitis (GAE), caused by *Acanthamoeba* or *Balamuthia*, occurs more commonly in immunocompromised patients. Infection likely occurs by inhalation or direct contact with contaminated soil or water followed by hematogenous spread. This disease has an insidious onset of focal neurologic deficits, and approximately 50% of patients present with headache. Skin, sinus, or lung infections with *Acanthamoeba* precede many of the CNS infections and may still be present at the onset of neurologic disease. GAE progresses to fatal outcome over a period of weeks to months (average 6 weeks).

Acanthamoeba keratitis is a corneal infection associated with minor trauma or the use of contact lenses in otherwise healthy persons. Clinical findings of *Acanthamoeba* keratitis include radial keratoneuritis and stromal ring infiltrate. Amebic keratitis usually follows an indolent course that initially may resemble herpes simplex or bacterial keratitis; delay in diagnosis is associated with worse outcomes.

Clinical Findings & Differential Diagnosis

PAM should be included in the differential diagnosis of acute meningoencephalitis in children with a history of recent freshwater swimming. The CSF is usually hemorrhagic, with leukocyte counts that may be normal early in the disease but later range from 400/mL to 2600/mL with neutrophil predominance, low to normal glucose, and elevated protein. The etiologic diagnosis relies on finding trophozoites on a wet mount of the CSF. Immunofluorescent and PCR-based diagnostic assays are available through the CDC.

GAE is diagnosed by brain biopsy of CT-identified non-enhancing lucent areas. The CSF of these patients is usually nondiagnostic with a lymphocytic pleocytosis, mild to severe elevation of protein (> 1000 mg/dL), and normal or low glucose. *Acanthamoeba* and *Balamuthia* amebas have only rarely been found in the CSF; however, they can be visualized in brain biopsies or grown from brain or other infected tissues. Immunofluorescent and PCR-based diagnostic assays are available through the CDC.

Acanthamoeba keratitis is diagnosed by finding the trophozoites in corneal scrapings or by isolating the parasite from corneal specimens or contact lens cultures.

Prevention

Because PAM occurs infrequently, active surveillance of lakes for *N fowleri* is not warranted. However, in the presence of a documented case, it is advisable to close the implicated lake to swimming. Sterile or boiled water should be used for nasal irrigation. *Acanthamoeba* keratitis can be prevented by heat disinfection of contact lenses, storage of lenses in sterile solutions, the use of disposable daily lenses, and by not wearing lenses when swimming in freshwater or showering.

Treatment

Treatment of amebic encephalitis is complex and usually unsuccessful. Urgent consultation with the CDC is recommended for all cases (CDC Emergency Operations Center at 770-488-7100). Though treatment numbers are small, regimens containing miltefosine (an antiparasitic used for treatment of leishmania) may increase survival in *Balamuthia mandrillaris* and *Acanthamoeba* infections, in combination with a variety of other drugs. A handful of successful treatments of children with *Naegleria* meningoencephalitis has been reported using miltefosine in combination with amphotericin B, fluconazole, rifampin, azithromycin, dexamethasone, and whole-body cooling to 34°C.

Acanthamoeba keratitis responds well to surgical debridement followed by 3–4 weeks of topical treatment. A common combination therapy utilizes polyhexamethylene biguanide (PHMB) or chlorhexidine with or without propamidine or hexamidine.

Alkharashi M et al: Medical interventions for *Acanthamoeba* keratitis. Cochrane Database Syst Rev 2015 Feb 24;2015(2): CD010792. doi:10.1002/14651858.CD010792.pub2 [PMID: 25710134].

Centers for Disease Control and Prevention. Naegleria fowleri-Primary Amebic Meningoencephalitis (PAM) - Amebic Encephalitis. https://www.cdc.gov/parasites/naegleria/index.html. Accessed April 11, 2023.

Centers for Disease Control and Prevention. Parasites—Acanthamoeba—Granulomatous Amebic Encephalitis (GAE); Keratitis. https://www.cdc.gov/parasites/acanthamoeba/index.html. Accessed April 11, 2023.

Gharpure R et al: Epidemiology and clinical characteristics of primary amebic meningoencephalitis caused by *Naegleria fowleri*: a global review. Clin Infect Dis 2021 Jul 1;73(1). doi:10.1093/cid/ciaa520 [PMID: 32369575].

TRICHOMONIASIS

Trichomonas vaginalis infection is discussed in Chapter 44.

METAZOAL INFECTIONS

NEMATODE (ROUNDWORM) INFECTIONS

1. Enterobiasis (Pinworms)

ESSENTIALS OF DIAGNOSIS & TYPICAL FEATURES

► Anal pruritus.
► Worms in the stool or eggs on perianal skin.

General Considerations

This worldwide infection is caused by *Enterobius vermicularis*. The adult worms are about 5–10 mm long and live in the colon; females deposit eggs on the perianal area, primarily at night, which cause intense pruritus. Scratching contaminates the fingers and allows transmission back to the host (autoinfection) or to contacts through fecal-oral spread.

Clinical Findings

A. Symptoms and Signs

Pinworms are associated with intense localized pruritis of the anus and vulva. Adult worms may migrate within the colon or up the urethra or vagina in girls. They can be found within the bowel wall, in the lumen of the appendix (usually an incidental finding by the pathologist), in the bladder, and even in the peritoneal cavity of girls.

B. Laboratory Findings

The usual diagnostic test ("Scotch tape test" or "paddle test") consists of pressing a piece of transparent tape on the child's anus in the morning prior to bathing, then placing it on a drop of xylene on a slide. Multiple tests over subsequent days may improve diagnostic sensitivity. Microscopic examination under low power usually demonstrates the ova. Scrapings from under fingernails may also be positive. Parents may visualize adult worms in the perianal region, often at nighttime while the child is asleep. Though stool testing for pinworm is typically negative, incidental identification of the flagellate parasite *Dientamoeba fragilis* in a stool O&P examination may suggest the presence of *Enterobius*, though why these two organisms frequently coexist in a patient is incompletely understood.

Differential Diagnosis

Nonspecific irritation or vaginitis, streptococcal perianal cellulitis (usually painful with marked erythema), and vaginal or urinary bacterial infections may at times resemble pinworm infection, although the symptoms of pinworms are often so suggestive that a therapeutic trial is justified without a confirmed diagnosis.

Treatment

A. Specific Measures

Treat all household members at the same time to prevent reinfections.

Pyrantel pamoate, available without a prescription, is given as a single dose (11 mg/kg; maximum 1 g); it is safe, inexpensive, and very effective. Albendazole (400 or 200 mg in children 1–2 years of age) in a single dose is also highly effective for all ages (though not approved by the US FDA). Because the drugs are not active against the eggs, therapy should be repeated after 2 weeks to kill the recently hatched adults. Significant constipation may impair treatment responses. Ivermectin is active but less effective against pinworm.

B. General Measures

Personal hygiene must be emphasized. Nails should be kept short and clean. Children should wear undergarments in bed to diminish contamination of fingers; bedclothes should be laundered frequently; infected persons should bathe in the morning, thereby removing a large proportion of eggs.

Centers for Disease Control and Prevention. Parasites—Enterobiasis (also known as Pinworm Infection). https://www.cdc.gov/parasites/pinworm/index.html. Accessed April 11, 2023.

2. Ascariasis

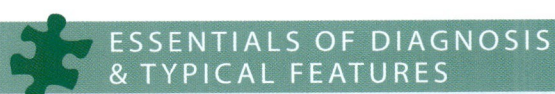

ESSENTIALS OF DIAGNOSIS & TYPICAL FEATURES

► Often asymptomatic but impacts micronutrient absorption.
► Abdominal cramps and discomfort.
► Large, white or reddish, round worms, or ova in the feces.

General Considerations

The whipworm, hookworms (see later), and *Ascaris* comprise the "soil-transmitted helminths." These parasites cause human infection through contact with eggs or larvae that thrive in the moist soil of the tropics and subtropics. Worldwide, more than a billion people are infected with at least one of these parasites, and, especially in less developed countries, it is not uncommon for children to be chronically and repeatedly infected with multiple worms. These parasites are strongly associated with poverty and poor sanitation. Children infected with these worms are at increased risk for malnutrition, stunted growth, intellectual disability, and cognitive and education deficits. Together, the soil-transmitted helminths are one of the world's most important causes of physical and intellectual impairment, with the majority of this burden falling on children.

Ascaris lumbricoides is a worldwide human parasite that is endemic in parts of the rural southeastern United States. Ova passed by carriers may remain viable for months under the proper soil conditions. The ova contaminate food or fingers and are subsequently ingested by a new host. The larvae hatch, penetrate the intestinal wall, enter the venous system, reach the alveoli, are coughed up the trachea and swallowed, returning to the small intestine, where they mature. The female lays thousands of eggs daily.

Clinical Findings

A. Symptoms and Signs

The majority of infections with *A lumbricoides* are asymptomatic, although moderate to heavy infections are associated with abdominal pain, weight loss, anorexia, diarrhea, and vomiting, and may lead to malnutrition. During the larval migratory phase, an acute transient eosinophilic pneumonitis (Löffler syndrome) may occur. Acute intestinal obstruction has been associated with heavy infections, which is more common in children due to their smaller intestinal diameter and higher worm burden. Worm migration can cause appendicitis, common bile duct obstruction (resulting in biliary colic, cholangitis, or pancreatitis), or peritonitis secondary to perforation.

B. Laboratory Findings

The diagnosis is made by observing the large roundworms (15–40 cm) in the stool or by microscopic detection of the ova on concentrated stool examination.

Treatment

Ascaris is treated with albendazole (400 mg in a single dose, or 200 mg in children 1–2 years of age), mebendazole (100 mg twice a day for 3 days or 500 mg once), or ivermectin (150–200 mcg/kg orally once). Nitazoxanide and pyrantel pamoate are also effective. In cases of intestinal or biliary obstruction, piperazine (150 mg/kg initially, followed by six doses of 65 mg/kg every 12 hours by nasogastric tube) can be used to paralyze the worms and help relieve obstruction. However, surgical removal is occasionally required. Because reinfection is common in areas of high worm burden, regular deworming programs are used to mitigate chronic nutritional and development impacts on children, although results have been disappointing in the setting of rapid reinfection.

Centers for Disease Control and Prevention. Parasites—Ascariasis. https://www.cdc.gov/parasites/ascariasis/index.html. Accessed April 11, 2023.

Clarke NE et al: Efficacy of anthelminthic drugs and drug combinations against soil-transmitted helminths: a systematic review and network meta-analysis. Clin Infect Dis 2019 Jan 1;68(1):96–105. doi:10.1093/cid/ciy423 [PMID: 29788074].

Conterno LO et al: Anthelmintic drugs for treating ascariasis. Cochrane Database Syst Rev 2020 Apr 14;4(4):CD010599. doi:10.1002/14651858.CD010599.pub2 [PMID: 32289194].

Jourdan PM et al: Soil-transmitted helminth infections. Lancet 2018 Jan 20;391(10117):252–265. doi:10.1016/S0140-6736(17)31930-X [PMID: 28882382].

Pullan RL et al: Effects, equity, and cost of school-based and community-wide treatment strategies for soil-transmitted helminths in Kenya: a cluster-randomised controlled trial. Lancet 2019; http://dx.doi.org/10.1016/S0140-6736(18)32591-1 [PMID: 31006575].

3. Trichuriasis (Whipworm)

Trichuris trichiura is a widespread human and animal parasite common in children living in warm, humid areas conducive to survival of the ova, and is one of the soil-transmitted helminths of major global health significance. Ingested infectious eggs hatch in the upper small intestine. The adult worms (30–50 mm long) live in the cecum and colon; the ova are passed and become infectious after several weeks in the soil. Unlike *Ascaris*, *Trichuris* does not have a migratory tissue phase. Symptoms are not present unless the infection is severe, in which case pain, diarrhea, iron-deficiency anemia, and mild abdominal distention are present. Massive infections may also cause rectal prolapse and dysentery. Detection of the characteristic barrel-shaped ova in the feces confirms the diagnosis. Mild to moderate eosinophilia may be present.

Treatment with mebendazole (100 mg orally twice a day for 3 days) or albendazole (400 mg in a single dose for 3 days, or 200 mg in children 1–2 years of age) tends to improve gastrointestinal symptoms when present. For heavy infections, longer duration of therapy, 5–7 days, can be considered. Combination therapy involving more than one drug may be more effective than single-drug therapy for refractory cases. Ivermectin is also effective.

Centers for Disease Control and Prevention. Parasites—Trichuriasis (also known as Whipworm Infection). https://www.cdc.gov/parasites/whipworm. Accessed April 12, 2023.

Matamoros G et al: Efficacy and safety of albendazole and high-dose ivermectin coadministration in school-aged children infected with *Trichuris trichiura* in Honduras: a randomized controlled trial. Clin Infect Dis 2021 Oct 5;73(7):1203–1210. doi:10.1093/cid/ciab365 [PMID: 33906234].

4. Hookworm

ESSENTIALS OF DIAGNOSIS & TYPICAL FEATURES

► Iron-deficiency anemia.
► Abdominal discomfort, weight loss, pruritic skin eruption.
► Ova in the feces.

► General Considerations

The common human hookworms are *Ancylostoma duodenale* and *Necator americanus*. Both are widespread in the tropics and subtropics, with an estimated 600–700 million people infected worldwide. The larger *A duodenale* is more pathogenic because it consumes more blood, up to 0.5 mL per worm per day.

The adults live in the jejunum. Eggs are passed in the feces and develop and hatch into infectious larvae in warm, damp soil within 2 weeks. The larvae penetrate human skin on contact, enter the blood, reach the alveoli, are coughed up and swallowed, and develop into adults in the intestine. The adult worms attach to intestinal mucosa, from which they suck blood. Anemia is the major sequela of infection; protein loss due to bleeding and disruption of the mucosal surface may also occur. Infection rates reach 90% in areas without sanitation.

Ancylostoma braziliense and *Ancylostoma caninum* (the dog and cat hookworm) cause cutaneous larva migrans, a creeping skin eruption in children and others who come in contact with soil contaminated with cat and dog feces. In the United States, the disease is most prevalent in the Southeast, but most cases are imported by travelers returning from tropical and subtropical areas.

► Clinical Findings

A. Symptoms and Signs

Patients with hookworm infection usually are asymptomatic. Chronic hookworm infection leads to blood loss and iron-deficiency anemia. Heavy infection may be associated with hypoproteinemia with edema. Chronic hookworm infection in children may lead to growth delay, deficits in cognition, and developmental delay. The larvae usually penetrate the skin of the feet and cause a stinging or burning sensation, followed by an intense local itching (ground itch) and a papulovesicular rash that may persist for 1–2 weeks. Pneumonitis associated with migrating larvae is uncommon and usually mild, except during heavy infections. Colicky abdominal pain, nausea, and/or diarrhea and marked eosinophilia may be observed.

In cutaneous larva migrans, larvae produce pruritic, reddish papules at the site of skin entry and intensely pruritic, serpiginous tracks or bullae appear as they migrate through the skin. These are pathognomonic for this disease. Larvae can move up to a few centimeters a day and activity can continue for several weeks, but eventually the rash is self-limiting. Systemic infection is less common but can be seen with *A caninum*.

B. Laboratory Findings

The large ova of both species of hookworm are found in feces and are indistinguishable. Microcytic anemia, hypoalbuminemia, eosinophilia, and hematochezia occur in severe cases.

▶ Prevention

Avoiding fecal contamination of soil and avoiding barefoot skin contact with potentially contaminated soil is recommended.

▶ Treatment

A. Specific Measures

Albendazole (400 mg orally in a single dose, or 200 mg in children 1–2 years of age) is significantly more efficacious than mebendazole or pyrantel pamoate and is considered the drug of choice for treatment of hookworm infections.

B. General Measures

Iron therapy and vitamin A supplementation in conjunction with deworming programs may help mitigate some of the negative nutritional and micronutrient effects of infection with hookworm and the other soil-transmitted helminths, particularly in settings where reinfection occurs rapidly.

Centers for Disease Control and Prevention. Parasites—Hookworm. https://www.cdc.gov/parasites/hookworm/. Accessed April 12, 2023.

Patel C et al: Efficacy and safety of albendazole in hookworm-infected preschool-aged children, school-aged children and adults in Cote d'Ivoire: a phase 2 randomized, controlled dose-finding trial. Clin Infect Dis 2021 Jul 15;73(2):e494–e502. doi: 10.1093/cid/ciaa989 [PMID: 32668456].

5. Strongyloidiasis

ESSENTIALS OF DIAGNOSIS & TYPICAL FEATURES

▶ Abdominal pain, diarrhea.

▶ Eosinophilia.

▶ Larvae in stools and duodenal aspirates.

▶ Serum antibodies.

▶ General Considerations

Strongyloides stercoralis is unique in having both parasitic and free-living forms; the latter can survive in the soil for prolonged periods. The parasite is found in most tropical and subtropical regions of the world, including some areas of the southeastern United States. The adults live in the submucosal tissue of the duodenum and occasionally elsewhere in the intestines. Eggs deposited in the mucosa hatch rapidly and thus the first-stage (rhabditiform) larvae are the predominant form found in duodenal aspirates and feces, rather than eggs. The larvae mature rapidly to the infectious tissue-penetrating filariform stage and initiate internal autoinfection within the intestine or in the perianal area. The filariform larvae passed in stool to the environment persist in soil and can penetrate the skin of another host, subsequently migrating into veins and pulmonary alveoli, reaching the intestine when coughed up and swallowed. Autoinfection can result in persistent infection for decades.

▶ Clinical Findings

A. Symptoms and Signs

Chronic *S stercoralis* infections can be asymptomatic or cause cutaneous, gastrointestinal, and/or pulmonary symptoms. At the site of skin penetration, a transient pruritic rash may occur. Autoinfection from larvae present in stool may result in severe itching in the perianal area and a rapidly migrating rash called larva currens. Migrating larvae in the lungs can cause wheezing, cough, shortness of breath, and hemoptysis. Although intestinal infections are often asymptomatic, the most prominent features of clinical strongyloidiasis include abdominal pain, distention, diarrhea, vomiting, and occasionally malabsorption.

Patients (primarily adults) with cellular immunodeficiencies and those on corticosteroids or chemotherapy may develop disseminated infection known as strongyloides hyperinfection syndrome, sometimes many years after the last exposure (eg, in immigrants living for prolonged periods in the United States), involving the intestine, the lungs, and the meninges. Gram-negative sepsis may complicate disseminated strongyloidiasis.

B. Laboratory Findings

A marked eosinophilia is common in strongyloidiasis. Definitive diagnosis can be difficult because of low parasite load and irregular larval output in stool. Finding larvae (not eggs) in the feces, duodenal aspirates, or sputum is diagnostic. IgG antibodies measured by ELISA or immunoblot are relatively sensitive (83%–93%). The presence of specific antibody does not distinguish between past and present infection. However, because prolonged, minimally symptomatic infections frequently occur, a person with a positive IgG test and no history of treatment should be considered infected. *Strongyloides* antibody assays can cross-react with other helminth infections. Patients with pulmonary symptoms with suspected *Strongyloides* infection should have sputum samples evaluated for *S stercoralis* in addition to antibody testing.

▶ Differential Diagnosis

Strongyloidiasis should be differentiated from peptic ulcer disease, celiac disease, regional or tuberculous enteritis, and hookworm infections. The pulmonary phase may mimic asthma or bronchopneumonia. Patients with severe infection can present with an acute abdomen.

▶ Prevention & Treatment

Ivermectin (two doses of 0.2 mg/kg given daily) is the drug of choice. To reduce the chances of treatment failure from autoinfection, a second two-dose course administered two weeks after the first course is often recommended. Albendazole is an alternative treatment (used when there is concomitant *Loa loa* infection, in which case ivermectin may provoke a fatal encephalopathy) but appears to have lower efficacy. Relapses are common. In the hyperinfection syndrome, 1–3 weeks of therapy with ivermectin may be necessary and multiple follow-up stool studies for 2 weeks after therapy are indicated to ensure clearance of larvae. Patients from endemic areas should be serotested and treated at the time of immigration or before undergoing immunosuppression, including short courses of corticosteroid therapy for conditions such as asthma.

Buonfrate D et al: Multiple-dose versus single-dose ivermectin for Strongyloides stercoralis infection (Strong Treat 1 to 4): a multicentre, open-label, phase 3, randomized controlled superiority trial. Lancet Infect Dis 2019 Nov;19(11):1181–1190. doi: 10.1016/S1473-3099(19)30289-0 [PMID: 31558376].

Centers for Disease Control and Prevention. Parasites—Strongyloides. https://www.cdc.gov/parasites/strongyloides/index.html. Accessed April 13, 2023.

Requena-Méndez A et al: Evidence-based guidelines for screening and management of strongyloidiasis in non-endemic countries. Am J Trop Med Hyg 2017 Sep 7;97(3):645–652 [PMID: 28749768].

6. Visceral Larva Migrans (Toxocariasis)

ESSENTIALS OF DIAGNOSIS & TYPICAL FEATURES

▶ Visceral involvement, including hepatomegaly, marked eosinophilia, and anemia.

▶ Posterior or peripheral ocular inflammatory mass.

▶ Elevated antibody titers in serum or aqueous fluid; demonstration of *Toxocara* larvae in biopsy specimen.

▶ General Considerations

Visceral larva migrans is a worldwide disease including all areas of the United States. The agent is the small intestinal roundworm (ascarid) of dogs and cats, *Toxocara canis* or *Toxocara cati*. The eggs passed by infected animals contaminate parks and other areas that young children frequent. Children with pica are at increased risk. Ingested eggs hatch and penetrate the intestinal wall, then migrate to the liver. Most of the larvae are retained in the liver, but some may pass through to reach the lungs, eyes, muscles, and/or the CNS, where they die and incite a granulomatous inflammatory reaction.

▶ Clinical Findings

A. Visceral Larva Migrans

Toxocariasis is usually asymptomatic, but young children (aged 1–5 years) sometimes present with anorexia, fever, fatigue, pallor, abdominal pain and distention, nausea, vomiting, and cough. Hepatomegaly is common, splenomegaly is unusual, and adenopathy is absent. Lung involvement, usually asymptomatic, can be demonstrated readily by radiologic examination. Seizures are common, but more severe neurologic abnormalities are infrequent. IgG antibody detection by ELISA is sensitive, specific, and useful in confirming the clinical diagnosis, with testing available through the CDC. Most patients recover spontaneously, but disease may last up to 6 months.

B. Ocular Larva Migrans

This condition occurs in older children and adults who present with a unilateral posterior or peripheral inflammatory eye mass. History of visceral larva migrans and eosinophilia are typically absent. Anti-*Toxocara* antibody titers are low in the serum but may be elevated in vitreous and aqueous fluids.

C. Diagnostic Findings

Leukocytosis with marked eosinophilia, anemia, and elevated liver function tests are typical. Hypergammaglobulinemia may be present. The diagnosis can be confirmed by finding larvae in granulomatous lesions. More often, positive serology and the exclusion of other causes of hypereosinophilia provide a presumptive diagnosis in typical cases.

Differential Diagnosis

Diseases associated with hypereosinophilia must be considered. Other parasitic infections include trichinosis (enlarged liver not common; muscle tenderness common), *Baylisascaris* (racoon roundworm, also encountered in US children), *Ascaris*, and *Strongyloides*. Noninfectious causes of significant eosinophilia in children include allergies and drug hypersensitivity syndromes, and rarely eosinophilic leukemia and collagen-vascular disease.

Prevention & Treatment

Treatment with albendazole (400 mg twice a day for 5 days) or mebendazole (100–200 mg twice a day for 5 days) is recommended for visceral infection. Aggressive anti-inflammatory treatment with systemic corticosteroids should accompany anti-parasitic treatment for ocular larva migrans. Treating any cause of pica, such as iron deficiency, is important. Corticosteroids are used to treat marked inflammation of lungs, eyes, or other organs. Pets should be dewormed routinely.

Bradbury RS, Hobbs CV: Toxocara seroprevalence in the USA and its impact for individuals and society. Adv Parasitol 2020;109:317–339 [PMID: 32381205].
Centers for Disease Control and Prevention. Parasites—Toxocariasis (also known as Roundworm Infection). https://www.cdc.gov/parasites/toxocariasis/index.html. Accessed April 13, 2023.

7. Trichinellosis (trichinosis)

ESSENTIALS OF DIAGNOSIS & TYPICAL FEATURES

- ► Vomiting, diarrhea, and abdominal pain within 1 week of eating infected meat.
- ► Fever, periorbital edema, myalgia, and marked eosinophilia.

General Considerations

Trichinella are small roundworms that infest hogs and several other meat-eating animals. Currently, there are eight recognized *Trichinella* species, of which *Trichinella spiralis* is the most common human pathogen, and most adapted to domestic and wild swine. The most important source of human infection worldwide is the domestic pig. Cases and outbreaks have been associated with numerous game animals. The human cycle begins with ingestion of viable larvae in undercooked meat. In the small intestine, the larvae develop into adult worms that mate and produce larvae, which enter the bloodstream and migrate to the striated muscle where they continue to grow and eventually encyst. Symptoms are caused by the inflammatory response in the intestines or muscle.

Clinical Findings

A. Symptoms and Signs

Most infections are asymptomatic. The severity of clinical disease is strongly correlated with the number of ingested larvae. Infection can be divided into two phases: an intestinal phase (typically within 1–2 days of cyst ingestion) and a muscular or systemic phase (typically 2 weeks after infection). The initial bowel penetration may cause fever, headache, chills, abdominal pain, nausea, vomiting, and diarrhea within 1 week after ingestion of contaminated meat. This may progress to the classic myopathic form, which consists of fever, eyelid or facial edema, myalgia, and weakness. Other signs may include maculopapular exanthem, subungual bleeding, conjunctivitis and subconjunctival hemorrhages, headaches, dry cough, and painful movement of the eye muscles. Rare complications include myocarditis, thromboembolic disease, and encephalitis, which can be fatal. Symptoms usually peak after 2–3 weeks but may last for months. Children typically have milder clinical and laboratory findings than adults.

B. Diagnosis

Nonspecific laboratory findings (particularly marked eosinophilia, elevated muscle enzymes) in the setting of a potential exposure should raise suspicion for trichinellosis. Confirmation depends primarily on demonstration of *Trichinella*-specific IgG antibody that is present after about 3 weeks. Sensitivity and specificity of serologic testing may be enhanced by serial testing to demonstrate a rise in titer. Muscle biopsy may demonstrate encysted larvae, which are diagnostic.

Differential Diagnosis

Manifestations of the intestinal phase of trichinosis are similar to many acute gastrointestinal infections; obtaining a history of recent dietary exposure to a potential source of *Trichinella* is essential if the diagnosis is to be considered at this stage. The systemic phase may mimic the fever and myalgias of influenza but marked eosinophilia is often present. The classic symptoms are pathognomonic if one is aware of this disease. Facial swelling may mimic complicated sinusitis.

Prevention

Meat in the United States is not inspected for trichinosis; all states require the cooking of hog swill, but hog-to-hog or hog-to-rat cycles may continue. All pork and sylvatic meat (eg, bear or walrus) should be cooked at least greater than 160°F followed by a 3-minute rest. Freezing meat to at least 5°F for 3 weeks may also prevent transmission, though *Trichinella* species infecting wild game may be more resistant to freezing. Animals used for food should not be fed or allowed access to raw meat. Careful cleaning and disinfection of meat-grinding equipment is essential, particularly after processing of wild game.

► Treatment

Albendazole (400 mg twice daily for 8–14 days) is the drug of choice for trichinosis; mebendazole is also effective. Concurrent corticosteroids (prednisone 30–60 mg/day for 10–15 days) are used for treatment of severe symptoms. Administration of analgesics is sometimes required. Relapses occur, particularly when treatment occurs late in the myopathic stage.

► Prognosis

Prognosis for severe cases with cardiac and cerebral complications is poor, with a mortality rate around 5%. In milder cases, prognosis is good, and most patients' symptoms disappear within 2–6 months.

Centers for Disease Control and Prevention. Parasites—Trichinellosis (also known as Trichinosis). https://www.cdc.gov/parasites/trichinellosis/index.html. Accessed April 14, 2023.

8. Raccoon Roundworm Infections

ESSENTIALS OF DIAGNOSIS & TYPICAL FEATURES

- ► Eosinophilic meningoencephalitis or encephalopathy.
- ► Ocular larva migrans.
- ► Contact with raccoons or raccoon feces.

► General Considerations

Human infections with *Baylisascaris procyonis*, the raccoon roundworm, though rare, may result in a severe and potentially fatal CNS illness. Humans who ingest the eggs excreted in raccoon feces become accidental hosts when the larvae penetrate the gut and disseminate via the bloodstream to the brain, eyes, viscera, and muscles. Pica and exposure to raccoon latrines (location of communal raccoon defecation) represent the main risk factors. Most infections are asymptomatic, but cases of severe encephalitis (neural larva migrans), endophthalmitis (ocular larva migrans), and visceral larva migrans may occur. Symptoms typically begin 2–4 weeks after inoculation. CNS infections present as acute, rapidly progressive encephalitis with eosinophilic pleocytosis of the CSF (varies from 4% to 68% eosinophils in mild

pleocytosis). Death or severe neurologic injury is common. Ocular infections resemble other larva migrans infections such as toxocariasis; therefore, *B procyonis* should be considered in the differential diagnosis of these infections when *Toxocara* serology is negative. The diagnosis of *B procyonis* is established by observing the larvae on examination of tissue biopsies or by serology (serum or CSF) and should be considered in the differential diagnosis in anyone with CSF eosinophilia. Anthelmintic drugs have not been shown to have any beneficial effect for the treatment of baylisascariasis, since they lack larvicidal effects in human tissues. Nevertheless, albendazole (20–40 mg/kg/day for 1–4 weeks) has been used to treat most cases, together with anti-inflammatory drugs. The prognosis is poor. Immediate prophylactic treatment with albendazole (25 mg/kg daily for 20 days) should be considered for those with known ingestion of raccoon feces.

Centers for Disease Control and Prevention. Parasites—Baylisascaris infection. https://www.cdc.gov/parasites/baylisascaris/index.html. Accessed April 14, 2023.

Sircar AD et al: Raccoon roundworm infection associated with central nervous system disease and ocular disease—six states, 2013–2015. MMWR Morb Mortal Wkly Rep 2016 Sep 9;65(35):930–933. doi: 10.15585/mmwr.mm6535a2 [PMID: 27608169].

CESTODE (TAPEWORM) INFECTIONS

1. Taeniasis & Cysticercosis

ESSENTIALS OF DIAGNOSIS & TYPICAL FEATURES

- ► Mild abdominal pain; passage of worm segments (taeniasis).
- ► Focal seizures, headaches (neurocysticercosis).
- ► Cysticerci present in biopsy specimens, on plain films (as calcified masses), or on CT scan or magnetic resonance imaging (MRI).
- ► Proglottids and eggs in feces; specific antibodies in serum or CSF.

► General Considerations

Cysticercosis affects as many as 100 million people globally, and neurocysticercosis is the leading cause of seizures in many developing countries. In the United States, cases are most often noted in individuals who have resided in Latin America. Pigs are the usual intermediate host of the tapeworm *Taenia solium*. Importantly, cysticercosis cannot be acquired by eating pork; rather, ingestion of pork may result in adult tapeworm infection (taeniasis) because infected pork contains the larval cysts that develop into the adult tapeworm but does not contain the eggs that lead to cysticercosis. Human cysticercosis occurs when the eggs, which are excreted in the feces of a human infected with the parasite, are ingested. It is possible for an individual with taeniasis to auto-ingest eggs from their own intestinal tapeworm, and thus develop cysticercosis.

Larvae released from ingested eggs enter the circulation to encyst in a variety of tissues, especially muscle and brain (neurocysticercosis). Full larval maturation occurs in 2 months, but the cysts cause little inflammation until the larvae die months to years later. Inflammatory edema ensues followed by calcification or disappearance of the cyst. A slowly expanding mass of sterile cysts at the base of the brain may cause obstructive hydrocephalus (racemose cysticercosis).

T solium and the beef tapeworm (*Taenia saginata*), which can cause taeniasis but not cysticercosis, are distributed worldwide. Contamination of food by eggs in human feces allows person-to-person spread without travel to endemic areas.

► Clinical Findings

A. Symptoms and Signs

1. Taeniasis—In most tapeworm infections, the only clinical manifestation is the passage of fecal proglottids, which are white, motile segments of tapeworm 1–2 cm in size. In contrast to the soil-transmitted helminths (hookworms, ascaris) tapeworms are not associated with significant nutritional deficiencies. Children may harbor the adult worm for years and complain of abdominal pain, anorexia, and diarrhea. As they are often longer (up to 30 feet) *T saginata* may cause more symptoms than *T solium*.

2. Neurocysticercosis (NCC)—In the parenchymatous (located in brain or spinal cord tissue) form, the parasite lodges as single or multiple cysts. Granuloma formation results with eventual pericystic inflammation, which is the cause of seizures in most patients. The initial stage of the cyst is viable, where the scolex exists within the cyst and there is minimal or no enhancement due to a limited host immune response. As the scolex dies, either due to the host immune response or cysticidal treatment there is a strong immune response, characterized by enhancement on CT or MRI. As the cyst further degenerates, it calcifies, leading to punctuate calcifications on CT scan. Brain cysts may remain clinically silent or cause seizures, headache, hydrocephalus, and basilar meningitis. Systemic signs and symptoms are uncommon and make a diagnosis of NCC unlikely. Rarely, the spinal cord is involved. NCC manifests an average of 5 years after exposure but may cause symptoms within the first year. Cysts forming in the eye can cause bleeding, retinal detachment, and uveitis. Definitive diagnosis requires histologic demonstration of larvae or cyst membrane. Presumptive diagnosis is often made by the characteristics of the cysts seen on CT scan or MRI. The presence of *T solium* eggs in feces is uncommon with cysticercosis (see above) but can support the diagnosis.

B. Laboratory Findings

Neuroimaging is the mainstay of diagnosis of NCC. The diagnosis should be suspected in any patient who has lived in an endemic area and presents with a compatible clinical picture (eg, seizures, elevated intracranial pressure) and suggestive lesions on neuroimaging. It is not uncommon for lesions of cysticercosis to be noted incidentally on neuroimaging performed for other reasons (eg, trauma).

Eggs or proglottids may be found in feces or on the perianal skin (using the tape method used for pinworms). Eggs of both *Taenia* species are identical. The species are identified by examination of proglottids.

Peripheral eosinophilia is minimal or absent. CSF eosinophilia is seen in 10%–75% of cases of NCC; its presence supports an otherwise presumptive diagnosis. Antibody testing of serum with enzyme-linked immunotransfer blot (EITB) is the preferred method for diagnosis when neuroimaging is abnormal. Titers are eventually positive in up to 98% of serum specimens. The sensitivity of CSF antibody and antigen testing is lower than in serum but may correlate with viable cysticerci. Solitary cysts or calcified cysts are associated with seropositivity less often than are multiple cysts. CSF titers are higher if cysts are near the meninges.

C. Differential Diagnosis

The differential diagnosis of neurocysticercosis includes tuberculous granuloma, echinococcosis, microabscesses, arachnoid cyst, neoplasms, and vascular lesions. Identification of a scolex is pathognomonic for NCC.

► Treatment

A. Taeniasis

Oral praziquantel (5–10 mg/kg once) can be used for treatment of tapeworm carriers. Caution should be used in patients from endemic areas for *T solium* as treatment can precipitate neurologic symptoms in those with asymptomatic NCC. Stool should be reexamined 3 months after treatment to document cure as praziquantel does not kill *Taenia* eggs. Niclosamide (50 mg/kg once, maximum 2 g) is an alternative treatment but is not available in the United States.

B. Cysticercosis

The treatment modalities for NCC include cysticidal agents (to kill larvae), corticosteroids (to decrease or prevent the inflammatory reaction), antiepileptic drugs (to control seizures if present), and surgery (to remove cysts or for placement of a shunt for hydrocephalus). Treatment should be tailored based on location, number, and stage of observed cysts. Treatment with a cysticidal agent is indicated in most cases of NCC, except in patients with inactive, calcified lesions. In patients with viable parenchymal cysts, cysticidal therapy decreases the burden of parasites and the number of seizures. Similarly, cysticidal therapy is associated with more complete and faster resolution on imaging and fewer seizures in patients with a single, small enhancing lesion. Ophthalmic examination should be conducted prior to cysticidal therapy to rule out intraocular cysts; the presence of these may require surgical removal and/or the use of steroids to prevent inflammatory responses to antiparasitic treatment.

Albendazole, 15 mg/kg/day (maximum, 800 mg for single enhancing lesions or 1200 mg for viable non-calcified cysts) divided in two doses daily for 8–15 days, is the treatment of choice. Larval death may result in clinical worsening because of inflammatory edema. A concurrent course of dexamethasone (0.1 mg/kg/day to a maximum of 6 mg/day) or prednisolone (1 mg/kg/day to a maximum of 40–60 mg) is recommended to decrease these symptoms. Patients with greater than two intraparenchymal lesions may benefit from co-administration of albendazole and praziquantel (50 mg/kg/day) in addition to corticosteroids. Corticosteroids are mandatory treatment for large intraventricular cysts and encephalitis (dexamethasone 0.1 mg/kg/day or prednisolone 1 mg/kg/day for as long as needed). Giant subarachnoid cysts may require more than one cycle of therapy or surgery (or both). Minimally invasive neurosurgery (neuroendoscopy) is recommended for removal of intraventricular cysts. Follow-up scans every several months help assess the response to therapy. Calcified lesions are considered nonviable and do not require treatment with antiparasitics. Patients with seizures related to NCC should also receive anti-epileptic drugs.

Prevention

Prevention of taeniasis requires proper cooking of meat; freezing will also inactivate viable cysts. Neurocysticercosis is prevented by careful washing of raw vegetables and fruits, treating intestinal carriers, avoiding the use of human excrement for fertilizer, and providing proper sanitary facilities. In patients with NCC acquired in nonendemic areas, household members should be screened for tapeworm carriage.

Prognosis

The prognosis is good in intestinal taeniasis. Symptoms associated with a few cerebral cysts may disappear in a few months; heavy brain infections may cause death or chronic neurologic impairment. Seizures may persist even in those patients with only calcified lesions and anticonvulsants may be needed indefinitely.

Bustos JA et al: Frequency and determinant factors for calcification in neurocysticercosis. Clin Infect Dis 2021;73(9):e2592 [PMID: 32556276].

Centers for Disease Control and Prevention. Parasites—Cysticercosis. http://www.cdc.gov/parasites/cysticercosis/. Accessed April 21, 2023.

White AC Jr et al: Diagnosis and treatment of neurocysticercosis: 2017 clinical practice guidelines by the Infectious Diseases Society of America (IDSA) and the American Society of Tropical Medicine and Hygiene (ASTMH). Clin Infect Dis 2018;66(8):1159–1163 [PMID: 29481580].

2. Echinococcosis

ESSENTIALS OF DIAGNOSIS & TYPICAL FEATURES

▶ Cystic tumors of the liver and lungs, rarely kidneys, bones, brain, and other organs.

▶ Eosinophilia.

▶ Urticaria and pruritus if cysts rupture.

▶ Protoscoleces or daughter cysts in the primary cyst.

▶ Positive serology.

▶ Epidemiologic evidence of exposure.

▶ General Considerations

Two species of *Echinococcus*, *Echinococcus granulosus* and *Echinococcus multilocularis*, can cause disease in humans. The two forms of echinococcus, cystic and alveolar, cause significant morbidity and mortality worldwide. Cystic echinococcus is endemic in many areas of the developing world, and alveolar echinococcus is typically found in far northern latitudes. Dogs and other canids are the definitive host for *E granulosis* and become infected through ingestion of infected organs of numerous herbivorous animals (especially sheep, but also goats, swine, horses, cattle, and camels) that serve as intermediate hosts. For *E multilocularis*, foxes are the principle definitive hosts and rodents are the intermediate hosts. Human infection occurs following incidental ingestion of eggs in canid stool. When ingested by humans, the eggs hatch and the larvae penetrate the intestinal mucosa and disseminate via the bloodstream to produce cysts in multiple organs. The primary sites of involvement are the liver (60%–70%) and the lungs (20%–25%). A unilocular cyst is most common. Cysts grow slowly over several years and may reach 25 cm in diameter, although most are much smaller. The cysts of *E multilocularis* are multilocular and demonstrate more rapid growth.

▶ Clinical Findings

A. Symptoms and Signs

The clinical manifestations of echinococcosis are variable and depend primarily on the site, size, and condition of the cysts. The rates of growth of cysts are variable, and range between 1 and 5 cm in diameter per year. In cystic echinococcus, a slowly growing single cyst often goes unnoticed until it causes dysfunction due to its size. Hepatomegaly, right upper quadrant pain, nausea, and vomiting may occur. Cysts may cause biliary obstruction. Most hepatic cysts are in the right lobe. Alveolar echinococcus typically begins in the liver but is characterized by a tumor-like lesion that can invade, necrose, and metastasize. If a cyst ruptures, the sudden release of its contents can result in a severe allergic reaction and death.

Rupture of a pulmonary cyst causes coughing, dyspnea, wheezing, urticaria, chest pain, and hemoptysis; cyst and worm remnants are found in sputum. Brain cysts may cause focal neurologic signs and convulsions; renal cysts cause pain and hematuria; bone cysts cause pain.

B. Laboratory Findings

Antibody assays are useful to support the diagnosis following identification of a cystic lesion on imaging, and available ELISA tests have high sensitivity. Immunoblot assays and direct parasitologic examination are necessary to confirm the presence of echinococcosis. Eosinophilia is present in only about 25% of patients. Abnormal liver enzymes may suggest biliary obstruction.

C. Imaging

The presence of a cyst-like mass in a person with appropriate epidemiologic exposure supports the diagnosis. Visualization of daughter cysts (cysts within a larger cyst) is highly suggestive of echinococcosis. CT, MRI, and ultrasonography are useful for the diagnosis of deep-seated lesions. Abdominal ultrasonography is the most widely used diagnostic tool and can be used to classify and stage abdominal cysts. Pulmonary or bone cysts may be visible on plain films.

▶ Differential Diagnosis

Tumors, bacterial or amebic abscess, cavitary pulmonary tuberculosis, mycoses, and benign cysts must be considered.

▶ Treatment

There is no "best" treatment option for cystic echinococcus, and no clinical trial has compared all the different treatment modalities. Treatment recommendations for cystic echinococcosis vary with staging based on WHO classification. Chemotherapy alone cures about one-third of patients. Albendazole (15 mg/kg/day divided in two doses for 3 months, max 400 mg twice daily), sometimes with the addition of praziquantel, is the regimen of choice. Definitive therapy of *E multilocularis* may require meticulous surgical removal of the cysts. Albendazole chemotherapy should be initiated for several days prior to surgery. A third treatment option is a four-step procedure (PAIR: puncture, aspiration, injection, and reaspiration). This procedure consists of (1) percutaneous puncture using ultrasound guidance, (2) aspiration of liquid contents, (3) injection of a protoscolicidal agents (95% ethanol or hypertonic saline for at least 15 minutes), and (4) reaspiration. PAIR is indicated for uncomplicated cases, or those not amenable to surgery. If the cyst leaks or ruptures during surgical or percutaneous drainage a severe, potentially life-threatening allergic reaction may occur. For alveolar echinococcus, radical surgery for complete resection of the cyst is the goal. In some patients (particularly in whom complete resection is not possible), lifetime chemotherapy may be required.

▶ Prognosis

Patients with large liver cysts may be asymptomatic for years. Surgery is often curative for lung and liver cysts, but not always for cysts in other locations.

Brunetti E et al: Expert consensus for the diagnosis and treatment of cystic and alveolar echinococcosis in humans. Acta Trop 2010;114(1):1–16. doi:10.1016/j.actatropica/2009.11.001 [PMID: 19931502].

Centers for Disease Control and Prevention. Parasites—Echinococcosis. http://www.cdc.gov/parasites/echinococcosis/. Accessed April 14, 2023.

Velasco-Tirado V et al: Medical treatment of cystic echinococcosis: systematic review and meta-analysis. BMC Infect Dis 2018;18:306. doi:10.1186/s12879-018-3201-y [PMID: 29976137].

Wen H et al: Echinococcosis: advances in the 21st century. Clin Microbiol Rev 2019;32(2):e00075-18. doi:10.1128/CMR.00075-18 [PMID: 30760475].

TREMATODE (FLUKE) INFECTIONS

Schistosomiasis

ESSENTIALS OF DIAGNOSIS & TYPICAL FEATURES

- ▶ Transient pruritic rash after exposure to freshwater.
- ▶ Fever, urticaria, arthralgias, cough, lymphadenitis, and eosinophilia.
- ▶ Weight loss, anorexia, hepatosplenomegaly, or hematuria.
- ▶ Eggs in stool, urine, or rectal biopsy specimens.

▶ General Considerations

One of the most common serious parasitic diseases, schistosomiasis, is caused by several species of *Schistosoma* flukes. *Schistosoma japonicum*, *Schistosoma mekongi*, and *Schistosoma mansoni* involve the intestines, and *Schistosoma haematobium* involves the urinary tract. The first two species are found in eastern and southeastern Asia; *S mansoni* in tropical Africa, the Caribbean, and parts of South America; and *S haematobium* in Africa.

Infection is caused by free-swimming larvae (cercariae), which emerge from freshwater snails that serve as the intermediate host. The cercariae penetrate human skin, migrate to the liver, and mature into adults, which then migrate through the portal vein to lodge in the bladder veins (*S haematobium*), superior mesenteric veins (*S mekongi* and *S japonicum*), or inferior mesenteric veins (*S mansoni*). Clinical disease results primarily from inflammation caused by the many eggs that are laid in the perivascular tissues or that embolize to the liver. Escape of ova into bowel or bladder lumen allows microscopic visualization and diagnosis from stool or urine specimens, as well as contamination of freshwater and infection of the snail hosts that ingest them.

▶ **Clinical Findings**

Much of the population in endemic areas is infected but asymptomatic. Only heavy infections produce symptoms.

A. Symptoms and Signs

Schistosomiasis is characterized by both acute and chronic disease states. The cercarial penetration may cause a maculopapular, pruritic rash, comprising discrete, erythematous, raised lesions that vary in size from 1 to 3 cm. The symptoms of acute schistosomiasis (Katayama syndrome) can last from days to weeks, and can include fever, malaise, cough, diarrhea, hematuria, and right upper quadrant pain. The chronic stages of gastrointestinal disease are characterized by hepatic fibrosis, portal hypertension, splenomegaly, ascites, and bleeding from esophageal varices. The chronic stages of genitourinary tract disease may result in obstructive uropathy, stones, infection, bladder cancer, fistulas, and anemia due to chronic hematuria. Terminal hematuria in children from an endemic region is a red flag for urinary schistosomiasis. Urogenital schistosomiasis in young girls can lead to chronic pelvic pain, infertility, ectopic pregnancies and increase the risk of contracting human immunodeficiency virus. Spinal cord granulomas and paraplegia due to egg embolization into the Batson plexus have been reported. Epidemiologic studies demonstrate a negative impact of schistosomiasis on educational and cognitive development among school-age children. An isolated dermatitis syndrome ("swimmer's itch") is caused by nonhuman *Schistosoma* species that die after penetrating the skin.

B. Laboratory Findings

The diagnosis is made by finding the species-specific eggs in feces (*S japonicum*, *S mekongi*, *S mansoni*, and occasionally *S haematobium*) or urine (*S haematobium* and occasionally *S mansoni*). If no eggs are found, concentration methods should be used. Because the shedding of eggs can vary, three specimens should be obtained. Urine specimens should be collected between 10 AM and 2 PM when maximal egg secretion occurs. Postexposure testing in asymptomatic patients should wait until 2 months after the last known freshwater contact as this is the time required for worms to start producing eggs following infection. Serologic tests are also useful, especially for making the diagnosis in patients who are not excreting eggs. Peripheral eosinophilia is common, and eosinophils may be seen in urine.

▶ **Prevention**

The best prevention is to avoid contact with contaminated freshwater in endemic areas. Efforts to destroy the snail hosts have been successful in areas of accelerated economic development.

▶ **Treatment**

A. Specific Measures

Praziquantel is the treatment of choice for schistosomiasis. A dosage of 40 mg/kg/day in two divided doses (*S mansoni* or *S haematobium*) over 1 day or 60 mg/kg/day in three divided doses (*S japonicum* or *S mekongi*) over 1 day is very effective and nontoxic. Praziquantel has limited effect on eggs and immature worms, and therefore a repeat dose 4–6 weeks later is sometimes needed. Eosinophilia may take several weeks to resolve after treatment.

B. General Measures

The patient's urinary tract should be evaluated carefully in *S haematobium* infection; reconstructive surgery may be needed. Hepatic fibrosis requires careful evaluation of the portal venous system and medical and surgical management of portal hypertension when appropriate.

▶ **Prognosis**

Therapy decreases the worm burden and liver size, despite continued exposure in endemic areas. Early disease responds well to therapy, but once significant scarring or severe inflammation has occurred, changes may not be reversible with anti-parasitic treatment.

Centers for Disease Control and Prevention. Parasites—Schistosomiasis. http://www.cdc.gov/parasites/schistosomiasis/. Accessed April 14, 2023.

Ezeamama AE et al: Cognitive deficits and educational loss in children with schistosome infection—a systematic re-view and meta-analysis. PLoS Negl Trop Dis 2018 Jan 12;12(1):e0005524. doi:10.1371/journal.pntd.0005524 [PMID: 29329293].

Kramer CV et al: Drugs for treating urinary schistosomiasis. Cochrane Database Syst Rev 2014;8:CD000053. doi:10.1002/14651858.CD000053.pub3 [PMID: 25099517].

MYCOTIC INFECTIONS

Fungi can be classified as yeasts, which are unicellular and reproduce by budding; as molds, which are multicellular and consist of tubular structures (hyphae) and grow by elongation and branching; or as dimorphic fungi, which can exist either as yeasts or molds depending on environmental conditions. Categorization according to anatomic and epidemiologic features is shown in Table 43–3. Fungal cells are taxonomically distinct from plant and animal cells. These differences, especially cell wall and cell membrane components, are utilized for diagnosis and are the basis of specific therapy.

In the United States, systemic fungal disease in normal hosts is commonly caused by three endemic organisms—*Coccidioides*, *Histoplasma*, and *Blastomyces*—which are restricted to certain geographic areas. Prior residence in or travel to these areas, even for a brief time, is a prerequisite for inclusion in a differential diagnosis.

Immunosuppression (especially depressed T-cell–mediated immunity), foreign bodies (eg, urinary and central catheters for *Candida*), ulceration of gastrointestinal and respiratory mucosa, severe burns, broad-spectrum antimicrobial therapy, malnutrition, HIV infection, and neutropenia or neutrophil defects are major risk factors for fungal infections (termed "opportunistic fungal infections"). Fungi, particularly *Candida*, are frequent causes of nosocomial infection; *Candida auris* is a highly resistant hospital-acquired infection that represents an emerging global health threat.

Laboratory diagnosis may be difficult because of the small number of fungi present in some lesions, slow growth of some organisms, and difficulty in distinguishing normal colonization of mucosal surfaces from infection. A tissue biopsy with fungal stains and culture is the best method for diagnosing some systemic fungal disease. Repeat blood cultures may be negative even in the presence of intravascular infections. Serologic tests are useful for diagnosing coccidioidomycosis and histoplasmosis, and antigen detection in urine and blood is useful for diagnosing blastomycosis, histoplasmosis, cryptococcosis, and aspergillosis.

The common superficial fungal infections of the hair and skin are discussed in Chapter 15.

Casadevall A: Fungal diseases in the 21st century: the near and far horizons. Pathog Immun 2018;3(2):183–196. doi:10.20411/pai.v3i2.249 [PMID: 30465032].
Centers for Disease Control and Prevention: Fungal diseases: https://www.cdc.gov/fungal/index.html. Accessed June 25, 2021.

Table 43–3. Pediatric fungal infections.

Type	Agents	Incidence	Diagnosis	Diagnostic Tests	Therapy	Prognosis
Superficial	*Candida*[a] Dermatophytes *Malassezia*	Very common	Simple	KOH prep	Topical/Oral	Good
Subcutaneous	*Sporothrix*[a]	Uncommon	Simple[b]	Culture	Oral	Good
Systemic: normal host (endemic)	*Coccidioides* *Histoplasma* *Blastomyces*	Common: regional	Often presumptive	Chest radiograph; serology, antigen detection; tissue biopsy, culture	None[c] or systemic	Good
Systemic: opportunistic infection	*Candida*[a] *Pneumocystis*[d] *Aspergillus* Mucorales *Malassezia* *Pseudallescheria* *Cryptococcus*[c]	Uncommon	Difficult[e]	Tissue biopsy, culture, antigen/ fungal product/ DNA detection and NMR for *Candida*	Systemic, prolonged	Poor if therapy is delayed and patient is severely immune compromised

KOH, potassium hydroxide; NMR, nuclear magnetic resonance.
[a]*Candida* and *Sporothrix* in immunocompromised patients may cause severe, rapidly progressive disease and require systemic therapy.
[b]Sporotrichosis may require biopsy for diagnosis.
[c]Can be self-limited in normal host.
[d]Asymptomatically infects many normal hosts.
[e]Except *Cryptococcus*, which is often diagnosed by antigen detection.

Candidiasis

ESSENTIALS OF DIAGNOSIS & TYPICAL FEATURES

▶ In normal or immunosuppressed individuals: superficial infections (oral thrush or ulcerations, vulvovaginitis, erythematous intertriginous rash with satellite lesions); candidemia related to intravascular devices.

▶ In immunosuppressed individuals: systemic infections (candidemia with renal, hepatic, splenic, pulmonary, or cerebral abscesses); chorioretinitis; cutaneous nodules.

▶ In either patient population: budding yeast and pseudohyphae are seen in biopsy specimens, body fluids, or scrapings of lesions; positive culture and PCR methods for diagnosing *Candida* in body fluids.

▶ General Considerations

Disease due to *Candida* is caused by *Candida albicans* in greater than 50% of cases in children; severe systemic infection may also be caused by *Candida tropicalis*, *Candida parapsilosis*, *Candida glabrata*, *Candida krusei*, and a few other *Candida* species. *C auris* is frequently highly drug-resistant, has been associated with outbreaks in health care settings, and is a growing global health threat. Speciation is important because of differences in pathogenicity and susceptibility to antifungal therapy.

C albicans frequently colonizes the skin, mucous membranes, and intestinal tract. Normal bacterial flora, intact epithelial barriers, neutrophils, and macrophages, in conjunction with antibody and complement and normal lymphocyte function, are factors in preventing invasion. Disseminated infection is almost always preceded by prolonged broad-spectrum antibiotic therapy, instrumentation (including intravascular catheters), and/or immunosuppression. Patients with diabetes mellitus are prone to superficial *Candida* infection; thrush and vaginitis are most common. *Candida* is the fourth most common blood isolate in hospitals in the United States and is a common cause of catheter-related urinary tract infection.

▶ Clinical Findings

A. Symptoms and Signs

1. Oral candidiasis (Thrush)—Adherent creamy white plaques on the buccal, gingival, or lingual mucosa are seen. Lesions may be few and asymptomatic, or they may be extensive and painful, extending into the esophagus. Thrush is very common in immune-normal infants in the first weeks of life and may last weeks despite topical therapy. Spontaneous thrush in older children is unusual unless they have recently received antimicrobials. Corticosteroid inhalation for asthma predisposes patients to thrush. HIV infection or other immune deficiency should be considered if there is no other reason for oral thrush, especially when it is persistent or recurrent. Angular cheilitis is the name given to painful erythematous fissures caused by *Candida* at the corners of the mouth, occasionally in association with vitamin or iron deficiencies.

2. Vaginal infection (Details in Chapter 44; *Sexually Transmitted Diseases*)— Risk factors for vulvovaginitis in girls include being sexually active, diabetes, recent antibiotic use, oral contraception and pregnancy. Thick, odorless, cheesy discharge with intense pruritus is typical. The vagina and labia are usually erythematous and swollen. Episodes are more frequent before menses.

3. Skin infection

A. DERMATITIS—Diaper dermatitis is often due entirely or partly to *Candida*. Pronounced erythema with a sharply defined margin and satellite lesions is typical. Pustules, vesicles, papules, or scales may be seen. Weeping, eroded lesions with a scalloped border are common. Any moist area, such as axillae, under breasts, and inguinal or neck folds, may be involved.

B. SCATTERED RED PAPULES OR NODULES—Such findings in immunocompromised patients may represent cutaneous dissemination.

C. PARONYCHIA AND ONYCHOMYCOSIS—These conditions occur in immunocompetent children but more commonly with immunosuppression, hypoparathyroidism, or adrenal insufficiency (*Candida* endocrinopathy syndrome). The selective absence of specific innate and T-cell responses to *Candida* can lead to marked, chronic skin and nail infections called chronic mucocutaneous candidiasis.

D. CHRONIC DRAINING OTITIS—*Candida* may contribute to chronic otorrhea among patients with tympanostomy tubes and otitis externa, particularly after exposure to multiple antibiotic courses.

4. Enteric infection—Esophageal involvement in immunocompromised patients is the most common enteric manifestation, resulting in substernal pain, dysphagia, and painful swallowing. Most patients do not have thrush. Stomach or intestinal ulcers also occur. Candidal peritonitis can occur following intestinal perforation.

5. Pulmonary infection—Because the organism frequently colonizes the upper respiratory tract, it is commonly isolated from respiratory secretions. Thus, demonstration of tissue invasion is needed to diagnose *Candida* pneumonia or tracheitis. It is rare, seen mainly in immunosuppressed patients and patients intubated for long periods, usually while taking antibiotics or from septic emboli in the setting of high burden candidemia. The infection may cause abscesses, nodular infiltrates, and effusion.

6. Renal infection—Most often, candiduria is associated with instrumentation, an indwelling catheter, or anatomic abnormality of the urinary tract. Symptoms of cystitis may be present. Masses of *Candida* ("fungal balls") may obstruct ureters and cause obstructive nephropathy. *Candida* casts in the urine suggest renal tissue infection. Occasionally, candiduria may be the only manifestation of disseminated disease.

7. Other infections—Meningitis, and osteomyelitis usually occur only in immunocompromised patients or neonates, generally in those with high-grade candidemia. Endocarditis may occur on an artificial or abnormal heart valve, especially when an intravascular line is present.

8. Disseminated candidiasis—Skin and mucosal colonization precedes but does not predict dissemination. Disseminated candidiasis may resemble bacterial sepsis. Extremely premature and low-birth weight infants are particularly susceptible. Infants present with feeding intolerance, cardiovascular instability, apnea, new or worsening respiratory failure, glucose intolerance, thrombocytopenia, or hyperbilirubinemia. In addition to prematurity, indwelling venous catheters, broad spectrum antibiotics, parenteral lipid infusions, and immune compromise are common risk factors for invasive disease. A careful search in immunocompromised patients should be carried out for lesions suggestive of disseminated *Candida* (retinal cotton-wool spots or chorioretinitis; nodular dermal abscesses).

Hepatosplenic candidiasis is a form of chronic disseminated candidiasis. This diagnosis should be suspected in patients with recent severe neutropenia who develop chronic fever, abdominal pain, and abnormal liver function tests, particularly when no bacterial pathogen is isolated and there is no response to antibiotics. Imaging of the liver, spleen, and kidney demonstrates multiple, small, round hypodense lesions.

B. Laboratory Findings

Budding yeast cells are easily seen in scrapings or other samples. A wet mount preparation of vaginal secretions is 50%–70% sensitive with the addition of 10% potassium hydroxide to the sample. The use of a Gram-stained smear is 70%–100% sensitive. Stains for fungal cell walls will increase sensitivity. The presence of pseudohyphae suggests tissue invasion. Positive cultures from nonsterile sites or drawn from indwelling urinary catheters may reflect colonization and need to be carefully evaluated, but *Candida* should never be considered a contaminant in cultures from normally sterile sites. Standard blood culture liquid media will support

growth of *Candida* spp., but 10%–40% of cultures may remain negative even with disseminated disease or endocarditis. The presence of germ tubes when incubated in human serum gives a presumptive speciation for *C albicans*. Newly available nuclear magnetic resonance spectroscopy and PCR methods greatly shorten the delay in diagnosis and speciation.

▶ Differential Diagnosis

Thrush may resemble milk or formula (which can be easily wiped away with a tongue blade or swab, revealing normal mucosa without underlying erythema or erosion), other types of ulcers (including herpes), or oral changes induced by chemotherapy. Skin lesions may resemble contact, allergic, chemical, or bacterial dermatitis; miliaria; folliculitis; or eczema. Vulvovaginitis needs to be distinguished from other causes of vaginal discharge and discomfort. Candidemia is difficult to differentiate from bacterial sepsis and should be considered in any seriously ill patient with the risk factors previously mentioned.

▶ Complications

Candidal endophthalmitis can occur as a result of candidemia. It is recommended all patients with candidemia receive a dilated fundoscopic examination. Arthritis and meningitis occur more often in neonates than in older children. Abscesses can occur in any organ and should be suspected with on-going candidemia. The greater the length or extent of immunosuppression and the longer the delay before therapy, the more likely that complications will occur.

▶ Treatment

A. Oral Candidiasis

In infants, oral nystatin suspension (100,000 units four to six times a day in the buccal fold after feeding for 2–3 days after resolution) usually suffices. Nystatin must come in contact with the lesions because it is not absorbed systemically. Older children may use it as a mouthwash (200,000–500,000 units five times a day), although it is poorly tolerated because of its taste. Clotrimazole troches (10 mg) four times a day are an alternative in older children. Prolonged therapy with either agent or more frequent dosing may be needed. Painting the lesions with a cotton swab dipped in gentian violet (0.5%–1%) is visually dramatic and messy but may help refractory cases. Eradication of *Candida* from pacifiers, bottle nipples, toys, or the mother's breasts (if the infant is breast-feeding and there is candidal infection of the nipples) may be helpful.

Oral azoles, such as fluconazole (6 mg/kg/day), are effective in older children with candidal infection refractory to nystatin. Discontinuation of antibiotics or corticosteroids is advised when possible. Esophageal candidiasis should be treated with systemic therapy as described later.

B. Skin Infection

Cutaneous infection usually responds to a cream or lotion containing nystatin, amphotericin B, or an imidazole (miconazole, clotrimazole, naftifine, and others). Associated inflammation such as severe diaper dermatitis is helped by the concurrent use of a topical low concentration corticosteroid cream, such as 1% hydrocortisone. It may help to keep the involved area dry. Suppression of intestinal *Candida* with nystatin and eradicating thrush may speed recovery and prevent recurrence of diaper dermatitis.

C. Vaginal Infections

Vulvovaginal candidiasis (see Chapter 44) is treated with clotrimazole, miconazole, triazoles, or nystatin (cheapest if generic is used) suppositories or creams, usually applied once nightly for 3–7 days. A high-dose topical clotrimazole formulation can be given for only a single night. Oral azole therapy is equally effective. A single 150-mg oral dose of fluconazole is effective for vaginitis in older girls. Frequent recurrent infections (often with *C glabrata*) may require elimination of risk factors, the use of oral therapy, or prophylactic antifungal therapy, such as a single dose of fluconazole weekly for 6 months.

D. Renal Infection

Candiduria in an immunocompetent host with a urinary catheter may respond to catheter removal. Candiduria should be treated in all high-risk patients, usually with 14-day course of fluconazole (3–6 mg/kg/day), which is concentrated in the urine. Amphotericin B is required for patients with fluconazole-resistant organisms. Echinocandins are generally avoided given poor concentration in the urine, though they penetrate the renal parenchyma well. Renal abscesses or ureteral fungus balls may require surgical intervention in addition to systemic antifungal therapy. Removal of an indwelling catheter is imperative.

E. Systemic Infection

1. Disseminated *Candida* infection—Systemic infection is dangerous and resistant to therapy. Surgical drainage of abscesses and removal of all infected tissue (eg, a heart valve) are required for cure. It is essential to be aware that candidal species vary in susceptibility patterns, and even among species that are more broadly susceptible, prior antifungal exposure may increase the risk of a resistant organism; consultation with an infectious disease specialist is recommended. For most disseminated candidal infections, an echinocandin is the preferred initial therapy. Micafungin and caspofungin are currently FDA-approved for pediatric patients. The initial dose and maintenance dosing varies with the drug chosen. Fluconazole may be substituted after 5–7 days if the response to therapy is satisfactory. Fluconazole as initial therapy is an alternative for selected patients who are not critically ill and who are likely to have a sensitive organism. Lipid formulations of amphotericin are alternatives when other drugs are not tolerated or when the isolate has an unfavorable resistance pattern.

Susceptibility testing for *Candida* species is available to guide antifungal decisions, and some susceptibility patterns can be inferred by species identification. *C glabrata* and *C krusei* are common isolates that may be resistant to fluconazole; these are often susceptible to the newer azoles and echinocandins. *Candida lusitaniae* is usually resistant to amphotericin. Many isolates of *C auris* are azole and amphotericin resistant; in the United States, most isolates remain susceptible to the echinocandins.

To prevent recurrence, hepatosplenic candidiasis is often treated until all lesions have disappeared or calcified. Selected patients with prolonged immunosuppression (eg, after hematopoietic stem cell transplantation) should receive prophylactic azole or echinocandin prophylaxis.

2. Candidemia—Infected central venous lines should be removed as soon as possible. If the infection is considered limited to the line and environs, a 14-day course (after the last positive culture) of a systemic antifungal agent following line removal is recommended for nonneutropenic patients. An echinocandin is preferred, with completion of therapy with fluconazole when sensitivity is established. Persistent fever and candidemia suggest infected thrombus, endocarditis, or tissue infection. All such patients should be examined by an ophthalmologist.

3. Very-low-birth-weight infants—Rates of severe *Candida* infection can exceed 5%–10% in some nurseries. Infected infants should receive intravenous amphotericin B (1 mg/kg/day) until demonstration of clinical improvement and then can be switched to fluconazole (12 mg/kg IV or PO) if the isolate is susceptible. Treatment should continue until 2 weeks after the last positive culture. Lumbar puncture and eye examination should be performed. Prophylaxis with fluconazole (3 mg/kg twice weekly) or oral nystatin (100,000 units three times daily) for 6 weeks should be considered for very-low-birth-weight neonates in nurseries with rates of invasive candidiasis greater than 10%.

▶ Prognosis

Superficial disease in normal hosts has a good prognosis; in abnormal hosts, it may be refractory to therapy. Early therapy of systemic disease is often curative if the underlying immune response is adequate. The outcome is poor when therapy is delayed or when host response is inadequate. Candidemia in the severely premature neonate increases the chance of death and poor neurodevelopmental outcome.

Candidiasis. In: Kimberlin DW et al (eds): Red Book: 2021 Report of the Committee on Infectious Diseases. 32nd ed. Elk Grove Village, IL: American Academy of Pediatrics; 2021:246–252.

Forsberg K et al: *Candida auris*: the recent emergence of a multi-drug-resistant fungal pathogen. Med Mycol 2019 Jan;57(1):1–12 [PMID: 30715430].

Pappas PG et al: Executive summary: clinical practice guideline for the management of candidiasis: 2016 update by the Infectious Diseases Society of America. Clin Infect Dis 2016 Feb 15;62(4):409–417 [PMID: 26810419].

Endemic mycoses

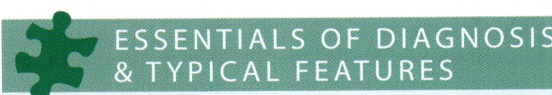

ESSENTIALS OF DIAGNOSIS & TYPICAL FEATURES

▶ Residence in, or travel to, an endemic area.

▶ In immunocompetent patients, most often subclinical infection or self-limited respiratory illness; acute pneumonia in a minority of cases.

▶ Severe pneumonia, extrapulmonary manifestations and disseminated disease typically occur in heavily immunocompromised patients.

▶ Diagnosis by histopathology with characteristic appearance, culture from tissue, bronchoalveolar lavage fluid or serologic testing.

▶ General Considerations

The most common endemic mycoses in the United States are blastomycosis, coccidioidomycosis, and histoplasmosis. The etiology of these mycoses are thermally dimorphic fungi that exist in the environment as nonpathogenic molds, but at body temperature within the human host they become pathogenic yeast. Each is localized to specific geographic regions.

Blastomycosis: The responsible fungi, *Blastomyces dermatitidis* or *Blastomyces gilchristii*, are found in soil primarily in the Mississippi and Ohio River valley, southeastern and south- central states, and states bordering the Great Lakes. *Blastomyces helices* is a rare but emerging pathogen in western regions of North America and is morphologically distinct from *B dermatitidis*.

Coccidioidomycosis: Coccidioidomycosis is caused by *Coccidioides immitis* or *posadasii*, endemic to the Sonoran Desert areas of the American Southwest and northern Mexico, southern California, eastern Oregon and Washington, and South America. The vast majority of reported cases in the United States come from Arizona and California. Arthospores are highly contagious and readily airborne in dry, windy climates.

Histoplasmosis: *Histoplasma capsulatum*, the causative fungus of histoplasmosis, is found in the central and eastern United States (Ohio, Mississippi, and Missouri River Valleys) and likely has a wide global distribution. Soil contamination is enhanced by the presence of bat or bird feces. Prior residence in or travel to these areas, even for a brief time, is a prerequisite for inclusion in a differential diagnosis.

Though each of these endemic fungal infections has unique epidemiologic and clinical characteristics, they share many features. Infections primarily results from inhalation of spores in the environment. Occasionally, direct inoculation of spores can cause disease in coccidioidomycosis. Human-to-human transmission does not occur except in the case of donor-derived infections associated with organ transplantation, particularly in the case of coccidioidomycosis. The extent of symptoms with primary infection or reinfection is influenced by the size of the infecting inoculum and immune status of the host. The majority of cases in immunocompetent individuals are asymptomatic or mild and self-limited. Symptomatic disease most often manifests as pneumonia that can be difficult to distinguish from other causes of community acquired and atypical pneumonia. Progressive pneumonia, extrapulmonary manifestations and disseminated disease are more likely to occur in immunocompromised hosts, particularly those with impaired cell-mediated immunity.

▶ Clinical Findings

A. Symptoms and Signs

Primary infection is subclinical in the majority of cases. Clinically apparent disease in immunocompetent patients most often manifests acute pulmonary disease that can mimic bacterial and viral pneumonia. This is typically self-limited. Subacute pulmonary infection may resemble tuberculosis with cough, weight loss, night sweats and pleurisy. Physical examination may be normal or rales may be heard. Less commonly, patients may have immune-mediated signs such as arthritis, pericarditis and erythema nodosum. Severe disease and disseminated infection is more likely to occur in immunocompromised patients. CNS disease can complicate any of the endemic mycoses.

Blastomycosis: Clinical disease due to *Blastomyces* typically includes cough with purulent sputum, chest pain, headache, weight loss, night sweats, and fever; some patients may progress to ARDS. Indolent progressive pulmonary disease is accompanied by extrapulmonary disease in approximately 25% of patients with blastomycosis. Cutaneous lesions are the most common extrapulmonary manifestation and are typically slowly progressive and ulcerative. Lytic bone disease can mimic chronic osteomyelitis and can affect any bone. Total body imaging should be pursued when extrapulmonary blastomycosis is diagnosed.

Coccidioidomycosis: Symptoms associated with primary infections due to *Coccidioides* vary from mild fever and arthralgia to severe influenza-like illness with high fever, nonproductive cough, pleuritic chest pains, arthralgias, headache, night sweats. Less than 5% of cases result in severe pulmonary disease. Chronic pulmonary infection is rare in children but may manifest as chronic cough, weight loss, and radiographic abnormalities. Up to 10% of children with coccidioidomycosis develop erythema nodosum or erythema multiforme. These manifestations imply a favorable host response to the organism. Sites of primary skin inoculation develop indurated ulcers with local adenopathy. Contiguous involvement of skin from deep infection in nodes or bone also occurs. The presence of chronic skin lesions should lead to a search for internal infection. Disseminated disease is more common in adults than children. Those at higher risk for disseminated coccidioidomycosis include neonates, pregnant women (especially during the third trimester), African Americans, Filipinos, Native Americans, and patients with HIV or other cellular immunity defects. The most common extrapulmonary sites involved are bone or joint (usually a single bone or joint; subacute or chronic inflammation), lymph nodes, and meninges (slowly progressive meningeal signs, ataxia, vomiting, headache, and cranial neuropathies).

Histoplasmosis: In endemic regions, over two-thirds of children are infected with *Histoplasma*. The majority of infections (90%) are asymptomatic and diagnosed incidentally when scattered calcifications are noted on imaging of the lungs or spleen. Approximately 5% of patients have mild-to-moderate pneumonia, which is often mistaken for influenza or another respiratory viral pneumonia. Acute pulmonary disease may present with fever, malaise, myalgia, arthralgia, and nonproductive cough occur 1–3 weeks after a heavy exposure. The subacute form may resemble other infections, such as tuberculosis, with cough, weight loss, night sweats, and pleurisy. Chronic disease is unusual in children. Immune-mediated signs such as arthritis, pericarditis, and erythema nodosum can occur less commonly. The usual duration of the disease is less than 2 weeks, followed by complete resolution, but without treatment, symptoms may occasionally last several months. Fungemia during primary infection is complicated by disseminated disease in approximately 5% of patients. Heavy exposure, severe underlying pulmonary disease, and immunocompromise are risk factors for progressive infection characterized by anemia, fever, weight loss, organomegaly, CNS or bone marrow involvement, and death. Adrenal gland involvement is common with systemic disease and the pericardium, intestines, skin and eyes can also be impacted.

B. Laboratory Findings

Definitive diagnosis of the endemic mycoses requires isolation or visualization of fungus in bodily fluid or tissue specimens. Each fungal organism has a characteristic appearance on histopathology.

Blastomycosis: *Blastomyces* infection is often associated with non-caseating granulomas and respiratory specimens may be positive using fungal cell wall stains. The budding

yeasts have refractile thick walls and are very large and distinctive (figure-of-eight appearance). The fungus can be readily isolated in most laboratories, but a week is often required. Sputum specimens are positive in more than 80% of cases and in almost all bronchial washings, and skin lesions are positive in 80%–100%.

Coccidioidomycosis: Respiratory secretions, pus, CSF, and tissue specimens may reveal large *Coccidioides* spherules (30–60 μm) containing endospores. Characteristic colonies grow within 2–5 days on routine fungal media. *Coccidioides* is a biohazard in culture so the laboratory should be informed prior to sending samples. Eosinophilia may occur prior to dissemination and is unique to coccidioidomycosis among the endemic mycoses.

Histoplasmosis: *Histoplasma* yeast forms are small and usually found in macrophages, but infrequently in sputum, urine, or CSF. Cultures of infected fluids or tissues may yield the organism after 1–4 weeks of incubation on fungal media but may be negative even in 15% of immunocompromised patients. Pancytopenia is common in patients with disseminated histoplasmosis and organisms may be seen infiltrating the bone marrow on biopsy.

Given the difficulty and potential hazards of growing endemic mycoses on culture, serologic antigen and antibody testing are often used to diagnose endemic mycoses. Detection of antigen in blood, urine, CSF, and bronchoalveolar lavage fluid is more sensitive in patients with disseminated disease and in immunocompromised hosts. Combining specimens may improve test performance. Cross-reactions with other fungal infections, including other endemic mycoses can occur.

Antibody testing is less helpful in **blastomycosis** but immunodiffusion, enzyme immunoassay (EIA), and complement fixation methods are often used in the diagnosis of coccidioidomycosis and histoplasmosis. For **coccidioidomycosis**, a sequential approach using the more sensitive EIA assay followed by confirmatory testing with the more specific immunodiffusion assay is often used. IgM antibodies arise early in infection but should be confirmed with IgG because of poor specificity. CSF and serum antibody titers correlate with disease progression and response to therapy. In **histoplasmosis**, EIA titers rise in the first 2–6 weeks of illness and fall thereafter unless dissemination occurs. A single high titer or a rising titer indicates a higher likelihood of disease. Antibody testing is less reliable in immunocompromised patients who cannot mount an antibody response and cross-reactions with other endemic fungi can occur. Molecular methods for detecting fungal DNA can be performed on multiple specimen types and may expedite the diagnosis.

C. Imaging

Each endemic mycosis has characteristic pulmonary radiographic presentations, though these vary between acute and chronic disease.

Blastomycosis: Radiographic features include lobar consolidations and fibronodular interstitial and patchy alveolar infiltrates in cases with progressive pneumonia. The paucity of cavitation and absence of hilar adenopathy distinguishes blastomycosis from coccidioidomycosis, histoplasmosis, and tuberculosis. Miliary patterns can occur with acute infection. Chronic disease can develop in the upper lobes, with cavities and fibronodular infiltrations similar to those seen in tuberculosis; however, these lesions rarely caseate or calcify.

Coccidioidomycosis: Approximately half of symptomatic infections with coccidioidomycosis are associated with abnormal chest radiographs—usually infiltrates with hilar adenopathy. Pulmonary consolidation, effusion, and thin-walled cavities may be seen. About 5% of infected patients have asymptomatic nodules or cysts after recovery. Unlike tuberculosis reactivation and histoplasmosis, apical disease is not prominent.

Histoplasmosis: Scattered pulmonary calcifications in a well-child are typical of past histoplasmosis. Acute histoplasmosis typically has focal mid-lung infiltrates, often with hilar and mediastinal adenopathy, occasionally with nodules, but seldom with effusion. Apical cavitation occurs with chronic infection, often on the background of preexisting pulmonary infection.

▶ Differential Diagnosis

Primary pulmonary infection is difficult to distinguish from other causes of atypical community acquired pneumonia. Endemic mycoses should be considered when a significant pulmonary infection in an endemic area fails to respond to antibiotic therapy. Subacute infection is similar among the major endemic mycoses and differentiation relies on epidemiologic exposures. Tuberculosis can mimic any of the endemic mycoses in clinical and radiographic presentation. Chronic pulmonary or disseminated disease must be differentiated from tuberculosis, cancer, or other fungal infections.

▶ Treatment

Blastomycosis: One view is that all children with proven blastomycosis should receive antifungal therapy to reduce disseminated disease; imperative if immunocompromised. Itraconazole (5–10 mg/kg/day; divided into two doses [maximum = 400 mg] for 6–12 months) is the preferred drug for mild to moderate infections. Mild-to-moderate blastomycosis is typically treated for 6–12 months. Bone disease is generally treated for 12 months. For severe, disseminated, or CNS disease, treatment with lipid or liposomal amphotericin B (3–5 mg/kg intravenously) should be initiated until clinical improvement. This is followed by prolonged therapy with an oral azole. Voriconazole should be used over itraconazole for CNS disease because of better drug penetration. Serum levels of itraconazole and voriconazole should be measured and optimized. Surgical debridement is required for devitalized bone and drainage of large abscesses or for pulmonary lesions not responding to medical therapy.

Coccidioidomycosis: In contrast to infections due to *Blastomyces* and *Histoplasma*, mild pulmonary infections due to *Coccidioides* in most immune competent patients do not require therapy, although some experts argue for treatment of all infections. Neonates, pregnant women, patients with high-risk racial backgrounds, and those with high antibody titers should also receive treatment. Untreated patients should be assessed for 1–2 years to document resolution and to identify any complications. Fluconazole is the preferred therapy for most forms of coccidioidomycosis, including meningeal disease. Use of amphotericin B intravenously (or sometimes intrathecally for CNS disease) is considered for refractory cases. Meningeal disease requires lifelong suppressive therapy. Surgical intervention should be considered for cavitary pulmonary lesions not responding to medical therapy and in patients with vertebral involvement. Neurosurgical evaluation and placement of a ventriculoperitoneal shunt should be considered in patients with who develop hydrocephalus from *Coccidioides* meningitis.

Histoplasmosis: Patients with acute pulmonary disease due to *Histoplasma* will benefit from oral itraconazole (3–5 mg/kg/day for 6–12 weeks). Those with subacute disease who remain symptomatic at the time of diagnosis should also receive oral therapy. Posaconazole is an alternative agent with good activity against all the endemic mycoses. Disseminated, CNS and chronic pulmonary histoplasmosis usually requires 4–6 weeks of IV therapy with lipid or liposomal amphotericin B followed by at least a year of oral azole therapy. Relapse of infection can occur in 15% of immunosuppressed patients with chronic pulmonary disease despite treatment. Chronically immunosuppressed patients may require lifelong maintenance therapy. Surgical excision of chronic pulmonary lesions is rarely required in patients with histoplasmosis.

▶ Prognosis

Patients with mild and moderately severe infections have a good prognosis. Disseminated and CNS disease portends a worse prognosis and may be fatal, especially in those with risk factors. With early diagnosis and treatment, children with disseminated disease usually recover; the prognosis worsens if the immune response is poor. Patients who are chronically immunosuppressed may have relapses of disease during or after treatment and may require lifetime antifungal suppressive therapy.

Frost HM et al: Blastomycosis in children: analysis of clinical, epidemiologic, and genetic features. J Pediatric Infect Dis Soc 2017;6:49 [PMID: 26703241].

Galgiani JN et al: 2016 Infectious Diseases Society of America (IDSA) Clinical Practice Guideline for the treatment of coccidioidomycosis. Clin Infect Dis 2016 Sep 15;63(6):e112–e146. https://doi.org/10.1093/cid/ciw360 [PMID: 27470238].

Maza-Morales M et al: Coccidioidomycosis in children and adolescents: an update. Curr Fungal Infect Rep 2020;14:106–114. doi: 10.1007/s12281-020-00381-8.

Oulette CP et al: Pediatric histoplasmosis in an area of endemicity: a contemporary analysis. J Pediatric Infect Dis Soc 2019 Nov 6;8(5):400–407. doi: 10.1093/jpids/piy073 [PMID: 30124985].

Rodrigues AM et al: The global epidemiology of emerging Histoplasma species in recent years. Stud Mycol 2020 Sep;97:100095 [PMID: 33335607].

Schwartz IS et al: Blastomyces helices, a new dimorphic fungus causing fatal pulmonary and systemic disease in humans and animals in Western Canada and the United States. Clin Infect Dis 2019 Jan;68(2):188–195 [PMID: 29878145].

Sporotrichosis

ESSENTIALS OF DIAGNOSIS & TYPICAL FEATURES

► Subacute cutaneous ulcers.

► New lesions appearing proximal to existing lesions along a draining lymphatic.

► Absence of systemic symptoms.

► Isolation of *Sporothrix schenckii* from wound drainage or biopsy.

General Considerations

Sporotrichosis is caused by *S schenckii*, a dimorphic fungus present as a mold in soil, plants, and plant products from most areas of North and South America. Spores of the fungus can cause infection when they breach the skin at areas of minor trauma. Zoonotic transmission has been reported, mostly associated with handling cats in South America.

Clinical Findings

Cutaneous disease is by far the most common manifestation. Typically, at the site of inapparent skin injury, an initial painless papular lesion will slowly become nodular and ulcerate. Subsequent new lesions develop in a similar fashion proximally along lymphatics draining the primary lesion and this pattern is strongly suggestive of the diagnosis. Solitary lesions may exist and some lesions may develop a verrucous character. Systemic symptoms are absent and laboratory evaluations are normal, except for acute-phase reactants. The fungus rarely disseminates in immunocompetent hosts. Cavitary pneumonia is a rare manifestation when patients inhale the spores. Immunocompromised patients, especially those with HIV infection, may develop disseminated skin lesions and multiorgan disease with extensive pneumonia.

Differential Diagnosis

The differential diagnosis of nodular lymphangitis (sporotrichoid infection) includes other endemic fungi and some bacteria, especially nontuberculous mycobacteria and nocardiosis, dermal leishmaniasis, pyoderma gangrenosum, and syphilis. Diagnosis is made by culture. Biopsy of skin lesions is the best source for laboratory isolation and will demonstrate granulomatous inflammation and occasionally characteristic yeast.

Treatment & Prognosis

Treatment is with itraconazole (200 mg/day or 5 mg/kg/day divided BID) for 2–4 weeks after lesions heal, usually 3–6 months. Prognosis is excellent with lymphocutaneous disease in immunocompetent children. Pulmonary or osteoarticular disease, especially in immunocompromised individuals, requires longer therapy. Amphotericin B may be required for disseminated disease, CNS disease, and severe pulmonary disease. Surgical debridement may be required.

Gremiao IDB et al: Zoonotic epidemic of sporotrichosis: cat to human transmission. PLoS Pathog 2017 Jan 19;13(1):e1006077. doi:10.1371/journal.ppat.1006077 [PMID: 28103311].

Sporotrichosis. In: Kimberlin DW et al (eds): *Red Book: 2021 Report of the Committee on Infectious Diseases*. 32nd ed. Elk Grove Village, IL: American Academy of Pediatrics; 2021:676–677.

PNEUMOCYSTIS & OTHER OPPORTUNISTIC FUNGAL INFECTIONS

The title of this section indicates that fungi that are normally not pathogenic, or do not cause severe disease, may do so when given the *opportunity* by changes in host defenses. They occur most commonly when patients are treated with corticosteroids, antineoplastic drugs, biological modifiers, or radiation, thereby reducing the number and function of neutrophils and B and T cells. Inborn errors in immune function (such as combined immunodeficiency or chronic granulomatous disease) may also be complicated by these fungal infections. Opportunistic infections are facilitated by altering the normal flora with antibiotics and by disruption of mucous membranes or skin with antineoplastic therapy or indwelling lines and tubes. Many children who will have depressed phagocytic and T-cell–mediated immune function for long periods (eg, after hematopoietic stem cell transplants) should receive prophylaxis against fungal infection during the period of severe immune suppression, most often with fluconazole or an echinocandin.

Opportunistic fungal infections should always be included in the differential diagnosis of unexplained fever or pulmonary infiltrates in immunocompromised patients. These pathogens should be aggressively pursued with imaging studies and with tissue sampling when clues are available. Treatment should be undertaken with consultants who are expert in managing these infections.

Table 43–4 indicates that filamentous fungi are prominent causes of severe systemic fungal disease in immunocompromised patients. The most important opportunistic fungi are further described here.

Aspergillosis: *Aspergillus* species (usually A *fumigatus*) can cause subacute pneumonia and sinusitis and should be considered when these conditions do not respond to antibiotics in immunocompromised patients. *Aspergillus* species also commonly cause invasive disease in patients with chronic granulomatous disease. Imaging may suggest the etiology, but this is best diagnosed by aspiration or biopsy of infected tissues. A characteristic CT finding is the "halo sign," which is a ground-glass opacity surrounding a pulmonary nodule or mass. Detection of galactomannose and β-D-glucan in blood and alveolar fluid may be useful for the diagnosis of presumptive of aspergillosis. Interpretation of these results may be difficult, with greater uncertainty in pediatric patients. *Aspergillus* can also be diagnosed by detecting fungal cell wall components or by PCR. Voriconazole is the drug of choice for many *Aspergillus* infections, but both echinocandins and amphotericin B formulations are good alternatives in certain scenarios. Serum levels of voriconazole should be determined to guide therapy.

Mucormycosis: The *Mucoromycota* (usually *Mucorales*) similarly may cause a subacute pneumonia in immunocompromised patients. Poorly controlled diabetics with acidosis are at particular risk for severe sinusitis due to *Mucoromycota*, which can extend to the orbit and brain. Mucormycosis is also more common in patients receiving iron chelation or intensive chemotherapy. On imaging, the "reversed halo sign" of a focal rounded ground-glass opacity surrounded by a crescent or complete ring of consolidation may be seen. Notably, the fungal antigens galactomannose and β-D-glucan are absent in the Mucoromycota and are not useful for diagnosis. Newer broad range next generation sequencing assays may provide an earlier diagnosis for many invasive opportunistic fungal infections. Amphotericin B formulations are recommended as initial therapy for mucormycosis. Posaconazole and isavuconazole may be as effective and better tolerated, though data in children are limited, and these are most often used as step-down therapy once a patient has demonstrated sufficient clinical improvement or for refractory cases. The role of combination therapy is unclear in children but the addition of an echinocandin may be of some benefit in adult studies.

Cryptococcosis: Although *Cryptococcus*, particularly *C gattii*, can cause disease in the immunocompetent hosts living in the Pacific Northwest, it is more likely to be clinically apparent or more severe in immunocompromised patients. Though pneumonia occurs in one-third of patients, meningitis is the most common clinical presentation following hematogenous spread from a pulmonary focus. Symptoms of elevated intracranial pressure and fever occur over days to months. Patients with poorly controlled HIV are at especially high risk for cryptococcal meningitis. Focal mass lesions (cryptococcomas) may be detected in the CNS on neuroimaging. Cutaneous disease with papules and ulcerating nodules can also occur in the setting of disseminated disease. Though any organ can be impacted, eye involvement is especially common, with disseminated disease. *Cryptococcus* may be demonstrated with specific antigen testing. Patients with severe cryptococcosis should receive liposomal amphotericin B formulations. Cryptococcal meningitis requires the addition of flucytosine or fluconazole. Induction therapy for at least 2 weeks is followed by several weeks of consolidation therapy with fluconazole and prolonged reduced dose maintenance therapy, sometimes lifelong in immunocompromised hosts.

Invasive *Malassezia* infection: *Malassezia furfur* is a yeast that normally causes the superficial skin infection known as tinea versicolor (see Chapter 15). This organism is considered an opportunist when fungemia is associated with prolonged intravenous therapy, especially with central lines used for hyperalimentation. The yeast, which requires skin lipids for its growth, can infect lines when lipids are present in the infusate. Some species will grow in the absence of lipids. Unexplained fever and thrombocytopenia are common. Pulmonary infiltrates may be present. The diagnosis is facilitated by using special culture techniques. The infection will respond to removal of the line or the lipid supplement. Amphotericin B may hasten resolution.

Cornely OA et al: Global guideline for the diagnosis and management of mucormycosis: an initiative of the European Confederation of Medical Mycology in cooperation with the Mycoses Study Group Education and Research Consortium. Lancet Infect Dis 2019;19(12):e405–e421 [PMID: 31699664].

Huppler AR et al: Role of molecular biomarkers in the diagnosis of invasive fungal diseases in children. J Pediatric Infect Dis Soc 2017;6(S1):S32–S44 [PMID: 28927202].

Panel on Opportunistic Infections in HIV-Exposed and HIV-Infected Children: Guidelines for the Prevention and Treatment of Opportunistic Infections in HIV-Exposed and HIV-Infected Children: Department of Health and Human Services: https://clinicalinfo.hiv.gov/sites/default/files/guidelines/documents/pediatric-oi/guidelines-pediatric-oi.pdf. Accessed July 8, 2021.

Patterson TF et al: Practice guidelines for the diagnosis and management of aspergillosis: 2016 update by the Infectious Diseases Society of America. Clin Infect Dis 2016;63:e1–e60 [PMID: 27365388].

Table 43–4. Unusual fungal infections in children.

Organism	Predisposing Factors	Route of Infection	Clinical Disease	Diagnostic Tests	Therapy and Comments
Aspergillus species	None	Inhalation of spores	Allergic bronchopulmonary aspergillosis; wheezing, cough, migratory infiltrates, eosinophilia	Organisms in sputum; positive skin test; specific IgE antibody; elevated IgE levels.	Hypersensitivity to fungal antigens. Use steroids. Antifungals may not be needed.
	Immunosuppression	Inhalation of spores	Progressive pulmonary disease: consolidation, nodules, abscesses Sinusitis	Disseminated disease: usually lung, brain; occasionally intestine, kidney, heart, bone. Invades blood vessels. Demonstrate fungus in tissues by stain or culture; septate hyphae branching at 45-degree angle; detecting antigen/fungal components in blood or respiratory samples may be useful; PCR available at some sites.	Amphotericin B, voriconazole, and oral caspofungin are equally effective; these can be used in combination.
Cryptococcus species	Immunosuppression, HIV; residence in Pacific Northwest for *Cryptococcus gattii*	Inhalation	CNS disease: meningitis, mass lesion (cryptococcoma) Pneumonia Disseminated disease: papules, ulcerating nodules, lytic bone changes, eye involvement	Capsule easily visualized with methenamine silver staining. Culture: routine media; high volume for CSF culture recommended. Serum and CSF antigen testing highly sensitive and specific. Some CSF multiplex PCR panels include.	Amphotericin B for severe disease. Add flucytosine for meningitis. Followed by long-term consolidation and maintenance therapy with fluconazole. Lumbar drain for intracranial hypertension.
Malassezia furfur, M pachydermatis	Central venous catheter, usually lipid infusion (can occur in the absence of lipid)	Line infection from skin colonization	Sepsis Pneumonitis Thrombocytopenia Rash	Culture of catheter or blood on lipid-enriched media (for *M furfur; M pachydermatis* does not need lipid). Fungus may be seen in buffy coat.	Discontinuation of lipid may be sufficient. Remove catheter. Short-term amphotericin B may be added. Organism ubiquitous on normal skin; requires long-chain fatty acids for growth.
Mucorales (*Mucor, Rhizopus, Absidia*)	Immunosuppression, diabetic acidosis, iron overload	Inhalation, mucosal colonization	Rhinocerebral: sinus, nose, necrotizing vasculitis; central nervous system spread Pulmonary Disseminated: any organ	Demonstrate broad aseptate hyphae branching at 90-degree angles in tissues by stain. Culture: rapidly growing, fluffy fungus. Detecting antigen/fungal components in blood or respiratory samples may be useful.	Amphotericin B, surgical debridement; voriconazole and posaconazole also often effective or can be used as a second agent for combined therapy. Poor prognosis.
Scedosporium spp.	Immunosuppression Minor trauma Also near drowning events	Inhalation Cutaneous	Disseminated abscesses (lung, brain, liver, spleen, other) Mycetoma (most common)	Culture of pus or tissue. Yellow-white granules in pus. Culture.	Surgical drainage; voriconazole or caspofungin. Aggressive surgery.

CNS, central nervous system; CSF, cerebrospinal fluid; HIV, human immunodeficiency virus; IgE, immunoglobulin E; PCR, polymerase chain reaction.

PNEUMOCYSTIS JIROVECI INFECTION

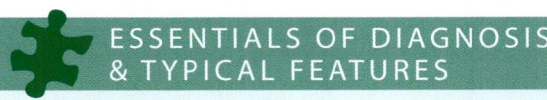

ESSENTIALS OF DIAGNOSIS & TYPICAL FEATURES

► Significant immunosuppression.

► Fever, tachypnea, cough, dyspnea.

► Hypoxemia; diffuse interstitial infiltrates.

► Detection of the organism in specimens of pulmonary origin.

► General Considerations

Although classified as a fungus on the basis of structural and nucleic acid characteristics, *Pneumocystis* responds readily to antiprotozoal drugs and antifolates. It is a ubiquitous pathogen. Initial infection is presumed to occur asymptomatically via inhalation, usually in early childhood, and to become a clinical problem upon reactivation associated with immune suppression. Person-to-person transmission may contribute to symptomatic disease in immunocompromised individuals. Clinical disease rarely occurs in the normal host. Whether by reactivation or new exposure, severe signs and symptoms occur chiefly in patients with abnormal T-cell function, such as hematologic malignancies and organ transplantation. *Pneumocystis* also causes severe pneumonia in patients with γ-globulin deficiency and is an AIDS-defining illness for children with advanced HIV infection. Prolonged, high-dose corticosteroid therapy for any condition is a risk factor. Prophylaxis usually prevents this infection (see Chapter 41).

Severely malnourished infants with no underlying illness may also develop this infection, as can those with congenital immunodeficiency. The incubation period is usually at least 1 month after onset of immunosuppressive therapy.

► Clinical Findings

A. Symptoms and Signs

In most patients, a gradual onset of fever, tachypnea, dyspnea, and mild, nonproductive cough occurs over 1–4 weeks. Initially the chest is clear, although retractions and nasal flaring are present. At this stage the illness is nonspecific. Hypoxemia out of proportion to the clinical and radiographic signs is an early finding; however, even minimally decreased arterial oxygen pressure values should suggest this diagnosis in immunosuppressed children. Tachypnea, nonproductive cough, and dyspnea progress. Respiratory failure and death occur without treatment. Acute dyspnea with pleuritic pain may indicate the complication of pneumothorax.

The general examination is unremarkable except for tachypnea and tachycardia; rales may be absent. Upper respiratory signs are absent.

B. Laboratory Findings

Laboratory findings reflect the underlying illness and are not specific. Serum lactate dehydrogenase levels may be elevated markedly as a result of pulmonary damage. In moderately severe cases, the arterial oxygen pressure is less than 70 mm Hg or the alveolar-arterial gradient is less than 35 mm Hg.

C. Imaging

Early chest radiographs are normal. The classic pattern in later films is bilateral, interstitial, lower lobe alveolar disease starting in the perihilar regions, without effusion, consolidation, or hilar adenopathy. High-resolution CT scanning may reveal extensive ground-glass attenuation or cystic lesions. Older HIV-infected patients present with other patterns, including nodular infiltrates, lobar pneumonia, cavities, and upper lobe infiltrates.

D. Diagnostic Findings

Diagnosis requires finding characteristic round (6–8 mm) cysts in a lung biopsy specimen, bronchial brushings, alveolar washings, induced sputum, or tracheal aspirates. Tracheal aspirates are less sensitive but are more rapidly and easily obtained. They are more often negative in children with leukemia compared with those with HIV infection; presumably, greater immunosuppression permits replication of a larger numbers of organisms. Because pneumonia in immunosuppressed patients may have many causes, negative results from tracheal secretions in suspected cases should prompt more aggressive diagnostic attempts. Bronchial washing using fiberoptic bronchoscopy is usually well tolerated and rapidly performed.

Several rapid stains—as well as the standard methenamine silver stain—are useful. The indirect fluorescent antibody method is more sensitive. These methods require competent laboratory evaluation, because few organisms may be present and many artifacts may be found. PCR methods are an important alternative but can reflect airways colonization and must be interpreted in the clinical context. Though 1,3-beta-D-glucan is a component of the organism's cell wall, sensitivity of serum testing for this antigen varies and it is more likely to be positive in the setting of high burden of disease and in patients with HIV.

► Differential Diagnosis

In immunocompetent infants, *C trachomatis* pneumonia is the most common cause of the afebrile pneumonia syndrome described for *Pneumocystis*. In older immunocompromised children, the differential diagnosis includes influenza, respiratory syncytial virus, cytomegalovirus, adenovirus, and other viral infections; bacterial and fungal pneumonia; pulmonary emboli or hemorrhage; congestive heart failure; and *Chlamydophila pneumoniae* and *Mycoplasma pneumoniae* infections. Lymphoid interstitial pneumonitis, which occurs in older infants with untreated HIV infection, is more indolent and the lactate dehydrogenase level is normal (see Chapter 41). *Pneumocystis* pneumonia is rare in children who are complying with prophylactic regimens.

▶ Prevention

Children at high risk for developing *Pneumocystis* infection should receive prophylactic therapy. Children at risk include those receiving chemotherapy for malignancy or high-dose corticosteroids, as well as those with organ or hematopoietic stem cell transplant or advanced HIV infection. All children born to HIV-infected mothers should receive prophylaxis against *Pneumocystis* starting at age 6 weeks unless HIV infection has been ruled out by tests for HIV in serum or the infant is presumed to be low risk for HIV. HIV-infected infants should receive therapy for the first year of life (see Chapter 41). The prophylaxis of choice is trimethoprim-sulfamethoxazole (150 mg/m²/day of trimethoprim and 750 mg/m²/day of sulfamethoxazole) for three consecutive days of each week. Alternatives to this prophylaxis regimen for children who cannot tolerate trimethoprim-sulfamethoxazole include atovaquone, dapsone, or aerosolized pentamidine, though these may be associated with more breakthrough infections. Intravenous pentamidine is sometimes considered for children with hematopoietic stem cell transplants.

▶ Treatment

A. General Measures

Supplemental oxygen and nutritional support may be needed. The patient should be in respiratory isolation.

B. Specific Measures

Trimethoprim-sulfamethoxazole (20 mg/kg/day of trimethoprim and 100 mg/kg/day of sulfamethoxazole in four divided doses is the treatment of choice. Intravenous treatment is indicated for moderate to severe disease with transition to oral after improvement, which may not be seen for 3–5 days. Duration of treatment is 3 weeks in HIV-infected children. Methylprednisolone (2–4 mg/kg/day in four divided doses intravenously) should also be given to patients with moderate to severe infection (partial oxygen pressure < 70 mm Hg or alveolar-arterial gradient > 35) for the first 5 days of treatment. The dosage is reduced by 50% for the next 5 days and further by 50% until antibiotic treatment is completed. If trimethoprim-sulfamethoxazole is not tolerated or there is no clinical response in 5 days, pentamidine isethionate (4 mg/kg once daily by slow intravenous infusion) should be given. Clinical efficacy is similar with pentamidine, but adverse reactions are more common. These reactions include dysglycemia, pancreatitis, nephrotoxicity, and leukopenia. Other effective alternatives utilized in adults include atovaquone, trimethoprim plus dapsone, and primaquine plus clindamycin.

▶ Prognosis

The mortality rate is high in immunosuppressed patients who receive treatment late in the illness.

Panel on Opportunistic Infections in HIV-Exposed and HIV-Infected Children: Guidelines for the Prevention and Treatment of Opportunistic Infections in HIV-Exposed and HIV-Infected Children: Department of Health and Human Services: https://clinicalinfo.hiv.gov/en/guidelines/hiv-clinical-guidelines-pediatric-opportunistic-infections/whats-new. Accessed April 21, 2023.

Sexually Transmitted Infections

Christiana Smith, MD, MSc
Ann-Christine Nyquist, MD, MSPH

INTRODUCTION

The rate of sexually transmitted infections (STIs) acquired during adolescence remains high despite widespread educational programs and increased access to health care. By senior year in high school, up to one-third of youth will have had sexual intercourse. The highest age-specific rates for gonorrhea, chlamydia, and human papillomavirus (HPV) infection occur in adolescents and young adults (15–24 years of age). While this age group accounts for only 25% of the sexually active population, it accounts for almost half of incident STIs. Adolescents contract STIs at a higher rate than adults because of sexual risk taking, age-related biologic factors (eg, cervical ectropion, maturing immune system), and barriers to health care access. In every state and the District of Columbia, adolescents can consent for the diagnosis and treatment of STIs. In many states, adolescents can also consent for human immunodeficiency virus (HIV) counseling and testing. Since individual state laws vary, health care providers should be knowledgeable about the legal definitions regarding age of consent and confidentiality requirements in their state.

Providers should routinely screen adolescents for STIs and discuss risk reduction. Since not all adolescents receive regular preventive care, providers should use acute care visits to offer screening and education. Health education counseling should be nonjudgmental and appropriate for the developmental level, yet sufficiently thorough to identify risk behaviors because many adolescents may not readily acknowledge engaging in certain behaviors.

ADOLESCENT SEXUALITY

The trend in the past decade is that high school students were less likely to have ever engaged in sexual activity, were less likely to have had four or more sexual partners, and were less likely to be currently sexually active. The most recent Youth Risk Behavior Survey (2021) reports that 30% of high school students have had sexual intercourse. Twenty-one percent of students had sex in the 3 months prior to the survey and 6% reported having had four or more lifetime sexual intercourse partners. Among youth currently sexually active, 52% reported that either they or their partner had used a condom during their last sexual intercourse. Substance use contributes to an increase in risky sexual activity; 21% of sexually active youth report that they used alcohol or drugs prior to their last intercourse.

Oral sex is common in adolescents, with approximately two-thirds of 15- to 24-year-olds reporting oral sexual activity. Adolescents may engage in oral sex instead of vaginal sex because they believe it to be less risky for sexually transmitted disease transmission and pregnancy. Approximately 11% of adolescents 15- to 19-year-olds have engaged in anal sex. Additionally, condom use is relatively uncommon during oral and anal sex, thus increasing the risk for acquisition of an STI. Sexual minority youth (SMY) are defined as those who identify as lesbian, gay, or bisexual; who are not sure of their sexual identity; or who have had sexual contact with people of the same sex. Adolescents struggling with their emerging sexual orientation and associated stigma may engage in sexual activity with partners of both sexes and may use substances to cope, thereby impairing their decision-making abilities. Stigma, discrimination, and other factors put these youth at a higher risk of suicide, depression, and substance use disorder than their non-SMY peers.

Guttmacher Institute: https://www.guttmacher.org/state-policy/explore/overview-minors-consent-law. Accessed May 1, 2023.

Marcell AV, Burstein GR; AAP Committee on Adolescence: Sexual and reproductive health care services in the pediatric setting. Pediatrics 2017;140(5):e20172858 [PMID: 29061870].

Youth Risk Behavior Survey Data Summary & Trends Report: 2011–2021. https://www.cdc.gov/healthyyouth. Accessed May 1, 2023.

RISK FACTORS

Certain factors increase the risk for STI acquisition. These include early age at sexual debut, lack of condom use, multiple partners, prior STI, history of STI in a partner, and sex with a partner who is at least 3 years older. The type of sex affects risk as well, with vaginal or anal sex being riskier than oral sex. The adolescent female is especially predisposed to chlamydia, gonorrhea, and HPV infection because the cervix during adolescence has an exposed squamocolumnar junction (ectropion). The rapidly dividing cells in this area are especially susceptible to microorganism attachment and infection. During early to mid-puberty, this junction slowly invaginates as the uterus and cervix mature, and by the late teens to the early 20s, the squamocolumnar junction is inside the cervix.

PREVENTION OF SEXUALLY TRANSMITTED INFECTIONS

Efforts to reduce STI risk behavior should begin before the onset of sexual experimentation: first by helping youth personalize their risk for STIs and encouraging positive behaviors that minimize these risks, and then by enhancing communication skills with sexual partners about STI prevention, abstinence, and condom use.

Primary prevention focuses largely on education and risk-reduction techniques. Health care providers should routinely address sexuality as part of well-adolescent checkups. Although more than 90% of students are taught about HIV and other STIs in school, adolescents have a difficult time personalizing risk. Discussing prevalence, symptoms, and sequelae of STIs can raise awareness and help teenagers make informed decisions about initiating sexual activity and the use of safer sex techniques. Abstinence is theoretically an effective method of preventing STIs; however, many studies have failed to show sustainable protection. Instead, discussing condoms, dental dams, and the proper use of lubrication facilitates safer sex practices. Barrier protection prevents infections with HIV, HPV, gonorrhea, Chlamydia, and herpes simplex virus (HSV). In addition, preexposure vaccination against hepatitis B virus (HBV), hepatitis A virus (HAV), and HPV reduces the risk of acquiring these STIs.

Secondary prevention requires identifying and treating STIs (see the next section, Screening for Sexually Transmitted Infections) before infected individuals transmit infection to others. Access to confidential medical care is critical to this objective. Cooperation with the state or county health departments is valuable because they assume responsibility for locating the contacts of infected persons and ensuring appropriate treatment.

Tertiary prevention is directed toward complications of a specific illness. Examples of tertiary prevention include treating cervicitis to prevent pelvic inflammatory disease (PID), treating PID before infertility develops, or treating syphilis in early stages to prevent progression.

SCREENING FOR SEXUALLY TRANSMITTED INFECTIONS

The ability of the health care provider to obtain an accurate sexual history is crucial in prevention and control efforts. Questions must be clear to the youth, so choose language that the adolescent will understand. If the adolescent has ever engaged in sexual activity, the provider needs to determine what kind of sexual activity (mutual masturbation or oral, anal, or vaginal sex); whether partners have been of opposite sex, same sex, or both; whether birth control or condoms were used; and whether it has been consensual or forced. During the interview, the clinician should take the opportunity to discuss risk-reduction techniques regardless of the history obtained from the youth.

A routine laboratory screening process is warranted if the patient has engaged in intercourse, presents with STI symptoms (Table 44–1), or reports a partner with an STI. Some centers screen all youth for STIs as part of routine well-adolescent care, regardless of their reported sexual activity. Annual screening for Chlamydia trachomatis and Neisseria gonorrhoeae is recommended by the Centers for Disease Control and Prevention (CDC) for all sexually active females aged 25 years or younger, as well as older women at increased risk of infection (ie, new sex partner, more than one sex partner). Routine chlamydial testing should be considered

Table 44–1. Signs and symptoms of sexually transmitted infections.

Common signs and symptoms in males
- Penile discharge
- Hematuria
- Testicular pain, redness, or swelling
- Pruritis in urethra or pubic region

Common signs and symptoms in females
- Vaginal discharge
- Vaginal pruritis
- Irregular menses/spotting
- Post coital bleeding
- Pelvic pain
- Abdominal pain
- Dyspareunia
- Vomiting

Common signs and symptoms in both sexes
- Dysuria
- Genital or oral ulcerations
- Inguinal adenopathy
- Genital warts
- Anorectal pain
- Rectal discharge
- Pharyngitis
- Fever
- Skin rash

for all adolescent males, especially for males who have sex with men (MSM), have new or multiple sex partners, or are in correctional facilities. For MSM, consideration should be given to testing oropharyngeal and rectal sites, as asymptomatic infections of these sites are common.

Cervical cancer screening should begin at age 21 with cervical cytology performed every 3 years. In areas that have a relatively high rate of syphilis and for MSM, a screening rapid plasma reagin (RPR) antibody test should be performed at least yearly or up to every 3–6 months if there are multiple partners or other high-risk behaviors. HIV antibody testing is recommended at least once per lifetime for all patients and repeat testing should be performed when an STI is present, or the history includes multiple partners and high-risk behaviors.

American Academy of Pediatrics Adolescent Health Care Campaign Toolkit: https://services.aap.org/en/news-room/campaigns-and-toolkits/adolescent-health-care/. Accessed May 1, 2023.

THE MOST COMMON BACTERIAL SEXUALLY TRANSMITTED INFECTIONS

CHLAMYDIA TRACHOMATIS INFECTION

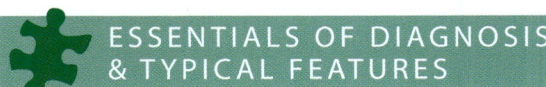

ESSENTIALS OF DIAGNOSIS & TYPICAL FEATURES

▶ *Chlamydia* is the most common bacterial STI in the United States; asymptomatic adolescents are the primary reservoir.

▶ Nucleic acid amplification testing (NAAT) is the most sensitive way to diagnose chlamydia and can be performed on multiple sample types, including urine and swabs of the cervix, vagina, urethra, rectum, and oropharynx.

▶ Prompt treatment is necessary to prevent serious sequelae, including PID, ectopic pregnancy, and infertility in females.

▶ General Considerations

C trachomatis is the most common bacterial cause of STIs in the United States, where over 1.6 million cases were reported in 2021. Almost two-thirds (65.9%) of all reported chlamydia cases occurred among adolescents and young adults aged 15–24 years. *C trachomatis* is an obligate intracellular bacterium with at least 15 different serologic variants: serovars A-K cause oculogenital disease and serovars L1, L2, and L3 cause lymphogranuloma venereum (LGV).

▶ Clinical Findings

A. Symptoms and Signs

Clinical infection in females manifests as dysuria, urethritis, vaginal discharge, cervicitis, irregular vaginal bleeding, or PID. The presence of mucopus at the cervical os (mucopurulent cervicitis) can be a sign of either chlamydial infection or gonorrhea. Chlamydial infection is asymptomatic in 75% of females.

Chlamydial infection may be asymptomatic in 70% of males or manifest as dysuria, urethritis, or epididymitis. Some patients complain of urethral discharge. On clinical examination, a clear white discharge may be found after milking the penis. Proctitis or proctocolitis from *Chlamydia* may occur in adolescents practicing receptive anal intercourse.

B. Laboratory Findings

NAAT is the most sensitive (92%–99%) way to detect *Chlamydia*. Enzyme-linked immunosorbent assay (ELISA) or direct fluorescent antibody (DFA) tests are less sensitive but may be the only testing option in some centers.

A cervical or vaginal swab in women, a urethral swab in men, or first-void urine specimen (the first 10–20 mL of voided urine collected after not voiding for 2 hours) in either sex, are ideal sample types for NAAT. For urine screening, sensitivity is improved with larger volumes of urine and longer duration of time since the prior void. NAAT should be performed at all anatomic sites of exposure, including the rectum and oropharynx. Many commercially available NAATs are Food and Drug Administration (FDA)-cleared for use on rectal and oropharyngeal swabs. The performance of NAATs on self-collected vaginal and rectal swabs is comparable to clinician-collected swabs and may be more acceptable to some patients. Often a single swab can be tested for both *C trachomatis* and *N gonorrhoeae*.

▶ Complications

Serious reproductive sequelae can occur in females, including PID, ectopic pregnancy, and infertility. Pregnant women with chlamydial infections can transmit *C trachomatis* to their neonate at birth, resulting in chlamydia ophthalmia and/or pneumonia. Epididymitis is a complication in males. Reactive arthritis can occur in association with chlamydial urethritis. This should be suspected in male patients who are sexually active and present with low back pain (sacroiliitis), arthritis (polyarticular), characteristic mucocutaneous lesions, and conjunctivitis.

▶ Treatment

Infected patients and their contacts, regardless of the extent of signs or symptoms, require treatment (Table 44–2). In 2021, the CDC began recommending a 7-day course of doxycycline as first-line treatment for uncomplicated

Table 44–2. Treatment regimens for sexually transmitted infections.

Syndrome	Organisms/Diagnoses	Recommended Regimens	Pregnancy [Category][a]
Urethritis and Cervicitis: Inflammation of urethra and/or cervix with erythema and/or mucoid, mucopurulent, or purulent discharge	*Neisseria gonorrhoeae*	45–150 kg: Ceftriaxone, 500 mg, IM, in a single dose[b] > 150 kg: Ceftriaxone, 1 g, IM, in a single dose[b] If chlamydial infection has not been excluded, also treat for *Chlamydia trachomatis* (see next row)	Safe [B]
	Chlamydia trachomatis	Doxycycline, 100 mg, orally, twice a day for 7 days (recommended) OR	Contraindicated [D]
		Azithromycin, 1 g, orally, in a single dose (alternative) OR	Safe [B]
		Levofloxacin, 500 mg, orally, once daily for 7 days (alternative)	Contraindicated [C]
	Nongonococcal urethritis[c] or cervicitis	Doxycycline, 100 mg, orally, twice a day for 7 days (recommended)	Contraindicated [D]
		Azithromycin, 1 g, orally, in a single dose (alternative)	Safe [B]
	Mycoplasma genitalium	*Recommended two-stage approach:* Doxycycline, 100 mg, orally, twice a day for 7 days	Contraindicated [D]
		Followed by Azithromycin, 1 g, orally, as a single dose, followed by 500 mg, orally, daily for 3 additional days (if resistance testing is available and macrolide susceptible)	Safe [B]
		Otherwise Moxifloxacin, 400 mg, orally, daily for 7 days (if resistance testing is not available or shows macrolide resistance)	Contraindicated [C]
	Trichomonas vaginalis (in males who have sex with females)	Metronidazole, 2 g, orally, in a single dose[d,e] OR	Safe [B]
		Tinidazole, 2 g, orally, in a single dose[d,e]	Contraindicated [C]
Vulvovaginitis	*T vaginalis*	Metronidazole, 500 mg, orally, twice daily for 7 days[d,e] OR	Safe [B]
		Tinidazole, 2 g, orally, in a single dose[d,e]	Contraindicated [C]
	Bacterial vaginosis	Metronidazole, 500 mg, orally, twice daily for 7 days[d,e] OR	Safe [B]
		Metronidazole gel 0.75%, 1 full applicator (5 g), intravaginally, once a day for 5 days[d,e] OR	Safe [B]
		Clindamycin cream 2%, 1 full applicator (5 g), intravaginally at bedtime, for 7 days	Safe [B]
	Candida albicans (and occasionally other *Candida* species or yeasts)	**Over-the-Counter Intravaginal Agents**[b] Clotrimazole 1% cream, 5 g, intravaginally, for 7–14 days OR	Safe [B]
		Clotrimazole 2% cream, 5 g, intravaginally, for 3 days OR	
		Miconazole 2% cream, 5 g, intravaginally, for 7 days OR	Contraindicated [C]
		Miconazole 4% cream, 5 g, intravaginally, for 3 days OR	
		Miconazole, 100-mg vaginal suppository, 1 suppository for 7 days OR	
		Miconazole, 200-mg vaginal suppository, 1 suppository for 3 days OR	
		Miconazole, 1200-mg vaginal suppository, 1 suppository for 1 day OR	
		Tioconazole, 6.5% ointment, 5 g, intravaginally, in a single application	Safe [B]

(Continued)

Table 44–2. Treatment regimens for sexually transmitted infections. (*Continued*)

Syndrome	Organisms/Diagnoses	Recommended Regimens	Pregnancy [Category][a]
		Prescription Intravaginal Agents[b]	
		Butoconazole 2% cream (single-dose bioadhesive product), 5 g intravaginally in a single application	Contraindicated [C]
		OR	
		Terconazole 0.4% cream, 5 g, intravaginally, daily for 7 days	Contraindicated [C]
		OR	
		Terconazole 0.8% cream, 5 g, intravaginally, for 3 days	
		OR	
		Terconazole, 80-mg vaginal suppository, 1 suppository for 3 days	
		Oral Agent	
		Fluconazole, 150-mg oral tablet, 1 tablet in single dose	Contraindicated [C]
PID[f]		**Recommended Parenteral Regimens:**	
		Ceftriaxone, 1 g, IV, every 24 h	Safe [B]
		PLUS	
		Doxycycline, 100 mg, orally or IV, every 12 h	Contraindicated [D]
		PLUS	
		Metronidazole, 500 mg, orally or IV, every 12 h	Safe [B]
		OR	
		Cefotetan, 2 g, IV, every 12 h **OR** Cefoxitin, 2 g, IV, every 6 h	Safe [B]
		PLUS	
		Doxycycline, 100 mg, orally or IV, every 12 h	Contraindicated [D]
		Recommended Intramuscular/Oral Regimens[g,h]:	
		One of the following:	
		Ceftriaxone, 500 mg, IM, once	Safe [B], Safe [B], Safe [B]
		OR Cefoxitin, 2 g, IM, **and** Probenecid, 1 g, orally, in a single dose concurrently	
		OR Other parenteral third-generation cephalosporin (eg, ceftizoxime, cefotaxime)	Safe [B]
		PLUS	
		Doxycycline, 100 mg, orally, twice a day for 14 days	Contraindicated [D]
		WITH	
		Metronidazole, 500 mg, orally, twice a day for 14 days[d]	Safe [B]
Genital ulcer disease	*Treponema pallidum* (primary or secondary syphilis)	Penicillin G benzathine, 2.4 million U, IM, in a single dose	Safe [B]
	Genital HSV—1st clinical episode[i]	Acyclovir, 400 mg, orally, 3 times/day for 7–10 days	Safe [B]
		OR	
		Valacyclovir, 1 g, orally, twice daily for 10 days	Safe [B]
		OR	
		Famciclovir, 250 mg, orally, 3 times/day for 7–10 days	Safe [B]
	Genital HSV—episodic treatment of recurrences	Acyclovir, 800 mg, orally, twice daily for 5 days	Safe [B]
		OR	
		Acyclovir, 800 mg, orally, 3 times daily for 2 days	Safe [B]
		OR	
		Famciclovir, 1 g, orally, 2 times daily for 1 day	Safe [B]
		OR	
		Famciclovir, 500 mg, orally, once, followed by 250 mg, orally, twice daily for 2 days	Safe [B]
		OR	
		Famciclovir, 125 mg, orally, twice daily for 5 days	Safe [B]
		OR	
		Valacyclovir, 500 mg, orally twice daily for 3 days	Safe [B]
		OR	
		Valacyclovir, 1 g, orally, once daily for 5 days	Safe [B]

(*Continued*)

Table 44–2. Treatment regimens for sexually transmitted infections. (*Continued*)

Syndrome	Organisms/Diagnoses	Recommended Regimens	Pregnancy [Category][a]
	Genital HSV—suppressive therapy	Acyclovir, 400 mg, orally, twice daily **OR**	Safe [B]
		Valacyclovir, 500 mg, orally, once daily **OR**	Safe [B]
		Valacyclovir, 1 g, orally, once daily **OR**	Safe [B]
		Famciclovir, 250 mg, orally, twice daily	Safe [B]
	Haemophilus ducreyi (chancroid)	Azithromycin, 1 g, orally, in a single dose **OR**	Safe [B]
		Ceftriaxone, 250 mg, IM, in a single dose **OR**	Safe [B]
		Ciprofloxacin, 500 mg, orally, twice daily for 3 days **OR**	Contraindicated [D]
		Erythromycin base, 500 mg, orally, 3 times/day for 7 days	Safe [B]
	Klebsiella granulomatis (granuloma inguinale [donovanosis])	Azithromycin, 1 g, orally, once/wk or 500 mg, orally, daily, for at least 3 wk and until all lesions have healed completely	Safe [B]
	C trachomatis serovars L1, L2, or L3; also known as Lymphogranuloma venereum (LGV)	Doxycycline, 100 mg, orally, twice a day for 21 days	Contraindicated [D]
Epididymitis	*C trachomatis, N gonorrhoeae*	Ceftriaxone, 500 mg, IM, in a single dose **PLUS**	Safe [B]
		Doxycycline, 100 mg, orally, twice daily for 10 days	Contraindicated [D]
	Enteric organisms (eg, *Escherichia coli*), *C trachomatis, N gonorrhoeae* among males who practice insertive anal sex	Ceftriaxone, 500 mg, IM, in a single dose **PLUS**	
		Levofloxacin, 500 mg, orally, once a day for 10 days	Contraindicated [C]
Proctitis	*C trachomatis, N gonorrhoeae,* HSV	Ceftriaxone, 500 mg, IM, in a single dose **PLUS**	Safe [B]
		Doxycycline, 100 mg, orally, twice daily for 7 days; extend to 21 days for presence of bloody discharge, perianal or mucosal ulcers, or tenesmus and a positive rectal *C trachomatis* test	Contraindicated [D]
		PLUS in the presence of rectal ulcers	Safe [B] Safe [B]
		Valacyclovir, 1 g, orally, twice daily **OR** acyclovir, 400 mg, orally, three times daily **OR** famciclovir, 250 mg, orally, three times daily for 7–10 days	Safe [B]
External anogenital warts (ie, penis, groin, scrotum, vulva, perineum, external anus, and perianus)	Human papillomavirus	*Patient-applied:* Imiquimod 3.75% or 5% cream[j] **OR**	Contraindicated [C]
		Podofilox 0.5% solution or gel **OR**	Contraindicated [C]
		Sinecatechins 15% ointment	Unknown safety
		Provider-administered: Cryotherapy with liquid nitrogen or cryoprobe **OR**	Safe
		Surgical removal either by tangential scissor excision, tangential shave excision, curettage, laser, or electrosurgery **OR**	Safe
		Trichloroacetic acid or bichloracetic acid 80%–90% solution	Safe

(Continued)

Table 44–2. Treatment regimens for sexually transmitted infections. (*Continued*)

Syndrome	Organisms/Diagnoses	Recommended Regimens	Pregnancy [Category][a]
Scabies[k]		Permethrin cream 5%: apply to entire body from the neck down, wash off after 8–14 h	Safe [B]
		or	
		Ivermectin, 200 mcg/kg orally, repeat in 7–14 days (take with food)	Contraindicated [C]
Pubic Lice[k]		Permethrin 1% creme rinse: wash off after 10 min	Safe [B]
		or	
		Pyrethrins with piperonyl butoxide: apply, wash off after 10 min	Safe [B]

IM, intramuscularly; PID, pelvic inflammatory disease; STI, sexually transmitted infection.

[a]FDA use in pregnancy ratings: [A] *Controlled studies show no risk*. Adequate, well-controlled studies in pregnant women have failed to demonstrate a risk to the fetus in any trimester of pregnancy. [B] *No evidence of risk in humans*. Adequate, well-controlled studies in pregnant women have not shown increased risk of fetal abnormalities despite adverse findings in animals, in the absence of adequate human studies, animal studies show no fetal risk. The chance of fetal harm is remote but remains a possibility. [C] *Risk cannot be ruled out*. Adequate, well-controlled human studies are lacking, and animal studies have shown a risk to the fetus or are lacking as well. There is a chance of fetal harm if the drug is administered during pregnancy; but the potential benefits outweigh the potential risk. [D] *Positive evidence of risk*. Studies in humans, or investigational or postmarketing data, have demonstrated fetal risk. Nevertheless, potential benefits from the use of the drug may outweigh the potential risk. For example, the drug may be acceptable if needed in a life-threatening situation or serious disease for which safer drugs cannot be used or are ineffective. [X] *Contraindicated in pregnancy*. Studies in animals or humans, or despite adverse findings in animals, or investigational or postmarketing reports have demonstrated positive evidence of fetal abnormalities or risk that clearly outweighs any possible benefit to the patient.

[b]If ceftriaxone is not feasible, may substitute cefixime, 800 mg, orally, in a single dose.

[c]Nongonococcal urethritis (NGU) is diagnosed when microscopy indicates inflammation without gram-negative intracellular diplococci (on Gram stain) or purple intracellular diplococci (on methylene blue or gentian violet staining) on urethral smear.

[d]In areas where *T vaginalis* is prevalent, males who have sex with females and have persistent or recurrent urethritis should be presumptively treated for *T vaginalis*.

[e]Alcohol consumption should be avoided during treatment with metronidazole or tinidazole; breastfeeding should be deferred for 72 hours after mother has received a 2-g dose of tinidazole.

[f]Hospitalization and parenteral treatment is recommended if patient has severe illness such as tubo-ovarian abscess, is pregnant, or is unable to tolerate or follow ambulatory regimens.

[g]Patients with inadequate response to outpatient therapy after 72 hours should be reevaluated for possible misdiagnosis and may require parenteral therapy.

[h]The recommended third-generation cephalosporins are limited in the coverage of anaerobes. Therefore, the addition of metronidazole to treatment regimens with third-generation cephalosporins should be considered.

[i]Treatment can be extended if healing is incomplete after 10 days of therapy.

[j]Wash treatment area with soap and water 6–10 hours after application.

[k]Bedding and clothing need to be decontaminated by washing in hot water or by dry-cleaning. Regimen may be repeated in 1 week if complete response is not achieved in pregnancy.

Data from Workowski KA et al: Sexually Transmitted Infections Treatment Guidelines, 2021. MMWR Recomm Rep. 2021 Jul 23;70(4):1–187.

anogenital chlamydia, rather than a single dose of azithromycin. The primary reason for this change is the improved efficacy of doxycycline for rectal chlamydia, which can occur in men and women and cannot be reliably predicted by reported sexual activity. When nonadherence to doxycycline is a significant concern, azithromycin can be given by direct observed therapy as an alternative treatment option, but these patients may require posttreatment evaluation and testing, especially in those with known rectal infection. Reinfection within several months of the first infection occurs commonly and is caused by failure of contacts to receive treatment or the initiation of sexual activity with a new infected partner. Because of this increased risk, all infected females and males should be retested approximately 3 months after treatment.

Wiesenfeld HC: Screening for *Chlamydia trachomatis* infections in women. N Engl J Med 2017;376(8):765–773 [PMID: 282225683].

NEISSERIA GONORRHOEAE INFECTION

ESSENTIALS OF DIAGNOSIS & TYPICAL FEATURES

▶ Gonorrhea is the second most common bacterial STI in the United States; a large proportion of cases occur among MSM.

▶ NAATs are the most sensitive way to diagnose gonorrhea and can be performed on many sample types; however, culture allows for antimicrobial susceptibility testing.

▶ Prompt treatment is necessary to prevent serious sequelae, including PID, ectopic pregnancy, and infertility in females.

General Considerations

Gonorrhea is the second most common bacterial STI in the United States, where over 710,000 new *N gonorrhoeae* infections were reported in 2021. MSM are disproportionately impacted by *N gonorrhoeae* infections, and (43.3%) of all reported cases in 2021 occurred among adolescents and young adults aged 15–24 years.

Sites of infection include the cervix, urethra, rectum, and pharynx. Humans are the natural reservoir. Gonococci are present in the exudate and secretions of infected mucous membranes.

Clinical Findings

A. Symptoms and Signs

In uncomplicated gonococcal cervicitis, females are symptomatic 23%–57% of the time, presenting with vaginal discharge and dysuria. Urethritis and pyuria may be present. Mucopurulent cervicitis with a yellowish discharge may be found, and the cervix may be edematous and friable. Other symptoms may include abnormal menstrual periods and dyspareunia. Approximately 15% of females with endocervical gonorrhea have signs of involvement of the upper genital tract. Compared with chlamydial infection, pelvic inflammation with gonorrhea has a shorter duration, but an increased intensity of symptoms, and is more often associated with fever. Symptomatic males usually present with a yellowish-green urethral discharge and dysuria, but most males (55%–67%) with *N gonorrhoeae* are asymptomatic. Both males and females can develop gonococcal proctitis and pharyngitis after appropriate exposure.

B. Laboratory Findings

Culture and NAAT are available for the detection of *N gonorrhoeae*. The sensitivity of NAAT is superior to culture,

but culture allows for antimicrobial susceptibility testing of organisms with suspected antibiotic resistance. Gram stain of urethral discharge showing gram-negative intracellular diplococci is diagnostic of gonorrhea in a symptomatic male. Gram stain of conjunctival exudate, synovial fluid, and cerebrospinal fluid (CSF) can be similarly useful. Cultures can be performed on samples from sterile (blood, synovial fluid, CSF) and non-sterile (cervix, vagina, rectum, urethra, pharynx) sites; samples from non-sterile sites require selective media that inhibit the growth of normal flora. NAAT are FDA-approved for use on cervical or vaginal swabs in women, urethral swabs in men, or urine specimens in either sex. Many commercially available NAATs are FDA cleared for use on rectal and oropharyngeal swabs. The performance of NAATs on self-collected vaginal and rectal swabs is comparable to clinician-collected swabs, and this approach may be more acceptable to some patients. In cases of treatment failure, both NAAT and culture with susceptibility testing should be performed at affected sites. Patients testing positive for gonorrhea should be screened for other STIs, including chlamydia, syphilis, and HIV.

Differential Diagnosis

Chlamydial infections can present very similar to gonococcal infections in men and women. Gonococcal pharyngitis needs to be differentiated from pharyngitis caused by streptococcal infection, herpes simplex, adenovirus, infectious mononucleosis (Epstein-Barr virus), and acute retroviral syndrome caused by HIV.

Complications

Disseminated gonococcal infection occurs in a minority (0.5%–3%) of patients with untreated gonorrhea. Arthritis and dermatitis can result from hematogenous spread. The joints most frequently involved are the wrist, metacarpophalangeal joints, knee, and ankle. Skin lesions are typically tender, with hemorrhagic or necrotic pustules or bullae on an erythematous base occurring on the distal extremities. Disseminated disease occurs more frequently in females than in males. Risk factors include pregnancy and gonococcal pharyngitis. Gonorrhea is complicated very infrequently by perihepatitis, endocarditis, and/or meningitis.

Serious reproductive sequelae can occur in females with gonococcal infection, including PID, ectopic pregnancy, and infertility. Pregnant women can transmit *N gonorrhoeae* to their neonate at birth, resulting in gonococcal ophthalmia, neonatal sepsis, septic arthritis, meningitis, or localized skin abscess (eg, at the site of a fetal scalp electrode).

Treatment (See Table 44–2)

In 2020, the CDC made significant changes to gonorrhea treatment recommendations to include a higher intramuscular (IM) dose of ceftriaxone regardless of anatomic site involved and removal of the recommendation for dual treatment with azithromycin. These changes reflect data demonstrating that high doses of ceftriaxone are needed for eradication of gonorrhea, especially from the pharynx, and increasing concern for the rising incidence of azithromycin resistance. In cases where chlamydial infection has not been excluded, the addition of doxycycline for 7 days is recommended. Quinolones should not be used to treat gonorrhea due to high levels of quinolone resistance in the United States, and oral cefixime should not be used except in cases where IM ceftriaxone is not available or for expedited partner therapy. Oral cefixime has limited efficacy for pharyngeal gonorrhea.

Uncomplicated urogenital or rectal gonorrhea does not require a test of cure when treated with first-line medications unless the patient remains symptomatic. However, a test of cure is recommended 7–14 days after treatment of pharyngeal gonorrhea, regardless of treatment regimen. In addition, retesting 3 months after treatment is indicated for gonococcal infection at any site due to high rates of reinfection, even among patients who believe their sex partners were treated. Patients should be advised to abstain from sexual intercourse for 7 days after both they and their partners have completed a course of treatment. In cases of suspected treatment failure after ceftriaxone, providers should obtain a gonorrhea culture to assess for antibiotic resistance and report the case to the CDC through local public health authorities within 24 hours.

St Cyr S et al: Update to CDC's Treatment Guidelines for Gonococcal Infection, 2020. MMWR Morb Mortal Wkly Rep 2020;69(50):1911–1916 [PMID: 33332296].

SYNDROMIC PRESENTATIONS OF SEXUALLY TRANSMITTED INFECTIONS

The patient presenting with an STI usually has one or more of the signs or symptoms described in this section. Treatment of each STI is detailed in Table 44–2.

CERVICITIS

ESSENTIALS OF DIAGNOSIS & TYPICAL FEATURES

▶ Cervicitis is characterized by endocervical exudates and friability or bleeding of the cervix.

▶ Treatment for cervicitis typically targets *C trachomatis* and *N gonorrhoeae*, but often no causative organism is identified.

▶ General Considerations

In most cases of cervicitis, no organism is isolated. The most common causes include *C trachomatis* or *N gonorrhoeae*. HSV, *Trichomonas vaginalis*, and *Mycoplasma genitalium* are less common causes. Bacterial vaginosis is recognized as a cause of cervicitis. Cervicitis may also be caused by chemical irritants (eg, douching) or idiopathic inflammation.

▶ Clinical Findings

A. Symptoms and Signs

Two major diagnostic signs characterize cervicitis: (1) purulent or mucopurulent endocervical exudate visible in the endocervical canal or on an endocervical swab and (2) easily induced bleeding with the passage of a cotton swab through the cervical os. Cervicitis is often asymptomatic, but many patients with cervicitis have an abnormal vaginal discharge or postcoital bleeding.

B. Laboratory Findings

Although endocervical Gram stain may show an increased number of polymorphonuclear leukocytes, this finding has a low positive predictive value and is not recommended for diagnosis. Patients with cervicitis should be tested for *C trachomatis*, *N gonorrhoeae*, trichomoniasis, and bacterial vaginosis using the most sensitive and specific tests available at the site.

▶ Complications

Persistent cervicitis is difficult to manage and requires reassessment of the initial diagnosis and evaluation for possible re-exposure to an STI. Cervicitis can persist despite repeated courses of antimicrobial therapy. The presence of a large ectropion can contribute to persistent cervicitis.

▶ Treatment

Empiric treatment for both *C trachomatis* and *N gonorrhoeae* is recommended in women at increased risk of STIs (eg, those aged < 25 years and those with a new sex partner). If the patient is at lower risk of STIs, treatment may wait until diagnostic test results are available (see Table 44–2). Patients should be instructed to abstain from sexual intercourse until they and their sex partners have completed treatment.

PELVIC INFLAMMATORY DISEASE

ESSENTIALS OF DIAGNOSIS & TYPICAL FEATURES

▶ PID may present with a wide variety of signs and symptoms (including abdominal pain, fever, vomiting, vaginal discharge); providers must have a low threshold for diagnosis and treatment of this disease.

▶ Prevention of serious sequelae, including infertility, is dependent on early administration of appropriate antibiotics.

General Considerations

PID is defined as inflammation of the upper female genital tract and may include any combination of endometritis, salpingitis, tubo-ovarian abscess, and pelvic peritonitis. It is the most common gynecologic disorder necessitating hospitalization for female patients of reproductive age in the United States. The incidence is highest in teenage girls. Predisposing risk factors include multiple sexual partners, younger age of initiating sexual intercourse, prior history of PID, and lack of condom use. Lack of protective antibody from previous exposure to sexually transmitted organisms and cervical ectropion also contribute to the development of PID. Many adolescents with subacute or asymptomatic PID are never identified.

PID is often a polymicrobial infection. Causative agents include *N gonorrhoeae*, *C trachomatis*, anaerobic bacteria including *Gardnerella vaginalis*, and genital mycoplasmas. Vaginal douching and other mechanical factors such as intrauterine devices or prior gynecologic surgery increase the risk of PID by providing access of lower genital tract organisms to pelvic organs. Recent menses and bacterial vaginosis have also been associated with the development of PID.

Clinical Findings

A. Symptoms and Signs

PID is challenging to diagnose because of the wide variation in presentation. No single historical, clinical, or laboratory finding has both high sensitivity and specificity for the diagnosis. Diagnosis of PID is usually made clinically (Table 44–3). Typical patients present with lower abdominal pain, pelvic pain, or dyspareunia. Systemic symptoms such fever, nausea, or vomiting may be present. Vaginal discharge is variable. Cervical motion tenderness, uterine or adnexal tenderness, or signs of peritonitis are often present. Mucopurulent cervicitis is present in 50% of patients. Tubo-ovarian abscesses can often be detected by careful physical examination (feeling a mass or fullness in the adnexa).

B. Laboratory Findings

Laboratory findings may include peripheral leukocytosis with a left shift and elevated acute-phase reactants (erythrocyte sedimentation rate or C-reactive protein). A positive genitourinary test for *N gonorrhoeae* or *C trachomatis* is supportive of the diagnosis of PID, although 25% of the time neither are detected. Pregnancy needs to be ruled out, both because the differential diagnosis of abdominal pain in a female includes ectopic pregnancy, and because pregnant women with PID are at high risk of complications. All

Table 44–3. Diagnostic criteria for pelvic inflammatory disease.

Minimum criteria
Empiric treatment of PID should be initiated in sexually active young women and others at risk for sexually transmitted infections if both of the following minimum criteria are present:
- Pelvic or lower abdominal pain with no other identifiable cause(s) for the illness, AND
- Cervical motion tenderness or uterine tenderness or adnexal tenderness on pelvic examination

Additional supportive criteria
Oral temperature > 38.3°C (101°F)
Abnormal cervical or vaginal mucopurulent discharge or cervical friability
Presence of abundant white blood cells on microscopic evaluation of vaginal secretions diluted in saline
Elevated erythrocyte sedimentation rate or elevated C-reactive protein
Laboratory documentation of infection with *Neisseria gonorrhoeae* or *Chlamydia trachomatis*

Definitive criteria (selected cases)
Histopathologic evidence of endometritis on endometrial biopsy
Tubo-ovarian abscess, fluid-filled tubes, or tubal hyperemia on sonography or other radiologic tests
Laparoscopic abnormalities consistent with PID

Adapted from Centers for Disease Control and Prevention: Sexually transmitted diseases treatment guidelines 2015.

women who have acute PID should be screened for other STIs, including HIV.

C. Diagnostic Studies

Laparoscopy is the gold standard for detecting salpingitis. It is used if the diagnosis is in question or to help differentiate PID from an ectopic pregnancy, ovarian cysts, or adnexal torsion. Endometrial biopsy should be performed in women undergoing laparoscopy who do not have visual evidence of salpingitis because some women may have isolated endometritis. Pelvic ultrasonography also is helpful in detecting tubo-ovarian abscesses, which are found in almost 20% of teens with PID. Transvaginal ultrasound is more sensitive than abdominal ultrasound.

Differential Diagnosis

Differential diagnosis includes other gynecologic illnesses (ectopic pregnancy, threatened or septic abortion, adnexal torsion, ruptured and hemorrhagic ovarian cysts, dysmenorrhea, endometriosis, or mittelschmerz), gastrointestinal illnesses (appendicitis, cholecystitis, hepatitis, gastroenteritis, or inflammatory bowel disease), and urinary tract illnesses (cystitis, pyelonephritis, or urinary calculi).

Complications

Scarring of the fallopian tubes with loss of ciliated epithelial cells is one of the major sequelae of PID. After one episode of PID, 17% of patients become infertile, 17% develop chronic pelvic pain, and 10% will have an ectopic pregnancy. Infertility rates increase with each episode of PID; three episodes of PID result in a 73% infertility rate. Duration of symptoms appears to be the largest determinant of infertility. Hematogenous or lymphatic spread of organisms from the fallopian tubes can rarely cause inflammation of the liver capsule (perihepatitis) resulting in symptoms of pleuritic right upper quadrant pain and elevation of liver enzymes.

Treatment

The objectives of treatment are both to achieve a clinical cure and to prevent long-term sequelae. Treatment should be initiated quickly because prevention of sequelae is dependent on early administration of antibiotics. Among women with PID of mild to moderate clinical severity, there are no differences in short- and long-term clinical and microbiologic response rates resulting from parenteral versus oral therapy. PID is frequently managed at the outpatient level, although some clinicians argue that all adolescents with PID should be hospitalized because of the frequency of complications. Severe systemic symptoms and toxicity, signs of peritonitis, inability to tolerate oral fluids, pregnancy, nonresponse or intolerance of oral antimicrobial therapy, and tubo-ovarian abscess favor hospitalization. In addition, if the health care provider believes that the patient will not adhere to treatment, hospitalization is warranted. Pregnant women with PID should be admitted and treated with parental antibiotics to reduce the risk of increased morbidity. Surgical drainage may be required for adequate treatment of tubo-ovarian abscesses.

The broad-spectrum antibiotic regimens described in Table 44–2 cover the numerous microorganisms associated with PID. All treatment regimens should be effective against *N gonorrhoeae* and *C trachomatis* because negative endocervical screening tests do not rule out upper reproductive tract infection with these organisms. The use of treatment regimens with anaerobic activity are recommended by the CDC. Patients with PID who receive outpatient treatment should be reexamined within 24–48 hours, with phone contact in the interim, to assess for persistent disease or treatment failure. Patients should have substantial improvement within 48–72 hours. Adolescents should be reexamined 7–10 days after the completion of therapy to ensure the resolution of symptoms. Patients who are diagnosed with chlamydial or gonococcal PID should be retested for these pathogens 3 months after treatment.

Brunham RC, Gottlieb SL, Paavonen J: Pelvic inflammatory disease. N Engl J Med 2015;372(21):2039–2048 [PMID: 25992748].

URETHRITIS

ESSENTIALS OF DIAGNOSIS & TYPICAL FEATURES

▶ Dysuria and urethral discharge is common in over half of patients.

▶ Treatment for urethritis typically targets *C trachomatis* and *N gonorrhoeae*.

General Considerations

The most common bacterial causes of urethritis in males are *N gonorrhoeae* and *C trachomatis*. Additionally, *T vaginalis*, HSV, *Ureaplasma urealyticum*, and *M genitalium* cause urethritis. Enteric organisms may cause urethritis in males practicing insertive anal intercourse. Mechanical manipulation or contact with irritants can also cause transient urethritis. Urethritis in both males and females is frequently asymptomatic.

Females often present with symptoms of a urinary tract infection and "sterile pyuria" (no enteric bacterial pathogens isolated), which reflects urethritis caused by the organisms described above.

Clinical Findings

A. Symptoms and Signs

If symptomatic, males present most commonly with a clear or purulent discharge from the urethra, dysuria, or urethral pruritus. Hematuria and inguinal adenopathy can occur. Most infections caused by *C trachomatis* and *T vaginalis* are asymptomatic, while 70% of males with *M genitalium* and 23%–90% with gonococcal urethritis are symptomatic.

B. Laboratory Findings

In a symptomatic male, a positive leukocyte esterase test on first-void urine, or microscopic examination of first-void urine demonstrating more than 10 white blood cells (WBCs) per high-power field, is suggestive of urethritis. Gram stain of urethral secretions demonstrating more than 2 WBCs per high-power field is also suggestive. Gonococcal urethritis is established by documenting the presence of WBCs containing intracellular gram-negative diplococci. Urethral swab or first-void urine for NAAT should be sent to the laboratory to detect *N gonorrhoeae*, *C trachomatis*, and *T vaginalis*. Specific NAAT testing of urine is also available for *Mycoplasma* and *Ureaplasma*.

Complications

Complications include recurrent or persistent urethritis, epididymitis, prostatitis, and reactive arthritis.

Treatment (See Table 44–2)

Patients with objective evidence of urethritis should receive empiric treatment for gonorrhea and chlamydial infection. Due to increasing resistance among *M genitalium* isolates, current recommendations include two-stage therapy with initial empiric treatment with doxycycline followed by either moxifloxacin or azithromycin (if known to be susceptible). If the infection is unresponsive to initial treatment and NAAT is negative, trichomoniasis should be ruled out and nongonococcal, nonchlamydial urethritis should be suspected and treated. Sexual partners should either be evaluated or treated for gonorrhea and chlamydial infection.

EPIDIDYMITIS

ESSENTIALS OF DIAGNOSIS & TYPICAL FEATURES

► Gradual onset of scrotal pain may be accompanied by dysuria and urinary frequency.
► Treatment for urethritis typically targets *C trachomatis* and *N gonorrhoeae*.

General Considerations

Epididymitis in a male who is sexually active is most often caused by *C trachomatis* or *N gonorrhoeae*. Epididymitis caused by *Escherichia coli* and other enteric organisms occurs among males who are the insertive partners during anal intercourse and in males who have urinary tract abnormalities.

Clinical Findings

A. Symptoms and Signs

Epididymitis presents as a constellation of pain, swelling, and inflammation of the epididymis. In many cases, the testis is also involved.

B. Laboratory and Diagnostic Studies

Diagnosis is generally made clinically. Color Doppler ultrasound can help make the diagnosis. Laboratory evaluation is the same as for suspected urethritis and should include urine culture if NAAT is negative.

Differential Diagnosis

Acute epididymitis must be distinguished from orchitis due to infarct, testicular torsion, or viral infection. Less common and more chronic illnesses include testicular cancer, tuberculosis, or fungal infection.

Complications

Infertility is rare, and chronic local pain is uncommon.

Treatment

Empiric therapy (see Table 44–2) is indicated before culture results are available. As an adjunct to therapy, bed rest, scrotal elevation, and analgesics are recommended until fever and local inflammation subside. Sex partners should be evaluated and treated for gonorrhea and chlamydial infections.

PROCTITIS, PROCTOCOLITIS, & ENTERITIS

ESSENTIALS OF DIAGNOSIS & TYPICAL FEATURES

► Anorectal itching, pain, and mucopurulent discharge around the anal canal are common symptoms.
► The majority of rectal chlamydia and gonococcal infections are asymptomatic.

General Considerations

Proctitis occurs predominantly among persons who participate in anal intercourse. Enteritis occurs among those whose sexual practices include oral-fecal contact. Proctocolitis can be acquired by either route depending on the pathogen. Common sexually transmitted pathogens causing proctitis or proctocolitis include *C trachomatis* (including LGV serovars), *Treponema pallidum*, HSV, *N gonorrhoeae*, *Giardia lamblia*, and enteric organisms. As many as 85% of rectal infections with *N gonorrhoeae* and *C trachomatis* are asymptomatic. The presence of symptomatic or asymptomatic proctitis may facilitate the transmission of HIV infection.

Clinical Findings

A. Symptoms and Signs

Proctitis, defined as inflammation limited to the distal 10–12 cm of the rectum, is associated with anorectal pain, tenesmus, and rectal discharge. Acute proctitis among persons who have recently practiced receptive anal intercourse is most often sexually transmitted. The symptoms of proctocolitis combine those of proctitis, plus diarrhea or abdominal cramps (or both), because of inflamed colonic mucosa more than 12 cm from the anus. Enteritis usually results in diarrhea and abdominal cramping without signs of proctitis or proctocolitis.

B. Laboratory and Diagnostic Studies

Evaluation may include anoscopy or sigmoidoscopy, stool examination, culture or NAAT for appropriate organisms, and serology for syphilis.

▶ Treatment

Management will be determined by the etiologic agent (see Table 44–2 and Chapter 42). Reinfection may be difficult to distinguish from treatment failure.

VAGINAL DISCHARGE

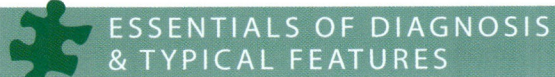

ESSENTIALS OF DIAGNOSIS & TYPICAL FEATURES

- ▶ Vaginal irritation, itching, discomfort with sexual intercourse and discharge are associated with vaginitis.
- ▶ Appropriate treatment depends on the etiology of vaginitis.

Adolescent girls may have a normal physiologic leukorrhea, secondary to turnover of vaginal epithelium. Infectious causes of discharge include *T vaginalis*, *C trachomatis*, *N gonorrhoeae*, and bacterial vaginosis pathogens. Candidiasis is a yeast infection that produces vaginal discharge but is not usually sexually transmitted. Vaginitis in general may cause vaginal discharge, vulvar itching, and irritation. Discharge may be white, gray, or yellow. Physiologic leukorrhea is usually white, homogeneous, and not associated with itching, irritation, or foul odor. Mechanical, chemical, allergic, or other noninfectious irritants of the vagina may cause vaginal discharge.

1. Bacterial Vaginosis

▶ General Considerations

Bacterial vaginosis is a polymicrobial infection of the vagina caused by an imbalance of the normal bacterial vaginal flora. The altered flora has a paucity of hydrogen peroxide-producing lactobacilli and increased concentrations of anaerobic bacteria (*Prevotella* spp. and *Mobiluncus* spp.), *G vaginalis*, *Ureaplasma*, and *Mycoplasma*. It is unclear whether bacterial vaginosis is sexually transmitted, but it is associated with having multiple sex partners and women with bacterial vaginosis are at increased risk for other STIs.

▶ Clinical Findings

A. Symptoms and signs

The most common symptom is a copious, malodorous, homogeneous thin gray-white vaginal discharge. Patients may report vaginal itching or dysuria. A fishy odor may be most noticeable after intercourse or during menses, when the high pH of blood or semen volatilizes the amines.

B. Laboratory Findings

Bacterial vaginosis is most often diagnosed using clinical criteria, which include: (1) presence of thin, white discharge that smoothly coats the vaginal walls; (2) fishy (amine) odor before or after the addition of 10% potassium hydroxide (KOH) to the discharge (whiff test); (3) pH of vaginal fluid greater than 4.5 determined with narrow-range pH paper; and (4) presence of "clue cells" on microscopic examination. Clue cells are squamous epithelial cells that have multiple bacteria adhering to them, making their borders irregular, and giving them a speckled appearance. A microscopy guide published by the CDC is available online and includes images of clue cells from vaginal wet preps (https://www.cdc.gov/labquality/docs/PMP_Booklet_7252019.pdf). Diagnosis requires three out of four criteria, although many female patients who fulfill these criteria have no discharge or other symptoms.

▶ Complications

Bacterial vaginosis during pregnancy is associated with adverse outcomes such as premature labor, preterm delivery, intra-amniotic infection, and postpartum endometritis. In the nonpregnant individual, it may be associated with PID and urinary tract infections.

▶ Treatment

All female patients who have symptomatic disease should receive treatment (see Table 44–2). Treatment in pregnancy prevents adverse outcomes of pregnancy. Because some studies associate bacterial vaginosis and PID, providers should have a low threshold for treating asymptomatic bacterial vaginosis. Recurrence of bacterial vaginosis is common. Follow-up examination 1 month after treatment for high-risk pregnant patients is recommended. Treatment of sex partners is unnecessary for males but is recommended for women who have sex with women.

Bradshaw CS, Sobel JD: Current treatment of bacterial vaginosis-limitations and need for innovation. J Infect Dis 2016;214 (Suppl 1):S14–S20 [PMID: 27449869].

CDC Provider-Performed Microscopy Procedures: A Focus on Quality Practices Appendix K1, K2. https://www.cdc.gov/labquality/docs/PMP_Booklet_7252019.pdf, Accessed May 1, 2023.

2. Trichomoniasis

▶ General Considerations

Trichomoniasis is caused by *T vaginalis*, a flagellated protozoan that infects 3.7 million people annually in the United States.

▶ Clinical Findings

A. Symptoms and Signs

Fifty percent of females with trichomoniasis develop a symptomatic vaginitis with vaginal itching, a green-gray malodorous frothy discharge, and dysuria. Occasionally postcoital bleeding and dyspareunia may be present. The vulva may be erythematous and the cervix friable.

B. Laboratory Findings

Mixing the discharge with normal saline facilitates detection of the flagellated protozoan on microscopic examination (wet preparation). This has a sensitivity of only 60%–70% even with immediate evaluation of the slide. More sensitive testing methods include NAAT and point-of-care antigen-based detection assays.

▶ Complications

Trichomonas infection in females has been associated with adverse pregnancy outcomes. Male partners of females diagnosed with trichomoniasis have a 22% chance of having trichomoniasis and should receive empiric therapy. Rescreening for *T vaginalis* at 3 months following initial infection is indicated for women due to the high rate of reinfection.

▶ Treatment

See Table 44–2 for treatment recommendations.

Meites E et al: A review of evidence-based care of symptomatic trichomoniasis and asymptomatic *Trichomonas vaginalis* infections. Clin Infect Dis 2015;61 (Suppl 8):S837–S848 [PMID: 26602621].

3. Vulvovaginal Candidiasis

▶ General Considerations

Vulvovaginal candidiasis is caused by *Candida albicans* in 85%–90% of cases. Most females will have at least one episode of vulvovaginal candidiasis in their lifetime, and almost half will have two or more episodes. The highest incidence is between ages 16 and 30 years. Predisposing factors include recent use of antibiotics, diabetes, pregnancy, and HIV. Risk factors include vaginal intercourse, especially with a new sexual partner, use of oral contraceptives, and use of spermicide. This disease is usually caused by unrestrained growth of *Candida* that normally colonizes the vagina asymptomatically or is acquired from the GI tract. Recurrences reflect reactivation of colonization.

▶ Clinical Findings

A. Symptoms and Signs

Typical symptoms include pruritus and a white, cottage cheese-like vaginal discharge without odor. The itching is more common midcycle and shortly after menses. Other symptoms include vaginal soreness, vulvar burning, vulvar edema and redness, dyspareunia, and dysuria (especially after intercourse).

B. Laboratory Findings

The diagnosis is usually made by visualizing yeast or pseudohyphae with 10% KOH (90% sensitive) or Gram stain (77% sensitive) of the vaginal discharge. Fungal culture can be used if symptoms and microscopy are not definitive or if disease is unresponsive or recurrent. However, culture is not specific as colonization is common in asymptomatic females. Vaginal pH is normal with yeast infections.

▶ Complications

The only complication of vulvovaginal candidiasis is recurrent infection. Most females with recurrent infection have no apparent predisposing or underlying conditions.

▶ Treatment

Short-course topical formulations effectively treat uncomplicated vaginal yeast infections (see Table 44–2). The topically applied azole drugs are more effective than nystatin. Treatment with azoles results in relief of symptoms and negative cultures in 80%–90% of patients who complete therapy. Oral fluconazole as a one-time dose is an effective oral treatment. Six-month prophylaxis regimens have been effective in many female patients with persistent or recurrent yeast infection. Recurrent disease is usually due to *C albicans* that remains susceptible to azoles and should be treated for 14 days with oral azoles. Some nonalbicans *Candida* will respond to itraconazole or boric acid gelatin capsules (600 mg daily for 14 days) intravaginally. Treatment of sex partners is not recommended.

GENITAL ULCERATIONS

ESSENTIALS OF DIAGNOSIS & TYPICAL FEATURES

▶ Ulcerative STIs can be generally distinguished by their clinical appearance, tenderness of ulcers, and associated lymphadenopathy.

▶ The most common ulcerative STIs in the United States include HSV and syphilis.

▶ Syphilis is typically diagnosed using serologic testing.

Table 44–4. Sexually transmitted causes of genital ulcerations.

	Causative Organism	Description of Ulcers	Ulcer Tenderness	Regional Lymphadenopathy
Herpes simplex virus	HSV1 or HSV2	Multiple, small, shallow	Painful	Occasionally present, tender, not suppurative
Syphilis	*Treponema pallidum*	Single, indurated, nonpurulent "chancre" with a clean base	Not painful	Nontender, firm adenopathy
Chancroid	*Haemophilus ducreyi*	One or more, sharply demarcated, ragged edges, purulent base	Painful	Tender; suppurative
Granuloma inguinale (donovanosis)	*Klebsiella granulomatis*	Single, slowly progressive, beefy red vascular appearance	Not painful	None
Lymphogranuloma venereum	*Chlamydia trachomatis* serovars L1, L2, L3	Single small papule or ulcer that often resolves prior to presentation	Not painful	Unilateral, tender, suppurative inguinal or femoral nodes

In the United States, young, sexually active patients who have genital ulcers usually have genital herpes or syphilis. The relative frequency of each disease differs by geographic area and patient population. More than one of these diseases can be present simultaneously. All ulcerative diseases are associated with an increased risk for HIV infection. In addition, primary HIV infection (acute retroviral syndrome) may present with oral and genital ulcers.

Ulcers may be present in vaginal, vulvar, cervical, penile, rectal, or oral locations, depending on the type of sexual behavior. Oral lesions may occur concomitantly with genital ulcerations. Each etiologic agent has specific characteristics that are described in the following sections and in Table 44–4. Lesion pain, inguinal lymphadenopathy, and urethritis may be present in association with the ulcers.

1. Herpes Simplex Virus Infection (See Also Chapter 40)

▶ **General Considerations**

HSV is the most common cause of visible genital ulcers. Both HSV-1 and HSV-2 are transmitted sexually; both serotypes are equally capable of causing infections of the oropharyngeal and anogenital regions. HSV-1 infections are frequently established in children by age 5 through oral acquisition; lower socioeconomic groups have higher infection rates. In 2015–2016, the seroprevalence among US adults was 47.8% for HSV-1 and 11.9% for HSV-2. HSV infections are lifelong as a result of latent infection of sensory ganglia, although many individuals infected with either type of HSV may not be aware of their infection because of mild or nonspecific symptoms when they were infected. Nevertheless, these individuals can still asymptomatically shed virus and thereby unknowingly transmit the infection, and they can reactivate the virus to cause clinical infection in themselves.

▶ **Clinical Findings**

A. Symptoms and Signs

Symptomatic initial genital HSV infection begins with vesicles on the vulva, vagina, cervix, penis, rectum, or urethra, which quickly progress to shallow, painful ulcerations. An atypical presentation of HSV infection includes vulvar erythema and fissures. Urethritis may occur. Initial infection can be severe, lasting up to 3 weeks, and be associated with fever and malaise, as well as localized tender adenopathy. The pain and dysuria can be extremely uncomfortable, requiring sitz baths, topical anesthetics, and occasionally catheterization for urinary retention.

Symptoms tend to be more severe in females. Recurrence in the genital area with HSV-2 is likely (65%–90%). Approximately 40% of individuals infected with HSV-2 will experience at least six recurrences per year in the early years after initial infection. Prodromal pain in the genital, buttock, or pelvic region is common prior to recurrences. Recurrent genital HSV is of shorter duration (5–7 days), with fewer lesions and usually no systemic symptoms. Commonly, the frequency of recurrences decreases over time, although approximately one-third of individuals fail to demonstrate this pattern. First-episode genital herpes infection caused by HSV-1 is usually the consequence of oral-genital sex. Primary HSV-1 infection may be as severe as HSV-2 infection, and treatment is the same. Recurrence of genital HSV-1 is much less frequent than genital HSV-2.

B. Laboratory Findings

Diagnosis of genital HSV infection is often made presumptively, but in one large series this diagnosis was incorrect for 20% of cases. NAAT is more sensitive and rapid than culture. Direct immunofluorescence assays are available but lack sensitivity. Serologic testing can be used to screen for HSV infection in asymptomatic patients and to distinguish serotypes.

Differential Diagnosis

Genital HSV infections must be distinguished from other ulcerative STI lesions (see Table 44–4). Non-STI causes of genital ulcers might include herpes zoster, Behçet syndrome, or lichen sclerosis.

Complications

Complications such as urinary retention and viral meningitis are usually associated with the first episode of genital HSV infection. Transmission to newborns can occur at birth.

Prevention

All patients with active lesions should be counseled to abstain from sexual contact. Almost all patients have very frequent periodic asymptomatic shedding of HSV, and most cases of genital HSV infection are transmitted from persons who are unaware that they have the infection or who are asymptomatic when transmission occurs. Individuals with prior symptomatic HSV should use barrier protection during sexual activity to protect susceptible partners. Antiviral prophylaxis for infected individuals reduces shedding and significantly reduces transmission to sexual partners.

Treatment

Antiviral drugs administered within the first 5 days of primary HSV infection decreases the duration and severity of symptoms (see Table 44–2). When used for recurrent disease, antiviral therapy should be started with the prodrome or during the first day of lesion onset for best results. Patients should have a prescription at home to initiate treatment. Episodic treatment of first or subsequent attacks will not prevent future attacks. If recurrences are frequent and cause significant physical or emotional discomfort, patients may elect to take antiviral prophylaxis daily to reduce the frequency (70%–80% decrease) and duration of recurrences.

2. Syphilis

General Considerations

Syphilis is an acute and chronic STI caused by *T pallidum*. The annual incidence of syphilis has been steadily increasing since reaching an all-time low in 2000. In 2021, 46.5% of all male primary and secondary syphilis cases in the United States occurred among MSM. Young MSM of color are disproportionately affected. Cases of primary and secondary syphilis also increased by 55.3% among women during 2020–2021, with associated increases in the rate of congenital syphilis.

Clinical Findings

A. Symptoms and Signs

Skin and mucous membrane lesions characterize the acute phase of primary and secondary syphilis. Primary syphilis usually presents as a painless solitary chancre at the point of inoculation, on the genitalia, anus, or oropharynx (see Table 44–4). The chancre appears on average 21 days (range: 3–90 days) after exposure and resolves spontaneously 4–8 weeks later. Because it is painless, it may go undetected, especially if the lesion is within the vagina, oropharynx, urethra, or rectum. Secondary syphilis occurs 4–10 weeks after the chancre appears, with generalized malaise, painless adenopathy, and a nonpruritic maculopapular rash that often includes the palms and soles. Secondary syphilis resolves in 1–3 months but can recur. Verrucous lesions known as condylomata lata may develop on the genitalia. These must be distinguished from genital warts. Lesions of the bone, viscera, aorta, and central nervous system predominate in the chronic phase (tertiary syphilis) (see Chapter 42). *T pallidum* can infect the central nervous system and result in neurosyphilis, which can occur at any stage. Manifestations of neurosyphilis can include altered mental status, cranial nerve dysfunction, meningitis, or stroke. Latent syphilis lacks any clinical manifestations and is diagnosed using serologic testing.

B. Laboratory Findings

T pallidum cannot be cultured and direct detection in lesion exudate or tissue (ie, by microscopic darkfield examination or NAAT) is not readily available in most laboratories. A presumptive diagnosis of syphilis requires two serologic tests, a nontreponemal test (ie, RPR or Venereal Disease Research Laboratory [VDRL] slide test), and a treponemal test (ie, *T pallidum* particle agglutination [TP-PA], fluorescent treponemal antibody absorption [FTA-ABS], *T pallidum* enzyme immunoassay [TP-EIA], or *T pallidum* chemiluminescence assay [TP-CIA]). Nontreponemal antibody titers typically correlate with disease activity and are used to follow treatment response. A fourfold change in nontreponemal antibody titers indicates a clinically significant difference. In contrast, treponemal antibody titers typically remain reactive for life and cannot be used to determine treatment response. The CDC and the US Preventive Services Task Force recommend serologic screening with a nontreponemal test, followed by confirmation with a treponemal test. However, some laboratories have adopted a "reverse-sequence" approach (Figure 44–1).

If a patient is engaging in high-risk sexual behavior or is living in an area in which syphilis is endemic, RPRs should be drawn yearly to screen for asymptomatic infection. Annual RPR testing among high-risk groups is essential to distinguish between early latent syphilis (1 year or less postinfection) and late latent syphilis (> 1 year postinfection), as treatment recommendations vary. Syphilis is reportable to state health departments, and all sexual contacts need to be evaluated. Patients with syphilis need to be evaluated for other STIs, especially HIV.

Testing of CSF, including cell count, protein, and CSF VDRL, is indicated in patients with neurologic signs and symptoms who may have neurosyphilis, patients with ocular

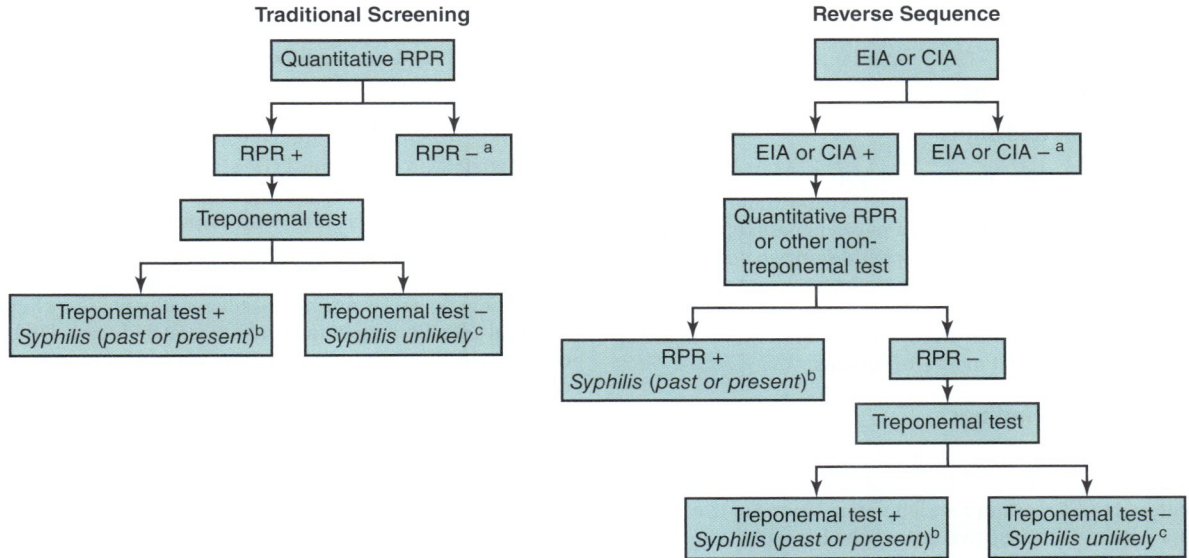

Traditional Screening

Quantitative RPR

RPR +   RPR – [a]

Treponemal test

Treponemal test +
Syphilis (past or present)[b]   Treponemal test –
Syphilis unlikely[c]

Reverse Sequence

EIA or CIA

EIA or CIA +   EIA or CIA – [a]

Quantitative RPR
or other non-
treponemal test

RPR +
Syphilis (past or present)[b]   RPR –

Treponemal test

Treponemal test +
Syphilis (past or present)[b]   Treponemal test –
Syphilis unlikely[c]

▲ **Figure 44–1.** Approaches to syphilis screening. The CDC recommends the traditional algorithm. If reverse sequence screening is used, it recommends that a specimen with reactive EIA/CIA results be tested reflexively with a quantitative nontreponemal test (RPR or VDRL). If test results are discordant, the specimen should be tested reflexively using a treponemal test for confirmation. EIA/CIA, enzyme immunoassay/chemiluminescence immunoassay; RPR, rapid plasma regain; VDRL, Venereal Disease Research Laboratory.
[a]If incubating or primary syphilis is suspected, treat with benzathine penicillin G 2.4 million units intramuscularly in a single dose.
[b]Evaluate clinically, determine whether treated for syphilis in the past, assess risk for infection, and administer therapy if indicated, based on stage of infection.
[c]If at risk for syphilis, repeat RPR in several weeks.
(Adapted from: Centers for Disease Control and Prevention (CDC): Discordant results from reverse sequence syphilis screening—five laboratories, United States, 2006–2010. MMWR Morb Mortal Wkly Rep 2011;60(5):133–137.)

manifestations such as uveitis, iritis, neuroretinitis, or optic neuritis, and patients who experience treatment failure. Follow-up CSF evaluation is indicated every 6 months in patients with neurosyphilis until the CSF cell count normalizes.

Complications

Untreated syphilis can lead to tertiary complications with serious multiorgan involvement, including aortitis and neurosyphilis. Transmission to the fetus can occur from an untreated pregnant woman (see Chapters 2 and 42). Syphilitic mucosal lesions can facilitate transmission of HIV. In addition, people with HIV who acquire syphilis may have unusual serologic responses (ie, false-negative results, delayed sero-reactivity), may be at increased risk of neurologic complications, and may have increased rates of treatment failure.

Treatment

See Table 44–2 for treatment recommendations. Parenteral penicillin G is the preferred drug for all stages of syphilis,

although the preparation, dose, and duration of treatment vary depending on clinical manifestations. While there are alternatives for use in penicillin-allergic patients, data on their efficacy are limited, and in some scenarios (ie, pregnancy), desensitization and treatment with penicillin are recommended. Patients should be reexamined and serologically evaluated with nontreponemal tests at 6 and 12 months after treatment. If signs or symptoms persist or recur, or patients do not have a fourfold decrease in their nontreponemal test titer, they should be considered to have failed treatment or be reinfected and need retreatment.

3. Chancroid

General Considerations

Chancroid is caused by *Haemophilus ducreyi*. It is relatively rare outside of the tropics and subtropics but is endemic in some urban areas in the United States, and has been associated with HIV infection, drug use, and sex work. Coinfection with syphilis or HSV occurs in as many as 17% of patients.

A detailed history, including travel, can be important in identifying this infection.

Clinical Findings

A. Symptoms and Signs

The typical lesion begins as a papule that erodes after 24–48 hours into an ulcer. The ulcer is painful and has ragged, sharply demarcated edges and a purulent base (unlike syphilis). The ulcer is typically solitary and somewhat deeper than HSV infection. The lesions may occur anywhere on the genitals and are more common in men than in women. Tender, fluctuant (differentiates from syphilis and HSV) inguinal adenopathy is present in 50% of patients.

B. Laboratory Findings

Culture, which has a sensitivity of less than 80%, can be performed on a special medium that is available in academic centers. NAAT may improve laboratory diagnosis if available. In a patient with negative test results for syphilis and HSV, with painful genital ulcers and regional adenopathy, a presumptive diagnosis of chancroid should be considered.

Treatment

Symptoms improve within 3 days after therapy (see Table 44–2). Most ulcers resolve in 7 days, although large ulcers may take 2 weeks to heal. Fluctuant adenopathy may require needle aspiration or incision and drainage. All sexual contacts need to be examined and treated, even if asymptomatic. Individuals with HIV coinfection may have slower rates of healing or treatment failures.

4. Lymphogranuloma Venereum

General Considerations

LGV, which is caused by *C trachomatis* serovars L1, L2, or L3, is rare in the United States. The disease is endemic in Southeast Asia, the Caribbean, Latin America, and areas of Africa. Since 2003, an increased number of cases in the United States, Western Europe, and Canada have occurred primarily among MSM and has been associated with HIV coinfection.

Clinical Findings

A. Symptoms and Signs

Patients with LGV present with a painless papule or ulcer that heals spontaneously, followed by the development of tender adenopathy that is typically unilateral. A classic finding is the groove sign—an inguinal crease created by concomitant involvement of inguinal and femoral nodes. These nodes become matted and fluctuant and may rupture. LGV can cause proctocolitis with rectal ulceration, purulent anal discharge, fever, tenesmus, and lower abdominal pain, primarily in MSM.

B. Laboratory Findings

Diagnosis of LGV can be difficult. It requires a clinical suspicion based on physical examination findings. Lesion swabs and lymph node aspirates can be tested for *Chlamydia* by culture, DFA, or NAAT. Additional genotyping is necessary to differentiate LGV from non-LGV serovars of *Chlamydia*. In the absence of laboratory testing to confirm the diagnosis, one should treat for LGV if clinical suspicion is high.

Differential Diagnosis

Differential diagnosis during the adenopathy phase includes bacterial adenitis, lymphoma, and cat-scratch disease. Differential diagnosis during the ulcerative phase encompasses all causes of genital ulcers (see Table 44–4).

Treatment

See Table 44–2 for treatment recommendations. Despite the effectiveness of azithromycin for non-LGV chlamydial infections, there have been no controlled treatment trials to recommend its use in LGV. Individuals with HIV are treated the same as those without HIV but should be monitored closely to assess response to treatment.

Stoner BP, Cohen SE: Lymphogranuloma venereum 2015: clinical presentation, diagnosis, and treatment. Clin Infect Dis 2015 Dec 15;61 (Suppl 8):S865–S873. doi: 10.1093/cid/civ756 [PMID: 26602624].

5. Granuloma Inguinale

Granuloma inguinale, or donovanosis, is caused by *Klebsiella granulomatis*, a gram-negative bacillus that is rare in the United States but is endemic in India, the Caribbean, and southern Africa. An indurated subcutaneous nodule erodes to form a painless, friable ulcer with granulation tissue. Diagnosis is based on clinical suspicion and supported by a Wright or Giemsa stain of the granulation tissue that reveals intracytoplasmic rods (Donovan bodies) in mononuclear cells. See Table 44–2 for treatment recommendations. Relapse may occur 6–18 months after apparently effective treatment.

GENITAL WARTS & HUMAN PAPILLOMAVIRUS

ESSENTIALS OF DIAGNOSIS & TYPICAL FEATURES

► Ninety percent of anogenital warts are caused by HPV and are usually diagnosed by visual inspection.

► Cervical cancer is caused by oncogenic types of HPV. Screening for cervical abnormalities and cancer should begin at age 21. HPV nucleic acid testing is available for detecting oncogenic types of HPV infection.

General Considerations

Condylomata acuminata, or genital warts, are caused by HPV, which can also cause cervical dysplasia and cervical cancer, and oropharyngeal and anal cancers. HPV is transmitted sexually. An estimated 20 million people in the United States are infected annually with HPV. The majority (74%) of new HPV infections occurs among those 15–24 years of age. It is estimated that 32%–50% of adolescent females having sexual intercourse in the United States have HPV infections, though only 1% may have visible lesions. Thirty to 60% of males whose partners have HPV have evidence of genital warts on examination.

Although there are almost 100 serotypes of HPV, types 6 and 11 cause approximately 90% of genital warts, and HPV types 16 and 18 cause more than 70% of cervical dysplasia and cervical cancer. The infection is more common in persons with multiple partners and in those who initiate sexual intercourse at an early age. See HPV vaccination in Chapter 10.

Clinical Findings

A. Symptoms and Signs

For males, verrucous lesions are found on the shaft or corona of the penis. Lesions also may develop in the urethra or rectum. Lesions do not produce discomfort. They may be single or found in clusters. Females develop verrucous lesions on any genital mucosal surface, either internally or externally, and often develop perianal lesions.

B. Laboratory Findings

External, visible lesions have unique characteristics that make the diagnosis straightforward. Condylomata acuminata can be distinguished from condylomata lata (syphilis), skin tags, and molluscum contagiosum by application of 5% acetic acid solution. Blanching of skin or mucous membranes, after application of 3%–5% acetic acid solution, termed *acetowhitening*, is used to indicate the extent of HPV infection.

Cervical cancer screening recommendations are published by the US Preventive Services Task Force. Cervical cytology with a Papanicolaou (Pap) smear is recommended every 3 years from age 21 to 29. Beginning at age 30, screening may include cytology alone, HPV NAAT, or a combination of both. Pap smears detect cervical abnormalities caused by HPV and are graded by the atypical nature of the cervical cells. These changes range from atypical squamous cells of undetermined significance (ASCUS) to low-grade squamous intraepithelial lesions (LSIL) and high-grade squamous intraepithelial lesions (HSIL). Consensus guidelines for the management of Pap smear results are published by the American Society of Colposcopy and Cervical Pathology (http://www.asccp.org/management-guidelines).

Differential Diagnosis

The differential diagnosis of genital warts includes normal anatomic structures (pearly penile papules, vestibular papillae, and sebaceous glands), molluscum contagiosum, seborrheic keratosis, and condyloma lata (syphilis).

Complications

Because genital warts can proliferate and become friable during pregnancy, many experts advocate their removal during pregnancy. HPV types 6 and 11 can cause laryngeal papillomatosis in infants who are infected during vaginal delivery. Complications of appropriate treatment include scarring with changes in skin pigmentation or pain at the treatment site. Cervical dysplasia may require biopsy and/or resection, which may result in cervical abnormalities that complicate pregnancy. Cervical, oral, and anal cancer is the most common and important sequela of oncogenic HPV infections.

Prevention

The use of condoms significantly reduces, but does not eliminate, the risk for transmission to uninfected partners. The 9-valent HPV vaccine is 96%–100% effective in preventing HPV-6 and 11-related genital warts and HPV-16 and 18-related cervical dysplasia and many of the cervical lesions caused by less common serotypes. It is recommended for females and males aged 9–26 years. The vaccine protects males against genital warts and anal cancer, which has a significantly increased incidence in males who practice anal sex (see Chapter 10).

Treatment

Penile and external vaginal or vulvar lesions can be treated topically. An experienced practitioner should treat internal and cervical lesions (see Table 44–2). Treatment may clear the visible lesions, but not reduce the presence of virus, nor is it clear whether transmission of HPV or subsequent development of cancer is reduced by treatment.

Warts may resolve or remain unchanged if left untreated or they may increase in size or number. Treatment can induce wart-free periods in most patients. Most recurrences occur within the 3 months following completion of a treatment regimen. Appropriate follow-up of abnormal Pap smears is essential to detect any progression to malignancy.

ASCCP Consensus Guidelines for Management of Abnormal Cervical Cytology: http://www.asccp.org/management-guidelines. Accessed May 1, 2023.
United States Preventative Services Task Force: Screening for Cervical Cancer. JAMA 2018;320(7):674–686. doi:10.1001/jama/2018.10897 [PMID: 30140884]

OTHER VIRAL INFECTIONS

ESSENTIALS OF DIAGNOSIS & TYPICAL FEATURES

► Hepatitis A, B, and C can be transmitted sexually; although vaccines are available to prevent HAV and HBV infections.

► Acute HIV infection often presents with an acute retroviral syndrome, which mimics other viral infections.

► Antiretroviral drugs can be used to prevent HIV acquisition when given before (as preexposure prophylaxis [PrEP]) or after (as postexposure prophylaxis [PEP]) HIV exposure.

1. Hepatitis (See Also Chapter 22)

► General Considerations

In the United States, viral hepatitis is caused primarily by three viruses: HAV, HBV, and hepatitis C virus (HCV). Each virus has the potential to spread through sexual activity. HAV spreads via fecal-oral transmission and oral-anal contact. Both HBV and HCV spread through contact with blood or body fluids. Sexual transmission of HBV is believed to be much more efficient than that of HCV, although some data suggest increased transmission of HCV in MSM.

Universal immunization recommendations for HAV and HBV have contributed to the decline in the prevalence of these diseases. Individuals born before implementation of routine vaccination, especially those in high-risk groups (multiple sexual partners, MSM, or people who inject drugs) should receive HAV and HBV vaccines. Serologic screening for HCV is recommended for all adults older than 18 years, for all women during each pregnancy, for persons with newly diagnosed HIV or HBV infection, and annually for persons with ongoing risk factors (ie, engaging in high-risk sexual practices or injecting drug use).

2. Human Immunodeficiency Virus (See Also Chapter 41)

► General Considerations

In 2020, there were 28,600 youth aged 13–24 years living with HIV in the United States, of whom only 56% were aware of their diagnosis, compared to 85% of adults. Young MSM continue to be the highest-risk group for HIV acquisition in the United States, particularly young men of color. Risk factors for contracting HIV include a prior STI (especially syphilis and rectal gonorrhea), infrequent condom use, practicing insertive or receptive anal sex (among both males and females), prior genital ulcerative STIs, trading sex for money or drugs, recreational drug use, homelessness, and being the victim of sexual abuse.

All adolescents being screened for other STIs should be screened for HIV infection, whether they have sex with males, females, or both. The CDC and the US Preventive Services Task Force recommend that all adults older than 13 years be screened for HIV at least once, with annual or more frequent screening recommended for those at higher risk for HIV acquisition. HIV screening can be performed in association with STI screening, pregnancy testing, and routine health evaluations. Opt-out screening (notifying the patient that HIV testing will be performed unless the patient declines) is recommended. Specific consent for HIV testing is not required. Most states allow minors to participate in HIV testing and treatment without parental notification, but providers should be aware of their state's laws.

► Clinical Findings

A. Symptoms and Signs

After a recent HIV infection, adolescents may be asymptomatic or may present with the acute retroviral syndrome, which occurs 2–6 weeks after exposure. This acute clinical syndrome, which occurs in about 50% of patients, is often indistinguishable from other viral illnesses (Table 44–5) and may include oral or genital ulcers. After the acute illness resolves, signs and symptoms of HIV are typically

Table 44–5. Symptoms of acute retroviral syndrome after HIV infection.

Common symptoms (> 50% of patients)
Fever
Fatigue
Pharyngitis
Headache
Myalgia
Anorexia
Less common (< 50%) symptoms
Weight loss
Diarrhea
Skin rash
Arthralgia
Oral ulcerations
Nausea/vomiting
Adenopathy
Uncommon (< 10%) but distinguishing symptoms
Odynophagia
Genital ulcer
Oral or vaginal candidiasis
Neurologic symptoms (ie, aseptic meningitis)

absent for many years, until life-threatening immunodeficiency develops.

B. Laboratory Findings

Laboratory testing for HIV is described in detail in Chapter 41. The current testing algorithm for serum or plasma recommends the use of an HIV 1/2 antigen/antibody combination immunoassay, which detects both established infections and acute infections as recent as 2–3 weeks after exposure. If acute HIV infection is suspected, HIV NAAT should also be performed.

▶ Treatment

Treatment for HIV is described in detail in Chapter 41. The most important aspect of identifying adolescents and young adults with HIV infection is linking them to care. Data support the treatment of youth with HIV infection in care settings that provide comprehensive, multidisciplinary care. These settings will be best equipped to provide emotional support, preventive care, risk reduction for contacts, access to research, and guidance on antiretroviral therapies.

Centers for Disease Control and Prevention: HIV and Youth. https://www.cdc.gov/hiv/group/age/youth/index.html. Accessed April 25, 2023.

3. HIV Postsexual Exposure Prophylaxis

Adolescents may present to health care providers seeking nonoccupational HIV postexposure prophylaxis (nPEP) following an assault or a high-risk sexual encounter. The risk for HIV transmission depends on the probability that the source is infected with HIV, the viral load of an infected source, and the type of exposure. The risk of transmission from an HIV-infected source per episode of receptive penile-anal sexual exposure is estimated at 0.5%–3%; the risk per episode of receptive vaginal exposure is estimated at less than 0.1%–0.2%. Transmission rates are higher in scenarios of sexual assault or abuse associated with trauma, bleeding, or tissue injury than with consensual sexual contact. The presence of an STI, particularly genital ulcerative lesions, in either partner also increases risk of transmission. HIV transmission from receptive oral exposure is rare, but the presence of oral sores or mucosal injuries increases risk. HIV transmission is greatly reduced if the source is receiving antiretroviral therapy and is essentially zero if the source has an undetectable viral load.

Providers who offer nPEP should consider the likelihood that exposure to HIV occurred, the potential benefits and risks of such therapy, and the interval between the exposure and initiation of therapy. There are no data that show nPEP is effective when more than 72 hours have passed since exposure. If the patient decides to initiate nPEP, clinical

management should be implemented according to published CDC guidelines. Providers should be aware that structural barriers exist to obtaining nPEP, and that adolescent assault victims have a high discontinuation rate due to adverse effects from the medication.

Centers for Disease Control and Prevention: Updated Guidelines for Antiretroviral Postexposure Prophylaxis After Sexual, Injection Drug Use, or Other Nonoccupational Exposure to HIV—United States, 2016. https://www.cdc.gov/hiv/pdf/programresources/cdc-hiv-npep-guidelines.pdf. Accessed May 1, 2023.

4. HIV Preexposure Prophylaxis

PrEP involves the use of antiretrovirals by people at high risk of HIV to prevent HIV acquisition. The CDC PrEP guidelines contain indications for PrEP use in MSM, heterosexual men and women, and people who inject drugs. The FDA has approved two co-formulated combinations of oral antiretroviral drugs that are taken daily, and one injectable antiretroviral drug administered every 8 weeks, as options for PrEP in individuals of any age who weigh greater than or equal to 35 kg. When used consistently, PrEP reduces the risk of HIV transmission through sex by 99%. Providers considering the use of PrEP in a minor at risk of HIV acquisition should consult with an experienced prescriber and understand the laws of their state with respect to providing preventive HIV medication without parental consent.

Centers for Disease Control and Prevention: US Public Health Service: preexposure prophylaxis for the prevention of HIV infection in the United States—2017 update: a Clinical practice guideline. https://www.cdc.gov/hiv/pdf/risk/prep/cdc-hiv-prep-guidelines-2017.pdf. Published March 2018. Accessed May 1, 2023.
Hosek S, Pettifor A: HIV Prevention interventions for adolescents. Curr HIV/AIDS Rep 2019;16(1):120–128 [PMID: 30707399].
Hosek SG et al: An HIV Preexposure prophylaxis demonstration project and safety study for young MSM. J Acquir Immune Defic Syndr 2017;74(1):21–29 [PMID: 27632233].

ECTOPARASITIC INFECTIONS

ESSENTIALS OF DIAGNOSIS & TYPICAL FEATURES

▶ Pubic lice is transmitted by close contact. Itching is common.

▶ Scabies is transmitted by close skin-to skin contact. Infection starts with severe itching that worsens at night. Treat all household members and close contacts.

1. Pubic Lice

Pthirus pubis, the pubic louse, lives in pubic hair. The louse or the nits can be transmitted by close contact from person to person. Patients complain of itching and may report having seen the insect. Examination of the pubic hair may reveal the louse crawling around or attached to the hair. Closer inspection may reveal the nit or sac of eggs, which is a gelatinous material (1–2 mm) stuck to the hair shaft. See Table 44–2 for treatment recommendations.

2. Scabies

Sarcoptes scabiei, the causative organism in scabies, is smaller than the louse. It can be identified by the classic burrow, which is created by the organism laying eggs and traveling just below the skin surface. Scabies can be sexually transmitted by close skin-to-skin contact and can be found in the pubic region, groin, lower abdomen, or upper thighs. The rash is intensely pruritic, especially at night, erythematous, and scaly. See Table 44–2 for treatment options. Ivermectin is an oral therapeutic option for scabies that may hold promise in the treatment of severe infestations or in epidemic situations. When treating with lotion or shampoo, the entire area needs to be covered for the time specified by the manufacturer. Two (or more) applications, each about a week apart, may be necessary to eliminate all mites. Bed sheets and clothes must be washed in hot water. Both sexual and close personal or household contacts within the preceding month should be examined and treated and considered for prophylactic therapy.

Leone PA: Scabies and pediculosis pubis: an update of treatment regimens and general review. Clin Infect Dis 2007;44:S153 [PMID: 17342668].

REFERENCES

Centers for Disease Control and Prevention: National Overview— Sexually Transmitted Disease Surveillance, 2021. https://www.cdc.gov/std/statistics/2021/default.htm. Accessed April 25, 2023.

Centers for Disease Control and Prevention. Sexually Transmitted Infections Treatment Guidelines, 2021. MMWR 2021;70:4. https://www.cdc.gov/std/treatment-guidelines/STI-Guidelines-2021.pdf [PMID: 34292926].

Snook ML et al: Adolescent gynecology: special considerations for special patients. Clin Obstet Gynecol 2012;55:651 [PMID: 22828097].

Travel Medicine

Suchitra Rao, MBBS, MSCS

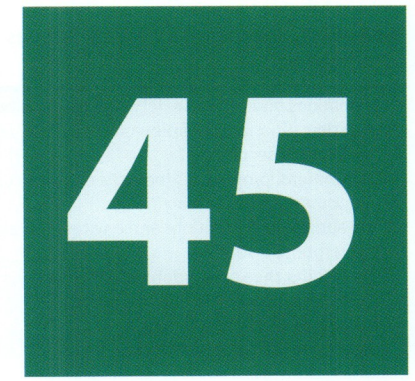

INTRODUCTION

Approximately 50%–70% of travelers become ill during their travel overseas. The number of children traveling with families continues to increase. Children who travel are especially susceptible to infectious diseases, trauma, and other health problems, which vary with the destination. Preparation for travel with children and infants includes consideration of destination-specific risks, underlying medical problems, and administration of both routine and travel-related vaccines. Pretravel counseling should ideally take place at least 1 month prior to travel, given the need to develop an effective immune response from any travel-associated vaccinations. The physician involved in pretravel counseling should focus on the issues listed in Table 45–1.

PREPARING CHILDREN & INFANTS FOR TRAVEL

▶ Travel Plans

Parents and care providers should be advised that travel with children and infants is much more enjoyable when the number of journeys in a single trip is limited, travel time is kept relatively short, and travel delays are anticipated. Planning for delays and other problems should include bringing new or favorite toys or games for distraction and carrying extra food and drink, changes of clothing, and fever medications.

Medical Care During Travel

It is useful to obtain names and addresses of local health care providers at the family's destination. This is available from travel medicine practitioners or from the membership directory of the International Society of Travel Medicine. The International Association for Medical Assistance to Travelers website (www.iamat.org) is another useful resource with a worldwide directory of providers proficient in English. Travel insurance, which is highly encouraged, should not only cover medical care at the destination but also provide 24-hour helplines with information regarding English-speaking physicians and hospitals, and arrange and pay for evacuation to a medical facility that provides necessary treatment that is not available locally. In emergencies, parents and caretakers should take their children to the largest medical facility in the area, which is more likely to have a pediatric unit and trauma services.

Trauma

Trauma is a common cause of morbidity and mortality in traveling children. Parents should rent larger, safer vehicles, and use car seats whenever possible. However, in many developing countries, car seats are not available, so caretakers may need to travel with their own. Taxis often do not have seatbelts, so it may be necessary to request taxis with seatbelts by calling in advance.

Air Travel

As the altitude increases the partial pressure of oxygen in the atmosphere decreases, resulting in aircraft passengers at cruising altitude breathing the equivalent of 15%–16% of fractional inspired oxygen (FIO_2) at sea level. This lower oxygen environment elicits little or no clinically relevant effects in healthy term infants and children, who can travel by commercial pressurized airplane. However, children at higher risk of complications from hypoxia during air travel may include premature infants and those with chronic cardiac, pulmonary disease and sickle cell disease, so appropriate counseling with their specialist is indicated. Many parents request advice regarding sedation of their child during travel. While this is not recommended, the most widely used agent is diphenhydramine. It is advisable to try a test dose prior to travel as idiosyncratic reactions and overdosing can lead to an anticholinergic syndrome or a paradoxical stimulating effect.

Table 45–1. Preparing for travel—issues specific to travel as indicated.

Vaccinations (indications, safety, and tolerability)
Insect precautions (use of protective clothing, repellants, bed nets, insecticides)
Malaria chemoprophylaxis (benefits of a particular regimen vs potential adverse reactions)
Food and water precautions and environmental risks from waterborne disease
Traveler's diarrhea precautions and medications for self-treatment
Health insurance/evacuation insurance
Trauma prevention and car seats
Access to medical care during travel
Altitude sickness
Disease outbreaks in destination
Climate
Jetlag
Animal exposure, trauma from animals
General health and routine illness
Clothing and footwear
Copies of prescriptions, vaccination documentation, physician's letter, list of medications
Travel-specific medications
Safe sex counseling
First-aid kits
Crime and safety

Ear Pain

Children and infants often have pain during ascent and descent of commercial airplanes due to changes in middle ear pressure causing retraction or protrusion of the tympanic membrane. Methods that can alleviate or minimize ear pain during these times include chewing, swallowing, nursing, and bottle feeding.

Motion Sickness

Almost 60% of children will experience motion sickness during travel. While older children have symptoms similar to those in adults (such as nausea, epigastric discomfort, headache, general discomfort), children younger than 5 years may have gait abnormalities as the predominant symptom. Non-pharmacologic preventive strategies include eating a light meal at least 3 hours before travel; avoiding dairy products and foods high in calories, protein, and sodium before travel; sitting in the middle of the back seat or in the front seat if age-appropriate; focusing on a stable object in the distance or the horizon; avoiding reading or other visual stimuli; eye closure; fresh air; and limiting excessive head movement. Pharmacologic intervention has not been well studied in children, but if necessary, antihistamines such as diphenhydramine are recommended for children younger than 12 years and scopolamine is acceptable for children older than 12 years. These measures, however, are not evidence based.

High Altitude

Acute mountain sickness is as common in children as in adults, but it may go unrecognized due to its subtle presentation, such as unexplained mental fussiness or change in appetite and sleep patterns. High-altitude pulmonary edema (HAPE) is seen in children traveling to high altitudes; it also occurs in children who live at high altitude, descend for an extended period, and return to altitude. Mild symptoms of altitude sickness can be treated with rest and hydration, or analgesics such as ibuprofen or acetaminophen. High-altitude sickness is milder and resolves much more quickly in children compared to adults, so prophylaxis is usually not required. Acetazolamide has not been studied in children for acute mountain sickness, but it is safe in this age group and has been used for both prophylaxis and treatment. The pediatric dose is 5 mg/kg/day (125 mg maximum) divided twice daily, starting 1 day before ascent and continued for 2 days at high altitude. An alternative treatment includes dexamethasone 0.15 mg/kg/dose orally every 6 hours.

Medications/First-Aid Kit

A small medical kit is useful when traveling, and suggested items are outlined in Table 45–2. Medications should be

Table 45–2. First-aid kit for international travel.

Medications
Malaria prophylaxis
Acetaminophen and ibuprofen
Antibiotics
Antihistamines
Topical formulations
Hydrocortisone ointment
Antibiotic and antifungal ointment
Insect repellants
Sunscreen
Antibacterial soap/alcohol-based hand sanitizer
Antiseptic wipes
Other
Bed nets
Thermometer
Medicine spoon and cup
Oral rehydration salts in powder form
Sterile cotton balls, cotton tip applicators
Tweezers, scissors, safety pins
Water purification tablets
Gauze bandages
Tape—hypoallergenic, waterproof
Triangular bandage/sling/splint
Tongue depressor
Adhesive bandages
Flashlight
First-aid book
Copies of prescriptions, list of medications, copy of insurance coverage

purchased prior to travel, as those obtained at some destinations may be of poor quality or contain toxic substances.

Chehab H, Fischer PR, Christenson JC: Preparing children for international travel. Pediatr Rev 2021 Apr;42(4):189–202 [PMID: 33795465].

Leung DT, LaRocque RC, Ryan ET: Travel medicine. Ann Intern Med 2018 Jan 2;168(1):ITC1–ITC16 [PMID: 29297035].

Stauffer W, Christenson JC, Fischer PR: Preparing children for international travel. Travel Med Infect Dis 2008;6(3):101–113 [PMID: 18486064].

VACCINATIONS—ROUTINE CHILDHOOD VACCINES MODIFIED FOR TRAVEL

International travelers to countries with high prevalence rates or outbreaks of vaccine-preventable diseases are at risk for infection and may contribute to disease importation into their native countries. The schedule for some vaccines can be accelerated for travel, and some vaccines can be given earlier than the recommended age. Vaccination pertaining to children traveling follows the routine vaccination schedule as outlined in Chapter 10. The recommended intervals balance the high-risk age for disease with infant immunologic responses. The recommended minimum interval between doses is listed in Table 45–3. Barriers to some early immunizations are antibody from the mother interfering with an infant's ability to mount an antibody response, particularly to live vaccines, and the lack of a T-cell–dependent immune response to certain immunogens in those younger than 2 years. Minor febrile illnesses are not a contraindication to routine or travel vaccines and should not lead to their postponement. Live vaccines should be given together or separated by 30 days or more.

VACCINATIONS—TRAVEL-SPECIFIC

Cholera Vaccine

Cholera is an acute, watery diarrheal illness caused by *Vibrio cholerae* (O1 or O139 serogroups). Global pandemics continue to occur in developing countries. The oral cholera vaccine is recommended for those 2 to 64 years of age traveling to areas of active cholera transmission. Vaccination is effective for at least 3-6 months. The only cholera vaccine available in the United States is the CVD 103-HgR (Vaxchora), which is a live vaccine against serogroup O1.

Japanese Encephalitis Vaccine

Japanese encephalitis (JE) is caused by a flavivirus transmitted by the night-biting Culex mosquito. The risk of contracting severe JE is low, especially for travelers who will have a brief stay in an endemic area, as the infection rate in Culex mosquitoes is 3% or lower, and only 1 in 200 infections with

Table 45–3. Accelerated vaccinations schedule.

Vaccine	Minimum Age for First Dose	Minimum Time to Second Dose (wk)	Minimum Time to Third Dose (wk)	Minimum Time for Fourth Dose (wk)
MMR	12 mo[a]	4	—	—
Hepatitis B	Birth	4	8[b]	—
DTaP	6 wk	4	4	6 mo
Hib	6 wk	4	4	8[c]
IPV	6 wk	4	4	6 mo[d]
MCV	6 wk[e]	8	[e]	[e]
MPS4	2 y[e]	5 y	[e]	[e]
PCV	4 wk	4	4	8
Varicella	12 mo	4	—	—
Rotavirus	4 wk[f]	4	4[g]	—
Hepatitis A	1 y	6 mo	—	—

DTaP, diphtheria-tetanus-acellular pertussis; Hib, *Haemophilus influenzae* type b; IPV, inactivated polio vaccine; MCV, meningococcal conjugate vaccine; MMR, measles-mumps-rubella; MPS4, meningococcal polysaccharide; PCV, pneumococcal conjugate vaccine.
[a]Children traveling abroad may be vaccinated as early as 6 months of age. Before departure, children aged 6–11 months should receive the first dose of MMR vaccine. This will not count toward their series, and they will still require two doses after 12 months of age.
[b]The third dose should be given at least 4 months after the first dose and at a minimum of 6 months of age.
[c]If third dose is given after 4 years, the fourth dose is not required.
[d]Recommended at 6–18 months of age, minimum age 4 years for final dose.
[e]Minimum 6 weeks for Hib-MenCY, 9 months for Menactra (MCV4-D), 2 years for Menveo (MCV4-CRM). Repeat vaccination depends on host status and ongoing risk factors.
[f]This differs from the package insert but is validated by data held by the manufacturer.
[g]No third dose is required if Rotarix is given.

JE leads to neuroinvasive disease. The case fatality rate is 30% in those with severe disease. Most symptomatic cases occur in children younger than 10 years and in the elderly, but travel-associated JE can occur at any age. The areas at risk are within Asia, Eastern Russia, some areas of the Western Pacific, and the Torres Strait Islands of Australia. The peak season is between April and October, during and just after the rainy season. The JE vaccine licensed and available for use in the United States is Ixiaro, an inactivated Vero cell culture–derived vaccine approved for use in children aged 2 months or older. The JE vaccine is recommended for travelers who plan to spend at least 1 month in endemic areas during the JE transmission season and frequent travelers to JE endemic areas. Vaccination should also be considered in the following scenarios: (1) short-term travelers to nonurban areas who will participate in outdoor activities; (2) travelers to an area with an ongoing JE outbreak; and (3) travelers to endemic areas who are uncertain of specific destinations, activities, or duration of travel.

Rabies Vaccine

Rabies is found worldwide and contracted through the bite or saliva-contaminated scratch of infected animals. Canine rabies is highly endemic in parts of Africa, Asia, and Central and South America (RabNet—www.who.int/rabies/rabnet/en/—provides country-specific animal and human data), where 40% of rabies occurs in children younger than 14 years. This increased risk is because children are attracted to animals, are more likely to be bitten and may not report minor encounters with animals. Most cases of rabies in travelers occur through the bite of an infected dog, cat, or monkey (particularly those that live near temples in parts of Asia). Bats, mongooses, and foxes are other animals that can transmit disease.

Rabies vaccine is available for pre- and postexposure prophylaxis. It is recommended for travelers to areas in which rabies is endemic and for those who will have occupational or recreational exposure (such as cavers), especially if access to medical care will be limited when traveling. The risk of a bite from a potentially rabid animal is up to 2% for travelers to the developing world. The three types of inactivated virus vaccine available are administered prior to exposure in two doses at days 0 and 7. Those with ongoing risk should check titers at least 1 year following the two-dose vaccination or receive a one-dose booster at least 21 days following the first vaccine. Vaccination prior to exposure may not be completely protective; further doses are required if a high-risk bite occurs. The minimum age of administration is 1 year and duration of protection is 2 years. Malaria chemoprophylaxis with mefloquine or chloroquine should begin 1 month after completing the rabies vaccine series to avoid interference with the immune response.

It is important to counsel travelers about animal avoidance and thorough cleansing of a bite wound with irrigation for at least 5 minutes. In the event of a bite in a nonvaccinated individual, rabies immunoglobulin ideally within 24–48 hours after contact and four doses of vaccine at days 0, 3, 7, and 14 are required. In a fully vaccinated child exposed to rabies, two booster doses should be given on days 0 and 3 of exposure, and rabies immunoglobulin is not required.

Tick-borne Encephalitis

Most infections with tick-borne encephalitis virus are asymptomatic, but acute neuroinvasive disease and febrile illness can occur. In 2021, the tick-borne encephalitis (TBE) vaccine was approved for use in the United States for those visiting endemic regions of Asia or Europe who may participate in outdoor activities with risk of exposure, especially during times when ticks are most active (April through November). The TBE vaccine is available for individuals aged 1 year and older as a three-dose series. For children 1–15 years of age, the primary vaccination schedule is at day 0, 1–3 months, and 5–12 months. For those 16 years and older, the schedule is at day 0, 14 days to 3 months, and 5–12 months. A fourth dose may be given at least 3 years after completion of the primary vaccination schedule if ongoing exposure or reexposure to TBE is expected.

Tuberculosis

Tuberculosis risk is increased for travelers, especially when visiting Africa, Asia, Latin America, and the former Soviet Union. The risk is higher in long-term travelers to countries with a high incidence of tuberculosis. Bacillus Calmette-Guérin (BCG) vaccination, which is given soon after birth in many countries but not in the United States, protects against miliary and meningeal tuberculosis, but not against pulmonary disease. Efficacy is only established in children younger than 1 year. It may be considered in children younger than 5 years who will be in a high-risk area for a prolonged period and have a negative test for tuberculosis (tuberculin skin test [TST] or interferon-γ release assay [IGRA]). It should not be given to immunosuppressed individuals. BCG is not widely available in the United States but may be administered in the destination country. A preferred alternative is that travelers to high-prevalence areas have a test for tuberculosis prior to travel and 3 months after return. It should be noted that live virus vaccines can create an anergic state, in which tuberculosis testing can be falsely negative. Therefore, testing should be performed on the same day as any live vaccine administration or at least 28 days later.

Typhoid Vaccine

The risk of typhoid fever in travelers is 1–10:100,000, depending on the destination. Areas at risk include South Asia, West and North Africa, South America, and Latin America. Travelers to the Indian subcontinent are at greatest risk. The vaccine is recommended for long-term travelers to an endemic area, those traveling off standard tourist routes, immuno-compromised travelers, those of south Indian ancestry, and patients with cholelithiasis. There are two vaccines available: a capsular polysaccharide (ViCPS) and a live attenuated (Ty21a) vaccine. The ViCPS is given intramuscularly 2 weeks prior to travel. The minimum age of administration for this vaccine is 2 years; efficacy is 75% over 2 years. Fever, headache, and severe local pain and swelling are reported with the ViCPS more frequently than with other vaccines. The Ty21a is an oral vaccine in capsule form given every other day for four doses. The schedule needs to be completed more than 1 week prior to travel to be effective. The capsules should be refrigerated but not frozen and should not be taken with liquids warmer than 37°C. It is licensed for children older than

6 years; efficacy is 80% over 5 years. It is contraindicated in immunodeficient populations. Doses should be delayed for more than 72 hours after receipt of antibiotics, as they interfere with growth of the vaccine strain bacteria. Mefloquine, chloroquine, and prophylactic doses of atovaquone-proguanil can be given concurrently with the typhoid vaccine.

Yellow Fever Vaccine

Yellow fever is a flavivirus transmitted by mosquitoes, found in urban and rural areas in sub-Saharan Africa and equatorial South America. Of those infected with the virus, 15% have moderate to severe infection. The licensed 17D strain is highly effective. It must be administered 10 days before travel to an endemic region to allow for the development of protective antibodies. It is required by many countries for reentry after travel to an endemic area, and receipt of the vaccine should be documented in the International Certificate of Vaccination that became available in December 2007 (wwwnc.cdc.gov/travel/yellowbook provides an updated list of countries in which yellow fever vaccination is recommended). For this reason, it is administered only at certified clinics. The vaccine is given subcutaneously, and a single dose confers lifelong immunity. As of July 1, 2016, a completed International Certificate of Vaccination or Prophylaxis is valid for the entire lifetime of the vaccines, and countries cannot require proof of revaccination as a condition of entry, even if the last vaccination was more than 10 years prior. However, a booster dose may be considered for travelers going to higher-risk settings, and travelers should still review the entry requirements for their destination. The recommended minimum age of administration is 9 months. The vaccine should not be administered to at-risk infants younger than 6 months, because of the increased risk of encephalitis (0.5–4 per 1000 vaccines). The risk of severe vaccine-related disease is also higher in adult caretakers older than 60 years. The decision to immunize infants who are 6–8 months of age must balance the infant's risk for exposure with the risk for vaccine-associated encephalitis. The vaccine is contraindicated in individuals with egg allergy or immunosuppression (including human immunodeficiency [HIV] syndrome with CD4 T-lymphocyte counts < 200 cells/mm^3 or a history of thymus disorder or thymectomy). A letter of medical exemption may be required for these travelers. In addition to age limitations, precautions to vaccination include asymptomatic HIV infection and CD4 T-lymphocyte count of 200–499 cells/mm^3, pregnancy, and breast-feeding. Adverse effects include encephalitis (15 per million doses for those aged > 60 years) and multisystem disease (5 per million doses in older people).

Angelo KM et al: The rise in travel-associated measles infections—GeoSentinel, 2015–2019. J Travel Med 2019 Sep 2;26(6):taz046 [PMID: 31218359].

CDC Traveler's Health Yellow Book: https://wwwnc.cdc.gov/travel/yellowbook/2018/international-travel-with-infants-children/traveling-safely-with-infants-children.

Clemens JD, Nair GB, Ahmed T, Qadri F, Holmgren J: Cholera. Lancet 2017 Sep 23;390(10101):1539–1549 [PMID: 28302312].

Hill DR et al: The practice of travel medicine: guidelines by the Infectious Diseases Society of America. Clin Infect Dis 2006 Dec 15;43(12):1499–1539 [PMID: 17109284].

TRAVELER'S DIARRHEA

Diarrhea is one of the most common illnesses in travelers to the developing world. Children are at highest risk, usually having more severe and prolonged illness than adults. A useful definition of diarrhea for traveling children is a change in normal stool pattern, with an increase in frequency (at least three stools per 24 hours) and a decrease in consistency to an unformed state. Most illnesses resolve over a 3- to 5-day period and occur in the first 2 weeks of travel. Enterotoxigenic *Escherichia coli* (ETEC) is the most common cause, accounting for up to one-third of cases. Other pathogens implicated are listed in Table 45–4. Counseling prior to travel includes education and caution with food handling and food and water consumption and provision for self-treatment in the event of illness.

▶ Prevention

Travelers should seek restaurants with a good safety reputation; eat hot, thoroughly cooked food; eat fruits and vegetables that can be peeled; and avoid tap water. They should

Table 45–4. Pathogens causing traveler's diarrhea.

Bacterial
Enterotoxigenic *Escherichia coli* (ETEC)
Enteroaggregative *E coli*
Salmonella spp
Shigella spp
Campylobacter jejuni
Aeromonas spp
Plesiomonas spp
Vibrio cholera
Noncholerae *Vibrio* spp
Enterotoxigenic *Bacteroides fragilis*
Viral
Rotavirus
Noroviruses
Sapoviruses
Parasitic
Giardia lamblia
Cyclospora cayetanensis
Cryptosporidium hominis
Entamoeba histolytica

also avoid ice cubes, fruit juices, fresh salads, unpasteurized dairy products, cold sauces and toppings, open buffets, undercooked foods, and food or beverages from street vendors. They should check the integrity of caps before buying bottled water to avoid bottles filled with tap water. It is also useful to remind travelers about hand washing after using the toilet and before eating. Families can consider using alcohol-containing hand sanitizers as an alternative to soap and water when access is limited during travel. Pasteurized or boiled milk is considered safe provided that it is stored at the appropriate temperature. It may be necessary to bring powdered milk to mix it with safe drinking water if the quality of milk is questionable. While these measures seem logical and should be recommended, there is little evidence that they prevent traveler's diarrhea, either in adults or in children.

Chemoprophylaxis & Treatment

The principles of treatment include adequate hydration and a short course of antibiotics when warranted; medical attention should be sought for severe or prolonged disease.

For mild disease, hydration may be all that is necessary, without any diet restriction. This can be achieved with oral rehydration therapy to supplement a regular diet. Packets of dry rehydration powder to be mixed with water are available from pharmacies, either prior to travel or at the destination. If this is not available, parents can be instructed on how to make oral rehydration solution (Table 45–5) or to use a sports drink such as Gatorade as a suitable alternative in older children and toddlers. The breast-fed infant should continue to breast-feed, in addition to receiving oral rehydration therapy.

The vomiting child is at greater risk of dehydration, so aggressive rehydration is crucial. Parents should be reassured that some fluid will be absorbed even if vomiting is ongoing. This is best achieved with small amounts of fluid, given often, to prevent further vomiting.

The antimotility agent loperamide, which is often used in adults to minimize symptom duration, is not advised for children because of the risk of adverse events such as toxic megacolon, ileus, extrapyramidal signs, hallucinations, and coma. Bismuth subsalicylate decreases the number of unformed stools in adults. Its routine use is not recommended in pediatrics, as aspirin is contraindicated in children younger than 18 years because of the risk of Reye syndrome, and dosing of bismuth has not been established for children.

Table 45–5. Recipe for oral rehydration solution.

- ¼ Teaspoon (1.25 cc) salt
- ¼ Teaspoon (1.25 cc) bicarbonate of soda[a]
- 2 Tablespoons (30 cc) sugar
- 1 L of water

[a]If bicarbonate of soda is not available, substitute an additional ¼ teaspoon (1.25 cc) of salt.

For children with signs and symptoms of bacterial gastroenteritis, such as fever or blood in the stool, empiric antibiotic therapy should be considered. The drug of choice in children is azithromycin (10 mg/kg orally once a day for 3 days). It is available in a powdered form that can be reconstituted and stored without refrigeration. It is an ideal choice because of the growing resistance of many gastroenteritis-causing bacteria to ciprofloxacin. There are no published pediatric trials of empiric azithromycin, so the dosing recommendations are based on pharmacokinetic data and studies involving the treatment of diarrhea in Africa and Thailand. Ciprofloxacin is currently not recommended for treatment of traveler's diarrhea in children, though it is used for treatment in adults.

Rifaximin, a nonabsorbable derivative of rifamycin, is effective in treating ETEC and other noninvasive enteropathogens. Since it is not absorbed, high concentrations are achieved in the intestinal lumen and it has a good safety profile. It is licensed for patients 12 years and older at a treatment dose of 200 mg three times a day for 3 days.

The use of prophylactic antibiotics in children is not recommended because of the risk of adverse events to prevent a disease of limited morbidity, as well as the potential for emergence of antibiotic resistance. Rifaximin, based on adult studies, is a useful chemoprophylactic agent, but it is expensive and requires further study in pediatrics. Probiotics showed no benefit for prevention of traveler's diarrhea, based on a recent meta-analysis of five randomized controlled trials.

Ashkenazi S, Schwartz E, O'Ryan M: Travelers' diarrhea in children: what have we learnt? Pediatr Infect Dis J 2016 Jun;35(6):698–700 [PMID: 26986771].
Giddings SL, Stevens AM, Leung DT: Traveler's diarrhea. Med Clin North Am 2016 Mar;100(2):317–330 [PMID: 26900116].

MALARIA PROPHYLAXIS & PREVENTION (SEE ALSO CHAPTER 43)

Malaria is the most common preventable infectious cause of death among travelers, and a common cause of fever in the returned traveler. Children comprise 20% of imported cases of malaria. It is largely a preventable disease in travelers through personal protective measures and chemoprophylaxis. However, no method is 100% protective. The risk of acquiring malaria varies with the season, climate, altitude, number of mosquito bites, and destination, with the highest risk in Oceania, Africa, the Indian subcontinent, and the Amazon.

▶ Prevention of Mosquito Bites

Malaria is transmitted via the night-biting *Anopheles* mosquitoes. Mosquito bites are avoided by staying in well-screened and air-conditioned rooms from dusk until dawn, wearing clothing covering the arms and legs, and avoiding scented soaps, shampoos, and perfumes. Mosquito nets are highly effective and can be used over beds, cribs, playpens, car seats, and strollers. Repellants containing DEET (30% or less) are also recommended, as this concentration confers 5–8 hours of protection. When used appropriately, DEET is safe for infants and children older than 2 months. It should not be applied to children's hands, mouth, or near the eyes, and is best washed off upon returning indoors. There have been case reports of seizures and toxic encephalopathy with the use of DEET, but these cases occurred with misapplication. Icaridin (also known as picaridin) is an alternative to DEET available in many countries. A concentration of 20% icaridin is as effective as DEET-containing products. It lacks the corrosiveness and greasy texture of DEET and is advised as safe for children by the American Academy of Pediatrics. However, because it is relatively new, it lacks the safety profile of DEET, especially for children. PMD is a plant-based repellant derived from lemon eucalyptus, and at a 30% concentration is equally effective as DEET. It may be used on children older than 6 months. It is considered safe if directions are followed and has been advocated for use by the Centers for Disease Control and Prevention. Clothing and bed nets may be sprayed with insecticides such as permethrin, which confers protection for 2–6 weeks, even with regular washing. Further studies are needed to establish its safety profile in children. The combination of DEET every 8–12 hours and permethrin on clothing is over 99% effective in preventing mosquito bites.

▶ Chemoprophylaxis

Prophylactic medications suppress malaria by killing asexual blood stages of the parasite before they cause disease, so protective levels of medication must be present in the blood before developing parasites are released from the liver. Therefore, it is necessary to start prophylaxis before the first possible exposure and to continue it for a sufficient period after return to a safe area.

The choice of antimalarial depends on the age of the child, resistance patterns, restrictions on the agent of choice, the child's ability to swallow tablets, the frequency of dosing, cost, availability of medication, and access to a compounding pharmacy for adequate dispensing of medication. For most children, once-weekly mefloquine is preferable and approved for children of any age. Atovaquone/proguanil is available in pediatric dosing, although only in tablet formulation. It is currently approved in most countries for children weighing greater than 5 kg. Doxycycline is another alternative and can be used in children younger than 8 years for durations of 21 days or less given reassuring data suggesting that it is not likely to cause visible teeth staining in this age group. Chloroquine is the drug of choice in areas of chloroquine sensitivity (Mexico, Hispaniola, Central America, west and north of the Panama Canal, and parts of North Africa, the Middle East, and China). Tafenoquine is a newer antimalarial, but its use for prophylaxis is currently restricted to those 18 years

or older. The pediatric and adult dosing, side effects, and other information about malaria chemoprophylaxis are in Table 45–6.

Antimalarial medications (with the exception of atovaquone/proguanil) are bitter, so it may be necessary to grind the medication into a very sweet food, such as chocolate syrup or sweetened condensed milk. Infants may need to have their medication prepared by a compounding pharmacy, where the appropriate dose can be placed in a gelatin capsule, which can then be opened by the caregiver and mixed into food or liquid.

Genton B, D'Acremont V: Malaria prevention in travelers. Infect Dis Clin North Am 2012 Sep;26(3):637–654 [PMID: 22963775].
Kafai NM, Odom John AR: Malaria in children. Infect Dis Clin North Am 2018 Mar;32(1):189–200 [PMID: 29269188].

OTHER TRAVEL-RELATED TOPICS

Visits to Friends & Relatives (VFR) in High-Risk Areas

Individuals who return to their home country are at the highest risk of travel-related infectious diseases. Sixty percent of malaria cases and over 75% of typhoid cases occur in these travelers, and VFR children are at highest risk of hepatitis A. The reasons for this include longer stays, travel to remote areas, intimate contact with the local population, and decreased likelihood of seeking (or following) pretravel advice because of familiarity with their home country.

Thus, certain issues need to be emphasized when discussing travel for VFRs. For example, visiting families should boil water and milk if other safe drinking water is expensive; consume only piping hot foods and beverages; and follow proper hand-washing techniques at all times.

Feja KN, Tolan RW Jr: Infections related to international travel and adoption. Adv Pediatr 2013;60(1):107–139 [PMID: 24007842].
Hendel-Paterson B, Swanson SJ: Pediatric travelers visiting friends and relatives (VFR) abroad: illnesses, barriers and pre-travel recommendations. Travel Med Infect Dis 2011 Jul;9(4):192–203 [PMID: 21074496].

FEVER IN THE RETURNED TRAVELER

More than one-half of travelers to the developing world experience a health-related travel problem during their trip; 8% require medical attention on return. The majority will develop common medical problems, such as upper respiratory tract infections, pneumonia, urinary tract infections, and otitis media, with the remainder developing travel-related infections. The most common travel-related diseases are malaria (21%), acute traveler's diarrhea (15%), dengue fever (6%), and typhoid/enteric fever (2%). Children

Table 45–6. Malaria prophylaxis.

Drug	Usage	Adult Dose	Pediatric Dose	Directions	Comments
Atovaquone/proguanil	Prophylaxis in areas with chloroquine-resistant or mefloquine-resistant *Plasmodium falciparum*.	Adult tabs contain 250 mg atovaquone and 100 mg proguanil hydrochloride.	Pediatric tabs contain 62.5 mg atovaquone and 25 mg proguanil hydrochloride.	Begin 1–2 days before travel to malarious areas. Take daily at the same time each day while in the area and for 7 days after leaving such areas.	Contraindicated in persons with severe renal impairment (creatinine clearance < 30 mL/min). Atovaquone/proguanil should be taken with food or a milky drink.
		1 Adult tab orally, daily.	5–8 kg: 1/2 pediatric tablet daily > 8–10 kg: 3/4 pediatric tablet daily > 10–20 kg: 1 pediatric tablet daily > 20–30 kg: 2 pediatric tablets daily > 30–40 kg: 3 pediatric tablets daily > 40 kg: 1 adult tablet daily.		Not recommended for prophylaxis for children < 5 kg, pregnant women, and women breast-feeding infants weighing 5 kg, but consider if drug-resistant area (call CDC). Do not take with tetracycline, metoclopramide, rifampin, or rifabutin (all reduce atovaquone concentration).
Chloroquine phosphate	Prophylaxis only in areas with chloroquine-sensitive *P falciparum*.	150 and 300 mg base tabs (300 and 500 mg salt) orally, once per week (any age or size).	5 mg/kg base (8.3 mg/kg salt) orally, once per week, up to max adult dose. Tabs not scored.	Begin 1–2 wk before travel to malarious areas. Take weekly on the same day of the week while in the area and for 4 wk after leaving such areas.	Contraindicated in persons with prior retinal or visual field changes. May exacerbate psoriasis. Bitter taste. Interferes with rabies vaccine response. Not contraindicated in pregnancy.
Doxycycline	Prophylaxis in areas with chloroquine-resistant or mefloquine-resistant *P falciparum*.	100 mg orally, daily.	8 y of age: 2 mg/kg up to adult dose of 100 mg/day. Syrup available.	Begin 1–2 days before travel to malarious areas. Take daily at the same time each day while in the area and for 4 wk after leaving such areas.	Contraindicated in children < 8 y of age and pregnant women. May decrease oral contraceptive efficacy. Photosensitivity.
Hydroxychloroquine sulfate	An alternative to chloroquine in areas with chloroquine-sensitive *P falciparum*.	310 mg base (400 mg salt) orally, once per week.	5 mg/kg base (6.5 mg/kg salt) orally, once per week, up to max adult dose. Tabs not scored.	Begin 1–2 wk before travel to malarious areas. Take weekly on the same day of the week while in the area and for 4 wk after leaving such areas.	

Drug	Indication	Adult dose	Pediatric dose	Timing	Comments
Mefloquine	Prophylaxis in areas with chloroquine-resistant *P falciparum*.	228 mg base (250 mg salt) orally, once per week.	5–9 kg: 4.6 mg/kg base (5 mg/kg salt), once per week. Tabs scored. 10–19 kg: ¼ tab once per week 20–30 kg: ½ tab once per week 31–45 kg: ¾ tab once per week: > 46 kg: 1 tab once per week.	Begin 1–2 wk before travel to malarious areas. Take weekly on the same day of the week while in the area and for 4 wk after leaving such areas (start 2 wk prior if want to evaluate for side effects that may necessitate change).	Contraindicated in persons allergic to mefloquine or related compounds (eg, quinine and quinidine) and in persons with active depression, a recent history of depression, generalized anxiety disorder, psychosis, schizophrenia, other major psychiatric disorders, or seizures. Use with caution in persons with psychiatric disturbances. Not recommended for persons with cardiac conduction abnormalities. Not contraindicated in pregnancy. Bitter taste.
Primaquine (posttravel prophylaxis for long-term *Plasmodium vivax* and *Plasmodium ovale* exposure)	Used for presumptive antirelapse therapy (terminal prophylaxis) to decrease the risk of relapses of *P vivax* and *P ovale*.	30 mg base (52.6 mg salt) orally, once per day for 14 days after departure from the malarious area.	0.6 mg/kg base (1.0 mg/kg salt) up to adult dose orally, once per day for 14 days after departure from the malarious area.	Primaquine presumptive antirelapse therapy is administered for 14 days after the traveler has left a malarious area. When chloroquine, doxycycline, or mefloquine is used for prophylaxis, primaquine is usually taken during the last 2 wk of postexposure prophylaxis, but may be taken immediately after those medications are completed. When atovaquone/proguanil is used for prophylaxis, primaquine may be taken either during the final 7 days of atovaquone/proguanil and then for an additional 7 days, or for 14 days after atovaquone/proguanil is completed.	Indicated for persons who have had prolonged exposure to *P vivax* and *P ovale* or both (eg, missionaries or peace corps volunteers). All persons who take primaquine should have a documented normal G6PD (glucose-6-phosphate dehydrogenase) level prior to starting this medication. Contraindicated in persons with G6PD1 deficiency. Also contraindicated during pregnancy and lactation unless the breast-fed infant has a documented normal G6PD level. Also an option for prophylaxis in special circumstances.
Tafenoquine	Prophylaxis in areas with chloroquine-resistant *P falciparum*.	200 mg orally, once per week	Not indicated for prophylaxis for children younger than 18 years of age	Begin 3 days prior to travel to malarious areas. Take weekly while in the area and for 1 week after leaving such areas.	Useful for shorter trips. Need to test for G6PD prior to use. Not for use by pregnant women. Not recommended in those with psychotic disorders.

who travel with caretakers visiting friends and relatives are at greatest risk. New pathogens and the changing epidemiology of some infectious diseases pose new risks to travelers—such as Ebola, avian influenza, multidrug-resistant TB, chikungunya virus, zika, and leishmaniasis.

Symptomatic returning travelers should be urgently and thoroughly evaluated for travel-related illness to prevent serious life-threatening disease and transmission to close contacts. The initial evaluation should include questions directed toward the travel itinerary, with dates of arrival and departure, specific activities, rural versus urban location, and accommodations. Specific information should be obtained regarding freshwater contact (eg, schistosomiasis, leptospirosis in some areas), sexual contacts, animal exposures, activities or hobbies, ill person contacts, and sources of food and water. A complete medication and vaccination history should be sought. Despite malaria chemoprophylaxis and protection against mosquitoes, no regimen is 100% protective. A thorough physical examination should include dermatologic examination, eye examination for scleral icterus, conjunctival injection or petechiae, and evaluation for hepatosplenomegaly or lymphadenopathy. Routine laboratory evaluation includes a complete blood count with differential, erythrocyte sedimentation rate (ESR), C-reactive protein (CRP), serum chemistry, liver enzyme profile, and urinalysis. The laboratory evaluation should also focus on diseases that are life threatening, with thick and thin smears for malaria (ideally three that are 12 hours apart), and blood cultures for typhoid fever. Specific testing should be done as directed by findings on history, physical examination, and preliminary laboratory test findings (Table 45–7). It may be necessary to seek the opinion of individuals with experience in international travel medicine.

Fever is the most common complaint in a child who becomes ill after international travel. The most common travel-related infectious causes of fever are summarized in Table 45–8. A more detailed description of the symptoms, signs, diagnosis, and treatment of these diseases that can occur in the returning traveler is presented in Chapters 40–43.

KEY POINTS/SUMMARY

- Preparation for travel with children and infants includes consideration of destination-specific risks, underlying medical problems, general travel safety, and administration of both routine and travel-related vaccines.

- Pretravel counseling should ideally take place at least 1 month prior to travel, given the need to develop an effective immune response from any travel-associated vaccinations.

- Given the prevalence of vaccine-preventable diseases in many countries worldwide, children should receive all routine childhood vaccines prior to travel, following the catch-up schedule as necessary.

Table 45–7. Diagnostic evaluations to consider for fever in the returned traveler.

Routine
Hematologic
Complete blood count and differential
Thick and thin blood smear (ideally collect three at 12-h intervals)
Sedimentation rate
C-reactive protein
Electrolytes
Liver function tests
Blood culture
Urine
Urinalysis
Culture
Specific to presentation
Hematologic
Serologies for specific pathogens
Stool
Culture or polymerase chain reaction (PCR)
Fecal leucocytes
Giardia and *Cryptosporidium* antigen test
Clostridium difficile toxin (if antibiotic exposure)
Ova and parasite examination
Special studies (eg, stool for Entamoeba histolytica antigen, special stains)
Cerebrospinal fluid
Cell count with differential, protein, glucose, culture, freeze extra sample
Antibody and polymerase chain reaction tests as appropriate
Imaging studies
Chest radiography and abdominal ultrasound imaging as appropriate
Other specialized tests
Placement of PPD (purified protein derivative) or IGRA (interferon-γ release assay)
Morning gastric aspirates (culture) or sputum (culture or PCR) and AFB (acid-fast bacilli) stain
Bronchoscopy
Sigmoidoscopy, colonoscopy
Skin biopsy
Bone marrow aspirate
Skin snips (eg, for *Onchocerciasis*)

- Travel-specific vaccines should be considered based on the traveler's underlying medical conditions, the travel itinerary, duration, purpose, and activities, all of which determine the potential risk of exposure and infection. These include rabies, JE, yellow fever, and typhoid vaccines.

- Counseling prior to travel includes education regarding food and water consumption and provision of self-treatment in the event of traveler's diarrhea.

- Malaria prevention for travelers includes repellants for skin and clothing, bed nets, and chemoprophylaxis with

Table 45–8. Illnesses in the returning traveler.

Disease	Etiology	Common Presenting Symptoms and Signs	Usual Incubation Period	Geographic Location	Mode of Transmission
Malaria	*Plasmodium falciparum*	Fever Headache Myalgias Chills Rigors	7–30 days	More prevalent in sub-Saharan Africa than in other regions of the world, also South East (SE) Asia, South America, Mexico	Bite from *Anopheles* mosquito
Malaria	*Plasmodium vivax*	As for *P falciparum*	10–17 days and up to 1 y	SE Asia, sub-Saharan Africa, South America, Central America	As for *P falciparum*
Malaria	*Plasmodium ovale*	As for *P falciparum*	16–18 days	West Africa, the Philippines, eastern Indonesia, and Papua New Guinea. It has been reported from Cambodia, India, Thailand, and Vietnam	As for *P falciparum*
Malaria	*Plasmodium malariae*	As for *P falciparum*	16–59 days	Sub-Saharan Africa, much of southeast Asia, Indonesia, on many of the islands of the western Pacific and in areas of the Amazon Basin of South America	As for *P falciparum*
Malaria	*Plasmodium knowlesi*	As for *P falciparum*	10–12 days	SE Asia	As for *P falciparum*
Dengue	Dengue virus	Fever Myalgias Maculopapular or petechial rash Arthralgias	2–7 days	Northern Australia, SE Asia, Mexico, Central America, South America, Puerto Rico, Florida Keys	Bite from *Aedes aegypti* mosquito
Typhoid fever	*Salmonella enterica* serovar *typhi*	Fever Malaise Anorexia Abdominal pain	10–14 days	South Asia, West and North Africa, South America, and Latin America	Ingestion of contaminated food/ water
Paratyphoid fever	*S enterica* serovar *paratyphi*	Same as for typhoid fever	Same as for typhoid fever	Same as for typhoid fever	Same as for typhoid fever
Schistosomiasis	*Schistosoma mansoni, Schistosoma hematobium, Schistosoma japonicum*	Urticarial rash Fever Headache Myalgia Respiratory symptoms	23–70 days (average 1 mo)	*S mansoni*—South America, Caribbean; *S hematobium*— Africa, Middle East *S japonicum*—Far East	Contaminated water containing freshwater snails
African tick typhus	*Rickettsia conorii*	Fever Headache Myalgia Maculopapular rash Malaise	5–7 days	Africa, Middle East, India, and Mediterranean Basin	Bite from hard ticks

(Continued)

Table 45–8. Illnesses in the returning traveler. (*Continued*)

Disease	Etiology	Common Presenting Symptoms and Signs	Usual Incubation Period	Geographic Location	Mode of Transmission
Scrub typhus	*Orientia tsutsugamushi*	Fever Headache Myalgia Possibly a maculopapular rash	10–12 days	"Tsutsugamushi triangle"—from northern Japan and Eastern Russia in the North, to Northern Australia in the South, to Pakistan and Afghanistan in the west	From chigger bites (the larval stage of the biculid mites)
Leptospirosis	*Leptospira* spp	Fever Headache Chills Myalgia Nausea Diarrhea Abdominal pain Uveitis Adenopathy Conjunctival suffusion	5–14 days (average 10 days)	Worldwide	Contact with urine from domestic and wild animals contaminating water and soil
Babesiosis	*Babesia microti, Babesia divergens, Babesia duncani*	Fevers Chills Symptoms similar to malaria	1–4 wk	Europe, United States, sporadic cases in Asia, Mexico, Africa	Bite of *Ixodes* ticks
Yellow fever	Yellow fever virus	Fever Chills Headache Jaundice Backache Myalgias Prostration Nausea Vomiting	3–6 days	Tropical and sub-Tropical Africa and South America, Caribbean (countries that lie within a band 15 degrees north to 10 degrees south of the Equator)	Bite of mosquitoes (*Aedes aegypti* and others)
Chikungunya	CHIK virus	Fever Joint pain Maculopapular rash Headache Nausea Vomiting Myalgias	2–12 days (usually 2–4 days)	Tropical Africa and Asia (SE Asia and India)	Bite from *Aedes* mosquitoes
Zika	Zika virus (ZIKV)	Fever Red eyes Joint pain Headache Maculopapular rash	3–12 days	Central, South America, Africa, Asia, South Pacific	Bite from *Aedes* mosquitoes
Amebiasis	*Entamoeba histolytica*	Fever Diarrhea Right upper quadrant pain	7–28 days	Worldwide, but higher incidence in developing countries	Contaminated food and water

mefloquine, doxycycline, atovaquone/proguanil, chloroquine, or tafenoquine.

- Individuals who return to their home country are at the highest risk of travel-related infectious diseases, and certain issues need to be emphasized when discussing travel for this group.

- Fever in a returning traveler requires immediate medical evaluation. The most common reasons for fever in a returned pediatric traveler are upper respiratory tract infections, pneumonia, urinary tract infections, and otitis media, with the remainder developing travel-related infections such as malaria, acute traveler's diarrhea, dengue fever, and typhoid/enteric fever.

Centers for Disease Control and Prevention (CDC) Yellow Book: https://wwwnc.cdc.gov/travel/page/yellowbook-home. Accessed November 30, 2017.
Feja KN1, Tolan RW Jr: Infections related to international travel and adoption. Adv Pediatr 2013;60(1):107–139 [PMID: 24007842].
Thwaites GE, Day NPJ: Approach to fever in the returning traveler. New Engl J Med 2017;376(6):548–560 [PMID: 28467877].

REFERENCES

Web Resources

CDC Yellow Book: http://wwwnc.cdc.gov/travel/content/yellow-book/home-2010.aspx.
Centers for Disease Control and Prevention (CDC): http://www.cdc.gov/travel/index.htm.
International Association for Medical Assistance to Travellers: http://www.iamat.org.

International Society of Travel Medicine: http://www.istm.org.
International SOS: http://www.internationalsos.com.
Malaria information specific to country: www.cdc.gov/malaria/risk_map.
ProMED: http://www.promedmail.org.
Rabies information specific to country: http://www.who.int/rabies/rabnet/en.
Royal Society of Tropical Medicine and Hygiene: http://www.rstmh.org.
WHO for maps of vaccine preventable diseases: http://www.who.int.ith.
Yellow fever vaccine clinics: https://wwwnc.cdc.gov/travel/page/search-for-stamaril-clinics.

General References

Feja KN, Tolan RW Jr: Infections related to international travel and adoption. Adv Pediatr 2013;60(1):107–139 [PMID: 24007842].
Giddings SL, Stevens AM, Leung DT: Traveler's diarrhea. Med Clin North Am 2016 Mar;100(2):317–330 [PMID: 26900116].
Greenwood CS, Greenwood NP, Fischer PR: Immunization issues in pediatric travelers. Expert Rev Vaccines 2008 Jul;7(5):651–661 [PMID: 18564019].
Myers AL, Christenson JC: Approach to immunization for the traveling child. Infect Dis Clin North Am 2015 Dec;29(4):745–757 [PMID: 26610424].
Rebaza A, Lee PJ: One more shot for the road: a review and update of vaccinations for pediatric international travelers. Pediatr Ann 2015 Apr;44(4):e89–e96 [PMID: 25875985].
Stauffer W, Christenson JC, Fischer PR: Preparing children for international travel. Travel Med Infect Dis 2008 May;6(3):101–113 [PMID: 18486064].
Thwaites GE, Day NP: Approach to fever in the returning traveler. N Engl J Med 2017 Feb 9;376(6):548–560 [PMID: 28177860].

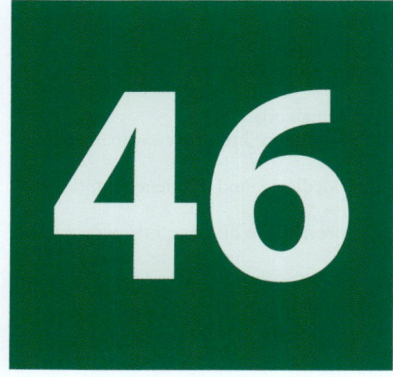

46

Chemistry & Hematology Reference Intervals

Melkon G. DomBourian, MD

Louise Helander, MBBS

Alice Campbell, MT (ASCP)

Laboratory tests provide valuable information necessary to evaluate a patient's condition and to monitor recommended treatment. Chemistry and hematology test results are compared with those of healthy individuals or those undergoing similar therapeutic treatment to determine clinical status and progress. In the past, the term *normal ranges* conveyed some ambiguity because, statistically, the term *normal* also implied a specific (Gaussian or normal) distribution and, epidemiologically, it implied the state of the majority, which is not necessarily the desirable or targeted population. This is most apparent in cholesterol levels, where values greater than 200 mg/dL are common but not desirable. Use of the term *reference range* or *reference interval* is therefore recommended by the International Federation of Clinical Chemistry (IFCC) and the Clinical and Laboratory Standards Institute (CLSI) to indicate that the values relate to a reference population and clinical condition.

Reference ranges are established for a specific age, biological sex, and level of sexual maturity; they are also defined for dietary restrictions, a specific pharmacologic status, and stimulation protocol. Similarly, diurnal variation is a factor, as is degree of obesity. Some reference ranges are particularly meaningful when combined with other test results (eg, parathyroid hormone and calcium) or when an entire set of substances being measured by clinical tests, commonly termed analytes, is evaluated.

Laboratory tests are becoming more specific and measure much lower concentrations than ever before. Therefore, reference ranges should reflect the analytical procedure as well as reagents and instrumentation used for a specific analysis. As test methodology continues to evolve, reference ranges are modified and updated.

CHALLENGES IN DETERMINING & INTERPRETING PEDIATRIC REFERENCE INTERVALS

The establishment of reference ranges is a complex process. However, the pediatric environment is particularly challenging for reference interval determination since growth and developmental stages do not have distinct and finite boundaries by which test results can be tabulated. Reference ranges may overlap and, in many cases, complicate diagnosis and treatment. Additionally, ethical concerns may exist related to blood draws in infants and young children to establish these reference ranges. A particular difficulty also lies in establishing pediatric reference ranges for analytes whose levels are changed under scheduled stimulation conditions. The common glucose tolerance test is such an example, but more complex endocrinology tests require skill and extensive experience to interpret in pediatric populations. Reference ranges for these serial tests are established over a long period of time and are not easily transferable between test methodologies. Despite these challenges, there have been multicenter studies to improve the quality and availability of pediatric reference ranges for laboratory testing. These efforts are important as clinical test instrument manufacturers routinely conduct large studies to identify reference intervals, but often focus on adult populations.

Adeli K: Special issue on laboratory reference intervals. eJIFCC. September 2008. http://www.ifcc.org/PDF/190201200801.pdf.

C28A3: *Defining, Establishing, and Verifying Reference Intervals in the Clinical Laboratory: Approved Guideline.* 3rd ed. http://www.clsi.org/source/orders.

Higgins V et al: Marked influence of adiposity on laboratory biomarkers in a healthy cohort of children and adolescents. J Clin Endocrinol Metab 2020 Apr 1;105(4):e1781–e1797 [PMID: 31845996].

Ozarda Y: Reference intervals: current status, recent developments and future considerations. Biochem Med (Zagreb) 2016;26(1):5–16 [PMID: 26981015].

GUIDELINES FOR USE OF DATA IN A REFERENCE RANGE STUDY

The College of American Pathologists provides guidelines for the adoption of reference ranges used in hospitals and commercial clinical laboratories. It recognizes the enormous task of establishing a laboratory's own reference ranges and recommends alternatives to the process. A laboratory may determine reference ranges by the following:

1. Conducting its own study to evaluate a statistically significant number of "healthy" volunteers. It is a monumental task for a laboratory to develop its own pediatric reference ranges due to the need for parental consent, approval by review boards, and the numerous age categories that need to be evaluated.

2. Adopting ranges established by the manufacturer of a particular analytical instrument. The laboratory must validate the data by analyzing a sample of 20 subjects representing that specific population to confirm that the adopted range is truly representative of that group.

3. Using reference data in the general medical literature and conferring with physicians to make sure the data agree with their clinical experience. A validation study is also recommended.

4. Analyzing hospital patient data. Laboratory test results from hospital patients have been used to compute reference ranges provided they fulfill stated clinical criteria. Patient records need to indicate that the patient's specific medical condition does not influence the analyte whose reference range is being determined. For example, a child undergoing surgery for bone fracture repair is expected to have normal electrolytes and thyroid function, whereas a child examined for precocious puberty should not be included in a reference range study for luteinizing hormone.

Statistically, the sample size of a hospital patient study should be considerably larger than that of a healthy group. A study from a healthy population may require 20 subjects to be statistically significant, whereas a hospital population should evaluate a minimum of 120 patients.

> Biological Variation Database Reference List: https://www.westgard.com/biodatabase3.htm.
> College of American Pathologists publication: https://www.cap.org/laboratory-improvement/accreditation/accreditation-checklists.
> Schnabl K, Chan MK, Gong Y, Adeli K: Closing the gap on paediatric reference intervals: the CALIPER initiative. Clin Biochem Rev 2008 Aug;29(3):89–96 [PMID: 19107221].

STATISTICAL COMPUTATION OF REFERENCE INTERVALS

The establishment of reference intervals is based on a statistical distribution of test results obtained from a representative population. The CLSI recommendation for data collection and statistical analysis provides guidelines for managing the data. For clinicians, it is not important that they can reproduce the calculation. It is far more critical to understand the benefits and restrictions provided by the described statistical

approaches and to evaluate patient results with these limitations in mind.

The reference range includes 95% of all results obtained from a representative population. Note that 5% of that population will have "abnormal" results, when in fact they are "healthy" and an integral part of the reference group study. Similarly, an equivalent 5% of the "ill" population will have laboratory results within the reference range. These are inherent features of the statistical computation. Taking that analysis one step further, the probability of a healthy patient having a test result within a calculated reference range is

$$P = .95$$

When multiple tests or panels of tests are used, the combined probability of all the test results falling in their respective reference ranges drops dramatically. For example, the probability of all results from 10 tests in the complete metabolic panel being in the reference range is

$$P = (.95)^{10} = .60$$

Therefore, about one-third of healthy patients will have one test result in the panel that is outside the reference range. Clinical judgment is needed to determine the significance of test results falling outside the reference range.

A. Parametric Method of Computation

The parametric method of establishing reference intervals is simple, though not always representative, since it assumes that the data have a Gaussian distribution. A mean (x) and standard deviation (SD) are calculated; test results of 95% of that specific population will fall within the mean ±1.96 SD, as shown in Figure 46–1.

Where the distribution is not Gaussian, a mathematical manipulation of the values (eg, plotting the log of the value, instead of the value itself) may give a Gaussian distribution.

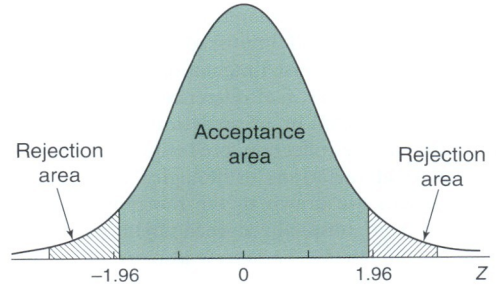

▲ **Figure 46–1.** Gaussian distribution and parametric calculation using $x \pm 1.96$ SD to define the range.

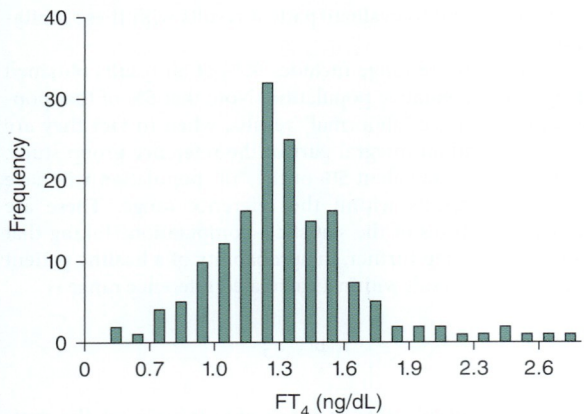

▲ **Figure 46–2.** Histogram of free thyroxine (FT$_4$) using clinic and hospital patients at Children's Hospital Colorado.

The mean and SD are then converted back to give a usable reference range.

B. Nonparametric Method of Computation

The nonparametric method of establishing reference ranges is currently recommended by CLSI, since it defines outliers as those in the extreme 2.5 percentile of the upper and lower limits of data, respectively. The number of data points excluded at the limits depends on the skew of the curve, and so the computation accommodates a non-Gaussian distribution. A histogram depicting the non-Gaussian distribution of data from a free thyroxine reference range study conducted at Children's Hospital Colorado in Aurora, Colorado, is shown in Figure 46–2.

Ichihara K, Boyd JC; IFCC Committee on Reference Intervals and Decision Limits (C-RIDL): An appraisal of statistical procedures used in derivation of reference intervals. Clin Chem Lab Med 2010 Nov;48(11):1537–1551 [PMID: 21062226].

WHY REFERENCE INTERVALS VARY

Recent modifications to reference ranges are due to the introduction of new and improved analytical procedures, advanced automated instrumentation, and standardization of reagents and certified reference materials. Reference ranges are also affected by preanalytical variations that can occur during sample collection, processing, and storage.

Preanalytical variations of biological origin can occur when specimens are drawn in the morning versus in the evening, or from hospitalized recumbent patients versus ambulatory outpatients. Variations also may be caused by metabolic and hemodynamic factors. Preanalytical factors may be a product of the socioeconomic environment or ethnic background (eg, genetic or dietary).

Analytical variations are caused by differences in analytical measurements and depend on the analytical tools as well as an inherent variability in obtaining a quantitative value. Furthermore, new reagents, instruments, and improved testing procedures added to the clinical laboratory can result in an element of variability between tests.

1. **Antigen-antibody reactions** have revolutionized clinical chemistry but have also added a degree of variability because biologically derived reagents have different specificity and sensitivity. In addition to the targeted analyte, some of its metabolites are also measured, and these may or may not be biologically active.

2. **Certified reference materials** continue to be reviewed and evaluated by organizations such as the World Health Organization and the National Institute for Standards and Technology.

3. **Analytical instrumentation** with advanced electronics and robotics has improved the accuracy of results and increased throughput. However, they have added an element of variability among instruments from different manufacturers.

4. **Analytical detection methods** have also made big strides as they have expanded from simple ultraviolet-visible spectrophotometry to fluorescence, nephelometry, radioimmunoassay, and chemiluminescence.

Jung B, Adeli K: Clinical laboratory reference intervals in pediatrics: the CALIPER initiative. Clin Biochem 2009 Nov;42 (16–17): 1589–1595. Epub 2009 Jul 7 [PMID: 19591815].
Tahmasebi H, Higgins V, Bohn MK, Hall A, Adeli K: CALIPER hematology reference Standards (I). Am J Clin Pathol 2020 Aug 5; 154(3):330–341 [PMID: 32561916].

SENSITIVITY, SPECIFICITY, & PREDICTIVE VALUES

Despite its statistical derivation, a reference interval does not necessarily provide a finite and clear-cut guideline as to whether a patient has a condition. There will always be a segment of the population whose test values fall within the reference interval yet have clinical manifestations that indicate disease is present. Similarly, a segment of the population will have test values outside the reference interval, but no clinical signs of disease. The ability of a test and corresponding reference interval to detect individuals with disease is defined by the diagnostic sensitivity of the test. Similarly, the ability of a test to detect individuals without disease is described by the diagnostic specificity. These characteristics are governed by the analytical quality of the test as well as the numerical parameters (reference interval) that define the presence of disease. The tolerance level for the desired sensitivity and specificity of a test requires significant input from clinicians.

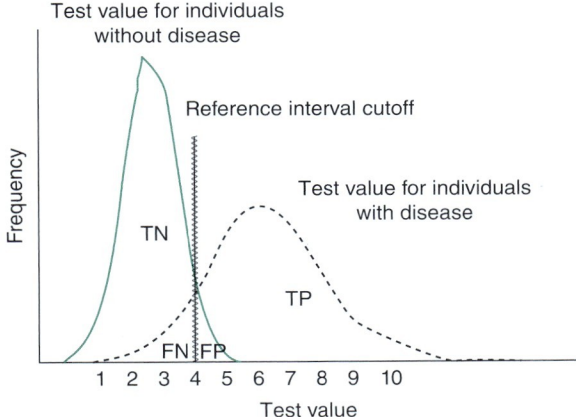

▲ **Figure 46–3.** Frequency distribution of test results for patients with and without disease. FN, false negative; FP, false positive; TN, true negative; TP, true positive.

Generally, specificity increases as sensitivity decreases. A typical distribution of test results, shown in Figure 46–3, provides information on individuals without disease (solid line) and individuals with the disease (dashed line). As with most tests, there is an overlap area. A patient with a test result of 1 is likely healthy, and the result indicates a true negative (TN) for the presence of disease. A patient with a test result of 9 is likely to have the disease, and the test result is a true positive (TP). There is a small, but significant, population with a test result of 2–5 in whom the test is not 100% conclusive. A statistical analysis may determine the most likely cutoff for healthy individuals, but the clinically acceptable cutoff depends on the test as well as clinical correlation.

If cutoff values for the reference interval are such that a test result indicates that a healthy patient has the disease, the result is a false positive (FP). Conversely if a test result indicates that a patient is well when in fact, he or she has the

disease, the result is a false negative (FN). To define the ability of the test and reference interval to identify a disease state, the diagnostic sensitivity and specificity are measured.

$$\text{Diagnostic sensitivity} = TP/(TP + FN)$$

$$\text{Diagnostic specificity} = TN/(TN + FP)$$

In the example shown in Figure 46–3, a reference interval of 0.5–3 will provide more TN results and minimize FP results. Alternatively, a reference interval of 0.5–4 will increase the rate of FN. Thus, an increase in sensitivity leads to a decrease in specificity. A medical condition that requires aggressive treatment may necessitate a test and corresponding reference interval with a high sensitivity, which is a measure of the TP rate. This is accomplished at the expense of lowering specificity.

One must also consider that both diagnostic sensitivity and specificity as derived do not take into account disease prevalence. As shown in Figure 46–4, diagnostic sensitivity is calculated exclusively within a diseased population and the converse is true for diagnostic specificity. In a clinical setting, one is screening a population of individuals with and without disease. Therefore, positive predicative value (PPV) and negative predictive value (NPV) must also be used to better understand test screening performance and are defined as follows:

$$PPV = TP/(TP + FP)$$

$$NPV = TN/(TN + FN)$$

A reference interval is a statistical representation of test results from a finite population, but it is by no means inclusive of every member of the group. It is merely one component in the measure of a patient's status to be viewed in relation to several other testing factors (Tables 46–1 to 46–3).

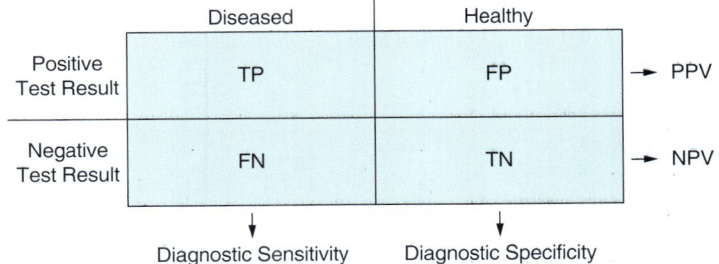

▲ **Figure 46–4.** Sensitivity, specificity, and predictive values of a test. FN, false negative; FP, false positive; NPV, negative predictive value; PPV, positive predictive value; TN, true negative; TP, true positive.

Table 46–1. General chemistry.

Analyte, Units Specimen Type	Age	Instrument	Male Range	Female Range
A$_{1C}$ hemoglobin (%) B	0 day–Adult	DCA Vantage	Normal: < 5.7% Prediabetes: 5.7%–6.4% Diabetes: > 6.5%	Normal: < 5.7% Prediabetes: 5.7%–6.4% Diabetes: > 6.5%
α-Fetoprotein (ng/mL) S, P	0–30 days 1–3 mo 4 mo–17 y ≥ 18 y	Vitros 5600	50–100,000 40–1000 0–12 < 7.5	50–100,000 40–1000 0–12 < 7.5
α$_1$-Antitrypsin (mg/dL) S, P	0–1 mo 1–5 mo 6 mo–2 y 2–18 y ≥ 19 y	Vitros 5600	79–223 71–190 60–161 70–179 88–183	79–223 71–190 60–161 70–179 88–183
Antistreptolysin O (IU/mL) S, P	0–18 y ≥ 19 y	Vitros 5600	< 241 < 200	< 241 < 200
Albumin (g/dL) S, P	0–7 days 8–30 days 1–2 mo 3–5 mo 6–12 mo 1–3 y 4–6 y 7–18 y ≥ 19 y	Vitros 5600	2.3–3.8 2.0–4.5 2.0–4.8 2.1–4.9 2.1–4.7 3.4–4.2 3.5–5.2 3.7–5.6 3.5–5.0	1.8–3.9 1.8–4.4 1.9–4.2 2.2–4.4 2.2–4.7 3.4–4.2 3.5–5.2 3.7–5.6 3.5–5.0
ALP (U/L) S, P	0–7 days 8–30 days 1–3 mo 4–6 mo 7–12 mo 1–3 y 4–6 y 7–9 y 10–11 y 12–13 y 14–15 y 16–18 y ≥ 19 y	Vitros 5600	77–265 91–375 60–360 55–325 60–300 129–291 134–346 156–386 120–488 178–455 116–483 58–237 38–126	65–270 65–365 80–425 80–345 60–330 129–291 134–346 156–386 116–515 93–386 62–209 45–116 38–126
ALT (U/L) S, P	0–3 y 4–13 y 14–18 y ≥ 19 y	Vitros 5600	12–45 10–41 11–26 < 50	14–45 11–28 10–35 5–34
Ammonia (μmol/L) P	0–1 day 1–13 y 14 d–17 y ≥ 18 y	Vitros 5600	64–107 56–92 21–50 9–33	64–107 56–92 21–50 9–33
Amylase (U/L) S, P	0–2 mo 3–5 mo 6–11 mo 1–18 y ≥ 19 y	Vitros 5600	0–30 0–50 0–80 30–100 30–110	0–30 0–50 0–80 30–100 30–110
Anticardiolipin IGA (CU) S	0 day–Adult	Inova Bio-Flash	< 20	< 20

(Continued)

Table 46–1. General chemistry. (*Continued*)

Analyte, Units Specimen Type	Age	Instrument	Male Range	Female Range
Anticardiolipin IGG (CU) S	0 day–Adult	Inova Bio-Flash	< 20	< 20
Anticardiolipin IGM (CU) S	0 day–Adult	Inova Bio-Flash	< 20	< 20
AST (U/L) S, P	0–7 days	Vitros 5600	30–100	24–95
	8–30 days		20–70	24–72
	1–3 mo		22–63	20–64
	4–6 mo		13–65	20–63
	7–12 mo		25–55	22–63
	1–3 y		20–60	20–60
	4–6 y		15–50	15–50
	7–9 y		15–40	15–40
	10–11 y		10–60	10–40
	12–15 y		15–40	10–30
	16–18 y		15–45	5–30
	≥ 19 y		17–59	14–36
Bilirubin direct (mg/dL) S, P	0–30 days	Vitros 5600	0–0.6	0–0.6
	> 1 mo		0–0.3	0–0.3
Bilirubin total (mg/dL) S, P	0–1 days	Vitros 5600	0.1–5.8	0.1–5.8
	1–2 days		0.1–8.5	0.1–8.5
	3–14 days		0.1–11.5	0.1–11.5
	15–30 days		< 11.5	< 11.5
	> 1 mo		0.2–1.2	0.2–1.2
BNP (ng/L) B	0 day–Adult	I-STAT	0–99	0–99
Pro-BNP (pg/mL) S, P	0 day–Adult	Vitros 5600	0–125	0–125
BUN (mg/dL) S, P	0–7 days	Vitros 5600	2–13	2–13
	8–30 days		2–16	2–15
	1–3 mo		2–12	2–14
	4–6 mo		1–14	1–13
	7–12 mo		2–14	1–13
	1–3 y		5–17	5–17
	4–13 y		7–17	7–17
	14–18 y		8–21	8–21
	≥ 19 y		9–20	7–17
C3 (mg/dL) S, P	0–1 mo	Vitros 5600	55–129	55–129
	1–2 mo		61–155	61–155
	2–3 mo		67–136	67–136
	3–4 mo		64–182	64–182
	4–5 mo		67–174	67–174
	5–6 mo		77–178	77–178
	6–9 mo		78–173	78–173
	9–11 mo		76–187	76–187
	11–12 mo		87–181	87–181
	1–2 y		84–177	84–177
	2–3 y		80–178	80–178
	3–5 y		89–173	89–173
	5–8 y		92–161	92–161
	8–10 y		93–203	93–203
	10–11 y		86–184	86–184
	> 11 y		88–165	88–165

(*Continued*)

Table 46–1. General chemistry. (*Continued*)

Analyte, Units Specimen Type	Age	Instrument	Male Range	Female Range
C4 (mg/dL) S, P	0–1 mo	Vitros 5600	9.2–33	9.2–33
	1–2 mo		9.7–37	9.7–37
	2–3 mo		11–35	11–35
	3–4 mo		11–50	11–50
	4–5 mo		9.3–47	9.3–47
	5–6 mo		11–55	11–55
	6–9 mo		12–48	12–48
	9–11 mo		16–51	16–51
	11–12 mo		16–52	16–52
	1–2 y		12–45	12–45
	2–3 y		13–47	13–47
	3–5 y		17–42	17–42
	5–8 y		16–42	16–42
	8–10 y		13–52	13–52
	10–11 y		10–40	10–40
	> 11 y		14–44	14–44
Ca (mg/dL) S, P	0–7 days	Vitros 5600	7.3–11.4	7.5–11.3
	8–30 days		8.6–11.7	8.4–11.9
	1–3 mo		8.5–11.3	8.0–11.1
	3–6 mo		8.3–11.4	7.7–11.5
	6–12 mo		7.7–11.0	7.8–11.1
	1–3 y		8.7–9.8	8.7–9.8
	4–9 y		8.8–10.1	8.8–10.1
	10–11 y		8.9–10.1	8.9–10.1
	12–13 y		8.8–10.6	8.8–10.6
	14–15 y		9.2–10.7	9.2–10.7
	16–18 y		8.9–10.7	8.9–10.7
	≥ 19 y		8.4–10.2	8.4–10.2
iCa (mmol/L) B	0–1 day	Radiometer ABL 90 flex	1.1–1.4	1.1–1.4
	1–3 days		1.1–1.5	1.1–1.5
	4–7 days		1.2–1.5	1.2–1.5
	8 days–1 mo		1.3–1.6	1.3–1.6
	1 mo–17 y		1.2–1.4	1.2–1.4
	≥ 18 y		1.2–1.3	1.2–1.3
Chloride (mmol/L) S, P	0–7 days	Vitros 5600	96–111	96–111
	8 days–6 mo		96–110	96–110
	6–12 mo		96–108	96–108
	1–18 y		96–109	96–109
	≥ 19 y		98–107	98–107
Cholesterol (mg/dL) S, P	0 day–2 mo	Vitros 5600	45–177	63–198
	2–6 mo		60–197	66–218
	7–12 mo		89–208	74–218
	1–2 y		44–181	44–181
	2–18 y		< 170	< 170
	≥ 19 y		< 200	< 200
Creatine kinase (U/L) S, P	0–3 mo	Vitros 5600	28–300	42–470
	3–12 mo		24–170	26–240
	1–2 y		27–160	24–175
	2–11 y		30–150	24–175
	11–14 y		30–150	30–170
	15–19 y		33–145	27–140

(Continued)

Table 46–1. General chemistry. (*Continued*)

Analyte, Units Specimen Type	Age	Instrument	Male Range	Female Range
Creatinine (mg/dL) S, P	0–3 days 3–10 days 10–17 days 17 days–1 y 1–11 y 11–17 y ≥ 18 y	Vitros 5600	0.33–1.08 0.15–0.90 0.15–0.61 0.15–0.52 0.23–0.61 0.42–0.90 0.71–1.18	0.33–1.08 0.15–0.90 0.15–0.61 0.15–0.52 0.23–0.61 0.42–0.90 0.52–0.99
Cystatin C (mg/L) S, P	0–3 mo 4–12 mo > 1 y	Vitros 5600	0.8–2.3 0.7–1.5 0.5–1.3	0.8–2.3 0.7–1.5 0.5–1.3
Ferritin (ng/mL) S,P	0–6 wk 7 wk–1 y 1–9 y 10–18 y 19–50 y > 18 y > 50 y	Vitros 5600	< 400 10–95 10–60 10–300 n/a 18–444 n/a	< 400 10–95 10–60 10–70 6–137 n/a 11–264
Anti-deamidated gliadin peptide IgA (S/CO)	0 day–Adult	Bio-Flash	< 20	< 20
Anti-deamidated gliadin peptide IgG (S/CO)	0 day–Adult	Bio-Flash	< 20	< 20
GGT (U/L) S, P	0–7 days 8–30 days 1–3 mo 4–6 mo 7–12 mo 1–3 y 4–6 y 7–9 y 10–11 y 12–13 y 14–15 y 16–18 y ≥ 19 y	Vitros 5600	25–148 23–153 17–130 8–83 10–35 5–16 8–18 11–21 14–25 14–37 10–28 9–29 15–73	19–131 17–124 17–124 15–109 10–54 5–16 8–18 11–21 14–23 12–21 12–22 9–23 12–43
Glucose (mg/dL) S, P	0–30 days > 1 mo	Vitros 5600	40–80 60–105	40–80 60–105
Glucose–CSF (mg/dL) CSF	0 day–Adult	Vitros 5600	40–75	40–75
HDL (mg/dL) S, P	0–2 y 2 y–Adult	Vitros 5600	8–61 45–60	8–61 45–60
β_2-Glycoprotein 1-antibody, IgA (CU) S	0 day–Adult	Inova Bio-Flash	0–20	0–20
β_2-Glycoprotein 1-antibody, IgG (CU) S	0 day–Adult	Inova Bio-Flash	0–20	0–20
β_2-Glycoprotein 1-antibody, IgM (CU) S	0 day–Adult	Inova Bio-Flash	0–20	0–20

(Continued)

Table 46–1. General chemistry. (*Continued*)

Analyte, Units Specimen Type	Age	Instrument	Male Range	Female Range
IgA (mg/dL) S, P	0–30 days 1–6 mo 6–12 mo 1–3 y 4–6 y 7–9 y 10–12 y 13–15 y 16–18 y ≥ 19 y	Vitros 5600	0–11 0–40 1–82 9–137 44–187 58–204 46–218 29–251 68–259 70–400	0–10 0–42 6–68 15–111 33–146 28–180 55–193 62–241 69–262 70–400
IgE (kUA/L) S	0–12 mo 1–2 y 2–3 y 3–9 y 10 y–Adult	Phadia ImmunoCAP	0–29 0–49 0–45 0–52 0–87	0–29 0–49 0–45 0–52 0–87
IgG (mg/dL) S, P	0–30 days 1–6 mo 6–12 mo 1–3 y 4–6 y 7–9 y 10–12 y 13–15 y 16–18 y ≥ 19 y	Vitros 5600	197–833 140–533 130–823 413–1112 468–1328 582–1441 685–1620 590–1600 522–1703 700–1600	162–872 311–664 325–647 421–1202 560–1319 485–1473 586–1609 749–1640 804–1817 700–1600
IgM (mg/dL) S, P	0–30 days 1–6 mo 6–12 mo 1–3 y 4–6 y 7–9 y 10–12 y 13–15 y 16–18 y ≥ 19 y	Vitros 5600	0–65 6–84 15–117 30–146 31–151 21–140 27–151 26–184 28–179 40–230	1–57 0–127 0–130 35–184 42–184 30–165 42–211 34–225 42–224 40–230
Iron (mcg/dL) S, P	0–7 days 7 d–1 y 1–10 y > 10 y	Vitros 5600	100–250 40–100 50–120 49–181	100–250 40–100 50–120 37–170
Iron-binding capacity (mcg/dL) S	0 day–Adult	Vitros 5600	261–462	265–497
LDH (U/L) S, P	0–5 days 6 days–3 y 4–6 y 7–9y 10–11 y 12–13 y 14–15 y 16–18 y ≥ 19 y	Vitros 5600	416–957 223–409 209–401 187–334 192–312 209–334 160–325 151–295 139–275	416–957 223–409 209–401 187–334 169–343 169–285 174–258 151–298 139–275

(Continued)

Table 46–1. General chemistry. (*Continued*)

Analyte, Units Specimen Type	Age	Instrument	Male Range	Female Range
LDL measured (mg/dL) S, P	0–2 y 2–19 y ≥ 19 y	Vitros 5600	<100 < 110 <120	<100 < 110 <120
Magnesium (mg/dL) S, P	0–6 days 7–30 days 1 mo–1 y 2–5 y 6–9 y 10–14 y > 14 y	Vitros 5600	1.2–2.6 1.6–2.4 1.6–2.6 1.5–2.4 1.6–2.3 1.6–2.2 1.5–2.3	1.2–2.6 1.6–2.4 1.6–2.6 1.5–2.4 1.6–2.3 1.6–2.2 1.5–2.3
Non-HDL cholesterol (mg/dL) S, P	0–19 y > 19 y	Vitros 5600 (calculated)	< 120 < 150	< 120 < 150
Potassium (mmol/L) S, P	0–6 days 7 days–2 mo 3 mo–17 y ≥ 18 y	Vitros 5600	3.7–5.9 4.1–5.3 3.4–4.7 3.5–5.0	3.7–5.9 4.1–5.3 3.4–4.7 3.5–5.0
Prealbumin (mg/dL) S, P	0–1 mo 1–5 mo 6 mo–3 y 4–5 y 6–13 y 14–18 y ≥ 19 y	Vitros 5600	7–22 8–34 7–32 12–30 12–42 22–45 17–42	7–22 8–34 7–32 12–30 12–42 22–45 17–42
Phosphorus (mg/dL) S, P	0–15 days 15 days–1 y 1–4 y 5–12 y 13–15 y 16–18 y ≥ 19 y	Vitros 5600	5.85–10.9 5.05–8.76 4.52–7.09 4.37–6.25 3.78–6.47 3.19–5.29 2.5–5.0	5.85–10.9 5.05–8.76 4.52–7.09 4.37–6.25 3.41–5.82 3.19–5.29 2.5–5.0
Procalcitonin (ng/mL) S, P	0 day–6 h 6–12 h 12–18 h 18–30 h 30–36 h 36–42 h 42 h–2 days 2 days–Adult	Vitros 5600	<2.0 <8.0 <15 <21 <15 <8 <2 ≤0.1	<2.0 <8.0 <15 <21 <15 <8 <2 ≤0.1
Prolactin (ng/mL) S, P	0 day–Adult	Vitros 5600	3.7–17.9	3.0–18.6
Sodium (mmol/L) S, P	0–7 days 8–30 days 1–6 mo 6–12 mo 1–18 y ≥ 19 y	Vitros 5600	133–146 134–144 134–142 133–142 134–143 137–145	133–146 134–144 134–142 133–142 134–143 137–145

(*Continued*)

Table 46–1. General chemistry. (*Continued*)

Analyte, Units Specimen Type	Age	Instrument	Male Range	Female Range
Anti–human tissue transglutaminase IgA (S/CO)	0 day–Adult	Inova Bio-Flash	< 20	< 20
Anti–human tissue transglutaminase IgG (S/CO)	0 day–Adult	Inova Bio-Flash	< 20	< 20
Troponin I (ng/mL) S, P	0 day–Adult	Vitros 5600	< 0.12	< 0.12
Total protein (g/dL) S, P	0–2 mo 2–6 mo 6–12 mo 1–3 y 4–6 y 7–9 y 10–19 y ≥ 20 y	Vitros 5600	3.9–7.6 4.1–7.9 3.9–7.9 5.9–7.0 5.9–7.8 6.2–8.1 6.3–8.6 6.2–8.2	3.4–7.0 3.9–7.6 4.5–7.8 5.9–7.0 5.9–7.8 6.2–8.1 6.3–8.6 6.2–8.2
Triglycerides (mg/dL) S, P	0–7 days 8–30 days 1–3 mo 3–6 mo 6–12 mo 1–2 y 2–9 y 10–18 y ≥ 19 y	Vitros 5600	21–182 30–184 40–175 45–291 45–501 27–125 < 75 < 90 < 115	28–166 30–165 35–282 50–355 36–431 27–125 < 75 < 90 < 115
Bicarb (mmol/L) S, P	0–7 days 7–30 days 1–6 mo 6–12 mo 1–18 y ≥ 19 y	Vitros 5600	17–26 17–27 17–29 18–29 20–31 22–30	17–26 17–27 17–29 18–29 20–31 22–30
Uric acid (mg/dL) S, P	0–30 days 1–12 mo 1–9 y 10–11 y 12–13 y 14–15 y 16–17 y ≥ 18 y	Vitros 5600	2.0–5.2 2.5–9.0 1.8–5.0 2.3–5.4 2.7–6.7 2.4–7.8 4.0–8.6 3.5–8.5	2.0–5.2 2.5–9.0 1.8–5.0 3.0–4.7 3.0–5.9 3.0–5.9 3.0–5.9 2.5–7.5
Vitamin B$_{12}$ (pg/mL) S, P	0 day–Adult	Vitros 5600	163–949	163–949

ALP, alkaline phosphatase; ALT, alanine aminotransferase; AST, aspartate aminotransferase; B, whole blood; BNP, brain natriuretic peptide; BUN, blood urea nitrogen; Ca, calcium; CSF, cerebrospinal fluid; GGT, γ-glutamyl transpeptidase; HDL, high-density lipoprotein; iCa, ionized calcium; IgA, immunoglobulin A; IgE, immunoglobulin E; IgG, immunoglobulin G; IgM, immunoglobulin M; LDH, lactic dehydrogenase; P, plasma; S, serum; U, urine.
Data from Children's Hospital Colorado Chemistry Laboratory Procedure Manuals.

Table 46–2. Endocrine chemistry.

Analyte, Units, Specimen Type, Source	Age	Methodology	Male Range	Female Range
Cortisol (mcg/dL) S, P	0 day–Adult (AM values)	Vitros 5600	4.5–22.7	4.5–22.7
	0 day–Adult (PM values)		1.7–14.1	1.7–14.1
FSH (mIU/mL) S	4 wk–11 mo	Abbott Alinity-i	0.16–4.1	0.24–14.2
	12 mo–8 y		0.26–3.0	1.0–4.2
	Tanner 1 (< 9.2 y)		0.26–3.0	1.0–4.2
	Tanner 2 (9.2–13.7 y)		1.8–3.2	1.0–10.8
	Tanner 3 (10.0–14.4 y)		1.2–5.8	1.5–12.8
	Tanner 4 (10.7–15.6 y)		2.0–9.2	1.5–11.7
	Tanner 5 (11.8–18.6 y)		2.6–11.0	1.0–9.2
	Adult		2.0–9.2	
	Follicular			1.8–11.2
	Midcycle			6.0–35.0
	Luteal phase			1.8–11.2
LH (mIU/mL) S, P	4 wk–11 mo	Abbott Alinity-i	0.01–5.7	0.01–5.7
	12 mo–8 y		0.01–0.24	0.01–0.24
	Tanner 1 (< 9.8 y)		0.01–0.24	0.01–0.14
	Tanner 2 (9.8–14.5 y)		0.16–4.0	0.16–3.8
	Tanner 3 (10.7–15.4 y)		0.16–4.1	0.08–9.8
	Tanner 4 (11.8–16.2 y)		0.3–5.7	0.3–9.5
	Tanner 5 (12.8–17.3 y)		0.3–5.7	0.3–9.5
	Adult		1.2–7.38	
	Follicular			1.6–7.38
	Midcycle			14.7–40.1
	Luteal			1.6–9.0
T$_4$, total (mcg/dL) S, P	0–3 days	Abbott Alinity-i	8–20	8–20
	3–30 days		5–15	5–15
	31 days–1 y		6–14	6–14
	1–5 y		4.5–12.5	4.5–12.5
	6–18 y		4.5–11.5	4.5–11.5
	≥ 19 y		4.5–11.5	5.5–11.5
T$_4$, free (ng/dL) S, P	0–3 days	Abbott Alinity-i	2.0–5.0	2.0–5.0
	3–30 days		0.9–2.2	0.9–2.2
	31 days–18 y		0.8–2.0	0.8–2.0
	≥ 19 y		0.78–2.19	0.78–2.19
TSH (mcIU/mL) S, P	0–3 days	Vitros 5600	1.0–20.0	1.0–20.0
	3–30 days		0.5–6.5	0.5–6.5
	31 days–5 y		0.5–6.0	0.5–6.0
	5–12 y		0.5–5.5	0.5–5.5
	≥ 13 y		0.5–5.0	0.5–5.0
Testosterone, total (ng/dL) S, P	Premature	Vitros 5600	37–198	5–22
	Newborn		75–400	20–64
	Prepubertal		1–10	1–10
	Tanner 1		1–10	1–10
	Tanner 2		18–150	7–28
	Tanner 3		100–320	15–35
	Tanner 4		200–620	13–32
	Tanner 5		350–970	20–38
	Adult		132–813	5–77

FSH, follicle-stimulating hormone; LH, luteinizing hormone; T$_3$, triiodothyronine; T$_4$, thyroxine; TSH, thyroid-stimulating hormone.
Data from Children's Hospital Colorado Chemistry Laboratory Procedure Manuals.

Table 46–3. Hematology.

Analyte, Units, Specimen Type, Source	Age	Methodology	Male Range	Female Range
WBC ($\times10^3$/µL) EDTA whole blood	0–1 mo 1–24 mo 2–12 y 12–18 y > 18 y	Sysmex XN-Series	6.5–16.7 7.7–13.7 5.7–10.5 5.2–9.7 5.8–10.3	6.5–16.7 7.7–13.7 5.7–10.5 5.2–9.7 5.8–10.3
RBC ($\times10^6$/µL) EDTA whole blood	0–14 days 15–30 days 1–2 mo 2–6 mo 6 mo–6 y 6–12 y 12–18 y > 18 y	Sysmex XN-Series	3.7–5.1 3.25–4.62 3.0–4.3 3.3–4.7 3.75–4.9 3.9–5.0 4.1–5.4 4.1–5.4	3.7–5.1 3.25–4.62 3.0–4.3 3.3–4.7 3.75–4.9 3.9–5.0 3.9–5.0 3.7–4.8
Hemoglobin (g/dL) EDTA whole blood	0–3 days 4–7 days 8–14 days 15–30 days 1–6 mo 6 mo–6 y 6–12 y 12–18 y > 18 y	Sysmex XN-Series	12.8–18.1 12.5–17.0 11.9–16.3 10.5–14.8 9.5–13.3 10.3–13.8 11.1–14.5 11.8–15.8 11.8–16.4	12.8–18.1 2.5–17.0 11.9–16.3 10.5–14.8 9.5–13.3 10.3–13.8 11.1–14.5 11.3–14.7 11.2–14.3
HCT (%) EDTA whole blood	0–3 days 4–7 days 8–14 days 15–30 days 1–6 mo 6 mo–6 y 6–12 y 12–18 y > 18 y	Sysmex XN-Series	36.5–51.4 35.0–47.5 33.6–45.0 30.0–40.9 27.0–38.5 30.5–39.7 32.9–41.5 34.0–46.0 34.0–48.0	36.5–51.4 35.0–47.5 33.6–45.0 30.0–40.9 27.0–38.5 30.5–39.7 32.9–41.5 33.0–42.6 33.0–42.6
MCV (fL) EDTA whole blood	0–3 days 4–7 days 8–30 days 1–2 mo 2–6 mo 6 mo–12 y 12–18 y > 18 y	Sysmex XN-Series	97.0–106.0 90.0–101.0 87.0–96.5 86.5–92.1 82.0–87.0 75.6–85.2 80.8–87.7 83.5–90.2	97.0–106.0 90.0–101.0 87.0–96.5 86.5–92.1 82.0–87.0 75.6–85.2 80.8–87.7 83.5–90.2
Polys ($\times10^3$/µL) (absolute) EDTA whole blood	0–3 days 4–30 days 1 mo–2 y 2–10 y 10–18 y > 18 y	Sysmex XN-Series	4.33–9.11 3.33–9.42 1.5–6.0 1.8–5.4 2.0–5.8 2.5–6.0	4.43–11.4 3.18–9.43 1.5–6.0 1.8–5.4 2.0–5.8 2.5–6.0
Immature granulocytes ($\times10^3$/µL) (absolute) EDTA whole blood	0–1 mo 1 mo–2 y 2–12 y 12–18 y > 18 y	Sysmex XN-Series	0–0.28 0–0.14 0.0–0.06 0.0–0.03 0.0–0.09	0–0.28 0–0.14 0.0–0.06 0.0–0.03 0.0–0.09

(Continued)

Table 46–3. Hematology. (*Continued*)

Analyte, Units, Specimen Type, Source	Age	Methodology	Male Range	Female Range
Lymphs (×10³/µL) (absolute) EDTA whole blood	0–15 days 15–30 days 1 mo–2 y 2–6 y 6–12 y > 12 y	Sysmex XN-Series	1.35–4.09 1.68–5.25 2.22–5.63 1.33–3.47 1.23–2.69 1.03–2.18	1.35–4.09 1.68–5.25 2.22–5.63 1.33–3.47 1.23–2.69 1.03–2.18
Monos (×10³/µL) (absolute) EDTA whole blood	0–15 days 16 days–6 mo 6 mo–2 y 2 y–Adult	Sysmex XN-Series	0.52–1.77 0.28–1.38 0.25–1.15 0.18–0.94	0.52–1.77 0.28–1.38 0.25–1.15 0.18–0.94
EOS (×10³/µL) (absolute) EDTA whole blood	0–1 mo 1 mo–2 y > 2 y	Sysmex XN-Series	0.03–0.51 0.01–0.42 0.02–0.23	0.03–0.51 0.01–0.42 0.02–0.23
Basos (×10³/µL) (absolute) EDTA whole blood	0–15 days 16 days–Adult	Sysmex XN-Series	0.02–0.11 0.01–0.07	0.02–0.11 0.01–0.07
Platelet (×10³/µL) EDTA whole blood	0 days–Adult	Sysmex XN-Series	150–500	150–500
MPV (fL) EDTA whole blood	0 days–Adult	Sysmex XN-Series	8.9–11.3	8.9–11.3
MCH (pg) EDTA whole blood	0–3 days 4–60 days 2 mo–18 y > 18 y	Sysmex XN-Series	31.7–36.4 29.8–33.4 26.0–30.7 28.3–31.4	31.7–36.4 29.8–33.4 26.0–30.7 28.3–31.4
MCHC (g/dL) EDTA whole blood	0 day–Adult	Sysmex XN-Series	33.5–36.0	33.5–36.0
RDW (%) EDTA whole blood	0–3 days 4–60 days 2 mo–Adult	Sysmex XN-Series	16.3–18.2 14.6–17.5 13.0–15.5	15.8–17.8 14.2–16.7 12.8–14.8

Data from Children's Hospital Colorado Hematology Laboratory Procedure Manual.

Index

Note: Page numbers followed by *f* or *t* denote figures or tables, respectively.